ENDOCRINOLOGY

VOLUME 1
ENDOCRINOLOGY

THIRD EDITION

Edited by

LESLIE J. DeGROOT

MICHAEL BESSER
HENRY G. BURGER
J. LARRY JAMESON
D. LYNN LORIAUX
JOHN C. MARSHALL
WILLIAM D. ODELL
JOHN T. POTTS, Jr.
ARTHUR H. RUBENSTEIN

Consulting Editors

GEORGE F. CAHILL, Jr.
LUCIANO MARTINI
DON H. NELSON

W.B. SAUNDERS COMPANY

A Division of Harcourt Brace & Company

PHILADELPHIA   LONDON   TORONTO   MONTREAL   SYDNEY   TOKYO

W.B. SAUNDERS COMPANY
A Division of
Harcourt Brace & Company

The Curtis Center
Independence Square West
Philadelphia, Pennsylvania 19106

Library of Congress Cataloging-in-Publication Data

Endocrinology / edited by Leslie J. DeGroot . . . [et al.] ; consulting editors, George F. Cahill, Jr., Luciano Martini, Don H. Nelson.—3rd ed.

p.   cm.

Includes bibliographical references and index.

ISBN 0–7216–4262–4 (set). ISBN 0–7216–4263–2 (v.1).—ISBN 0–7216–4264–0 (v.2).—ISBN 0–7216–4265–9 (v. 3)

1. Endocrine glands—Diseases.   2. Endocrinology.   I. DeGroot, Leslie J.
   [DNLM: 1. Endocrine Diseases.   2. Endocrine Glands.   3. Hormones.   WK 100 E5345 1995]

RC648.E458   1995

616.4—dc20

DNLM/DLC   93–8208

ENDOCRINOLOGY

Set   ISBN 0–7216–4262–4
Volume 1   ISBN 0–7216–4263–2
Volume 2   ISBN 0–7216–4264–0
Volume 3   ISBN 0–7216–4265–9

Printed in the United States of America.

Last digit is the print number: 9   8   7   6   5   4   3   2   1

Contributors

NOBUYUKI AMINO, M.D.
Professor of Medicine, Department of Laboratory Medicine, Osaka University Medical School, Staff Physician, Osaka University Hospital, Osaka, Japan.
Autoimmune Thyroid Disease/Thyroiditis

JOSEPHINE ARENDT, Ph.D.
Professor of Endocrinology, School of Biological Sciences, University of Surrey, Surrey, England.
The Pineal Gland: Basic Physiology and Clinical Implications

ANDREW ARNOLD, M.D.
Associate Professor of Medicine, Harvard Medical School. Chief, Laboratory of Endocrine Oncology, Massachusetts General Hospital, Boston, Massachusetts.
Hyperparathyroidism; Hypoparathyroidism

LOUIS V. AVIOLI, M.D.
Schoenberg Professor of Medicine and Director, Division of Bone and Mineral Diseases, Washington University School of Medicine. Director, Division of Endocrinology and Metabolism, The Jewish Hospital of St. Louis, St. Louis, Missouri.
Disorders of Calcification: Osteomalacia and Rickets

SAMI T. AZAR, M.D.
Formerly Instructor in Medicine, Boston University School of Medicine. Presently Assistant Professor in Medicine, American University in Beirut, Beirut, Lebanon.
Hypoaldosteronism and Mineralocorticoid Resistance

DAVID T. BAIRD, M.B., D.Sc.
M.R.C. Clinical Research Professor, University of Edinburgh. Consultant Gynaecologist, Royal Infirmary, Edinburgh, Scotland.
Amenorrhea, Anovulation, and Dysfunctional Uterine Bleeding

H. W. GORDON BAKER, M.D., B.S., Ph.D., FRACP
Senior Research Fellow, Department of Obstetrics and Gynaecology, University of Melbourne. Andrologist, The Royal Women's Hospital and Austin Hospital; Senior Research Associate, Prince Henry's Institute of Medical Research, Monash Medical Centre, Clayton, Victoria, Australia.
Male Infertility

RANDALL B. BARNES, M.D.
Associate Professor, Department of Obstetrics and Gynecology, University of Chicago Pritzker School of Medicine. Attending Physician, Chicago Lying-in Hospital, Chicago, Illinois.
Hyperandrogenism, Hirsutism, and the Polycystic Ovary Syndrome

GEORGE B. BARTLEY, M.D.
Associate Professor of Ophthalmology, Mayo Medical School. Chair, Department of Ophthalmology, Mayo Clinic, Rochester, Minnesota.
Ophthalmopathy

ETIENNE-EMILE BAULIEU, M.D., Ph.D.
Professor, Collège de France. Chef de Service de Biochimie Hormonale, Hôpital de Bicêtre, Bicêtre, France.
Nuclear Receptor Superfamily

PETER H. BAYLIS, B.Sc., M.D., FRCP
Professor, The Medical School, University of Newcastle-Upon-Tyne. Consultant Physician, Royal Victoria Infirmary, Newcastle-Upon-Tyne, England.
Vasopressin and Its Neurophysin

GREGORY P. BECKS, M.D., FRCPC
Assistant Professor, Department of Medicine, Division of Endocrinology and Metabolism, University of Western Ontario. Attending Staff, Department of Medicine, Endocrine Division, St. Joseph's Health Centre of London, London, Ontario, Canada.
Diagnosis and Treatment of Thyroid Disease During Pregnancy

GRAEME I. BELL, Ph.D.
Professor of Biochemistry and Molecular Biology, and Medicine, University of Chicago Pritzker School of Medicine, Chicago, Illinois.
Chemistry and Biosynthesis of the Islet Hormones: Insulin, Islet Amyloid Polypeptide (Amylin), Glucagon, Somatostatin, and Pancreatic Polypeptide

RICHARD M. BERGENSTAL, M.D.
Clinical Associate Professor, University of Minnesota Medical School. Senior Vice President, International Diabetes Center, and Chairman, Endocrinology, Park Nicollet Medical Center, Minneapolis, Minnesota.
Diabetes Mellitus: Therapy

MICHAEL BESSER, M.D., D.Sc., FRCP
Professor of Medicine and Endocrinology, and Head, Departments of Medicine and Endocrinology, Medical College of St. Bartholomew's Hospital, University of London. Honourary Consultant Physician in Charge, Department of Endocrinology, St. Bartholomew's Hospital, London, England
Tests of Pituitary Function

DENNIS M. BIER, M.D.
Professor of Pediatrics, Baylor College of Medicine. Director, Children's Nutrition Research Center; Attending Physician, Texas Children's Hospital, Houston, Texas.
Metabolic Aspects of Fuel Homeostasis in the Fetus and the Neonate

HÅKAN BILLIG, M.D., Ph.D.
Assistant Professor, Department of Physiology, Göteborg University, Göteborg, Sweden.
Ovarian Hormone Synthesis and Mechanism of Action

MARC R. BLACKMAN, M.D.
Associate Professor of Medicine, Johns Hopkins University School of Medicine. Chief, Division of Endocrinology and Metabolism, and Associate Program Director, General Clinical Research Center, Francis Scott Key Medical Center, Baltimore, Maryland.
Endocrinology and Aging

STEPHEN R. BLOOM, M.A., M.D., D.Sc., FRCP
Professor of Endocrinology, Royal Postgraduate Medical School, Hammersmith Hospital, London, England.
Hormones of the Gastrointestinal Tract

GEORGE A. BRAY, M.D.
Professor of Medicine, Louisiana State University School of Medicine. Executive Director, Pennington Biomedical Research Institute, Baton Rouge, Louisiana.
The Syndromes of Obesity: An Endocrine Approach

H. BRYAN BREWER, Jr., M.D.
Chief, Molecular Disease Branch, National Heart, Lung, and Blood Institute, National Institutes of Health, Bethesda, Maryland.
Disorders of Lipoprotein Metabolism

F. RICHARD BRINGHURST, M.D.
Associate Professor of Medicine, Harvard Medical School. Associate Physician, Massachusetts General Hospital, Boston, Massachusetts.
Parathyroid Hormone: Physiology, Chemistry, Biosynthesis, Secretion, Metabolism, and Mode of Action; Calcium and Phosphate Distribution, Turnover, and Metabolic Actions

ARTHUR E. BROADUS, M.D., Ph.D.
Professor and Chairman, Division of Endocrinology, Yale University School of Medicine. Staff Physician, Yale-New Haven Hospital, New Haven, Connecticut
Malignancy-Associated Hypercalcemia

HENRY G. BURGER, M.D., FRACP, FCP(SA), FRACOG
Honorary Professor of Medicine, Monash University. Director, Prince Henry's Institute of Medical Research, and Director, Endocrine Unit, Monash Medical Centre, Clayton, Victoria, Australia.
Gonadal Regulatory Peptides

GERARD N. BURROW, M.D.
Dean and Professor of Internal Medicine, Yale University School of Medicine. Attending Physician, Department of Internal Medicine, Yale-New Haven Hospital, New Haven, Connecticut.
Diagnosis and Treatment of Thyroid Disease During Pregnancy

ROBERT K. CAMPBELL, Ph.D.
Executive Research Director, Ares Advanced Technology, Randolph, Massachusetts.
Gonadotropins

ERNESTO CANALIS, M.D.
Professor of Medicine and Orthopedics, University of Connecticut School of Medicine. Director of Research, St. Francis Hospital and Medical Center, Hartford, Connecticut.
Metabolic Bone Disease: Introduction and Classification

JOSÉ F. CARA, M.D.
Assistant Professor, University of Chicago Pritzker School of Medicine. Attending Physician, Wyler Children's Hospital, Chicago, Illinois.
Somatic Growth and Maturation

DON H. CATLIN, M.D.
Associate Professor, Departments of Medicine and of Molecular and Medical Pharmacology, University of California Los Angeles School of Medicine. Attending Physician, UCLA Hospital and Clinics, Los Angeles, California.
Anabolic Steroids

WILLIAM W. CHIN, M.D.
Professor of Medicine, Harvard Medical School. Investigator, Howard Hughes Medical Institute; Chief, Division of Genetics, and Senior Physician, Brigham and Women's Hospital, Boston, Massachusetts.
Hormonal Regulation of Gene Expression

JACK W. COBURN, M.D.
Adjunct Professor of Medicine, University of California Los Angeles School of Medicine. Staff Physician, Veterans Affairs Hospital, Los Angeles, California.
The Renal Osteodystrophies

NANCY E. COOKE, M.D.
Associate Professor of Medicine and Genetics, University of Pennsylvania School of Medicine. Staff Physician, Hospital of the University of Pennsylvania, Philadelphia, Pennsylvania.
Prolactin: Basic Physiology

ELIZABETH ANNE COWDEN, B.Sc.(Hons), M.B.Ch.B., FRCP (Glasgow), M.D. (Hons)
Acting Head, University Section of Endocrinology and Metabolism, University of Manitoba. Head, Section of Endocrinology and Metabolism, St. Boniface General Hospital, Winnipeg, Manitoba.
Endocrinology of Lactation and Nursing: Disorders of Lactation

MICHAEL J. CRONIN, Ph.D.
Visiting Associate Professor of Physiology, University of Virginia. Adjunct Professor of Physiology, University of Southern California, San Francisco, California.
Growth Hormone–Releasing Hormone: Basic Physiology and Clinical Implications

WILLIAM F. CROWLEY, Jr., M.D.
Professor of Medicine, Harvard Medical School. Chief, Reproductive Endocrine Sciences Center and National Center for Infertility Research, Massachusetts General Hospital, Boston, Massachusetts.
Gonadotropins and the Gonad: Normal Physiology and Their Disturbances in Clinical Endocrine Diseases

PHILIP E. CRYER, M.D.
Professor of Medicine and Director, Division of Endocrinology, Diabetes and Metabolism, Washington University School of Medicine. Physician, Barnes Hospital, St. Louis, Missouri.
Orthostatic (Postural) Hypotension

GARY C. CURHAN, M.D., M.S.
Instructor in Medicine, Harvard Medical School. Chief, Clinical Nephrology, Brockton/West Rox-

bury Veterans Administration Medical Center, West Roxbury, Massachusetts.
Calcium Nephrolithiasis

GORDON B. CUTLER, Jr., M.D.
Chief, Section on Developmental Endocrinology, Developmental Endocrinology Branch, National Institute of Child Health and Human Development, and Senior Staff Physician, Warren Grant Magnuson Clinical Center, National Institutes of Health, Bethesda, Maryland.
Cushing's Syndrome

DAVID L. DANIELS, M.D.
Professor of Radiology, Medical College of Wisconsin. Neuroradiologist, Froedtert Memorial Lutheran Hospital, Consultant in Radiology, Veterans Administration Medical Center, Milwaukee, Wisconsin.
Radiographic Evaluation of the Pituitary and Anterior Hypothalamus

DOMINIQUE DARMAUN, M.D., Ph.D.
Visiting Associate Professor of Pediatrics, University of Florida/Health Sciences Center. Attending Physician, Nemours Children's Clinic, Jacksonville, Florida.
Metabolic Aspects of Fuel Homeostasis in the Fetus and the Neonate

WILLIAM H. DAUGHADAY, M.D.
Irene M. and Michael E. Karl Professor Emeritus of Medicine, Washington University School of Medicine. Physician, Barnes Hospital, St. Louis Jewish Hospital, St. Louis, Missouri.
Growth Hormone, Insulin-Like Growth Factors, and Acromegaly

VAL DAVAJAN, M.D.†
Professor, Department of Obstetrics and Gynecology, Los Angeles County/University of Southern California Medical Center, Los Angeles, California.
Infertility: Causes, Evaluation, and Treatment

RALPH A. DeFRONZO, M.D.
Professor of Medicine and Chief, Diabetes Division, University of Texas Health Science Center, San Antonio, Texas.
Regulation of Intermediary Metabolism During Fasting and Feeding

LESLIE J. DeGROOT
Professor of Medicine, University of Chicago Pritzker School of Medicine. Staff Physician, University of Chicago Medical Center, Chicago, Illinois.
Mechanisms of Thyroid Hormone Action; Thyroid Neoplasia; Congenital Defects in Thyroid Hormone Formation and Action

---

†Deceased 7/13/93.

DAVID M. de KRETSER
Professor and Director, Institute of Reproduction and Development, Monash University. Consultant, Reproductive Biology Unit, Monash Medical Centre, Clayton, Victoria, Australia.
Basic Endocrinology of the Testis

MARIE B. DEMAY, M.D.
Assistant Professor of Medicine, Harvard Medical School. Assistant in Medicine, Massachusetts General Hospital, Boston, Massachusetts.
Hereditary Defects in Vitamin D Metabolism and Vitamin D Receptor Defects

ROBERTO Di LAURO, M.D.
Professor of Genetics, Dipartimento Di Scienze e Biotecnologie Mediche, Universita di Udine. Head, Laboratory of Biochemistry and Molecular Biology, Stazione Zoologica Anton Dohrn, Naples, Italy.
Biosynthesis and Secretion of Thyroid Hormones

JOHN L. DOPPMAN, M.D.
Director of Radiology, Department of Radiology, National Institutes of Health, Bethesda, Maryland.
Adrenal Imaging

J. E. DUMONT, M.D., Ph.D.
Professor of Biochemistry, School of Medicine and School of Sciences, University of Brussels. Consultant in Endocrinology, University Hospital Erasme, Brussels, Belgium.
Thyroid Regulation

CHRISTOPHER R. W. EDWARDS, M.D.
Professor of Clinical Medicine, Department of Medicine, University of Edinburgh. Honourary Consultant Physician, Western General Hospital, Edinburgh, Scotland.
Primary Mineralocorticoid Excess Syndromes

EDWARD N. EHRLICH, M.D.
Professor Emeritus, Section of Endocrinology and Metabolism, Department of Medicine, University of Wisconsin Medical School. Attending Physician, University of Wisconsin Hospital and Clinics, Madison, Wisconsin.
Hormonal Regulation of Electrolyte and Water Metabolism

DAVID A. EHRMANN, M.D.
Assistant Professor, Section of Endocrinology, Department of Medicine, University of Chicago Pritzker School of Medicine. Attending Physician, University of Chicago Hospitals, Chicago, Illinois.
Hyperandrogenism, Hirsutism, and the Polycystic Ovary Syndrome

RAGNAR EKHOLM, M.D., Ph.D.
Professor Emeritus of Anatomy, Department of Anatomy, University of Göteborg, Göteborg, Sweden.
Thyroid Gland: Anatomy and Development

DARIUSH ELAHI, Ph.D.
Associate Professor of Medicine, Department of Medicine, University of Maryland School of Medicine Veterans Affairs Medical Center, Geriatrics and Guest Researcher, NIH/NIA, Laboratory of Clinical Physiology, Baltimore, Maryland.
Endocrinology and Aging

ERIC A. ESPINER, M.B., M.D., FRACP, FRSNZ
Professor in Medicine, Christchurch School of Medicine, University of Otago. Head, Department of Endocrinology, Christchurch Hospital, Christchurch, New Zealand.
Hormones of the Cardiovascular System

STEFAN S. FAJANS, M.D.
Professor Emeritus (Active) of Internal Medicine, Division of Endocrinology and Metabolism, University of Michigan Medical School, Ann Arbor, Michigan.
Diabetes Mellitus: Definition, Classification, Tests

ELEUTERIO FERRANNINI, M.D.
Chief, Metabolic Branch, CNR Institute of Physiology, Pisa, Italy.
Regulation of Intermediary Metabolism During Fasting and Feeding

DELBERT A. FISHER, M.D.
Professor Emeritus, Pediatrics and Medicine, University of California Los Angeles School of Medicine. Senior Scientist, Research and Education Institute, Harbor-UCLA Medical Center, Torrance, California.
Thyroid Disease in the Fetus, Neonate, and Child; Fetal and Neonatal Endocrinology

LORRAINE A. FITZPATRICK, M.D.
Associate Professor of Medicine, Mayo Graduate School of Medicine, Mayo Clinic and Mayo Foundation. Consultant in Endocrinology, Mayo Clinic, St. Mary's Hospital, Rochester Methodist Hospital, Rochester, Minnesota.
Hypoparathyroidism

JEFFREY S. FLIER, M.D.
Professor of Medicine, Harvard Medical School. Chief, Division of Endocrinology, Beth Israel Hospital, Boston, Massachusetts.
Syndromes of Insulin Resistance and Mutant Insulin

MAGUELONE G. FOREST, M.D.
Director of Research, INSERM. Hôpital Debrousse, Lyons, France.
Diagnosis and Treatment of Disorders of Sexual Development

DANIEL W. FOSTER, M.D.
Donald W. Seldin Distinguished Chair and Chairman, Department of Internal Medicine, University of Texas Southwestern Medical School, Dallas, Texas.
Diabetes Mellitus: Acute Complications, Ketoacidosis, Hyperosmolar Coma, Lactic Acidosis

AARON L. FRIEDMAN, M.D.
Professor, Nephrology Section, Department of Pediatrics, University of Wisconsin Medical School. Attending Physician, University of Wisconsin Hospital and Clinics, Madison, Wisconsin.
Hormonal Regulation of Electrolyte and Water Metabolism

ELI A. FRIEDMAN, M.D.
Distinguished Teaching Professor of Medicine, State University of New York Health Science Center at Brooklyn. Attending Physician and Director, Division of Renal Disease, University Hospital of Brooklyn and Kings County Hospital Center, Brooklyn, New York.
Diabetes Mellitus: Late Complications, Nephropathy

HENRY G. FRIESEN, M.D.
President, Medical Research Council of Canada, Ottawa, Ontario, Canada.
Endocrinology of Lactation and Nursing: Disorders of Lactation

JOHN W. FUNDER, M.D.
Director, Baker Medical Research Institute, Prahran, Victoria, Australia.
Aldosterone Action: Biochemistry

MATS E. GÅFVELS, M.D., Ph.D.
Visiting Assistant Professor, Department of Obstetrics and Gynecology, University of Pennsylvania School of Medicine, Philadelphia, Pennsylvania.
Placental Hormones

ROBERT F. GAGEL, M.D.
Professor of Medicine, University of Texas M.D. Anderson Cancer Center; Associate Professor of Medicine, Baylor College of Medicine, Houston, Texas.
Multiple Endocrine Neoplasia Type 2

HENRIK GALBO, M.D., D.M.Sc.
Professor, Exercise Physiology, Department of Medical Physiology, University of Copenhagen. Chief Physician, Internal Medicine and Rheumatology, University Hospital, Copenhagen, Denmark.
Integrated Endocrine Responses and Exercise

STEEN GAMMELTOFT, M.D.
Professor, University of Copenhagen. Medical Director, Glostrup Hospital, Copenhagen, Denmark.
Hormone Signaling via Membrane Receptors

THOMAS GARDELLA, Ph.D.
Assistant Professor of Medicine, Harvard Medical School. Assistant Professor in Biochemistry, Massachusetts General Hospital, Boston, Massachusetts.
Parathyroid Hormone: Physiology, Chemistry, Biosynthesis, Secretion, Metabolism, and Mode of Action

EDWARD P. GELMANN, M.D.
Professor of Medicine, Georgetown University School of Medicine. Chief, Division of Medical Oncology, Vincent T. Lombardi Cancer Research Center, Washington, D.C.
Endocrine Management of Malignant Disease

FABRIZIO GENTILE, M.D., Ph.D.
Investigator, Centro di Endocrinologia e Oncologia Sperimentale del Consiglio Nazionale delle Ricerche, Naples, Italy.
Biosynthesis and Secretion of Thyroid Hormones

HANS GERBER, M.D.
Privatdozent, University of Bern School of Medicine. Head of Division, Department of Clinical Chemistry, University Hospital, Inselspital, Bern, Switzerland.
Multinodular Goiter

MARVIN C. GERSHENGORN, MD.
Abby Rockefeller Mauze Distinguished Professor of Endocrinology in Medicine, and Chief, Division of Molecular Medicine; Cornell University Medical College. Attending Physician, The New York Hospital, New York, New York.
Second Messenger Signaling Pathways: Phosphatidylinositol and Calcium

MOHAMMAD A. GHATEI, Ph.D.
Lecturer, Division of Endocrinology and Metabolism, Royal Postgraduate Medical School, Hammersmith Hospital, London, England.
Hormones of the Gastrointestinal Tract

STEVEN R. GOLDRING, M.D
Associate Professor of Medicine, Harvard Medical School. Chief of Rheumatology, New England Deaconess Hospital; Clinical Associate, Massachusetts General Hospital, Boston, Massachusetts
Disorders of Calcification: Osteomalacia and Rickets

LOUIS J. G. GOOREN, M.D., Ph.D.
Professor of Medicine, Free University, Amsterdam. Head of Division of Andrology, Department of Endocrinology, Free University Hospital, Amsterdam, The Netherlands.
Normal and Abnormal Sexual Behavior

COLUM A. GORMAN, M.B., B.Ch., Ph.D.
Professor of Medicine, Mayo Medical School. Consultant, Mayo Clinic, Rochester, Minnesota.
Ophthalmopathy

NICHOLAS M. GOUGH, Ph.D.
Head, Molecular Hematology Laboratory, The Walter and Eliza Hall Institute of Medical Research, Royal Melbourne Hospital, Melbourne, Australia.
Hormones and Blood Cell Production

ANDREW J. GREEN, M.D.
Medical Director, Diabetes Center of Excellence, Overland Park Regional Medical Center, Overland Park, Kansas.
The Neuropathies of Diabetes

ASHLEY GROSSMAN, B.A., B.Sc., M.D., FRCP
Professor of Neuroendocrinology, St. Bartholomew's Hospital Medical College, University of London. Honourary Consultant Physician, St. Bartholomew's Hospital, London, England.
Corticotropin-Releasing Hormone: Basic Physiology and Clinical Applications

JOEL F. HABENER, M.D.
Professor of Medicine, Harvard Medical School. Investigator, Howard Hughes Medical Institute; Chief, Laboratory of Molecular Endocrinology, and Associate Physician, Massachusetts General Hospital, Boston, Massachusetts.
Cyclic AMP Second Messenger Signaling Pathway; Hyperparathyroidism

JANET E. HALL, M.D.
Assistant Professor in Medicine, Harvard Medical School. Assistant in Medicine, Massachusetts General Hospital, Boston, Massachusetts.
Gonadotropins and the Gonad: Normal Physiology and Their Disturbances in Clinical Endocrine Diseases

REGINALD HALL, B.Sc., M.D., FRCP, OBE
Professor Emeritus of Medicine, University of Wales College of Medicine, Cardiff, Wales.
Thyrotropin-Releasing Hormone: Basic and Clinical Aspects

DAVID J. HANDELSMAN, M.B., B.S., Ph.D., FRACP
Associate Professor, Departments of Obstetrics and Gynaecology and of Medicine, University of Sydney. Director, Andrology Unit and Department of Endocrinology, Royal Prince Alfred Hospital, Sydney, Australia.
Testosterone and Other Androgens: Physiology, Pharmacology, and Therapeutic Use; Contraception in the Male

HISATO HARA, M.D.
Visiting Research Associate, University of Chicago Hospitals, Chicago, Illinois.
Developmental Abnormalities of the Thyroid; Surgery of the Thyroid

S. MITCHELL HARMAN, M.D., Ph.D.
Associate Professor, Department of Medicine, Johns Hopkins University School of Medicine. Section Chief, Endocrinology Section, Gerontology Research Center, National Institute on Aging, National Institutes of Health. Attending Physician, Francis Scott Key Medical Center, Baltimore, Maryland.
Endocrinology and Aging

VICTOR M. HAUGHTON, M.D.
Professor of Radiology and Director of MRI Research, Medical College of Wisconsin. Radiologist, Milwaukee County Medical Complex, Froedtert Memorial Lutheran Hospital; Consultant in Radiology, Veterans Administration Medical Center, Milwaukee, Wisconsin.
Radiographic Evaluation of the Pituitary and Anterior Hypothalamus

MOREY W. HAYMOND, M.D.
Professor of Pediatrics, Mayo Medical School. Medical Director, Nemours Children's Clinic, Jacksonville, Florida.
Metabolic Aspects of Fuel Homeostasis in the Fetus and the Neonate

DAVID HEBER, M.D., Ph.D.
Professor of Medicine and Chief, Division of Clinical Nutrition, Department of Medicine, University of California Los Angeles School of Medicine. Director, Clinical Nutrition Research Unit, University of California Los Angeles, Los Angeles, California.
Endocrine Responses to Starvation, Malnutrition, and Illness

KEVAN C. HEROLD, M.D.
Assistant Professor, Department of Medicine, University of Chicago Pritzker School of Medicine. Attending Physician, Chicago Children's Diabetes Center and LaRabida Children's Hospital, Chicago, Illinois.
Immunological Mechanisms Causing Autoimmune Endocrine Disease

ARMIN E. HEUFELDER, M.D.
Instructor in Internal Medicine and Endocrinology, and Molecular Thyroid Research Laboratory Director, Medizinische Klinik, Klinikum Innenstadt, Ludwig-Maximilians-University, Munich, Germany.
Ophthalmopathy

RICHARD A. HIIPAKKA, Ph.D.
Senior Research Associate, Ben May Institute, University of Chicago, Chicago, Illinois.
Androgen Receptors and Action

GARY D. HODGEN, Ph.D.
Professor and President, The Jones Institute for Reproductive Medicine, Department of Obstetrics and Gynecology, Eastern Virginia Medical School, Norfolk, Virginia
Ovarian Follicular Maturation, Ovulation, and Ovulation Induction

JEFFREY M. HOEG, M.D.
Head, Section of Cell Biology, Molecular Disease Branch, National Heart, Lung, and Blood Institute, National Institutes of Health, Bethesda, Maryland.
Disorders of Lipoprotein Metabolism

J. J. HOET, M.D.
Professor of Medicine, University of Louvain, Louvain, Belgium.
Anatomy, Developmental Biology, and Pathology of the Pancreatic Islets

MICHAEL F. HOLICK, Ph.D., M.D.
Professor of Medicine, Physiology and Dermatology, Boston University School of Medicine. Chief, Endocrinology, Diabetes, and Metabolism Section, Boston University Medical Center and Boston City Hospital and Veterans Administration Hospital; Director, General Clinical Research Center, and Director, Vitamin D, Skin, and Bone Research Laboratory, Boston University School of Medicine, Boston, Massachusetts
Vitamin D: Photobiology, Metabolism, and Clinical Applications

EVA HORVATH, Ph.D.
Associate Professor of Pathology, University of Toronto. Research Associate, St. Michael's Hospital, Toronto, Ontario, Canada.
Anatomy and Histology of the Normal and Abnormal Pituitary Gland

AARON J. W. HSUEH, Ph.D.
Professor, Division of Reproductive Biology, Stanford University Medical Center, Stanford, California
Ovarian Hormone Synthesis and Mechanism of Action

HIROO IMURA, M.D.
President, Kyoto University, Kyoto, Japan.
Adrenocorticotropic Hormone

KARL L. INSOGNA, M.D.
Associate Professor, Endocrinology, Yale University School of Medicine. Attending Physician, Yale-New Haven Hospital, New Haven, Connecticut.
Malignancy-Associated Hypercalcemia

ROBERT ISRAEL, M.D.
Professor, University of Southern California School of Medicine, Los Angeles. Attending Physician, Women's Hospital; Hospital of the Good Samaritan, Los Angeles, California.
Infertility: Causes, Evaluation, and Treatment

KOICHI ITO, M.D.
Visiting Research Associate, University of Chicago Hospitals, Chicago, Illinois.
Developmental Abnormalities of the Thyroid; Surgery of the Thyroid

J. LARRY JAMESON, M.D., Ph.D.
Charles F. Kettering Professor of Medicine; Chief, Division of Endocrinology, Metabolism, and Molecular Medicine, Northwestern University Medical School. Chief, Section of Endocrinology and Metabolism, Northwestern Memorial Hospital, Chicago, Illinois.
Applications of Molecular Biology in Endocrinology; Mechanisms of Thyroid Hormone Action

JONATHAN B. JASPAN, M.D.
Tullis-Tulane Alumni Chair in Diabetes, and Professor of Medicine, Tulane University Medical Center School of Medicine. Attending Physician, Endocrinology and General Internal Medicine, Tulane University Medical Center and Clinics; Medical Center of Louisiana; and Veterans Administration Medical Center, New Orleans, Louisiana.
The Neuropathics of Diabetes

NATHALIE JOSSO, M.D.
Research Director, Institut de la Santé et de la Recherche Médicale, Ecole Normale Supérieure. Hôpital Saint-Vincent de Paul, Paris, France.
Anatomy and Endocrinology of Fetal Sex Differentiation

C. RONALD KAHN, M.D.
Mary K. Iacocca Professor of Medicine, Harvard Medical School. Research Director, Elliott P. Joslin Research Laboratory, Joslin Diabetes Center, Boston, Massachusetts.
Hormone Signaling via Membrane Receptors; the Molecular Mechanism of Insulin Action

EDWIN L. KAPLAN, M.D.
Professor of Surgery, University of Chicago Pritzker School of Medicine and University of Chicago Hospitals, Chicago, Illinois.
Developmental Abnormalities of the Thyroid; Surgery of the Thyroid

JOSEPHINE Z. KASA-VUBU, M.D.
Assistant Professor of Pediatrics, University of Michigan Medical School. Assistant Professor of Pediatrics, University of Michigan Medical Center, Ann Arbor, Michigan.
Precocious and Delayed Puberty: Diagnosis and Treatment

HARRY R. KEISER, M.D.
Clinical Professor of Medicine, Georgetown University School of Medicine, Washington, D.C. Clinical Director, National Heart, Lung, and Blood Institute, National Institutes of Health, Bethesda, Maryland.
Pheochromocytoma and Related Tumors

ROBERT P. KELCH, M.D.
Professor of Pediatrics, Department of Pediatrics, University of Michigan Medical School. Chairman, Department of Pediatrics, University of Michigan Medical Center, and Physician-in-Chief, C.S. Mott Children's Hospital, Ann Arbor, Michigan.
Precocious and Delayed Puberty: Diagnosis and Treatment

DANIEL KENIGSBERG, M.D.
Clinical Associate Professor, State University of New York at Stony Brook. Chief, Section of Reproductive Endocrinology, John T. Mather Memorial Hospital, Fort Jefferson, New York.
Ovarian Follicular Maturation, Ovulation, and Ovulation Induction

JEFFREY B. KERR, Ph.D.
Associate Professor, Department of Anatomy, Monash University, Clayton, Victoria, Australia.
Basic Endocrinology of the Testis

BARRY F. KING, Ph.D.
Professor of Cell Biology and Human Anatomy, University of California School of Medicine, Davis, California.
Placental Hormones

RONALD KLEIN, M.D., M.P.H.
Professor, Department of Ophthalmology and Visual Sciences, University of Wisconsin Medical School. Attending Physician, University of Wisconsin Hospitals and Clinics, Madison, Wisconsin.
Diabetes Mellitus: Late Complications, Oculopathy

STANLEY G. KORENMAN, M.D.
Professor of Medicine and Associate Dean, University of California Los Angeles. Chief of Endocrinology, Center for the Health Sciences; Attending Physician, University of California Los Angeles Medical Center, Los Angeles, California.
Male Impotence

KALMAN KOVACS, M.D., Ph.D.
Professor of Pathology, University of Toronto. Pathologist, St. Michael's Hospital, Toronto, Ontario, Canada.
Anatomy and Histology of the Normal and Abnormal Pituitary Gland

STEPHEN M. KRANE, M.D.
Persis, Cyrus and Marlow B. Harrison Professor of Medicine, Harvard Medical School. Physician and Chief of Arthritis Unit, Massachusetts General Hospital, Boston, Massachusetts
Metabolic Bone Disease: Introduction and Classification; Disorders of Calcification: Osteomalacia and Rickets

HENRY KRONENBERG, M.D.
Professor of Medicine, Harvard Medical School. Chief, Endocrine Unit, Massachusetts General Hospital, Boston, Massachusetts.
Parathyroid Hormone: Physiology, Chemistry, Biosynthesis, Secretion, Metabolism, and Mode of Action

A. H. LAUBER, M.D.
Laboratory of Neurobiology and Behavior, The Rockefeller University, New York, New York.
Hypothalamus and Hormone–Regulated Behaviors

VALERIANO LEITE, M.D.
Post-doctoral Fellow, Department of Physiology, University of Manitoba, Winnipeg, Canada. Endocrinologist, Department of Endocrinology, Portuguese Cancer Institute, Lisbon, Portugal.
Endocrinology of Lactation and Nursing: Disorders of Lactation

ÅKE LERNMARK, Ph.D.
Professor in Experimental Endocrinology, and Chairman, Department of Endocrinology and Clinical Genetics, Karolinska Institute, Stockholm, Sweden.
Insulin-Dependent (Type I) Diabetes: Etiology, Pathogenesis, and Natural History

MICHAEL A. LEVINE, M.D.
Professor of Medicine and Pathology, Johns Hopkins University School of Medicine. Physician, Johns Hopkins Hospital, Baltimore, Maryland.
Pseudohypoparathyroidism

SHUTSUNG LIAO, Ph.D.
Professor, Ben May Institute and the Department of Biochemistry and Molecular Biology, University of Chicago.
Androgen Receptors and Action

GRAHAM C. LIGGINS, M.D., Ph.D.
Professor Emeritus, University of Auckland. Director, Research Centre in Reproductive Medicine, National Women's Hospital, Auckland, New Zealand.
Endocrinology of Parturition

DENNIS W. LINCOLN, D.Sc.
Director, MRC Reproductive Biology Unit, Edinburgh, Scotland.
Gonadotropin-Releasing Hormone (GnRH): Basic Physiology

MARC E. LIPPMAN, M.D.
Professor of Medicine and Pharmacology, Georgetown University School of Medicine. Director, Vincent T. Lombardi Cancer Research Center, Washington, D.C.
Endocrine Management of Malignant Disease

JONATHAN S. LoPRESTI, M.D., Ph.D.
Assistant Professor of Medicine, University of Southern California School of Medicine. Attending Physician, Los Angeles County/USC Medical Center, Los Angeles, California.
Nonthyroidal Illnesses

D. LYNN LORIAUX, M.D.
Professor of Medicine, University of Oregon School of Medicine. Head, Division of Endocrinology, Oregon Health Sciences University, Portland, Oregon.
An Introduction to Endocrinology; Adrenal Insufficiency

IAIN MacINTYRE, M.D., D.Sc., FRCP
Associate Director, The William Harvey Research Institute, St. Bartholomew's Hospital Medical College, London, England.
Calcitonin: Physiology, Biosynthesis, Secretion, Metabolism, and Mode of Action

NOEL K. MACLAREN, M.D.
Professor and Chairman, Department of Pathology and Laboratory Medicine, University of Florida College of Medicine. Attending Physician, Shands Hospital, Gainesville, Florida.
Polyglandular Failure Syndromes

WILLY J. MALAISSE, M.D., Ph.D.
Professor of Chemical Pathology and Director of the Laboratory of Experimental Medicine, Brussels Free University, Brussels, Belgium.
Insulin Secretion and Beta Cell Metabolism

CARL D. MALCHOFF, M.D., Ph.D.
Associate Professor of Surgery and Medicine, University of Connecticut Health Center. Associate Professor of Surgery and Medicine, John Dempsey Hospital, Farmington, Connecticut.
Glucocorticoid Resistance

DIANA M. MALCHOFF, Ph.D.
Assistant Professor of Surgery and Medicine, University of Connecticut Health Center, Farmington, Connecticut
Glucocorticoid Resistance

LEIGHTON P. MARK, M.D.
Associate Professor of Radiology, Medical College of Wisconsin. Neuroradiologist, Froedtert Memorial Lutheran Hospital, Consultant in Radiology, Veterans Administration Medical Center, Milwaukee, Wisconsin.
Radiographic Evaluation of the Pituitary and Anterior Hypothalamus

JOHN C. MARSHALL, M.D., Ph.D.
Professor and Chair, Department of Internal Medicine, University of Virginia School of Medicine. Physician in Chief, University of Virginia Hospitals, University of Virginia Health Sciences Center, Charlottesville, Virginia.
Regulation of Gonadotropin Secretion; Hormonal Regulation of the Menstrual Cycle and Mechanisms of Anovulation

JOSEPH B. MARTIN, M.D., Ph.D.
Professor of Neurology, University of California San Francisco School of Medicine, San Francisco, California.
Functional Anatomy of the Hypothalamic–Anterior Pituitary Complex

T. J. MARTIN, M.D., D.Sc., FRACP
Professor of Medicine, Department of Medicine, University of Melbourne. Director, St. Vincent's Institute of Medical Research, St. Vincent's Hospital, Melbourne, Australia.
Parathyroid Hormone–Related Protein

DIANA MARVER, M.D.
Associate Professor of Internal Medicine, Division of Nephrology, Department of Internal Medicine, University of Texas Southwestern Medical Center, Dallas, Texas.
Aldosterone Action: Biochemistry

WALTER J. McDONALD, M.D.
Associate Dean for Education; Oregon Health Sciences University. Active Staff, University Hospital, Portland, Oregon.
Adrenal Insufficiency

J. DENIS McGARRY, Ph.D.
Professor of Internal Medicine and Biochemistry, University of Texas Southwestern Medical School, Dallas, Texas.
Diabetes Mellitus: Acute Complications, Ketoacidosis, Hyperosmolar Coma, Lactic Acidosis

J. MAXWELL McKENZIE, M.D.
Kathleen and Stanley Glaser Professor and Chairman, Department of Medicine; Professor, Department of Physiology and Biophysics, University of Miami School of Medicine. Chief, Medical Services, Jackson Memorial Hospital; Staff Physician, University of Miami Hospital and Clinics, Miami, Florida.
Hyperthyroidism

GERALDO MEDEIROS-NETO, M.D.
Associate Professor of Endocrinology, University of São Paulo Medical School. Chief, Thyroid Laboratory, Division of Endocrinology, Department of Medicine, Hospital das Clinicas, São Paulo, Brazil.
Iodide Deficiency Disorders

CHRISTOPH A. MEIER, M.D.
Instructor, University Hospital. Research Associate, Thyroid Unit, Department of Endocrinology, University Hospital, Geneva, Switzerland.
Thyroid-Stimulating Hormone in Health and Disease

A. WAYNE MEIKLE, M.D.
Professor of Medicine, Division of Endocrinology, University of Utah School of Medicine. University of Utah Hospital, and Associated Regional and University Pathologists, Director of Endocrine Testing, Salt Lake City, Utah.
Endocrinology of the Prostate and of Benign Prostatic Hyperplasia

JAMES C. MELBY, M.D.
Professor of Medicine, Boston University School of Medicine, Boston, Massachusetts.
Hypoaldosteronism and Mineralocorticoid Resistance

SHLOMO MELMED, M.D.
Professor of Medicine, University of California Los Angeles School of Medicine. Director, Cedars-Sinai Medical Center Research Institute, Los Angeles, California.
Tumor Mass Effects of Lesions in the Hypothalamus and Pituitary; General Aspects of the Management of Pituitary Tumors by Surgery or Radiation Therapy

JAN MESTER, M.D.
Unité de Recherches sur les Peptides, Neurodigestifs et le Diabète, Institut Nationel de la Santé et de la Recherche Médicale, Paris, France.
Nuclear Receptor Superfamily

DONALD METCALF, M.D.
Research Professor of Cancer Biology, The Walter and Eliza Hall Institute of Medical Research, Royal Melbourne Hospital, Melbourne, Australia.
Hormones and Blood Cell Production

BOYD E. METZGER, M.D.
Professor of Medicine, Division of Endocrinology and Metabolism, Northwestern University Medical School. Attending Physician, Northwestern Memorial Hospital, Chicago, Illinois.
Diabetes Mellitus and Pregnancy

ROGER L. MIESFELD, Ph.D.
Associate Professor of Biochemistry, University of Arizona, Arizona Cancer Center, Tucson, Arizona.
Glucocorticoid Action: Biochemistry

DANIEL R. MISHELL, Jr., M.D.
Lyle T. McNeile Professor and Chairman, Department of Obstetrics and Gynecology, University of Southern California School of Medicine. Chief of Professional Services, Los Angeles County/University of Southern California Medical Center, Women's Hospital, Los Angeles, California.
Contraception

MARK E. MOLITCH, M.D.
Professor of Medicine, Center for Endocrinology, Metabolism and Molecular Medicine, Northwestern University Medical School. Attending Physician, Northwestern Memorial Hospital; Consultant, Lakeside Veterans Administration Hospital, Chicago, Illinois.
Pitfalls in Endocrine Tests and Testing in Pregnancy

JOHN MONEY, M.D.
Professor Emeritus of Medical Psychology and Professor Emeritus of Pediatrics, Johns Hopkins University and Johns Hopkins University School of Medicine. Director, Psychohormonal Research Unit, Johns Hopkins Hospital, Baltimore, Maryland
Normal and Abnormal Sexual Behavior

THOMAS J. MOORE, M.D.
Associate Professor of Medicine, Harvard Medical School. Director, Ambulatory Clinical Center, and Director, Cardiac Risk Reduction Center, Brigham and Women's Hospital, Boston, Massachusetts.
Hormonal Aspects of Hypertension

RICHARD M. MORTENSEN, M.D., Ph.D.
Assistant Professor of Medicine, Harvard Medical School. Associate Physician, Brigham and Women's Hospital, Boston, Massachusetts.
Aldosterone Action: Physiology

J. M. MOSELEY, Ph.D.
Senior Research Fellow, University of Melbourne. Department of Medicine, St. Vincent's Hospital, Melbourne, Australia.
Parathyroid Hormone–Related Protein

WILLIAM R. MOYLE, Ph.D.
Professor of Obstetrics and Gynecology, University of Medicine and Dentistry of New Jersey–Robert Wood Johnson Medical School, Piscataway, New Jersey.
Gonadotropins

ANDREW MUIR, M.D.
Assistant Professor, Department of Pathology and Laboratory Medicine, Department of Pediatrics, University of Florida College of Medicine. Attending Physician, Shands Hospital, Gainesville, Florida.
Polyglandular Failure Syndromes

EUGENIO E. MÜLLER, M.D.
Professor and Chairman, Department of Pharmacology, School of Medicine, University of Milan. Professor of Pharmacology, University of Milan, Milan, Italy.
Role of Neurotransmitters and Neuromodulators in the Control of Anterior Pituitary Hormone Secretion

ALLAN MUNCK, Ph.D.
Third Century Professor of Physiology, Dartmouth Medical School, Lebanon, New Hampshire.
Glucocorticoid Action: Physiology

ANIKÓ NÁRAY-FEJES-TÓTH, M.D.
Associate Professor of Physiology, Dartmouth Medical School, Lebanon, New Hampshire.
Glucocorticoid Action: Physiology

ROBERT M. NEER, M.D.
Associate Professor of Medicine, Harvard Medical School. Director, Osteoporosis Center, Massachusetts General Hospital, Boston, Massachusetts.
Medical Management of Hyperparathyroidism and Hypercalcemia; Osteoporosis

DON H. NELSON, M.D.
Professor Emeritus of Medicine, University of Utah Medical School. Attending Physician, University Hospital, Salt Lake City, Utah.
A Historical Overview of the Adrenal Cortex

MARIA I. NEW, M.D.
Professor and Chairman, Department of Pediatrics, Cornell University Medical College. Chairman, Department of Pediatrics, The New York Hospital, New York, New York.
Congenital Adrenal Hyperplasia

NICOS A. NICOLA, Ph.D.
Head, Laboratory for Molecular Regulators, The Walter and Eliza Hall Institute of Medical Research, Royal Melbourne Hospital, Melbourne, Australia.
Hormones and Blood Cell Production

JOHN T. NICOLOFF, M.D.
Professor of Medicine, University of Southern California School of Medicine. Attending Physician, Los Angeles County/USC Medical Center, Los Angeles, California.
Thyroid Hormone Transport and Metabolism; Nonthyroidal Illnesses

LYNNETTE K. NIEMAN, M.D.
Chief, Unit on Reproductive Medicine, Developmental Endocrinology Branch, and Senior Staff Physician, National Institute of Child Health and

Human Development, National Institutes of Health, Bethesda, Maryland.
Cushing's Syndrome

JEFFREY A. NORTON, M.D.
Professor of Surgery, Chief of Endocrine and Oncologic Surgery, Washington University School of Medicine. Attending Surgeon, Barnes Hospital, St. Louis, Missouri.
Surgical Management of Hyperparathyroidism

SAMUEL R. NUSSBAUM, M.D.
Associate Professor of Medicine, Harvard Medical School. Director, Endocrine Associates, Massachusetts General Hospital, Boston, Massachusetts.
Parathyroid Hormone: Physiology, Chemistry, Biosynthesis, Secretion, Metabolism, and Mode of Action; Medical Management of Hyperparathyroidism and Hypercalcemia

WILLIAM D. ODELL, M.D., Ph.D.
Professor of Medicine and Physiology, University of Utah School of Medicine. Chairman, Department of Internal Medicine, University of Utah, Salt Lake City, Utah.
Genetic Basis of Sexual Differentiation; Endocrinology of Sexual Maturation; The Menopause and Hormonal Replacement

JERROLD M. OLEFSKY, M.D.
Professor of Medicine and Chief, Endocrinology and Metabolism Section, University of California San Diego School of Medicine, La Jolla. Attending Physician, University Hospital, and Veterans Administration Medical Center, San Diego, California.
Diabetes Mellitus (Type II): Etiology and Pathogenesis

NIALL M. O'MEARA, M.D.
Consultant Physician/Endocrinologist, Department of Diabetes and Endocrinology, Mater Misericordiae Hospital, Dublin, Ireland.
Secretion and Metabolism of Insulin, Proinsulin, and C-Peptide

LELIO ORCI, M.D.
Professor, Histology and Cell Biology, Department of Morphology, University of Geneva Medical School, Geneva, Switzerland.
Glucagon Secretion, Alpha Cell Metabolism, and Glucagon Action

LAWRENCE N. PARKER, M.D.
Professor of Medicine, University of California at Irvine College of Medicine. Assistant Chief of Endocrinology, Veterans Administration Medical Center, Long Beach, California.
Adrenal Androgens

JEFFREY H. PERLMAN, M.D.
Senior Fellow in Medicine, Cornell University Medical College. Clinical Fellow, New York Hospital, and Memorial Sloan-Kettering Cancer Center, New York, New York.
Second Messenger Signaling Pathways: Phosphatidylinositol and Calcium

D. W. PFAFF, M.D.
Professor of Neurobiology and Behavior, The Rockefeller University, New York, New York.
Hypothalamus and Hormone-Regulated Behaviors

RICHARD L. PHELPS, M.D.
Assistant Clinical Professor of Medicine, Northwestern University Medical School. Attending Physician, Northwestern Memorial Hospital, Chicago, Illinois.
Diabetes Mellitus and Pregnancy

BRIAN T. PICKERING, B.Sc, Ph.D, D.Sc.
Professor of Anatomy, University of Bristol, Bristol, England.
Oxytocin

DANIEL H. POLK, M.D.
Associate Professor, Department of Pediatrics, University of California Los Angeles School of Medicine, Los Angeles, California. Physician Specialist, Harbor-UCLA Medical Center, Torrance, California.
Thyroid Disease in the Fetus, Neonate, and Child; Fetal and Neonatal Endocrinology

KENNETH S. POLONSKY, M.D.
Professor of Medicine and Chief, Section of Endocrinology. Director, Diabetes Research and Training Center, University of Chicago Pritzker School of Medicine, Chicago, Illinois.
Secretion and Metabolism of Insulin, Proinsulin, and C-Peptide

JOHN T. POTTS, Jr., M.D.
The Jackson Professor of Clinical Medicine, Harvard Medical School. Physician-in-Chief, Massachusetts General Hospital, Boston, Massachusetts.
Parathyroids: Introduction; Parathyroid Hormone: Physiology, Chemistry, Biosynthesis, Secretion, Metabolism, and Mode of Action; Hyperparathyroidism; Differential Diagnosis of Hypercalcemia; Medical Management of Hyperparathyroidism and Hypercalcemia

EDWIN L. PRIEN, Jr., M.D.
Instructor in Medicine, Harvard Medical School. Assistant Physician, Massachusetts General Hospital, Boston, Massachusetts.
Calcium Nephrolithiasis

LISA P. PURDY, M.D., C.M., FRCP(C)
Fellow in Endocrinology, Northwestern University Medical School, Chicago, Illinois.
Diabetes Mellitus and Pregnancy

JOSÉ QUINTANS, M.D., Ph.D.
Professor, Department of Pathlogy, Committee on Immunology and the College, University of Chicago and University of Chicago Cancer Center, Chicago, Illinois.
Immunological Mechanisms Causing Autoimmune Endocrine Disease

JORGE A. RAMIREZ, M.D.
Assistant Director, Medical Education, Arnold Palmer Hospital for Women and Children, Orlando, Florida.
The Renal Osteodystrophies

MICHAEL B. RANKE, M.D.
Professor of Pediatrics, University of Tübingen. Head, Department of Endocrinology, Children's Hospital, University of Tübingen, Tübingen, Germany.
Growth Hormone Insufficiency: Clinical Features, Diagnosis, and Therapy

SAMUEL REFETOFF, M.D.
Professor of Medicine and Pediatrics, University of Chicago Pritzker School of Medicine. Attending Physician, University of Chicago Hospitals, Chicago, Illinois.
Thyroid Hormone Transport and Metabolism; Thyroid Function Tests

SEYMOUR REICHLIN, M.D., Ph.D.
Professor of Medicine, Tufts University School of Medicine. Senior Endocrinologist, New England Medical Center, Boston, Massachusetts.
Endocrine-Immune Interaction

CLAUDE REMACLE, Ph.D.
Professor of Biology, University of Louvain, Louvain, Belgium.
Anatomy, Developmental Biology, and Pathology of the Pancreatic Islets

IVANA PAVLIC RENAR, M.D.
Institute Vuk Vrhovac, Zagreb, Croatia
Neuroendocrine Tumors of Carcinoid Variety

B. REUSENS, Ph.D.
Department of Biology, University of Louvain, Louvain, Belgium.
Anatomy, Developmental Biology, and Pathology of the Pancreatic Islets

GAIL P. RISBRIDGER, Ph.D.
NH and MRC Senior Research Fellow, Institute of Reproduction and Development, Monash University, Melbourne, Australia.
Basic Endocrinology of the Testis

PETER N. RISKIND, M.D., Ph.D.
Assistant Professor of Neurology, Harvard Medical School. Assistant Neurologist, Massachusetts General Hospital, and Spaulding Rehabilitation Hospital, Boston, Massachusetts.
Functional Anatomy of the Hypothalamic–Anterior Pituitary Complex

ROBERT L. ROSENFIELD, M.D.
Professor of Pediatrics and Medicine, University of Chicago Pritzker School of Medicine. Head, Section of Pediatric Endocrinology, Wyler Children's Hospital, Chicago, Illinois.
Hyperandrogenism, Hirsutism, and the Polycystic Ovary Syndrome; Somatic Growth and Maturation

ZEV ROSENWAKS, M.D.
Professor, Department of Obstetrics and Gynecology, Cornell University Medical College. Director, The Center for Reproductive Medicine and Infertility, The New York Hospital-Cornell Medical Center, New York, New York.
Ovarian Follicular Maturation, Ovulation, and Ovulation Induction

ARTHUR H. RUBENSTEIN, M.D.
Professor and Chairman, Department of Medicine, University of Chicago Pritzker School of Medicine, Chicago, Illinois.
Chemistry and Biosynthesis of the Islet Hormones: Insulin, Islet Amyloid Polypeptide (Amylia), Glucagon, Somatostatin, and Pancreatic Polypeptide; Diabetes Mellitus: Therapy

WILLIAM E. RUSSELL, M.D.
Associate Professor of Pediatrics and Cell Biology, Vanderbilt University. Attending Physician, Vanderbilt Children's Hospital, Nashville, Tennessee.
Peptide Growth Factors

ISIDRO B. SALUSKY, M.D.
Professor of Pediatrics, University of California Los Angeles School of Medicine. Director, Pediatric Dialysis Program, and Program Director, General Clinical Research Center, UCLA Medical Center, Los Angeles, California.
The Renal Osteodystrophies

GAETANO SALVATORE, M.D.
Full Professor, Dipartimento di Biologia e Patologia Cellulare e Molecolare, Universita di Napoli Federico II. Dean, Medical School, Universita di Napoli Federico II. President, Stazione Zoologica Anton Dohrn, Naples, Italy.
Biosynthesis and Secretion of Thyroid Hormones

SALVIA SANTAMARINA-FOJO, M.D.
Head, Section of Molecular Biology, National Heart, Lung, and Blood Institute, National Institutes of Health, Bethesda, Maryland.
Disorders of Lipoprotein Metabolism

RICHARD J. SANTEN, M.D.
Professor of Medicine, and Chairman, Department of Internal Medicine, Wayne State University School of Medicine. Physician-in-Chief, Detroit Medical Center, Detroit, Michigan.
Gynecomastia

DAVID H. SARNE, M.D.
Associate Professor of Medicine, University of Illinois at Chicago. Physician, University of Illinois at Chicago Medical Center, Veterans Administration Center–Westside, Chicago, Illinois.
Thyroid Function Tests

MAURICE F. SCANLON, B.Sc., M.D., FRCP
Professor of Endocrinology, University of Wales College of Medicine. Consultant Physician, University Hospital of Wales, Cardiff, Wales.
Thyrotropin-Releasing Hormone: Basic and Clinical Aspects

DESMOND A. SCHATZ, M.D.
Associate Professor, Department of Pediatrics, University of Florida College of Medicine. Attending Physician, Shands Hospital, Gainesville, Florida.
Polyglandular Failure Syndromes

ALAN L. SCHILLER, M.D.
Irene Heinz Given and John LaPorte Given Professor of Medicine, Mount Sinai School of Medicine. Chairman of Pathology, Mount Sinai Medical Center and Mount Sinai Hospital, New York, New York.
Metabolic Bone Disease: Introduction and Classification

ROBERT E. SCULLY, M.D.
Professor Emeritus of Pathology, Harvard Medical School. Pathologist, Massachusetts General Hospital, Boston, Massachusetts.
Ovarian Tumors with Endocrine Manifestations; Testicular Tumors with Endocrine Manifestations

GINO V. SEGRE, M.D.
Associate Professor of Medicine, Harvard Medical School. Associate Physician and Director, Endocrine Clinical Laboratory, Massachusetts General Hospital, Boston, Massachusetts.
Parathyroid Hormone: Physiology, Chemistry, Biosynthesis, Secretion, Metabolism, and Mode of Action; Differential Diagnosis of Hypercalcemia

F. JOHN SERVICE, M.D., Ph.D.

Professor of Medicine, Mayo Medical School. Consultant in Endocrinology and Metabolism, Mayo Clinic, Rochester, Minnesota.

Hypoglycemia, Including Hypoglycemia in Neonates and Children

YORAM SHENKER, M.D.

Associate Professor, Section of Endocrinology and Metabolism, Department of Medicine, University of Wisconsin Medical School. Attending Physican, William S. Middleton Memorial Veterans Administration Hospital and University of Wisconsin Hospital and Clinics, Madison, Wisconsin.

Hormonal Regulation of Electrolyte and Water Metabolism

LOUIS M. SHERWOOD, M.D.

Adjunct Professor of Medicine, University of Pennsylvania School of Medicine. Visiting Professor of Medicine, Albert Einstein College of Medicine. Senior Vice President, Medical and Scientific Affairs, U.S. Human Health Division, Merck & Co., West Point, Pennsylvania. Attending Physician, Montefiore Medical Center, Bronx Municipal Hospital Center, Bronx, New York.

Paraneoplastic Endocrine Disorders (Ectopic Hormone Syndromes)

MANAN SHUKLA, M.D.

Visiting Research Associate, University of Chicago Hospitals, Chicago, Illinois.

Developmental Abnormalities of the Thyroid; Surgery of the Thyroid

EVAN R. SIMPSON, Ph.D.

Professor of Obstetrics/Gynecology and Biochemistry, The University of Texas Southwestern Medical Center, Dallas, Texas.

Steroid Hormone Biosynthesis in the Adrenal Cortex and its Regulation by Adrenocorticotropin

FREDERICK R. SINGER, M.D.

Clinical Professor of Medicine, University of California Los Angeles School of Medicine. Medical Director, Osteoporosis/Metabolic Bone Disease Program, St. John's Hospital and Health Center, Santa Monica, California.

Paget's Disease of Bone

PETER J. SNYDER, M.D.

Professor of Medicine, University of Pennsylvania School of Medicine. Attending Physician, Hospital of the University of Pennsylvania, Philadelphia, Pennsylvania.

Gonadotroph Adenomas

ALLEN M. SPIEGEL, M.D.

Chief, Molecular Pathophysiology Branch, National Institute of Diabetes and Digestive and Kidney Diseases, National Institutes of Health, Bethesda, Maryland.

Pseudohypoparathyroidism

DONALD F. STEINER, M.D.

Professor of Biochemistry and Molecular Biology and Medicine, University of Chicago Pritzker School of Medicine, Chicago, Illinois.

Chemistry and Biosynthesis of the Islet Hormones: Insulin, Islet Amyloid Polypeptide (Amylin), Glucagon, Somatostatin, and Pancreatic Polypeptide

ANDREW F. STEWART, M.D.

Professor of Medicine and Endocrinology, Yale University School of Medicine. Chief, Endocrinology, West Haven Veterans Administration Medical Center; Attending Physician, Yale-New Haven Hospital, New Haven, Connecticut.

Malignancy-Associated Hyercalcemia

JEROME F. STRAUSS III, M.D., Ph.D.

Luigi Mastroianni, Jr. Professor, and Director, Center for Research in Women's Health and Reproduction and Associate Chairman, Department of Obstetric and Gynecology, University of Pennsylvania School of Medicine. Attending Physician, Hospital of the University of Pennsylvania, Philadelphia, Pennsylvania.

Placental Hormones

HUGO STUDER, M.D.

Full Professor of Medicine, University of Bern. Head, Department of Medicine, University Hospital, Inselspital, Bern, Switzerland.

Multinodular Goiter

SONIA L. SUGG, M.D.

Medical Staff Fellow, Surgery Branch, National Cancer Institute, National Institutes of Health, Bethesda, Maryland.

Surgical Management of Hyperparathyroidism

HISATO TADA, M.D.

Research Associate, Department of Laboratory Medicine, Osaka University Medical School. Staff Physician, Osaka University Hospital, Osaka, Japan.

Autoimmune Thyroid Disease/Thyroiditis

HOWARD S. TAGER, Ph.D.

Professor of Biochemistry and Molecular Biology and Medicine, University of Chicago Pritzker School of Medicine, Chicago, Illinois.

Chemistry and Biosynthesis of the Islet Hormones: Insulin, Islet Amyloid Polypeptide (Amylin), Glucagon, Somatostatin, and Pancreatic Polypeptide

RAJESH V. THAKKER, M.A., FRCP

M.R.C. Clinical Scientist and Senior Lecturer, Royal Postgraduate Medical School. Honourary Consultant Physician and Endocrinologist, The Hammersmith Hospital, London, England.

Multiple Endocrine Neoplasia Type 1

MICHAEL O. THORNER, M.B., B.S., D.Sc., FRCP

Kenneth R. Crispell Professor of Medicine; Chief, Division of Endocrinology and Metabolism, University of Virginia Health Sciences Center, Charlottesville, Virginia.

Growth Hormone–Releasing Hormone: Basic Physiology and Clinical Implications; Prolactin: Hyperprolactinemic Syndromes and Management

FRED W. TUREK, Ph.D.

Professor and Chairman, Department of Neurobiology and Physiology, Northwestern University Medical School, Chicago, Illinois.

Endocrine and Other Biological Rhythms

ROGER H. UNGER, M.D.

Touchstone/West Distinguished Chair in Diabetes Research and Professor of Internal Medicine, University of Texas Southwestern Medical School. Senior Medical Investigator, Veterans Administration Medical Center; Director, Center for Diabetes Research, University of Texas Southwestern Medical Center, Dallas, Texas.

Glucagon Secretion, Alpha Cell Metabolism, and Glucagon Action

ROBERT D. UTIGER, M.D.

Clinical Professor of Medicine, Harvard Medical School. Attending Physician, Brigham and Woman's Hospital, Boston, Massachusetts.

Hypothyroidism

EVE VAN CAUTER, Ph.D.

Research Associate (Professor); University of Chicago Pritzker School of Medicine, Chicago, Illinois.

Endocrine and Other Biological Rhythms

JUDSON J. VAN WYK, M.D.

Kenan Professor of Pediatrics, University of North Carolina School of Medicine. Attending Pediatrician, University of North Carolina Children's Hospital, Chapel Hill, North Carolina.

Peptide Growth Factors

MARY LEE VANCE, M.D.

Associate Professor of Medicine, University of Virginia School of Medicine. Staff Physician, University of Virginia Hospital, Charlottesville, Virginia.

Prolactin: Hyperprolactinemic Syndromes and Management

G. VASSART, M.D., Ph.D.

Professor of Medical Genetics, Free University of Brussels, Faculty of Medicine. Director, Department of Medical Genetics, Erasme Hospital, Brussels, Belgium.

Thyroid Regulation

AARON VINIK, M.D.

Professor of Internal Medicine and Anatomy/Neurobiology and Director, Diabetes Research Institute, Eastern Virginia Medical School, Norfolk, Virginia.

Neuroendocrine Tumors of Carcinoid Variety

ROBERT VOLPÉ, M.D., FRCP(C), FACP, FRCP (Edin)

Professor Emeritus, Division of Endocrinology and Metabolism, Department of Medicine, University of Toronto. Active Staff and Director of Endocrinology Research Laboratory, The Wellesley Hospital; Consultant, Department of Medicine, Princess Margaret Hospital (Ontario Cancer Institute), Toronto, Ontario, Canada.

Subacute and Sclerosing Thyroiditis

MICHELLE P. WARREN, M.D.

Associate Professor of Clinical Obstetrics and Gynecology and Clinical Medicine, Columbia College of Physicians and Surgeons. Head, Reproductive Endocrinology, Roosevelt Site, St. Luke's–Roosevelt Hospital Center, New York, New York.

Anorexia Nervosa

JOHN A. H. WASS, M.D., FRCP

Professor of Clinical Endocrinology, St. Bartholomew's Hospital Medical College. Honourary Consultant Physician, St. Bartholomew's Hospital, London, England.

Somatostatin; Tests of Pituitary Function

MICHAEL R. WATERMAN, Ph.D.

Professor and Chairman, Department of Biochemistry, Vanderbilt University School of Medicine, Nashville, Tennessee.

Steroid Hormone Biosynthesis in the Adrenal Cortex and its Regulation by Adrenocorticotropin

BRUCE D. WEINTRAUB, M.D.

Director, NIH Interinstitute Endocrinology Training Program. Chief, Molecular and Cellular Endocrinology Branch, National Institute of Diabetes and Digestive and Kidney Diseases, National Institutes of Health, Bethesda, Maryland.

Thyroid-Stimulating Hormone in Health and Disease

MORRIS F. WHITE, Ph.D.

Associate Professor of Biological Chemistry, Department of Medicine, Harvard Medical School. Investigator, Elliott P. Joslin Research Laboratory, Joslin Diabetes Center, Boston, Massachusetts.

Molecular Mechanism of Insulin Action

JOHN F. WILBER, M.D.

Professor of Medicine, University of Maryland School of Medicine. Staff Physician, University of Maryland Systems, Baltimore, Maryland.

Control of Thyroid Function: The Hypothalamic-Pituitary-Thyroid Axis

JOHN P. H. WILDING, B.M., MRCP
Senior Registrar, Division of Endocrinology and Metabolism, Hammersmith Hospital, London, England.
Hormones of the Gastrointestinal Tract

E. DILLWYN WILLIAMS, M.D.
Professor of Histopathology, University of Cambridge. Consultant Histopathologist, Addenbrookes Hospital, Cambridge, England.
Medullary Carcinoma of the Thyroid

GORDON H. WILLIAMS, M.D.
Professor of Medicine, Harvard Medical School. Senior Physician and Chief, Endocrine-Hypertension Service, Brigham and Women's Hospital, Boston, Massachusetts.
Aldosterone Action: Physiology; Hormonal Aspects of Hypertension

STEPHEN J. WINTERS, M.D.
Professor of Medicine, University of Pittsburgh School of Medicine, Pittsburgh, Pennsylvania.
Clinical Disorders of the Testis

ROBERT J. WITTE, M.D.
Assistant Professor, University of Nebraska School of Medicine. Radiologist, University of Nebraska Medical Center, Omaha, Nebraska
Radiographic Evaluation of the Pituitary and Anterior Hypothalamus

FREDRIC E. WONDISFORD, M.D.
Assistant Professor of Medicine, Harvard Medical School. Chief, Thyroid Unit, Division of Endocrinology and Metabolism, Beth Israel Hospital, Boston, Massachusetts.
Thyroid-Stimulating Hormone in Health and Disease

MARGITA ZAKARIJA, M.D.
Professor, Department of Medicine and Department of Microbiology and Immunology, University of Miami School of Medicine. Staff Physician, University of Miami Hospital and Clinics, and Jackson Memorial Hospital, Miami, Florida.
Hyperthyroidism

Preface

One of the most awe-inspiring experiences in medicine occurs on meeting each new patient. In the course of an hour an individual, previously quite unknown, allows the physician total access to his innermost problems, fears, and secrets, and to his body. A good physician must accept this gift with humility and respond with candor, empathy, and responsibility. The opportunity presented to help a fellow human suffering from illness provides the most fundamental satisfaction in being a physician. The physician must bring to bear on the problem his knowledge of pathophysiology, presented with an understanding of human interactions.

To prepare for this task, doctors subject themselves to a demanding education and a long apprenticeship. They then must almost totally relearn their art and science every decade in order to stay abreast of advances. Endocrinology shares in this development of knowledge, perhaps even leads in the change, as the constant stream of new clinical and laboratory observations forces us to update our prior ideas. It is the challenge to encompass this evolving field of endocrinology—and bring it to clinicians and researchers in a useful manner—that we address in the third edition of ENDOCRINOLOGY.

Our goals remain as stated in the first edition:

- To review basic knowledge of endocrine physiology and biochemistry in a complete and up-to-date manner
- To provide a thorough clinical discussion of each topic
- To integrate the basic and clinical material around human endocrinology
- To make clear the integration of the endocrine system in a gland-by-gland manner, as well as the important multi-hormonal integration in relation to physiological functions
- To have our presentations made by the most accomplished endocrinologists throughout the world.

Reflecting these goals, our book is divided into three complementary sections. The first six chapters provide a foundation for understanding contemporary molecular endocrinology, emphasizing the function of cell membrane and nuclear receptors, and "second messengers". The second section provides a traditional gland-oriented presentation of basic endocrine physiology and clinical problems. The third section integrates contemporary knowledge around important physiological or pathological functions, such as feeding, obesity, rhythms, and polyglandular autoimmunity.

Our book is in every sense the product of a joint effort by eight distinguished co-editors. They have taken the responsibility for organizing each of the sections, which are in a real sense equal to whole books in themselves. In keeping with our plan to bring the most current concepts to our readers, we have the privilege of introducing three new section editors for this edition. Dr. Lynn Loriaux now edits the chapters on Adrenal Disease, Dr. Larry Jameson has organized the introductory chapters and "Integrated Endocrinology," and in an acknowledgment of the "One World" of endocrinology, Dr. Henry Burger of Melbourne has taken responsibility for the section on Male Reproduction.

We are blessed by having experts from around the world write our chapters, and even to submit them more or less promptly. Readers will note many totally new chapters including those on the application of molecular biological techniques to endocrine disease, the molecular basis of insulin action, adrenal imaging, adrenal androgens, glucocorticoid resistance, gonadal regulatory peptides, endocrine testing in pregnancy, male contraception, multiple endocrine neoplasias, hormones of the cardiovascular system, and endocrine hypertension, to name a few. And the rest of the chapters have been largely rewritten as well.

It is with a sense of accomplishment and excitement that we bring this edition to the endocrine community. We believe it will provide students, fellows, clinical endocrinologists, academicians, and researchers around the world with a complete source to which they can turn to find answers to their questions. The chief editor is continually awed by the brilliance displayed by the authors in each section. To these distinguished scientists and clinicians, I express my great respect and most sincere thanks. It is their knowledge and hard work that make this volume possible and unique in its scope and contribution.

LESLIE J. DeGROOT, M.D.

Contents

PART III   THYROID GLAND

VOLUME 2

PART IV   PARATHYROIDS

PART VI   ADRENAL CORTEX

VOLUME 3

PART IX ENDOCRINOLOGY OF PREGNANCY

PART X MALE REPRODUCTION

†Deceased.

PART XI   INTEGRATED ENDOCRINE SYSTEMS

PART I

PRINCIPLES OF HORMONE ACTION

An Introduction to Endocrinology

LYNN D. LORIAUX

Endocrinology is the study of cell-to-cell communication by messenger molecules traversing an extracellular space. In this way cells communicate with themselves, with nearest neighbors, with distant cells via a circulatory system, and with separate organisms across an intervening "environment." These types of cell-to-cell communication are designated as autocrine, paracrine, endocrine, and "pherocrine," respectively. The biological beginnings of these processes probably occurred with the transition from unicellular to multicellular organisms having sufficient size to prohibit direct communication among all constituent cells. The process, in its generic sense, provided the framework that permitted cooperation among cells and ultimately the striking biological diversity inherent in the natural tendency of cells to differentiate toward specialized function. Because of this early deployment in the process of evolution, endocrine systems play important roles in many of the most basic biological activities of complex organisms—food seeking and satiety, metabolism and caloric economy, growth and differentiation, reproduction, homeostasis, response to environmental change, arousal, defense, flight, and secluding behaviors.

As cell-to-cell communication provided survival advantage, evolutionary pressure across the last billion years layered complexity upon complexity in extant endocrine systems. Old systems were scrapped and new ones invented. Old hormones took on new functions as new receptor molecules evolved, and new ligands were devised for old receptors. Systems began to subserve different specialized functions in different species.

Attempts to unravel this tangled skein began a mere 2500 years ago with the beginning of free inquiry in the city-states of Greece. The development of our understanding of the endocrine system closely parallels the evolution of the physical and biological sciences across the intervening years. The earliest allusions to an endocrine system came from Aristotle, who, in 400 BC, described the effects of castration on the songbird.[1] Galen, 400 years later, described and named the thyroid gland in dissections of great apes and, perhaps, of humans.[2] Galen's monumental contributions to medicine and biology were unchallenged across the 1000 years of the Middle Ages, an incubation that culminated in the Renaissance and its efflorescence of art and science. Attention to anatomical detail, heightened by artists like Leonardo and Michelangelo, proved to be a focus that energized the landmark collaboration of Vesalius and Kalkar and its product, *De Humanis Corporis Fabrica*,

published in 1543.[3] This work, one of the true inflection points in biological science, provided the first accurate account of human anatomy and, along with it, descriptions of many human endocrine organs. More importantly, *De Fabrica* lifted the cloak of infallibility from the teachings of Galen and set the trajectory of modern scientific enquiry as no other single event has done.

In short order anatomists such as Eustachius and Fallopius,[4] primarily of the Paduan school, precisely described the structure of the endocrine system in humans. The physiologists followed. Bernard demonstrated the process of "internal secretion,"[5] and Bayliss and Starling showed that the epithelium of the small intestine contained a substance that could, when injected into the bloodstream of dogs, stimulate the exocrine secretion of the pancreas.[6] They called the substance *secretin*. Molecules with this property, stimulating a response in a distant organ via the bloodstream, were first referred to as *hormones*, from the greek hormao (to arouse), by Professor Starling in 1905 in his Croonian Lectures to the Royal College, "The Chemical Correlation of the Functions of the Body."

The work of the physiologists was vested with a clinical relevance by the observations of the great physicians: Addison on adrenal insufficiency,[7] Graves and von Basedow on goiter and hyperthyroidism,[8, 9] Minkowski and von Mering on diabetes,[10] Marie on acromegaly,[11] Cushing on glucocorticoid excess,[12] and Albright on hyperparathyroidism,[13] among others. These "untreatable diseases" spurred on the efforts of the biochemists who followed to isolate and purify the hormones; thyroxine by Harrington,[14] cortisone by Kendall[15] and Reichstein,[16] insulin and parathormone by Collip,[17, 18] growth hormone and ACTH by Li,[19] and the hypothalamic-releasing hormones by Guillemin.[20] Medicine was advanced by these discoveries. Examples include the successful treatment of hypothyroidism by Murray,[21] adrenal insufficiency by Thorn,[22] growth hormone deficiency by Rabin,[23] and diabetes mellitus by Joslin. In addition, the purification of the various hormones permitted the development of measurements for them, culminating in the development of radioimmunoassay by Berson and Yallow in 1969.[24] This advance greatly stimulated the study of endocrine physiology, particularly "feedback regulation" of hormone secretion. Our understanding of endocrine pathophysiology was also greatly enhanced by this advance, as was the clinical management of diseases of the endocrine system. Finally, the "receptor" concept was advanced in endocrinology primarily by the example of the syndrome of pseudohypoparathyroidism, a receptor-mediated resistance to the effects of parathormone described by Fuller Albright in 1944.[26] This finding ushered in the current era of investigation in endocrinology including the cell biology of hormone action, receptor structure and function, signal transduction, gene regulation, peptide processing, and the mechanisms of hormone secretion.

Emerging from this accumulated body of knowledge is our current concept of the basic attributes of the "endocrine system." There are nine classic glands (hypothalamus, pineal, pituitary, thyroid, parathyroid, pancreas, adrenal, testis, and ovary) and an ever-increasing number of nonclassical glands (thymus, heart, gut, kidney, placenta, skin) that secrete hormones. These hormones are divided into two categories: lipid soluble and water soluble. Examples of lipid-soluble hormones are steroids and iodothyronines. Examples of water-soluble hormones are glycoprotein hormones (luteinizing hormone, follicle-stimulating hormone, and human chorionic gonadotropin) and the catecholamines (epinephrine and norepinephrine).

The synthesis and secretion of hormones is not different from that of other molecules in the same general class. The peptide hormones, for example, are generally derived from larger precursor molecules that are the first products of translation. These large molecules are sequentially processed by "cleavage" enzymes, often yielding a number of biologically active products. A good example of this is the biosynthesis of ACTH. In the anterior pituitary gland, the precursor molecule, pro-opiomelanocortin (POMC), is first cleaved to β lipotropic hormone (LPH), ACTH, a "junction peptide" (JP), and an inactive carboxyl terminal peptide, POMC 1-74. In the intermediate lobe, further processing cleaves β LPH into γ LPH and β-endorphin, and ACTH is cleaved into corticotropin-like intermediate lobe peptide (CLIP) and ACTH 1-13. Several of these products are biologically active. Prohormones exist for insulin, somatostatin, glucagon, enkephalin, antidiuretic hormone, gastrin, parathyroid hormone, and calcitonin, among others. The steroid hormones are metabolic products of cholesterol, and both the iodothyronines and catecholamines are derived from tyrosine.

Water-soluble hormones, such as insulin, can be transported in plasma as is, while the lipid soluble hormones must be "solubilized" by noncovalent binding to transport proteins. Testosterone, dihydrotestosterone, and estradiol circulate in a bound complex with sex-hormone binding protein (SHBG), a 90-kDa glycoprotein. Cortisol, progesterone, and aldosterone circulate largely bound to cortisol-binding globulin (CBG), a 52-kDa α-2 globulin. Thyroxine and to a much lesser extent triiodothyronine circulate bound to thyroxine-binding globulin, a 54-kDa glycoprotein. In addition to permitting vascular transport in an aqueous medium, the "binding proteins" retard the metabolic clearance of the bound hormones and serve as a reservoir of bound protein to defend the circulating free, and presumably biologically active, concentration.

Lipid-soluble hormones gain entry into cells passively by virtue of miscibility with the lipid component of the cell membrane. These hormones interact with cytosol or nuclear receptors that recognize and interact with specific gene regulatory sequences. This interaction leads to a "hormone action" mediated by new protein synthesis. Water-soluble hormones are, by themselves, excluded from the interior of the cell and must interact with cell surface or "membrane-bound" receptors. These hormones must interact with the nucleus through the medium of a second messenger. Second messengers are not single entities but represent a cascade of events set in motion by a hormone-receptor interaction that leads to an alteration in the concentration of molecular species interacting with "hormone-responsive" gene regulatory elements (GRE). The best understood of the second messengers is the adenyl cyclase system. In this system the hormone receptor is linked to adenyl cyclase and, hence, cAMP production. The hormone receptor is linked to the enzyme by two G proteins, one that can suppress and one that can enhance adenyl cyclase activity. In this way, cAMP alone can mediate more than one hormone response in a given cell. cAMP regulates the "activation," via phosphorylation, of enzymes in the kinase family that, in turn, catalyze the activation of a cAMP response element–binding protein (CREB). CREB is the effector of hormone action in this second messenger system. Other second messengers depend on the modulation of guanylate cyclase, tyrosine kinase, phosphoinositol turnover, calcium flux, and, in some cases, ion channel activity.

In the classic endocrine system, one or more consequences of hormone action are "sensed" at some level, and the hormone secretory process is modulated to preserve a given "normal" level of hormone action. This is the phenomenon of *negative feedback*. It can be conceptualized most readily in the form of a home heating system. The typical home heating system consists of fuel source, furnace, and thermostat. The temperature set on the thermostat is the independent variable in the system. As the temperature in the house falls below that set on the thermostat, the furnace is switched on, consuming fuel and heating the house until the temperature exceeds that set on the thermostat. Thus, the actual temperature oscillates around a mean temperature that approximates that set on the thermostat. The furnace will burn more or less depending upon open windows and people coming and going through the various portals to the outside. Most endocrine systems function in an analogous way. The plasma concentration of calcium, for example, is tightly regulated in the human. As the calcium concentration falls, parathormone is secreted to raise it; as the calcium concentration rises, parathormone secretion is curtailed and the calcium concentration falls. The "thermostat" is in the parathyroid glands where parathormone is synthesized and secreted. The "fuel source" is the skeletal reserve of calcium, and the furnace is the parathormone-responsive cadre of bone cells—osteoclasts and osteocytes. Feedback systems are inherently rhythmic. There is a basal fluctuation around the independent variable, but more complicated rhythms can be superimposed such as in a house that has the thermostat turned down for the night. The endocrine rhythms have been named for the period duration. Circhoral rhythms are "about an hour," circadian rhythms are "about a day" (*circa*, about; *dies*, a day), circatrigantan rhythms are "about a month," and circannual rhythms are "about a year." Examples are the 90-minute periods of gonadotropin secretion, the daily rhythm of plasma cortisol concentration, the monthly period of the reproductive cycle in women, and the annual period of seasonal breeding in ungulates.

Gland, hormone, transport, action, and feedback—these are the fundamental attributes of the endocrine system.

This book attempts to distill into a single-source reference work the accumulated understanding of these processes in the human endocrine system, as well as the diseases that emanate from their disordered function. The authors have attempted to walk the fine line that separates "encyclopedic from pedantic" and "comprehensive from irrelevant." This necessitates selectivity; everything cannot be presented. The book is current as of the time of publishing. This means that considerable material of a "research" nature will be found here. It is well to remember that Medicine is differentiated from the other healing arts primarily by its scientific base, and endocrinology is foremost in this regard. The inclusion of this material is necessary to round out the picture of "where we are now." Nonetheless, the reader is advised to keep in mind the current pace of discovery. The most recent material in this book is the least likely to stand the test of time. Fuller Albright said it best: "Hypotheses are subject to change without notice!" This is the essence of endocrinology.

REFERENCES

1. Aristotle: Historia Animalium, Book 9, Volume 4.
2. Sarton G: Galen of Pergamon. Lawrence, University of Kansas Press, 1954.
3. Vesalius A: De Humanis Corporis Fabrica, Basel, 1543.
4. Eustachius B: Opuscula Anatomica, Venice, 1563.
5. Loriaux DL: Claude Bernard. The Endocrinologist 1:362–363, 1991.
6. Bayliss WM, Starling EH: The mechanism of pancreatic secretion. J Physiol 28:325–353, 1902.
7. Addison T: On the Constitutional and Local Effects of Disease of the Suprarenal Glands. London, Highly, 1855.
8. Graves RJ: Clinical Lectures. London Medical and Surgical Journal (Renshaw's) 7:599, 1835.
9. von Basedow V: Exophthalmos durch Hypertrophie des Zellegewebes in der Augenhohle. Wochenschrift für die Gesammte Heikunde 6:197–204, 1840.
10. von Mering J, Minkowski O: Arch Exp Path Pharmakol 26:371–387, 1890.
11. Marie P, de Souza-Leite JD: Essays on Acromegaly. London, New Sydenham Society, 1891.
12. Cushing H: The basophil adenomas of the pituitary body and their clinical manifestations (pituitary basophilism). Bull Johns Hopkins Hosp 50:137–195, 1932.
13. Albright F, Aub J, Bauer W: Hyperparathyroidism—a common and polymorphic condition as illustrated by seventeen proven cases from one clinic. JAMA 102:1276–1287, 1934.
14. Sawin CT, Kendall EC: The Endocrinologist 1:291–293, 1991.
15. Kendall EC, Mason HL, McKenzie BF, et al: Proceedings of the Mayo Clinic 9:245–250, 1934.
16. Grollman A: Physiological and chemical studies on the adrenal cortical hormone. Symp Quant Biol 5:313, 1937.
17. Collip JB: The original method as used for the isolation of insulin in semi-pure form for the treatment of the first clinical cases. J Biol Chem 55:50–51, 1923.
18. Collip JB: The extraction of a parathyroid hormone that will prevent or control parathyroid tetany and which regulates the level of blood calcium. J Biol Chem 63:395–438, 1925.
19. Li CH, Evans HM, Simpson ME: Isolation and properties of the anterior hypophyseal growth hormone. J Biol Chem 159:353–366, 1945.
20. Burgus R, Guilleman R, et al: Structure moleculaire du facteur hypothalamique hypophysiotrope TRF d'orngne ovine: Mise en evidence par spectrometrie de masse de la sequence PCA-His-Pro-NH2. Compt Rendu 269:226–228, 1969.
21. Murray GR: Note on the treatment of myxedema by hypodermic injections of an extract of the thyroid gland of sheep. Br Med J 2:796–797, 1891.
22. Thorn GW, Firor WM: Desoxycorticosterone acetate therapy in Addison's disease: Clinical consideration. JAMA 231:76, 1940.
23. Raben MS: Recent Prog Horm Res 15:71, 1959.
24. Berson SA, Yalow RS: Radioimmunoassays of peptide hormones in plasma. N Engl J Med 277:640–647, 1967.
25. Albright F, Burnett CH, Smith PH, Parson W: Pseudohypoparathyroidism: An example of the "Seabright-Bantam" syndrome. Endocrinology 30:922–932, 1942.

2

Hormonal Regulation of Gene Expression

WILLIAM W. CHIN

Traditionally, hormones are defined as substances produced by glandular organs within the body, which are introduced into the bloodstream to affect the activity and function of specific distant target tissues. However, recent studies indicate that this family of substances may be expanded to include those that act locally. Together they participate in the control of general cellular growth and the immune and hematopoietic systems and the activities of nonclassic endocrine target cells. Thus hormones serve as messengers to coordinate or orchestrate a multitude of cellular events throughout the body.

It is the pervasive nature of hormones that makes the understanding of their modes of action compelling. We know that the action of hormones is mediated by specific receptors present on the surface of and/or within these cells. This initial interaction starts a cascade of events that leads to the ultimate activation of specific genes within the cell, resulting in effects on cellular activity and function. We also know that a major effect of hormones on cells is the regulation of gene expression. However, it should be emphasized that hormones may also exert their effects on events other than those at the gene transcriptional level. These include post-transcriptional, translational, and post-translational events. In addition, these effects may also involve the alteration of secretion. The recent developments in molecular and cellular biology and genetics have provided a deeper understanding of mechanisms of gene regulation by hormones.[1–3] They form the basis for the discussion in this chapter.

PATHWAYS OF GENE EXPRESSION AND PROTEIN SYNTHESIS

The production of a functional protein is the crucial goal in the flow of information from the genome. These proteins include molecules that are important for cellular structure (including membrane and cytoskeletal components), enzymes active in the production of energy and the synthesis of nonpolypeptide substances such as steroids, as well as transported or secreted molecules such as polypeptide hormones. Each protein is encoded by a gene, defined functionally as a transcriptional unit, and the first step in the synthesis of a protein is the transcription of its gene.[4]

There are approximately 100,000 genes in the typical haploid genome of a eukaryotic cell.[1–3] With the exception of variation among genes present in cells of the immune system, all somatic cells contain the identical set of genetic information. As a result, one major question is how specific cells develop certain phenotypes given the same set of genes. Hence, the tissue-specific expression of genes is an area of major interest and research. It is clear that a given cell expresses only a relatively small percentage of the full array of genes. For instance, the liver cell may express only 10 to 30 per cent of these 100,000 genes. In contrast, another cell such as a brain cell may express as many as 50 to 75 per cent of these genes. There are two major groups of expressed genes: one that is expressed in common among these cells, encoding the so-called housekeeping proteins that are involved in the maintenance of membrane structure, cytoskeleton, energy production, and other general cellular functions; and the other that is expressed only in limited tissue types and that dictates tissue-specific phenotypes.

The flow of information in the pathway of gene expression is shown in Figure 2–1. The gene undergoes *transcription* in the nucleus to yield a precursor ribonucleic acid (RNA), known as *heteronuclear RNA*. At this point, the first transduction of information occurs. Data in the form of a polymer of deoxyribonucleotides (DNA) is transformed into information stored as a polymer of ribonucleotides (RNA). This RNA precursor is short-lived in the nucleus, having a half-life of several minutes while undergoing a number of alterations, including *RNA processing* or splicing, with the removal of intervening or intron sequences, as well as 5′- and 3′ modifications. After processing of the precursor RNA, the mature messenger RNA (mRNA) is transported from the nucleus to the cytoplasm. Soon thereafter, the mRNA interacts with the protein synthetic machinery composed of ribosomal RNA/protein complexes located in the cytoplasm in either membrane or non–membrane-associated forms.

The nucleic acid information is then transferred into protein form, encoded in a polymer of amino acids and known as the polypeptide precursor, by *translation*. The initial precursor of a number of proteins destined for secretion or membrane insertion contains a 20–30 amino acid residue segment at the extreme amino-terminal end. This segment typically contains a core of hydrophobic amino acids flanked by several charged residues. Although no consensus primary sequence has emerged for this region, it likely possesses a common secondary/tertiary struc-

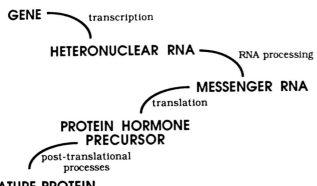

GENE ⟶ transcription

HETERONUCLEAR RNA ⟶ RNA processing

MESSENGER RNA

translation

PROTEIN HORMONE
PRECURSOR

post-translational
processes

MATURE PROTEIN
HORMONE

FIGURE 2–1. **The informational flow from gene to mature protein.** This schematic diagram reviews the flow of information in the cell from the gene to its encoded mature protein, e.g., the synthesis of a protein hormone. The first step is the transfer of information in the gene to heteronuclear RNA via the process of transcription. This heteronuclear RNA is rapidly modified in the nucleus via RNA processing to yield a mature mRNA. The mRNA is then transferred from the nucleus to the cytoplasm where it encounters ribosomes, associated in this instance with the endoplasmic reticulum. At this site translation occurs to yield the protein hormone precursor. In a series of co-translational steps, the leader or signal peptide located at the N-terminus of the precursor allows its vectorial transport from the cytoplasm into the cisternae of the endoplasmic reticulum via interactions with signal recognition particles and docking proteins located in the endoplasmic reticulum. Soon thereafter the leader peptide is cleaved by signal peptidase, and N-glycosylation occurs in the case of glycoproteins. The immature protein hormone precursor is then transported through the Golgi apparatus, where further post-translational processes occur before yielding the mature hormone, which enters secretory vesicles.

ture. This hydrophobic sequence, also known as a *leader* or *signal peptide*, is apparently required for appropriate transfer of the protein to the correct compartment, namely, the endoplasmic reticulum (ER), within the cell. Hence secretory proteins containing such sequences and destined for membranes leave the cytoplasm (in a topological sense) and enter the extracytoplasmic or cisternal space. Even before translation is complete, this precursor molecule is rapidly altered by the removal of the signal peptide and possibly glycosylated by the addition of N-linked carbohydrate moieties.

This partially processed protein then enters the Golgi complex where further *post-translational processes* or modifications may occur. These events include additional protein cleavage, phosphorylation, further glycosylation (trimming and addition of N-terminal sugars, and O-glycosylation), acetylation, sulfation of carbohydrate moieties, lipidation, and other events. Also important is protein folding and protein-protein interactions at the tertiary and quaternary

levels. Thus major events occur at this level prior to complete synthesis and to final assignment to a cellular compartment. In the case of polypeptide hormones, the nearly mature molecule is then sequestered in the secretory granule, where it is concentrated and stored until the appropriate extracellular signals are received to indicate its release. Even at this late step of hormone synthesis and secretion, alterations of proteins may occur.

GENE STRUCTURE

Important advances in our understanding of eukaryotic gene structure and organization have been made over the last decade or so. First, DNA, and the genes therein, is present in the cell nucleus as a highly organized structure in vivo, known as *chromatin*.[5, 6] A notable feature is the 30-nm chromatin fiber with its key repeating component, the nucleosome. The nucleosome is composed of 160 nucleotides of DNA wrapped twice around a protein octamer core (H2A, H2B, H3 and H4; two molecules each). Linker DNA, which binds to yet another histone protein, H1, connects the nucleosomes together. Recent work suggests a regulatory role of chromatin structure in gene expression. In the "quiescent" state, the DNA engaged as chromatin is not accessible to various nuclear regulatory factors and gene activity and is said to be repressed. Activation results in alterations of chromatin structure in addition to de novo synthesis or modification of regulatory proteins. Since further evidence suggests that the nucleosome remains largely unperturbed during transcription, it is not yet known how the transcription initiation and elongation steps can successfully accommodate the apparent restrictive nature of the chromatin fiber.

Second, the gene or transcriptional unit, by definition, contains all of the information required for the determination of the ultimate protein product. While much is known about genes in prokaryotes or unicellular organisms, the eukaryotic gene is expectedly more complex. In prokaryotic genes, information is co-linear with that present in the mRNA molecule. Hence, there is a one-to-one relationship between the information present in the DNA of the prokaryotic gene and that of the eventual polypeptide translation product. In contrast, the eukaryotic gene contains pieces of DNA interspersed between coding regions. In this sense, the information present in the gene itself is usually not co-linear with that which eventually reaches the protein. Such interspersed sequences, known as *introns* or *intervening sequences*, have been discovered in most eukaryotic genes (Fig. 2–2). The function of such

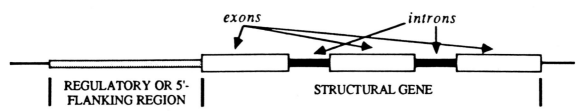

exons   *introns*

REGULATORY OR 5'-
FLANKING REGION

STRUCTURAL GENE

FIGURE 2–2. **The molecular anatomy of the structural gene.** The structural gene, which consists of coding and noncoding regions known as exons and introns, encodes information retained in its corresponding mRNA and protein. The exons contain information ultimately retained in mRNA and its encoded protein. In addition, the 5'-regulatory region is shown to the left of the structural gene. Exons are indicated by open boxes and introns by solid bars interspersed between exons; regulatory or 5'-flanking regions are indicated by a narrow hatched bar.

apparently extraneous information is not yet clear, although apparently introns separate functional domains in some genes and often serve to enrich the diversity of the resultant mRNA transcripts.[7]

In general, the gene is composed of two major components, the structural region and the regulatory or promoter region (Fig. 2–3). The structural region possesses the information that will be retained by mRNA and hence by the encoded protein. However, the structural region is essentially nonfunctional without the presence of the regulatory region. The latter domain determines the basal and regulated expression of the structural gene. For the purpose of further discussion, the regulatory region is considered to be present at the 5′ end of the transcriptional unit. It should be emphasized that such regulatory domains may, in fact, be present within the 3′ end or other parts of the gene.

A great deal of information has been acquired recently about the regulatory regions. The major breakthrough, however, has developed from the ability to study the structure and function of the 5′ or regulatory region of genes utilizing gene-transfer experiments. Basically, the approach involves the ability to place various sections of either naturally occurring or in vitro mutagenized regulatory regions attached to "reporter" genes. These new recombinant genes are then placed into foreign cells via the process of gene transfer. If one utilizes a reporter gene whose product is not normally found in mammalian cells, then the ability to detect such a reporter gene product either enzymatically or immunologically indicates the presence of transcriptional activity of the particular recombinant DNA construct. Hence, any change in the amount of protein is assumed to be directly proportional to the activity of the regulatory region. Furthermore, any changes in the regulatory regions that result in alterations in the quantity of the reporter gene product reflect those changes that affect areas of the regulatory region crucial to transcriptional regulation. In this manner, it has been learned that the regulatory region is in some respects complex in detail but yet simple in general organization and hence similar to that found in prokaryotic genes.

These studies have shown that regulatory regions contain three major components: (1) minimal or basal promoter, (2) upstream regulatory or proximal promotor elements, and (3) enhancers (Fig. 2–4). The basal promoter contains sufficient information to dictate basal gene transcription and usually has two features, the TATA motif or box and/or the initiator (Inr). The TATA box is located 25 to 30 nucleotides upstream of the 5′ end of the structural region (Fig. 2–4). At this sequence the transcription machinery and particularly RNA polymerase II—the enzyme that synthesizes the RNA precursor—begin their interaction with DNA. This A-T–rich region forms a less stable hybrid that presumably allows basal factor binding and RNA polymerase II interaction, and transcription initiation with a nucleotide placed 25 to 30 bases downstream from the TATA box at the Inr site. Hence the TATA box is fixed in both position and orientation relative to the start site of transcription. Although this sequence is not strictly required inasmuch as it is absent in a few (especially housekeeping) genes, its alteration results in decreased efficiency of transcription and inaccuracy in start site choice. However, naturally occurring TATA-less minimal promoters usually possess an Inr site.[8–10]

Recent studies have provided new insight into the biochemical nature of the protein complex formed over the TATA box and the site of transcription initiation.[8–10] At least seven major basal transcription factors (TFIIA, TFIIB, TFIID, TFIIE, TFIIF, TFIIH, and TFIIJ), in addition to RNA polymerase II, are involved (Fig. 2–5). The key player in the formation of the transcription initiation complex is TFIID, which is itself a large multisubunit complex (>700 kDa) consisting of at least eight proteins. The TATA-binding protein (TBP) is the major component of TFIID that permits the binding of TFIID to the promoter. Closely associated with TBP are seven additional factors, known as coactivators or TBP-associated proteins (TAF's), that are

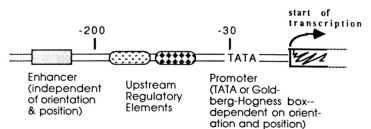

FIGURE 2–4. **The 5′-flanking or regulatory region of a typical eukaryotic gene.** Several cis-DNA elements are present in the regulatory region of the eukaryotic genes. This schematic diagram depicts such a region. The arrow indicates the start of transcription of the structural gene. Such regulatory regions, although shown in the 5′-flanking region, may also be present in introns or 3′-flanking regions of the gene. Such elements may be placed with several thousand bases upstream of the start of transcription. The first element is the promoter (TATA box) indicated by the sequence TATA. This A-T-rich region is located 25 to 30 bases upstream from the start of transcription. It is at this site that the eukaryotic RNA polymerse II first interacts to begin the process of transcription. Alterations in the sequence of this TATA box result in decreased efficiency and accuracy of transcription start sites, and hence this element depends on orientation and position. Another cis-DNA element is illustrated by two ovals that are designated upstream regulatory elements. These sequences bind to nuclear proteins or transacting factors that may augment transcription in a non-tissue-specific manner. Also, there is a DNA element known as an enhancer which binds to similar cellular factors and serves to increase or decrease general rates of transcription, depending on the interaction of these factors with DNA and other factors, including RNA polymerase II, located in its vicinity. Interestingly, as noted above, enhancer elements may be placed many thousands of nucleotides away from the start of transcription and hence appear to be independent of both orientation and position. It is this element that may be important in dictating tissue-specific and development-stage-specific expression. A subclass of enhancers includes the hormone regulatory elements that are discussed in the text.

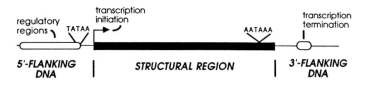

FIGURE 2–3. **The transcriptional unit.** Each protein is encoded by a transcriptional unit. This genetic element contains three major regions: the structural gene, which is bounded at the 5′-end by the site of transcriptional initiation and near the 3′-end by the polyadenylation signal, AA-TAA, and the 5′- and 3′-flanking DNA regions. In the 5′-flanking DNA region are usually located elements responsible for the regulation of transcription including the promoter element, TATAA. The 3′-flanking region contains elements that determine transcriptional termination.

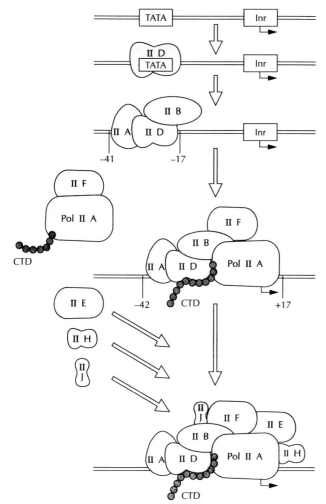

FIGURE 2–5. Schematic diagram of the assembly of the basal transcription machinery. The first interaction in the production of a transcription complex using RNA polymerase II is the binding of TFIIB to the TATA box. Thereafter, TFIIB and TFIIA associate to form the DAB complex. Then, RNA polymerase II (shown with its carboxy-terminal domain [CTD]) along with TFIIF form the DABpolF complex. Subsequent addition of TFIIE, TFIIH, and TFIIJ complete the basal transcription complex. Inr represents the initiator site. (From Zawel L, Reinberg D: Advances in RNA polymerase II transcription. Curr Op Cell Biol 4:488–495, 1992.)

necessary for communication with the basal transcriptional machinery and regulation of resultant gene activity by upstream regulatory elements. The nature of the set of TAF's associated with TBP is variable, depending on specific minimal promoters and tissues. Figure 2–5 illustrates the pathway of initiation complex formation in basal transcription; note that RNA polymerase II enters into the complex only after the formation of the TFIID-TFIIA-TFIIB (DAB) multimer on DNA. The carboxy-terminal domain (CTD) of RNA polymerase II contains repeating tandem heptapeptide sequences, Tyr-Ser-Pro-Thr-Ser-Pro-Ser, and is soon phosphorylated after association with DAB, perhaps to permit transcription elongation. Finally, for TATA-less promoters, specific Inr-binding proteins may substitute for TBP.

The next important regulatory region contains upstream elements, which are *cis*-DNA regions or sequences that apparently bind and interact with other specific nuclear and cytoplasmic *trans*-acting protein factors.[11, 12] The binding of these proteins to the DNA apparently results in protein-

protein interactions that involve the basal initiation complex and increase or decrease specific RNA transcription. Among such sequences are the CAAT- and GC-rich boxes that bind to CAAT-box binding proteins and Spl, respectively. In general, these interactions alter gene transcription in a non–tissue-specific manner.

The third crucial *cis*-DNA element in the regulatory region is the *enhancer*. Enhancers consist of 6- to 20-base pair DNA sequences that also bind to specific proteins within the cell. The interaction of these specific proteins with enhancers again apparently facilitates either protein-protein or protein-DNA interactions including productive interactions with the basal transcriptional machinery, causing dramatic changes in transcription. Such enhancer sequences were first described in viral systems, specifically SV40, but soon were described in other genes, including those encoding immunoglobulins and hormones. Enhancers may also mediate negative effects on transcription and have been designated silencer or repressor sequences.

Enhancers may be located in many sites within and around the transcriptional unit and hence are position-independent. Curiously, they may also be orientation-independent. The enhancers are the *cis*-DNA sequences that may mediate tissue- and development-stage–specific activation of gene expression.[13-15] Another type of enhancer is the locus control region or LCR, initially described in the far upstream region of the human β-globin locus.[16] It corresponds to a stable DNase I-hypersensitive site that mediates expression of the gene locus independent of the site of integration and is devoid of nucleosomes. Functionally, it is defined by its ability to confer upon a transgene the property of expression independent of the genomic location. Finally, a subset of enhancer-type elements involving DNA sequences that interact with various hormone receptors has recently been demonstrated. These hormone-regulatory elements (HRE) mediate the regulation of gene expression by steroid (estrogen, progesterone, glucocorticoid, testosterone, and others) and thyroid hormone, vitamin D, and retinoid receptors.[17, 18] These hormone receptors, either bound or unbound to their respective ligands, interact with the HRE's again either to increase or to decrease transcriptional activity.

For example, the ability of glucocorticoid receptor to bind with high affinity to specific sequences within eukaryotic genes was first demonstrated in several genes expressed in mouse mammary tumor (MMTV) and murine sarcoma viruses, which are regulated by glucocorticoids, and within the metallothionein II_A, tyrosine aminotransferase, tryptophan oxygenase, and growth hormone genes. In the long terminal repeat of MMTV, at least five such HRE's were defined. Subsequently, a "consensus" sequence for the glucocorticoid GRE was established[19]:

$$5'\text{-}\underline{\text{GGTACA}}\text{NNN}\underline{\text{TGTTCT}}\text{-}3'$$

where N = A, C, G, or T. Of note is the relatively high degree of variability in these sequences as well as the evident lack of a two-fold axis of symmetry. Such dyad symmetry in DNA-binding sites had been described in detail for sites of protein interactions in bacteriophage λ-DNA with repressor and cro proteins.[20, 21] These DNA-binding proteins are homopolymeric dimers with subunits possessing an α-helix–turn–α-helix structural motif. Interactions with DNA occur primarily through binding at the major groove over several turns of DNA. Recent crystallographic studies have shown that the glucocorticoid receptor interacts with DNA in a similar manner. In addition, the glucocorticoid receptor like other transcription factors possesses a transactivational domain in addition to the DNA-binding region. These domains are variable in nature, as acidic, proline, and glutamine residue–rich regions have been noted.

In summary, within a several thousand base pair region upstream of the structural region, there are multiple regulatory *cis*-DNA elements. It is also evident that such enhancer sequences may be present in downstream regions such as intronic as well as 3'-flanking regions. For example, a hormone-regulatory element for the glucocorticoid receptor is apparently present in the first intron of the human growth hormone gene. Further, most of these elements are often *not* position- or orientation-specific, in contrast to the TATA box. These elements and their cognate binding proteins play integral roles in the hormonal regulation of gene expression.

TRANSCRIPTION

As stated at the outset, the major effect of hormones apparently is exerted at the transcriptional level. Clearly, modulation of gene activity by altering transcriptional rates of genes can significantly alter the amount of protein ultimately produced in a cell by determining the level of mRNA in the cytoplasm.[4] The crucial step in transcription appears to reside in the initiation step. In other words, the interaction of the transcriptional machinery with a specific gene is often the rate-limiting step in gene expression. Hence, the frequency of RNA polymerase II initiation of transcription of a given gene determines the rate of transcription of its structural region. Further, the binding of proteins to other regions of the regulatory portion of the gene may alter the initial RNA polymerase/promoter interaction to influence the rate of transcription initiation. Thus, enhancers, silencers, and HRE's within the gene, and their interactions with their respective nuclear-binding proteins, ultimately determine the level of gene activity[16, 17] (Fig. 2–6). These effects are manifested either as tissue-, development-stage-specific expression, or hormone-regulation of the rates of gene transcription.

In addition, it should be noted that other processes are involved in the complete transcription of the structural region. They include transcription, elongation, and termination.[22] In prokaryotes, these two events play important roles in determining the rate of gene transcription. However, the importance of these two steps in the regulation of eukaryotic gene expression is still ill-defined, although the necessary components and sequences involved in such processes are being elucidated.

mRNA MATURATION

The initial product of gene transcription is a heteronuclear RNA that represents a complete copy of the structural gene, including exons and introns (Fig. 2–7). This precursor RNA is relatively short-lived, so that within minutes a number of RNA-processing steps occur. The 5' end of the RNA precursor is modified by the addition of a 7-methylguanosine via a 5'-5' triphosphate bond by guanylyl- and methyltransferases. This reaction, referred to as 5' capping, is finished after only 25 to 30 nucleotides are incorporated in the nascent RNA and is essential for optimal translational efficiency and increased RNA stability. This requirement is not universal, however, inasmuch as the mRNA's of several eukaryotic viruses, including poliovirus, do not contain 5' caps but are apparently well-translated. In addition, a cap-binding protein has been described that binds the 5' cap of mRNA's and stimulates their translation, presumably by facilitating the formation of a stable 40S initiation complex.[23, 24]

Another process involves polyadenylation (poly A) of the

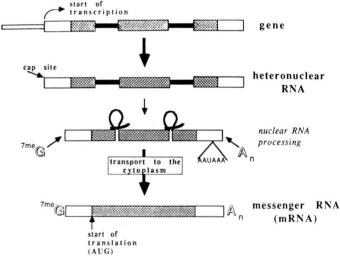

FIGURE 2–7. **Gene transcription.** The steps in gene transcription leading to the production of mature mRNA are shown. On the first line the typical eukaryotic gene is illustrated, with the structural region depicted including three exons and two introns. The hatched areas within the exons designate regions that ultimately encode the protein precursor. The small hatch bar to the left of the structural gene represents a portion of the 5'-regulatory region. Transcription of this gene results in heteronuclear RNA shown on the second line. Note that both exon and intron sequences are transcribed. However, modifications occur in the nucleus known as nuclear RNA processing steps. Major events include formation of the 5'-cap by addition of [7]methyl G (^{7me}G) and trimming of the 3'-end of the initial transcript near the AAUAAA polyadenylation site, followed by addition of a homopolymeric tract of A residues yielding a poly A tail (An). Lastly, the intron sequences are removed via RNA-splicing events. The modified RNA is now equivalent to mature mRNA, which is then transported to the cytoplasm where it may be translated. The small arrow in the mRNA shown in the fourth line indicates the start of translation at the initiation codon (AUG).

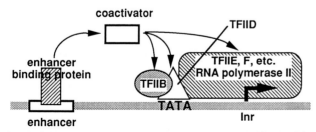

FIGURE 2–6. **Interaction of the basal transcription machinery with enhancer binding proteins.** A co-activator to mediate the communication of the "activated" enhancer with specific components of the basal transcription machinery is also shown.

3′ end of the heteronuclear RNA. Most eukaryotic mRNA's contain a polyadenylic acid tract of 200 to 250 As. The site of the poly A tract has been well characterized and lies approximately 20 to 25 nucleotides downstream from a canonical AAUAAA sequence present near the 3′ end of the eukaryotic mRNA. This polyadenylation signal is virtually invariant among mRNA's. The precise mechanisms involved in determining the location of the poly A tract are not completely known. However, transcription likely continues several hundred nucleotides downstream of this site. Hence, the 3′ end of the heteronuclear RNA requires 3′-endonucleolytic cleavage prior to polyp A addition by poly A polymerase.[25] The role of the poly A tract is also unclear, although it may be important in increased RNA stability, improved translational efficiency by interaction with the poly A–binding protein, and in nuclear-cytoplasmic transport. Thus, both the 5′ and 3′ ends of the mRNA are modified to increase its stability and perhaps translational efficiency.

The other major process involved in the maturation of heteronuclear RNA in the nucleus involves the removal of intron sequences via the process of RNA splicing. Considerable information has been obtained over the last several years concerning the mechanisms by which the precise cleavage of intervening sequences is achieved.[26, 27] Briefly, the intron contains consensus-type sequences at either end and internal sequences that allow cleavage at exon-intron boundaries and religation at exon-exon borders, with the formation of an intron "lariat" intermediate that is then rapidly degraded.[27, 28] This RNA splicing process must be painstakingly accurate. If not, subtle errors may be introduced into the mRNA and leading to premature translation termination, or frameshift. Such control is entrusted to small nuclear riboprotein complexes (snRNP's), which possess RNA's complementary to several of the conserved sequence regions of exon-intron junctions and introns. The snRNP's interact with the growing RNA transcript to form a spliceosome, the RNA splicing "factor." Since genes often contain multiple introns, it is important to know how the sequence of intron removal is determined. The nature of the splice junction sequences, the activities of general and specific splicing factors, and the presence of splicing inhibitors such as hnRNA binding proteins all play roles.

The necessity to remove intron sequences allows the interesting possibility of alternative splicing. Since every intron has a donor and acceptor site for its splicing, it is possible that adjacent exons may not be spliced together in the "usual" manner. Instead, exons may be spliced together while removing intervening exons. Hence, transcriptional units may be complex, and it may be possible to obtain different mRNA's from the same initial heteronuclear RNA precursor. While there is a "default" splicing pattern discernible for most hnRNA's, numerous tissue-specific, development-specific, and regulated factors, likely involving RNA-binding proteins, participate to produce an alternate RNA-splicing pathway.[29]

A dramatic example of such an event is described by the work of Rosenfeld et al.[30, 31] involving the synthesis of calcitonin/calcitonin gene–related peptide (CGRP), as illustrated in Figure 2–8. During the transcription of the major calcitonin/CGRP gene, two heteronuclear RNA transcripts are formed, exons 1 → 4 and exons 1 → 6, each apparently terminated by distinct polyadenylation and associated tran-

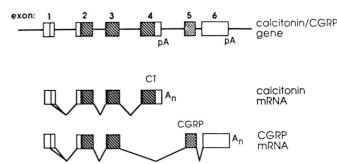

FIGURE 2–8. **Alternate RNA processing.** A simple transcriptional unit will result in the production of a single protein. Alternatively, a complex transcriptional unit may produce multiple mRNA's from a single gene that will encode different polypeptides or polypeptide precursors. This figure depicts alternate splicing of the mRNA encoded by the calcitonin/calcitonin gene-related peptide (CGRP) gene. The calcitonin/CGRP gene contains six exons. Note that exons 4 and 6 contain polyadenylation (pA) signals. Presumably the initial heteronuclear RNA or calcitonin/CGRP gene transcripts contain either exons 1-2-3-4 or 1-2-3-4-5-6. The first transcript yields calcitonin mRNA and contains exon 4, which encodes calcitonin. If, however, the second transcript is alternatively spliced to exclude exon 4, then a CGRP mRNA is produced encoding CGRP and exon 5. These mRNA's are expressed in a tissue-specific manner so that calcitonin mRNA is expressed in the C cell of the thyroid gland and CGRP mRNA is expressed in the central nervous system. Note also that exon 1 may be alternatively spliced in both calcitonin and CGRP transcripts.

scriptional termination signals in exons 4 and 6. Note that exons 4 and 5 encode the calcitonin and CGRP precursors, respectively. Exon 1 → 4 mRNA encodes calcitonin, but alternative splicing of exon 4 from the exon 1 → 6 transcript results in CGRP mRNA. This process is not stochastic but rather involves tissue-specific RNA processing enzymes and factors, inasmuch as calcitonin mRNA is expressed primarily in C cells of the thyroid gland and CGRP mRNA in the brain. Alternate growth hormone forms in human pituitary gland, and substance P–substance K expression mRNA splicing can yield mRNA variants to produce altered coding regions. Rat α-amylase is encoded by a single gene but by nonidentical mRNA's in salivary gland and liver with differences in the 5′-untranslated regions. This results from alternative splicing of two 5′ exons, each containing a promoter element and a cap site that occurs in a tissue-specific manner. Thus, promoter choice is yet another mechanism for the generation of mRNA diversity.

The final product of these various processing steps is a mature, functional mRNA that is destined for transport to the cytoplasm. The potential for hormone regulation of protein synthesis at any of these steps is real. Finally, the stability of heteronuclear RNA and mRNA in the cytoplasm and nucleus may vary from gene to gene and may depend on specific *cis*-RNA elements.[32] For example, A-U–rich sequences in the 3′-untranslated regions of certain cytokine and early-response gene mRNA's and the iron-response element (IRE) in the 3′-untranslated region of the transferrin receptor mRNA may each dictate altered stability.[33]

mRNA TRANSLATION

The mature mRNA enters the cytoplasm via an unknown transport process. There it encounters the protein synthetic machinery involving ribosomes that are free or membrane-bound. The membrane-bound ribosomes present in the endoplasmic reticulum are sites for synthesis of most polypeptides destined for extracellular transport or membrane locations. The mRNA with specific sequences, presumably just 5'- of the translation initiation codon (AUG), initially binds to the 40S ribosomal complex containing 18S ribosomal RNA as well as many ribosomal proteins.[34, 35] After this initial interaction, the 60S ribosomal complex and other factors facilitate protein translation. In this process the information encoded in the ribonucleotide bases of the mRNA is decoded into the language of amino acids in the protein (Fig. 2–9). The details of this process may be obtained in any standard textbook of molecular biology and biochemistry.

The rate of initiation of translation of mRNA's is a key determinant of the rate at which peptide chains are synthesized.[36, 37] However, polypeptide chain elongation and termination may occasionally be rate-limiting steps. It is conceivable that any of these steps also may be hormonally regulated, although it should be emphasized again that the step most likely to be regulated by hormones, in analogy to transcriptional initiation, is translation initiation. While data supporting hormone control of translation as an important step in the hormonal regulation of protein synthesis and gene expression are not plentiful, there are sufficient examples of modulation at this level to ensure its likelihood. Such control could be exerted at the global (affecting all mRNA's in a cell) or specific mRNA levels. Clearly, attack of general translational initiation, elongation, or termination factors would lead to global control, whereas the IRE-binding protein interaction with the 5'-untranslated region of the ferritin mRNA, for example, would result in specific mRNA regulation.[38, 39] Other less well-known mechanisms of translational control include post-transcriptional editing of mRNA and readthrough of termination condons.

Other important events occur during the translational process. In the case of secretory or membrane proteins, the characteristic hydrophobic leader or signal sequence, which is present at the amino-terminal end of the polypeptide precursor, is rapidly cleaved in a co-translational manner by an enzyme, signal peptidase. In addition, carbohydrate moieties are added to asparagine (Asn) residues in the process of N-glycosylation. The asparagine residue that is subjected to carbohydrate addition in glycopeptides is usually associated with the sequences, Asn-X-Thr or Asn-X-Ser. This consensus sequence is a necessary but not sufficient condition for N-glycosylation to occur. Oligosaccharide-linked dolichol lipid intermediates transfer oligosaccharide moieties to these sites on glycoprotein in the endoplasmic reticulum, presumably during translation. These events have been substantiated in great detail in various viral and glycoprotein hormone systems.

The interaction of the secretory or membrane polypeptide precursor with the ribosome soon after translation has been described in detail.[40, 41] The process of protein translocation to and through the ER involves two major steps: (1) targeting of protein to the ER and (2) the transport of the protein into the ER lumen.[42] The leader peptide initially binds to a signal recognition particle (SRP), which consists of small RNA's and proteins. This SRP/signal peptide interaction actually halts translation momentarily. This pause allows the SRP/signal peptide complex to associate with an appropriate docking protein (SRP receptor) present as an integral membrane protein in the endoplasmic reticulum. This interaction then permits the "threading" or vectorial transport of the signal peptide through the membrane via an unknown mechanism. Presumably, the ribosome is associated at the ER with a receptor (ribosome receptor) that may serve to maintain the "open" state of an hydrophilic protein channel. Once these steps have occurred, the SRP dissociates from the complex, allowing translation to continue. The energy generated by translation of the mRNA apparently allows for further movement of the precursor peptide through the membrane. It is unknown presently whether these events are targets of hormone regulation.

PROTEIN PRECURSOR PROCESSING/ POST-TRANSLATIONAL EVENTS

The partially processed precursor polypeptide is further matured during its transport from the ER through the Golgi complex. Recent data indicate that there are multiple components within this organelle, including cis- and trans-compartments.[25] Early in the transport through the Golgi complex, events such as protein folding, disulfide linkage formation, and subunit interactions may occur with the assistance of molecular chaperones such as heat shock proteins 70 and 90.[44, 45] In addition, glycosylation continues in a complex manner. The initial carbohydrate moieties are whittled down to high mannose cores by a number of glycosidases. However, soon thereafter, other enzymes place distal sugars onto this original carbohydrate backbone. This carbohydrate maturation process takes place during transport through the Golgi complex.

In addition, other events may occur inside or outside the Golgi complex, including phosphorylation either on Ser/Thr or Tyr residues. These events are regulated by the

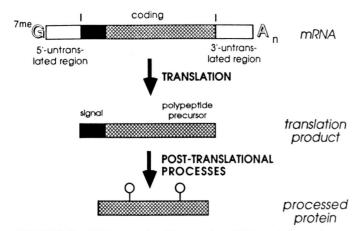

FIGURE 2–9. mRNA translation. The steps in mRNA translation and post-translational processes are shown. The mRNA encounters ribosomal complexes in either membrane- or nonmembrane-bound regions in the cytoplasm where translation occurs. The information present in the coding region of the mRNA is transduced into the translation product, which consists of the polypeptide precursor. Shown is protein destined for secretion or membrane insertion. It contains a prototypical signal or leader peptide sequence at the N-terminus of the polypeptide precursor. In a number of co- and post-translational processes, this initial precursor is modified to yield the processed protein. The "lollipop" structures depict typical structures (carbohydrate moiety) that result from a post-translational process, glycosylation.

activity of specific serine/threonine and/or tyrosine kinases, respectively. Conversely, specific phosphatases may be involved in gene regulation by similar mechanisms.[46] The roles of these enzymes in intracellular signaling and hormone action are discussed further in another chapter. In addition, other events such as acetylation, sulfation, and lipid addition may transpire.

All these events also may be regulated functions, although the magnitude of their importance is not yet known. Two major examples exist of how hormonal factors may influence post-translational processing events. TRH and its stimulation of thyrotropin biosynthesis and secretion and GnRH and its stimulation of gonadotropin biosynthesis and secretion both result in alterations of the carbohydrate moieties of the subunits of their respective regulated glycoprotein hormones. The major effect of these changes is an alteration in the biological activity of the resultant thyrotropin and gonadotropins. Hence, stimulation of secretion by specific hypothalamic releasing factors results in the production of more biologically potent glycoprotein hormones. These observations indicate that post-translational events may indeed be regulated. In addition, the ability of various proteins to be phosphorylated by C kinases, cAMP-dependent protein kinases, or membrane-bound tyrosine kinases provides the means to produce important secondary or tertiary messenger molecules within the cell to serve as a major point of regulation in cellular metabolism.

Another important feature of post-translational events includes tissue-specific and perhaps hormone-regulated alternate protein processing of polypeptide precursors. A classic example of alternate protein cleavage of a protein precursor is the processing of the precursor of ACTH, proopiomelanocortin (POMC) (Fig. 2–10). From a number of elegant studies by Roberts and Herbert, and Mains and Eipper, it is known that ACTH is derived from a larger precursor, POMC, with an approximate size of 31,000 daltons.[47] It is intriguing to note that the POMC precursor is synthesized in both the anterior and intermediate lobes of the pituitary glands of a number of species. However, the products from the various tissues, as shown in Figure 2–10, vary greatly. The anterior pituitary corticotrope produces ACTH, β-LPH, and N-terminal peptide. In contrast, the intermediate lobe produces α-MSH, corticotropin-like intermediate lobe peptide (CLIP), γ-MSH, γ-LPH, and β-endorphin. It is apparent that each tissue has enzymes that modify the pattern in which proteins are cleaved, yielding different sets of biologically active peptides. In addition, recently an enzyme that adds a C-terminal amide linkage has been described and may also be biologically important. This α-amidation enzyme is crucial for the ultimate biological activity of a number of hypothalamic and gastrointestinal peptides. In addition to being expressed in a tissue-specific manner, it is possbile that these various enzymes may be hormonally regulated.

SECRETORY GRANULE

All secretory polypeptides eventually are either stored in secretory granules or are constitutively released into the extracellular space.[48, 49] It is unclear at this point how these two pathways are regulated, although consensus secondary/tertiary structures of transported precursors must be involved in the sorting process. The stored polypeptides remain in the granules until the appropriate extracellular signals are received by the cell to indicate that such stored hormones or peptides are to be released. Large amounts of data have been gathered over the last several years concerning the biochemical and biophysical nature of the secretory granules. In most instances, polypeptide hormones are stored in near-crystalline form in these granules. This concentration of molecules in these organelles apparently is crucial for the function of endocrine cells whose major object is to be able to respond to extracellular stimuli with release of important regulatory peptides or hormones.

SECRETION

Secretion is the final common pathway taken by proteins destined for export. The various molecular mechanisms involved in secretion are discussed in another chapter. Briefly, extracellular signals interact with cellular membrane receptors to produce secondary and tertiary messengers, which include increases in cytosolic calcium and inositol triphosphate, and activation of specific intracellular kinases, including C-kinase and cAMP-dependent protein kinase. These kinases, in turn, phosphorylate other proteins within the cell, which then presumably interact rapidly with secretory granules to participate in its eversion and hence release of stored contents.

REGULATION OF GENE TRANSCRIPTION

From this rather general overview of the flow of information from the gene to the secretory granule in the bio-

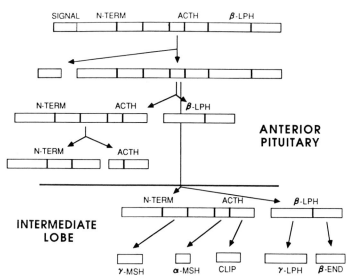

FIGURE 2–10. **Alternate polypeptide precursor processing.** Diversity of final polypeptide products may be achieved by alternative protein processing of polypeptide precursors. The precursor to ACTH is approximately 31,000 Da and is known as pro-opiomelanocortin (POMC). A number of biologically active peptides including ACTH and β-lipotropin (β-LPH) are flanked by pairs of dibasic residues. In the anterior pituitary gland, the POMC polypeptide precursor is cleaved by trypsin-like enzymatic activity to yield ACTH and β-LPH. In contrast, in the intermediate lobe, this same POMC precursor is processed differently to yield other peptides, including CLIP, α-MSH, and endorphin-like peptides. Thus, the POMC polypeptide precursor is differently processed in a tissue-specific fashion.

synthesis of a polypeptide hormone or other product, it is clear that there are potentially multiple sites of regulation by factors such as hormones. I have stressed that a major locus of regulation is the initiation of transcription. In this section, I will delve further into this area. It has long been known that a number of hormones such as glucocorticoids, estrogen, progesterone, androgens, and thyroid hormones regulate cellular activity by altering gene expression. However, only with the advent of new tools in recombinant DNA technology and molecular biology has further dissection of the structure-function relations of genes with respect to hormone action been accomplished.

As already described, a major example is elucidation of DNA sequences that modulate or mediate glucocorticoid hormone action.[50, 51] Work with glucocorticoid-responsive virus, MMTV, and glucocorticoid-responsive genes encoding tyrosine aminotransferase and metallothionein II$_A$ has provided evidence that such glucocorticoid-response elements (GRE's) exist.[16, 17] In particular, a small region of the long terminal repeat (LTR) region of the RNA tumor virus has been shown to confer glucocorticoid regulation upon heterologous genes. The major conclusion from these studies is that there is a consensus 15-bp DNA sequence present in single and multiple copies in regulatory regions of these genes. Alteration of any of these sequences may result in loss of responsivity to glucocorticoids. In addition, swapping or transfer of such putative GRE's to a heterologous gene confers upon that new gene the phenotype of regulation by glucocorticoid hormones.

Presumably the glucocorticoids enter the cell to interact with the cytoplasmic form of glucocorticoid receptor, with the resultant activation of the receptor. This newly activated glucocorticoid receptor is then transported to the nucleus, where it serves as a *trans*-acting factor and binds directly to specific GRE's via its Cys-rich zinc finger DNA binding domain.[52, 53] This latter finding was obtained using a number of DNA binding assays including DNA filter binding, gel-shift analysis, and DNA sequence footprinting techniques. Hence these GRE's are specialized enhancers. Unlike the typical enhancer that binds to a specific nuclear protein, which then increases the activity of the promoter to which it is associated, the activity of these HRE's depends on the interaction of a particular ligand to its cognate receptor prior to and along with receptor-DNA interactions. The only detail that requires further elucidation in this scheme is the mechanism by which a ligand-bound nuclear receptor/DNA complex communicates with the basal transcriptional machinery to modulate gene transcription.

Thus we understand in greater detail the molecular mechanisms involved in how hormones such as steroid and thyroid hormone regulate gene expression. It has been shown that polypeptide hormones regulate gene activity in a similar way. In particular, polypeptide hormones interact with membrane receptors to induce new secondary and tertiary messenger molecules that often are newly phosphorylated or dephosphorylated products.[54] Prime examples are cAMP response element binding protein (CREB),[55] and c-*jun*/c-*fos* in the A-kinase and C-kinase signaling systems respectively. These molecules then interact directly with the DNA, much as the steroid hormone/steroid hormone receptor complexes do with their respective regulatory elements.[56] Thus the mechanisms of action may share a common pathway. Indeed, recent evidence indicates that

a rich network of communication encompassing various signaling pathways results in abundant molecular "cross-talk."[57]

Although much emphasis has been placed on the interaction of such complexes to regulatory elements within genes to provide a *positive* effect, it is likely that there are as many examples of *negative* effects (Fig. 2–11). Thus, in addition to enhancer-type sequences, silencer or repressor sequences with negative effects exist.[58–60] Clearly, the ability to stimulate gene transcription alone is not enough in a complex regulatory system; it is necessary to have negative regulatory effects as well.

REGULATION OF OTHER PROCESSES

Although we have focused our attention on events occurring at the gene transcriptional level, it is evident from our previous discussion that other sites of protein synthesis pathway may be points at which regulation by hormones may occur (Fig. 2–12). In particular, regulation of heteronuclear RNA and mRNA stabilities is likely to involve highly controlled events. Estrogen has been shown to stabilize chicken liver vitellogenin mRNA's, and prolactin can increase the half-life of casein mRNA's in breast tissue. New data concerning the sequence requirements that may dictate stability of mRNA's, and hence cytoplasmic or nucleoplasmic factors responsible for RNA degradation, lead us to believe that this may be another crucial focus for regulation.

As already described, RNA splicing may also be regulated. In addition to tissue-specific RNA-splicing events, it is possible that such processes are hormonally regulated

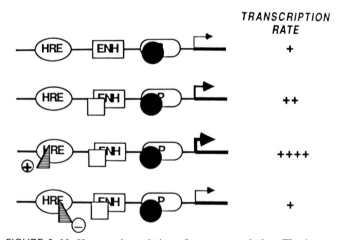

TRANSCRIPTION
RATE

+

++

++++

+

FIGURE 2–11. **Hormonal regulation of gene transcription.** The interactions of a number of trans-acting factors in the fine regulation of transcriptional rate are depicted. In the first line, a RNA polymerase II molecule (solid circle) is shown interacting with the promoter element P. In this instance, a basal transcription rate is observed. In the second line, this gene is shown to have bound yet another factor, which interacts with an enhancer. This augments further the rate of transcription seen at the basal level. In the next line, a third factor has bound to the hormone regulatory element (HRE), resulting in a positive effect that further increases the transcription rate. Alternatively, as shown in line 4, interaction of an HRE with a negative regulatory hormone-receptor hormone complex may result in decreased transcription rates, returning the original enhanced levels of transcription back to basal levels. In this manner, the combination of multiple factors may result in a "fine tuning" of the rate of gene transcription.

initiation
elongation
termination

HETERONUCLEAR RNA
alternative RNA splicing
degradation

mRNA
degradation

TRANSLATION
initiation
elongation
termination

POST-TRANSLATION
alternative protein processing
other modifications
non-covalent--folding, etc.
covalent--phosphorylation,
glycosylation, etc
degradation

STORAGE
SECRETION

FIGURE 2–12. **Potential sites of hormonal regulation of gene expression.** The major locus of hormonal regulation of gene expression is transcriptional initiation. However, it is clear that other loci are affected by hormones, including alternative RNA splicing of heteronuclear RNA, mRNA stability, initiation of mRNA translation, post-translational events including alternative protein processing, polypeptide modifications, and degradation, as well as storage and secretion.

not only to yield different mRNA's by alternative exon and polyadenylation site choice but also to alter the expression of one versus another mRNA by alternative promoter choice. In addition, it is possible that transcription elongation and termination may be other foci for hormonal regulation.

As previously suggested, translation may be regulated by hormones. For example, glucose regulates insulin mRNA translation. Other examples are certain to be forthcoming. Finally, protein processing with its attendant changes in the ultimate product may also be regulated by various hormonal factors. Such events are less well understood and will be a source of greater attention and study in the near future.

SUMMARY

Hormones influence the quantity and quality of protein synthesis by altering a number of steps in the process in a striking manner. Large amounts of data have been gathered over the last several years concerning the hormonal regulation of gene activity. The general molecular mechanisms involved in such processes are now fairly well established. Indeed, steroid and thyroid hormones bind to their respective intracellular receptors, which in turn may interact directly with specific DNA's that are tagged by hormone-response elements to regulate gene activity. Polypeptide hormones interact indirectly by first binding to their specific cell-surface receptor, which ultimately produces secondary or tertiary intracellular messenger molecules. These then impinge directly upon the gene to alter its

activity. It is clear that such regulatory effects are complex and involve the interactions of many different molecules in combination to cause a regulatory event at the transcriptional level. In addition, it is evident that hormones also regulate the biosynthesis of polypeptide at post-transcriptional, translational, and post-translational levels. Thus hormones play important roles in the regulation of cellular metabolism by influencing a number of steps in the flow of information from the gene to the ultimate biologically active protein. Such insight into hormone regulation provides a broader understanding of the control of gene expression in general.

REFERENCES

1. Lewin BM: Genes IV. New York, John Wiley and Sons, 1990.
2. Darnell J, Lodish H, Baltimore D: Molecular Cell Biology. New York, Scientific American Books, 1990.
3. Alberts B, Dray D, Lewis J, et al: Molecular Biology of the Cell. New York, Garland Publishing, Inc, 1989.
4. Darnell JE Jr: Variety in the level of gene control in eukaryotic cells. Nature 297:365–371, 1982.
5. Felsenfeld G: Chromatin as an essential part of the transcriptional mechanism. Nature 355:219–224, 1992.
6. Wolffe AP: New insights into chromatin function in transcriptional control. FASEB J 6:3354–3361, 1992.
7. Sharp PA: Splicing of messenger RNA precursors. Science 253:766–771, 1987.
8. Zawel L, Reinberg D: Advances in RNA polymerase II transcription. Curr Op Cell Biol 4:488–495, 1992.
9. Pugh BF, Tjian R: Diverse transcriptional functions of the multisubunit eukaryotic TFID complex. J Biol Chem 267:679–682, 1992.
10. Conaway RC, Conaway JW: General initiation factors for RNA polymerase II. Annu Rev Biochem 62:161–190, 1993.
11. Beato M: Gene regulation by steroid hormones. Cell 56:335–344, 1989.
12. Mitchell PJ, Tjian R: Transcriptional regulation in mammalian cells by sequence-specific DNA binding proteins. Science 245:371–378, 1989.
13. Hanahan D: Heritable formation of pancreatic β-cell tumours in transgenic mice expressing recombinant insulin/simian virus 40 oncogenes. Nature 315:115–122, 1985.
14. Walker MD, Edlund T, Boulet AM, Rutter WJ: Cell-specific expression controlled by the 5'-flanking region of insulin and chymotrypsin genes. Nature 306:557–561, 1983.
15. Edlund T, Walker MD, Barr PJ, Rutter WJ: Cell-specific expression of the rat insulin gene: Evidence for role of two distinct 5' flanking elements. Science 230:912–916, 1985.
16. Yamamoto KR: Steroid receptor regulated transcription of specific genes and gene networks. Ann Rev Genet 19:209–252, 1985.
17. Evans RM: The steroid and thyroid hormone receptor superfamily. Science 240:889–895, 1988.
18. Dillon N, Grosveld F: Transcriptional regulation of multigene loci: Multilevel control. Trends Genet 9:134–137, 1993.
19. Jantzen HM, Strahle U, Gloss B, et al: Cooperativity of glucocorticoid response elements located far upstream of the tyrosine aminotransferase gene. Cell 49:29–38, 1987.
20. Ptashne M: How eukaryotic transcription activators work. Nature 335:683–689, 1988.
21. Pabo CO: Transcription factors: Structural families and principles of DNA recognition. Annu Rev Biochem 61:1053–1095, 1992.
22. Greenblatt J, Nodwell JR, Mason SW: Transcriptional antitermination. Nature 354:401–406, 1993.
23. Nevins JR: The pathway of eukaryotic mRNA formation. Annu Rev Biochem 52:441–466, 1983.
24. Shatkin AJ: mRNA cap binding proteins: essential factors for initiating translation. Cell 40:223–224, 1985.
25. Wahle E, Keller W: The biochemistry of 3'-end cleavage and polyadenylation of messenger RNA precursors. Annu Rev Biochem 61:419–440, 1992.
26. Padgett RA, Grabowski PJ, Konarska MM, et al: Splicing of messenger RNA precursors. Annu Rev Biochem 55:1119–1150, 1986.

27. Keller W: The RNA lariat: A new ring to the splicing of mRNA precursors. Cell 39:423–425, 1984.

28. Maniatis T: Mechanisms of alternative pre-mRNA splicing. Science 251:33–34, 1991.

29. Mattox W, Ryner L, Baker BS: Autoregulation and multifunctionality among trans-acting factors that regulate alternative pre-mRNA processing. J Biol Chem 267:19023–19026, 1992.

30. Leff SE, Rosenfeld MG: Complex transcriptional units: diversity in gene expression by alternative RNA processing. Annu Rev Biochem 55:1091–1117, 1986.

31. Smith CWJ, Patton JG, Nadal-Ginard B: Alternative splicing in the control of gene expression. Annu Rev Genet 25:527–577, 1989.

32. Nielsen DA, Shapiro DJ: Insights into hormonal control of messenger RNA stability. Mol Endocrinol 4:953–957, 1990.

33. Atwater JA, Wisdom R, Verma IM: Regulated mRNA stability. Ann Rev Genetics 24:519–541, 1990.

34. Kozak M: Compilation and analysis of sequences upstream from the translational start site in eukaryotic mRNAs. Nucleic Acids Res 12:857–872, 1984.

35. Kozak M: Selection of initiation sites by eucaryotic ribosomes: Effect of inserting AUG triplets upstream from the coding sequence for preproinsulin. Nucleic Acids Rex 12:3873–3892, 1984.

36. London IM, Levin DH, Matts RL et al: Regulation of protein synthesis. The Enzymes 18:359–380, 1987.

37. Melefors O, Hentze MW: Translational regulation by mRNA/protein interactions in eukaryotic cells: ferritin and beyond. BioEssays 15:85–90, 1993.

38. Gesteland RF, Weiss RB, Atkins JF: Recording: Reprogrammed genetic decoding. Science 257:1640–1641, 1992.

39. Hershey JWB: Translational control in mammalian cells. Annu Rev Biochem 60:717–755, 1991.

40. Wickner WT, Lodish HF: Multiple mechanisms of protein insertion into and across membranes. Science 230:400–408, 1985.

41. Sanders SL, Schekman R: Polypeptide translocation across the endoplasmic reticulum membrane. J Biol Chem 267:13791–13794, 1992.

42. Hong W, Tang BL: Protein trafficking along the exocytotic pathway. BioEssays 15:231–238, 1993.

43. Rothman JE, Orci L: Molecular dissection of the secretory pathway. Nature 355:409–415, 1992.

44. Matthews CR: Pathways of protein folding. Annu Rev Biochem 62:653–683, 1993.

45. Ellis RJ, van der Vies SM: Molecular chaperones. Annu Rev Biochem 60:321–347, 1991.

46. Walton KM, Dixon JE: Protein tyrosine phosphatases. Annu Rev Biochem 62:101–120, 1993.

47. Douglass J, Civelli O, Herbert E: Polyprotein gene expression: Generation of diversity of neuroendocrine peptides. Annu Rev Biochem 53:665–715, 1984.

48. Kelley RB, Grote E: Protein targeting in the neuron. Annu Rev Neurosci 16:95–127, 1993.

49. Moore HH, Kelly RB: Re-routing of a secretory protein by fusion with human growth hormone sequences. Nature 321:443–446, 1986.

50. Lucas PC, Granner DK: Hormone response domains in gene transcription. Annu Rev Biochem 61:1131–1173, 1992.

51. Gronemeyer H: Control of transcription activation by steroid hormone receptors. FASEB J 6:2524–2529, 1992.

52. Johnson PF, McKnight SL: Eukaryotic transcriptional regulatory proteins. Ann Rev Biochem 58:799–839, 1989.

53. Harrison SC: A structural taxonomy of DNA-binding domains. Nature 353:715–719, 1991.

54. Hunter T, Karin M: The regulation of transcription by phosphorylation. Cell 70:375–387, 1992.

55. Habener JF. Cyclic AMP response element binding proteins: a cornucopia of transcription factors. Mol Endocrinol 4:1087–1094, 1990.

56. Murdoch GH, Franco R, Evans RM, Rosenfeld MG: Polypeptide hormone regulation of gene expression. Thyrotropin-releasing hormone rapidly stimulates both transcription of the prolactin and the phosphorylation of a specific nuclear protein. J Biol Chem 258:15329–15335, 1983.

57. Diamond MI, Miner JN, Yoshinaga SK, Yamamoto KR. Transcriptional factor interactions: selectors of positive and negative regulation from a single DNA element. Science 249:1266–1272, 1990.

58. Jones NC: Negative regulation of enhancers. Nature 321:202–204, 1986.

59. Brent R: Repression of transcription in yeast. Cell 42:3–4, 1985.

60. Guarente L: Yeast promoters: Positive and negative elements. Cell 36:799–800, 1984.

3

Hormone Signaling Via Membrane Receptors

STEEN GAMMELTOFT
C. RONALD KAHN

INTRODUCTION

Regulatory Molecules and Intercellular Communication

Regulation of metabolic processes, control of cell growth and differentiation, and appropriate integration of normal physiological function in multicellular organisms depend upon communication between cells. Cell-cell communication is mediated in large part by the action of regulatory molecules of the endocrine, nervous, hematopoietic, and immune systems. In these systems the primary signals of intercellular communication are hormones, growth factors, cytokines, and neurotransmitters, which act by endocrine, paracrine, autocrine, juxtacrine, or neurotransmitter mechanisms. The regulatory substances can be divided chemically into peptides, amino acids, amino acid derivatives, fatty acids, amines, and steroids. Although hormones, growth factors, cytokines, and neurotransmitters show a great diversity in structure and physiological actions, their cellular and molecular mechanism of action show many common features.

Humans and higher mammals possess over 500 known different regulatory molecules that have the capability of interacting with a large number of different cell types variably distributed in tissues throughout the body. This poses a tremendous challenge to any system of information exchange in terms of both specificity and sensitivity. The specificity of informational transfer between cells is gov-

erned by the type and concentration of regulatory molecule and by the capacity of each target cell to specifically respond to this molecular signal but not to others. In addition, specificity is controlled by the space of distribution of the active substance. Some regulatory molecules such as hormones act on cells located at a distance (endocrine effect), whereas others such as growth factors act on adjacent cells (paracrine or juxtacrine effect) or the secretory cell itself (autocrine effect). Finally, neurotransmitters are released from nerve endings and act on adjacent cells (neurotransmitter effect). Growth factors and hormones acting by paracrine or autocrine mechanisms, as well as neurotransmitters, may have the capability of stimulating multiple tissues, but their action is limited by the fact that the concentrations of substance required for biological response are achieved only within the limited space of a synapse or on cells adjacent to the same extracellular space.

The major factor determining the tissue response to a regulatory molecule is the presence of a cellular receptor and the postreceptor effector systems to which that receptor is coupled. For peptide hormones, growth factors, neurotransmitters, catecholamines, and prostaglandins, the receptors are present on the plasma membrane of the cell. For steroid hormones, iodothyronines, retinoic acid, and vitamin D, the receptors and initial sites of action are in the cytoplasm or nucleus of the cell. All cellular receptors serve two crucial functions: (1) recognition of the regulatory molecule as an entity distinct from all of the other substances present in the extracellular fluid; this is accomplished by specific, high-affinity binding. (2) transformation of this binding into a signal that ultimately modifies cellular functions (e.g., metabolism, growth, secretion, and contraction). Although many of the concepts of receptor function are similar for membrane and nuclear receptors, this chapter focuses on the mechanism of action of regulatory substances that act at the cell surface and the nature

---

The use of abbreviations in this chapter is limited in order to make the text more comprehensive. Some abbreviations have been inserted to conform to the style of the book. Abbreviations that are generally accepted in the original literature are mentioned once.

In view of the broad scope of this review the reference list is not complete and the references included should be considered only as representative.

of some of the proteins involved in this action. The mechanism of action of steroid and thyroid hormones is discussed in Chapter 6.

Development of the Receptor Concept

The concept that cells possess specific receptors for regulatory molecules was first proposed in the early 1900's by Langley from studies on the actions of nicotine and curare[1] and by Paul Ehrlich, who was investigating the actions of certain toxins and antitrypanocidal drugs.[2] The concept of receptors actually preceded the concept of an endocrine system and work of Starling, in which he described the actions of circulating substances, ''hormones,'' that could be produced in one cell and act at a distance on another cell. Taken together, these authors concluded that drugs, toxins, and hormones have a specificity of action that is governed by the presence of specific ''receptive substances'' on or in the target cell. This idea was quickly captured by pharmacologists as a model for the effects of drugs. However, early attempts to demonstrate receptors for hormones were largely inconclusive, and it remained uncertain whether cells possessed specific receptors for hormones, and, if they did, whether these receptors were inside or on the surface of the cell.

The first convincing evidence that some hormones may act by means of surface membrane receptors came through indirect studies which revealed that antibodies to peptide hormones, such as TSH and insulin, could reverse the actions of these hormones once they had begun.[3] This was consistent with the notion that the hormone was still on the cell surface and accessible to the antibody at the time of its biological action. Similar conclusions were reached in studies showing that treatment of cells with proteolytic enzymes, at concentrations that did not disrupt cell integrity, specifically blocked action of some peptide hormones[4] and that peptide hormones remained active after being covalently coupled to large polymeric beads that prevented their entrance into the cell,[5] again suggesting a protease-sensitive receptor on the cell surface. Most important, how-

ever, was the discovery by Sutherland and his co-workers of an intracellular messenger of hormone action, cAMP.[6, 7] On the basis of the preceding studies, these workers proposed the ''second-messenger concept'' of hormone action. In this scheme, the hormone is the first messenger of intercellular communication and is secreted in the bloodstream, where it is free to interact with surface membrane receptors on target cells. This interaction results in generation of a secondary messenger inside the cell that mediates the hormone's effects on intracellular enzymes, membrane transport, contractile proteins, secretory vesicles, and gene expression (Fig. 3–1). The second messenger or secondary signal may be a small organic molecule such as cAMP, cGMP, or an inositol triphosphate; it may be an ion such as calcium or magnesium or it may be activation of a protein kinase that results in covalent modification of intracellular proteins by phosphorylation causing a change in their activity. This model represents a paradigm on which most concepts of the mechanism of action of hormones, growth factors, and neurotransmitters have been based, although, as will become apparent, it is probably too simplistic to account for the full spectrum of actions of most regulatory molecules. The era of molecular biology has introduced new paradigms for the mechanism of hormone action. These emphasize two simplifying principles of redundancy and diversity in hormone signaling. On the one hand simple mechanisms or modules are used over and over again in many organisms and cellular systems. On the other hand there are many ways of achieving the same effect on cellular regulation. A limited number of signal transduction systems are widespread in organisms from bacteria to eukaryotic cells involving similar receptors, signaling molecules, and enzymes. They show, however, an extensive heterogeneity of the individual components at each level from membrane receptors to final effectors. The combination of redundancy and diversity results in a signaling network that allows the sophisticated regulation of cellular functions.

The specific details of the mechanism of hormone, growth factor, or neurotransmitter action are usually studied at the cellular and molecular level. However, physiolog-

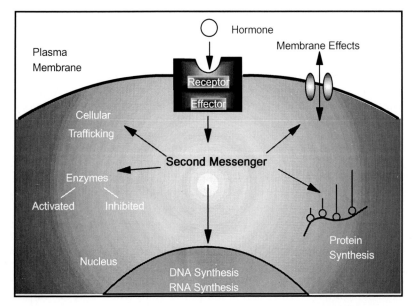

FIGURE 3–1. **A general model for the action of hormones, growth factors, and neurotransmitters via membrane receptors.** The hormone in the extracellular fluid interacts with the receptor and activates an associated effector system (which may or may not be in the same molecule). This activation results in generation of an intracellular signal or second messenger that, through a variety of common and branched pathways, produces the final effects of the hormone on metabolic enzyme activity, protein synthesis, membrane transport, cellular trafficking, DNA and RNA synthesis, and cellular growth and differentiation. (From Kahn CR, Smith RJ, Chin WW: Mechanism of action of hormones that act at the cell surface. *In* Wilson JD, Foster DW: Williams Textbook of Endocrinology. Philadelphia, WB Saunders Co, 1992, p 92.)

ically it is important to recognize the mechanism of action as an interaction between extracellular, diffusible molecules and complex tissues. This process can be visualized at the whole-body level through studies of the distribution and fate of hormones, growth factors, or neurotransmitters in intact animals. With use of hormones and neurotransmitters in a radioactively labeled tracer form, the fate of these substances can be determined by direct measurement of tissue uptake of radioactivity[8] or with use of noninvasive techniques such as external scintillation scanning with high-energy gamma emitters (e.g., ^{123}I)[9] or positron emission tomography.[10]

An example is the study of in vivo kinetics of insulin by scintillation scanning.[9] After intravenous injection, the insulin tracer is rapidly cleared from the circulation as it is distributed into the extracellular fluid space and is bound to receptors on liver, muscle, and adipose tissue. Within the first 15 minutes most of the insulin is bound, internalized, and degraded. In addition, some uptake of hormone and of degradation fragments occurs in nontarget tissues, such as the kidney and the spleen, through receptor-independent mechanisms. By 30 minutes after the injection all that remains are some degradation products of insulin in the kidney and the bladder. Although the exact details of the distribution may vary between injected and physiologically secreted insulin, because the latter first enters the portal rather than the systemic circulation, the basic principles are the same. It is important to remember that there is a lag in the onset of hormone action compared with these distribution kinetics. This lag is determined by the time required for distribution of the hormone, transport of the hormone across the vascular endothelium, diffusion of the hormone in the extracellular space, binding of the hormone to receptors on the target cell, and generation of intracellular signals by the hormone-receptor complex.[11]

PROPERTIES OF THE LIGAND-RECEPTOR INTERACTION

Direct Studies of Membrane Receptors

Direct studies of the interaction of ligands with membrane receptors were first achieved in 1970 using radiolabeled angiotensin[12] and ACTH.[13] Similar ligand-binding studies have now been performed for virtually all of the regulatory molecules: hormones, growth factors, and neurotransmitters. The basic approach for such studies is depicted in Figure 3–2. Typically a radioactively labeled ligand (peptides are labeled with ^{125}I; amines, fatty acids, and amino acids with ^{3}H) is incubated with isolated intact cells, cell membranes, or solubilized receptors in the presence or absence of unlabeled ligand until steady-state is obtained.[14–17] The receptor-bound ligand is then separated from the free ligand by centrifugation, precipitation, or filtration, and the percentage of ligand bound to the receptor is determined by counting the radioactive tracer in a gamma or β-scintillation counter. Unlabeled ligand competes with the labeled ligand for binding to the receptor, producing a competition, inhibition, or displacement curve. The use of receptors to detect labeled ligands is referred to as *radioreceptor assay*. Labeled ligand binding to receptors is a saturable process, and the residual binding

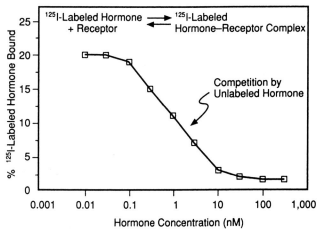

FIGURE 3–2. **Displacement curve of ligand binding to receptor.** ^{125}I-labeled hormone is incubated with receptor and increasing concentrations of unlabeled hormone. After separation of bound and free hormone, the percentage of bound ^{125}I activity is calculated and plotted against the total hormone concentration (labeled plus unlabeled hormone). The result is a competition (or inhibition) curve. Note that even at extremely high concentrations there is some binding of hormone. This binding is considered to be nonspecific and is subtracted from the total to give the specific binding. (From Kahn CR, Smith RJ, Chin WW: Mechanism of action of hormones that act at the cell surface. *In* Wilson JD, Foster DW: Williams Textbook of Endocrinology. Philadelphia, WB Saunders Co, 1992, p 92.)

in the presence of a large excess of unlabeled hormone is considered "nonspecific." Improvement of labeling and separation techniques has yielded tracer ligands that are identical with the native ligand except for the addition or substitution of the radioactive atom. With such tracers, the residual "nonspecific binding" can be almost totally accounted for by trapping of free tracer in the cell or membrane pellet.[17] In some cases it is necessary to use ligand analogues if the native substance is difficult or impossible to label radioactively, if it has a low affinity, or if it is easily degraded. For some receptors—especially neurotransmitter receptors—the labeled ligand is often a receptor antagonist, since the antagonist binds to the receptor with higher affinity and specificity than the normal agonist. Antireceptor antibodies have also been used as ligands for receptor detection.[18, 19] Such antibodies may recognize domains of the receptor distinct from the physiological ligand-binding domain and thus allow detection of receptors that are altered in their ligand-binding region. Although the basic technique of radioreceptor assay is similar to that of radioimmunoassay, there are several important differences. Since the receptor interaction requires biological specificity, it is crucial that the ligand be labeled in a manner that does not alter its biological activity. In addition, since the receptors are part of a cell membrane, the receptor is usually in a particulate or cell-associated form rather than in aqueous solution. Solubilization of the receptors requires detergent treatment. Using these systems appropriately, many of the properties of the ligand-receptor interaction can be characterized.

Since peptide hormones and growth factors are present at very low concentrations (picomolar to nanomolar, i.e., 10^{-12} to 10^{-9} M), receptors must have appropriately high affinities (i.e., K_d 10^{-12} to 10^{-9} M) to achieve significant binding at physiological concentrations. The high affinity of hormone and growth factor receptors is reflected in low dissociation rate constants and relatively longer half-lives of the ligand-receptor complex, whereas the association between hormone or growth factor and receptor is rapid. In contrast, neurotransmitters are released in high amounts into the synaptic cleft or neuromuscular junction to achieve higher concentrations. The affinity of neurotransmitter receptors is accordingly generally lower (i.e., K_d 10^{-4} to 10^{-7} M). Neurotransmitter action is characterized by rapid onset and offset, and dissociation rate constants are higher.[19–21]

On any cell there are a finite number of receptors for each hormone, growth factor, or neurotransmitter to which the cell responds, the number varying from fewer than 100 to greater than 100,000 receptors per cell. Generally, "target" cells possess a high number of receptors, whereas "nontarget" cells have none or a low number of receptors consistent with the specificity requirements of the system. Interestingly, exceptions to this rule have led to the discovery of previously unrecognized hormone, growth factor, or neurotransmitter actions on cells not thought to be a classic target tissue. For example, insulin receptors are present in relatively high concentration not only on liver, muscle, and fat cells but also on lymphocytes, gonadal cells, and even brain tissue. Similarly, thyroid-stimulating hormone (TSH) receptors are found on both thyroid cells and adipocytes, and prolactin receptors are present on mammary cells and hepatocytes.

Receptor-Binding Theory

The simplest model of receptor-binding of ligands is based on three assumptions: reversibility of the interaction between receptor and ligand, bimolecularity of the binding reaction, and noncooperativity of receptors.[17] These assumptions are expressed in the reaction scheme:

$$R + L = RL$$

(R is free receptor, L free ligand, and RL is receptor-bound ligand).

At steady-state the binding reaction is described by two equations. First, the *steady-state equation* based on the law of mass action:

$$[R][L]/[RL] = k_2/k_1 = K_d = 1/K_a$$

(K_d and K_a are the dissociation and association constants at steady-state; k_1 and k_2 are the association rate and dissociation rate constants). Second, the *conservation equation* of total receptor concentration (R_T):

$$[R_T] = [R] + [RL]$$

By combining the steady-state and conservation equations, a relationship between the concentrations of receptor-bound ligand (or ligand-occupied receptor), [RL], and free ligand, [L], is obtained:

$$[RL] = [R_T][L]/([L] + K_d)$$

The most common graphic representation of steady-state binding data is the displacement, inhibition, or competition curve (see Fig. 3–2). This plot is based on a simple transformation of the concentration relationship:

$$[RL]/[L] = [R_T]/([L] + K_d)$$

The presence of nonspecific binding is easily detected in this plot as a constant value of [RL]/[L] at ligand concentrations above 10^{-7} to 10^{-4} M and can be subtracted to give receptor-bound ligand.

For calculation of binding affinity, K_d, and total receptor number, [R_T], the Scatchard plot of steady-state binding data has been widely used.[20] This linear plot is based on a transformation of the concentration relationship:

$$[RL]/[L] = [R_T]/K_d - [RL]/K_d$$

The abscissa-intercept equals [R_T] and the slope $-1/K_d$ (Fig. 3–3). Many receptors exhibit two or more classes of binding sites of different affinity and others exhibit negative or positive cooperative interactions. Both phenomena can result in curvilinear Scatchard plots.[21–23] Receptor-binding affinity may also be determined by estimation of the rate constants of association, k_1, and dissociation, k_2, from measurements of transient-state kinetics.[24]

Ligand Specificity

The most important characteristic and essential feature of receptors is to recognize specific ligand(s) and to discriminate them from the large number of other regulatory molecules. In general, receptors show a high degree of molecular specificity in their ligand binding. The physiological ligand is bound with high affinity, whereas ligands with similarities in their structure bind with lower affinity, and unrelated substances do not interact. For example, insulin binds to the insulin receptor with 100 times the affinity of insulin growth factor-I (IGF-I) and > 10,000 the affinity of glucagon. Affinity and specificity of the receptor binding determine the bioactivity of hormones, growth factors, and neurotransmitters (Fig. 3–4). Most of the differences observed in potency of various analogues or derivatives are due to differences in binding affinity of the receptor. Regulatory substances may also differ in their ability to initiate signal transduction after binding, i.e., their intrinsic activity, although this is less common. Competitive antagonists are ligands that bind to the receptor with high affinity but have no intrinsic activity.

The structural features of regulatory molecules that define their receptor-binding affinity and intrinsic bioactivity are only partially understood. Analysis of the relationship between structure and activity of a bioactive substance requires the synthesis of a large number of structural analogues, resolution of their three-dimensional structure by x-ray crystallography or nuclear magnetic resonance, and measurements of their bioactivity in appropriate test systems. This has been feasible for small organic molecules such as epinephrine, acetylcholine, and γ-aminobutyric acid (GABA), and for these substances the structure-function relationship has been described in great detail. In addition, these analogues have been used in the functional characterization of receptor subtypes such as the different classes of adrenergic and GABA receptors.[25, 26]

Small single-chain peptide hormones and neuropeptides such as ACTH, glucagon, substance P, cholecystokinin, and others do not seem to have an ordered structure in solution, and their receptor-binding affinity and intrinsic activity appear to be governed by short linear domains of the molecule of 5 to 10 amino acids.[27, 28] For these molecules it is possible to produce peptide fragments as well as nonpep-

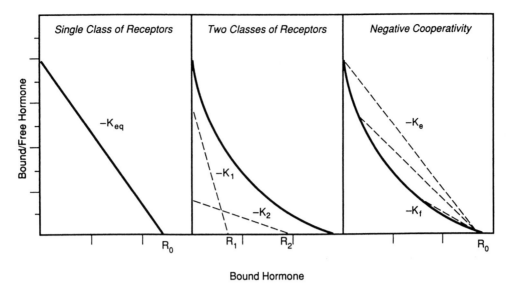

FIGURE 3–3. Scatchard analysis of ligand-receptor interaction. When the bound/free ratio is plotted against the bound hormone for a single class of noninteractive sites (an ideal bimolecular reversible reaction), a straight line is obtained (*left*). The slope of the line is the negative value of the association constant $-K_a$ (or $-1/K_d$), and the intercept on the abscissa is the total receptor concentration (R_T). Curvilinear Scatchard plots may arise as the result of two classes of sites (*middle*) or the presence of negative cooperativity (*right*). In the two-class model, the curve is the sum of two straight lines representing a high-affinity, low-capacity site ($-K_1$, R_1) and a low-affinity, high-capacity site ($-K_2$, R_2). In the negative cooperativity model, there is a single class of interactive sites. The total receptor concentration is R_0 (or R_T). The high-affinity state is $-K_e$ (the affinity of the empty receptor). As the sites are filled, the affinity falls, eventually reaching a low-affinity state $-K_{fl}$ (the affinity of the filled receptor). (From Kahn CR, Smith RJ, Chin WW: Mechanism of action of hormones that act at the cell surface. *In* Wilson JD, Foster DW: Williams Textbook of Endocrinology. Philadelphia, WB Saunders Co, 1992, p 95.)

tide agonists and competitive antagonists that bind to the receptor but lack intrinsic activity.[29–31] For larger peptide hormones and growth factors that have a complex three-dimensional structure, such as insulin, growth hormone, epidermal growth factor (EGF), and others, the binding and activity domain is formed by residues from different parts of the molecule that come together to form a bioactive surface.[24, 32] Chemical synthesis, chemical modification of native peptides, and biosynthesis using recombinant DNA techniques have been used for the production of analogues; structural analysis by x-ray crystallography or nuclear magnetic resonance and bioactivity studies have been successfully applied to describe the receptor-binding region of such molecules as insulin and growth hormone.[24, 33] For this latter group of peptide hormones and growth factors, however, synthesis of smaller bioactive "molecular cores," nonpeptide agonists, and competitive antagonists has not been possible to date.

RECEPTOR STRUCTURE

Cloning of Membrane Receptors

Receptors for hormones, growth factors, and neurotransmitters are integral membrane proteins. The prototype is composed of extracellular, transmembrane, and cytoplasmic domains that are involved in different functions: ligand binding, receptor aggregation, intracellular signaling, and internalization. By definition a transmembrane domain is common to all membrane receptors. It is composed of 21 to 23 predominantly hydrophobic amino acids

that form an α-helix with 7 turns, a length (approximately 30 nm) sufficient to span the lipid membrane bilayer. Apart from the hydrophobic nature of the amino acids, no consensus sequence has been described. On both sides of the transmembrane domain are hydrophilic amino acids presumably to lock the hydrophobic sequence into its membrane-bound position and prevent the receptor from sliding across the membrane. In addition to the insertion in the lipid bilayer, the membrane-spanning α-helix may be capable of forming aggregates with other membrane-spanning α-helices in the same receptor or in other receptor molecules, a feature that may be important in signaling.

Receptor structures have been determined from the full-length nucleotide sequences of mRNA molecules encoding membrane receptors for hormones, growth factors, and neurotransmitters. The first membrane receptors to be sequenced were the nicotinic acetylcholine receptor[34] and the EGF receptor.[35] Because transmembrane receptors are nonabundant molecules, their characterization involved a combination of both biochemical and molecular biological techniques. Thus the receptor proteins were first purified in small amounts and short stretches of amino acid sequence were determined. Oligonucleotide probes corresponding to the amino acid sequence were synthesized for screening of a cDNA library derived from a tissue or cell expressing mRNA for the receptor. Positive clones were selected by hybridization under stringent conditions, and the cDNA insert of the phage was sequenced and the amino acid sequence deduced.

In addition to this basic approach, three other techniques for cloning and sequencing of other receptors have been applied. The first is homology screening, in which receptors with similar sequences are detected by screening

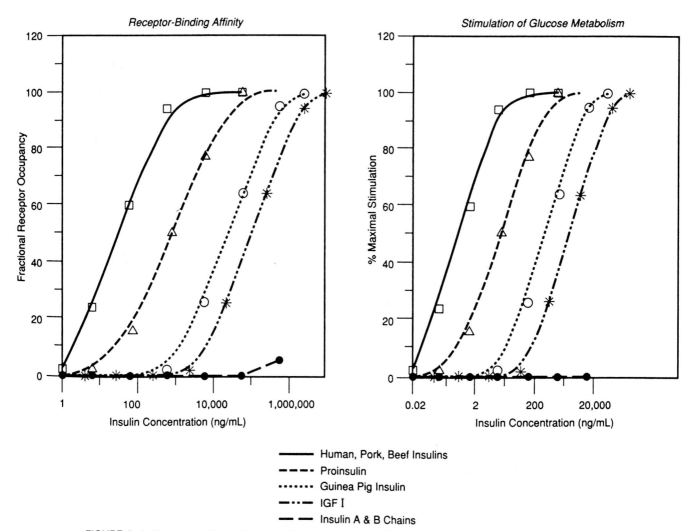

FIGURE 3–4. **Ligand specificity of receptor binding.** Correlation between binding and bioactivity. The left panel shows the binding of a series of insulin analogues to the receptor in rat liver plasma membranes. The right panel shows the ability of the same analogues to stimulate glucose metabolism in isolated adipocytes. There is an almost perfect correlation between receptor affinity *(left)* and relative bioactivity *(right)*. Also note that the bioactivity scale reflects increased insulin sensitivity because of the presence of spare receptors. (IGF-I, insulin-like growth factor 1.) To convert insulin values from nanograms per milliliter to nanomoles per liter, multiply by 0.1722. (Adapted from Freychet P, Roth J, Neville DM Jr: Insulin receptors in the liver: Specific binding of [¹²⁵I]-insulin to the plasma membrane and its relation to insulin bioactivity. Proc Natl Acad Sci USA 68:1833–1837, 1971.)

the cDNA library with a known receptor cDNA probe under low-stringency conditions. One example is the human EGF receptor homologue HER-2, which was cloned and sequenced by screening with a cDNA probe for the viral oncogene v-*erb* B.[36] The sequence is similar to that of the rat cellular oncogene c-*neu*[37, 38]; however, because the ligand was initially unknown, the receptor was designated an "orphan receptor." The ligand of this receptor was later identified by various groups and termed either *neu* differentiation factor, heregulin, or neuregulin.[39] A second approach to receptor cloning involves the polymerase chain reaction technique. Based on a presumed sequence similarity with a known receptor, synthetic oligonucleotide primers that are directed toward conserved domains are used for amplification of the unknown receptor cDNA. This cDNA fragment can then be used as a specific probe for screening of cDNA libraries under stringent conditions. This technique has been applied in the cloning of many of

the G protein–coupled receptors including the TSH receptor.[40] Furthermore, receptors have been identified by expression cloning. This approach is the most laborious but has been used for cloning of neurotransmitter receptors such as the substance K receptor[41] and peptide hormone receptors such as the TSH-releasing hormone (TRH) receptor.[42] In each case, there was expression of mRNA in a frog oocyte and screening of ligand-induced membrane ion flux or depolarization followed by selection, amplification, and sequencing of the relevant cDNA. Finally, expression cloning in the Cos cell line has been used for identification and sequencing of hormone receptors such as the parathyroid hormone (PTH) receptor and the glucagon receptor.[43, 44]

The elucidation of the amino acid sequences has clarified the idea that membrane receptors possess multiple functional domains. Experiments utilizing in vitro mutagenesis to form a chimeric receptor that possesses specific domains derived from different receptors has provided a better understanding of their structure and function. In addition to the ligand-binding and transmembrane domains, membrane receptors may contain cytoplasmic domains that (1) interact with G proteins to activate effector systems (i.e., adenylate cyclase); (2) possess inherent enzyme activity (i.e., quanylate cyclase or tyrosine kinases); (3) associate with an active enzyme (i.e., tyrosine kinases); (4) bind cytoplasmic proteins containing specific src homology 2 (SH2) domains (i.e., phosphoinositol 3-kinase); (5) determine membrane insertion (phospholipid interaction); (6) interact with other receptors or subunits to form oligomers (i.e., active receptor dimers); (7) initiate internalization; and (8) regulate receptor activity.

The amino-terminus of the peptide chain is generally extracellular and contains the ligand-binding domain. These regions are often glycosylated and may contain sulfate and phosphate groups. They may also have sites of fatty acid acylation, as well as complex disulfide linkages. The receptor may contain one, four, or seven transmembrane-spanning domains. In addition to serving as ''anchors'' to the membrane, these transmembrane domains may play important roles in receptor oligomerization and interaction with ligands. Finally, there is the carboxyl-terminal domain. This cytoplasmic region may be the direct effector domain of the molecule, as in the case of the receptor tyrosine kinases, or may play a role in modulation of receptor activity and/or internalization. For the seven-transmembrane segment receptors, the third intracytoplasmic loop may also act as the site of interaction with G proteins (see below). The ability of receptors to bind to different ligands and to transduce these signals by yet other sets of effectors resides in structural subtleties of the specific domains.

Families of Membrane Receptors

Membrane receptors can be classified structurally and functionally into three main families which differ in the number and arrangement of membrane-spanning segments and signal transduction[45]: seven-transmembrane segment receptors coupled to G proteins; single-transmembrane segment receptors directly or indirectly coupled to intracellular enzymes; and four-transmembrane segment receptors that form ligand-gated ion channels (Table 3–1). Receptors for hormones, growth factors, and neurotransmitters are represented in all three groups, indicating that the ligand binding and signal transduction involved in their biological actions show significant variation (Fig. 3–5).

The largest family of membrane receptors is the seven-transmembrane segment receptors that utilize G proteins to couple to adenylate cyclase or phospholipase C that catalyze formation of intracellular signaling molecules (second messengers) (e.g., cAMP or inositol triphosphate and diacylglycerol) (Table 3–2). More than 100 members of this family have been identified, including adrenergic, dopaminergic, serotonergic, muscarinic, cholinergic, peptidergic, dietary chemical, odorant, and retinal receptors.[46] These receptors are composed of an extracellular amino-terminal domain of varying length, which is characteristically glycosylated, seven hydrophobic transmembrane domains connected by three extracellular and three intra-

TABLE 3–1. FAMILIES OF MEMBRANE RECEPTORS: STRUCTURAL AND FUNCTIONAL CLASSIFICATION

FAMILY/CLASS	SUBUNIT COMPOSITION	TRANSDUCTION SYSTEM	LIGANDS

1. Seven-transmembrane segment receptors
  I. Rhodopsin-like receptors
  II. Glucagon and calcitonin receptors
  III. Metabotropic glutamate receptors
	Monomers or homodimers or post-translational heterodimers	Via a G protein
		(A) Plus a diffusible messenger, cAMP, inositol 3-phosphate
		
		(B) Acting directly on a channel
		
		(C) After receptor cleavage by a polypeptide hormone acting as a site-specific protease (and not as a classic agonist) to form a self-activating receptor
			(A) All the small transmitters (except glycine); peptides; neuropeptides; odorants; certain cytokines (e.g., IL-8); lipid and related agonists (e.g., eicosanoids)
			(B) Atrial muscarinic; neuronal α_1-adrenergic, etc.
			(C) Thrombin is the only case so far known

2. Single-transmembrane segment receptors
  I. Tyrosine kinase receptors
  II. Guanylate cyclase receptors
  III. Serine/threonine kinase receptors
  IV. Tyrosine phosphatase receptors
  V. Multisubunit receptors
	Monomers or homodimers or post-translational heterotetramers or native heterodimers or heterotrimers	The binding subunit itself is:
		(A) a ligand-stimulated tyrosine kinase
		(B) a ligand-stimulated guanylate cyclase
		(C) a ligand-stimulated serine/threonine kinase
		(D) intrinsic tyrosine phosphatase
		(E) not of known enzymatic activity associating with a cytoplasmic tyrosine kinase
			All are polypeptides:
			(A) mitogenic growth factors, insulin
			(B) natriuretic peptides
			(C) transforming growth factor β
			(D) unknown
			(E) neurotrophins; growth hormone, prolactin, and many cytokines

3. Four-transmembrane segment receptors	Heteromeric or homomeric	Transmitter-gated ion channels (A) Extracellularly activated (B) Intracellularly activated	(A) GABA$_A$, glycine, acetylcholine (nicotinic), glutamate, serotonin, ATP (B) cGMP, cAMP, ATP, inositol-triphosphate, Ca^{2+}

Modified from Barnard EA: Receptor classes and transmitter-gated ion channels. Trends Biochem Sci 17:368–374, 1992.

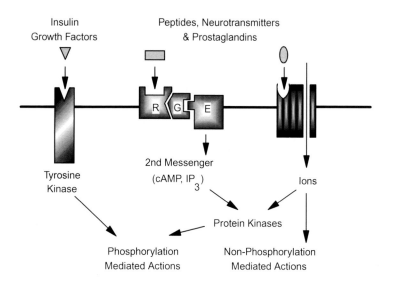

FIGURE 3–5. **Three major classes of membrane receptors.** Growth factors, including insulin, bind to a major class of receptors with a single transmembrane segment that act as protein tyrosine kinases stimulating the phosphorylation of proteins on tyrosine residues. A second major class of agonists binds to receptors (R) with seven transmembrane segments, which are coupled to separate effector (E) molecules by G proteins (G). The third major class of receptors includes ligand-gated ion channels, which are composed of five subunits each with four transmembrane segments. Protein tyrosine phosphorylations, second messengers, or ions activate distinct protein serine-threonine kinases that elicit phosphorylation-mediated actions. Ion fluxes may induce nonphosphorylation-mediated actions such as membrane depolarization. (Modified from Kahn CR, Smith RJ, Chin WW: Mechanism of action of hormones that act at the cell surface. *In* Wilson JD, Foster DW: Williams Textbook of Endocrinology. Philadelphia, WB Saunders Co, 1992, p 96.)

cellular hydrophilic loops, and a cytoplasmic C-terminal domain that contains potential phosphorylation sites involved in regulation of receptor activity. The extracellular parts of the receptor form a ligand-binding site, whereas the intracellular parts form a G protein–coupling site.[46]

Members of the second family of membrane receptors have a single transmembrane segment and include receptors that contain or couple with catalytic activity (e.g., tyrosine kinase, serine-threonine kinase, guanylate cyclase, and phosphotyrosine phosphatase) (Table 3–3). Activation of

TABLE 3–2. SEVEN-TRANSMEMBRANE SEGMENT RECEPTORS

RHODOPSIN FAMILY

Retinal
Odorants
Epinephrine: α-1, α-2, β-1, β-2
Acetylcholine (muscarinic): M1, M2, M3, and M4
Serotonin: 1A, 1B, 1C, 2
Dopamine: D1, D2
Angiotensin
Vasopressin
Substance K
Substance P (neurokinin): types 1, 2, 3
Neuromedin K
Neuropeptide Y
Cholecystokinin
Gastrin
Prostaglandins
Adenosine
Luteinizing hormone
Follicle-stimulating hormone
Chorion gonadotropin
Thyroid-stimulating hormone
Adrenocorticotropic hormone
Interleukin-8
Thrombin

GLUCAGON-CALCITONIN RECEPTOR FAMILY

Glucagon
Vasoactive intestinal polypeptide
Calcitonin
Secretin
Pituitary adenylate cyclase–activating peptide
Growth hormone–releasing factor

GLUTAMATE METABOTROPIC RECEPTOR FAMILY

Glutamate: MG1–MG7

these receptors and their intrinsic or associated enzymes induces intracellular signals via phosphorylation or dephosphorylation of proteins or by formation of cGMP. More than 50 members of this family are known and include polypeptide growth factor, cytokine, and peptide hormone receptors.[47, 48] These receptors have a large extracellular domain with either a characteristic disulfide cross-linked region or an IgG-like domain, a single hydrophobic transmembrane domain, and a large cytoplasmic domain. The family can be subdivided depending on the structure of the cytoplasmic domain that specifies the nature of the intracellular signaling mechanism. Protein tyrosine kinase–containing receptors are typified by the EGF, insulin, IGF-I, platelet-derived growth factor (PDGF), fibroblast growth factor (FGF), and nerve growth factor (NGF) receptors. Receptors with intrinsic serine-threonine kinase activity include the transforming growth factor β (TGF-β) receptor types 1 and 2. Receptors that contain guanylate cyclase activity bind atrial natriuretic peptide (ANP). Membrane receptors for growth hormone (GH), prolactin, erythropoietin, granulocyte-macrophage, and granulocyte colony–stimulating factors, interferon-α, -β, and -γ, and interleukins (IL) IL-2, IL-3, IL-4, IL-5, IL-6, and IL-7 are devoid of intrinsic enzyme activity in the cytoplasmic domain but associate with cytoplasmic tyrosine kinases such as those of the Janus family of kinases (JAK) and other membrane proteins to form multisubunit receptor complexes. The tumor necrosis factor (TNF) p55 receptor and NGF p75 receptor are also devoid of intrinsic enzyme activity, and their signaling mechanism is yet unknown. Finally, a class of membrane proteins has a receptor-like structure that contains phosphotyrosine phosphatase activity in their cytoplasmic domain, but no extracellular ligands have yet been identified. Of note, several members of this receptor family may also may be expressed as a nonmembrane-associated form, as a result of either alternative splicing of a membrane-spanning–domain-encoding exon or proteolytic cleavage of the extracellular domain close to the plasma membrane. These circulating receptor forms act as serum-binding proteins for the ligands.[47, 48]

The third family of membrane receptors has four transmembrane segments and includes ligand-gated ion channels (Table 3–4). These receptors are composed of homologous subunits that can assemble in a pentamer

TABLE 3–3. SINGLE-TRANSMEMBRANE SEGMENT RECEPTORS

PROTEIN TYROSINE KINASE RECEPTOR FAMILY

Epidermal growth factor
Neu-differentiation factor (human EGF receptor 2)
Insulin
Insulin-like growth factor I
Fibroblast growth factors
Platelet-derived growth factors A and B
Colony-stimulating factor-1 (macrophage colony–stimulating factor)
Nerve growth factors (neurotrophins)
Hepatocyte growth factor (scatter factor)

GUANYLATE CYLASE RECEPTOR FAMILY

Atrial natriuretic peptide: types A, B, and C

SERINE/THREONINE KINASE RECEPTOR FAMILY

Transforming growth factor β: types I and II
Activin
Inhibin

MULTISUBUNIT RECEPTOR FAMILY

Growth hormone
Prolactin
Placental lactogen
Erythropoietin
Interleukin-2, 3, 4, 5, 6, 7
Granulocyte-macrophage colony–stimulating factor
Granulocyte colony–stimulating factor
Interferons α, β, and γ
Tumor necrosis factor: p75
Leukemia inhibitory factor
Oncostatin
Ciliary neurotrophic factor

TUMOR NECROSIS FACTOR–NERVE GROWTH FACTOR RECEPTOR FAMILY

Tumor necrosis factor p55
Nerve growth factor p75

PHOSPHOTYROSINE PHOSPHATASE RECEPTOR FAMILY

Ligands unknown

PLASMAPROTEIN RECEPTOR FAMILY

Low-density lipoprotein
Transferrin
Asialoglycoproteins
Polymeric immunoglobulin A/Immunoglobulin M
Mannose-6-phosphate/insulin-like growth factor II
Urokinase plasminogen activator
α_2-Macroglobulin

surrounding a membrane pore. Signal transduction in this case is by means of the opening of a cation or an anion channel.[45] Ligand-gated ion channels include nicotinic acetylcholine, GABA$_A$, glycine, glutamate, serotonin, and adenosine triphosphate (ATP) receptors. A related class of ligand-gated channels is activated intracellularly by cGMP, cAMP, ATP, inositol triphosphate, cADP-ribose and Ca^{2+} (ryanodine receptor). The ligand-gated ion channels perform fast signaling, since their transduction is independent of any intracellular or membrane-diffusible factor. Their ion selectivity varies between Na$^+$, K$^+$, Ca^{2+}, Mg^{2+}, Cl$^-$, and HCO$_3^-$. A large number of receptor subtypes with varying composition of different subunit isoforms exist; these show marked differences in ligand specificity, signal transduction, pharmacology, and distribution.[45]

Some hormones, growth factors, and neurotransmitters are known to be related and have overlapping structural features and biological activities. Classic examples include the families of (1) prolactin, GH, and placental lactogen;

(2) insulin, IGF-I, and IGF-II; (3) secretin, glucagon, and vasoactive intestinal polypeptide (VIP); (4) gastrin and cholecystokinin; (5) luteinizing hormone (LH), follicle-stimulating hormone (FSH), and human chorionic gonadotropin (hCG); and (6) ACTH, melanocyte-stimulating hormone (MSH), and other derivatives of pro-opiomelanocortin. Many of these families of hormones are related by evolution and are derived from similar or identical precursors.

Families of related hormones often interact with families of related receptors. For example, the prolactin and GH receptors have ~30 per cent overall similarity, with four highly homologous regions in the extracellular domain and one in the cytoplasmic domain. The receptors for insulin and IGF-I are virtually identical in overall structure and have about 50 per cent sequence identity throughout their length. Receptors for secretin, glucagon, and VIP show a high degree of structural similarity, and receptors for LH and hCG are related.

Structural similarities of hormone receptors may extend beyond these families of related hormones and indicate receptors that utilize similar effector pathways. The receptors for insulin and IGF-I, EGF, and PDGF have highly homologous intracellular tyrosine kinase domains that possess the enzymatic activity required for signal transduction but very different extracellular domains, which are responsible for ligand binding. Receptors for GH, prolactin, hematopoeitic growth factors, and cytokines show homology in their structure and interact with cytoplasmic tyrosine kinases of the JAK family, although their binding domains are different. Likewise, receptors that act through G proteins show similar overall structure with seven transmembrane segments, although the ligands they bind are quite different, ranging from polypeptide hormones (e.g., TSH) to small molecules (e.g., catecholamines). In the case of receptors coupled to G proteins, the signal transduction mechanisms are similar, but the final effects of the hormones are quite different.

There are some striking exceptions to the general rule that homologous hormones have structurally related receptors. For example, IGF-II is a peptide growth factor with a structure closely related to that of insulin and IGF-I and which also binds to the insulin and IGF-I receptor. However, the primary receptor for IGF-II is a large single-chain polypeptide that bears no resemblance to the tetrameric receptors for IGF-I or insulin. Furthermore, unlike the receptors for IGF-I and insulin, the IGF-II receptor has no

TABLE 3–4. LIGAND-GATED ION CHANNEL RECEPTOR FAMILY

EXTRACELLULAR ACTIVATED

GABA$_A$
Acetylcholine (nicotinic): muscle, neuronal
Glycine
Glutamate: AMPA, kainate, NMDA
Serotonin (5-HT$_3$)
ATP (purinergic receptor)

INTRACELLULAR ACTIVATED

Inositol-triphosphate and Ca^{2+} (endoplasmic reticulum)
cADP-ribose and Ca^{2+} (ryanodine receptor)
cGMP
cAMP
ATP

intrinsic tyrosine kinase activity, nor is it phosphorylated on tyrosine residues. The IGF-II receptor appears to be a bifunctional receptor that has a binding site for IGF-II and a binding site for mannose-6-phosphate–containing glycoproteins (e.g., lysosomal enzymes). The function of the IGF-II/mannose-6-phosphate receptor appears to be transport of these ligands to lysosomes, either for degradation or activation.

A single hormone or neurotransmitter may also interact with two different types of receptors differing in structure. Acetylcholine binds to a nicotinic receptor composed of four different subunits that form an ion channel and a muscarinic receptor that is coupled to phospholipid turnover through a G protein. Glutamate binds to different isoforms of ligand-gated ion channels, as well as to the metabotropic receptor that couples to G proteins. In addition, many receptors for neurotransmitters, hormones, and growth factors are present as multiple closely related isotypes that are products of distinct genes or result from alternative splicing of mRNA. The receptor isoforms have ligand binding sites that differ in affinity for any given group of ligand agonists and antagonists.

The existence of families of related hormones and receptors has significance physiologically. This is evidenced, for example, by the almost interchangeable biological effects of LH and chorionic gonadotropin (CG) and by the similar effects of growth hormone and prolactin on breast tissue. Other examples of overlap of hormone action are most often observed under circumstances in which one hormone is elevated to pathologically high levels and mimics the action of another hormone by binding to its receptor with a low affinity, i.e., receptor cross-reactivity.

Functional Domains of Membrane Receptors

Seven-Transmembrane Segment Receptors

This family is characterized by two structural features: most of the molecular mass is packed within the seven membrane-spanning segments and each receptor carries a G protein recognition sequence on its intracellular face (Fig. 3–6). Although most members of this class share some areas of sequence identity, it is only the overall structure with seven membrane-spanning segments that is common to all of them.[40–44, 49–59]

RHODOPSIN/NEUROTRANSMITTER FAMILY. The largest class of seven-transmembrane segment receptors is the family homologous to the visual pigment receptor rhodopsin,[49] and includes receptors for external signals such as light, odorants, and dietary chemicals and receptors for diverse internal signals such as hormones, neurotransmitters, and growth factors. It is remarkable that one class of receptors with the same fundamental structure can interact with such a broad spectrum of ligands. The number of odorant and dietary chemical receptors that have been cloned from the olfactory bulb and the taste buds exceeds more than 100 and seems to relate to the great number of signals perceived.[50] This class includes a large number of receptors for small hormones, neurotransmitters, and neuropeptides (e.g., epinephrine, dopamine, serotonin, acetyl-choline (muscarinic), prostaglandins, adenosine, substance K, substance P, neuromedin K, neuropeptide Y, angiotensin, vasopressin, gastrin, and cholecystokinin).[51–56] For each of these ligands several receptor subtypes have been identified, which show differences in binding kinetics, signal transduction, and tissue distribution, thus giving a clue to the variation in the cellular biology and physiology for each of these hormones and neurotransmitters. Finally, this class of seven-transmembrane receptors includes receptors for large polypeptide hormones (e.g., TSH, LH, FSH, and hCG).[40, 57, 58] These receptors are distinguished by their large extracellular amino-terminus involved in binding of the ligand. A special case of ligand binding and activation of the receptor has been described for the thrombin receptor. Thrombin specifically cleaves the receptor in its relatively long extracellular domain to liberate a new amino-terminal segment therein that acts as a ligand. This leads to self-activation of the receptor and hence intracellular signaling events.[59]

GLUCAGON-CALCITONIN RECEPTOR FAMILY. The second class of the seven-transmembrane receptors includes receptors for polypeptide hormones and neuropeptides (e.g., glucagon, secretin, growth hormone–releasing factor, pituitary adenylate cyclase–activating peptide, calcitonin, and VIP. This class is distinguished by homology in the sequence of the seven-transmembrane domains as well as the amino-terminus.[44]

METABOTROPIC GLUTAMATE RECEPTOR FAMILY. Finally, the metabotropic glutamate receptor is structurally distinct, as it shows no sequence homology with other seven-transmembrane segment receptors. Seven isoforms of the metabotropic glutamate receptor have been identified by cloning of their cDNA. All have a long extracellular amino-terminus and couple with G proteins. They can, however, be divided into three subgroups on the basis of ligand specificity toward glutamate receptor agonists and signal transduction involving stimulation of inositol triphosphate and inhibition of cAMP formation. So far the metabotropic glutamate receptors have been detected exclusively in the central nervous system.[60]

ADRENERGIC RECEPTORS. The structure and functional domains of seven-transmembrane receptors coupled to G proteins were first elucidated for the adrenergic receptors and later for the serotonin, dopamine, and muscarinic cholinergic receptors.[51–54] The adrenergic receptors exist as six different isoforms, α_1, α_2, α_3, β_1, β_2, and β_3, which share considerable protein sequence homology. Each is a single polypeptide with approximate molecular weights of 64 to 80 kDa; for example, the human β_1- and β_2-adrenergic receptors are 477 and 413 amino acid residues in size, respectively. The biological activity of the isolated polypeptide chain has been proved utilizing reconstitution-type experiments. Hydropathy plots of the deduced amino sequence were used to predict that the receptors possess seven hydrophobic, α-helical regions that correspond to the seven transmembrane domains previously observed in rhodopsin. Comparing the human β_1- and β_2-adrenergic receptors, these domains are more conserved than the overall molecule between (71 per cent versus 54 per cent, respectively). Comparison of transmembrane domains between β-adrenergic and muscarinic cholinergic receptors suggests that the most conserved regions involve the half

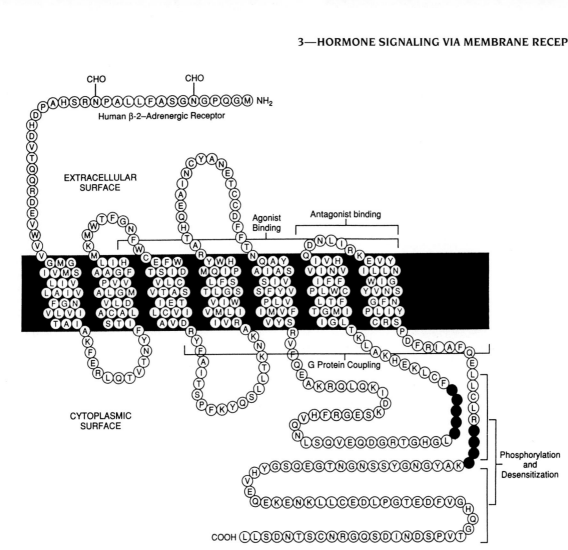

FIGURE 3–6. **Structure of a seven-transmembrane segment receptor, the β₂-adrenergic receptor.** The seven clusters of residues in the black rectangle representing the plasma membrane represent hydrophobic, α-helical membrane spanning domains. CHO indicates probable glycosylation sites in the extracellular domain of the receptor. The residues in the intracellular domain of the receptor indicated in the filled circles represent phosphorylation sites of the specific β-adrenergic receptor kinase. Domains of putative agonist and antagonist binding, G protein coupling, phosphorylation, and desensitization are shown. (Modified with permission from Dohlman HG, Caro MG, Lefkowitz RJ: A family of receptors coupled to guanine nucleotide regulatory proteins. Biochemistry 26:2657–2664, 1987. Copyright 1987 American Chemical Society.)

of each α-helix closest to the cytoplasm. The great variability in these helices near the extracytoplasmic region between different receptors suggests a role in specificity.[46]

The identification of functional domains among the adrenergic receptors has been facilitated by the ability to produce chimeric receptor forms by combining regions of the different adrenergic receptor subtypes. It has been shown that, although ligands interact with transmembrane regions 2 to 7, adrenergic agonist specificity lies primarily in transmembrane region 4, whereas antagonist interactions may involve transmembrane regions 6 and 7. Thus the catecholamine apparently interacts with its receptor primarily via a pocket formed by the transmembrane domains as they appear at the extracytoplasmic face.

An important domain in receptor function is one required for G protein coupling. It is located in the second and third cytoplasmic loops, as well as the carboxy-terminal tail of the receptor. Yet another domain is one that mediates receptor desensitization, a process in which a rapid diminution of effector response is observed after brief ex-

posure of receptor to agonist. In the adrenergic receptor system, homologous desensitization involves the phosphorylation on serine-threonine residues in the carboxy-terminal tail or the third cytoplasmic loop of the receptor by the cytoplasmic enzymes, cAMP-dependent protein kinase and β-adrenergic receptor kinase. This uncouples the receptor from its associated G protein. A molecule known as β-arrestin further modulates the interaction between the β-adrenergic receptor and β-adrenergic receptor kinase.[61, 62] In view of the domain organization of the adrenergic receptors, it is noteworthy that the genes for these receptors lack introns within the protein coding regions. In many eukaryotic genes, the exon-intron structure of the gene is reflected by the functional domain structure of the protein.

Single-Transmembrane Segment Receptors

This family is characterized by a structure with only one transversal of the bilayer, a characteristic that provides a minimum exposure of the receptor to the membrane lipids and facilitates receptor mobility, aggregation, and internalization. This family consists of several subfamilies that are functionally related by having intrinsic catalytic activity: tyrosine kinase, serine-threonine kinase, and guanylate cyclase, whereas one subfamily of single-transmembrane segment receptors has no enzymatic activity but apparently associates with cytoplasmic tyrosine kinases.

PROTEIN TYROSINE KINASE RECEPTOR FAMILY. The tyrosine kinase–containing receptors constitute a large group of receptors which can be divided into seven classes on the basis of comparison of their individual structures.[47, 63, 64] These include EGF and neu (or HER-2) receptors, insulin and IGF-I receptors, PDGF receptors α and β, CSF-1 and kit receptors, FGF receptors, NGF (or trk) receptors, and hepatocyte growth factor (HGF) (or scatter factor) receptors. Figure 3–7 shows the three classes of receptor tyrosine kinases that were the first to be cloned: EGF receptors, insulin receptors, and PDGF receptors. In spite of the existence of multiple receptors and oncogene products with tyrosine kinase activity, phosphorylation of cellular proteins on tyrosine residues is a much less common event than serine phosphorylation, comprising less than 1 per cent of all protein phosphorylation in the cell under normal conditions.

The first class is represented by the EGF receptor, in which the hormone binding and tyrosine kinase domains are contained in a single transmembrane peptide chain.[35–38]

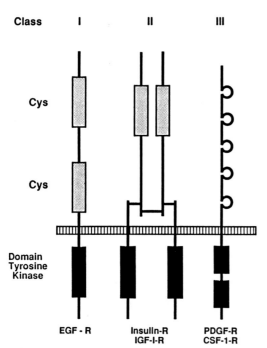

Class   I   II   III

Cys

Cys

Domain
Tyrosine
Kinase

EGF - R   Insulin-R   PDGF-R
            IGF-I-R   CSF-1-R

FIGURE 3–7. **Structure of single-transmembrane segment receptors, receptor tyrosine kinases.** Three classes are shown: class I is represented by the EGF receptor; class II by insulin and IGF-I receptors; class III by PDGF and CSF-1 receptors. The shaded rectangles in EGF and insulin receptors represent cysteine-rich regions (Cys). Disulfide bonds in these regions are thought to have an important role in establishing the structure of the ligand binding site. The circles in the PDGF receptor represent IgG-like repeats. The black rectangles in all three classes represent the tyrosine kinase domain, which is interrupted by an insert in PDGF receptors. (Modified from Kahn CR, Smith RJ, Chin WW: Mechanism of action of hormones that act at the cell surface. *In* Wilson JD, Foster DW: Williams Textbook of Endocrinology. Philadelphia, WB Saunders Co, 1992, p 113.)

The configuration of the ATP binding site and the tyrosine kinase domain is generally similar to that of other members of the src tyrosine kinase superfamily. The extracellular domain contains cysteine-rich domains that appear to be important for hormone binding, although these exist in two interrupted regions in the EGF receptor. There is evidence that the EGF receptor is inactive in its monomeric form and that transmission of the ligand signal requires receptor dimerization.[65]

A second class including the homologous insulin and IGF-I receptors are the most complex, with a heterotetrameric structure consisting of two α and two β subunits joined by disulfide cross-bridges. The α subunits are entirely extracellular and contain a cysteine-rich region that is believed to be involved in hormone binding. The β subunits possess an extracellular domain, a transmembrane domain, and an intracellular domain that contains an ATP-binding site and a catalytic kinase domain. The α and β subunits are synthesized as part of a single receptor precursor molecule that undergoes proteolytic processing to form the two subunits in a manner analogous to synthesis of insulin from proinsulin.[66–69]

The PDGF receptors form a third structural group of tyrosine kinase receptors. They contain binding and tyrosine kinase activities in a single peptide chain but possess a different type of extracellular cysteine-rich structure that is believed to form IgG-like repeats. In addition, the tyrosine kinase domain is interrupted by an insert of about 100 amino acids that are unrelated to other tyrosine kinases. Two types of PDGF receptors have been cloned: PDGF receptor α and PDGF receptor β.[69, 70] They show about 60 per cent sequence identity and different binding specificity toward the three types of PDGF dimers: PDGF AA, AB, and BB. The monomeric PDGF receptor is inactive but is activated after ligand-induced dimerization; this results in formation of three PDGF receptor dimers: αα, ββ, and αβ. PDGF AA binds only to PDGF receptor αα, whereas PDGF BB binds with high affinity to PDGF receptor ββ and with lower affinity to PDGF receptor αα. PDGF AB interacts with all three PDGF receptor dimeric complexes. PDGF receptor α and receptor β show differences in their cellular actions. The PDGF receptor ββ is more potent in stimulating cell division and chemotaxis than is the PDGF αα. Thus the existence of three PDGF dimers, as well as the three dimeric PDGF receptor complexes, gives possibilities for varying the cellular effects.

The group of FGF receptors includes four single-chain receptors that show some relationship with the PDGF receptor class. They are characterized by an extracellular domain with three IgG-like repeats, one transmembrane domain, and a cytoplasmic domain with a tyrosine kinase interrupted by a small insert of 14 amino acids. The sequence of the extracellular domain may vary depending on alternative splicing resulting in several receptor subtypes with varying ligand specificity. Ligands for these receptors include nine members of the FGF family that are widespread in the organism.[71, 72]

The group of CSF-1 receptors, including the c-*kit* oncogene product, are distantly related to PDGF and FGF receptors. They have IgG-like domains in their extracellular portion and kinase insert in their cytoplasmic portion.[73]

The NGF receptor group includes three members: trk A, trk B, and trk C, named after the c-*trk* oncogene product, which was found to bind NGF. Trk receptors are single-chain polypeptides with cysteine-rich, leucine-rich, and IgG-like regions in the extracellular domain, a single transmembrane domain, and a cytoplasmic domain with a tyrosine kinase interrupted by an insert.[74] Trk receptors bind five members of the NGF (or neurotrophin) family: NGF, brain-derived neurotrophic factor (BDNF), neurotrophin-3, -4, and -5, which are widespread in the nervous system.

HGF binds to the c-*met* oncogene product. This is a two-chain disulfide-linked polypeptide with an extracellular α-subunit and a transmembrane β subunit with a cytoplasmic tyrosine kinase domain, a structure that is reminiscent of the insulin receptor.[75] The HGF receptor is synthesized as a single polypeptide chain inactive precursor that is cleaved to an active two-chain molecule.

GUANYLATE CYCLASE RECEPTOR FAMILY. Guanylate cyclase receptors form a small but distinct group characterized by the self-contained guanylate cyclase in the cytoplasmic domain.[76, 77] Guanylate cyclase catalyzes the formation of cGMP from guanosine triphosphate (GTP) and exists in cells in both soluble and membrane-associated forms. In mammals three types of guanylate cyclase receptors have been cloned, of which receptor type A binds ANP and receptor types B and C bind peptides homologous to ANP, i.e., natriuretic peptides B and C (abbreviated BNP and CNP). In sea urchin eggs two proteins, resact and speract, activate guanylate cyclases by binding to membrane receptor.[78] The deduced amino acid sequence of guanylate cyclase derived from cloned cDNA's predicts a single transmembrane domain. The carboxyl-terminal domain is intracellular, is highly conserved from sea urchins to mammals, and has two repeats of the guanylate cyclase. In contrast, the extracellular domain is variable, contains the amino-terminus, and may serve as a ligand-binding domain. The receptor guanylate cyclases are members of a superfamily of proteins that includes the cytoplasmic form of the guanylate cyclase.

SERINE-THREONINE KINASE RECEPTOR FAMILY. Serine-threonine kinase receptors represent a newly discovered group of receptors with self-contained enzymatic activity.[79–81] These receptors are single-chain peptides with large extracellular domains containing a cysteine-rich region, a transmembrane domain, and a cytoplasmic serine-threonine kinase with two inserted sequences. The kinase is homologous to other serine-threonine kinases such as protein kinases A and C. Six members of this receptor group have been cloned and characterized, including TGF-β receptors I and II, activin, inhibin, müllerian-inhibiting substance, and bone morphogen receptors. Ligand-activated serine-threonine kinase is involved in the signaling of these substances, although the signal pathway is not yet clear.

PHOSPHOTYROSINE PHOSPHATASES. A group of membrane-bound phosphotyrosine phosphatases with receptor-like structures has been cloned.[82] They are single-chain peptides with a large extracellular domain containing a cysteine-rich glycosylated region that forms a putative ligand-binding site, a single transmembrane domain, and a cytoplasmic domain with two tandem tyrosine phosphatases. Eight members with some sequence homology have been cloned, including CD45, a leukocyte common antigen. No extracellular ligands for these receptor-like membrane proteins have yet been identified. The extracellular

domain has regions with similarity to cell adhesion molecules, suggesting that they may be involved in cell aggregation. The protein tyrosine phosphatases have potential importance in dephosphorylation of proteins phosphorylated on tyrosine in response to insulin and growth factor receptor tyrosine kinases.

MULTISUBUNIT RECEPTORS FAMILY. A large group of single-transmembrane segment receptors is characterized by the absence of enzymatic activity in the binding subunit. Receptors for GH, prolactin, cytokines, hematopoietic factors, and ciliary neurotrophic factor (CNTF) are related by sequence homology of the extracellular domain, whereas known motifs of signaling proteins such as kinases and phosphatases are absent in the cytoplasmic domain.[83–89] These receptors are composed of several subunits that form active homologous or heterologous oligomers. The complex of two identical or different subunits binds their ligands with high affinity, whereas the single subunits bind with lower affinity.[90–92] The high-affinity multisubunit receptors induce tyrosine phosphorylation by coupling with cytoplasmic tyrosine kinases of the Janus family of kinases (abbreviated JAK), of which four different members are known.[93, 94]

The GH receptor is a 130-kDa protein consisting of 620 amino acids divided into a 246-residue extracellular domain, a single-transmembrane domain of 24 amino acids, and an intracellular domain of about 350 residues (Fig. 3–8). The extracellular domain possesses several potential sites of N-linked and O-linked glycosylation, as in most membrane receptors, but there are no cysteine-rich regions or obvious repeating structures. Although the GH receptor is tyrosine-phosphorylated,[93] the elucidation of its primary structure showed that the intracellular domain bears no resemblance to receptors of known functional type. The difference between the apparent molecular weight (130 kDa) and the predicted amino acid molecular weight by composition (70 kDa) is thought to be caused by a high level of glycosylation and covalent association of the

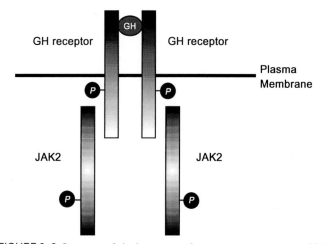

FIGURE 3–8. **Structure of single-transmembrane segment receptors which form homologous dimers; the growth hormone receptor.** One GH molecule binds to identical binding sites on the extracellular domains of two GH receptors that form a homodimer. The intracellular domains associate with a tyrosine kinase of the Janus family of kinases. Encircled P denotes potential tyrosine phosphorylation sites on the intracellular portion of GH receptor.

receptor with ubiquitin. When expressed in mammalian cells, the human GH receptor binds only human GH, whereas the rabbit receptor binds human GH, bovine GH, and ovine prolactin. This correlates well with the known species specificity of GH.[83, 84] The extracellular domain of the GH receptor has been expressed in a soluble, secreted form and its three-dimensional structure determined by x-ray crystallography.[95] The GH receptor was crystallized in its ligand-bound form, and the structure revealed that the extracellular domain forms a symmetrical dimer that associates with one GH molecule. GH has two distinct receptor-binding sites that interact with the same ligand-binding region on the two receptors in the dimer. It appears that formation of the GH receptor homodimer is needed for high-affinity binding of GH and activation of cellular responses. This was supported by the finding that a GH mutant with inactivation of one of the two binding sites acted as an antagonist to GH.

The prolactin receptor is also a single-transmembrane polypeptide with 209 amino acids on the extracellular face but only 58 amino acids in the cytoplasm.[84] It has four homologous regions in the extracellular domain but only one homologous region in the intracellular domain. Like the GH receptor, the prolactin receptor has no known functional signaling elements. In mammalian tissues there is a larger form of the prolactin receptor, highly homologous to the GH receptor. Also as a result of alternative splicing, secretory forms of both the GH receptor and the prolactin receptor exist that contain no transmembrane or intracellular domains.[83, 84]

Cytokines and hematopoietic growth factors, a large family of protein mediators, regulate proliferation, differentiation, and functions of various lineages in the immune and hematopoietic system of receptors. Cloning of the receptors for erythropoietin, IL-2, IL-3, IL-4, IL-5, IL-6, and IL-7, colony-stimulating factors for granulocytes and macrophages (abbreviated GM-CSF, G-CSF, M-CSF), leukemia-inhibiting factor, oncostatin, CNTF, TNF p 75, and interferon-α, -β, and -γ revealed that they consist of two distinct subunits, α subunits and β subunits (Fig. 3–9).[85–89] For two groups of cytokine receptors including IL-3, IL-5, and GM-CSF as well as IL-6, leukemia-inhibiting factor, oncostatin, and CNTF receptors the α-subunit is cytokine-specific, whereas the β subunit is common among the three members of each group.[90–92] The α subunits have a typical sequence motif possessed by the hematopoietic growth factor receptors in their extracellular domains consisting of four conserved cysteine residues and a conserved tryptophane-serine-X-tryptophane-serine sequence. There is a short stretch of a conserved amino acid sequence, arginine-phenylalanine-leucine-proline in the cytoplasmic domain of these α subunits. The mature α subunits are glycoproteins of 60 to 80 kDa with a short cytoplasmic domain of about 50 amino acids. Each α subunit binds its specific cytokine with low affinity (K_d = 2-100 nM). The β subunit, a glycoprotein of about 120 to 140 kDa, has an extracellular domain with two segments of the conserved motif of the hemopoietic growth factor receptors and a large cytoplasmic domain without any known motif of signaling proteins. Only one type of β subunit (common Iβ or $β_c$) is present in IL-3, IL-5, and GM-CSF receptors. Although $β_c$

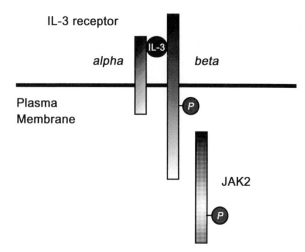

FIGURE 3–9. **Structure of single-transmembrane segment receptors that form heterologous dimers; the interleukin-3 receptor.** IL-3 binds to the IL-3 receptor complex composed of α subunit, β subunit, and a cytoplasmic tyrosine kinase. Encircled P is a potential tyrosine phosphorylation site.

does not bind any cytokine by itself, it forms high-affinity receptors (K_d = 100 pM) with an α subunit. IL-6, leukemia-inhibiting factor, and CNTF receptors have specific α-subunits with an IgG-like domain and the common motif of the hematopoietic growth factor receptors of four cysteines. A 130-kDa glycoprotein known as gp130 is involved in the formation of the high-affinity receptor and represents a common subunit in these receptors.[90–92]

TNF AND NGF RECEPTOR FAMILY. Two receptors for TNF α and β (p55), and NGF (p75) are related by structural homology. These are single transmembrane segment and monomeric receptors with no known signaling sequence in their cytoplasmic portion.[96, 97] It should be emphasized that TNF binds also to a p75 receptor, a member of the cytokine receptor family and that NGF binds to the trk receptor tyrosine kinase, both of which are involved in signal transduction of TNF and NGF, respectively. The role of the p55 TNF receptor and p75 NGF receptor has been an enigma. Recent studies suggest that they may be involved in cell apoptosis and mediate the cytotoxic actions of TNF and effects of NGF on programmed cell death in development of the nervous system.[98, 99]

PLASMA PROTEIN RECEPTOR FAMILY. Several membrane receptors for various plasma proteins including low-density lipoprotein (LDL), transferrin, asialoglycoproteins, polymeric IgA and IgM, $α_2$-macroglobulin, and phosphomannosylated proteins have been cloned.[100–103] These receptors are characterized by a short cytoplasmic domain with no known signaling sequence and large diverse extracellular domains with resemblance to hormone and growth factor receptors. Cloning of the LDL receptor revealed that it consists of five domains: ligand-binding, EGF precursor homology, 0-linked sugars, hydrophobic plasma membrane spanning region, and a short cytoplasmic tail that contains the information necessary for concentrating the LDL receptor in coated pits and facilitating its rapid endocytosis. The human transferrin receptor is a disulfide-linked dimer with a hydrophobic membrane-spanning region located 61 amino acids from the N-terminus. This predicts that the transferrin receptor is oriented in the membrane with a cytoplasmic amino-terminus and an extracellular carboxy-terminus like the asialoglycoprotein receptor but different from other membrane receptors. The cation-independent mannose-6-phosphate receptor is a large membrane protein of 2455 amino acid residues of which only 163 is in the carboxy-terminal cytoplasmic domain. The sequence is identical to the IGF-II receptor, indicating that it is a multifunctional protein involved in the internalization of both phosphomannosylated proteins (lysosomal enzymes) and IGF-II.[103]

Four-Transmembrane Segment Receptors

This family includes the extracellular ligand-gated ion channels that are regulated by neurotransmitters such as acetylcholine (nicotinic), GABA$_A$, glycine, glutamate, serotonin (5-HT$_3$) and ATP.[34, 104–106] The property that defines this family is that five receptor subunits with sequence similarity form an ion channel. Figure 3–10 shows a cross-section of the GABA$_A$ receptor ion channel with two of the five subunits forming the ion channel. The transmitter molecule itself operates the opening or closing of the channel by binding to sites on the receptor. These receptors perform fast signaling, since their transduction is independent of any intracellular or membrane-diffusible factor. In addition to the usual case of receptor activation by a presynaptically released transmitter, the transmitter may arrive on the intracellular side. The latter subdivision includes those receptors in which the signaling occurs across an organelle membrane (e.g., the ryanodine receptor and inositol triphosphate receptor in which Ca^{2+} ions are transferred from an intracellular store in response to the binding of inositol triphosphate, cADP-ribose, or Ca^{2+}).

The extracellular ligand-gated ion channels control flux of cations, Na$^+$, K$^+$, Mg^{2+}, or Ca^{2+}, and anions, HCO$_3^-$, or Cl$^-$ across the plasma membrane and are functionally and structurally related to the voltage-gated ion channels that are regulated by charge gradients across the cell membrane.[107, 108]

The best studied ligand-gated ion channel is the nicotinic acetylcholine receptor first described in *Torpedo californica*.[34] Five glycosylated subunits, two of which are identical, form an Na$^+$ channel inherent in the nicotinic acetylcholine receptor structure. Although these subunits are encoded by four separate genes, they possess a high degree of sequence similarity, including four transmembrane spanning domains. The molecular weights of the α, β, γ, and δ subunits are 40, 48, 58, and 64 kDa, respectively. As a pentameric complex, the α$_2$βγδ ligand-gated ion channel has a molecular weight of approximately 250 kDa. Each receptor requires two acetylcholine molecules, each binding to an α-subunit, to induce a rapid conductance change. The second transmembrane spanning domain in each subunit may form the lining for the ion pore.[109]

The subunits of the ligand-gated ion channels are homologous. The GABA$_A$ and glycine receptors, which mediate inhibitory activity in the central nervous system, contain structurally similar subunits. The α-subunits of the GABA$_A$ have 75 per cent homology, while the α, β, γ, and δ subunits share 30 to 40 per cent homology. In addition,

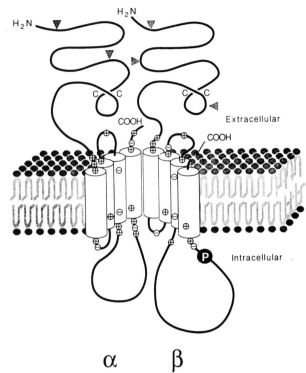

FIGURE 3–10. **Structure of a four-transmembrane segment receptor.** The GABA$_A$ receptor is composed of five subunits (2α, β, γ, δ) that form an ion channel across the membrane. α and β Subunits are shown in a cross-section of the GABA$_A$ receptor inserted in the membrane. Four membrane-spanning domains in each subunit are shown as cylinders. The structure in the extracellular domain is drawn in an arbitrary manner. Potential extracellular sites for *N*-glycosylation are indicated by triangles. Constant cysteine residues (C) are also shown: the pair 15 residues are apart in Cys-Cys loop in all the receptor subunits of this class. The encircled P denotes that sites for phosphorylation by protein kinases are present in the intracellular loop in certain receptor GABA$_A$ subunits: for protein kinase A, on all β and some α subunits, for protein kinase C on some α and γ subunits, and for tyrosine kinase on γ subunits. Those charged residues that can be located close to the ends of the membrane-spanning domains are shown as circles with positive charges marked, or as open squares for negative charges. Note the large excess of positive charge that will be at the mouth of the channel when five of the GABA$_A$ subunits are assembled to form a receptor. (Adapted from Barnard EA: Receptor classes and the transmitter-gated ion channels. Trends Biochem Sci 17:368–374, 1992.)

the GABA$_A$ subunit shares 35 per cent similarity with the 48-kDa subunit of the glycine receptor.[104, 105] Thus it appears that the ligand-gated ion channels are derived from a common ancestral gene. Furthermore, each subunit contains an extensive extracellular amino-terminal domain with multiple sites of glycosylation. This structure is reminiscent of that observed in a number of G protein–linked receptors. There is a large intracytoplasmic loop located between transmembrane regions 3 and 4 that contains multiple sites for phosphorylation, suggesting a role for regulation by cellular protein kinases. The carboxy-terminus of most subunits is short and is located in the extracellular space. It should be added that ion channels may also be operated by members of the seven-transmembrane segment receptor family via G proteins as signal transducers. For instance, the muscarinic cholinergic receptor and the β-adrenergic receptor in the heart regulate K$^+$ channels and Ca^{2+} channels, respectively, and the α$_1$-adrenergic receptor in neurons regulates K$^+$ channels.

BIOSYNTHESIS AND TURNOVER OF MEMBRANE RECEPTORS

Like all components of the cell, membrane receptors are in a constant state of turnover. As for other membrane and secretory proteins, receptor synthesis begins on the rough endoplasmic reticulum.[110, 111] In the endoplasmic reticulum proteins destined for the plasma membrane are sorted from other proteins by the presence of a signal sequence and certain conformational determinants. The endoplasmic reticulum also provides a form of quality control, sorting out incompletely folded or misfolded proteins, unassembled protein subunits, and proteins whose transport is post-translationally regulated. The immature receptors then pass through the Golgi complex, where they are modified by glycosylation, fatty acid acylation, disulfide bond formation, and, in some cases, cleavage into subunits. The mature receptors are inserted into the plasma membrane by a poorly understood process involving membrane fusion.[112]

Once inserted into the plasma membrane, the receptors are available for ligand binding and signal transduction. In the basal state, most hormone and growth factor receptors are distributed diffusely over the surface of the cell. Following ligand binding, receptors aggregate in coated pits that are lined on the intracellular surface with the protein clathrin.[113] The coated pits invaginate and pinch off to form vesicles called endosomes, or receptosomes, which are acidified. In the acidic environment the ligand dissociates from the receptor and undergoes degradation.[114] This process is termed *receptor-mediated endocytosis* (see below). In general, hormone receptors are recycled to the cell surface, whereas growth factor receptors are degraded following endocytosis. Hormone receptors make 50 or more cycles into the cell and back to the surface membrane before degradation. Thus the half-time for degradation of receptors varies from a few hours to about 24 hours. Under normal circumstances, the half-time for receptor synthesis matches the half-time for degradation so that the receptor pool remains in steady-state. Alterations in synthesis or degradation rate can result in changes in receptor number and altered biological response. Such changes may play a crucial role in certain pathophysiological states.

RECEPTOR-MEDIATED ENDOCYTOSIS

In addition to signaling at the cell surface, receptors for polypeptide hormones, growth factors, and neuropeptides are internalized from the cell surface to intracellular organelles. The receptor-mediated endocytosis serves at least two different functions: (1) cellular degradation of the regulatory polypeptide whereby the substance is cleared from the extracellular space and the signal mediated by the receptor is terminated; and (2) cellular desensitization to regulatory substances by reduction of the receptor concentration on the cell surface.[115–117] These processes are similar to the receptor-mediated uptake of nutrients (e.g., cholesterol, iron) and plasma proteins (e.g., asialoglycoproteins, phosphomannosylated proteins) which brings these substances to specific intracellular organelles for degradation or utilization.[118] Although the cellular phenomenon of receptor-mediated endocytosis was discovered about 15 years ago, the molecular mechanisms have been elucidated only recently. In these studies, site-directed mutagenesis and transfection of receptors into cell lines have been applied. In addition, naturally occurring mutations in patients with defects in receptor internalization have cast light on the molecular events in receptor-mediated endocytosis. Physiologically, it is important to recognize that processes of receptor-mediated endocytosis and intracellular degradation of polypeptide hormones, growth factors, and neuropeptides represent the major pathway in the breakdown of these substances. Thus receptor binding is rate-limiting in the turnover of hormones in vivo and determines the metabolic clearance rate. For example, proinsulin, which binds to the insulin receptor with only 2 per cent affinity relative to insulin, shows a significantly longer half-life in the organism.

Receptor-mediated endocytosis of extracellular ligands should be distinguished from other processes of internalization of extracellular material such as phagocytosis and fluid-phase pinocytosis.[119] Although the three processes are similar in that extracellular particles, substances, or fluid are internalized within an invagination of the plasma membrane, the molecular mechanisms involved, the intracellular sorting, and the final destination in cellular organelles are different. Phagocytosis describes the internalization of particulate matter visible by light microscopy (i.e., larger than 0.1 to 0.2 μm in diameter [like bacteria, virus, or immune complexes]) and involves attachment of the particle to the cell surface, internalization, and delivery of the material to lysosomes for degradation. Fluid-phase pinocytosis is used to describe a constitutive process in which smaller substrates including insoluble particles or solutes enter the cell in the fluid content of the endocytic vesicle. The internalized fluid and its content may be trancytosed to the opposite surface of a polarized cell or may be delivered to the lysosome for degradation. Fluid-phase pinocytosis is also involved in turnover of membrane lipids and proteins including receptors. By this process 50 to 200 per cent of the cell surface area is internalized per hour.[119]

Cellular Mechanism of Receptor-Mediated Endocytosis

Receptor-mediated endocytosis of extracellular ligands involves binding to the receptor on the cell surface, lateral diffusion of receptor-ligand complexes in the membrane, and aggregation in clathrin-coated pits (Fig. 3–11). The receptor and ligand are internalized in a clathrin-coated vesicle that is transformed into an uncoated endosome.[113] These vesicles have been shown to have pH of 5.0 to 6.5 and to be capable of acidification because of the activity of a H^+-ATPase, which exchanges cations in the endosomal lumen with H^+. The pH is lowered to pH of 4.5 to 5.0 in the endosomes forming a prelysosome, which eventually fuses with the lysosome to form a multivesicular body. In the acid environment the peptide ligand dissociates from the receptor and is subsequently degraded by specific and unspecific proteases. Some receptors also undergo degradation in the lysosome, whereas other receptors return to the plasma membrane by recycling in endosomal vesicles.[115–117]

CLATHRIN-COATED PITS. An essential component of the

endocytic mechanism is the clathrin-coated pit. These specialized regions of the plasma membrane are lined on the intracellular surface with the protein clathrin and a heterodimeric adaptor protein as well as other proteins involved in interaction with the receptor.[120, 121] The fraction of the cell surface area occupied by coated pits varies between ~4 per cent in human fibroblasts and 0.4 per cent in adipocytes. The large majority of receptors for plasma proteins such as transferrin and LDL are located in coated pits in the absence of ligand, whereas receptors for polypeptide hormones and growth factors are located outside coated pits and their aggregation is induced by the ligand.

In addition, some receptors possess a specific amino acid sequence (glutamine-proline-X-tyrosine, where X is any amino acid) located in the region of the receptor protein just inside the cell membrane, which seems to be crucial for internalization.[118] This applies to the LDL receptor, the transferrin receptor, the IgA/IgM receptor, the insulin receptor and the EGF receptor. For some receptors, covalent modification by enzymes such as phosphorylation on serine, threonine, and tyrosine residues may also play a role in stimulating internalization.

The intracellular recycling phase shows significant differences among receptors varying from 15 minutes or less for the LDL and transferrin receptor up to 5 hours for the insulin receptor. The plasma membrane phase can be as short as a few minutes depending on whether the receptor on the cell surface is inside or outside the clathrin-coated pits and whether the ligand is present. LDL receptors are, for example, localized preferentially in coated pits even in the absence of ligand and recycle rapidly, whereas insulin receptors move into the coated pits of the cell surface only when they are associated with ligand and their basal recycling is low.

Intracellular Routes of Membrane Receptors

Although all endocytic receptors enter cells in the same coated pits and are delivered to the same acidified endosomes, the receptor-ligand complex may follow one of four routes involving either recycling or degradation of ligand and/or receptor. Examples of receptors that follow these routes are given in Table 3–5.

Route 1: Receptor recycling and ligand degradation. As described above, polypeptide hormones (e.g., insulin, growth hormone, LH, and TSH) and plasma proteins (e.g., LDL and asialoglycoproteins) dissociate from their respective receptors within the acidified endosome and are degraded in the lysosome. The receptor leaves the endosome via a vesicle that buds off the endosome and fuses with the plasma membrane. Route 1 allows reuse of receptors. One LDL receptor can make up to 150 trips through the endosome without losing its function and mediate the uptake of hundreds of ligands during its usual life span of 10 to 30 hours.[118] Recycling of insulin receptors maintains a constant receptor level on the cell surface and normal hormone sensitivity of the cell. Insulin stimulates short-term metabolic responses during which the cell remains responsive to insulin. The cell may, however, be desensitized to insulin by down-regulation of receptors following chronic exposure to insulin for more than 24 hours.[117, 122–125]

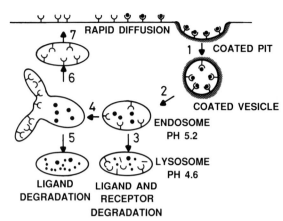

FIGURE 3–11. **Model of receptor-mediated endocytosis.** (1) Receptors bind their ligand and aggregate in coated pits, which bud off to a coated vesicle. (2) Coated vesicles lose their clathrin-coat and form acidified endosomes where ligands are dissociated from receptor. (3) Endosomes fuse with lysosomes where ligand and receptor are degraded. (4) Endosomes form multivesicular bodies. (5) Prelysosomal vesicles are formed and the ligand is degraded. (6) Vesicles with unoccupied receptors are formed. (7) Recycling of receptors in the plasma membrane. (From Schlessinger J: The epidermal growth factor receptor as a multifunctional allosteric protein. Biochemistry 27:3119, 1988.)

Route 2: Receptor degradation and ligand degradation. Growth factors (e.g., EGF, PDGF, and NGF) and pituitary hormones (hCG) dissociate from their receptors in the acidic endosome, but the receptor does not return to the cell surface. Both ligand and receptor are transported to the lysosome and degraded. Degradation of receptors leads to depletion of receptors from the cell surface and resistance to the action of growth factors.[122, 126] Growth factors initiate a number of effects, a process that leads to cell

TABLE 3–5. ENDOCYTOSIS OF RECEPTORS: FOUR INTRACELLULAR PATHWAYS

ROUTE 1: RECEPTOR RECYCLING AND LIGAND DEGRADATION

Insulin
Glucagon
Somatostatin
Follicle-stimulating hormone
Luteinizing hormone
Chorionic gonadotropin
Insulin-like growth factor I and II
Transforming growth factor β
Erythropoietin
Vasoactive intestinal polypeptide
Low-density lipoprotein
Asialoglycoproteins
α_2-Macroglobulin

ROUTE 2: RECEPTOR DEGRADATION AND LIGAND DEGRADATION

Epidermal growth factor
Platelet-derived growth factor
Nerve growth factor
Interleukin-2
Growth hormone

ROUTE 3: RECEPTOR RECYCLING AND LIGAND RECYCLING

Transferrin (to plasma membrane)
Mannose-6-phosphate–containing proteins (to Golgi)

ROUTE 4: RECEPTOR AND LIGAND TRANSCYTOSIS

Insulin (vascular endothelium)
Polymeric IgA and IgM (intestinal epithelium)

TABLE 3–6. DIVERGENT SIGNAL TRANSDUCTION

I. Multiple receptors and receptor isoforms
II. Multiple coupling mechanisms
    1. G proteins: multiple α-, β-, and γ-subunit isoforms
    2. SH2 domains: enzyme, adaptor, and cytoskeletal proteins
    3. Ion channels: different ion selectivity
III. Multiple effector systems
    1. Adenylate cyclase: several isoforms
    2. Phospholipases: multiple enzymes
    3. Protein kinases and phosphatases (Ser-Thr or Tyr): multiple enzymes
    4. Lipid kinases: several enzymes
    5. Fatty acid acylation: several forms
    6. ADP-ribosylation
IV. Multiple signaling molecules
    1. Cyclic nucleotides: cAMP, cGMP, cADP-ribose
    2. Phosphatidylinositols: InsP$_3$, InsP$_4$, DAG
    3. Eicosanoids: multiple factors
    4. Ions: Ca^{2+}, Mg^{2+}
    5. Small GTP-binding proteins: ras, rho, rab, rac, ral
    6. Transcription factors: AP-1, CREB, IFSG-3, SIF-A

division, a long-term response during which the cell remains desensitized. In certain cells, however, a fraction of EGF receptors escape degradation and recycle.

Route 3: Recycling of receptor and recycling of ligand. The complex of the transferrin receptor and Fe^{3+}-transferrin is stable in the acidic endosome, whereas the iron atom is stripped from transferrin at pH 5. The apotransferrin/receptor complex returns to the cell surface and dissociates at neutral pH. Like the LDL receptor, the transferrin receptor recycles every 15 to 20 minutes for more than 100 times.[128] Polypeptide hormones (insulin and GH) may also follow route 3 in addition to route 1. Following endocytosis the major fraction of receptor-bound hormone is sorted into a degradative pathway as already described, whereas a minor fraction is sorted into a nondegradative or retroendocytotic pathway. In adipocytes and hepatocytes about 25 per cent of internalized insulin and growth hormone is recycled and released in intact form at the cell surface, whereas 75 per cent is degraded in the lysosome.[117] It is possible that receptor-bound hormones can recycle in endosomes defective in the acidification mechanism or that endosomes fuse with the plasma membrane before acidification occurs. Recycling of intact hormone may be important for propagating the signal within a tissue.

Route 4: Transcytosis of receptor and ligand. In polarized cells such as mammary epithelial cells the receptor that carries IgA and IgM is transported from the basolateral to the apical cell surface. The extracellular domain of the receptor is cleaved off and the ligand released. In endothelial cells receptor-mediated transcytosis of hormones, such as insulin, is used to carry the hormone across the vascular barrier to the extracellular space.[129, 130] This transendothelial transport may be very important in bringing the hormone to the receptor on the target cell, since in many tissues the capillary network possesses tight junctions that block access of the hormone to its target cell. In the endothelial cell during the process of transcytosis, there is little or no fusion of the endosome bearing the hormone-receptor complex with lysosomes and thus little or no degradation.

RECEPTOR SIGNALING MECHANISMS

Three Levels of Receptor Signaling

To appreciate the process of hormone, growth factor, and neurotransmitter action at the cellular level it is easiest to think of signaling by membrane receptor as occurring at three levels or in three stages (Fig. 3–12 and Table 3–6). The *first level* is composed of the initial events at the plasma membrane related to the receptor itself and formation of intracellular mediators. For the seven-transmembrane segment receptors this includes binding of ligand, G protein coupling, and activation of membrane-bound enzymes (adenylate cyclases, phospholipases), and formation of the second messengers (cAMP, inositol triphosphate, and diacylglycerol). Ligand binding to single-transmembrane segment receptors leads to a conformational change, receptor dimerization, activation of intrinsic or associated tyrosine or serine-threonine kinases, substrate binding, and phosphorylation. Four-transmembrane segment receptors respond to ligand binding by conformational changes of the five subunits and opening of the ion channel with flux of Na^+, K^+, Ca^{2+}, Mg^{2+}, HCO_3^- or Cl^-.

The *second level* is a cascade of protein phosphorylation and dephosphorylation reactions induced by a network of at least five serine-threonine protein kinases including cAMP-activated protein kinase (abbreviated PKA), cGMP-activated protein kinases, diacylglycerol-activated protein kinase C (abbreviated PKC), ras-activated raf kinase, and calmodulin-activated kinases.

The *third level* is the final biological effectors of the lig-and-receptor–induced signaling cascade. These include membrane transport molecules (glucose transporters, amino acid carriers, and Na^+, K^+-ATPase) that are translocated to the plasma membrane from intracellular stores or activated following hormone stimulation; enzymes for glycogen, and lipid synthesis (glycogen synthase, pyruvate dehydrogenase, acetyl CoA carboxylase, triacylglycerol lipase) that are activated by phosphorylation or dephosphoryla-

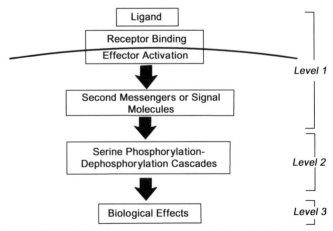

FIGURE 3–12. Three levels of receptor signaling. *First level:* activation of receptor and effector including ligand binding, transmembrane signal transfer, protein interactions, enzyme activation, and second messenger formation. *Second level:* protein kinase and protein phosphatase reactions. *Third level:* final actions on cellular transporters, enzymes, filaments, vesicles, ribosomes, and genes.

tion; ribosomal proteins involved in protein synthesis (S6 protein, elongation factor); contractile proteins in muscle (myosin, actin); secretory proteins in endocrine and exocrine cells (secretory vesicle proteins); transcription factors in regulation of gene expression; and cell cycle proteins involved in induction of cell growth.

Level 1: Receptor and Effector Activation

Ligand binding to receptor is common to all hormone, growth factor, and neurotransmitter receptors, although the chemical reaction shows differences depending on the chemical properties of the ligand. In general, the ligand interacts with the receptor by means of hydrogen bonds, ionic bonds, hydrophobic interactions, or Van der Waals forces. Receptor binding of small organic ligands such as acetylcholine and epinephrine involves primarily ionic bonds, whereas hydrogen bonds and hydrophobic interactions are important in binding of peptide ligands.

Ligand binding initiates different molecular signals depending on the receptor family. Two major signaling pathways exist, one initiated by the family of G protein–linked receptors and the other by receptors linked by tyrosine kinases either directly or indirectly. These separate mechanisms are coupled to energy-requiring (GTP or ATP) transducing mechanisms utilizing either G protein–activated enzymes and formation of second messengers or phosphotyrosine-binding proteins and activation of enzymes directly or via intermediary steps. These mechanisms appear to represent two fundamental molecular interactions in cell regulation.[46–48, 63–65, 130]

Signaling by seven-membrane transmembrane segment receptors involves interaction of at least three membrane molecules, the receptor itself, a trimeric G protein composed of α, β, and γ subunits, and an effector enzyme, adenylate cyclase, or phospholipase C. These enzymes catalyze the formation of such second messengers as cAMP, diacylglycerol, and inositol triphosphate via the G protein GDP-GTP cycle. The ligand-activated receptor acts as a G protein exchange factor (or guanine nucleotide–releasing factor) and promotes dissociation of GDP from the G protein α-subunit in exchange for GTP. The G protein is then released from the hormone-receptor complex and dissociates in the α-subunit and the βγ dimer. The complex between the α-subunit and GTP interacts with the effector enzyme and regulates its activity. In some systems the free βγ dimer may also interact directly with an effector. The α-subunit possesses intrinsic GTPase activity. Hydrolysis of GTP leaves GDP in the binding site and causes dissociation of the α subunit from the effector. The α-subunit loaded with GDP reassociates with the βγ dimer, and the system returns to the basal state.

Receptor-linked tyrosine kinases transmit their signals via a two-step mechanism involving autophosphorylation and interaction with phosphotyrosine-binding proteins. Ligand-induced dimerization of the receptor activates the tyrosine kinase that phosphorylates selected tyrosine residues in the kinase domain of the other receptor in the dimer. Thus, receptor auto-phosphorylation actually involves a trans-phosphorylation reaction within the dimer. The tyrosine residues occur in specific tetrapeptide motifs such as tyrosine-methionine-proline-methionine or tyrosine-glutamic acid-isoleucine-glutamic acid, which in their phosphorylated form interact with phosphotyrosine-binding proteins. This class of cellular proteins is characterized by specific regions termed src homology 2 (SH2) domains. SH2 domains were originally recognized as loosely conserved motifs in the sequences of *src* tyrosine kinase and other viral oncogenes. It appears that the phosphotyrosine-binding protein interaction is based on the specific recognition of phosphotyrosine motifs by SH2 domains. SH2 domains have been identified in a variety of cellular proteins with different functions. These include enzymes such as phospholipase C-γ and the ras GTPase-activating protein (abbreviated GAP); adaptor molecules such as growth factor receptor–binding protein-2 (abbreviated GRB2) and the regulatory subunit (p85) of phosphatidylinositol 3-kinase; and structural proteins such as myosin and spectrin. SH2-containing proteins propagate the signal by means of at least three pathways involving activation of phospholipase C-γ and formation of inositol triphosphate and diacylglycerol, activation of phosphoinositol 3-kinase, and activation of the small G protein ras following interaction with GRB2.

Most receptor tyrosine kinases such as EGF, PDGF, FGF, and NGF receptors contain several autophosphorylation sites in their cytoplasmic domain that interact with various SH2 domain-containing proteins. The insulin and IGF-I receptor tyrosine kinases represent an exception that an additional cytoplasmic protein, insulin receptor substrate-1, is phosphorylated and serves as a docking site for the SH2 domain proteins. GH, hematopoietic growth factor, and cytokine receptors without intrinsic kinase activity form homo- or heterodimeric complexes that activate cytoplasmic tyrosine kinases belonging to the family of JAK's leading to SH2 domain protein interaction.

Receptors with intrinsic guanylate cyclase activity like that of the ANP receptor, or serine-threonine kinase activity like that of the TGF-β receptor, represent new paradigms in cellular signaling. Activation of the ANP receptor leads to cGMP formation and stimulation of the cGMP-dependent protein kinase.[76–78] The signaling mechanism of the TGF-β receptor is still unclear.[79–81] Finally, ligand binding to ion channel receptors results in flux of cations such as Na^+, K^+ or anions such as Cl^- or HCO_3^-, which may change the membrane potential leading to either depolarization or hyperpolarization, or the ion may act as an intracellular mediator in the case of Ca^{2+}, Mg^{2+}.[45, 131, 132] Only the two major signaling systems in hormone action, G-protein coupling and phosphotyrosine-binding protein interactions, are described in more detail.

G PROTEINS. The seven-transmembrane segment receptors couple with G proteins, which are the crucial signal transducers that lie between receptors and effectors in the plasma membrane both topologically and functionally (Fig. 3–13). The G proteins are part of a larger superfamily of more than 50 GTP-binding and -hydrolyzing proteins that share structural homology. These can be divided in two groups on the basis of their molecular size.[133, 134] Low-molecular-weight G proteins (20 to 25 kDa), also called ras-like G proteins, are monomeric and are involved in diverse cellular processes such as receptor tyrosine kinase signaling (ras proteins), vesicular transport (rab proteins), membrane ruffling (rac proteins), stress fiber formation, and focal adhesion (rho proteins).[135–138] High-molecular-weight G proteins exist as heterotrimers consisting of three differ-

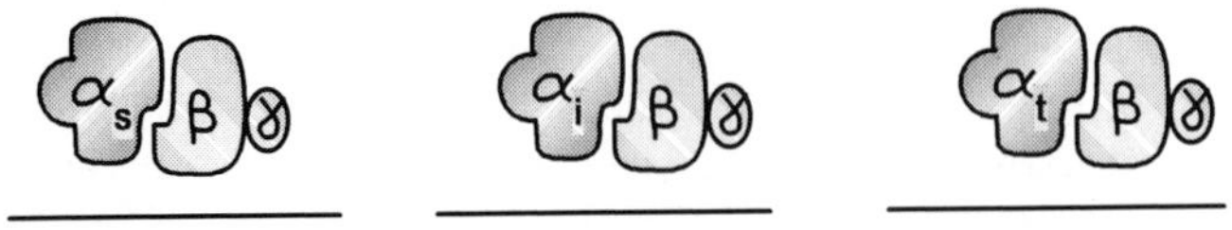

	G_s-Protein	G_i-Protein	Transducin
Receptors	β-adrenergic Glucagon ACTH, LH, etc.	α-adrenergic Muscarinic Somatostatin, etc.	Rod and cone opsins
Effectors	Adenylyl cyclase Ca^{2+} channels	Adenylyl cyclase K^+/Ca^{2+} Channels	Cyclic GMP PDE
ADP-ribosylation	Cholera toxin	Pertussis toxin	Cholera toxin Pertussis toxin

FIGURE 3–13. **Structure and properties of G_s protein, G_i protein, and transducin.** Subunits are α, β, and γ. (Modified from Kahn CR, Smith RJ, Chin WW: Mechanism of action of hormones that act at the cell surface. *In* Wilson JD, Foster DW: Williams Textbook of Endocrinology. Philadelphia, WB Saunders Co, 1992, p 110.)

ent subunits, α (molecular mass 39- to 46-kDa), β (37-kDa), and γ (8-kDa) and serve signal transduction functions. The ability of various receptors to either stimulate or decrease cAMP production resides in the interaction of these receptors with stimulatory G proteins (G_s) or inhibitory G proteins (G_i). Members of a subclass of heterotrimeric G proteins are involved in protein synthesis and serve as peptide chain elongation factors.[139]

The α subunits of the G proteins are activated by binding GTP in the presence of Mg^{2+}, a step that allows interaction with the appropriate effector system such as adenylate cyclase. All α subunits are themselves enzymes and possess intrinsic GTPase activity hydrolyzing GTP to GDP and free inorganic phosphate (P_i). The β and γ subunits of the G proteins exist as a tightly associated complex and serve as a functional dimer that interact with the α subunit. The heterotrimer is bound to the plasma membrane by lipid modifications that serve to anchor the subunits to the membrane.

The general mechanism of G protein–mediated trans-

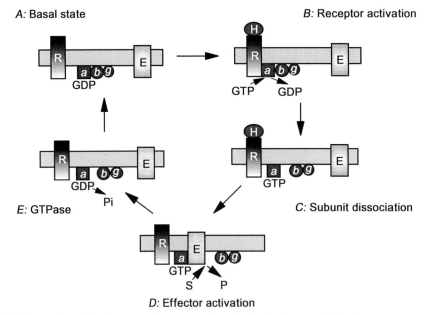

D: Effector activation

FIGURE 3–14. **G protein-mediated transmembrane signaling.** In the basal state *(A)*, the hormone receptor (R) is unoccupied and the effector (E) is inactive. Upon hormone binding and receptor activation *(B)*, the receptor interacts with the αβγ heterotrimer *(abg)* to promote a conformational change and dissociation of GDP from the guanine-nucleotide-binding site; at normal cellular concentrations of guanine nucleotides, GTP fills the site immediately. Binding of GTP has two consequences *(C)*. The G protein dissociates from the H-R complex, reducing the affinity of hormone for receptor and, in turn, freeing the receptor for another liaison with a neighboring quiescent G protein. GTP binding also reduces the affinity of α for βγ, and subunit dissociation occurs. This frees α-GTP to fulfill its primary role as a regulator of effectors that catalyse conversion of substrate (s) to product (p) *(D)*. At least in some systems, the free βγ subunit complex may also interact directly with an effector E_1 and modulate the activity of the active complex, or it may act independently at a distinct effector (E_2). The α subunits possess intrinsic GTPase activity *(E)*. The rate of this GTPase determines the lifetime of the active species and the associated physiological response. The α subunit catalyzes hydrolysis of GTP, leaves GDP in the binding site, and causes dissociation and deactivation of the active complex. The GTPase activity of αs is, in essence, an internal clock that controls an on/off switch. The GDP bound form of α has high affinity for βγ; subsequent reassociation of αGDP with βγ returns the system to the basal state *(A)*. (Modified from Hepler JR, Gilman AG: G proteins. Trends Biochem Sci 17:383–387, 1992.)

membrane signaling is well understood (Fig. 3–14). In the absence of ligand, the hormone receptor interacts directly with the heterotrimeric G protein and the rate of GDP dissociation from the α subunit limits GTPase activity. Presence of the hormonal ligand and formation of the hormone-receptor complex promotes GDP dissociation from the α subunit of the heterotrimer allowing intracellular GTP to bind to the α subunit. This results in (1) dissociation of the α subunit from βγ, (2) lowering of the affinity of the receptor for the ligand, (3) production of an activated α subunit that can interact with an effector molecule such as adenylate cyclase, and (4) induction of the inherent GTPase activity in the α subunit. But as in all signaling events, the presence of ligand results in a rapid but short-lived intracellular response. The increased ability of the ''activated'' α subunit to hydrolyze GTP and thus to increase GDP-GTP ratios results in a brake on activation. Thus a G protein signal transduction cycle can be produced and regulated.[140–145]

To date, cDNA's that encode 21 distinct G protein α subunits have been cloned. These can be divided into four major subfamilies according to amino acid sequence relationships, i.e., those represented by G_s, G_i, G_q, and G_{12} (Table 3–7). G protein α subunits show considerable structural homology with molecular sizes ranging from 39 to 46 kDa. Hormone and odorant receptors interact with members of the G_s subfamily (G_s and G_{olf}) to stimulate adenylate cyclase and thus enhance the rate of cAMP synthesis. Because of alternative splicing of exon 3 in the $α_s$ gene, there are $α_s$ subunit variants that differ in size and GDP dissociation rate. Six distinct isoforms of adenylate cyclase have been described to date, all of which are activated by the $α_s$ subunit. The $α_{olf}$ subunit protein is expressed exclusively in the olfactory neuroepithelium and serves to link odorant receptors with an olfactory-specific form of adenylate cyclase. In addition to activation of adenylate cyclase, purified $α_s$-subunits regulate at least two ion channels, stimulating voltage-gated Ca^{2+} channels in skeletal muscle and inhibiting cardiac Na^+ channels.

The $α_i$ subunit of the G protein exists in at least eight forms, each derived from a different gene. When present in the αβγ heterotrimer, the $α_i$ subunit results in a G protein that mediates the inhibition of adenylate cyclase among other potential functions. The $α_{0A}$ and $α_{0B}$ subunits are splice variants and present in the brain. Other $α_i$ subunits include $α_t$ or transducin, which is activated by light-activated rhodopsin in the photoreceptor rod outer segments. A transducin-like G protein named gusducin (G_g) has been described recently and is apparently expressed only in taste buds. Other $G_α$ families have been cloned, including G_q (five members) and G_{12} (two members). The $α_q$ subunit is linked to muscarinic acetylcholine receptors

TABLE 3–7. PROPERTIES OF MAMMALIAN G PROTEINS

FAMILY	SUBUNIT	TISSUE	RECEPTORS	EFFECTOR (ACTION)
G_S	$α_{s/S}$	Ubiquitous	β-Adrenergic, TSH, glucagon, others	Adenylate cyclase (+)
	$α_{s/L}$	Ubiquitous		Ca^{2+} channels (+)
	$α_{olf}$	Olfactory	Odorant	Adenylate cyclase (+)
G_i	$αi_1$	Nearly ubiquitous	Muscarinic M_2,	K^+ channels (+)
	$α_{i2}$	Ubiquitous	$α_2$-adrenergtic,	Ca^{2+} channels (−)
	$α_{i3}$	Nearly ubiquitous	others	Adenylate cyclase (−) ?
	$α_{0A}$	Brain, others	Met-enkephalin,	Phospholipase C (+) ?
	$α_{0B}$	Brain, others	$α_2$-adrenergic, others	Phospholipase A_2 (+) ?
	$α_{t1}$	Retinal rods	Rhodopsin	cGMP-specific
	$α_{t2}$	Retinal cones	Cone opsin	phosphodiesterase (+)
	$α_g$	Taste buds	Taste ?	?
	$α_Z$	Brain, adrenal, platelets	Muscarinic M_2 ?, others ?	Adenylate cyclase (−) ? others ?
G_q	$α_q$	Nearly ubiquitous	Muscarinic M_1,	Phospholipase C-β1,
	$α_{11}$	Nearly ubiquitous	$α_1$-adrenergic,	-β2, -β3 (+), others ?
	$α_{14}$	Lung, kidney, liver	?	?
	$α_{15}$	B cells, myeloid cells	?	?
	$α_{16}$	T cells, myeloid cells	?	Phospholipase C-β1, β2, -β3 (+)
G_{12}	$α_{12}$	Ubiquitous	?	?
	$α_{13}$	Ubiquitous	?	?
β	$β_1$	Ubiquitous	−	Required for $G_α$-receptor interaction
	$β_2$	Nearly ubiquitous	−	Inhibition of $G_α$ activation
	$β_3$	Nearly ubiquitous	−	
	$β_4$	Nearly ubiquitous	−	
				Modulate activation of certain adenylate cyclases
γ	$γ_1$	Retina, other ?	−	by $G_{sα}$ or calmodulin
	$γ_2$	Brain, adrenal, other ?	−	
	$γ_3$	Brain, testis, other ?	−	
	$γ_4$	Kidney, retina	−	Phospholipase C (+)
	$γ_5$	Liver, other ?	−	K^+ channels ?
	$γ_6$	Brain, other ?	−	Phospholipase A_2 ?

+, stimulation; −, inhibition.
?: receptor, effector or action is unknown.
−: receptor is not revelant as the βγ dimer does not interact with the receptor alone, but only as part of the trimeric $G_{αβγ}$.
Modified from Hepler JR, Gilman AG: G proteins. Trends Biochem Sci 17:383–387, 1993.

and α_1-adrenergic receptors and stimulate phospholipase C-β. The function of the others is still unknown. All of the α subunits are organized in four domains: (1) a Mg^{2+}-dependent GTP binding site, (2) a GTPase domain, (3) receptor binding and effector interaction domains located in the C-terminal end of the α subunit, and (4) a domain involved in $\beta\gamma$ interaction located in the N-terminal region of the α subunit.

At least four distinct β and six γ subunits have been described; it is a safe bet that these numbers will increase.[133] The β subunit exists in four highly related forms of almost the same molecular mass (37 kDa) encoded by four different genes. The γ subunit family is more heterogeneous and includes six forms, with apparent molecular size of 7.3 to 8.5 kDa and large sequence variation. β and γ Subunits are usually observed in tight association with the formation of a $\beta\gamma$ dimer, although each subunit apparently can also function as a homodimer. In addition, γ subunits are prenylated and serve to anchor the G protein to plasma membrane. Normally the $\beta\gamma$ subunits are required for regulation of the α subunit by hormone-receptor complexes. An independent regulatory role of the $\beta\gamma$ dimer has recently been demonstrated.[145–147] Type I adenylate cyclase (α_s subunit and calmodulin-activated) is inhibited by the $\beta\gamma$ complex, whereas phospholipase C-$\beta2$ is stimulated. Types II and IV adenylate cyclases are activated by the $\beta\gamma$ dimer only when the α_s subunit is also present. Recent findings indicate that the $\beta\gamma$ subunits play an obligatory role in agonist-induced receptor phosphorylation and desensitization. Taken together, these observations suggest that dissociation of G protein subunits in the membrane can generate parallel and interactive signals via both α subunits and $\beta\gamma$ subunits representing a mechanism for cross-talk between signaling pathways.

ACTIVATION OF ADENYLATE CYCLASE. The major effector enzyme of the G protein–coupled receptor system is the adenylate cyclase.[148] This enzyme is a single-chain membrane glycoprotein (molecular size = 115 to 150 kDa) with two clusters of six transmembrane domains separated by two cytoplasmic loops. Two repeats of the catalytic domain are present in each of two cytoplasmic loops, both of which are necessary for enzyme activity. Six isoforms of adenylate cyclase have been identified with varying tissue distribution, α subunit specificity, interaction with $\beta\gamma$ subunits, and regulation by Ca^{2+}-calmodulin.[149, 150] The catalytic activity of adenylate cyclase is regulated by interaction with the α subunits of stimulatory or inhibitory G proteins (Fig. 3–15). Binding of activated α_s results in augmented enzyme activity rapidly converting ATP to cAMP. cAMP, in turn, reacts with the two regulatory subunits of cAMP-dependent protein kinase resulting in their dissociation from two catalytic subunits and an increase in the kinase activity. cAMP-dependent protein kinase then may phosphorylate other proteins and initiate a phosphorylation-dephosphorylation cascade (see Ch. 4). The intracellular level of cAMP may be reduced in two ways: inhibition of the activity of adenylate cyclase by interaction with α_i or conversion of cAMP to inactive 5'AMP by the action of phosphodiesterase.[151]

Two bacterial toxins have been shown to interact with G proteins and cellular cAMP levels. Pertussis toxin treatment of cells stimulates ADP-ribosylation of α subunits of the G_i protein family at a carboxy-terminal cysteine residue. This results in receptor uncoupling and constitutive activation of adenylate cyclase. Cholera toxin, on the other hand, stimulates ADP-ribosylation of α subunits of the G_s protein family at an arginine residue. This constitutively activates the G_s proteins by inhibiting the GTPase activity and stabilizing the GTP-bound conformation with the result of prolongation of their ability to stimulate effector systems such as adenylate cyclase. Thus both pertussis toxin and cholera toxin produce increased cAMP levels.

The heterogeneity of G protein structure and function is increased further by "cassette" design (Fig. 3–15). For example, multiple G proteins may interact with a single receptor-hormone complex resulting in activation and inhibition of different effector systems in response to a single agonist. Similarly, multiple receptors may interact with a single G protein. This flexibility of interaction at the receptor–G protein and G protein–effector interfaces results in a potentially complex regulatory network. Major examples of such heterogeneity lie in the observation that the β adrenergic receptor, in reconstitution studies, can activate G_s and G_i, and G_s has been shown to interact with both adenylate cyclase and calcium channel in atrial tissues. Fur-

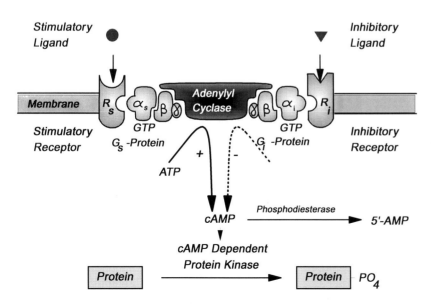

FIGURE 3–15. **Schematic depiction of the adenylate cyclase system.** Stimulatory or inhibitory ligands interact with their respective receptors, R_s and R_i. The stimulatory or inhibitory receptors act via G_s protein or G_i protein on adenylyl cyclase. When adenylyl cyclase is stimulated (+), ATP is converted to cAMP, which in turn activates cAMP-dependent protein kinase, and this results in protein phosphorylation. Inhibition of adenylyl cyclase (−) decreases the cAMP production. cAMP is metabolized to inactive 5' AMP by phosphodiesterase. (Modified from Kahn CR, Smith RJ, Chin WW: Mechanism of action of hormones that act at the cell surface. *In* Wilson JD, Foster DW: Williams Textbook of Endocrinology. Philadelphia, WB Saunders Co, 1992, p 106.)

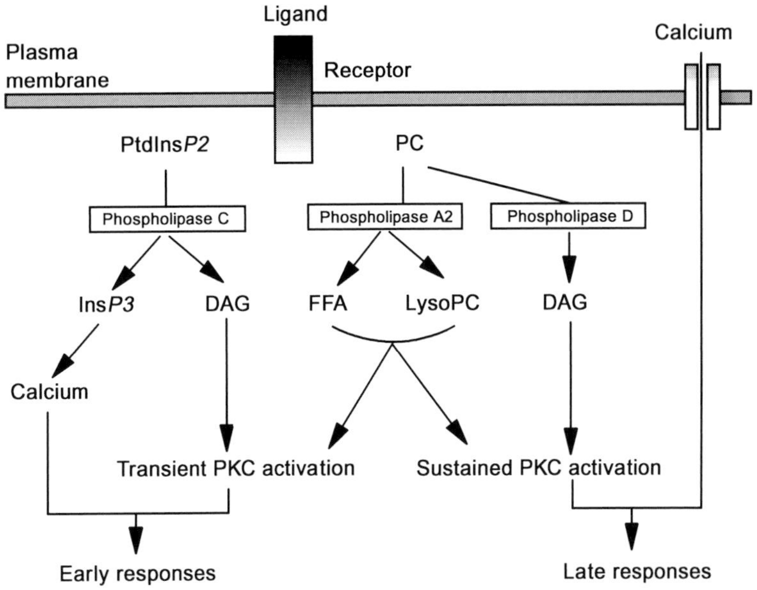

FIGURE 3–16. **Signal-induced degradation of membrane phospholipids and cellular responses.** $PtdInsP_2$, phosphatidylinositol 4,5-bisphosphate; PC, phosphatidylcholine; $InsP_3$, inositol 1,4,5-triphosphate; DAG, diacylglycerol; FFA, *cis*-unsaturated fatty acid; lysoPC, lysophosphatidylcholine; PKC, protein kinase C. (From Asaoka Y, Nakamura S, Yoshida K, Nishizuka Y: Protein kinase C, calcium and phospholipid degradation. Trends Biochem Sci 17:414–417, 1992.)

thermore, it has been shown that various G proteins are expressed in a tissue-specific manner and their levels may be hormonally regulated.

Another important feature of this signal transduction system is its ability to amplify signals. Because activation of G proteins results in dissociation of the G proteins from hormone-receptor complexes, a single complex can activate multiple G proteins. For instance, in the β adrenergic receptor system, one agonist-receptor interaction can activate up to 20 G proteins. Similarly, light activation of rhodopsin can result in a thousand-fold increase in the stimulation of G_t.

PHOSPHATIDYLINOSITOLS AND CALCIUM. A number of hormones, neurotransmitters, and growth factors mediate their cellular actions by means of inositol triphosphate and diacylglycerol as their second messengers.[152, 153] Inositol triphosphate controls cellular processes by generating internal calcium signals.[154–156] This bifurcating messenger system can be activated by two major pathways, one initiated by the G protein–linked receptors and the other by receptors linked by tyrosine kinases either directly or indirectly. These separate receptor mechanisms coupled to G proteins or phosphotyrosine proteins activate phospholipase C to hydrolyze phosphatidylinositol 4,5-bisphosphate stored in the plasma membrane to give both diacylglycerol and inositol triphosphate (Fig. 3–16).[156] Diacylglycerol activates protein kinase C in the plasma membrane. Inositol triphosphate released into the cytoplasm binds to the inositol triphosphate receptor on the endoplasmic reticulum to release calcium ions. The phospolipase C superfamily is now known to comprise at least 16 isoenzymes classified into three families: phospholipases C-β, -γ, and -δ.[157] The mechanism of activation is best understood for phospholipases C-β and -γ, which involve interactions with G proteins and tyrosine kinases, respectively. Phospholipase C-β is activated by the α subunits of the G_q and G_{12} families of G proteins and by the βγ dimer of the G_i family. Examples of receptors utilizing this signaling system include acetylcholine (muscarinic), histamine, $α_1$-adrenergic, serotonin, ATP, prostaglandins, vasopressin, cholecystokinin, GHRH, TRH, angiotensin II, oxytocin, substance P, neuropeptide

Y, thrombin, PTH, odorants, and light. Phospholipase C-γ is activated by receptor tyrosine kinases such as the EGF and PDGF receptors by means of a two-step mechanism: (1) interaction between a phosphotyrosine motif in the kinase domain, phosphotyrosine-leucine-asparticacid-leucine and two SH2 domains in the regulatory domain of phospholipase C-γ; and (2) phosphorylation of three tyrosine residues in phospholipase C-γ. Examples of receptors utilizing this signaling system are PDGF, EGF, FGF, NGF, and cytokines as well as the T-cell receptor.

Inositol triphosphate operates through receptors whose molecular and physiological properties closely resemble the calcium-mobilizing ryanodine receptors of muscle.[155, 157] A family of five inositol triphosphate receptors has now been identified with molecular diversity arising from both alternative splicing and the existence of separate genes. The inositol triphosphate receptor is a very large homotetrameric protein (molecular size = 313 kDa) in which sequences near the carboxy-terminal domain are thought to form eight membrane-spanning helices that together comprise the Ca^{2+} channel. The large N-terminal lies free in the cytoplasm with the inositol triphosphate binding site located at its end, a long way from the channel-forming carboxy-terminal region. Upon binding inositol triphosphate, the receptor undergoes a conformational change that leads to channel opening and Ca^{2+} release (Fig. 3–17).

The other major intracellular calcium channel, the ryanodine receptor, is approximately twice as large as the inositol triphosphate receptor but shows considerable structural and functional homology (Table 3–8). The ryanodine receptor does not bind inositol triphosphate; however, it responds to membrane depolarization in two ways. In the sarcoplasmic reticulum of skeletal muscle the dihydropyridine receptor in the surface membrane senses a change in voltage which is transmitted to the ryanodine receptor. In cardiac muscle a voltage-operated calcium channel gates a small amount of trigger calcium, which then activates the ryanodine receptor. Recent evidence suggests that the ryanodine receptor is regulated by a new second messenger: cyclic ADP-ribose.[158–160] The formation

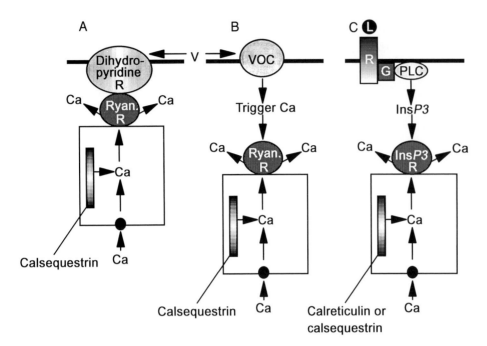

FIGURE 3–17. **Calcium signaling.** Control of calcium release by intracellular tetrameric calcium channels. *A,* Ryanodine receptors located in the sarcoplasmic reticulum of skeletal muscle contribute to the T-tubule foot structure responsible for excitation-contraction coupling. The dihydropyridine receptor in the surface membrane senses a change in voltage and undergoes a conformational change which is transmitted through the bulbous head of the ryanodine receptor to open the calcium channel in the sarcoplasmic reticulum. *B,* Calcium-induced calcium release in cardiac muscle and perhaps also in neurons. A voltage-operated channel (VOC) responds to the change in voltage by gating a small amount of trigger calcium, which then activates the ryanodine receptor to release stored calcium. *C,* Agonist-induced calcium release. Signal transduction at the cell surface generates inositol triphosphate (InsP₃), which diffuses into the cell to release calcium by binding to the InsP₃ receptor. Calsequestrin and calreticulin represent calcium stores in the endoplasmic reticulum. (From Berridge MJ: Inositol triphosphate and calcium signalling. Nature 361:315–325, 1993.)

of cADP-ribose is enhanced by cGMP, suggesting a possible link with the local hormone nitric oxide, which activates the cytoplasmic guanylate cyclase.[161] Thus the ryanodine receptor may be controlled by conventional extracellular signals such as hormones and neurotransmitters via stimulation of nitric oxide release, cGMP production and cADP-ribose formation. cADP-Ribose sensitizes the ryanodine receptor to the stimulatory effect of Ca^{2+}, a phenomenon well known for the inositol triphosphate receptor and its ligand.

The membrane stores from which calcium is released contain three major components: pumps to sequester calcium; binding proteins (e.g., calsequestrin and calreticulin) to store calcium; and the specific inositol triphosphate and ryanodine channels to release calcium back into the cytosol. The inositol triphosphate and ryanodine receptors are normally located on modified portions of the endoplasmic reticulum, termed calciosomes. Calcium contained within the intracellular stores is released to the cytosol when inositol triphosphate binds to its receptor and opens the calcium channel or when plasma membrane depolarization activates the dihydropyridine receptor channel and opens the ryanodine channel. The distribution of the two receptors varies considerably from cell to cell. About 50 per cent of the Ca^{+2} in the calciosomes is releasable upon inositol triphosphate or ryanodine receptor stimulation, whereas the remainder is discharged only in the presence of ionophores. The inositol triphosphate–induced transient increase in cytoplasmic Ca^{2+} levels may be further propagated by a Ca^{2+} induced calcium release. Like the ryanodine receptor, the inositol triphosphate receptor is sensitive to Ca^{2+}, and the initial inositol triphosphate–induced Ca^{2+} release is enhanced by positive feedback. The Ca^{2+} is soon curtailed as the cytoplasmic accumulation of calcium activates the negative feedback component. The latter may depend upon the receptor switching from an active state that can gate calcium to an inactive state. Once the concentration of calcium returns to its resting level, the inactive receptor converts back to the inositol triphosphate–sensitive state in about one second, thus setting the state for another Ca^{2+} spike. The action of inositol triphosphate is also attenuated by metabolism of inositol triphosphate to an inactive inositol bisphosphate.

Ca^{2+}-CALMODULIN-DEPENDENT KINASE AND PROTEIN KINASE C. Calcium binds to calmodulin, triggering conformational changes in this protein that allow it to activate many enzymes, including a number of protein kinases.[162] Calmodulin-dependent protein kinases can be divided into two classes, termed "multifunctional" and "dedicated." As implied by the name multifunctional, these calmodulin-dependent protein kinases, like protein kinase A, phosphorylate many intracellular proteins. The best characterized is the calmodulin-dependent multiprotein kinase. By contrast, dedicated calmodulin-dependent protein kinases phosphorylate a single substrate and include myosin light

TABLE 3–8. COMPARISON OF RYANODINE AND INOSITOL TRIPHOSPHATE RECEPTORS

PROPERTY	RYANODINE	INSP₃
Structure	4 × 565 kDa	4 × 313 kDa
Regulators		
Inositol triphosphate	No effect	+
Cyclic ADP-ribose	+	No effect
Cytosolic Mg^{2+}	−	−
Cytosolic Ca^{2+}	+	±
Luminal Ca^{2+}	+	+
Adenine nucleotides	+	±
Calmodulin	−	No effect
cAMP-dependent kinase	?	±
Pharmacology		
Ryanodine	±	No effect
Ruthenium red	−	No effect
Procaine	−	No effect
Caffeine	+	Slight −
Heparin	No effect	−

+, stimulatory; −, inhibitory.
Modified from Taylor CW, Marshall ICB: Calcium and inositol 1,4,5-triphosphate receptors: a complex relationship. Trends Biochem Sci 17:403–407, 1992.

chain kinase, phosphorylase kinase, and elongation factor 2 kinase, which regulate muscle contraction, glycogenolysis, and protein synthesis, respectively.

Protein kinase C represents a family of related isozymes (molecular size = 67 to 83 kDA) that are encoded by 10 different genes.[163–166] Furthermore, alternative splicing may result in greater complexity of these forms. These protein kinase C isozymes show different enzymological characteristics and tissue expression (Table 3–9). They are divided into three groups of four classical or conventional protein kinase C subspecies (α, β1, β2, and γ), four new protein kinase C subspecies (δ, ϵ, η (L), and θ) and two atypical protein kinase C subspecies (ξ, λ). All members of the protein kinase C family are dependent on phosphatidylserine but show different requirements for Ca^{2+} and phospholipid metabolites for their activation. Classic protein kinase C enzymes are activated by Ca^{2+} and diacylglycerol, and this activation is further enhanced by *cis*-unsaturated fatty acids including oleic, linoleic, linolenic, and arachidonic. On the other hand, "new" protein kinase C enzymes are insensitive to Ca^{2+}, although they respond well to diacylglycerol and phorbol esters. One of the atypical protein kinase C enzymes does not respond to Ca^{2+}, diacylglycerol, or phorbol esters, but it requires phosphatidylserine and is activated by *cis*-unsaturated fatty acids.

Protein kinase C mediates early responses to neurotransmitters and hormones (e.g., secretion and mast cell release) which are induced by transient activation of protein kinase C by diacylglycerol and Ca^{2+} after phosphatidylinositol 4,5 bisphosphate hydrolysis by the phospholipase C-β or -γ. Late responses to growth factors and hormones (such as proliferation and differentiation) are induced by sustained activation of protein kinase C by *cis*-unsaturated fatty acids and lysophosphatidylcholine after phosphatidylcholine hydrolysis by phospholipase A_2 as well as by diacylglycerol after phosphatidylcholine hydrolysis by phospholipase D.

TYROSINE KINASES IN HORMONE AND GROWTH FACTOR ACTION. Tyrosine kinase activation is involved in the intracellular signal transduction of receptor tyrosine kinases such as EGF, PDGF, FGF, NGF, IGF-I and insulin receptors and receptors linked with cytoplasmic tyrosine kinases such as GH, prolactin, cytokine, and hematopoietic growth fac-

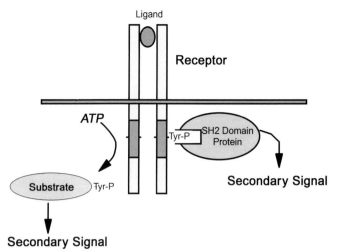

FIGURE 3–18. **Mechanism of signaling by receptor tyrosine kinase.** Ligand binding to the extracellular portion of the receptor induces receptor dimerization and activation of the tyrosine kinase in the intracellular portion. Tyrosine residues in the receptor and substrate are phosphorylated. SH2 domain protein interacts with phosphotyrosine peptide motif in the receptor. Tyrosine-phosphorylated substrate and SH2 domain protein induces secondary signals.

tor receptors.[63–65, 167, 168] Two steps are involved in the initial signal transduction of these receptors: dimerization and tyrosine kinase activation (Fig. 3–18). The single-transmembrane segment receptors exist as inactive monomers in the plasma membrane with the exception of the insulin and IGF-I receptors that are inactive disulfide-linked heterotetramers. Upon ligand binding active receptor dimers are formed by three different mechanisms: (1) a monomeric, monovalent ligand (e.g., EGF) binds to one receptor leading to conformational changes of the extracellular domain and association with another ligand-receptor complex; (2) a dimeric, bivalent ligand (e.g., PDGF) binds sequentially two receptors that associate in a dimer; (3) a monomeric, bivalent ligand (e.g., GH) binds two receptors through different receptor-binding regions leading to formation of a dimer.[95] There is preliminary evidence that insulin acts as a monomeric, bivalent ligand that associates with each of the two halves in the covalent heterotetrameric receptor. The ligand-induced dimerization is essential for activation of the tyrosine kinase as evidenced by the rapid autophosphorylation of the tyrosine kinase and phosphorylation of intracellular substrates.

Autophosphorylation appears to occur through a *trans*-mechanism in which one tyrosine kinase phosphorylates the other in the dimer. The role of autophosphorylation in signal transfer has been studied in great detail for the EGF, PDGF, FGF, CSF-1, and insulin receptor tyrosine kinases. In receptor tyrosine kinases such as EGF, PDGF, FGF, and CSF-1 receptors the main function of the autophosphorylation is to phosphorylate individual tyrosine residues in the cytoplasmic domain of the receptor.[169, 170] These phosphotyrosines appear to serve as highly selective docking sites that bind cytoplasmic signaling molecules. These signaling molecules mediate the pleiotrophic responses of cells to growth factors and insulin. The insulin receptor represents an exception that autophosphorylation of three regulatory tyrosine residues in the two tyrosine

TABLE 3–9. PROTEIN KINASE C SUBSPECIES IN MAMMALIAN TISSUES

GROUP	TYPE	ACTIVATORS	TISSUE
cPKC	α	Ca^{2+}, DAG, PS, FFA, LysoPC	Ubiquitous
	βI	Ca^{2+}, DAG, PS, FFA, LysoPC	Some tisues
	βII	Ca^{2+}, DAG, PS, FFA, LysoPC	Many tissues
	γ	Ca^{2+}, DAG, PS, FFA, LysoPC	Brain only
nPKC	δ	DAG, PS	Ubiquitous
	ϵ	DAG, PS, FFA	Brain and others
	η	?	Lung, skin, heart
	θ	?	Skeletal muscle
aPKC	λ	PS, FFA	Ubiquitous
		?	Ovary, testis and others

Abbreviations: DAG, diacylglycerol; PS, phosphatidylserine; FFA, *cis*-unsaturated fatty acid; LysoPC, lysophosphatidylcholine.

Modified from Asaoka Y, Nakamura S, Yoshida K, Nishizuka Y: Protein kinase C, calcium and phospholipid degradation. Trends Biochem Sci 17:414–417, 1993.

kinases of the receptor heterotetramer leads to a 20-fold increase of the kinase activity (see Ch. 80). This is also true for the homologous IGF-I receptor as well as for the unrelated HGF receptor. The active insulin and IGF-I receptor tyrosine kinases phosphorylate the insulin receptor substrate-1, which serves as a docking protein and interacts with a number of signaling molecules.[171] The receptor tyrosine kinase is a classical allosteric enzyme, in which the extracellular domain is the regulatory subunit and the cytoplasmic domain the catalytic subunit. In the unoccupied state the extracellular domain of the receptor inhibits the tyrosine kinase activity intrinsic to the cytoplasmic domain; this inhibition is released after ligand binding, after removal of the extracellular domain by proteolytic cleavage, or by expression of isolated tyrosine kinases as in oncogenes.[172] The extracellular and intracellular domains are linked by the transmembrane domain. Mutations in the transmembrane region can activate the tyrosine kinase.[173] This suggests that ligand binding induces a propagated conformational change through the transmembrane domain to the cytoplasmic domain of the receptor, a phenomenon that has been confirmed using conformationally sensitive antibodies.[174]

Four lines of evidence indicate that receptor tyrosine kinase activation is necessary for signal transduction by growth factors and insulin. Overexpression of normal receptor tyrosine kinases in cells which have low numbers of endogenous receptors increases the sensitivity and responsiveness of a number of biological effects.[175] Receptor tyrosine kinases is mutated at the ATP binding lack kinase activity. These receptor mutants retain ligand binding activity, are internalized, and mediate ligand degradation; however, they fail to stimulate biological actions including membrane transport, cytoskeletal organization, ribosomal protein S6 activation, glycogen synthesis, and DNA synthesis.[176] Monoclonal antibodies to the kinase domain of the insulin and EGF receptors have been microinjected into cells and have been shown to decrease the effects of insulin and EGF on both the kinase activity and biological responses.[177] Finally, the association between receptor tyrosine kinase activity and biological actions is supported by observations in humans or experimental animals with genetic or acquired alterations of tyrosine kinase activity. Loss of function results in developmental defects or hormone resistance.[178, 179] Gain of function results in hyperplastic or malignant growth disorders.[180]

The signal transduction of receptor tyrosine kinases involves two rate-limiting steps (Fig. 3–18). One is binding of signaling molecules with SH2 domains to specific phosphotyrosine-containing peptide sequences in the tyrosine kinase. The SH2 domain proteins include src tyrosine kinase, phospholipase C-γ, the regulatory subunit p85 of phosphatidylinositol 3-kinase, ras GTPase-activating protein, SH2-containing sequence protein (abbreviated SHC), growth factor receptor-binding protein-2 (abbreviated GRB2), SH2 domain phosphotyrosine phosphatases -1 and -2 (abbreviated SHPTP-1 and -2). A second mechanism is tyrosine phosphorylation of signaling molecules such as phospholipase C-γ, src tyrosine kinase, SH2-containing sequence protein, and SH2 domain phosphotyrosine phosphatase-1. Autophosphorylation on specific tyrosine residues allows the receptor tyrosine kinase to select a reper-

toire of SH2 domain-containing proteins. For example, the EGF receptor contains five tyrosine residues in the carboxy-terminal tail of the receptor that are phosphorylated.[169] Each individual phosphotyrosine residue binds specifically SH2 domain-containing regulatory molecules.[181, 182] The structural basis for the specificity of the interaction between tyrosine-phosphorylated proteins and SH2 domain proteins has established a general principle: phosphotyrosine-containing peptides as short as four amino acids bind to SH2 domains with high affinity. For example, the p85 subunit of phosphatidylinositol 3-kinase binds to phosphotyrosine-methionine-proline-methionine in PDGF and CSF-1 receptors and insulin receptor substrate-1; GRB2 binds phosphotyrosine-isoleucine-asparagine-glutamine in EGF and CSF-1 receptors and insulin receptor substrate-1; phospholipase C-γ binds phosphotyrosine-leucine-isoleucine-proline in EGF and PDGF receptors.[183] The binding affinity of different phosphopeptides for a given SH2 domain vary by 100-fold. The x-ray crystallographic structures of the SH2 domains in a complex with the specific phosphotyrosine tetrapeptides have provided an exact structural model of the interaction.[184–188]

SH2 AND SH3 DOMAIN PROTEINS. Domains homologous to two regions in the src tyrosine kinase are found in an increasing number of cellular proteins.[189] These have been termed the SH2 and SH3 domains (Fig. 3–19). The SH1 domain is the domain homologous to the catalytic region of the src tyrosine kinase that is common to the superfamily of tyrosine kinases.[190] Based on their function SH2 domain-containing proteins can be divided into three classes: (1) enzymes such as src tyrosine kinase, abl tyrosine kinase, phospholipase C-γ, ras GTPase-activating protein, and SH2 domain phosphotyrosine phosphatases-1 and -2; (2) adaptor molecules such as p85-subunit of phosphatidylinositol 3-kinase, growth factor receptor-binding protein, SH2-containing sequence protein and interferon-stimulated gene factor-3 (abbreviated IFSG-3); and (3) structural proteins such as spectrin, myosin, and tensin (Fig. 3–20). The interaction with specific phosphotyrosine motifs on receptors activates the SH2 domain protein leading to an increase of its enzymatic activity, molecular interactions, or cytoskeletal changes. One of the SH2 domain adaptor proteins, the p91 subunit of the interferon-γ–stimulated gene factor-3

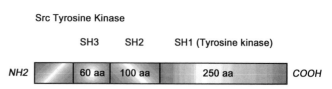

Src Tyrosine Kinase

SH3   SH2   SH1 (Tyrosine kinase)

NH2 | 60 aa | 100 aa | 250 aa | COOH

FIGURE 3–19. **Src homology domains.** Src contains three domains that have been found in a variety of cellular proteins involved in intracellular signal transduction. The SH1 domain is 250 amino acids (aa) and represents the catalytic domain of the tyrosine kinase that is common to the superfamily of src-like tyrosine kinases including membrane receptors, cytoplasmic and nuclear tyrosine kinases. The SH2 domain of approximately 100 amino acids and the SH3 domain of 60 amino acids are common to proteins with putative signaling functions. The SH2 domain binds tyrosine-phosphorylated regions of target proteins, frequently linking activated growth factor receptors to signal molecules. The SH3 domain binds proline-rich motifs in proteins often connected with small G proteins.

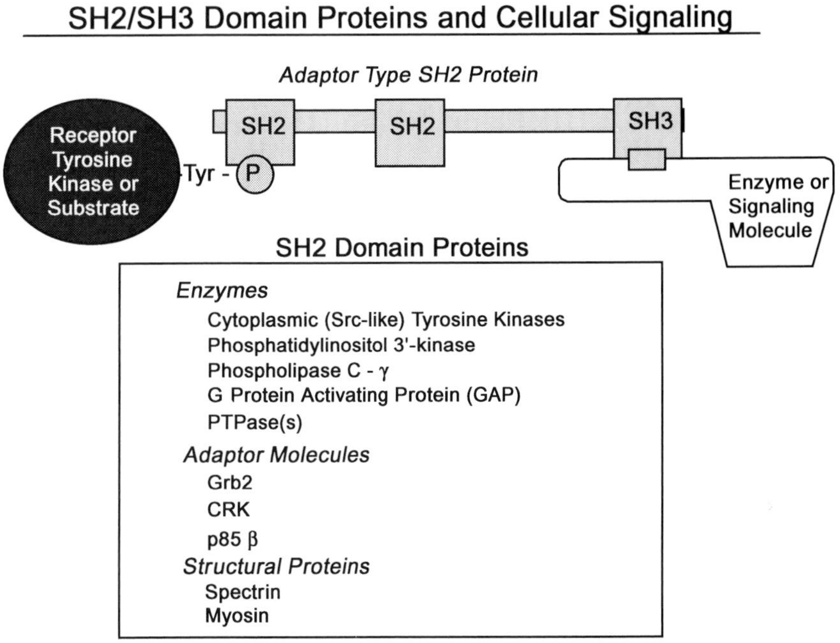

SH2/SH3 Domain Proteins and Cellular Signaling

FIGURE 3–20. **SH2-SH3 domain proteins and cellular signaling.** The adaptor type SH2 protein contains two SH2 domains and one SH3 domain. The SH2 domain binds a specific phosphotyrosine motif on receptor tyrosine kinase or substrate. SH3 domain binds an enzyme or signaling molecule. SH2 domain proteins can be divided in three groups consisting of enzymes, adaptor molecules, and structural proteins.

complex, is tyrosine-phosphorylated in response to interferon-γ, as well as other growth factors (e.g., EGF, PDGF, CSF-1, and IL-10.) The phosphorylated p91 subunit is then translocated from the cytoplasm to the nucleus and activates gene transcription by way of interaction with the interferon-γ–response element (see p. 49). Several of the proteins contain two repeats of the SH2 domain, indicating that they are capable of binding two phosphotyrosine peptide sequences. Thus it is possible that one protein with two SH2 domains such as the p85 regulatory subunit of phosphatidylinositol 3-kinase binds the two receptor tyrosine kinases in the active dimer conformation.

The interaction between phosphotyrosine peptide and SH2 domain determines the selectivity of the signal transduction pathway in a large repertoire of SH2 domain-containing proteins. The different phosphotyrosine docking sites on a receptor tyrosine kinase may bind multiple SH2 proteins in a "signal transfer complex" and the signaling function of the receptor will be determined by the sum of phosphotyrosine-SH2 domain interactions. As SH2 domains show overlapping specificity toward phosphotyrosine motifs, they may compete for the same docking sites on a receptor. Some SH2 domain proteins such as the SH2-containing sequence protein and the SH2 domain phosphotyrosine phosphatases-1 and -2 are phosphorylated on tyrosine residues and may propagate the signal by way of interaction with other SH2 domain proteins.[191–194] Several SH2 domain proteins contain one or more SH3 domains (Fig. 3–20). The function of SH3 domains is less clear, but recent evidence suggests that they are involved in the interaction with small ras-like G proteins.[195–198] GRB2 has two SH3 domains that interacts with two characteristic polyproline sequences in ras guanine nucleotide–releasing protein leading to activation of ras.[199–201] The elucidation of the x-ray crystallographic structure of the SH3 domain may lead to further understanding of this interaction.[196] Thus two steps of protein-protein interactions involving SH2 and SH3 domains transmit the signal from the active receptor tyrosine kinase to ras activation.[198]

RAS AND TYROSINE KINASE SIGNAL TRANSDUCTION. The ras genes are a ubiquitous eukaryotic gene family, including H-ras, K-ras, and N-ras.[200] A large number of related genes have been identified that have 30 to 55 per cent homology to ras, including rho, ral, rab, rac, and rap.[134–138] All ras-related proteins bind guanine nucleotides (GTP and GDP) and possess intrinsic GTPase activity. The biochemical properties of ras resemble closely those of G proteins involved in the modulation of signal transduction through seven-transmembrane segment receptors. Ras is anchored to the plasma membrane via prenylation at its carboxy-terminus.[201] Ras is active in its GTP-bound form and inactive in its GDP-bound form (Fig. 3–21). Activation of ras by exchange of bound GDP for GTP is facilitated by a ras guanine nucleotide–releasing factor (also called GDP-GTP exchange factor or GDP-releasing factor). Inactivation of ras by hydrolysis of bound GTP to GDP and P_i is catalyzed by the intrinsic GTPase following its activation by a ras GTPase-activating protein (ras-GAP).

Experimental evidence has now revealed a role for ras in signal transduction of receptor tyrosine kinases in mammalian cells.[202, 203] Microinjection of neutralizing ras antibodies reverses the transformed phenotype of H-ras–transformed cells and blocked PDGF- and insulin-induced mitogenesis. A dominant negative mutant of ras inhibits EGF, PDGF, FGF, NGF, and insulin actions. Overexpression of c-ras increases the sensitivity to several growth factors and insulin. Another line of evidence was obtained in two lower animal species: the nematode *Caenorhabditis elegans* and the fruitfly *Drosophila melanogaster*. Genetic and developmental studies revealed that activation of receptors homologous with the mammalian EGF receptor in these species leads to activation of ras via interaction with two molecules homologous to mammalian GRB2 and ras guanine nucleotide–releasing protein (GNRP). The latter was named "son of sevenless" (abbreviated SOS) because the protein mediates the signal of the "sevenless" receptor tyrosine kinase in *Drosophila* during eye development. The direct interaction between GRB2 and the GNRP/SOS pro-

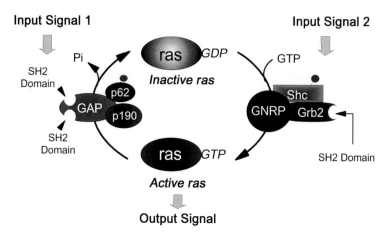

FIGURE 3–21. **The ras cycle and receptor signaling.** The conversion of inactive ras-GDP to active ras-GTP is facilitated by interaction with guanine nucleotide–releasing protein (GNRP). GNRP (also called SOS) is under control of input signal 2 via interaction with two SH2 domain-containing proteins: growth factor receptor-binding protein-2 (GRB2) and SH2-containing sequence protein (SHC) (phosphorylated on tyrosine). GRB2 and SHC are activated by interaction with tyrosine-phosphorylated receptors via their SH2 domains. Active ras-GTP mediates the output signal. The conversion of active ras-GTP to inactive ras-GDP is facilitated by GTPase-activating protein (GAP) that activates the intrinsic ras-GTPase and hydrolysis of GTP to GDP and P_i. GAP, a SH2 domain-containing protein, forms a complex with two proteins, p62 (phosphorylated on tyrosine) and p110, and is under control of input signal 1 probably via interaction between its two SH2 domains and yet unknown phosphotyrosine proteins.

tein in EGF receptor activation of ras has also been demonstrated in mammalian systems.[204–206]

Growth factors and insulin stimulate a group of intracellular protein kinases that includes raf kinase, mitogen-activated protein (abbreviated MAP) kinase-kinase, and mitogen-activated protein kinase. Activation of raf kinase is essential for induction of cell proliferation and appears to result from a direct interaction between activated ras and raf kinase.[207, 208] This represents one signal transduction pathway by receptor-linked tyrosine kinases (Fig. 3–22). Growth factor, cytokines, or insulin activate receptor-linked tyrosine kinases and protein phosphorylations at the membrane level. GRB2 binds to specific phosphotyrosine motifs in the kinase domains. ras guanine nucleotide–releasing protein (i.e., son of sevenless protein) is translocated to the membrane in a pre-existing complex with the GRB2 and activates membrane-bound ras by GDP-GTP exchange. ras activates raf kinase, which initiates a phosphorylation cascade including activation of MAP kinase-kinase, MAP kinase, and S6 protein kinase.

In summary, the signal transduction by receptor tyrosine kinases can be described by four paradigms: (1) *Activation by tyrosine phosphorylation.* Phosphorylation of a single tyrosine residue on phospholipase C-γ increases its hydrolysis of phosphatidylinositol 4,5-bisphosphate to inositol triphosphate and diacylglycerol. (2) *Activation by conformational change.* Interaction with a specific phosphotyrosine peptide changes the conformation of the regulatory p85 subunit of phosphatidylinositol 3-kinase and activates its catalytic subunit p110. (3) *Activation by translocation to the plasma membrane.* The ras guanine nucleotide–releasing protein, son of sevenless, is associated with GRB2 and translocated to the plasma membrane, where it activates ras. (4) *Activation by phosphorylation and translocation to the nucleus.* The p91 subunit of the interferon-γ–stimulated gene factor-3 is tyrosine-phosphorylated and initiates gene expression. These four paradigms represent concurrent signaling pathways which are cooperative as well as redundant. For example, activation of both ras and p91 transcription factor is involved in the EGF receptor–induced cell growth and transformation. Mutation of the five carboxy-terminal tyrosines in the EGF receptor blocks EGF-induced ras activation, whereas p91 activation is increased and cell transformation is unchanged. It is possible that both positive and negative signals activated by the EGF are eliminated in the receptor mutant resulting in an unchanged response.

The signal transduction of receptor tyrosine kinases involves a combination of signaling molecules that interacts in a complex molecular network of cooperative and inhibitory reactions. Furthermore, the signal transduction based on the simple interaction between phosphotyrosine tetrapeptide motifs and SH2 domains illustrates two simplifying principles of biology: the principle of redundancy and the principle of diversity.[209] The principle of redundancy means that a simple mechanism or module is selected as a building block and used over and over in other systems. The principle of diversity utilizes the concept that there are many ways of achieving the same goal—for example, stimulating glycogen metabolism or generating cell division. It is clear that the SH2 domain-signaling mechanism is highly redundant in evolution and that the SH2 domain-

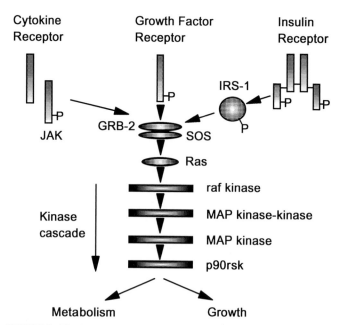

FIGURE 3–22. **Signal pathway of receptor-activated tyrosine kinase receptors.** Activation of receptor-linked tyrosine kinases by cytokines, growth factors, and insulin induces receptor autophosphorylation. The complex of GRB2 and son of sevenless (SOS) guanine nucleotide–releasing protein is recruited to the plasma membrane by the receptor via SH2 domain-phosphotyrosine interaction. SOS activates raf kinase that initiates a phosphorylation cascade: mitogen-activated protein (MAP) kinase-kinase, MAP-kinase and p90[rsk] leading to cellular effects on metabolism and cell growth.

containing proteins and interactions show a rich diversity in cellular regulation.

PHOSPHOTYROSINE PHOSPHATASES. The net level of phosphotyrosine proteins in the cell is the result of two opposite reactions: phosphorylation and dephosphorylation. The phosphorylation reaction is catalyzed by tyrosine kinases and the dephosphorylation reaction by a class of enzymes called phosphotyrosine phosphatases. Although so far the characterization of tyrosine kinases and protein phosphorylation has received the greatest attention, several phosphotyrosine phosphatases have now been cloned and defined at the molecular level.[82] Two groups of phosphotyrosine phosphatases have been identified: (1) large transmembrane proteins which resemble receptors, some with two tandem repeats of the catalytic domain in the intracellular portion; (2) smaller intracellular enzymes with a single catalytic domain (Fig. 3–23). The phosphotyrosine phosphatase catalytic domain is not structurally related to the serine-threonine-specific phosphatases.

More than 10 transmembrane phosphotyrosine phosphatases have been cloned and their structures show considerable variation in the extracellular portion, whereas the cytoplasmic portion is characterized by one or two catalytic domain(s). Several are receptor-like structures, but the nature of the extracellular ligands is a puzzle. The first phosphotyrosine phosphatase to be cloned was the leukocyte common antigen, CD45, the function of which is still unknown. Another member of the group has an extracellular region with similarity to carbonic anhydrase, suggesting that low-molecular-weight ligands may be involved. Two membrane phosphatases show homology with the extracellular portion of the cell adhesion molecules and may be involved in cell aggregation.

The intracellular phosphotyrosine phosphatases are a large group of proteins with structural and functional diversity. Two SH2 domain-containing phosphotyrosine phosphatases-1 and -2 (also known as phosphotyrosine phosphatases 1C and 1D or syp) interact with tyrosine-phosphorylated proteins, suggesting a potential role in receptor tyrosine kinase signaling.[191–193] SH2 domain phosphotyrosine phosphatase-1 is found predominantly in hematopoietic cells, whereas type 2 is present in other cell types. Both may be involved in modulating signals from cytokine and growth factor receptors after binding to specific phosphotyrosine motifs on receptor-linked tyrosine kinases. Four possible functions of SH2 domain phosphotyrosine phosphatases are as follows: (1) reduction of signaling by dephosphorylation of phosphorylation sites on receptor tyrosine kinases; (2) inactivation of tyrosine-phosphorylated signaling molecules (e.g., phospholipase C-γ and src tyrosine kinase) by dephosphorylation; (3) signal amplification via binding of other tyrosine-phosphorylated signaling proteins to one of the two SH2 domains; (4) signal transmission via interaction between another SH2 domain protein and the phosphorylated tyrosine residue in the carboxy-terminus of SH2 domain phosphotyrosine phosphatase-1. So far these mechanisms are speculative and the role of cytoplasmic phosphotyrosine phosphatases in cellular signaling remains unclear. Phosphatases specific for various receptor tyrosine kinases await identification.

REGULATION BY SERINE-THREONINE PHOSPHORYLATION. Several tyrosine kinase receptors are phosphorylated not only on tyrosine residues but also on serine and threonine

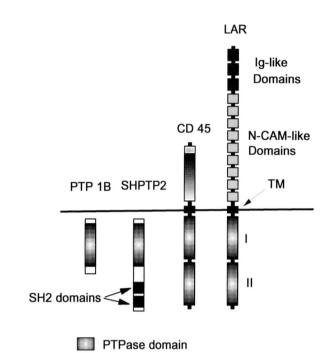

FIGURE 3–23. Structures of phosphotyrosine phosphatases. Two cytoplasmic phosphotyrosine phosphatases (PTP) are shown: PTPase 1B and SHPTP2. Both have one catalytic domain. SHPTP2 contains two SH2 domains. Two transmembrane (TM) phosphotyrosine phosphatases are shown: CD45 (a leukocyte common antigen) and LAR (leukocyte common antigen-related). Both have two tandem catalytic domains in the cytoplasmic portion. The extracellular portions are diverse and contain Ig-like and N-CAM–like domains.

residues. There is evidence that the extent of receptor serine phosphorylation is modulated and that this may decrease the tyrosine kinase activity and autophosphorylation of the receptors. For example, protein kinase C has been shown to phosphorylate the EGF receptor on serine residues and to decrease the EGF-stimulated tyrosine kinase activity.[210] The insulin receptor is also phosphorylated on serine residues in response to phorbol esters, presumably through their effects on protein kinase C activity.[211] As with the EGF receptor, serine phosphorylation of the insulin receptor is associated with decreased tyrosine kinase activity and insulin action. Insulin itself, in addition to its effects on tyrosine autophosphorylation, leads to increased phosphorylation of the insulin receptor on serine residues, and this may also have a role in modulating insulin action. Recent work indicates that there may also be a specific insulin receptor-associated serine kinase, although this enzyme has not yet been well characterized.[212] In regard to the possible role of serine phosphorylation in reversing hormone action, it is interesting to note that insulin-stimulated serine phosphorylation of insulin receptors does not occur in cells with mutant receptors that cannot undergo tyrosine autophosphorylation.

Level 2: Signal Transduction

PROTEIN KINASE AND PROTEIN PHOSPHATASE REACTIONS. The initial activation of membrane receptors and effectors controls the formation of signal molecules. The latter then activates the second level of hormone, growth factor, and

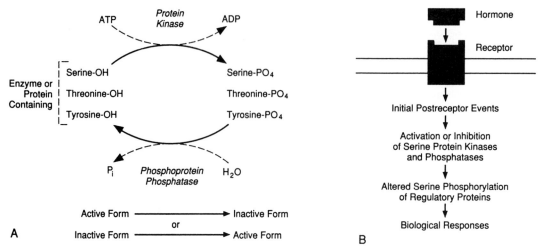

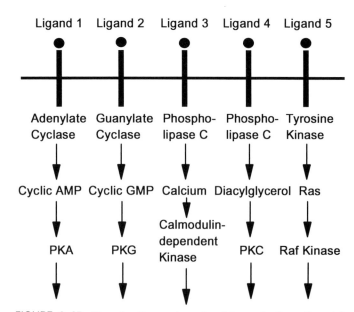

FIGURE 3–24. **Protein phosphorylation cascades in hormone action.** *A,* Regulation of enzymes and other proteins by phosphorylation and dephosphorylation. In phosphorylation of a protein, a protein kinase stimulates the transfer of a phosphate group from ATP to a hydroxyl group on the side chain of a serine, threonine, or tyrosine residue. The phosphate group can be removed by the action of phosphoprotein phosphatases. This process usually results in conversion of an active protein or enzyme to an inactive form or vice versa (see Table 3–10). *B,* Role of phosphorylation and dephosphorylation of serine in mediating the effects of peptide hormones on metabolic pathways. (Modified from Kahn CR, Smith RJ, Chin WW: Mechanism of action of hormones that act at the cell surface. *In* Wilson JD, Foster DW: Williams Textbook of Endocrinology. Philadelphia, WB Saunders Co., 1992, p 104.)

neurotransmitter action through a cascade of protein kinases and protein phosphatases.[213] Phosphorylation or dephosphorylation of serine, threonine, and (occasionally) tyrosine residues triggers conformational changes in regulated proteins which alter their activity, leading to the physiological responses that are evoked by particular agonists (Fig. 3–24). Protein phosphorylation as a mechanism for regulating protein activity was first recognized with glycogen phosphorylase. It is clear that this mechanism for the reversible modification of proteins is widespread and affects nearly all aspects of growth and homeostasis in the eukaryotic cell. The enzymes catalyzing this transfer of the γ-phosphate of ATP to a protein substrate, the protein kinases, constitute a large and diverse family of enzymes. The superfamily of protein kinases consists of serine-threonine protein kinases and tyrosine kinases, which show amino acid sequence homology but differ in their substrate specificity and cellular abundance. The general consensus sequence recognized by serine-threonine protein kinases contains serine or threonine surrounded by basic amino acids (e.g., arginine-arginine-X-serine [γ or threonine]-Z, where X is any small residue and Z is a large hydrophobic group). Serine-threonine protein kinases are much more common than tyrosine protein kinases. In resting cells phosphoserine and phosphothreonine account for almost 99.9 per cent of phosphorylated proteins. In proliferating cells, however, the proportion of proteins with phosphotyrosine increases and may reach a value of 10 per cent in growth factor– or oncogene-transformed cell lines. This reflects the importance of tyrosine protein kinases in initiating and transmitting signals from growth factors, hormones, and cytokines during activation of cell proliferation. The serine-threonine protein kinases, on the other hand, are involved in the signal transduction of all regulatory pathways of both resting and growing cells. The diverse actions of different agonists are largely explained by the pleiotrophic actions of the serine-threonine protein kinases and phosphatases that they regulate and by the

presence (or absence) in cells of the particular target on which they act.[214]

Five principal signaling systems operate by means of activation of serine-threonine protein kinases in eukaryotic cells (Fig. 3–25). cAMP exerts nearly all its effects by activating cAMP-dependent kinase, which is ubiquitous and phosphorylates many intracellular proteins involved in a

FIGURE 3–25. **Five signaling systems involving activation of protein serine-threonine kinases.** Extracellular agonists activate either G protein–linked receptors, guanylate cyclase receptors, or receptor protein tyrosine kinases leading to formation of cAMP, cGMP, or diacylglycerol (DAG), release of Ca^{2+} or activation of ras. Each of these signaling molecules activate in turn cAMP-dependent protein kinase (PKA), cGMP-dependent protein kinase (PKG), protein kinase C (PKC), calmodulin-dependent kinases, or raf kinase. These serine-threonine kinases phosphorylate enzymes and proteins resulting in cellular actions. (Modified from Cohen P: Signal integration at the level of protein kinases, protein phosphatases and their substrates. Trends Biochem Sci 17:408–413, 1992).

large array of responses. cGMP activates a specific cGMP-dependent protein kinase that has a more restricted role, since it is located in smooth muscle and the cerebellum. Calcium ions bind to calmodulin and activate many enzymes, including a number of Ca^{2+}/calmodulin-dependent protein kinases. These protein kinases are involved in regulation of functions as diverse as muscle contraction, glycogenolysis, and protein synthesis. Diacylglycerol activates protein kinase C, which causes multiple physiological responses (e.g., secretion, proliferation, and differentiation). The Raf protein kinase, which seems to be involved in the stimulation of many actions such as glycogen synthesis, protein synthesis, and cell division, is activated by ras. These signaling systems are key components in the signal transduction of a large number of extracellular agonists and their receptors and elicit a large array of cellular responses. Although the pathways are outlined as being independent of each other, they actually interact at every level so that different signals have additive, synergistic, or antagonistic effects. Two major levels at which this signal integration takes place are the level of protein kinases and protein phosphatases and their substrates.

Many regulatory enzymes exist in alternative phosphorylated and dephosphorylated states that differ markedly in their catalytic activity (Table 3–10). The level of enzyme phosphorylation is determined by the activities of opposing serine-threonine protein kinases and phosphatases that may be limited in their actions to a single target enzyme or may act on multiple regulatory enzymes. A large number of serine-threonine protein kinases are activated during hormone and growth factor stimulation, e.g., cAMP- and cGMP-dependent protein kinases, protein kinase C, calmodulin-dependent protein kinase II, myosin light chain kinase, phosphorylase kinase, raf kinase, acetyl-CoA carboxylase kinase, ATP-citrate lyase kinase, casein kinase II, mitogen-activated protein kinases, and ribosomal S6 kinases.[121, 122] Many of the effects of hormones and growth factors are brought about by activation of protein phosphatases and dephosphorylation of serine or threonine residues. These protein phosphatases (e.g., protein phosphatase-1 and calmodulin-regulated protein phosphatase-2B) regulate the activity of a number of metabolic enzymes including the stimulation of glycogen synthase, pyruvate kinase, and pyruvate dehydrogenase and the inhibition of triacylglycerol lipase, phosphorylase, and phosphorylase kinase.[119] In general, protein kinase and phosphatase reactions are involved in all aspects of cellular physiology. Three examples are discussed here.

Glycogenolysis in mammalian muscle is a system in which protein phosphorylation was first identified as a reg-

ulatory device.[213] Glycogenolysis is activated during muscle contraction by calcium. Ca^{2+} is released from endoplasmic reticulum in response to membrane depolarization and influx of trigger calcium. In resting muscle, glycogenolysis is activated by cAMP following activation of the β-adrenergic receptor. The effects of these two signal molecules are integrated at the level of phosphorylase kinase by two different mechanisms. The enzyme is composed of four subunits, α, β, γ, and δ; α and β are the regulatory subunits, γ is the catalytic subunit, and δ is calmodulin. In its dephosphorylated state, the activity of phosphorylase kinase is suppressed by the interaction of γ subunit with α, β, and δ subunits. The inhibition is partially relieved by interaction of Ca^{2+} with the δ subunit and by interaction of the contractile protein troponin C with the β subunit, allowing the γ subunit of phosphorylase kinase to activate glycogen phosphorylase. This initiates glycogenolysis to provide ATP required to sustain contraction. Phosphorylation of the α and β subunits by cAMP-dependent protein kinase in response to cAMP relieves their inhibitory constraints on the γ subunit. The phosphorylated form of phosphorylase kinase still has an absolute requirement for Ca^{2+} but is activated at lower concentrations than the dephosphorylated enzyme.

Insulin and epinephrine exert opposite effects on storage of glucose into glycogen.[215] Insulin stimulates glycogen synthesis and inhibits glycogenolysis in skeletal muscle by causing activation dephosphorylation of glycogen synthase and dephosphorylation and inhibition of glycogen phosphorylase, simultaneously. The dephosphorylation of both enzymes is catalyzed by protein phosphatase-1. This enzyme is activated by insulin through phosphorylation of a serine residue on the G subunit, termed site 1. Phosphorylation of site 1 is catalyzed by an insulin-stimulated serine-threonine kinase, p90[rsk], which is a mammalian homologue of ribosomal protein S6 kinase II. Epinephrine activates cAMP-dependent protein kinase, which phosphorylates the G subunit at site 2, triggering dissociation of protein phosphatase-1 from the G subunit and its release from glycogen. This prevents protein phosphatase-1 from dephosphorylating the glycogen-associated enzymes, such as glycogen synthase and glycogen phosphorylase. Thus the activating effect of site 1 phosphorylation is abolished by site 2 phosphorylation; this explains how epinephrine overrides the effect of insulin on glycogen metabolism.

An important serine-threonine protein kinase in the signaling pathway of several growth factors and hormones is the mitogen-activated protein kinase (abbreviated MAP kinase), originally named microtubule-associated protein-2 kinase based on a substrate used in a phosphorylation assay in vitro.[216] The enzyme is also known as extracellular signal-regulated kinase (abbreviated ERK) because it is activated by a variety of extracellular ligands.[217] Two forms of mitogen-activated protein kinase have been purified from fibroblasts and cloned, p42[mapk] and p44[mapk]. Mitogen-activated kinases are stimulated by phosphorylation on threonine and tyrosine residues and were originally thought to be direct substrates for receptor tyrosine kinases. Several recent reports indicate that a protein kinase termed mitogen-activated protein kinase-kinase is responsible for activation of mitogen-activated protein kinase.[218] This kinase (also known as MEK for MAP-ERK kinase) has dual specificity as it appears to catalyze the phosphorylation of both threo-

TABLE 3–10. METABOLIC ENZYMES ACTIVATED BY PHOSPHORYLATION OR DEPHOSPHORYLATION

ACTIVATION BY PHOSPHORYLATION	ACTIVATION BY DEPHOSPHORYLATION
Phosphorylase kinase	Pyruvate dehydrogenase
Protein phosphatase-1	Pyruvate kinase
Glycogen phosphorylase	Glycogen synthase
Triglyceride lipase	
ATP citrate lyase	
Ribosomal S6 kinase	

nine and tyrosine residues of mitogen-activated protein kinase. A molecular link between the receptor tyrosine kinases at the membrane and mitogen-activated protein kinase in the cytoplasm has recently been described. Mitogen-activated protein kinase-kinase is activated by phosphorylation on serine indicating the existence of a specific mitogen-activated protein kinase-kinase-kinase that has been identified as raf kinase. Raf kinase is activated by growth factors via interaction with ras. In intact cells, the mitogen-activated protein kinases appear to be the activator of p90[rsk]. In skeletal muscle, insulin-stimulated p90[rsk] phosphorylates the G subunit of protein phosphatase-1, which increases its rate of dephosphorylation of glycogen synthase and phosphorylase kinase. Thus mitogen-activated protein kinase may be a direct intermediate in the regulation of glycogen synthesis by insulin by causing the stimulation of glycogen synthase and inhibition of glycogen phosphorylase. In addition, mitogen-activated kinase can phosphorylate the transcription factor jun. This places mitogen-activated kinase at a branch point in hormone and mitogen signaling.

Level 3: Cellular Actions

The activation of receptors, signaling molecules, second messengers, and protein kinase cascades leads to the third level in hormone, growth factor, and neurotransmitter action. This includes the final cellular responses on metabolism, transport, biosynthesis, secretion, contraction, growth, and differentiation. The molecular mechanisms involved are diverse, including activation of enzymes, regulation of contractile or cytoskeletal proteins, translocation of intracellular vesicles, stimulation of ribosomal translation and protein synthesis, and initiation of gene transcription. These processes have been studied in great detail. A complete survey of the third level of hormone action is outside the scope of this chapter; however, two examples are discussed.

REGULATION OF MEMBRANE TRANSPORT. An important action of peptide hormones and growth factors is to regulate the influx of nutrients, including amino acids and glucose. This involves regulation of specific transport systems for these molecules (Fig. 3–26). Amino acids are transported by at least five different carrier systems in the plasma membrane of mammalian cells.[219] Each of these is believed to depend on the function of a specific transport protein that recognizes a group of closely related amino acids. Most of these amino acid transports function as cotransport systems or "symporters," bringing in Na^+ in conjunction with the amino acid. The neutral amino acid transport system, which favors alanine, glycine, and proline, termed *system A*, is the most active of the hormonally regulated systems.[220] Hormonal stimulation of transport requires a number of intermediate steps.[221] There is usually a lag of 5 to 15 minutes before the increase in transport is observed, and then the cell is committed to the increase in transport (for some period of time) even if the hormone is removed. Hormones or growth factors acting through G protein–coupled receptors as well as receptor tyrosne kinases have been shown to increase amino acid transport. This indicates that the two major signal transduction systems are involved. In almost all cases, the increase in trans-

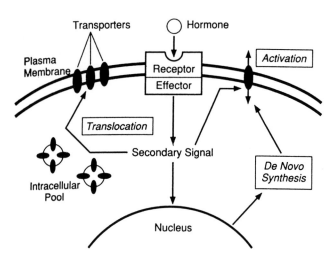

FIGURE 3–26. **Model of hormone action on membrane transport.** Possible mechanisms of hormone stimulation of membrane transport. Hormones act on amino acid and glucose transport by a number of mechanisms including de novo synthesis, activation, and translocation of transporters from an intracellular pool to the plasma membrane. (From Kahn CR, Smith RJ, Chin WW: Mechanism of action of hormones that act at the cell surface. *In* Wilson JD, Foster DW: Williams Textbook of Endocrinology. Philadelphia, WB Saunders Co., 1992, p 107.)

port activity is associated with an increase in the V_{max} of the transporter. Possible mechanisms for this increase in V_{max} include de novo synthesis of the transporter molecules, translocation of active transporters to the membrane, posttranslational conversion of inactive transporters to an active form, or an increase in membrane potential that might secondarily increase transport as a result of the dependence of these systems on the co-transport of sodium ions. The accumulated amino acids are either metabolized or build into proteins.

Glucose transport is regulated by several hormones including insulin, growth hormone, and epinephrine. Seven distinct mammalian glucose transporters (abbreviated GLUT-1–GLUT-7) have been identified by cDNA cloning and sequencing.[222] All of the transporters are proteins of molecular weight 45 to 50 kDa and possess 12 membrane-spanning domains. Two are the Na^+-dependent glucose transporters 6 and 7 involved in active transport of glucose by intestinal epithelium and renal tubular cells. Five glucose transporters are involved in Na^+-independent facilitative transport of glucose into various cells. These transporters show tissue-specific and developmentally regulated expression. Two glucose transporters, 1 and 4, are expressed in many tissues and their regulation by various hormones has been extensively studied.[223–225] GLUT-4 is the primary insulin-sensitive transporter present in skeletal muscle, cardiac muscle, and adipose tissue. GLUT-1 is expressed in red cells, brain, kidney, liver, muscle and so on and shows variable response to hormones. Hormonal regulation of glucose transport involves two processes: (1) translocation of glucose transporters from intracellular vesicles to the plasma membrane and (2) changes in transport activity.[226] Upon insulin stimulation, glucose transport in adipose cells and muscle is increased 10- to 20-fold after a lag period of 30 seconds. This effect depends primarily on an increase in V_{max} with little or no effect on the K_m. The major component of insulin stimulation of glucose transport is an energy-dependent translocation of intracellular vesicles containing GLUT-4 to the plasma membrane, whereas insulin has a minor effect on the intrinsic transporter activity.[227] The effect is reversible, and following removal of insulin from its receptor, GLUT-4 returns to the intracellular pool. Insulin does not stimulate glucose uptake in liver and erythrocytes that express GLUT-1 and not 4. Adrenergic agents and phorbol esters inhibit glucose transport by reversible suppression of the intrinsic activity of the transporters residing at the plasma membrane with little or no effect on translocation. These effects may be mediated by activation of cAMP-dependent protein kinase and protein kinase C and serine phosphorylation of GLUT-4.

REGULATION OF GENE EXPRESSION BY MEMBRANE RECEPTORS.

Transient signals generated by activation of membrane receptors are converted into long-term changes in gene expression by signal-regulated transcription factors that mediate the effects of polypeptide hormones, cytokines, and neurotransmitters. Rapid advances in our knowledge about transcription factors have been achieved over the last several years, but the steps leading from the cell surface to the nucleus have proved far more elusive, this despite clear evidence that extracellular ligands activate distinct genetic programs and diverse cellular responses. Three important signal transduction pathways that regulate gene expression by modulating the activity of nuclear transcription factors have been identified.[228–231] These include AP-1, cAMP-response element-binding protein, and interferon-γ–stimulated gene factor-3 (Fig. 3–27).

AP-1 was originally defined as a DNA-binding activity recognizing the 12-O-tetradecanoylphorbol-13-acetate response element. Molecular cloning revealed that AP-1 consists of a collection of structurally related transcription factors, which belong to the jun and fos families.[232] AP-1 is responsible for transcriptional induction of a number of genes in response to activation of protein kinase C by receptor tyrosine kinases. cAMP response element binding protein (CREB) binds to the cAMP response element within promoters of cAMP-inducible genes. cAMP response element binding protein mediates the induction of genes in response to activation of cAMP-dependent protein kinase by G protein–coupled receptors.[233] Interferon-stimulated gene factor-3 (IFSG-3) is a DNA-binding activity that interacts with the interferon-γ activation sequence of interferon-γ–responsive genes. IFSG-3 is related to sis-inducible factors (SIF) that interact with a sis-inducible element in the c-fos gene promoter. sis represents an oncogenic form of PDGF. Both interferon- and sis-induced factors regulate transcriptional activity in response to receptor-linked tyrosine kinases activated by growth factors and cytokines.

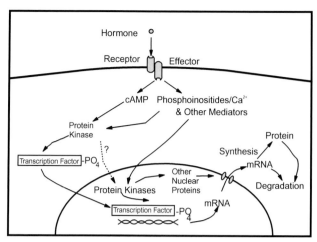

FIGURE 3–27. **Mechanisms of hormone action on gene expression.** Interaction of hormone with its receptor results in the production of cAMP, phosphoinositides (inositol triphosphate and diacylglycerol), Ca²⁺, and other mediators. These signaling molecules activate protein kinases in the cytoplasm or in the nucleus that in turn phosphorylate transcription factors. In the nucleus activated transcription factor-PO₄ can then bind to response elements in promoter regions of responsive genes and regulate gene expression. Increased gene transcription leads to formation of mRNA and protein synthesis. Phosphorylation of other nuclear proteins may be involved in translocation of mRNA to the cytoplasm. (Modified from Kahn CR, Smith RJ, Chin WW: Mechanism of action of hormones that act at the cell surface. *In* Wilson JD, Foster DW: Williams Textbook of Endocrinology. Philadelphia, WB Saunders Co., 1992, p 107.)

AP-1 (jun-fos) and CREB proteins belong to the group of signal-regulated transcription factors with conserved DNA binding and dimerization domains (Fig. 3–28). These factors have a modular structure consisting of three distinct and separable domains involved in DNA binding with a high content of basic amino acid residues, dimerization with a leucine zipper, and transcriptional activation with regulatory phosphorylation sites. Like all members of the basic domain/leucine zipper domain family, the jun and fos proteins must dimerize prior to DNA binding. The jun proteins bind DNA as either homodimers or heterodimers of members of the jun family, whereas fos proteins must heterodimerize with one of the jun proteins. Combinatorial interactions between the jun and fos proteins give rise to dimers with different activities, although their DNA sequence specificity *(TGACTCA)* appears to be very similar. All of these dimers are thought to contribute to AP-1 activity and participate in its regulation by extracellular factors. AP-1 should be regarded as a nuclear messenger that mediates the actions of signal transduction pathways stimulated by growth factors, cytokines, hormones, and neurotransmitters, most of which are initiated by the activation of either tyrosine kinases or phospholipid turnover. The

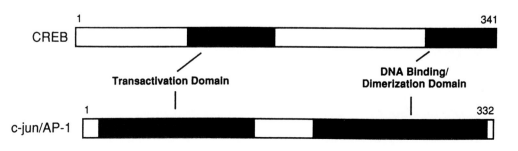

FIGURE 3–28. Schematic diagram of two transcription factors: CREB and AP-1. (From Kahn CR, Smith RJ, Chin WW: Mechanism of action of hormones that act at the cell surface. *In* Wilson JD, Foster DW: Williams Textbook of Endocrinology. Philadelphia, WB Saunders Co., 1992, p 108.)

DNA-binding activity of jun is regulated by serine-threonine phosphorylations of amino-terminal (stimulatory) and carboxy-terminal (inhibitory) residues. Two signaling pathways lead to activation of jun. Stimulation of raf kinase and mitogen-activated protein kinase by receptor-linked tyrosine kinases results in phosphorylation of the stimulatory sites of jun by an unidentified kinase, whereas protein kinase C stimulates phosphatase activity, which dephosphorylates the inhibitory sites.[234]

The family of CREB proteins consists of at least eight members, with the same DNA sequence specificity (*TGACTCA*), of which only one has been established as a mediator of cAMP action. CREB protein forms transcriptionally active homodimers as well as heterodimers with members of the jun/fos family. CREB protein contains three phosphorylation sites in its amino-terminal half, of which at least one, serine,[133] is known to be involved in regulation of the DNA-binding activity. CREB protein is activated in response to extracellular signals that elevate cAMP levels. cAMP binds to the regulatory subunit of cAMP-dependent protein kinase, allowing the catalytic subunit to dissociate and translocate into the nucleus, where it phosphorylates cAMP response element protein on Ser[133]. Protein phosphatase-1 has been implicated in dephosphorylation and inactivation of CREB protein.

SIF and IFSG-3 are related transcription factors that are induced by PDGF (v-*sis* encodes the PDGF B-chain) and interferon-γ, respectively. The DNA binding activities bind to two DNA response elements, *sis*-inducible element and interferon-γ–activated site.[231] Sequence similarities between the two DNA elements suggest that IFSG-3 and SIF represent similar if not identical transcription factors. These two transcription factors consist of complexes of three or more proteins and one subunit p91 is common to both. A latent form of p91 is present in the cytoplasm and becomes phosphorylated on tyrosine in cells stimulated with interferon-γ, EGF, PDGF, CSF-1, or IL-10. The presence of an SH2 domain on p91 suggests that this protein may interact directly with the receptor-linked tyrosine kinases. The phosphorylated active form of p91 subunit is translocated to the nucleus and binds to the specific DNA sequences.[235–237] As discussed above, this pathway may represent an alternative mechanism for growth factor-induced cell proliferation.

RECEPTOR SIGNALING NETWORK

Most of the fundamental concepts of receptor signaling have been based on the cascade or second messenger model of hormone action. However, difficulty exists in explaining the specificity of hormone action with this classical model, because components of signal transduction are shared or activated by different classes of signaling molecules (see Table 3–6). For example, in any single cell several peptide hormones, catecholamines, and other ligands with different functions may be capable of stimulating adenylate cyclase. This is further confused by the finding that many of the proteins in this pathway of hormone action exist in a number of isoforms. Thus many receptors belong to closely related families and/or exist in several isoforms. There is a very large and complex family of G proteins,

different isoforms of adenylate cyclase, multiple phospholipases, and several forms of cAMP-dependent protein kinase and protein kinase C that can be activated or inhibited by different receptors with types of signaling mechanisms. Likewise, the intracellular serine-threonine phosphorylation and dephosphorylation cascade, involving enzymes such as the mitogen-activated kinases, is activated by ligands as divergent as growth factors (EGF, PDGF, FGF), hormones (insulin, GH), cytokines (IL, interferons), lectins, and antigens, which use different receptors and different intracellular signal transduction systems. On the other hand, it appears that many complex cellular responses, such as cell proliferations, depend on activation of multiple pathways. Finally it has become clear that cross-talk between signaling pathways is not simply the result of counteracting forces on the level of second messengers or stimulation of counteracting enzymes (e.g., kinases and phosphatases) but involves subtle complexities of interaction that could not easily be accommodated in the classic models of hormone action.

MULTIPLE SIGNALING AND INTERACTING SIGNAL PATHWAYS. An important clue to how these complex and interacting signaling pathways could provide both specificity and necessary divergent signals required for complex mitogenic processes has begun to emerge through studies of the phosphotyrosine-SH2 domain interaction involved in signaling by the receptor tyrosine kinases. Whereas proteins as diverse as enzymes, adaptor molecules, and structural proteins all contain SH2 domains, all SH2 domains are equivalent to or bind to the same types of phosphorylation motifs. Indeed, each SH2 domain and each phosphorylation motif appears to dictate a specific type of protein-protein interaction, in many ways similar to that of an intracellular ligand interacting with an intracellular receptor. Different phosphotyrosine-containing receptors and receptor substrates possess different types of phosphorylation sites capable of engaging different SH2 domain proteins. The structural features of the phosphorylation motifs confer varying degrees of SH2 domain specificity and binding affinity. The PDGF receptor, for example, is capable of binding p85 subunit of phosphatidylinositol 3-kinase, ras GTPase-activating protein, and phospholipase C-γ at different sites on the receptor, whereas the phosphorylation motifs of insulin receptor substrate-1 bind p85 subunit of phosphatidylinositol 3-kinase, GRB2, and SH2 domain phosphotyrosine phosphatase-2 but not phospholipase C-γ or ras GTPase-activating protein. Furthermore, in some cases the noncovalent interaction activates the associated enzymes (e.g., phosphatidylinositol 3-kinase), whereas in other cases the binding is not activating (PDGF receptor and phospholipase C-8).

These recent observations provide an important refinement of our previous models of receptor signaling. The basic concept of a receptor ligand interaction being the lock and key to activation of a linear, amplifying cascade of reactions leading to the final biological effects of the ligand is clearly oversimplified and thus usually untrue. More often, the ligand receptor interaction produces several types of intracellular signals through noncovalent interaction as well as direct chemical modification (i.e., SH2 domain binding and substrate phosphorylation by a tyrosine kinase). Diverse ligands and diverse receptors produce similar types of early activating signals. This accounts for the finding that many of these ligands activate a number of similar or identical intracellular enzymatic pathways. The difference in the final biological response depends not only on the nature of tissue distribution of the receptors and their intracellular signaling components but also on the exact "combination" of signals generated. In the case of the tyrosine kinases, which act through phospholipase C-γ, ras GTPase-activating protein, phosphatidylinositol 3-kinase, and other enzymes, we might postulate that different ligands produce different combinations of effect. For example, PDGF has a combination of 25-50-25-0, whereas insulin has a combination of 0-0-50-25. Thus, even in a cell expressing each of these signaling molecules, the exact combination of events allows for overlapping, but distinct physiological effects. This system may be further fine-tuned by the molecular anatomy of the cell, i.e., compartmentalization, as well as by back-up or alternative pathways that may activate the same final effector system.

IMPLICATIONS FOR THE SIGNALING NETWORK. The notion of a network of quantitatively distinct signals, rather than a simple pathway or cascade of qualitative signals, has a number of implications with regard to ligand signaling (Fig. 3–29). First, it is clear that, in such a model, convergent as well as divergent pathways of intracellular signaling are important in generating the final biological response. This response to ligand stimulation is activation of multiple signaling enzymes and/or generation of several signaling molecules; the final response depends on some quantitative combination of these signals. The fact that signaling systems form a closely linked network of very different types of signaling molecules helps explain the cross-talk that occurs between different signaling systems within the cell. The ability of one ligand to affect, both positively and negatively, the actions of another ligand is accommodated by their ability not only to have similar or different effects on one pathway of hormone action but also to have differ-

ing effects on different components of this integrated network.

How many different pathways or systems may be involved in the actions of a single ligand is difficult to predict. Even pathways that thus far have been difficult to link to biological responses such as receptor internalization, and the impact of covalent or noncovalent modifications, may play important roles in modifying the quantity of the signal, even when they do not modify the quality of the signal. Indeed, multicomponent signaling may be required to generate specific metabolic responses, as well as the complex growth response. Finally, this type of networking may explain some of the complex signaling phenomena observed with hormones and growth factors acting through conventional second messenger systems, such as the adenylate cyclase system. As with the receptors acting through intracellular kinases and serine, threonine, or tyrosine phosphorylations, the G protein–coupled receptors may also undergo covalent modification by phosphorylation, which may affect association with other signaling molecules, effectiveness of coupling and/or desensitization, and subcellular distribution.

RECEPTOR REGULATION AND MECHANISMS OF DESENSITIZATION

Relationship Between Receptor and Effect

The quantitative relationship and stoichiometry between the molecules involved in signaling is complex. Since the concentration of hormones and growth factors is usually very low (between 10^{-12} and 10^{-10} M) and the K_d of the receptor is higher (in the range of 10^{-10} to 10^{-8} M), the receptor will not reach full occupancy under physiological conditions. Furthermore, the receptor concentration on the cell surface is generally low (between 10^{-12} and 10^{-10} M) compared with the intracellular concentration of effectors and second messengers, which is between 10^{-8} and 10^{-6} M, indicating that maximal activation will not be achieved. Consequently, target cells must amplify the signal in order to control cellular processes that operate on substrates in the concentration range of 10^{-6} to 10^{-3} M. This amplification occurs at both the receptor and effector levels and includes the spare "receptor" and "nonlinear coupling" phenomena described below. It should be emphasized, however, that although the signal amplification is functionally well characterized, the underlying molecular mechanisms are not clear.

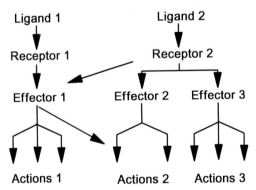

FIGURE 3–29. **Network of receptor signaling.** Convergent as well as divergent pathways of intracellular signaling are important in generating the final biological response. One ligand interacts with its receptor and activates multiple signaling enzymes with generation of several signaling molecules. A second ligand interacts with its receptor and affects, both positively and negatively, the actions of the other ligand. This cross-talk between different signaling systems within the cell is accommodated by the ability of the ligands not only to have similar or different effects on one signaling pathway but also by having differing effects on different components of this integrated network. The final biological actions depend on quantitative combination of these signals. (Modified from Kahn CR, Smith RJ, Chin WW: Mechanism of action of hormones that act at the cell surface. *In* Wilson JD, Foster DW: Williams Textbook of Endocrinology. Philadelphia, WB Saunders Co., 1992, p 102.)

Spare Receptors and Effector Coupling

At the level of the receptor, many hormones and transmitters produce a maximal biological response with only a fraction of the total cell surface receptors occupied (Fig. 3–30). For example, insulin stimulation of glucose transport in adipocytes is maximal when only about 2 per cent of all insulin receptors are occupied.[238, 239] Similar observations have been made for the actions of ACTH on glucocorticoid production in the adrenal and gonadotropins on steroidogenesis in the ovary and testis.[240] This phenomenon has given rise to the term *spare receptors*. The concept

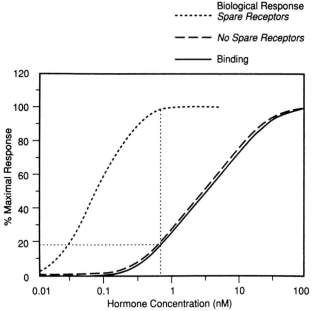

FIGURE 3–30. Correlation between agonist binding and cellular response. Effect of spare receptors to amplify signal. The solid line represents a hormone binding to its receptor. The dashed line indicates a biological response in which there are no spare receptors. The dotted line indicates a response for which there are spare receptors. In the last case, the maximal biological response occurs with less than 20 per cent receptor occupancy. (Modified from Kahn CR, Smith RJ, Chin WW: Mechanism of action of hormones that act at the cell surface. *In* Wilson JD, Foster DW: Williams Textbook of Endocrinology. Philadelphia, WB Saunders Co., 1992, p 100.)

of spare receptors implies that the maximal hormonal response occurs with less than maximal receptor occupancy. A second, more subtle dissociation between occupancy and action may also occur in the form of *nonlinear coupling*. In this case, there is amplification of the signal such that the half-maximal effect occurs with less than 50 per cent of the occupancy required for a maximal effect. Often nonlinear coupling and spare receptors occur together.

These phenomena play important physiological roles in both the kinetics of hormone action and the potential for regulation in disease states. Since the value of K_d of most membrane receptors is somewhat higher than the concentration of the hormone, the reaction of hormone binding to its receptor would proceed slowly if it were not for the presence of a relative excess of receptors on the cell surface. These excess receptors drive the reaction forward, especially at low ligand concentrations. Likewise, as the concentration of hormones and growth factors in the extracellular fluid fluctuates, the presence of the spare receptors that have been occupied by the hormone allows the signal to persist as the concentration decreases. Similar types of signal amplification occur at intracellular effectors of hormone action. For example, hormones that act through stimulation of adenylyl cyclase and accumulation of cAMP usually produce much more cAMP than is required for maximal activation of cAMP-dependent protein kinase. Likewise, cAMP-dependent protein kinase is usually activated beyond the level required for maximal substrate phosphorylation. Thus there is a series of increasingly sensitive dose-response curves as the hormonal signal is amplified at each step in its action pathway.

Spare receptors and signal amplification defines hormone and neurotransmitter response patterns in physiological and pathological states in which one or more steps in the signaling pathway are altered. In a system that has no spare receptors or effector amplification, a 50 per cent decrease in receptor number would result in a parallel 50 per cent decrease in the final biological response. By contrast, a 50 per cent fall in receptor number in a system that has many spare receptors produces only a small (two-fold) rightward shift in the dose-response curve for hormone action (i.e., decreased sensitivity with no change in maximal response). A decrease in maximal response occurs only when receptor concentration falls to very low levels (Fig. 3–31). Analysis of the relationship between the concentration and action of an agonist in a pathological state can provide insights into the mechanism of the altered response. In states of hormone or neurotransmitter resistance there may be decreased sensitivity to the agonists (i.e., a rightward shift in the dose-response curve with no change in maximal response) (Fig. 3–32). This implies a defect at a step that is not rate-limiting. This is the case often at the level of the receptor in cells with spare receptors but may also be at the level of effector involved in amplification. In states of decreased sensitivity, increasing the agonist concentration will overcome the resistance and eventually produce a normal biological response. In some states of hormone or neurotransmitter resistance, there is a decrease in the maximal response—that is, decreased responsiveness, occurring with or without a concomitant decrease in sensitivity. Decreased responsiveness implies a defect at some rate-limiting step in the signaling pathway. Usually, but not always, this is at the level of intracellular effectors. In such states, increasing agonist concentrations produce increasing response only up to a point, such that maximal response is never normal.[241]

HOMOLOGOUS RECEPTOR REGULATION. A number of physiological and pathological factors can affect the binding affinity, number, and signal transmission ability of membrane receptors and play a role in disease (Table 3–11). These regulators of receptor binding and signal transduction may result in desensitization or hypersensitization of a cellular response. The regulatory response may be classified by the site of regulatory action (i.e., factors that alter receptor binding versus factors affecting receptor or effector signaling and by the nature of the regulatory factor: homologous regulation referring to effects of the agonist itself and heterologous regulation caused by effects of other agonists such as hormones, neurotransmitters, or drugs.)

Desensitization of signal transduction may occur through a variety of processes, including receptor internalization or receptor uncoupling mediated by receptor phosphorylation. In many target cells, ligand-induced internalization of the receptor produces an increase in the fraction of receptors located intracellularly and undergoing degradation.[123, 125] Ultimately, the degradation of receptors leads to *down-regulation* of receptor number on the cell surface. This negative homologous regulation is characteristic for polypeptide hormones and growth factors.[242, 243] Teleologically it can be viewed as a simple negative feedback loop that functions to decrease receptor concentration when agonist concentrations are chronically elevated, thus "protecting" the cell against the excessive hormone

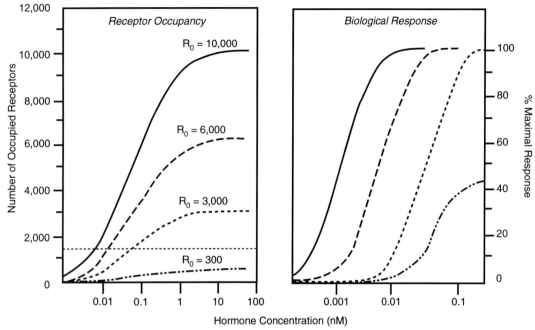

FIGURE 3–31. **Effect of spare receptors on signaling after reduction of receptors.** The original hormone binding curve *(solid line)* for receptors with K_d = 0.1 nM and total receptor concentration, R_0 = 10,000 per cell corresponds to a biological response curve *(solid line)* with ED_{50} = 0.001 nM and a maximal response with about 18 per cent receptor occupancy. When the number of receptors per cell is gradually reduced, there is at each hormone concentration a proportional reduction in the concentration of hormone-receptor complex and in biological response and a shift in the dose-response curve to the right *(stipled lines)*. Because only about 18 per cent receptor occupancy is needed to achieve a maximal response, the maximal biological response is reduced only when the total receptor concentration R_0 falls below the level of about 1800/cell. (Modified from Kahn CR, Smith RJ, Chin WW: Mechanism of action of hormones that act at the cell surface. *In* Wilson JD, Foster DW: Williams Textbook of Endocrinology. Philadelphia, WB Saunders Co, 1992, p 101.)

or neurotranmitter actions. In reality, the regulation process is often imperfect, with a small increase in agonist concentration producing a relatively large amount of down-regulation, thus leading to a hormone-resistant state.

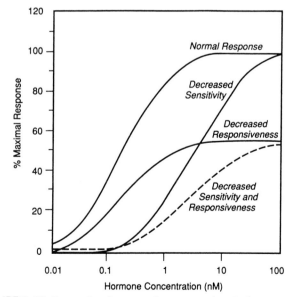

FIGURE 3–32. **Types of resistance to hormone action.** In hormone-resistant states there may be a rightward shift of the dose-response curve (decreased sensitivity), a decrease in maximal response (decreased responsiveness), or a combination of the two. (Adapted from Kahn CR: Insulin resistance, insulin sensitivity and insulin unresponsiveness: A necessary distinction. Metabolism 27(Suppl 2):1893–1902, 1978.)

Although most agonists produce down-regulation of their receptors, some hormones or growth factors such as prolactin may act as homologous positive regulators. In this case exposure of cells to prolactin increased receptor synthesis.[244] This in turn results in increased receptor number and cellular responsiveness to the hormone and provides a positive feedback loop in hormonal response.

The other form of homologous regulation of receptors is agonist-induced desensitization of G protein–coupled receptors.[61, 245] It was first described for the β-adrenergic receptors that the agonist-stimulated signal attenuates rapidly even in the continual presence of the stimulus. Homologous desensitization of the $β_2$-adrenergic receptor occurs through agonist-activated receptor phosphorylation that is catalyzed by a specific receptor kinase called β-adrenergic receptor kinase. This kinase recognizes only the ligand-occupied receptor, phosphorylates it on serine residues, and alters the subsequent coupling of the receptor with G proteins leading to cellular desensitization to β-agonists.[62] Originally it was believed that β-adrenergic receptor phosphorylation and desensitization were due to the action of cAMP-dependent protein kinase that is stim-

TABLE 3–11. FACTORS AFFECTING RECEPTOR BINDING AND SIGNALING

Homologous agonist	Membrane lipids
Heterologous agonists	Cell growth and differentiation
Ions and small molecules	Viral infection
Drugs	Antibodies to receptor
Covalent modifications	

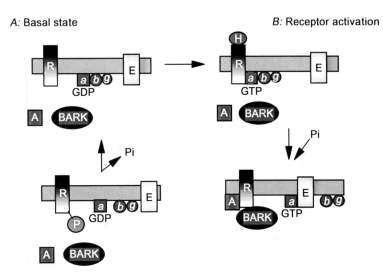

A: Basal state

B: Receptor activation

D: Receptor desensitization

C: Receptor phosphorylation

FIGURE 3–33. **Homologous desensitization of the β_2-adrenergic receptor.** Agonist binding to the β_2-adrenergic receptor activates a specific β-adrenergic receptor kinase (BARK) that phosphorylates serine residues in the cytoplasmic domains of the ligand-occupied receptor. The phosphorylation alters the subsequent coupling of the receptor with G protein (abg) leading to cellular desensitization to β-agonists. Binding of β-arrestin (A) to phosphorylated receptors further quenches signal transduction.

ulated by β-adrenergic agonists. Further quenching of signal transduction requires the binding of the protein β-arrestin to phosphorylated receptors (Fig. 3–33). Three receptor kinases (rhodopsin kinase and β-adrenergic receptor kinase-1 and -2) have been identified, and three arrestins are known (arrestin, arrestin-1, and arrestin-2). The β-adrenergic receptor kinase and arrestin isoforms are widely distributed, suggesting that they may have broad receptor specificity regulating several G protein–coupled receptors. The molecular mechanism involved has been elucidated with mapping of serine phosphorylation sites in the cytoplasmic domains of the β_2-adrenergic receptor.

HETEROLOGOUS RECEPTOR REGULATION. There are many examples that positive heterologous regulation of receptors plays an essential role in the intercellular communication characteristic of the endocrine and paracrine systems. FSH stimulates the production of LH receptors in the ovary leading to normal maturation of the ovum.[246] Prolactin also potentiates LH action in the Leydig cell, in part by increasing the number of LH receptors. Thyroid hormone augments the expression of β-adrenergic receptors, and this accounts for some of the findings of a hyperadrenergic state in hyperthyroid patients.[247] Estrogens cause an increase in the number of oxytocin receptors in the uterus and also augment the effect of prolactin on increasing expression of prolactin receptor number in mammary tissues.[248] Examples of negative heterologous regulation include β-adrenergic agents and growth factors such as PDGF, which down-regulate the EGF receptor by activation of protein kinases A and C and serine phosphorylation of the EGF receptor.[249] Some hormones exert both positive and negative effects by acting at different points in the hormone action cascade and thus produce a complex combination of effects. Glucocorticoids, for example, lower insulin receptor binding affinity in adipose tissue but increase receptor expression at a transcriptional level in lymphoid tissue.[250] Glucocorticoids also increase the synthesis of many insulin counter-regulatory enzymes at the transcriptional level. A variety of other factors, including ions, covalent modifications, drugs, membrane lipids, cell growth and differentiation, viral infection, and antibodies may also alter receptor binding and signal transduction properties

(Table 3–11). Although our knowledge of receptor regulation is still quite incomplete, it is apparent that physiological effects of hormones, growth factors, and neurotransmitters are regulated as much at the level of signal transduction in the target cell as at the level of alterations in their biosynthesis or secretion.

MEMBRANE RECEPTORS AND DISEASE

In pathological states, alterations of receptor function and signal transduction can lead to abnormalities in cellular responsiveness to hormones or neurotransmitters that cause or contribute to the clinical disorder. Most of these clinical disease states are characterized by hormone resistance rather than increased hormone responsiveness. Five conditions affecting receptors and signaling molecules can be involved in the pathogenesis of various clinical disorders: genetic defects in receptors and effector molecules, abnormal receptor regulation, antibodies to receptors, receptor specificity crossover, and receptor oncogenes. These conditions affect all three major signal transduction pathways: G protein–coupled receptors, receptor tyrosine kinases, and ligand-gated ion channels, leading to a variety of diseases. Because of the broad scope of this review, we focus on representative examples. These should be considered, however, simply as model systems that may be representative of the role of membrane receptors in diseases in general.

GENETIC DEFECTS IN RECEPTORS. An increasing number of receptor mutations have been described in various disorders following the cloning of receptor cDNA's and genes that rendered molecular genetic analysis possible. Most of these mutants are found in autosomal inherited disorders, although somatic mutations in receptor genes have been described. These mutations range from missense mutations with substitution of a single amino acid to nonsense mutations with amino acid chain termination and truncation of the receptor polypeptide chain or in rare cases complete absence of receptor. Depending on the location of the mutated amino acid residue in the receptor protein, receptor function may be affected and various functional disturbances may emerge. These include loss of function mutations with impairment of receptor biosynthesis, trafficking, and signaling, and gain of function mutations with constitutive activation of receptor signaling. Mutations that affect the post-translational modification of the receptor (glycosylation, peptide chain cleavage, oligomerization, folding) or receptor trafficking (internalization, recycling, degradation) may lead to reduced receptor expression at the cell surface. Mutations that affect receptor function (ligand binding, oligomerization, G protein coupling, tyrosine kinase activation, ion channel opening) may lead to impaired signaling. It should be emphasized, however, that the largest number of receptor mutations, some of which represent natural DNA polymorphism among individuals, are silent and without functional significance. A limited number of clinically significant mutations affecting members of the three major receptor families and their signaling systems have been described leading to endocrinological, neurological, immunological, or developmental disorders. Six receptor gene defects are discussed here (Table 3–12).

More than 20 mutations of different residues in the insulin receptor have been described that are associated with varying degrees of insulin resistance.[251–253] These mutations are located in all portions of the insulin receptor and affect receptor functions with regard to biosynthesis, trafficking, and signaling (Fig. 3–34). Three syndromes of severe insulin resistance appear to result from genetic defects in the insulin receptor or insulin action pathways; these are the Type A syndrome of insulin resistance, leprechaunism, and lipoatrophic diabetes. In addition to insulin resistance and glucose intolerance or overt diabetes, these syndromes share a number of common features, including variable degrees of acanthosis nigricans and hyperandrogenism. The *Type A syndrome of insulin resistance* has been described as extreme insulin resistance, acanthosis nigricans, and hyperandrogenism occurring in the absence of obesity or lipoatrophy. It is distinguished from Type B insulin resistance by the lack of antibodies to the insulin receptor or other evidence of autoimmune disease. Identification of the molecular and biochemical defects in patients with Type A insulin resistance indicates that this is a heterogeneous group of disorders. Patients have been observed to have reduced to normal levels of insulin receptor mRNA, expression of abnormal, unprocessed receptors, and markedly decreased number of normal insulin receptors or receptors with decreased tyrosine kinase activity. This apparent heterogeneity is explained as specific mutations in patients with the Type A syndrome of insulin resistance. In one patient, a genetic recombination event appeared to

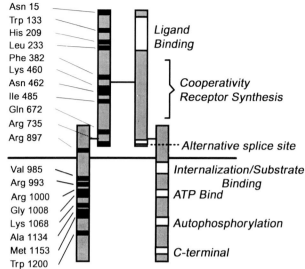

FIGURE 3–34. **Insulin receptor mutants in patients with insulin resistance.** Mutations of amino acid residues in the extracellular α subunit of the insulin receptor affect ligand binding, cooperative receptor interactions, and receptor synthesis. Alternative splicing of the carboxy-terminal end of the α subunit modifies receptor binding affinity. Mutations of residues in the cytoplasmic portion of the β subunit affects internalization, substrate binding, and tyrosine kinase activation (ATP binding, autophosphorylation). (Modified from Kahn CR, Smith RJ, Chin WW: Mechanism of action of hormones that act at the cell surface. *In* Wilson JD, Foster DW: Williams Textbook of Endocrinology. Philadelphia, WB Saunders Co, 1992, p 123.)

have resulted in the loss of the tyrosine kinase domain of the insulin receptor.[254] In another patient, a point mutation resulted in the substitution of valine for glycine in a part of the ATP-binding site of the receptor β subunit and a decrease in tyrosine kinase activity.[255] Both of these patients had decreased receptor number, suggesting that there may be an abnormality in the second insulin receptor allele or a suppressive effect of the mutant receptor. In a third patient with the Type A syndrome of insulin resistance, there was a point mutation that converted the sequence of the prereceptor cleavage site from arginine-lysine-arginine-arginine to arginine-lysine-arginine-serine.[256] This resulted in the accumulation of unprocessed receptor which binds insulin ineffectively and shows decreased tyrosine kinase activation.

The syndrome of *leprechaunism* also results from heterogeneous genetic defects. In addition to insulin resistance, patients with leprechaunism are characterized by intrauterine and neonatal growth retardation and a clinical course complicated by paradoxical fasting hypoglycemia that is usually fatal within the first year of life. In one of these patients, insulin resistance was shown to result from a compound heterozygous state with two mutant insulin receptor alleles. In one allele there was a missense mutation that converted Lys[460] to Glu[460] in the receptor α-subunit, and in the second allele there was a nonsense mutation in the α-subunit that led to chain termination.[257] The specific mechanisms through which these mutations lead to the leprechaun phenotype have not yet been defined.

The syndrome of *Laron dwarfism* is characterized by markedly decreased somatic growth evident from the first months of life and other clinical features similar to those in patients with isolated GH deficiency.[258] In contrast to the GH-deficient patients, high circulating levels of GH are

TABLE 3–12. GENETIC DEFECTS IN MEMBRANE RECEPTORS

RECEPTOR	EFFECT	DISORDER
Insulin	Decreased activity	Insulin resistance, leprechaunism, lipoatrophic diabetes
GH	Decreased activity	Laron dwarfism
LH	Constitutive activity	Precocious puberty
GHRF	Decreased activity	*Little* mouse
TSH	Constitutive activity	Thyrotoxicosis
α-MSH	Increased or constitutive activity	Darkened coat color

seen in Laron dwarfism, whereas the GH-dependent IGF-I appears to be deficient. Several mutations have been identified in these patients, including nonsense and missense mutations of GH receptor gene resulting in synthesis of nonfunctional GH receptor proteins, and the level of functionally active GH receptors in liver as well as circulating GH binding protein has been shown to be markedly decreased in affected patients.[259, 260]

Familial male precocious puberty is a gonadotropin-independent disorder that is inherited in an autosomal dominant male-limited pattern. Affected males exhibit signs of puberty by age 4 and have prepubertal levels of LH, testosterone, and Leydig cell hyperplasia. A single mutation of glycine to aspartate in the sixth transmembrane helix of the LH receptor was found in affected individuals from eight different families. This mutation was accompanied by increased cAMP production in the absence of agonist, suggesting that autonomous Leydig cell activity is caused by a constitutively activated LH receptor.[261]

GHRF is a hypothalamic regulatory peptide that controls GH production by the pituitary gland via interaction with specific GHRF receptors on somatotrophs. A genetically transmitted dwarfism in mice known as the *little* mouse has a phenotype with anterior pituitary hypoplasia and a marked decrease in glandular GH mRNA and protein. GH secretion in *little* mice can be stimulated by pharmacological agents that increase intracellular levels of cAMP. Analysis of the GHRF receptor gene in the *little* mouse revealed a point mutation that alters Asp^{60} to Gly^{60}, involving an amino acid conserved in the amino-terminal extracellular region of all the members of this family of seven-transmembrane segment, G_s protein-coupled receptors. Transfection studies of this receptor mutant showed that it was functionally defective and unable to transduce GRF-dependent increases in intracellular cAMP levels as in the normal receptor.[262]

The pituitary hormone TSH stimulates the function, expression, differentiation, and growth of thyroid cells by cAMP-dependent mechanisms. Thyroid hyperplasia and hyperthyroidism result from increased activity of the adenylate cyclase–cAMP pathway. In a group of 11 humans with hyperfunctioning thyroid adenomas, somatic mutations of the third cytoplasmic loop of the TSH receptor were identified in three cases. The mutations were restricted to the tumor tissue and involved two different residues, aspartic acid 619 to glycine in two cases, and alanine 623 to isoleucine in one case. The mutant receptors confer constitutive activation of adenylate cyclase.[263]

α-MSH is a pituitary hormone that stimulates melanin production in melanocytes and regulates hair pigmentation in mammals. α-MSH activation of the melanocortin receptor (type 1) and adenylate cyclase in cells of melanocytic origin in hair follicles results in a darkened coat color. Two point mutations in the second transmembrane domain and first cytoplasmic loop of the melanocortin receptor cause constitutive activation or hyper-responsiveness of the receptors, respectively. These mutations lead to phenotypes with dark coat color in brown mice, in the black panther, and in the black Labrador dog. Another mutation in the melanocortin receptor leads to α-MSH resistance and a phenotype with yellow coat color as in the fox and the Golden Retriever.[264]

RECEPTOR REGULATION. Cell surface receptor number is down-regulated or desensitized in response to acute exposure to extracellular agonists. Chronic exposure, however, leads to markedly decreased receptor concentrations on the cell surface and cellular resistance to the action of hormones or neurotransmitters. The binding affinity of receptors is affected by many factors including the agonist, hormones, fasting, exercise, and diet composition. In contrast to changes in receptor number, which appear to derive from modifications in the normal pathways of receptor synthesis and degradation, the molecular mechanisms that lead to altered binding affinity are less well defined. Reduction in receptor number and affinity are often associated with alterations in the signal transduction pathway leading to decreased hormone sensitivity and responsiveness.

Two conditions, obesity and non–insulin-dependent diabetes mellitus (Type II) are characterized by insulin resistance that appears to result from alterations in both receptor number and signal transduction.[265] Lower numbers of insulin-binding sites have been observed in monocytes and adipocytes from obese and Type II diabetic patients and in animal models of obesity. Characteristically, the decrease in insulin receptor number correlates inversely with the elevation in circulating insulin levels found in obese and some diabetic patients.[266] If insulin levels are lowered by diet or drugs that interfere with insulin secretion, receptor number returns to normal.[267, 268] This suggests that the decreased number of insulin receptors in insulin-resistant patients may result from receptor down-regulation induced by chronic excess of insulin. In nonobese Type II diabetic patients who do not have elevated insulin levels, receptor number is not markedly decreased, and insulin resistance appears to result primarily from abnormalities in the signaling pathway, but these have not yet been identified. In addition, coexistent defects in insulin receptor number and intracellular signaling of insulin are found in obese patients. Independent of obesity, there appear to be defects in insulin action in Type II diabetes that may result from both decreased receptor tyrosine kinase activity and more distal steps in insulin action.[269–271] The observation that insulin receptor number can be restored to normal if insulin levels are decreased in obese patients suggests that the changes in receptor number are secondary to the cellular insulin resistance and not a primary causal factor. Possibly, the intracellular alterations in insulin action initiate resistance to the hormone, insulin levels rise as a compensatory response, and this results in a decrease in insulin receptor number and even greater insulin resistance.

ANTIRECEPTOR ANTIBODIES. In a subgroup of autoimmune disorders antireceptor antibodies are generated and play an important role in the pathogenesis of the clinical state of deficient or excess agonist action. Disorders resulting from either inhibitory or stimulatory antibodies have been described for insulin, TSH, and β-adrenergic and acetylcholine receptors (see Table 3–13, p. 58). Although the basis for disorders with antireceptor antibodies has not been defined, it is likely related to some alteration in specific immune response genes because some patients exhibit more than one type of autoimmune disease.

The most common endocrine disorder in which antireceptor antibodies play an important role is *Graves' disease*.[272] Patients with Graves' disease have circulating antibodies to diverse thyroid cell surface antigens including the TSH receptor that was originally described more than

30 years ago as the "long-acting thyroid stimulator" (LATS).[273] The stimulatory activity of LATS on thyroid cell growth and hormone production results from anti-TSH receptor antibodies. These antibodies activate the TSH receptor and thyroid secretion of triiodothyronine (T_3) and thyroxine (T_4), resulting in the thyrotoxicosis that occurs in Graves' disease (Fig. 3–35). In occasional patients, anti-TSH receptor antibodies are inhibitory rather than stimulatory and lead to myxedema. In the course of the disease in a single patient, the nature of receptor antibodies in the circulating pool can shift over time from stimulatory to inhibitory and back to stimulatory. Anti-TSH receptor antibodies are important not only in defining the pathogenesis for abnormal thyroid function in Graves' disease but also in monitoring response to therapy.[274]

Antibodies to the insulin receptor were first identified in

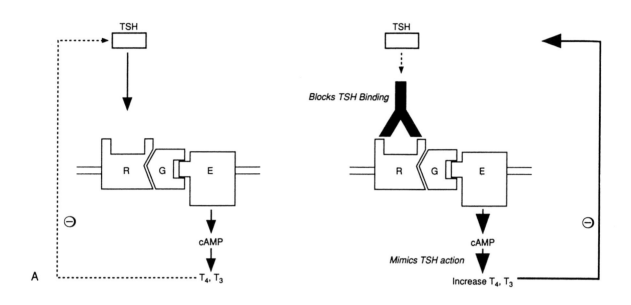

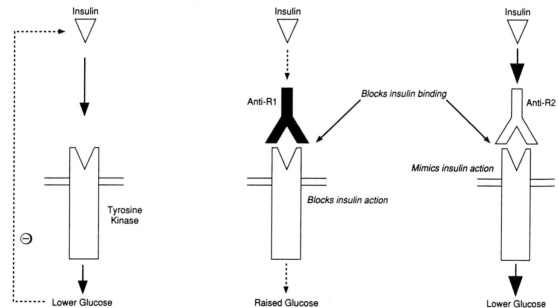

FIGURE 3–35. *A,* TSH receptor antibodies in patients with Graves' disease. In normal individuals TSH binds to its specific receptor (R) on thyroid cells coupled to a stimulatory G protein (G) and activates adenylate cyclase (E). Increase in cAMP leads to release of T_3 and T_4. Thyroid hormones reduce TSH secretion from the pituitary by a negative feedback effect on the hypothalamus. In patients with Graves' disease, blocking autoantibodies bind to the TSH receptor and stimulate cAMP production as TSH, which results in release of T_3 and T_4. Elevated levels of thyroid hormones suppress TSH secretion but have no effect on circulating levels of TSH receptor antibodies. *B,* In normal individuals insulin binds to its specific receptor and activates the intrinsic tyrosine kinase. Increased glucose metabolism lowers circulating glucose levels. Two types of insulin receptor antibodies (anti-R1 and anti-R2) block insulin binding and block or mimic insulin action. These antibodies produce hyperglycemia or hypoglycemia and are associated with low, normal, or high plasma insulin levels. (From Kahn CR, Smith RJ, Chin WW: Mechanism of action of hormones that act at the cell surface. *In* Wilson JD, Foster DW: Williams Textbook of Endocrinology. Philadelphia, WB Saunders Co, 1992, p 126.)

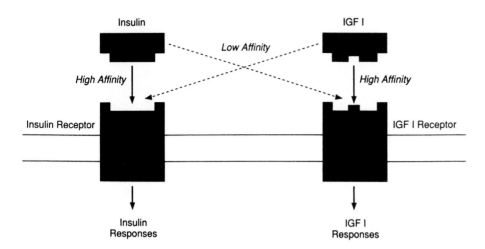

FIGURE 3–36. **Specificity crossover between insulin and IGF-I.** Insulin and IGF-I bind to and activate the specific receptor for the other with approximately 100-fold lower potency than its own receptor. (From Kahn CR, Smith RJ, Chin WW: Mechanism of action of hormones that act at the cell surface. *In* Wilson JD, Foster DW: Williams Textbook of Endocrinology. Philadelphia, WB Saunders Co, 1992, p 126.)

patients with a rare syndrome (Type B) of severe insulin resistance characterized by glucose intolerance, diabetes mellitus, extreme hyperinsulinemia, insulin resistance, acanthosis nigricans, as well as evidence of autoimmune disease.[275, 276] Most patients have high levels of polyclonal IgG antibodies that bind to the insulin receptor and block hormone binding (Fig. 3–35). Antibody binding to the receptor is followed initially by the stimulation of metabolic effects that mimic the response to insulin binding. Subsequently, the antibodies appear to induce receptor down-regulation and insulin resistance. It is of interest that these antibodies only mimic hormone effects when present in a bivalent form. Monovalent (F_{ab}) antibody fragments bind to receptors and block hormone binding but do not evoke responses. This indicates the important role for receptor-receptor interactions in the initiation of insulin action. In some patients, the stimulatory anti-insulin receptor antibodies result in clinically significant hypoglycemia rather than insulin resistance. Hypoglycemia can be the presenting finding or can evolve in the course of a disease that initially presents with insulin resistance.[277]

A second form of rare insulin resistance secondary to anti-insulin receptor antibodies has been described in patients with *ataxia telangiectasia*.[278] This is an inherited autosomal recessive disorder with multisystem disease including progressive ataxia, telangiectasias, immune system abnormalities, increased incidence of neoplasia, and insulin-resistant diabetes. Most patients have decreased or undetectable IgA and IgE, and the anti-receptor antibodies belong to an unusual low-molecular-weight form of IgM.

RECEPTOR CROSS-REACTIVITY. Receptors and their ligands are classified into families with structural similarities that reflect their evolution from common ancestral molecules.[279] These structural homologies can result in the binding of a given agonist, albeit with lower affinity, to the receptors for another agonist. This cross-reactivity of hormone binding is illustrated for insulin and IGF-I and their respective receptors in Figure 3–36. In diseases in which there are elevated hormone levels, receptor crossover can result from the activation of receptors for one hormone through low-affinity binding of another hormone.

Examples of clinical disorders with receptor cross-reactivity are described in Table 3–14. In acromegaly, high levels of GH lead to abnormal tissue growth through the activation of GH receptors.[280] In a significant number of patients, there is also evidence of excess prolactin activity, with resulting galactorrhea, amenorrhea, and infertility. In some cases, this results from concurrent elevations of both GH and prolactin levels; however, in the majority of patients prolactin levels are normal and the hyperprolactinemia syndrome is explained by binding of GH to prolactin receptors. Similar hormone receptor cross-reactivity appears to explain the occurrence of hyperthyroidism in some patients with trophoblastic tumors. Trophoblastic tumor tissue not only produces large quantities of CG, which can bind with low affinity to the TSH receptor, but also in many cases variants of CG are produced which exhibit even greater affinity for TSH receptors than the CG of normal pregnancy.[281] Nonpancreatic neoplasms that produce large quantities of IGF-II can lead to clinically significant hypoglycemia, although it is not clear whether this results from IGF-II binding to insulin receptors or IGF-I receptors or both.[282, 283] Other disorders that may represent receptor crossover include the hyperandrogenism of certain forms of severe insulin resistance resulting from cross-reactivity of insulin with ovarian IGF-I receptors and possibly macrosomia in infants of diabetic mothers insulin cross-reactivity with IGF-I receptors in somatic tissues.

RECEPTORS AND ONCOGENES. A number of genes have been identified whose products are involved in regulating normal cell growth. In addition, more than 50 genes have been identified that are capable of inducing a transformed,

TABLE 3–13. CLINICAL DISORDERS ASSOCIATED WITH AUTOANTIBODIES TO MEMBRANE RECEPTORS

SYNDROME	RECEPTOR	CLINICAL FEATURES
Graves' disease	TSH	Thyrotoxicosis (stimulatory antibody; phases of hypothyroidism due to inhibitory antibodies)
Type B insulin resistance	Insulin	Insulin-resistant diabetes, acanthosis nigricans, evidence of autoimmune disease
Ataxia telangiectasia	Insulin	Insulin-resistant diabetes, progressive ataxia, telangiectasia
Myasthenia gravis	Acetylcholine	Muscle weakness

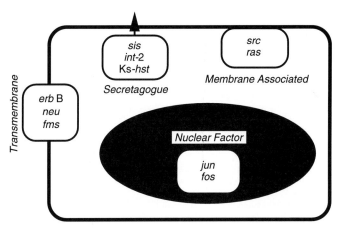

FIGURE 3–37. **Cellular localization of oncogenes.** Oncogenes encode four categories of constitutively active cellular proteins: secretagogue (autocrine growth factors), transmembrane (receptors tyrosine kinases), membrane-associated (small G proteins or tyrosine kinases), and nuclear factors (transcription factors). (From Kahn CR, Smith RJ, Chin WW: Mechanism of action of hormones that act at the cell surface. *In* Wilson JD, Foster DW: Williams Textbook of Endocrinology. Philadelphia, WB Saunders Co, 1992, p 128.)

TABLE 3–14. RECEPTOR CROSS-REACTIVITY INVOLVING PEPTIDE HORMONES

CROSS-REACTING HORMONE	RECEPTOR	CLINICAL DISORDER
GH	Prolactin	Galactorrhea (with acromegaly)
hCG	TSH	Hyperthyroidism (with trophoblastic tumors)
Insulin	IGF-I (in ovary)	Hyperandrogenism (with insulin resistance)
Insulin	IGF-I	Macrosomia (in newborn infants of diabetic mothers)
IGF-II	Insulin	Hypoglycemia (with certain tumors)

cellular phenotype and that have been termed oncogenes.[284–286] It is now clear that growth control genes on the one hand and oncogenes on the other hand are largely one and the same. Although unequivocal evidence for this idea was obtained only recently, the concept itself emerged gradually beginning with the discovery of viral oncogenes (v-*onc* genes) and the fact that these genes represent cell-derived sequences (termed proto-oncogenes, cellular oncogenes, or c-*onc*). Oncogenic viruses have developed the potential of cell transformation by means of acquiring a proto-oncogene and changing it into a viral oncogene by various mutations of the gene, resulting in amino acid substitutions and deletions in the oncogene protein that increase its transforming activity. Furthermore, an oncogene under the control of a viral promoter may be abnormally regulated and the oncogene protein product overexpressed, leading to increased mitogenic signaling. Retroviral oncogenes have been identified as a cause of cancer in a variety of animal species, but not in humans.

In human cancer somatic mutations of proto-oncogenes that lead to gene amplification, overexpression, aberrant expression, or constitutive activation of oncogene proteins have been detected. The increased activity of these oncogene products may contribute to the development and maintenance of the tumor.

Several proto-oncogenes encoding growth factors, receptors, signaling molecules, and transcription factors involved in normal growth control have turned out to have oncogenic potential.[286, 287] Oncogene products can act at all levels in cellular signal transduction from the cell surface to the nucleus (Fig. 3–37). Examples include growth factors such as PDGF and FGF, receptor tyrosine kinases (EGF and CSF-1 receptors), signaling molecules (ras and src), and transcription factors (jun-fos and myc) (Table 3–15). Each of these oncogenes may be overexpressed, aberrantly expressed, or constitutively activated, leading to uncontrolled cell growth.[288, 289] The simian sarcoma virus contains a retroviral oncogene, v-*sis*, that encodes the β subunit of PDGF. This subunit forms an active dimer that is a potent mitogen, and overexpression of v-*sis* in a variety of cells leads to cell transformation and tumor growth.[290] Two oncogenes, *int*-2 and *hst*, are detected in murine and human tumors that encode proteins of the FGF family.[291]

The avian erythroblastosis virus contains an oncogene, v-*erb* B, that encodes a form of the EGF receptor truncated in the amino-terminal, in the ligand-binding domain, and in the carboxy-terminal, regulatory domain.[292] The v-*erb* B

TABLE 3–15. GROWTH FACTOR RECEPTORS AND ONCOGENES

ONCOGENE	ACTIVITY	SOURCE	MODE OF ACTIVATION
v-*sis*	PDGF β-chain	Simian retrovirus	Retroviral activation
int-2	βFGF	Murine mammary tumors	Amplification
hst	βFGF	Human tumors	Amplification
v-*erb* B	EGF-receptor	Avian retroviruses	Truncation; point mutations
neu	Human EGF-receptor 2	Rat neuroblastoma	Point mutation
v-*fms*	CSF-1 receptor	Feline retrovirus	Point mutations; truncation
trk	NGF receptor	Human colon carcinoma	Truncation
v-*src*	Tyrosine kinase	Avian retrovirus	Point mutations
v-*abl*	Tyrosine kinase	Murine retrovirus	Rearrangement
v-*H-ras*	GTPase	Murine retrovirus	Point mutations
v-*K-ras*	GTPase	Murine retrovirus	Point mutations
v-*N-ras*	GTPase	Human neuroblastoma	Point mutation
v-*raf*	Serine-threonine kinase	Mouse sarcoma virus	Truncation
v-*jun*	Transcription factor	Avian retrovirus	Truncation; point mutations
v-*fos*	Transcription factor	Murine retrovirus	Truncations
v-*myc*	Transcription factor	Retroviruses	Amplification

product is constitutively active and induces cellular transformation. v-*fms* encodes an oncogenic form of the CSF-1 receptor with a carboxy-terminal truncation and point mutations described originally in feline sarcoma virus.[293] *neu* and *trk* are two receptor oncogenes originally found in rat neuroblastoma and human colon carcinoma, respectively. *neu* corresponds to HER-2 (erb B-2) and is activated by a point mutation in the transmembrane domain.[294] *trk* represents an amino-terminally truncated form of the NGF receptor that is constitutively active.[74]

v-*src* and v-*abl* are examples of retroviral oncogenes encoding cytoplasmic tyrosine kinases that are constitutively activated by deletions of carboxy-terminal and amino-terminal domains, respectively.[295] The *ras* family of oncogenes consists of v-H-*ras* and v-K-*ras* originally discovered in mouse sarcoma virus and N-*ras* detected in human neuroblastoma.[296] Oncogenic activation of *ras* results from single-point mutations and correlates with a decrease in the ability to hydrolyze GTP. v-*raf* comes from a mouse sarcoma virus, and its serine-threonine kinase activity is increased by amino-terminal truncation.[297]

v-*fos* and v-*jun* are two retroviral oncogenes that encode transcription factors of the AP-1 family and are activated by carboxy-terminal and amino-terminal deletions, respectively.[298] The v-*myc* gene was originally found in various retroviruses and encodes a nuclear DNA-binding phosphoprotein with a leucine zipper domain. *Myc* is induced by growth factors as an early gene response, but its function is not clear. Different forms of *myc* are amplified in several human tumors.[299] Finally, suppressor or recessive oncogenes encode proteins that inhibit the transformed cellular phenotype. The retinoblastoma (Rb) susceptibility gene encodes a 105-kDa nuclear protein involved in the regulation of the cell cycle apparently by binding to and regulating cellular transcription factors such as E2F.[300] Mutations of both copies of the Rb gene occur in a wide variety of tumors, yielding cells that no longer express a functional Rb protein.

REFERENCES

Introduction

1. Langley JN: On nerve endings and on special excitable substances. Proc R Soc Lond 78:170–194, 1906.
2. Ehrlich P: Nobel lecture (1908) on partial functions of the cell. *In* Himmelwelt M, Marquardt M, Dale H (eds): The Collected Papers of P. Ehrlich. Vol. 3. Oxford, Pergamon, 1956, pp 183–194.
3. Pastan I, Roth J, Macchia V: Binding of hormone to tissue: The first step in polypeptide hormone action. Proc Natl Acad Sci USA 56:1802–1809, 1966.
4. Kono T: Destruction of insulin effector system of adipose tissue cells by proteolytic enzymes. J Biol Chem 244:1772–1778, 1969.
5. Cuatrecasas P: Interaction of insulin with the cell membrane: The primary action of insulin. Proc Natl Acad Sci USA 63:450–454, 1969.
6. Sutherland EW: Studies on the mechanism of hormone action (Nobel lecture). Science 177:401–408, 1972.
7. Ross EM, Gilman AG: Biochemical properties of hormone-sensitive adenylate cyclase. Annu Rev Biochem 49:533–565, 1980.
8. Zeleznik AJ, Roth J: Demonstration of the insulin receptor in vivo in rabbits and its possible role as a reservoir for the plasma hormone. J Clin Invest 61:1363–1367, 1978.
9. Sodoyez JC, Sodoyez-Goffaux F, Giullaume M, Merchi G: ^{123}I-insulin metabolism in normal rats and humans: External detection by a scintillation camera. Science 219:865–867, 1983.
10. Eckelman WC, Reba RC, Rzeszotarski WJ, et al: External imaging of cerebral muscarinic acetylcholine receptors. Science 223:291–293, 1984.
11. Bergman RN: Toward physiological understanding of glucose tolerance. Minimal-model approach. Diabetes 38:1512–1517, 1989.

Properties of Ligand-Receptor Interaction

Direct Studies of Membrane Receptors

12. Lin SY, Goodfriend TL: Angiotensin receptors. Am J Physiol 218:1319–1328, 1970.
13. Lefkowitz RJ, Roth J, Pricer W, Pastan I: ACTH receptors in the adrenal: Specific binding of ACTH-^{125}I and the relation to adenyl cyclase. Proc Natl Acad Sci USA 65:745–752, 1970.
14. Kahn CR: Membrane receptors for hormones and neurotransmitters. J Cell Biol 70:261–286, 1976.
15. Hollenberg MD, Nexo E: Receptor binding assays. *In* Jacobs S, Cuatrecasas P (eds): Receptors and Recognition, Series B. Vol. II. London, Chapman and Hall, 1981, pp 1–31.
16. Venter C, Harrison LC: Receptor Biochemistry and Methodology, Vols. I–II. New York, Alan R. Liss, 1980–1989.
17. Gammeltoft S: Peptide Hormone Receptors. *In* Hutton JC, Siddle K (eds): Peptide Hormone Action: A Practical Approach. Oxford, Oxford University Press, 1990, pp 1–41.
18. Maron R, Taylor SI, Jackson R, Kahn CR: Analysis of insulin receptors on human lymphoblastic cell lines by flow cytometry. Diabetologia 22:118–129, 1984.
19. Katoh M, Raguet S, Zachwieja J, Djiane J, Kelly PA: Hepatic prolactin receptors in the rat: Characterization using monoclonal anti-receptor antibodies. Endocrinology 120:739–749, 1987.

Receptor-Binding Theory

20. Scatchard C: The attraction of proteins for small molecules and ions. Ann NY Acad Sci 51:660–672, 1949.
21. Kahn CR, Freychet P, Neville DM Jr, Roth J: Quantitative aspects of the insulin-receptor interaction in liver plasma membranes. J Biol Chem 249:2249–2257, 1974.
22. DeLean A, Rodbard D: Kinetics of cooperative binding. *In* O'Brien J (ed): The Receptor. Vol. II. New York, Plenum Publishing Corp., 1970, pp. 143–192.
23. DeMeyts P, Bianco AR, Roth J: Site-site interactions among insulin receptors: Characterization of the negative cooperativity. J Biol Chem 241:1877–1888, 1976.
24. Gammeltoft S: Insulin receptors: Binding kinetics and structure-function relationship of insulin. Physiological Rev 64:1321, 1984.

Ligand Specificity

25. Lefkowitz RJ, Caron MG, Stiles GL: Mechanisms of membrane-receptor regulation: Biochemical, physiological, and clinical insights derived from studies of the adrenergic receptors. N Engl J Med 310:1570, 1984.
26. Levitan ED, Schofield PR, Burt DR, et al: Structural and functional basis for GABA_A receptor heterogeneity. Nature 328:221–227, 1988.
27. Hoffman K, Wingender W, Finn FM: Correlation of adrenocorticotropic activity ACTH analogous with degree of binding to an adrenal cortical particulate preparation. Proc Natl Acad Sci USA 67:829–836, 1970.
28. Rorstad OP, Wanke I, Coy DH, et al: Selectivity of binding of peptide analogs to vascular receptors for vasoactive intestinal peptide. Mol Pharmacol 37:971–977, 1990.
29. Gether U, Johansen TE, Snider RM, et al: Different binding epitopes for substance P and a non-peptide antagonist. Nature 362:345–348, 1993.
30. Beinborn M, Lee Y-M, McBride EW, et al: A single amino acid of the cholecystokinin-B/gastrin receptor determines specificity for non-peptide antagonists. Nature 362:348–350, 1993.
31. Fong TM, Cascieri MA, Yu H, et al: Amino-aromatic interaction between histicine 197 of the neurokinin-1 receptor and CP 96345. Nature 362:350–353, 1993.
32. Blundell T, Wood S: The conformation, flexibility, and dynamics of polypeptide hormones. Annu Rev Biochem 51:123–154, 1982.
33. Abdel-Meguid SS, Shieh HS, Smith WW, et al.: Three-dimensional structure of a genetically engineered variant of porcine growth hormone. Proc Natl Acad Sci USA 84:6434–6437, 1987.

Receptor Structure: Cloning of Receptors

34. Mishina M, Kurosaki T, Tobimatsu T, et al: Expression of functional acetylcholine receptor from cloned cDNAs. Nature 307:604, 1984.

35. Ullrich A, Coussens L, Hayflick JS, et al: Human epidermal growth factor receptor cDNA sequence and aberrant expression of the amplified gene in A 431 epidermoid carcinoma cells. Nature 309:418, 1984.
36. Coussens L, Yang-Feng TL, Liao Y-C, et al: Tyrosine kinase receptor with extensive homology to EGF receptor shares chromosomal location with *neu* oncogene. Science 230:1132, 1985.
37. Schechter AL, Stern DF, Vaidyanathan L, et al: The *neu* oncogene: An *erb*-B-related gene encoding a 185,000-M, tumour antigen. Nature 312:513, 1984.
38. Yamamoto T, Ikawa S, Akiyama T, et al: Similarity of protein encoded by the human c-*erb*-B 2 gene to epidermal growth factor receptor. Nature 319:230, 1986.
39. Marchionni MA, Goodearl ADJ, Chen MS, et al: Glial growth factors are alternatively spliced *erb*2 ligands expressed in the nervous system. Nature 362:312–318, 1993.
40. Parmentier M, Libert F, Maenhaut C, et al: Molecular cloning of the thyrotropin receptor. Science 246:1620, 1989.
41. Masu Y, Nakayama K, Tamaki H, et al: cDNA cloning of bovine substance-K receptor through oocyte expression system. Nature 329:836, 1987.
42. Straub RE, Frech GC, Joho RH, Gershengorn MC: Expression cloning of a cDNA encoding the mouse pituitary thyrotropin-releasing hormone receptor. Proc Natl Acad Sci USA 87:9514–9518, 1990.
43. Abou-Samra A, et al: Expression cloning of the PTH receptor. Proc Natl Acad Sci USA 89:2732, 1992.
44. Jelinek LJ, Lok S, Rosenberg GB, et al: Expression cloning and signaling properties of the rat glucagon receptor. Science 259:1614–1616, 1993.

Families of Membrane Receptors

45. Barnard EA: Receptor classes and transmitter-gated ion channels. Trends Biochem Sci 17:368–374, 1992.
46. O'Dowd BR, Lefkowitz RJ, Caron MG: Structure of the adrenergic and related receptors. Ann Rev Neurosci 12:67–83, 1989.
47. Schlessinger J, Ullrich A: Receptor tyrosine kinases. Neuron 9:1–, 1992.
48. Nicola NA: Hemopoietic cell growth factors and their receptors. Annu Rev Biochem 58:45, 1989.

Functional Domains of Membrane Receptors

49. Nathans J, Hogness DS: Isolation, sequence analysis, and intron-exon arrangement of the gene encoding bovine rhodopsin. Cell 34:307, 1983.
50. Raming K, Krieger J, Strotman J, et al: Cloning and expression of odorant receptors. Nature 361:353–356, 1993.
51. Kobilka BK, Dixon RAF, Frielle T, cDNA for the human β2-adrenergic receptor: A protein with multiple membrane-spanning domains and encoded by a gene whose chromosomal location is shared with that of the receptor for platelet-derived growth factor, roc. Natl Acad Sci USA 84:46, 1987.
52. Kubo T, Fukuda K, Mikami A, et al: Cloning, sequencing and expression of complementary DNA encoding the muscarinic acetylcholine receptor. Nature 323:411, 1986.
53. Julius D, MacDermott AB, Axel R, Jessell TM: Molecular characterization of a functional cDNA encoding the serotonin 1c receptor. Science 241:558, 1988.
54. Bunzow JR, Van Tol HHM, Grandy DK, et al: Dopamine receptors. Cloning and expression of a rat D2 dopamine receptor cDNA. Nature 336:783, 1988.
55. Jackson TR, Blair LAC, Marshall J, et al: Angiotensin receptor. The *mas* oncogene encodes an angiotensin receptor. Nature 335:437, 1988.
56. Yokota Y, Sasai Y, Tanaka K, et al: Molecular characterization of a function cDNA for rat substance P receptor. J Biol Chem 264:17649, 1989.
57. McFarland KC, Sprengel R, Phillips HS, et al: Lutropin-choriongonadotropin receptor: An unusual member of the G protein coupled receptor family. Science 245:494–499, 1989.
58. Loosfelt H, Misrahi M, Atger M, et al: Cloning and sequencing of porcine LH-hCG receptor cDNA: Variants lacking transmembrane domain. Science 245:525–528, 1989.
59. Vu T-KH, Hung DT, Wheaton VI, Coughlin SR. Cloning of thrombin receptor. Cell 64:1057–1068, 1991.
60. Masu M, Tanabe Y, Tsuchida K, Shigemoto R, Nakanishi S: Sequence and expression of a metabotropic glutamate receptor. Nature 349:760–765, 1991.

61. Benovic JL, Bouvier M, Caron MG, Lefkowitz RJ: Regulation of adenylyl cyclase-coupled beta and adrenergic receptors. Ann Rev Cell Biol 4:405–420, 1988.
62. Dawson TM, Arriza JL, Jaworsky DE, et al: β-adrenergic receptor kinase-2 and β-arrestin-2 as mediators of odorant-induced desensitization. Science 259:825–829, 1993.
63. Yarden Y, Ullrich A: Molecular analysis of signal transduction by growth factors. Biochemistry 27:3113, 1988.
64. Ullrich A, Schlessinger J: Receptor tyrosine kinase family. Cell 61:203–200, 1990.
65. Schlessinger J: The epidermal growth factor receptor as a multifunctional allosteric protein. Biochemistry 27:3119, 1988.
66. Ullrich A, Bell JR, Chen EY, et al: Human insulin receptor and its relationship to the tyrosine kinase family of oncogenes. Nature 313:756–700, 1985.
67. Ebina Y, Ellis L, Jarnagin K, et al: The human insulin receptor cDNA: The structural basis for hormone-activated transmembrane signaling. Cell 40:747, 1985.
68. Ullrich A, Gray A, Tam AW: Insulin-like growth factor I receptor primary structure: Comparison with insulin receptor suggests structural determinants that define functional specificity. EMBO J 5:2503, 1986.
69. Yarden Y, Escobedo JA, Kuang W-J: Structure of the receptor for platelet-derived growth factor helps define a family of closely related growth factor receptors. Nature 323:226, 1986.
70. Claesson-Welsh L, Eriksson A, Westermark B, Heldin C-H: cDNA cloning and expression of the human A type PDGF receptor establishes structural similarity to the B type PDGF receptor. Proc Natl Acad Sci USA 86:4917, 1989.
71. Lee PL, Johnson DE, Cousens LS, et al: Purification and complementary DNA cloning of a receptor for basic fibroblast growth factor. Science 245:57, 1989.
72. Dionne CA, Crumley FB, Bellot F: Cloning and expression of two distinct high-affinity receptors cross-reacting with acidic and basic fibroblast growth factors. EMBO J 9:2685, 1990.
73. Sherr CJ, Rettenmier CW, Sacca R: The c-*fms* proto-oncogene product is related to the receptor for the mononuclear phagocyte growth factor, CSF-1. Cell 41:665, 1985.
74. Klein R, Jing S, Nanduri KV, et al: The *trk* encodes a receptor for nerve growth factor. Cell 65:189–197, 1991.
75. Naldini L, Weidner KM, Vigna E, et al: Scatter factor and hepatocyte growth factor are indistinguishable ligands for the MET receptor. EMBO J 10:2867–2878, 1991.
76. Garbers DL: Guanylate cyclase, a cell surface receptor. J Biol Chem 264:9103, 1989.
77. Lowe DG, Chang MS, Hellmiss R, et al: Human atrial natriuretic peptide receptor defines a new paradigm for second messenger signal transduction. EMBO J 8:1377–1384, 1989.
78. Thompson DK, Garbers DL: Guanylyl cyclase in cell signaling. Curr Opin Cell Biol 2:206–211, 1993.
79. Wrana JL, Attisano L, Carcamo J, et al: TGFβ signals through a heteromeric protein kinase receptor complex. Cell 71:1003–1014, 1992.
80. Chen R-H, Ebner R, Derynck R: Inactivation of the type II receptor reveals two receptor pathways for the diverse TGF-β activities. Science 260:1335–1338, 1993.
81. Ebner R, Chen R-H, Shum L, et al: Cloning of a type I TGF-β receptor and its effect on TGF-β binding to the type II receptor. Science 260:1344–1348, 1993.
82. Fischer EH, Charbonneau H, Tonks NK: Protein tyrosine phosphatases: A diverse family of intracellular and transmembrane enzymes. Science 253:401–406, 1991.
83. Leung DW, Spencer SA, Cachianes G: Growth hormone receptor and serum binding protein: purification, cloning and expression. Nature 330:537, 1987.
84. Edery M, Jolicoeur C, Levi-Meyrueis C, et al: Identification and sequence analysis of a second form of prolactin receptor by molecular cloning of complementary DNA from rabbit mammary gland. Proc Natl Acad Sci USA 86:950, 1989.
85. D'Andrea AD, Lodish HF, Wong GG: Expression cloning of the murine erythropoietin receptor. Cell 57:277, 1989.
86. Hatakeyama M, Tsudo M, Minamoto S, et al: Interleukin-2 receptor β chain gene: Generation of three receptor forms by cloned human α and β chain cDNA's. Science 244:551, 1989.
87. Yamasaki K, Taga T, Hirata Y, et al: Cloning and expression of the human interleukin-6 (BSF-2/IFNβ) receptor. Science 241:825, 1988.
88. Gearing DP, King JA, Gough NM, Nicola NA: Expression cloning of a receptor for human granulocyte-macrophage colony-stimulating factor. EMBO J 8:3667, 1989.

89. Uzé G, Lutfalla G, Gresser I: Genetic transfer of a functional human interferon α receptor into mouse cells: Cloning and expression of its cDNA. Cell 60:225, 1990.

90. Miyajima A, Hara T, Kitamura T: Common subunits of cytokine receptors and the functional redundancy of cytokines. Trends Biochem Sci 17:378–382, 1992.

91. Davis S, Aldrich TH, Stahl N, et al: LIFRβ and gp 130 as heterodimerizing signal transducers of the tripartite CNTF receptor. Science 260:1805–1808, 1993.

92. Murakami M, Hibi M, Nakagawa N, et al: IL-6 homodimerization of gp130 and associated activation of a tyrosine kinase. Science 260:1808–1810, 1993.

93. Argetsinger LS, Campbell GS, Yang X, et al: Identification of JAK2 as a growth hormone receptor-associated tyrosine kinase. Cell 74:237–244, 1993.

94. Velazquez L, Fellous M, Stark GR, Pellegrini S: A protein tyrosine kinase in the interferon α/β signaling pathway. Cell 70:313–322, 1992.

95. de-Vos AM, Ultsch M, Kossiakoff AA: Human growth hormone and extracellular domain of its receptor: Crystal structure of the complex. Science 255:306–312, 1992.

96. Radeke MJ, Misko TP, Hsu C, et al: Gene transfer and molecular cloning of the rat nerve growth factor receptor. Nature 325:593, 1987.

97. Smith CA, Davis T, Anderson D, et al: A receptor for tumor necrosis factor defines an unusual family of cellular and viral proteins. Science 248:1019, 1990.

98. Van Ostade X, Vandenabeele P, Everaerdt B, et al: Human TNF mutants with selective activity on the p55 receptor. Nature 361:266–269, 1993.

99. Rabizadeh S, Oh J, Zhong L, et al: Induction of apoptosis by the low-affinity NGF receptor. Science 261:345–348, 1993.

100. Yamamoto T, Davis CG, Brown MS: The human LDL receptor: A cysteine-rich protein with multiple alu sequences in its mRNA. Cell 39:27, 1984.

101. McClelland A, Kühn LC, Ruddle FH: The human transferrin receptor gene: Genomic organization, and the complete primary structure of the receptor deduced from a cDNA sequence. Cell 39:267, 1984.

102. Lobel P, Dahns NM, Kornfeld S: Cloning and sequence analysis of the cation-independent mannose-6-phosphate receptor. J Biol Chem 263:2563, 1988.

103. Morgan DO, Edman JC, Standring DN, et al: Insulin-like growth factor II receptor as a multifunctional binding protein. Nature 329:301, 1987.

104. Schofield PR, Darlison MG, Fujita N, et al: Sequence and functional expression of the GABA receptor shows a ligand-gated receptor super-family. Nature 328:221, 1987.

105. Schmieden V, Grenningloh G, Schofield PR, Betz H: Functional expression in Xenopus oocytes of the strychnine binding 48 kd subunit of the glycine receptor. EMBO J 8:695–700, 1989.

106. Hollmann, M, O'Shea-Greenfield A, Rogers SW, Heinemann S: Cloning by functional expression of a member of the glutamate receptor family. Nature 342:643, 1989.

107. Jan LY, Jan YN: Voltage-sensitive ion channels. Cell 56:13–25, 1989.

108. Catterall WA: Structure and function of voltage-sensitive ion channels. Science 242:50–61, 1988.

109. Changeux JP: The acetylcholine receptor: Its molecular biology and biotechnological prospects. Bioessays 10:48–54, 1989.

Biosynthesis and Turnover

110. Goldstein JL, Brown MS: Regulation of low-density lipoprotein receptors: Implications for pathogenesis and therapy of hypercholesterolemia and atherosclerosis. Circulation 76:504–507, 1987.

111. Hedo JA, Kahn CR, Hayashi M, et al: Biosynthesis and glycosylation of the insulin-receptor evidence for a single-polypeptide precursor of the two major subunits. J Biol Chem 258:10020–10026, 1983.

112. Ronnett GV, Knutson VP, Kohanski RA, et al: Role of glycosylation in the processing of the newly translated insulin proreceptor in 3T3-L1 adipocytes. J Biol Chem 259:4566–4572, 1984.

113. Pearse BMF, Bretscher MS: Membrane recycling by coated vesicles. Annu Rev Biochem 50:85–101, 1981.

114. Mellman I, Fuchs R, Helenius A: Acidification of the endocytic and exocytic pathways. Annu Rev Biochem 55:663, 1986.

Receptor-Mediated Endocytosis

115. Gorden P, Carpentier J-L, Freychet P, Orci L: Internalization of polypeptide hormones: Mechanism, intracellular localization and significance. Diabetologia 18:263, 1980.

116. Pastan IH, Willingham MC: Receptor-mediated endocytosis of hormones in cultured cells. Annu Rev Physiol 43:239–250, 1981.

117. Sonne O: Receptor-mediated endocytosis and degradation of insulin. Physiol Rev 68:1129, 1988.

118. Goldstein JL, Brown MS, Anderson RGW, et al: Receptor-mediated endocytosis: Concepts emerging from the LDL receptor system. Annu Rev Cell Biol 1:1, 1985.

119. Besterman JM, Low RB: Endocytosis: A review of mechanisms and plasma membrane dynamics. Biochem J 210:1, 1983.

Cellular Mechanism of Receptor-Mediated Endocytosis

120. Glickman JN, Conibear E, Pearse BMF: Specificity of binding of clathrin adaptors to signals on the mannose-6-phosphate/insulin-like growth factor II receptor. EMBO J 8:1041–1047, 1989.

121. Sorkin A, Carpenter G: Interaction of activated EGF receptors with coated pit adaptins. Science 261:612–614, 1993.

Intracellular Routes of Membrane Receptors

122. Schlessinger J, Shechter Y, Willingham MC, Pastan I: Direct visualization of binding, aggregation and internalization of insulin and epidermal growth factor on living fibroblastic cells. Proc Natl Acad Sci USA 75:2659–2663, 1978.

123. Knutson VP, Ronnett GV, Lane MD: Rapid, reversible internalization of cell surface insulin receptors. Correlation with insulin-induced down-regulation. J Biol Chem 158:12139, 1983.

124. Fehlmann M, Carpentier J-L, Van Obberghen E, et al: Internalized insulin receptors are recycled to the cell surface in rat hepatocytes. Proc Natl Acad Sci USA 79:1187, 1982.

125. Posner BI, Khan MN, Kay DG, Bergeron JJ: Internalization of hormone receptor complexes: Route and significance. Adv Exp Med Biol 205:185–201, 1986.

126. Carpenter G, Cohen S: Epidermal growth factor. Annu Rev Biochem 48:193, 1979.

127. Ascoli M: Lysosomal accumulation of the hormone-receptor complex during receptor-mediated endocytosis of human choriogonadotropin. J Cell Biol 99:1242–1250, 1984.

128. Klausner RD, Ashwell G, Van Renswoude J, Harford JB, Bridges KR: Binding of apotransferrin to K562 cells: Explanation of the transferrin cycle. Proc Natl Acad Sci USA 80:2263, 1983.

129. King GL, Johnson SM: Receptor-mediated transport of insulin across endothelial cells. Science 227:1583–1586, 1985.

130. Dernovsek K, Bar R, Ginsberg B, Lioubin M: Rapid transport of biologically intact insulin through cultured endothelial cells. J Clin Endocrinol Metab 58:761–765, 1984.

Receptor Signaling Mechanisms

Three Levels of Receptor Signaling
Level 1: Receptor and Effector Activation

130. Gilman AG: G proteins: Transducers of receptor-generated signals. Annu Rev Biochem 56:615, 1987.

131. Dingledine R, Myers SJ, Nicholas RA: Molecular biology of mammalian amino acid receptors. FASEB J 4:2636–2645, 1990.

132. Bolton TB, Beech DJ, Komori S, Prestwich SA: Voltage- and receptor-gated channels. Prog Clin Biol Res 327:229–243, 1990.

133. Hepler JR, Gilman AG: G proteins. Trends Biochem Sci 17:383–387, 1992.

134. Bourne HR, Sanders DA, McCormick F: The GTPase superfamily: Conserved structure and molecular mechanism. Nature 349:117–127, 1991.

135. Bokoch GM, Der CJ: Emerging concepts in the Ras superfamily of GTP-binding proteins. FASEB J 7:750–759, 1993.

136. Hall A: The cellular functions of small GTP-binding proteins. Science 249:635–640, 1990.

137. Ridley AJ, Paterson HF, Johnston CL, et al: The small GTP-binding protein rac regulates growth factor-induced membrane ruffling. Cell 70:401–410, 1992.

138. Ridley AJ, Hall A: The small GTP-binding protein rho regulates the assembly of focal adhesions and actin stress fibers in response to growth factors. Cell 70:389–399, 1992.

139. Schimmel P: GTP hydrolysis in protein synthesis: Two for Tu. Science 259:1264–1265, 1993.

140. Johnson GL, Dhanasekaran N: The G-protein family and their interaction with receptors. Endocr Rev 10:317–331, 1989.

141. Freissmuth M, Casey PH, Gilman AG: G proteins control diverse pathways of transmembrane signalling. FASEB J 3:1906–1914, 1989.

142. Neer EJ, Clapham DE: Roles of G protein subunits in transmembrane signalling. Nature 333:129–134, 1988.

143. Ross EM: Signal sorting and amplification through G protein coupled receptors. Neuron 5:141–152, 1990.

144. Casey PJ, Gilman AG: G protein involvement in receptor-effector coupling. J Biol Chem 263:2577–2580, 1988.

145. Clapham DE, Neer EJ: New roles for G-protein δγ-dimers in transmembrane signaling. Nature 365:403–406, 1993.

146. Birnbaumer L: Receptor-to-effector signaling through G proteins: roles for βγ dimers as well as α subunits. Cell 71:1069–1072, 1992.

147. Katz A, Wu D, Simon MI: Subunits βγ of heterodimeric G protein activate β2 isoform of phospholipase C. Nature 360:686–689, 1992.

148. Gilman AG: G-proteins and regulation of adenylyl cyclase. JAMA 262:1819–1825, 1989.

149. Salter RS, Krinks MH, Klee CB, Neer EJ: Calmodulin activates the isolated catalytic subunit of brain adenylate cyclase. J Biol Chem 256:9830–9833, 1981.

150. Glat CE, Snyder SH: Cloning and expression of an adenylyl cyclase localised to the corpus striatum. Nature 361:536–538, 1993.

151. Limbird LE: Receptors linked to inhibition of adenylate cyclase: Additional signalling mechanisms. FASEB J 2:2686–2695, 1988.

152. Catt KJ, Balla T: Phosphoinositide metabolism and hormone action. Annu Rev Med 40:487–509, 1989.

153. Exton JH: Signalling through phosphatidylcholine breakdown. J Biol Chem 265:1–4, 1990.

154. Williamson JR, Monck JR: Hormone effects on cellular Ca^{2+} fluxes. Annu Rev Physiol 51:107–124, 1989.

155. Berridge MJ: Inositol triphosphate and calcium signaling. Nature 361:315–325, 1993.

156. Liscovitch M: Crosstalk among multiple signal-activated phospholipases. Trends Biochem Sci 17:393–399, 1992.

157. Taylor CW, Marchall ICB: Calcium and inositol 1,4,5-triphosphate receptors. Trends Biochem Sci 17:403–407, 1992.

158. Berridge MJ: A tale of two messengers. Nature 365:388–389, 1993.

159. Meszaros LG, Bak J, Chu A: Cyclic ADP-ribose as an endogenous regulator of the non-skeletal type ryanodine receptor Ca^{2+} channel. Nature 364:76–79, 1993.

160. Galione A, White A, Willmott, et al: cGMP mobilizes intracellular Ca^{2+} in sea urchin eggs by stimulating cyclic ADP-ribose synthesis. Nature 365:456–459, 1993.

161. Knowles RG, Moncada S: Nitric oxide as a signal in blood vessels. Trends Biochem Sci 17:399–402, 1992.

162. Manalan AS, Klee CB: Calmodulin. Adv Cyclic Nucleotide Protein Phosphorylation Res 18:227–278, 1984.

163. Asaoka Y, Nakamura S, Yoshida K, Nishizuka Y: Protein kinase C, calcium and phospholipid degradation. Trends Biochem Sci 17:414–417, 1992.

164. Bell RM: Protein kinase C activation by diacylglycerol second messengers. Cell 45:631–632, 1986.

165. Nishizuka Y: The molecular heterogeneity of protein kinase C and its implications for cellular regulation. Nature 334:661–665, 1988.

166. Putney JW Jr: The molecular heterogeneity of protein kinase C and its implications for cellular regulation. Nature 334:661–665, 1988.

167. Pazin MJ, Williams LT: Triggering signaling cascades by receptor tyrosine kinases. Trends Biochem Sci 17:374–378, 1992.

168. Carpenter G: Receptors for epidermal growth factor and other polypeptide mitogens. Annu Rev Biochem 56:881, 1987.

169. Margolis BL, Lax I, Kris R, et al: All autophosphorylation sites of epidermal growth factor (EGF) receptor and HER2/neu are located in their carboxyl-terminal tails. J Biol Chem 264:10667–10671, 1989.

170. Fantl WJ, Escobedo JA, Martin GA, et al: Distinct phosphotyrosines on a growth factor receptor bind to specific molecules that mediate different signalling pathways. Cell 69:413–423, 1992.

171. Myers MG Jr, White MF: The new elements of insulin signaling. Insulin receptor substrate-1 and proteins with SH2 domains. Diabetes 42:643–650, 1993.

172. Shoelson SE, White MF, Kahn CR: Tryptic activation of the insulin receptor. J Biol Chem 263:4852–4860, 1988.

173. Longo N, Shuster RC, Griffin LD, et al: Activation of insulin receptor signaling by a single amino acid substitution in the transmembrane domain. J Biol Chem 267:12416–12419, 1992.

174. Perlman R, Bottaro D, White MF, Kahn CR: Conformational changes in the α- and β-subunits of the insulin receptor identified by anti-peptide antibodies. J Biol Chem 264:8946–8950, 1989.

175. Murakami MS, Rosen OR: The role of insulin receptor autophosphorylation in signal transduction. J Biol Chem 266:22653–22660, 1991.

176. Chou CK, Dull TJ, Russel DS, et al: Human insulin receptors mutated at the ATP-binding site lack protein tyrosine kinase activity and fail to mediate postreceptor effects of insulin. J Biol Chem 262:1842–1847, 1987.

177. Morgan DO, Roth RA: Acute insulin action requires insulin receptor kinase activity: Introduction of an inhibitory monoclonal antibody into mammalian cells blocks the rapid effects of insulin. Proc Natl Acad Sci USA 84:41–45, 1987.

178. Freidenberg GR, Henry RR, Klein HH, et al: Decreased kinase activity of insulin receptors from adipocytes of non-insulin-dependent diabetic subjects. J Clin Invest 79:240–250, 1987.

179. Kadowaki T, Kasuga M, Akanuma Y, et al: Decreased autophosphorylation of the insulin receptor-kinase in streptozotocin-diabetic rats. J Biol Chem 259:14208–14216, 1984.

180. Roussel MF, Downing JR, Rettenmeir CW, Sherr CJ: A point mutation in the extracellular domain of the human CJF-1 receptor (c-fms) proto-oncogene product 1 activates its transforming potential. Cell 55:979–988, 1988.

181. Ruff-Jamison S, McGlade J, Pawson T, et al: Epidermal growth factor stimulates the tyrosine phosphorylation of SHC in the mouse. J Biol Chem 268:7610–7612, 1993.

182. Fanti WJ, Escobedo JA, Martin GA, et al: Distinct phosphotyrosines on a growth factor receptor bind to specific molecules that mediate different signaling pathways. Cell 69:413–423, 1992.

183. Songyang Z, Shoelson SE, Chaudhuri M, et al: SH2 domains recognize specific phosphopeptide sequences. Cell 72:767–778, 1993.

184. Waksman G, Kominos D, Robertson SC, et al: Crystal structure of the phosphotyrosine recognition domain SH2 of v-src complexed with tyrosine-phosphorylated peptides. Nature 358:646–653, 1992.

185. Musacchio A, Noble M, Pauptit R, et al: Crystal structure of a Src-homology 3 (SH3) domain. Nature 359:851–855, 1992.

186. Booker GW, Breeze AL, Downing AK, et al: Structure of an SH2 domain of the p85α subunit of phosphatidylinositol-3-OH kinase. Nature 358:684–687, 1992.

187. Eck MJ, Shoelson SE, Harrison SC: Recognition of a high affinity phosphoryl peptide by the Src homology-2 domain of p56^{lck}. Nature 362:87–91, 1993.

188. Waksman G, Shoelson SE, Pant N, et al: Binding of a high affinity phosphotyrosyl peptide to the src SH2 domain: crystal structures of the complexed and peptide-free forms. Cell 72:779–790, 1993.

189. Pawson T, Gish GD: SH2 and SH3 domains: From structures to function. Cell 71:358–362, 1992.

190. Hanks SK, Quinn AM, Hunter T: The protein kinase family: Conserved features and deduced phylogeny of the catalytic domain. Science 241:42–52, 1990.

191. Shen S-H, Bastien L, Posner BI, Chretien P: A protein-tyrosine phosphatase with sequence similarity to the SH2 domain of the protein-tyrosine kinases. Nature 352:736–739, 1991.

192. Feng G-S, Hui C-C, Pawson T: SH2-containing phosphotyrosine phosphatase as a target of protin-tyrosine kinase. Science 259:1607–1611, 1993.

193. Vogel W, Lammers R, Huang J, Ullrich A: Activation of a phosphotyrosine phosphatase by tyrosine phosphorylation. Science 259:1611–1614, 1993.

194. Pelicci G, Lanfrancone L, Grignani F, et al: A novel transforming protein (SHC) with an SH2 domain is implicated in mitogenic signal transduction. Cell 70:93–104, 1993.

195. Ren R, Mayer BJ, Cichetti P, Baltimore D: Identification of a ten-amino acid proline-rich SH3 binding site. Science 259:1157–1161, 1993.

196. Yu H, Rosen MK, Shin TB, et al: Solution structure of the SH3 domain of src and identification of its ligand-binding site. Science 258:1665–1668, 1992.

197. Duchesne M, Schweighoffer F, Parker F, et al: Identification of the SH3 domain of GAP as an essential sequence for ras-GAP-mediated signaling. Science 259:525–528, 1993.

198. Egan SE, Weinberg RA: The pathway to signal achievement. Nature 365:781–783, 1993.

199. Chardin P, Camonis JH, Gale NW, et al: Human SOS1: a guanine nucleotide exchange factor for ras that binds to GRB2. Science 260:1338–1343, 1993.

200. Barbacid M: ras Genes. Ann Rev Biochem 56:779–827, 1987.

201. Marshall CJ: Protein prenylation: A mediator of protein-protein interactions. Science 259:1865–1866, 1993.

202. Burgering BM, Medema RH, Maassen JA, et al: Insulin stimulation of gene expression mediated by p21ras activation. EMBO J 10:1103–1109, 1991.

203. Medema RH, Wubbolts R, Bos JL: Two dominant inhibitory mutants of p21ras interfere with insulin-induced gene expression. Mol Cell Biol 11:5963–5967, 1991.

204. Rozakis-Adcock M, Fernley R, Wade J, et al: The SH2 and SH3 domains of mammalian Grb2 couple the EGF receptor to the Ras activator mSos1. Nature 363:83–85, 1993.

205. Li N, Batzer A, Daly R, et al: Guanine-nucleotide-releasing factor hSos1 binds to Grb2 and links receptor tyrosine kinases to Ras signaling. Nature 363:85–88, 1993.

206. Lowenstein EJ, Daly RJ, Batzer AG, et al: The SH2 and SH3-domain containing protein GRB2 links receptor tyrosine kinases to ras signaling. Cell 70:93–104, 1993.

207. Moodie SA, Willumsen BA, Weber MJ, Wolfman A: Complexes of ras-GTP with Raf-1 and mitogen-activated protein kinase kinase. Science 260:1658–1661, 1993.

208. Zhang X-F, Settleman J, Kyriakis JM, et al: Normal and oncogenic p21^{ras} proteins bind to the aminoterminal regulatory domain of c-Raf-1. Nature 364:308–313, 1993.

209. Koshland DE Jr: The two-component pathway comes to eukaryotes. Science 261:532, 1993.

210. Cochet C, Gill GN, Meisenhelder J, et al: C-kinase phosphorylates the epidermal growth factor receptor and reduces its epidermal growth factor-stimulated tyrosine protein kinase activity. J Biol Chem 259:2553–2558, 1984.

211. Takayama S, White MF, Kahn CR: Phorbol ester-induced serine phosphorylation of the insulin receptor decreases its tyrosine kinase activity. J Biol Chem 263:3440–3447, 1988.

212. Lewis RE, Wu GP, MacDonald RG, Czech MP: Insulin-sensitive phosphorylation of serine 1293/1294 on the human insulin receptor by a tightly associated serine kinase. J Biol Chem 265:947–954, 1990.

Level 2: Signal Transduction

213. Cohen P: Signal integration at the level of protein kinases, protein phosphatases and their substrates. Trends Biochem Sci 17:408–413, 1992.

214. Hanks SK, Quin AM, Hunter T: The protein kinase family: conserved features and deduced phylogeny of the catalytic domains. Science 241:42–52, 1988.

215. Dent P, Lavoinne A, Nakielny S, et al: The molecular mechanisms by which insulin stimulates glycogen synthesis in mammalian skeletal muscle. Nature 348:302–307, 1990.

216. Seger R, Ahn NG, Boulton TG, et al: Microtubule-associated protein 2 kinases, ERK1 and ERK2, undergo autophosphorylation on both tyrosine and threonine residues: Implications for their mechanism of activation. Proc Natl Acad Sci USA 88:6142–6146, 1991.

217. Boulton TG, Nye SH, Robbins DJ, et al: A family of protein-serine/threonine kinases that are activated and tyrosine phosphorylated in response to insulin and NGF. Cell 65:663–675, 1991.

218. Ahn NG, Seger R, Bratlien RL, et al: Multiple components in an epidermal growth factor-stimulated protein kinase cascade. In vitro activation of a myelin basic protein/microtubule-associated protein 2 kinase. J Biol Chem 266:4220–4227, 1991.

Level 3: Cellular Actions

219. Shotwell MA, Kilberg MS, Oxender DL: The regulation of neutral amino acid transport in mammalian cells. Biochim Biophys Acta 737:267–284, 1983.

220. Cariappa R, Kilberg MS: Hormone-induced system A amino acid transport activity in rat liver plasma membrane and Golgi vesicles. J Biol Chem 265:1470–1475, 1990.

221. Fehlmann M, LeCam A, Freychet P: Insulin and glucagon stimulation of amino acid transport in isolated rat hepatocytes. J Biol Chem 254:10431–10437, 1979.

222. Bell GI, Kayano T, Buse JB, et al: Molecular biology of mammaliam glucose transporters. Diabetes Care 13:198–208, 1990.

223. Mueckler M, Caruso C, Baldwin SA, et al: Sequence and structure of a human glucose transporter. Science 229:941–945, 1985.

224. Birnbaum MB: Identification of a novel gene encoding an insulin-responsive glucose transport protein. Cell 57:305–315, 1989.

225. Charron MJ, Brosius FC III, Alper SL, Lodish HF: A glucose transport protein expressed predominantly in insulin responsive tissues. Proc Natl Acad Sci USA 86:2535–2539, 1989.

226. Simpson IA, Cushman SW: Hormonal regulation of mammalian glucose transport. Ann Rev Biochem 55:1059–1089, 1986.

227. Suzuki K, Kono T: Evidence that insulin causes translocation of glucose transport activity of the plasma membrane from an intracellular storage site. Proc Natl Acad Sci USA 77:2542–2545, 1980.

228. Karin M, Smeal T: Control of transcription factors by signal transduction pathways: the beginning of the end. Trends Biochem Sci 17:418–422, 1992.

229. Hunter T, Karin M: The regulation of transcription by phosphorylation. Cell 70:375–387, 1992.

230. Montminy MR, Gonzalez GA, Yamamoto KK: Regulation of cAMP inducible genes by CREB. Trends Neurosci 18:184–188, 1990.

231. Montminy M: Trying a new pair of SH2s. Science 261:1694–1695, 1993.

232. Angel P, Allegretto EA, Okino ST, et al: Oncogene *jun* encodes a sequence-specific trans-activator similar to AP-1. Nature 332:166–169, 1988.

233. Montminy MR, Sevarino KA, Wagner JA, et al: Identification of a cyclic-AMP responsive element within the rat somatostatin gene. Proc Natl Acad Sci USA 83:6682–6686, 1986.

234. Pulverer BJ, Kyriakis JM, Avruch J, et al: Phosphorylation of *c-jun* mediated by MAP kinases. Nature 353:670–674, 1991.

235. Sadowski HB, Shuai K, Darnell JE Jr, Gilman MZ: A common nuclear signal transduction pathway activated by growth factors and cytokine receptors. Science 261:1739–1744, 1993.

236. Ruff-Jamison S, Chen K, Cohen S: Induction by EGF and interferon-γ of tyrosine phosphorylated DNA binding proteins in mouse liver nuclei. Science 261:1733–1736, 1993.

237. Fu X-Y: A transcription factor with SH2 and SH3 domains is directly activated by an interferon α-induced cytoplasmic protein tyrosine kinase(s). Cell 70:323–335, 1992.

Receptor Signaling Network

238. Kono T, Barham FW: The relationship between the insulin binding capacity of fat cells and the cellular response to insulin. J Biol Chem 246:6210–6216, 1971.

239. Gliemann J, Gammeltoft S, Vinten J: Time course of insulin receptor binding and insulin-induced lipogenesis in isolated rat fat cells. J Biol Chem 250:3368–3374, 1975.

240. Dufau ML: Endocrine regulation and communicating functions of the Leydig cell. Ann Rev Physiol 50:483–508, 1988.

241. Kahn CR: Insulin resistance, insulin insensitivity and insulin unresponsiveness: A necessary distinction. Metabolism 27(Suppl. 2):1893–1902, 1978.

242. Kasuga M, Kahn CR, Hedo JA, et al: Insulin-induced receptor loss in cultured lymphocytes is due to accelerated receptor degradation. Proc Natl Acad Sci USA 78:6917–6921, 1981.

243. Hinkle DM, Tashijian AH Jr: Thyrotropin-releasing hormone regulates the number of its own receptors in GH₃ strain of pituitary cells in culture. Biochemistry 14:3845–3851, 1975.

244. Posner BI, Kelley PA, Friesen HG: Prolactin receptor in rat liver: Possible induction by prolactin. Science 188:57–59, 1978.

245. Hausdorff WP, Caron MG, Lefkowitz RJ: Turning off the signal: Desensitization of β-adrenergic receptor function. FASEB J 4:2881–2889, 1990.

246. Nimrod A, Tsafriri A, Linder HR: In vitro induction of binding sites for HCG in rat granulosa cells by FSH. Nature 267:632–633, 1977.

247. Williams LT, Lefkowitz RJ, Watanabe AM, et al: Thyroid hormone regulation of β-adrenergic receptor number. J Biol Chem 252:2787–2789, 1977.

248. Posner BI, Kelley PA, Friesen HG: Induction of lactogenic receptor in rat liver: Influence of estrogen and the pituitary. Proc Natl Acad Sci USA 71:2407–2410, 1974.

249. Wrann M, Fox CF, Ross R: Modulation of epidermal growth factor receptors on 3T3 cells by platelet-derived growth factor. Science 210:1363–1365, 1980.

250. McDonald AR, Goldfine ID: Glucocorticoid regulation of insulin receptor gene transcription in IM9 cultured lymphocytes. J Clin Invest 81:499–504, 1988.

251. O'Rahilly S, Moller DE: Mutant insulin receptors in syndromes of insulin resistance. Clin Endocrinol 36:121–132, 1992.

252. Taylor SI, Kadowaki T, Kadowaki H, et al: Insulin receptor mutants. Diabetes Care 13:257–279, 1992.

253. O'Rahilly S, Choi WH, Patel P, et al: Detection of mutations in insulin-receptor gene in NIDDM patients by analysis of single-stranded conformation polymorphisms. Diabetes 40:777–782, 1991.

254. Taira M, Taira M, Hashimoto N, et al: Human diabetes associated with a deletion of the tyrosine kinase domain of the insulin receptor. Science 245:63–66, 1989.

255. Odawara M, Kadowaki T, Yamamoto R, et al: Human diabetes associated with a mutation in the tyrosine kinase domain of the insulin receptor. Science 245:66–68, 1989.
256. Yoshimasa Y, Seino S, Whittaker J, et al: Insulin-resistant diabetes due to a point mutation that prevents insulin proreceptor processing. Science 240:784–787, 1988.
257. Kadowaki T, Bevins CL, Cama A, et al: Two mutant alleles of the insulin receptor gene in a patient with extreme insulin resistance. Science 240:787–790, 1988.
258. Laron Z, Pertzelan A, Mannheimer S: Genetic pituitary dwarfism with high serum concentration of growth hormone. A new inborn error of metabolism? Isr J Med Sci 2:152–155, 1966.
259. Eshet R, Laron Z, Pertzelan A, et al: Defect of human growth hormone receptors in the liver of two patients with Laron-type dwarfism. Isr J Med Sci 20:8–11, 1984.
260. Daughaday WH, Trivedi B: Absence of serum growth hormone binding protein in patients with growth hormone receptor deficiency (Laron dwarfism). Proc Natl Acad Sci USA 84:4636–4640, 1987.
261. Shenker A, Laue L, Kosugi S, et al: A constitutively activating mutation of the luteinizing hormone receptor in familial male precocious puberty. Nature 365:652–654, 1993. `
262. Lin S-C, Lin CR, Gukovski I, et al: Molecular basis of the *little* mouse phenotype and implications of cell type-specific growth. Nature 364:208–213, 1993.
263. Parma J, Duprez L, Van Sande J, et al: Somatic mutations in the thyrotropin receptor gene causing hyperfunctioning thyroid adenomas. Nature 365:649–651, 1993.
264. Robbins LS, Nadeau JH, Johnson KR, et al: Pigmentation phenotypes of variant extension locus alleles result from point mutations that alter MSH receptor function. Cell 72:827–834, 1993.
265. Truglia JA, Livingston JN, Lockwood DH: Insulin resistance: Receptor and post-binding defects in human obesity and non-insulin dependent mellitus. Am J Med 79:13–22, 1985.
266. Olefsky JM, Reaven GM: Insulin binding in diabetes: Relationships with plasma insulin levels and insulin sensitivity. Diabetes 26:680–688, 1977.
267. Archer JA, Gorden P, Roth J: Defect in insulin binding to receptors in obese man: amelioration with caloric restriction. J Clin Invest 55:166–174, 1975.
268. Neufeld ND, Ezrin C, Corbo L, et al: Effects of caloric restriction and exercise on insulin receptors in obesity: Association with changes in membrane lipids. Metabolism 34:580–587, 1993.
269. Häring H, Obermaier-Kusser B: Insulin receptor kinase defects in insulin-resistant tissues and their role in the pathogenesis of NIDDM. Diabetes/Metab Rev 5:431–441, 1989.
270. Kolterman OG, Gray RS, Griffin J, et al: Receptor and postreceptor defects contribute to the insulin resistance in non-insulin-dependent diabetes mellitus. J Clin Invest 68:957–969, 1993
271. Caro JF, Ittoop O, Pories WJ, et al: Studies on the mechanism of insulin resistance in the liver from humans with noninsulin-dependent diabetes. J Clin Invest 78:249–258, 1986.
272. Smith BR, McLachlan SM, Furmaniak J: Autoantibodies to the thyrotropin receptor. Endocr Rev 9:106–121, 1988.
273. Adams DD: The presence of an abnormal thyroid stimulating hormone in the serum of some thyrotoxic patients. J Clin Endocrinol Metab 18:699–712, 1958.
274. Madec AM, Laurent MC, Lorcy Y, et al: Thyroid stimulating antibodies: An aid to the strategy of treatment of Graves' disease? Clin Endocrinol 21:247–255, 1984.
275. Flier JS, Kahn CR, Roth J, Bar RS: Antibodies that impair insulin receptor binding in an unusual diabetic syndrome with severe insulin resistance. Science 190:63–65, 1975.
276. Kahn CR, Flier JS, Bar RS, et al: The syndromes of insulin resistance and acanthosis nigricans. Insulin-receptor disorders in man. N Engl J Med 294:739–745, 1976.
277. Taylor SI, Grunberger G, Marcus-Samuels B, et al: Hypoglycemia associated with antibodies to the insulin receptor. N Engl J Med 307:1422–1426, 1982.
278. Bar RS, Levis WR, Rechler MM, et al: Extreme insulin resistance in ataxia telangiectasia: Defect in affinity of insulin receptors. N Engl J Med 298:1164–1171, 1978.
279. Fradkin JE, Eastman RC, Lesniak MA, Roth J: Specificity spillover at the hormone receptor—exploring its role in human disease. N Engl J Med 320:640–645, 1989.
280. De Pablo F, Eastman RC, Roth J, Gorden P: Plasma prolactin in acromegaly before and after treatment. J Clin Endocrinol Metab 53:344–352, 1981.
281. Carayon P, Lefort G, Nisula B: Interaction of human chorionic gonadotropin and human luteinizing hormone with human thyroid membranes. Endocrinology 106:1907–1916, 1980.
282. Gorden P, Hendricks CM, Kahn CR, et al: Hypoglycemia associated with non-islet-cell tumor and insulin-like growth factors: A study of the tumor types. N Engl J Med 305:1452–1455, 1981.
283. Daughaday WH, Emanuele MA, Brooks MH, et al: Synthesis and secretion of insulin-like growth factor II by a leiomyosarcoma with associated hypoglycemia. N Engl J Med 319:1434–1440, 1988.
284. Bishop JM: The molecular genetics of cancer. Science 235:305–311, 1987.
285. Hunter T: The functions of oncogene products. Prog Clin Biol Res 288:25–34, 1989.
286. Leutz A, Graf T: Relationships between oncogenes and growth control. *In* Sporn MB, Roberts AB: Peptide Growth Factors and Their Receptors. Vol. II. New York, Springer-Verlag, 1990, pp 655–703.
287. Kraux MH, Pierce JH, Fleming TP, et al: Mechanisms by which genes encoding growth factors and growth factor receptors contribute to malignant transformation. Ann NY Acad Sci 551:320–335, 1988.
288. Cantley LC, Auger KR, Carpenter C, et al: Oncogenes and signal transduction. Cell 64:281–302, 1991.
289. Weinberg RA: Oncogenes, antioncogenes and the molecular basis of multistep carcinogenesis. Cancer Res 49:3713–3721, 1989.
290. Doolittle RF, Hunkapiller MW, Hood LE, et al: Simian sarcoma virus onc gene, v-sis, is derived from the gene (or genes) encoding a platelet derived growth factor. Science 221:275–277, 1983.
291. Dickson C, Peters G: Potential oncogene products related to growth factors. Nature 326:833–800, 1987.
292. Downward J, Yarden Y, Mayes E, et al: Close similarity of epidermal growth factor receptor and v-erbB oncogene protein sequences. Nature 311:483–485, 1984.
293. Sherr CJ, Rettenmeier CW, Sacca R, et al: The c-fms proto-oncogene product is related to the receptor for the mononuclear phagocyte growth factor. Cell 41:665–676, 1985.
294. Coussens L, Yang-Feng TL, Liao Y-C, et al: Tyrosine kinase receptor with extensive homology to EGF receptors shares chromosomal location with the neu oncogene. Science 230:1132–1139, 1985.
295. Cooper JA: The src-family of protein-tyrosine kinases. *In* Kemp B, Alewood PF (eds): Peptides and Protein Phosphorylation. Boca Raton, CRC Press, 1993.
296. McCormick F: Ras GTPase activating protein: Signal transmitter and signal terminator. Cell 56:5–8, 1989.
297. Rapp UR, Goldsborough MD, Mark GE, et al: Structure and biological activity of v-raf, a unique oncogene in lung carcinogenesis. Proc Natl Acad Sci USA 80:42:4218–4222, 1993.
298. Curran T, Franza BR Jr: Fos and jun: the AP1 connection. Cell 55:395–397, 1988.
299. Klein G, Klein E: Conditioned tumorigenicity of activated oncogenes. Cancer Res 46:3211–3224, 1986.
300. Helin K, Lees JA, Vidal M, et al: A cDNA encoding a pRB-binding protein with properties of the transcription factor E2F. Cell 70:337–350, 1992.

4

Second Messenger Signaling Pathways: Phosphatidyl Inositol and Calcium

MARVIN C. GERSHENGORN
JEFFREY H. PERLMAN

Extracellular regulatory molecules, such as hormones, neurotransmitters, and growth factors, interact with cells by binding to specific cell surface receptors. As a result of this interaction, the receptor may be activated to lead to the generation of second messenger molecules intracellularly. A ubiquitous second messenger system utilizes the hydrolysis of phosphoinositides (PPI's), phospholipids that contain the sugar *myo*-inositol as the polar head group. The primary PPI hydrolyzed is phosphatidylinositol 4,5-bisphosphate (PI(4,5)P$_2$) to generate two molecules that serve as second messengers, inositol-1,4,5-trisphosphate (I-1,4,5-P$_3$) and 1,2-diacylglycerol (1,2-DAG).[1, 2] Closely related to the actions of these messengers are changes in the concentration of free (or ionized) calcium in the cytoplasm ([Ca^{2+}]$_i$). Because the same signaling pathway is used in many different cell types to stimulate distinct responses, for example, secretion from endocrine cells and contraction of smooth muscle cells, it is evident that there are cell-specific factors required to elicit the final responses. The major aim of this chapter is to discuss the mechanisms by which these second messengers are generated, regulated, and metabolized, and their proximate effects. (The more distal steps that lead to specific cellular responses will not be discussed.) It has become apparent that other membrane phospholipids, such as phosphatidylcholines, can be hydrolyzed by specific phospholipases to generate 1,2-DAG; these systems as well as interactions between second messenger systems are described also.

PHOSPHOINOSITIDES

PPI's, or inositol lipids, are composed of a glycerol backbone containing fatty acyl groups at the 1- and 2-positions and a phosphate group coupled via a phosphodiester linkage at the 3-position to *myo*-inositol (Fig. 4–1). The *myo*-inositol head group may have additional phosphates, usually at the 4-position or 4- and 5-positions. A minor subclass of PPI's, which may be important in the action of growth

factors and insulin and in signaling by oncogenes,[3] has been described that contains a phosphate at the 3-position of *myo*-inositol. PPI's are minor lipids in cells constituting on average 5 to 10 per cent of the total phospholipid. Phosphatidylinositol (PI) is the parent lipid and is phosphorylated by a specific enzyme, PI 4-kinase, to yield PI 4-monophosphate (PI-(4)P), which is in turn phosphorylated by PI(4)P 5-kinase to PI(4,5)P$_2$ (Fig. 4–2). There are lipid phosphatases within cells that de-phosphorylate PI(4)P and PI(4,5)P$_2$ to PI. De-phosphorylation of PI(4)P and PI(4,5)P$_2$ has been termed a "futile cycle" to distinguish it from the PPI cycle (see below), because it does not generate intracellular messenger molecules. These phosphatases are active and limit the levels of PI(4)P and PI(4,5)P$_2$ in unstimulated cells. PI accounts for 85 to 95 per cent of PPI's, whereas PI(4,5)P$_2$, which is the primary substrate in cells for second messenger generation, constitutes only 2 to 3 per cent. An agonist, such as a hormone, binds to its receptor, which in turn activates a PPI-specific phospholipase C (PPI-PLC) that hydrolyzes PI(4,5)P$_2$ to I-1,4,5-P$_3$ and 1,2-DAG. I-1,4,5-P$_3$ is water-soluble; it is released into the cytoplasm and diffuses away from the membrane, whereas 1,2-DAG remains membrane-bound. I-1,4,5-P$_3$ leads to release of Ca^{2+} from intracellular stores into the cytoplasm and elevates [Ca^{2+}]$_i$, and 1,2-DAG activates protein kinase C (PKC).

Phosphoinositide-Specific Phospholipase C

Phospholipase C (PLC) is a family of enzymes that hydrolyze phospholipids at the 3-position phosphodiester bond of the glycerol backbone. When PI(4,5)P$_2$ is the substrate, PLC action leads to the formation of I-1,4,5-P$_3$ and 1,2-DAG (Fig. 4–3). PPI-specific PLC (PPI-PLC) is a subfamily of PLC that acts specifically on inositol-containing lipids and does not hydrolyze other phospholipids, such as phosphatidylcholine (PC). PPI-PLC can be divided into three types (PPI-PLC-β, PPI-PLC-γ, and PPI-PLC-δ),

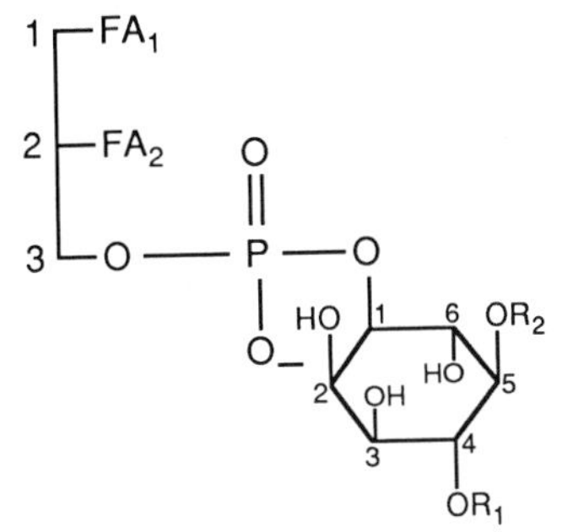

FIGURE 4–1. **Structures of the major phosphoinositides.** The glycerol backbone is esterified at positions 1 and 2 to fatty acids FA_1 and FA_2, respectively. FA_1 is usually a saturated fatty acid whereas FA_2 may be arachidonic acid. The phosphate head group is coupled to *myo*-inositol at the 3-position of glycerol. PI, phosphatidylinositol; PI(4)P, phosphatidylinositol 4-monophosphate; $PI(4,5)P_2$, phosphatidylinositol 4,5-bisphosphate.

which are distinct proteins that exhibit only a small amount of sequence identity.[4] There are also isoenzyme subtypes designated by a Roman numeral after the Greek letter, e.g., PPI-PLC-βI and PPI-PLC-βII, which are closely related proteins that share a high degree of sequence identity. PPI-PLC enzymes are single polypeptide chains that do not have separate regulatory subunits. PPI-PLC-β and PPI-PLC-γ are approximately the same molecular size (~150 kDa) whereas PPI-PLC-δ is smaller (~85 kDa).

All PPI-PLC isoenzymes catalyze hydrolysis of PI, PI(4)P, and $PI(4,5)P_2$ in vitro, and it appears that PI, and perhaps PI(4)P, may serve as substrates for these enzymes in certain cells even though $PI(4,5)P_2$ is the primary substrate in vivo. (PPI's that are phosphorylated at the 3-position of the *myo*-inositol head group, such as PI3-monophosphate, are not substrates for these enzymes.) In cells, PPI-PLCβ and PPI-PLCγ isoenzymes appear to be the ones involved in receptor-activated $PI(4,5)P_2$ hydrolysis, but the mechanisms of their activation are different. A difference in the primary amino acid sequences between PPI-PLCβ and PPI-PLCγ, which is related to their mechanisms of activation, is that PPI-PLCγ contains *src* homology (SH2 and SH3) domains, whereas PPI-PLC-β does not. SH2 and SH3 domains, which were found originally in proteins of the *src* oncogene family of tyrosine kinases, mediate binding to other proteins that contain phosphorylated tyrosine residues, for example, growth factor receptors (see below).

Receptor Activation of PPI-PLC

A partial list of receptors that can activate the PPI cascade is presented in Table 4–1 to demonstrate the large variety of regulatory molecules that use this signaling pathway. The list is divided into two major classes on the basis of the mechanism of receptor activation of PPI-PLC. In one class, agonist-occupied receptor is coupled to activation of PPI-PLC-β by a guanine nucleotide–binding regu-

latory (G) protein. In the other class, activation of PPI-PLC-γ involves protein tyrosine phosphorylation and G proteins are not involved.

A large number of receptors have been found to activate PPI-PLC by means of coupling to a G protein. This is analogous to the most common mechanism of receptor activation of adenylyl cyclase, in which the agonist-occupied receptor binds to $G_{stimulatory}$ (G_s) and the receptor-G_s complex then activates adenylyl cyclase[5] (see Ch. 5B). Initial indications that a G protein was involved in receptor activation of PPI-PLC were that observations made in this system using plasma membrane preparations isolated from several cell types[6] were similar to findings in the receptor-G_s-adenylyl cyclase system. Guanine nucleotides were found to change the receptor affinity for some ligands that activate PPI-PLC. This occurs because guanine nucleotides affect receptor–G protein coupling, and association of receptor with G protein affects the affinity of ligand binding to receptor. Secondly, agonist stimulation of hydrolysis of PIP_2 was noted to be synergistically enhanced by guanine triphosphate (GTP) analogues. This occurs because binding of GTP to the G protein is a necessary step in G protein activation (see ref. 5 for a description of G-protein activation). G proteins are heterotrimers consisting of α, β, and γ subunits. The α subunit binds guanine nucleotides and appears to play the major role in activating effector enzymes or ion channels. A role for the β and γ subunits, which bind avidly to each other, in activating or modifying the activation of some effectors has been found in a limited number of cases. However, it is primarily the α subunit of the G protein that has been shown to activate PPI-PLC.

During the last several years, the complementary DNA's (cDNA's) for a number of G proteins have been cloned and the specificity of their interactions with effector enzymes, such as PLC or adenylyl cyclase, or ion channels has begun to be elucidated.[7] There are four G protein subfamilies that have been identified: G_s, $G_{inhibitory}$ (G_i), G_q, and G_{12}. There appear to be two classes of G proteins that can activate PPI-PLC, pertussis toxin–sensitive and pertussis toxin–insensitive G proteins. This classification is based on observations that for some agonists activation of PPI-PLC can be inhibited by pretreating cells with pertussis toxin, whereas with other agonists pertussis toxin does not affect receptor activation of PPI-PLC. By analogy to the mecha-

TABLE 4–1. RECEPTORS THAT CAN ACTIVATE THE PHOSPHOINOSITIDE PATHWAY

EFFECT OF RECEPTOR OCCUPANCY	RECEPTOR
I. A. Activate PPI-PLCβ predominantly	TRH
	GnRH
	Angiotensin II
	Muscarinic m_2
B. Activate PPI-PLCβ and inhibit AC	Neuropeptide Y Y_1
	TSH
C. Activate PPI-PLCβ and AC	PTH
	Calcitonin
	LH
	EGF
II. Activate PPI-PLCγ	PDGF

Examples are given of receptors that activate PPI-PLCβ or PPI-PLCγ. Some receptors may couple to two G-proteins and thereby stimulate more than one signaling cascade. Examples are given of receptors that predominantly stimulate PPI-PLCβ or stimulate PPI-PLCβ in addition to either inhibiting or stimulating adenylyl cyclase.

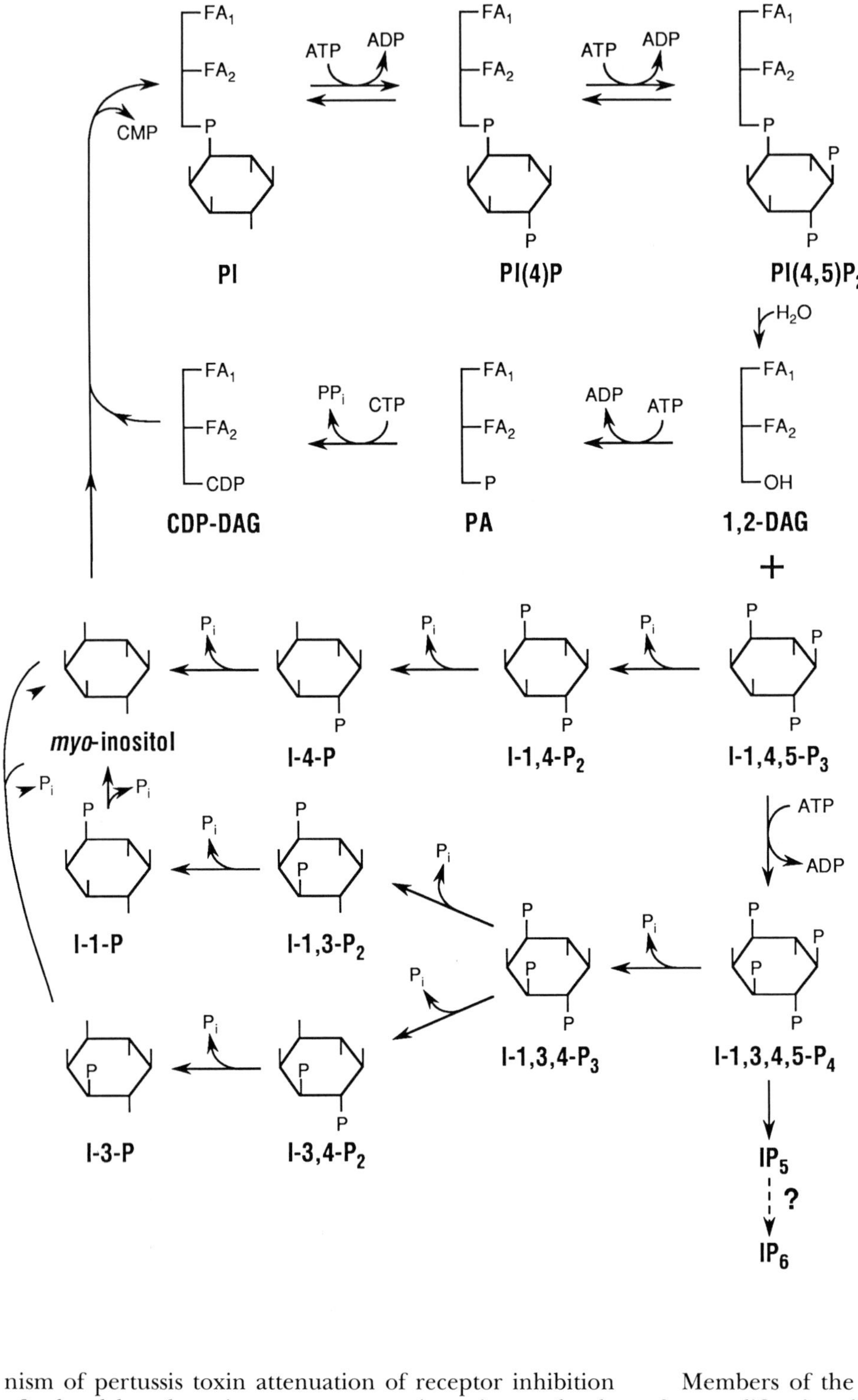

FIGURE 4–2. **The phosphoinositide cycle.** The major products and pathways of the phosphoinositide cycle in animal cells are shown. Functional groups on *myo*-inositol are hydroxyl groups unless otherwise indicated as P, phosphate. Ins, *myo*-inositol; PI, phosphatidylinositol; PI(4)P, phosphatidylinositol 4-monophosphate; PI(4,5)P$_2$, phosphatidylinositol 4,5-bisphosphate; FA$_1$, fatty acid at 1-position; FA$_2$, fatty acid at 2-position; 1,2-DAG, 1,2-diacylglycerol; PA, phosphatidic acid; I-1,4,5-P$_3$, inositol-1,4,5-trisphosphate; I-1,3,4-P$_3$, inositol-1,3,4-trisphosphate; Ins-1,3,4,5-P$_4$, inositol-1,3,4,5-tetrakisphosphate; IP$_5$, inositol pentakisphosphate; IP$_6$, hexakisphosphate; I-1,4-P$_2$, inositol-1,4-bisphosphate; I-1,3-P$_2$, inositol-1,3-bisphosphate; I-3,4-P$_2$, inositol-3,4-bisphosphate; I-4-P, inositol-4-monophosphate; I-1-P, inositol-1-monophosphate; I-3-P, inositol-3-monophosphate; ATP, adenosine 5'-triphosphate; ADP, adenosine 5'-diphosphate; CTP, cytidine 5'-triphosphate; CMP, cytidine 5'-monophosphate; PP$_i$, pyrophosphate; P$_i$, inorganic phosphate.

nism of pertussis toxin attenuation of receptor inhibition of adenylyl cyclase, it appears pertussis toxin covalently modifies some G proteins and thereby prevents those G proteins from coupling to receptor and activating PPI-PLC.[8] Pertussis toxin catalyzes the addition of adenosine diphosphate (ADP)-ribose to a cysteine residue in a region in the carboxyl-terminus of the G protein α subunit that is involved in binding to receptor. Although the G protein α subunit that mediates pertussis toxin–sensitive activation of PPI-PLC has not been definitively identified, it is likely to be a member of the G$_i$ subfamily because these G proteins are substrates for pertussis toxin–mediated ADP-ribosylation.

Members of the G$_q$ subfamily, which are not substrates for modification by pertussis toxin, have recently been found to activate PPI-PLC in reconstitution experiments in vitro.[9, 10] Indeed, G$_q$ proteins were shown to activate PPI-PLC-βI but not PPI-PLC-γI or PPI-PLC-δI.[11] In experiments using isolated plasma membranes and antibodies against G$_q$ proteins to specifically inhibit G$_q$ action, receptor activation by a number of agonists, including bradykinin, angiotensin, and histamine, has been shown to activate PLC via coupling to G$_q$.[12] Therefore, these proteins appear to be the pertussis toxin–insensitive activators of PPI-PLC.

Receptors that couple via a G protein to activate PPI-PLC-β are members of a large family of receptors that

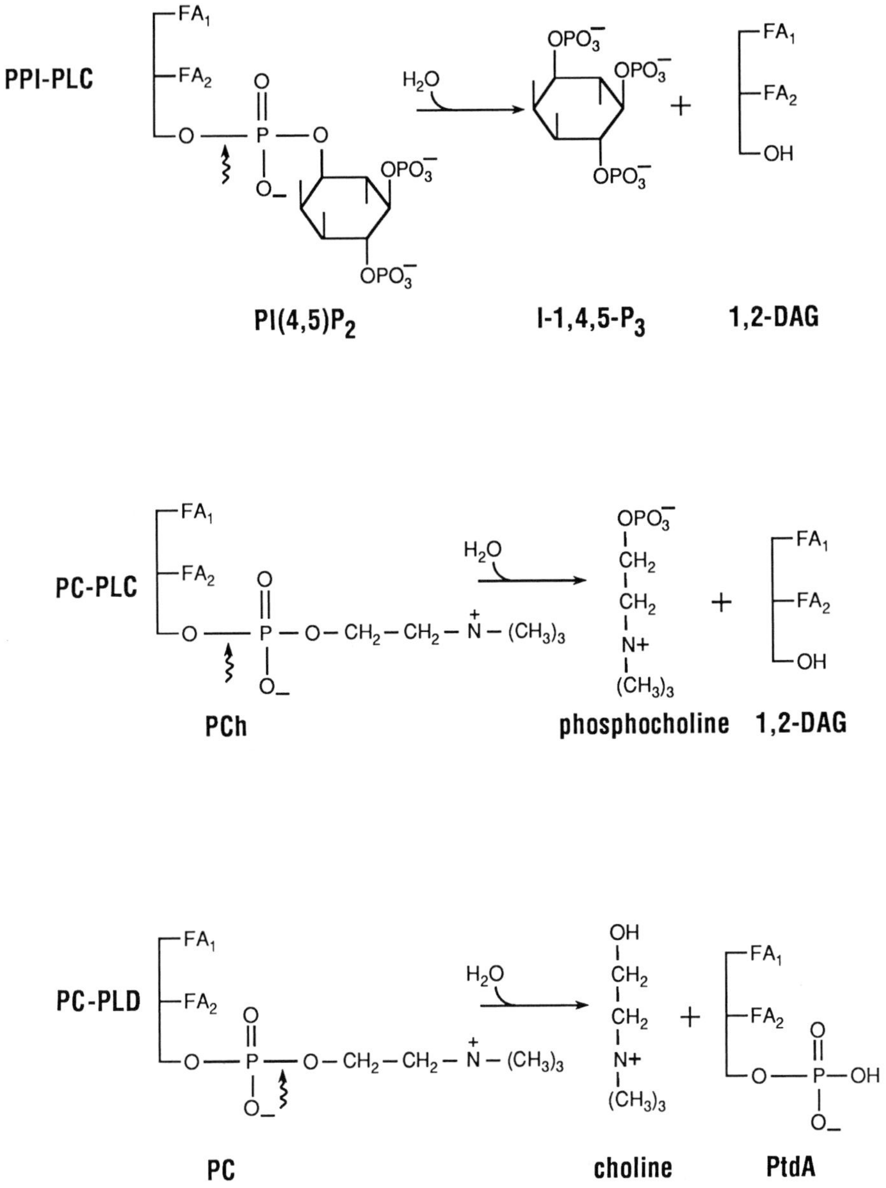

FIGURE 4–3. **Enzymatic hydrolysis of phospholipids.** The sites of hydrolysis are indicated by a wavy line. PPI-PLC, phosphoinositide-specific phospholipase C; PC-PLC, phosphatidylcholine-specific phospholipase C; PC-PLD, phosphatidylcholine phospholipase D; PI(4,5)P_2, phosphatidylinositol 4,5-bisphosphate; I-1,4,5-P_3, inositol-1,4,5-trisphosphate; 1,2-DAG, 1,2-diacylglycerol.

couple by means of interaction with G proteins.[13, 14] These receptors share a common putative topology in the cell surface membrane in which they span the bilayer of this membrane seven times. Much current research is directed toward understanding the domains within these receptors that interact with G proteins. See Chapter 5 for a complete discussion of these receptors.

PPI-PLC-γI, in contrast to PPI-PLC-βI, has been shown to associate with and be activated by agonist-occupied receptors that possess intrinsic tyrosine kinase activity.[15] These receptors for growth factors, such as epidermal growth factor, platelet-derived growth factor, and fibroblast growth factor, do not appear to couple to G proteins. Their putative topology in the plasma membrane is different from that proposed for G protein–coupled receptors in that they span the cell surface membrane a single time (see Ch. 3). Growth factor–stimulated PPI-PLC activation appears to be dependent on the tyrosine kinase activity of the receptor. Growth factor receptor activation leads to an increase in PPI-PLC-γI activity but not PPI-PLC-βI or PPI-PLC-δI activity. The agonist-occupied receptor phosphory-

lates itself on tyrosine residues, which results in increased association with PPI-PLC-γI through the *src* homology domains. Upon association with the agonist-occupied receptor, PPI-PLC-γI is phosphorylated at specific tyrosine residues; this causes enzyme activation. Hydrolysis of PI(4,5)P_2 appears to be made more favorable by the association of PPI-PLC-γI (which is present in unstimulated cells in the cytoplasm) with the receptor because this may position PPI-PLC-γI closer to its plasma membrane–bound substrate. PPI-PLC-βI may, in contrast, be membrane-bound in unstimulated cells, but this has not been definitively proved.

Phosphoinositide Cycle

After hydrolysis of PI(4,5)P_2, both I-1,4,5-P_3 and 1,2-DAG serve as intracellular messengers and then are rapidly metabolized. I-1,4,5-P_3 undergoes a series of metabolic conversions that generate a large number of inositol phosphate derivatives, some of which may be active in generating calcium signals.[16, 17] This is currently an area of intensive research. As shown in Figure 4–2, I-1,4,5-P_3 can be hydrolyzed by a series of phosphatases to *myo*-inositol or it can be phosphorylated by a specific kinase to inositol-1,3,4,5-tetrakisphosphate (I-1,3,4,5-P_4). Although it has not been proved, some investigators think that I-1,3,4,5-P_4 is biologically active and can influence cell Ca^{2+} homeostasis by acting with I-1,4,5-P_3 to stimulate influx of extracellular Ca^{2+}. I-1,3,4,5-P_4 can be de-phosphorylated to inositol-1,3,4-trisphosphate (I-1,3,4-P_3), which does not affect Ca^{2+} fluxes and can be converted by successive de-phosphorylations to *myo*-inositol. Alternatively, I-1,3,4,5-P_4 can be phosporylated to inositol pentakisphosphate (IP_5) and possibly to inositol hexakisphosphate (IP_6). It is not known whether IP_5 or IP_6 has second messenger activity. Thus I-1,4,5-P_3 is metabolized in a series of de-phosphorylation reactions that constitute a degradative pathway, whereas phosphorylation of I-1,4,5-P_3 may be an activatory pathway.

1,2-DAG may be phosphorylated by 1,2-DAG kinase to phosphatidic acid (PA). (1,2-DAG and PA are central intermediates in the synthesis of many cellular phospholipids.) PA can be condensed with cytidine triphosphate (CTP) to form CDP-diacylglycerol (CDP-DAG), a reaction catalyzed by PA: cytidylyl transferase. CDP-DAG and *myo*-inositol are utilized by PI synthase to form PI; cytidine monophosphate (CMP) is a by-product of this reaction. PI synthase is the only enzyme specific for the synthesis of PI. PI may then be successively phosphorylated to PI(4)P and PI (4,5)P_2 by PI 4-kinase and PI(4)P 5-kinase, respectively.

During stimulation of PPI hydrolysis, there is increased synthesis of PI, PI(4)P and PI(4,5)P_2 to replenish the pool of PI(4,5)P_2 that would otherwise be rapidly depleted.[18] For example, the amount of inositol phosphates formed in cells during a 15-minute stimulation by agonist can be the equivalent of 10 times the original content of PI(4,5)P_2. Therefore, during agonist stimulation there is a marked activation of PI synthase and of the PI 4-kinase and PI(4)P 5-kinase. The mechanism(s) through which synthesis of these lipids is increased has not been conclusively demonstrated. There is no evidence of direct activation of the synthetic enzymes by the receptor or by the second messengers generated. A mechanism for activation of PI synthase has been proposed[19]; however, data supporting it have been obtained in only a few cell types. This hypothesis is based on the observation that PI inhibits the activity of PI synthase, a phenomenon that has been termed *product inhibition*. It was proposed that during agonist-stimulated hydrolysis of PPI's and synthesis of PI(4)P and PI(4,5)P_2 the decrease in the level of PI releases the PI synthase from product inhibition and increases its activity. A similar mechanism does not account for the increase in the activities of the PPI kinases because there is only a transient decrease in PI(4)P or PI(4,5)P_2 during stimulation. Another circumstance in which PI synthesis can be diminished in some cell types in tissue culture is when they are deprived of the precursor, *myo*-inositol. This situation does not seem to be operative in the intact animal or human because the levels of *myo*-inositol in blood do not vary widely enough to affect PI synthesis under normal physiological conditions. It has been suggested, however, that *myo*-inositol depletion may occur in patients with diabetes mellitus[20] or that intracellular *myo*-inositol depletion could occur in cells of the CNS in patients who are receiving lithium therapy for manic-depressive illness.[21] Lithium may deplete cellular *myo*-inositol by inhibiting several of the

phosphatases that dephosphorylate the inositol polyphosphates.

The principal cellular site of synthesis of PI appears to be within the endoplasmic reticulum, but there is evidence that it also occurs in the plasma membrane.[22] Phosphorylation of PI to PI(4)P and then to PI(4,5)P_2 occurs predominantly in the plasma membrane. Because the majority of PPI hydrolysis occurs at the cell-surface membrane, PI synthesized within the endoplasmic reticulum would have to be transferred to the plasma membrane. Although transport proteins for phospholipids have been found,[23] there is no evidence that transport via these binding proteins is increased during stimulation of PPI hydrolysis. Another process that could account for the transfer of PI from the endoplasmic reticulum to the plasma membrane is membrane cycling. Receptor activation stimulates internalization (or endocytosis) and recycling (or retroendocytosis) of receptors[24] and may stimulate exocytosis in secretory cells. These movements of membrane-delimited vesicles from within the cell to the cell surface could serve to replenish some of the PI lost secondary to PPI hydrolysis. PI synthesis within the plasma membrane could be activated also.

CALCIUM SIGNALING

Regulated changes in intracellular calcium have been found to mediate some processes—for example, secretion, contraction, and transcription. Therefore, it is clear that events that lead to changes in $[Ca^{2+}]_i$ constitute an important signaling mechanism for a diverse number of cellular functions. The $[Ca^{2+}]_i$ in unstimulated cells is approximately 100 nanomolar (1×10^{-7}M), which is about 10,000-fold lower than the ambient extracellular Ca^{2+} concentration (Fig. 4–4). This low Ca^{2+} concentration is maintained by the concerted effects of a number of cellular processes. The major barrier to Ca^{2+} influx is the cell surface membrane, which is highly impermeable to Ca^{2+}. Ion channels in the plasma membrane through which Ca^{2+} can flow are predominantly inactive (or "closed") in unstimulated cells. In some cells, especially excitable cells such as neurons and neuroendocrine cells, these channels can exhibit brief activations ("Ca^{2+} spikes") spontaneously that allow significant basal Ca^{2+} influx. These channels can be activated (or "opened") to permit a large Ca^{2+} influx. In addition to preventing Ca^{2+} influx, the plasma membrane contains two energy-dependent processes that limit elevations of $[Ca^{2+}]_i$ by extruding Ca^{2+} from the cell. These are the Ca^{2+}-Mg^{2+} ATPase (or plasma membrane "Ca^{2+} pump") and the Na^+-Ca^{2+} exchange mechanism, which is dependent on the Na^+ gradient established by the Na^+-K^+ ATPase. Within the cell, several organelles sequester Ca^{2+} from the cytoplasm and thereby contribute to the maintenance of a low $[Ca^{2+}]_i$. The major organelles involved in this process are the endoplasmic reticulum and mitochondria. The endoplasmic reticulum is a high-affinity, low-capacity Ca^{2+}-sequestering organelle that plays a major role in maintaining $[Ca^{2+}]_i$ in the nanomolar range, whereas mitochondria, which have a lower affinity but higher capacity for Ca^{2+}, seem to serve a protective function against larger increases in $[Ca^{2+}]_i$. Ca^{2+} is sequestered within the endoplasmic reticulum because of the action of a mem-

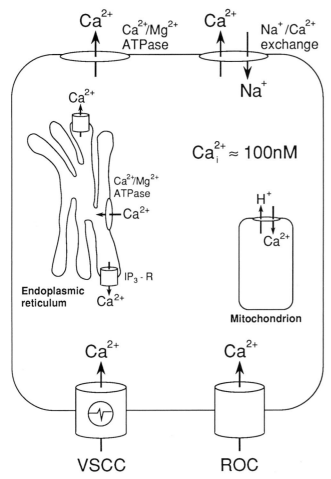

FIGURE 4–4. **Schematic depiction of a cell illustrating mechanisms of regulation of intracellular ionized calcium.** The concentration of ionized, or free, intracellular Ca^{2+} (Ca^{2+}_i) in the unstimulated cell is approximately 100 nM. The plasma membrane contains Ca^{2+}/Mg^{2+} ATPases, or plasma membrane "Ca^{2+} pumps," and Na^+/Ca^{2+} antiporters that extrude Ca^{2+} from the cell as well as voltage-sensitive calcium channels (VSCC's) and receptor-operated channels (ROC's), through which Ca^{2+} can enter the cell. VSCC's are present in excitable cells. The endoplasmic reticulum contains Ca^{2+}/Mg^{2+} ATPases, which are different from those present in the plasma membrane and allow sequestration of Ca^{2+}, and I-1,4,5-P_3-sensitive (I-1,4,5-P_3 receptor, IP_3-R) and I-1,4,5-P_3-insensitive mechanisms to allow for mobilization of Ca^{2+}. The mitochondria sequester calcium at high $[Ca^{2+}]_i$ through Ca^{2+}/H^+ antiporters.

brane-bound Ca^{2+}-Mg^{2+} ATPase, which is distinct from the Ca^{2+} pump in the plasma membrane and which "pumps" Ca^{2+} into the vesicular lumen. A different mechanism, which is based on the mitochondrial proton gradient, is involved in Ca^{2+} sequestration by mitochondria. $[Ca^{2+}]_i$ can be elevated during the action of agonists that signal via the PPI cascade by the release of Ca^{2+} from the endoplasmic reticulum. Thus $[Ca^{2+}]_i$ can rise either through entry of extracellular Ca^{2+} via the plasma membrane or through release of Ca^{2+} from endoplasmic reticulum stores. Elevations from either source, which range usually from 0.5 to 10 micromolar (5×10^{-7}M to 10^{-5}M), may take the form of oscillations or of sustained changes (see below). Extracellular Ca^{2+} influx occurs primarily through voltage-sensitive channels (in excitable cells) or through receptor-operated channels. Regulated mobilization of intracellular Ca^{2+} is thought to be from I-1,4,5-P_3-sensitive and -insensitive stores (see below).

The elevation of $[Ca^{2+}]_i$ leads in turn to the activation of a number of cellular processes. The central aspect of this process is an increase in binding of Ca^{2+} to a number of specific regulatory proteins (or protein subunits) that upon binding Ca^{2+} undergo a conformational change and are thereby activated. For example, in skeletal muscle cells, Ca^{2+} binds to troponin C and stimulates contraction. A ubiquitous Ca^{2+}-binding protein is calmodulin,[25] which is a protein that regulates a number of processes, including macromolecular synthesis, secretion, cytoskeletal function, carbohydrate metabolism, and ion transport. Ca^{2+}-calmodulin complexes bind to and activate several enzymes. Activation by Ca^{2+}-calmodulin complexes of some enzymes leads directly to the response, for example, activation of Ca^{2+}-Mg^{2+} ATPase leads to Ca^{2+} transport. Ca^{2+}-calmodulin complexes also activate a number of protein kinases that in turn phosphorylate other regulatory proteins on serine and threonine residues.[26] Some of these Ca^{2+}-calmodulin–dependent protein kinases, such as myosin light chain kinase (which regulates cytoskeletal function) and phosphorylase kinase (which regulates carbohydrate metabolism), phosphorylate a limited number of proteins and regulate specific processes. In contrast, Ca^{2+}-calmodulin–dependent multifunctional protein kinase phosphorylates a broad array of proteins and may mediate many of the more diverse actions caused by elevation of $[Ca^{2+}]_i$, for example, regulation of gene transcription, protein synthesis, and secretion in many different cells. Thus, subsequent to the elevation of $[Ca^{2+}]_i$, Ca^{2+} binds to regulatory proteins which in turn amplify and propagate the signal by activating a number of enzymes that activate other distal steps in the signaling cascade.

I-1,4,5-P_3 Mobilization of Calcium

Agonist stimulation of $PI(4,5)P_2$ hydrolysis leads to a rapid (within seconds) formation of I-1,4,5-P_3 that causes an elevation of $[Ca^{2+}]_i$.[27] I-1,4,5-P_3 is generated on the intracellular side of the plasma membrane and diffuses in the cytoplasm to bind to receptors on localized regions of the endoplasmic reticulum. The I-1,4,5-P_3 receptor is a Ca^{2+} channel that upon binding I-1,4,5-P_3 undergoes a conformational change through which the channel is "opened" and stored Ca^{2+} is released.[28]

The I-1,4,5-P_3 receptor is composed of four noncovalently bound identical subunits. It has been postulated that the membrane-spanning domains of the four subunits form a single central transmembrane pore. Cloning of the receptor subunit revealed it to be a large protein (molecular weight of greater than 250,000 kDa) with several putative membrane spanning domains near the carboxyl-terminus.[29, 30] The carboxyl-terminus is on the lumenal side of the membrane and a larger N-terminal region is on the cytoplasmic side of the membrane. Neuronal cells contain at least three specific subtypes of I-1,4,5-P_3 receptors that are generated through alternative splicing of a single gene, which occurs in a tissue-specific and developmental-specific manner.[31] Thus a variety of Ca^{2+} release responses may be possible in different cell types because of the presence of distinct receptor proteins.

It has been demonstrated that the binding of at least 3 molecules of I-1,4,5-P_3 is required for the opening of these calcium channels.[32] It has been postulated that binding of I-1,4,5-P_3 to a site on each subunit may induce a conformational change that, after binding of three or four I-1,4,5-P_3 molecules, would lead to an open ion channel. This requirement for binding of multiple I-1,4,5-P_3 molecules may affect the kinetics and magnitude of the release response.

An interesting finding is that there is sequence homology in the putative membrane regions of the I-1,4,5-P_3 receptor and the skeletal muscle ryanodine receptor, a calcium channel in the muscle sarcoplasmic reticulum that is involved in stimulus-contraction coupling.[30, 33] The ryanodine receptor appears to be responsible for calcium-induced calcium release in muscle cells. Calcium-induced calcium release in nonmuscle cells may occur via a ryanodine receptor–like protein that could sustain a Ca^{2+} response or generate Ca^{2+} oscillations stimulated by agonists that signal via PPI hydrolysis (see below).

Receptor Activation of Calcium Influx

Cell surface calcium channels can be viewed as pores in the plasma membrane that when opened permit the rapid influx of a large number of Ca^{2+} ions.[34, 35] Ca^{2+} channels have been divided into two large classes: voltage-sensitive calcium channels (VSCC's) and receptor-operated calcium channels (ROC's). It may be, however, that a single channel can be activated by depolarization or receptor activation without a change in membrane potential difference or that receptor activation can modify the opening of VSCC's caused by depolarization.

Much more is known about the structures and pharmacology of VSCC's than of ROC's; multiple subtypes have been described in different tissues. In general, the different types of VSCC's display differences in the membrane potential (or voltage) at which they are activated and the magnitude and duration of their conductances. The three major subtypes of VSCC's have been designated as L-type (long-lasting), T-type (transient), and N-type (neither long-lasting nor transient) channels. The N-type channel is primarily found in neuronal tissue. Important pharmacological tools for the study of these channels are antagonists that block Ca^{2+} flux. Dihydropyridine drugs, such as nifedipine, are used to discriminate between L- and T-type channels because L-type channels are inhibited by these agents, whereas T-type channels are not. L- and T-type channels have been found in neuroendocrine cells—for example, cells of the anterior pituitary gland.[36] In these cells, receptor activation leads to membrane depolarization that in turn opens VSCC's, causing a large influx of extracellular Ca^{2+}.

There are several mechanisms that lead to opening of ROC's.[37] Some cell surface receptors are themselves ion channels that are activated upon binding agonist. The best examples of receptors that are ion channels are not, however, selective Ca^{2+} channels. The nicotinic acetylcholine receptor, for example, is a cation channel that primarily allows Na^+ influx, but Ca^{2+} may transit the channel also. A second mechanism is activation of Ca^{2+} channels by G proteins.[38, 39] G protein activation has been observed, for example, for Ca^{2+} and K^+ channels. In addition to activation by depolarization, VSCC's in cardiac and skeletal mus-

cle cells have been shown to be directly activated by G_s, the activator of adenylyl cyclase. The receptor/Gs/Ca^{2+} channel, therefore, constitutes a complex that is activated upon agonist binding that is very similar to receptor/Gq/PPI-PLC-β. (A K^+ channel has been found to be opened by a member of the G_i family.[40])

Another mechanism involved in receptor activation of Ca^{2+} channels is mediation by second messenger molecules. For example, in cardiac myocytes, activation of the β-adrenergic receptor leads to generation of cAMP that activates cAMP-dependent protein kinase (protein kinase A) (see Ch. 5B), which phosphorylates the VSCC. Phosphorylation of the VSCC does not in itself activate the channel; rather, it increases the Ca^{2+} flux when the channel is activated by depolarization. Receptor activation of Ca^{2+} channels in cardiac cells is a good example of dual control of channel function by a direct G protein effect and by phosphorylation resulting from second messenger stimulation of a protein kinase (see below).

Receptor-Mediated Changes in [Ca^{2+}]$_i$

This section describes the changes in [Ca^{2+}]$_i$ that result from agonist action. In many cells, the majority of agonists stimulate release of intracellular Ca^{2+} and influx of extracellular Ca^{2+} simultaneously or in temporal sequence. Techniques for monitoring [Ca^{2+}]$_i$ have improved in sensitivity so that changes in [Ca^{2+}]$_i$ in individual cells can be measured. This has revealed a pattern of response that was obscured in the past by the averaging of changes in many cells. In addition to elevations of ionized Ca^{2+} in the cytoplasm to constant higher levels, an oscillatory pattern of changes in [Ca^{2+}]$_i$ is found in some cell types in response to certain agonists. Oscillatory changes in [Ca^{2+}]$_i$ had been known to occur in excitable cells, such as pacemaker cells of the sinoatrial node, but were not recognized in nonexcitable cells, such as hepatocytes. Oscillations in [Ca^{2+}]$_i$ can occur secondary to periodic changes in either Ca^{2+} influx or mobilization from cellular stores.[41, 42] A model has been presented to explain regulation of Ca^{2+}-dependent processes by a mechanism dependent on the frequency of Ca^{2+} oscillations,[43] rather than the better recognized amplitude-dependent mechanism (see above).

In excitable cells, agonists that signal via PPI hydrolysis often stimulate elevations in [Ca^{2+}]$_i$ that are caused both by release of Ca^{2+} from endoplasmic reticulum stores and influx of Ca^{2+} through VSCC's. These elevations can be oscillatory or nonfluctuating. In mammotrophs and gonadotrophs of the anterior pituitary, it has been found that receptor activation by thyrotropin-releasing hormone (TRH) and gonadotropin-releasing hormone (GnRH), respectively, stimulates biphasic elevations of [Ca^{2+}]$_i$, with the initial rise being caused by I-1,4,5-P_3 mobilization of endoplasmic reticulum Ca^{2+} followed by a secondary and more sustained rise caused by influx of extracellular Ca^{2+} through VSCC's (Fig. 4–5).[36, 44] The initial spike phase of these elevations may fluctuate or be nonoscillatory and is caused by I-1,4,5-P_3 release of cellular Ca^{2+}. These different patterns of elevation of [Ca^{2+}]$_i$ have been noted even among individual cells of cloned cell lines. Ca^{2+} influx does not contribute to these oscillations directly, although it is needed to replenish stores during prolonged stimula-

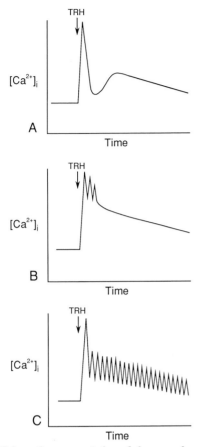

FIGURE 4–5. **Schematic representation of the several patterns of elevations in [Ca^{2+}]$_i$ in mammotrophs stimulated by TRH.** Examples of responses to TRH, administered at the indicated time. *A,* A biphasic nonoscillatory response consisting of an initial spike followed by a sustained plateau. *B,* An initial oscillatory spike phase followed by a non-oscillatory sustained phase. *C,* An initial spike followed by an oscillatory sustained phase. [Ca^{2+}]$_i$, concentration of ionized intracellular calcium.

tion. (This is in contrast to the better understood spontaneous or stimulated oscillations seen in neuronal cells that are caused by periodic Ca^{2+} influx through VSCC's.) The elevations of [Ca^{2+}]$_i$ are limited in magnitude and duration. This is caused by the transient nature of the activating mechanisms, which are inhibited by negative feedback regulation (see below), and by counterregulatory mechanisms that cause Ca^{2+} extrusion from cells and sequestration into cellular stores (see above).

Elevations of [Ca^{2+}]$_i$ in nonexcitable cells stimulated by agonists that signal via PPI hydrolysis can also be oscillatory or nonfluctuating. For example, stimulation of hepatocytes can lead to Ca^{2+} oscillations or nonfluctuating increases in [Ca^{2+}]$_i$. The oscillations in nonexcitable cells, as those found in neuroendocrine cells, are caused by I-1,4,5-P$_3$-mediated release of cellular Ca^{2+} and Ca^{2+} influx is necessary only to prevent depletion of cellular stores.

The mechanism of I-1,4,5-P$_3$-mediated Ca^{2+} oscillations is not known. A number of models based on observations in different cell types have been proposed to explain this phenomenon.[45] It is likely that none of these mechanisms is operative in all cell types but rather that different mechanisms mediate these changes in different cells. The four models are distinguished by two major characteristics: the presence or absence of fluctuation of I-1,4,5-P$_3$ concentra-

tion and positive or negative feedback by Ca^{2+}. In the first model it is proposed that I-1,4,5-P$_3$ oscillates and Ca^{2+} feedback is positive. I-1,4,5-P$_3$ formation fluctuates in parallel with the changes in [Ca^{2+}]$_i$ because Ca^{2+} may increase the activity of some PPI-PLC isoenzymes. When [Ca^{2+}]$_i$ increases, more I-1,4,5-P$_3$ is formed, and when Ca^{2+} decreases, I-1,4,5-P$_3$ formation is diminished. The decrease in Ca^{2+} is caused by transient depletion of I-1,4,5-P$_3$-sensitive Ca^{2+} stores. In the second model it is proposed that I-1,4,5-P$_3$ oscillates and Ca^{2+} feedback is negative. Activation of PKC is proposed to inhibit formation of I-1,4,5-P$_3$ by inhibiting receptor–G protein coupling or activation of PPI-PLC (see below). The effect of PKC may be caused by phosphorylation of the receptor, G protein, or PPI-PLC. Therefore, in this model negative feedback regulation causes the transient inhibition of I-1,4,5-P$_3$ formation and establishes I-1,4,5-P$_3$ fluctuations. A third model proposes that the level of I-1,4,5-P$_3$ does not oscillate and that Ca^{2+} feeds back negatively on Ca^{2+} release. In this model, after a time delay, Ca^{2+} inhibits I-1,4,5-P$_3$-induced Ca^{2+} release by affecting the I-1,4,5-P$_3$ receptor. When [Ca^{2+}]$_i$ is sufficiently decreased, Ca^{2+} release is initiated again. In the fourth model it is proposed that I-1,4,5-P$_3$ does not oscillate and Ca^{2+} feeds back positively on Ca^{2+} release. In this model there are two cellular stores of Ca^{2+}, one of which is I-1,4,5-P$_3$-sensitive and the other is insensitive. The elevation of [Ca^{2+}]$_i$ caused by I-1,4,5-P$_3$ in turn releases Ca^{2+} from the I-1,4,5-P$_3$-insensitive store, and decreases in Ca^{2+} occur when this store is transiently depleted. This model is therefore based on the concept of Ca^{2+}-induced Ca^{2+} release that was first observed in muscle cells. This mechanism of Ca^{2+}-induced Ca^{2+} release has also been postulated to account for the "wave" of elevation of [Ca^{2+}]$_i$ observed in some cells that is initiated in one part of a cell and then traverses across the entire cell.[1]

1,2-DAG and Protein Kinase C

The other limb of the PPI pathway is activated by 1,2-DAG.[46] 1,2-DAG, in combination with phosphatidylserine (PS) and, depending on the isoenzyme subtype (see below), with or without an elevation of [Ca^{2+}]$_i$, activates the phospholipid-dependent PKC.[47, 48] PKC in turn phosphorylates a number of regulatory proteins leading to more distal effects such as stimulation of secretion and of transcription. In unstimulated cells, the level of 1,2-DAG in membranes is very low but accumulates transiently in response to an agonist. Phorbol esters, such as phorbol myristate acetate (12-O-tetradecanoylphorbol-13-acetate), are potent tumor promoters that can mimic 1,2-DAG and activate PKC. Phorbol esters (or synthetic 1,2-DAG's such as 1-oleoyl-2-acetylglycerol) have been used widely in studies of this limb of the PPI signaling pathway because they activate PKC without involving receptors or requiring hydrolysis of PPI's.

PKC is a serine and threonine kinase, that is, it phosphorylates serine and threonine residues in protein substrates but does not phosphorylate tyrosine residues. PKC activation is thought to require translocation from a cytosolic location to membranes. Although it was initially thought that PKC was activated only when it became associated with the plasma membrane, there is evidence that PKC can also associate with and be activated within the membrane of the nucleus.[49]

PKC has been found to be a family of at least eight isoenzymes. In vitro, PKC isoenzymes α, βI, βII, and γ are Ca^{2+}- and phospholipid-dependent enzymes, whereas isoenzymes δ, ϵ, ζ, and η are Ca^{2+}-independent but phospholipid-dependent.[50] The Ca^{2+}-dependent protein kinase C may require involvement of both limbs of the PPI pathway for activation in vivo, whereas the Ca^{2+}-independent isoenzymes may be activated by 1,2-DAG alone. As is discussed later, there are receptor-activated phospholipases that can hydrolyze phospholipids other than PPI's to generate 1,2-DAG without forming I-1,4,5-P_3 or stimulating increases in $[Ca^{2+}]_i$. It has been suggested that activation of different PKC isoenzymes in vivo may lead to distinct cellular responses. This could occur if different isoenzymes phosphorylated distinct proteins. This has not been shown as yet, but this aspect of signaling is undergoing intensive investigation. Differential activation of PKC isoenzymes could be caused, for example, by differences in agonist effects on $[Ca^{2+}]_i$. It is also possible that activation of different isoenzymes may occur because they are present in different cellular compartments. Differential regulation of PKC isoenzymes has been shown to occur during stimulation of a single cell type by a single agonist. For example, TRH stimulates three phases of 1,2-DAG elevation in GH_3 pituitary cells in culture at 15 seconds, 10 minutes, and 6 to 12 hours, respectively.[51] The early peak causes the redistribution of PKC isoenzymes α, β, δ, and ϵ; the second peak does not stimulate PKC; and the third peak corresponds to down-regulation (and perhaps activation) of PKC ϵ but not of α, β, and δ. Thus elevations in 1,2-DAG can have differential effects on PKC isoenzymes that may lead to distinct cellular responses.

An important proximate effect of activation of PKC is one of negative feedback to inhibit PPI signaling, which has been observed in several cell types.[52] This effect, which could be mediated by phosphorylation of the receptor,[53] G protein,[54] or PPI-PLC,[4] can inhibit continued activation of the PPI-PLC and thereby limit the response. Activation of PKC has also been found to inhibit Ca^{2+} influx by phosphorylation of Ca^{2+} channels.[35] The more distal effects of activation of PKC, which are primarily mediated by phosphorylation of regulatory proteins, include stimulation of secretion from endocrine, exocrine, and blood cells, of steroidogenesis in adrenal and Leydig cells, of lipogenesis in adipocytes, of glycogenolysis in hepatocytes, and of contraction of smooth muscle cells. PKC is also a mediator of cellular growth and proliferation and may be abnormally activated in some forms of tumorigenesis.[47]

Although it appears that the primary role of 1,2-DAG is to activate PKC, 1,2-DAG has other actions in signal transduction. 1,2-DAG appears to activate and translocate other enzymes involved in cell signaling such as 1,2-DAG kinase and phospholipase A_2.[55] Further, 1,2-DAG is an important precursor for the production of arachidonic acid and its active metabolites, the eicosanoids,[56] through the action of 1,2-DAG lipase.[57] (Another important signaling pathway that generates eicosanoids more directly involves the activation of phospholipase A_2. Phospholipase A_2 hydrolyzes phospholipids at the 2-position of the glycerol backbone to release arachidonic acid.[58])

Formation of 1,2-DAG Without I-1,4,5-P_3

There are other phospholipases that appear to be involved in signal transduction, although they are not as well understood as the pathway activated by PPI-PLC. Activation of a phosphatidylcholine-specific phospholipase C (PC-PLC), which hydrolyzes PC to yield 1,2-DAG and phosphocholine (see Fig. 4–3), has been implicated in signaling in hepatocytes and several other cell types by a number of agonists that may also activate PPI hydrolysis.[59] There are several differences between the signals generated by PC hydrolysis versus $PI(4,5)P_2$ hydrolysis. PC-PLC activation does not lead to a second messenger that can elevate $[Ca^{2+}]_i$ because phosphocholine does not affect cellular Ca^{2+} homeostasis. Because $[Ca^{2+}]_i$ does not increase, Ca^{2+}-dependent processes are not activated and the Ca^{2+}-independent PKC isoenzymes may be activated specifically (see above). Different PKC isoenzymes may also be more activated during PC hydrolysis than during PPI hydrolysis because the fatty acid composition of PC's and PPI's is different,[60] and 1,2-DAG's with different fatty acyl groups may activate PKC isoenzymes differently. Further, the magnitude and duration of formation of 1,2-DAG are markedly greater with activation of PC-PLC than with PPI-PLC. This appears to be so because the cell content of PC (35 to 40 per cent of phospholipids) is greater than that of PPI's, and negative feedback to inhibit PC hydrolysis is not as marked as with $PI(4,5)P_2$ hydrolysis. This suggests that stimulation of PC hydrolysis may be involved with processes such as cell growth and differentiation that are dependent on persistent activation of PKC.

Another pathway leading indirectly to 1,2-DAG formation has recently begun to be elucidated, but its physiologic role is not certain. This involves receptor activation of a phospholipase D that hydrolyzes phospholipids to yield phosphatidic acid (PA) and the de-phosphorylated polar head group (see Fig. 4–3). PA can in turn be de-phosphorylated to 1,2-DAG by PA phosphohydrolase. The specific phospholipids hydrolyzed by receptor-activated phospholipase D are not well defined, although PC is a substrate for this enzyme. These reactions, therefore, not only produce 1,2-DAG but also PA, which may have separate effects in signal transduction.[61]

INTERACTIONS BETWEEN SIGNALING PATHWAYS

It is important to consider that agonist stimulation of the PPI signaling cascade often occurs in a physiological setting in which the cell is receiving input from multiple extracellular regulatory factors; therefore, several signaling pathways are being activated simultaneously. In fact, it is now clear that several of the hormones, neurotransmitters, and growth factors that activate the I-1,4,5-P_3/1,2-DAG/Ca^{2+} signaling pathway activate other pathways concomitantly. This may occur because a cell may exhibit more than one receptor (or receptor subtype) that can bind a given agonist (see Ch. 3). For example, adrenergic agonists can bind to different receptors that can activate PPI hydrolysis (α-1 receptors), or stimulate (β receptors) or inhibit (α-2 receptors) adenylyl cyclase by coupling to different G proteins.[62, 63] Alternatively, a single receptor can couple to two different G proteins and regulate two different signaling pathways.[13] The advent of molecular cloning techniques has made it possible to transfect a cell with a specific receptor and distinguish whether a single receptor can activate more than one G protein. Examples of coupling of a receptor to more than one G protein are shown in Table 4–1. For example, activation of the m2 muscarinic receptor causes marked inhibition of adenylyl cyclase and weak stimulation of PPI hydrolysis[64] by interacting with G_i and G_q, respectively, whereas binding of agonist to the receptor for thyroid-stimulating hormone (thyrotropin, TSH) simultaneously stimulates adenylyl cyclase and PPI hydrolysis apparently by activating G_s and G_q, respectively.[65] A single receptor for growth factors such as epidermal growth factor or platelet-derived growth factor, which contain intrinsic protein tyrosine kinase activity, activates PPI hydrolysis by phosphorylating PPI-PLC-γI simultaneously with stimulation of other components of the tyrosine kinase cascade.[15]

When two or more transduction cascades are activated simultaneously, either because of being initiated by the same agonist or by different agonists, the intracellular signaling molecules can affect similar processes and the cellular response(s) can thereby be varied. There are examples in which two (or more) distinct pathways affect the same response in which the two pathways interact to produce an additive or synergistic response, or in which activation of one pathway inhibits the response stimulated by the other. These interactions may occur at one or several steps in the signaling cascade. For example, secretion from the anterior pituitary gland can be stimulated by elevations of $[Ca^{2+}]_i$ and cAMP.[66] In prolactin-secreting cells, TRH stimulates prolactin secretion by activating the PPI signaling cascade, whereas vasoactive intestinal peptide (VIP) stimulates prolactin secretion by elevating cAMP. When TRH and VIP are added simultaneously at maximally effective concentrations, stimulation of prolactin secretion is additive and the kinetics of stimulated prolactin secretion is a composite of the two agonist effects. When TRH is added hours before, the amount of prolactin secreted in response to VIP is increased because TRH stimulates prolactin synthesis as well as secretion. Angiotensin II (AII), like TRH, stimulates prolactin secretion by activating the PPI signaling cascade. When both TRH and AII are added simultaneously at maximum concentrations, stimulation of prolactin secretion is not fully additive. If cells are exposed to TRH before addition of AII, stimulation of prolactin secretion by AII is attenuated. This diminished response to AII may be caused by feedback inhibition caused by TRH, which might be mediated by PKC-mediated phosphorylation of the AII receptor, G protein, or PPI-PLC (see above). Attenuation of the response to TRH is also observed when pituitary cells are stimulated persistently by TRH.[67] This attenuation of response to agonist has been termed *desensitization*.[68] It is evident, therefore, that not only are cellular responses varied by which agonists are acting but also by the kinetics of their action. These interactions are common and are required for the differences observed in the actions of these extracellular regulatory factors under different physiological conditions.

CONCLUDING REMARKS

A fundamental aspect of cell regulation is the capacity to elicit specific responses to different extracellular regulatory molecules in a single cell using the same signal transduction pathway. For receptors that signal through phospholipid hydrolysis, specificity is in part the result of the interactions among the three intracellular messengers: I-1,4,5-P_3, 1,2-DAG, and Ca^{2+}. These messengers interact in positive and negative ways to modulate initiation and propagation of the signaling cascade. Because different receptors cause distinct patterns of generation of these messengers, distinct interactions occur and varied responses are elicited. This contrasts with another ubiquitous signaling system, adenylyl cyclase–cAMP, in which a single messenger is generated. Thus, signaling via phospholipid hydrolysis appears to generate a broader range of specific responses than can be elicited by receptors that signal via cAMP.

REFERENCES

1. Berridge MJ, Irvine RF: Inositol phosphates and cell signaling. Nature 341:197–205, 1989.
2. Majerus PW, Ross TS, Cunningham TW, et al: Recent insights in phosphatidylinositol signaling. Cell 63:459–465, 1990.
3. Cantley LC, Auger KR, Carpenter C, et al: Oncogenes and signal transduction. Cell 64:281–302, 1991.
4. Rhee SG, Choi KD: Regulation of inositol phospholipid-specific phospholipase C isozymes. J Biol Chem 267:12393–12396, 1992.
5. Gilman AG: Regulation of adenylyl cyclase by G proteins. Adv Second Messenger Phosphoprotein Res 24:51–57, 1990.
6. DeVivo M, Gershengorn MC: G proteins and phospholipid turnover, ADP-ribosylating Toxins and G Proteins. *In* Moss J, Vaughan M (eds): Insights into Signal Transduction. Washington, D.C., American Society for Microbiology, 1990, p 267.
7. Simon MI, Strathmann MP, Gautam N: Diversity of G proteins in signal transduction. Science 252:802–808, 1991.
8. Ui M: Pertussis Toxin as a Valuable Probe for G-Protein Involvement in Signal Transduction, ADP-ribosylating Toxins and G Proteins. *In* Moss J, Vaughan M (eds): Insights into Signal Transduction. Washington, D.C., American Society for Microbiology, 1990, p 45.
9. Smrcka AV, Hepler JR, Brown KO, Sternweis PC: Regulation of polyphosphoinositide-specific phospholipase C activity by purified G_q. Science 251:804–807, 1991.
10. Wu D, Lee CM, Rhee SG, Simon MI: Activation of phospholipase C by the α subunits of the G_q and G_{11} proteins in transfected Cos-7 cells. J Biol Chem 267:1811–1817, 1992.
11. Taylor SJ, Chae HZ, Rhee SG, Exton JH: Activation of the β1 isozyme of phospholipase C by α subunits of the G_q class of G proteins. Nature 350:516–518, 1991.
12. Gutowski S, Smrcka A, Nowak L, et al: Antibodies to the α_q subfamily of guanine nucleotide-binding regulatory protein α subunits attenuate activation of phosphatidylinositol 4,5-bisphosphate hydrolysis by hormones. J Biol Chem 266:20519–20524, 1991.
13. Dohlman HG, Thorner J, Caron MG, Lefkowitz RJ: Model systems for the study of seven-transmembrane-segment receptors. Annu Rev Biochem 60:653–688, 1991.
14. Kaziro Y, Itoh H, Kozasa T, et al: Structure and function of signal-transducing GTP-binding proteins. Annu Rev Biochem 60:349–400, 1991.
15. Ullrich A, Schlessinger J: Signal transduction by receptors with tyrosine kinase activity. Cell 61:203–212, 1990.
16. Irvine RF, Moor RM, Pollock WK, et al: Inositol phosphates: proliferation, metabolism and function. Philos Trans R Soc Lond (Biol) 320:281–298, 1988.
17. Bansal VS, Majerus PW: Phosphatidylinositol-derived precursors and signals. Annu Rev Cell Biol 6:41–67, 1990.

18. Monaco ME, Gershengorn MC: Subcellular organization of receptor-mediated phosphoinositide turnover. Endocr Rev 13:707–718, 1992.

19. Imai A, Gershengorn MC: Regulation by phosphatidylinositol of rat pituitary plasma membrane and endoplasmic reticulum phosphatidyl-inositol synthase activities. A mechanism for activation of phosphoinositide resynthesis during cell stimulation. J Biol Chem 262:6457–6459, 1987.

20. Zhu X, Eichberg J: A *myo*-inositol pool utilized for phosphatidylinositol synthesis is depleted in sciatic nerve from rats with streptozotocin-induced diabetes. Proc Natl Acad Sci USA 87:9818–9822, 1990.

21. Berridge MJ, Downes CP, Hanley MR: Neural and developmental actions of lithium: A unifying hypothesis. Cell 59:411–419, 1989.

22. Imai A, Gershengorn MC: Independent phosphatidylinositol synthesis in pituitary plasma membrane and endoplasmic reticulum. Nature 325:726–728, 1987.

23. Wirtz KWA: Phospholipid transfer proteins. Annu Rev Biochem 60:73–99, 1991.

24. Goldstein JL, Brown MS, Anderson RGW, et al: Receptor-mediated endocytosis: Concepts emerging from the LDL receptor system. Annu Rev Cell Biol 1:1–39, 1985.

25. Klee CB, Crouch TH, Richman PG: Calmodulin. Annu Rev Biochem 49:489–515, 1980.

26. Hanson PI, Schulman H: Neuronal Ca^{2+}/calmodulin-dependent protein kinases. Annu Rev Biochem 61:559–601, 1992.

27. Berridge MJ: Inositol trisphosphate as a second messenger in signal transduction. Ann NY Acad Sci 494:39–51, 1987.

28. Ferris CD, Snyder SH: Inositol 1,4,5-trisphosphate-activated calcium channels. Annu Rev Physiol 54:469–488, 1992.

29. Ferris CD, Huganir RL, Supattapone S, Snyder SH: Purified inositol 1,4,5-trisphosphate receptor mediates calcium flux in reconstituted lipid vesicles. Nature 342:87–89, 1989.

30. Furuichi T, Yoshikawa S, Miyawaki A, et al: Primary structure and functional expression of the inositol 1,4,5-trisphosphate-binding protein P$_{400}$. Nature 342:32–38, 1989.

31. Nakagawa T, Okano H, Furuichi T, et al: Novel subtypes of the mouse inositol 1,4,5-trisphosphate receptor are expressed in a tissue- and developmentally specific manner. Proc Natl Acad Sci USA 88:6244–6248, 1991.

32. Meyer T, Holowka D, Stryer L: Highly cooperative opening of calcium channels by inositol 1,4,5-trisphosphate. Science 240:653–656, 1988.

33. Takeshima H, Nishimura S, Matsumoto T, et al: Primary structure and expression from complementary DNA of skeletal muscle ryanodine receptor. Nature 339:439–445, 1989.

34. Catterall WA: Structure and function of voltage-sensitive ion channels. Science 242:50–61, 1988.

35. Hosey MM, Lazdunski M: Calcium channels: Molecular pharmacology, structure and regulation. J Membr Biol 104:81–105, 1988.

36. Stojilkovic SS, Catt KJ: Calcium oscillations in anterior pituitary cells. Endocr Rev 13:256–280, 1992.

37. Brown AM: A cellular logic for G protein-coupled ion channel pathways. FASEB J 5:2175–2179, 1991.

38. Birnbaumer L, Perez-Reyes E, Bertrand P, et al: Molecular diversity and function of G proteins and calcium channels. Biol Reprod 44:207–224, 1991.

39. Brown AM, Birnbaumer L: Ionic channels and their regulation by G protein subunits. Annu Rev Physiol 52:197–213, 1990.

40. Brown AM, Birnbaumer L: Direct G protein gating of ion channels. Am J Physiol 254:H401–10, 1988.

41. Berridge MJ: Calcium oscillations. J Biol Chem 265:9583–9586, 1990.

42. Berridge MJ: Cytoplasmic calcium oscillations: A two pool model. Cell Calcium 12:63–72, 1991.

43. Goldbeter A, Dupont G, Berridge MJ: Minimal model for signal-induced Ca^{2+} oscillations and for their frequency encoding through protein phosphorylation. Proc Natl Acad Sci USA 87:1461–1465, 1990.

44. Gershengorn MC: Mechanism of thyrotropin releasing hormone stimulation of pituitary hormone secretion. Annu Rev Physiol 48:515–526, 1986.

45. Harootunian AT, Kao JPY, Paranjape S, Tsien RY: Generation of calcium oscillations in fibroblasts by positive feedback between calcium and IP$_3$. Science 251:75–78, 1991.

46. Bishop WR, Bell RM: Functions of diacylglycerol in glycerolipid metabolism, signal transduction and cellular transformation. Oncogene Res 2:205–218, 1988.

47. Nishizuka Y: The role of protein kinase C in cell surface signal transduction and tumour promotion. Nature 308:693–698, 1984.

48. Rooney DE, MacLachlan N, Smith J, et al: Early amniocentesis: A cytogenetic evaluation. Br Med J 298:25, 1989.

49. Divecha N, Banfic H, Irvine RF: The polyphosphoinositide cycle exists in the nuclei of Swiss 3T3 cells under the control of a receptor (for IGF-I) in the plasma membrane, and stimulation of the cycle increases nuclear diacylglycerol and apparently induces translocation of protein kinase C to the nucleus. EMBO J 10:3207–3214, 1991.

50. Nishizuka Y: The molecular heterogeneity of protein kinase C and its implications for cellular regulation. Nature 334:661–665, 1988.

51. Kiley SC, Parker PJ, Fabbro D, Jaken S: Differential regulation of protein kinase C isozymes by thyrotropin-releasing hormone in GH$_4$C$_1$ cells. J Biol Chem 266:23761–23768, 1991.

52. Kikkawa U, Nishizuka Y: The role of protein kinase C in transmembrane signaling. Annu Rev Cell Biol 2:149–178, 1986.

53. Leeb-Lundberg LMF, Cotecchia S, Lomasney JW, et al: Phorbol esters promote α$_1$-adrenergic receptor phosphorylation and receptor uncoupling from inositol phospholipid metabolism. Proc Natl Acad Sci USA 82:5651–5655, 1985.

54. Pyne NJ, Murphy GJ, Milligan G, Houslay MD: Treatment of intact hepatocytes with either the phorbol ester TPA or glucagon elicits the phosphorylation and functional inactivation of the inhibitory guanine nucleotide regulatory protein G$_i$. FEBS Lett 243:77–82, 1989.

55. Bell RM, Coleman RA: Enzymes of glycerolipid synthesis in eukaryotes. Annu Rev Biochem 49:459–487, 1980.

56. Smith WL, Borgeat P: The eicosanoids: Prostaglandins, thromboxanes, leukotrienes, and hydroxyeicosaenoic acids. *In* Vance DE, Vance JE: Biochemistry of Lipids and Membranes. Menlo Park, CA, Benjamin-Cummings, 1985, p 325.

57. Irvine RF: How is the level of free arachidonic acid controlled in mammalian cells? Biochem J 204:3–16, 1982.

58. Waite M: The Phospholipases. New York, Plenum Press, 1987.

59. Exton JH: Signaling through phosphatidylcholine breakdown. J Biol Chem 265:1–4, 1990.

60. Holub BJ, Kuksis A: Metabolism of molecular species of diacylglycerophospholipids. Adv Lipid Res 16:1–125, 1978.

61. Putney JW, Jr: Recent hypotheses regarding the phosphatidylinositol effect. Life Sci 29:1183–1194, 1981.

62. Emorine LJ, Feve B, Pairault J, et al: Structural basis for functional diversity of β$_1$-, β$_2$- and β$_3$-adrenergic receptors. Biochem Pharmacol 41:853–859, 1991.

63. Lomasney JW, Cotecchia S, Lefkowitz RJ, Caron MG: Molecular biology of α-adrenergic receptors: Implications for receptor classification and for structure-function relationships. Biochim Biophys Acta Mol Cell Res 1095:127–139, 1991.

64. Hosey MM: Diversity of structure, signaling and regulation within the family of muscarinic cholinergic receptors. FASEB J 6:845–852, 1992.

65. Vassart G, Parmentier M, Libert F, Dumont J: Molecular genetics of the thyrotropin receptor. Trends Endocrinol Metab 2:151–156, 1991.

66. Mason WT, Rawlings SR, Cobbett P, et al: Control of secretion in anterior pituitary cells—linking ion channels, messengers and exocytosis. J Exp Biol 139:287–316, 1988.

67. Perlman JH, Gershengorn MC: Thyrotropin-releasing hormone stimulation of phosphoinositide hydrolysis desensitizes. Evidence against mediation by protein kinase C or calcium. Endocrinology 129:2679–2686, 1991.

68. Hausdorff WP, Caron MG, Lefkowitz RJ: Turning off the signal: Desensitization of β-adrenergic receptor function. FASEB J 4:2881–2889, 1990.

Cyclic AMP Second Messenger Signaling Pathway

JOEL F. HABENER

The discovery of the cAMP second messenger signaling pathway made a major impact in understanding how growth, development, and metabolism of cells is regulated in response to environmental cues. Studies that led to an elucidation of the mechanisms involved in the important cAMP-directed signaling pathway have spanned nearly five decades. The historical aspects of the key research discoveries are reviewed briefly. Lessons can be learned by appreciating the conceptualization and experimentation that systematically led to further conclusions, modifications of hypotheses, and additional experimentation carried out successively by the Coris,[1] Rall and Sutherland,[2] Fischer,[3] and Krebs,[4] all of whom were awarded the Nobel Prize in physiology and medicine. Several excellent reviews of various aspects of the cAMP-dependent signaling system have appeared.[5–12]

Historical Perspectives

In the early 1940's, the Coris established the basic biochemistry of glycogenolysis by the identification of the key enzymes of glycogen metabolism, namely, glycogen phosphorylase, phosphoglucomutase, and glucose-6-phosphatase.[13] Most importantly, they demonstrated that glycogen breakdown is stimulated by the hormones glucagon and epinephrine. A key finding was that glycogen phosphorylase was interconvertible from an inactive form (phosphorylase b) to an active form (phosphorylase a), a discovery for which the Coris were jointly awarded the Nobel Prize in 1951.[1] These pioneering studies were further pursued by Sutherland and his co-workers, who, using broken liver

cell preparations, showed that glucagon and epinephrine stimulated the activity of glycogen phosphorylase, a rate-limiting step in the conversion of glycogen to glucose.[2] Further, they demonstrated that although the hormonally responsive enzymatic activity resided in the particulate fraction, the generation of activity required the re-addition of the soluble fraction contained in the broken cell preparation.[14] These seminal observations led Sutherland to the isolation and identification of the essential factor in the soluble fraction as an adenine ribonucleotide, subsequently established to be 3′,5′-monophosphate, otherwise known as cAMP.[15] The work of this group culminated in the isolation and characterization of adenylyl cyclase and phosphodiesterase, the two key enzymes responsible for the synthesis and degradation of cAMP, respectively. Identification of cAMP was an essential step for the consequent conceptualization of the "second messenger" hypothesis by which hormones, acting on receptors located on the cell surface, lead to the synthesis of the second messenger (cAMP), which in turn regulates cellular activity. This concept provided a model to explain how extracellular signals such as hormones can transduce their informational cues to the interior of the cell. For this series of brilliant discoveries Sutherland was awarded the Nobel Prize in 1971.

During the time that Sutherland and his co-workers were characterizing adenylyl cyclase and phosphodiesterase, Fischer and Krebs pursued further the identification of the targets in the signal transduction pathway on which cAMP exerts its effects. In the late 1950's they discovered that the activity of glycogen phosphorylase is altered by a reversible phosphorylation mediated by phosphorylase kinase and opposing phosphatases, and that the phosphorylation required cAMP.[10, 16, 17] In 1968, the laboratories of Krebs and Greengard independently isolated the enzyme responsible for the activation of phosphorylase kinase.[18, 19] The enzyme was called *phosphorylase kinase kinase*, because it phosphorylated phosphorylase kinase; however, it was soon discovered to be the key enzyme activated by cAMP and was renamed *cAMP-dependent protein kinase A* (cPK, PKA) because of its widespread importance in the phosphorylation of many substrate proteins other than phosphorylase kinase.[10] As discussed below, PKA is a heterotetrameric protein consisting of two regulatory and two catalytic subunits. cAMP binds to the regulatory subunit and thereby relieves inhibition of the catalytic subunit by releasing the activated catalytic subunit from the inactive complex with the regulatory subunit. The catalytic subunit is then free to phosphorylate specifically certain serine and threonine residues in proteins whose functions are regulated by PKA. Krebs and Fischer shared the Nobel Prize in 1992 for their work on this critically important pathway of phosphorylation (and dephosphorylation) initiated by cAMP-dependent protein kinase A.[3, 4]

Pleiotropic Actions of cAMP

The cellular actions of cAMP are numerous (Fig. 5–1). Notably, with few exceptions, all of the actions of cAMP are mediated by PKA. One exception appears to be that cAMP binds to and directly regulates the activity of olfactory receptor–regulated ion channels.[20] cAMP, via its actions on PKA, activates certain enzymes and inactivates others. For example, phosphorylase kinase[10] and type II PKA[6, 7] are activated, and glycogen synthase is inactivated phosphorylations by PKA[10] (see below). Certain receptors, e.g., β-adrenergic receptors[23, 24] and ion channels, e.g., cystic fibrosis transmembrane conductance regulator (CFTR),[25] are regulated by phosphorylation by PKA. In addition, the structural proteins tubulin[26] and microtubule-associated proteins[27] are modified by PKA-induced phosphorylation. An important function of PKA is the phosphorylation and consequent activation of nuclear transcription factors that bind to cAMP-responsive enhancer elements of many genes. These proteins are known variously as cAMP response-element binding proteins (CREB's) or activating transcription factors (ATF's).[28–30] PKA also stimulates glucocorticoid receptor–mediated gene transcription, but this effect of PKA may be indirect via the phosphorylation of

an intermediate factor.[31] The regulatory subunit of PKA is a homologue of the prokaryotic catabolite activating protein,[21] and the regulatory subunit has been shown by fluorescence assays to bind DNA in vitro.[23] There is, however, as yet no clear evidence to support a functional role for the regulatory subunit in animal cells apart from its important actions as an inhibitor of the catalytic subunit.

The mechanism by which phosphorylation activates or inactivates the biological functions of a protein most often involves a change in the conformation or folding of the protein.[32, 33] The change in conformation is considered to be allosteric when the change in the shape of the protein occurs at a distance from the site that is phosphorylated by a specific protein kinase, for example, by PKA. Examples of the involvement of PKA in the allosteric regulation of protein activities are discussed later in this chapter.

cAMP Cross-Talk with Other Signaling Pathways

The cAMP-dependent signaling pathway is frequently coupled to, and works in concert with, other cellular signaling pathways. Such pathways include (1) the phospholipase C–mediated production of the second messengers diacylglycerol and inositol triphosphate that activate protein kinase C and intracellular receptors responsible for the mobilization of ionic calcium from intracellular stores, respectively[34, 35]; (2) the calcium-calmodulin kinases[36]; and (3) the receptor-kinases that include the insulin, epidermal growth factor (EGF), insulin-like growth factor I (IGF-I), and platelet-derived growth factor (PDGF) receptors,[37, 38] among others.[39, 40]

Cross-talk among the different signaling pathways can occur by at least two mechanisms involving either intermolecular or intramolecular phosphorylation cascades. A classic example of an intermolecular cascade is the activation of an isoform of type II PKA in which the catalytic subunit "autophosphorylates" the regulatory subunit and thereby is at least partially responsible for the activation of the catalytic subunit (discussed below). Active PKA then phosphorylates and activates phosphorylase kinase, which in turn phosphorylates and activates glycogen phosphorylase, the key enzyme in converting glycogen to glucose-1-phosphate. Intramolecular phosphorylation cascades involve multisite and hierarchical protein phosphorylation by the participation of several so-called "processive" kinases that

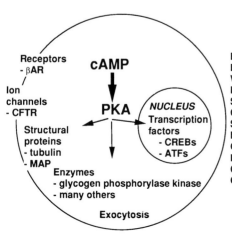

FIGURE 5–1. The cAMP-dependent second messenger pathway modifies many different cellular functions. Almost all functions of cAMP are mediated by the activation of protein kinase A (PKA). Some of the known functions modulated by PKA are shown on the right. Representative proteins, whose functions are regulated by PKA-directed phosphorylation, are depicted in the diagram of the cell shown on the left. βAR, adrenergic receptor; CFTR, cystic fibrosis transmembrane conductance regulator; MAP, microtubule-associated protein; CREB, cAMP response element binding protein; ATF, activating transcription factor.

act synergetically with other kinases by successive phosphorylations of closely adjacent sites on the same protein.[41, 42] For example, glycogen synthase is regulated (inactivated) by such a cascade, in which an initial phosphorylation by PKA (the primary kinase) is required for phosphorylation on a close-by serine or threonine by casein kinase isotype I. Casein kinases (CK) I and II preferentially phosphorylate serines or threonines in proteins that contain acidic amino acids within two to three residues aminoproximal (CKI) or carboxy-proximal (CKII) to the serine or threonine that is phosphorylated. The phosphorylation of a serine, threonine (or tyrosine), converts a neutral or hydrophobic amino acid to a negatively charged amino acid because of the highly negative charge imparted by the phosphate. To fully inactivate glycogen synthase, yet another intramolecular processive phosphorylation by casein kinase II, followed by a secondary phosphorylation by glycogen synthase kinase-3, is required.[43] The intricacies of the signaling pathways involved in the activation of these multiple kinases are not fully understood. However, a potent activator of CKII is the activated (ligand-bound) EGF-receptor kinase, a finding pointing to a cross-talk of signaling pathways between a receptor-tyrosine kinase and cAMP-dependent protein kinase.[44]

COMPONENTS OF THE cAMP-DEPENDENT CELLULAR SIGNALING PATHWAY

The cAMP-dependent signaling pathway consists of several intermolecular interactions leading to the generation of an active catalytic subunit of PKA capable of phosphorylating target sites on protein substrates. A generalized overall schematic illustration of this pathway is given in Figure 5–2. The detailed molecular mechanisms at work in the cascade of molecular interactions have yet to be completely elucidated. However, some interpretations can be made regarding how the individual components of the pathway are linked together.

Model of Activation of Protein Kinase A by cAMP

The initiating event in the pathway of cAMP-dependent signaling is the binding of a hormone (ligand) to its receptor. This type of interaction appears to be a crucial first step in the signaling cascade resulting in the eventual formation of cAMP. The binding of the hormone ligand to its receptor, which occurs specifically and with a high affinity (in the range of nanomolar concentrations of ligand), results in a change in the conformation of the receptor reflected within the transmembrane and cytoplasmic domains. The second step in the signaling cascade is the receptor-directed conversion of an associated guanine-binding protein (G protein) from an inactive to an active form. The cycling of G protein from an inactive to an active state and back to inactive form is described in greater detail below in reference to the model shown in Figure 5–3. The activated G protein, the guanosine triphosphate (GTP)-bound derivative of the G protein α-subunit, activates the enzyme adenylyl cyclase referred to earlier, leading to the conversion of ATP to $3'5'$ AMP, otherwise known as cAMP. The degradation of cAMP to $5'$AMP is effected by the enzyme phosphodiesterase (see Fig. 5–2). The key role of cAMP is to bind to the regulatory subunits of the inactive heterotetrameric complex of protein kinase A, thereby eliciting an allosteric change in the complex resulting in the liberation of the active catalytic subunits from the inactive complex. The catalytic subunits, once freed from their regulatory subunits, are available to phosphorylate sites on protein substrates, resulting in the modification of the biological actions of the proteins (see Fig. 5–2). A more detailed explanation of the cAMP-stimulated activation of PKA is given later in this chapter.

The G-Protein Cycle

The coupling of G proteins is of critical importance in transmitting the signal generated by hormone receptor interactions to the formation of cAMP (Fig. 5–3). The G proteins consist of complex families of α, β, and γ subunits that in the inactive state form heterotrimeric complexes with guanosine diphosphate (GDP) bound to the α-subunit.[11, 45–48] Much attention has been focused on the regulatory functions of the α-subunit, various isotypes of which can be either stimulatory ($G\alpha_s$) or inhibitory ($G\alpha_i$).

Binding of a ligand to its receptor effects a conformational change in the receptor and its associated G protein leading to the exchange of GTP for GDP and concomitant

FIGURE 5–2. cAMP-dependent signal transduction pathway. The diagram depicts the essential components of the cellular signaling pathway mediated by the second messenger cAMP. The "first" messenger or activator is the hormone/receptor/G-protein complex. The "second" messenger effector is cAMP. The "third" messenger is the protein kinase A that phosphorylates crucial protein substrates, resulting in the generation of the final bioactive "fourth" messenger. See text for a more detailed explanation.

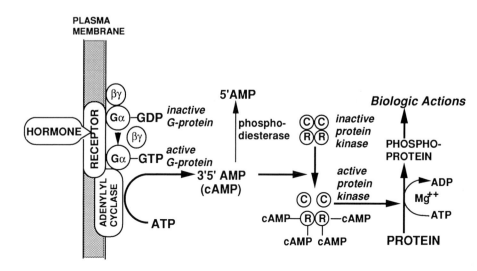

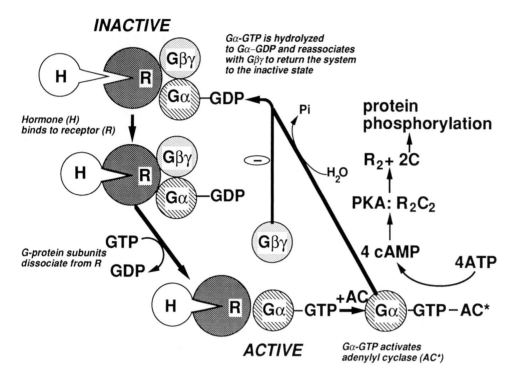

FIGURE 5–3. The guanine nucleotide–binding protein (G-protein) cycle. The diagram is a more detailed depiction of the G-protein function shown in Figure 5–2. The Gα-subunit can be either stimulatory (Gs) or inhibitory (Gi), depending on the isotype of the subunit involved. The activated Gα-GTP complex modulates the activity of adenylyl cyclase leading to the activation of protein kinase A and the resultant phosphorylation of key protein substrates that manifest the cellular response. Gα-GTP is inactivated by hydrolysis of GTP to GDP by the intrinsic GTPase activities of the Gα subunit.

dissociation of the GTP-bound α-subunit from the βγ-subunit dimeric complex. This GTP-activated Gα then binds to adenylyl cyclase to either activate or inhibit the enzyme, depending upon whether the type of Gα is stimulatory (Gαs) or inhibitory (Gαi). The extent of activated adenylyl cyclase formed depends on the relative amounts of stimulatory or inhibitory Gα subunits present in a given location within the cell at a given time. The pharmacological distinction between the actions of stimulatory and inhibitory G proteins has been facilitated by the use of two bacterial toxins that adenosine diphosphate (ADP)-ribosylate Gα subunits. Cholera toxin activates Gαs and pertussis toxin inhibits Gαi and Gαo ("other"), a G protein enriched in brain but whose functions are poorly understood. The use of nonhydrolyzable analogues of GTP, such as GPP(NH)P and GTPγS, has also been of great value in dissecting the G-protein pathways. These GTP analogues constitutively activate Gα proteins because they cannot be hydrolyzed to GDP.

Following the activation of adenylyl cyclase, the G proteins return to the inactive state. GTP is hydrolyzed to GDP by the intrinsic GTPase activity contained in the Gα-subunit. Gα dissociates from adenylyl cyclase and the βγ-subunits reassociate with the α-subunit. It is unknown to what extent the inactivation of G protein is due to the hydrolysis of GTP to GDP or to the reassociation of the α and βγ-subunits. It appears that the βγ complex may control certain effectors directly. It has been proposed that βγ can inhibit adenylyl cyclase directly or indirectly through interactions with calmodulin. Studies in vitro have shown that βγ inhibits type I adenylyl cyclase and stimulates the type II enzyme, whereas Gαs stimulates both enzyme isotypes.[49] In addition, βγ may regulate the activities of K+ channels and certain isotypes of phospholipase C. The inhibitory or stimulatory actions of βγ appear to reside in the particular isotype of the γ-subunit involved, of which a minimum of eight have been identified so far. The unraveling of the complex interactions of the G protein subunits is at the forefront of molecular and cellular research.

Investigators are just now beginning to understand the complex nature of the G proteins. In addition to the Gs and Gi heterotrimeric complexes, there are Gq and Go complexes that are coupled to phospholipid/Ca²⁺ and brain-specific pathways of signal transduction, respectively. Specific G-protein isotypes exist in the retina (Gt) and the olfactory epithelium (Golf). Twenty or more isotypes of Gα and at least a dozen isotypes of the Gβ (four) and Gγ (eight) subunit have been identified by sequencing of cloned recombinant cDNA's.[11] Many of the primary transcripts derived from the subunit genes are alternatively spliced, resulting in the formation of mRNA's that encode yet additional isoforms of the subunit proteins.[11] The precise functions of most of the large number of G-protein subunit isoforms are unknown, because at present they are proteins identified only by recombinant DNA cloning technology; investigators are in search of their cellular functions. An additional important function, however, of the class of G proteins that has been shown to couple to receptors is to regulate ion channels. Gs directly modulates the activity of voltage-dependent calcium channels, and evidence has been presented supporting a role for the pertussis-sensitive Gi and Go in the coupling of receptors of a variety of hormones and neurotransmitters to potassium and calcium channels,[50] resulting in either stimulatory or inhibitory control, depending on the type of channel affected.[51, 52] Further, the receptor-coupled and channel-coupled G proteins represent merely a subfamily of a much larger family of GTP-binding proteins involved in such diverse functions as the control of protein synthesis, e.g., elongation factor (EF-Tu), protein translocation across membranes, and ADP ribosylation (ADP-ribosylation factors, ARF's).[45] In addition, there exists an entire complex family of small GTP-binding proteins known as the Ras proteins involved in growth and differentiation, regulation of adenylyl cyclase, vesicular transport, as well as many other functions that have yet to be defined.[45]

The Adenylyl Cyclases

The adenylyl cyclases consist of a diverse family of membrane-associated enzymes of which at least eight distinct isotypes have been identified.[53] The distribution of the various enzyme isotypes among different tissues is highly variable. Most tissues contain several different isotypes, but in many tissues one or more of the isotypes are absent.

The structures of the adenylyl cyclases are remarkable inasmuch as they consist of two alternating hydrophobic and hydrophilic domains (Fig. 5–4). The hydrophobic domains contain six membrane-spanning domains, and the cytoplasmic hydrophilic domains each contain 250 residues that are homologous to the putative catalytic domains of the guanylyl cyclases. This overall structure of adenylyl cyclase is similar to those of the glucose transporters and to the P glycoprotein, the product of the multidrug resistance gene. This structure suggests that, in addition to its catalytic function of converting ATP to cAMP, the enzyme serves as the transporter that exports cAMP from the cell. The disposal of cAMP appears to involve two mechanisms: degradation by phosphodiesterase in the cell and transport out of the cell. Both mechanisms may in turn be regulated as a means for titrating the amount of cAMP available in the cell during the time that the catalytic activity of the enzyme is turned on by the active G protein, G_α-GTP. The differences in functions of the various isoforms of the adenylyl cyclases have not yet been determined.

Structures of the R and C Subunits of Protein Kinase A

The heterotetrameric complex that constitutes the holoenzyme of PKA consists of two catalytic and two regulatory subunits.[5–8] Thus far, three isotypes have been identified for the catalytic subunit (C_α, C_β, C_γ), apparent molecular weights (Mr) = 40,800, and two types for the regulatory subunit (RI, RII), each of which has two isotypes (RI_α, RI_β, RII_α, RII_β), Mr's of 92,000 to 108,000 (Table 5–1). The sequences of both the catalytic and the regulatory subunits are highly conserved. For example, the amino acid sequences of C_α and C_β are 93 per cent identical. The C_γ subunit is somewhat less well conserved: 79 and 83 per cent identical to C_α and C_β, respectively.[6] Conservation of the sequences among the four regulatory subunits is likewise quite high. As discussed below in more detail, certain of

TABLE 5–1. cAMP-Dependent Protein Kinase A

Heterotetrameric complex	
Subunits:	2 regulatory (R)
	2 catalytic (C)
Isoforms:	R: RIα, RIβ, RIIα, RIIβ
	C: Cα, Cβ, Cγ

the various types and isotypes of subunits have distinct subcellular distributions and functions.

The Catalytic Subunits

The catalytic subunit contains a region that is highly conserved in the catalytic core of many different protein kinases. This region contains several motifs involved in ATP-binding, substrate recognition, and phosphotransfer (Fig. 5–5). The structure of C_α has been partially solved by x-ray crystallography both with and without a bound pseudosubstrate, so that the relevant contacts between ATP, Mg^{2+}, and substrate are relatively well understood.[54, 55]

The ATP-binding fold resides in the amino-terminal region and contains a glycine loop motif GXGXXG followed carboxy proximal by a lysine (K-72) and an acidic residue, glutamic acid (E-91), common to a variety of proteins that bind nucleotides. The glycine loop, lysine-72, glutamic acid-91, and aspartic acid-184 are all involved in the coordinate binding of Mg^{2+}-ATP. For reasons as yet unknown, Mg^{2+}-ATP binds more tightly to the catalytic subunit when complexed with the type I as opposed to the type II regulatory subunit.

The catalytic subunit of PKA phosphorylates serines or threonines in protein substrates when the serine or threonine is located in a motif RRXS/TY (where X and Y are usually hydrophobic amino acids) that is accessible to the kinase on the surface of the protein substrate. The catalytic subunit can also bind to (but cannot phosphorylate) pseudosubstrate motifs in which the serine or threonine are replaced by any other amino acid. Both phosphorylatable (RII) substrates and pseudosubstrates (RI) are present in the regulatory subunits and serve as so-called autoinhibitory domains[56] (Fig. 5–5 and Table 5–2). In addition to the regulatory subunits, the catalytic subunits can be inhibited by endogenous cellular proteins known as *protein kinase inhibitors* (PKI's). At least four isoforms of PKI's have been cloned from skeletal muscle and testis, all of which contain a pseudosubstrate site for interaction with the catalytic subunits of PKA.[57] As such, the PKI's bind more or less irreversibly to catalytic subunits, thereby inhibiting their catalytic functions. The precise roles that PKI's have in regard to their competition with R subunits to bind to and to

FIGURE 5–4. Diagram of the cellular location and orientation of adenylyl cyclase predicted from its primary amino acid sequence. The cyclase contains two symmetrical regions that span the plasma membrane six times. Two large cytoplasmic loops share sequence similarities with guanylyl cyclase.

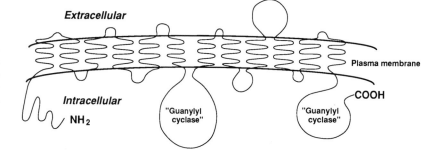

**TABLE 5–2. PSEUDOSUBSTRATE AND AUTOINHIBITOR SEQUENCES
IN PROTEIN KINASE A**

RIα	K G R R -	R R G A I	S A E V
RIβ	K A R R -	R R G C V	S A E V
RIIα	P G R F D	R R V S* V	C A E T
RIIβ	I N R F T	R R A S* V	C A E A
PKI	S G R T G	R R N A I	H D I L
Consensus	X X R X X	R R X X X	X A E X
Phosphorylation		R R X S̲* Y	
Motif		T̲*	

*Serines or threonines phosphorylated by protein kinase A.

inhibit catalytic subunits are unknown. Clearly, however, the diversity of PKI isoforms and their specific expression widely among different tissues attests to their importance in modulating the regulation and the activity of the PKA's.

The substrate recognition domain overlaps the Mg^{2+} ATP-binding and R-subunit binding regions and appears to consist of a hydrophobic pocket in which key acidic residues such as glutamic acids—170, 322, and 346 (E-170, E-322, E-346)—form ionic interactions with one of the arginines in the substrate recognition motif RRXS/TY. Threonine-197 is phosphorylated and the negatively charged phosphothreonine seems to likewise potentiate interaction with the positively charged arginines in substrate recognition motifs. The R-subunit binding domain is not yet clearly delineated but appears to involve the carboxyl terminal region of the catalytic subunit as well as an inhibitory region. The catalytic subunits undergo at least two types of posttranslational modifications, phosphorylations[58] and myristylation[59] at the amino terminus, the functional consequences of which are entirely unknown.

The Regulatory Subunits

The structures of the regulatory subunits are highly asymmetrical proteins of apparent Mr's ranging from 92,000 to 108,000 and consist of functionally distinct domains (Fig. 5–5). The amino-terminal domain is responsible for protein-protein interactions, i.e., dimerization of the two R subunits, binding to the catalytic subunit, and binding to anchoring proteins that target the inactive holoenzyme to specific subcellular locations. The carboxyl-terminal domain consists of two tandem repeated sequences that bind cAMP and thereby allosterically regulate the affinity of association of the R with the C subunit (see below).

The two regulatory subunits form antiparallel dimers through binding interactions at the amino terminal regions of the proteins. The RI subunits are covalently cross-linked by two disulfide linkages between cysteines, Cys16, and Cys37. Dimerization of the RII subunits, however, does not involve covalent linkages. Rather, the dimerization of RII involves strong noncovalent interactions of β-sheet–like secondary structure contained within the first 30 amino acids of the RII subunits. The contrast in the biochemical mechanisms of dimer formation between RI and RII subunits may reflect important differences in the biological functions of the RI and RII subunit isotypes. The type II regulatory subunit differs from the type I subunit in several respects. The autophosphorylation of RII by the catalytic subunits facilitates its release from the catalytic subunit. The phosphorylated type II holoenzyme dissociates at a lower concentration of cAMP than dephosphorylated holoenzyme. Unlike RI, RII is located in particulate fractions of cells and readily binds to membrane-located anchoring proteins, AKAP's (A-kinase anchor protein).[6, 60–63] In addition, RII associates much more tightly with the catalytic subunits compared with RI, and much higher concentrations of cAMP are required to effect the allosteric change in conformation necessary to release the catalytic from the regulatory subunits.

In addition to the ''autophosphorylation'' of the type II regulatory subunit by the catalytic subunit of PKA, both the

Catalytic Subunit

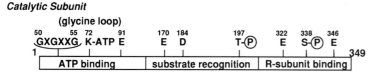

Regulatory Subunit

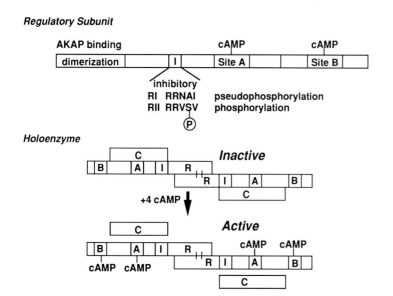

FIGURE 5–5. Diagrammatic representations of the catalytic and regulatory subunits of protein kinase A. Shown are the catalytic subunit (*upper*), regulatory subunit (*middle*), and the holoenzyme (*lower*) consisting of the heterotetrameric complex of catalytic and regulatory subunits (*lower*). The holoenzyme is depicted in both the inactive, fully complexed form, and the active, dissociated form. As is described in detail in the text, the catalytic subunit consists of three (overlapping) domains responsible for the binding of Mg^{2+}-ATP, recognition of and binding to substrate, and binding to dimerization with the regulatory (R) subunit. The regulatory subunits consist of dimerization domains that also function as sites for binding to anchoring proteins (AKAPs), domains that serve as inhibitory domains, and two cAMP-binding sites designated as sites A and B.

type I and II regulatory subunits are phosphorylated by protein kinases other than PKA. The biological relevance, however, of the phosphorylations is unknown. RI_α is phosphorylated by cGMP-dependent protein kinase but requires the presence of cAMP. Both isotypes of the RII subunit (RII_α and RII_β) are phosphorylated by the synergistic actions of the processive protein kinases, glycogen synthase kinase-3 (GSK-3), and casein kinase II (CKII).[41] Although the functional significance of these multiple phosphorylations is unclear, it seems certain that they represent important posttranslational modifications of the subunits that in some way alters their biological functions.

Allosteric Regulation of the Activation of Protein Kinase A by cAMP

Each regulatory subunit monomer contains two high-affinity cAMP binding sites, termed A and B, located in the carboxyl-terminal region of the subunit.[6, 7] The domain A and B regions share sequence similarities and probably arose by gene duplications. Analyses of the kinetics of dissociation of the catalytic subunit from the regulatory subunit in response to cAMP indicate that the binding of cAMP to sites A and B of the holoenzyme shows positive cooperativeness. cAMP first binds to site B on the regulatory subunit leading to a partial conformational change in R that loosens its association with C, rendering site A more accessible for binding of a second molecule of cAMP. Occupancy of sites A and B by cAMP results in the complete dissociation of the catalytic subunits from the heterotetrameric enzyme complex.

The A and B sites have different exchange rates for cAMP: site A has a faster rate of cAMP dissociation than does site B. Further, sites A and B have different binding preferences for cAMP analogues. Site A preferentially binds N-6 and C-6 substituted cAMP analogues such as dibutryl cAMP, whereas site B prefers C-8 substituted analogues such as 8-bromo-cAMP and 8-chlorophenylthio-cAMP.[63] In addition, there are differences in the preferential selectivities of cAMP analogues between the type I and type II regulatory subunits.[63] Certain of the analogues bind more tightly to sites A or B of RI than RII and vice versa. These differences in the relative potencies and selectivities of cAMP analogues for RI versus RII further indicate that the biological roles of the subunits must differ significantly.

Two particularly useful analogues of cAMP have been developed, of which one is an agonist (Sp-cAMP) and the other an antagonist (Rp-cAMP) for the activation of PKA.[64] The analogues contain alterations of the two exocyclic oxygens. The two chiral isomers of 3′, 5′-monophosphothioate contain sulfur at either the equatorial (Rp) or axial (Sp) position. Rp-cAMP is the first bona fide cAMP antagonist, and its actions can be compared directly with the Sp-cAMP agonist.

Functions of the Isotypes of R and C Subunits of Protein Kinase A

As discussed earlier, compared with the extensive complexities of the isotypes of the G proteins and adenylyl cyclases, the isoforms of the PKA subunits appear to be relatively limited in numbers. There are two major types of regulatory subunits, RI and RII, each of which has two subtypes: RI_α, RI_β, and RII_α, RII_β. Three isotypes of the catalytic subunit have been identified so far: C_α, C_β, and C_γ. The differences in functions of the various isotypes of the subunits are not fully understood. Their relative expression, however, appears to depend on the type of tissue involved, and they differ in their distributions among different subcellular compartments. In general, the α isotypes RI_α, RII_α, and C_α are expressed uniformly in a wide variety of tissues, whereas the expression of the β isotypes RI_β, RII_β, and C_β is more restricted to brain and neuroendocrine and endocrine tissues.[6] The RI_α and RI_β subunits are located in the cytoplasm and soluble fractions of broken cell preparations in contrast to RII_α and RII_β, which are in the particulate, membranous fraction. A substantial fraction of RII_β has been localized to the nucleus and perinuclear regions, suggesting a special role for this subunit in the targeting of the associated catalytic subunit close to substrate sites for phosphorylation in the nucleus.[65] In particular, the RII subunits associate with high affinities with A-kinase anchoring proteins (AKAP's) that are located at specific sites within the cell and are proposed to target the PKA holoenzyme to specific subcellular locations by binding to the RII subunits.[61] No distinctions have been made between the substrate recognition properties or actions of C_α and C_β. However, C_γ apparently has a higher affinity for histone than for kemptide, LRRASLG, the high-affinity standard substrate for phosphorylation by C_α and C_β.[66] Further, the activity of C_γ is not inhibited by the protein kinase inhibitor peptide (5-24amide), which is widely used as a PKA-specific inhibitor. The expression of C_γ appears to be restricted to the testis, from which a unique testis inhibitor isoform has been cloned.[67] It is possible that C_γ may have novel kinase activities distinct from those of C_α and C_β, and that by analogy subtle differences in functions of Cα and C_β exist also but have not yet been discovered.

Regulation of Subunit Gene Expression, Stability, Translocation, and Reassociation

The complexities of the interactions, regulation, and even autoregulation of the expression of the subunits of PKA are only now beginning to be understood. The regulation of the expression of many of the subunits in a specific phenotype of cell under a certain circumstance can involve changes in gene transcription, RNA processing and export from the nucleus, mRNA stability, translocation, and protein stability. In spite of the complexities of the regulation, some generalizations can be made. First, free subunits are less stable than the subunits in the intact holoenzyme complex; i.e., the free subunits are more susceptible to proteolysis compared to the bound subunits. Second, the type II regulatory subunit (RII) binds catalytic subunits more tightly than does RI. Higher cellular levels of cAMP are required to dissociate RII from C than RI from C. Thus, at relatively low levels of cAMP, RI will preferentially dissociate and be susceptible to degradation. Third, in certain cells, such as Sertoli cells of the testis, sustained high levels of cAMP increase the RII_β subunit by increasing the half-lives of both RII_β mRNA and protein, whereas mRNA's for RI_α, RII_α, and C_α are increased only two- to four-fold.[68] Fourth, it is likely that the induction of mRNA for certain of the subunits, e.g., RI_α, involves increased gene transcription mediated by activation of cAMP-responsive transcription factors such as cAMP response-element binding protein (CREB), whose transcriptional activity is stimulated by phosphorylation by C_α or C_β (see below). PhosphoCREB stimulates the transcription of many genes by binding to cAMP response elements located in their promoters.[28–30]

Increased RII_β can serve as a "trap" to inactivate C. For example, overexpression of C_α programmed by an expression plasmid transfected into rat pheochromocytoma cells results in a 50-fold enhanced stimulation of a co-transfected reporter plasmid consisting of the VIP promoter containing a cAMP-response element and the chloramphenicol acetyltransferase gene.[69] Co-transfection, however, with an expression plasmid encoding the RII_β subunit, inhibits stimulation by the C_α subunit to 10 per cent of control levels.[69] Because RII_β associates more tightly to C subunits than does RI_α or RI_β, all free C subunits will be complexed with RII_β, resulting in the liberation of RI subunits, which are then degraded. Thus increased RII_β levels not only lower levels of C subunits but also lower levels of RI subunits.

Paradoxically, in some circumstances, RII_β can also stimulate or restore cAMP-dependent gene transcription.[70] The cAMP-unresponsive pheochromocytoma cell line, A126-1B2, is incapable of activating a transfected somatostatin gene promoter containing a cAMP response element. However, co-transfection of a vector expressing the RII_β, but not RII_α or RI_α, subunit restores cAMP responsivity of the transcription driven by the somatostatin gene promoter. Although the role of RII_β in the restoration of cAMP-responsive transcription is unknown, it is possible that RII_β may target the catalytic subunit in a holoenzyme complex to the nucleus or to a perinuclear location.[65] Activation of PKA by cAMP releases catalytic subunit, which phosphorylates and activates nuclear transcription factor CREB. Localization of RII to the perinuclear Golgi apparatus has been demonstrated by immunocytochemical techniques.[65] It seems unlikely that RII has a direct role in the activation of transcription, but such a possibility cannot be totally discarded. Evidence has been presented that RII can bind to cAMP-response elements.[22]

The type I regulatory subunit of PKA can also inhibit the transcription of cAMP-responsive genes.[71] Several liver-specific genes are transcriptionally regulated by cAMP-dependent mechanisms likely involving CREB's. In the course of carrying out studies of cell fusions between hepatocytes and fibroblasts, extinction of the transcription of the hepatic genes was observed.[71] By genetic and recombinant DNA approaches, the gene encoding the tissue specific extinguisher was isolated and shown to be RI_α.[71] Further analyses revealed that in hepatic cells RI_α levels are unusually low but are at normal levels in most other tissues, including fibroblasts. Thus fusion of fibroblasts to hepatocytes introduced RI_α into the hepatocyte, thereby binding C subunit and preventing phosphorylation of CREB's necessary for the activation of the transcription of the liver-specific genes. It appears that the regulation of both the translocation and the activities of the PKA subunit isotypes plays a major role in the cAMP-dependent signal transduction pathway.

REPRESENTATIVE CELLULAR ACTIONS OF cAMP-DEPENDENT PROTEIN KINASE A

The targets for the biological actions of cAMP mediated by PKA are multiple. In almost every instance phosphorylation of a protein substrate results in a change in the biological activity of the protein, either stimulatory or inhibitory. Phosphorylation evokes crucial changes in the conformation of the proteins, often by allosteric mechanisms. Four representative examples of how PKA-directed phosphorylation regulates the activities of proteins are given below: An enzyme, glycogen phosphorylase; a receptor, β-adrenergic receptor (βAR); an ion channel, the cystic fibrosis transmembrane conductance regulator (CFTR), which is a chloride channel; and a DNA-binding transcription factor, CREB.

Glycogen Phosphorylase

As discussed earlier, glycogen phosphorylase was important historically as the model protein for investigations that led to defining the important roles of cAMP and phosphorylation in the transmission of hormone action to modulation of the biologic activity of a protein.[2, 10] In the 1940's it was recognized that glycogen phosphorylase existed in both active (phosphorylase a) and inactive (phosphorylase b) forms.[1] Subsequent studies of the phosphorylation of glycogen phosphorylase in both skeletal muscle and liver showed that phosphorylase b was activated to phosphorylase a by a phosphorylase kinase and inactivated by a phosphorylase phosphatase.

$$\text{Phosphorylase b} \xrightarrow[\substack{\text{phosphatase} \\ \text{Pi} \leftarrow H_2O}]{\substack{ATP \rightarrow ADP \\ \text{kinase}}} \text{Phosphorylase a}$$
$$\text{(inactive)} \qquad\qquad\qquad \text{(active)}$$

Next, it was demonstrated that the activity of phosphorylase kinase was reversible, and although the kinase was capable of autophosphorylation, its activation was mediated by phosphorylation by yet another kinase, phosphorylase kinase kinase, subsequently renamed cAMP-dependent protein kinase A (PKA)[10] (Fig. 5–6).

The enzymatic cycle of glycogen breakdown represents a classic example of regulation by successive phosphorylations, a so-called kinase cascade. PKA activates phosphorylase kinase, which then activates glycogen phosphorylase. In addition, both a negative and a positive counterregulatory phosphorylation is effected by PKA. Phosphorylations initiated by PKA but followed by an additional phosphorylation by the processive kinase, casein kinase I, inhibit glycogen synthase, the biosynthetic enzyme in the cycle (Fig. 5–6). Phosphorylation by PKA activates a phosphatase-inhibitor protein, resulting in inhibition of protein phosphatase, thereby enhancing the PKA-mediated phosphorylation.[72]

β-Adrenergic Receptor

The mechanism of the rapid agonist-induced desensitization of the β-adrenergic receptor appears to involve phosphorylations by PKA and an additional cAMP-inde-

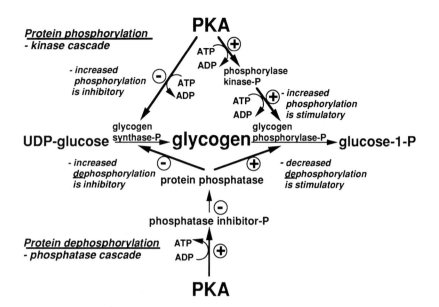

FIGURE 5–6. The enzymatic cycle of glycogen breakdown (conversion of glycogen to glucose). Phosphorylations of key enzymes in the cycle by cAMP-dependent protein kinase A (PKA) regulate the formation of glucose (glucose-1-phosphate) by the breakdown of glycogen in muscle tissue. PKA stimulates by phosphorylation of the activity of the enzyme phosphorylase kinase that, in turn, phosphorylates and activates glycogen phosphorylase. At the same time, PKA phosphorylates and so inactivates the glycogen synthetic enzyme, glycogen synthase. Protein phosphatases (protein ptase) provide counterregulatory influences imposed by the protein kinases. Further, phosphatase inhibitor proteins (ptase-inhibitor) and protein kinase A proteins (PKI) modulate the phosphorylation-dependence cascade of regulation and counterregulation of the enzymes involved in glycogen breakdown.

pendent protein kinase known as βARK (β-adrenergic receptor kinase) (Fig. 5–7).[23, 24] These phosphorylations are important for the rapid desensitization that occurs within 30 minutes after the receptor is occupied by ligand. The rapid phase of receptor desensitization is to be distinguished from the slow desensitization that takes place during longer (several hours) periods of exposure to ligand.[23] The rapid desensitization is reversible, does not require ongoing protein synthesis, and almost certainly involves an "uncoupling" of the receptor to G protein (see below). In contrast, the slow desensitization results from sequestration and internalization of the receptor and recovery requires new protein synthesis.

The mechanisms of the desensitization appear to be distinct for the two different kinases; phosphorylation by PKA occurs at low (nanomolar) and by βARK at high (micromolar) concentrations of ligand. βARK was discovered by analyses of the β-adrenergic receptor expressed in two distinct mutant S49 mouse lymphosarcoma cell lines.[23] The CYC⁻ mutant line lacks G protein (G_sα) and the Kin⁻ mutant line lacks PKA. In both cell lines, rapid desensitization occurred (albeit somewhat less than in wild-type cells), pointing to the existence of a relevant kinase other than PKA. The agonist-induced desensitization of receptors can be either homologous or heterologous. In the former, the agonist specifically desensitizes the distinct receptors that are occupied. In the latter, a liganded receptor desensitizes other distinctly different receptors on the cell surface.

βARK appears to induce homologous and PKA heterologous desensitization of the β-adrenergic receptor.[23] Although the reasons for the dependence of these two kinases on different concentrations of agonist are not known, it appears that a functionally significant level of phosphorylation of the receptor by βARK occurs only when a substantial number of receptors in a cell are occupied by agonist. The physiological implications of this circumstance are unknown. It has been proposed that the PKA-mediated desensitization may be tuned to receptors that respond to low concentrations of circulating hormones, whereas the βARK-induced desensitization occurs in locally acting paracrine or autocrine systems such as receptors located at nerve synapses, where concentrations of agonist are relatively high.[23]

That agonist-induced rapid desensitization of the β-adrenergic receptor involves phosphorylation by either PKA or βARK was shown in reconstitution experiments using isolated receptors incorporated into phospholipid vesicles.[73] Receptors prepared from desensitized cells or from cells that had not been treated with agonist and were phosphorylated in vitro with either PKA or βARK were all resistant to desensitization. Evidence that the phosphorylation of the receptor uncouples it from G_sα was likewise shown in reconstitution experiments in which phosphorylation of the receptor by PKA or βARK attenuated agonist-induced GTPase activity.[74] The cloning of the β-adrenergic receptor has allowed analyses of the effects of mutations in the receptor on its function. The serines and threonines that

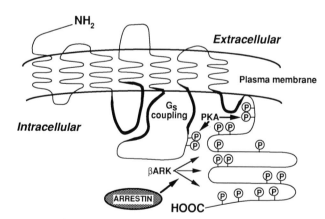

FIGURE 5–7. The human β₂-adrenergic receptor (βAR). The structure of the amino acid sequence of βAR was determined by cloning the cDNA encoding the receptor. The model shown is deduced from the structure of the receptor as well as from analyses of the perturbations in function induced by mutations introduced into the receptor. The βAR is a member of a large family of receptors that are coupled to G proteins. It consists of seven membrane-spanning segments and three cytoplasmic domains that are believed to be involved in the interactions of the receptor with G proteins (highlighted by the thickened lines). The cytoplasmic domains are phosphorylated by both protein kinase A (PKA) and a β-adrenergic receptor kinase (βARK). The phosphorylations mediate, in some way, the desensitization or uncoupling of the receptor from the G proteins (see text). Arrestin is a protein that is involved in the modulation of phosphorylations by PKA and βARK.

are phosphorylated by PKA and βARK reside in the third cytoplasmic loop and the cytoplasmic C-terminal tail of the receptor (Fig. 5–7). PKA phosphorylates at least two sites, one in the cytoplasmic loop and the other in the tail, whereas βARK phosphorylates several sites, all of which reside in the tail. The integrity of both the loop and the tail have been shown to be important in the coupling of the G protein to the receptor. Mutations of the sites for phosphorylation by either PKA or βARK reduced the level of phosphorylation of the receptor and the agonist induced desensitization by 50 per cent of the wild-type receptor.[23] Mutations of both PKA and βARK sites extinguished phosphorylation and markedly attenuated desensitization.

The mechanisms by which phosphorylation of the β-adrenergic receptor result in the uncoupling of the G protein from the receptor are not yet understood. At least two mechanisms have been proposed, however, and are under investigation: phosphorylation-induced modification of amphipathic α-helices in the receptor and inhibition of G protein–receptor coupling by an effector protein, arrestin.[23] Amphipathic α-helices are well known to be structured motifs in proteins that are utilized in protein-protein interactions. The introduction of a highly negatively charged phosphoserine in place of a neutral serine residue may in some way perturb the helicity and/or amphipathy of the helix, thereby impairing interaction with the G protein. Arrestin is a protein that has been proposed to competitively inhibit the interaction of G protein with the receptor.[75] It was first identified as an inhibitor of the interaction of transducin, a retinal G protein, to phosphorylated rhodopsin.[76] Later, a cDNA encoding a homologue of retinal arrestin was cloned from a bovine brain library. The brain and retinal arrestins are 59 per cent identical in their amino acid sequences. Further, when the brain and retinal arrestins, prepared by cDNA-directed expression and isolation from COS-7 cells, were tested in a reconstitution assay containing G_s and β-adrenergic receptor phosphorylated by βARK, the brain arrestin was much more effective than the retinal arrestin in facilitating desensitization. Conversely, the retinal arrestin was more effective than the brain arrestin in reversing the light activation of the rhodopsin receptor.[23] Thus, it seems likely that the arrestins are important regulatory effectors whose actions are integrated with both the PKA and βARK phosphorylations of the receptors and the interactions of G proteins with the receptors.

Cystic Fibrosis Transmembrane Conductance Regulator (CFTR)

The CFTR is a regulated chloride channel located in the apical membranes of secretory epithelia.[25] The channel regulates the transepithelial secretion of chloride. cDNA's and genes encoding the channel have been cloned.[77] It is now determined that mutations in the gene impair the normal functioning of the channel and cause the inborn error of metabolism known as cystic fibrosis.[78] Defective secretion of chloride and accompanying water leads to increased viscosity of epithelial cell secretions, culminating in the development of impaired airway and gastrointestinal functions. The mutations in the CFTR gene result in the

synthesis of defective CFTR chloride channels that do not open in response to intracellular signaling pathways.

Activation of the CFTR (opening of the channel) is mediated by phosphorylation by PKA and is enhanced by the binding of ATP at two sites located on the cytoplasmic face of the channel. cAMP-dependent signaling is crucial for the activation (opening) of the CFTR channel. It has been shown that cAMP agonists increase the permeability of apical membranes to chloride of normal epithelia but not epithelia of patients with cystic fibrosis.[79]

The CFTR chloride channel is composed of five distinct domains: two transmembrane spanning domains, each of which spans the membrane six times and forms the pore that conducts the chloride ions, two nucleotide binding domains that regulate the channel by binding and/or hydrolysis of ATP, and an R-domain phosphorylated on at least four serines by PKA[25, 77] (Fig. 5–8). These serines in the R-domain are phosphorylated by PKA in vitro and by cAMP agonists in vivo.[78] Furthermore, mutation of the serines to alanines results in a loss of channel activation, and mutational deletion of the R-domain results in a constitutively active channel that is only partially responsive to increases in cAMP. The dephosphorylation of the serines phosphorylated by PKA appears to involve protein phosphatase 2A and not phosphatases 1 or 2B.[80] Evidence has been presented that the R-domain may also be phosphorylated by both calcium-dependent and calcium-independent isotypes of protein kinase C.

Activation of CFTR chloride channels also requires ATP; once phosphorylated by PKA, the channels require cytosolic ATP to open. The ATP binds to single sites on each of the nucleotide-binding domains (Fig. 5–8). Notably, the nonhydrolyzable analogue of ATP, ATPγS, does not open CFTR channels, whereas the hydrolyzable analogues ATP>GTP>CTP (order of potency) reversibly open the channels phosphorylated by PKA. Thus, both phosphorylation of the R-domain and binding of ATP to the nucleotide binding domains are required to fully activate (open) the channels.

These observations on the effects of phosphorylation and ATP binding on the function of the CFTR have led to the proposal of a model to explain how the channel might work.[25, 77] The membrane spanning domains constitute a hollow cylinder with a central pore or channel created by 12 α-helical structures inserted transversely through the membrane (Fig. 5–8). The nucleotide binding domains, located on the cytoplasmic face adjacent to the opening of the channel, change conformation upon binding of ATP so as to enlarge the "diameter" of the pore. In the unphosphorylated state the R-domain, presumed to be globular in shape, "plugs" the pore and when phosphorylated (by PKA) is repelled from the region of the opening (perhaps by electrostatic forces), thereby opening the pore to allow the passage of chloride ions through the channel.

Phosphorylation by cAMP-dependent PKA is clearly an important step in the regulation of the activity CFTR chloride channel. It is highly likely that PKA is of tantamount importance in the regulation of many other ion channels as well. Evidence has been presented suggesting a role of PKA in the modulation of the activity of ATP-sensitive potassium channels on pancreatic β cells, again in concert with the binding and/or hydrolysis of ATP.[81, 82]

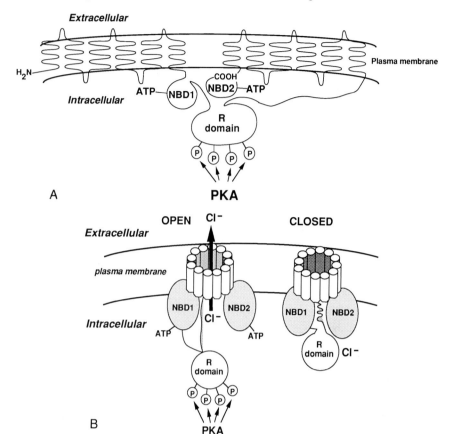

FIGURE 5–8. Models of the cystic fibrosis transmembrane conductance regulator (CFTR), a chloride channel whose defective functioning causes the disease cystic fibrosis. *A*, Overall topography of the CFTR. The channel spans the plasma membrane 12 times and thereby forms a 12-sided cylinder creating the pore through which chloride ions flow as shown schematically in *B*. The two nucleotide binding domains (NBD1 and NBD2) located on the cytoplasmic face of the channel bind ATP and as such are believed to conformationally widen the channel opening. The globular regulatory domain (R-domain) is phosphorylated on at least four sites by cAMP-dependent protein kinase A (PKA). It has been proposed that in the unphosphorylated state, the R-domain plugs the pore of the channel and thereby closes the channel. When phosphorylated, the R-domain is repelled by electrostatic forces away from the channel pore and thereby opens the channel, allowing for export of chloride ions from the inside to the outside of the cell.

Activation of Gene Transcription by Protein Kinase A

A major discovery during the past several years has been the identification of DNA-binding proteins whose transcriptional functions are activated by phosphorylation by PKA.[28–30, 83] These proteins bind specific DNA elements located in the promoters of many genes. These elements, and the DNA-binding proteins that interact with them, are referred to as cAMP response elements (CRE's) and CREB's, respectively.[28–30] The term *activating transcription factor* (ATF) is also used to describe proteins that bind to CRE's because the nomenclature derived from virological research in which viral proteins activate cellular proteins that bind to CRE's.[28] Not all ATF's mediate cAMP responses. A representative example of the role of PKA and CREB in the regulation of proinsulin gene transcription in pancreatic beta cells is shown in Figure 5–9.[84]

The CREB DNA-binding protein, and its structurally closely related homologues CREM and ATF-1, have all been cloned. Numerous isoforms of CREB and CREM exist that arise by way of the alternative splicing of exons.[85–88] The structural components responsible for the functions of CREB and CREM have been characterized in considerable detail. These proteins are members of a subfamily of a large superfamily of DNA-binding proteins known collectively as the bZIP proteins, so named because of the similar structures of their DNA-binding domains that consist of a basic region (b) involved in recognition and binding to DNA and a leucine zipper (ZIP), a coiled-coil structure with heptad repeats of leucines responsible for dimeriza-

tion[30] (Fig. 5–10). Additional information is contained in several reviews on CREB and bZIP proteins.[28–30, 89]

The transcriptional activities of CREB and the proteins that most closely resemble it in their structures are intensely regulated by the cAMP-dependent signaling pathway and appear to be unique in this regard. Given that the bZIP transcriptional proteins now identified constitute a large family, members of which compete for binding to their enhancer DNA's, it is understandable that nature would evolve only a limited set of these proteins for activation by cAMP-dependent protein kinase A, with the other proteins responsive to other non–cAMP-directed pathways. Thus, as far as is known, CREB, CREM, and ATF-1 represent the final communicative link in the regulation of gene expression in response to the activation of cAMP-dependent signaling systems.[30]

The primary amino acid sequences of the bZIP proteins diverge considerably outside their DNA-binding and dimerization domains—i.e., their domains that activate transcription (transactivation) have evolved so as to mediate signal transduction, each factor in response to distinct stimuli. For example, of the known bZIP transcription factors, only CREB, CREM, and ATF-1 are activated upon phosphorylation by cAMP-dependent PKA, and also in some circumstances CREB is activated by calcium-calmodulin kinase.[90, 91] By contrast, the protein kinase C (PKC) signal transduction pathway regulates the phosphorylation of the Jun-Fos (AP-1) complex.[40] Consistent with the role of CREB in the cAMP pathway, there is a consensus site, RRPSY (A-kinase box), for phosphorylation by PKA at serine-119 in CREB327 and at the corresponding serine 133 in CREB341

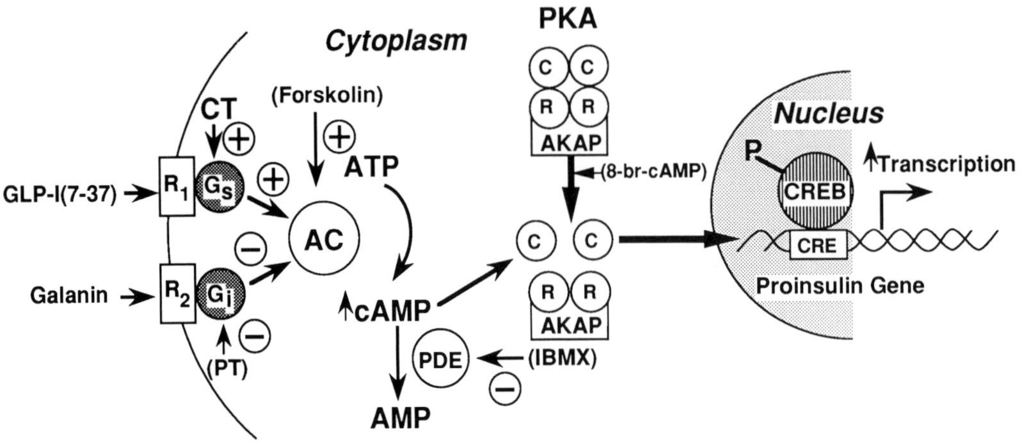

FIGURE 5–9. Hypothetical model of a pancreatic β-cell showing opposing actions of the hormones glucagon-like peptide-1(7–37) [GLP-I(7–37)] and galanin in the regulation of the cAMP-dependent signaling pathway. The receptor for GLP-1(7–37) is coupled to a stimulatory G protein (G_s), whereas the receptor for galanin is coupled to an inhibitory G protein (G_i) (see Fig. 5–3). Thus, the extent of activation of adenylyl cyclase (AC) is a result of the relative activities of G_s and G_i. The final response in the signaling pathway is the activation of the DNA-binding transcription factor CREB that binds to cAMP-response elements located in the promoters of genes such as the proinsulin gene and thereby stimulates transcription of the gene. The pharmacological agents cholera toxin (CT) and pertussis toxin (PT) activate G_s and G_i, respectively. Forskolin directly stimulates the activity of adenyl cyclase. Isobutyl methyl xanthine (IBMX) inhibits phosphodiesterase (PDE) and 8-br-cAMP is a cell permeable cAMP agonist. AKAP, A-kinase anchoring protein (see text).

(Fig. 5–10). The two CREB isoforms differ by an alternatively spliced exon of 14 amino acids. The identical A-kinase box, RRPSY, is present in the corresponding location in CREM and ATF-1. The PKA site in CREB is surrounded by a cluster of potential phosphorylated serine and threonine residues (kinase-inducible domain [KID] or phosphorylation, P-Box) over a stretch of about 50 residues. Consensus sites for potential phosphorylations by PKC, casein kinase II (CKII), and glycogen synthase kinase-3 (GSK-3) reside in the P-Box. The protein kinases CKII and GSK-3 are known to be processive or hierarchical kinases, inasmuch as phosphorylation of one site facilitates the successive phosphorylation of adjacent sites.[41] Phosphorylation of the PKA site may trigger a cascade of phosphorylations by the other kinases (Fig. 5–10B). Studies have shown that phosphorylation of the PKA site (serine-119) is essential for the activation of CREB.[93] However, phosphorylation of the serine-119 of CREB327 or the corresponding serine-133 in CREB341 is necessary, but it is not sufficient to generate the transactivation functions of CREB. Sequences located carboxy-proximal to serine-119 are required to confer transcriptional transactivation func-

tions of CREB.[94] Phosphorylation of the P-Box may allosterically alter CREB to reveal the protein conformational structure required for transactivation.[94] It has been proposed that the regions involved in transactivation are the glutamine-rich regions that flank the kinase-inducible domain.[92, 94] Furthermore, this model predicts that this allosteric effect would be potentiated by the insertion of the alternatively spliced 14 amino acids that constitute the difference between CREB327 and CREB341.[95] Whether or not, however, these extra 14 amino acids enhance the transactivation of CREB341 over CREB327 is uncertain. In addition to the kinase-inducible domain that is crucial for transcriptional transactivation, evidence has been presented that the additional spliced 14 amino acids are important for transactivation in some but not all cell lines.[92–95]

The importance in vivo of the requirement for phosphorylation of CREB by PKA to generate its transactivational functions was shown by Struthers et al.,[96] who produced dwarfism in transgenic mice expressing a CREB with a serine to alanine substitution mutation at the site (residue serine-133) phosphorylated by PKA. The transgene

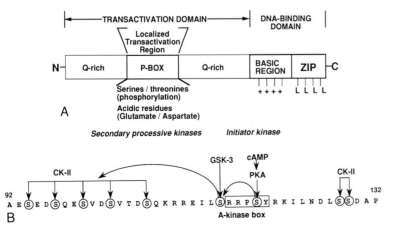

FIGURE 5–10. Diagram of the structure of CREB, cAMP response element binding protein. A, CREB belongs to the superfamily of transcription factors known as the bZIP proteins, so named because the DNA-binding region consists of a basic region (b) responsible for DNA recognition and a leucine zipper coiled–coil (ZIP) involved in dimerization. B, The transcriptional transactivation domain of CREB consists of a region of approximately 50 residues and contains multiple sites that are phosphorylated by protein kinases, among the most important of which is cAMP-dependent protein kinase A.

consisted of the promoter of the rat growth hormone gene fused to the coding sequence of the point-mutated CREB. Thus, expression of the mutated CREB was directed to the somatotrophs of the pituitary during development. Because the mutated CREB still dimerized with wild-type CREB and bound to CRE's but could not transactivate gene transcription, the mutated CREB competed the actions of wild-type CREB, resulting in atrophied pituitary glands deficient in somatotrophs and the production of growth hormone. Because CREB proteins are expressed at relatively high levels in testis,[89] it would be interesting to learn the effects upon mice that have been rendered transgenic with mutation CREB Ser 133 Ala under the regulation of testes-specific promoters.

Notably, in certain circumstances CREB appears to activate gene transcription independent of its phosphorylation by PKA. In the pancreatic islet cell line, Tu6, both wild-type CREB and CREB with a mutation in the PKA-regulated Ser-133 phosphorylation site of a somatostatin CRE-reporter plasmid activate transcription equally in the presence of cAMP-activated PKA.[97] In this case, the activation of transcription of the CRE required a second promoter element, which appears to bind an islet cell factor Isl-1. Thus, in the absence of phosphorylation by PKA, CREB may activate transcription via other non–phosphorylation-dependent mechanisms. CREB also has been reported to lack transactivational activity on somatostatin and vasoactive intestinal peptide (VIP)-CRE reporters in undifferentiated F9 embryonal carcinoma cells, but in differentiated cells. This is not the case.[98] Both undifferentiated and differentiated cells appeared to contain equivalent amounts of functionally active PKA, suggesting the possibility that an inhibitor of CREB transactivation is present in the undifferentiated cells. Because the state of phosphorylation of CREB in undifferentiated versus differentiated cells was not examined in these studies, the mechanism(s) for the inhibition remain(s) unknown.

Whereas most research on the regulation of CREB transactivation has been directed toward mechanisms involving protein kinases, relatively little is known about phosphatase-mediated inactivation of CREB. Recently, however, Hagiwara et al.[99] have provided compelling evidence that protein phosphatase-1 (PP-1) selectively dephosphorylates the serine-133 in CREB341 (serine-119 in CREB327) and correspondingly attenuates the transactivational activity of CREB. Although both PP-1 and PP2A will dephosphorylate this site in CREB, examination of the relative inhibition constants of PP-1 and PP2A for the phosphatase inhibitor okadaic acid, IC_{50} of 20 nM and 0.2 nM, respectively, strongly suggests that PP-1 is the relevant phosphatase in vivo.[99] Further, the PP-1-specific phosphatase inhibitor protein-1 (IP-1) abrogated the activity of PP-1. Thus, an interesting model for regulation is proposed because the activity of IP-1 depends on phosphorylation by either PKA or calcium-calmodulin kinase. In this model, activation of PKA by cAMP would result in the phosphorylation and activation of CREB and IP-1, the latter leading to the inhibition of PP-1.

The effects of phosphorylation on the dimerization and DNA-binding of CREB are less certain than the effects on transactivation. Yamamoto et al.[100] originally reported that phosphorylation of a partially purified CREB or CREB-like protein by protein kinase C, but not protein kinase A, enhanced dimerization and binding to a CRE. The studies, however, relied on analyses of the effects of phosphorylation on the transition of CREB from a monomer to a dimer as assessed by binding to a CRE-containing oligonucleotide using an electrophoretic mobility shift assay. Because it is now generally believed that bZIP proteins including CREB bind to DNA only as dimers and not as monomers, these observations of Yamamoto et al.[100] may have to be reinterpreted in a different light. Recently, Nichols et al.[101] provided evidence that phosphorylation of CREB by PKA enhances binding to asymmetrical CRE's such as the CRE in the tyrosine amino transferase gene (TGACGCAG), but not to symmetrical CRE's such as those found in the promoters of the somatostatin (TGACGTCA) gene. These observations are interesting because they indicate that phosphorylation of a site approximately 150 amino acids distant from the bZIP DNA-binding domain can influence binding. Such a mechanism must involve a phosphorylation-induced folding or stabilization of CREB. Such effects of phosphorylation on distant sites have also been observed for the transcription factors jun, myb, and SRF. The binding of CREB to CRE's may also be enhanced by phosphorylation through a non–cAMP-dependent signaling pathway. TGFβ induces phosphorylation of CREB or a CREB-like protein, resulting in increased binding to a fibronectin gene CRE and collagenase gene tetraphorbol acetate (TPA)-response element.[102] The studies suggest that the CREB-like protein binds to these DNA elements as a heterodimer with a Fos-like protein, but the identity of the DNA-binding complex remains to be determined.

It has been proposed that negatively charged amphipathic helices of the DNA-binding proteins GAL4 and GCN4 interact with the basal transcriptional machinery to stimulate transcription.[103–105] It is likely that the negatively charged residues and phosphorylation of the CREB P-Box serve to transactivate transcription in a manner similar to the way in which the yeast GAL4 and GCN4 transcription factors transactivate RNA polymerase II.

SUMMARY

The cAMP-dependent signal transduction pathway is one of several such signaling pathways whose function is to convey information from the environment outside of cells to the complex metabolic activities that take place within the cell. Essentially all of the many actions of cAMP are conveyed by way of its activation of the enzyme, cAMP-dependent protein kinase A. The inactive holoenzyme is a heterotetrameric complex consisting of two regulatory and two catalytic subunits. The allosteric regulator cAMP binds to two sites on each of the two regulatory subunits, thereby dissociating the two catalytic subunits from the complex. The free catalytic subunits bind Mg^{2+}-ATP and are phosphotransferases that phosphorylate protein substrates on serines and threonines in the sequence motif RRXS/T. Two isoforms of the regulatory subunit have been identified (RI and RII), each of which has two isotypes (RI_{α}, RI_{β}, and RII_{α}, RII_{β}). Three isotypes of the catalytic subunit are known (C_{α}, C_{β}, C_{γ}). The RI and RII isoforms are located predominantly in the cytoplasm and associated with membranous organelles, respectively. The α isotypes are distributed ubiquitously in most all tissue types, whereas the β isotypes appear to be restricted to brain, endocrine glands, and testes. The RII subunits are targeted to specific subcellular locations by binding to A-kinase anchoring proteins, perhaps to bring the catalytic subunits in close proximity to their substrates. Functional differences among the three catalytic subunits have not yet been found, except that C_γ is enriched in testis and phosphorylates substrates with other than the standard motif. The relative cellular levels of subunits of protein kinase A are autoregulated in a complex manner at levels of gene transcription, subunit mRNA and protein stability, and subunit interactions. Phosphorylations by protein kinase A of substrate proteins such as enzymes, receptors, ion channels, and DNA-binding transcription factors alter the conformation and thereby the functional activities of the proteins.

ACKNOWLEDGMENTS: I thank George Holz, IV, Mario Vallejo, and Christopher Miller for helpful suggestions and Townley Budde for preparation of the manuscript.

REFERENCES

1. Coris' Nobel Address, Science, 1951.
2. Sutherland EW: Studies on the mechanism of hormone action. Science 177:401–408, 1972.
3. Fischer, Nobel Address, Science, 1993.
4. Krebs, Nobel Address, Science, 1993.
5. Edelman AM, Blumenthal DK, Krebs EG: Protein serine/threonine kinases. Ann Rev Biochem 56:567–613, 1987.
6. Scott JK: Cyclic nucleotide-dependent protein kinases. Pharmacol Ther 50:123–145, 1991.
7. Taylor ST, Buechler JA, Yonemoto W: cAMP-dependent protein kinase: Framework for a diverse family of regulatory enzymes. Annu Rev Biochem 59:971–1005, 1990.
8. Taylor SS: cAMP-dependent protein kinase: Model for an enzyme family. J Biol Chem 264:8443–8446, 1989.
9. Harper JF, Haddox MK, Johanson RA, et al: Compartmentation of second messenger action: immunocytochemical and biochemical evidence. Vitam Horm 42:197–252, 1985.
10. Krebs EG: Role of the cyclic AMP-dependent protein kinase in signal transduction. JAMA 262:1815–1818, 1989.
11. Gilman AG: G proteins and regulation of adenylyl cyclase. JAMA 262:1819–1825, 1989.
12. Hanks SK, Quinn AM, Hunter T: The protein kinase family: Conserved features and deduced phylogeny of the catalytic domains. Science 241:42–52, 1988.
13. Cori GT, Cori CF: The enzymatic conversion of phosphorylase a to b. J Biol Chem 158:321–345, 1945.
14. Rall TW, Sutherland EW, Berthet J: The relationship of epinephrine and glucagon to liver phosphorylase IV. Effect of epinephrine and glucagon on the reactivation of phosphorylase in liver homogenates. J Biol Chem 224:463–475, 1957.
15. Sutherland EW, Rall TW: Fractionation and characterization of a cyclic adenine ribonucleotide formed by tissue particles. J Biol Chem 232:1077–1091, 1958.
16. Fischer EH, Krebs EG: Conversion of phosphorylase b to phosphorylase a in muscle extracts. J Biol Chem 216:121–132, 1955.
17. Krebs EG, Graves DJ, Fischer EH: Factors affecting the activity of phosphorylase b kinase. J Biol Chem 234:2867–2873, 1959.
18. Kuo EG, Greengard P: An adenosine 3′, 5′-monophosphate-dependent protein kinase from E. coli. J Biol Chem 244:3417–3419, 1969.
19. Walsh DA, Perkins JP, Krebs EG: An adenosine 3′, 5′ monophosphate-dependent protein kinase from rabbit skeletal muscle. J Biol Chem 243:3763–3765, 1968.
20. Nakamura T, Gold GH: A cyclic nucleotide-gated conductance in olfactory receptor cilia. Nature 325:442–444, 1987.
21. Weber IT, Steitz TA, Bubis J, Taylor SS: Predicted structures of cAMP binding domains of type I and type II regulatory subunits of cAMP-dependent protein kinase. Biochemistry 26:343–351, 1987.
22. Wu JC, Wang JH: Sequence-selective DNA binding to the regulatory subunit of cAMP-dependent protein kinase. J Biol Chem 264:9989–9993, 1989.
23. Hausdorff WP, Caron MG, Lefkowitz RJ: Turning off the signal: Desensitization of β-adrenergic receptor function. FASEB J 4:2881–2889, 1990.
24. Okamoto T, Murayama Y, Hayashi Y, et al: Identification of a G_s activator region of the β2-adrenergic receptor that is autoregulated via protein kinase A-dependent phosphorylation. Cell 67:723–730, 1991.
25. Collins FS: Cystic fibrosis: Molecular biology and therapeutic implications. Science 256:774–779, 1992.
26. Sandoval IV, Cuatrecasas P: Opposing effects of cyclic AMP and cyclic GMP on protein phosphorylation in tubulin preparations. Nature 262:511–514, 1976.
27. Lohmann SM, DeCammilli P, Einig I, Walter U: High-affinity binding of the regulatory subunit (RII) of cAMP-dependent protein kinase to microtubule-associated and other cellular proteins. Proc Natl Acad Sci USA 81:6723–6727, 1984.
28. Habener, JF: Cyclic AMP response element binding proteins: A cornucopia of transcription factors. Mol Endocrinol 4:1087–1093, 1990.
29. Meyer TE, Habener JF: Cyclic AMP-dependent transactivation of gene transcription mediated by the CREB phosphoprotein. In Mond JJ, Cambier JC, Weiss A (eds): Advances in Regulation of Cell Growth, Vol 2; Cell Activation: Genetic Approaches. New York, Raven Press, 1991, pp 61–81.
30. Meyer TE, Habener JF: Cyclic AMP response element binding protein (CREB) and related transcription-activating DNA-binding proteins. Endocr Rev 14:269–290, 1993.
31. Rangarajan PN, Umesono K, Evans RM: Modulation of glucocorticoid receptor function by protein kinase A. Mol Endocrinol 6:1451–1457, 1992.
32. Johnson LN, Barford D: Glycogen phosphorylase. The structural basis of the allosteric response and comparison with other allosteric proteins. J Biol Chem 265:2409–2412, 1990.
33. Sprang SR, Acharya KR, Goldsmith EJ, et al: Structural changes in glycogen phosphorylase induced by phosphorylation. Nature 336:215–221, 1988.
34. Berridge MJ: 1993 Inositol trisphosphate and calcium signalling. Nature 361:315–325, 1988.
35. Nishizuka Y: The role of protein kinase C in cell surface signal transduction and tumour promotion. Nature 308:693–698, 1984.
36. Schulman H, Lou LL: Multifunctional C^{2+}/calmodulin-dependent protein kinase: Domain structure and regulation. Trends Biol Sci 14:62–66, 1989.
37. Hunter T, Cooper JA: Protein-tyrosine kinases. Ann Rev Biochem 54:897–930, 1985.
38. Blackshear PJ, Nairn AC, Kuo JF: Protein kinases 1988: A current perspective. FASEB J 2:2957–2969, 1988.
39. Karin M: Signal transduction from cell surface to nucleus in development and disease. FASEB J 6:2581–2590, 1992.
40. Hunter T, Karin M: The regulation of transcription by phosphorylation. Cell 70:375–387, 1992.
41. Roach PJ: Multisite and hierarchical protein phosphorylation. J Biol Chem 266:14139–14142, 1991.
42. Roach PJ: Control of glycogen synthase by hierarchical protein phosphorylation. FASEB J 4:2961–2968, 1990.
43. Woodgett JR: A common denominator linking glycogen metabolism, nuclear oncogenes, and development. Trends Biol Sci 16:177–181, 1991.
44. Ackerman P, Glover CVC, Osheroff N: Stimulation of casein kinase II by epidermal growth factor: Relationship between the physiological activity of the kinase and the phosphorylation state of its β subunit. Proc Natl Acad Sci USA 87:821–825, 1990.
45. Bourne HR, Sanders DA, McCormick F: The GTPase superfamily: Conserved structure and molecular mechanism. Nature 349:117–127, 1991.
46. Johnson GL, Dhanasekaran N: The G-protein family and their interaction with receptors. Endocr Rev 10:317–331, 1989.
47. Neer EJ, Clapham DE: Roles of G protein subunits in transmembrane signalling. Nature 333:129–134, 1988.
48. Birnbaumer L: Transduction of receptor signal into modulation of effector activity by G proteins: The first 20 years or so. FASEB J 4:3068–3078, 1990.
49. Taussig R, Quarmby LM, Gilman AG: Regulation of purified type I and type II adenylylcyclases by G protein β_γ subunits. J Biol Chem 268:9–12, 1993.
50. Holz GG, Rane SG, Dunlop K: GTP-binding proteins mediate transmitter inhibition of voltage-dependent calcium channels. Nature 319:670–672, 1986.

51. Yatani A, Codina J, Brown AM, Birnbaumer L: Direct activation of mammalian muscarinic potassium channel by GTP regulatory protein G_K. Science 235:207–211, 1987.
52. Hescheler J, Rosenthal W, Trautwein W, Shultz G: The GTP-binding protein, G_o, regulates neuronal calcium channels. Nature 325:445–447, 1987.
53. Krupinski J, Lehman TC, Frankenfield CD, et al: Molecular diversity in the adenylyl cyclase family. J Biol Chem 267:24858–24862, 1992.
54. Knighton DR, Zheng J, Eyck LFT, et al: Crystal structure of the catalytic subunit of cyclic adenosine monophosphate–dependent protein kinase. Science 253:407–414, 1991.
55. Knighton DR, Zheng J, Eyck LFT, et al: Structure of a peptide inhibitor bound to the catalytic subunit of cyclic adenosine monophosphate–dependent protein kinase. Science 253:414–420, 1991.
56. Soderling TH: Regulation by autoinhibitory domains. J Biol Chem 265:1823–1826, 1990.
57. Van Patten SM, Howard P, Walsh DA, Maurer RA: The α- and β-isoforms of the inhibitor protein of the 3′,5′-cyclic adenosine monophosphate–dependent protein kinase: Characteristics and tissue- and developmental-specific expression. Mol Endocrinol 6:2114–2122, 1992.
58. Toner-Webb J, Van Patten SM, Walsh DA, Taylor SS: Autophosphorylation of the catalytic subunit of cAMP-dependent protein kinase. J Biol Chem 267:25174–25180, 1992.
59. Clegg CH, Ran W, Uhler MD, McKnight GS: A mutation in the catalytic subunit of protein kinase A prevents myristylation but does not inhibit biological activity. J Biol Chem 264:20140–20146, 1989.
60. Scott JD, Stofko RE, McDonald JR, et al: Type II regulatory subunit dimerization determines the subcellular localization of the cAMP-dependent protein kinase. J Biol Chem 265:21561–21566, 1990.
61. Carr DW, Stofko-Hahn RE, Fraser IDC, et al: Interaction of the regulatory subunit (RII) of cAMP-dependent protein kinase with RII-anchoring proteins occurs through an amphipathic helix binding motif. J Biol Chem 266:14188–14192, 1991.
62. Hirsch AH, Glantz SB, Li Y, et al: Cloning and expression of an intron-less gene for ADAP75, an anchor protein for the regulatory subunit of cAMP-dependent protein kinase IIβ. J Biol Chem 267:2131–2134, 1992.
63. Ally S, Tortora G, Clair T, et al: Selective modulation of protein kinase isozymes by the site-selective analog 8-chloroadenosine 3′,5′-cyclic monophosphate provides a biologic means for control of human colon cancer cell growth. Proc Natl Acad Sci USA 85:6319–6322, 1988.
64. Rothermel JD, Stec WJ, Baronisk J, et al: Inhibition of glycogenolysis in isolated rat hepatocytes by the Rp diastereomer of adenosine cyclic 3′,5′-phosphorothioate. J Biol Chem 258:12125–12128, 1983.
65. Nigg EA, Schafer G, Hilz H, Eppenberger HM: Cyclic-AMP–dependent protein kinase type II is associated with the golgi complex and with centrosomes. Cell 41:1039–1051, 1985.
66. Beebe SJ, Salomonsky P, Jahnsen T, Li Y: The $C_γ$ subunit is a unique isozyme of the cAMP-dependent protein kinase. J Biol Chem 267:25505–25512, 1992.
67. Van Patten SM, Ng DC, Th'ng JPH, et al: Molecular cloning of a rat testis form of the inhibitor protein of the cAMP-dependent protein kinase. Proc Natl Acad Sci USA 88:5383–5387, 1991.
68. Knutsen HK, Tasken KA, Eskild W, Hansson V: Inhibitors of RNA and protein synthesis stabilize messenger RNA for the RIIβ subunit of protein kinase A in different cellular compartments. Biochem Biophys Res Comm 183:632–639, 1992.
69. Buchler W, Meinecke M, Chakraborty T, et al: Regulation of gene expression by transfected subunits. Eur J Biochem 188:253–259, 1990.
70. Tortora G, Cho-Chung YS: Type II regulatory subunit of protein kinase restores cAMP-dependent transcription in a cAMP-unresponsive cell line. J Biol Chem 265:18067–18070, 1990.
71. Jones KW, Shapero MH, Chevrette M, Fournier REK: Subtractive hybridization cloning of a tissue-specific extinguisher: TSE1 encodes a regulatory subunit of protein kinase A. Cell 66:861–872, 1991.
72. Cohen P, Cohen PTW: Protein phosphatases come of age. J Biol Chem 264:21435–21438, 1989.
73. Hausdorff WP, Bouvier M, O'Dowd BF, et al: Phosphorylation sites on two domains of the β2-adrenergic receptor are involved in distinct pathways of receptor desensitization. J Biol Chem 264:12657–12665, 1989.
74. Sibley DR, Benovic JL, Caron MG, Lefkowitz RJ: Regulation of transmembrane signalling by receptor phosphorylation. Cell 48:913–922, 1987.
75. Benovic JL, Kuhn H, Weyand I, et al: Functional desensitization of the isolated β-adrenergic receptor kinase: Potential role of an analog for the retinal protein arrestin (48-kDa protein). Proc Natl Acad Sci USA 84:8879–8882, 1987.
76. Wilden U, Hall SW, Kuhn H: Phosphodiesterase activation by photoexcited rhodopsin is quenched when rhodopsin is phosphorylated and binds the intrinsic 48-kDa protein of rod outer segments. Proc Natl Acad Sci USA 83:1174–1178, 1986.
77. Cheng SH, Rich DP, Marshall J, et al: Phosphorylation of the R domain by cAMP-dependent protein kinase regulates the CFTR chloride channel. Cell 66:1027–1036, 1991.
78. Anderson MP, Berger HA, Rich DP, et al: Nucleotide triphosphates are required to open the CFTR chloride channel. Cell 67:775–784, 1991.
79. Riordan JR, Rommens JM, Kerem B-S, et al: Identification of the cystic fibrosis gene: Cloning and characterization of complementary DNA. Science 245:1066–1073, 1989.
80. Berger HA, Travis SM, Welsh MJ: Regulation of the cystic fibrosis transmembrane conductance regulator Cl⁻ channel by specific protein kinases and protein phosphatases. J Biol Chem 268:2037–2047, 1993.
81. Holz GG IV, Kuhtreiber WM, Habener JF: Pancreatic beta cells are rendered glucose-competent by the insulinotropic hormone glucagon-like peptide-1(7-37). Nature 361:362–365, 1993.
82. Holz GG IV, Habener JF: Signal transduction crosstalk in the endocrine system: Pancreatic β-cells and the glucose competence concept. Trends Biol Sci 17:388–393, 1992.
83. Montminy MR, Gonzalez GA, Yamamoto KK: Regulation of cAMP-inducible genes by CREB. Trends Neurosci 13:184–188, 1990.
84. Fehmann H-C, Habener JF: Galanin inhibits proinsulin gene expression stimulated by the insulinotropic hormone glucagon–like peptide-I(7-37) in mouse insulinoma βTC-1 cells. Endocrinol 130:2890–2896, 1992.
85. Hoeffler JP, Meyer TE, Yun Y, et al: Cyclic AMP-responsive DNA-binding protein: Structure based on a cloned placental cDNA. Science 242:1430–1433, 1988.
86. Gonzalez GA, Yamamoto KK, Fischer WH, et al: A cluster of phosphorylation sites on the cyclic AMP-regulated nuclear factor CREB predicted by its sequence. Nature 337:749–752, 1989.
87. Foulkes NS, Mellstrom B, Benusiglio E, Sassone-Corsi P: Developmental switch of CREM function during spermatogenesis: From antagonist to activator. Nature 355:80–84, 1992.
88. Meyer TE, Habener JF: Cyclic AMP response element binding protein CREB and modulator protein CREM are products of distinct genes. Nucl Acids Res 20:6106, 1992.
89. de Groot RP, Sassone-Corsi P: Hormonal control of gene expression: Multiplicity and versatility of cAMP-responsive nuclear regulators. Mol Endocrinol 7:145–153, 1993.
90. Dash PK, Karl KA, Colicos MA, et al: cAMP response element-binding protein is activated by Ca^{2+}/calmodulin- as well as cAMP-dependent protein kinase. Proc Natl Acad Sci USA 88:5061–5065, 1991.
91. Sheng M, Thompson MA, Greenberg ME: CREB: A Ca^{2+}-regulated transcription factor phosphorylated by calmodulin-dependent kinases. Reports 252:1427–1430, 1991.
92. Lamph WW, Dwarki VJ, Ofir R, et al: Negative and positive regulation by transcription factor cAMP response element-binding protein is modulated by phosphorylation. Proc Natl Acad Sci USA 37:4320–4324, 1990.
93. Gonzalez FA, Montminy MR: Cyclic AMP stimulates somatostatin gene transcription by phosphorylation of CREB at serine 133. Cell 59:675–680, 1989.
94. Gonzalez GA, Menzel P, Leonard J, et al: Characterization of motifs which are critical for activity of the cyclic AMP-responsive transcription factor CREB. Mol Cell Biol 11:1306–1312, 1991.
95. Yamamoto KK, Gonzalez GA, Menzel P, et al: Characterization of a bipartite activator domain in transcription factor CREB. Cell 60:611–617, 1990.
96. Struthers RS, Vale WW, Arias C, et al: Somatotroph hypoplasia and dwarfism in transgenic mice expressing a non-phosphorylatable CREB mutant. Nature 350:622–625, 1991.
97. Leonard J, Serup P, Gonzalez G, et al: The LIM family transcription factor Isl-1 requires cAMP response element binding protein to promote somatostatin expression in pancreatic islet cells. Proc Natl Acad Sci USA 89:6247–6251, 1992.
98. Masson N, Ellis M, Goodbourn S, Lee KAW: Cyclic AMP response element-biding protein and the catalytic subunit of protein kinase A are present in F9 embryonal carcinoma cells but are unable to activate the somatostatin promoter. Mol Cell Biol 12:1096–1106, 1992.
99. Hagiwara M, Alberts A, Brindle P, et al: Transcriptional attenuation

following cAMP induction requires PP-1–mediated dephosphorylation of CREB. Cell 70:105–113, 1992.

100. Yamamoto KK, Gonzalez GA, Biggs WH III, Montminy MR: Phosphorylation-induced binding and transcriptional efficacy of nuclear factor CREB. Nature 334:494–498, 1988.

101. Nichols M, Weih F, Schmid W, et al: Phosphorylation of CREB affects its binding to high and low affinity sites: implications for cAMP-induced gene transcription. EMBO J 11:3337–3346, 1992.

102. Kramer IM, Koornneef I, de Laat W, van den Eljnden-van Raaij AFM: TGF-β1 induces phosphorylation of the cyclic AMP responsive element binding protein in ML-CC164 cells. EMBO J 10:1083–1089, 1991.

103. Weinmann R: The basic RNA polymerase II transcriptional machinery. Gene Expr 2:81–91, 1992.

104. Pugh BF, Tjian R: Diverse transcriptional functions of the multi-subunit eukaryotic TFIID complex. J Biol Chem 267:679–682, 1992.

105. Rigby PWJ: Three in one and one in three: it all depends on TBP. Cell 72:7–10, 1993.

106. Denner LA, Weigel NL, Maxwell BL, Schrader WT, O'Malley BW. Regulation of progesterone receptor-mediated transcription by phosphorylation. Science 250:1740, 1992.

6

Nuclear Receptor Superfamily

JAN MESTER
ETIENNE-EMILE BAULIEU

Somatic cells are subjected to a multitude of external signals that rule their behavior: expression of specialized functions, cell division cycle, and often simple survival. Most of the external signals are detected by specific receptor molecules situated on the cell membrane and interpreted by a cascade of molecular events triggered by the signal-receptor interaction. Induction or repression of the expression of specific genes frequently is a part of the cellular response to the activation of membrane receptors.

A particular category of signaling molecules (including steroid and thyroid hormones and active vitamin metabolites such as retinoids—vitamin A derivatives and calcitriol—derived from vitamin D_3) traverse the cell membrane and thus short-circuit membrane-associated transducing systems and directly activate intracellular receptor molecules that are mainly located in the nucleus. Alterations in the specific gene expression are then a quasi-immediate consequence of the exposure of the cells to this type of signal.

Progress in research on the family of nuclear receptors, accomplished mainly over the last decade, is reviewed in this chapter. The interested reader may consult our chapter Steroid Hormone Receptors in the second edition of this book, published in 1989, which contains comments and references on hormone binding, the beginning of the story of steroid membrane receptors presently continuing with neurosteroid action,[1] and some pathophysiological concepts not further reviewed in this chapter. Excellent reviews on the contemporary developments in the moving field of nuclear receptors recently have been published.[2–9]

FROM PROTEIN TO GENE

The existence of specific cellular components, "receptors," serving to detect the external signaling molecules and transmit the relevant information, has been postulated since the beginning of this century. They remained elusive until radioactively labeled hormones of high specific activity became available, permitting binding studies of hormones whose physiological concentrations at the target level are very low, of the order of $10^{-9 \pm 1}$ M.

The earliest experimental demonstration of such cellular components interacting with a hormone was obtained in the early sixties, when several groups demonstrated the presence of a high-affinity binding protein specific for estrogen in the cytosoluble fraction of the mammalian uterus. Similar intracellular binding proteins for all five categories of steroid hormones, and later also for certain other signaling molecules such as thyroid hormones and fat-soluble vitamin-active metabolites (Fig. 6–1), subsequently were found in numerous tissues and species.[10–15]

Within a short time, indirect arguments postulated that the intracellular high-affinity steroid-binding proteins are actually involved in the action of steroid hormones and therefore qualify as "receptors."[14] A powerful argument was the fact that natural steroids as well as synthetic analogues displayed affinity for the appropriate receptors that

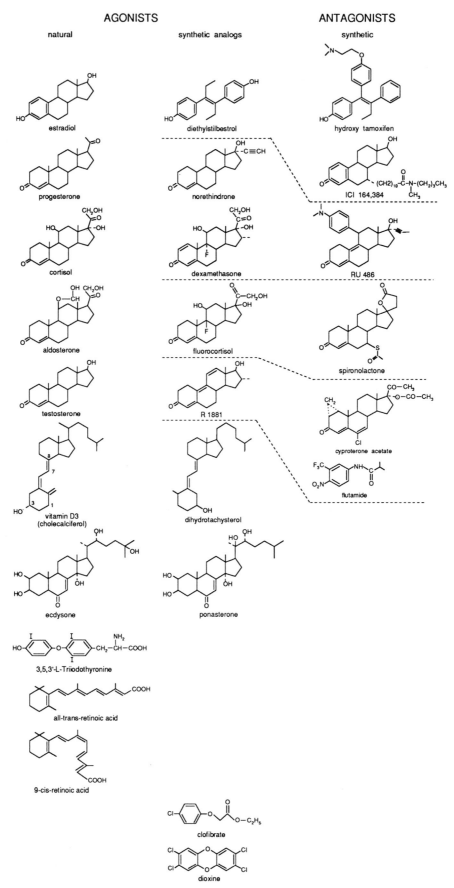

FIGURE 6-1 *See legend on opposite page*

correlated with their biological activities, whether agonist or antagonist.[14–18]

Characterization of Steroid Hormone Receptors: Nontransformed and Transformed Forms

Steroid receptors were the first to be discovered. All steroid hormone target tissues contain the appropriate receptor, which can be detected either in the soluble fraction of the homogenate, cytosol (before exposure of the tissue to the hormone, as with estrogen receptor [ER] in the immature rodent uterus), or in the cell nuclei when the receptor has been complexed in vivo with its ligand (e.g., after injection of estradiol).[14–18] This observation led to a long-lasting image of "cytoplasmic" ligand-free receptors "translocated" to the nucleus upon binding of the hormone.[19] In fact, later studies showed that ligand-free sex steroid hormone receptors are predominantly nuclear, but their association with chromatin becomes tighter after binding of the hormone (see later discussion). The binding of the hormone leads to changes in the behavior and physicochemical properties of the receptor. The term *activation,* or more appropriately *transformation,* is used to denote the combination of these changes. The transformed receptors, which are of sedimentation coefficient approximately "4S," are smaller than nontransformed ones of sedimentation coefficient approximately "8S" and bind tightly to DNA as well as to phosphocellulose (indicating a different surface charge distribution as compared with the nontransformed receptors). Their affinity for the hormone is greater as judged by the longer half-life of dissociation of the hormone-receptor complexes (Fig. 6–2). Heterogeneity of transformed steroid hormone receptors has been reported but often relates to post-translational modifications or to proteolytic degradation occurring in crude tissue extracts, with the notable exception of the chicken and human progesterone receptors (PR), which exist in two forms (A and B), differing by size and charge, which are

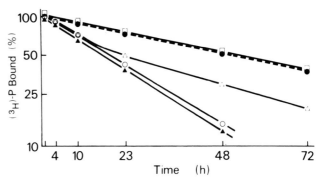

FIGURE 6–2. **Dissociation kinetics of nontransformed vs. transformed PR-³H-progesterone complexes.** The nontransformed complexes were formed by incubation of the labeled hormone with the chick oviduct cytosol either at 0°C (○, △), or at 25°C in the presence of molybdate (▲). The transformed complexes were formed at 25°C in the absence of molybdate. The dissociation kinetics was studied by "chase" with excess unlabeled progesterone at 0°C, either in the presence (□, ○) or in the absence of molybdate (●, ▲, △). First-order kinetics of dissociation is observed for both nontransformed and transformed complexes, with half-lives of 17 h and 56 h, respectively. If nontransformed complexes are allowed to dissociate in the absence of molybdate, a biphasic curve is observed reflecting transformation of the complexes in the course of the experiment (△).[230]

readily separated by DEAE cellulose or phosphocellulose chromatography.[20] There are several genes as well as post-transcriptional modifications for receptors of thyroid hormones and retinoids, resulting in extensive diversity.[21, 22]

The process of transformation can be triggered in vitro by a number of mild treatments such as incubation of the nontransformed (cytosoluble) receptor with the hormone at an elevated temperature (25°C) or (at 0°C) with heparin[23] or adenosine triphosphate (ATP),[24] or in a medium of high ionic strength (≥0.3M NaCl).[25] Although the presence of the hormone at its binding site is not necessary, it accelerates the process of transformation.[23, 24] In fact, it seems that the nontransformed receptor-hormone complex is in a thermodynamically metastable state, waiting for the first stimulus to become transformed. Study of the nontransformed receptors was therefore considerably facil-

---

FIGURE 6–1. **Ligands for DNA-binding receptors.** The most important *natural agonist* corresponding to a cognate-specific receptor is represented. Among natural agonists, there are five steroidal hormonal ligands in most animals. In rodents such as rats and mice, the most abundant glucocorticosteroid is corticosterone and not cortisol. The most active androgen in all species is 5α-dihydrotestosterone and not the secreted testosterone. 1,25-dihydroxycholecalciferol and β-ecdysone are the active metabolites of vitamin D₃ and ecdysone, respectively. There are two retinoic acids, metabolites of vitamin A, which bind to two different specific receptors. Among synthetic agonists, we have selected one example (when available). Clofibrate and dioxine receptors have no known natural ligands. Besides synthetic *antihormones,* there are a few natural antagonists such as progesterone, which has antimineralocorticosteroid activity.

DNA-binding receptors with known ligands:

estradiol receptor	ER
progesterone receptor	PR
glucocorticosteroid receptor	GR
mineralocorticosteroid receptor	MR
androgen receptor	AR
vitamin D₃ (1,25-dihydroxycholecalciferol) receptor	VDR
ecdysone receptor	ECR
thyroid hormone receptor	TR
retinoic acid receptor	RAR
retinoic acid X receptor	RXR
peroxisome proliferator activator receptor	PPAR
dioxine receptor	

itated by the observation that oxyanions of the type MeO_4^{2-} (where Me = Mo, V, W, and probably also other metals of the group Vb and VIb of the periodic system) inhibit the transformation very efficiently.[26–28] It has been shown that nontransformed receptors are hetero-oligomers containing a non–hormone-binding component, the stress protein hsp90.[29–31] A prominent feature of the process of transformation in vitro is the release of the hormone-binding subunits ("true" receptor) from the complex with hsp90.

It appears plausible that more subtle, conformational changes are associated with or follow the binding of the ligand and the release of hsp90 and produce receptor-ligand complexes that can then perform different biological functions. Evidence for such conformational changes has recently been produced for the human PR (hPR) on the basis of the formation of proteolysis-resistant fragments.[32] (The existence of a small, ~20-kDa proteolysis-resistant fragment of the PR has been known since the early 1970's.[33–35]) In addition, the conformational alterations are different when agonistic as opposed to antagonistic ligand binds to the receptor, supporting the concept that the ligand plays an active role in receptor transformation.

Purification of Steroid Hormone Receptors: A Classical (Outdated?) Art

Further progress in the understanding of the mechanism of cellular signaling by steroid hormones has required efficient methods yielding highly purified receptors, both transformed and nontransformed, in amounts sufficient for analysis and for immunization of animals in order to obtain specific antibodies. Since receptors represent ≤ 0.1 per cent of total protein, it was necessary to develop methods based on affinity chromatography; the efforts in this direction were complicated by the high specificity of the receptor-ligand interaction so that chemically modified molecules (linked to a solid support) often failed to bind the receptor. Systematic studies of the affinities of steroid hormone receptors for natural and synthetic analogues had to be carried out in order to design derivatives that could be coupled to the support and retain their binding to the appropriate receptor. PR from the chick oviduct was the first to be purified to near-homogeneity, as both the nontransformed and transformed varieties,[36, 37] so that several antibodies reacting with the individual components could be produced. This helped elucidate the structural relationships of these proteins. Estrogen receptors from the calf uterus were also purified by affinity chromatography[38] and by ligand bioaffinity methods using chemically modified ligands covalently bound to soluble selectable molecules: high molecular weight dextran[39] or biotin.[40]

Another successful strategy was based on the tight binding of transformed steroid hormone receptors to DNA; columns of nonspecific DNA coupled to cellulose allow purification by loading the hormone-receptor complexes and eluting them with a high salt buffer. (Instead of DNA cellulose, phosphocellulose can be used.) Evidently, nontransformed receptors cannot be purified by this approach. Rat liver glucocorticosteroid receptors and chick oviduct progesterone receptors were purified by methods including DNA cellulose or phosphocellulose chromatog-

raphy.[20, 41] Partially purified receptors were often sufficient for immunization and production of highly specific monoclonal antibodies, which turned out to be the key instrument in molecular cloning of the corresponding cDNA's. New species of mRNA have been identified by cloning homologous sequences. This approach has led to the detection of more than 50 new "receptors," corresponding, or not, to known regulatory ligands. Often, all that is known of these receptors is the deduced primary sequence. In the absence of a known ligand, these receptor proteins are referred to as "orphan" receptors.

The procedures used for the purification of steroid hormone receptors are illustrated in Figure 6–3.

The identities of receptor proteins were established by three methods, the first being *affinity labeling*. This method is convenient as it can be applied with nonpurified tissue extracts. It relies on the use of ligands that can form a covalent bond with the receptor (either spontaneously or after exposure to UV light) and was used to label the PR using (^{3}H) promegestone;[42] ER (with [^{3}H] aziridine tamoxifen)[43]; and glucocorticosteroid receptor (GR) (with [^{3}H] dexamethasone mesylate).[44] Electrophoresis in denaturing (sodium dodecyl sulphate) polyacrylamide gel (SDS-PAGE) and fluorography revealed that bovine ER migrated as a single band of 65 kDa[38] and rat GR also as a single band (estimated at 85 kDa),[44] whereas chick oviduct PR was detected as two protein bands of 79 and 110 kDa.[45] These two polypeptides correspond to the forms A and B, respectively, of the receptor.

A second method of receptor protein identification is *analysis of highly purified receptor preparations*. Purified transformed receptors for estrogens, progesterone, and glucocorticosteroids were found by SDS-PAGE analysis to be identical to the proteins detected by affinity labeling with

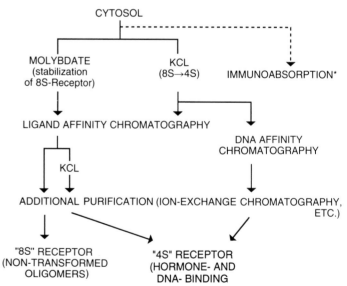

FIGURE 6–3. Methods of purification of steroid receptors. The flow chart illustrates the procedures successfully employed to purify ER, PR, and GR from various human, rabbit, and chicken tissues. Following the production of antibodies, the immunoadsorption-based procedures can be used as the affinity step, either for the nontransformed or for the transformed receptors. Affinity chromatography may not be necessary if the source of receptor is sufficiently rich, as it is in the case with cloned (fragments of) receptors expressed in suitable host systems (for instance, baculovirus-based constructs).

the appropriate ligands.[38, 46] Analysis of the nontransformed, highly purified chick oviduct progesterone receptor revealed the same hormone-binding proteins as did the nontransformed preparations, plus another protein migrating at 90 kDa, suggesting that nontransformed receptors are hetero-oligomers including hormone-binding as well as non–hormone-binding subunits. Chemical crosslinking supported this conclusion.[37] Similar observations were subsequently also made with the nontransformed ER[38] and GR,[47] androgen (AR),[29, 30] and mineralocorticosteroid receptors (MR).[48]

A third identification method is *immunochemistry*. As in the case of affinity labeling, there is no need to purify the receptor. It was satisfactory if not surprising that, in immunoblots, specific antibodies visualized the same proteins as those detected by the preceding methods.

Analysis of the nontransformed receptors by incubation with a monoclonal antibody directed against the non–hormone-binding 90-kDa subunit and sucrose gradient centrifugation confirmed the presence of the 90-kDa protein complexed with the hormone-binding subunits. The 90-kDa protein was found to be identical in all the steroid receptors of the chick oviduct; by subsequent studies it has been shown to be the heat-shock protein hsp90.[29, 30] There are two isoforms of hsp90, α and β, products of two different genes. Both seem to be present in steroid receptors. Methods used for the identification of the components of oligomeric receptors of steroid hormones are illustrated in Figure 6–4.

While for instance the progesterone receptors exist in diluted solution as monomers after transformation, the estrogen receptors have a strong tendency to form homodi-

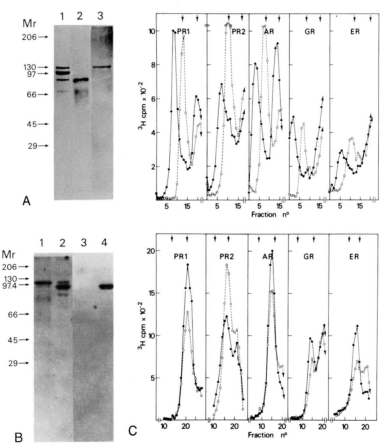

FIGURE 6–4. **Identification of the components of the non-transformed and transformed receptors from the chick oviduct.** *A*, The chick oviduct progesterone receptor was purified by ligand-affinity chromatography followed by fractionation on DEAE-cellulose. Electrophoretic analysis (SDS-PAGE, silver-stained) is shown for the nontransformed receptor (lane 1) and for the subunits A (lane 2) and B (lane 3), separated by DEAE-cellulose chromatography. The nontransformed receptor preparation reveals the presence of both A and B subunits as well as the non–ligand-binding hsp90.[36] *B*, The purified B-subunit of the chick PR was loaded in lanes 1 and 3 and the nontransformed PR in lanes 2 and 4. Lanes 1 and 2 were immunoblotted with the polyclonal antibody prepared against the nontransformed receptor: all components of the receptor are revealed. Immunoblotting of the lanes 3 and 4 with the monoclonal antibody, which reacts exclusively with the hsp90, reveals the hsp90 band in the nontransformed receptor but yields no signal in the B-subunit preparation.[29, 37] *C*, Analysis of complexes of different receptors present in the chick oviduct cytosol with anti-hsp90 antibody by ultracentrifugation is sucrose gradient. *Upper panel*, nontransformed receptors (molybdate-stabilized); *lower panel*, transformed receptors. PR1, progesterone receptor; AR, androgen receptor; GR, glucocorticosteroid receptor; ER, estrogen receptor; labeled by appropriate tritiated ligands. *Solid line*, incubation with the monoclonal anti-hsp90 antibody BF4; *dashed line*, incubation without the antibody. PR2 represents an experiment where nonimmune rat IgG fraction was included in the control incubation *(dashed line)*. The arrows indicate the sedimentation constant markers (horseradish peroxidase: 3.6S; glucose oxidase: 7.9S). The BF4 antibody binds to all nontransformed receptors, forming heavy complexes (11-13S), but does not affect the rate of sedimentation of the transformed receptors.[29]

mers.[49] This is also reflected in the molecular composition of the nontransformed forms: progesterone receptors are hetero-oligomers containing one hormone-binding polypeptide (A or B) in association with a dimer of hsp90, while the nontransformed estrogen receptor contains two hormone-binding subunits and two molecules of hsp90.

Besides hsp90, a protein of 59 kDa has also been found to be present in nontransformed receptors for steroid hormones.[50, 51] The 59-kDa protein does not associate directly with steroid hormone receptors but forms a complex with the hsp90 dimer.[52] Sequence studies suggested that the p59 protein is an immunophilin, and it has been effectively confirmed that it binds immunosuppressants such as FK506 and rapamycin.[51]

Subcellular Localization of Steroid Hormone Receptors

As already mentioned, early studies done with tissue homogenates led to the detection of unliganded steroid hormone receptors in the cytosoluble fraction and were interpreted as evidence of their cytoplasmic localization. A notable exception was the case of the estrogen receptor of chick[53] and amphibian[54] liver, which are bound to the nucleus even in the absence of the hormone.

Binding of the hormone and the ensuing tight association with the cell nucleus (concomitantly with receptor transformation and acquisition of affinity for DNA) were presented as the two-step mechanism of steroid hormone action.[55] Later research demonstrated that in fact unliganded receptors of steroid hormones are predominantly nuclear (Fig. 6–5). This conclusion was based on experiments in which cells were enucleated with cytochalasin instead of their structure being destroyed in diluting buffers,[56] as well as by immunohistochemical detection of receptor proteins.[57] Nonetheless, binding the hormone and the subsequent structural changes of the receptor may well be seen as the two initial steps in steroid action. In the case of GR, cytoplasmic localization of the nonliganded form has been supported by immunocytochemistry in certain cells[58, 59]; therefore, it remains possible that at least this receptor may conform to the original version of the two-step model. The situation is not simple, and the results not completely clear for two reasons. First, it has been shown that the apparent distribution between the nucleus and the cytoplasm compartments of the immunocytochemically detected receptor depends on the fixation technique.[60, 61] Second, besides the obvious cytoplasmic synthesis of receptors as that of any protein, implying a transfer to the nucleus, there may be an energy-dependent shuttle mechanism governing the subcellular distribution of steroid receptors.[62]

In contrast with the hormone binding components of the receptor, the hsp90 protein is predominantly cytoplasmic and also generally much more abundant. These facts cast some doubt on the hypothetical structure of the nontransformed receptor oligomer: the association of the hsp90 dimer with the nontransformed receptor could in principle occur after the destruction of the cell. However, most studies carried out in different laboratories support the concept that the receptor-hsp90 complexes pre-exist in the living cell.[63–66] The nuclear localization of a portion of the cellular pool of hsp90 has also been demonstrated[67, 68] (Fig. 6–5). In addition, it has been recently shown that expression of a recombinant hsp90, equipped with a strong nuclear addressing sequence, leads to nuclear localization of steroid receptor mutants locking nuclear localization signals.[68a]

Under appropriate conditions of extraction, the oligomeric complexes of steroid hormone receptors and hsp90 are found associated with several other proteins including hsp70[69] and the 59-kDa immunophilin; for these two proteins, a nuclear localization has been reported.[52, 69] Whether these and possibly still other proteins interact with the nontransformed receptors in the living cell remains to be documented. Also the question of whether the nontransformed hetero-oligomeric receptor is synthesized in the cytoplasm and transferred as such into the nucleus or assembled in the nucleus is still unanswered.

Molecular Cloning of Steroid Hormone Receptors

The availability of specific antibodies that could recognize the steroid receptor molecules was crucial for screen-

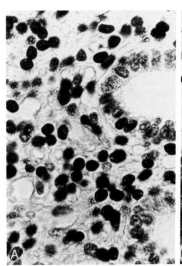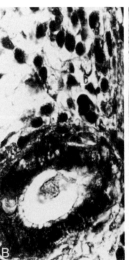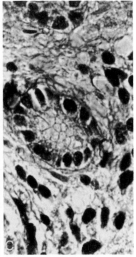

FIGURE 6–5. **Immunodetection of the components of nontransformed receptors.** Paraffin sections of the rabbit uterus were incubated with monoclonal antibodies directed against: *A,* β subunit of the chick oviduct, crossreacting with mammalian PR. *B,* Chicken hsp90 (reacting with mammalian hsp90). *C,* Rabbit p59. The presence of antibodies was revealed by the immunoperoxidase procedure.[60]

ing expression libraries for cDNA's corresponding to the mRNA's coding for the receptors.

The first cloned were the human GR[70] and ER[71]; other cDNA clones came in rapid succession. Their sequences have shown considerable homology not only within the steroid receptor family but also with receptors for several other lipophilic ligands and other nuclear proteins.[72] Whereas the isolation of the first cDNA clones depended on the production of specific antibodies, cDNA's coding for other receptors were subsequently isolated by different methods that made use of the high degree of sequence conservation of the DNA-binding domain and of the receptors' modular structure (see later discussion).

Apart from the receptors of steroid hormones, the "nuclear receptor superfamily," as defined by primary structure homologies, includes at present the receptors of thyroid hormones (TR), retinoids (RAR and RXR), and vitamin D–active metabolite calcitriol (VDR) as well as those of the insect hormone ecdysone, and a large number of proteins for which no regulatory ligand has been identified. As noted, they are frequently called orphan receptors, although their receptor function is only a hypothesis. Indeed, many of these "receptors" simply may be transcription factors among others that happen to display homology with the nuclear receptor superfamily but are subject to other types of regulation. (For a comprehensive classification of nuclear receptors according to sequence homologies, see ref. 72.)

In addition to the "recruitment by sequence," several other candidates for membership in the nuclear receptor club are pending, on the basis of analogies in the mechanism of regulation. These are proteins known—or supposed—to bind lipophilic molecules such as dioxin,[73] vitamins E and K, and possibly even plant hormones such as abscissic acid, brassinosteroids, and gibberelins.[74] However, analogy of function does not necessarily imply analogy of structure. In particular, although the dioxin receptor is a transcription factor regulated by a small lipophilic molecule (and forms complexes with hsp90), it belongs to the helix-loop-helix family of transcription factors that includes, for instance, MYOD.[73a, 73b]

STRUCTURE AND FUNCTION

On the basis of sequence conservation, several structural segments originally noted for the ER[75] can be distinguished along the consensus amino acid sequence representing "the" nuclear receptor molecule (Fig. 6–6). The considerable size variability of the different family members is mostly due to the differences in the length of the amino-terminal portion. The DNA-binding domain (DBD) and the ligand-binding domain (LBD) have been defined by sequence analogies and functional studies. A portion between the DBD and the LBD serves as a "hinge" and may have crucial significance for the spatial configuration of the receptor. The DBD and the LBD are approximately of constant length in all receptors (~70 and ~250 amino acids, respectively).

The functional features of the nuclear receptors assigned to the individual structural domains are evidently approximate and not always exactly the same for the differ-

ent members of the superfamily. Moreover, several functions are partially coincident, and it seems logical to assume that there are interactions between the hormone-binding and transcription transactivation functions.

The division of labor between the individual receptor domains ("modular structure" of the nuclear receptors) has been verified in experiments in which domains from different receptors were swapped; as predicted, the LBD proved to determine the ligand regulation of transcriptional activation, whereas the DBD directed the gene (i.e., promoter) specificity.

There is a certain correspondence between the functional domains of nuclear receptors and the exon and intron structure of the corresponding genes.[75] In nearly all genes, the N-terminal portion of the molecule and each of the two zinc fingers of the DBD (see below) are encoded by separate exons (Fig. 6–7). It seems plausible that all nuclear receptors have evolved from a single ancestral gene. A putative evolutionary tree of the nuclear receptor superfamily has been proposed[72] (Fig. 6–8).

The function of the nuclear receptors concerns the regulation of the expression of particular categories of genes. This regulation is exerted by interaction with specific DNA sequences and with other proteins involved in gene expression control; both these modes of action of the nuclear receptors have been amply demonstrated. More subtle effects of nuclear receptors may exist at the level of chromatin architecture and nucleosome positioning (see below); such effects could be important in the cell type–specific regulation of gene expression.

Other possible modes of action of steroid hormone receptors have been suggested in the past but did not receive further attention: interaction with nuclear RNA/RNP particles,[76] effect on the stability of mRNA, initiation of translation, and elongation of the growing polypeptide chain.[77–79] Such post-transcriptional effects may be a consequence of changes in the expression of genes coding for proteins that participate in the regulation of mRNA contents and translation.[80] In this context, it is interesting to note that the induction of the expression of the progesterone receptor gene by estrogens (a fairly universal, physiologically important event) is apparently due, at least in part, to post-transcriptional processes.[81]

Interaction with DNA: Hormone Response Elements (HRE's) and DNA-Binding Domain (DBD)

Early studies of steroid hormone receptors have demonstrated that the ligand-induced transformation "activates" the binding to nonspecific DNA. The existence of specific DNA sequences for which the receptors would bind with high affinity and selectivity was implicitly assumed, but the confirmation of this working hypothesis had to await development of suitable analytical methods as well as cloning of genomic fragments of the steroid-regulated genes. For the study of specific DNA-protein interaction, there are three essential methodological approaches: (1) DNA protection ("footprinting"), (2) retardation of migration of oligodeoxynucleotides in gel electrophoresis (electrophoretic mobility shift assay [EMSA]), and (3) an assay of the transcriptional regulation in the conditions of transient trans-

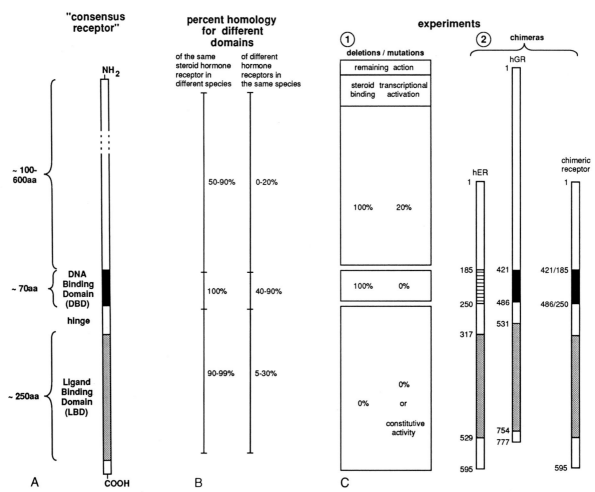

FIGURE 6–6. **Steroid hormone receptors.** In *A,* the drawing represents a consensus receptor. The DNA-binding domain (DBD), ligand-binding domain (LBD), and the hinge between them are of similar length for all receptors. The NH2-terminal region of these receptors is poorly conserved. In *B,* homologies of different domains for the same hormone receptor in different species and for different hormone receptors in the same species are indicated. In *C,* two types of experiments are presented: First, the hormonal response is decreased after alterations in the NH2-terminal region, and abolished if DBD is modified. Alteration in the LBD affects steroid binding, and in most cases abolishes the hormonal response. However, truncation of the LBD may lead to constitutive activity (with no hormonal response). Second, chimera experiments consist in switching the DBD of hER and hGR. The chimeric receptor can trigger a glucocorticosteroid-specific response via GR-DBD induced by an estrogenic steroid (via the ER-LBD).

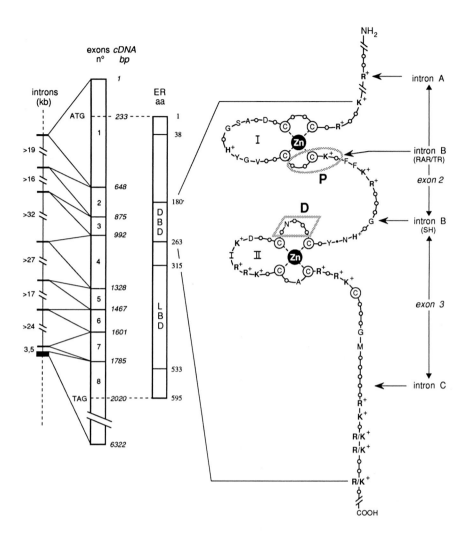

FIGURE 6-7. **DNA binding domain.** Zinc (Zn) fingers, D- and P-boxes, and genomic organization of receptors. The two characteristic Zn fingers of steroid receptors are represented. Note the coordination of Zn with 4 cysteines, and also the conserved fifth cysteine in the C-terminal extremity of the second finger. The conserved amino acids are indicated, as well as proximal (P) and distal (D) boxes. The two Zn fingers are coded by separate exons (2 and 3); the portions of the intervening introns are also shown for steroid hormone receptors (SH) and for RAR/TR. In the left part of the figure, the receptor domains are indicated for hER (amino acid numbers). The corresponding exons are numbered, and the cDNA numbers of bp and the approximate sizes of introns are shown.

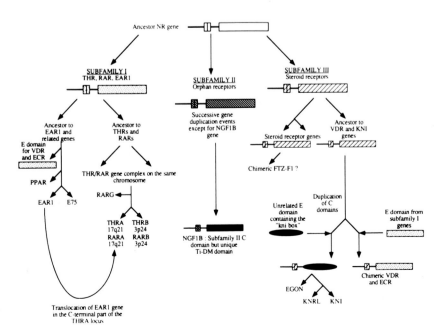

FIGURE 6-8. **Hypothetical evolutionary scenario for the nuclear receptor genes.** The evolution history of nuclear receptors has been deduced[72] on the basis of conserved amino acids in two regions: 1, DBD ("C-domain," containing the two zinc fingers), represented as a square box on the left; 2, LBD ("E-domain," including TAF-2 and hydrophobic surfaces presumably involved in dimerization), represented by the rectangle on the right. Three subfamilies have evolved from a postulated ancestral gene. Since in each subfamily there are both human and *Drosophila* genes, they apparently diverged before the separation of vertebrates and arthropods >500 million years ago. ECR is the ecdysone receptor; EAR1, PPAR, E75, NGF1B, FTZ-F1, KNI, KNRL, and EGON are different orphan receptors. VDR and ECR genes appear to result from a fusion of two domains that have evolved separately.

fection of constructs expressing an indicator gene (most commonly chloramphenicol acetyl transferase [CAT] or luciferase). These methods are illustrated in Figure 6–9.

Hormone Response Elements

The DNA sequences required for the specific binding of nuclear receptors (hormone response elements; HRE's) are generally situated upstream of the transcription initiation site and present two short (5 to 6 base pairs) segments of a very similar or identical sequence (in opposite orientation for most nuclear receptors), interspersed or not by a short nonconserved segment. It has been demonstrated for GR[82] that each hexanucleotide binds one receptor molecule, and the two juxtaposed receptor molecules interact with each other, forming a more or less stable dimer (see below). This mode of protein-DNA binding is currently presented as an interaction of receptor molecules (monomers or subunits of a dimer) with "half-sites" of the recognition sequence. A schematic model as proposed by Schwabe and colleagues[83] is shown in Figure 6–10.

A somewhat unexpected conclusion of the studies of the HRE's used by diverse nuclear receptors was the apparently high degree of cross-recognition. Thus, a different GRE and PRE (glucocorticosteroid vs. progesterone response element) does not seem to exist; both GR and PR specifically bind to the same elements, corresponding to the "consensus" sequence AGAACA(N_3)TGTTCT. The bind-

ing is "functional" and leads to transcriptional activation of reporter genes in transfected cells. The productive interaction with different receptor-hormone complexes is not restricted to the artificial consensus sequences, as the "real" GRE of the long terminal repeat (LTR) of the mouse mammary tumor virus (MMTV) is also responsive (in transient expression assay) not only to GR and PR but also to AR.[84–86] Given the similarities between the GR and MR in terms of primary sequence and hormone specificity, it is then no wonder that these two receptors do not seem to display DNA sequence specificity either. There is a difference between the GRE and ERE ((A)GGTCA(n_3)TGACC(T)) consensus sequences, but the degree of similarity is remarkable. RAR, TR, and vitamin D receptor (VDR) cross-recognize the same palindromic DNA sequences (GGTCATGACC) that also bear a strong resemblance to the ERE; however, there is a structural feature that precludes productive (i.e., efficient in transcriptional activation) cross-recognition—namely, absence of the spacer segment of three base pairs between the half-sites of the TRE/RARE. In natural HRE's, one half-site can be considerably different from the consensus. It appears that after binding of one receptor subunit to the "good" half-site, the other subunit will be able to accommodate deviations in the HRE sequence, resulting from the stabilizing interactions between the monomers.[86a]

In contrast with steroid hormone receptor HRE's, TRE/RARE half-sites are functional also as direct repeats.[87]

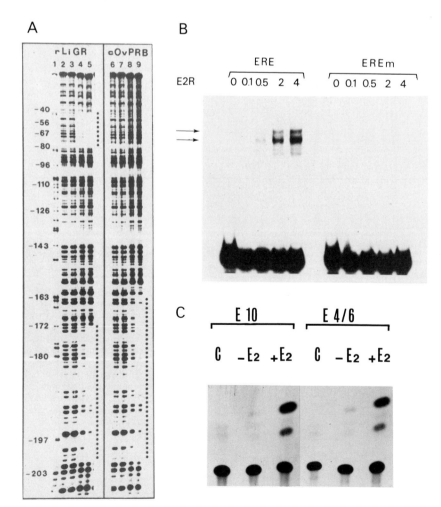

FIGURE 6–9. **Specific interactions between nuclear receptors and DNA.** *A,* DNAse I protection assay ("DNA footprinting"). The ^{32}P-labeled promoter-containing fragment of the chicken lysozyme gene was subjected to a limited digestion with DNAse I either in the absence of added receptors (lanes 2, 3, 6, and 7), or in the presence of purified rat liver GR (LiGR; 1.5 and 3 μg, respectively; lanes 4 and 5) or chick oviduct PR, B-subunit (cOvPRB; 0.75 and 1.5 μg, respectively; lanes 7 and 8), complexed with the appropriate ligands, and subsequently analyzed by sequencing polyacrylamide gel electrophoresis. Lane 1-size markers; the numbers indicate the distance from the transcription site. The regions protected by the bound receptors are revealed by the absence of digestion fragments within the appropriate length margins (dots).[233] *B,* Detection by retardation in gel electrophoresis ("gel shift"). Two 37-base pair deoxyoligonucleotides (^{32}P-labeled) containing either the ERE sequences of the *Xenopus* vitellogenin A2 gene (ERE wt) or the mutated, nonfunctional ERE (EREm) were incubated with different amounts of hormone-complexes ER (0 to 4 ng). Free DNA (fast-migrating band) and two protein-DNA complexes (arrows) were resolved by polyacrylamide gel electrophoresis.[234] *C,* Activation of indicator gene transcription. Balb/C fibroblasts were stably transfected with human ER, and two of the clones expressing the receptor were analyzed by transient ERE-CAT (chloramphenicol acetyltransferase) transfection assay. After transfection and incubation with or without estradiol (E), the CAT activity was determined using ^{14}C-labeled chloramphenicol; the substrate (slowly migrating spot) and two differently acetylated forms were separated by thin layer chromatography. Control (C): mock-transfection.[209]

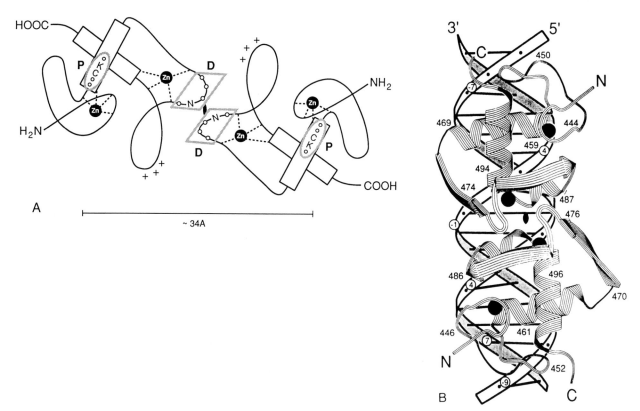

FIGURE 6–10. **Schematic representation of the dimer DBD.** *A*, Relative orientation of the ER DBD monomers as indicated by two-dimensional ^{1}H NMR.[83] Each monomer contains two helices perpendicular to each other *(rectangles)*. The zinc atoms *(discs)* are coordinated by four cysteines *(dashed lines)*. EGA amino acid residues are parts of the P-box sequences; the dimerization surfaces overlapping with the D-box are indicated by parallelograms. The postulated relative orientation of the monomers is such that the recognition helices are antiparallel, to fit in successive major grooves 34 A apart. The conserved basic side chains are also indicated (+ + +). *B*, Interaction with DNA. The DBD subunits bind to successive major grooves, whereas the dimerization surfaces are positioned over the minor grooves. This model is based on a crystallographic analysis[111] using the GR DBD and an artificial GRE where the two half-sites are separated by four (instead of three) nucleotides. As a consequence, only one subunit faces the target half-site, and the second subunit faces a noncognate DNA sequence, shifted by one base pair.

In this arrangement, the two half-sites are separated by a spacer whose length influences the specificity of recognition. Three nucleotides for VDR, four nucleotides for TR, and five for RAR/RXR appear to recognize the same sequences spaced by a single nucleotide[88] (Table 6–1). However, systematic experiments with synthetic oligonucleotides have led to the conclusion that no simple and rigorous rules with which the RAR/RXR-HRE recognition would be defined by spacing or orientation of the half-sites can be established; the actual sequences of the HRE's as well as the flanking bases appear to be important in defining the receptor-binding efficiencies.[86]

Clearly, in cells that express several types of nuclear receptors, the selectivity of receptor-promoter interactions is insufficient to ensure cell-specific regulation of gene expression, which relies on numerous other processes (see below).

Binding of a nuclear receptor molecule to the HRE sequences usually leads to the *enhancement* of transcription; however, the opposite effect, *inhibition* of transcription, is also frequent. Glucocorticosteroids down-regulate the expression of numerous genes, often by inducing the binding of the receptor to specific DNA sequences (termed nGRE), which are structurally similar to GRE's but do not correspond to the GRE consensus sequence. Moreover,

different nGRE's display considerable sequence variability, so that there is no clear consensus. In order to observe the inhibitory effect of the receptor, obviously there must be a sufficiently high basal transcription, directed by a strong enhancer. Therefore, it seems plausible to propose that in fact the inhibition of transcription observed is often a consequence of the fact that the nGRE acts as a weak enhancer and attenuates the effect of the strong basal enhancer—for instance, by steric hindrance of the binding of the basal enhancer–activating transcription factor. In agreement with this interpretation, the same nGRE's may actually act as glucocorticosteroid-inducible transcriptional activators or inhibitors, according to the cell type. In the promoters of genes negatively regulated by glucocorticosteroids, there is frequently an overlap between the (basal) enhancer and the nGRE, so that the hormone-dependent transcriptional inhibition could be due to a mutually exclusive binding of the receptor or the corresponding enhancer-binding proteins. This is the case for the mouse proliferin gene, in which nGRE overlaps with the AP-1 binding site (recognized by *fos/jun* heterodimer and *jun/jun* homodimer).[89] In other genes, overlapping nGRE/AP-2 (regulated by the cAMP signal transducer protein CREB) recognition sequences have been found.[90] The weak (or absent) transcription-activating effect of the GR bound to nGRE may

TABLE 6–1. RECEPTOR-DNA INTERACTIONS: CONSTRAINTS ON SPECIFICITY

| RECEPTOR | STRUCTURAL FEATURES OF THE RECEPTOR | | CONSENSUS HRE SEQUENCE | |
	P-box	D-box	Direct Repeats	Inverted Repeats
"GR subfamily":				
GR, PR, MR	GSCKV	AGRND		AGAACA(n₃)TGTTCT
AR	GSCKV	ASRND		
"ER/TR subfamily":				
ER	EGCKA	PATNQ		AGGTCA(n₃)TGACCT
TRα	EGCKG	KYDSC	AGGTCA(n₄)AGGTCA	AGGTCATGACCT
TRβ	EGCKG	KYEGK	AGGTCA(n₄)AGGTCA	AGGTCATGACCT
RARα,RARβ	EGCKG	HRDKN	AGGTCA(n₅)AGGTCA	
VD₃R	EGCKG	PFNGD	AGGTCA(n₃)AGGTCA	
RXR	EGCKG	RDNKD	AGGTCA(n)AGGTCA	
v-erbA	EGCKG	TYDGC		

The HRE sequences present in the promoters of the different hormone-regulated genes often present considerable deviations from the "consensus," as shown in this table. Moreover, HRE sequences with spacers of different lengths responding to RAR[231] or to VDR[232] recently have been found.

be a consequence of a (hypothetical) nonproductive conformation of the receptor protein, in contrast with the productive conformation resulting from binding to a GRE site; in this hypothesis, GRE and nGRE would act as allosteric ligands.[91] Another interesting feature of the interaction of GR with the nGRE from the POMC gene promoter is the fact that apart from the usual GR homodimer, an additional GR monomer binds on the opposite side of the double helix.[92]

The effects of the GR on transcription of complex promoters (containing another enhancer sequence besides that recognized by the receptor) are also influenced by the interactions between the receptor and the enhancer-binding proteins. Diamond et al.[89] have shown that glucocorticosteroids can either stimulate or inhibit transcription directed by the mouse proliferin promoter, which contains AP1-like sequences as well as an element recognized by the GR. The activation of transcription by the GR is observed in transient transfection experiments if the recipient cells express the c-jun protein (in the absence of c-fos), whereas in the presence of both c-jun and c-fos (forming a heterodimer which strongly activates the AP1-directed promoter function), the GR inhibits the "basal" transcription. In the absence of both c-jun and c-fos, glucocorticosteroids fail to interact with the nGRE element of the mouse proliferin promoter and consequently do not affect its activity. These data can be interpreted by a model in which the interaction of the GR with the proliferin nGRE is stabilized by the presence of the adjacent Jun molecule. Protein-protein interaction between the GR and c-jun has indeed been demonstrated[93, 94] in support of this model. As another example, the glucocorticosteroid receptor-mediated inhibition of the TPA-induced collagenase gene transcription relies on the interaction between the receptor and the AP1 complex. However, this does not prevent the AP1 complex from binding to the TRE sequence in the promoter.[95]

An additional complication arises from the fact that the transcriptional activity of complex promoters is strongly regulated by post-translational modifications of the fos/jun proteins. The inhibition of transcription directed by such promoters (e.g., the promoter of the c-jun gene[96]) can thus be overcome by the modulation of the fos/jun activity by phorbol esters.

TR presents another case of transcriptional repression by a nuclear receptor in which the repression can be exercised by the unoccupied form of the receptor. Upon binding of the hormone, the receptor becomes an activator of transcription.[97–99] A particular case is the viral oncogenic homologue of the TR, the v-erb A gene product. As a consequence of deletions and point mutations, this protein has lost its ability to bind T3; it binds to the thyroid hormone response element (TRE; present in the promoter regions of T3-regulated genes), but binding of v-erb A is characterized by a considerably lower affinity than that of the TR/TRE interaction and is not "productive" (i.e., does not lead to gene transcription).[100] Thus, the v-erb A gene may act as a dominant repressor of gene expression and blocks the growth-inhibitory action of the T3-inducible proteins. A variant "TRE," which confers transcriptional repression upon binding of the T3-TR complex, has also been described. Such an "nTRE" element, with a sequence that differs from that of the palindromic TRE by three out of 10 bases, is found for instance in the promoter of the keratin 14 gene.[101] The transcription of epidermal keratin genes is repressed by the T3-TR complex but also by RAR's, α, β, as well as γ. Similarly, the expression of the EGF-receptor as well as of the c-erbB2/neu genes is negatively regulated by the liganded TR and RAR's, while the unliganded forms of these receptors release the transcriptional inhibition.[102]

DNA Binding Domain

The portion of the receptor that interacts with the specific DNA sequences (HRE) is situated in the internal portion of the protein (domain C). It is not surprising that this region has the highest degree of conservation within the nuclear receptor superfamily (see Fig. 6–6). Structural analysis of this region reveals the presence of two loops, each containing four cysteines that form coordination bonds with Zn^{2+} ion ("zinc fingers"). This general structure was first reported for the Xenopus laevis transcription factor IIIA, in which the zinc-binding configuration is of the type C_2-H_2,[103] and is found in many DNA-binding proteins. The implication of the two zinc-finger structures of the GR in the DNA binding has been confirmed by studies in which short peptides comprising the "fingers" have been shown to bind to DNA in a sequence-specific, Zn^{2+}-

dependent manner.[104] Zn^{2+} ions are also required for the sequence-specific DNA binding of the bovine estrogen receptor.[105] NMR analysis of recombinant peptides that encompass the DNA-binding domain of GR and ER expressed in *E. coli*[83, 106] shows that a sequence of around 70 amino acids forms a compact domain, particularly the portion comprising the first zinc finger, while the second zinc finger seems to be less well ordered and more flexible in solution. Despite the primary sequence similarity, the spatial structure of the steroid hormone receptor DNA-binding domain is distinctly different from that of the "classical" zinc fingers of the transcription factor III A-type.

DNA sequence specificity is determined, at least in part, by three amino acids within a short element of five amino acid residues at the end of the N-terminal (proximal) finger, termed P-box. Seven different sequences of the P-box have been found[72] (Table 6–1) by analysis of the genes coding for the numerous members of the nuclear receptor family, including orphan receptors. Another short segment, named D-box, situated at the N-terminal end of the C-terminal (distal) finger, is important for the specificity of HBD-HRE recognition and in particular appears to detect the spacing between the two half-sites. Therefore, the D-box sequence is decisive, for instance, for the difference between the ER and TR binding to their HRE's, which differ only by the presence or absence of a three-nucleotide spacer.[87] This segment has also been shown to be necessary for cooperative binding of the GR-LBD to the GRE sequence,[107] in agreement with the hypothesis that the D-box may participate in protein-protein interaction between receptor monomers. The DNA binding domain also appears to contain a dimerization signal.[108, 109]

Portions of the receptor outside the zinc fingers also participate in the receptor-DNA binding. Thus, a basic region situated on the C-terminal part of the molecule (amino acids 256 to 270) is important for the efficient binding of the estrogen receptor to ERE sequences.[3] Estrogen binding to the LBD also favors the interaction between DBD and ERE, probably by influencing the spatial configuration of the receptor molecule. In the case of PR, high-affinity binding to PRE requires additional sequences, in both the N-terminal region and LBD.[109]

The binding of the receptor to the HRE sequences implies cooperative interaction between two receptor molecules. This conclusion was reached by means of study of the interaction of the GR with the response element GRE, which regulates the tyrosine aminotransferase gene expression.[82, 85] In polyacrylamide gel electrophoresis, two retarded bands of the labeled DNA fragment were observed after incubation with the DBD of the receptor (recombinant, expressed in *E. coli*). A point mutation in one of the two half-sites of GRE (TGTTCT) eliminated the binding of the receptor, while, when a mutation was introduced into the other half-site (TGTACA), only the slower of the two retarded complexes was abolished (presumably representing a complex between two DBD's and both half-sites). This observation indicates that the DBD polypeptide has a higher affinity for the TGTTCT hexanucleotide and that binding of a DBD molecule to this half-site strongly increases the affinity of DBD for the other half-site. Changing the distance between the two half-sites abolished the facilitated binding to the lower-affinity half-site, indicating a cooperative interaction between the two DBD molecules.

The DNA sequences of other steroid HRE also present configurations of two half-sites, implying associations with receptor dimers. HRE-binding studies have confirmed strong cooperative interactions between monomers bound to the DNA half-sites (e.g., progesterone receptor).[6] Cooperative interaction of dimer-forming transcription factors with adjacent "half-sites" in the gene promoter is a common phenomenon.[110]

The interaction between two receptor molecules is favored by their binding to HRE half-sites,[111] but at least in certain cases can be also visualized in the absence of DNA. Thus, ER forms particularly stable dimers in solution. In the nontransformed oligomers, two estrogen-binding receptor subunits are already present.[38] In the case of PR, the nontransformed oligomers contain only one hormone-binding subunit, A or B. Transformation releases this subunit, which then can form homo- or heterodimers, less stable than those of the ER but detectable under appropriate conditions.[112] The apparent molecular size of purified transformed PR's (illustrated by the sedimentation constant 4S in sucrose gradient centrifugation) is that of a mixture of monomers but in crude tissue extracts a larger form (6S; corresponding approximately to the dimer) has also been found.[113] Components other than receptor itself may therefore participate in dimer formation and stabilization. Dimerization of PR's appears to be hormone-induced in vivo.[114] Studies of solution structure indicate the existence of a dimerization interface of GR and ER in the N-terminal domain of the CII finger (D-box)[83, 106] (Fig. 6–10). However, there is indirect evidence that ER contains a second, strong dimerization interface in the LBD domain, since a 22-amino acid peptide of the mouse ER HBD is sufficient to confer high-affinity DNA binding to an LBD-truncated mouse ER.[115] The presence in the LBD domain of conserved hydrophobic amino acids supports the possibility that this region is involved in protein-protein interaction and presumably dimerization.[72]

Efficient binding of some classes of receptors (e.g., TR, RAR, VDR) to their cognate HRE sequences requires accessory proteins present in eukaryotic cells; one such protein has been purified from yeast and shown to be a single-stranded DNA-binding protein.[3, 116–119] The interaction between receptors and HRE sequences is regulated by accessory proteins expressed in a cell-specific manner (see ref. 98); thus, the gene expression depends on the presence of both receptors and appropriate accessory factors, conferring an additional constraint to ensure the cell-specific regulation. Remarkably, unliganded RXR has been shown to act as an accessory protein for RAR as well as TR and VDR, favoring their productive interactions with the cognate response elements.[120] This additional activity of RXR augments the possibilities of cell-specific regulation of gene expression by nuclear receptors.

Other accessory proteins may also turn out to be transcription factors in their own right, not necessarily able to form heterodimers with nuclear receptors but rather interacting with the dimers themselves.

Nuclear Receptors and Transcription Factors: Synergistic and Antagonistic Interactions

In many of the genes regulated by the proteins of the nuclear receptor superfamily, several copies of HRE sequences are present, both near and at a considerable distance from the promoter.[2, 121] There is strong experimental evidence indicating that receptor dimers that bind to the HRE sequences interact with each other in a cooperative manner, so that the resulting enhancement of transcription is greater than the sum of the contributions of the individual HRE-receptor elements.[122–124]

The nuclear receptors interact not only with their (identical) counterparts but also with other categories of nuclear receptors and with other transcription factors.[99, 125] This is not surprising if one admits the hypothesis that the enhancement of transcription relies on the stabilization of a preinitiation complex at the promoter sequence. It has been shown that the HRE sequences alone (placed at a short distance upstream from the TATA box of a reporter gene) are sufficient to induce gene transcription in the presence of the appropriate hormone-receptor complexes.[84] The same HRE sequences are ineffective if inserted far from the TATA box. These observations support the idea of interaction between the receptor-HRE structure and the preinitiation complex including RNA polymerase II and TATA binding protein. However, a distant HRE regains its efficiency as a hormone-inducible enhancer of transcription if another enhancer element—identical or different (for example CCAAT or CCCAC)—is inserted in its proximity, illustrating the existence of cooperative interactions between different categories of enhancer-binding proteins.[84] The image of a multimeric protein-DNA structure, sufficiently strong to maintain a correctly folded DNA string and allow the formation of the preinitiation complex, is perhaps too trivial but helps to visualize the mode of action of nuclear receptors and other enhancer-binding proteins. In this context, it is of interest that binding of the estrogen receptor to the ERE element induces bending of the DNA segment.[126, 127] DNA bending by a transcription factor may well be a universal feature, as it has been also observed with the *E. coli* catabolite activator protein-cAMP complex.[128]

Synergistic interactions involving HRE-receptor structures were confirmed also by the mutational approach, both in "natural" genes and in constructs.[124, 129–131]

Inhibition of gene expression by nuclear receptors can also result from protein-protein interactions. The inhibition of AP1/TRE-dependent transcription by GR has been extensively studied (see earlier). The AP1/TRE-regulated transcription is also inhibited by retinoids[132] and thyroid hormones.[98]

Transcription Activation Functions (TAF's) and Transcription Intermediary Factors (TIF's)

Mutational analysis of receptors has brought about arguments for the presence of two domains that can activate transcription initiation at promoters linked to HRE. One such domain (TAF1) is situated in the N-terminal region (A/B) and the other (TAF2) is in the HBD of ER,[133] PR,[134] and GR, in which two acidic segments termed "τ1" and "τ2" are involved in transactivation function[135] (Table 6–2). Although either of these two TAF domains alone can activate transcription, the presence of both confers to the receptor a greater activity than the sum of the two, indicat-

TABLE 6–2. DNA-BINDING RECEPTORS: TRANSACTIVATION DOMAINS

	TAF-1 N-terminal	TAF-2 C-terminal (overlapping LBD)
Activity	• Constitutive (irrespective of ligand) • Cell- and promoter-dependent	• Hormone-dependent • Activated by agonists • Inhibited by antagonists • Cell- and promoter-dependent

ing cooperation of the transcription-activating domains. Several copies of the GRτ1 present in tandem fashion in a chimeric protein also lead to a greater transcriptional response than a single τ1.[135] The TAF/τ sequences are not conserved, and therefore no consensus has been defined. A short (30-amino acid) peptide (τ2) within the TAF2 region of the GR has been found to activate specific gene transcription when fused to the yeast transcription factor Gal4,[135] but the corresponding fragments of the PR and ER lacked transcription-activating properties. The short transcription-activating sequences identified in TAF1 of ER and PR do not show similar characteristics and do not resemble prototypical acidic-activating domains.[3] The TAF2 domain coincides with the LBD and appears to consist of a number of dispersed elements brought together upon hormone binding.[136] One short sequence important for TAF2 activity (15 amino acids situated between residues 538 and 552 of the mouse ER) has been found to be well conserved among many members of the nuclear receptor family, including GR (but different from the τ2 element).[137] It is to be noted that this 15-amino acid conserved sequence is absent in several nuclear receptors without known regulatory ligand, in agreement with the possibility that these receptors may be true orphans.

The efficiency of the TAF1 and TAF2 domains of the different receptors studied turned out to be dependent on both cellular and promoter contexts. For instance, the LBD-deleted PR remained functional in CV1 cells, in which its TAF2 activity is low, but not in HeLa cells, in which both TAF1 and TAF2 are active.[3, 134, 138] Similarly, the A/B region (containing TAF1) of ER linked to the Gal4-DBD activated Gal4 promoter-directed transcription in chicken embryo fibroblasts but not in HeLa cells.[139, 140] The configuration of the TAF domain is evidently decisive for its activity. While the active configuration of the TAF1 and TAF2 domains in intact receptors or in chimeric constructs requires the presence of an agonist ligand at the LBD, the TAF1 domain appears to possess constitutive activity when separated from the rest of the receptor molecule[3, 139]; the efficiency of transcriptional activation by isolated TAF1 domain of the ER is strongly influenced by other cellular proteins (see further on). These observations are consistent with the possibility that LBD-deleted receptors can become constitutively active in target cells and cause, for instance, deregulated growth of cells that are normally hormone-dependent, such as those of mammary epithelium. Such truncated receptors could participate in tumorigenesis.[141, 142]

Identification of the TAF domains made it possible to study the homo- and heterosynergistic interactions involving different nuclear receptor categories as well as other

		ER		GR		AAD (VP16)	Ad2MLP UE
		TAF-1	TAF-2	TAF-1	TAF-2		
ER	TAF-1	1	25	25	16	40	1
	TAF-2	25	3	6	6	1	25
GR	TAF-1	25	6	3	4	25	ND
	TAF-2	16	6	4	10	5	ND
AAD(VP16)		40	1	25	5	5	75

A

		ACTIVATOR					
		ER		GR		AAD	
COMPETITOR		TAF-1	TAF-2	TAF-1	TAF-2	VP16	GAL4
ER	TAF-1	++	+	+++	+++	+++	+++
	TAF-2	++	+	++	+++	++	+++
GR	TAF-1	+	⊖	++	⊖	⊖	+
	TAF-2	+	+	+	+	⊖	+
AAD VP16(N)		⊖	⊖	+++	+/-	+++	+++

B

FIGURE 6–11. **Synergism between TAF's.** *A,* Homosynergism and hetero-synergism between the hER activation functions TAF-1 and TAF-2, the hGR activation functions TAF-1 and TAF-2, and the AAD of VP16.[140] The results are expressed as fold stimulation of transcription taking one for additive stimulation. *B,* Transcriptional interference and squelching be-tween TAF's. The stimulation in the absence of coexpression of competi-tor is taken as 100%; the effect of competitor is represented in terms of residual activity: + + + (9–22%), + + (30–36%), + (52–70%), and − (92–103%).[143]

enhancer-binding proteins. The intricate specificities of these interactions are illustrated in Figure 6–11*A*.[143] While the TAF1 and TAF2 of ER strongly synergize, there is only a weak synergy between the two TAF domains of GR. The TAF1 domains of both GR and ER strongly heterosynergize with the acidic activation domain (AAD) VP16 of the herpes simplex virus; in contrast, the synergy between the VP16 AAD and the TAF2 regions of these receptors was much weaker (TAF2 of GR) or absent (TAF2 of ER). These observations underline the differences between the TAF1 and TAF2 domains of nuclear receptors.

Transcriptional activation requires participation of *cellular factors* available in *limited quantities*[144] and utilized by different categories of enhancers. The existence of such factors follows, for instance, from the bell-shaped dose response curves of transcriptional activation in cells transfected with increased amounts of hER[134]; at high con-centrations of hER, the cellular factors mediating transcrip-tional activation (transcription intermediary factors or TIF's) are titrated out (squelched). The same or structur-ally and functionally similar TIF's are used by different enhancer-binding proteins that can squelch transcription directed by noncognate enhancers. Thus, the ER-TAF1 in-terferes with activation functions not only of ER-TAF1 but also of ER-TAF2, GR-TAF1 and 2, as well as of the VP16

and GAL4 AAD's[144, 145] (see Fig. 6–11). While the coopera-tion of transactivation functions of the different nuclear receptors/enhancer binding proteins presents a coherent pattern of reciprocity, the transcriptional interference phe-nomenon is frequently unidirectional; thus, VP16 AAD did not affect the transcription activation functions of ER-TAF1 or 2, separated or present within the intact estrogen recep-tor molecule (while both of these TAF regions squelched the transcription activation function of VP16 AAD). Several possible explanations of the "noncommutativity" of squelching can be considered[143] but need to be verified. It is likely that the identification of TIFs will provide some surprises and may help to explain better the apparently inextricable tangle of true receptors, orphan receptors, and accessory proteins—at least some of these categories do converge, as has been seen with RXR.

The existence of several mechanisms that control the transcriptional regulation activity of nuclear receptors—hormone binding, DNA sequence recognition, distinct sep-arate transcription activation domains interacting with multiple intermediary factors—increases the possibilities by which the cell ensures the appropriate rate of transcrip-tion of specific genes. The individual genes regulated by the same nuclear receptor thus present a great diversity of sequence elements recognized by different transcription regulatory factors. The presence, structure, and organiza-tion of the different regulatory elements are characteristic of a given gene and define its hormone response unit (HRU).[146] Examples of HRU are shown in Figure 6–12.

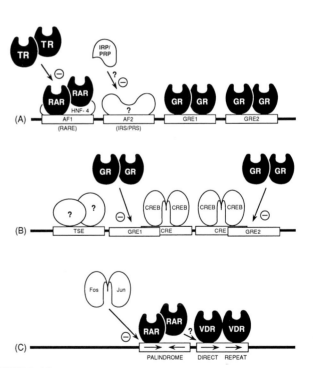

FIGURE 6–12. **Multifunctional regulatory domains of protein promoters.** Factors depicted as bound to DNA elements mediate stimulatory effects on gene transcription. When shown above promoters, they mediate nega-tive effects by either displacing the bound factors or by interfering with the activity of the bound factors solely through protein-protein interac-tions. *A,* PEPCK gene; *B,* The glycoprotein hormone α-subunit gene; *C,* The osteocalcin gene; GR, glucocorticosteroid receptor; VDR; vitamin D receptor; IRP/BRP; insulin response protein/phorbol ester response pro-tein.[146]

Nuclear Receptors and Chromatin Structure

Most studies of the mechanism of transcriptional regulation by nuclear receptors have been carried out in transiently transfected cells. Under such conditions, the exogenous DNA fragments are not integrated in chromosomes but function as episomes, so that chromatin proteins normally positioned along cellular DNA may not interfere with receptor/HRE/preinitiation complex/promoter interactions, as when endogenous genes are involved. Evidently, in this manner the complete image of cellular regulations cannot be obtained.

In vivo, the same receptor will be able to induce the expression of different genes in a totally *cell-specific* manner, which is determined by the state of cell differentiation. An obvious example is the regulation of egg protein synthesis in the chicken. In the liver, estrogens induce the synthesis of the proteins of the yolk (mainly vitellogenin), whereas in the oviduct they regulate the synthesis of the proteins of egg white (mainly ovalbumin). However, the egg white protein synthesis induction requires previous exposure of the oviduct to estrogens ensuring terminal differentiation of the tubular gland cells; after a subsequent estrogen withdrawal, the cells remain differentiated and ready to respond to a secondary estrogen stimulation by an immediate resumption of egg white protein synthesis. Early studies have demonstrated that the availability of genes for the induction of transcription by hormones correlates with their pattern of accessibility to nuclease digestion, implying the role of the chromatin organization in the regulation of gene expression by nuclear receptors. Nonhistone proteins are likely to be responsible for the "specialized" chromatin structure, and much remains to be learned about how such structures can develop during embryonal and neonatal tissue differentiation and hormone-dependent differentiation and be subsequently maintained.

Another aspect of gene regulation in the living cell concerns the role of nucleosomes. Nucleosome-free stretches of DNA are present in transcribed genes as revealed by DNAse 1 hypersensitivity studies.[147] However, precisely positioned nucleosomes have been found in the regulatory regions of several genes.[148] It has been shown that the presence of nucleosomes drastically reduces the binding of the GR to nonspecific DNA but not to the upstream GRE of the mouse mammary tumor virus (MMTV) promoter[149]; nucleosome positioning may therefore help to direct the receptor to its cognate sequences in the regulated promoters.

Another function of nucleosomes concerns the *availability* of the promoter for binding of the preinitiation complex; the role of nuclear receptors/enhancer binding proteins would be to allow the initiation of transcription by nucleosome displacement. In the case of steroid-regulated genes, DNAse 1 hypersensitive sites located over HRE's become detectable after hormone treatment and disappear again after hormone withdrawal, suggesting that the receptor modifies the structure and displaces nucleosomes from the DNA sequences implicated in transcription regulation. The importance of nucleosome displacement is indicated by the fact that the transcription factor NFI (a candidate for the role of a TIF in the MMTV-LTR glucocorticoid-dependent transcription) binds to the MMTV GRE sequences only in cells treated with a glucocorticosteroid agonist; NFI cannot bind to DNA before removal of the nucleosome[150] (Fig. 6–13).

Regulation of the Function of Nuclear Receptors

Ligand-Receptor Interaction and Ligand Binding Domain

It should be remembered that the nuclear receptor superfamily members are defined only by sequence homologies; therefore, regulation of their function may not always involve the binding of a small regulatory molecule. For recognized functional receptors, mutational analysis has shown that ligand binding and specificity are determined by sequences in the LBD. For example, single amino acid mutations cause resistance to glucocorticosteroids,[151] androgens,[152, 153] vitamin D,[154] and thyroxine[155, 156] in humans. Apart from a mutation Asp 641 → Val, identified by sequence analysis of the glucocorticosteroid-resistant receptor, a conserved cysteine has been detected by chemical modification with a covalently attached dexamethasone mesylate at position 638. The two incriminated amino acid residues lie within a relatively hydrophobic region, as expected for the steroid-binding pocket. Other structural features may have their importance in the binding of the regulatory ligand. For instance, deletion of the last 12 C-terminal amino acids abolished hormone binding by the human androgen receptor.[157] This sort of modification of the receptor molecule may affect binding either by deleting a peptide sequence interacting with the ligand or by canceling the functional spatial configuration of the receptor. In the human PR, the presence of amino acids interacting with progesterone in the extreme C-terminal portion of the LRD is indicated by the loss of binding upon deletion of this region (42 amino acids). Surprisingly, such truncated receptor retained its affinity for the antagonist ligand RU486, and the truncated receptor–RU486 complex efficiently activated PRE/GRE–driven transcription, in contrast with the wild-type receptor.[158] These observations agree with a model in which the C-terminal portion of the LBD region prevents the transcriptional activation function; agonist binding and receptor transformation liberate the TAF domains of the integral receptor molecule, whereas the antagonist does not fully relieve the inhibitory effect of the C-terminal LBD domain of the integral receptor molecule.

A single amino acid change can alter the specificity of a receptor for a given ligand; an example of such a change is the mutation Cys 575 → Gly, which confers on the chicken PR the capacity to bind the antagonistic ligand RU486 (the wild-type chicken PR does not bind RU486). In the human PR, the mutation in the opposite direction (Gly → Cys) abrogates binding of RU486 but not that of an agonist. The corresponding mutation in the human GR results in a loss of binding of both dexamethasone and RU486.[159]

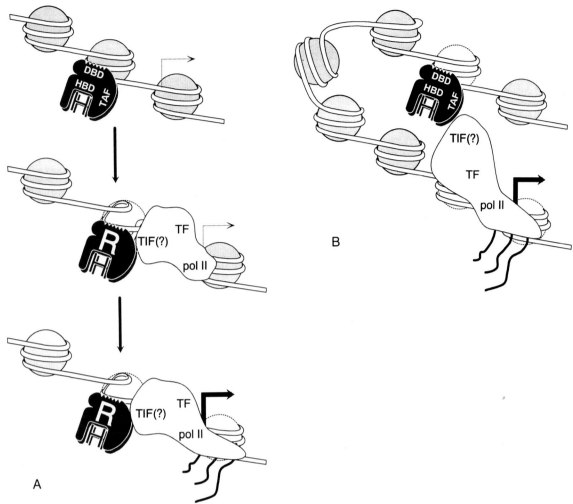

FIGURE 6–13. **DNA-binding receptor, chromatin structure, and transcription.** *A,* The receptor binds the hormone H at the hormone-binding domain (HBD) level, interacts with DNA by the DNA-binding domain (DBD), and has several transcription activation functions (TAF's), which may interact with transcription factors. The HRE (hormone response element) is situated on a nucleosome; after binding of receptor to DNA, the nucleosome is modified or displaced. The binding of the receptor to HRE thus allows the preinitiation complex to be placed at the transcription initiation site. In *B,* HRE is located far away from the initiation site of transcription, and intermediary protein factors (TIF's) are probably involved.

Molecular Mechanism of Action of Hormone Antagonists

Lipophilic molecules specifically recognized by nuclear receptors regulate their transcriptional activity. Certain categories of such molecules bind to the same receptor but differ in their agonistic potency (for instance, estrone and estriol are less efficient than estradiol). The existence of weak agonists has led to the idea of competitive inhibition of hormone action. Subsequently, synthetic compounds were developed that act as potent agonists or as antagonists that are partially or totally devoid of agonist activity. These compounds bear a structural resemblance to the natural agonist but carry also modifications that have to be compatible with binding to the receptor but preclude one or more of the essential functional properties of the complex. The complex formed between the antagonist and the receptor is thus "nonproductive," i.e., it fails to activate transcription of certain or all genes normally regulated by the receptor. The best known examples of such pure antagonists are described.

ANTIESTROGENS. Tamoxifen and its derivatives are pure antiestrogens in the chicken and partial agonists (which are able to induce the expression of certain genes) in mammalian cells but lack growth-promoting activity in human breast cells.[17, 160–162] Tamoxifen is an efficient hormonal anticancer agent in the hormone-dependent subset of breast cancer patients. ICI164, 384, a recently developed antagonist, is apparently totally devoid of estrogenic activity in all species tested.[163, 164]

ANTIGLUCOCORTICOSTEROIDS AND ANTIPROGESTATIVES. RU486 forms nonproductive complexes with both GR and PR of mammalian (but not chicken; see above) cells. Its medical use as an alternative contraceptive drug is accepted in several countries. Dexamethasone mesylate has been also shown to behave as a pure antagonist toward the GR.[44]

ANTIANDROGENS. Flutamide, a pure synthetic androgen

antagonist, is currently used in the management of metastatic prostate cancer.[165] Nilutamide[166] has similar properties and applications.

The possibilities of hormonal manipulations of diverse pathologies are not yet exhausted. For instance, a compound that selectively counteracts the effects of retinoic acid mediated by the RARα has been recently described.[167] Moreover, there are multiple molecular mechanisms that are potential targets for modulation by hormone antagonists (Table 6–3).

The underlying molecular causes of the nonproductive character of antagonist-receptor complexes may be related to one or more of the processes that lead to the formation of the activated receptor and/or the interaction of the receptor with DNA, with TIF's, or with the preinitiation complex. Transformation of the ER (see earlier) as well as tight binding to the nucleus appears to take place normally with pure antagonists such as tamoxifen (or 4-OH tamoxifen, a highly potent antiestrogen) in the chicken oviduct.[168] Similarly, transformed receptor-dexamethasone mesylate complexes become tightly associated with cell nucleus in vivo but do not activate GRE-dependent transcription.[169] In contrast, in mouse lymphoid cells, the glucocorticoid-receptor complex with RU486 does not become tightly associated with the nuclear fraction.[170, 171] GR complexed with RU486 displays sequence-specific binding to GRE sequences but fails to induce transcription.[172] According to another study,[173] human PR-RU486 complex does activate transcription in a cell-free system, although to a lesser extent than does the PR-agonist complex. This would strengthen the importance of the interference of RU486 with the receptor transformation process in vivo. The biological activities of certain steroid antagonists sometimes present a paradox (for instance, tamoxifen), which is easier to understand given the complexity of transcriptional regulation by nuclear receptors and the involvement of diverse cellular proteins needed for the formation of receptor-preinitiation complexes. It is probable that different cellular TIF's are needed for the induction of transcription of different genes.

The efficiency in vivo of low concentrations of hormone antagonists may be boosted by formation of (unproductive) heterodimers, in which one of the receptor monomers is occupied by the (endogenous) agonist, whereas the other binds the antagonist. The existence of such hetero-

TABLE 6–3. ANTIHORMONE ACTION: POTENTIAL CELLULAR AND MOLECULAR TARGET (CELLULAR AND MOLECULAR TARGETS OF ANTIHORMONE ACTION)

Entry into the target cell
Intracellular transport
Metabolic activation
Receptor binding
  • Competition by antagonists
  • Down-regulation of the receptor
Receptor transformation/activation
  • Stabilization of the nontransformed receptor
  • Interference with dimerization
  • Interference with transcription activating function(s).

Not all hormones and receptors follow the same sequence of events to produce a response. In particular, there are differences at the level of intracellular transport and metabolic activation.

dimers has been demonstrated for the PR: they can form in solution and also on imperfectly palindromic HRE's, and therefore on most natural HRE's.[174, 175]

Nuclear Localization, Hsp90 Binding, and Association with Cellular Proteins

Contrary to models based on early studies, the biologically inactive, ligand-free steroid hormone receptors (nontransformed form) are largely localized in the cell nucleus although not tightly bound to DNA. The transport of the neosynthesized receptor molecule to the nucleus relies on short amino acid sequences rich in Lys/Arg residues.[176, 177] Several such sequences are present in steroid receptors; their cooperation is necessary to ensure nuclear localization of each receptor.[178] For instance, in the human ER, three constitutive and one estrogen-inducible nuclear localization sequence (NLS) have been identified. The region of ER containing NLS is involved in the interaction with hsp 90.[179] Therefore, the transport of ER into the nucleus may precede the assembly of hetero-oligomers containing ER and hsp90. The spatial configuration of the receptor molecule can be decisive for its subcellular localization. Thus, a strong constitutive NLS of GR is masked by the LBD in a ligand-free receptor; this may be the cause of the observed predominantly cytoplasmic localization of this steroid receptor.

The question of the precise "address" of the receptor in the nucleus has not been definitively answered. In fact, there are two questions, one concerning the nontransformed receptor molecules and the other concerning the "excess" pool of transformed receptor-hormone complexes. (There are 10^3-10^4 receptor molecules per cell, whereas the number of the HRE sequences is unlikely to exceed the order of 10^2.) The transformed chick oviduct PR molecules have been shown to interact with a specific nonhistone protein considered to be the "acceptor,"[180] which may serve to bind the PR molecules that have not found a place on a promoter. Interaction with the "acceptor" may also channel the receptor molecule for destruction (see earlier).

Nontransformed steroid hormone receptors do not bind in vivo to their cognate HRE's, possibly because of their association with hsp90. There are only indirect but strong arguments to support this statement: (1) the weak association of ligand-free receptors with the nucleus, (2) absence of transcription-stimulating activity; and (3) absence of transcription inhibitory activity in those situations in which it is observed after the addition of the hormone such as dexamethasone (see earlier). The hsp90 interaction domain, situated in the C-terminal region, coincides with the TAF2 domain (and with LBD).[179, 181, 182] However, the tridimensional structure of the receptor-hsp90 complex may interfere with the receptor-HRE binding. Indeed, the presence of the ligand is not necessary for the receptor molecule, separated from hsp90, to bind specifically to the HRE sequences.[183–187] In contrast with steroid hormone receptors, TR does not complex with hsp90 and binds to TRE in vivo in the absence of ligand. This fact supports the hypothesis that hsp90 negatively regulates receptor-DNA interactions. Direct evidence for a role of hsp90 in the modulation of the interaction of ER with its cognate DNA as revealed by EMSA has recently been obtained.[188a] Other possible functions of the receptor-hsp90 association are correct folding, protection against degradation, and transport (for discussion, see ref. 188).

The hsp90 protein is abundant in nearly all cells of higher organisms and clearly has other cellular functions apart from its interaction with steroid hormone receptors. One of the first characteristics observed with this protein was its binding to the c-src oncoprotein.[189] In addition, several other proteins were detected in immune precipitates of hsp90, including some also associated with steroid hormone receptors (proteins of Mr 56-59 kDa)[50, 51] (Fig. 6–14), and hsp70, which associates also with the transformed receptor.[190] The importance of these proteins for the receptor function is unknown.

Post-transcriptional Modifications

The only confirmed post-transcriptional modifications of nuclear receptors are of the most common kind, namely phosphorylations; their significance remains largely unknown and may differ according to the receptor. With the exception of ER, which is phosphorylated on tyrosine, in other steroid hormone receptors serine residues are phosphorylated in intact cells.[191] As an example, it has been shown[192] that GR has to be phosphorylated in order to be able to bind the steroid ligand. (Because dephosphorylated receptor is "inactive," the acquisition of binding capacity has been termed *activation*.) Dephosphorylation has been shown to cause loss of hormone-binding capacity also for ER and PR.[193] For PR, phosphorylation has been correlated with nuclear localization, but, surprisingly, while it is the cytosoluble (i.e., weakly bound to the nucleus) chick PR that is phosphorylated,[194] the opposite is true for rabbit PR.[195] Moreover, the phosphorylation of the rabbit PR is hormone-dependent, suggesting functional significance. Conversely, the loss of tight nuclear binding of the ER by dephosphorylation has also been observed.[196] For the GR, a role of phosphorylation in nuclear binding has also been documented.[197]

Indirect evidence exists that receptor phosphorylation is implicated in the regulation of the transcription activating function. This follows from experiments showing that the progesterone and estrogen receptor-dependent, HRE-directed transcription of an indicator gene (in transient transfection assay) can be induced by dopamine, a neurotransmitter that acts via a cell membrane receptor.[198] A serine residue in the PR (Ser 628 of the chicken PR) has been identified that is necessary for the dopamine activation of the receptor-dependent transcription (but not for its activation by progesterone). The transcriptional activities of PR and ER were also inducible by okadaic acid (a protein phosphatase inhibitor), suggesting the role of receptor phosphorylation in the transcription activating function of these receptors; however, the Ser 628 residue of the chicken PR was not necessary for the effect of okadaic acid. (Remarkably, GR was not activated either by dopamine or by okadaic acid.)

It seems safe to conclude that phosphorylation is involved in the function of steroid hormone receptors. The same may be true for other nuclear receptors; for instance, the stimulation of transcription of several genes by triiodo-

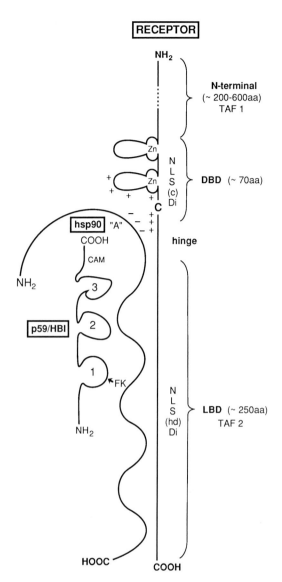

FIGURE 6–14. **Steroid hormone receptors and associated proteins (hsp90 and p59/HBI).** The organization of the steroid *receptor* domains is represented, with the fifth cysteine after the second finger and the conserved positively charged amino acids at the N-terminal end of the DBD. Hsp90 interacts in a multipoint arrangement with LBD, and the negatively charged A region of the heat shock protein can interact with the positively charged receptor segment and obliterate the DBD function. p59/HBI (hsp-binding immunophilin) is made of three FKBP12-like domains. The NH2-terminal FKB-like domain can bind immunosuppressant drugs FK 506 and rapamycin. The interaction with hsp90 takes place at the second FKBP-like domain. There is at least one calmodulin (CAM) binding domain. TAF, transcriptional activation function; NLS, nuclear localization signal; C, constitutive; hd, hormone-dependent; Di, dimerization interface; FK, FK506.

thyronine was selectively blocked by inhibitors of protein kinases.[199] The enzymes that modulate the phosphorylation state of nuclear receptors have not been identified. Copurification of protein kinases with PR[200, 201] suggests that specific enzymes may preferentially associate with steroid hormone receptors.

The receptor-associated hsp90 is also a phosphoprotein, phosphorylated on serine residues[202] and displaying ATPase activity.[202a] Neither the receptors nor hsp90 possesses intrinsic kinase activities.

NUCLEAR RECEPTORS AND CELLULAR AND PHYSIOLOGICAL REGULATIONS

The vast range of biological functions of nuclear receptors is not discussed here. Instead, we have tried to summarize the subject briefly.

Tissue Differentiation; Hormone-Dependent Cancers

In the lower species, two well-studied examples of differentiation dependent on nuclear receptors are seen in insects (molting hormone: ecdysone). In mammals, one function of glucocorticosteroids is in the maturation of the fetal lung. Of course, sex steroids control sex determination during fetal age. In addition, retinoids are known for their role in morphogenesis and in differentiation of several tissues, including skin and cartilage, as well as the hematopoietic and nervous systems.[203, 204] At puberty, sex steroid secretion ensures further development and differentiation of target tissues equipped with the appropriate receptors and other accessory proteins, at least some of which, as we have seen, display various degrees of cell specificity. Exactly how the differentiated functions become established and perpetuated is a subject for further study. Among other methods, molecular studies of development defects may help to make further advances.

A particular aspect of hormone regulation of differentiated cells is the growth control by sex steroids in normal and malignant target tissues. Certain reproductive organs (uterus, oviduct, prostate) as well as other tissues (muscles) are markedly induced to grow by secretion or administration of estrogens or of androgens. It has been shown[205] that the "immediate early" cell cycle–related gene c-*fos* is estrogen-inducible in the human breast cancer–derived cell line MCF7, via an ERE element in its promoter. However, in these cells estradiol also induces the expression of genes coding for growth factors,[206] and it is not clear to what extent autocrine and paracrine mechanisms are responsible for the induction of cell proliferation by sex steroids.

In breast and prostate cancer patients, elimination of the agonistic steroid (or the use of an antihormone) often offers an efficient therapeutic possibility; however, the remissions are usually transient, as the tumors evolve to a hormone-independent stage. In an estrogen-dependent experimental model (GR mouse mammary carcinoma), the acquisition of estrogen independence is accompanied by the partial or complete replacement of the normal ER (65 kDa) by truncated (50- and 35-kDa) forms,[207] supporting the possibility that mutations in the ER gene underlie the loss of hormone requirement. This possibility would imply constitutively active ER mutants, acting via the TAF1 domain[141]; the existence of such mutants has been documented.[142] Progression to a hormone-independent state can probably also result from alterations of the expression of proto-oncogenes and antioncogenes,[208] without mutations in the receptor gene, circumventing the need for estrogen-induced cell growth.

Given the growth-promoting activity of estrogen in normal and malignant target cells, it was surprising to find that the introduction of the ER into cells derived from breast cancer cells that lost their hormone dependence, or into nonestrogen-target cells, can produce cell lines in which estrogens act as growth inhibitors.[209, 209a] Squelching of transcription-mediating factors required for the expression of cell cycle–related genes may account for this observation.

Regulation of the Cell Content and Function of Receptors

There are essentially three modes of regulation of the cell content of a given receptor: (1) tissue differentiation (establishment of a basal rate of transcription of the receptor gene and of genes coding for proteins modulating its expression and function); (2) homologous regulation by the ligand; and (3) heterologous regulation by other cell-signaling processes.

Practically nothing is known about the mechanism by which the target cell for a given lipophilic regulatory molecule acquires the capacity to express the appropriate receptor. The presence of receptors of hormones such as estrogens in fetal tissues (e.g., uterus) at fetal age has been well documented, but the initial stimulus that triggers the expression of the receptor gene remains to be identified.

The function of nuclear receptors is by definition regulated by the *homologous ligand;* however (as discussed earlier in this chapter), the existence of "true" orphan receptors, for which there is no regulatory ligand, cannot be excluded. Both positive and negative modes of regulation of the *cellular content* of a receptor by its own ligand have been described. In general, the estrogen receptor gene expression is induced by estrogens. At the same time, a transient down-regulation of the functional estrogen receptor is observed in certain tissues (uterus)[210, 211] but not in others (chick oviduct).[160] Other examples of such homologous down-regulation are the progesterone receptor of the mammalian uterus[212] as well as chick oviduct,[213] and the GR (ubiquitous).[214] At least in part, the down-regulation of the GR appears to result from transcriptional repression due to an nGRE element in the promoter.[215] However, this mechanism probably does not account for the rapid down-regulation observed. Accelerated turnover of the receptor protein following hormone binding, transformation, and interaction with DNA may be involved. Similarly, the down-regulation of the PR gene expression by progestins includes (but probably is not entirely explained by) inhibition of transcription of the PR gene.[161] In the case of the ER, contradictory results have been reported concerning the effect of ligands on its turnover: the agonist ligand (estradiol) appears to lengthen the half-time of ER, whereas the "pure" steroidal antiestrogen ICI 164384 accelerates the ER turnover. However, the nonsteroidal antiestrogens tamoxifen and nafoxidine had little or no effect on the cellular turnover of the estrogen receptor.[216] (All these studies have been carried out with cell cultures, and the conclusions cannot necessarily be extrapolated to normal tissues.) The loss of function of the receptor may precede the actual destruction of the protein, and such desensitized receptors still may be reutilizable or at least able to bind the hormone.[217] Receptor recycling has been shown, in the case of GR, to depend on the phosphorylation of specific aminoacid residues: inhibition of serine/threonine phosphatases by okadaic acid blocked the recycling of GR along with a site-specific hyperphosphorylation.[197]

Heterologous regulation by extracellular signals is also common. The induction of the PR by estrogens is virtually universal in the appropriate target tissues and results from accumulation of PR mRNA.[218] Conversely, the ER can be induced by progesterone, both in the endometrium of the rodent uterus and in the chick oviduct.[219, 220] At the same time, antiestrogenic activity of progesterone is also common and is manifested both in inhibition of the estrogen-induced accumulation of the ER and of estrogen-induced growth and specific protein synthesis in the target tissue.[220–222]

Cell signaling transmitted by membrane receptors is another mode of regulation of the expression of genes coding for nuclear receptors. Although it seems reasonable to expect that such regulations are numerous and complex, at present only sporadic information is available on this subject. One example is the down-regulation of the transcriptional activation by GR in cells expressing the oncogenes *ras* or *mos*. The effect of *mos* correlates with the inhibition of nuclear retention of the receptor and with its reutilization. The effect of *ras* on GR turnover/activity may well result from the *ras* activation of the cellular *mos* (or related) protein. Although the *mos* protein is a serine/threonine kinase, the idea that it may prevent recycling by maintaining the receptor in a phosphorylated state could not be confirmed.[217] Instead, *mos* appears to act via induction of c-*fos* gene expression; this rather unexpected observation is well supported by experimental data[223, 224] and accounts also for the observation that exposure of cells to phorbol esters (which activate protein kinase C and induce the expression of TRE-driven genes including c-*fos*) also down-regulates GR.[225] The GR down-regulation by *fos* may be a consequence of the protein-protein interaction, which would target GR for inactivation.[223, 224] Down-regulation by phorbol esters is not restricted to GR. In cultured human breast cancer cells, the content of estrogen receptor mRNA was extensively decreased by exposure to TPA.[226]

Another aspect of heterologous regulation of the function of nuclear receptors concerns their interaction with components of the "nontransformed" oligomer, namely, proteins hsp90 and p59 (and possibly others). The hsp90-receptor interaction may be implicated in the negative regulation of transcriptional activation in the absence of the agonist ligand but also possibly in protection against degradation and in "addressing" of the neosynthesized receptor molecules.[52] For the p59, it is interesting that this protein has been shown to specifically bind immunosuppressors FK 506 and rapamycin.[227] Cloning of the p59 cDNA has led to its identification as an immunophilin, highly homologous to the FK 206-binding protein FKBP 12.[228] The role of p59 in the regulation of the function of steroid receptors is suggested by the fact that, in the presence of immunosuppressants (FK 206, rapamycin), ligand binding by the nontransformed receptor preparations is increased by approximately 25 per cent.[229] With transformed receptor preparations (receptor separated from the non–hormone-binding proteins), no effect of immunosuppressants is seen. However, a definitive explanation of the physiological role of p59 in the regulation of nuclear receptor function is not yet available.

Regulation of the Activity of Nuclear Receptors: Implications for Disease and Therapy

In order to precisely adjust the expression of nuclear receptor-regulated genes to the requirements of the moment, the cell uses a number of "fine-tuning" mechanisms.

SIGNALING MOLECULE. This mode of modulation is the chemical form (estradiol vs estrone; cortisol vs corticosterone, and so on); mode of secretion (endocrine/paracrine/autocrine mechanisms); delivery (humoral transport mechanisms; plasma binding proteins; entry into the target cell; intracellular metabolic activation/inactivation).

RECEPTOR. This involves transcription of the receptor gene, generation of mRNA isoforms by alternative splicing, synthesis of the receptor protein and its post-translational activation and inactivation, and subcellular compartmentalization and formation of complexes with cellular proteins (hsp90; immunophilin p59; hsp70).

REGULATION OF TRANSCRIPTION. This is characterized by accessibility of the receptor-regulated promoter (chromatin structure related to the differentiation state); sequences, number, and positions of the HRE elements; accessory proteins, intermediary factors; and interaction with other enhancer-binding proteins.

POST-TRANSCRIPTIONAL PROCESSES. This controls translation and post-translational modifications required for the formation of active gene products coded by the receptor-regulated gene, and feedback loops including receptor down-regulation.

The complexity of these regulatory mechanisms has at least two important implications: first, inevitably the machine will display failures that will produce diverse pathology; and second, the study of the nuclear receptor–regulated processes has to be reductionist, with all the risks for the interpretation of the experimental data.

ACKNOWLEDGMENTS: We would like to acknowledge the editorial work of Philippe Leclerc and the contribution to the manuscript of Françoise Boussac, Jean-Claude Lambert, Corinne Legris, and Luc Outin.

REFERENCES

1. Baulieu EE: Neurosteroids: a function of the brain. *In* Costa E, Paul SM (eds): Neurosteroids and Brain Function. New York, Thieme, 1991, pp 63–73.
2. Beato M: Gene regulation by steroid hormones. Cell 56:335–344, 1989.
3. Gronemeyer H: Transcription activation by estrogen and progesterone receptors. Ann Rev Genet 25:89–123, 1991.
4. Fuller PJ: The steroid receptor superfamily: Mechanisms of diversity. FASEB J 5:3092–3099, 1991.
5. Parker MG (ed): Nuclear Hormone Receptors—Molecular Mechanisms, Cellular Functions, Clinical Abnormalities. London, Academic Press, 1991.
6. O'Malley BW, Tsai SY, Bagchi M, et al: Molecular mechanism of action of a steroid hormone receptor. Recent Prog Horm Res 47:1–24, 1991.
7. Funder JW: Steroids, receptors, and response elements: The limits of signal specificity. Recent Prog Horm Res 47:191–207, 1991.
8. Cato ACB, Ponta H, Herrlich P: Regulation of gene expression by steroid hormones. Progr Nucl Acid Res Molec Biol 43:1–36, 1992.

9. Wahli W, Martinez E: Superfamily of steroid nuclear receptors—positive and negative regulators of gene expression. FASEB J 5:2243–2251, 1991.

10. Jensen EV, Jacobson HI: Basic guide to mechanism of estrogen action. Recent Prog Horm Res 18:387–414, 1962.

11. Talwar P, Segal SJ, Evan A, Davidson DW: The binding of estradiol in the uterus: a mechanism for depression of RNA synthesis. Proc Natl Acad Sci USA 52:1059–1066, 1964.

12. Toft D, Gorski J: A receptor molecule for estrogen: Isolation from the rat uterus and preliminary characterization. Proc Natl Acad Sci USA 55:1574–1581, 1966.

13. Baulieu EE, Alberga A, Jung I: Récepteurs hormonaux: Liaison spécifique de l'oestradiol à des protéines utérines. CR Acad Sci Paris 265:354–357, 1967.

14. Raspé G (ed): Schering workshop on steroid hormone receptors. Advances in the Biosciences, Vol III. New York, Pergamon Press, 1970.

15. Korenman SG: Comparative binding affinity of estrogens and its relation to estrogenic potency. Steroids 13:163–177, 1968.

16. Raynaud JP, Ojasoo T: The relevance of structure-affinity relationships in the study of steroid. In Eriksson H, Gustafsson JA (eds): Steroid Hormone Receptors: Structure and Function. Amsterdam, Elsevier, 1983, pp 141–170.

17. Sutherland RL, Jordan VC (eds): Non-steroidal antiestrogens. New York, Academic Press, 1981.

18. Baulieu EE, Atger M, Best-Belpomme M, et al: Steroid hormone receptors. Vitam Horm 33:649–731, 1975.

19. Jensen EW, DeSombre ER: Estrogens and progestins. In Litwack G (ed): Biochemical Actions of Hormones, Vol II. New York, Academic Press, 1972.

20. Schrader WT, Birnbaumer ME, Hughes MR, et al: Studies on the structure and function of chicken progesterone receptor. Recent Prog Horm Res 37:583–633, 1981.

21. Mangelsdorf DJ, Borgmeyer U, Heyman RA, et al: Characterization of three RXR genes that mediate the action of 9-cis retinoic acid. Genes Dev 6:329–344, 1992.

22. Mendelsohn C, Ruberte E, Chambon P: Retinoid receptors in vertebrate limb development. Dev Biol 152:50–61, 1992.

23. Yang CR, Mester J, Wolfson A, et al: Activation of the chick oviduct progesterone receptor by heparin in the presence or absence of hormone. Biochem J 208:399–406, 1982.

24. Moudgil VK, Eessalu TE, Buchou T, et al: Transformation of chick oviduct progesterone receptor in vitro: Effect of hormone, salt, heat, and adenosine triphosphate. Endocrinology 116:1267–1274, 1985.

25. Milgrom E, Atger M, Baulieu EE: Acidophilic activation of steroid hormone receptors. Biochemistry 12:5198–5205, 1973.

26. Leach KL, Dahmer MD, Hammond ND, et al: Molybdate inhibition of glucocorticoid receptor in activation and transformation. J Biol Chem 254:11884–11890, 1979.

27. Nishigori H, Toft D: Inhibition of progesterone receptor activation by sodium molybdate. Biochemistry 19:77–83, 1980.

28. Dahmer MK, Housley PR, Pratt WB: Effects of molybdate and endogenous inhibitors on steroid-receptor inactivation, transformation and translocation. Ann Rev Physiol 46:67–81, 1984.

29. Joab I, Radanyi C, Renoir JM et al: Immunological evidence for a common non-hormone binding component in non-transformed chick oviduct receptors of four steroid hormones. Nature 308:850–853, 1984.

30. Catelli MG, Binart N, Jung-Testas I, et al: The common 90-kd protein component of non-transformed "8S" steroid receptors is a heat-shock protein. EMBO J 4:3131–3135, 1985.

31. Schuh S, Yonemoto W, Brugge J, et al: A 90,000-dalton binding protein common to both steroid receptors and the Rous sarcoma virus transforming protein, pp60v-src. J Biol Chem 260:14292–14296, 1985.

32. Allan GF, Leng X, Tsai SY, et al: Hormone and antihormone induce distinct conformational changes which are central to steroid receptor activation. J Biol Chem 267:19513–19520, 1992.

33. Sherman MR, Tuazon FB, Diaz SC, Miller LK: Multiple forms of oviduct progesterone receptors analyzed by ion exchange filtration and gel electrophoresis. Biochemistry 15:980–988, 1976.

34. Sherman MR, Pickering LA, Rollwagen FM, Miller LK: Mero-receptors: Proteolytic fragments of receptors containing the steroid-binding site. Fed Proc 37:167–173, 1978.

35. Rochefort H, Baulieu EE: Effect of KCl, CaCl2, temperature and oestradiol on the uterine cytosol receptor of oestradiol. Biochimie 53:893–907, 1971.

36. Renoir JM, Mester J, Buchou T, et al: Purification by affinity chromatography and immunological characterization of a 110 kDa component of the chick oviduct progesterone receptor. Biochem J 217:685–692, 1984.

37. Renoir JM, Buchou T, Mester J, et al: Oligomeric structure of the molybdate-stabilized, non-transformed "8S" progesterone receptor from chicken oviduct cytosol. Biochemistry 23:6016–6023, 1984.

38. Redeuilh G, Moncharmont B, Secco C, Baulieu EE: Subunit composition of the molybdate-stabilized "8-9S" non-transformed estradiol receptor purified from calf uterus. J Biol Chem 262:6869–6875, 1987.

39. Hubert P, Mester J, Dellacherie E, et al: Soluble biospecific macromolecule for purification of estrogen receptor. Proc Natl Acad Sci USA 75:3143–3147, 1978.

40. Redeuilh G, Secco C, Baulieu EE: The use of the biotinyl estradiol-avidin system for the purification of "non-transformed" estrogen receptor by biohormonal affinity chromatography. J Biol Chem 260:3996–4002, 1985.

41. Gustafsson JA, Okret S, Wiström AC, et al: On the use of poly- and monoclonal antibodies in studies on the structure and function of the glucocorticosteroid receptor. In Eriksson H, Gustafsson JA (eds): Steroid Hormone Receptors: Structure and Function. Amsterdam, Elsevier, 1983, pp 355–389.

42. Dure LS, Schrader WT, O'Malley BW: Covalent attachment of a progestational steroid to chick oviduct progesterone receptor by photoaffinity labelling. Nature 283:784–786, 1980.

43. Katzenellenbogen JA, Carlson KE, Heiman DF, et al: Efficient and highly selective covalent labeling of the estrogen receptor with [³H]tamoxifen aziridine. J Biol Chem 258:3487–3495, 1983.

44. Simmons SS, Thompson EB: Dexamethasone 21-mesylate: An affinity label of glucocorticoid receptors from rat hepatoma tissue culture cells. Proc Natl Acad Sci USA 78:3541–3545, 1981.

45. Mester J, Renoir JM, Buchou T, et al: Structure of the chick oviduct progesterone receptor. In Sluyser M (ed): Interaction of Steroid Hormone Receptors with DNA. Chichester, Ellis Horwood, 1985, pp 126–154.

46. Okret S, Carlstedt-Duke J, Wikström AC, et al: Glucocorticoid receptor structure and function. In Sluyser M (ed): Interaction of Steroid Hormone Receptors with DNA. Chichester, Ellis Horwood, 1985, pp 155–189.

47. Denis M, Poelling L, Wikstöm AC, Gustafsson JA: Requirement of hormone for thermal conversion of the glucocorticoid receptor to a DNA-binding state. Nature 333:686–688, 1988.

48. Rafestin-Oblin ME, Couette B, Radanyi C, et al: Mineralocorticosteroid receptor of the chick intestine: Oligomeric structure and transformation. J Biol Chem 264:9304–9309, 1989.

49. Notides AC, Nielsen S: The molecular mechanism of the in vitro 4S to 5S transformation of the uterine estrogen receptor. J Biol Chem 249:1866–1873, 1974.

50. Tai PKK, Maeda Y, Nakao K, et al: A 59-kilodalton protein associated with progestin, estrogen, androgen and glucocorticoid receptors. Biochemistry 25:5269–5275, 1986.

51. Lebeau MC, Binart N, Cadepond F, et al: Steroid receptor associated proteins: heat shock protein 90 and p59 immunophilin. In Mougdil VK (ed): Meadowbrook Conference, October 1992, Boston, Springer-Verlag, in press.

52. Renoir JM, Radanyi C, Faber LE, Baulieu EE: The non–DNA-binding heterooligomeric form of mammalian steroid hormone receptors contains a hsp90-bound 59-kilodalton protein. J Biol Chem 265:10740–10745, 1990.

53. Mester J, Baulieu EE: Nuclear estrogen receptor of chick liver. Biochim Biophys Acta 261:236–244, 1972.

54. Ozon R, Belle R: Récepteurs de l'oestradiol-17β dans le foie de poule et de l'amphibien Discoglossus pictus. Biochim Biophys Acta 297:155–163, 1973.

55. Jensen EV, Suzuki T, Kawashima T, et al: A two step mechanism for the interaction of estradiol with rat uterus. Proc Natl Acad Sci USA 59:632–638, 1968.

56. Welshons WV, Lieberman ME, Gorski J: Nuclear localization of unoccupied estrogen receptors. Nature 307:747–749, 1984.

57. King WJ, Greene GL: Monoclonal antibodies localise oestrogen receptor in the nuclei of target cells. Nature 307:745–747, 1984.

58. Govindan MV: Immunofluorescence microscopy of the intracellular translocation of glucocorticoid-receptor complexes in rat hepatoma (HTC) cells. Exp Cell Res 127:293–297, 1980.

59. Papmichail M, Tsokos N, Tsawdaroglou N, Sekeris CE: Immunocytochemical demonstration of glucocorticoid receptor in different cell

types and their translocation from the cytoplasma to the cell nucleus in the presence of dexamethasone. Exp Cell Res 125:490–493, 1980.

60. Gasc JM, Delahaye F, Baulieu EE: Compared intracellular localization of the glucocorticoid and progesterone receptors: An immunocytochemical study. Exp Cell Res 181:492–504, 1989.

61. Brink M, Humbel BM, De Kloet ER, Van Driel R: The unliganded glucocorticoid receptor is localized in the nucleus, not in the cytoplasm. Endocrinology 130:3575–3581, 1992.

62. Perrot-Applanat M, Logeat F, Groyer-Picard MT, et al: Immunocytochemical study of mammalian progesterone receptor using monoclonal antibodies. Endocrinology 116:1473–1483, 1985.

62a. Tuohimaa P, Pekki A, Blaüer M, et al: Nuclear progesterone receptor is mainly heat shock protein 90-free in vivo. Proc Natl Acad Sci USA 90:5848–5852, 1993.

63. Rexin M, Busch W, Gehring U: Chemical cross-linking of heteromeric glucocorticoid receptors. Biochemistry 27:5593–5601, 1988.

64. Howard KJ, Distelhorst CW: Evidence for intracellular association of the glucocorticoid receptor with the 90-kDa heat shock protein. J Biol Chem 263:3474–3481, 1988.

65. Baulieu EE: Steroid hormone antagonists at the receptor level. A role for the heat-shock protein MW 90,000 (hsp90). J Cell Biochem 35:161–174, 1987.

66. Pratt WB: Transformation of glucocorticoid and progesterone receptors to the DNA-binding state. J Cell Biochem 35:51–68, 1987.

67. Gasc JM, Renoir JM, Faber LE, et al: Nuclear localization of two steroid-associated proteins, hsp90 and p59. Exp Cell Res 186:362–367, 1990.

68. Berbers GAM, Kunnen R, Van Bergen EN, et al: Localization and quantitation of hsp84 in mammalian cells. Exp Cell Res 177:257–271, 1988.

68a. Kang KI, Devin J, Cadepond F, et al: In vivo functional protein-protein interaction: Nuclear targeted hsp 90 shifts cytoplasmic steroid receptor mutants into the nucleus. Proc Natl Acad Sci USA, in press.

69. Sanchez ER, Hirst M, Scherrer LC, et al: Hormone-free mouse glucocorticoid receptors overexpressed in Chinese hamster ovary cells are localized to the nucleus and are associated with both hsp70 and hsp90. J Biol Chem 265:20123–20130, 1990.

70. Hollenberg SM, Weinberger C, Ong ES, et al: Primary structure and expression of a functional human glucocorticoid receptor cDNA. Nature 318:635–641, 1985.

71. Green S, Walter P, Kumar V, et al: Human oestrogen receptor cDNA: Sequence, expression and homology to v-erb-A. Nature 320:134–139, 1986.

72. Laudet V, Hänni C, Coll J, et al: Evolution of the nuclear receptor gene superfamily. EMBO J 11:1003–1013, 1992.

73. Poland A, Glover E, Ebetino FH, et al: Photoaffinity labelling of the Ah receptor. J Biol Chem 261:6352–6365, 1986.

73a. Ema M, Sogawa K, Watanabe N, et al: cDNA cloning of a putative Ah receptor. Biochem Biophys Res Commun 184:246–253, 1992.

73b. Burbach K, Poland A, Bradfield CA: Cloning of the Ah receptor cDNA reveals a distinctive ligand-activated transcription factor. Proc Natl Acad Sci USA 89:8185–8189, 1992.

74. Weinberger C, Bradley DJ: Gene regulation by receptor binding lipid-soluble substances. Annu Rev Physiol 52:823–840, 1990.

75. Ponglikitmongkol M, Green S, Chambon P: Genomic organization of the human oestrogen receptor gene. EMBO J 7:3385–3388, 1988.

76. Liang T, Liao S: Association of the uterine 17β-estradiol–receptor complex with ribonucleoprotein in vitro and in vivo. J Biol Chem 249:4671–4678, 1974.

77. Palmiter RD, Carey NH: Rapid inactivation of ovalbumin messenger ribonucleic acid after acute withdrawal of gene. Proc Natl Acad Sci USA 71:2357–2361, 1974.

78. Palmiter RD: Rate of ovalbumin messenger ribonucleic acid synthesis in the oviduct of estrogen primed chicks. J Biol Chem 248:8260–8270, 1973.

79. Franceschi RT, Romano PR, Park KY: Regulation of type I collagen synthesis by 1,25-dihydroxyvitamin D$_3$ in human osteosarcoma cells. J Biol Chem 263:18938–18945, 1988.

80. Pierce RA, Kolodziej ME, Park WC: 1.25-Dihydroxy-vitamin D3 represses tropomyosin expression by a posttranscriptional mechanism. J Biol Chem 267:11593–11599, 1992.

81. Turcotte B, Meyer ME, Bellard M, et al: Control of transcription of the chicken progesterone receptor gene. In vitro and in vivo studies. J Biol Chem 266:2582–2589, 1991.

82. Dahlman-Wright K, Siltala-Roos H, Carlstedt-Duke J, Gustafsson JA: Protein-protein interactions facilitate DNA binding by the glucocorticoid receptor DNA-binding domain. J Biol Chem 265:14030–14035, 1990.

83. Schwabe JWR, Neuhaus D, Rhodes D: Solution structure of the DNA-binding domain of the oestrogen receptor. Nature 348:458–461, 1990.

84. Strähle U, Klock G, Schütz G: A DNA sequence of 15 base pairs is sufficient to mediate both glucocorticoid and progesterone induction of gene expression. Proc Natl Acad Sci USA 84:7871–7875, 1987.

85. Tsai SY, Carlstedt-Duke J, Weigel NL, et al: Molecular interactions of steroid hormone receptor with its enhancer element: Evidence for receptor dimer formation. Cell 55:361–369, 1988.

86. Mader S, Leroy P, Chen J-Y, Chambon P: Multiple parameters control the selectivity of nuclear receptors for their response elements. J Biol Chem 268:591–600, 1993.

86a. Scheidereit C, Westphahl HM, Carlson C, et al: Molecular model of the interaction between the glucocorticoid receptor and the regulatory elements of inducible genes. DNA 5:383–391, 1986.

87. Umesono K, Evans RM: Determinants of target gene specificity for steroid/thyroid hormone receptors. Cell 57:1139–1146, 1989.

88. Mangelsdorf DJ, Umesono K, Kliewer SA, et al: A direct repeat in the cellular retinol-binding protein type II gene confers differential regulation by RXR and RAR. Cell 66:555–561, 1991.

89. Diamond MI, Miner JN, Yoshinaga SK, Yamamoto K: Transcription factor interactions: Positive or negative regulation from a single DNA element. Science 249:1266–1272, 1990.

90. Akerblom IE, Slater EP, Beato M, et al: Negative regulation by glucocorticoids through interference with a cAMP responsive enhancer. Science 241:350–353, 1988.

91. Sakai DD, Helm S, Carlstedt-Duke J, et al: Hormone-mediated repression: A negative glucocorticoid response element from the bovine prolactin gene. Genes Dev 2:1144–1154, 1988.

92. Drouin J, Sun YL, Chamberland M, et al: Novel glucocorticoid receptor complex with DNA element of the hormone-repressed POMC gene. EMBO J 12:145–156, 1993.

93. Yang-Yen H-F, Chambard J-C, Sun Y-L, et al: Transcriptional interference between c-jun and the glucocorticoid receptor: mutual inhibition of DNA binding due to direct protein-protein interaction. Cell 62:1205–1215, 1990.

94. Schüle R, Ranggarajan P, Kliewer S, et al: Functional antagonism between oncoprotein c-jun and the glucocorticoid receptor. Cell 62:1217–1226, 1990.

95. König H, Ponta H, Rahmsdorf HJ, et al: Interference between pathway-specific transcription factors: glucocorticoids antagonize phorbol ester-induced AP-1 activity without altering AP-1 site occupation in vivo. EMBO J 11:2241–2246, 1992.

96. Fagot D, Buquet-Fagot C, Mester J: Antimitogenic effects of dexamethasone in chemically transformed mouse fibroblasts. Endocrinology 129:1033–1041, 1991.

97. Koenig RJ, Lazar MA, Hodin RA, et al: Inhibition of thyroid hormone action by a non-hormone binding c-erbA protein generated by alternative mRNA splicing. Nature 337:659–661, 1989.

98. Zhang XK, Wills KN, Husmann M, et al: Novel pathway for thyroid hormone receptor action through interaction with jun and fos oncogene activities. Mol Cell Biol 11:6016–6025, 1991.

99. Damm K, Thompson CC, Evans RM: Protein encoded by v-erbA functions as a thyroid-hormone receptor antagonist. Nature 339:593–597, 1989.

100. Sap J, Munez A, Schmitt J, et al: Repression of transcription mediated at a hormone response element by the v-erbA oncogene product. Nature 340:242–244, 1989.

101. Tomic M, Jiang CK, Epstein HS, et al: Nuclear receptors for retinoic acid and thyroid-hormone regulate transcription of keratin genes. Cell Reg 1:965–973, 1990.

102. Hudson LG, Santon JB, Glass CK, et al: Ligand-activated thyroid hormone and retinoic acid receptors inhibit growth factor receptor promoter expression. Cell 62:1165–1175, 1990.

103. Berg JM: Zinc fingers and other metal-binding domains. J Biol Chem 265:6513–6516, 1990.

104. Archer TK, Hager GL, Omichinski JG: Sequence-specific DNA binding by glucocorticoid receptor "zinc finger peptides." Proc Natl Acad Sci USA 87:7560–7564, 1990.

105. Sabbah M, Redeuilh G, Secco C, et al: DNA and hsp90 binding activity of estrogen receptor is dependent on receptor bound metal. J Biol Chem 262:8631–8635, 1987.

106. Härd T, Kellenbach E, Boelens R, et al: Solution structure of the glucocorticoid receptor DNA-binding domain. Science 249:157–160, 1990.

107. Dahlman-Wright K, Wright A, Gustafsson JA, et al: Interaction of the glucocorticoid receptor DNA-binding domain with DNA as a dimer is mediated by a short segment of five amino acids. J Biol Chem 266:3107–3112, 1991.

108. Kumar V, Green S, Stack G, et al: Functional domains of the human estrogen receptor. Cell 51:941–951, 1987.

109. Meyer ME, Quirin-Stricker C, Lerouge T, et al: A limiting factor mediates the differential activation of promoters by the human progesterone receptor isoforms. J Biol Chem 267:10882–10887, 1992.

110. Kim B, Little JW: Dimerization of a specific DNA-binding protein on the DNA. Science 255:203–209, 1992.

111. Luisi BF, Xu WX, Otwinowski Z, et al: Crystallographic analysis of the interaction of the glucocorticoid receptor with DNA. Nature 352:497–505, 1991.

112. DeMarzo AM, Beck CA, Onate SA, et al: Dimerization of mammalian progesterone receptors occurs in the absence of DNA and is related to the release of the 90-kDa heat shock protein. Proc Natl Acad Sci USA 88:72–76, 1991.

113. Schrader WT, Birnbaumer ME, Hughes MR, et al: Studies on the structure and function of the chicken progesterone receptor. Recent Prog Horm Res 37:583–629, 1981.

114. Guiochon-Mantel A, Loosfelt H, Lescop P, et al: Mechanisms of nuclear localization of the progesterone receptor: Evidence for interaction between monomers. Cell 57:1147–1154, 1989.

115. Lees JA, Fawell SE, White R, et al: A 22-amino acid peptide restores DNA-binding activity to dimerization defective mutants of the estrogen receptor. Mol Cell Biol 10:5529–5531, 1990.

116. Morray MB, Towle HC: Identification of nuclear factors that enhance binding of the thyroid hormone receptor to thyroid hormone response element. Mol Endocrinol 9:1434–1442, 1989.

117. Burnside J, Darling DS, Chin WW: A nuclear factor that enhances binding of thyroid hormone response elements. J Biol Chem 265:2500–2504, 1990.

118. Glass CK, Lipkin SM, Devary OV, et al: Positive and negative regulation of gene transcription by a retinoic acid–thyroid hormone receptor heterodimer. Cell 59:697–708, 1989.

119. Liao J, Ozono K, Sone T, McDonnell DP, Pike JW: Vitamin D receptor interaction with specific DNA requires a nuclear protein and 1,25-dihydroxyvitamin D. Proc Natl Acad Sci USA 87:9751–9755, 1990.

120. Williams GR, Brent GA: Commentary: specificity of nuclear hormone receptor action: who conducts the orchestra? J Endocrinol 135:191–194, 1992.

121. Evans RM: The steroid and thyroid hormone receptor superfamily. Science 240:889–895, 1988.

122. Ankenbauer W, Strähle U, Schütz G: Synergistic action of glucocorticoid and estradiol responsive elements. Proc Natl Acad Sci USA 85:7526–7530, 1988.

123. Cato ACB, Heitlinger E, Ponta H, et al: Estrogen and progesterone receptor-binding sites on the chicken vitellogenin II gene: Synergism of steroid hormone action. Mol Cell Biol 8:5323–5330, 1988.

124. Klein-Hitpass L, Kaling M, Ryffel GU: Synergism of closely adjacent estrogen-responsive elements increases their regulatory potential. J Mol Biol 201:537–544, 1988.

125. Brüggemeyer U, Kalff M, Franke S, et al: Ubiquitous transcription factor OTF-1 mediates induction of the MMTV promoter through synergistic interaction with hormone receptors. Cell 64:565–572, 1991.

126. Nardulli A, Shapiro DJ: Binding of the estrogen receptor DNA-binding domain to the estrogen response element induces DNA bending. Mol Cell Biol 12:2037–2042, 1992.

127. Sabbah M, Le Ricousse S, Redeuilh G, et al: Estrogen receptor–induced bending of the Xenopus vitellogenin A2 gene hormone response element. Biochem Biophys Res Commun 185:944–952, 1992.

128. Schultz SC, Shields GC, Steitz TA: Crystal structure of a CAP-DNA complex: The DNA is bent by 90°. Science 253:1001–1007, 1991.

129. Jantzen HM, Strähle U, Gloss B, et al: Cooperativity of glucocorticoid response elements located far upstream of the tyrosine aminotransferase gene. Cell 49:29–38, 1987.

130. Buetti E, Kühnel B: Distinct sequence elements involved in the glucocorticoid regulation of the mouse mammary tumor virus promoter identified by linker scanning mutagenesis. J Mol Biol 190:379–389, 1986.

131. Miksicek R, Borgmeyer U, Nowock J: Interaction of the TGGCA-binding protein with upstream sequences is required for efficient transcription of mouse mammary tumor virus. EMBO J 6:1355–1360, 1987.

132. Schüle R, Rangarajan P, Na Yang, et al: Retinoic acid is a negative regulator of AP-1 responsive genes. Proc Natl Acad Sci USA 88:6092–6096, 1991.

133. Kumar V, Chambon P: The estrogen receptor binds tightly to its responsive element as a ligand-induced homodimer. Cell 55:145–156, 1988.

134. Bocquel MT, Kumar V, Stricker C, et al: The contribution of the N- and C-terminal regions of steroid receptors to activation of transcription is both receptor and cell-specific. Nucl Acids Res 17:2581–2595, 1989.

135. Hollenberg SM, Evans RM: Multiple and cooperative transactivation domains of the human glucocorticoid receptor. Cell 55:899–906, 1988.

136. Webster NJG, Green S, Tasset D, et al: The transcriptional activation function located in the hormone-binding domain of the human oestrogen receptor is not encoded in a single exon. EMBO J 8:1441–1446, 1989.

137. Danielian PS, White R, Lees JA, et al: Identification of a conserved region required for hormone dependent transcription activation by steroid hormone receptors. EMBO J 11:1025–1033, 1992.

138. Carson MA, Tsai MJ, Conneely OM, et al: Structure-function properties of the chicken progesterone receptor A synthesized from complementary deoxyribonucleic acid. Mol Endocrinol 1:791–801, 1987.

139. Berry M, Metzger D, Chambon P: Role of the two activating domains of the oestrogen receptor in the cell-type and promoter-context dependent agonistic activity of the anti-oestrogen 4-hydroxytamoxifen. EMBO J 9:2811–2818, 1990.

140. Tora L, White J, Brou C, et al: The human estrogen receptor has two independent non acidic transcriptional activation functions. Cell 59:477–487, 1989.

141. Sluyser M: Steroid/thyroid receptor-like proteins with oncogenic potential: A review. Cancer Res 50:451–458, 1990.

142. Fuqua SAW, Fitzgerald SD, Chamness GC, et al: Variant human breast tumor estrogen receptor with constitutive transcriptional activity. Cancer Res 51:105–109, 1991.

143. Tasset D, Tora L, Fromental C, et al: Distinct classes of transcriptional activating domains function by different mechanisms. Cell 62:1177–1187, 1990.

144. Sadowski I, Ma J, Trizenberg S, et al: Gal4-VP16 is an unusually potent transcriptional activator. Nature 335:563–564, 1988.

145. Meyer ME, Gronemeyer H, Turcotte B, et al: Steroid hormone receptors compete for factors that mediate their enhancer function. Cell 57:433–442, 1989.

146. Lucas C, Granner DK: Hormone response domains in gene transcription. Annu Rev Biochem 61:1131–1173, 1992.

147. Garel A, Axel R: Selective digestion of transcriptionally active ovalbumin genes from oviduct nuclei. Proc Natl Acad Sci USA 73:3966–3970, 1976.

148. Richard-Foy H, Hager G: Sequence-specific positioning of nucleosomes over the steroid inducible MMTV promoter. EMBO J 6:2321–2328, 1987.

149. Perlmann T: Glucocorticoid receptor DNA-binding specificity is increased by the organization of DNA in nucleosomes. Proc Natl Acad Sci USA 89:3884–3888, 1992.

150. Adom J, Carr KD, Gouilleux F, et al: Chromatin structure of hormono-dependent promoters. J Steroid Biochem Mol Biol 40:325–332, 1991.

151. Hurley DM, Accili D, Stratakis CA, et al: Point mutation causing a single amino acid substitution in the hormone binding domain of the glucocorticoid receptor in familial glucocorticoid resistance. J Clin Invest 86:680–686, 1991.

152. Tilley WD, Marcelli M, Wilson JD, McPhaul MJ: Characterization and expression of a cDNA encoding the human androgen receptor. Proc Natl Acad Sci USA 86:327–331, 1989.

153. Lubahn DB, Brown TR, Simental JA, et al: Sequence of the intron/exon junctions of the coding region of the human androgen receptor gene and identification of a point mutation in a family with complete androgen insensitivity. Proc Natl Acad Sci USA 86:9534–9538, 1989.

154. Ritchie HH, Hughes MR, Thompson ET, et al: An ochre mutation in the vitamin D$_3$-resistant rickets in three families. Proc Natl Acad Sci USA 86:3783–3787, 1989.

155. Usala SJ, Tennyson GE, Bale AE, et al: A base mutation of the c-erbA β thyroid hormone receptor in a kindred with generalized thyroid hormone resistance. J Clin Invest 85:93–100, 1990.

156. Sakurai A, Takeda K, Ain K, et al: Generalized resistance to thyroid hormone associated with a mutation in the ligand-binding domain of the human thyroid hormone receptor β. Proc Natl Acad Sci USA 86:8977–8991, 1989.

157. Jenster G, Van Der Korput HAGM, Van VroonHoven C, et al: Domains of the human androgen receptor involved in steroid binding, transcriptional activation, and subcellular localization. Mol Endocrinol 5:1396–1404, 1991.

158. Vegeto E, Allan GF, Schrader WT, et al: The mechanism of RU486 antagonism is dependent on the conformation of the carboxy-terminal tail of the human progesterone receptor. Cell 69:703–713, 1992.

159. Benhamou B, Garcia T, Lerouge T, et al: A single amino acid that determines the sensitivity of progesterone receptors to RU486. Science 255:206–209, 1992.

160. Sutherland R, Mester J, Baulieu EE: Tamoxifen is a potent "pure" anti-oestrogen in chick oviduct. Nature 267:434–435, 1977.

161. Alexander IE, Clarke CL, Shine J, Sutherland RL: Progestin inhibition of progesterone receptor gene expression in human breast cancer cells. Mol Endocrinol 3:1377–1386, 1989.

162. Lippman M, Bolan G, Huff R: The effects of oestrogens and antioestrogens on hormone-responsive breast cancer in long-term tissue culture. Cancer Res 36:4595–4601, 1976.

163. Wakeling AE, Bowler J: Biology and mode of action of pure antioestrogens. J Steroid Biochem 30:141–147, 1988.

164. Bowler J, Lilley TJ, Pittam JD et al: Novel steroidal pure antiestrogens. Steroids 54:71–99, 1989.

165. Crawford ED, Eisenberger MA, McLeod DG, et al: A controlled trial of leuprolide with and without flutamide in prostatic carcinoma. N Engl J Med 321:419–424, 1989.

166. Moguilewsky M, Fiet J, Tournemine C, Raynaud J-P: Pharmacology of an antiandrogen, Anandron, used as an adjuvant therapy in the treatment of prostate cancer. J Steroid Biochem 24:139–146, 1986.

167. Apfel C, Bauer F, Crettaz M, et al: A retinoic acid receptor α antagonist selectively counteracts retinoic acid effects. Proc Natl Acad Sci USA 89:7129–7133, 1992.

168. Mester J, Sutherland RL, Binart N, et al: Steroid receptors and hormone action in the chick oviduct. In Dumont JE, Nunez J (eds): Hormones and Cell Regulation, Vol 5. Amsterdam, Elsevier, 1981, pp 221–240.

169. Richard-Foy H, Sistare FD, Riegel AT, et al: Mechanism of dexamethasone 21-mesylate antiglucocorticoid action. II. Receptor-antiglucocorticoid complexes are unable to interact productively with MMTV LTR chromatin in vivo. Mol Endocrinol 1:659–665, 1987.

170. Segnitz B, Gehring U: Mechanism of action of a steroidal antiglucocorticoid in lymphoid cells. J Biol Chem 265:2789–2796, 1990.

171. Sablonnière B, Danze PM, Formstecher P, et al: Physical characterization of the activated and non-activated forms of the glucocorticoid-receptor complex bound to the steroid antagonist [³H] RU486. J Steroid Biochem 25:605–614, 1986.

172. Guiochon-Mantel A, Loosfelt H, Ragot T, et al: Receptors bound to antiprogestin form abortive complexes with hormone responsive elements. Nature 336:695–698, 1988.

173. Bagchi MK, Elliston JF, Tsai S, et al: Identification of a functional intermediate in receptor activation in progesterone-dependent cell-free transcription. Nature 345:457–460, 1990.

174. Meyer ME, Pornon A, Ji J, et al: Agonistic and antagonistic activities of RU486 on the functions of the human progesterone receptor. EMBO J 9:2923–2932, 1990.

175. DeMarzo AM, Oñate SA, Nordeen SK, et al: Effects of the steroid antagonist RU486 on dimerization of the human progesterone receptor. Biochemistry 31:10491–10501, 1992.

176. Picard D, Kumar V, Chambon P, et al: Signal transduction by steroid hormones: nuclear localization is differentially regulated in estrogen and glucocorticoid receptors. Cell Regul 1:291–299, 1990.

177. Picard D, Khursheed B, Garabedian MJ, et al: Reduced levels of hsp90 compromise steroid receptor action in vivo. Nature 348:166–168, 1990.

178. Ylikomi T, Bocquel MT, Berry M, et al: Cooperation of proto-signals for nuclear accumulation of estrogen and progesterone receptors. EMBO J 11:3681–3694, 1992.

179. Chambraud B, Berry, M, Redeuilh G, et al: Several regions of human estrogen receptor are involved in the formation of receptor heat shock protein 90 complexes. J Biol Chem 265:20686–20691, 1990.

180. Spelsberg TC, Littlefield BA, Seelke R, et al: Role of specific chromosomal proteins and DNA sequences in the nuclear binding sites for steroid receptors. Recent Prog Horm Res 39:463–517, 1983.

181. Pratt WB, Jolly DJ, Pratt DV et al: A region in the steroid binding domain determines formation of the non–DNA-binding, 9S glucocorticoid receptor complex. J Biol Chem 263:267–273, 1988.

182. Cadepond F, Schweizer-Groyer G, Segard-Maurel I, et al: Heat shock protein 90 as a critical factor maintaining glucocorticosteroid receptor in a nonfunctional state. J Biol Chem 266:5834–5841, 1991.

183. Bailly A, Le Page C, Rauch M, Milgrom E: Sequence-specific DNA binding of the progesterone receptor to the uteroglobin gene: Effects of hormone, antihormone and receptor phosphorylation. EMBO J 5:3235–3241, 1986.

184. Fawell SE, Lees JA, White R, Parker MG: Characterization and colocalization of steroid binding and dimerization activities in the mouse estrogen receptor. Cell 60:953–962, 1990.

185. Rodriguez R, Carson MA, Weigel NL, et al: Hormone-induced changes in the in vitro DNA-binding activity of the chicken progesterone receptor. Mol Endocrinol 3:356–362, 1989.

186. Tora L, Mullick A, Metzger D, et al: The cloned human estrogen receptor contains a mutation which alters its hormone binding properties. EMBO J 8:1981–1986, 1989.

187. Willmann T, Beato M: Steroid-free glucocorticoid receptor binds specifically to mouse mammary tumour virus DNA. Nature 324:688–691, 1986.

188. Pratt WB: Interaction of hsp 90 with steroid receptors: organizing some diverse observations and presenting the newest concepts. Mol Cell Endocrinol 74:C69–C76, 1990.

188a. Sabbah M, Radanyi C, Redeuilh G, Baulieu EE: The heat shock protein Mr 90000 (HSP 90) modulates the binding of the estrogen receptor to its cognate DNA (in preparation).

189. Brugge JS: Interaction of the Rous sarcoma virus protein pp60src with the cellular proteins pp50 and pp90. Curr Top Microbiol Immunol 123:1–22, 1986.

189a. Oppermann H, Levinson W, Bishop JM: A cellular protein that associates with the transforming protein of Rous sarcoma virus. Proc Natl Acad Sci USA 78:1067–1071, 1981.

190. Sanchez ER, Hirst M, Scherrer LC, et al: Hormone-free mouse glucocorticoid receptors overexpressed in Chinese hamster ovary cells are located to the nucleus and are associated with both hsp70 and hsp90. J Biol Chem 265:20123–20130, 1990.

191. Auricchio F: Phosphorylation of steroid receptors. J Steroid Biochem 32:613–622, 1989.

192. Sando JJ, Hammond ND, Statford CA, Pratt WB: Activation of thymocyte glucocorticoid receptors to the steroid binding form. J Biol Chem 254:4779–4789, 1979.

193. Migliaccio A, Lastoria S, Moncharmont B, et al: Phosphorylation of calf uterus 17β-esradiol receptor by endogenous Ca²⁺-stimulated kinase activating the hormone binding of the receptor. Biochem Biophys Res Commun 109:1002–1010, 1982.

194. Garcia T, Jung-Testas I, Baulieu EE: Tightly bound nuclear progesterone receptors is not phosphorylated in primary chick oviduct cultures. Proc Natl Acad Sci USA 83:7573–7577, 1986.

195. Logeat F, Le Cunff M, Pamphile R, et al: The nuclear-bound form of the progesterone receptor is generated through a hormone-dependent phosphorylation. Biochem Biophys Res Commun 131:421–427, 1985.

196. Auricchio F, Migliaccio A, Castoria G, et al: Evidence that in vivo estradiol receptor translocated into nuclei is dephosphorylated and released into cytoplasm. Biochem Biophys Res Commun 106:149–157, 1982.

197. De Franco DB, Qi M, Borror KC, et al: Protein phosphatase types 1 and/or 2A regulate nucleocytoplasmic shuttling of glucocorticoid receptors. Mol Endocrinol 5:1215–1228, 1991.

198. Power RF, Mani SK, Codina J, et al: Dopaminergic and ligand-independent activation of steroid hormone receptors. Science 254:1636–1639, 1991.

199. Swierczynski J, Mitchell DA, Reinhold DS, et al: Triiodothyronine-induced accumulations of malic enzyme, fatty acid synthase, acetyl-coenzyme A carboxylase, and their mRNAs are blocked by protein kinase inhibitors. J Biol Chem 266:17459–17466, 1991.

200. Garcia T, Buchou T, Renoir JM, et al: A protein kinase copurified with chick oviduct progesterone receptor. Biochemistry 25:7937–7942, 1986.

201. Miller-Diener A, Schmidt TJ, Litwack G: protein kinase activity associated with the purified rat hepatic glucocorticoid receptor. Proc Natl Acad Sci USA 82:4003–4007, 1985.

202. Garcia T, Tuohimaa P, Mester J, et al: Protein kinase activity of purified components of the chicken oviduct progesterone receptor. Biochem Biophys Res Commun 113:960–966, 1983.

202a. Nadeau K, Das A, Walsh CT: Hsp 90 chaperonins possess ATPase activity and bind heat shock transcription factors and peptidyl prolyl isomerases. J Biol Chem 268:1469–1487, 1993.

203. Delescluse C, Cavey MT, Martin B, et al: Selective high affinity retinoic acid receptor α and β-γ ligands. Mol Pharmacol 40:556–562, 1991.

204. Felli MP, Vacca A, Meco D, et al: Retinoic acid–induced down-regulation of the interleukin-2 promoter via *cis*-regulatory sequences containing an octamer motif. Mol Cell Biol 11:4771–4778, 1991.

205. Weisz A, Rosales R: Identification of an estrogen response element upstream of the human c-*fos* gene that binds the estrogen receptor and the AP-1 transcription factor. Nucl Acids Res 18:5097–5106, 1990.

206. Dickson RL, Lippman ME (eds): Breast Cancer: Cellular and Molecular Biology. Boston, Kluwer, 1988.

207. Moncharmont B, Ramp G, De Goeij CCJ, Sluyser M: Comparison of estrogen receptors in hormone-dependent and hormone-independent grunder strain mouse mammary tumors. Cancer Res 51:3843–3848, 1991.

208. Lippman ME, Dickson RB: Mechanisms of growth control in normal and malignant breast epithelium. Recent Prog Horm Res 45:383–435, 1989.

209. Gaben A-M, Mester J: Balb/C mouse 3T3 fibroblasts expressing human estrogen receptor: effect of estradiol on cell growth. Biochem Biophys Res Commun 176:1473–1481, 1991.

209a. Garcia M, Derocq Q, Freiss G, Rochefort H: Activation of estrogen receptor transfected into a receptor-negative breast cancer cell line decreases the metastatic and invasive potential of the cells. Proc Natl Acad Sci USA 89:11538–11542, 1992.

210. Sarff M, Gorski J: Control of estrogen binding protein concentration under basal conditions and after estrogen administration. Biochemistry 10:2557–2563, 1971.

211. Mester J, Baulieu EE: Dynamics of oestrogen receptor distribution between the cytosol and nuclear fractions of immature rat uterus following oestradiol administration. Biochem J 146:617–623, 1975.

212. Milgrom E, Luu Thi M, Atger M, Baulieu EE: Mechanisms regulating the concentration and the conformation of progesterone receptor(s) in the uterus. J Biol Chem 248:6388–6394, 1973.

213. Mester J, Baulieu EE: Progesterone receptors in the chick oviduct: Determination of the total concentration of binding sites in the cytosol and nuclear fraction and effect of progesterone on their distribution. Eur J Biochem 72:405–414, 1977.

214. Baxter JD, Rousseau GG, Benson MC, et al: Role of DNA and specific cytoplasmic receptors in glucocorticoid action. Proc Natl Acad Sci USA 69:1892–1896, 1972.

215. Govindan MV, Pothier F, Leclerc S, et al: Human glucocorticoid receptor gene promoter-homologous down regulation. J Steroid Biochem Mol Biol 40:317–323, 1991.

216. Dauvois S, Danielian PS, White R, et al: Antiestrogen ICI 164,384 reduces cellular estrogen receptor content by increasing its turnover. Proc Natl Acad Sci USA 89:4037–4041, 1992.

217. Qi M, Hamilton BJ, De Franco D: v-*mos* oncoproteins affect the nuclear retention and reutilization of glucocorticoid receptors. Mol Endocrinol 3:1279–1288, 1989.

218. Nardulli AM, Greene GL, O'Malley BW, Katzenellenbogen BS: Regulation of progesterone receptor messenger ribonucleic acid and

protein level in MCF-7 cells by estradiol: Analysis of estrogen effect on progesterone receptor synthesis and degradation. Endocrinology 122:939–944, 1988.

219. Mester J, Martel D, Psychoyos A, Baulieu EE: Hormonal control of oestrogen receptor in uterus and receptivity for ovoimplantation in the rat. Nature 250:776–778, 1974.

220. Sutherland RL, Geynet C, Binart N, et al: Steroid receptors and effects of oestradiol and progesterone on chick oviduct proteins. Eur J Biochem 107:155–164, 1980.

221. Clark JH, Hsueh AJW, Peck EJ: Regulation of estrogen receptor replenishment by progesterone. Ann NY Acad Sci 286:161–176, 1977.

222. Mester J, Baulieu EE: Effects of progesterone: Synergy and antagonism with oestrogen. Trends Biochem Sci 9:56–59, 1984.

223. Touray M, Ryan F, Saurer S, et al: mos-induced inhibition of the glucocorticoid receptor function is mediated by Fos. Oncogene 6:211–217, 1991.

224. Touray M, Ryan F, Jaggi R, Martin F: Characterisation of functional inhibition of the glucocorticoid receptor by Fos/Jun. Oncogene 6:1227–1234, 1991.

225. Vacca A, Screpanti I, Maroder M, et al: Tumor-promoting phorbol ester and ras oncogene expression inhibit the glucocorticoid-dependent transcription from the mouse mammary tumor virus long terminal repeat. Mol Endocrinol 3:1659–1665, 1989.

226. Lee CSL, Koga M, Sutherland RL: Modulation of estrogen receptor and epidermal growth factor receptor by phorbol ester in MCF7 breast cancer cells. Biochem Biophys Res Commun 162:415–421, 1989.

227. Tai PKK, Albers MW, Chang H, et al: Association of a 59-kilodalton immunophilin with the glucocorticoid receptor complex. Science 256:1315–1318, 1992.

228. Callebaut I, Renoir J-M, Lebeau M-C, et al: An immunophilin that binds Mr 90,000 heat shock protein: Main structural features of a mammalian p59 protein. Proc Natl Acad Sci USA 89:6270–6274, 1992.

229. Renoir JM, Radanyi C, Baulieu EE: Un effet des immunosuppresseurs FK506 et rapamycine sur le fonctionnement du récepteur de la progestérone: la protéine "p59-HBI," au carrefour de l'immunologie et de l'endocrinologie? CR Acad Sci Paris 315:421–428, 1992.

230. Wolfson A, Mester J, Chang-Ren Y, Baulieu EE: "Non-activated" form of the progesterone receptor from chick oviduct: Characterization. Biochem Biophys Res Commun 95:1577–1584, 1980.

231. Durand B, Saunders M, Leroy P, et al: All-*trans* and 9-*cis* retinoic acid induction of CRABPII transcription is mediated by RAR-RXR heterodimers bound to DR1 and DR2 repeated motifs. Cell 71:73–85, 1992.

232. Carlberg C, Bendik I, Wyss A, et al: Two nuclear signalling pathways for vitamin D. Nature 361:657–660, 1993.

233. Von der Ahe D, Renoir J-M, Buchou T, et al: Receptors for glucocorticosteroid and progesterone recognize distinct features of DNA regulatory element. Proc Natl Acad Sci USA 83:2817–2821, 1986.

234. Sabbah M, Gouilleux F, Sola B, et al: Structural differences between the hormone and antihormone estrogen receptor complexes bound to the hormone response element. Proc Natl Acad Sci USA 88:390–394, 1991.

Applications of Molecular Biology in Endocrinology

J. LARRY JAMESON

Recombinant DNA technology is revolutionizing our understanding of cell biology. Although expertise in these techniques was once restricted to a few specialized research groups, the last decade has seen rapid dissemination of fundamental molecular biology protocols. Because many recent advances rely on recombinant DNA methods, a basic understanding of these approaches is relevant for clinicians as well as scientists engaged in laboratory investigation. A recurring theme throughout this book is the synergism derived from combining information from traditional studies of pathophysiology with new insights from molecular biology. Nowhere is this more apparent than in studies of inherited endocrine disorders such as MEN I and II (see Ch. 151).

In addition to providing a new means for the diagnosis of inherited disorders, the identification of mutations in endocrine genes also enhances our understanding of pathophysiology.[1-6] Mutations have been described at multiple different steps in the pathways of hormone action. There are now examples of mutations in hormones themselves, hormone receptors, second messenger signaling pathways, and the transcription factors that transduce hormone signals. One can predict continued rapid advances in this field with the transfer of genetic testing into clinical practice in the near future.

In the first half of this chapter, fundamental methods in molecular biology are reviewed to provide a brief overview of recombinant DNA terminology and the experimental approaches that are used elsewhere in the book. Because the purpose of this chapter is to provide an overview for readers outside of the molecular biology field, general and specific references should be consulted for a more comprehensive review of topics. In the second half of the chapter, a selected group of well-characterized disorders has been used to show how molecular biology techniques are being used to study endocrine diseases.

RECOMBINANT DNA METHODS USED TO ANALYZE GENE STRUCTURE

The Structure of DNA and RNA

The genetic blueprint of cells is defined by DNA. An important feature of DNA is its complementarity. The fact that DNA is double-stranded with complementary strands allows it to undergo duplication during DNA synthesis and cell division and to transcribe RNA that is complementary to one of its strands. The complementarity of DNA is an inherent property of nucleotide base pairing. DNA is composed of a linear sequence of four different nucleic acids: adenine (A), guanine (G), thymidine (T), and cytosine (C)

(Fig. 7–1). The nucleotide, A, forms a specific pair with T, and G forms a specific pair with C. Many recombinant DNA techniques make use of the specific bonds formed by nucleic acid pairs to allow detection of specific genes or mRNA's. For example, hybridization procedures such as the Southern blot or the Northern blot (see below) take advantage of the fact that radiolabeled nucleic acids anneal with high affinity and specificity only to sequences that are complementary.

The structure of DNA is predominantly in the form of a double helix, as initially described by Watson and Crick in 1953.[7] The complementary strands of nucleic acid sequences are arranged in an antiparallel manner (Fig. 7–1): that is, the upper or sense strand is designated 5′ to 3′, whereas the lower or antisense strand is oriented 3′ to 5′. Inside the cell, DNA is wrapped around histone protein complexes referred to as *nucleosomes*. DNA can be packaged further into a compact form in chromosomes. During times of DNA replication or active transcription, DNA is unpacked to allow an access of regulatory factors and enzymes.

RNA differs from DNA by the addition of a hydroxyl group in the sugar ring. In addition, RNA uses the nucleic acid uridine (U) instead of thymidine (T). The complementarity of nucleic acid sequences is preserved between DNA and RNA. This allows RNA polymerase to transcribe RNA sequences that reflect the sequence of the template DNA. RNA is always transcribed in a 5′ to 3′ direction from the DNA template. By definition, the transcribed RNA is referred to as the ''sense strand,'' reflecting the fact that this sequence can subsequently be translated into proteins. There are several types of RNA, including ribosomal RNA (rRNA), messenger RNA (mRNA), and transfer RNA (tRNA). rRNA is by far the most abundant of these and comprises a major part of the ribosomal complexes that

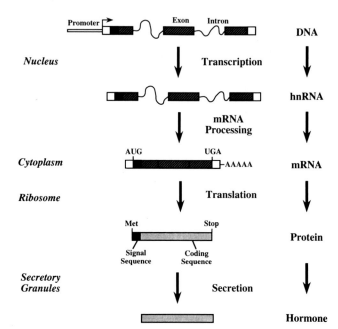

FIGURE 7–2. **Flow of genetic information.** Genes are transcribed into mRNA, which is translated into protein. The cellular locations and processing steps involved in hormone biosynthesis are illustrated schematically.

are used for protein translation. mRNA refers to a relatively small proportion of cellular RNA that is specifically translated into proteins. As its name implies, tRNA is involved in the recognition of specific codons in mRNA and the transfer of the aminoacyl amino acids to the translation complex.

The flow of genetic information from DNA to RNA to protein is shown schematically in Figure 7–2. The information in DNA is divided into small units of three nucleotides that are called *codons*. The concept of the triplet codon is a crucial feature of nucleic acid sequences. The three nucleotides in a codon ultimately define which amino acid will be translated from an mRNA sequence. Altogether, there are 64 different codons that can be created from combinations of the four different nucleotides (Fig. 7–3). The great majority of codons specify one of the 20 different amino acids. There is considerable degeneracy in the codons that can determine a particular amino acid. For example, glycine (Gly) can be encoded by four different codons. In general, for any amino acid, the sequence of the first two nucleotides tends to be the same, with the most variation occurring in the third position. This phenomenon, referred to as ''wobble'' in the third position, has several important implications. Mutations that occur in the third position are less likely to cause amino acid substitutions than those which occur in one of the first two positions. Moreover, a common problem in molecular biology is the need to clone a gene based on protein sequence. The degeneracy in nucleic acids that can encode a given amino acid makes it very difficult to predict nucleic acid sequence from amino acid sequence. In these circumstances, one ideally designs DNA probes based on stretches of amino acids that have minimal degeneracy (e.g., Met, Trp). In addition to defining amino acid sequence, some codons have special functions. For example, when preceded by appropriate ribosomal recognition sequences, the codon AUG is most frequently used to initiate translation

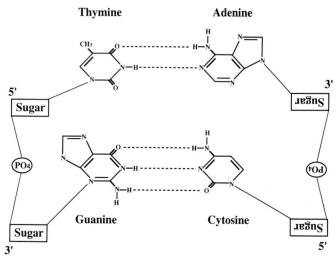

FIGURE 7–1. **Structure of DNA.** The DNA double helix is formed by hydrogen bonds *(dotted lines)* between pairs of pyrimidines (thymine, cytosine) and purines (adenine, guanine). Thymine (T) pairs with adenine (A) and guanine (G) pairs with cytosine (C). Each nucleotide is attached to a sugar residue (deoxyribose) that is linked to the next nucleic acid in the chain by a phosphate group (PO₄). The two strands of DNA are oriented antiparallel with one chain in the 5′ to 3′ direction and the other in the 3′ to 5′ direction. Because pyrimidines always pair with a purine, the spacing along the phosphate backbone (10.7 Å) is constant along the helix.

Second Position

		U	C	A	G	
U		Phe	Ser	Tyr	Cys	U
		Phe	Ser	Tyr	Cys	C
		Leu	Ser	Stop	Stop	A
		Leu	Ser	Stop	Trp	G
C		Leu	Pro	His	Arg	U
		Leu	Pro	His	Arg	C
		Leu	Pro	Gln	Arg	A
		Leu	Pro	Gln	Arg	G
A		Ile	Thr	Asn	Ser	U
		Ile	Thr	Asn	Ser	C
		Ile	Thr	Lys	Arg	A
		Met	Thr	Lys	Arg	G
G		Val	Ala	Asp	Gly	U
		Val	Ala	Asp	Gly	C
		Val	Ala	Glu	Gly	A
		Val	Ala	Glu	Gly	G

*(Left margin: **First Position**; Right margin: **Third Position**)*

FIGURE 7–3. **Triplet codons for amino acids.** Each amino acid is coded by a group of three nucleotides, referred to as *codons*. Because of degeneracy, many amino acids can be encoded by more than one codon. The frequency of amino acid usage in proteins roughly correlates with the number of different codons. Certain codons also serve as signals for control of translation. For example, AUG, which encodes methionine, is used most commonly for the start of translation. Other codons, such as UGA, serve as stop codons.

and specifies that a protein begin with the amino acid methionine. Other codons such as UAA, UGA, and UAG do not specify a particular amino acid but rather indicate that translation should be stopped. In rare circumstances, the stop translation sequence of UGA can be overridden by other regulatory elements in mRNA, causing insertion of the unusual amino acid, selenocysteine, and continuation of translation. In eukaryotes, this phenomenon was first recognized in type II deiodinase, an enzyme involved in thyroid hormone metabolism.[8]

The Structure of Genes

A *gene* refers to an individual transcription unit that encodes either a single protein or perhaps a protein subunit. Genes are divided structurally into exons and introns (Fig. 7–2) (see Ch. 2). Exons refer to the portion of genes that are eventually incorporated into RNA, whereas introns refer to the spacing regions between the exons that are spliced out of precursor RNA's. The upstream 5' flanking regions of endocrine genes typically contain hormone response elements and other regulatory regions including sequences involved in the initiation of transcription. This regulatory region of the gene is also referred to as the *promoter*. At the 3' end of the gene, there are regulatory sequences involved in transcriptional termination, and in some instances hormone- or tissue-specific regulatory elements may also reside downstream of the gene or in introns.

Transcription of a gene by the enzyme RNA polymerase results in the synthesis of a precursor RNA, which is subsequently processed to splice out intronic sequences. RNA is processed further before transfer out of the nucleus, including the addition of 100 to 250 adenine residues (polyadenylation) to the 3' end of the mRNA. RNA processing provides several opportunities for regulatory steps. In some genes, alternate exon splicing allows substitution of some exons for others or splicing out and removal of particular exons.[9] In this manner, the protein that is ultimately produced can have blocks of sequences that are variable, depending on which exons are included in the mRNA. A well-studied example of alternate processing is found in the case of the calcitonin gene in which alternate splicing allows production of either calcitonin or calcitonin gene–related peptide (CGRP).[9] In this instance, alternate splicing occurs in a tissue-specific manner and the encoded proteins have different biologic functions.[10, 11] There are many other examples of alternate processing of endocrine genes and receptors. In some cases, such as the thyroid hormone receptor α gene, alternate splicing results in the production of either a normal receptor protein or a variant that cannot bind hormone (c-*erb*A α II) because a crucial region of the hormone-binding domain has been substituted with a different exon[12, 13] (see Ch. 37).

Specific signals such as the AAUAAA sequence at the 3' end of the mRNA are involved in designating the site for polyadenylation (poly-A tail). There are also examples in which the poly-A tail can be added to alternative sites of the RNA transcript.[14] The exact role of alternate poly-A addition has not been well defined. However, it may be involved in either transfer of mRNA from the nucleus to the cytoplasm or possibly in translational efficiency. There are several examples in which hormonal manipulations cause specific changes in the length of the poly-A tail.[15–19] Moreover, RNA sequences in the 3' region that lie between the coding sequence and the poly-A tail are frequently involved in either RNA stabilization or destabilization.[20] Thus, one effect of adding poly-A sequences to more distal regions of the mRNA is that potential regulatory sequences are retained in the mRNA transcript.

After transport from the nucleus to the cytoplasm, mRNA is available for translation by ribosomes. The cellular mechanisms that control translation efficiency are not well understood. Multiple ribosomes may be attached to and translate a single mRNA template into separate proteins. The complex that includes mRNA and several ribosomes is referred to as a *polysome*. In the case of secretory proteins and membrane receptors that ultimately reside in the extracellular environment, the proteins are synthesized in the ribosome and then undergo a series of post-translational modifications including glycosylation and translocation across membranes (see Ch. 2). Current evidence suggests that much of the control of RNA stability may take place at the level of the ribosome and possibly in conjunction with protein translation.[21, 22]

Approaches for Cloning and Sequencing Genes and cDNA's

Preparation and Screening DNA Libraries

A first step for analyses of endocrine gene expression is to obtain a cDNA clone for the gene in question. There are a number of different technical approaches for cloning

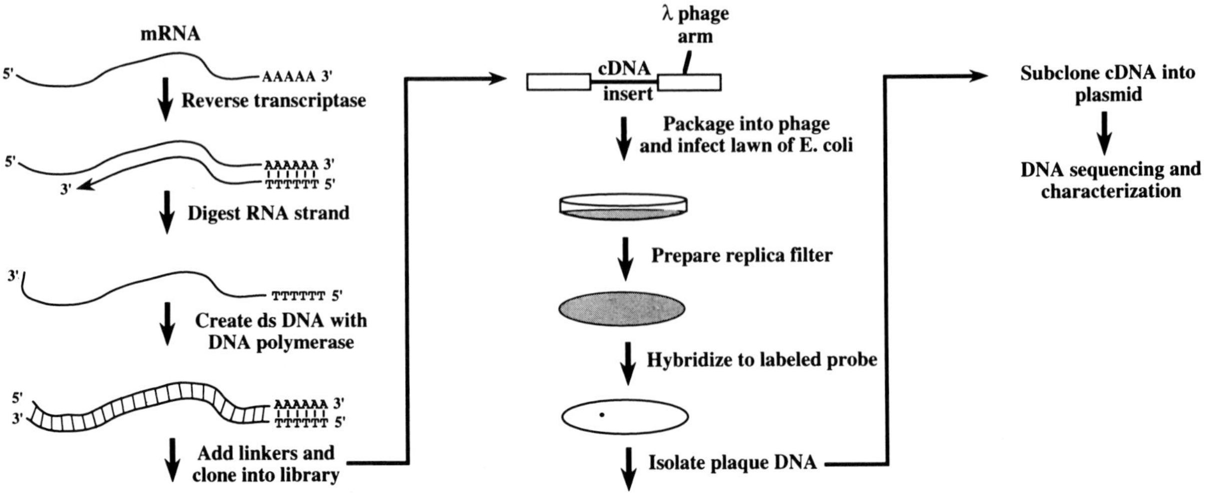

FIGURE 7–4. **Preparation and screening of DNA libraries.** Libraries are used for cloning genes or cDNA's. In the example shown for a cDNA library, a series of enzymatic steps are used to prepare double-stranded cDNA from mRNA. The cDNA's are inserted into a modified λ phage that can be used to infect a lawn of *E. coli.* After phage-induced lysis of the *E. coli,* DNA from the lytic plaques is transferred to a membrane and hybridized with radiolabeled probes. Identified plaques are rescreened, and DNA from positive clones is subcloned into plasmids for further characterization. See text for details and for variations on the procedure.

genes; a complete description of these alternatives is beyond the scope of this chapter (see ref. 23). Nevertheless, it is useful to consider a typical cloning strategy to illustrate some of the principles involved. The first step in the cloning of a cDNA is to prepare a library (Fig. 7–4). This involves making a complementary copy of mRNA using the enzyme reverse transcriptase. This complementary DNA or cDNA is then replicated to create a double-stranded sequence that can be inserted into λ phage vectors,[23] or occasionally into plasmid[24, 25] or cosmid vectors.[26] The λ phage thus contains a population of cDNA's that reflects the composition of mRNA in a given tissue or cell type. Thus, mRNA's that are more abundant will be represented more frequently in the library. A crucial aspect of cDNA cloning is to prepare libraries from tissues that have either abundant levels of a given mRNA or have been treated to induce expression of a specific mRNA.

Having created a library, the next step is to screen it for a specific clone (Fig. 7–4). Library screening is typically done using one of two methods, although alternative strategies are available. In one approach, the λ phage is used to infect a lawn of *E. coli* to create phage plaques from which DNA can be transferred to replicate filters to allow screening with radioactive hybridization probes.[27] This strategy requires knowledge of the DNA sequence that is being sought either from information derived from protein sequence or perhaps derived from a homologous gene sequence from a related species. A second strategy for library screening uses antibodies to detect the protein that is being sought. In this approach, the phage library is created so that the cDNA's are linked to a β-galactosidase fusion gene that can be induced after the phage have infected *E. coli.* In this manner, the infected *E. coli* can be used to express large quantities of proteins encoded by the cDNA and expressed as fusion proteins. Analogous to screening by DNA hybridization, these fusion proteins can be transferred to replicate membranes but are then screened with specific antibodies raised against the protein in question.[23]

Subcloning DNA into Plasmids

In general, it is necessary to screen approximately 1×10^6 plaque-forming units to identify a single clone. Once potential clones have been identified in the library, individual phage containing a specific cDNA clone are isolated and the cDNA insert can be subcloned into plasmid DNA for further analyses[28] (Fig. 7–5). Subcloning into plasmids takes advantage of restriction enzymes that cut DNA at specific recognition sites. In many cases, the restriction enzymes cut DNA asymmetrically to result in DNA "overhangs." Because the DNA overhangs involve a specific DNA sequence, the same enzyme will generate cohesive ends if used to excise the DNA insert and to open the plasmid cloning vector. In this manner, the complementary nature of the cohesive DNA ends is used to greatly increase the efficiency of fragment insertion into the plasmid and ligation by the enzyme DNA ligase. In practice, many plasmids contain a series of restriction enzyme sites clustered in a region referred to as a *polylinker.* The polylinker allows insertion of DNA fragments that have been cut with different types of restriction enzymes, allowing flexibility in the choice of enzyme and the capability to insert fragments directionally by using different enzymes at each end of the DNA insert.

DNA Sequencing

A great advantage of transferring cDNA's into plasmids is that it allows rapid and large-scale amplification of cloned DNA in *E. coli.*[29] It is then possible to perform recombinant DNA manipulations with larger quantities of DNA and to rapidly analyze the DNA sequence of the cDNA insert. A variety of methods are available for DNA

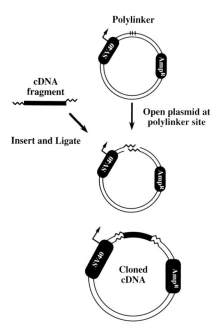

FIGURE 7–5. Subcloning DNA into plasmids. Fragments of DNA can be amplified by cloning into plasmids that are propagated in *E. coli*. The most common cloning strategy involves using restriction enzymes that create cohesive or compatible ends on the DNA fragment and in the circular plasmid. After annealing the cohesive ends of the DNA insert to the complementary ends of the plasmid, the DNA fragments are ligated and the recombinant plasmid is introduced into *E. coli* by the process of transformation. Growth of the *E. coli* in the presence of antibiotics allows selection of bacterial colonies that contain the plasmid antibiotic resistance gene. Large amounts (mg quantities) of recombinant plasmid can be produced in *E. coli*. A variety of plasmids are now available, allowing expression of cloned genes that are driven by bacterial, viral or eukaryotic promoters. In the example shown, the cDNA has been inserted downstream of the simian virus 40 (SV40) promoter to allow expression in mammalian cell lines.

sequencing. Initially, the Maxam-Gilbert procedure was used for most DNA sequencing.[30] It is based on selective chemical modification of the different nucleotides (G, A, T, C) followed by cleavage and electrophoresis on a gel that allows DNA fragments to be resolved at a single base level. This procedure for DNA sequencing has largely been supplanted by protocols derived from the Sanger method for chain termination.[31] Chain termination protocols are based on the principle that dideoxynucleotides can be used to terminate DNA polymerization (Fig. 7–6). By establishing four different reactions, each containing a dideoxynucleotide for each base, the DNA sequence can be ran-

domly terminated at specific nucleotides (e.g., T). When the four reactions are run in parallel on a DNA-sequencing gel, the sequence can be determined by "reading" the base that terminates the sequence at each new position. DNA sequencing is readily amenable to automation. There are now protocols that allow robotic handling of the sequencing reactions as well as automated reading of the sequencing gels. With the DNA sequence in hand, computer programs are used to convert DNA sequence into predicted amino acid codons and to identify characteristic restriction enzyme sites and other structural features that are useful for further studies of the clone.

Uses of Cloned cDNA's and Genes

A cDNA clone is a crucial first step for a number of subsequent studies. For example, the cloned cDNA can be used to isolate the gene that encodes it. In a manner somewhat analogous to cDNA library screening, genomic libraries can be screened using radiolabeled cDNA's.[32] Isolation of genes allows detailed analyses of genomic organization and promoter structure. The promoters of endocrine genes are of particular interest because they often contain the regulatory elements that allow modulation by hormonal and second messenger signaling systems. For example, regulatory elements for glucocorticoid receptors and transcription factors that respond to cAMP (via protein kinase A) often reside in the promoter regions of genes (see Chs. 5 and 6). Cloned cDNA's also allow detailed structure-function analyses of hormones or their receptors. The cDNA's can be translated in vitro using reticulocyte lysates[33] or overexpressed in *E. coli*[34] or tissue culture cells[35] to allow analyses of structure by physical methods or by mutagenesis.

METHODS USED TO ANALYZE GENE EXPRESSION

Perhaps the most widespread use of cloned cDNA's is to analyze patterns of gene expression in different tissues and in response to various hormonal manipulations. The Northern blot is the most common procedure used for analyses of mRNA expression[36] (Table 7–1). In this technique, total mRNA is extracted from a tissue or cell line and subjected to electrophoresis to fractionate the mRNA according to size. The fractionated mRNA is then transferred and bound to a membrane followed by hybridiza-

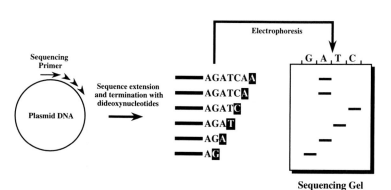

FIGURE 7–6. DNA sequencing. A variety of methods are available for sequencing DNA. In the example shown, the chain termination procedure[31] is illustrated schematically. Single-stranded DNA is first prepared either by denaturing the double-stranded plasmid or using M13 phage that infect *E. coli*. A sequencing primer complementary to the DNA is used to synthesize radiolabeled DNA. By establishing four separate reactions that contain dideoxynucleotides for each base (G,A,T,C), the sequences are terminated randomly. Electrophoresis and autoradiography of each of the reactions run in parallel create a "sequencing ladder." In the example shown, the sequence reads G-A-T-C-A-A from the bottom to the top of gel (5' to 3').

TABLE 7–1. SUMMARY OF BLOTTING PROCEDURES

PROCEDURE	SUBSTANCE DETECTED	PROBE	MAJOR APPLICATION
Southern blot	DNA	Nucleic acid	Gene structure
Northern blot	RNA	Nucleic acid	Gene expression
Western blot	Protein	Antibody	Protein levels
Southwestern blot	Protein	DNA	DNA-protein interactions
Farwestern blot	Protein	Protein	Protein-protein interactions

tion to a radiolabeled cDNA probe. Because the radioactive probe is complementary to its corresponding mRNA, a radioactive hybridization signal is seen only for this specific mRNA and in proportion to its abundance.

A number of other methods are available for analyzing mRNA expression. RNase protection is a particularly sensitive method that relies on solution hybridization of the mRNA of interest to a radiolabeled cRNA.[37] Hybridization of the mRNA to the probe allows it to be protected from digestion by RNase, an enzyme that destroys single-stranded RNA but not the double-stranded probe after it is annealed to the mRNA. The amount of mRNA in the sample can be determined by analyzing the amount of protected probe. Although RNase protection is very sensitive, it can be technically difficult and it does not allow repeated analyses of the same mRNA sample as is possible with a Northern blot membrane. Recently, a reaction combining reverse transcriptase and the polymerase chain reaction (RT-PCR) has gained favor as a highly sensitive method for measuring mRNA.[38] In this procedure, mRNA is first copied into cDNA by reverse transcriptase, a step that is analogous to the method used for producing a cDNA library. Subsequently, the PCR is used to amplify the cDNA product (see below). If PCR is carried out under carefully controlled conditions, the amount of amplified product will reflect the amount of a specific mRNA that was present in the starting material. Through the use of radiolabeled primers or nucleotides in the PCR reaction, the method is readily amenable to quantitation. In situ hybridization is a procedure that combines analyses of mRNA expression with histology.[39] Tissue samples are hybridized with radiolabeled probes, allowing patterns as well as levels of gene expression to be determined. In situ hybridization is particularly useful for tissues with complex or heterogeneous arrangements of cell types (e.g., ovary, brain) because it allows identification of which cells are producing a given mRNA transcript (Fig. 7–7).

TRANSCRIPTIONAL AND POST-TRANSCRIPTIONAL REGULATION OF GENES

Nuclear Run-on Assays

Having demonstrated regulation of a given mRNA by Northern blot or alternative methods for quantitating mRNA levels, it is often important to know whether steady-state mRNA levels are altered because of changes in transcription of the gene or as a consequence of changes in mRNA stability. A classic approach for studies of transcrip-

tional regulation involves the nuclear "run-on assay."[40] In this procedure, nuclei are isolated after a specific stimulus and allowed to carry out mRNA synthesis in vitro. Because the amount of mRNA synthesis under these conditions reflects the number of transcripts initiated before isolation of nuclei, one can estimate the transcription rate by determining the amount of elongated mRNA. Radiolabeled mRNA is hybridized to immobilized DNA to allow quantitation.

Post-transcriptional Regulation

mRNA stability can be assessed in a number of ways. Actinomycin D, which inhibits RNA synthesis, is often used to assess whether a specific treatment alters the stability of mRNA. Although widely used, actinomycin D can be toxic to cells and can block the synthesis of proteins that may be involved in mRNA stabilization or degradation, thereby confounding the results in some instances. Pulse-chase analyses provide an alternative procedure for studies of mRNA stability.[41] In this technique, RNA is labeled with a pulse of radioactive uridine followed by a prolonged incubation (chase) with nonradioactive ribonucleotides. The

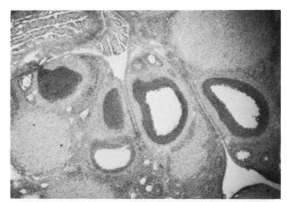
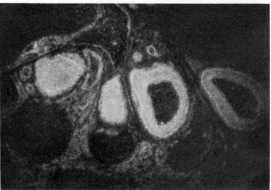

FIGURE 7–7. **In situ hybridization.** Expression of inhibin α-subunit mRNA in the rat ovary on the day of proestrus. The top panel shows a hematoxylin-eosin stained section and the bottom panel shows the paired darkfield micrograph of silver grains produced by the radioactive probe that hybridizes to α-inhibin mRNA. Expression of α-inhibin is seen in the granulosa cells of healthy follicles and there is little or no expression in interstitial cells, the corpus luteum, or atretic follicles. Original photographs were ×40 magnification. (Adapted with permission from Woodruff TK, D'Agostino J, Schwartz NB, Mayo KE: Dynamic changes in inhibin messenger RNAs in rat ovarian follicles during the reproductive cycle. Science 239:1296. Copyright 1988 by the American Association for the Advancement of Science.)

nonradioactive chase prevents further incorporation of radioactive uridine into newly transcribed mRNA. Thus, the stability of a specific mRNA is reflected by the length of time that the radioactive pulse is retained. The amount of labeled RNA is quantitated by hybridization to DNA immobilized on filters analogous to the procedure used in nuclear run-on assays.

Transient Gene Expression Studies in Transfected Cells

Transient gene expression studies provide an alternative technique for examining transcriptional control (Fig. 7–8). In addition, this method allows detailed mutagenesis of cloned promoter sequences before their introduction into cells.[42] In this procedure, the promoter sequences of genes are typically fused to a reporter gene that can be assayed readily.[43] Common reporter genes include chloramphenicol acetyltransferase (CAT), luciferase (LUC), and β-galactosidase (β-GAL). In each case, these reporter genes represent enzymes whose activities are not normally found in eukaryotic cells. Thus, in the absence of gene transfer, the background activity of these reporter enzymes is negligible.

The promoter-reporter fusion gene constructs are introduced into cells using a process referred to as *transfection*.[42] Transfected genes are transcriptionally active over 24 to 72 hours, allowing relatively rapid analyses of promoter func-

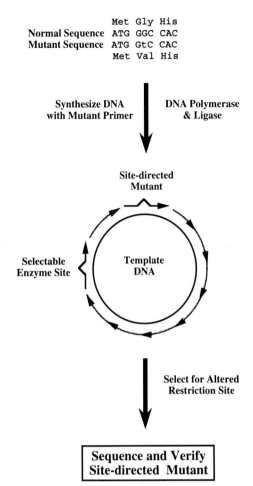

FIGURE 7–9. **Strategy for site-directed mutagenesis.** Site-directed mutagenesis is used to introduce specific mutations into DNA. Common uses include promoter mutagenesis to identify DNA regulatory elements or changes in coding sequences that result in specific amino acid substitutions in proteins, enzymes, or receptors. A variety of methods are available for site-directed mutagenesis. Most current procedures use an oligonucleotide primer harboring a site-directed mutation to initiate template replication by a DNA polymerase or to initiate the polymerase chain reaction. In the example shown, a G to t substitution converts a glycine to valine. The mutant primer is used to synthesize a new copy of the plasmid that will now incorporate the mutant sequence. By including a second primer that contains a selectable restriction enzyme site, it is possible to screen rapidly for recombinant clones that are likely to contain the expected mutation.

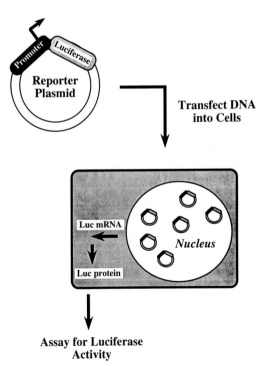

FIGURE 7–8. **Transient gene expression.** Plasmids are transfected into mammalian cell lines for transient expression studies. The transfected plasmids are transcribed for several days after which the DNA is either degraded or becomes integrated into the host cell genome. If a selectable marker (e.g., neomycin resistance) is included in the transfection, it is possible to isolate stably transfected clones of cells. A common experimental paradigm uses transient expression to measure the activity and regulation of a promoter. In the example shown, the promoter drives expression of a luciferase reporter gene. The amount of luciferase enzyme produced is proportionate to the transcriptional activity of the promoter.

tion. Alternatively, transfected genes can be stably introduced into cells by selecting for a resistance marker such as neomycin or dihydrofolate reductase. The principal goal of transfection experiments is to define DNA sequences that are required for promoter function or which respond to a specific hormone signal or second messenger pathway. A variety of methods are now available to allow deletion or site-directed mutagenesis of promoter elements (Fig. 7–9). This approach has been crucial for defining DNA sequences that regulate tissue specific expression, basal promoter activity, and a variety of hormone response elements such as cAMP-responsive elements (CRE's) and sequences that mediate responses to steroid and thyroid hormone receptors. Identification of these DNA regulatory sequences is often a first step toward characterization of the transcription factors that interact with these elements.

ANALYSES OF TRANSCRIPTION FACTOR INTERACTIONS WITH DNA

The regulatory DNA sequences in genes function by binding transcription factors (see Ch. 2). These proteins are generally classified into three groups: general transcription factors, enhancer-binding proteins, and transcription activation factors (TAF's) (Fig. 7–10). Because this is a relatively nascent area of research, our understanding of these proteins and their classification is changing rapidly. General transcription factors include proteins that bind to the proximal regions of genes near the start site of transcription. These proteins include the TATA-binding protein (TBP), also referred to as TFIID, as well as a series of other general transcription factors (GTF's) such as TFIIA, B, and E that comprise a complex group of proteins that regulate transcription initiation.[44, 45] Enhancer-binding proteins typically interact with DNA sequences located upstream of the basal transcription complex. Enhancer-binding proteins are usually bipartite, having a DNA-binding domain and a separate domain involved in protein-protein contacts and transcriptional activation. This group of proteins includes transcription factors with a broad range of regulatory functions. For example, proteins such as Pit-1 are involved in cell-specific expression. Pit-1 is a homeodomain class (related to homeobox genes involved in *Drosophila* embryonic development) of transcription factor that is expressed specifically in somatotrophs, lactotrophs, and thyrotrophs in which it is involved in transcription of the growth hormone and prolactin genes.[46, 47] As described below, mutations in the Pit-1 gene cause deficiencies of GH, Prl, and TSH.[48–50] Other enhancer proteins bind to second messenger signal response elements such as CRE's. CRE's bind a large family of transcription factors referred to as CRE-binding (CREB) proteins or activating transcription factors (ATF's) (see Ch. 5).[51] Structurally related DNA sequences bind members of the *jun/fos* family of transcription factors that are involved in cell signaling by protein kinase C and a variety of growth factor signaling pathways.[52] Other enhancer proteins include nuclear receptors such as the glucocorticoid, estrogen, and thyroid hormone receptors (see Chs. 6 and 37). These receptors bind to hormone response elements in target genes to activate or repress transcription. Enhancer proteins in each of these groups typically bind to DNA with high affinity (e.g., Kd less than 10^{-9} M). How they alter transcription remains an area of active investigation. In some cases, they may alter nucleosome phasing to allow additional transcription factors to have access to DNA.[53, 54] In other cases, they may form direct protein-protein contacts with components of the basal transcription complex such as TBP or TFIIB.[55–57] Finally, interactions between enhancer binding proteins and general transcription factors appear to frequently require members of the third class of transcription factors, the TAF's.[58, 59] Because TAF proteins do not bind to DNA with high affinity, their identification and characterization have lagged behind that of other groups of transcription factors. TAF's likely serve as bridging proteins that link enhancer binding proteins to the basal transcription complex through protein-protein contacts. For any given gene, the array of different transcription factors that bind to the promoter is relatively large (usually more than 20). This large repertoire of proteins provides an important means for regulatory control at the level of transcription. Consequently, when considering the role of any given regulatory DNA element and its cognate transcription factor, it is important to recognize that specific combinations of transcription factors may result in unique properties that are not necessarily applicable to another gene. It is apparent that the complexity of "basal" transcription factors is only beginning to be appreciated.

Two techniques have been particularly useful for identifying protein interactions with DNA. *DNase I footprinting* is a method that relies on the ability of bound protein to protect DNA from digestion by the enzyme DNase I[60] (Fig. 7–11). Consequently, protein-bound regions of DNA appear as a "footprint" on the DNA sequence ladder that is created after partial digestion of radiolabeled DNA with the enzyme. DNase I footprinting is most useful for screening 100 to 300 base pair regions of DNA for the locations of protein-binding sites. After identification of protein-binding sites by footprinting or functional studies in which promoter mutations have localized a regulatory element, the *electrophoretic gel mobility shift assay* (EMSA) is useful for more detailed analyses of protein-DNA interactions.[61] The EMSA is based on the fact that the mobility of short DNA fragments (usually 20 to 200 base pairs) is markedly reduced during nondenaturing gel electrophoresis when protein is bound[62] (Fig. 7–12). The degree of mobility shift is approximately proportional to the size of the bound protein complex. Therefore, the EMSA is also useful for detecting the presence of proteins as monomers, homodimers, and heterodimers. It provides a sensitive measure of protein-DNA interactions, allowing detection of specific binding proteins even in crude nuclear extracts. The method is also relatively simple technically and allows an array of competition assays to be performed to demonstrate specificity and binding affinity.

Studies of protein-DNA interactions not only localize binding sites in promoters but also provide a useful assay for monitoring purification of transcription factors. Once a discrete DNA-binding site has been localized, it can be used for purification by DNA affinity chromatography.[63] If enough pure protein can be obtained, protein sequence

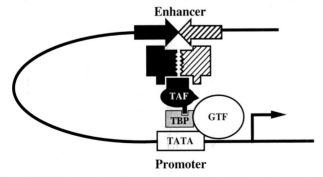

FIGURE 7–10. Formation of an active transcription complex. Interactions between enhancer binding proteins and components of the basal transcription complex is illustrated schematically. There is evidence that many enhancer binding proteins interact with the basal transcription machinery via adaptor or bridging proteins. The TATA binding protein (TBP) also forms contacts with a large group of general transcription factors as well as RNA polymerase II. Implicit in this model is that specific protein-protein contacts as well as protein-DNA contacts are involved in the assembly of transcription complexes on individual promoters.

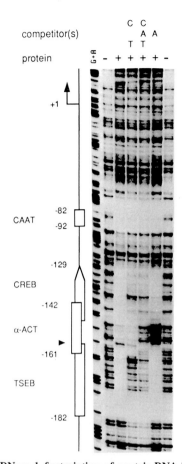

FIGURE 7–11. **DNase 1 footprinting of protein-DNA interactions.** Proteins that bind to specific DNA sites with high affinity can be detected as a "footprint" by exposing the DNA-protein complex to DNase 1, an enzyme that digests DNA. When DNA fragments are radiolabeled, areas bound by proteins are protected from DNase 1 digestion and appear as footprints when the partially digested DNA is subjected to denaturing electrophoresis. In the example shown, the glycoprotein hormone α-subunit gene promoter has been footprinted by nuclear proteins extracted from a placental cell line (JEG-3) that expresses the α and β subunit genes of hCG. Typical of most promoters, a number of transcription factors bind to DNA regulatory elements. Distinct protein binding sites can be detected by the presence of separate footprints as well as the ability to compete for protein binding with short oligonucleotides that correspond to the DNA recognition sequence. Labeled DNA was incubated without (−) or with (+) nuclear extracts from JEG-3 cells before partial digestion with DNase I. A G + A Maxam-Gilbert sequencing ladder is shown on the left. Sequences protected from DNase I digestion are indicated by boxes on the left. Competitor oligonucleotides (~1000-fold excess) that correspond to the individual protected regions are indicated above the lanes. The competitors are: C, cAMP response element (CRE); A, α-activating element (α-ACT); T, trophoblast specific element (TSE). (Adapted with permission from Steger DJ, Altschmied J, Buscher M, Mellon PL: Evolution of placenta-specific gene expression: Comparison of the equine and human gonadotropin α-subunit genes. Mol Endocrinol 5:243, 1991.)

radiolabeled DNA is used to probe proteins immobilized on a membrane in a manner otherwise analogous to a Western blot[65] (see Table 7–1). Cloning transcription factors is extremely valuable for studying mechanisms of gene transcription because it allows their production in large quantities in *E. coli* or other expression systems for detailed structure-function analyses.

RECOMBINANT DNA APPROACHES TO PROTEIN STRUCTURE AND FUNCTION

Protein Expression Systems

It is now possible to express recombinant proteins using a variety of different expression systems. The development of these expression systems represents an important example of how fundamental investigation of bacterial and viral life cycles can have unexpected practical applications that could not have been readily anticipated at the outset of the

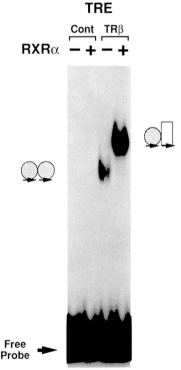

FIGURE 7–12. **Gel shift analyses of protein-DNA interactions.** Protein interactions with DNA can be detected by analyzing the ability of DNA bound proteins to shift (decrease) the mobility of radiolabeled DNA during nondenaturing gel electrophoresis. The gel shift technique is very sensitive and is particularly useful for detailed analyses of the DNA sequence determinants for specific protein binding. In the example shown, binding of the thyroid hormone receptor β (TRβ) to a thyroid hormone response element (TRE) is demonstrated. The thyroid hormone receptor binds to this element as a homodimer (2 circles bound to DNA) or as a heterodimer (circle and square bound to DNA) with the retinoic acid X receptor α (RXRα). The mobility of the unbound DNA is very rapid, whereas the mobility of the TRβ-TRE complex is shifted up in the gel. The TRβ/RXRα heterodimers cause an even greater mobility shift of the DNA, probably because of the increased molecular mass of the heterodimeric protein complex. (Adapted with permission from Nagaya T, Jameson JL: Thyroid hormone receptor dimerization is required for dominant negative inhibition by mutations that cause thyroid hormone resistance. J Biol Chem 268:15766, 1993.)

analysis can be performed to provide a strategy for cloning the transcription factor cDNA based on predicted nucleic acid sequences. Alternatively, radiolabeled DNA sequences that bind proteins can sometimes be used to screen cDNA expression libraries directly.[64] This strategy requires that expressed protein bind to DNA without the requirement for another protein co-factor and that the *E. coli*–expressed protein fold in a manner that still allows DNA binding. The capacity of transcription factors to bind radiolabeled DNA under the conditions similar to library screening can usually be demonstrated in the Southwestern blot, in which studies. Most expression systems take advantage of strong viral promoters that drive expression selectively in *E. coli*, insect cells, or mammalian cells. For example, the viral T7 promoter is very active in certain strains of *E. coli* (e.g., BL21), allowing recombinant proteins that are cloned downstream of this promoter to be expressed in milligram quantities in an inexpensive culture system.[34] By attaching sequences that encode artificial epitopes to the amino-terminal or carboxy-terminal ends of the recombinant proteins, it is often possible to purify the expressed proteins rapidly by affinity chromatography using appropriate antibodies against the epitope. The *baculovirus system* has also gained favor because it allows extraordinarily efficient expression in insect cell lines (e.g., Sf9) that are susceptible to infection by the baculovirus.[66] In this case, the recombinant protein of interest is inserted in place of the viral polyhedrin protein, allowing expression to approach 10 to 30 per cent of total cellular protein. As described above (see Fig. 7–5), promoters derived from viruses that infect mammalian cells (e.g., SV40) can be used to drive expression in these cell lines. The choice of these or other expression systems (e.g., yeast) depends on the goal of the study as well as the characteristics of the specific protein being expressed. For example, proteins that require glycosylation cannot be post-translationally modified in *E. coli*. Overexpressed proteins are sometimes insoluble (e.g., inclusion bodies) or folded incorrectly, often necessitating empirical trials with different expression systems. Although mammalian cell lines generally do not express proteins at the high level seen in *E. coli* or baculovirus systems, they are more amenable to studies of physiological processing or post-translational modification.

Overexpression of recombinant proteins has been invaluable for detailed studies of proteins that are scarce in natural sources. For example, the capacity to express recombinant activin and inhibin has allowed their physiological functions to be examined in a manner that would have proved difficult if natural sources were used for their purification.[67, 68] Moreover, natural sources often produce multiple proteins with overlapping or antagonistic activities,[69, 70] whereas recombinant proteins can be produced under conditions in which contamination is unlikely. In addition to experimental applications, recombinant proteins are finding their way into clinical use. Examples include recombinant insulin, growth hormone, and gonadotropins.

Site-Directed Mutagenesis of Proteins

The development of expression systems for recombinant proteins has made it feasible to rapidly perform structure-function studies using site-directed mutagenesis. Analogous to strategies described above for site-directed mutagenesis of promoter elements, it is equally feasible to alter the coding sequences of proteins (Fig. 7–9). Mutagenesis might involve large deletions of amino acids to grossly define critical domains. Alternatively, a common initial strategy is to exchange domains between related proteins to define specific functional regions. For example, by swapping different regions of the estrogen and glucocorticoid receptors, it is possible to define domains that bind specific hormonal ligands or DNA sequences.[71] Specific mutagenesis of individual amino acids or small regions of proteins allows functional domains to be defined at high resolution. For example, mutations of putative glycosylation or phosphorylation sites allow the roles of these modifications to be tested relatively rapidly.

APPLICATIONS OF TRANSGENIC MODELS

Expression of Endocrine Genes in Transgenic Animals

Transgenic mice provide an opportunity to examine developmental and hormonal regulation of transferred genes in vivo. Transgenic mice are most commonly produced by microinjection of genes into one of the pronuclei of a fertilized mouse egg[72–74] (Fig. 7–13). The microinjected eggs are then implanted into a pseudopregnant foster mother. The next step is to identify progeny that have actually incorporated the transgene. Typically, this involves Southern blot analysis of tail DNA to determine whether the transgene has been incorporated. Alternatively, it is possible to use the polymerase chain reaction to analyze DNA from biopsies of one or more tissues.

The selection of promoter sequences used to drive the expression of the transgene is a crucial aspect of the transgenic strategy. For studies that are primarily used to address regulation of a given promoter, these sequences are often linked to reporter genes such as β-galactosidase to allow rapid histological analyses. It is frequently necessary to use relatively long fragments of promoter sequences or additional intronic or 3′ gene sequences to obtain appropriate developmental and tissue-specific expression. An example of using transgenes that function in a manner that recapitulates physiology is illustrated by insertion of the normal GnRH gene into a strain of hypogonadal mouse (hpg/hpg) that contains a deletion of the native GnRH gene.[75, 76] The GnRH transgene is expressed in the hypothalamus and corrects the hypogonadotropic hypogonadism, providing a model of "gene therapy" in which both the pattern of expression and the physiological function of the abnormal gene are replicated. Promoter mutagenesis studies can be used to delineate functional regulatory elements in vivo. For example, some of the regulatory elements required for cell-specific expression of the pro-opiomelanocortin (POMC) promoter have been defined using transgenic approaches.[77, 78] Alternatively, when the goal is to overexpress a hormone or enzyme, it is sometimes preferable to use a widely expressed and strong promoter such as the metallothionein or actin promoters. A dramatic example of the effects of hormone expression in transgenic mice is provided by overexpression of growth hormone resulting in a model of gigantism.[79]

Targeted Oncogenesis and Development of Endocrine Tumors

There has been great interest in using transgenic animals to ablate specific cell lineages or to perform targeted oncogenesis by expressing strong transforming genes in specific cell types.[80] Each of these techniques requires that a promoter drive expression of the transgene in selected

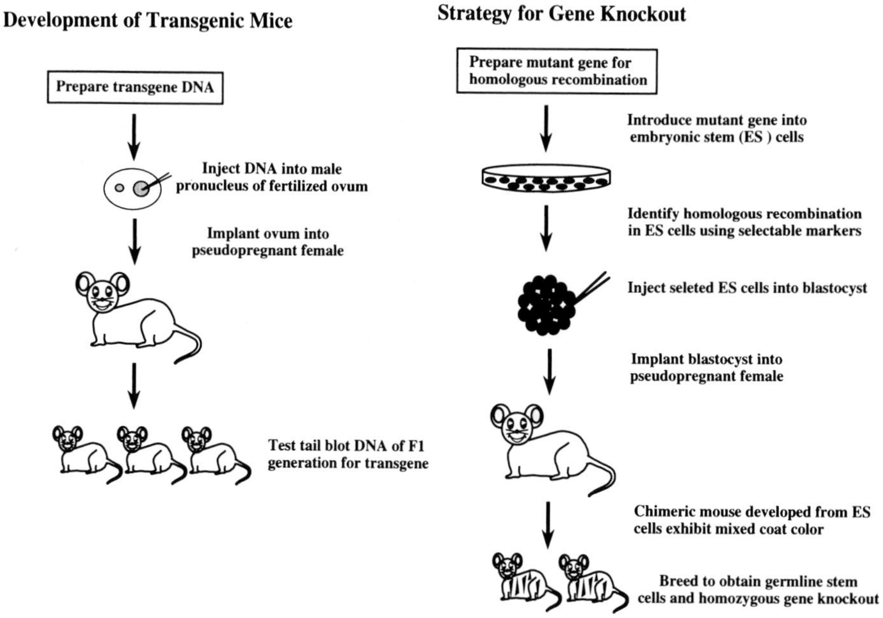

FIGURE 7–13. **Transgenic models.** Transgenic mice allow studies of recombinant genes in vivo. On the left, a strategy is shown for introducing transgenes into fertilized eggs with subsequent implantation into surrogate females. In this approach, the purpose of the transgenes may be to overexpress a hormone (e.g., growth hormone) from an active promoter (e.g., metallothionein). Alternatively, the transgene may use a specific promoter (e.g., insulin) to target expression of a different gene (e.g., large T antigen) in specific cells (β cells of the islets). On the right, a strategy for "gene knockout" is illustrated. In this approach, homologous recombination is used to mutate the endogenous gene in embryonic stem (ES) cells. After selection of ES cells containing the altered gene, the cells are injected into blastocysts which are introduced into a surrogate female. Mixed coat color identifies progeny that contain the ES cells. Additional breeding of heterozygous mice allows production of mice that are homozygous for the gene knockout.

Development of Transgenic Mice

Prepare transgene DNA

Inject DNA into male pronucleus of fertilized ovum

Implant ovum into pseudopregnant female

Test tail blot DNA of F1 generation for transgene

Strategy for Gene Knockout

Prepare mutant gene for homologous recombination

Introduce mutant gene into embryonic stem (ES) cells

Identify homologous recombination in ES cells using selectable markers

Inject seleted ES cells into blastocyst

Implant blastocyst into pseudopregnant female

Chimeric mouse developed from ES cells exhibit mixed coat color

Breed to obtain germline stem cells and homozygous gene knockout

cell types in a very specific manner. For ablation experiments, reagents such as diphtheria toxin or other agents have been used to eliminate specific cell types.[81, 82] Targeted oncogenesis has been performed using several oncogenes, most frequently the SV40 large T-antigen.[83–85] In several instances, tumors from transgenic mice have been adapted to cell culture to provide new cell lines for detailed studies in vitro.[85]

Homologous Recombination and Gene Knockout Approaches

More recently, it has been possible to perform "gene knockout" experiments to generate null mutations in transgenic mice.[86] This strategy uses homologous recombination and embryonic stem cells in culture to mutagenize a specific target gene (Fig. 7–13). Homologous recombination implies that the exogenous mutant form of a gene identifies homologous genomic sequences and undergoes recombination at a rate that greatly exceeds random insertion. Selectable markers attached to the exogenous gene are used to identify cells efficiently that have undergone homologous recombination. After selection of cells containing a mutated, nonfunctional target gene, the ES cells are injected into mouse blastocysts, where they are incorporated into a variety of normal tissues, including the germ line. Mice subsequently can be bred such that the gene knockout is carried in a heterozygous or homozygous form. In principle, this approach allows the null phenotype to be analyzed for essentially any gene. An example in endocrinology of information derived from a gene knockout experiment is illustrated by the developmental and physiological consequences of eliminating the gene encoding the α-subunit of inhibin.[87] Deletion of the inhibin α-subunit gene caused a high incidence of gonadal tumors, suggesting an important role for inhibin as a biological repressor of gonadal cell proliferation and transformation. Gene knockout experiments such as this create biological models that would occur rarely in nature and allow detailed analyses of the physiological role of deleted genes.

It is notable that the physiological effects of gene knockout experiments are often less dramatic than predicted based on foregoing studies of the function of a given gene. This situation often occurs in the setting of large gene families, and the lack of dramatic physiological consequences is attributed to biological redundancy of residual family members. For example, homozygous deletion of transcription factor CREB has minimal phenotypic effects, presumably because other members of the CREB/ATF family can replace its function (see Ch. 5). On the other hand, when a dominant negative mutant of CREB is created such that it retains the ability to bind to DNA, but without the capacity to mediate transactivation, the results are quite different from the gene knockout approach. Transgenic mice expressing the dominant negative form of CREB targeted into GH-producing cells exhibit dramatic somatotrope hypoplasia and dwarfism.[88] Presumably, the dominant negative form of CREB binds to target sequences for an array of CREB/ATF family members to functionally "knock out" the activity of multiple related transcription factors.

MOLECULAR GENETIC APPROACHES TO ENDOCRINE DISEASE

The technical aspects of the foregoing discussion of recombinant DNA methodology may raise questions concerning how such techniques can be useful to the practicing endocrinologist. In large measure, molecular biology is already transforming the practice of endocrinology and will continue to do so for the near term. In addition to improving our understanding of hormone and receptor structure-function, these techniques have allowed the production of large quantities of recombinant insulin, growth hormone, and gonadotropins. There is also an increasing reliance on recombinant DNA methods to identify new growth factors, cytokines, and hormones, as well as their physiological functions. An overview of recent progress in the molecular basis of endocrine diseases foreshadows the future role of these methods in clinical practice.

Several hundred endocrine disorders exhibit an inheritance pattern suggestive of a primary gene defect.[89] Gene mutations have now been identified in many of these disorders (Table 7–2). Some common themes emerge even from the relatively small number of mutations that have been described to date. First, the phenotypic variability that characterizes many endocrine diseases is often reflected in genetic heterogeneity. Some clinical phenotypes that were thought previously to represent distinct diseases can now be interpreted as manifestations of different types of mutations within a single gene. For example, the clinical variants of congenital adrenal hyperplasia can be attributed to distinct mutations in 21-hydroxylase or other enzymes involved in steroid biosynthesis.[5] Second, the propensity of

TABLE 7–2. SUMMARY OF MUTATIONS THAT CAUSE ENDOCRINE DISEASES

SITE OF ENDOCRINE MUTATION	DISORDER	MODE OF INHERITANCE	CHROMOSOME LOCATION	TYPE OF MUTATION	REFERENCE
Hormone Mutations					
Insulin	Hyperproinsulinemia	AR	11p15.5	P	106
Growth hormone	Dwarfism	AR	17q22-q24	D,P	91
Parathyroid hormone	Hypoparathyroidism	AD	11p15.3-15.1	P	107
Thyroid-stimulating hormone	Hypothyroidism	AR	1p22	D,P	109
Thyroglobulin	Hypothyroidism; goiter	AR	8q24.2-q24.3	P	199
Luteinizing hormone	Hypogonadism	AR	19q13.32	P	103
Vasopressin/Neurophysin II	Central diabetes insipidus	AD	20p12.21	P	108
Binding Protein Mutations					
Thyroxine-binding globulin	Euthyroid hypothyroxinemia	XL	Xq21-22	D,P	112
Transthyretin	Euthyroid hyperthyroxinemia	AD	18q11.2-12.1	P	114
Albumin	Euthyroid hyperthyroxinemia	AD	4q11-q13	?	200
Membrane Receptor Mutations					
Insulin receptor	Insulin resistance	AR,AD	19p13.3-13	P	4
Growth hormone receptor	Laron dwarfism	AR	5p13-p12	P	116
TSH receptor	Hypothyroidism, TSH resist.	AR	14q31	?	120
Vasopressin V2 receptor	Nephrogenic diabetes insipidus	XL	Xq27-q28	P	118
Nuclear Receptor Mutations					
Vitamin D	Vitamin D resistance	AR	?	P	130
Thyroid hormone	Thyroid hormone resistance	AD,AR	3p24.3	P,D	201
Glucocorticoid	Glucocorticoid resistance	AR	5q31	P	132
Androgen	Androgen resistance	XL	Xcen-q13	P,D	202
Signal Pathway Mutations					
Ras P21	Tumorigenesis	S	20q12-13.2	P	188
Gsα	Acromegaly	S	20q13.2-13.3	P	184
Gsα	Albright osteodystrophy	AD,S	20q13.2-13.3	P	186
Gsα	McCune-Albright	AD,S	20q13.2-13.3	P	185
Giα	Tumorigenesis	S	3p21	P	183
p53	Tumorigenesis	S	17p13	D,P	203
Retinoblastoma	Tumorigenesis	S	13q14	D,P	204
PRAD-1 (Cyclin D1)	Tumorigenesis	S	11q13	Transloc.	197
PTC (papillary thyroid carcinoma)	Tumorigenesis	S	10q	Transloc.	176
Transcription Factor Mutations					
SRY translocation	XX male	XL	Ypter	Transloc.	139
SRY mutation	XY female	YL	Ypter	P	205
Pit-1	GH, PRL, TSH deficiency	AR,AD	?	D,P	49
Endocrine Syndromes					
Kallmann	Hypogonadotropic hypogonadism	XL,AR,AD	Xp22.3	D,P,Transloc.	206
Prader-Willi	Hypogonadism, obesity	AD	15q11	D	155
MEN I	Neoplasia: pit, pancr, parathy	AD	11q13	?	169
MEN II (*ret* mutations)	Neoplasia: parathy, pheo, MTC	AD	10q21.1	P	174
MEN IIb	MEN II and neurofibromas	AD	10q21.1	?	207
Adren. Hypoplasia/Hypogonadism	Adrenal insuf., hypogonadism	XL	Xp21.3-21.2	D	159
Enzyme Mutations					
Thyroid peroxidase	Goiter, hypothyroidism	AR	2pter-12	P	167
21-hydroxylase	CAH, androgen excess, salt wasting	AR	6p21	P,D	5
17α-hydroxylase	Androgen def., HTN	AR	10	P	164
11β-hydroxylase	Androgen excess, HTN	AR	8q21	P	163
3β-hydroxysteroid dehydrogenase	Androgen excess, often lethal	AR	1p13	?	208
5α-reductase type 2	Male pseudohermaphroditism	AR	2p23	D,P	166
Aldosterone Synthase	Glucocorticoid, remediable HTN	AD	8q21	D,Transloc.	168

AD, autosomal dominant; AR, autosomal recessive; S, somatic cell mutation; XL, X-linked; YL, Y-linked; P, point mutation; D, deletion; transloc, translocation; ?, unknown. Representative references are provided. Please see additional citations in the indicated references.
Modified with permission from Jameson JL, Hollenberg AN: Recent advances in studies of the molecular basis of endocrine disease. Horm Metab Res 24:201, 1992.

certain genes to be targets for frequent mutations may be explained in part by gene structure and organization. Genes such as growth hormone that have been duplicated to form gene clusters are predisposed to undergo recombination and deletion.[90, 91] Third, although many of the mutations reported initially have been associated with severely affected patients, it is likely that mutations with less severe consequences will also be identified. For example, the phenotype of androgen insensitivity includes a spectrum of disorders that ranges from severe resistance in the case of testicular feminization to milder resistance in Reifenstein's syndrome and other syndromes of mild androgen resistance associated with gynecomastia and infertility.[6] These disorders are each caused by mutations in the androgen receptor, but the mutations result in different degrees of receptor dysfunction. In some cases, the receptor is deleted or mutated in such a manner that it is completely inactive. In other examples, mutations perturb the amount or stability of the receptor, causing partial resistance. An extension of this concept is that genetic polymorphisms (DNA sequence variants) in the normal population could also cause subtle differences in hormone or receptor activity, thereby constituting part of the basis for variability that is seen in the normal range of hormone levels and activity.

Methods Used to Detect Gene Deletions and Point Mutations

Recombinant DNA approaches that are used initially to investigate a particular disorder are usually based on clues derived from its clinical and pathophysiological characteristics, which in some cases allow one to predict the gene that harbors a defect. For example, it is reasonable to postulate that selective GH deficiency in several members of a family might be due to a defect in the gene encoding GH or perhaps GHRH. In other cases, however, there are no obvious candidate genes. For example, in the multiple endocrine neoplasia syndromes it is difficult to predict a gene that causes proliferation of selected lineages of endocrine cells. In this case, the most expeditious approach is to first identify an abnormal genetic locus using cytogenetics, if large genetic alterations are present, or linkage analyses to localize chromosomal regions carrying markers associated with the disease phenotype (see below). After candidate genes are identified, they can be analyzed for mutations in affected patients to verify that they cause a given disorder. A summary of approaches useful for identifying mutations is listed in Table 7–3.

Use of Southern Blots to Analyze Gene Structure

After identification of a disease gene, a number of different types of molecular techniques are available for defining specific mutations. To define the gross structure of the gene, a useful first approach is to use Southern blot analyses to detect large gene deletions or rearrangements[92] (Fig. 7–14). In this method, genomic DNA is digested with one or more restriction endonucleases creating an array of DNA fragments that are separated according to length using agarose gel electrophoresis. After transfer of the DNA fragments to a membrane, a radiolabeled probe that is specific for the gene of interest is hybridized to the DNA

TABLE 7–3. APPROACH TO MUTATIONAL ANALYSES

Detailed clinical characterization
    Establish phenotypes and heterogeneity
    Identify possible candidate genes
Major deletions and rearrangements
    Cytogenetics
    Southern blot analyses
Small deletions or point mutations
    SSCP or DGGE to determine regions of gene with
        mutations
    Cloning and sequencing of the abnormal gene
    PCR coupled to DNA sequencing
Inherited disorders caused by an unknown gene
    Linkage by RFLP or VNTR
    Chromosome walking, and cloning of candidate genes
Functional properties of identified gene mutations
    In vitro analyses of mutant proteins
    In vivo and transgenic analyses of mutant proteins

Modified with permission from Jameson JL, Hollenberg AN: Recent advances in studies of the molecular basis of endocrine disease. Horm Metab Res 24:201, 1992.

on the membrane. Under appropriate conditions of hybridization stringency, the probe will detect only the few DNA fragments that are complementary in sequence. Gene deletions would be detected as absent fragments or by fragments with reduced size. Gene rearrangements result in complex patterns of DNA fragments with increased and/or decreased lengths. It is important to use several different restriction enzymes for these types of analyses because polymorphisms in the DNA sequence of a restriction enzyme site would also alter the length of the DNA fragments without necessarily affecting the gene of interest. If the gene appears to be intact when analyzed using multiple restriction enzymes, a single base mutation or a small deletion that alters the final protein product is more likely than a gross alteration in gene structure.

The Polymerase Chain Reaction and Detection of Point Mutations

The PCR has greatly improved the efficiency of detecting single base changes by allowing rapid amplification and analyses of a particular gene or a portion of the gene[93] (Fig. 7–15). The PCR technique is a very powerful tool for molecular diagnostics for the following reasons. First, the dramatic amplification of DNA allows diagnostic analyses using very small amounts of initial starting tissue. For example, sufficient DNA for PCR is routinely extracted from lymphocytes or from cells present in saliva, hair, amniotic fluid, chorionic villi, or other accessible tissue sources. Second, because PCR uses short synthetic oligonucleotides to prime the reaction, it can be readily applied to any gene as long as the DNA sequence is known. Even when the gene sequence is not known, PCR is useful for linkage studies because highly polymorphic sequences (variable number tandem repeats [VNTR]) occurring near the gene can be amplified to allow linkage analyses without relying on the presence of specific alterations in restriction enzyme sites.[94] VNTR's represent repeated elements that are interspersed throughout the genome. Specific distances between the repeats allow them to be used as markers in linkage analyses. Finally, the PCR technique is straightforward enough that it can be readily transferred to different medical centers and laboratories.

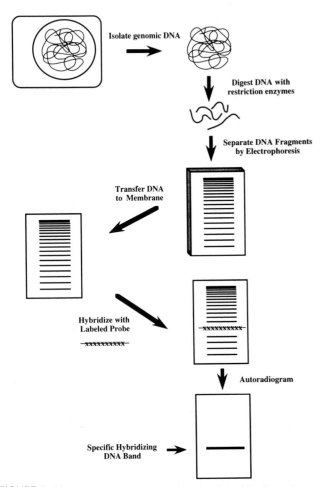

FIGURE 7–14. Southern blot method. The Southern blot is used to analyze gene structure. Genomic DNA is isolated and digested into an array of fragments using restriction enzymes. The DNA is separated according to length by agarose gel electrophoresis and transferred to a membrane. The immobilized DNA is hybridized with a radiolabeled probe that binds only to its complementary sequence. Specific hybridizing bands are detected by autoradiography. In addition to its use for analyzing gene structure, the Southern blot is also used to detect restriction fragment length polymorphisms (RFLP's). RFLP's occur when the sequence of the restriction enzyme site is polymorphic or variable in the population. Consequently, the length of the resulting DNA fragment detected by the probe will be altered by the absence or presence of an RFLP. RFLP's are often used to analyze whether a given phenotype is linked to a marker gene (see Fig. 7–17).

In many cases, the PCR is the starting point for more detailed characterization of a mutation. In early studies to identify a specific mutation, the PCR product is often used for DNA sequencing to establish the location and base change that is present in the gene. Because the amount of DNA provided by PCR is relatively large, it usually is not difficult to subclone the amplified fragment into a plasmid to allow subsequent DNA sequencing. Alternatively, recent protocols and automated DNA sequencing methods allow direct sequencing of the DNA fragment without an intervening subcloning step.[95] In addition to efficiency, direct sequencing has the additional advantage that the sequence analysis is based on a large population of amplified DNA molecules rather than on individual clones that may contain PCR-generated sequence errors (occur approximately 1/3000 bases). Direct DNA sequencing of the PCR product has the advantage that a heterozygous mutation can be detected by the presence of two different nucleotides at the mutant position.

After characterization of specific mutations, several techniques allow more rapid screening for the mutation in other patients. In some methods, the crucial regions of a gene can be screened for mutations by detecting altered mobility during gel electrophoresis. In denaturing gradient gel electrophoresis (DGGE), the PCR primers contain a long stretch of G's and C's that anneal to create a GC clamp.[96] In this manner, the double-stranded DNA can be partially melted during electrophoresis but will be clamped at the end because of the relatively high melting temperature of G-C bonds (three hydrogen bonds for G-C versus two for A-T; see Fig. 7–1). Consequently, the GC clamp emphasizes differences in melting temperatures that result from sequence mismatches caused by mutations. If a mutation is present, a mismatch with the wild-type sequence lowers the melting point of the DNA hybrid, resulting in strand separation and altered mobility in the gel. A similar technique, referred to as *single-stranded conformational polymorphism* (SSCP), is based upon the ability of mutations to cause altered conformation and mobility of single-stranded DNA during nondenaturing electrophoresis.[97] Both DGGE and SSCP can be applied to the PCR products to screen large regions of a gene for mutations and to screen large numbers of patients in separate reactions. At present, SSCP appears to be more readily applied to a wide array of sequences. Both of these methods require that the reaction conditions be established rigorously to avoid false-negative results. It should also be noted that polymorphisms would appear as mutations even if they do not alter amino acid sequence. Thus, it is necessary to sequence the putative mutant regions to definitively establish the presence of a mutation.

After a particular mutation has been identified, oligonucleotide-specific hybridization (OSH) can be useful to es-

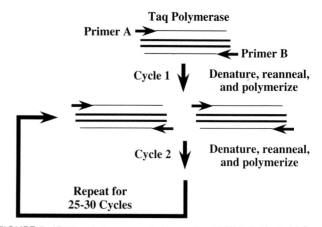

FIGURE 7–15. The polymerase chain reaction (PCR). In the initial cycle of PCR, the double-stranded DNA template is heat denatured to allow primers A and B to anneal and initiate synthesis of a new copy of each strand of DNA. Because Taq polymerase is heat stable, the reaction mixture can be immediately subjected to another round of heat denaturation and new DNA synthesis. In each cycle of PCR, the number of DNA molecules is doubled, resulting in a rapid expansion in the amount of DNA as the cycle number progresses. In a typical reaction of 30 cycles, the amount of DNA is theoretically amplified by about 10^9. PCR has broad applications including DNA diagnostics from small amounts of tissue, quantitative mRNA analysis, cloning, construction of plasmids, and site-directed mutagenesis.

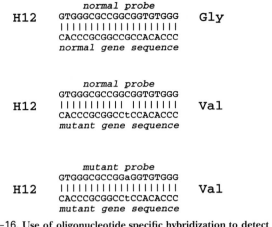

```
        normal probe
H12   GTGGGCGCCGGCGGTGTGGG       Gly
      ||||||||||||||||||||
      CACCCGCGGCCGCCACACCC
       normal gene sequence


        normal probe
H12   GTGGGCGCCGGCGGTGTGGG       Val
      |||||||||| |||||||||
      CACCCGCGGCCtCCACACCC
       mutant gene sequence


        mutant probe
H12   GTGGGCGCCGGaGGTGTGGG       Val
      ||||||||||||||||||||
      CACCCGCGGCCtCCACACCC
       mutant gene sequence
```

FIGURE 7–16. **Use of oligonucleotide specific hybridization to detect *ras* mutations.** Rapid screening for mutations is desirable as the number of different mutants increases and their functional importance is documented. A number of procedures for mutant screening are available. Most of these procedures are based upon the fact that the melting temperature of a mutant wild-type DNA hybrid is reduced relative to that of a wild-type double-stranded DNA hybrid. Oligonucleotide-specific hybridization (OSH) is based on the fact that sequence mismatches cause marked alterations in the melting temperatures of short oligonucleotides (14–25 mers). Consequently, a radiolabeled oligonucleotide probe that contains a common mutation can be hybridized to DNA under conditions in which it hybridizes to mutant but not wild-type sequences. For example, mutations that cause activation of the *ras* genes occur specifically in codons 12 and 61. These mutations prevent GTP hydrolysis, causing the *ras* protein to remain in a constitutively active state. In the example shown, a C to t mutation causes a glycine to valine substitution. If one screens DNA from tumor specimens with the radiolabeled probe for a Val mutation in the Harvey *ras* gene at codon 12 (H12), hybridization occurs only when the complementary mutant sequence is present. *ras* mutations analyzed by this technique have been identified in approximately 30 per cent of thyroid neoplasms.

tablish whether this nucleotide change is present in other family members or in other unrelated patients[98] (Fig. 7–16). For example, specific mutations have been identified that cause constitutive activation of the GTP-binding *ras* and Gsα proteins that are involved in cellular signaling. These mutations prevent GTP hydrolysis that is necessary to inactivate signaling by these proteins. In the case of the *ras* genes (H-*ras*, K-*ras*, N-*ras*), mutations in two different regions of the proteins (codons 12/13 or codon 61) cause constitutive activation. Because the number of nucleotide changes at these positions is limited, it is possible to use oligonucleotides that are complementary to the mutant allele to screen for specific mutations (Fig. 7–16). In this case, it is often practical to amplify samples of DNA from a large number of specimens and apply them to a membrane to screen for different mutations. This technique is based upon the principle that single base pair mismatches cause alterations in hybridization efficiency when short oligonucleotides are used as probes. Consequently, hybridization conditions and control specimens have to be established for each mutant sequence. Oligonucleotide-specific hybridization is most useful when the number of potential mutations is small and when it is necessary to screen large numbers of specimens for mutations. As described below, mutations in proto-oncogenes are being actively investigated to better understand the molecular basis of endocrine neoplasia.

Restriction Fragment Length Polymorphisms and Linkage Studies

Although these techniques and others (see Table 7–3) allow relatively rapid analyses of mutations in specific genes, the genes that cause disorders such as MEN 1 have not been characterized. In this situation, one attempts first to identify the chromosomal location of the responsible gene using cytogenetic techniques or linkage analyses (Fig. 7–17). For inherited disorders, restriction fragment length polymorphisms (RFLP's) can be used to establish whether a candidate gene is near (linked to) a marker gene with a known chromosomal location.[99] The object of these analyses is to develop an accurate method of screening for the familial syndrome and to move progressively closer to the involved gene to allow it to be identified and cloned. An important principle of linkage studies is that the frequency of recombination events is approximately proportionate to the genetic distance between the RFLP marker and the disease gene. Thus, when a series of genetic markers is used to establish linkage to a disease phenotype in large informative kindreds, markers that are closest to the true locus of the disease gene are less likely to undergo recombination events and will attain a higher linkage score. Linkage is usually expressed as a lod score, which is a ratio that reflects the probability that the disease and marker loci are linked rather than unlinked.[100] Lod scores are expressed as the logarithm to the base 10 such that positive numbers favor linkage and negative scores support nonlinkage. Lod scores of +3 are generally accepted as supporting linkage, whereas a score of −2 is consistent with the absence of linkage. When candidate genetic regions have been identified by linkage, more detailed analyses can be performed with anonymous genetic markers. It is often reasonable at this stage to attempt cloning by chromosome walking techniques[101] using traditional genomic libraries or yeast artificial chromosomes, in which large regions of specific chromosomes can be analyzed.[102] *Chromosomal walking* involves using a series of genetic markers to progressively "walk" toward a gene locus based on linkage or structural proximity as defined by mapping techniques. Using these approaches, many of the endocrine diseases with an uncertain molecular pathology should be defined in the next few years (see Table 7–2). The application of different molecular diagnostic procedures to various types of genetic mutations is summarized in Table 7–4.

Functional Studies of Mutant Hormones and Receptors

Identification of a DNA sequence alteration alone is not sufficient to establish that it is responsible for the disease phenotype. First, nucleotide substitutions could represent polymorphisms that are DNA sequence variations that occur in the population as a whole. If the base change occurs in the coding sequence but does not alter an amino acid, it is most likely a polymorphism. However, even if the amino acid sequence is changed, it is still possible that the amino acid substitution is "physiologically silent" and does not significantly alter protein function. One approach for addressing the issue of polymorphisms is to screen a large number (e.g., 100) of normal individuals for the putative

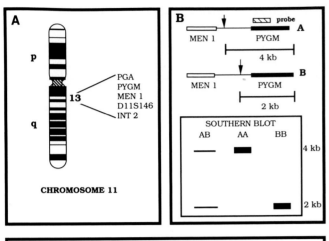

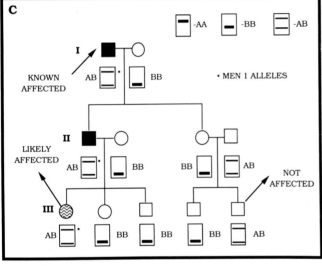

FIGURE 7–17. **Use of restriction fragment length polymorphisms to define the MEN 1 locus.** *A,* Schematic representation of human chromosome 11 and the putative position of the MEN 1 gene at band q13 with surrounding linked genes. Correlation of disease phenotype and inheritance of a specific RFLP allows analysis of linkage. Linkage implies that a given marker gene (e.g., PYGM) is close to a second gene (e.g., MEN 1 locus). Because chromosomes undergo rearrangement in a manner that is proportionate to physical distance separating two loci, a low recombination frequency suggests that the two genes are located near one another. *B,* The use of restriction fragment length polymorphisms is depicted. Separate alleles can be identified through the appearance of a second restriction site on one allele that generates a different sized fragment on a Southern blot when a probe homologous to a gene closely linked to the MEN 1 locus is used. In this case, PYGM, the muscle phosphorylase gene, is depicted. *C,* A hypothetical pedigree of a family with MEN 1 is shown. Alleles of family members are denoted by schematic illustrations of Southern blots. Within the affected family, the disease is carried on the "A" allele (*). Those affected or carrying the disease are shaded. Note that the male in generation II, who is not part of the original family, also possesses the "A" allele polymorphism, but is not affected, indicating that this RFLP analysis is only relevant within a family, not in the general population. (Adapted with permission from Jameson JL, Hollenberg AN: Recent advances in studies of the molecular basis of endocrine disease. Horm Metab Res 24:201, 1992.)

mutation. If the amino acid substitution is found in normals, it is by definition a polymorphism. Codons that are highly conserved across species (presumably implying functional importance) have a higher chance of being mutations. Finally, mutations tend to be "linked" to the disease phenotype when examined in several family members, whereas polymorphisms should sort randomly unless they are located close to the disease locus. Although these determinations of polymorphisms are not entirely reliable,

they are of practical importance because the next steps in assessing the functional importance of a "candidate mutation" can require significant experimental effort.

Assuming there is evidence against a polymorphism, it is almost always possible using recombinant techniques to assess the effect of a mutation in a functional assay. As illustrated in Figure 7–18, recombinant mutant and wild-type proteins can be expressed and subjected to a variety of functional assays. In the example shown, mutant LHβ

TABLE 7–4. MOLECULAR GENETIC DIAGNOSTIC PROCEDURES

METHOD	GENE DELETIONS	GENE REARRANGEMENTS	LOSS OF HETEROZYGOSITY	LINKAGE	POINT MUTATIONS
Cytogenetics			+		
Southern blot	+	+			
RFLP			+	+	
VNTR			+	+	
PCR	+	+			+
Direct DNA sequencing					+
RNase cleavage					+
OSH					+
DGGE					+
SSCP					+

RFLP, restriction fragment length polymorphism; VNTR, variable number tandem repeat; PCR, polymerase chain reaction; OSH, oligonucleotide specific hybridization; DGGE, denaturing gradient gel electrophoresis; SSCP, single-stranded conformational polymorphism.

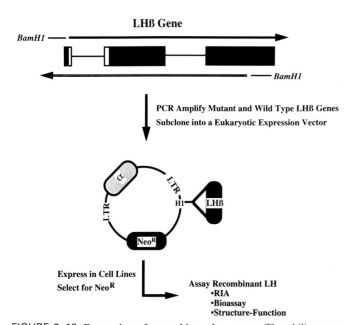

FIGURE 7–18. **Expression of recombinant hormones.** The ability to express recombinant hormones is an important application of molecular biology techniques. Recombinant insulin, growth hormone, and glycoprotein hormones are among many hormones that have found a role in clinical medicine. A variety of expression systems are available including *E. coli*, baculovirus, vaccinia virus, and mammalian cells. The choice of expression system is dictated by a variety of issues including characteristics of the protein, desired production level, and cost. A strategy for producing recombinant LH is illustrated for the purpose of analyzing the functional consequences of mutations in the LHβ gene.[103] The LHβ gene is amplified by PCR from genomic DNA and inserted into a eukaryotic expression vector. The presence of a viral long terminal repeat (LTR) provides a strong promoter to drive expression in transfected mammalian cell lines. Because LH is a heterodimer containing an α and β subunit, the vector is designed to contain a copy of the α gene to allow the genes to be coexpressed from the same plasmid. A third gene encoding neomycin resistance allows selection and isolation of clonal cell lines that have been successfully transfected with the expression vector. Secreted LH can be analyzed by structural methods and for its functional properties. This approach allows delineation of hormone domains important for α-β subunit dimerization, receptor binding, and activation. When scaled up for bioreactors, similar strategies can be used for the production of large quantities of hormones.

can be assessed for its ability to form an α-β heterodimer, to undergo glycosylation, to bind to its receptor, and to activate receptor signaling pathways.[103] Mutant enzymes such as 21-hydroxylase can be analyzed for their ability to bind substrate or to carry out catalysis.[5] Mutant receptors such as the insulin receptor have been subjected to an array of functional tests including insulin binding, receptor autophosphorylation, receptor internalization, and receptor stability.[4] Nuclear receptors, such as the thyroid hormone receptor, can be analyzed not only for their ability to bind thyroid hormone and to identify DNA target sequences, but also for their capacity to function as transcription factors in transient gene expression assays (see Ch. 37).[3] These types of studies not only establish whether a given mutation is of functional importance but also provide insight into protein structure-function and hormone action. In most instances, these "experiments of nature" provide rapid identification of crucial functional domains because identification of the mutations is biased by the presence of a recognizable clinical phenotype.

Overview of Inherited Endocrine Disorders

Because the number of mutations in different endocrine genes is already staggering,[1, 2] it is not practical to describe each of these disorders in a comprehensive manner. The interested reader is referred to individual chapters and to the references in Table 7–2. It is, nevertheless, useful to provide an overview of mutations that occur at different steps in endocrine pathways if for no other reason than to indicate the breadth and heterogeneous nature of disorders caused by gene defects.

Hormone Mutations

One might have expected that mutations in hormones would represent a common molecular basis for endocrine disorders. However, this does not appear to be the case. For the most part, causes of hormone deficiency syndromes remain enigmatic. For example, growth hormone deficiency rarely involves deletions or mutations in the growth hormone gene.[104] Rather, most cases can be attributed to an inherited or acquired hypothalamic defect that could involve GHRH, the GHRH-producing neuron, or one of the regulatory pathways that control GHRH secretion. Attempts to attribute GH deficiency to GHRH mutations have not been successful, and most patients respond to exogenous GHRH, implying that GHRH receptor mutations may also be uncommon. In some respects, GH deficiency is reminiscent of idiopathic hypogonadotropic hypogonadism, which is not due to a GnRH gene defect but rather to defects in a gene that controls migration of the GnRH-producing neurons.[1, 2] A relatively rare form of GH deficiency does involve a deletion of the GH gene (about 35 cases),[90] and to date represents one of the few well-studied hormone mutations. In early studies, Southern blot analyses of DNA from affected children demonstrated a homozygous deletion of the GH gene, consistent with the autosomal recessive inheritance pattern (Fig. 7–19). On the other hand, heterozygous carriers had a single copy of the GH gene with no apparent clinical manifestations of growth hormone deficiency.

The GH gene is a member of a large gene cluster that also includes a growth hormone variant gene as well as several structurally related chorionic somatomammotropin genes and pseudogenes (highly homologous but functionally inactive relatives of a normal gene). Because such gene clusters contain multiple homologous DNA sequences arranged in tandem, they are particularly prone to undergo recombination, leading to gene duplication or deletion. It has been proposed that mispairing of areas with sequence homology can lead to unequal crossover during meiosis with resultant gene duplication on one chromosome and gene deletion on the other chromosome.[91, 105] Thus, the frequency of growth hormone gene deletions might have been increased by having a number of related gene sequences arranged in tandem. Aside from applications in family studies to detect affected individuals or carrier states, there are potential clinical implications for recognizing the subgroup of patients with GH gene deletions. Many of these children develop antibodies after administration of exogenous GH, perhaps because that antigen was not present during development of immunocompetence.

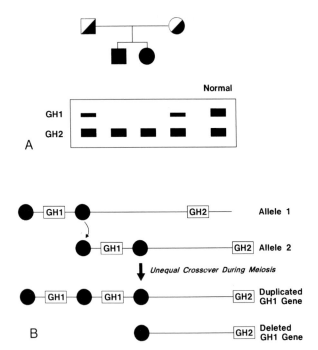

FIGURE 7–19. **Use of Southern blots to detect GH gene deletions.** *A,* Southern blot analysis of a pedigree with deletion of the GH gene. Heterozygous parents are denoted by half-shaded symbols and homozygous children are shown with fully shaded symbols. The GH gene is a member of a gene cluster that also includes a GH variant gene and several chorionic somatomammotropin genes. The Southern blot shows the appearance of the detected GH genes in a schematic fashion. GH1 refers to the GH gene and GH2 refers to the GH variant gene. For clarity, hybridization to the related chorionic somatomammotropin genes is not shown. The blot is consistent with all family members having a GH2 gene on each chromosome. Each parent has only one copy of the GH1 gene. The children have each inherited the parental chromosome that lacks the GH1 gene. In a larger pedigree, the disorder would sort in an autosomal recessive manner. Deletion of the GH gene probably occurs by unequal crossing over during meiosis *(B),* a phenomenon that is made more likely by the presence of repetitive copies of the GH genes.[90] (Adapted with permission from Jameson JL, Arnold A: Clinical Review 5: Recombinant DNA strategies for determining the molecular basis for endocrine disorders. J Clin Endocrinol Metab 70:301, 1990. Copyright © by the Endocrine Society.)

Other mutations that have been described in hormones are listed in Table 7–2. Even with this short list, it is apparent that a number of important insights can be gained from such studies. The mutations in preproinsulin indicate that mutations that prevent processing of the preproinsulin precursor molecule cause secretion of biologically inactive insulin molecules.[106] A mutation in the signal sequence of PTH causes hypoparathyroidism, even when only one of the two PTH genes is affected.[107] It has been shown that this mutation interferes with hormone transport and processing, leading to the hypothesis that the mutant molecule could block the transport of other cellular proteins, including the normal PTH protein. Mutations in the vasopressin gene appear to be somewhat analogous to the PTH mutation. An autosomal dominant form of diabetes insipidus is caused by heterozygous mutations in neurophysin, the precursor protein for vasopressin.[108] The fact that the amino acid changes occur in the carboxy-terminal precursor protein rather than in vasopressin itself suggests that abnormalities in protein processing may prevent vasopressin synthesis or result in cellular toxicity such that the remaining

normal allele is unable to produce enough vasopressin to maintain normal water homeostasis. Homozygous mutations in the TSHβ and LHβ subunits cause hypothyroidism and hypogonadism, respectively. One TSHβ-subunit mutation defines a region of the molecule that is required for heterodimerization with the α subunit,[109] whereas others either truncate the protein or interfere with its biological activity.[110] The LHβ-subunit mutation defines a region that is crucial for binding to the LH receptor.[103] In these and other autosomal recessive disorders, there is an opportunity to examine the effect of a "gene knockout" in humans. Thus, elimination of functional hormones such as growth hormone, LH, or TSH allows one to attribute specific physiological roles to the hormone that may be difficult to discern in normal individuals. For example, complete elimination of LH, with retention of normal FSH, allows the functions of these hormones to be discriminated. As described above, creation of gene knockouts by homologous recombination in transgenic mice is an active area of research that allows creation of animal models for studying hormone and receptor function.

Binding Protein Mutations

The binding protein mutations cause little in the way of clinical disease, but if not recognized they often lead to unnecessary treatment. Knowledge of the molecular basis of these disorders is useful to better understand the physiology of the hormone system involved as well as to gain insight into hormone-protein interactions. As shown in Table 7–2, these defects are largely confined to proteins that bind thyroid hormone (see Ch. 52).

Thyroxine-binding globulin (TBG) is the major thyroid hormone transport protein in the serum. Abnormalities in its production are not rare, occurring in approximately 1/2500 male births.[111] Complete TBG deficiency is X-linked and is clinically apparent in males who are euthyroid but have very low levels of thyroid hormone in the serum. These patients are often mistakenly treated for hypothyroidism. Although large deletions of the TBG gene have not been found,[112] a number of different point mutations can cause functional loss of TBG by either alterations in protein structure or glycosylation.[111]

In addition to TBG, thyroid hormone binds in the serum to albumin and transthyretin (thyroxine-binding prealbumin). Euthyroid hyperthyroxinemia can result from either an altered form of binding protein or excess production of one of the binding proteins. TBG excess most commonly results from effects of drugs or hormones, although familial examples have been described. Familial dysalbuminemic hyperthyroxinemia is an autosomal dominant condition in which albumin has an increased affinity for thyroid hormone.[113] It is characterized by elevated levels of total T_4 with normal levels of free T_4 and TSH. The presence of abnormal binding proteins can be detected using electrophoretic analyses of serum thyroid hormone binding proteins. Transthyretin can be overproduced, usually in patients with pancreatic endocrine tumors, or it can be present in a mutant form that has an increased affinity for thyroxine caused by a single amino acid substitution.[114] The mutant form of transthyretin also causes a form of dysalbuminemic hyperthyroxinemia resulting in elevated total T_4 without apparent clinical consequences. Patients with this and similar thyroid hormone binding protein disorders need to be distinguished from individuals who are truly hyperthyroid.

Membrane Receptor Mutations

In Laron-type dwarfism, a receptor or postreceptor defect had been proposed because growth hormone levels were high, IGF levels were low, and patients failed to respond to growth hormone therapy. Such hormone resistance is characteristic of many receptor mutations, although alterations in signaling pathways can result in a similar phenotype (e.g., pseudohypoparathyroidism). After the putative growth hormone receptor was initially cloned, two patients with Laron dwarfism were found to have mutations of the gene.[115] This finding confirmed that the clone for the receptor was correct in addition to demonstrating that defects in the GH receptor can cause Laron dwarfism. In further studies, a number of different point mutations have been identified in the growth hormone receptor.[116]

Mutations in the insulin receptor have been characterized extensively in patients with severe hormone resistance. Multiple missense and nonsense mutations have been described in different regions of the receptor, causing different insulin resistance phenotypes such as leprechaunism, the Rabson-Mendenhall syndrome, and Type A insulin resistance.[4] The mechanisms of insulin receptor inactivation and their relationship to these syndromes and others are summarized in Chapter 91.

An X-linked form of vasopressin resistance has now been attributed to mutations in the vasopressin 2 receptor on the long arm of the X chromosome.[117–119] Like many other genetic disorders, vasopressin receptor mutations include a wide array of different mutants, suggesting that because the disorder does not significantly alter viability, spontaneous mutations have arisen independently to result in similar clinical phenotypes. Defects in other membrane receptors in the endocrine system have not been well defined to date at the molecular level. There have also been descriptions of thyroid-stimulating hormone[120] and ACTH resistance syndromes.[121]

Nuclear Receptor Mutations

In addition to the mutations in membrane receptors (i.e, insulin resistance), hormone resistance syndromes also occur as a consequence of defects in nuclear receptors (i.e., resistance to thyroid hormone). The syndrome of resistance to thyroid hormone (RTH) is representative of nuclear receptor resistance syndromes, but it also illustrates some unique aspects of a disease that is inherited in a dominant manner (see Chs. 37 and 52). RTH, which was first described by Refetoff et al.,[122] is characterized by elevated circulating levels of free thyroid hormone, inappropriately normal or increased levels of TSH, and the absence of clinical manifestations of thyrotoxicosis. Two thyroid hormone receptor genes, designated TRα and TRβ, encode highly homologous proteins with different tissue distributions. Genetic analyses show linkage between the RTH syndrome and the β-receptor gene locus in several kindreds.[123, 124] This observation has since been extended by sequencing β-receptor genes in multiple different families with this disorder. In the families that have a

dominant mode of transmission, affected individuals have mutations in one allele of the β-receptor gene together with a second normal allele.[125, 126] Interestingly, these and additional mutations are clustered in two different regions of the receptor carboxy-terminal, ligand-binding domain (Fig. 7–20). The mutant receptors fail to bind thyroxine or bind hormone with reduced affinity. Consequently, their ability to modulate target gene expression is impaired.[127] Because the affected individuals possess a second normal β-receptor allele and two normal α-receptor alleles, the mutant receptor has been proposed to inhibit the activity of normal receptors. In support of this concept, the receptor mutants have been shown to block the action of the wild-type receptors in transient gene expression assays, probably by binding to DNA target sites where the mutant receptors function as antagonists.[128]

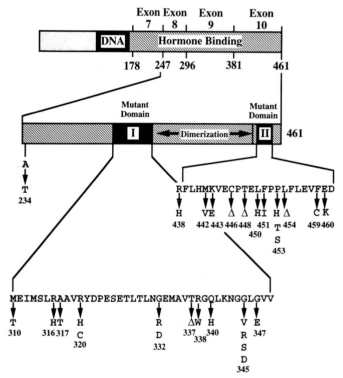

FIGURE 7–20. **Locations of mutations in the thyroid hormone receptor that cause resistance to thyroid hormone.** The thyroid hormone receptor β is illustrated schematically, including the central DNA binding (*hatched*) and carboxy-terminal ligand binding domains. The locations of hydrophobic repeats in the putative dimerization domain are indicated by arrows. The ligand binding domain is expanded to allow illustration of the sites of mutations. Mutations are shown in single letter amino acid code. Note that in some locations (e.g., amino acids 345, 453) more than one type of mutation has occurred. In addition, certain mutations have occurred in several apparently unrelated kindreds (not shown). Deletions and frameshift mutations are shown as Δ and fs, respectively. It is notable that no naturally occurring mutations have occurred in the DNA binding domain. In addition, the mutations appear to be clustered into two relatively restricted areas that reside on either side of the putative dimerization domain. The locations of the mutations are consistent with current models for how the mutant receptor acts in a dominant manner to antagonize normal receptor function.[3] According to this model, the mutant receptor retains the ability to dimerize with cofactors and bind to DNA with high affinity to block the ability of normal receptors to bind to DNA target sites. (Adapted with permission from Nagaya T, Jameson JL: Thyroid hormone receptor dimerization is required for dominant negative inhibition by mutations that cause thyroid hormone resistance. J Biol Chem 268:15766, 1993.)

Mutations have also been identified in several other members of the nuclear hormone receptor family. Syndromes of androgen resistance represent one of the more common and well-studied receptor defects.[6] These disorders exhibit sex-linked transmission, consistent with the location of the androgen receptor on the X chromosome. One of the striking features of this syndrome is its broad phenotypic spectrum that includes at one end complete testicular feminization and at the other end men with subtle defects in virilization. Coupled to this phenotypic spectrum, a number of different receptor-binding defects have been described ranging from undetectable or reduced binding activity to normal androgen binding with qualitative defects in receptor stability. The androgen receptor gene has now been sequenced in a relatively large number of affected individuals, although primarily those with severe forms of resistance.[6] Many mutations result in premature termination codons, although gene deletions and single amino acid substitutions have also been found. No clinical effects of the heterozygous condition have been noted in females with androgen receptor mutations. In female carriers of the mutation, X inactivation would likely allow expression of only one of the receptor alleles within a given cell, and the dominant negative activity seen with the thyroid hormone receptor may not be possible.

Hypocalcemic vitamin D–resistant rickets is a rare inherited form of rickets that is unresponsive to treatment with 1,25-dihydroxyvitamin D.[129, 130] The disease has a recessive pattern of inheritance and most cases, if not all, have involved consanguineous families. A variety of mutations have been identified in different kindreds including amino acid substitutions in the zinc-finger DNA binding domains as well as nonsense mutations that cause premature termination. The naturally occurring mutations in the vitamin D receptor have been useful for providing insights into the biological role of vitamin D in skin differentiation, hair growth, and lymphocyte function.[131, 132]

In familial glucocorticoid resistance, serum concentrations of cortisol and cortisol production rates are elevated without the characteristic clinical manifestations of glucocorticoid excess. ACTH levels are inappropriately increased, indicating reduced feedback inhibition at the level of the hypothalamic-pituitary axis. Because ACTH also stimulates adrenal androgens and mineralocorticoids, precocious puberty and hypertension can be features of this syndrome. Sequencing of the glucocorticoid receptor cDNA in one family revealed a single amino acid substitution in the ligand-binding domain.[132] The mutation reduced the affinity of glucocorticoids and prevented transcriptional activation by the mutant receptor in transient gene expression assays. An autosomal codominant mode of inheritance has been suggested in view of the fact that heterozygotes are mildly affected. By analogy with mutations in the ligand binding domain of the thyroid hormone receptor, it is possible that the mutant GR can function in a dominant negative manner to block the activity of the normal receptor.

It is notable that inherited mutations have not been described for the estrogen or progesterone receptors. It is possible that mutations in these receptors would not be compatible with life, and almost certainly they would interfere with reproductive potential, thereby limiting transmission from one generation to the next. Estrogen receptor variants and mutations have been described in breast cancers, although a role in pathogenesis has not been clearly defined.[133, 134]

Transcription Factor Mutations

One of the final steps in hormone action involves effects on gene expression, mediated via transcription factors. Even though the characterization of transcription factors is still a nascent area of research, defects have already been identified. In principle, the nuclear hormone receptors could be classified as transcription factors and described under this category. Not surprisingly, some of the other transcription factor mutations have involved developmental pathways. Elucidation of mutations in the testis-determining factor (TDF) gene provides a dramatic example of one these developmental mutations.[135] The Y chromosome determines male sex by virtue of encoding the TDF. In the absence of a Y chromosome, ovaries form, and a female develops. The TDF gene was located by examining rare cases of phenotypic females with an XY genotype. It was hypothesized that these individuals might have deleted or mutated TDF genes on the Y chromosome. The sex-determining region on the short arm of the Y chromosome was initially delineated by mapping large deletions or translocations of the Y chromosome that resulted in a female phenotype. This region of the human Y chromosome contained a candidate gene, termed SRY, that is highly conserved in mammals and is expressed in gonadal tissue during a developmental window that corresponds to the period when the testis begins to form. Three lines of evidence support the view that SRY is the testis-determining gene. First, in two XY females who did not have large deletions of the Y chromosome, mutations were found in SRY which were not present in their fathers.[135] Second, there is a deletion in the mouse homologue of SRY in sex-reversed mice.[136] Third, expression of SRY in transgenic mice is sufficient to induce testis development in females.[137] Although these data indicate that SRY is the crucial gene for an early step in male sex determination, it is likely that SRY is only one of several developmental switches that initiate a cascade of sex-specific gene expression. Mutations in other genes in such a cascade could also give rise to the female phenotype in cases in which SRY is normal.

XX males have been shown to have translocations of Y chromosome–specific sequences onto the pseudoautosomal region of the X chromosome.[138, 139] These translocated Y chromosome sequences contain SRY. Sterility in XX males may reflect the presence of two X chromosomes (analogous to Klinefelter's syndrome) or the absence of additional Y chromosome sequences that are required for fertility.

The transcription factor, Pit-1, was first identified on the basis of its binding to multiple sites in the growth hormone and prolactin promoters.[46, 47] Pit-1 expression is restricted to the pituitary gland, and the protein is found only in somatotrophs, lactotrophs, and thyrotrophs.[140] Pit-1 mutations have been identified in several strains of mice that have specific deficits of GH, Prl, and TSH.[141] These data confirm a central role for Pit-1 in the development of these cell types and/or the expression of these genes. Similar patterns of pituitary hormone deficiencies have been described in humans[142] who have also been shown to have mutations in Pit-1. Interestingly, different Pit-1 mutations result in autosomal recessive[48, 50] and autosomal dominant[49] inheritance patterns; this suggests that the distinct mutations have different effects on Pit-1 function. For example, it is possible that the recessive mutation involves an inactivated form of Pit-1, whereas the dominant disorder may involve a dominant negative mutation analogous to that for the thyroid hormone receptor.

Endocrine Syndromes

In addition to the MEN syndromes (see below), progress has been made recently for several other classic endocrine syndromes. Kallmann's syndrome, or idiopathic hypogonadotropic hypogonadism (IHH) associated with anosmia, is an inherited disorder that is caused by GnRH deficiency. Several different inheritance patterns have been described, including autosomal recessive, X-linked, and autosomal dominant with incomplete penetrance.[143, 144] In contrast to an animal model of this disorder (the hypogonadal mouse), in which there is a GnRH gene deletion,[102] all IHH patients examined to date appear to have an intact GnRH gene.[145] Furthermore, the sequence of the GnRH gene in several different individuals with IHH has been shown to be normal.[146, 147] Thus, it appears that IHH in the human, unlike the hypogonadal mouse model, may involve defects in the processes that regulate development of GnRH-producing neurons or expression of the GnRH gene rather than defects in the gene itself.[148, 149] Genetic linkage studies provided evidence for a candidate gene on the short arm of the X chromosome (Xp22.3) in some patients with the X-linked form of Kallmann's syndrome[150, 151] and mutations in the KAL gene have been found in several individuals with the syndrome.[148, 149] Coupled with the recent finding that GnRH neurons migrate into the hypothalamus from the olfactory placode,[148, 152] it is plausible that the KAL gene on the X chromosome is involved in the migration of the GnRH neurons as well as development of the olfactory tract.[153] These observations are consistent with a model in which a defect in this gene causes Kallmann's syndrome and might account for some of its phenotypic variants in that different degrees of developmental aberrations in neuronal migration could lead to isolated anosmia, IHH, or both.

Prader-Willi syndrome is characterized by developmental delay, hypotonia, hypogonadism, and obesity. It is caused by deletions of chromosome 15q11-13.[154] Interestingly, Angelman's syndrome is associated with cytogenetically indistinguishable deletions of chromosome 15, but it is phenotypically distinct, resulting in severe mental retardation, hypotonia, ataxia, and inappropriate laughter. Genetic imprinting (alterations in genomic expression that occur during development) has been proposed to explain the phenotypic differences in these two syndromes.[155, 156] Specifically, Prader-Willi syndrome is associated with a paternally derived chromosome 15 containing the deletion, whereas Angelman's syndrome occurs when the deletion resides on the maternally derived chromosome 15.[157, 158] These findings, along with other observations that occur in uniparental disomy, support the hypothesis of genetic imprinting at this locus, suggesting that certain genes are differentially silenced during gametogenesis in males and females. Identification of the gene or genes involved in these syndromes should help to clarify the effects of imprinting.

Congenital adrenal hypoplasia with hypogonadism is an X-linked recessive disorder that causes adrenal insufficiency in infancy or early childhood.[159] Through study of patients with interstitial deletions of the X chromosome, the AH locus has been mapped in the region Xp21.3-p21.2. The disease is associated with hypogonadotropic hypogonadism, but it is distinct from Kallmann's syndrome, which has been localized to a nearby region on the X chromosome. In contrast to individuals with Kallmann's syndrome, patients with AH exhibit subnormal gonadotropin responses after administration of pulsatile GnRH. The gene defect in AH has not been determined, but it may cause a defect in pituitary gland function.

Steroidogenic Enzyme Mutations

Because a number of enzymatic steps are required for steroid hormone biosynthesis and metabolism, it is not surprising that defects occur in multiple different enzymes, giving rise to distinct clinical syndromes. Deficiency of 21-hydroxylase is the most common cause of CAH.[160] 21-Hydroxylase is responsible for conversion of progesterone to corticosterone in the mineralocorticoid pathway and for conversion of 17-hydroxyprogesterone to 11-deoxycortisol in the glucocorticoid pathway. Because of decreased cortisol production, excess ACTH is secreted, leading to stimulation of the adrenal gland and overproduction of precursor steroids, including adrenal androgens.

Deficiency of 21-hydroxylase encompasses a broad phenotypic spectrum. The severe classic form occurs in approximately 1/5000 to 1/20,000 births; less severe nonclassic forms occur as frequently as 1/30 to 1/100 births in certain genetic populations. In females affected with the classic form of the disease, hypersecretion of adrenal androgens during fetal development causes ambiguous external genitalia, whereas in males the classic form is usually recognized because of severe salt wasting due to combined mineralocorticoid and glucocorticoid deficiency. In the nonclassic form, prenatal virilization does not occur, but virilization of variable severity occurs postnatally.

Many of the earlier clinical observations regarding CAH are now well explained by the molecular basis for the disease.[5] The 21-hydroxylase locus is on the short arm of chromosome 6, adjacent to the HLA locus, explaining previous findings that HLA typing was useful for predicting disease risk (the HLA locus is linked to the 21-hydroxylase locus). There are two 21-hydroxylase genes, A and B. The 21A gene is a functionally inactive pseudogene, whereas the adjacent 21B gene is the active copy. The 21-hydroxylase genes appear to have been duplicated along with the adjacent C4A and C4B complement genes. A large number of different types of deletions and point mutations of the 21B gene have been described. Large deletions and rearrangements probably occur in 10 to 20 per cent of cases. On the other hand, small deletions and point mutations are relatively common. Interestingly, many of the mutations in the 21B gene correspond to sequences in the inactive 21A gene. These data have been interpreted as evidence for gene conversion in which sequences from the adjacent 21A gene are substituted for sequences in 21B, probably as a consequence of a mispairing and DNA repair mechanism. The inheritance of CAH is autosomal recessive. Heterozygotes are typically unaffected clinically and are detected only by hormonal testing. The classic form of the disease is due to large deletions or severe mutations of both 21B alleles, whereas the nonclassic form of the disease is caused by one of several combinations of severe and mildly affected 21B alleles. Thus, the variability in clinical phenotype appears to be the consequence of a high degree of heterogeneity at the genetic level. Prenatal testing for CAH is now possible using either HLA typing or DNA analyses.[161, 162] It is important to recognize the disorder during the first trimester for glucocorticoids to ameliorate prenatal virilization in females.

Mutations in the 11β-hydroxylase and 17α-hydroxylase genes are also classified under CAH because impaired production of cortisol causes elevation of ACTH and consequently adrenal stimulation. Mutations in 11β-hydroxylase cause androgen excess and virilization but are distinguished clinically from 21-hydroxylase mutations by mineralocorticoid excess, which causes hypertension in about two-thirds of patients.[163] In contrast, defects in 17α-hydroxylase cause sex steroid deficiency with overproduction of mineralocorticoids, resulting in hypertension and hypokalemia. Recognition of mutations in the P450c17 gene led to the finding that a single protein had two different enzymatic activities (17α-hydroxylase and 17,20 lyase) that were previously thought to represent different proteins.[164]

Defects in the enzyme 5α-reductase result in a complex phenotype of male pseudohermaphroditism.[165] 5α-Reductase causes conversion of testosterone to dihydrotestosterone, an androgen that plays an important role in development of male external genitalia. These individuals have an XY karyotype and are born with ambiguous genitalia characterized as pseudovaginal perineoscrotal hypospadias. At puberty, there is masculinization with good muscle development and enlargement of the phallus, but the prostate remains small and beard growth is scanty. In some cultures where the prevalence of the disease is high, affected individuals are raised as girls but change gender identity at puberty.[165] 5α-Reductase is encoded by two enzymes designated 1 and 2. 5α-Reductase 2 is the major enzyme in genital tissue and is the site of mutations that cause male pseudohermaphroditism. As with 21-hydroxylase deficiency, a number of different sites in the enzyme have been mutated in different families, and many affected individuals are compound heterozygotes.[166]

Defects in thyroid peroxidase are characterized by hypothyroidism and goiter, presumably as a result of prolonged thyroid gland stimulation by TSH. The disorder is manifested in the homozygous state. In one individual, there is a short insertion in the eighth exon of the thyroid peroxidase gene.[167] Based on previous biochemical studies, defects in thyroid peroxidase may represent a relatively common cause of inborn errors of thyroid hormone synthesis (see Ch. 52).

Glucocorticoid remediable hypertension is characterized by high levels of abnormal adrenal steroids 18-oxocortisol and 18-hydroxycortisol and a variable degree of hyperaldosteronism. Because production of these steroids occurs in a region of the adrenal cortex that is under the control of ACTH, their production is reduced by administration of glucocorticoids. This disorder is now known to result from an interesting gene rearrangement (see Ch. 155).[168] The genes encoding aldosterone synthetase and steroid 11β-hydroxylase are normally arranged in tandem on chromosome 8q. Aldosterone synthetase is expressed in the zona glomerulosa, where it is involved in aldosterone production, whereas 11β-hydroxylase is expressed in the ACTH-dependent fasciculata as well as in the glomerulosa. These two genes are 95 per cent identical, predisposing to gene duplication by unequal crossing over. Because the fusion gene contains the regulatory regions of 11β-hydroxylase and the coding sequence of aldosterone synthetase, the latter enzyme is subjected to an abnormal pattern of expression in the ACTH-dependent zone of the adrenal gland, resulting in overproduction of mineralocorticoids.

SOMATIC MUTATIONS THAT CAUSE ENDOCRINE NEOPLASIA

Multiple Endocrine Neoplasia Syndromes

Multiple endocrine neoplasia syndromes have long been recognized as predispositions to endocrine tumor development that are transmitted in an autosomal dominant manner. Both syndromes involve the parathyroid glands. However, MEN 1 is associated with adenomas of the pituitary and pancreas (see Ch. 151, first part) whereas MEN 2 is associated with adrenal (pheochromocytomas) and thyroid C cell (medullary carcinoma) neoplasia (see Ch. 151, second part).

The MEN syndromes represent good examples of the experimental approaches that are required to identify and characterize unknown genes that cause well-characterized phenotypes. A crucial first step is to determine the chromosome on which a candidate MEN gene resides. Subsequently, the position of the disease-causing gene can be more precisely mapped in relation to known genes and other DNA markers on that chromosome. For MEN 1 and 2, candidate genes have been mapped to chromosomes 11 and 10, respectively, using linkage analyses.[169, 170] To perform linkage studies, maternally or paternally derived allelic variants (DNA polymorphisms, RFLP's) need to be distinguished and their inheritance tracked within a family. As described above, after identification of a polymorphism, the degree of correlation between inheritance of a specific DNA variant and inheritance of the disease can be assessed. The application of linkage analysis to the MEN problem is illustrated in Figure 7–17. The MEN 1 locus has been found to be near the muscle phosphorylase gene (PYGM), which is known to be located on chromosome 11, band q13.[169, 171] Digestion of DNA with an enzyme that contains a polymorphic site near the PYGM allows the maternal and paternal alleles to be distinguished. In this manner, it is possible to determine whether the MEN phenotype is linked to a particular PYGM polymorphism. As shown in Figure 7–17, the affected grandfather in generation 1 is heterozygous for the polymorphism, and one can assume that one of the two alleles carries the mutant form of the MEN 1 gene. Analysis of his descendants allows determination of whether the A or the B allele is responsible for the syndrome in this family. In the second generation, a son receives the A allele from his affected father and acquires the syndrome, whereas a daughter receives the B allele from her affected father and is unaffected. The assignment of the disease gene to the A allele is verified in the third generation.

Several caveats are illustrated by this family. First, phenotypic assignments for MEN 1 cannot be made reliably until an individual is in the third or fourth decade, and there is always the possibility of making a false-negative phenotypic assignment of someone who will develop the disease at a later date or at a subclinical level. Second, linkage studies require relatively large families as well as the presence of informative polymorphic markers. Finally, the information derived from such a linkage analysis is applicable only to the family under investigation. Note that other individuals in the population with the A type allele are not likely to carry the MEN gene, as the polymorphism is only a marker of which chromosome the mutant MEN gene is carried on in this particular kindred. Each of these points emphasizes the importance of identifying the actual MEN 1 disease gene so that molecular diagnostics can be performed directly.

Speculation on the function of the MEN 1 gene has centered on its role as a possible tumor suppressor gene. Tumor tissue from patients with MEN 1 has been shown to have loss of heterozygosity at the putative MEN 1 location.[169] In this situation, it is hypothesized that the inherited (presumably defective) MEN 1 allele remains and that somatic loss of the normal MEN 1 gene represents a "second hit" at the suppressor gene locus, thereby leading to tumorigenesis. This scenario is analogous to the two-hit model for loss of retinoblastoma gene function, a well-characterized example of a tumor suppressor gene.[172] Further analyses of the deletions that occur in the normal chromosome can provide valuable information concerning the minimal sequence that is required to alter the MEN gene.[171]

Unlike MEN 1, loss of heterozygosity is not seen in tumors from patients with MEN 2 at the proposed loci on chromosome 10, suggesting that a different pathophysiology exists for MEN 2.[173] In the case of MEN 2, affected individuals often have thyroid C-cell hyperplasia in childhood before the development of medullary thyroid carcinoma. This observation is consistent with a model in which the MEN 2 gene predisposes to hyperplastic growth with a second and perhaps distinct somatic mutation leading to tumorigenesis and clonal proliferation. Recently, mutations in the *ret* proto-oncogene, a putative tyrosine kinase receptor, have been identified as the probable cause of MEN 2a.[174] In several MEN 2 kindreds, distinct *ret* mutations were found in a cluster of cysteines located at the juncture of the extracellular and transmembrane domains of the protein. The functional effects of these mutations are not currently understood. Interestingly, rearrangements of *ret* had previously been identified in papillary thyroid carcinoma, leading to its designation as a "PTC" oncogene[175, 176] (see below). Identification of MEN 2 gene carriers is particularly important because of the consequences of nonrecognition of medullary thyroid carcinoma or pheochromocytoma. In the future, screening for *ret* mutations may allow high-risk individuals to undergo more intense endocrine screening, whereas low-risk individuals

may not require such extensive hormone testing (see Ch. 151, second part).

Concept of Clonality in Endocrine Tumors

As noted above, in MEN 2, there is clear hyperplasia of thyroid C cells before the development of medullary thyroid carcinoma. Examples of autonomous hyperplastic growth have also been described as a rare cause of Cushing's disease, in nesidioblastosis, and in adrenal tumors. However, the phenomenon of hyperplasia leading to tumorigenesis is rare in most other endocrine tumors. Almost all pituitary, thyroid, and parathyroid tumors are clonal in origin[177–181]; that is, the tumor tissue represents an expansion of a single cell as opposed to polyclonal proliferation of multiple cells. The concept of clonality is important because clonal tumors presumably arise as a result of a somatic mutation that either provides a growth advantage to the precursor tumor cell or prevents the cells from reaching terminal differentiation and senescence. In contrast, polyclonal expansion implies that an exogenous stimulus such as a growth factor is stimulating cell proliferation. Of course, these models are not mutually exclusive. For example, a growth factor could cause hyperplasia and predispose cells to the acquisition of a somatic mutation that would subsequently cause clonal expansion. Similarly, an early somatic mutation might result in overproduction of a growth factor that is capable of causing polyclonal responses.

Despite these theoretical areas of overlap between monoclonal and polyclonal models for tumorigenesis, it is apparent that most clinically relevant endocrine tumors studied to date are monoclonal. Several lines of investigation establish monoclonal origin. For example, because of X-chromosome inactivation in females (Lyon's hypothesis), it is possible to determine whether tumors have arisen from a single cell, which would result in all tumor cells showing the same pattern of X-inactivation. Alternatively, multiple-cell origin would result in an even distribution of X-inactivated chromosomes. In practice, this method involves using a polymorphic site on the X chromosome to distinguish the maternal and paternal alleles in combination with a procedure that takes advantage of differential sensitivity of certain restriction enzymes to the methylation patterns that occur on activated and inactivated X-chromosomes.[182] This technique reveals a single X chromosome allele in clonal tumors, whereas both alleles are seen in polyclonal tumors. A second line of evidence for clonal origin is that gene rearrangements or chromosomal losses are seen uniformly in the tumor cells; this suggests that these defects either contribute to tumorigenesis or were fortuitously present in the original tumor cell. In either case, these alterations support monoclonal expansion. Given the probable monoclonal origin of most endocrine tumors, it is reasonable to seek the somatic mutations that lead to clonal expansion. This issue is of particular interest in endocrine tumors, many of which produce symptoms because of the overproduction of hormones as well as by their mass and invasive characteristics. Thus, somatic mutations in functioning endocrine tumors might be predicted to involve hormone-signaling pathways or to at least preserve the differentiated phenotype of the endocrine cell such that hormone biosynthesis continues.

Signaling System Mutations

Mutations at several steps along signaling pathways are theoretically capable of contributing to tumorigenesis if they impinge upon cell cycle regulation or alter the ability of the cell to grow independent of the usual constraints of contact inhibition. One can envision mutations occurring in membrane receptors, in the G proteins that they couple with, in enzymes that mediate receptor signaling, and in the targets of these kinases such as nuclear transcription factors. There is a growing list of examples of mutations at each of these steps. Mutations or oncogenic homologues of growth factor receptors such as v-*erb* B (homologue of EGF receptor) and v-*sis* (homologue of PDGF receptor) mimic pathways that normally control cell growth and represent a potent step in tumorigenesis. There is now evidence that somatic mutations in membrane receptors, such as the TSH receptor, can lead to constitutive activation of downstream signaling pathways, resulting in altered cell growth.

For many peptide hormone receptors, signals are transduced via G proteins. G proteins are GTPases that are active when GTP is bound and inactivated after GTP hydrolysis to GDP. Mutations in G proteins have been described in several different types of endocrine neoplasia.[183] For example, mutations in the Gsα subunit have been identified in somatotroph adenomas, either at codon 201 or 227.[184] Both of these mutations inhibit GTP hydrolysis and thereby cause constitutive activation of the Gsα subunit. Activation of Gsα in this cell type stimulates adenylate cyclase, leading to elevated cAMP levels, a situation that may mimic GHRH stimulation. As a result, the Gsα mutation may cause excess GH secretion and possibly contribute to abnormal cell growth as well. Importantly, these mutations are somatic rather than inherited, as evidenced by the fact that G proteins from other tissues do not contain the amino acid substitution. Gsα mutations have also been identified in autonomous thyroid adenomas, and mutations in the Gi2 subunit have been found in adrenal and ovarian tumors.[183]

It is interesting to note that Gsα mutations identical to those described in somatotroph adenomas also occur in McCune-Albright syndrome.[185] In McCune-Albright, the mutations occur early in development such that the tissue distribution of the mutation is broad rather than being restricted to somatotroph cells. Nevertheless, patients with McCune-Albright are predisposed to somatotroph adenomas along with the more typical clinical features of polyostotic fibrous dysplasia, autonomous ovarian function, café au lait spots, and autonomous thyroid or adrenal nodules. Each of these features is caused by the Gsα mutation, and the variable clinical phenotype is thought to result in part from the point during development when the Gsα mutation arises, leading to different degrees of mosaicism. In some respects, the clinical phenotype of McCune-Albright appears to reflect the ability of a constitutively active Gsα mutation to cause abnormal cell growth and function in specific tissues. Thus, one might predict that spontaneous Gsα mutations can also cause tumors in these same tissues

in the patients without McCune-Albright syndrome. If this is the case, then it may be most reasonable to consider the effects of Gsα mutations in terms of a spectrum. At one end is McCune-Albright, in which multiple tissues are affected. Mosaics with Gsα mutations that occur later in development may have only a subset of tissues affected. At the other end of the spectrum, Gsα mutations that occur in fully developed tissues may lead to thyroid or pituitary nodules without other manifestation of McCune-Albright syndrome.

Albright hereditary osteodystrophy (AHO) is also caused by a Gsα mutation, although in this case the mutation eliminates Gsα function rather than causing constitutive activity. AHO is characterized by short stature, obesity, and skeletal abnormalities. Resistance to several Gsα protein coupled hormones such as PTH, TSH, LH, and FSH is characteristic. Different Gsα mutations have been described in several families with AHO.[186, 187] Interestingly, the disease is inherited in an autosomal dominant manner, and patients with the same mutation can exhibit different clinical phenotypes of hormone resistance. This suggests that the heterozygous deficiency in Gsα is sufficient to cause the disease and that other variables dictate its clinical expression.

ras is also a GTPase and it is structurally related to the G proteins. The *ras* P21 proteins are involved in the control of cell growth and differentiation. Somatic mutations in the three *ras* genes have been identified in a number of different human malignancies, including tumors of the endocrine system.[188] *ras* mutations at two specific loci (codons 12/13, codon 61) convert the proteins into oncogenes. Like the G protein mutations just described, mutations at either site in *ras* inhibit GTPase activity. *ras* mutations occur in approximately 30 per cent of thyroid tumors[189] but appear to be uncommon in other endocrine tumors such as pituitary and parathyroid.[180]

The thyroid gland is a relatively good model for studies of multistep tumorigenesis because of the well-characterized histological subtypes and extensive clinical information concerning risk factors and prognosis (Fig. 7–21)[189, 190] (see Ch. 50). Gsα mutations have been described in a limited group of thyroid tumors, including some autonomous nodules. Thus, by analogy with the Gsα mutations associated with GH producing pituitary adenomas, constitutive activation of the adenylate cyclase pathway in the thyroid might be expected to mimic some of the effects of TSH, which is known to stimulate production of cAMP. In this manner, the Gsα mutation may bypass the requirement of TSH stimulation, resulting in autonomy. *Ras* mutations are seen in benign as well as malignant thyroid tumors, and there is not a clear predilection for papillary versus follicular cancers.[191–193] Thus, *ras* mutations do not appear to be sufficient for transformation, but they may contribute to abnormal growth control in combination with other somatic mutations. A gene rearrangement has been described in papillary carcinomas that appears to be relatively specific for this type of tumor.[175] This rearrangement involves an intrachromosomal inversion on the long arm of chromosome 10.[176] The result of the inversion is that a gene encoding a putative tyrosine kinase (*ret*) is brought under the control of a new promoter, presumably altering its pattern and/or level of expression. The rearranged oncogene is referred to as PTC for papillary thy-

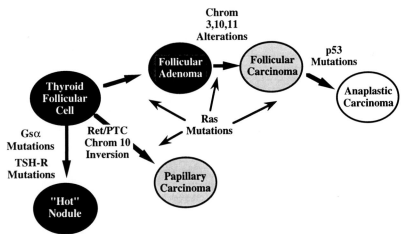

FIGURE 7–21. **Different types of somatic mutations associated with thyroid neoplasia.** Most endocrine neoplasms are monoclonal in origin, implying the presence of one or more somatic mutations. Among endocrine tumors, mutations associated with the progression of thyroid neoplasia have been studied in the most detail.[189] The thyroid follicular cell is shown to progress to an autonomous nodule upon acquisition of a Gsα mutation that activates the cAMP pathway. Papillary carcinoma is often associated with an inversion on chromosome 10 that juxtaposes a tyrosine kinase *(ret)* under the control of a new promoter to create the PTC oncogene. Progression of follicular adenomas to carcinomas appears to correlate with selected chromosomal losses, presumably because of the loss of tumor suppressor genes. *Ras* mutations have been found in benign and malignant thyroid tumors perhaps representing one of multiple "hits" that accumulate during tumor progression. The appearance of p53 mutations accompanies the formation of anaplastic carcinomas. None of these mutations has been proved to be sufficient for thyroid tumorigenesis and many additional types of mutations remain to be identified. Nevertheless, these correlations represent an initial step toward understanding the biological basis for tumor progression.

roid carcinoma and is observed in approximately 20 per cent of papillary carcinomas.[194] As already noted, mutations in *ret* have also been identified in patients with MEN IIa, indicating that this oncogene can be activated in several different ways.[174] Other mutations, including potential point mutations, must also be capable of causing transformation to the papillary tumor phenotype, as most tumors do not contain the rearranged PTC oncogene. Studies of loss of heterozygosity, presumably involving tumor suppressor genes, have revealed deletions on several different chromosomes. Deletions on chromosomes 3, 10, and 11 occur with greatest frequency and are particularly associated with follicular carcinomas. Not surprisingly, anaplastic carcinomas have accumulated the largest array of oncogene "hits," including a high prevalence of mutations in the p53 tumor suppressor gene.[190] Thus, thyroid tumorigenesis is not unlike the situation that is evolving with other well-studied models such as colon and lung carcinomas in which a stepwise accumulation of different mutations is associated with more invasive tumor types.[195] Additional studies may clarify whether specific types of mutations are correlated with characteristic histologic tumor types. Ultimately, it is hoped that characterization of oncogene mutations will provide biological markers of diagnostic and prognostic value.

A novel mechanism for tumorigenesis has been provided by studies of parathyroid adenomas. A subset of parathyroid tumors were found to contain rearrangements of the PTH gene.[196] Analysis of the translocation revealed that the PTH promoter was fused to a member of the cyclin D family.[197] The translocation involved an intrachromosomal rearrangement on chromosome 11. The fusion gene is referred to as PRAD for parathyroid adenomatosis. Because cyclins regulate progress through the cell cycle, it is likely that expression of cyclin D1 from the PTH promoter

rather than its native promoter causes the tumor cell to have altered growth regulation. This particular somatic rearrangement is an interesting example of how monoclonal expansion could occur because the mutation involves a gene that is directly involved in cell proliferation. In addition to playing a role in the development of a subset of parathyroid adenomas, there is emerging evidence that cyclin D1 may be involved in the development of some breast tumors and lymphomas.[198]

In summary, endocrine neoplasms, while not necessarily representing the most aggressive forms of cancer, are providing important models for identification of new oncogenes as well as the steps involved in the progression of tumors from the benign to the malignant phenotype. Because many oncogenes involve alterations of cellular signaling pathways that have been well characterized in hormone-secreting cells, it is likely endocrine tumors will provide important models for the pathophysiology of neoplasia in future studies.

ACKNOWLEDGMENTS: The author is grateful to Anthony Hollenberg and Andrew Arnold for their contributions to earlier versions of this subject matter. This work was supported by NIH grants DK 42144, HD 23519, and HD 29164.

REFERENCES

1. Jameson JL, Arnold A: Clinical Review 5: Recombinant DNA strategies for determining the molecular basis for endocrine disorders. J Clin Endocrinol Metab 70:301–307, 1990.
2. Jameson JL, Hollenberg AN: Recent advances in studies of the molecular basis of endocrine disease. Horm Metab Res 24:201–209, 1992.
3. Jameson JL: Thyroid hormone resistance: pathophysiology at the molecular level. J Clin Endocrinol Metab 74:708–711, 1992.

4. Taylor SI, Cama A, Accili D, et al: Genetic basis of endocrine disease. 1. Molecular genetics of insulin resistant diabetes mellitus. J Clin Endocrinol Metab 73:1158–1163, 1991.

5. White PC, New MI: Genetic basis of endocrine disease 2: Congenital adrenal hyperplasia due to 21-hydroxylase deficiency. J Clin Endocrinol Metab 74:6–11, 1992.

6. McPhaul MJ, Marcelli M, Zoppi S, et al: Genetic basis of endocrine disease. 4. The spectrum of mutations in the androgen receptor gene that causes androgen resistance. J Clin Endocrinol Metab 76:17–23, 1993.

7. Watson JD, Crick FHC: Molecular structure of nucleic acids: A structure for deoxynucleic acids. Nature 171:737–738, 1953.

8. Berry MJ, Banu L, Chen YY, et al: Recognition of UGA as a selenocysteine codon in type I deiodinase requires sequences in the 3′ untranslated region. Nature 353:273–276, 1991.

9. Rosenfeld MG, Emeson RB, Yeakley JM, et al: Calcitonin gene-related peptide: a neuropeptide generated as a consequence of tissue-specific, developmentally regulated alternative RNA processing events. Ann N Y Acad Sci 657:1–17, 1992.

10. Jonas V, Lin CR, Kawashima E, et al: Alternative RNA processing events in human calcitonin/calcitonin gene-related peptide gene expression. Proc Natl Acad Sci U S A 82:1994–1998, 1985.

11. Delsert CD, Rosenfeld MG: A tissue-specific small nuclear ribonucleoprotein and the regulated splicing of the calcitonin/calcitonin gene-related protein transcript. J Biol Chem 267:14573–14579, 1992.

12. Izumo S, Mahdavi V: Thyroid hormone receptor alpha isoforms generated by alternative splicing differentially activate myosin HC gene transcription. Nature 334:539–542, 1988.

13. Mitsuhashi T, Tennyson GE, Nikodem VM: Alternative splicing generates messages encoding rat c-erbA proteins that do not bind thyroid hormone. Proc Natl Acad Sci U S A 85:5804–5808, 1988.

14. Leff SE, Rosenfeld MG, Evans RM: Complex transcriptional units: diversity in gene expression by alternative RNA processing. Annu Rev Biochem 55:1091–1117, 1986.

15. Carrazana EJ, Pasieka KB, Majzoub JA: The vasopressin mRNA poly(A) tract is unusually long and increases during stimulation of vasopressin gene expression in vivo. Mol Cell Biol 8:2267–2274, 1988.

16. Robinson BG, Frim DM, Schwartz WJ, Majzoub JA: Vasopressin mRNA in the suprachiasmatic nuclei: daily regulation of polyadenylate tail length. Science 241:342–344, 1988.

17. Zingg HH, Lefebvre DL, Almazan G: Regulation of poly(A) tail size of vasopressin mRNA. J Biol Chem 263:11041–11043, 1988.

18. Krane IM, Spindel ER, Chin WW: Thyroid hormone decreases the stability and the poly(A) tract length of rat thyrotropin beta-subunit messenger RNA. Mol Endocrinol 5:469–475, 1991.

19. Weiss J, Crowley W Jr., Jameson JL: Pulsatile gonadotropin-releasing hormone modifies polyadenylation of gonadotropin subunit messenger ribonucleic acids. Endocrinology 130:415–420, 1992.

20. Shyu AB, Greenberg ME, Belasco JG: The c-fos transcript is targeted for rapid decay by two distinct mRNA degradation pathways. Genes Dev 3:60–72, 1989.

21. Pachter JS, Yen TJ, Cleveland DW: Autoregulation of tubulin expression is achieved through specific degradation of polysomal tubulin mRNAs. Cell 51:283–292, 1987.

22. Yen TJ, Machlin PS, Cleveland DW: Autoregulated instability of beta-tubulin mRNAs by recognition of the nascent amino terminus of beta-tubulin. Nature 334:580–585, 1988.

23. Huynh TV, Young RA, Davis RW: Constructing and screening cDNA libraries in λgt10 and λgt11. In Glover DM (ed): DNA Cloning Techniques: A Practical Approach. Vol 2. New York, IRL Press, 1985, pp 49–78.

24. Okayama H, Berg P: High-efficiency cloning of full-length cDNA. Mol Cell Biol 2:161–170, 1982.

25. Okayama H, Berg P: A cDNA cloning vector that permits expression of cDNA inserts in mammalian cells. Mol Cell Biol 3:280–289, 1983.

26. Ish-Horowitz D, Burke JF: Rapid and efficient cosmid cloning. Nucleic Acids Res 9:2989–2998, 1981.

27. Benton WD, Davis RW: Screening λgt recombinant clones by hybridization to single plaques in situ. Science 196:180, 1977.

28. Dugaiczyk A, Boyer HW, Goodman HM: Ligation of EcoRI endonuclease-generated DNA fragments into linear and circular structures. J Mol Biol 96:174–184, 1975.

29. Birnboim HC, Doly J: A rapid alkaline extraction method for screening recombinant plasmid DNA. Nucleic Acids Res 7:1513–1523, 1979.

30. Maxam AM, Gilbert W: A new method for sequencing DNA. Proc Natl Acad Sci USA 74:560–564, 1977.

31. Sanger F, Nicklen S, Coulson AR: DNA sequencing with chain-terminating inhibitors. Proc Natl Acad Sci USA 74:5463–5467, 1977.

32. Maniatis T, Hardison RC, Lacy E, et al: The isolation of structural genes from libraries of eucaryotic DNA. Cell 15:687–701, 1978.

33. Lodish HF, Rose JK: Relative importance of 7-methylguanosine in ribosome binding and translation of vesicular stomatitis virus mRNA in wheat germ and reticulocyte cell-free systems. J Biol Chem 252:1181–1188, 1977.

34. Studier FW, Moffatt BA: Use of bacteriophage T7 RNA polymerase to direct selective high-level expression of cloned genes. J Mol Biol 189:113–130, 1986.

35. Mulligan RC, Berg P: Expression of a bacterial gene in mammalian cells. Science 209:1422–1427, 1980.

36. Alwine JC, Kemps DJ, Stark GR: Method for detection of specific RNAs in agarose gels by transfer to diazobenzyloxymethyl-paper and hybridization with DNA probes. Proc Natl Acad Sci USA 74:5350–5354, 1977.

37. Melton DA, Krieg PA, Rebagliati MR, et al: Efficient in vitro synthesis of biologically active RNA and RNA hybridization probes from plasmids containing a bacteriophage SP6 promoter. Nucleic Acids Res 12:7035–7056, 1984.

38. Wang AM, Doyle MV, Mark DF: Quantitation of mRNA by the polymerase chain reaction. Proc Natl Acad Sci U S A 86:9717–9721, 1989.

39. Pardue ML: In situ hybridization. In Higgins BD, Ha SJ (eds): Nucleic Acid Hybridization: A Practical Approach. Oxford, IRL Press, 1985, pp 179–202.

40. McKnight GS, Palmiter RD: Transcriptional regulation of the ovalbumin and conalbumin genes by steroid hormones in chick oviduct. J Biol Chem 254:9050–9058, 1979.

41. Rodgers JR, Johnson ML, Rosen JM: Measurement of mRNA concentration and mRNA half-life as a function of hormonal treatment. Methods Enzymol 109:572–592, 1985.

42. Graham FL, van der Eb AJ: A new technique for the assay of infectivity of human adenovirus 5 DNA. Virology 52:456, 1973.

43. Gorman CM, Moffat LF, Howard BH: Recombinant genomes which express chloramphenicol acetyltransferase in mammalian cells. Mol Cell Biol 2:1044–1051, 1982.

44. Rigby PW: Three in one and one in three: it all depends on TBP. Cell 72:7–10, 1993.

45. Zawel L, Reinberg D: Initiation of transcription by RNA polymerase II: a multi-step process. Prog Nucleic Acid Res Mol Biol 44:67–108, 1993.

46. Ingraham HA, Chen RP, Mangalam HJ, et al: A tissue-specific transcription factor containing a homeodomain specifies a pituitary phenotype. Cell 55:519–529, 1988.

47. Castrillo JL, Bodner M, Karin M: Purification of growth hormone-specific transcription factor GHF-1 containing homeobox. Science 243:814–817, 1989.

48. Pfaffle RW, DiMattia GE, Parks JS, et al: Mutation of the POU-specific domain of Pit-1 and hypopituitarism without pituitary hypoplasia. Science 257:1118–1121, 1992.

49. Radovick S, Nations M, Du Y, et al: A mutation in the POU-homeodomain of Pit-1 responsible for combined pituitary hormone deficiency. Science 257:1115–1118, 1992.

50. Tatsumi K, Miyai K, Notomi T, et al: Cretinism with combined hormone deficiency caused by a mutation in the PIT1 gene. Nat Genet 1:56–58, 1992.

51. Habener JF: Cyclic AMP response element binding proteins: A cornucopia of transcription factors. Mol Endocrinol 4:1087–1094, 1990.

52. Hunter T, Karin M: The regulation of transcription by phosphorylation. Cell 70:375–387, 1992.

53. Richard-Foy H, Hager GL: Sequence-specific positioning of nucleosomes over the steroid-inducible MMTV promoter. EMBO J 6:2321–2328, 1987.

54. Archer TK, Lefebvre P, Wolford RG, Hager GL: Transcription factor loading on the MMTV promoter: a bimodal mechanism for promoter activation. Science 255:1573–1576, 1992.

55. Ing NH, Beekman JM, Tsai SY, et al: Members of the steroid hormone receptor superfamily interact with TFIIB (S300-II). J Biol Chem 267:17617–17623, 1992.

56. Lin YS, Ha I, Maldonado E, et al: Binding of general transcription factor TFIIB to an acidic activating region. Nature 353:569–571, 1991.

57. Hagemeier C, Bannister AJ, Cook A, Kouzarides T: The activation domain of transcription factor PU.1 binds the retinoblastoma (RB) protein and the transcription factor TFIID in vitro: RB shows sequence similarity to TFIID and TFIIB. Proc Natl Acad Sci U S A 90:1580–1584, 1993.

58. Ruppert S, Wang EH, Tjian R: Cloning and expression of human TAFII250: a TBP-associated factor implicated in cell-cycle regulation. Nature 362:175–179, 1993.

59. Hoey T, Weinzierl RO, Gill G, et al: Molecular cloning and functional analysis of Drosophila TAF110 reveal properties expected of coactivators. Cell 72:247–260, 1993.

60. Galas D, Schmitz A: DNase footprinting: A simple method for the detection of protein-DNA binding specificity. Nucl Acids Res 5:3157–3170, 1978.

61. Singh H, Sen R, Baltimore D, Sharp PA: A nuclear factor that binds to a conserved sequence motif in transcriptional control elements of immunoglobulin genes. Nature 319:154–158, 1986.

62. Fried M, Crothers DM: Equilibria and kinetics of lac repressor-operator interactions by polyacrylamide gel electrophoresis. Nucleic Acids Res 9:6505–6525, 1981.

63. Kadonaga JT, Tjian R: Affinity purification of sequence-specific DNA binding proteins. Proc Natl Acad Sci U S A 83:5889–5893, 1986.

64. Singh H, LeBowitz JH, Baldwin AS, Sharp PA: Molecular cloning of an enhancer binding protein: Isolation by screening of an expression library with a recognition site DNA. Cell 52:415–423, 1988.

65. Hoeffler JP, Meyer TE, Yun Y, et al: Cyclic AMP-responsive DNA-binding protein: structure based on a cloned placental cDNA. Science 242:1430–1433, 1988.

66. Smith GE, Summers MD, Fraser MJ: Production of human beta interferon in insect cells infected with a baculovirus expression vector. Mol Cell Biol 3:2156–2165, 1983.

67. Schwall RH, Nikolics K, Szonyi E, et al: Recombinant expression and characterization of human activin A. Mol Endocrinol 2:1237–1242, 1988.

68. Schmelzer CH, Burton LE, Tamony CM, et al: Purification and characterization of recombinant human activin B. Biochim Biophys Acta 1039:135–141, 1990.

69. Vale W, Rivier J, Vaughan J, et al: Purification and characterization of an FSH releasing protein from porcine ovarian follicular fluid. Nature 321:776–779, 1986.

70. Ling N, Ying SY, Ueno N, et al: Pituitary FSH is released by a heterodimer of the beta-subunits from the two forms of inhibin. Nature 321:779–782, 1986.

71. Umesono K, Evans RM: Determinants of target gene specificity for steroid/thyroid hormone receptors. Cell 57:1139–1146, 1989.

72. Erickson RP: Creating animal models of genetic disease. Am J Hum Genet 43:582–586, 1988.

73. Hanahan D: Transgenic mice as probes into complex systems. Science 246:1265–1275, 1989.

74. Lipes MA, Eisenbarth GS: Transgenic mouse models of type I diabetes. Diabetes 39:879–884, 1990.

75. Mason AJ, Pitts SL, Nikolics K, et al: The hypogonadal mouse: reproductive functions restored by gene therapy. Science 234:1372–1378, 1986.

76. Mason AJ, Hayflick JS, Zoeller RT, et al: A deletion truncating the gonadotropin-releasing hormone gene is responsible for hypogonadism in the hpg mouse. Science 234:1366–1371, 1986.

77. Tremblay Y, Tretjakoff I, Peterson A, et al: Pituitary-specific expression and glucocorticoid regulation of a proopiomelanocortin fusion gene in transgenic mice. Proc Natl Acad Sci U S A 85:8890–8894, 1988.

78. Liu B, Hammer GD, Rubinstein M, et al: Identification of DNA elements cooperatively activating proopiomelanocortin gene expression in the pituitary glands of transgenic mice. Mol Cell Biol 12:3978–3990, 1992.

79. Palmiter RD, Brinster RL, Hammer RE, et al: Dramatic growth of mice that develop from eggs microinjected with metallothionein-growth hormone fusion genes. Nature 300:611–615, 1982.

80. Hanahan D: Oncogenes in transgenic mice. Nature 312:503–504, 1984.

81. Behringer RR, Mathews LS, Palmiter RD, Brinster RL: Cell lineage ablation in transgenic mice by cell-specific expression of a toxin gene. Dwarf mice produced by genetic ablation of growth hormone-expressing cells. Cell 62:609, 1990.

82. Kendall SK, Saunders TL, Jin L, et al: Targeted ablation of pituitary gonadotropes in transgenic mice. Mol Endocrinol 5:2025–2036, 1991.

83. Hanahan D: Heritable formation of pancreatic beta-cell tumours in transgenic mice expressing recombinant insulin/simian virus 40 oncogenes. Nature 315:115–122, 1985.

84. Mellon PL, Windle JJ, Goldsmith PC, et al: Immortalization of hypothalamic GnRH neurons by genetically targeted tumorigenesis. Neuron 5:1–10, 1990.

85. Windle JJ, Weiner RI, Mellon PL: Cell lines of the pituitary gonadotrope lineage derived by targeted oncogenesis in transgenic mice. Mol Endocrinol 4:597–603, 1990.

86. Mansour SL, Thomas KR, Capecchi MR: Disruption of the proto-oncogene int-2 in mouse embryo-derived stem cells: a general strategy for targeting mutations to non-selectable genes. Nature 336:348–352, 1988.

87. Matzuk MM, Finegold MJ, Su JG, et al: Alpha-inhibin is a tumour-suppressor gene with gonadal specificity in mice. Nature 360:313–319, 1992.

88. Struthers RS, Vale WW, Arias C, et al: Somatotroph hypoplasia and dwarfism in transgenic mice expressing a non-phosphorylatable CREB mutant. Nature 350:622–624, 1991.

89. McKusick VA: Mendelian Inheritance in Man. Baltimore, The Johns Hopkins University Press, 1988, pp 1–1626.

90. Vnencak-Jones CL, Phillips JA 3rd, Chen EY, Seeburg PH: Molecular basis of human growth hormone gene deletions. Proc Natl Acad Sci U S A 85:5615–5619, 1988.

91. Vnencak-Jones CL, Phillips JA: Hot spots for growth hormone gene deletions in homologous regions outside of Alu repeats. Science 250:1745–1748, 1990.

92. Southern EM: Detection of specific sequences among DNA fragments separated by gel electrophoresis. J Mol Biol 98:503–517, 1975.

93. Saiki RK, Gelfand DH, Stoffel S, et al: Primer-directed enzymatic amplification of DNA with a thermostable DNA polymerase. Science 239:487–491, 1988.

94. Nakamura Y, Leppert M, O'Connell P, et al: Variable number of tandem repeat (VNTR) markers for human gene mapping. Science 235:1616–1622, 1987.

95. Zhang X, Kousoulas KG: Direct sequencing of PCR-amplified high GC DNA. Biotechniques 14:376–377, 1993.

96. Top B: A simple method to attach a universal 50-bp GC-clamp to PCR fragments used for mutation analysis by DGGE. PCR Methods Appl 2:83–85, 1992.

97. Poduslo SE, Dean M, Kolch U, O'Brien SJ: Detecting high-resolution polymorphisms in human coding loci by combining PCR and single-strand conformation polymorphism (SSCP) analysis. Am J Hum Genet 49:106–111, 1991.

98. Verlaan-de Vries M, Bogaard ME, van den Elst H, et al: A dot-blot screening procedure for mutated ras oncogenes using synthetic oligodeoxynucleotides. Gene 50:313–320., 1986.

99. Davies KE, Read A: Molecular Basis of Inherited Disease. Oxford, IRL Press, 1988, pp 1–77.

100. Ott J: Estimation of the recombination fraction in human pedigrees: efficient computation of the likelihood for human linkage studies. Am J Hum Genet 26:588–597, 1974.

101. Lacks SA, Greenberg B: Sequential cloning by a vector walking along the chromosome. Gene 104:11–17, 1991.

102. Capecchi MR: Mouse genetics. YACs to the rescue. Nature 362:205–206, 1993.

103. Weiss J, Axelrod L, Whitcomb RW, et al: Hypogonadism caused by a single amino acid substitution in the β-subunit of luteinizing hormone. N Engl J Med 326:179–183, 1991.

104. Rogol AD, Blizzard RM, Foley T Jr, et al: Growth hormone releasing hormone and growth hormone: genetic studies in familial growth hormone deficiency. Pediatr Res 19:489–492, 1985.

105. Vnencak-Jones, CL, Phillips JA 3rd, Wang DF: Use of polymerase chain reaction in detection of growth hormone gene deletions. J Clin Endocrinol Metab 70:1550–1553, 1990.

106. Steiner DF, Tager HS, Chan SJ, et al: Lessons learned from molecular biology of insulin-gene mutations. Diabetes Care 13:600–609, 1990.

107. Arnold A, Horst SA, Gardella TJ, et al: Mutation of the signal peptide-encoding region of the preproparathyroid hormone gene in familial isolated hypoparathyroidism. J Clin Invest 86:1084–1087, 1990.

108. Ito M, Mori Y, Oiso Y, Saito H: A single base substitution in the coding region for neurophysin II associated with familial central diabetes insipidus. J Clin Invest 87:725–728, 1991.

109. Hayashizaki Y, Hiraoka Y, Endo Y, et al: Thyroid-stimulating hor-

mone (TSH) deficiency caused by a single base substitution in the CAGYC region of the beta-subunit. EMBO J 8:2291–2296, 1989.

110. Dacou-Voutetakis C, Feltquate DM, Drakopoulou M, et al: Familial hypothyroidism caused by a nonsense mutation in the thyroid-stimulating hormone beta-subunit gene. Am J Hum Genet 46:988–993, 1990.

111. Mori Y, Seino S, Takeda K, et al: A mutation causing reduced biological activity and stability of thyroxine-binding globulin probably as a result of abnormal glycosylation of the molecule. Mol Endocrinol 3:575–579, 1989.

112. Mori Y, Refetoff S, Flink IL, et al: Detection of the thyroxine-binding globulin (TBG) gene in six unrelated families with complete TBG deficiency. J Clin Endocrinol Metab 67:727–733, 1988.

113. Yeo PP, Yabu Y, Etzkorn JR, et al: A four generation study of familial dysalbuminemic hyperthyroxinemia: diagnosis in the presence of an acquired excess of thyroxine-binding globulin. J Endocrinol Invest 10:33–38, 1987.

114. Moses AC, Rosen HN, Moller DE, et al: A point mutation in transthyretin increases affinity for thyroxine and produces euthyroid hyperthyroxinemia. J Clin Invest 86:2025–2033, 1990.

115. Godowski PJ, Leung DW, Meacham LR, et al: Characterization of the human growth hormone receptor gene and demonstration of a partial gene deletion in two patients with Laron-type dwarfism. Proc Natl Acad Sci U S A 86:8083–8087, 1989.

116. Amselem S, Sobrier ML, Duquesnoy P, et al: Recurrent nonsense mutations in the growth hormone receptor from patients with Laron dwarfism. J Clin Invest 87:1098–1102, 1991.

117. Merendino J Jr., Speigel AM, Crawford JD, et al: Brief report: a mutation in the vasopressin V2-receptor gene in a kindred with X-linked nephrogenic diabetes insipidus. N Engl J Med 328:1538–1541, 1993.

118. Holtzman EJ, Harris H Jr., Kolakowski L Jr., et al: Brief report: a molecular defect in the vasopressin V2-receptor gene causing nephrogenic diabetes insipidus. N Engl J Med 328:1534–1537, 1993.

119. Lightman SL: Molecular insights into diabetes insipidus. N Engl J Med 328:1562–1563, 1993.

120. Stanbury JB, Rocmans P, Buhler UK, Ochi Y: Congenital hypothyroidism with impaired thyroid response to thyrotropin. N Engl J Med 279:1132–1136, 1968.

121. Verhoeven GF, Wilson JD: The syndromes of primary hormone resistance. Metabolism 28:253–289, 1979.

122. Refetoff S, DeWind LT, DeGroot LJ: Familial syndrome combining deaf-mutism, stuppled epiphyses, goiter and abnormally high PBI: possible target organ refractoriness to thyroid hormone. J Clin Endocrinol Metab 27:279–294, 1967.

123. Refetoff S, Weiss RE, Usala SJ: The syndromes of resistance to thyroid hormone. Endocr Rev 14:348–399, 1993.

124. Usala SJ, Weintraub BD: Thyroid hormone resistance syndromes. Trends Endocrinol Metab 2:140–144, 1991.

125. Sakurai A, Takeda K, Ain K, et al: Generalized resistance to thyroid hormone associated with a mutation in the ligand-binding domain of the human thyroid hormone receptor beta. Proc Natl Acad Sci U S A 86:8977–8981, 1989.

126. Usala SJ, Tennyson GE, Bale AE, et al: A base mutation of the C-erbA beta thyroid hormone receptor in a kindred with generalized thyroid hormone resistance. Molecular heterogeneity in two other kindreds. J Clin Invest 85:93–100, 1990.

127. Chatterjee VK, Nagaya T, Madison LD, et al: Thyroid hormone resistance syndrome. Inhibition of normal receptor function by mutant thyroid hormone receptors. J Clin Invest 87:1977–1984, 1991.

128. Nagaya T, Madison LD, Jameson JL: Thyroid hormone receptor mutants that cause resistance to thyroid hormone. Evidence for receptor competition for DNA sequences in target genes. J Biol Chem 267:13014–13019, 1992.

129. Hughes MR, Malloy PJ, Kieback DG, et al: Point mutations in the human vitamin D receptor gene associated with hypocalcemic rickets. Science 242:1702–1705, 1988.

130. Malloy PJ, Hochberg Z, Tiosano D, et al: The molecular basis of hereditary 1,25-dihydroxyvitamin D3 resistant rickets in seven related families. J Clin Invest 86:2071–2079, 1990.

131. Feldman D, Malloy PJ: Hereditary 1,25-dihydroxyvitamin D resistant rickets: molecular basis and implications for the role of 1,25(OH)2D3 in normal physiology. Mol Cell Endocrinol 72:C57–62, 1990.

132. Hurley DM, Accili D, Stratakis CA, et al: Point mutation causing a single amino acid substitution in the hormone binding domain of the glucocorticoid receptor in familial glucocorticoid resistance. J Clin Invest 87:680–686, 1991.

133. McGuire WL, Chamness GC, Fuqua SA: The importance of normal and abnormal oestrogen receptor in breast cancer. Cancer Surv 14:31–40, 1992.

134. Fuqua SA, Chamness GC, McGuire WL: Estrogen receptor mutations in breast cancer. J Cell Biochem 51:135–139, 1993.

135. Berta P, Hawkins JR, Sinclair AH, et al: Genetic evidence equating SRY and the testis-determining factor. Nature 348:448–450, 1990.

136. Gubbay J, Collignon J, Koopman P, et al: A gene mapping to the sex-determining region of the mouse Y chromosome is a member of a novel family of embryonically expressed genes. Nature 346:245–250, 1990.

137. Koopman P, Gubbay J, Vivian N, et al: Male development of chromosomally female mice transgenic for Sry. Nature 351:117–121, 1991.

138. Petit C, de la Chapelle A, Levilliers J, et al: An abnormal terminal X-Y interchange accounts for most but not all cases of human XX maleness. Cell 49:595–602, 1987.

139. Page DC, Brown LG, la Chapelle A: Exchange of terminal portions of X- and Y-chromosomal short arms in human XX males. Nature 328:437–440, 1987.

140. Simmons DM, Voss JW, Ingraham HA, et al: Pituitary cell phenotypes involve cell-specific Pit-1 mRNA translation and synergistic interactions with other classes of transcription factors. Genes Dev 4:695–711, 1990.

141. Li S, Crenshaw EB 3rd, Rawson EJ, et al: Dwarf locus mutants lacking three pituitary cell types result from mutations in the POU-domain gene pit-1. Nature 347:528–533, 1990.

142. Wit JM, Drayer NM, Jansen M, et al: Total deficiency of growth hormone and prolactin, and partial deficiency of thyroid stimulating hormone in two Dutch families: a new variant of hereditary pituitary deficiency. Horm Res 32:170–177, 1989.

143. Santen RJ, Paulsen CA: Hypogonadotropic eunuchoidism. I. Clinical study of the mode of inheritance. J Clin Endocrinol Metab 36:47–54, 1973.

144. White BJ, Rogol AD, Brown KS, et al: The syndrome of anosmia with hypogonadotropic hypogonadism: A genetic study of 18 new families and a review. Am J Med Genet 15:417–435, 1983.

145. Weiss J, Crowley WF, Jameson JL: Structure of the GnRH gene in patients with idiopathic hypogonadotropic hypogonadism. J Clin Endocrinol Metab 69:299–303, 1989.

146. Nakayama Y, Wondisford FE, Lash RW, et al: Analysis of gonadotropin-releasing hormone gene structure in families with familial central precocious puberty and idiopathic hypogonadotropic hypogonadism. J Clin Endocrinol Metab 70:1233–1238, 1990.

147. Weiss J, Adams E, Whitcomb RW, et al: Normal sequence of the GnRH gene in patients with idiopathic hypogonadotropic hypogonadism. Biol Repro 45:743–747, 1991.

148. Schwanzel-Fukuda M, Bick D, Pfaff DW: Luteinizing hormone-releasing hormone (LHRH)-expressing cells do not migrate normally in an inherited hypogonadal (Kallmann) syndrome. Brain Res Mol Brain Res 6:311–326, 1989.

149. Crowley WF, Jameson JL: Clinical counterpoint: Gonadotropin-releasing hormone deficiency: Perspectives from clinical investigation. Endocr Rev 13:635–640, 1993.

150. Ballabio A, Bardoni B, Carrozzo R, et al: Contiguous gene syndromes due to deletions in the distal short arm of the human X chromosome. Proc Natl Acad Sci USA 86:10001–10005, 1989.

151. Meitinger T, Heye B, Petit C, et al: Definitive localization of X-linked Kallman syndrome (hypogonadotropic hypogonadism and anosmia) to Xp22.3: close linkage to the hypervariable repeat sequence CRI-S232. Am J Hum Genet 47:664–669, 1990.

152. Wray S, Nieburgs A, Elkabes S: Spatiotemporal cell expression of luteinizing hormone-releasing hormone in the prenatal mouse: Evidence for an embryonic origin in the olfactory placode. Brain Res Dev Brain Res 46:309–318, 1989.

153. Bick D, Curry CJ, McGill JR, et al: Male infant with ichthyosis, Kallmann syndrome, chondrodysplasia punctata, and an Xp chromosome deletion. Am J Med Genet 33:100–107, 1989.

154. Mascari MJ, Gottlieb W, Rogan PK, et al: The frequency of uniparental disomy in Prader-Willi syndrome. Implications for molecular diagnosis. N Engl J Med 326:1599–1607, 1992.

155. Nicholls RD, Knoll JH, Butler MG, et al: Genetic imprinting suggested by maternal heterodisomy in nondeletion Prader-Willi syndrome. Nature 342:281–285, 1989.

156. Hall JG: Genomic imprinting and its clinical implications. N Engl J Med 326:827–829, 1992.

157. Knoll JH, Wagstaff J, Lalande M: Cytogenetic and molecular studies

in the Prader-Willi and Angelman syndromes: An overview. Am J Med Genet 46:2–6, 1993.

158. Nicholls RD: Genomic imprinting and uniparental disomy in Angelman and Prader-Willi syndromes: a review. Am J Med Genet 46:16–25, 1993.

159. Kletter GB, Gorski JL, Kelch RP: Congenital adrenal hypoplasia and isolated gonadotropin deficiency. Trends Endocrinol Metab 2:123–128, 1991.

160. New MI: Basic and clinical aspects of congenital adrenal hyperplasia. J Steroid Biochem 27:1–7, 1987.

161. Speiser PW, Laforgia N, Kato K, et al: First trimester prenatal treatment and molecular genetic diagnosis of congenital adrenal hyperplasia (21-hydroxylase deficiency). J Clin Endocrinol Metab 70:838–848, 1990.

162. Pang S, Pollack MS, Marshall RN, Immken L: Prenatal treatment of congenital adrenal hyperplasia due to 21-hydroxylase deficiency. N Engl J Med 322:111–115, 1990.

163. White PC, Dupont J, New MI, et al: A mutation in CYP11B1 (Arg-448—His) associated with steroid 11 beta-hydroxylase deficiency in Jews of Moroccan origin. J Clin Invest 87:1664–1667, 1991.

164. Kagimoto K, Waterman MR, Kagimoto M, et al: Identification of a common molecular basis for combined 17 alpha-hydroxylase/17,20-lyase deficiency in two Mennonite families. Hum Genet 82:285–286, 1989.

165. Imperato-McGinley J, Gautier T, Peterson RE, Shackleton C: The prevalence of 5 alpha-reductase deficiency in children with ambiguous genitalia in the Dominican Republic. J Urol 136:867–873, 1986.

166. Thigpen AE, Davis DL, Milatovich A, et al: Molecular genetics of steroid 5 alpha-reductase 2 deficiency. J Clin Invest 90:799–809, 1992.

167. Abramowicz MJ, Targovnik HM, Varela V, et al: Identification of a mutation in the coding sequence of the human thyroid peroxidase gene causing congenital goiter. J Clin Invest 90:1200–1204, 1992.

168. Lifton RP, Dluhy RG, Powers M, et al: A chimaeric 11 beta-hydroxylase/aldosterone synthase gene causes glucocorticoid-remediable aldosteronism and human hypertension. Nature 355:262–265, 1992.

169. Larsson C, Skogseid B, Oberg K, et al: Multiple endocrine neoplasia type 1 gene maps to chromosome 11 and is lost in insulinoma. Nature 332:85–87, 1988.

170. Mathew CG, Chin KS, Easton DF, et al: A linked genetic marker for multiple endocrine neoplasia type 2A on chromosome 10. Nature 328:527–528, 1987.

171. Bystrom C, Larsson C, Blomberg C, et al: Localization of the MEN1 gene to a small region within chromosome 11q13 by deletion mapping in tumors. Proc Natl Acad Sci U S A 87:1968–1972, 1990.

172. Friend SH, Bernards R, Rogelj S, et al: A human DNA segment with properties of the gene that predisposes to retinoblastoma and osteosarcoma. Nature 323:643–646, 1986.

173. Kidd KK, Simpson NE: Search for the gene for multiple endocrine neoplasia type 2A. Recent Prog Horm Res 46:305–341, 1990.

174. Mulligan LM, Kwok JBJ, Healey CS, et al: Germ-line mutations of the RET proto-oncogene in multiple endocrine neoplasia type 2A. Nature 363:458–460, 1993.

175. Fusco A, Grieco M, Santoro M, et al: A new oncogene in human thyroid papillary carcinomas and their lymph-nodal metastases. Nature 328:170–172, 1987.

176. Grieco M, Santoro M, Berlingieri MT, et al: PTC is a novel rearranged form of the ret proto-oncogene and is frequently detected in vivo in human thyroid papillary carcinomas. Cell 60:557–563, 1990.

177. Arnold A, Staunton CE, Kim HG, et al: Monoclonality and abnormal parathyroid hormone genes in parathyroid adenomas. N Engl J Med 318:658–662, 1988.

178. Alexander JM, Biller BM, Bikkal H, et al: Clinically nonfunctioning pituitary tumors are monoclonal in origin. J Clin Invest 86:336–340, 1990.

179. Biller BM, Alexander JM, Zervas NT, et al: Clonal origins of adrenocorticotropin-secreting pituitary tissue in Cushing's disease. J Clin Endocrinol Metab 75:1303–1309, 1992.

180. Friedman E, Bale AE, Marx SJ, et al: Genetic abnormalities in sporadic parathyroid adenomas. J Clin Endocrinol Metab 71:293–297, 1990.

181. Namba H, Matsuo K, Fagin JA: Clonal composition of benign and malignant human thyroid tumors. J Clin Invest 86:120–125, 1990.

182. Vogelstein B, Fearon ER, Hamilton SR, Feinberg AP: Use of restriction fragment length polymorphisms to determine the clonal origin of human tumors. Science 227:642–645, 1985.

183. Lyons J, Landis CA, Harsh G, et al: Two G protein oncogenes in human endocrine tumors. Science 249:655–659, 1990.

184. Landis CA, Masters SB, Spada A, et al: GTPase inhibiting mutations activate the alpha chain of Gs and stimulate adenylyl cyclase in human pituitary tumours. Nature 340:692–696, 1989.

185. Weinstein LS, Shenker A, Gejman PV, et al: Activating mutations of the stimulatory G protein in the McCune-Albright syndrome. N Engl J Med 325:1688–1695, 1991.

186. Patten JL, Johns DR, Valle D, et al: Mutation in the gene encoding the stimulatory G protein of adenylate cyclase in Albright's hereditary osteodystrophy. N Engl J Med 322:1412–1419, 1990.

187. Weinstein LS, Gejman PV, Friedman E, et al: Mutations of the Gs alpha-subunit gene in Albright hereditary osteodystrophy detected by denaturing gradient gel electrophoresis. Proc Natl Acad Sci U S A 87:8287–8290, 1990.

188. Bos JL: Ras oncogenes in human cancer: a review. Cancer Res 49:4682–4689, 1989.

189. Fagin JA: Genetic basis of endocrine disease 3: Molecular defects in thyroid gland neoplasia. J Clin Endocrinol Metab 75:1398–1400, 1992.

190. Fagin JA, Matsuo K, Karmakar A, et al: High prevalence of mutations of the p53 gene in poorly differentiated human thyroid carcinomas. J Clin Invest 91:179–184, 1993.

191. Suarez HG, du Villard JA, Severino M, et al: Presence of mutations in all three ras genes in human thyroid tumors. Oncogene 5:565–570, 1990.

192. Lemoine NR, Mayall ES, Wyllie FS, et al: High frequency of ras oncogene activation in all stages of human thyroid tumorigenesis. Oncogene 4:159–164, 1989.

193. Karga H, Lee JK, Vickery AL, et al: Ras oncogene mutations in benign and malignant thyroid neoplasia. J Clin Endocrinol Metab 73:832–836, 1991.

194. Santoro M, Carlomagno F, Hay ID, et al: Ret oncogene activation in human thyroid neoplasms is restricted to the papillary cancer subtype. J Clin Invest 89:1517–1522, 1992.

195. Fearon ER, Vogelstein B: A genetic model for colorectal tumorigenesis. Cell 61:759–767, 1990.

196. Arnold A, Kim HG, Gaz RD, et al: Molecular cloning and chromosomal mapping of DNA rearranged with the parathyroid hormone gene in a parathyroid adenoma. J Clin Invest 83:2034–2040, 1989.

197. Motokura T, Bloom T, Kim HG, et al: A novel cyclin encoded by a bcl11-linked candidate oncogene. Nature 350:512–515, 1991.

198. Williams ME, Swerdlow SH, Rosenberg CL, Arnold A: Characterization of chromosome 11 translocation breakpoints at the bcl-1 and PRAD1 loci in centrocytic lymphoma. Cancer Res 52:5541–5544, 1992.

199. Ieiri T, Cochaux P, Targovnik HM, et al: A 3′ splice site mutation in the thyroglobulin gene responsible for congenital goiter with hypothyroidism. J Clin Invest 88:1901–1905, 1991.

200. Ruiz M, Rajatanavin R, Young RA, et al: Familial dysalbuminemic hyperthyroxinemia: a syndrome that can be confused with thyrotoxicosis. N Engl J Med 306:635–639, 1982.

201. Weiss RE, Refetoff S: Thyroid hormone resistance. Annu Rev Med 43:363–375, 1992.

202. Zoppi S, Marcelli M, Deslypere JP, et al: Amino acid substitutions in the DNA-binding domain of the human androgen receptor are a frequent cause of receptor-binding positive androgen resistance. Mol Endocrinol 6:409–415, 1992.

203. Vogelstein B, Kinzler KW: p53 function and dysfunction. Cell 70:523–526, 1992.

204. Weinberg RA: Tumor suppressor genes. Science 254:1138–1146, 1991.

205. Jager RJ, Anvret M, Hall K, Scherer G: A human XY female with a frame shift mutation in the candidate testis-determining gene SRY. Nature 348:452–454, 1990.

206. Bick D, Franco B, Sherins RJ, et al: Brief report: intragenic deletion of the KALIG-1 gene in Kallmann's syndrome. N Engl J Med 326:1752–1755, 1992.

207. Norum RA, Lafreniere RG, O'Neal LW, et al: Linkage of the multiple endocrine neoplasia type 2B gene (MEN2B) to chromosome 10 markers linked to MEN2A. Genomics 8:313–317, 1990.

208. Pang S, Levine LS, Stoner E, et al: Nonsalt-losing congenital adrenal hyperplasia due to 3 β-hydroxysteroid dehydrogenase deficiency with normal glomerulosa function. J Clin Endocrinol Metab 56:808–818, 1983.

PART II

NEURO-ENDOCRINOLOGY

Functional Anatomy of the Hypothalamic–Anterior Pituitary Complex

PETER N. RISKIND
JOSEPH B. MARTIN

The hypothalamus is a phylogenetically ancient structure forming a rostral extension of the brain stem reticular formation. Extensive links with other brain areas important for visceral, autonomic, and behavioral functions contribute to the vital role of the hypothalamus in homeostasis. A unique aspect of hypothalamic function is its role as the ultimate purveyor of brain influence upon the pituitary gland.

Hypothalamic control of the pituitary is mediated by two distinct but not completely separate systems. The hormones of the hypothalamic-neurohypophyseal system are released into the systemic circulation by axon terminals arising from large, magnocellular hypothalamic neurons. In contrast, control of the anterior pituitary hormone secretion is mediated by hypothalamic releasing (and release-inhibiting) hormones, which are secreted from axon terminals of small, parvocellular neurons. The releasing hormones are secreted into a specialized portal system of veins that drain to the anterior pituitary. Secretory products of CNS neurons, both releasing hormones and neurohypophyseal hormones, stimulate target cells after transport through the blood, mimicking classic actions of hormones found in the periphery. This chapter describes the anatomical basis for hypothalamic regulation of the anterior pituitary. A discussion of neural control of the posterior pituitary can be found in Chapters 25 and 26.

HISTORY AND BACKGROUND

Clinicians at the turn of the century first ascribed various endocrine abnormalities to the presence of tumors of the pituitary region.[1] Frohlich reported the case of a boy with a pituitary tumor, obesity, and failure of sexual development (adiposogenital dystrophy, or Frohlich's syndrome[2]). In 1904, Erdheim[3] described a case of Frohlich's syndrome in a patient with a suprasellar tumor deforming the diencephalon. Aschner[4] subsequently reported experiments in dogs which proved that adiposogenital dystrophy does not require direct damage to the pituitary and concluded that the essential damage involves the base of the brain.

The hypophyseal-portal blood vessels, now known to be the conduit of the hypothalamic hypophysiotropic hormones, were first described in 1930 by Popa and Fielding,[5] who noted a distinctive group of capillary loops at the inferior extent of the hypothalamus. These vessels leave the brain to form the long portal veins, which descend along the pituitary stalk to terminate in the pituitary gland. Popa and other workers originally concluded that blood flows upward from the pituitary to the brain, a controversy that persisted into the modern era of neuroendocrinology. On the other hand, Wislocki and King[6] described the portal vessels of the monkey and suggested, on the basis of their anatomical findings, that the direction of blood flow is also downward in this animal. Green and Harris[7] subsequently visualized downward flow from the hypothalamus to the pituitary in the rat and proposed that the portal vessels form a conduit for specific regulatory substances secreted from the hypothalamus to the anterior pituitary. This proposal, termed the *portal vessel chemotransmitter hypothesis,* is now regarded as proven.

Evidence supporting the portal vessel chemotransmitter hypothesis sparked a highly competitive and prolonged research effort to identify the chemical structures of the hypothalamic releasing factors. Early studies confirmed that acid extracts of hypothalami from various species have specific stimulatory or inhibitory effects on secretion of pituitary hormones.[8-10] The task of identifying the chemical structures of the hypophysiotropic hormones was most successfully taken up by Andrew Schally and Roger Guillemin and their collaborators, beginning in the mid-1950's. Both groups recognized that massive amounts of hypothalamic tissue would have to be analyzed. Obtaining their material from nearby slaughterhouses, Guillemin's group[11] used sheep hypothalami as their research material, whereas Schally's group[12] used hypothalami from the pig. The success of both groups depended on the development of convenient and reliable hormone assays and the application of innovative techniques of peptide chemistry. To date, five hypothalamic peptides having specific and potent effects on anterior pituitary hormone release have been identified. Once identified, such releasing factors are generally termed *releasing hormones* (e.g., thyrotropin-releasing hormone).

The structure of thyrotropin-releasing hormone (TRH), a tripeptide, was reported virtually simultaneously by two laboratories in 1969.[11, 12] In 1971, Schally and co-workers characterized luteinizing hormone–releasing hormone (LHRH, now preferentially termed *gonadotropin-releasing hormone*, GnRH),[13] a decapeptide. Guillemin and his collaborators subsequently identified somatostatin (SS, also termed *somatotropin* or *growth hormone release–inhibiting hormone*, SRIF),[14] a tetradecapeptide that inhibits growth hormone release. The structures of TRH, GnRH, and SS were found to be identical in pigs and sheep. Vale and co-workers[15] identified the sequence of ovine corticotropin-releasing hormone (oCRH, or oCRF), a 41–amino acid peptide that stimulates corticotropin (ACTH) and β-endorphin (β-END) release from the anterior pituitary. Two related growth hormone–releasing hormone (GRH) peptides (differing in the carboxy-terminal amino acids) were both initially isolated from human pancreatic adenomata removed from patients with acromegaly.[16, 17] The 44–amino acid peptide, human pancreatic GRH (hpGRH 1-44), and the 40–amino acid peptide (hpGRH 1-40) are present within the human hypothalamus, both presumably derived from a single prohormone.

Current evidence indicates that prolactin secretion is primarily under the inhibitory control of dopamine, acting as a prolactin release–inhibiting factor (PIF).[18] There is also evidence for prolactin release–stimulating factor(s) [(PRF), the principal candidates being vasoactive intestinal polypeptide (VIP),[19] peptide histidine isoleucine (PHI),[20] and TRH[21]].

Recent molecular biological analyses have revealed that the neuropeptide-releasing hormones are synthesized as part of larger prohormones and are then cleaved from the prohormones during post-translational enzymatic processing. Thus, TRH is cleaved from preprothyrotropin-releasing hormone,[22] GnRH is derived from pre-proGnRH,[23] somatostatin from pre-prosomatostatin,[24] GRH from pre-proGRH,[25] and CRH from pre-proCRH.[26]

ANATOMY OF THE HYPOTHALAMUS

Gross Anatomy

The ventral aspect of the hypothalamus forms a convex bulge, the tuber cinerum (gray eminence), which lies at the base of the brain above the pituitary gland.[27] The median eminence (infundibulum) is readily recognized as a richly vascular band that runs longitudinally along the midline of the tuber cinerum. The median eminence forms the floor of the third ventricle and extends ventrally to become continuous with the pituitary stalk.

The boundaries of the hypothalamus are imprecise and have been somewhat arbitrarily defined.[28] Its anterior limit has classically been defined as the optic chiasm and lamina terminalis. However, the preoptic area (which lies immediately rostral to the chiasm) is functionally and developmentally similar to the hypothalamus. Posteriorly the hypothalamus is bounded by an imaginary coronal plane lying between the posterior aspect of the mammillary bodies and the posterior commissure. Dorsally it is bounded by a horizontal plane at the level of the hypothalamic sulcus on the medial wall of the third ventricle. Its lateral limits are defined by the internal capsule and basis pedunculi.

Nuclear Groups

A satisfactory description of hypothalamic topography is complicated by the lack of clear boundaries between many of the cellular nuclei and the fact that many hypothalamic regions contain diffuse collections of cells without distinct cell groupings.[28] Furthermore, endocrine, autonomic, and behavioral functions of the hypothalamus correspond poorly to morphologically defined nuclei.

In their classic review of hypothalamic anatomy, Nauta and Haymaker[27] promoted Crosby and Woodburne's[29] earlier division of the hypothalamus into three longitudinal zones—a lateral, a medial, and a periventricular zone. The lateral zone is divided from the medial zone by the plane of the fornix. Traversing the lateral zone longitudinally is the medial forebrain bundle (MFB), a prominent fiber system connecting limbic and brain stem regions. In primates the medial zone is differentiated into a homogeneous periventricular zone and a medial hypothalamic zone. Nuclear groups within the hypothalamus generally lie within one of these zones. The lateral hypothalamic zone is richly interconnected with the medial hypothalamic areas. This anatomical arrangement underscores the apparent function of the lateral zone as a relay station connecting limbic and brain stem areas with each other and with the medial hypothalamus. In contrast, the medial and periventricular zones appear to be more specialized for neuroendocrine and visceral functions. The major hypothalamic nuclei and hypothalamic areas (regions less clearly defined than nuclei) are indicated in Table 8–1.

The Median Eminence

The median eminence (ME) is a specialized region of the floor of the third ventricle which gives rise to the

TABLE 8–1. MAJOR HYPOTHALAMIC CELL GROUPS*

PERIVENTRICULAR ZONE	MEDIAL ZONE	LATERAL ZONE
Preoptic periventricular area	Medial preoptic area	Lateral preoptic area
Anterior periventricular nucleus	Medial preoptic nucleus	Lateral hypothalamic area
Suprachiasmatic nucleus	Anterior hypothalamic area	Supraoptic nucleus
Paraventricular-periventricular nucleus	Paraventricular nucleus	
Arcuate nucleus (infundibular nucleus)	Ventromedial nucleus	
Dorsomedial nucleus	Perifornical nucleus	
Tuberal magnocellular nucleus	Posterior hypothalamic area	
	Medial mamillary nucleus	

*Adapted from Bleir R, Cohn P, Siggelkkow IR: A cytoarchitectonic atlas of the hypothalamus and hypothalamic third ventricle of the rat. *In* Morgane PJ, Panskeep J (eds): Handbook of the Hypothalamus, Vol 1. New York, Marcel Dekker, 1979, pp 137–220.

pituitary stalk. Together the upper stalk and ME form the contract zone between terminals of the tuberoinfundibular neurons and the capillaries of the hypophyseal portal circulation. Characteristic features of the ME are a high vascularity and blood flow, fenestrated endothelium, virtually complete lack of neuronal perikarya, and specialized ependymal cells, known as *tanycytes*.

The ME contains three zones, or layers: the inner ependymal zone, the inner palisade zone, and the outer, or external, palisade zone.

The inner ependymal zone lines the floor of the third ventricle. It contains a capillary plexus separate from that of the palisade zones and is composed primarily of the cell bodies of tanycytes, which line the ventral part of the third ventricle. Unlike the ependyma of the dorsal third ventricle, the ventricular surface of the tanycytes is covered with microvilli rather than cilia. The tanycytes are connected by tight junctions, forming a barrier between the ventricular CSF and the extracellular space of the ME. Long basal processes from the tanycytes pass through both palisade zones of the ME to end on capillary walls. Interestingly, terminal boutons of axons in the outer palisade zone occasionally make synapse-like contacts with tanycyte processes. The function of the tanycytes remains a matter of speculation. Because of their morphology, they have been invoked as potential conduits for transfer of hormones from CSF to capillaries of the ME,[30] or vice versa.[31] However, convincing evidence to support a conduit function is lacking.

The middle layer of the ME, the inner palisade zone, contains the unmyelinated axons of magnocellular neurosecretory neurons en route from the hypothalamus to the neurohypophysis. In addition, this zone contains nerve terminals originating from brain stem catecholaminergic and peptidergic neurons.[32]

The outer palisade zone (external zone) contains the nerve terminals of the tuberoinfundibular neurons, which secrete their products into the portal blood. Electron microscopy[33] shows this zone to be composed of unmyelinated nerve fibers, axon terminals, glial cells, and basal processes of tanycytes. The terminals are separated from the capillary lumen of the portal vessels by the fenestrated endothelium and by two basement membranes, one surrounding the capillary and the other the neuroepithelium. The releasing factors enter the portal blood by diffusion from the extracellular space defined by these basement membranes.

The Tuberoinfundibular Neurons

The location of neurons whose terminals project to the external zone of the ME (thus constituting the tuberoinfundibular neurons) has been studied using a variety of techniques. Recent studies of the ME using application of substances that are transported in a retrograde direction from nerve terminals to cell bodies have given the most direct results. For example, by applying wheat-germ agglutinin to the ME of rats, Lechan and co-workers[34] demonstrated a heavy ME projection from perikarya in the septal-preoptic area, anterior periventricular area, medial and rostral paraventricular nucleus (PVN), and arcuate nucleus. Rare positive cell staining was also seen in the ventro-

medial nucleus, dorsomedial nucleus, and supraoptic nucleus. Only a few labeled cells were seen in the medullary tegmentum, in a location perhaps corresponding to the A-1 noradrenergic group. The paucity of labeled brain stem cells may have resulted from methodological factors (e.g., brief survival times) rather than an actual sparseness of their projections. For the most part, the tuberoinfundibular neurons are parvocellular. However, some magnocellular neurons of the PVN project to the external layer of the ME, where their terminals end in apposition to portal capillaries.[35]

Hypothalamic-Hypophyseal Circulation

The blood supply of the hypothalamus varies somewhat between species, but in all mammals it is derived from small branches of the internal carotid, middle cerebral, anterior cerebral, anterior communicating, posterior cerebral, and posterior communicating arteries.[36] In general, each part of the hypothalamus is supplied by more than one arterial source. In humans the ME is supplied by the paired superior hypophyseal arteries. The anterior pituitary gland has the highest blood flow of any organ in the body (0.8 ml/g/min) but receives its blood supply indirectly after passage through the ME and portal vessels. Thus, complete interruption of the portal vessels can result in anterior pituitary infarction.[36] In contrast, the neurohypophysis receives a direct arterial blood supply from the inferior hypophyseal artery.

The long portal vessels (6 to 10 in number) originate dorsally from a confluence of capillary loops within the ME. They descend along the anterior surface of the pituitary stalk and drain into the adenohypophysis. They also anastomose with capillaries of the neurohypophysis. As noted earlier, the preponderance of blood flow is downward, from the brain to the pituitary gland. Page[37] directly visualized blood flow in the pig after injections of dye into the carotid arteries; blood flow between various regions of the neurohypophysis occurred, but blood flow from the neural lobe into the ME could not be documented. Interestingly, on some occasions blood from the neural lobe was observed to flow into the pars distalis.

The Blood-Brain Barrier (BBB)

The presence of high-resistance tight junctions between the endothelia and a paucity of pinocytotic vesicles in brain blood vessels serve to segregate most of the brain extracellular space from chemical substances within the systemic circulation. This BBB permits selective entry of circulating substances based on their lipid solubility, size, charge, and presence of specific carrier systems. This barrier has been operationally defined by exclusion of horseradish peroxidase (HRP), a small protein of molecular weight 43,000. Notably, certain of the circumventricular organs and part of the hypothalamus fail to exclude HRP or other proteins after intravenous injection.[38] Entry of HRP under these circumstances suggests that these brain regions lie outside the BBB.

Numerous investigations have confirmed the original observations of Wislocki and King[6] that the ME is freely permeable to intravascular substances and is therefore by definition outside the BBB. Furthermore, experiments with the direct application of HRP to the ME suggest the presence of a diffusion barrier between the ME and the remainder of the medial basal hypothalamus.[39] However, several recent studies suggest that additional hypothalamic regions are readily permeable to the systemic circulation. Van den Pol and Cassidy[40] found that HRP enters much of the arcuate nucleus within 15 minutes after systemic injection into rats. Interestingly, arcuate nucleus HRP labeling was found mainly within the area containing tanycytes, suggesting that the tanycyte processes act as a loose barrier to lateral diffusion.

Even more extensive hypothalamic entry of HRP was reported by Broadwell et al.[38] Two hours after a large injection of HRP into mice, labeling could be detected throughout much of the ventrobasal hypothalamus. This result is not supported by the findings of many other studies, which have demonstrated an integrity of the BBB within the hypothalamus exclusive of the ME. Direct and rapid access of circulating hormones to the ME (and possibly the mediobasal hypothalamus) could potentially modulate the release of hypothalamic releasing factors.

LOCALIZATION STUDIES

Hypothalamic Hypophysiotropic Hormones

Thyrotropin-Releasing Hormone (TRH)

TRH radioimmunoreactivity is widely distributed throughout much of the brain and gastrointestinal tract. The highest levels of TRH in the body are found in the ME.[41]

The densest collection of TRH-containing cell bodies is found in the medial, parvocellular division of the PVN.[42] Other hypothalamic regions rich in TRH-immunoreactive perikarya are the suprachiasmatic preoptic nucleus, the perifornical region, the dorsomedial hypothalamic nucleus, and the basolateral hypothalamus. These findings are in essential agreement with those reported by Hokfelt et al,[43] except for a denser collection of perikarya in the ventromedial hypothalamic nucleus found in the latter study.

TRH-containing fibers are widely distributed within the hypothalamus. The ME, dorsomedial hypothalamic nucleus, medial PVN, perifornical region, periventricular region, and organum vasculosum of the lamina terminalis (OVLT) are particularly rich. A dense meshwork of TRH-positive fibers is also seen in the posterior pituitary.

TRH-containing cell bodies within the medial, parvocellular division of the PVN are the probable cells of origin of the TRH axons projecting to the ME (Fig. 8–1). Lesions of this area decrease the concentration of TRH in the median eminence and lower plasma TSH levels.[44] Stimulation of this area releases thyroid-stimulating hormone from the pituitary.[45] Analysis of immunohistochemical staining for the TRH-prohormone in combination with retrograde labeling of neurons that project to the median eminence also supports the conclusion that the hypophysiotropic TRH-producing neurons are localized mainly to the medial, parvocellular PVN.[46] Lesion studies by Palkovits and co-workers[47] imply that the TRH-containing axons swing laterally from the PVN to pass through the lateral retro-chiasmatic area (immediately posterior to the caudal edge of the optic chiasm) before turning medially to the median eminence. TRH terminals in the external layer are distributed primarily in the medial part of the ME.

Gonadotropin Hormone–Releasing Hormone (GnRH)

The anatomic distribution of GnRH is much more restricted than that of TRH. In mammals, GnRH immunoreactivity is detectable within the hypothalamus, septum and preoptic area, amygdala, and midbrain.[48] In the rat the highest concentrations of GnRH are found in the ME, arcuate nucleus, and OVLT.[49] Recent studies have demonstrated that GnRH immunoreactivity is also present within a population of ganglion cells and axons along the course of the terminalis nerve, a cranial nerve that projects from the nasal septum into the ventromedial surface of the forebrain.[50] The presence of GnRH-immunopositive perikarya within the terminalis nerve has been confirmed in a variety of mammals, including humans. Furthermore, analysis of embryonic animals has demonstrated that GnRH-immunopositive cells originate within the epithelium of the medial olfactory pit and subsequently migrate along the terminalis nerve into the forebrain and hypothalamus.[51] These results suggest a logical explanation for the association of idiopathic hypothalamic hypogonadism with anosmia (Kallmann's syndrome), which can be associated with an X-chromosome deletion; indeed, analysis of a Kallmann fetus has demonstrated dense clusters of GnRH-immunopositive cells and fibers within the nose in the absence of GnRH-immunopositive cells within the brain, indicating that this syndrome may result from a failure of GnRH-neuronal migration from the nose into the brain.[52]

King and her co-workers[53] have described the distribution of GnRH-immunopositive perikarya in the rat. GnRH cells are diffusely aggregated in the nucleus of the vertical limb of the diagonal band of Broca (immediately rostral to the preoptic area), medial septal nuclei, medial preoptic nucleus, and anterior hypothalamic area. This rostral collection of GnRH cells also extends caudally such that a few cells are present in the lateral and basal hypothalamus. Two diffuse fiber systems are also seen: The lateral system forms part of the MFB, whereas the medial system is periventricular. These fiber groups are separated by the medial hypothalamic nuclei over most of their course, then converge in the basal hypothalamus close to their termination in the ME. These data are consistent with results of lesion experiments demonstrating that interruption of GnRH fibers lateral and caudal to the preoptic area decreases immunostaining and radioimmunoassayable GnRH within the ME.[54] The residual GnRH activity in the ME after laterally placed lesions suggests that the medial GnRH pathway may also contribute to ME GnRH content. ME GnRH terminals in the rat are concentrated in the lateral third of the external lamina.

Silverman and co-workers[55] used similar techniques to investigate GnRH perikarya in primates. GnRH-immunopositive cells were found in the preoptic area and in a periventricular zone extending from the anterior hypothalamus to the level of the premammillary nuclei. Cells were also seen in the infundibular (arcuate), supraoptic, and septal nuclei.

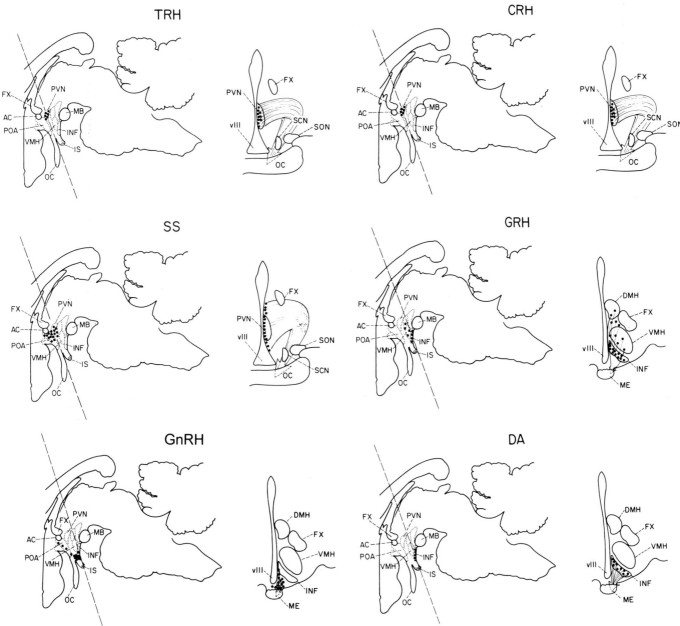

FIGURE 8–1. Schematic depiction of the location of tuberoinfundibular neurons that secrete TRH, CRH, SS, GRH, GnRH, and DA, based on human and animal studies (see text). Tuberoinfundibular neurons (solid dots) are shown in a coronal section (adapted from drawings by P. Marshall) through the plane of densest cell bodies, and in a sagittal section (adapted from DeArmond SJ, Fusco MM, Dewey MM: Structure of the Human Brain. New York, Oxford University Press, 1976). The projection pathway of tuberoinfundibular axons toward the median eminence is depicted by the solid lines forming a point. Abbreviations: OC, optic chiasm; IS, infundibular stalk; INF, arcuate nucleus (infundibular nucleus); MB, mammillary body; PVN, paraventricular nucleus; FX, fornix; AC, anterior commissure; POA, preoptic area; VMH, ventromedial hypothalamic nucleus; ME, median eminence; DMH, dorsomedial hypothalamic nucleus; vIII, third ventricle; SON, supraoptic nucleus; SCN, suprachiasmatic nucleus.

Most recently, the distribution of GnRH-immunopositive perikarya in humans has been ascertained.[56] GnRH cells were heavily concentrated in the most ventral aspect of the medial basal hypothalamus, between the third ventricle and the median eminence. Cells were not confined to distinct nuclear groups but were scattered throughout the periventricular infundibular region. Only a minority of cells were located in the rostral hypothalamus (Fig. 8–1).

The exact pattern of GnRH terminals in the ME also differs between species; Anthony et al[57] found that GnRH terminals in rats are primarily in the external layer of the ME, but in bats GnRH terminals are mainly in the internal zone. Humans, monkeys, and ferrets have intermediate patterns, with terminals in both the external and internal zones.

Somatostatin (SS)

Like TRH, SS has a much more widespread distribution in the mammalian brain and gut than GnRH. SS is present within various brain and spinal cord regions, the retina, and the gastrointestinal tract and pancreas.[58] The highest human brain concentration is found in the ME.[59] High levels are also found in the arcuate nucleus, the periventricular regions of the anterior hypothalamus and preoptic area, and the ventromedial hypothalamic nucleus. Moderate levels of SS are present in the remainder of the anterior hypothalamus.

The neuronal localization of SS immunoreactivity within the brain is coextensive with localization of prosomatostatin mRNA, as determined by in situ hybridization histochemistry combined with immunohistochemistry.[60] The heaviest concentration of positive cells is located within the periventricular region of the hypothalamus at the level of the PVN; SS-positive cells are also concentrated within the paraventricular, suprachiasmatic, and arcuate nuclei. Outside of the hypothalamus, heavy concentrations of SS-positive cells are localized within the anterior olfactory nuclei, hippocampus, amygdala, and cerebral cortex.

The tuberoinfundibular SS neurons are located in the anterior periventricular region (Fig. 8–1). Electrolytic lesions of the anterior periventricular hypothalamus reduce SS content of the ME by 80 to 90 per cent.[61, 62] Depletion of ME SS levels by either frontal hypothalamic deafferentation[62] or lateral parasagittal knife cuts[63] suggests that SS fibers loop laterally across the MFB before re-entering the ventromedial nucleus at the ME level.

The most numerous SS-positive fibers are located within the pituitary stalk and ME (external and inner layers) and in the arcuate nucleus, ventromedial hypothalamic nucleus, and suprachiasmatic nucleus. Numerous fibers also terminate near capillaries in the OVLT.

Corticotropin-Releasing Hormone (CRH)

CRH immunoreactivity has been found in multiple brain areas, the spinal cord, and the gastrointestinal tract.[64, 65] However, the great majority of CRH-containing cell bodies are located within the hypothalamus.[66, 67] The highest brain concentration of CRH is found within the ME.[68]

In the rat hypothalamus, the heaviest concentration of rCRH-positive perikarya is located in the medial, parvocellular part of the PVN. High concentrations of rCRH-positive cells are also localized within the preoptic periventricular hypothalamus, suprachiasmatic nucleus, posterior hypothalamic nucleus, dorsal and ventral parts of the premammillary nucleus, dorsal hypothalamic area, lateral hypothalamic area at the level of the ventromedial nucleus, and lateral parvocellular and magnocellular parts of the PVN. Scattered rCRH-positive cells are also seen in the supraoptic nucleus, in perifornical areas, and in the rostral lateral hypothalamus.[69] Within certain groups of cells, intracellular CRH positivity is co-localized with other hypothalamic peptides.[70]

Immunocytochemical labeling of peptides in combination with in situ hybridization of mRNA has demonstrated that a large proportion of enkephalin-positive cells in the parvocellular PVN contain mRNA encoding CRH, and that a smaller percentage of CRH-positive cells contain mRNA encoding enkephalin.[71]

A subpopulation of neurons in the medial, parvocellular PVN selectively increases CRH staining after adrenalectomy,[72] indicating the junctional anatomy for the selective feedback effect of adrenal corticosteroids upon these cells. That adrenalectomy also alters differential neuropeptide processing in these target neurons is indicated by the de novo development of positive staining for vasopressin in

almost 70 per cent of cells.[73] Following adrenalectomy, CRH is also co-localized with the potent opioid dynorphin (1-8) in a subpopulation of PVN cells.[74]

Hypothalamic deafferentation studies in the rat indicate that the tuberoinfundibular CRH neurons are located primarily in the medial, parvocellular PVN. Their fibers course laterally from the PVN, turn ventrally in the lateral hypothalamus, and curve medially within the lateral retrochiasmatic area toward the ME (Fig. 8–1).

Growth Hormone–Releasing Hormone (GRH)

The distribution of GRH is even more restricted than that of GnRH. In the rat, radioimmunoreactive GRH is highest in the ME, followed by the arcuate nucleus.[75]

Immunocytochemical studies demonstrate slight species differences in GRH distribution. There is unanimous agreement that the majority of GRH-positive perikarya in rat, monkey, and human are located within and contiguous to the arcuate nucleus.[76–79] Several studies in the rat also describe GRH-staining (rGRH) cells in the perifornical region of the anterior and lateral hypothalamus, medial and lateral borders of the ventromedial hypothalamic nucleus, PVN, dorsomedial hypothalamic nucleus, and lateral basal hypothalamus.[76]

GRH-positive fibers are seen in highest concentration in the ME, primarily within the external zone.[76–79] Fibers are also seen in the suprachiasmatic anterior hypothalamus, ventromedial hypothalamic nucleus, and mediodorsal hypothalamus.

Immunocytochemical studies in humans show a similar distribution of GRH-positive perikarya. All reports agree that GRH perikarya are located within, above, and lateral to the arcuate nucleus. In addition, some GRH-staining cells are found in the perifornical region and in the periventricular zone.

Lechan and co-workers[77] have described the topography of GRH cells in rhesus monkey using antisera to GRH 1-44. The distribution of positive cells is more restricted than in the rat and human, being limited primarily to the arcuate nucleus and ventromedial hypothalamic nucleus.

The location of the GRH-tuberinfundibular neurons has been deduced by experiments with a neurotoxin, monosodium glutamate (MSG). When given to neonatal rodents, MSG selectively destroys more than 90 per cent of perikarya within the arcuate nucleus, without significant injury to other hypothalamic regions or axons of passage.[80] Such lesions result in virtual abolition of ME GRH immunoreactivity, suggesting that the locus of GRH-tuberoinfundibular neurons is the arcuate nucleus. Continued pulsatile secretion of growth hormone (albeit much reduced in amplitude) in MSG-treated animals[81] is consistent with the existence of a small component of tuberoinfundibular-GRH neurons outside the arcuate nucleus.

Hypothalamic Neurotransmitters

Dopamine (DA)

Well known as a catecholaminergic neurotransmitter and precursor of norepinephrine, DA also serves as a prolactin-inhibiting factor (PIF). The highest hypothalamic concentrations of DA are found in the ME and arcuate nucleus.

On the basis of their histofluorescence studies, Dahlstrom and Fuxe[82] divided the hypothalamic dopaminergic neurons into the A12 (arcuate nucleus), A13 (zona incerta), and A14 (anterior periventricular) cell groups. The A12 dopaminergic neurons comprise only 3 to 5 per cent of the arcuate nucleus neurons but constitute the majority (and perhaps all) of the tuberoinfundibular dopaminergic (TIDA) cells. Deafferentation of the medial basal hypothalamus does not reduce ME DA concentration so long as the arcuate nucleus is preserved.[83] Neurotoxic lesions of the arcuate nucleus by MSG result in a 45 per cent reduction of ME DA,[84] consistent with a major dopaminergic projection to ME from the arcuate nucleus. Analyses of retrograde labeling in combination with immunohistochemistry for tyrosine hydroxylase have confirmed that a high proportion of arcuate nucleus dopaminergic neurons project to the ME.

Histofluorescence[85] and immunocytochemical studies[86] demonstrate a dense plexus of DA-containing terminals in the ME, primarily in the lateral third of the external layer. DA-containing cells in the anterior periventricular hypothalamus (A14 group)[82] may project to the preoptic area as well as to the internal layer of the ME.[87] Along with the DA-containing cells of the rostral arcuate nucleus, the A14 cell group sends axons to the neural and intermediate lobes of the pituitary in the rat.[88]

Norepinephrine (NE)

NE is ubiquitously, although unevenly, distributed throughout the hypothalamus. NE is found in highest concentrations in the PVN, retrochiasmatic area, ventromedial hypothalamic nucleus, and dorsomedial hypothalamic nucleus. ME NE concentrations are about one fifth those of DA. NE is chiefly localized within the inner layer, rather than the external lamina, of the ME. These observations are consistent with a role for NE as an intrahypothalamic neurotransmitter rather than a releasing hormone.

Deafferentation of the medial basal hypothalamus results in a 70 to 90 per cent reduction of hypothalamic NE levels,[83] indicating that hypothalamic NE is exclusively of extrahypothalamic origin. Selective lesion or knife-cut studies combined with biochemical assays implicate the NE cell groups in the lower brain stem as the source of hypothalamic NE. Cells in the lateral reticular nucleus of the medulla (A1 group) are the most important single contributors,[89] but cells surrounding the nucleus of the solitary tract (A2 group), locus ceruleus (A6), ventrolateral pons (A5), and mesencephalic reticular formation (A7) also project to the hypothalamus. Noradrenergic projections from the A2 and A6 cell groups are directed primarily toward parvicellular regions of the PVN (e.g., those areas that govern the anterior pituitary), whereas the A1 group projects most extensively to magnocellular regions, which control posterior pituitary secretion.[90] Most of the noradrenergic fibers are carried to the hypothalamus by the ventral noradrenergic bundle.

Epinephrine (Epi)

Epi concentrations within the hypothalamus are about 10 per cent of those of NE. Highest concentrations are found in the dorsomedial hypothalamic nucleus, PVN, periventricular region, arcuate nucleus, and supraoptic nucleus. Immunocytochemistry directed at phenylethylamine-N-transferase, the synthetic enzyme for Epi, stains terminals throughout the hypothalamus. The greatest concentration of immunopositive terminals is located in the dorsomedial hypothalamic nucleus, arcuate nucleus, medial parvocellular division of the PVN, perifornical region, and periventricular region. Only a few Epi terminals are seen in the ME, none in the external layer. All Epi-containing cells of the brain are thought to be located within the medulla, in the rostral ventrolateral (C1) or rostromedial (C2) medulla, or ventral to the floor of the fourth ventricle (C3). All three adrenergic cell groups project more heavily to the parvocellular, anterior hypophysiotropic parts of the PVN than to the magnocellular areas, which control posterior lobe secretions.[91] Interestingly, however, deafferentation of the medial basal hypothalamus produces only a 60 per cent overall decline in hypothalamic Epi content.[91]

Serotonin (5-HT)

5-HT is diffusely distributed throughout the hypothalamus, with its heaviest concentration (in the rat) in the suprachiasmatic nucleus.[92] High levels of 5-HT are also detectable in the arcuate nucleus and basal and posterior regions of the hypothalamus, with only moderate levels found in the ME. A recent immunohistochemical study indicates that the hypothalamic distribution of 5-HT may be species specific, as virtually no 5-HT fibers could be seen in the suprachiasmatic nucleus of macaque monkeys,[93] unlike previous findings in rat studies.

Hypothalamic deafferentation results in a 60 per cent fall in overall hypothalamic 5-HT content,[94] suggesting a combination of intrahypothalamic and extrahypothalamic sources of 5-HT. The major extrahypothalamic 5-HT projection to the hypothalamus comes from the midbrain raphe nuclei, but the question of the location of the intrahypothalamic 5-HT perikarya has been controversial.[95] Recently, immunocytochemical staining with specific 5-HT antisera has demonstrated 5-HT–positive perikarya adjacent to the third ventricle, primarily in the dorsomedial hypothalamic nucleus.

Portal blood 5-HT levels are not elevated compared with systemic blood values, but levels of the major 5-HT metabolite, 5-hyroxy-indole-3-acetic acid, are significantly increased in portal blood.[96] Thus it is possible, although unproved, that 5-HT or a 5-HT metabolite has a physiological role as a factor.

REFERENCES

1. Anderson E: Earlier ideas of hypothalamic function, including irrelevant concepts. In Haymaker W, Anderson E, Nauta WJH (eds): The Hypothalamus. Springfield, IL, Charles C Thomas, 1968, pp 1–12.
2. Frohlich A: Ein fall von tumor der hypophysis cerebri ohne akromegalie. Wien Klin Rundsch 15:883–886, 1901.
3. Erdheim J: Uber hypophysenganggeschwulste and hirncholesteratome. Sitzber Akad Wiss Wien 113:537–726, 1904.
4. Aschner B: Uber die funktion der hypophyse. Pfluegers Arch Ges Physiol 146:1–146, 1909.
5. Popa G, Fielding U: A portal circulation from the pituitary to the hypopthalamic region. J Anat 65:88, 1930.
6. Wislocki GB, King LS: Permeability of the hypophysis and hypothala-

mus to vital dyes, with study of hypophyseal blood supply. Am J Anat 58:421–472, 1936.

7. Green JD, Harris GW: Neurovascular link between neurohypophysis and adenohypophysis. J Endocrinol 5:136–146, 1947.
8. Saffran M, Schally AV: Release of corticotropin by anterior pituitary tissue in vitro. Can J Biochem 33:408–415, 1955.
9. Meites J, Talwalker PK, Nicoll CS: Intiation of lactation in rats with hypothalamic or cerebral tissue. Proc Soc Exp Biol Med 103:298–300, 1960.
10. Krulich L, Dhariwal APS, McCann SM: Stimulatory and inhibitory effects of purified hypothalamic extracts on growth hormone release from rat pituitary in vitro. Endocrinology 83:783–790, 1968.
11. Burgus R, Dunn T, Deisderio D, et al: Characterization of the ovine hypothalamic hypophysiotropic TSH-releasing factor. Nature 226:321–325, 1970.
12. Nair RMG, Barett JF, Bowers CY, Schally AV: Structure of porcine thyrotropin releasing hormone. Biochemistry 9:1103–1106, 1970.
13. Schally AV, Arimura A, Baba Y, et al: Isolation and properties of the FSH- and LH-releasing hormone. Biochem Biophys Res Commun 43:393–399, 1971.
14. Brazeau P, Vale W, Burgus R, et al: Hypopthalamic polypeptide that inhibits the secretion of immunoreactive pituitary growth hormone. Science 179:77–79, 1973.
15. Vale W, Spiess J, Rivier C, Rivier J: Characterization of a 41-residue ovine hypothalamic peptide that stimulates secretion of corticotropin and beta-endorphin. Science 213:1394–1397, 1983.
16. Guillemin R, Brazeau P, Bohlen P, et al: Growth hormone releasing factor from a human pancreatic tumor that caused acromegaly. Science 218:585–587, 1982.
17. Rivier J, Spiess J, Thorner M, Vale W: Characterization of a growth hormone releasing factor from a human pancreatic islet tumor. Nature 300:276–278, 1982.
18. MacLeod RM: Regulation of prolactin secretion. In Martini L, Ganong WF (eds): Frontiers in Neuroendrocrinology, Vol 4. New York, Raven Press, 1976, pp 169–194.
19. Abe H, Engler D, Molitch ME, et al: Vasoactive intestinal peptide is a physiological mediator of prolactin release in the rat. Endocrinology 116:1383–1390, 1985.
20. Werner S, Hulting AL, Hokfelt T, et al: Effect of the peptide PHI-27 on prolactin release in vitro. Neuroendrocrinology 37:476–478, 1983.
21. Tashijian AH Jr, Barowsky NJ, Jensen DK: Thyrotropin releasing hormone: Direct evidence for stimulation of prolactin production by pituitary cells in culture. Biochem Res Commun 43:516, 1971.
22. Lee SL, Steward K, Goodman RH: Structure of the gene encoding rat thyrotropin releasing hormone. J Biol Chemistry 263:16604–16609, 1988.
23. Seeberg PH, Andelman JP: Characterization of cDNA for precursor of human luteinizing hormone releasing hormone. Nature 311:666–668, 1984.
24. Montminy MR, Goodman RH, Horvitch SJ, et al: Primary structure of the gene encoding pre-prosomatostatin. Proc Natl Acad Sci USA 81:3337–3340, 1984.
25. Mayo KE, Vale W, Rivier J, et al: Expression-cloning and sequence of a cDNA encoding human growth hormone-releasing factor. Nature 306:86–88, 1983.
26. Shibahara S, Morimoto Y, Furatani Y, et al: Isolation and sequence analysis of the human corticotropin-releasing factor precursor gene. EMBO J 2:775–779, 1983.
27. Nauta WJH, Haymaker W: Hypothalamic nuclei and fiber connections. In Haymaker W, Anderson E, Nauta WJH (eds): The Hypothalamus. Springfield, IL, Charles C Thomas, 1969, pp 136–209.
28. Christ JF: Derivation and boundaries of the hypothalamus, with atlas of hypothalamic grisea. In Haymaker W, Anderson E, Nauta WJH (eds): The Hypothalamus. Springfield, IL, Charles C Thomas, 1969, pp 13–606.
29. Crosby EC, Woodburne RT: Comparative anatomy of preoptic area and hypothalamus, A. Res Nerv Ment Dis Proc 20:52–169, 1940.
30. Ben-Jonathon N, Mical RS, Porter JC: Transport of LRF from CSF to hypophysial portal and systemic blood and release of LH. Endocrinology 95:18–25, 1974.
31. Krieger DT, Liotta AS: Pituitary hormones in brain: Where, how, and why? Science 205:366–372, 1979.
32. Kizer JS, Palkovits M, Brownstein MJ: The projections of A8, A9 and A10 dopaminergic cell bodies: Evidence for a nigral hypothalamic–median eminence dopaminergic pathway. Brain Res 108:363–370, 1976.
33. Knigge KM, Scott DE: Structure and function of the median eminence. Am J Physiol 129:223–244, 1970.

34. Lechan RM, Nestler JL, Jacobson S: The tuberoinfundibular system of the rat as demonstrated by immunohistochemical localization of retrograde transported wheat germ agglutinin (WGA) from the median eminence. Brain Res 245:1–15, 1982.
35. Antunes JL, Carmel PW, Zimmerman EA: Projection from paraventricular nucleus to the zona externa of the median eminence of the rhesus monkey: An immunohistochemical study. Brain Res 137:1–10, 1977.
36. Dawson BH: The blood vessels of the human optic chiasma and their relation to those of the hypophysis and hypothalamus. Brain 81:201–217, 1958.
37. Page RB: Directional pituitary blood flow: A microcinephotographic study. Endocrinology 1123:157–165, 1983.
38. Broadwell RD, Oliver C, Brightman MW: Entry of peroxidase into neurons of the central and peripheral nervous system from extracerebral and cerebral blood. J Comp Neurol 166:257–284, 1976.
39. Lechan RM, Nestler JL, Jacobson S, Reichlin S: The hypothalamic tuberoinfundibular system of the rat as demonstrated by horse-radish peroxidase (HRP) microiontophoresis. Brain Res 195:13–27, 1980.
40. Van den Pol AN, Cassidy JR: The hypothalamic arcuate nucleus of rat: A quantitative Golgi analysis. J Comp Neurol 204:65–98, 1982.
41. Brownstein MJ, Palkovits M, Saavedra JM, et al: Thyrotropin-releasing hormone in specific nuclei of the rat brain. Science 185:267–269, 1974.
42. Lechan RM, Jackson IMD: Immunohistochemical localization of thyrotropin-releasing hormone in the rat hypothalamus and pituitary. Endocrinology 111:55–65, 1982.
43. Hokfelt T, Johansson O, Ljungdahl A, et al: Peptidergic neurons. Nature 284:515–521, 1980.
44. Aizawa T, Greer MA: Delineation of the hypothalamic area controlling thyrotropin secretion in the rat. Endocrinology 109:1731–1738, 1981.
45. Martin JR, Reichlin S: Plasma thyrotropin (TSH) response to hypothalamic electrical stimulation and to injection of synthetic thyrotropin releasing hormone (TRH). Endocrinology 90:1079–1085, 1972.
46. Kawano H, Tsuruo Y, Bando H, Daikoku S: Hypophysiotropic TRH-producing neurons identified by combining immunochemistry from Pro-TRH and retrograde tracing. J Comp Neurol 307:531–538, 1991.
47. Palkovits M, Eskay RL, Brownstein MJ: The course of thyrotropin-releasing hormone fibers to the median eminence in rats. Endocrinology 110:1526–1528, 1982.
48. Sternberger LA, Hoffman GE: Immunocytology of luteinizing hormone–releasing hormone. Neuroendocrinology 25:111–128, 1978.
49. Selmanoff MK, Wise PM, Barraclough CA: Regional distribution of luteinizing hormone–releasing hormone (LH-RH) in rat brain determined by microdissection and radioimmunoassay. Brain Res 192:421–432, 1980.
50. Schwanzel-Fukuda M, Soledadd Garcia M, Morrell JI, Pfaff DW: Distribution of luteinizing hormone releasing hormone in the nervus terminalis and brain of the mouse detected by immunocytochemistry. J Comp Neuro 255:231–244, 1987.
51. Schwanzel-Fukuda M, Pfaff DW: Migration of LHRH-immunoreactive neurons from the olfactory placode rationalizes olfactor-hormonal relationships. J Steroid Biochem Molec Biol 39:565–572, 1991.
52. Schwanzel-Fukuda M, Bick D, Pfaff DW: Luteinizing hormone (LHRH)–expressing cells do not migrate normally in an inherited hypogonadal (Kallmann) syndrome. Molec Brain Res 6:311–326, 1989.
53. King JC, Tobet SA, Snavely FL, Arimura AA: LHRH immunopositive cells and their projections to the median eminence and organum vasculosum of the lamina terminalis. J Comp Neurol 209:287–300, 1982.
54. Palkovits M, Pattou E, Herman JP, Kordon C: Mapping of LH-RH–containing projections to the mediobasal hypothalamus by differential deafferentation experiments. Brain Res 298:283–288, 1984.
55. Silverman AJ, Antunes JL, Abrams GM, et al: The luteinizing hormone–releasing hormone pathways in rhesus (Macaca mulatta) and pigtailed (Macaca nemestrina) monkeys: New observations on thick unembedded sections. J Comp Neurol 211:309–317, 1982.
56. King JL, Anthony ELP, Fitzgerald DM, Stopa EG: Luteinizing hormone–releasing hormone neurons in human preoptic/hypothalamus: Differential intraneuronal localization of immunoreactive forms. J Clin Endocrinol Metab 60:88–97, 1985.
57. Anthony ELP, King JC, Stopa EG: Immunocytochemical localization of the LH-RH in the median eminence, infundibular stalk, and neurohypophysis: Evidence for multiple sites of releasing hormone secretion in humans and other mammals. Cell Tiss Res 236:5–14, 1984.
58. Patel YC, Reichlin S: Somatostatin in hypothalamus, extrahypothalamic brain and peripheral tissues of the rat. Endocrinology 102:523–530, 1978.

59. Cooper PE, Fernstrom JD, Rorstad OP, et al: The regional distribution of somatostatin, substance P and neurotensin in human brain. Brain Res 218:219–232, 1981.
60. Fitzpatrick-Mcelligott S, Card JP, Lewis ME, Baldino R Jr: Neuronal localization of prosomatostatin mRNA in the rat brain with in situ hybridization histochemistry. J Comp Neurol 273:558–572, 1988.
61. Critchlow V, Rice RW, Abe K, Vale W: Somatostatin content of the median eminence in female rats with lesion-induced disruption of the inhibitory control of growth hormone secretion. Endocrinology 103:817–825, 1978.
62. Epelbaum J, Willoughby JO, Brazaua P, Martin JB: Effects of brain lesions and hypothalamic deafferentation on somatostatin distribution in the rat brain. Endocrinology 101:1495–1502, 1977.
63. Palkovits M, Kobayashi RM, Brown M, Vale W: Changes in hypothalamic, limbic and extrapyramidal somatostatin levels following various hypothalamic transections in rat. Brain Res 195:499–505, 1980.
64. Suda T, Tomori N, Tozawa F, et al: Distribution and characterization of immunoreactive corticotropin-releasing factor in human tissues. J Clin Endocrinol Metab 55:861–866, 1984.
65. Olschowka JA, O'Donahue TL, Mueller GP, Jacobowitz DM: Hypothalamic and extrahypothalamic distribution of CRF-like–immunoreactive neurons in the rat brain. Neuroendocrinology 35:305–308, 1982.
66. Bloom FE, Battenberg ELF, Rivier J, Vale WW: Corticotropin releasing factor (CRF): Immunoreactive neurons and fibers in rat hypothalamus. Regul Pept 4:43–83, 1982.
67. Merchenthaler I, Vigh S, Petrusz P, Schally AV: Immunocytochemical localization of corticotropin-releasing factor (CRF) in the rat brain. Am J Anat 165:385–396, 1982.
68. Hashimoto K, Ohno N, Aoki Y, et al: Distribution and characterization of corticotropin-releasing factor and arginine vasopressin in rat hypothalamic nuclei. Neuroendocrinology 34:32–37, 1982.
69. Sakanaka M, Shibasaki T, Lederis K: Corticotropin releasing factor–like immunoreactivity in the rat brain as revealed by a modified cobalt–glucose oxidase–diaminobenzidine method. J Comp Neurol 260:256–298, 1987.
70. Sawchenko PE, Swanson LW, Vale WW: Corticotropin-releasing factor: Co-expression within distinct subsets of oxytocin-, vasopressin-, and neurotensin-immunoreactive neurons in the hypothalamus of the male rat. J Neurosci 4:1118–1129, 1984.
71. Pretel S, Piekut D: Coexistence of corticotropin-releasing factor and enkephalin in the paraventricular nucleus of the rat. J Comp Neurol 294:192–201, 1990.
72. Bugnon C, Fellman D, Gouget A: Changes in corticolibrin and vasopressin-like immunoreactivities in the zona externa of the median eminence in adrenalectomized rats: Immunocytochemical study. Neurosci Lett 37:43–49, 1983.
73. Kiss JZ, Mezey E, Skirboll L: Corticotropin-releasing factor–immunoreactive neurons of the paraventricular nucleus become vasopressin positive after adrenalectomy. Proc Natl Acad Sci USA 81:1854–1858, 1984.
74. Roth KA, Weber E, Barchas JD, et al: Immunoreactive dynorphin (1-8) and corticotropin-releasing factor in subpopulation of hypothalamic neurons. Science 219:189–191, 1983.
75. Kita T, Chihara K, Abe H, et al: Regional distribution of rat growth hormone releasing factor–like immunoreactivity in rat hypothalamus. Endocrinology 116:259–262, 1985.
76. Merchenthaler I, Vigh S, Schally AV, Petrusz P: Immunocytochemical localization of growth hormone releasing factor in the rat hypothalamus. Endocrinology 114:1082–1085, 1984.
77. Lechan RM, Lin HD, Ling N, et al: Distribution of immunoreactive growth hormone releasing factor (1-44)NH2 in the tuberoinfundibular system of the rhesus monkey. Brain Res 309:55–61, 1984.
78. Bloch B, Brazeau P, Ling N, et al: Immunohistochemical detection of growth hormone–releasing factor in brain. Nature 301:607–608, 1983.
79. Bloch B, Gaillard RC, Brazeua P, et al: Topographical and ontogenetic study of the neurons producing growth hormone–releasing factor in human hypothalamus. Regul Pept 8:21–31, 1984.
80. Olney JW: Excitotoxic mechanisms of neurotoxicity. In Spencer PS, Schaumberg HH (eds): Experimental and Clinical Neurotoxicology. Baltimore, Williams & Wilkins, 1980, p 271.
81. Millard WJ, Martin JB Jr, Audet J, et al: Evidence that reduced growth hormone secretion observed in monosodium glutamate–treated rats is the result of a deficiency in growth hormone-releasing factor. Endocrinology 110:540–549, 1982.
82. Dahlstrom A, Fuxe K: Evidence for the existence of monoamine containing neurons in the central nervous system: Demonstration of monoamines in cell bodies of brainstem neurons. Acta Physiol Scand 62(Suppl 232):1–55, 1964.
83. Brownstein MJ, Palkovits M, Tappaz ML, et al: Effects of surgical isolation of the hypothalamus on its neurotransmitter content. Brain Res 117:287–295, 1976.
84. Antoni FA, Kanyicska B, Mezey E, Makara GB: Neonatal treatment with monosodium-L-glutamate: Differential effects on growth hormone and prolactin release induced by morphine. Neuroendocrinology 35:231–235, 1982.
85. Bjorklund A, Falck B, Hromek F, et al: Identification of terminals of the tubero-hypophyseal monoamine fiber system in the rat by means of stereotaxic and microspectrofluorometric techniques. Brain Res 17:1–23, 1970.
86. Hokfelt T, Elde R, Fuxe K, et al: Aminergic and peptidergic pathways in the nervous system with special reference to the hypothalamus. In Reichlin S, Baldessari RT, Martin JB (eds): The Hypothalamus. New York, Raven Press, 1978, pp 69–136.
87. Day TA, Blessing W, Willoughby JO: Noradrenergic and dopaminergic projections to the medial preoptic area of the rat: A combined horse-radish peroxidase/catecholamine histofluorescence study. Brain Res 193:543–548, 1980.
88. Moore RH, Bloom FE: Central catecholamine systems: Anatomy and physiology of the dopamine system. Ann Rev Neurosci 1:129–169, 1978.
89. Palkovits M, Zaborszky A, Feminger E, et al: Noradrenergic innervation of the rat hypothalamus: Experimental biochemical and electron microscopic studies. Brain Res 191:161–171, 1980.
90. Cunningham ET Jr, Sawchenko PE: Anatomical specificity of noradrenergic inputs to the paraventricular and supraoptic nuclei of the rat hypothalamus. J Comp Neurol 274:60–76, 1988.
91. Cunningham ET, Bohn MC, Sawchenko PE: Organization of adrenergic inputs to the paraventricular and supraoptic nuclei of the hypothalamus of the rat. J Comp Neurol 292:651–667, 1990.
92. Saavedra JM, Palkovits M, Brownstein MJ, Axelrod J: Serotonin distribution in the nuclei of the rat hypothalamus and preoptic region. Brain Res 77:157–165, 1974.
93. Kawata M, Takeuchi Y, Ueda S, et al: Immunohistochemical demonstration of serotonin-containing nerve fibers in the hypothalamus of the monkey, *Macaca uscata*. Cell Tiss Res 236:495–503, 1984.
94. Palkovits M, Saavedra JM, Jacobwitz DM, et al: Serotonergic innervation of the forebrain: Effects of lesions on serotonin and tryptophan hydroxylase levels. Brain Res 130:121–134, 1977.
95. Frankfurt M, Lauder JM, Azmitia E: The immunocytochemical localization of serotoninergic neurons in the rat hypothalamus. Neurosci Lett 24:227–232, 1981.
96. Johnston CA, Gibbs DM, Negro-Vilar A: High concentrations of epinephrine derived from a central source and of 5-hydroxyindole-3-acetic acid in hypophysial portal plasma. Endocrinology 113:819–820, 1983.

9

Anatomy and Histology of the Normal and Abnormal Pituitary Gland

EVA HORVATH
KALMAN KOVACS

ANATOMY AND HISTOLOGY OF THE NORMAL GLAND

The pituitary, surrounded by the sphenoid bone and covered with the sellar diaphragm, lies in the sella turcica, near the hypothalamus and optic chiasm.[1] The adult pituitary measures $12 \times 9 \times 6$ mm in diameter and weighs about 0.6 g; it enlarges during pregnancy[2] and may weigh 1 g or even more in multiparous women. The pituitary is capable of producing hormones at quite an early phase of fetal life. At about the end of the third month of gestation the pituitary is grossly apparent, and acidophil and basophil cells can be detected in the anterior lobe. From the eighth week of pregnancy, electron microscopy detects the presence of secretory granules in the cytoplasm of some adenohypophyseal cells, and storage of hormones can also be demonstrated by using immunocytological techniques.[3, 4]

The human pituitary is divided into two parts: (1) the adenohypophysis, which derives from the evagination of the stomodeal ectoderm, known as Rathke's pouch, and (2) the neurohypophysis, which arises from the neural ectoderm of the floor of the forebrain. It has been suggested that the adenohypophysis also is of neuroectodermal derivation, arising from the neural ridge.[5] Experimental evidence, obtained in quail-chick chimeras, supports this hypothesis, but data are not yet available in mammalian embryos.[3]

The adenohypophysis (lobus glandularis), which constitutes approximately 80 per cent of the entire pituitary, consists of the pars distalis (pars anterior, anterior lobe), the pars intermedia (intermediate lobe, intermediate zone), and the pars tuberalis (pars infundibularis, pars proximalis). The pars distalis is the largest and, from the functional point of view, the most important part of the adenohypophysis.

The pars intermedia in the human pituitary[6] is a poorly developed, rudimentary structure with no apparent endocrine significance. It lies between the anterior and poste-

rior lobes and consists of a few cystic cavities lined by cuboidal epithelium and filled with colloid material.

The pars tuberalis is the upward extension of the pars distalis along the pituitary stalk. It is composed of a few layers of chromophobe cells interspersed with occasional acidophil and basophil cells. Although immunocytological techniques reveal the presence of hormones, mainly FSH and LH in the cytoplasm of the pars tuberalis cells,[7] this part of the pituitary is assumed to play no major role in adenohypophyseal secretion.

Adenohypophyseal cells can be disclosed in two regions outside the adenohypophysis: (1) in the posterior lobe and (2) in the pharyngeal pituitary. Accumulation of basophil cells in the posterior lobe is known as basophil cell invasion[6] and is noted in more than 50 per cent of adult autopsies. It is not apparent before puberty, and it occurs more frequently in men and with advancing age. The cells are PAS-positive but smaller and less granular than those of the anterior lobe. In some cases, they are numerous and spread deeply into the posterior lobe. Basophil cell invasion is unassociated with any specific endocrine abnormality, disease, or therapy. Although immunocytological techniques have revealed the presence of ACTH and other proopiomelanocortin (POMC) peptides in these cells,[8] their principal function is unknown.

The pharyngeal hypophysis,[9, 10] usually less than 4 mm in diameter, is embedded in the sphenoid bone and consists of small clusters of poorly differentiated chromophobe cells and occasional acidophil and basophil cells. Unlike the pars distalis, it has a rich innervation but no portal blood supply; that is, the blood flowing through the pharyngeal hypophysis contains no hypothalamic-regulating hormones. Although immunocytological techniques have detected the presence of adenohypophyseal hormones in the cytoplasm of these cells and although it has been claimed that it can take over some of the functions of the anterior pituitary in cases of hypophysectomy or hypopituitarism, no direct evidence indicates that the pharyngeal hypophysis plays a major role in endocrine secretion.

A substantial knowledge of pituitary circulation[11-13] is of fundamental importance if one wishes to understand the functional correlations between the hypothalamus and pituitary and the details of how adenohypophyseal secretory activity is regulated by the hypophysiotropic area of the hypothalamus. The pituitary receives its blood supply from the superior and inferior hypophyseal arteries. The superior hypophyseal arteries arise from the internal carotid arteries. Some of their branches penetrate the infundibulum (the funnel-shaped upper end of the neural stalk attached to the bottom surface of the hypothalamus) and terminate either in gomitoli or in the capillary network around the gomitoli. The gomitoli lie in large numbers in the infundibulum and upper part of the neural stalk. They are about 1 to 2 mm long and 50 to 100 μm wide and consist of a long central artery with a strong muscular coat surrounded by a dense capillary plexus. Their function is not clearly understood, but they appear to regulate blood flow to the anterior lobe and also to the adjacent capillary network, thereby affecting the entry of hypothalamic-regulating hormones into the bloodstream. The hypothalamic-regulating hormones produced in various parts of the hypothalamus flow downward along the nerve fibers to the infundibulum. The perigomitolar capillary network is the site where they enter the circulation. Larger parallel veins are formed from these capillaries. These are the long portal vessels that run down in the pituitary stalk and terminate in the capillaries of the anterior lobe, carrying with them in high concentration the hypothalamic-regulating hormones. The short portal vessels, originating in the distal part of the stalk and in the posterior lobe, also penetrate the anterior lobe and transport substances from the posterior pituitary to the pars distalis.

The question of whether the anterior lobe receives blood exclusively from the portal circulation or has some additional direct arterial blood supply is not fully resolved. Some data[12] seem to indicate that 70 to 90 per cent of adenohypophyseal blood comes from the large portal vessels and the remainder from the short portal vessels. Early morphologic studies[12] show that the loral artery not only supplies the infundibulum and upper part of the stalk with blood but also gives rise to the artery of the fibrous core, which penetrates the anterior lobe without passing through the infundibulum and carries arterial blood to the adenohypophyseal cells. Conflicting evidence has been published by Bergland and Page,[14] denying the role of the loral artery in the blood supply of the pars distalis. Other sources of direct arterial blood to the adenohypophysis are the capsular arteries. These arteries arise from the inferior hypophyseal arteries and not only supply blood to the pituitary capsule but also penetrate the superficial portions of the adenohypophysis, transporting arterial blood to a few cell rows beneath the capsule. Recent studies of 182 human pituitaries, performed by Gorczyca and Hardy,[15] confirm the roles of the middle hypophyseal artery and small capsular arteries in supplying direct arterial blood to the anterior lobe. The inferior hypophyseal arteries, originating in the internal carotid arteries, supply blood to the posterior lobe and do not participate in adenohypophyseal circulation outside the capsular arteries. Venous blood is transported from the pituitary via the adjacent venous sinuses into the internal jugular vein. Observations[14] on vascular casts have led to the revelation that the volume of venous drainage from the pars distalis is considerably smaller than that of portal blood reaching the gland. This discrepancy prompted Bergland and Page[14] to postulate that the direction of blood flow within the common neurohypophyseal vascular bed may be reversed, causing the short portal vessels to serve as both afferent and efferent channels. Such a mechanism would indeed be of utmost importance in hypothalamic regulatory functions.

Electron microscopic studies revealed that the capillaries of the anterior lobe consist of fenestrated endothelium, subendothelial space, and a distinct basal lamina.[6] Hormones released from adenohypophyseal cells first have to pass through their own basal lamina and subsequently all the layers of the capillary walls before entering the circulation. Secretory granules, which contain the hormone within the adenohypophyseal cells, become invisible following their release. Thus, the process of hormone transport between the cell and the capillary lumen cannot be studied currently by morphological techniques, nor is sufficient information available on various factors that may affect this process.

Despite its close proximity to the brain, the anterior lobe contains no nerves except for a few sympathetic fibers that enter the adenohypophysis along the vessels. These fibers may influence blood flow to the anterior lobe, but innervation has no significance in regulating adenohypophyseal secretory activity. The hypothalamus influences adenohypophyseal function by the releasing and inhibiting hormones that are transported to the anterior lobe via the portal vessels. The posterior lobe,[11] which consists histologically of nerve fibers, nerve endings, glial cells (pituicytes), and neurosecretory granules containing vasopressin, oxytocin, and neurophysins, has a rich arterial blood supply independent of the anterior lobe. The inferior hypophyseal arteries, which arise in the internal carotid arteries, supply the posterior lobe with blood. The posterior lobe is richly innervated by the supraopticohypophyseal and the tuberohypophyseal tracts. The supraopticohypophyseal tract arises in the supraoptic and paraventricular nuclei, located in the anterior part of the hypothalamus.[11] The tuberohypophyseal tract originates in the central and posterior parts of the hypothalamus. Both tracts reach the posterior lobe via the pituitary stalk. The integrity of the neurohypophyseal structure depends upon its innervation: the posterior lobe undergoes marked atrophy following destruction of the pituitary stalk or various hypothalamic lesions interfering with the integrity of supraopticohypophyseal or tuberohypophyseal tracts.[11] The neurons of the supraoptic and paraventricular nuclei also atrophy if their axons are damaged.[16, 17]

Cytology of Normal and Abnormal Gland

Currently at least five distinct cell types are believed to exist in the human adenohypophysis,[6, 18] distinguished by their distribution, histology, ultrastructure, and hormone content. Based on the enduring one cell–one hormone theory, all these cell types are irreversibly committed to a single hormonal function. However, an increasing body of evidence suggests that populations of various pituitary cell types may consist of more than one plurihormonal and potentially multifunctional subpopulation.[18] The functional implications of such cytological variations are not yet appreciated, but a new perception of a more flexible, interconnected pituitary, regulated by a complex array of endocrine, paracrine, and autocrine influences, is already emerging. The existence of uncharacterized pituitary cell types is also likely, strongly supported by the occurrence of three pituitary adenoma types showing no apparent ties to any of the known cell types (see "Silent Adenomas").

Somatotrophs

Somatotrophs, or growth hormone (GH)–producing cells, constitute approximately 50 per cent of the adenohypophyseal cell population. The middle-sized ovoid cells, residing chiefly in the lateral wings of the anterior lobe, stain with acid dyes (acidophils) and show strong immunoreactivity for GH.[6, 8] The somatotroph population is not homogeneous. Apart from variations in secretory granule size and morphology, a contingent of GH-cell population is capable of producing prolactin (PRL) as well.[18, 19] These dual secretors, called mammosomatotrophs, are considered transitional cells with potential for alternating between somatotroph and lactotroph functions.[19] A subset of GH cells contains and probably secretes glycoprotein hormone α-subunit.[18] The full functional significance of these variants is poorly understood.

By electron microscopy[18] the majority of the somatotrophs are spherical or oval cells with a spherical nucleus; well-developed, lamellar, rough-surfaced endoplasmic reticulum (RER) located at the periphery of the cells; and a prominent Golgi complex, usually containing a few immature secretory granules (Fig. 9–1). Many GH cells are densely granulated, possessing a large number of spherical,

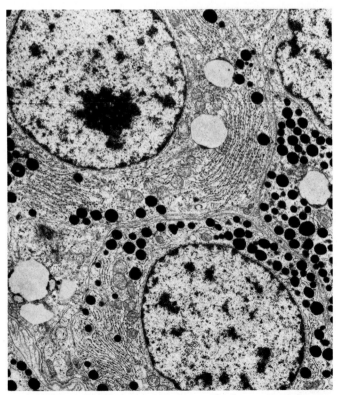

FIGURE 9–1. **Growth hormone cells.** Note the well-developed RER and the numerous dense secretory granules (×7,900).

evenly dense secretory granules measuring between 250 and 500 nm, the majority between 350 and 450 nm. Less densely granulated cells with lucent cytoplasm also occur.

The number, immunoreactivity, and ultrastructure of GH cells appear remarkably stable under various conditions. No distinct morphological appearance is recognized for the functionally suppressed somatotroph. Stimulation by growth hormone–releasing hormone (GRH), produced by various endocrine neoplasms, leads to a potentially massive GH cell hyperplasia causing acromegaly or gigantism.[18, 20] Such lesions usually are strongly acidophilic, consisting of densely granulated somatotrophs distinguished only by unusually prominent Golgi apparatus. Examples of the newly recognized idiopathic hyperplasia, inducing gigantism in infancy, produce both GH and PRL, representing mammosomatotroph lesions.[21] Both forms of hyperplasia may eventually lead to formation of adenoma.

Some cases of idiopathic hyposomatotropism are associated with a reduction of somatotrophs, but others seem to have a nearly normal growth hormone and somatotroph content, suggesting that the primary lesion resides outside of the pituitary.[22]

Prolactin Cells

Prolactin cells,[6, 18, 23] also called mammotrophs, lactotrophs, or luteotrophs, belong to the acidophil cell series and are less numerous than the somatotrophs, constituting 10 to 30 per cent of the total cell population. This cell type, scattered throughout the pars distalis and showing focal accumulation within the posterolateral areas, can be demonstrated by their strong PRL immunoreactivity, localized chiefly in the Golgi region. Only a small minority of PRL cells is granulated densely enough to display diffuse cytoplasmic staining.

By electron microscopy, the uncommon densely granulated prolactin cell is ovoid and contains parallel arrays of well-developed RER and a prominent Golgi complex. The spherical or ovoid secretory granules are numerous and measure in the range of 400 to 700 nm. The majority of prolactin cells have a middle-sized or small polyhedral cell body with long processes. The lucent cytoplasm contains abundant RER, a well-developed Golgi complex, and small (200 to 350 nm), sparse secretory granules (Fig. 9–2). The fine-structural marker of the prolactin cell is "misplaced exocytosis," that is, extrusion of secretory granules on the lateral cell membranes, distant from the capillaries.[18]

A sharp increase in the number of prolactin cells (hyperplasia) occurs in pregnancy and lactation[2, 18] and as a result of estrogen treatment. During development of gestational PRL cell hyperplasia (Fig. 9–3), some of the PRL-producing cells appear to be recruited from the bihormonal mammosomatotroph subset of GH cell population. PRL cell hyperplasia may accompany other neoplastic or non-neoplastic pituitary lesions, corticotroph adenomas, thyroid stimulating hormone cell hyperplasia, as well as any suprasellar mass of pituitary or nonpituitary origin impinging upon the pituitary stalk. The association of PRL cell adenoma and hyperplasia seldom occurs. Idiopathic PRL cell hyperplasia as a sole pathological lesion accounting for clinically evident hyperprolactinemia and its sequelae is exceptionally rare.[24] By morphology, it consists of enlarged, stimulated cells with excessively developed RER and Golgi

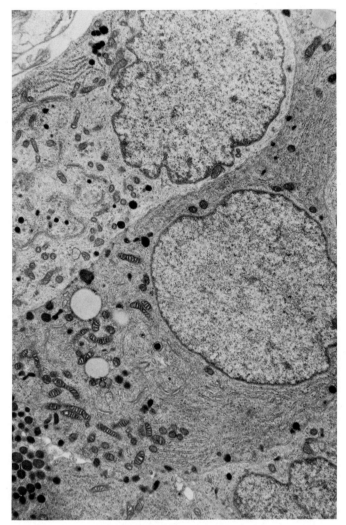

FIGURE 9–2. **Sparsely granulated prolactin cell** (top). The Golgi complex is prominent with numerous developing secretory granules (×7,100).

membranes, sparse secretory granules, and exocytosis similar to PRL cell hyperplasia caused by estrogen excess or loss of dopamine inhibition.

PRL cells show signs of suppression in glands harboring PRL cell adenoma or in cases of dopamine agonist treatment. Such cells are decreased in size, have dark heterochromatic nucleus, have lost most of their RER and Golgi membranes, but still show signs of exocytosis.[18]

Corticotrophs

Corticotrophs, or ACTH-producing cells,[6, 18] constitute approximately 20 per cent of adenohypophyseal cells and are basophilic and PAS-positive. Corticotrophs can also be identified with the immunoperoxidase technique by using specific antisera raised against 1-39 ACTH and some other derivatives of the POMC molecule such as β-lipotropin (β-LPH) and endorphins.[8] By electron microscopy[18] the elongated, angular cells have round or slightly irregular nuclei. The well-developed RER usually appears in the form of widely dispersed, slightly dilated profiles. The prominent Golgi complex may contain immature secretory granules. The cytoplasm usually harbors a large number of spherical or irregular, slightly dented, or heart-shaped secretory

granules having different electron density and measuring 250 to 400 nm in diameter (Fig. 9–4).[8, 18] Features facilitating the recognition of this cell type are morphology of secretory granules, frequent occurrence of large lysosomal bodies, and the presence of type 1 filaments (width about 70 Å) representing cytokeratin.[25, 26]

Idiopathic corticotroph hyperplasia is an uncommon cause of Cushing's disease.[18, 27–29] The proliferation of corticotrophs may be dispersed, not leading to changes in tissue architecture, or nodular, associated by expansion and distortion of reticulin network. Massive multinodular corticotroph hyperplasia may be seen in cases of ectopic production of corticotropin-releasing hormone.[30]

Untreated primary adrenal insufficiency is rarely seen today. In such cases, the enlarged pituitary corticotrophs contain little granulation. Massive diffuse nodular hyperplasia or adenoma may also be noted.[31]

The most common morphologic abnormality of human corticotrophs is Crooke's hyalinization (Fig. 9–5), constituted by the perinuclear accumulation of a faintly eosinophilic, glassy, homogeneous substance displacing the cytoplasmic granules to the cell periphery.[6, 18] Crooke's hyaline material is composed of type 1 filaments, contains no ACTH, and accumulates under conditions of endogenous or exogenous hypercortisolism.

Thyrotrophs

The cytoplasm of thyrotrophs, or thyroid-stimulating hormone (TSH)–producing cells, which constitute approximately 5 per cent of adenohypophyseal cells, stains with the PAS technique, aldehyde fuchsin, and aldehyde thionin. TSH cells can also be identified with the immunoperoxidase technique using specific antisera raised against TSHβ.[8]

Electron microscopy[18] reveals that the elongated, characteristically angular cells possess short profiles of slightly dilated RER and globular Golgi complex with numerous Golgi vesicles. The small secretory granules measure 100 to 300 nm, are mostly spherical, vary in electron opacity, and, especially in sparsely granulated cells, are often positioned near the plasmalemma.

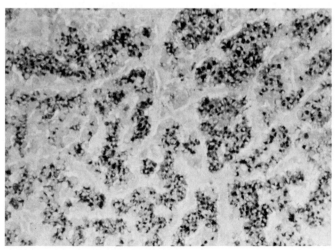

FIGURE 9–3. **Prolactin cell hyperplasia** in the pituitary of a woman who died during the third trimester of pregnancy. Immunoperoxidase method for prolactin (×100).

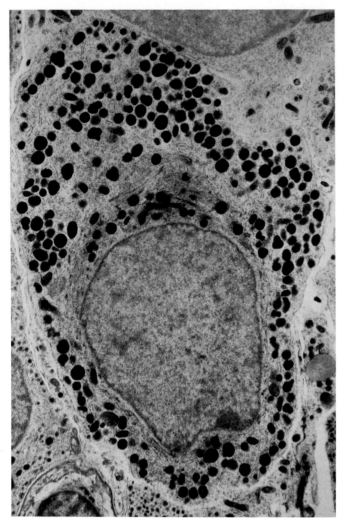

FIGURE 9–4. **Corticotroph cell.** Note the often indented or irregular secretory granules and bundles of type 1 microfilaments adjacent to the nucleus, the morphologic markers of this cell type (×9,400).

Gonadotrophs

According to current views, one cell type secretes both gonadotropic hormones (follicle-stimulating hormone [FSH] and luteinizing hormone [LH]). FSH/LH cells, or gonadotropin-producing cells, constitute approximately 15 per cent of the adenohypophyseal cell population. They are PAS-positive and contain immunoreactive FSH and LH. By electron microscopy,[18] the middle-sized or small ovoid cells always have a considerable surface area adjoining the capillaries. The cells possess uniform spherical or ovoid nuclei. The well-developed RER consists of slightly dilated meandering cisternae containing a fine granular substance of low electron density. The RER may occupy as much as 15 per cent of the cytoplasmic area. The mitochondria are rod-shaped and moderately dense, with numerous lamellar cristae. The large ring-shaped Golgi complex may contain immature secretory granules. The majority of the secretory granules measure between 250 and 300 nm, but larger granules with a diameter of 400 to 450 nm occur regularly as well. Following removal of the ovaries or testes and in various other forms of primary hypogonadism, gonadotrophs enlarge and become vacuolated (castration cells) (Fig. 9–6). By electron microscopy, the marked changes consist of a sharp increase in volume density of the dilated RER (up to 50 per cent) and hypertrophy of the Golgi complex. Many of these "castration cells" become sparsely granulated, with the margination of remaining secretory granules along the cell membrane.

An interesting finding is the juxtaposition of gonadotrophs and prolactin cells[18] in the human as well as rodent pituitary, suggesting a paracrine relationship between the two cell types.[35]

Follicular Cells

Follicular cells are epithelial cells joined by terminal bars and forming follicle or acinus-like structures, but they are not delimited by basement membrane as are true follicles.[18] Most of them are practically agranular. The function of follicles is unclear. They may be formed by different types

Thyrotrophs undergo hypertrophy and hyperplasia in various forms of primary hypothyroidism, such as chronic thyroiditis, surgical or radiation thyroidectomy, or prolonged treatment with goitrogens.[18, 32, 33] The markedly enlarged "thyroidectomy" cells contain immunoreactive TSH. The stimulated thyrotrophs possess extensively developed, dilated RER and prominent Golgi apparatus containing developing secretory granules. The number of secretory granules in the cytoplasm may be reduced. Accumulation of lysosomes, appearing as coarse PAS- and aldehyde thionin–positive globules in histological specimens, is common. Thyrotroph hyperplasia may be associated with significant enlargement of pituitary gland and sometimes with elevation of serum PRL levels, thereby mimicking PRL-producing adenoma.[32] Such a combination of signs is known to have led to unwarranted surgical exploration of the pituitary. Thyrotrophs regress following treatment with thyroxine or in cases of Graves' disease. The fine structure of suppressed thyrotrophs in the human pituitary has not been sufficiently explored.[34]

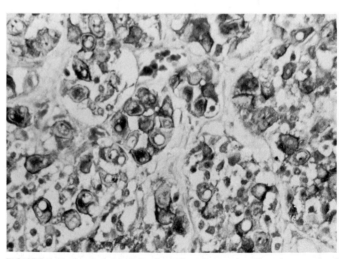

FIGURE 9–5. **Crooke's hyalinization of corticotrophs.** Note the unstained ring-like accumulation of Crooke's hyalin in a case of ectopic ACTH syndrome. Lead hematoxylin (×250).

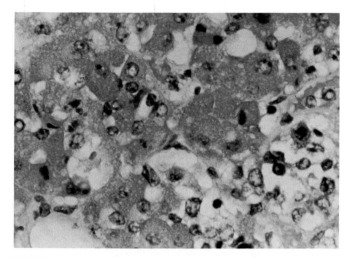

FIGURE 9–6. This large group of hypertrophied cells with finely vacuolated cytoplasm (positive for anti β-FSH and anti β-LH) represents gonadotroph cell hyperplasia in the pituitary of an elderly man with Klinefelter syndrome. PAS technique (×400).

of granulated cells, undergoing degranulation and other marked cytological changes, around the foci of ruptured glandular cells.[18, 36] Experimental evidence suggests possible paracrine connection between follicular cells and adjacent hormone-secreting cells.[37]

ANATOMY AND HISTOLOGY OF THE ABNORMAL GLAND

Although the pathological anatomy of the anterior lobe is not dealt with here in detail, it appears pertinent to give a brief account of some abnormalities that affect the structure of the anterior lobe and can be associated with changes in adenohypophyseal secretory activity and clinical symptoms. These lesions are not limited to a specific cell type; nevertheless, they have considerable importance in endocrine pathology. Pituitary neoplasms, mainly pituitary adenomas, are also discussed in this part of the chapter.

Lesions caused by circulatory disturbances constitute an important portion of adenohypophyseal pathology. Hemorrhages in the anterior lobe are uncommon. They are found in association with head injuries or with rapidly growing pituitary neoplasms. Proliferation of tumor cells may alter intrahypophyseal pressure, resulting in the compression of vascular walls and the redistribution of blood, and the vessels may undergo hypoxic injury. In cases of severe vascular damage, the vessel walls may be impaired to such an extent that they can no longer withstand rises in blood pressure and rupture. Pituitary apoplexy is the extreme variant of this process.[38] Occasionally, almost the entire tumor can undergo destruction. In cases of hormone-secreting adenomas, massive hemorrhage may cause striking amelioration of the clinical symptoms, even hypopituitarism.

Infarcts are due to interruption of blood supply to the anterior lobe. Smaller necrotic foci in the adenohypophysis are not uncommon findings at autopsies[39, 40] and occur in approximately 1 to 6 per cent of unselected autopsy material. Smaller infarcts remain unrecognized clinically and

can be noted only by histologic investigation. Severe hypopituitarism occurs only if more than 90 per cent of functional adenohypophyseal parenchyma is destroyed.

Adenohypophyseal infarcts can be found in association with various diseases.[39, 40] They can be detected more frequently in patients with diabetes mellitus, after head injury, and in association with cerebrovascular accidents, increased intracranial pressure, and epidemic hemorrhagic fever. Adenohypophyseal infarction develops following transection or destruction of the pituitary stalk, which interrupts blood flow to the anterior lobe. Frequent occurrences of adenohypophyseal necrosis have been reported in patients who, as a result of various diseases, are maintained on mechanical ventilators or respirators before they die.[41, 42] Histologically, the lesions correspond to coagulative infarcts and are frequently, but not always, accompanied by severe hypoxic lesions of the brain ("respirator brain").

A special form of pituitary infarction, rarely seen today in developed countries, is postpartum pituitary necrosis, which is found in women who die during the puerperium after a complicated labor.[43] These women usually suffer severe blood loss and are in shock around the time of delivery, the most common obstetric factors being retained placenta and postpartum hemorrhage. At the end of gestation the anterior lobe appears to be susceptible to ischemic necrosis because shock in men and in nonpregnant women is only rarely accompanied by pituitary infarction. The cause of the increased incidence of pituitary necrosis around the time of delivery is not known, nor is the pathogenesis of the lesion clear. Embolism, thrombosis, vasospasm, and vascular compression have all been suggested as possible causes.

Fibrous atrophy is the final phase of ischemic necrosis of the anterior lobe.[43] The necrotic areas are gradually replaced by fibrous tissue. Adenohypophyseal cells are not capable of sufficient regeneration, so permanent hypopituitarism may develop in cases of extensive infarction. Postpartum hypopituitarism due to massive adenohypophyseal ischemic infarction is called Sheehan's syndrome, giving credit to the Liverpool pathologist who described numerous details of this intriguing disease entity.

Massive destruction of the adenohypophysis[6, 44] may occur from various non-neoplastic conditions, possibly with associated circulatory disturbances. Tuberculosis, syphilis, sarcoidosis, and Langerhan's histiocytosis (histiocytosis X) may cause extensive damage to the anterior lobe with resultant hypopituitarism.

Suprasellar granulomas as well as similarly placed neoplasms may produce pituitary dysfunction (hypopituitarism or hyperprolactinemia) by interfering with the production or transport of hypothalamic adenohypophyseal–regulating factors into the portal circulation. An immune mechanism has been postulated in cases of lymphocytic hypophysitis.[45] This rare disorder occurs almost exclusively in women, associated with pregnancy and delivery in most cases,[46] and only two reported cases occurred in men.[45, 46]

PITUITARY NEOPLASMS

Pituitary neoplasms, which constitute approximately 10 per cent of all intracranial tumors, can be primary or secondary, benign or malignant, hormone-producing or functionally inactive. Only the most important forms are dealt with here.

Craniophyaryngiomas,[47] accounting for approximately 3 per cent of all intracranial neoplasms, arise in the remnants of Rathke's pouch. They are almost always benign, are more commonly suprasellar than intrasellar in location, and often show calcification, which enables them to be diagnosed by imaging techniques. They never produce pituitary hormones, but the presence of immunoreactive human chorionic gonadotropin has been reported in the cyst fluid of these neoplasms.[48] Craniopharyngiomas may cause hypopituitarism by compressing or destroying adenohypophyseal tissue or the hypophyseotropic area of the hypothalamus. They can compress the pituitary stalk and interfere with portal circulation and can affect pituitary function either by reducing the blood supply to the anterior lobe or by blocking the synthesis or flow of hypothalamic-regulating hormones to the adenohypophysis, in some cases causing hyperprolactinemia and PRL cell hyperplasia.

Primary carcinomas[6, 49, 50] of the anterior lobe are rare and originate in adenohypophyseal cells. They may produce growth hormone, ACTH, or PRL or may appear nonsecretory. In some cases, histological examination fails to establish the biological behavior of the tumor.

Secondary tumors[6, 51, 52] in the pituitary gland are infrequently found at autopsy and are rarely recognized clinically. In general, they are not accompanied by overt clinical symptoms except occasionally by diabetes insipidus, which may develop in patients with metastases to the posterior lobe. Hypopituitarism is extremely rare because a large part of the anterior lobe has to be replaced by tumor tissue before a decrease in secretion of adenohypophyseal hormones becomes clinically evident. Suprasellar metastases may produce clinical hypopituitarism by interfering with the production or transport of hypothalamic-regulating hormones to the portal circulations; in such cases, there may be little or no ischemic necrosis of the adenohypophysis. Pituitary metastases usually occur in the advanced phase of neoplastic disease, when several other organs are also affected by disseminated cancer. These patients usually do not survive long enough to develop hypopituitarism.

Studies on autopsy material indicate that secondary tumor deposits occur in the hypophysis in approximately 1 to 3 per cent of all cancer patients.[51] This figure is presumably somewhat lower than the real incidence because small foci of cancer metastases can easily be overlooked unless numerous sections are made from the gland. The breast is the most frequent site of primary neoplasm.[51, 52] Pituitary metastases, however, may also arise in patients with primary tumors in other locations, such as bronchus, prostate, and colon. The cause of increased incidence of pituitary metastases in breast cancer patients is not known.

Pituitary adenomas, the most frequent primary tumors of this gland, are benign neoplasms arising in adenohypophyseal cells[6, 53, 54] (Fig. 9–7). They used to be divided into chromophobe, acidophil, and basophil tumors, but this classification is misleading when correlation of structure is made with secretory activity.[6] Chromophobe adenomas are highly active tumors in some cases, capable of secreting various pituitary hormones, such as GH, PRL, and ACTH. Acidophil adenomas can produce GH or PRL or can be

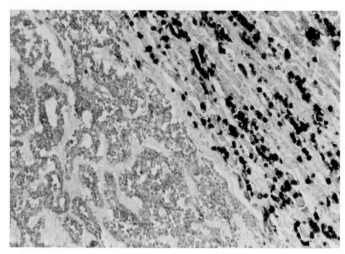

FIGURE 9–7. **Border of a "chromophobe" adenoma** and of surrounding nontumorous gland. The tumor contains no immunoreactive hormones. Immunoperoxidase technique for growth hormone (×100).

functionless. Basophil adenomas may secrete ACTH or may be inactive endocrinologically. Thus, the distinction of chromophobe, acidophil, and basophil adenomas discloses only the tinctorial characteristics of the cytoplasm of adenoma cells; it fails to shed light on their functional activity or on the hormones they produce.

According to current classification, based primarily on immunocytochemistry, electron microscopy, and endocrinological investigation, pituitary adenomas can be divided into the following entities (with the corresponding incidence in our unselected surgical material of more than 1700 adenomas, in parentheses):

1. Somatotroph (GH cell) adenomas (13 to 15 per cent)
2. Lactotroph (PRL cell) adenomas (25 to 28 per cent)
3. Mixed somatotroph and lactotroph adenomas (3 to 5 per cent)
4. Acidophil stem cell adenomas (1 to 3 per cent)
5. Mammosomatotroph adenomas (1 to 2 per cent)
6. Corticotroph adenomas (symptomatic) (8 to 10 per cent)
7. Silent adenomas (5 to 7 per cent)
8. Thyrotroph adenomas (1 per cent)
9. Gonadotroph adenomas (7 to 9 per cent)
10. Null cell adenomas (13 to 15 per cent)
11. Oncocytomas (10 to 12 per cent)
12. Plurihormonal adenomas (1 to 3 per cent)

Space does not permit discussion of all these entities in detail. What we intend to provide is a short, illustrated compendium on the subject, with extensive up-to-date references for the interested reader.

Somatotroph Adenomas

GH-producing tumors of the pituitary are clinically associated with acromegaly or gigantism. Two morphological variants are known to exist.[6, 53–55] The acidophilic, densely granulated GH cell adenoma is a highly differentiated tumor that usually exhibits a slow growth rate, often not expanding beyond the boundaries of the sella. The cytoplasm of adenoma cells shows a strong overall positivity for immunoreactive GH (Fig. 9–8).[8] Ultrastructurally,[53–55] the adenoma cells display a strong resemblance to nontumorous somatotrophs, possessing regular nuclei with light chromatin, prominent nucleolus, and well-developed cytoplasm (Fig. 9–9). The RER, arranged in parallel cisternae at the cell periphery, is prominent. The sacculi of the conspicuous Golgi apparatus consistently harbor developing secretory granules. The mitochondria show regular features. In the rest of the cytoplasm, the secretory granules are numerous and have closely fitted, limiting membrane and high electron opacity. They measure mostly 300 to 500 nm, but considerably larger granules may be noted as well. As an anomaly of granule formation, elongated, pointed, or rhomboid granules may be present occasionally.[54]

The sparsely granulated GH cell adenomas are mostly chromophobic, often displaying nuclear pleomorphism. These tumors are more likely to run an aggressive course characterized by faster growth rate, sellar erosion, and parasellar extension. At the time of pituitary surgery, the average age of patients harboring sparsely granulated GH cell adenoma is lower than the age of those with the densely granulated variant.[6] Immunocytochemistry reveals GH in the cytoplasm of adenoma cells. The positivity, however, is usually limited to the Golgi region owing to sparsity of secretory granules.[6, 8] Sparsely granulated adenomatous GH cells have a highly distinctive ultrastructure that has little in common with the well-differentiated, densely granulated type.[54, 55] They are irregular with strikingly pleomorphic, often crescent-shaped or multiple nuclei. The RER is fairly well developed in randomly scattered profiles. Sparsely granulated GH cell adenomas regularly contain smooth-surfaced endoplasmic reticulum (SER) in association with the fibrous bodies. The Golgi apparatus is well-developed. The most distinguishing diagnostic feature of this adenoma type is the occurrence of spherical fibrous bodies (Fig. 9–10).[6, 53–55] They are composed of concentrically arranged type 2 cytokeratin[56] filaments (average width 115 Å) and/or tubular SER and are invariably located in the Golgi region, often displacing the Golgi apparatus.

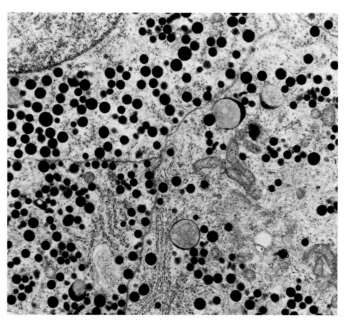

FIGURE 9–9. **Densely granulated growth hormone cell adenoma** (×9,300). (From Horvath E, Kovacs K: Ultrastructural classification of pituitary adenomas. Can J Neurol Sci 3:9–21, 1976; courtesy of Dr. R. T. Ross, editor and publisher of the journal.)

Various cytoplasmic components may be engulfed within the fibrous bodies. The incidence of these structures varies from case to case, but they are usually numerous. Fibrous bodies are diagnostic of GH-producing cells of the human pituitary, including bihormonal (GH and PRL) cells. Another characteristic mark of sparsely granulated GH cell adenomas is the frequent occurrence of supernumerary centrioles, which are usually located near or within the

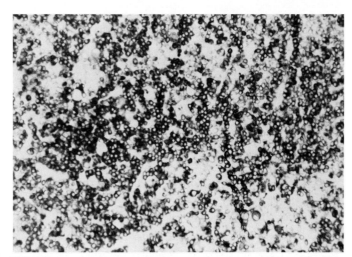

FIGURE 9–8. **Densely granulated growth hormone cell adenoma** exhibiting strong cytoplasmic immunostaining for anti–human growth hormone. Immunoperoxidase technique (×100).

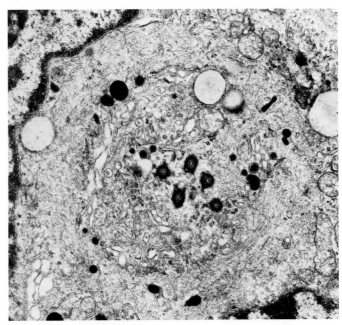

FIGURE 9–10. **Sparsely granulated growth hormone cell adenoma.** Group of five centrioles encircled by type 2 microfilaments of a fibrous body (×17,300). (From Kovacs K, Horvath E, Strattman IE, Ezrin C: Cytoplasmic microfilaments in the anterior lobe of the human pituitary gland. Acta Anat 87:414–426, 1974; courtesy of S. Karger A.G., Basel.)

fibrous bodies. The reason for the accumulation of centrioles, which occurs selectively in sparsely granulated GH cell adenomas and acidophilic stem cell adenomas, is unknown. The secretory granules are spherical and sparse and usually measure no more than 250 nm. Deposition of endocrine amyloid may be an additional feature in both densely and sparsely granulated GH cell tumors.[54, 57] In our surgical material, the incidence of the two types of GH cell adenomas is very close (within 0.5 per cent). Contrary to earlier claims, we found no correlation between serum GH level and morphological type of pituitary adenoma.

The medical treatment of GH-producing adenomas, often in a form of preoperative medication, is becoming increasingly common. At present, a long-acting analogue of somatostatin (Sandostatin, octreotide, SMS 201-995) is the most frequently used compound.[58, 59] The morphologic effects of the drug are variable and show no close correlations with the clinical effects of treatment. Varying degrees of perivascular and/or interstitial fibrosis is the most common change. A significant reduction of the volume of tumor or the number of tumor cells is infrequent. If it occurs, it is usually associated with increased size and volume density of secretory granules. Other morphological alterations, such as lysosomal accumulation with crinophagy or oncocytic change, are not consistently present either.

Lactotroph Adenomas

PRL cell adenoma is the most common endocrinologically active tumor type, accounting for about 27 per cent of symptomatic pituitary tumors in adult surgical material.[6, 53, 54, 60] In recent years, the number of operated cases has noticeably declined, owing to the wider use of dopaminergic agonists (bromocriptine, lisuride, quinagolide) in the management of PRL-producing tumors.

As with GH-producing tumors, two morphological variants of PRL cell adenomas are recognized. They cannot be distinguished clinically, as both forms are associated with signs and symptoms of hyperprolactinemia. The very rare densely granulated PRL cell adenoma is intensely acidophilic by histology and shows a strong all-over cytoplasmic positivity for immunoreactive PRL. The fine-structural appearance of adenoma cells displays a resemblance to those of nontumorous, densely granulated PRL cells, as well as to some of the adenomatous mammosomatotroph cells. The oval or elongated, well-differentiated cells possess prominent RER and Golgi apparatus and numerous spherical or pleomorphic, evenly electron-dense secretory granules in the range of 500 to 700 nm. Granule extrusions are noted regularly.

Nearly all PRL cell adenomas are sparsely granulated and chromophobic or slightly acidophilic by histology. They consistently give a strong positivity for immunoreactive PRL in the Golgi region.[6, 8] The positivity of sparse and small secretory granules may not be readily apparent at the resolution of the optical microscope. The fine structure of the tumor is very characteristic.[6, 60] The closely apposed polyhedral cells have oval or slightly irregular nuclei with light, finely dispersed chromatin and a dense, prominent nucleolus. The RER is extensively developed and often organized in parallel rows and concentric whorls called Nebenkerns. The Golgi complex occupies a large area of

the cytoplasm and regularly contains numerous developing secretory granules (Fig. 9–11). The sparse secretory granules are spherical or pleomorphic, are evenly electron dense, and measure 130 to 300 nm, the majority between 200 and 250 nm. The most characteristic feature of this tumor type is the extrusion of secretory granules on the lateral cell membranes, distant from the perivascular spaces and intercellular extensions of the basal lamina ("misplaced exocytosis"). It should be stressed that this form of secretion is the normal means of hormone discharge from PRL cells. Misplaced exocytosis is diagnostic of PRL production in both nontumorous and neoplastic human pituitary.

The ultrastructural diagnosis of typical sparsely granulated PRL cell adenomas is easy as well as reliable. Two additional features that occur relatively often in these tumors are calcification[6, 61] (about 15 per cent) and deposition of endocrine amyloid[57, 60] (5 to 6 per cent).

With the advent of medical treatment for PRL-producing adenomas, it must be kept in mind that the dopaminergic agonist bromocriptine, while reducing the volume of prolactinomas, exerts a profound effect on the morphology of

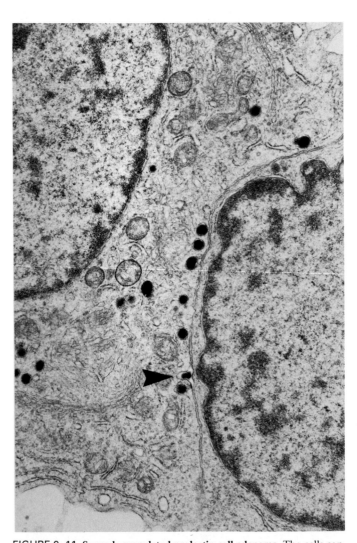

FIGURE 9–11. **Sparsely granulated prolactin cell adenoma.** The cells contain abundant RER and a large Golgi complex but relatively few and small secretory granules. Note granule extrusion (*arrowhead*) on lateral cell membrane (×16,100).

these tumors, including their ultrastructure.[60] The changes, which appear to be reversible in the majority of cases, are the reduction of the size of the cell, cytoplasmic area, nucleus, and nucleolus; increase of nuclear/cytoplasmic ratio; decrease in volume of cytoplasmic area, nucleus, and nucleolus; and decrease in volume density of RER and Golgi complex. The degree of change depends on the dose of bromocriptine, length of treatment, length of drug-free periods (if any) before surgery, and individual response to the drug.[62] All these variables make the fine-structural appearance of treated PRL-producing tumors quite incalculable and difficult to interpret without knowledge of relevant clinical data.

Mixed Somatotroph and Lactotroph Adenomas

In about 40 per cent of acromegalic patients, hypersecretion of GH is accompanied by simultaneous elevation of serum PRL levels.[55, 63, 64] In a number of cases, this finding signifies that the growing tumor, impinging upon the stalk, median eminence, and hypophysiotropic area of the hypothalamus, interferes with the production, release, and/or transport of PRL-inhibiting factor(s) (PIFs), resulting in increased PRL secretion from the nontumorous part of the pituitary. In other cases, hyperprolactinemia is caused by a bihormonal pituitary neoplasm. The morphologic, especially fine-structural analysis, is the only reliable way to reveal the exact nature of pituitary lesions in such cases. The bimorphous mixed (GH cell–PRL cell) adenomas are associated clinically with acromegaly or gigantism and varying degrees of hyperprolactinemia. By histology, they are acidophilic to chromophobic, depending on the number of cytoplasmic granules. The immunoperoxidase technique reveals GH and PRL in different cell populations.[6, 55] The distribution of the two cell types may be uneven in some tumors. The ultrastructural details of GH cells and PRL cells are identical to those described earlier in this chapter as either densely or sparsely granulated forms. Although every variant may occur in mixed adenomas, the combination of densely granulated GH cells and sparsely granulated PRL cells appears to be the most frequent (Fig. 9–12). It should be noted that some mixed tumors, especially those of children and adolescents, may contain some bihormonal cells, chiefly mammosomatotrophs, as well.[54]

Acidophil Stem-Cell Adenomas

These monomorphous, bihormonal tumors are likely to show a fast growth rate and invasion of parasellar, especially infrasellar areas.[65] They are associated clinically with signs and symptoms of hyperprolactinemia, although serum PRL levels are usually much lower than the values expected with well-differentiated PRL cell adenomas of comparable sizes. Occasionally physical stigmata of acromegaly may develop, usually without any apparent elevation of serum GH levels ("fugitive acromegaly"). Histologically, the tumor is chromophobic or, owing to mitochondrial accumulation, acidophilic. Immunocytochemistry detects PRL and, in some cases, also GH in the tumors. The two hormones may be present in the same cells. Electron microscopy[6, 53, 54, 65]

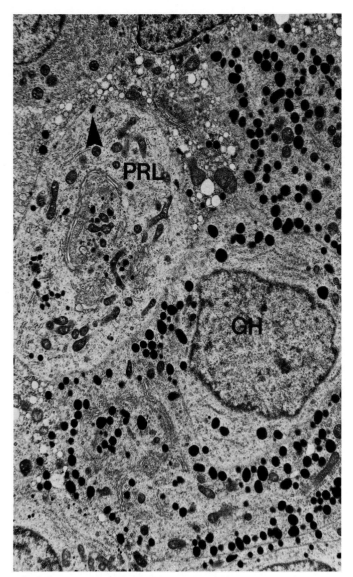

FIGURE 9–12. **Mixed adenoma** composed of densely granulated growth hormone cells (GH) and sparsely granulated prolactin cells (PRL). Note granule extrusion in the prolactin cell (*arrowhead*) (×6,900).

of the adenoma cells documents some fine-structural markers of both adenomatous PRL cells (granule extrusions) and adenomatous, sparsely granulated GH cells (fibrous bodies, tubular SER, multiple centrioles) coupled, in most cases, with oncocytic change and an unusual form of mitochondrial gigantism (Fig. 9–13). The latter appears to be specific and thus diagnostic of this tumor type. The acidophil stem-cell adenoma shows preponderance in women. Its course is especially aggressive in young individuals. To our knowledge, a few cases have been treated with bromocriptine with good response.

Mammosomatotroph Adenomas

These monomorphous, bihormonal adenomas are well-differentiated, slowly growing lesions associated with typical acromegaly and usually mild or moderate hyperprolactinemia.[66] The adenoma cells are acidophilic by histology and

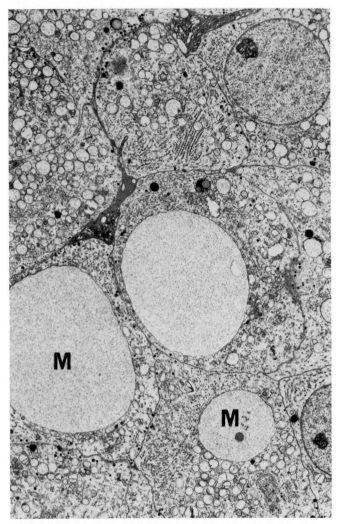

FIGURE 9–13. **Acidophil stem-cell adenoma** showing diffuse oncocytic change and mitochondrial gigantism (M) (×4,600).

show intense cytoplasmic positivity for immunoreactive GH. Immunostaining for PRL, present in the same cells, is usually much more subtle. The fine-structural appearance[6, 53, 54, 66] of the tumor shows a strong resemblance to that of highly differentiated, densely granulated GH cell adenomas. The secretory granules, however, are often pleomorphic and unusually large, measuring up to 2000 nm. Large, irregular secretory granules with a mottled core and large granule extrusions, with permanence of extruded secretory material in the intercellular spaces, are the fine-structural markers of this adenoma type (Fig. 9–14). Some of these tumors, beginning in childhood, may have less typical features.[67]

Corticotroph Adenomas

Corticotroph cell adenomas are either associated with Cushing's disease or occur in patients who have had bilaterally adrenalectomy to cure their hypercorticism (Nelson's syndrome).[6] Owing to the increased use of greatly improved imaging and neurosurgical techniques for operative removal of pituitary corticotroph cell microadenomas,

the frequency of Nelson's syndrome is now rare. The majority of corticotroph cell tumors are basophilic microadenomas, showing a characteristic sinusoidal pattern. The adenoma cells exhibit strong PAS positivity and contain, as demonstrated by the immunoperoxidase technique, ACTH and related peptides, β-LPH, and endorphins.[6, 68] The ultrastructural features of tumor cells resemble those of nontumorous corticotrophs.[6, 54, 68] The often angular cells have ovoid nuclei and relatively electron-dense cytoplasm. The well-developed, slightly dilated RER is randomly distributed in the cytoplasm; free ribosomes are numerous. The prominent Golgi complex regularly harbors developing secretory granules. The secretory granules are numerous, may be spherical or irregular (indented or heart-shaped), and exhibit varying electron density. They measure 250 to 450 nm, the majority being 300 to 350 nm. The diagnostic marker of corticotroph cell adenomas is the presence of type 1 filaments (Fig. 9–15). The fine (70 Å width) cytokeratin filaments form bundles, and their location is mainly perinuclear. The filaments are identical to those seen in normal corticotrophs and those forming Crooke's hyalin material in corticotrophs of patients with hypercortisolism.

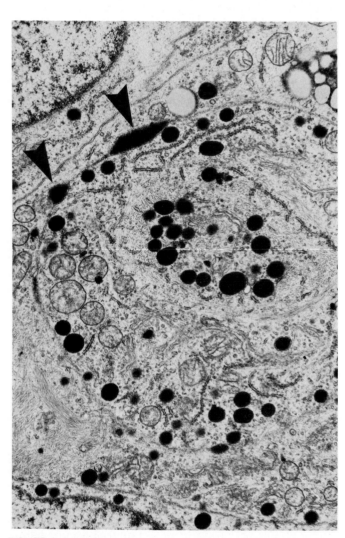

FIGURE 9–14. **Mammosomatotroph adenoma** possessing large secretory granules and deposits of secretory material in the intercellular space (*arrowheads*) (×11,900).

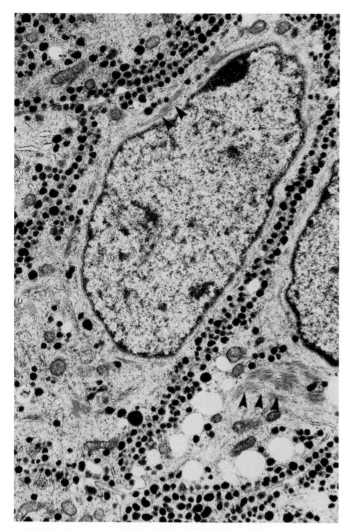

FIGURE 9–15. **Corticotroph adenoma associated with Cushing's disease.** The elongated, angular cells often have indented, irregular secretory granules with varying electron opacity and bundles of type 1 microfilaments *(arrowheads)* (×11,800).

Tumors in Nelson's syndrome contain a few or no filaments.

In a minority of corticotroph cell adenomas, excessive accumulation of type 1 filaments takes place, endowing the adenoma cells with the appearance of Crooke's cells (Fig. 9–16).[69, 70] In view of the variations in clinical presentation and morphologic features, Crooke's hyalinization cannot be explained satisfactorily in these cases.

A rare variant of corticotroph cell adenoma is chromophobic and PAS-negative, or contains only a few PAS-positive granules.[6] These tumors have a diffuse rather than sinusoidal pattern, and immunopositivity for ACTH and related peptides is scanty. Electron microscopy reveals considerably less differentiated tumors than the basophilic variant. The RER and Golgi apparatus are poorly developed, and the secretory granules are uncharacteristic, sparse, and small, measuring around 200 nm. A few type 1 filaments usually occur, aiding the pathological diagnosis. These tumors are likely to be macroadenomas at the time of surgery. It is not clear whether this is due to a faster growth rate or relatively low hormonal activity, allowing the tumors to remain undetected for a longer time.

Silent Adenomas

The term *silent adenoma* applies to a group of three well-differentiated pituitary adenomas having distinct, well-recognizable ultrastructure but no evidence of deriving from any of the known pituitary cell types.[71] Clinically, they present as seemingly nonfunctioning adenomas causing only symptoms due to tumor growth, or they may be accompanied by hyperprolactinemia.[71, 72]

Subtype 1 silent "corticotroph" adenomas are basophilic, contain immunoreactive ACTH, β-LPH, and endorphins, and possess an ultrastructural appearance indistinguishable from that of corticotroph cell adenomas in cases of Cushing's disease.[54, 71] This tumor type may arise in the posterior lobe basophils. These cells have the same morphology as anterior lobe corticotrophs and produce POMC but process the gene product differently.

Subtype 2 tumors[54, 71] show a striking male preponderance. By histology, they are chromophobic or contain a modest amount of basophilic and PAS-positive granulation. Immunopositivity for ACTH and related peptides is invariably present. By electron microscopy, the usually well-dif-

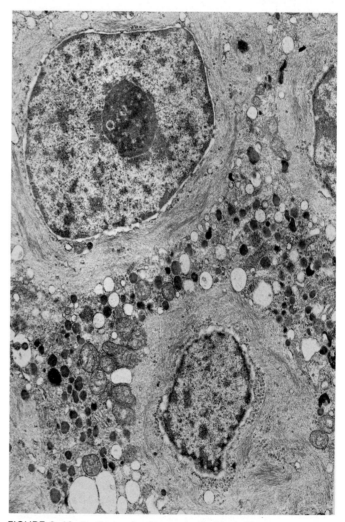

FIGURE 9–16. **Corticotroph adenoma in Cushing's disease, showing extensive Crooke's hyalinization.** The accumulating type 1 microfilaments displace secretory granules and other cytoplasmic components to the cell periphery. The cell membranes are not discernible, a common but unexplained finding in Crooke's cells (×9,700).

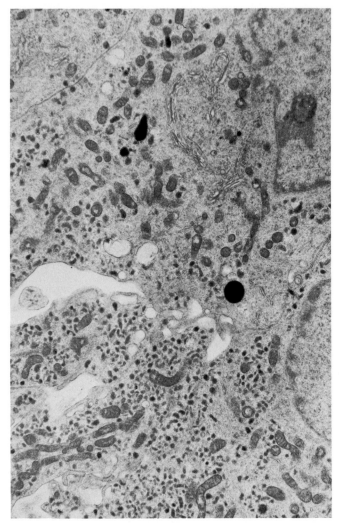

FIGURE 9–17. **Silent "corticotroph" adenoma, subtype 2.** The tumor contains immunoreactive ACTH and related peptides, but the only endocrine sign in the young male patient is hyperprolactinemia (×10,300).

ferentiated, angular cells possess well-developed RER and Golgi complex and a varying number of spherical, oval, or distinctly teardrop-shaped secretory granules measuring up to 450 nm, the majority being around 250 nm (Fig. 9–17). Microfilaments are not present.

Subtype 3 silent adenomas[71, 72] occur as nonfunctioning tumors in men, whereas in young women they are usually associated with oligomenorrhea, amenorrhea, galactorrhea, and mild to moderate hyperprolactinemia, thus mimicking prolactin-producing tumors. These fast-growing tumors are chromophobic or slightly acidophilic and may exhibit light PAS positivity. They may show positive immunostaining in a minority of cells with antisera raised against ACTH and endorphins and, in some cases, with antisera generated against other pituitary hormones as well, whereas the majority of cells remain negative. The highly differentiated fine-structural features of these tumors bear similarity to those of glycoprotein hormone–producing adenomas. The tumor cells, however, are often unusually large, containing well-developed RER, SER, and Golgi apparatus in the abundant cytoplasm. The small, chiefly spherical secretory granules measure up to 250 nm (Fig. 9–18).

The parent cells of subtype 1 and subtype 2 silent "corticotroph" adenomas may represent hitherto uncharacterized members of a POMC-producing cell line. All subtype 1 and some subtype 2 tumors express the POMC gene, as shown by in situ hybridization.[73, 74] Subtype 3 silent adenomas are mostly negative in this regard, and their derivation is entirely obscure.

Thyrotroph Adenomas

The rare thyrotroph adenomas[75–77] may be associated with long-standing untreated or insufficiently treated primary hypothyroidism or with hyperthyroidism characterized by high T_4 and T_3 as well as elevated serum TSH levels. In some cases, for reasons not understood at present, morphologically typical thyrotroph tumors may appear clinically silent in euthyroid patients.[75] By histology, thyrotroph adenomas are chromophobic with a sinusoidal pattern. Immunostaining demonstrates TSH in most of these tumors. In a few adenomas, however, the immunoperoxidase technique fails to detect the hormone, rendering the diagnosis

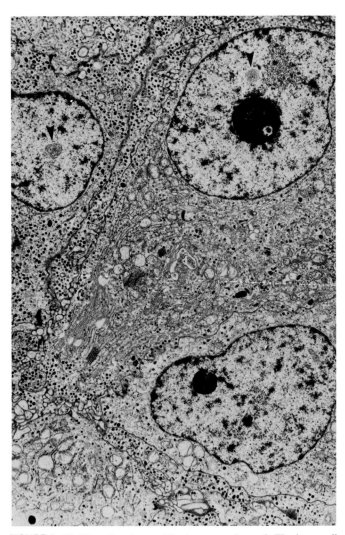

FIGURE 9–18. **Silent "corticotroph" adenoma, subtype 3.** The large cells have extensively developed endoplasmic reticulum, a Golgi complex, and a varying number of small secretory granules. Note nuclear spheridia (*arrowheads*) (×5,400).

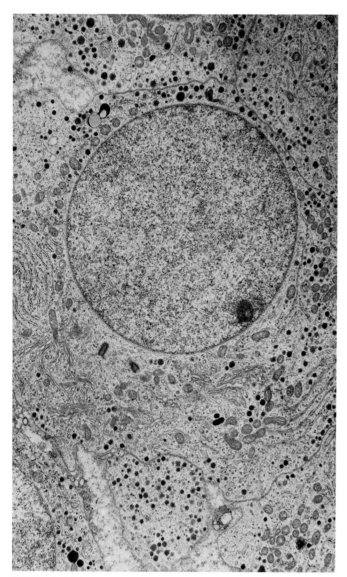

FIGURE 9–19. **Thyrotroph adenoma associated with hyperthyroidism.** The well-differentiated cells harbor prominent RER and Golgi apparatus, as well as numerous small (approx. 200 nm) secretory granules (×8,500).

of thyrotroph adenoma tentative. Electron microscopy may reveal well-differentiated tumors[6, 75, 76] consisting of middle-sized or large angular cells with uniform nuclei; prominent, slightly dilated RER; large Golgi area; and a varying number of small (100 to 350 nm) granules accumulating mainly in the cell processes (Fig. 9–19). In other instances,[6, 75] the tumors appear to be less differentiated, with irregular nuclei, small cytoplasm containing poorly or moderately developed RER, inconspicuous Golgi complex, and small, sparse, secretory granules. The appearance of this variant is rather similar to that of null cell adenoma. No close correlation exists between fine-structural features and hormonal activity of the tumors.

Gonadotroph Adenomas

The diagnosis of gonadotroph adenoma may prove to be very difficult, requiring the aid of hormone assays as well as immunocytochemistry and electron microscopy.[78, 79]

Most clinically diagnosed cases so far occur in men, as elevated serum FSH (and rarely LH) levels are detected in a large percentage of male patients with gonadotroph tumors.[80] On the other hand, in women with gonadotroph cell adenomas, serum FSH and LH levels rarely exceed the upper limit of the normal range for the patient's age. By histology, gonadotroph tumors display the same pattern as thyrotroph adenomas: mostly chromophobic with a sinusoidal structure. Cells showing basophilic staining and intense PAS positivity may occur rarely. In our experience, immunohistochemistry detects FSH and/or LH in about 85 per cent of tumors removed from men but gives positive results in less than half of the tumors of women. The fine structure of gonadotroph adenomas shows a consistent, easily recognizable sex-linked dichotomy, unparalleled so far in any other tumor type. Adenomas in men[78] often have indistinct electron microscopic features similar to those of null cell adenomas. Some tumors may be well-differentiated, displaying some similarity to normal gonadotrophs, but with no unusual features (Fig. 9–20). On the other hand, the majority of gonadotroph adenomas in women appear to be highly differentiated, with abundant, slightly dilated RER and prominent Golgi complex, exhibiting a

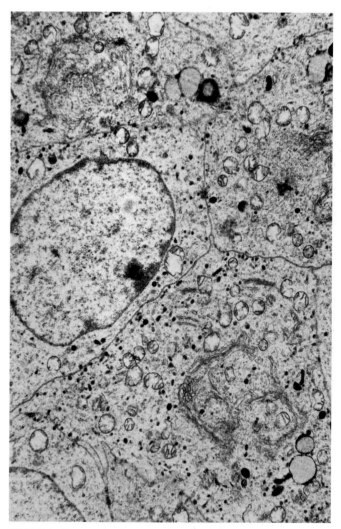

FIGURE 9–20. **Gonadotroph adenoma, male type.** The small, polyhedral cells possess prominent Golgi complexes but only moderately developed RER and sparse secretory granules (×10,400).

highly characteristic and unique vesicular dilation of the Golgi sacculi ("honeycomb Golgi")[78] (Fig. 9–21). The secretory granules, in tumors of both sexes, are small, usually less than 200 nm. The reason for the unique sex-related fine-structural variance in gonadotroph adenomas is unexplained.

Null Cell Adenomas and Oncocytomas

The term *null cell adenoma* denotes pituitary tumors that consist of cells provided with the general characteristics of endocrine secretory cells but lacking distinctive fine-structural and/or immunocytochemical markers that could assign them to a specific cell type.[81] Clinically, these neoplasms appear to be nonfunctional. They are chromophobic by histology, with a sinusoidal or diffuse pattern. By immunocytology, they are negative for all pituitary hormones or contain only scattered cells staining positively for one or more hormones, mainly glycoprotein hormones and their α-subunits.[81, 82] Electron microscopy[53, 54, 81] reveals tumors consisting of closely apposed, small polyhedral cells with

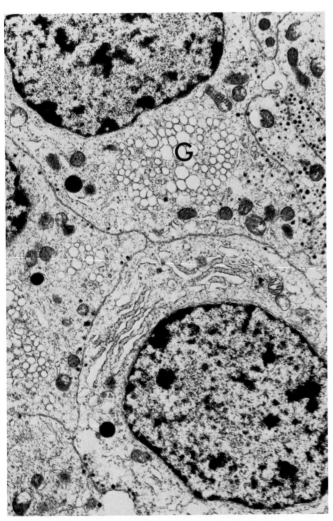

FIGURE 9–21. **Gonadotroph adenoma, female type.** The uniform cells possess abundant dilated RER and small (150 nm) secretory granules accumulating in the cell processes. Note the vesicular transformation of the Golgi complex (G, "honeycomb Golgi"), the hallmark of this tumor type (×10,000).

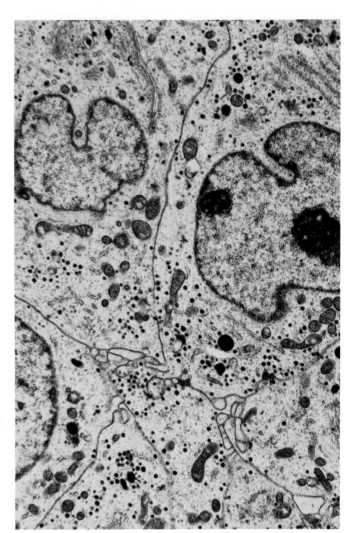

FIGURE 9–22. **Null cell adenoma.** The small cells have irregular nuclei and poorly developed cytoplasmic organelles (×10,400).

irregular nuclei. The small cytoplasm contains short, scattered profiles of poorly developed RER, clusters of free ribosomes, and a variable number of small, rod-shaped mitochondria (Fig. 9–22). The Golgi apparatus may be more prominent than the rest of the cytoplasmic organelles. The secretory granules are sparse and small, measuring 100 to 250 nm. They often have an irregular, dense core and a halo under the limiting membrane.

Oncocytic transformation—that is, the increase in number and volume density of mitochondria—may be evident in a variable proportion of cells of null cell adenomas. If oncocytic change is very extensive, involving practically every adenoma cell, we label the tumor pituitary oncocytoma. By histology, these tumors are either chromophobic or, owing to the accumulation of mitochondria, show various degrees of acidophilia over the coarsely granular cytoplasm. By immunohistochemistry, oncocytomas behave in the same manner as null cell adenomas, and the ultrastructure of cellular organelles is essentially the same in the two variants, with the exception of mitochondrial abundance, which is the sole fine-structural marker of oncocytomas (Fig. 9–23).[6, 83] The mitochondria, occupying up to 55 per cent of the cytoplasmic area, are either small and rod-shaped with numerous cristae ("dark" oncocytes, acido-

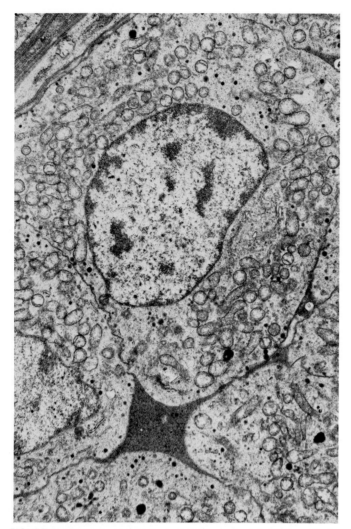

FIGURE 9–23. **Pituitary oncocytoma** showing marked abundance of mitochondria (×9,900).

philic by histology) or large and ovoid or spherical and rarefied with loss of cristae ("light" oncocytes, chromophobic by histology).

Null cell adenomas and oncocytomas are grouped together on the basis of absence or paucity of morphological markers. They most probably represent a heterogeneous group,[82] although the majority of clinically nonfunctioning adenomas express the genes for α- and β-subunits of glycoprotein hormones.[84]

It is important to note that oncocytic transformation may also occur in any type of clinically functioning adenomas, especially in older patients. In these tumors, however, the immunohistochemical and fine-structural markers of that particular adenoma type are retained, and these neoplasms should be classified according to their cytogenesis and hormonal function.

Plurihormonal Adenomas

The term *plurihormonal adenoma* designates pituitary tumors producing more than one hormone. Plurihormonal adenomas may consist of one cell type (monomorphous) or more cell types (plurimorphous) by electron micros-

copy.[53] The most common bihormonal adenomas, producing GH and PRL, are discussed earlier in this chapter. Here we wish to call attention to less frequent, sometimes very unusual, combinations. The occurrence of plurihormonal adenomas producing hormones of the "acidophil" and glycoprotein hormone cell lines is surprisingly common.[53, 85] They most often contain, by immunocytochemistry, GH and α-subunit, frequently associated by scattered immunoreactivity for PRL and TSH. Some tumors may show scanty LH- and FSH-like immunoreactivity as well. Discrepancies between the immunohistochemical profile, ultrastructure, and clinical presentation of these adenomas are not unusual because some of the hormones produced by the tumor are unassociated with clinical and biochemical abnormalities. GH is almost invariably symptomatic. Apart from the frequent simultaneous occurrence of increased GH and PRL levels, the most common association of endocrine disorders caused by the same pituitary adenoma is acromegaly and hyperthyroidism.[86, 87] The uncommon GH and PRL immunoreactivities in glycoprotein hormone–producing adenomas are rarely significant and are symptomatic only in exceptional cases.

Other combinations (e.g., ACTH + PRL, ACTH + α-subunit, ACTH + LH, PRL + FSH, TSH + PRL, PRL + α-subunit + endorphin, ACTH + PRL) are rare and not yet well classified.[53]

REFERENCES

1. Bergland RM, Ray BS, Torack RM: Anatomical variations in the pituitary gland and adjacent structures in 225 autopsy cases. J Neurosurg 28:93–99, 1968.
2. Scheithauer BW, Sano T, Kovacs K, et al: The pituitary gland in pregnancy: A clinicopathologic and immunohistochemical study of 69 cases. Mayo Clin Proc 65:461–474, 1990.
3. Dubois PM, Hemming FJ: Fetal development and regulation of pituitary cell types. J Electron Microsc Tech 19:2–20, 1991.
4. Asa SL, Kovacs K, Singer W: Human fetal adenohypophysis: Morphologic and functional analysis in vitro. Neuroendocrinology 53:562–572, 1991.
5. Pearse AGE, Takor T: Embryology of the diffuse neuroendocrine system and its relationship to the common peptides. Fed Proc 38:2288–2294, 1979.
6. Kovacs K, Horvath E: Tumors of the pituitary. In Atlas of Tumor Pathology, 2nd Series, Fascicle 21. Washington, DC, Armed Forces Institute of Pathology, 1986.
7. Asa SL, Kovacs K, Bilbao JM: The pars tuberalis of the human pituitary: A histologic, immunocytochemical, ultrastructural and immuno-electron microscopic analysis. Virchows Arch 399:49–59, 1983.
8. Kovacs K, Horvath E, Ryan N: Immunocytology of the human pituitary. In Sternberg S, DeLellis RA (eds): Diagnostic Immunocytochemistry. New York, Masson, 1981, pp 17–35.
9. Boyd JD: Observations on the human pharyngeal hypophysis. J Endocrinol 14:66–77, 1956.
10. McGrath P: The volume of the human pharyngeal hypophysis in relation to age and sex. J Anat 110:275–282, 1971.
11. Scheithauer BW: The hypothalamus and neurohypophysis. In Kovacs K, Asa SL (eds): Functional Endocrine Pathology. Boston, Blackwell Scientific Publications, 1991, pp 170–244.
12. Stanfield JP: The blood supply of the human pituitary gland. J Anat 94:257–273, 1960.
13. Daniel PM, Prichard MML: Studies of the hypothalamus and the pituitary gland with special reference to the effects of transection of the pituitary stalk. Acta Endocrinol 80 (Suppl) 201:1–216, 1975.
14. Bergland RM, Page RB: Pituitary-brain vascular relations: A new paradigm. Science 204:18–24, 1979.
15. Gorczyca W, Hardy J: Arterial supply of the human anterior pituitary gland. Neurosurgery 20:369–378, 1987.

16. Sheehan HL, Whitehead R: The neurohypophysis in postpartum hypopituitarism. J Pathol Bacteriol 85:145–169, 1963.
17. Sheehan HL, Kovacs K: The subventricular nucleus of the human hypothalamus. Brain 89:589–614, 1966.
18. Horvath E, Kovacs K: Fine structural cytology of the adenohypophysis in rat and man. J Electron Microsc Tech 8:401–432, 1988.
19. Frawley LS, Boockfor FR: Mammosomatotropes: Presence and functions in normal and neoplastic pituitary tissue. Endocr Rev 12:337–355, 1991.
20. Thorner MO, Perryman RL, Cronin MJ, et al: Somatotroph hyperplasia. J Clin Invest 70:965–977, 1982.
21. Moran A, Asa SL, Kovacs K, et al: Gigantism due to pituitary mammosomatotroph hyperplasia. N Engl J Med 323:322–327, 1990.
22. Schechter J, Kovacs K, Rimoin D: Isolated growth hormone deficiency: Immunocytochemistry. J Clin Endocrinol Metab 59:798–800, 1984.
23. Asa SL, Penz G, Kovacs K, Ezrin C: Prolactin cells in the human pituitary: A quantitative immunocytochemical analysis. Arch Pathol Lab Med 106:360–363, 1982.
24. Jay V, Kovacs K, Horvath E, et al: Idiopathic prolactin cell hyperplasia of the pituitary mimicking prolactin cell adenoma: A morphological study including immunocytochemistry, electron microscopy and in situ hybridization. Acta Neuropathol 82:147–151, 1991.
25. Neumann PE, Horoupian DS, Goldman JE, Hess MA: Cytoplasmic filaments of Crooke's hyaline change belong to the cytokeratin class. An immunocytochemical and ultrastructural study. Am J Pathol 116:214–222, 1984.
26. Halliday WC, Asa SL, Kovacs K, Scheithauer BW: Intermediate filaments in the human pituitary gland: An immunohistochemical study. Can J Neurol Sci 17:131–136, 1990.
27. McNicol AM: Patterns of corticotropic cells in the adult human pituitary in Cushing's disease. Diagn Histopathol 4:335–341, 1981.
28. Saeger W, Ludecke DK: Pituitary hyperplasia. Definition, light and electron microscopic structures and significance in surgical specimens. Virchows Arch (A) 399:277–287, 1983.
29. Lloyd RV, Chandler WF, McKeever PE, Schteingart DE: The spectrum of ACTH-producing pituitary lesions. Am J Surg Pathol 10:618–626, 1986.
30. Carey RM, Varma SK, Drake CR Jr, et al: Ectopic secretion of corticotropin-releasing factor as a cause of Cushing's syndrome. A clinical, morphologic, and biochemical study. N Engl J Med 311:13–20, 1984.
31. Scheithauer BW, Kovacs K, Randall RV: The pituitary in untreated Addison's disease: A histologic and immunocytologic study of 18 adenohypophyses. Arch Pathol Lab Med 107:484–487, 1983.
32. Khalil A, Kovacs K, Sima AAF, et al: Pituitary thyrotroph hyperplasia mimicking prolactin-secreting adenoma. J Endocrinol Invest 7:399–404, 1984.
33. Scheithauer BW, Kovacs K, Randall RV, Ryan N: Pituitary gland in hypothyroidism. Histologic and immunocytologic study. Arch Pathol Lab Med 109:499–504, 1985.
34. Scheithauer BW, Kovacs K, Young WF Jr, Randall RV: The pituitary in hyperthyroidism. Mayo Clin Proc 67:22–26, 1992.
35. Denef C: Paracrine interactions in the anterior pituitary. Clin Endocrinol Metab 15:1–32, 1986.
36. Marin F, Stefaneanu L, Kovacs K: Folliculo-stellate cells of the pituitary. Endocr Pathol 2:180–192, 1991.
37. Baes M, Allaerts W, Denef C: Evidence for functional communication between folliculo-stellate cells and hormone secreting cells in perifused anterior pituitary cell aggregates. Endocrinology 120:685–691, 1987.
38. Cardoso ER, Peterson EW: Pituitary apoplexy: A review. Neurosurgery 14:363–373, 1984.
39. Kovacs K: Necrosis of anterior pituitary in humans. Neuroendocrinology 4:179–199, 201–241, 1969.
40. Kovacs K: Adenohypophysial necrosis in routine autopsies. Endokrinologie 60:309–316, 1972.
41. McCormick WF, Halmi NS: The hypophysis in patients with coma depasse ("respirator brain"). Am J Clin Pathol 54:374–383, 1970.
42. Kovacs K, Bilbao JM: Adenohypophysial necrosis in respirator maintained patients. Pathol Microbiol 41:275–282, 1974.
43. Sheehan HL, Davis JC: Post-partum hypopituitarism. Springfield, IL, Charles C Thomas, 1982, pp 1–453.
44. Sano T, Kovacs K, Scheithauer BW, et al: Pituitary pathology in acquired immunodeficiency syndrome. Arch Pathol Lab Med 113:1066–1070, 1989.
45. Pestell RG, Best JD, Alford FP: Lymphocytic hypophysitis. The clinical spectrum of the disorder and evidence for an autoimmune pathogenesis. Clin Endocrinol 33:457–466, 1990.
46. Cosman F, Post KD, Holub DA, Wardlaw SL: Lymphocytic hypophysitis. Report of 3 new cases and review of the literature. Medicine 68:240–256, 1989.
47. Petito CK, De Girolami U, Earle KM: Craniopharyngioma: A clinical and pathological review. Cancer 37:1944–1952, 1976.
48. Harris PE, Perry L, Chard T, et al: Immunoreactive human chorionic gonadotrophin from the cyst fluid and CSF of patients with craniopharyngioma. Clin Endocrinol 29:503–508, 1988.
49. Scheithauer BW, Randall RV, Laws ER Jr, et al: Prolactin cell carcinoma of the pituitary: Clinicopathologic, immunohistochemical, and ultrastructural study of a case with intracranial and extracranial metastases. Cancer 55:598–604, 1985.
50. Mountcastle RB, Roof BS, Mayfield RK, et al: Case report: Pituitary adenocarcinoma in an acromegalic patient: Response to bromocriptine and pituitary testing. A review of the literature on 36 cases of pituitary carcinoma. Am J Med Sci 298:109–118, 1989.
51. Kovacs K: Metastatic cancer of the pituitary gland. Oncology 27:533–542, 1973.
52. Teears RJ, Silverman EM: Clinicopathologic review of 88 cases of carcinoma metastatic to the pituitary gland. Cancer 36:216–220, 1975.
53. Horvath E, Kovacs K: The adenohypophysis. In Kovacs K, Asa SL (eds): Functional Endocrine Pathology. Boston, Blackwell Scientific Publications, 1991, pp 245–281.
54. Horvath E, Kovacs K: Ultrastructural diagnosis of human pituitary adenomas. Microsc Res Tech 20:107–135, 1992.
55. Kovacs K, Horvath E: Pathology of growth hormone–producing tumors of the human pituitary. Semin Diag Pathol 3:18–33, 1986.
56. Neumann PE, Goldman JE, Horoupian DS, Hess MA: Fibrous bodies in growth hormone–secreting adenomas contain cytokeratin filaments. Arch Pathol Lab Med 109:505–508, 1985.
57. Landolt AM, Kleihues P, Heitz PU: Amyloid deposits in pituitary adenomas. Arch Pathol Lab Med 111:453–458, 1987.
58. Barkan AL, Lloyd RV, Chandler WF, et al: Preoperative treatment of acromegaly with long-acting somatostatin analog SMS 201-995: Shrinkage of invasive pituitary macroadenomas and improved surgical remission rate. J Clin Endocrinol Metab 67:1040–1048, 1988.
59. Beckers A, Kovacs K, Horvath E, et al: Effect of treatment with octreotide on the morphology of growth hormone–secreting pituitary adenomas: Study of 24 cases. Endocr Pathol 2:123–131, 1991.
60. Horvath E, Kovacs K: Pathology of prolactin cell adenomas of the human pituitary. Semin Diag Pathol 3:4–17, 1986.
61. Rilliet B, Mohr G, Robert F, Hardy J: Calcification in pituitary adenomas. Surg Neurol 15:249–255, 1981.
62. Kovacs K, Stefaneanu L, Horvath E, et al: Effect of dopamine agonist medication on prolactin producing adenomas. A morphological study including immunocytochemistry, electron microscopy and in situ hybridization. Virchows Arch (A) 418:439–446, 1991.
63. Melmed S, Braunstein GD, Horvath E, et al: Pathophysiology of acromegaly. Endocr Rev 4:271–290, 1983.
64. Scheithauer BW, Kovacs K, Randall RV, et al: Pathology of excessive production of growth hormone. Clin Endocrinol Metab 15:655–681, 1986.
65. Horvath E, Kovacs K, Singer W, et al: Acidophil stem cell adenoma of the human pituitary. Clinico-pathological analysis of 15 cases. Cancer 47:761–771, 1981.
66. Horvath E, Kovacs K, Killinger DW, et al: Mammosomatotroph cell adenoma of the human pituitary: A morphologic entity. Virchows Arch (A) 398:277–289, 1983.
67. Felix IA, Horvath E, Kovacs K, et al: Mammosomatotroph adenoma of the pituitary associated with gigantism and hyperprolactinemia. A morphological study including immunoelectron microscopy. Acta Neuropathol (Berl) 71:76–82, 1986.
68. Robert F, Hardy J: Human corticotroph cell adenomas. Semin Diag Pathol 3:34–41, 1986.
69. Felix IA, Horvath E, Kovacs K: Massive Crooke's hyalinization in corticotroph cell adenomas of the human pituitary: A histological, immunocytochemical, and electron microscopic study of three cases. Acta Neurochir 58:235–243, 1982.
70. Horvath E, Kovacs K, Josse R: Pituitary corticotroph cell adenoma with marked abundance of microfilaments. Ultrastruct Pathol 5:249–255, 1983.
71. Horvath E, Kovacs K, Killinger DW, et al: Silent corticotropic adenomas of the human pituitary gland: A histologic, immunocytologic and ultrastructural study. Am J Pathol 98:617–638, 1980.
72. Horvath E, Kovacs K, Smyth HS, et al: A novel type of pituitary adenoma: Morphological features and clinical correlations. J Clin Endocrinol Metab 66:1111–1118, 1988.

73. Lloyd RV, Fields K, Jin L, et al: Analysis of endocrine active and clinically silent corticotropic adenomas by in situ hybridization. Am J Pathol 137:479–488, 1990.

74. Stefaneanu L, Kovacs K, Horvath E, Lloyd RV: In situ hybridization study of pro-opiomelanocortin (POMC) gene expression in human pituitary corticotrophs and their adenomas. Virchows Arch (A) 419:107–113, 1991.

75. Saeger W, Ludecke DK: Pituitary adenomas with hyperfunction of TSH: Frequency, histological classification, immunocytochemistry and ultrastructure. Virchows Arch (A) 394:255–267, 1982.

76. Girod C, Trouillas J, Claustrat B: The human thyrotropic adenoma: Pathologic diagnosis in five cases and critical review of the literature. Semin Diag Pathol 3:58–68, 1986.

77. Beckers A, Abs R, Mahler C, et al: Thyrotropin-secreting pituitary adenomas: Report of seven cases. J Clin Endocrinol Metab 72:477–483, 1991.

78. Horvath E, Kovacs K: Gonadotroph adenomas of the human pituitary: Sex-related fine structural dichotomy. A histologic, immunocytochemical, and electron microscopic study of 30 tumors. Am J Pathol 117:429–440, 1984.

79. Trouillas J, Girod C, Sassolas G, Claustrat B: The human gonadotropic adenoma: Pathologic diagnosis and hormonal correlations in 26 tumors. Semin Diag Pathol 3:42–57, 1986.

80. Snyder PJ: Gonadotroph cell adenomas of the pituitary. Endocr Rev 6:552–563, 1985.

81. Kovacs K, Horvath E, Ryan N, Ezrin C: Null cell adenoma of the human pituitary. Virchows Arch (A) 387:165–174, 1980.

82. Kovacs K, Asa SL, Horvath E, et al: Null cell adenomas of the pituitary: Attempts to resolve their cytogenesis. In Lechago J, Kameya T (eds): Endocrine Pathology Update. New York, Field and Wood, 1990, pp 17–31.

83. Yamada S, Asa SL, Kovacs K: Oncocytomas and null cell adenomas of the human pituitary: Morphometric and in vitro functional comparison. Virchows Arch (A) 413:333–339, 1988.

84. Jameson JL, Klibanski A, Black PM, et al: Glycoprotein hormone genes are expressed in clinically nonfunctioning pituitary adenomas. J Clin Invest 80:1472–1478, 1987.

85. Scheithauer BW, Horvath E, Kovacs K, et al: Plurihormonal pituitary adenomas. Semin Diag Pathol 3:69–82, 1986.

86. Beck-Peccoz P, Piscitelli G, Amr S, et al: Endocrine, biochemical, and morphological studies of a pituitary adenoma secreting growth hormone, thyrotropin (TSH), and α-subunit: Evidence for secretion of TSH with increased bioactivity. J Clin Endocrinol Metab 62:704–711, 1986.

87. Malarkey WB, Kovacs K, O'Dorisio TM: Response of a GH- and TSH-secreting pituitary adenoma to a somatostatin analogue (SMS 201-995): Evidence that GH and TSH coexist in the same cell and secretory granules. Neuroendocrinology 49:267–274, 1989.

10

Role of Neurotransmitters and Neuromodulators in the Control of Anterior Pituitary Hormone Secretion

EUGENIO E. MÜLLER

BRAIN NEUROTRANSMITTERS AND NEUROPEPTIDES

Characteristic Features
Principal Locations of Neuronal Pathways
  Relevant to Neuroendocrine Function

NEUROTRANSMITTER REGULATION OF ANTERIOR PITUITARY HORMONES

ACTH
  Catecholamines
  Serotonin
  Acetylcholine
  Histamine
  GABA
Growth Hormone
  Catecholamines
  Serotonin
  Acetylcholine
  Histamine
  GABA
Gonadotropins
  Catecholamines
  Serotonin
  Acetylcholine
  Histamine
  Amino Acids
Prolactin
  Catecholamines
  Serotonin
  Histamine
  GABA
Thyroid-Stimulating Hormone
  Catecholamines

BRAIN PEPTIDES AND ANTERIOR PITUITARY HORMONES

Opioid Peptides
Other Neuropeptides

THERAPEUTIC IMPLICATIONS OF NEUROACTIVE DRUGS IN NEUROENDOCRINE DISORDERS

Growth Homone Deficiency and Excess
  States
Hypogonadotropic Hypogonadism
Cushing's Disease
Prolactinomas

It is now clear that the anterior pituitary gland (AP) is under the influence of hypothalamic and extrahypothalamic structures. A host of messenger substances, whose chemical identity has been now established,[1] are released from hypothalamic neurons and conveyed to the AP via a portal system of capillaries. The functional activity of hypothalamic neurosecretory neurons, which manufacture and deliver specific hypophysiotropic regulatory hormones (RH's) into the portal system, is in turn under the control of a host of neurotransmitters and neuropeptides.[2] The function of these substances is to relay to the hypophysiotropic neurosecretory neurons of the hypothalamus, via typical or atypical synaptic connections, neural or neurohormonal influences, which are translated into hormonal responses to be delivered to the AP. Consequently, pharmacologically induced manipulations of this neurotransmitter-neuropeptide system of control induce profound changes in the secretion of AP hormones, and RH's and CNS-acting compounds can be used to probe pituitary or hypothalamic function, respectively, and in humans to diagnose and treat neuroendocrine disorders.[2]

BRAIN NEUROTRANSMITTERS AND NEUROPEPTIDES

Neurotransmitter and peptidergic systems in the endocrine hypothalamus and related extrahypothalamic areas ensure the proper control of AP function. The widely held distinction between classic neurotransmitter communication and peptidergic communication is now blurred, and in spite of their recognized differences, the two systems can no longer be considered two entirely disparate entities. It is now clear that the same compound may have multiple, operationally distinct actions as transmitter (acting to elicit strictly localized short-lived responses at an easily identifiable locus, the synapse), neuromodulator (unable to directly dominate membrane excitability by altering a specific ionic conductance as a neurotransmitter does, but rather modulating the subsynaptic action of a neurotransmitter-coupled event), and neurohormone (acting at a relatively great distance from the site of release and not in synaptic contact with the synthesizing neurons), depending on the engagement of specific receptors.[3]

Another reason for breakdown of demarcation between these messenger substances is the recognition that they may coexist in the same neuron in different CNS areas as well as in the mediobasal hypothalamus (MBH). The functional role of these co-stored neurotransmitters and neuropeptides has yet to be completely clarified, although demonstration of co-storage also within nerve terminals of these neuronal systems at the median eminence (ME) level suggests a co-release at this site. It can be said that, in general, amines and amino acids are employed as neurotransmitters, whereas peptides function as neuromodulators and neurohormones.[4]

Discussion of the influences exerted by brain messengers on the neuroendocrine control of AP secretion requires at least a brief description of the characteristic features of these compounds, mention of the CNS-acting compounds capable of interfering with the different metabolic steps or with presynaptic and postsynaptic receptors, and, lastly, mention of the regional distribution of the main neuronal pathways in the CNS.

Characteristic Features

As a general rule, neurotransmitters are small molecules synthesized in a short series of steps from precursor amino acids in the diet. In general, each nerve cell contains the enzymes that synthesize a single transmitter. The one synthesized is stored in synaptic vesicles until a stimulus calls for release. Intraneuronal neurotransmitter levels are kept fairly constant by replacement of released transmitter by enzymatic synthesis in nerve endings, recapture of neurotransmitter from synaptic space, and/or supply of transmitter or its precursor in storage vesicles from the perikaryon. Neurotransmitters are found in brain in concentrations of nanograms to micrograms per gram and show high affinity for specific receptor sites.

The first substance to be established as a neurotransmitter was acetylcholine (ACh), and 5 to 10 per cent of brain synapses are thought to be cholinergic. Amino acids (γ-aminobutyric acid [GABA], glycine, glutamate, aspartate, and taurine) form the main group of central transmitters (estimated 25 to 40 per cent synapses). The monoamines (catecholamines, tryptamines, and histamine) account for only 1 to 2 per cent of brain synapses, but the monoamine pathways are widely distributed throughout the brain. The principal steps in the formation of neurotransmitters are depicted in Figure 10–1.

Many drugs are capable of inhibiting the functional activity of neurotransmitter neurons. They comprise biosynthesis inhibitors at the level of different enzymatic steps, depletors of the granular pool, and neurotoxic agents that destroy neurotransmitter terminals. Conversely, neurotransmitter precursors or inhibitors of metabolic degradation or uptake potentiate neurotransmitter mechanisms (Tables 10–1 to 10–4).

The pathways by which the neuropeptides are synthesized closely resemble those occurring in peripheral hormone-producing tissues. Peptides are produced only in the ribosomes of the cell body, in the form of a larger precursor molecule (prohormone) that provides a means for generating multiple biological activities from a single gene product. Whereas terminal stores of monoamine transmitters may be replenished by synthesis and by reuptake into nerve terminals, each peptide molecule released from a nerve ending must be replaced by axonal transport; there is no evidence for the existence of reuptake systems or other mechanisms for recycling peptide once it is released from nerve terminals. Peptides may be released intermittently rather than tonically, the amounts stored in terminals may be large relative to the amounts released, and the released peptide may activate receptors at much lower concentrations than the classic transmitters. Hence, in general, neuropeptides are present in the brain in concentrations of picograms to nanograms per gram.

Principal Locations of Neuronal Pathways Relevant to Neuroendocrine Function

Progress in the topographical localization of principal neurotransmitter systems has been made possible by many technical advances, especially histochemical and immunohistochemical methodologies, the introduction of steady-

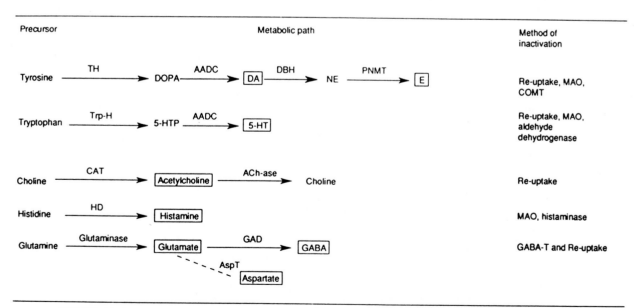

FIGURE 10–1. **Steps in the formation of classic neurotransmitters.** Abbreviations: AAAD, aromatic amino acid decarboxylase; ACh-ase, acetylcholine-esterase; AspT, mitochondrial aspartate transaminase; CAT, choline acetyltransferase; COMT, catechol-O-methyltransferase; DA, dopamine; DβH, dopamine β-hydroxylase; DOPA, dihydroxyphenylalanine; E, epinephrine; GABA-T, γ-aminobutyric acid transaminase; GAD, glutamic acid decarboxylase; HD, histidine decarboxylase; 5-HT, 5-hydroxytryptamine; 5-HTP, 5-hydroxytryptophan; MAO, monoamine oxidase; NE, norepinephrine; PNMT, phenylethanolamine-N-methyltransferase; TH, tyrosine hydroxylase; Trp-H, tryptophan hydroxylase.

TABLE 10–1. DRUGS ALTERING CATECHOLAMINE FUNCTION

DRUG	MECHANISMS OF ACTION	OBSERVATIONS
Apomorphine	Direct stimulation of pre- and postsynaptic DA receptors	Increase in brain 5-HT and 5-hydroxy-indoleacetic acid
Bromocriptine (2-Br-α-ergocriptine)	Direct stimulation of pre- and postsynaptic DA receptors	Action depending in part on brain CA stores
Lisuride	Direct stimulation of pre- and postsynaptic DA receptors	Peripheral antiserotoninergic activity
Cabergoline	Direct stimulation of pre- and postsynaptic DA receptors	Long-lasting action
Pergolide	Direct stimulation of pre- and postsynaptic DA receptors	Long-lasting action
CV 205-502 (quinagolide)	Direct stimulation of pre- and postsynaptic DA receptors	Long-lasting action
Piribedil	Direct and indirect stimulation of DA receptors	—
Amantadine	Direct and indirect stimulation of DA receptors	Blockade of DA reuptake
Nomifensine	Blockade of DA and NE reuptake	—
Clonidine	Direct stimulation of central and peripheral α_2-adrenoceptors	Stimulation of central histamine H_2-receptors
L-Dopa	Increased synthesis of DA and NE	Displacement of 5-HT by DA formed in serotoninergic neurons
α-MpT (α-methyl-paratyrosine)	Blockade of tyrosine hydroxylase and of DA, NE, and epinephrine synthesis	Conversion to α-methyl DA and α-methyl NE endowed with intrinsic receptor-stimulating activity
Reserpine	Release of intragranular pool of CA's and inhibition of granular uptake; some effect on 5-HT neurons	—
Carbidopa	Selective inhibition of peripheral aromatic L-amino acid decarboxylase	—
Chlorpromazine	Blockade of DA and NE receptors	Hypersensitivity to adrenergic stimulation
Haloperidol	Blockade of DA receptors	—
Pimozide	Blockade of DA receptors	At high doses, blockade of NE receptors
Phentolamine	Blockade of α_1- and α_2-adrenoceptors	Long-lasting action
Phenoxybenzamine	Blockade of α_1- and α_2-adrenoceptors	Long-lasting action; blockade also of 5-HT, histamine, and ACh receptors
Methoxamine	α_1-Adrenoceptor agonism	Slight β-blockade penetration of blood-brain barrier
Prazosin	Blockade of α_1-adrenoceptors	Slight β-blockade
Idazoxan	Blockade of α_2-adrenoceptors	Blockade also of DA receptors
Yohimbine	Blockade of α_2-adrenoceptors	—
Propranolol	Blockade of β_1- and β_2-adrenoceptors	—
Pindolol	Blockade of β_1- and β_2-adrenoceptors	Interaction with $5\text{-HT}_{1A/1B}$ receptors

Modified from Müller EE: Brain messengers and the pituitary gland. *In* Dulbecco R (ed): Encyclopedia of Human Biology, Vol 2. San Diego, Academic Press, 1991, with permission.

See text for abbreviations.

state or non–steady-state methods for measurement of turnover, enzymatic techniques for the determinations of neurotransmitters in selective hypothalamic nuclei, and in vivo and in vitro autoradiography.[2, 4, 5]

It is now clear that amine neurotransmitters, that is, catecholamines (dopamine [DA], epinephrine, norepinephrine [NE]), indoleamines (serotonin [5-HT]) and histamine), have perikarya in the brain stem that contribute ascending ventral and dorsal pathways to innervate limbic and hypothalamic structures, including the internal (NE, 5-HT) and external (DA) layers of the ME. Of particular relevance for neuroendocrine control is the tuberoinfundibular DA (TIDA) pathway, which projects from the arcuate nucleus to the ME and releases DA directly into the hypophyseal portal vessels. ACh-containing neurons are present in the supraoptic nucleus and in the lateral preoptic area, and a cholinergic tuberoinfundibular pathway, similar to the TIDA pathway, is envisaged.

Among the amino acid neurotransmitters, GABA-containing neurons are found in the mediobasal, posterior, and median hypothalamus, projecting nerve fibers into the external layer of the ME (TI–GABA-ergic pathway). Neurons containing acidic excitatory amino acids (EAA's) are present in discrete brain nuclei of rats, including many hypothalamic nuclei (arcuate, periventricular, ventromedial), and nerve terminals project to the ME.

All of these areas are potential sites for hypophysiotropic peptide–neurotransmitters interaction. These include the possibility of a direct action of neurotransmitters transported into hypophyseal vessels (DA, epinephrine, GABA), the still-elusive interactions of peptide-peptide, neurotransmitter-neurotransmitter, and peptide-neurotransmitter due to co-localizaton and co-release of two or more molecules in the same neuron (for further details see ref. 2).

Consequently, drugs that act as agonists or antagonists at neurotransmitter receptors or that alter different aspects of neurotransmitter function (Tables 10–1 to 10–4) may be useful as tools to study the physiology and pathophysiology of AP hormone secretion, as well as for diagnostic and therapeutic intervention.

Detailed mapping of the principal brain neuropeptides is beyond the scope of this chapter, and the reader is referred to reference 4. Some generalities can be expressed on the basis of these distribution studies. Thus, some brain

TABLE 10–2. DRUGS ALTERING SEROTONIN FUNCTION

DRUG	MECHANISM OF ACTION	OBSERVATIONS
L-Tryptophan	Selective increase in 5-HT synthesis, storage, and metabolism	—
5-Hydroxy-tryptophan	Increase in 5-HT synthesis	Decrease (by displacement) of brain DA and NE levels
8-OH-DPAT	5-HT$_{1A}$-receptor agonism	—
Ipsapirone	5-HT$_{1A}$-receptor antagonism	—
Fenfluramine	Release of 5-HT from vesicular stores	Blockade of 5-HT reuptake
pCPA (p-chloro-phenyl-alanine)	Blockade of tryptophan hydroxylase and of 5-HT synthesis	Release of CA's
Fluoxetine	Selective blockade of 5-HT reuptake	—
Methysergide	Blockade of 5-HT receptors	Potential dopaminergic, antidopaminergic, and antiserotoninergic activity
Cyproheptadine	Blockade of 5-HT receptors	Antihistamine, anticholinergic, and anticatecholaminergic activity
Metergoline	Blockade of 5-HT receptors	Potential dopaminergic activity

Modified from Müller EE: Brain messengers and the pituitary gland. *In* Dulbecco R (ed): Encyclopedia of Human Biology, Vol 2. San Diego, Academic Press, 1991; with permission.
See text for abbreviations.

areas are rich in both peptide-immunoreactive cell bodies and terminals. Other areas, such as the cerebellum, have low levels of most neuropeptides; the thalamus is also poor in neuropeptides.

Cortical areas are particularly rich in some neuropeptides, such as vasoactive intestinal peptide (VIP), cholecystokinin (CCK), somatostatin (SS), and corticotropin-releasing hormone (CRH). Peptides are present mainly in small interneurons, a notable exception being the long projections of endorphinergic neurons whose cell bodies in the arcuate nucleus send terminals to innervate various nuclei of the brain stem.

TABLE 10–3. DRUGS ALTERING CHOLINERGIC AND GABA-ERGIC FUNCTIONS

DRUG	MECHANISMS OF ACTION	OBSERVATIONS
Acetylcholine	Direct stimulation of muscarinic and nicotinic receptors	—
Pyridostigmine	Reversible inhibition of acetylcholinesterase	Does not cross the blood-brain barrier
Atropine	Antagonism at muscarinic M$_1$- and M$_2$-receptors	—
Pirenzepine	Antagonism at muscarinic M$_1$-receptors	Poor penetration of the blood-brain barrier
Aminooxyacetic acid	Inhibition of GABA catabolism	—
Sodium valproate	Inhibition of GABA catabolism	—
Muscimol	Direct stimulation of GABA$_A$-receptors	—
Baclofen	Direct stimulation of GABA$_B$-receptors	Action not antagonized by bicuculline
Bicuculline	Antagonism at GABA receptors	—

Modified from Müller EE: Brain messengers and the pituitary gland. *In* Dulbecco R (ed): Encyclopedia of Human Biology, Vol 2. San Diego, Academic Press, 1991; with permission.
See text for abbreviations.

TABLE 10–4. DRUGS ALTERING HISTAMINERGIC AND EXCITATORY ACIDIC AMINO ACID FUNCTION

DRUG	MECHANISMS OF ACTION	OBSERVATIONS
2-Methylhistamine	H$_1$-receptor agonism	—
Dimaprit	H$_2$-receptor agonism	—
N-Methylhistamine	H$_3$-receptor agonism	Limited selectivity
Thioperamide	H$_3$-receptor agonism	Good penetration of the blood-brain barrier
Diphenhydramine	H$_1$-receptor antagonism	Anticholinergic activity
Meclastine	H$_1$-receptor antagonism	No anticholinergic activity
Cimetidine	H$_2$-receptor antagonism	Poor penetration of the blood-brain barrier
Ranitidine	H$_2$-receptor agonism	Poor penetration of the blood-brain barrier
Quisqualic acid	EAAA*-receptor agonism	—
Glutamic acid	EAAA-receptor agonism	—
Aspartic acid	EAAA-receptor agonism	—
N-Methyl-D-aspartate	EAAA-receptor agonism	—
Kainic acid	EAAA-receptor agonism	—

Modified from Müller EE: Brain messengers and the pituitary gland. *In* Dulbecco R (ed): Encyclopedia of Human Biology, Vol 2. San Diego, Academic Press, 1991; with permission.
*EAAA = Excitatory acidic amino acids.
See text for other abbreviations.

Figure 10–2 depicts schematically the topography of some neurotransmitters and neuropeptides in the rat brain.

NEUROTRANSMITTER REGULATION OF ANTERIOR PITUITARY HORMONES

Table 10–5 lists the stimulatory and inhibitory effects on AP secretion of brain neurotransmitters in humans, as derived from the reviewed experimental evidence.

ACTH

Catecholamines

α_1- and α_2-Adrenoceptors are found in high density in the hypothalamus, particularly in the paraventricular nucleus (PVN), which contains the cell bodies of CRH and arginine vasopressin (AVP) neurons.[6] The density of β-adrenoceptors is lower in the hypothalamus than in other brain areas,[6] and even lower density is found in the AP, which in mammals does not receive an adrenergic innervation from the brain.[7]

The role of CA's on the hypothalamic-pituitary-adrenal (HPA) axis in experimental animals and humans has received much attention. It is now clear that in humans activation of α_1-adrenoceptors, for example, by methoxamine, a highly selective α_1-adrenergic agonist or following activation of endogenous CA function, stimulates the secretion of ACTH by an action within the blood-brain barrier (BBB), presumably on the PVN and not at the AP.[8a] Evidence has been provided in humans that combined blockade of opioid receptors by naloxone and α_2-adrenergic receptors by idazoxan is an effective method of activating NE neurons with ensuing ACTH secretion via α_1-adrenoceptors.[9] In contrast to methoxamine, infusion of NE at doses that increased systolic blood pressure did not result in any rise in plasma cortisol and was inhibitory at high infusion rates.[10, 11]

Growth Hormone

Catecholamines

α-Adrenergic mechanisms regulate GH secretion in both subprimate and primate species. Blockade of CA synthesis or depletion of CA storage granules by reserpine almost completely suppresses episodic GH secretion in conscious rats, an effect counteracted by the α_2-adrenergic agonist, clonidine.[2] In normal subjects, blockade of α_2-adrenoceptors by yohimbine lowers the clonidine-induced plasma GH rise[32]; administration of α-adrenergic antagonists also reduces GH response to hypoglycemia and L-dopa.[2] Apparently, α_2-adrenergic influences act by stimulating GRH release,[33] a proposition supported by the detection of specific α_2-adrenergic nerve terminals in the arcuate nucleus.[6] Findings in both dogs[34] and humans[35] suggest that clonidine may also act by inhibiting SS release. α_1-Adrenergic stimulation, which inhibits GH release in rats and dogs, occurs via an increased release of hypothalamic SS.[2] β-Adrenergic pathways are also inhibitory to GH release because propranolol potentiates the GH response to several stimuli, although it has no stimulatory effect on basal GH levels except in Asian subjects. Inferential evidence indicates that β-receptors regulate GH secretion via SS.[36]

Dopaminergic pathways are also involved in the control of GH secretion, although their role appears to be largely ancillary. Both direct- and indirect-acting DA agonists elevate GH levels in humans; however, DA and its agonists inhibit GH release in patients with acromegaly and also inhibit stimulated GH release.[36] These effects are due to direct activation of DA receptors located on the tumoral somatotrophs (acromegaly) and the demonstration that DA agonists trigger not only GRH but also SS release from the hypothalamus, respectively.[37]

Serotonin

The contribution of 5-HT pathways to GH secretion is controversial, both stimulation and inhibition having been suggested from human studies.[2] In humans, although variable results have been obtained with 5-hydroxytryptophan (5-HTP), oral or intravenous administration of the physiological 5-HT precursor tryptophan has been found to release only modest amounts of GH.[38] Fenfluramine, a potent stimulant of 5-HT neurotransmission, inhibits GH release induced by L-dopa/propranolol, but not arginine-stimulated GH release.[39] Fenfluramine probably induces release of hypothalamic SS.

Acetylcholine

Cholinergic neurotransmission is an important modulator of GH secretion. Studies in rats and dogs have shown that central or peripheral administration of muscarinic agonists or antagonists stimulates or suppresses, respectively, GH release. In humans, muscarinic agonists stimulate basal GH release, whereas muscarinic antagonists, regardless of whether or not they cross the BBB, abolish the rise in plasma GH induced by a host of GH secretagogues, except insulin hypoglycemia.[36] Cholinergic modulation appears to effect GH release via stimulation or inhibition of hypothalamic SS release.[40] This is the mechanism whereby, in humans, atropine and pirenzepine completely abolish the

GRH-induced GH rise, and, conversely, pyridostigmine greatly potentiates it.[41] In addition, studies in rats and humans have suggested the involvement of cholinergic mechanisms in the autofeedback regulation of GH secretion.[2]

Histamine

Histamine affects GH secretion indirectly, but different results are obtained depending on the route of administration. Central infusion of histamine into male rats inhibits the pulsatile GH secretion and the GH response to morphine.[42] The inhibitory effect seems to be mediated via H_1-receptors, as it is mimicked by H_1-receptor agonists and prevented by H_1-receptor antagonists.[42] Systemic administration of histamine increases basal or GRH-stimulated GH release in intact or estrogen/progesterone–primed male rats and in dogs, involving primarily activation of H_1 receptors, but also H_2 receptors.[43] In humans, histamine facilitates stimulated GH secretion. In normal subjects, H_1-receptor antagonists reduce the GH response to arginine but do not affect GH secretion elicited by insulin hypoglycemia.[44] H_1-receptor agonism induces a paradoxical response to TRH.[43] H_2-receptor antagonists have less effect on GH responses, likely because of poor penetration of the BBB.[36]

GABA

In healthy, psychiatric, or neurological subjects, distinct increments of plasma GH occurring 60 to 90 minutes after injection are induced by gram amounts of GABA or a few milligrams of muscimol,[45] a potent $GABA_A$ receptor agonist. Administration of the $GABA_B$ receptor agonist, baclofen, also stimulates basal GH levels but inhibits GH responses to arginine and hypoglycemia.[46] GABA-ergic pathways therefore seem to have a stimulatory effect on basal GH levels and an inhibitory one on stimulated GH secretion.[46a]

Gonadotropins

Catecholamines

Based on studies in rodents, central NE neurons clearly exert a facilitatory role in allowing GnRH neurons to produce and discharge their products on the afternoon of proestrus, the phase of the estrous cycle during which ovulation occurs. This activation, however, is not an absolute requirement, because in rats the estrous cycle is re-established a few days after severance of the ventral ascending NE bundle.[2] In ovariectomized rats or monkeys, pulsatile luteinizing hormone (LH) secretion is inhibited by the use of blockers of NE synthesis or of α-adrenergic receptors and is steadily re-established following acute administration of α-adrenergic agonists.[2] This suggests that central adrenergic systems provide a permissive environment in the hypothalamus for episodic discharge of GnRH and that rhythmicity underlying pulsatile LH secretion resides within the GnRH neurons.

In humans, the role played by CA's seems less prominent. DA might exert an inhibitory action on GnRH-producing neurons, as suggested by the existence of significant overlap between GnRH and DA nerve terminals in the lateral wings of the external layer of the ME.[47] Inhibition of pulsatile and phasic gonadotropin secretion by DA might be one of the mechanisms through which reproductive function is impaired in hyperprolactinemic states.[48]

Serotonin

The role of hypothalamic 5-HT in the regulation of LH secretion in experimental animals remains an area of controversy. However, some of the earlier apparent conflicts could perhaps be resolved by the view that 5-HT has a modulatory influence on LH secretion via a bimodal mechanism. Accordingly, a 5-HT mechanism inhibitory to LH secretion would be localized in the MBH and a stimulatory or facilitatory 5-HT mechanism in the preoptic–anterior hypothalamic area.[2] In humans no evidence exists for a role of 5-HT pathways in gonadotropin secretion.[49]

Acetylcholine

No definitive conclusions have been drawn as to the role of the cholinergic system in gonadotropin secretion. It can be said that compared with the major role of brain CA's, at least in rodents, that of ACh is only ancillary. No evidence has been given for a role for ACh in gonadotropin secretion in humans.[2]

Histamine

Histamine possesses a stimulatory action on LH but not follicle-stimulating hormone (FSH) release in female rats, but only when administered at proestrus, indicating that a particular steroid milieu is required and that the amine might participate in mechanisms underlying the ovulatory process.[50] In humans histamine had no effect on basal LH or FSH secretion, but it enhanced the LH response to GnRH in men[51] and in women during different phases of the menstrual cycle.[52] The action of histamine occurs in the hypothalamus, because it stimulated LH release from incubated pituitary fragments only in the presence of hypothalamic tissue.[43] In men, the enhancing effect of histamine on the GnRH-stimulated LH release was inhibited by H_1- and H_2-receptor antagonists.[51]

Amino Acids

GABA. The predominant effect of GABA appears to be inhibition of LH release. Administration of bicuculline, a GABA receptor antagonist, to conscious, ovariectomized rats induced a transient inhibition of plasma LH levels, which was followed by a persistent stimulation.[52] Consistent with these findings, but pointing to a pituitary site of action, are reports that administration of γ-vinyl-GABA blunted the elevation in plasma LH and FSH induced by GnRH in normal male subjects,[31] as did sodium valproate given to women during the luteal phase.[54] Neither drug caused significant changes in basal gonadotropin concentrations. Data pointing to a direct effect of GABA at the gonadotrophs have also been obtained in animal studies.[2]

GLUTAMATE. In vivo studies have shown that L-glutamate and, more potently N-methyl-D-aspartate (NMDA), induce acute elevation of plasma LH levels in prepubertal and adult rats[55] and rhesus monkeys.[56] In addition, kainic acid has been shown to exert clear LH-releasing activity.[55] Because EAA's do not have a direct action on the pituitary[57] and the effects of NMDA can be blocked by the administration of a GnRH antagonist,[58] the action of EAA's on LH secretion is evidently exerted via the CNS. In this respect, it has been reported that NMDA and kainic acid elicited GnRH release from the MBH in vitro.[59] Studies in which the potencies of EAA agonists and the selective antagonism of EAA effects were studied have provided evidence that non-NMDA receptors primarily mediate the excitatory action of L-glutamate on GnRH release from nerve terminals in the rat arcuate nucleus–ME region.[60] Data have also been presented suggesting that the establishment of excitatory inputs to GnRH neurons may play a fundamental role in initiating puberty. Conversely, administration of competitive or noncompetitive antagonists of NMDA receptors delayed the time of vaginal opening in the rat.[2] Based on the LH response to acute administration of L-glutamate, L-aspartic acid, and NMDA in prepubertal monkeys, the use of EAA's has been proposed as a clinical test of GnRH neuronal function,[61] although oral administration of glutamic acid failed to stimulate LH secretion in normal volunteers.[61a]

Prolactin

Catecholamines

The ability of DA to inhibit prolactin (PRL) secretion both in vitro and in vivo is well documented. DA released into the portal vasculature by the TIDA neurons of the hypothalamus exerts a tonic inhibition of prolactin (PRL) secretion from the lactotrophs of the AP gland. This inhibition is mediated by specific, high-affinity DA receptors located on the surface of AP cells. Of the subtypes of DA receptors characterized, only the D_2 subtype can be identified in the AP.[2] Data have also been provided that DA, at very low concentrations, can stimulate in vitro PRL secretion through a receptor that is similar to yet distinct from the D_2 receptor.[62] In addition to DA, a group of direct- and indirect-acting DA agonists is capable of inhibiting PRL secretion. Among them the most exciting group of compounds is the group of ergot derivatives, that is, peptide-containing ergot alkaloids and those showing the tetracyclic ergoline structure.[2] The PRL-inhibiting activity of these compounds provides the rationale for their use in suppressing puerperal lactation and in treating hyperprolactinemia (see also below). As a corollary of these findings, many types of neuroleptic agents (phenothiazines, butyrophenones, phenylbutylpiperidines, thioxanthenes, benzamides) that antagonize the action of DA at the pituitary receptor site increase serum PRL in laboratory animals and humans.[2] The ability of these compounds to induce persistent increases in PRL secretion plays a major role in the alterations of menstrual cycle, amenorrhea with or without galactorrhea, gynecomastia, decreased libido, and impotence seen in patients treated with these drugs. NE and epinephrine exert only an ancillary effect on the neural control of PRL secretion. In humans, administration of clonidine fails to affect plasma PRL levels.[63]

Serotonin

The 5-HT system exerts in rodents and monkeys an important facilitatory role in the stimulated PRL secretion (stress or suckling in lactating dams).[2] Central or systemic administration of 5-HTP increases PRL release. A similar stimulatory effect is obtained by 5-HT–releasing drugs, and 5-HT reuptake inhibitors enhance the stimulatory effect of 5-HTP.[2] In contrast, depletion of 5-HT stores[64] or destruction of 5-HT nerve terminals[65] decreases basal as well as stimulated PRL release. Likewise, lesions[65] or stimulation[66] of 5-HT neurons in the raphe nuclei of the brain stem reduces or increases PRL secretion, respectively. The action of 5-HT on PRL release would be mediated by a PRL-releasing factor (PRF), most likely VIP or peptide histidine isoleucine amide.[2] Studies in rodents have shown that combined activation of 5-HT_1, 5-HT_2, and 5-HT_3 receptors is required to obtain a maximal stimulatory effect of 5-HT.[67] In humans evidence has been provided for a facilitatory role of 5-HT, although it is not so clear-cut.[2]

Histamine

Data have been presented in rodents favoring the view that histamine releases PRL via activation of H_2 receptors and disproving previous data pointing to an inhibitory effect on PRL secretion of H_2 receptor activation.[43] Consistent with the view that activation of H_2 receptors would be inhibitory to PRL secretion is the finding that intravenous administration of bolus doses of cimetidine in humans produces clear-cut rises in plasma PRL,[68] an effect that is dose-dependent, is greater in females than in males, and can be abolished by pretreatment with DA agonists. In contrast, short- or long-term oral administration of cimetidine does not alter plasma PRL levels,[69] likely owing to its inability to attain sufficiently high blood levels and hence adequate penetration into the brain. A wealth of data suggest that the effect of cimetidine on PRL is a reflection of an intrinsic property of the drug unrelated to its H_2-receptor blocking activity, likely its well-documented antiandrogenic activity in animals and humans.[70]

GABA

GABA exerts an inhibitory control over PRL secretion in rodents.[2] Neurons of the TI-GABA system directly secrete the amino acid into the hypophyseal capillaries, from which it is transported to the lactotrophs to interact with specific binding sites. Both high-affinity, low-capacity and low-affinity, high-capacity binding sites have been detected in the rat AP.[71] GABA and benzodiazepine receptors but not glutamic acid decarboxylase activity also are present in human AP's.[72] The high-affinity GABA-binding site would be the one responsible for the GABA-induced inhibition of PRL secretion in the rat.[71] In addition to the inhibitory component of GABA action on PRL secretion, which is preferentially activated by systemically administered GABA or GABA-mimetic drugs, a central stimulatory component exerts its action via inhibition of TIDA neuronal function.[71] This stimulatory component is also evident from studies of systemic or intracisternal administration of GABA-ergic compounds in normal subjects or patients with cerebrovascular disorders.[45, 73] Interestingly, intravenous administration of GABA to normal women elicits a biphasic response

because a transient increase in plasma PRL levels is then followed by a sustained inhibition of PRL secretion.[74]

The similarity of this pattern to the biphasic effect on rat plasma PRL of peripherally administered muscimol is attractive. It suggests an initial phase of activation of CNS GABA receptors (stimulatory phase), followed by a more sustained activation of pituitary GABA receptors (inhibitory phase). Administration of sodium valproate induced a clear-cut lowering of basal plasma PRL in normal and idiopathically hyperprolactinemic women but failed to do so in patients with surgically proven prolactinomas.[75]

Thyroid-Stimulating Hormone

Catecholamines

Studies in rodents demonstrate that central NE transmission increases secretion of TSH by acting on α_2-adrenoceptors, likely located on thyroid-releasing hormone (TRH)–containing neurons within the PVN and dorsomedial nucleus areas.[2] Evidence relating the NE system to TSH secretion in humans is rather scanty.[8a] In contrast to the facilitatory effect exerted on TSH secretion by NE transmission is the inhibitory influence that the dopaminergic system exerts in both animals and humans.[76] In subjects with primary hypothyroidism, a single L-dopa dose lowers the elevated TSH levels, although it does not alter the response to TRH. Bromocriptine and DA are instead effective in lowering baseline levels and inhibiting the TSH response to TRH in hypothyroid subjects, and DA also in euthyroid subjects. As a logical counterpart to these studies, DA receptor antagonists elevate plasma TSH levels.[2]

BRAIN PEPTIDES AND ANTERIOR PITUITARY HORMONES

The effects on the hypothalamus and/or the pituitary of some neuropeptides are reported in Tables 10–6 and 10–7.

In addition to the known hypophysiotropic RH's, a cohort of CNS neuropeptides exert profound neuroendocrine effects. The presence of these compounds in nuclei of the endocrine hypothalamus, where they may coexist with RH's, their secretion from hypothalamic nerve endings, and detection in hypophyseal portal blood suggest a neurohormonal role and a hypophysiotropic function.[2] However, these peptides can alter endocrine function not only as hormones but also as neurotransmitters, neuromodulators,[3] and paracrine or autocrine factors[77]; moreover, their physiological role in the control of AP hormone secretion has yet to be unequivocally established.

Opioid Peptides

Among neuropeptides a major role in the neural control of pituitary function must be credited to endogenous opioid peptides (EOP's).[2, 78] EOP's used so far stimulate the secretion of GH in either subprimates and primates (met-enkephalin analogues but not β-END are effective in humans) acting on the hypothalamus to release GRF and inhibiting SS release. The physiological significance of

TABLE 10–6. Neuropeptides and Pituitary Hormone Release: Action on the CNS

PEPTIDE (DOSAGE)	HORMONE					
	ACTH	Prolactin	Growth Hormone	TSH	FSH	LH
Substance P (μg)	NT	+?	−?	0	0	+
Neurotensin (μg)	NT	−,+	+	0	0	+?
Vasoactive intestinal peptide (ng)	NT	+	+	0	0	+
Gastric inhibitory polypeptide (μg)	NT	0	+	0	−	0
Motilin (μg)	NT	NT	−*	NT	NT	NT
Galanin (ng)	0†	+†	+	0†	0†	0†
Cholecystokinin (ng)	+	+	+	−	0	+
Angiotensin II (μg)	+	−	−	0	NT	+
Neuropeptide Y (ng)	+	0‡	−	0‡	+*	+*
Bombesin (ng)	NT	+§	+	0	0†	0†
Calcitonin (μg)	+†	−?	−	NT	NT	NT
IL-1α (ng)	+	0	NT	NT	0	−
IL-1β (ng)	+	0	−	−	NT	−

Key to symbols: NT, not tested; +, stimulation; −, inhibition; 0, no effect; ?, controversial findings; IL, interleukin.
*Given intracerebroventricularly.
†Human data.
‡Data derived from the effect of bovine and avian pancreatic polypeptides.
§Blockade of stress-induced PRL release.
Modified from Müller EE, Nistico G: Brain Messengers and the Pituitary. San Diego, Academic Press, 1989.

EOP's for GH secretion, however, is not clear, because naloxone fails to alter basal and stimulated GH secretion. EOP's also stimulate PRL secretion via inhibition of TIDA neuronal function, but, at least in humans, do not exert a tonic stimulatory action on basal PRL secretion. Unequivocal evidence has been given that EOP's exert an important role in the control of gonadotropin secretion and, hence, reproductive function in both animals and humans. They act mainly by inhibiting GnRH release from the hypothalamus via decrease of excitatory adrenergic influences and also exert an important role in the inhibitory feedback effects of gonadal steroids on LH release, making hypothalamic neurons sensitive to gonadal steroids. Concerning their role on the HPA axis, their major effect is to tonically inhibit the secretion of ACTH. Naloxone, although at high doses, increases ACTH, and corticosterone secretion in rats and cortisol secretion in humans, and chronic administration of morphine inhibits stress-induced activation of the HPA axis.

Other Neuropeptides

An interesting feature of the neuroendocrine activity of CNS neuropeptides is the diversity of effects they can exert on the secretion of distinct hormones according to their

TABLE 10–7. Neuropeptides and Pituitary Hormone Release: Action on the Pituitary

PEPTIDE (DOSAGE)	HORMONE					
	ACTH	Prolactin	Growth Hormone	TSH	FSH	LH
Substance P (ng)	NT	+	0	0	−*	−*
Neurotensin (ng)	NT	+	0	+?	0	0
Vasoactive intestinal peptide (μg)	+†	+	+‡§	0	0	0
Peptide histidine isoleucine amide (μg)	NT	+	+‡§	NT	NT	NT
Gastric inhibitory polypeptide (μg)	NT	NT	−	NT	+	+
Motilin (μg)	NT	NT	+	NT	NT	NT
Galanin (ng)	NT	0	0	NT	NT	NT
Cholecystokinin (μg)	0	+**	0	0	0	0
Angiotensin II (ng)	+	+	0	0	NT	0
Neuropeptide Y (μg)	NT	NT	−†	NT	+	+
Bombesin (ng)	NT	+†	+†	NT	NT	NT
Calcitonin (μg)	NT	+	0	−	NT	−
IL-1α (μg)	+,0	0	0	−	NT	NT
IL-1β (μg)	+	0	0	−	NT	NT

Same symbols as in Table 10–6.
Inhibition of GnRH-stimulated release.
†Only on tumor cells.
‡In the presence of dexamethasone.
§On human somatotropinomas.
**At huge doses on the rat AP.
Modified from Müller EE, Nistico G: Brain Messengers and the Pituitary. San Diego, Academic Press, 1989.

target site of action, a fact compounding interpretation of their actual, physiological role. Thus, experimental evidence suggests for substance P in the rat a dual stimulatory and inhibitory role on the secretion of gonadotropins, exerted at the hypothalamic and pituitary levels,[79] respectively. VIP is an established PRF that appears to play a physiological role in the regulation of PRL synthesis, at least in the rat.[2, 80] This neurohormone originating in the PVN neurons has been demonstrated in the portal circulation, and via this pathway it would affect specific receptors located in the lactotrophs, increase intracellular concentrations of cAMP, and effect PRL release. But more recent observations suggest that VIP may arise within the AP as well. Anti-VIP immunoneutralization lowers PRL secretion of pituitary incubates,[81] suggesting a paracrine mechanism of control, and also lowers secretion of PRL by dispersed pituitary cells and a tumoral cell line, GH_3, which secretes PRL and GH,[82] suggesting an autocrine mechanism.

It is also apparent that different variables may greatly influence the effects of neuropeptides. The PRF effect of VIP subsides in ovariectomized rats, postmenopausal women, and women bearing a PRL-secreting tumor and is re-established in ovariectomized rats by estrogen treatment. These observations indicate that estrogens prompt the expression of VIP receptors in lactotrophs via genomic activation.[83] VIP is essentially ineffective in eliciting GH release from superfused rat pituitary cells but strongly stimulates GH release in the presence of dexamethasone in the culture medium. In addition, it effects direct stimulation of GH release from human somatotropinomas in vitro.[2] Species-related differences are also present. For instance, neurotensin with neuroendocrine actions in rodents (Tables 10–6 and 10–7) is ineffective to alter TSH, GH, PRL, and LH secretion in humans.[84]

To summarize from these and other data, a picture of extreme complexity emerges, with interaction either within different brain messengers or between them and pituitary and target gland hormones. Although the ultimate goal is ensuring proper functioning of the pituitary and the endocrine systems, these interactions are still poorly understood.

THERAPEUTIC IMPLICATIONS OF NEUROACTIVE DRUGS IN NEUROENDOCRINE DISORDERS

The notion that the secretion of RH's is not autonomous but is in turn regulated by brain neurotransmitters and neuropeptides leads to the conclusion that their dysfunction may be the trigger for specific neuroendocrine disorders. It is noteworthy in this context that so far no evidence has been provided for major alterations in RH gene structure in humans. Evidence for neurotransmitter-neuropeptide dysfunction as a cause for specific neuroendocrine disorders is considered and the potential of neuropharmacological approaches to therapy discussed.

Growth Hormone Deficiency and Excess States

The finding that most adults and children with GH deficiency show variable but unequivocal rises in plasma GH levels after administration of GRH would exclude the existence of a functional impairment of somatotrophs and favor instead a primary hypothalamic dysfunction.[85] Pituitary GH is present but not secreted, probably owing to lack of GRH synthesis and/or release. The presence of low but detectable GRH levels in the CSF of children with idiopathic GH deficiency[86] is suggestive of dysfunction of neurons regulating the release of GRH from GRH-containing neurons. No information is available on SS titers in the CSF of these subjects. In this context, recent attempts to stimulate GH release in children with idiopathic GH deficiency, intrauterine growth retardation, or constitutional growth delay by treatment with DA agonists (L-dopa, bromocriptine) or α_2-adrenergic agonists (clonidine) must be considered.[87, 88] The results seem to be promising, although diminution of the initial effect has been observed under long-term (12 months) treatment. Broadening and confirmation of these findings are awaited.

The clear GH-releasing effect of pyridostigmine prompted studies to verify whether this drug would be useful for the treatment of short stature. This does not seem to be the case because chronic oral treatment failed to improve spontaneous GH secretion and height velocity in short children with clinical symptoms peculiar to hypothalamic dysfunction.[88, 89] Cholinergic drugs are unable to alter GH hypersecretion in acromegaly, because pirenzepine fails to inhibit basal as well as GRH stimulated GH secretion, and pyridostigmine does not potentiate the GRH-induced GH rise.[90]

Thus, medical therapy of acromegaly with neuroactive compounds is restricted to the use of direct DA agonists.[2] These are members of the peptide or ergoline family of compounds (bromocriptine, lisuride, pergolide, cabergoline) whose administration induces a consistent suppression of the elevated GH levels in about 60 per cent of patients for a direct action on DA receptors. It is difficult to evaluate the percentage of patients who benefit from the treatment, owing mainly to the lack of common criteria for assessing treatment effectiveness, but bromocriptine seems to normalize GH levels in about 25 to 30 per cent of patients. Of equal importance is that drug withdrawal is followed 24 to 48 hours later by a sharp rise in GH levels, even after several years of treatment. Tumor shrinkage occurs in only 10 to 15 per cent of patients and is more frequent in hyperprolactinemic than in normoprolactinemic acromegalics. Apart from lowering plasma GH levels, clinical and metabolic improvements have been reported following the institution of medical therapy, although apparently patients benefit from but are not cured by chronic treatment with ergot drugs. The introduction of potent analogues of SS capable of long-lasting reductions in plasma GH levels will limit the therapeutic use of ergot derivatives in acromegaly.[91]

Both dopaminergic ergot and cholinergic antagonist drugs have been used in children with tall stature. Although bromocriptine reportedly reduced the growth rate in tall adolescent boys, further studies are warranted before conclusions about final height can be drawn.[92] In these subjects, chronic administration of pirenzepine only transiently suppressed GH secretion and failed to reduce growth velocity.[93] In contrast, the inhibitory effect of pirenzepine on GH secretion persisted when the drug was given chronically in patients with Type 1 diabetes mellitus and elevated plasma GH levels, implying that it may be useful for improvement of patient metabolic control.[94]

Hypogonadotropic Hypogonadism

Secondary amenorrhea is by far the most common symptom attributable to pituitary function in women. It is usually transient and unaccompanied by structural abnormalities of hypothalamus, pituitary, or ovary (hypothalamic amenorrhea). Evidence supporting a role of EOP's in the cause of amenorrhea is derived from studies of amenorrheic women treated with naloxone.[78] A clear increment in LH levels was observed in women with amenorrhea and/or hyperprolactinemia, suggesting that the acyclicity was due, at least in part, to the effect of an increased EOP tone on GnRH and gonadotropin secretion. Thus, long-acting opioid antagonists may represent a useful therapeutic approach in these cases, although their potential use would be hindered by their anorectic properties[95] and the well-known relation existing between weight loss and amenorrhea.

Cushing's Disease

The awareness that a host of neurotransmitters and neuropeptides are involved in the regulation of ACTH secretion and the evidence that some neuroactive drugs initially thought to act on the hypothalamus to decrease CRH activity actually may act at the pituitary level account for a medical approach to therapy in Cushing's disease. Drugs used in these contexts include cyproheptadine, whose use relies on the known stimulatory action of the 5-HT neuronal system on the HPA axis[96]; bromocriptine[97] and sodium valproate,[98] ultimately able to stimulate DA and GABA receptors located on the corticotrophs; and, more recently, reserpine coupled with pituitary irradiation.[99] Although in distinct cases some clinical and biochemical remission is evident, the role of the medical therapy in Cushing's disease is ancillary to transsphenoidal microsurgery.

Prolactinomas

PRL-secreting tumors, either 10 mm diameter or less (microprolactinomas) or larger (macroprolactinomas), are the most frequently occurring neoplasms in the human pituitary.[2] Clinically, hyperprolactinemia is associated with amenorrhea, galactorrhea, infertility, decreased libido, impotence, and in macroprolactinomas, visual disturbances. In patients with microprolactinomas, DA agonist-ergot–related drugs represent a primary medical therapy. Administration of these drugs causes immediate and sustained PRL suppression, with restoration of fertility in women and normalization of hyperprolactinemic hypogonadism in men. Usually within two months of the return of menstruation, ovulation and adequacy of the luteal phase are achieved and galactorrhea disappears. In men, libido and potency return to normal and, if reduced, the seminal volume also normalizes. When treatment is started, bromocriptine, the drug most commonly used, and other ergolines may cause different neurovegetative symptoms owing to activation of central and peripheral DA receptors. Thus, low doses of drugs that are increased slowly and taken during rather than after a meal or sustained-release preparations are mandatory to minimize the side effects.[100] Two long-acting injectable preparations of bromocriptine are available; their injection in patients with prolactinoma is followed by a prompt and steep PRL decrease lasting for weeks or months.[101] In many instances shrinkage of the pituitary tumor can also be documented. Only transient and mild side effects are noted. The effects of medical therapy are particularly noteworthy in macroprolactinomas because these tumors are rarely cured by surgery, and with radiation therapy subsequent hypopituitarism is common. It is now apparent that reduction of tumor size as documented by tomographic scan and amelioration of visual disturbances can be anticipated in 75 per cent of patients. From the foregoing evidence, medical treatment of macroprolactinomas appears to be more appropriate than neurosurgical transsphenoidal exploration for the primary treatment of the disease. Overall, only in some patients does long-term medical treatment seem to result in a persisting correction of the underlying cause of the adenoma. It is hoped that more prolonged drug regimens, different drugs, or newer DA agonists[102] will prove more effective in this context.

REFERENCES

1. Reichlin S: Neuroendocrinology. *In* Wilson JD, Foster DW (eds): Williams Textbook of Endocrinology. Philadelphia, WB Saunders, 1992, pp 135–219.
2. Müller EE, Nistico G: Brain Messengers and the Pituitary. San Diego, Academic Press, 1989.
3. Bloom FE: Neurohumoral transmission and the central nervous system. *In* Gilman A, Goodman LS, Rall TW, Murad F (eds): Goodman and Gilman's The Pharmacological Basis of Therapeutics. New York, Macmillan, 1985, pp 236–259.
4. Hökfelt T, Johansson O, Goldstein M: Chemical anatomy of the brain. Science 225:1326–1334, 1984.
5. McQueen JK: Classical transmitters and neuromodulators. *In* Flückiger E, Müller EE, Thorner MO (eds): Transmitter Molecules in the Brain, Basic and Clinical Aspects of Neuroscience, Vol 2. Springer Sandoz Advanced Texts. Heidelberg, Springer-Verlag, 1987, pp 7–16.
6. Leibowitz SF, Jhanwar-Unyal M, Dvarkin B, Makman MH: Distribution of alpha-adrenergic, beta-adrenergic and dopaminergic receptors in discrete hypothalamic areas of rat. Brain Res 233:97–114, 1982.
7. Saavedra JM, Palkovits M, Kizer JS, et al: Distribution of biogenic amines and related enzymes in the rat pituitary gland. J Neurochem 25:257–260, 1975.
8. Al-Damluji S: Measuring the activity of brain adrenergic receptors in man. J Endocrinol Invest 14:245–254, 1991.
8a. Al-Damluji S, Francis D: Activation of central α_1-adrenoceptors in humans stimulates secretion of prolactin and TSH, as well as ACTH. Am J Physiol 264:E208–E214, 1993.
9. Grossman A, Besser GM: Opiates control ACTH through a noradrenergic mechanism. Clin Endocrinol (Oxf) 17:287–290, 1982.
10. Al-Damluji S, Cunnah D, Grossman A, et al: Effect of adrenaline on basal and ovine corticotrophin-releasing factor–stimulated secretion in man. J Endocrinol 112:145–150, 1987.
11. Al-Damluji S, Perry L, Tombin S, et al: Alpha-adrenergic stimulation of corticotropin secretion by a specific central mechanism in man. Endocrinology 45:68–76, 1987.
12. Tilders FJH, Berkenbosch F, Smelik PG: Adrenergic mechanisms involved in the control of pituitary-adrenal activity in the rat: A β-adrenergic stimulatory mechanism. Endocrinology 110:114–120, 1982.
13. Fuller RW: Serotoninergic stimulation of pituitary-adrenocortical function in rats. Neuroendocrinology 32:118–127, 1981.

14. Petraglia F, Facchinetti F, Martignoni E, et al: Serotoninergic agonists increase plasma levels of β-endorphin and β-lipotropin in humans. J Clin Endocrinol Metab 59:1138–1142, 1984.

15. Gilbert F, Brazell C, Tricklebank MD, Stahl SM: Activation of the 5-HT1A receptor subtype increases rat plasma ACTH concentrations. Eur J Pharmacol 147:431–437, 1988.

16. Engel G, Gothert M, Hoyer D, et al: Identity of inhibitory presynaptic 5-hydroxytryptamine (5-HT) autoreceptors in the rat brain cortex with 5-HT1B binding sites. Naunyn Schmiedebergs Arch Pharmacol 332:1–7, 1986.

17. Lesch K-P, Söhnle K, Poten B, et al: Corticotropin and cortisol secretion after central 5-hydroxytryptamine-1A (5-HT$_{1A}$) receptor activation: Effects of 5-HT receptor and β-adrenoceptor antagonists. J Clin Endocrinol Metab 70:670–674, 1990.

18. Gibbs DM, Vale W: Effects of serotonin reuptake inhibitor fluoxetine on corticotropin-releasing factor and vasopressin secretion into hypophyseal portal blood. Brain Res 280:176–180, 1983.

19. Calogero AE, Bernardini R, Margioris AN, et al: Effects of serotoninergic agonists and antagonists on corticotropin-releasing hormone secretion by explanted rat hypothalami. Peptides 10:189–200, 1989.

20. Alper RH: Evidence for central and peripheral serotoninergic control of corticosterone secretion in the conscious rat. Neuroendocrinology 51:255–260, 1990.

21. Jones MT, Hillhouse EW: Neurotransmitter regulation of corticotropin-releasing factor in vitro. Ann NY Acad Sci 297:536–560, 1977.

22. Calogero EA, Gallucci WT, Bernardini R, et al: Effect of cholinergic agonists and antagonists on rat hypothalamic corticotropin-releasing hormone secretion in vitro. Neuroendocrinology 47:303–308, 1988.

23. Raskind MA, Peskind ER, Veith RC, et al: Differential effects of aging on neuroendocrine responses to physostigmine in normal men. J Clin Endocrinol Metab 70:1420–1425, 1990.

24. Knigge U, Bach FW, Matzen S, et al: Effect of histamine on the secretion of pro-opiomelanocortin derived peptides in rats. Acta Endocrinol (Copenh) 119:312–319, 1988.

25. Hashimoto K, Yonoki S, Takara S, Ofuji J: ACTH release in pituitary cell cultures. Effect of neurogenic peptides and neurotransmitter substances on ACTH release induced by hypothalamic corticotropin releasing factor (CRF). Endocrinol Jpn 26:103–109, 1979.

26. Itowi N, Yamatodani A, Cacabelos R, et al: Effect of histamine depletion on circadian variations of corticotropin and corticosterone in rats. Neuroendocrinology 50:187–192, 1989.

27. Knigge U, Matzen S, Hannibal T, et al: Involvement of histamine in the mediation of the stress-induced release of alpha-melanocyte-stimulating hormone in male rats. Neuroendocrinology 54:646–652, 1991.

28. Allolio B, Deuss U, Kaulen D, Winkelmann W: Effect of meclastine, a selective H$_1$-receptor antagonist, upon ACTH release. Clin Endocrinol (Oxf) 19:239–245, 1983.

29. Calogero AE, Gallucci WT, Chrousos GP, Gold PW: Interaction between GABAergic neurotransmission and rat hypothalamic corticotropin-releasing hormone secretion in vitro. Brain Res 463:28–36, 1988.

30. Anderson RA, Mitchell R: Effects of gamma-aminobutyric acid receptor agonists on the secretion of growth hormone, luteinizing hormone, adrenocorticotrophic hormone and thyroid-stimulating hormone from the rat pituitary gland in vitro. J Endocrinol 108:1–8, 1986.

31. Cavagnini F, Schechter PJ, Invitti C, et al: Effect of gamma-vynil-GABA mimetic compound on hypothalamic-pituitary function in man. In Endroczi E, Angelucci L, de Wied D, Scapagnini U (eds): Integrative Neurohumoral Mechanisms. Budapest, Akademiai Kiado, 1982, pp 529–537.

32. Camanni F, Ghigo E, Mazza E, et al: Aspects of neurotransmitter control of GH secretion: Basic and clinical studies. In Müller EE, Cocchi D, Locatelli V (eds): Advances in Growth Hormone and Growth Factor Research. New York, Springer-Verlag, 1989, pp 264–281.

33. Kabayama Y, Kato Y, Murakami Y, et al: Stimulation by alpha-adrenergic mechanisms of the secretion of growth-hormone releasing factor (GRF) from perfused rat hypothalamus. Endocrinology 119:432–434, 1986.

34. Arce V, Cella SG, Loche S, et al: Synergistic effect of growth hormone-releasing hormone (GHRH) and clonidine in stimulating GH release in young and old dogs. Brain Res 537:359–362, 1990.

35. Dieguez C, Valcavi R, Page MD, et al: L-Dopa releases GH via a GRF-dependent mechanism in normal human subjects, whereas arginine, clonidine and adrenalin plus propranolol do not. In Müller EE, MacLeod R (eds): Neuroendocrine Perspectives, Vol 6. New York, Springer-Verlag, 1989, pp 205–211.

36. Müller EE: Neural control of somatotropic function. Physiol Rev 67:962–1053, 1987.

37. Kitajima N, Chihara K, Abe K, et al: Effects of dopamine on immunoreactive growth-hormone releasing factor and somatostatin secretion from rat hypothalamic slices perfused in vitro. Endocrinology 124:69–76, 1989.

38. Müller EE, Brambilla F, Cavagnini F, et al: Slight effect of L-tryptophan on GH release in normal human subjects. J Clin Endocrinol Metab 39:1–6, 1974.

39. Casanueva FA, Villanueva L, Peñalva A, Cabezas-Cerrato J: Depending on the stimulus, central serotoninergic activation by fenfluramine blocks or does not alter growth hormone secretion in man. Neuroendocrinology 38:302–308, 1984.

40. Locatelli V, Torsello A, Redaelli M, et al: Cholinergic agonist and antagonist drugs modulate in the rat the growth hormone–releasing hormone–induced growth hormone release. Evidence for mediation by somatostatin. J Endocrinol 111:271–278, 1986.

41. Massara F, Ghigo E, Demislis K, et al: Cholinergic involvement in the growth hormone–releasing hormone–induced growth hormone release. Studies in normal and acromegalic subjects. Neuroendocrinology 43:670–675, 1986.

42. Netti C, Guidobono F, Olgiati VR, et al: Histamine agonist and antagonist drugs: Interference with CNS control of GH release in rats. Horm Res 14:180–191, 1981.

43. Knigge U, Warberg J: The role of histamine in the neuroendocrine regulation of pituitary hormone secretion. Acta Endocrinol (Copenh) 124:609–619, 1991.

44. Pontiroli AE, Viberti G, Vicari A, Pozza G: Effect of the antihistaminergic agents meclastine and deschlorpheniramine on the response of human growth hormone to arginine infusion and insulin hypoglycemia. J Clin Endocrinol Metab 43:582–586, 1976.

45. Tamminga C, Neophytides A, Chase TN, Frohman LA: Stimulation of prolactin and growth hormone secretion by muscimol, a γ-aminobutyric acid agonist. J Clin Endocrinol Metab 47:1348–1351, 1978.

46. Cavagnini F, Invitti C, Di Landro A, et al: Effects of a gamma-aminobutyric acid (GABA) derivate, baclofen, on growth hormone and prolactin secretion in man. J Clin Endocrinol Metab 45:579–584, 1977.

46a. Gillies G, Davidson K: Gabaergic influences on somatostatin secretion from hypothalamic neurons cultured in defined medium. Neuroendocrinology 55:248–256, 1992.

47. Selmanoff M: The lateral and medial median eminence distribution of dopamine, norepinephrine and luteinizing hormone–releasing hormone and the effect of prolactin on catecholamine turnover. Endocrinology 108:1716–1722, 1981.

48. Moore KE, Johnston CA: The median eminence: Aminergic control mechanisms. In Müller EE, MacLeod RM (eds): Neuroendocrine Perspectives, Vol 1. Amsterdam, Elsevier Biomedical, 1982, pp 23–68.

49. Parati EA, Zanardi P, Cocchi D, et al: Neuroendocrine effects of quipazine in man in health state or with neurological disorders. J Neural Transm 47:273–297, 1980.

50. Donoso AO: Induction of prolactin and luteinizing hormone release by histamine in male and female rats and the influence of brain transmitter antagonists. J Endocrinol 76:193–202, 1980.

51. Knigge U, Wollesen F, Dejgaard A, et al: Modulation of basal and LHRH-stimulated gonadotropin secretion by histamine in normal men. Neuroendocrinology 38:93–96, 1984.

52. Knigge U, Thuesen B, Wollesen F, et al: Effect of histamine on basal and TRH/LH-RH stimulated PRL and LH secretion during different phases on the menstrual cycle in normal women. Neuroendocrinology 41:337–341, 1985.

53. McCann SM, Mizunuma H, Samson WK, Lumpkin MD: Differential hypothalamic control of FSH secretion: A review. Psychoneuroendocrinology 8:299–308, 1983.

54. Elias AN, Szekeres AV, Stone S, Valenta LJ: A presumptive role for gamma-aminobutyric acid in the regulation of gonadotropin secretion in man. Am J Obstet Gynecol 144:72–76, 1982.

55. Price MT, Olney JW, Cicero TJ: Acute elevations of serum luteinizing hormone induced by kainic acid, N-methyl-aspartic acid and homocysteic acid. Neuroendocrinology 26:352–358, 1976.

56. Gay VL, Plant TM: N-methyl-D, L, aspartate elicits hypothalamic gonadotropin-releasing hormone release in prepubertal male rhesus monkeys (Macaca mulatta). Endocrinology 120:2289–2296, 1987.

57. Schainker BA, Cicero TJ: Acute central stimulation of luteinizing hormone by parenterally administered N-methyl-D, L-aspartic acid in the male rat. Brain Res 184:425–437, 1980.

58. Cicero TJ, Meyer ER, Bell RD: Characterization and possible opioid

modulation of N-methyl-D-aspartic acid induced increases in serum luteinizing hormone levels in the developing male rat. Life Sci 42:1725–1732, 1988.

59. Bourguignon J-P, Gerard A, Franchimont P: Direct activation of gonadotropin-releasing hormone secretion through different receptors to neuroexcitatory amino acids. Neuroendocrinology 49:402–408, 1989.

60. Donoso AO, Lopez FJ, Negro-Vilar A: Glutamate receptors of the non-N-methyl-D-aspartic acid type mediate the increase in luteinizing hormone-releasing hormone release by excitatory amino acids in vitro. Endocrinology 126:414–420, 1990.

61. Medhamurthy R, Dichek HL, Plant TM, et al: Stimulation of gonadotropin secretion in prepubertal monkeys after hypothalamic exicitation with aspartate and glutamate. J Clin Endocrinol Metab 71:1390–1392, 1990.

61a. Carlson HE, Miglietta JT, Roginsky MS, Stegin KLD: Stimulation of pituitary hormone secretion by neurotransmitter amino acids in humans. Metabolism 38:1179–1182, 1989.

62. Burris TP, Stringer LC, Freeman ME: Pharmacologic evidence that a D2 receptor subtype mediates dopaminergic stimulation of prolactin secretion from the anterior pituitary gland. Neuroendocrinology 54:175–183, 1991.

63. Lal S, Tolis G, Martin JB, et al: Effect of clonidine on growth hormone, prolactin, luteinizing hormone, follicle stimulating hormone and thyroid stimulating hormone in the serum of normal men. J Clin Endocrinol Metab 37:719–724, 1975.

64. Gil-Ad I, Zambotti F, Carruba MO, et al: Stimulatory role of brain serotoninergic system on prolactin secretion in male rat. Proc Soc Exp Biol Med 151:512–518, 1976.

65. Advis JP, Simpkins JW, Bennett J, Meites J: Serotoninergic control of prolactin release in male rats. Life Sci 24:359–366, 1979.

66. Schettini G, Quattrone A, Di Renzo G, Preziosi P: Serotoninergic involvement in neuroendocrine function. Pharmacol Res Commun 12:249–254, 1980.

67. Jørgensen H, Knigge U, Warberg J: Involvement of 5-HT1, 5-HT2 and 5-HT3 receptors in the mediation of the prolactin response to serotonin and 5-hydroxytryptophan. Neuroendocrinology 55:336–343, 1992.

68. Carlson HE, Ippoliti AF: Cimetidine, an H2-antihistamine, stimulates prolactin secretion in man. J Clin Endocrinol Metab 43:367–370, 1977.

69. Masala A, Alagna S, Faedda R, et al: Prolactin secretion in man following acute and long-term cimetidine administration. Acta Endocrinol (Copenh) 93:392–395, 1980.

70. Peden NR, Boyd EJS, Browning MCK, et al: Effect of two histamine H2-receptor blocking drugs on basal levels of gonadotropins, prolactin, testosterone and oestradiol-17-β-during treatment of duodenal ulcer in male patients. Acta Endocrinol (Copenh) 96:564–568, 1981.

71. Apud JA, Cocchi D, Masotto C, et al: Prolactin control by the tuberoinfundibular GABAergic system: Role of anterior pituitary GABA receptors. Psychoneuroendocrinology 9:125–133, 1984.

72. Grandison L, Cavagnini F, Schmid R, et al: γ-Aminobutyric acid- and benzodiazepine-binding sites in human anterior pituitary tissue. J Clin Endocrinol Metab 54:597–601, 1982.

73. Takahara J, Yunoki S, Yakushiji W, et al: Stimulatory effects of gamma-aminohydroxybutyric acid (GABOB) on growth hormone, prolactin and cortisol release in man. Horm Metab Res 12:31–34, 1980.

74. Melis GB, Paoletti AM, Mais V, Fioretti P: Interference of dopamine infusion on γ-aminobutyric acid (GABA)-stimulated prolactin increase. J Endocrinol Invest 4:445–448, 1980.

75. Melis GB, Paoletti AM, Mais V, et al: The effects of the GABAergic drug, sodium valproate, on prolactin secretion in normal and hyperprolactinemic subjects. J Clin Endocrinol Metab 54:485–489, 1982.

76. Krulich L: Neurotransmitter control of tyrotropin secretion. Neuroendocrinology 35:139–147, 1982.

77. Denef C, Baes M, Schramme C: Paracrine interactions in the anterior pituitary: Role in the regulation of PRL and growth hormone secretion. In Ganong WF, Martini L (eds): Frontiers in Neuroendocrinology, Vol 9. New York, Raven Press, 1986, pp 115–132.

78. Grossman A, Clement-Jones V, Besser GM: Clinical implications of endogenous opioid peptides. In Müller EE, MacLeod RM, Frohman LA (eds): Neuroendocrine Perspectives, Vol 4. Amsterdam, Elsevier, 1985, pp 242–294.

79. Vyayan E, McCann SM: In vivo and in vitro effects of substance P and neurotensin on gonadotropin and prolactin release. Endocrinology 105:64–71, 1979.

80. Abe H, Engler D, Molitch ME, et al: Vasoactive intestinal peptide is a physiological mediator of prolactin release in the rat. Endocrinology 116:1383–1390, 1985.

81. Hagen TC, Arnaout MA, Scherzer WZ, et al: Antisera to vasoactive intestinal peptide inhibit basal prolactin release from dispersed anterior pituitary cells. Neuroendocrinology 43:641–645, 1986.

82. Nagy G, Mulchahey JJ, Neill JD: Autocrine control of prolactin secretion by vasoactive intestinal peptide. Endocrinology 122:364–366, 1988.

83. Pizzi M, Rubessa S, Simonazzi E, et al: Requirement of oestrogens for the sensitivity of prolactin cells to vasoactive intestinal peptide in rats and man. J Endocrinol 132:311–316, 1992.

84. Blackburn AM, Fletcher DR, Adrian TE, Bloom SR: Neurotensin infusion in man: Pharmacokinetics and effect on gastrointestinal and pituitary hormones. J Clin Endocrinol Metab 51:1257–1261, 1980.

85. Thorner MO, Cronin MJ: Growth hormone releasing factor: Clinical and basic studies. In Müller EE, MacLeod RM, Frohman LA (eds): Neuroendocrine Perspectives, Vol 4. Amsterdam, Elsevier, 1985, pp 95–144.

86. Chihara K, Kashio Y, Abe H, et al: Idiopathic growth hormone deficiency and GH deficiency to hypothalamic germinoma: Effect of single and repeated administration of human-GH-releasing factor (hpGRF) on plasma GH level and endogenous hpGRF-like immunoreactivity level in cerebrospinal fluid. J Clin Endocrinol Metab 60:269–278, 1985.

87. Loche S, Lampis A, Cella SG, et al: Clonidine treatment in children with short stature. J Endocrinol Invest 11:763–767, 1988.

88. Müller EE, Locatelli V, Ghigo E, et al: Involvement of brain catecholamines and acetylcholine in growth hormone deficiency states. Pathophysiological, diagnostic and therapeutic implications. Drugs 41:161–177, 1991.

89. Ghigo E, Mazza E, Bellone J, et al: Neuroactive drugs in growth disorders. Acta Pediatr Scand (Suppl) 367:33–37, 1989.

90. Müller EE, Locatelli V, Cocchi D, et al: Aspects of growth hormone (GH) secretion in GH hypersecretory states. In Faglia G, Beck-Peccoz P, Ambrosi B, et al (eds): Amsterdam, Excerpta Medica, 1991, pp 29–38.

91. Chiodini PG, Cozzi R, Dallabonzana D, et al: Medical treatment of acromegaly—Dopaminergic agonists and long-acting somatostatin. In Müller EE, Cocchi D, Locatelli V (eds): Advances in Growth Hormone and Growth Factor Research. New York, Springer-Verlag, 1989, pp 423–436.

92. Schoenle R, Theintz G, Torresani G, et al: Lack of bromocriptine-induced reduction of predicted height in tall adolescents. J Clin Endocrinol Metab 65:355–358, 1987.

93. Hindmarsh PC, Pringle PJ, Brook CGD: Cholinergic muscarinic blockade produces short-term suppression of growth hormone secretion in children with tall stature. Clin Endocrinol (Oxf) 29:289–296, 1988.

94. Martina V, Maccario M, Tagliabue M, et al: Chronic treatment with pirenzepine decreases growth hormone secretion in insulin-dependent diabetes mellitus. J Clin Endocrinol Metab 68:392–396, 1989.

95. Trenchard E, Silverstone T: Naloxone reduces food intake of normal human volunteers. Appetite 4:43–50, 1983.

96. Krieger DT: Physiopathology of Cushing's disease. Endocr Rev 4:22–43, 1983.

97. Lamberts SJW: Cushing's disease. An overview. In Lamberts SJW, Tilders TJH, van der Veen EA, Assies J (eds): Trends in the Diagnosis and Treatment of Pituitary Adenomas. Baarn, Drukkery, 1984, pp 345–354.

98. Dornhorst A, Jenkins JS, Lamberts SWJ, et al: The evaluation of sodium valproate in the treatment of Nelson's syndrome. J Clin Endocrinol Metab 56:985–991, 1983.

99. Minamori Y, Murayama M, Yasuda K, Miura K: Effect of short-term and long-term reserpine treatment on hypothalamo-pituitary axis in patients with Cushing's disease. Abstract Book 74 Annu Meet Endocr Soc S. Antonio, Abs. no. 604, 1992.

100. Besser GM, Wass JAH, Grossman A, et al: Clinical and therapeutic aspects of hyperprolactinemia. In MacLeod RM, Thorner MO, Scapagnini U (eds): Prolactin. Padua, Liviana Press, 1985, pp 833–847.

101. Cavagnini F, Maraschini C, Moro M, et al: The use of two injectable long-acting bromocriptine preparations (Parlodel LA and Parlodel LAR, Sandoz) in patients with prolactinoma. In Genazzani AR, Petraglia F, Volpe A, Facchinetti F (eds): Advances in Gynecological Endocrinology. Casterton Hall, Carnforth, The Parthenon Publ Group, 1988, pp 39–50.

102. Khalfallah Y, Claustrat B, Grochowicki M, et al.: Effects of a new prolactin inhibitor, CV 205–502, in the treatment of human macroprolactinomas. J Clin Endocrinol Metab 71:354–359, 1990.

11

Thyrotropin-Releasing Hormone: Basic and Clinical Aspects

MAURICE F. SCANLON
REGINALD HALL

Although the existence of a thyrotropin-releasing hormone (TRH) was first suggested more than two decades ago,[1] it was not until 15 years later that a porcine hypothalamic extract with TSH-releasing properties was isolated.[2] Elucidation of the structure and subsequent synthesis of porcine[3] and ovine[4] TRH established its nature as the weakly basic tripeptide pyro-Glu-His-Pro-amide (Fig. 11–1). The biological activity of synthetic TRH is identical to that of the natural material; synthetic TRH exhibits a lack of phylogenetic specificity common to several other hypothalamic regulatory peptides. The importance of TRH in the maintenance of normal thyroid function and its interaction with other neuroregulators of TSH secretion is now well established and has been recently reviewed.[5] It should be remembered, however, that because of the lack of availability of human thyroid-stimulating hormone–producing cells, all the data concerning the pituitary effects of TRH in vitro have accrued from the use of animal tissue and cell lines. In addition to its role in the control of function of the thyrotroph, TRH has several other actions on the anterior pituitary. It is also widely distributed throughout the extrahypothalamic brain, spinal cord, and other body tissues and probably has important neuromodulatory and paracrine roles in these areas.

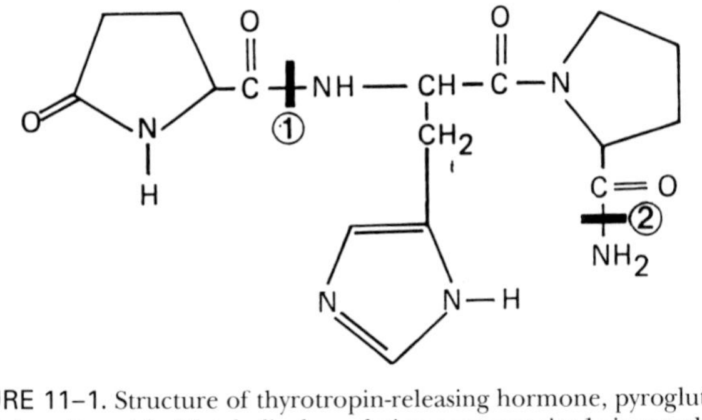

SYNTHESIS AND METABOLISM

TRH, like other more complex peptides, is derived from post-translational cleavage of a larger precursor molecule.[6–8] Investigation of the synthesis of TRH proved difficult for many years, in part because antibodies to this small peptide do not cross-react with precursor molecules. It was assumed, therefore, that any putative precursor should contain the sequence Glu-His-Pro-Gly, that the glutamine residue would cyclize during processing and maturation to yield pyroglutamic acid, and that the extra glycine would be required for the formation of the terminal amide. A synthetic oligonucleotide corresponding to Glu-His-Pro-Gly was used to screen a cDNA library prepared from total poly(A)RNA extracted from amphibian skin, which contains many peptides common to mammalian brain and the gastrointestinal tract, often (as for TRH) in much larger quantities.[9] The resultant polypeptide commenced with a grouping of hydrophobic amino acids (which is characteristic of signal peptides) and contained three complete and one incomplete copy of the sequence Lys-Arg-Glu-His-Pro-Gly-Lys-Arg-Arg. Processing at Lys-Arg residues and, subsequent cleavage by a carboxypeptidase-B–like enzyme would release several TRH precursors, which would then cyclize into TRH itself. Since TRH is highly conserved through the

FIGURE 11–1. Structure of thyrotropin-releasing hormone, pyroglutamyl-histidyl-prolinamide. Metabolic degradation occurs at site 1 via membrane-bound pyroglutamyl aminopeptidase and at site 2 via TRH deamidase. (From Scanlon MF: Thyroid stimulating hormone. *In* Braverman LC, Utiger RD (eds): The Thyroid: A Fundamental and Clinical Text. Philadelphia, JB Lippincott, 1991, pp 230–256.)

animal kingdom, it is likely that the putative precursor isolated from frog skin is similar to that in mammalian hypothalamus. Indeed, antibodies to a peptide sequence present in the pro-TRH molecule, deduced from cloned amphibian skin cDNA, cross-react with neuronal perikarya in the parvocellular division of the medulla oblongata of rats.[6] Similar antibodies have been used to characterize the mammalian (rat) TRH prohormone, and both TRH and pro-TRH have been found in neurons of the paraventricular nucleus, whereas only TRH is present in axon terminals in the median eminence.[6, 9] The cDNA sequence of the rat TRH precursor encodes a protein with a molecular size of 29,247 daltons that contains five copies of the sequence Glu-His-Pro-Gly.

These data confirm that a TRH precursor molecule analogous to that present in frog skin is also present in rat brain and that TRH in the mammalian nervous system is a product of ribosomal synthesis.[10] Indeed, rat pro-TRH is processed at paired basic residues to a family of peptides including TRH and flanking and intervening sequences. These peptides may prove to exert important intracellular or extracellular functions,[11, 12] and there may be preferential processing of pro-TRH to produce different peptides in different brain regions.[9] The gene encoding human prepro-TRH has now been isolated, cloned, and sequenced from a human lung fibroblast genomic DNA library using a rat prepro-TRH cDNA fragment. Exon 3 contains six copies of the TRH sequence compared with five copies in the rat, and human prepro-TRH contains 242 amino acids, whereas the rat molecule contains 255 amino acids. Corresponding homologies with the rat are 73.3 per cent and 59.5 per cent at the nucleic acid and amino acid levels, respectively.[13] Further studies have assigned the gene encoding human prepro-TRH to chromosome 3.[14]

TRH is rapidly degraded in tissues and serum to TRH free acid, the stable cyclized metabolite histidyl-proline-diketopiperazine (His-Pro-DKP; cyclo(His-Pro)), and its constituent amino acids.[15–18] TRH is hydrolyzed at the pyroGlu-His bond (see Fig. 11–1) by a particulate enzyme, pyroglutamyl aminopeptidase, which is present in synaptosomal and anterior pituitary membrane preparations.[19–21] This enzyme is similar to the serum-degrading enzyme[22] in that it has great specificity for TRH.[23] Since cyclo(His-Pro) has several pharmacological actions, it has been suggested that TRH may act as a prohormone for this molecule, although recent data suggest that cyclo(His-Pro) may arise independently in several tissues[24, 25] and can be absorbed in sufficient quantities from certain foods to achieve biologically significant levels.[26] The plasma half-life of TRH is short, ranging from about two minutes in thyrotoxic animals to six minutes in the hypothyroid[27–29]; the differences may be due to the effects of thyroid status on membrane-bound pyroglutamyl aminopeptidase (type 1), since the serum pyroglutamyl aminopeptidase (type 2), which also shows high stereospecificity for TRH, is independent of thyroid status.[30] This effect of thyroid status may also be mediated—at least in part—by TSH itself, which can promote the formation of cyclo(His-Pro) through inhibition of TRH amidase.[15] The activity of the anterior pituitary TRH-degrading enzyme is rapidly and potently stimulated by thyroid hormones, whereas brain-degrading activity is unaffected.[31, 32] This is entirely appropriate to the differing roles of TRH within the pituitary and brain. The potency of the thyroid hormone effect on the degradation of TRH

by anterior pituitary membranes indicates that this may be an important regulatory mechanism.

HYPOTHALAMIC AND PITUITARY DISTRIBUTION AND ACTIONS OF TRH AND METABOLITES

Immunoreactive TRH is widely distributed in the hypothalamus, particularly high concentrations being found in the median eminence and in the nuclei of the so-called thyrotropic area or paraventricular nucleus.[33–35] Lesions of the paraventricular nuclei reduce circulating TRH levels and TSH responses to primary hypothyroidism.[36–38] More recently the presence of TRH and pro-TRH perikarya has been demonstrated by means of immunohistochemical studies in the parvocellular division of this nucleus,[6, 39] and it is a major site of origin of the immunoreactive TRH in the median eminence. In contrast, lesions of the hypothalamic paraventricular nuclei cause increased TRH levels in the nucleus of the tractus solitarius[40]; this indicates that TRH fibers in this region do not arise in the hypothalamus. TRH and TRH-positive nerve fibers are present in posterior pituitary tissue,[41] and lesions of the thyrotropic area of the hypothalamus reduce TRH levels in both the anterior and posterior pituitary glands[42, 43]; these two observations indicate that the hypothalamus is the probable source of most immunoreactive TRH in these areas.[44] However, as with several other hypothalamic peptides, the TRH gene is expressed in both normal and adenomatous human anterior pituitary tissue, which can therefore synthesize and secrete very small amounts of immunoreactive TRH.[45, 46] The functional relevance of these observations is unknown, although a paracrine role in the control of pituitary function seems most likely.

The best defined physiological actions of hypothalamic TRH concern its role in the control of thyrotroph function, although it does act on the secretion of several other anterior pituitary hormones in a variety of physiological and pathophysiological settings (Fig. 11–2).

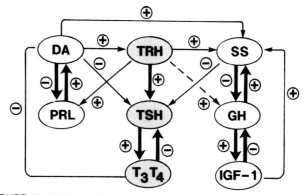

FIGURE 11–2. Schematic representation of the complex interactions that can occur between primary and secondary modulators of thyrotrope function. This represents a summary of data available from in vivo and in vitro studies in animals and in humans. DA, dopamine; SS, somatostatin; IGF-1, insulin-like growth factor 1. (From Scanlon MF: Thyroid stimulating hormone. *In* Braverman LC, Utiger RD (eds): The Thyroid: A Fundamental and Clinical Text. Philadelphia, JB Lippincott, 1991, pp 230–256.)

Control of Thyroid-Stimulating Hormone (TSH) Synthesis and Release

The dominant stimulatory role of the hypothalamus in the control of TSH synthesis and release is mediated by TRH. The direct dose-related action of TRH on TSH release is well known both in vivo and in vitro,[42, 47, 48] and decreased TSH release and hypothyroidism follow hypothalamic-pituitary dissociation with hypothalamic lesions and diseases.[38, 44, 49] This action of TRH occurs at nanomolar concentrations[50] and is mediated by specific high-affinity receptors.[51] TRH is released from nerve terminals in the median eminence into hypophyseal portal blood at physiologically relevant concentrations,[52] and, furthermore, sheep in which antibodies to TRH are raised have a decline in thyroid function.[53] Intravenous administration of 15 to 500 μg of TRH to normal humans causes a dose-related release of TSH from the pituitary. The serum TSH response to TRH, given intravenously to normal subjects, is detectable within two to five minutes after TRH administration, is maximal at 20 to 30 minutes, and serum TSH levels return to basal levels by two to three hours. An elevation in serum thyroid hormone levels follows, the peak serum T_3 and T_4 concentrations occurring about three and eight hours, respectively, after TRH. In addition to stimulating TSH release, TRH also stimulates TSH synthesis by promoting transcription and translation of the β-TSH gene.[54-57] More recent studies indicate that the transacting protein Pit-1 (or a closely related protein) probably mediates this stimulatory effect of TRH on the β-TSH gene.[58] Pit-1 is a pituitary-specific transactivating factor that regulates cell-specific expression of both prolactin (PRL) and growth hormone (GH) genes and mediates the action of TRH on PRL gene expression in GH_3 cells.[59, 60] The pattern of TSH release after prolonged intravenous infusion of TRH in humans is biphasic. The early phase may reflect the release of a readily releaseable pool of stored TSH within the thyrotrophs, whereas the later phase probably reflects release of newly synthesized TSH.[61] Glu-His-Pro-Gly, the immediate precursor of TRH, which is converted to pyro-Glu-His-ProNH₂ by an α-amidating enzyme, does not release TSH in normal or acromegalic subjects, although it elicits a small TSH response in patients with anorexia nervosa.[62, 63] It is likely that this molecule has only a very low affinity, if any, for the TRH receptor.

TRH plays an important role in the post-translational processing of the oligosaccharide moieties of TSH and hence exerts an important influence on the biological activity of the TSH that is secreted.[64, 65] Full glycosylation of TSH is required for complete biological activity as assessed by the stimulation of adenylate cyclase activity in thyroid membrane preparations or the generation of cAMP in functional rat thyroid (FRTL-5) cells.[66-68] Receptor binding, however, is not impaired by deglycosylation, indicating some alternative mechanism for reduced agonist activity.[69] In early studies TRH was found to have differential effects on the glycosylation of TSH and the translation of TSH gene products,[70] and subsequently several studies showed that TRH can modify the sialic acid, sulphate, and carbohydrate components of TSH.[71-76] These animal and in vitro data explain the clinical observation that some patients with central hypothyroidism and slightly elevated basal serum TSH levels secrete TSH with reduced biological ac-

tivity.[77] Long-term TRH administration increased TSH biological activity in some of these patients.[78, 79] It is likely that alterations in both hypothalamic TRH secretion and the response of thyrotrophs to TRH contribute to the variable biological activity of the TSH secreted in different thyroid disorders[80-83] and in patients with TSH-secreting pituitary adenomas.[84, 85]

Interactions Between TRH and Thyroid Hormones

Although TRH acts in concert with the inhibitory hypothalamic regulators somatostatin and dopamine (DA) in order to control TSH synthesis and release, thyroid hormones exert the most important negative feedback control via direct pituitary inhibition of the thyrotroph (Fig. 11-13). In this process local intrapituitary conversion of T_4 to T_3 is particularly important.

In addition to their direct inhibitory actions on TSH subunit gene expression and TSH release, thyroid hormones also modulate the number of TRH receptors on the thyrotrophs. There is a two-fold increase in TRH binding to anterior pituitary membranes from hypothyroid animals, and the increase can be reduced by thyroid hormone replacement.[86, 87] This effect is specific because epidermal growth factor and somatostatin receptors do not alter, indicating that the regulation of TRH receptors by thyroid hormones is not secondary to general changes in membrane structure.[88] T_3 also decreases TRH receptors in TSH-

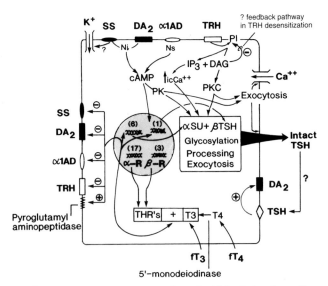

FIGURE 11–3. Thyroid hormones reduce the biological actions of somatostatin (SS), dopamine (DA), epinephrine, and TRH. This is due to a reduction in number rather than affinity of DA_2, TRH, and α₁-adrenergic (α₁-AD) receptors, and the same may well apply to SS receptors. These actions and the stimulation of pyroglutamyl aminopeptidase by T_3 are probably due to binding of the activated thyroid hormone receptor (TRH) to relevant parts of the genome. Diacylglycerol (DAG) may participate in feedback inhibition of the functional response to TRH receptor agonism causing apparent TRH desensitisation. TRH and α₁-AD agonism exert additive effects on TSH release, indicating separate intracellular pathways. The numbers in parentheses indicate the chromosomal origin of the α and β thyroid hormone receptors. (From Scanlon MF: Thyroid stimulating hormone. *In* Braverman LC, Utiger RD (eds): The Thyroid: A Fundamental and Clinical Text. Philadelphia, JB Lippincott, 1991, pp 230–256.)

secreting tumors in mice and GH/PRL–secreting GH$_3$ cells.[88, 89] Conversely, in GH$_4$C$_1$ cells TRH itself causes a dose-related reduction in T$_3$ receptors and T$_3$ responsiveness[90] that may represent a further site of feedback interaction between T$_3$ and TRH at the pituitary level.

In addition to their ability to inhibit TSH secretion, thyroid hormones exert powerful effects on hypothalamic function. Injection of nanomolar concentrations of T$_3$ into the hypothalamus of hypothyroid monkeys causes immediate inhibition of TSH release.[91] Whether this effect is due to inhibition of TRH secretion or to stimulation of somatostatin or dopamine secretion is unknown, although T$_3$ can stimulate immediate somatostatin release from hypothalamic tissue in vitro.[92] The effects of thyroid status on the hypothalamic content of TRH are controversial, but in general thyroid hormone excess or deficiency has little effect on the content of TRH in the hypothalamus as a whole. The situation has been clarified by the study of TRH gene expression in the paraventricular nuclei of the hypothalamus: TRH mRNA levels in this region increase in hypothyroidism and are reduced by thyroid hormone treatment.[93, 94] Furthermore, rats with bilateral lesions of the paraventricular nuclei did not have the normal rise of serum TSH and TSH subunit mRNA following induction of primary hypothyroidism,[95] an effect that presumably reflects depletion of TRH. These results indicate that the paraventricular nuclei of the hypothalamus are a target for the action of thyroid hormones and therefore contribute to the neuroregulation of TSH secretion.

Actions of TRH on Prolactin

TRH is a potent stimulator of PRL release, but it is still disputed whether TRH is a physiological PRL-releasing factor.[96] The threshold dose of exogenous TRH is the same for both TSH and PRL,[97] and the PRL response to suckling or mammary nerve stimulation in rats is accompanied by TSH release[98] and also by an increase of TRH in portal blood.[99, 100] Furthermore, in sheep immunized against TRH, the PRL response to heat exposure is reduced.[100] However, against a physiological PRL-releasing role for TRH in humans, physiological stimuli to PRL release such as suckling and stress do not increase TSH secretion, and the circadian rhythms of TSH and PRL are dissociated.[101] Administration of TRH antibodies to rats has no consistent effect on basal serum levels of PRL.[100] In summary therefore, TRH may play a physiological role in mediating certain PRL responses such as the response to suckling in rats but does not appear to have any important role in the control of PRL secretion in humans. Although the idea is often stated, there is no evidence that the hyperprolactinemia that is found in as many as 30 per cent of patients with primary hypothyroidism is due to increased TRH secretion. Indeed it may be more related to reduced lactotroph DA receptor number.[5] The immediate TRH precursor pyroGlu-His-Pro-Gly has no significant effects on PRL and TSH secretion in normal women or in patients with acromegaly, uremia, or prolactinoma. However, it does stimulate significant PRL and slight TSH release in patients with anorexia nervosa.[62] Whether this is due to the expression of specific receptors in this condition or is a reflection of other hypothalamic neurotransmitter changes remains

to be investigated. It does seem clear that this molecule does not act via the TRH receptor.

TRH free acid does not stimulate TSH or PRL release either in vivo or in vitro, whereas cyclo(His-Pro) inhibits PRL release both in vitro (in rat anterior pituitary and human prolactinoma cultures[102–105]) and in vivo in rhesus monkeys.[106] However, a wide dosage range of cyclo(His-Pro) did not alter basal or TRH-stimulated TSH and PRL release in normal subjects or in patients with hyperprolactinemia or primary hypothyroidism. This finding argues against any important physiological role for this dipeptide in the control of these hormones in humans.[107]

Actions of TRH on Growth Hormone

The actions of TRH on GH release are complex, but in normal subjects GH release does not follow TRH administration. In contrast, in certain pathophysiological conditions such as acromegaly and diabetes mellitus there can be quite striking serum GH responses to TRH administration. It seems likely that many if not all of these paradoxical serum GH responses to TRH are a consequence of functional or structural dissociation between the hypothalamus and the anterior pituitary somatotrophs, perhaps operating via reduced somatostatin activity (Table 11–1). Interestingly, a paradoxical serum GH response to TRH can be induced both in vivo and in vitro[108] by prior growth hormone-releasing hormone (GRH) administration. Also the GH responses to many stimuli including dopaminergic agonists, α$_2$-adrenergic agonists, insulin hypoglycemia, exercise, and arginine are reduced or abolished during the course of TRH administration, possibly due to a hypothalamic action of TRH to release somatostatin, because administration of antibodies to somatostatin abolishes these inhibitory actions of TRH.[109] In humans, however, TRH infusion does not affect the GH response to exogenous administration of pharmacological doses of GRH.[110] The TRH precursor peptide pyroGlu-His-Pro-Gly stimulated striking GH release in 8 out of 15 patients with acromegaly and this correlated well with the GH response to TRH. In contrast, this molecule had no effect on TSH or PRL release in these patients.[63] It remains to be investigated whether some adenomatous somatotrophs express receptors for this TRH precursor molecule.

Actions of TRH on Other Pituitary Hormones

In normal subjects TRH has no demonstrable effects on ACTH release, but a striking rise in serum ACTH levels

TABLE 11–1. PARADOXICAL GH RESPONSES TO TRH

Normal subjects	After GRH administration; after H$_1$ agonist drugs; full-term fetus
Endocrine	Acromegaly; primary hypothyroidism (children); diabetes mellitus; carcinoid syndrome; during GRH infusion
Neuropsychiatric	Anorexia nervosa; depression; schizophrenia
Metabolic	Chronic liver disease; chronic renal failure; protein-calorie malnutrition; thalassemia
Experimental (rats)	Hypothalamic destruction; ectopic pituitary transplantation; hypothyroidism

can follow TRH administration in some patients with Cushing's disease or Nelson's syndrome.[111] Exogenous TRH can also stimulate vasopressin secretion,[112] which suggests a possible function for the TRH neurons whose axons enter the posterior pituitary gland. TRH produces a small but consistent increase in serum FSH in men,[113] an action that is abolished by prior treatment with estrogens.[114] Neither the underlying mechanisms nor the possible physiological relevance of these findings is understood.

MECHANISMS UNDERLYING NEUROENDOCRINE ACTIONS OF TRH

TRH binds to specific high-affinity receptors on anterior pituitary membranes, and the mouse pituitary TRH receptor has recently been cloned. The TRH receptor is a member of the family of G protein–coupled receptors containing seven membrane spanning domains and an extracellular N-terminal region with N-glycosylation sites.[115] In TSH-secreting tumors in mice and in GH_3 cells, TRH can reduce the number of its own receptors after chronic exposure.[88, 116] In GH_3 cells this is preceded by a decrease in activity of TRH receptor mRNA.[117, 118] However, this finding has not been confirmed for normal anterior pituitary cells, and it is not known whether it has any physiological relevance in normal animals. Furthermore, no data are yet available concerning the human TRH receptor or the mechanism of action of TRH in human thyrotrophs. Continuous TRH administration both in vivo and in vitro causes marked homologous desensitization of TSH and PRL responses.[119–121] This secretory refractoriness probably occurs at a site beyond the TRH receptor[122] and, because it occurs in vitro, cannot be explained by the increase in serum T_4 and T_3 concentrations that accompanies TRH administration in vivo. Virtually all the work on the secondary message events involved in TRH action has been performed on GH_3 cells and mouse thyrotroph tumor cells. In these systems, TRH stimulates the activity of phospholipase C by coupling to the pertussis toxin–sensitive guanosine triphosphate–binding proteins G_q and G_{11}.[123] This causes rapid hydrolysis of phosphatidylinositol 4,5-bisphosphate to inositol 1,4,5 bisphosphate and 1,2-diacylglycerol.[124, 125] The latter in turn activates intracellular protein kinase C (PKC). PKC may participate in an intracellular feedback system to limit receptor-mediated hydrolysis of inositol phospholipids (see Fig. 11–2). This system may underlie the desensitization of hormonal responses to chronic TRH administration because staurosporine, a potent inhibitor of PKC, can block the TRH-induced refractoriness of inositol phospholipid hydrolysis in rat anterior pituitary tissue.[126] Furthermore, it seems likely that the TRH-induced decrease in TRH receptor mRNA levels in GH_3 cells is mediated by PKC.[118]

TRH causes an immediate, rapid increase in intracellular free calcium (which decays rapidly) followed by an extended plateau of elevated intracellular free calcium.[127–131] This biphasic action correlates with secretory activity, electrical changes, and the induction of ^{45}Ca fluxes in GH_3 cells.[128, 132–135] The first phase reflects increased release from intracellular stores caused by inositol triphosphate whereas the second phase is due to calcium influx[130, 131] and depends on the presence of slowly inactivating, L-type, voltage-sensitive calcium channels.[136] The biphasic pattern of

TSH response and intracellular free calcium levels to maximal doses of TRH in mouse thyrotrope tumor cells is determined by the TRH receptor number; downregulation of TRH receptors abolishes the early secretory burst of TSH release and the intracellular free calcium elevation.[137]

TRH increases cAMP levels in pituitary tissue, but the increase is probably secondary to stimulation of phosphatidylinositol turnover by TRH.[138] In different brain regions, TRH selectively stimulates either cAMP generation or phosphatidylinositol turnover.[139] These results indicate that TRH receptors are functionally linked to different intracellular pathways in different sites.

INTERACTIONS BETWEEN TRH AND OTHER NEUROREGULATORS

The neuroregulation of TSH is complex.[5] Although TRH mediates the dominant stimulation of the thyrotroph by the hypothalamus, there is now convincing evidence in both animals and humans for a stimulatory role of α_1-adrenergic pathways and for inhibitory roles of both dopaminergic pathways and somatostatin.[5] As a consequence of the specialized anatomical arrangements within the hypothalamus, each of these hypophysiotropic neuronal systems regulating TSH secretion is in turn influenced by networks of other neurons that project from several brain regions.[140] Without these projections basal TSH secretion (in rats and presumably in humans) and feedback regulation by thyroid hormones is relatively normal, suggesting that basal TRH secretion is regulated by intrinsic hypothalamic function. In contrast, circadian rhythms of TSH and pituitary-thyroid changes in response to stress and cold exposure in rats are mediated by nerve pathways that project to the medial basal hypothalamus.[141] These interacting pathways are illustrated diagrammatically in Figure 11–4.

Animal studies using central neurotransmitter agonist and antagonist drugs have indicated the existence of stimulatory α-noradrenergic and inhibitory dopaminergic pathways in the control of TSH secretion in rats.[142] Alpha-adrenergic agonists injected systemically or into the third ventricle stimulate TSH release and α-adrenergic antagonists or catecholamine depletors block TSH responses to cold.[47, 143–145] More precisely, it appears that α-2 pathways are stimulatory whereas α-1 pathways are inhibitory,[146] particularly in hypothyroidism.[147] It has been assumed from such in vivo studies that these neurotransmitter effects are mediated by the appropriate modulation of TRH and/or somatostatin release into hypophyseal portal blood. A clear example of this is that the acute TSH release following cold stress in rats can be abolished by pretreatment with either anti-TRH antibodies or α-adrenergic antagonists; this suggests that adrenergically stimulated TRH release mediates this effect.[42, 47, 48] Furthermore, lesions affecting the temperature-regulating center of the preoptic nucleus of the hypothalamus abolish the TSH response to cold stress but do not cause hypothyroidism,[200] presumably via interruption of this specific α-adrenergic/TRH pathway. However, in vitro studies using rat hypothalamic tissue have not produced data in keeping with this attractive and simple hypothesis. For example, dopamine and dopamine-agonist drugs stimulate both TRH and somatostatin release from rat hypothalamus, acting via the dopamine$_2$ (DA_2)

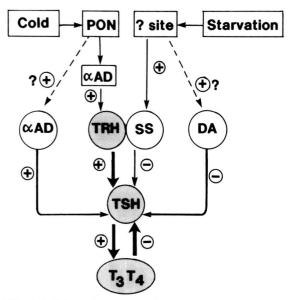

FIGURE 11–4. Schematic representation of probable pathways involved in secondary alterations in hypothalamic-pituitary-thyroid function in response to temperature and caloric restriction. PON represents the temperature-sensitive region of the hypothalamic preoptic nucleus. The hypothalamic site for integration of the metabolic signals resulting from caloric restriction is unknown. (From Scanlon MF: Thyroid stimulating hormone. *In* Braverman LC, Utiger RD (eds): The Thyroid: A Fundamental and Clinical Text. Philadelphia, JB Lippincott, 1991, pp 230–256.)

class of dopamine receptor.[148–151] This may reflect a general action of DA_2 receptors to mediate enhanced neuropeptide release at the level of the median eminence in contrast to the usual inhibitory action of DA_2 agonism at the level of the anterior pituitary. Similarly, in vitro studies using rat anterior pituitary cells have clearly demonstrable direct, stimulatory α_2-adrenergic, and inhibitory dopaminergic (via DA_2 receptors) actions on TSH synthesis, release, and subunit gene expression.[5]

TSH is secreted in a pulsatile manner throughout the day with increases in pulse amplitude and frequency at night.[152–156] Patients with severe primary hypothyroidism have increased pulse amplitude throughout the day but loss of the usual nocturnal increase in pulse amplitude,[157] in agreement with previous reports.[158] The secretory pulses of TSH, α subunit, and the gonadotropins show a high degree of concordance consistent with the operation of a common hypothalamic pulse generator.[157] The central mechanisms underlying TSH pulsatility and rhythmicity are unknown. They are probably mediated in part by signals from the suprachiasmatic nuclei of the hypothalamus. These nuclei are paired structures situated just above the optic chiasm that initiate intrinsic circadian rhythmicity, the timing of which can be influenced by nonvisual nerve impulses arising in the retina.[159] It is reasonable to suppose that TRH pulsatility may mediate pulsatile TSH release, but there is no definite evidence for this.[5]

EXTRAHYPOTHALAMIC DISTRIBUTION AND ACTIONS OF TRH AND ITS METABOLITES

The widespread distribution of TRH in extrahypothalamic brain and other tissues indicates the likelihood that

this small peptide functions as a neurotransmitter or neuromodulator in nervous tissue while possibly having a paracrine action as a local cellular regulator in other tissues. This is in accord with phylogenetic data indicating that TRH existed long before the development of the pituitary gland.[42] It should be stated clearly however that most of the present functional data have accrued from pharmacological studies, and although TRH may have widespread influences on cellular function, the importance of any such actions in relation to hierarchical signal mechanisms is largely unknown.

Nervous Tissue

Authentic TRH is widely distributed throughout extrahypothalamic brain areas including the nucleus accumbens septi, various cranial nerve motor nuclei, medulla oblongata, and ventral spinal cord,[34, 35, 41, 160, 161] and levels are unaltered by lesions of the thyrotrophic area of the hypothalamus.[34, 35, 39, 41, 43] TRH immunoreactivity is also present in human cerebellum, cortex, and thalamus[162, 163] and is found in higher concentrations in the basal ganglia of patients dying with Huntington's chorea[164] which may be of functional relevance to this disease. TRH, 5-hydroxytryptamine, and substance P coexist within neuronal projections from the medulla oblongata to the ventral spinal cord.[165–167] Furthermore, a structural (and presumably functional) interdependence of these two molecules has been demonstrated because destruction of serotoninergic neurons with the neurotoxin 5,7-dihydroxytryptamine (5,7-DHT) causes depletion of ventral spinal cord TRH levels[165, 168] and increased TRH receptor number, which is limited to the ventral spinal cord.[169] Cyclo(His-Pro) is also widely distributed throughout the extrahypothalamic brain and is present in concentrations greater than those of TRH.[170–172] However, this dipeptide is derived from other sources as well as TRH because TRH and cyclo(His-Pro) have very different ontogenetic patterns in the rat[24] and destruction of serotoninergic nerves with 5,7-DHT causes depletion of spinal cord TRH but not of cyclo(His-Pro) levels.[25]

Not surprisingly, in view of its distribution, pharmacological studies have demonstrated a wide variety of actions for TRH. At the neuronal level, TRH acts directly on the electrical activity of certain neurons and stimulates increased release and turnover of certain neurotransmitters. In addition TRH has been implicated in the control of arousal, appetite, thermoregulation, respiration, locomotion, and the neural control of gastrointestinal motility and secretion. It should be emphasized that several other neuropeptides have also been implicated in these functions and probably interact with TRH. Certain of these effects are immediate and transient in keeping with a classical neurotransmitter role whereas others are more prolonged, suggesting a neuromodulatory role on the actions of other neurotransmitters. In support of a physiological role for extrahypothalamic TRH, specific high-affinity TRH receptors are present in membrane preparations from a variety of brain regions but not always those with the highest concentrations of immunoreactive TRH.[173, 174] TRH is localized to synaptosomal preparations and can be released from various brain sites by several stimuli, including depolarization.[175–177]

The various CNS or CNS-mediated pharmacological actions of TRH are listed in Table 11–2. TRH causes increased norepinephrine and acetylcholine turnover[178–179] and stimulates dopamine release from the nucleus accumbens.[180] Microinjection of TRH or stable analogues into the nucleus accumbens stimulates increased locomotor activity, which may be a functional consequence of the release of endogenous dopamine by TRH from this area.[180–184] Injection of TRH into the nucleus accumbens also produces hyperthermia,[185] although the mechanism is unclear.

A variety of investigations have indicated that TRH antagonizes the narcosis induced by several central depressant drugs including pentobarbital and ethanol.[186–188] It appears that the septum is important in mediating this effect[189] but that TRH-induced dopamine release is not involved.[190] Central or peripheral administration of TRH or various stable analogues antagonizes the hypothermic and antinociceptive actions of neurotensin[191–193] and also antagonizes the hypothermic and cataleptic effects of opiates without affecting the analgesia.[194] Intracerebroventricular administration of TRH in the rat suppresses feeding and drinking behavior,[195, 196] an action that may be mediated by the induction of rhythmical electrical activity in nucleus tractus solitarius neurons by TRH.[197] The various actions of TRH on cardiorespiratory activity, temperature regulation, and other autonomic functions are probably mediated by other specific TRH-sensitive sites in the brain stem.[198, 199] TRH causes acute depolarization of spinal lower motor neurons (LMN's) in culture[200] and may be a trophic factor for motor neurons. It also stimulates choline acetyltransferase levels in ventral spinal cord.[201] Serum from patients with motor neuron disease stimulates TRH production by cultured fetal rat brain stem cells as does the motor neurotoxin L-BMAA,[202] providing further circumstantial evidence for a link between TRH and LMN function. Central

TABLE 11–2. CNS OR CNS-MEDIATED PHARMACOLOGICAL ACTIONS OF TRH

A. Basic neuronal actions
   1. Alters firing rate of certain neurons.
   2. Stimulates rhythmical electrical activity in nucleus tractus solitarius.
   3. Increases norepinephrine turnover.
   4. Increases acetylcholine turnover.
   5. Stimulates dopamine release in nucleus accumbens.
   6. Acute depolarization of cultured LMN's.
   7. LMN trophic factor.
B. Behavioral and vegetative actions
   1. Increased locomotor activity (nucleus accumbens).
   2. Stimulates respiration (brain stem).
   3. Hyperthermia (nucleus accumbens).
   4. Suppresses feeding and drinking behavior (ICV).
C. Brain-gut actions (vagal cholinergic mechanism)
   1. Stimulates gastrointestinal motility (ICV).
   2. Increases gastric acid, pepsin, and exocrine pancreatic secretion (ICV).
D. Interactions with other drugs and neuropeptides
   1. Antagonizes narcosis induced by certain depressant drugs (e.g., pentobarbital and ethanol [ICV and peripheral]).
   2. Antagonizes the hypothalamic and antionociceptive action of neurotensin (ICV and peripheral).
   3. Antagonizes the hypothalamic and cataleptic effects of opiates without affecting analgesia (ICV and peripheral).

ICV, Intracerebroventricular.

administration of TRH also stimulates gastrointestinal motility as well as increased gastric acid, pepsin, and exocrine pancreatic secretion.[203–206] These effects are mediated, at least in part, via activation of vagal cholinergic mechanisms.

In view of the likelihood that brain cyclo(His-Pro) may not arise totally from TRH, it is interesting that cyclo(His-Pro) causes hypothermia that is antagonized by TRH[207] while at the same time it has even greater potency than TRH in at least one parameter of behavioral activity in rats, namely the antagonism of ethanol-induced narcosis.[208] In addition, cyclo(His-Pro) causes a transient increase in brain cyclic GMP levels and inhibits sodium-dependent catecholamine transport into nerve endings.[209, 210] The physiological relevance of these observations is unclear at present.

Pancreas and Gastrointestinal Tract

Authentic TRH is present in the gastrointestinal tract and pancreatic islets[211–215]; functional studies have indicated that TRH may participate in the neural regulation of gastrointestinal secretion and motility. In a recent study TRH co-localized with gastrin in the antral cells of human fetuses but could not be identified in adult tissues.[216] Pancreatic TRH concentrations are high in the early neonatal period and decline thereafter to low concentrations in the adult.[215, 217, 218] In hypothyroidism pancreatic TRH is increased due to inhibition of pancreatic TRH-degrading activity,[219] and using this model it has been demonstrated that TRH immunoreactivity is present in insulin-containing β cells.[219] Administration of TRH enhances arginine-induced glucagon release in adult dogs[220] while destruction of β cells with streptozotocin reduces islet TRH levels.[212] Systemic administration of TRH in humans retards xylose and glucose absorption from the gut and inhibits pentagastrin-stimulated acid secretion.[221, 222] In addition, TRH has a direct action stimulating contraction of isolated guinea pig duodenal segments.[223] Despite these observations an integrated role for TRH in the control of gastrointestinal function is unclear. TRH may also be produced "ectopically" in the gastrointestinal tract. Significant quantities of immunoreactive TRH, which was biologically and chromatographically identical to TRH, were identified in a human pancreatic carcinoid tumor causing Cushing's syndrome.[224]

Genitourinary Tract

High levels of TRH-like immunoreactivity have been reported in reproductive tissues from a variety of species including rats and rabbits and in the human prostate, seminal vesicle, and semen.[225–230] Although these peptides are regulated by thyroid hormones,[230, 231] recent detailed characterization of the immunoreactive material has identified a closely related molecule, pyroGlu-Glu-ProNH$_2$, and a larger polypeptide containing TRH immunoreactivity at the C terminus.[229, 232–234] Furthermore, these peptides are not formed by expression of the TRH gene in rabbit and rat reproductive tissues.[229, 230] The present situation is somewhat unclear, since a recent report details the presence of high levels of authentic TRH and related peptides in human semen, which decline following vasectomy.[235] Further studies are necessary to clone the relevant genes and ascribe functions to these different TRH-like peptides.

Other Tissues

TRH-like immunoreactivity is present in the retina[236, 237] as well as in human placenta[238] and thyroid tissue, where the TRH gene is expressed in normal thyroid parafollicular cells.[239] Authentic TRH has also been detected in extracts of a variety of human tumors.[240]

CLINICAL RELEVANCE OF TRH

The availability of TRH led to the exploration and development of this peptide as an adjunct to diagnosis in a variety of endocrine disorders. However, recent understanding of its actions and role in extrahypothalamic brain areas and in spinal cord have promoted the exploratory use of TRH as a diagnostic and potential therapeutic agent in several nonendocrine disorders.

Diagnosis of Endocrine Disease

Since many factors interact at any given time to determine both basal TSH levels and responsiveness to TRH, it is hardly surprising that alterations in TSH responsiveness to TRH occur in a variety of different settings. Physiological and pharmacological alterations are listed in Table 11–3. In broad terms, pharmacological agents affecting TSH and TRH responses can be divided into two groups: those that act via alterations in thyroid status (thyroid hormones, antithyroid drugs, iodides, and iopanoic acid) and those that act via central alterations in hypothalamic-pituitary control. It should be emphasized that these latter agents do not necessarily lead to alterations in thyroid status. For example, although DA agonists lead to immediate suppression of basal and TRH-stimulated TSH release[241, 242] and DA

TABLE 11–3. ALTERATIONS IN TSH RESPONSES TO TRH

	TSH/TRH
Physiological	
Females vs males	↑
Follicular phase	↑
Circadian rhythm (nocturnal)	↑
Pharmacological	
DA and DA agonists	↓
Adrenergic antagonists	↓
Excess thyroid hormone	↓
Somatostatin	↓
Corticosteroids	↓
Phenytoin (in vitro data)	↓
Heroin addiction	↓
DA antagonists	↑
Antithyroid drugs	↑
Iodides	↑
Iopanoic acid	↑
Estrogens	↑
Theophylline (in vitro data)	↑

TABLE 11–4. ALTERATIONS IN TSH RESPONSE TO TRH IN DISEASE STATES

Primary thyroid disease	
Hyperthyroidism (any cause)	↓
Subclinical hyperthyroidism	↓
Diffuse nontoxic goiter (15%)	↓
Treated hyperthyroidism (3–12 months)	↓
Ophthalmic Graves' disease (30%)	N or ↓ or ↑
Hypothyroidism (any cause)	↑
Subclinical hypothyroidism	↑
Pituitary disease	
Acromegaly	N or ↓
Cushing's disease	N or ↓
Nelson's syndrome	N or ↓
Prolactinomas	N or ↓ or ↑
"Nonfunctional" adenomas	N or ↓
TSH feedback adenoma	↑
"TSH toxicosis" without adenoma	↑
"TSH toxicosis" with adenoma	↓
Familial hypopituitarism with enlarged sella in childhood	↑
Hypothalamic disease (any cause)	N or ↓ or ↑
Idiopathic GH deficiency	N or ↑
Idiopathic hypopituitarism in childhood	N or ↑
Neuropsychiatric disorders	
Anorexia nervosa	N or ↓
Unipolar depression	N or ↓
Other endocrine/metabolic disorders	
Chronic renal failure	N or ↓
Starvation	N or ↓
Elderly sick/euthyroid	N or ↓

antagonists cause immediate TSH release and may lead to slight enhancement of TSH responsiveness,[243] chronic administration of such agents does not lead to hypothyroidism[244] or hyperthyroidism, respectively. This implies that mechanisms exist whereby the hypothalamic-pituitary-thyroid axis can compensate to maintain euthyroidism, presumably via modulation of the activity of hypothalamic regulatory pathways.

When physiological and pharmacological alterations in TRH responsiveness have been excluded, there remain a variety of pathological states in which disturbances in control may occur. As is well known, the most clear-cut and consistent alterations in TSH control occur in primary thyroid disorders (Table 11–4). However, in the clinical setting the use of the "TRH test" has been superceded by the development of highly sensitive, two-site, third and fourth generation TSH assays. From such studies it is clear that the TSH response to TRH parallels the basal TSH level. The usefulness of TRH testing is now limited to the investigation of various hypothalamic/pituitary disorders.

The patterns of TSH response to TRH show broad overlaps in patients with different hypothalamic and pituitary diseases; nevertheless, some reliance is placed on the response to dynamic testing even when the basal TSH level is itself elevated as in so-called "TSH toxicosis" (see Table 11–3). In this condition the absence of a TSH response to TRH in the presence of elevated basal TSH and thyroid hormone levels points to the presence of a TSH-secreting pituitary adenoma.[5] This is not the case in patients with generalized resistance to thyroid hormones, who usually display an elevated basal TSH and a response to TRH that is proportional to the basal TSH level.[245] In most other pituitary disease states, the TSH response to TRH is usually normal or reduced and a flat TSH response strongly suggests a pituitary lesion. Occasional patients with large pituitary tumors may show a delayed pattern of TSH response, which is also seen in hypothalamic disease and which is probably due to reduction in the transport of TRH to the pituitary.[246] Indeed, some patients with hyperprolactinemia or prolactinomas may show exaggerated TSH responses to TRH,[246, 247] but the pattern of response is usually normal. It should be emphasized that factors other than tumor size may also determine the degree of TSH responsiveness to TRH. Recent studies indicate that patients with pituitary disease and GH deficiency show greater TSH responses to TRH than do pituitary disease patients with normal GH reserve.[248] At the other extreme, acromegalic patients with excess GH secretion frequently show reduced TSH responses to TRH. The implication here is that GH may modulate TSH directly or possibly via alterations in hypothalamic somatostatin release. In Cushing's disease the elevated circulating corticosteroid levels may also play a role in TSH suppression.

In hypothalamic disease of any etiology the TSH response to TRH may be suppressed or show a delayed and not infrequently exaggerated pattern, peak TSH levels being achieved at 60 minutes or later following TRH administration. However, such patterns of response may also be seen in patients with large pituitary lesions causing stalk compression.[246] In certain cases of hypothalamic-pituitary disease, basal TSH levels and responsiveness to TRH may be slightly elevated with secondary hypothyroidism. In this instance, excess immunoreactive TSH with reduced biological activity is produced[79]; the situation can be reversed by continuous TRH administration.[78]

The measurement of hormonal responses other than TSH to TRH has also been widely investigated. In patients with hyperprolactinemia a reduced or absent PRL response to TRH is consistent with but not diagnostic of a prolactinoma because reduced responses may also occur in stalk-compression hyperprolactinemia.[246] Nor does the presence of a considerable PRL response to TRH exclude the diagnosis of a prolactinoma. A paradoxical GH response to TRH can be useful in the detection of altered dynamics of GH regulation and, in the case of acromegaly, abolition of the GH response to TRH is used by some as a good parameter of successful transphenoidal surgery.[249]

As regards other endocrine conditions, TRH administration has been evaluated as a secretagogue for calcitonin, but it seems clear that pentagastrin stimulation—with or without calcium—causes a more reliable and consistent calcitonin response in the diagnosis of medullary carcinoma of the thyroid.[250, 251]

TRH in Nonendocrine Disease

The arousal, analeptic, locomotor, and opiate antagonist actions of TRH have stimulated research in patients with disorders relating to these particular functions. However, most neuropeptides, including TRH, penetrate the blood-brain barrier poorly. This circumstance may account in part for the considerable variability in results.

An extensive literature has developed concerning the patterns and degrees of hormonal responses to TRH in several neuropsychiatric disorders. Unfortunately the results have contributed little to the understanding of disease etiology, although there may be some minor prognostic benefit.[252–254] The TSH response to TRH is reduced, on a group mean basis, in patients with unipolar as opposed to bipolar depression,[255–259] schizophrenia,[260] and Alzheimer's disease.[261] As early as 1972 it was postulated that this finding in depressed patients might reflect reduced endogenous TRH–like activity. This indicated a therapeutic possibility for TRH supported by subsequent behavioral findings of arousal, ergotropic, or analeptic activity.[262] However, although early studies suggested a transient antidepressant action for TRH in patients,[255, 262] subsequent double-blind studies failed to confirm this effect.[263, 264] As of this writing there is no established value for TRH or any of its more stable analogues in the treatment of depression.

The presence of TRH in various cranial nerve motor nuclei, the cerebellum, and the ventral spinal cord prompted investigation in patients with various movement disorders. Clinical studies have indicated a small beneficial effect of administration of both intravenous TRH and the oral analogue RX77368 on motor function in patients with amyotrophic lateral sclerosis.[257–268] There also appears to be some improvement in the movement disorder in patients with spinocerebellar degeneration.[269] In the latter situation the authors suggest that TRH improves norepinephrine turnover in the brain stem and cerebellum. TRH treatment of 17 patients with idiopathic cerebellar degeneration caused subjective improvement in 47 per cent and objective improvement in 35 per cent.[270] However, these beneficial effects appear to be minor and transient, and the present findings are based largely on uncontrolled studies.

In view of the ability of TRH to antagonize some of the effects of opiates but not the analgesic activity, the effects of TRH have been studied in various forms of experimental shock in which opiate antagonism with naloxone has been found to be of benefit. Indeed, TRH is effective in maintaining blood pressure in hemorrhagic and endotoxic shock in the rat and in improving neurological recovery and survival after spinal trauma in cats.[198, 271–274] In keeping with these findings it has been reported recently that TRH causes a transient rise in blood pressure and stimulation of ventilation following intravenous administration in both animals and humans.[275–277] Although accompanied by elevation in circulating catecholamine levels, these cardiorespiratory effects of TRH do not occur entirely through this sympathoadrenal response.[198, 275, 278] It has been suggested that TRH-induced vasopressin release may be the relevant mediating factor.[274, 275] However, other investigators have found no effects of bolus administration of TRH on blood pressure in humans, whereas there appears to be an approximate doubling of circulating levels of atrial natriuretic peptide without changes in aldosterone or cortisol levels.[279] Whatever the underlying mechanisms, each of these interesting observations merits further evaluation in the clinical setting in order to delineate the potential regulatory mechanisms subserved by TRH in cardiorespiratory physiology.

An interesting recent development concerns exploration of the potential value of TRH in the treatment of the fetal respiratory distress syndrome (RDS). This syndrome results from immaturity of the fetal lungs, which fail to expand after delivery due to lack of a lipoprotein surfactant.[280, 281] Thyroid hormones enhance surfactant synthesis in immature lungs.[282] Since the placenta is permeable to TRH but not to TSH[283] and thyroid hormone transfer is limited, and since maternal TRH administration causes a rise in fetal thyroid hormones[284, 285] via the release of fetal TSH, TRH administration to the mothers of preterm infants may be of benefit in reducing the frequency or complications of fetal RDS.

When TRH was added to the standard RDS treatment with glucocorticoids to women at risk for delivering a premature child, there was a significant improvement in the lecithin/sphingomyelin ratio (an index of lung maturation) in amniotic fluid after one and two weeks of treatment and a slight but not significant reduction in the frequency of RDS.[286] There was also a significant reduction of time on the respirator in affected children and a decreased frequency of the major complication of RDS, bronchopulmonary dysplasia.[286] In a recent double-blind multicenter study 404 women with threatened preterm delivery at less than 32 weeks' gestation received betamethasone plus TRH or betamethasone plus placebo.[287] TRH treatment did not affect the total incidence of RDS, but chronic lung disease developed in significantly fewer TRH-treated infants, and there were fewer adverse outcomes in this group.[287] Although this therapeutic approach appears to be favorable, the results must be compared with the effects of synthetic surfactants such as colfosceril palmitate (Exosurf) and natural surfactants which are now becoming available.

REFERENCES

1. Greer MA: Evidence of hypothalamic control of the pituitary release of thyrotrophin. Proc Soc Exp Biol Med 77:603–608, 1951.
2. Schally AV, Bowers CY, Redding TW, Barrett JF: Isolation of thyrotropin releasing factor (TRF) from porcine hypothalamus. Biochem Biophys Res Commun 25:165–169, 1966.
3. Folkers K, Enzman F, Boler J, et al: Discovery of modification of the synthetic tripeptide sequence of the thyrotropin releasing hormone having activity. Biochem Biophys Res Commun 37:123–126, 1969.
4. Burgus R, Dunn TF, Desiderio D, et al: Characterisation of the hypothalamic hypophysiotropic TSH-releasing factor (TRF) of ovine origin. Nature 226:321–325, 1970.
5. Scanlon MF: Thyroid stimulating hormone. In Braverman LC, Utiger RD (eds): The Thyroid: A Fundamental and Clinical Text. Philadelphia, JB Lippincott Co., 1991, pp 230–256.
6. Jackson IMD, Wu P, Lechan RM: Immunohistochemical localisation in the rat brain of the precursor for thyrotropin-releasing hormone. Science 229:1097–1099, 1985.
7. McKelvy JF: Thyrotropin-releasing hormone synthesis. In Griffiths EC, Bennett GW (eds): Thyrotropin-Releasing Hormone. New York, Raven Press, 1983, pp 51–56.
8. Richter K, Kawashima E, Egger R, et al: Biosynthesis of thyrotropin releasing hormone in the skin of Xenopus laevis: Partial sequence of the precursor deduced from cloned cDNA. EMBO J 3:617–621, 1984.
9. Lechan RM, Wu P, Jackson IMD, et al: Thyrotropin releasing hormone precursor: Characterization in rat brain. Science 231:159–161, 1986.
10. Jackson IMD: Controversies in TRH biosynthesis and strategies toward the identification of a TRH precursor. Ann NY Acad Sci 553:7–10, 1989.
11. Wu P: Identification and characterization of TRH-precursor peptides. Ann NY Acad Sci 553:60–63, 1989.
12. Wu P, Jackson IM: Post-translational processing of thyrotropin-releasing hormone precursor in rat brain: Identification of 3 novel peptides derived from pro-TRH. Brain Res 456:22–26, 1988.
13. Yamada M, Radovick S, Wondisford FE, et al: Cloning and structure of human genomic DNA and hypothalamic cDNA encoding human prepro-thyrotropin-releasing hormone. Mol Endocrinol 4(4):551–556, 1990.
14. Yamada M, Wondisford FE, Radovick S, et al: Assignment of human prepro-thyrotropin-releasing hormone (TRH) gene to chromosome 3. Somat Cell Mol Genet 17(1):97–100, 1991.
15. Battaini F, Peterkofsky A: Inhibition of dopamine (DA) uptake and (Na⁺, K⁺)-ATPase in rat brain synaptosomes by histidyl-proline diketopiperazine [cyclo(His)pro], a metabolite of thyrotropin releasing hormone (TRH). Fed Proc 39:594–598, 1980.
16. Griffiths EC, Hooper KC, Jeffcoate SL, White N: Peptides in the rat hypothalamus inactivating thyrotropin-releasing hormone (TRH). Acta Endocrinol 79:209–216, 1975.
17. Jackson IMD, Papapetrou PD, Reichlin S: Metabolic clearance of thyrotropin-releasing hormone in the rat in hypothyroid and hyperthyroid states: Comparison with serum degradation in vitro. Endocrinology 104:1292–1298, 1979.
18. Yanagisawa T, Prasad C, Peterkofsky A: The subcellular and organ distribution and natural form of histidyl-proline-diketopiperazine in rat brain determined by a specific radioimmunoassay. J Biol Chem 255:10290–10298, 1980.
19. Garat B, Miranda J, Charli J-L, Joseph-Bravo P: Presence of a membrane bound pyroglutamyl aminopeptidase degrading thyrotropin releasing hormone in rat brain. Neuropeptides 6:27–40, 1985.
20. Horsthemke B, Leblanc P, Kordon C, et al: Subcellular distribution of particle bound neutral peptidases capable of hydrolyzing gonadoliberin, thyroliberin, enkephalin and substance P. Eur J Biochem 139:315–320, 1984.
21. O'Connor B, O'Cuinn G: Localization of a narrow specificity thyroliberin hydrolyzing pyroglutamyl aminopeptidase in synaptosomal membranes of guinea pig brain. Eur J Biochem 144:271–278, 1984.
22. Bauer K, Nowak P, Kleinkauf H: Specificity of a serum peptidase hydrolyzing thyroliberin at pyroglutamyl-histidine bond. Eur J Biochem 118:173–177, 1981.
23. O'Connor B, O'Cuinn G: Purification of and kinetic studies on a narrow specificity synaptosomal membrane pyroglutamate aminopeptidase from guinea pig brain. Eur J Biochem 150:47–53, 1985.
24. Lamberton RP, Lechan RM, Jackson IMD: Ontogeny of thyrotropin releasing hormone (TRH) and histidyl proline diketopiperazine (His-Pro-DKP) in the rat CNS and pancreas. Endocrinology 115:2400–2405, 1984.
25. Lechan RM, Jackson IMD: Thyrotropin-releasing hormone but not histidyl-proline-diketopiperazine is depleted from rat spinal cord following 5,7-dihydroxytryptamine treatment. Brain Res 326:152–155, 1985.
26. Hilton CW, Prasad C, Vo P, Mouton C: Food contains the bioactive peptide, cyclo(His-Pro). J Clin Endocrinol Metab 75(2):375–378, 1992.
27. Bauer K: Regulation of degradation of thyrotropin releasing hormone by thyroid hormones. Nature 259:591–593, 1976.
28. White N, Jeffcoate SL, Griffiths EC, Hooper KC: Effect of thyroid status on the thyrotrophin-releasing hormone-degrading activity of rat serum. J Endocrinol 71:13–17, 1976.
29. Iverson E: Pharmacokinetics of thyrotrophin-releasing hormone in patients in different thyroid states. J Endocrinol 128(1):153–159, 1991.
30. Yamada M, Mori M: Thyrotropin-releasing hormone-degrading enzyme in human serum is classified as type II of pyroglutamyl aminopeptidase: Influence of thyroid status. Proc Soc Exper Biol Med 194(4):346–351, 1990.
31. Bauer K: Adenohypophyseal degradation of thyrotropin releasing hormone regulated by thyroid hormones. Nature 330:375–377, 1987.
32. Ponce G, Charli J-L, Pasten JA, et al: Tissue-specific regulation of pyroglutamate aminopeptidase II activity by thyroid hormones. Neuroendocrinology 48:211–213, 1988.
33. Brownstein M, Palkovits M, Saavedra JM, et al: Thyrotropin releasing hormone in specific nuclei of the brain. Science 185:267–269, 1974.
34. Brownstein MJ, Utiger RD, Palkovits M, Kizer JS: Effect of hypothalamic deafferentation on thyrotropin releasing hormone levels in rat brain. Proc Natl Acad Sci USA 72:4177–4179, 1975.
35. Jackson IMD, Reichlin S: Thyrotropin releasing hormone (TRH). Distribution in the brain, blood and urine of the rat. Life Sci 14:2259–2266, 1974.
36. Aizawa G, Greer M: Delineation of the hypothalamic area controlling thyrotropin secretion in the rat. Endocrinology 109:1731–1738, 1981.
37. Greer MA: The role of the hypothalamus in the control of thyroid function. J Clin Endocrinol Metab 12:1259–1268, 1952.
38. Martin JB, Boshans R, Reichlin S: Feedback regulation of TSH secretion in rats with hypothalamic lesions. Endocrinology 87:1032–1040, 1970.
39. Lechan RM, Jackson IMD: Immunohistochemical localization of thy-

rotropin-releasing hormone in the rat hypothalamus and pituitary. Endocrinology 111:55–65, 1982.

40. Siaud P, Tapia-Arancibia L, Szafarczyk A, Alonso G: Increase of thyrotropin-releasing hormone immunoreactivity in the nucleus of the solitary tract following bilateral lesions of the hypothalamic paraventricular nuclei. Neurosci Lett 79:47–52, 1987.

41. Hokfelt T, Fuxe K, Johannsson O, et al: Distribution of thyrotropin-releasing hormone (TRH) in the central nervous system as revealed by immunohistochemistry. Eur J Pharmacol 34:389–392, 1975.

42. Jackson IMD: Thyrotropin releasing hormone. N Engl J Med 306: 145–155, 1982.

43. Jackson IMD: Thyrotropin-releasing hormone (TRH): distribution in mammalian species and its functional significance. In Griffiths EC, Bennett GW (eds): Thyrotropin-Releasing Hormone. New York, Raven Press, 1983, pp 3–18.

44. Jackson IMD, Reichlin S: Brain thyrotropin-releasing hormone is independent of the hypothalamus. Nature 267:853–854, 1977.

45. Le Dafniet M, Lefebvre P, Barret A, et al: Normal and adenomatous human pituitaries secrete thyrotropin-releasing hormone in vitro: Modulation by dopamine, haloperidol, and somatostatin. J Clin Endocrinol Metab 71(2):480–486, 1990.

46. Pagesy P, Croissandeau G, Le Dafniet M, et al: Detection of thyrotropin-releasing hormone (TRH) by mRNA by the reverse transcription-polymerase chain reaction in the human normal and tumoral anterior pituitary. J Biochem Biophys Res Commun 182(1):182–187, 1992.

47. Morley JE: Neuroendocrine control of thyrotropin secretion. Endocrine Rev 2:396–436, 1981.

48. Scanlon MF, Lewis M, Weightman DR, et al: The neuroregulation of human thyrotropin secretion. In Martini L, Ganong WF (eds). Frontiers in Neuroendocrinology. New York, Raven Press, 1980, pp 333–380.

49. Brolin SE: The importance of the stalk connexion for the power of the anterior pituitary of the rat to react structurally upon ceasing thyroid function. Acta Phys Scand 14:233–244, 1947.

50. Vale W, Grant G, Amoss M, et al: Culture of enzymatically dispersed anterior pituitary cells: Functional validation of a method. J Clin Endocrinol Metab 91:562–572, 1972.

51. Labrie F, DeLean A, Lagrace L, et al: Interactions of TRH, LHRH and somatostatin in the anterior pituitary gland. In Bimbanmer L, O'Malley BW (eds): Receptors and Hormone Action (vol 3). London, Academic Press, 1978.

52. Sheward WJ, Harmar AJ, Fraser HM, Fink G: TRH in rat pituitary stalk blood and hypothalamus. Studies with high performance liquid chromatography. Endocrinology 113:1865–1869, 1983.

53. Fraser HM, McNeilly AS: Effect of chronic immunoneutralization of thyrotropin-releasing hormone on the hypothalamic-pituitary thyroid axis, prolactin and reproductive function in the ewe. Endocrinology 111:1964–1974, 1982.

54. Carr FE, Shupnik MA, Burnside J, Chin WW: Thyrotropin-releasing hormone stimulates the activity of the rat thyrotropin β-subunit gene promoter transfected into pituitary cells. Mol Endocrinol 3:717–724, 1989.

55. Franklyn JA, Wilson M, Davis JR, et al: Demonstration of thyrotropin β-subunit messenger RNA in primary culture: Evidence for regulation by thyrotropin-releasing hormone and forskolin. J Endocrinol 111:R1–R4, 1986.

56. Kourides IA, Gurr JA, Wolf O: The regulation and organization of thyroid stimulating hormone genes. Recent Prog Horm Res 40:79–120, 1984.

57. Shupnik MA, Greenspan SL, Ridgway EC: Transcriptional regulation of thyrotropin subunit genes by thyrotropin-releasing hormone and dopamine in pituitary cell culture. J Biol Chem 261:12675–12679, 1986.

58. Steinfelder HJ, Hauser P, Nakayama Y, et al: Thyrotropin-releasing hormone regulation of human TSHB expression: Role of a pituitary-specific transcription factor (Pit-1/GHF-1) and potential interaction with a thyroid hormone–inhibitory element. Proc Nat Acad Sci USA 88(8):3130–3134, 1991.

59. Guo-zai Y, Pan WT, Bancroft C: Thyrotropin-releasing hormone action on the prolactin promoter is mediated by the POU protein Pit-1. Mol Endocrinol 5:535–541, 1991.

60. Guo-zai Y, Bancroft C: Mediation by calcium of thyrotropin-releasing hormone action on the prolactin promoter via transcription factor Pit-1. Mol Endocrinol 5:1488–1497, 1991.

61. Chan V, Wang C, Yeung TT: Thyrotropin, alpha and beta-subunits of thyrotropin and prolactin response to four hour constant infusions of thyrotropin releasing hormone in normal subjects and pa-

tients with pituitary-thyroid disorders. J Clin Endocrinol Metab 49:127–132, 1979.

62. Mori M, Murakami M, Satoh T, et al: A possible direct precursor of thyrotropin-releasing hormone, pGlu-His-Pro-Gly, stimulates prolactin secretion in anorexia nervosa. J Clin Endocrinol Metab 71(1):252–255, 1990.

63. Mori M, Satoh T, Miyashita K, et al: TRH-Gly, a precursor of TRH, alters GH secretion in acromegaly. Life Sci 49(14):1031–1037, 1991.

64. Magner JA: Thyroid-stimulating hormone: Biosynthesis, cell biology and bioactivity. Endocr Rev 11:354–385, 1990.

65. Magner JA, Kane J, Chou ET: Intravenous thyrotropin (TSH)-releasing hormone releases human TSH that is structurally different from basal TSH. J Clin Endocrinol Metab 74(6):1306–1311, 1992.

66. Amir SM, Kubota K, Tramontano D, et al: The carbohydrate moiety of bovine thyrotropin is essential for full bioactivity but not for receptor recognition. Endocrinology 120:345–352, 1987.

67. Berman MI, Thomas CG, Manjunath P, et al: The role of the carbohydrate moiety in thyrotropin action. Biochem Biophys Res Commun 133:680–687, 1985.

68. Nissim M, Lee KO, Petrick PA, et al: A sensitive thyrotropin (TSH) bioassay based on iodide uptake in rat FRTL-5 thyroid cells: Comparison with the adenosine 3′,5′-monophosphate response to human serum TSH and enzymatically deglycosylated bovine and human TSH. Endocrinology 121:1278–1287, 1987.

69. Amir S, Menezes-Ferreira MM, Shimohigashi Y, et al: Activities of deglycosylated thyrotropin at the thyroid membrane receptor–adenylate cyclase system. J Endocrinol Invest 8:537–541, 1986.

70. Wilber JF: Stimulation of ^{14}C-glucosamine and ^{14}C-alanine incorporation into thyrotropin by synthetic thyrotropin-releasing hormone. Endocrinology 89:873–877, 1971.

71. Gesundheit N, Weintraub BD: Mechanisms and regulation of TSH glycosylation. Adv Exp Med Biol 205:87–95, 1986.

72. Gesundheit N, Fink DL, Silverman LA, Weintraub BD: Effect of thyrotropin-releasing hormone on the carbohydrate structure of secreted mouse thyrotropin: Analysis by lectin affinity chromatography. J Biol Chem 262:5197–5203, 1987.

73. Menezes-Ferreira MM, Petrick PA, Weintraub BD: Regulation of thyrotropin (TSH) bioactivity by TSH-releasing hormone and thyroid hormone. Endocrinology 118:2125–2130, 1986.

74. Taylor T, Weintraub BD: Thyrotropin (TSH)-releasing hormone regulation of TSH subunit biosynthesis and glycosylation in normal and hypothyroid rat pituitaries. Endocrinology 116:1968–1976, 1985.

75. Taylor T, Gesundheit N, Weintraub BD: Effects of in vivo bolus versus continuous TRH administration on TSH secretion, biosynthesis and glycosylation in normal and hypothyroid rats. Mol Cell Endocrinol 46:253–261, 1986.

76. Taylor T, Gesundheit N, Gyves PW, et al: Hypothalamic hypothyroidism caused by lesions in rat paraventricular nuclei alters the carbohydrate structure of secreted thyrotropin. Endocrinology 122:283–290, 1988.

77. Faglia G, Bitensky L, Pinchera A, et al: Thyrotropin secretion in patients with central hypothyroidism: Evidence for reduced biological activity of immunoreactive thyrotropin. J Clin Endocrinol Metab 48:989–998, 1979.

78. Beck-Peccoz P, Amir S, Menezes-Ferreira MM, et al: Decreased receptor binding of biologically inactive thyrotropin in central hypothyroidism: Effect of treatment with thyrotropin-releasing hormone. N Engl J Med 312:1085–1090, 1985.

79. Faglia G, Beck-Peccoz P, Ballabio M, Nava C: Excess of β-subunit of thyrotropin (TSH) in patients with idiopathic central hypothyroidism due to the secretion of TSH with reduced biological activity. J Clin Endocrinol Metab 56:908–914, 1983.

80. DeCherney GS, Gesundheit N, Gyves PW, et al: Alterations in the sialylation and sulfation of secreted mouse thyrotropin in primary hypothyroidism. Biochem Biophys Res Commun 159:755–762, 1989.

81. Miura Y, Perkel VS, Papenberg KA, et al: Concanavalin-A, lentil and ricin affinity binding characteristics of human thyrotropin: Differences in the sialylation of thyrotropin in sera of euthyroid, primary and central hypothyroid patients. J Clin Endocrinol Metab 69:985–995, 1988.

82. Wide L: Median charge and charge heterogeneity of human pituitary FSH, LH and TSH. Acta Endocrinol (Copenh) 109:181–186, 1985.

83. Yora T, Matsuzaki S, Kondo Y, Ui N: Changes in the contents of multiple components of rat pituitary thyrotropin in altered thyroid states. Endocrinology 104:1682–1685, 1979.

84. Beck-Peccoz P, Piscitelli G, Amir S, et al: Endocrine, biochemical and morphological studies of a pituitary adenoma secreting growth hormone, thyrotropin (TSH), and α-subunit: Evidence for secretion of

TSH with increased bioactivity. J Clin Endocrinol Metab 62:704–711, 1986.

85. Gesundheit N, Petrick PA, Nissim M, et al: Thyrotropin-secreting pituitary adenomas: Clinical and biochemical heterogeneity. Ann Intern Med 111:827, 1989.

86. DeLean A, Ferland L, Drouin J, et al: Modulation of pituitary thyrotropin releasing hormone receptor levels by estrogens and thyroid hormones. Endocrinology 100:1496–1504, 1977.

87. Hinkle PM, Perrone MH, Schonbrunn A: Mechanism of thyroid hormone inhibition of thyrotropin-releasing hormone action. Endocrinology 108:199–205, 1981.

88. Hinkle PM, Tashjian AH: Thyrotropin-releasing hormone regulates the number of its own receptors in the GH_3 strain of pituitary cells in culture. Biochemistry 14:3845–3851, 1975.

89. Hinkle PM, Goh KBC: Regulation of thyrotrophin releasing hormone receptors and responses by L-triiodothyronine in dispersed rat pituitary cell cultures. Endocrinology 110:1725–1731, 1982.

90. Kaji H, Hinkle PM: Regulation of thyroid hormone receptors and responses by thyrotropin-releasing hormone in GH_4C_1 cells. Endocrinology 121:1697–1704, 1987.

91. Belchetz PE, Gredley G, Bird D, Himsworth RL: Regulation of thyrotropin secretion by negative feedback of triiodothyronine on the hypothalamus. J Endocrinology 76:439–448, 1977.

92. Berelowitz M, Maeda K, Harris S, Frohman LA: The effect of alterations in the pituitary-thyroid axis on hypothalamic content and in vitro release of somatostatin-like immunoreactivity. Endocrinology 107:24–29, 1980.

93. Koller KJ, Wolff RS, Warden MK, Zoeller RT: Thyroid hormones regulate levels of thyrotropin-releasing hormone mRNA in the paraventricular nucleus. Proc Natl Acad Sci USA 84:7329–7333, 1987.

94. Segerson TP, Kauer J, Wolfe HC, et al: Thyroid hormone regulates TRH biosynthesis in the paraventricular nucleus of the rat hypothalamus. Science 238:78–80, 1987.

95. Taylor T, Wondisford FE, Blaine T, Weintraub BD: The paraventricular nucleus of the hypothalamus has a major role in thyroid hormone feedback regulation of thyrotropin synthesis and secretion. Endocrinology 126:317–323, 1990.

96. Leong DA, Frawley LS, Neill JD: Neuroendocrine control of prolactin secretion. Annu Rev Physiol 45:109–127, 1983.

97. Noel GL, Dimond RC, Wartofsky L, et al: Studies of prolactin and TSH secretion by continuous infusion of small amounts of thyrotropin-releasing hormone (TRH). J Clin Endocrinol Metab 39:6–17, 1974.

98. Burnet FR, Wakerley JB: Plasma concentrations of prolactin and thyrotrophin during suckling in methane-anaesthetized rats. J Endocrinol 70:429–437, 1976.

99. De Greef WJ, Visser TJ: Evidence for the involvement of hypothalamic dopamine and thyrotropin-releasing hormone in suckling-induced release of prolactin. J Endocrinology 91:213–223, 1981.

100. Fraser HM, McNeilly AS: Inhibition of thyrotropin-releasing hormone by antibodies. In Griffiths EC, Bennett GW (eds): Thyrotropin-Releasing Hormones. New York, Raven Press, 1983, pp 179–190.

101. Peters JR, Foord SM, Dieguez C, Scanlon MF: TSH neuroregulation and alterations in disease states. Clin Endocrinol Metab 12:669–694, 1983.

102. Bauer K, Graf KJ, Fiavre-Baumann A, et al: Inhibition of prolactin secretion by histidyl-proline-diketopiperazine. Nature 274:174–175, 1978.

103. Enjalbert A, Ruberg N, Arancibia S, et al: Inhibition of in-vitro prolactin secretion by histidyl-proline-diketopiperazine, a degradation production of TRH. Eur J Pharmacol 58:97–98, 1979.

104. Lamberts SWJ, Visser TJ: The effects of histidyl-proline-diketopiperazine a metabolite of TRH on prolactin release by the rat pituitary gland in vitro. Eur J Pharmacol 71:337–341, 1981.

105. Melmed S, Carlson HE, Hershman JM: Histidyl-proline-diketopiperazine suppressing prolactin secretion in human pituitary tumor cell cultures. Clin Endocrinol 16:97–100, 1982.

106. Brabant G, Wickings EJ, Nieschlag E: The TRH-metabolite histidyl-proline-diketopiperazine (DKP) inhibits PRL secretion in male rhesus monkeys. Acta Endocrinol 98:189–194, 1981.

107. Peters JR, Foord SM, Dieguez C, et al: Lack of effect of the TRH related dipeptide histidyl-proline-diketopiperazine on TSH and PRL secretion in normal subjects, in patients with microprolactinomas and in primary hypothyroidism. Clin Endocrinol 23:289–293, 1985.

108. Borges JLC, Uskavitch DR, Kaiser DL, et al: Human pancreatic growth hormone releasing factor-40 (hpGRF-40) allows stimulation of GH release by TRH. Endocrinology 113:1519–1521, 1983.

109. Katakamitt H, Arimura A, Frohman LA: Hypothalamic somatostatin mediates the suppression of growth hormone secretion by centrally administered thyrotropin-releasing hormone in conscious rats. Endocrinology 117:1139–1144, 1985.

110. Jordan V, Dieguez C, Rodriguez-Arnao MD, et al: Influence of dopaminergic, adrenergic and cholinergic blockade and TRH administration on GH responses to GRF 1–29. Clin Endocrinol 24:291–298, 1986.

111. Krieger DT, Luria M: Plasma ACTH and cortisol responses to TRH, vasopressin or hypoglycemia in Cushing's disease and Nelson's syndrome. J Clin Endocrinol Metab 44:361–369, 1977.

112. Sowers JR, Hershman JM, Skowsky WR, Carlson HE: Effects of TRH on serum arginine vasopressin in euthyroid and hypothyroid subjects. Horm Res 7:232–237, 1976.

113. Mortimer CH, Besser GM, McNeilly AS, et al: Interaction between secretion of the gonadotrophins, prolactin, growth hormone, thyrotrophin and corticosteroids in man: The effects of LH/FSH-RH, TRH and hypoglycemia alone and in combination. Clin Endocrinol 2:317–322, 1973.

114. Mortimer CH, Besser GM, Goldie DJ, et al: The TSH, FSH and prolactin responses to continuous infusion of TRH and the effects of estrogen administration in normal males. Clin Endocrinol 3:97–102, 1974.

115. Straub RE, Frech GC, Joho RH, Gershengorn MC: Expression cloning of a cDNA encoding the mouse pituitary thyrotropin releasing hormone receptor. Proc Natl Acad Sci USA 87:9514–9518, 1990.

116. Gershengorn MC: Bihormonal regulation of the thyrotropin-releasing hormone receptor in mouse pituitary thyrotropic tumor cells in culture. J Clin Invest 62:937–943, 1978.

117. Oron Y, Straub RE, Traktman P, Gershengorn MC: Decreased TRH receptor mRNA activity precedes homologous downregulation: Assay in oocytes. Science 238:1406–1408, 1987.

118. Fujimoto J, Straub RE, Gershengorn MC: Thyrotropin-releasing hormone (TRH) and phorbol myristate acetate decrease TRH receptor messenger RNA in rat pituitary GH_3 cells: Evidence that protein kinase-C mediates the TRH effect. Mol Endocrinol 5:1527–1532, 1991.

119. Judd AM, Canonico PL, MacLeod RM: Prolactin release from MtTW15 and 731a pituitary tumors is refractory to TRH and VIP stimulation. Mol Cell Endocrinol 36:221–226, 1984.

120. Mongioli A, Aliffi A, Vicari E, et al: Down-regulation of prolactin secretion in men during continuous thyrotropin-releasing hormone infusion: Evidence for induction of pituitary desensitization by continuous TRH administration. J Clin Endocrinol Metab 56:904–908, 1983.

121. Sheppard MC, Shennan KJ: Desensitization of rat anterior pituitary gland to thyrotropin releasing hormone. J Endocrinol 101:101–105, 1984.

122. Mori M, Yamada M, Kobayashi S: Role of the hypothalamic TRH in the regulation of its own receptors in rat anterior pituitaries. Neuroendocrinology 48:153–158, 1988.

123. Hsieh K-P, Martin TFJ: Thyrotropin-releasing hormone and gonadotropin-releasing hormone receptors activate phospholipase C by coupling to the guanosine triphosphate-binding proteins G_q and G_{11}. Mol Endocrinol 6:1673–1681, 1992.

124. Drummond AH: Inositol lipid metabolism and signal transduction in clonal pituitary cells. J Exp Biol 124:337–342, 1986.

125. Gershengorn MC: Thyrotropin-releasing hormone action: Mechanism of calcium-mediated stimulation of prolactin secretion. Recent Prog Horm Res 41:607–653, 1985.

126. Iriuchijima T, Mori M: Inhibition by staurosporine of TRH-induced refractoriness of inositol phospholipid hydrolysis by rat anterior pituitaries. J Endocrinol 124:75–79, 1990.

127. Albert PR, Tashjian AH: Thyrotropin-releasing hormone-induced spike and plateau in cytosolic free Ca^{2+} concentrations in pituitary cells. J Biol Chem 259:5827–5832, 1984.

128. Geras EJ, Gershengorn MC: Evidence that TRH stimulates secretion of TSH by two calcium-mediated mechanisms. Am J Physiol 242:109–114, 1981.

129. Akerman SN, Zorec R, Cheeck TR, et al: Fura-2 imaging of thyrotropin-releasing hormone and dopamine effects on calcium homeostasis of bovine lactotrophs. Endocrinology 129:475–488, 1991.

130. Tornquist K: Evidence for TRH-induced influx of extracellular Ca^{2+} in pituitary GH4C1 cells. Biochem Biophys Res Commun 180:860–866, 1991.

131. Law GJ, Pachter JA, Thastrup O, et al: Thapsigargin, but not caffeine, blocks the ability of thyrotropin-releasing hormone to release Ca^{2+} from an intracellular store in GH_4C_1 cells. Biochem J 267:359–364, 1990.

132. Gershengorn MC: Thyrotropin releasing hormone stimulation of prolactin release: Evidence for a membrane potential-independent, Ca^{2+}-dependent mechanism of action. J Biol Chem 255:1801–1803, 1980.

133. Gershengorn MC, Thaw C: TRH stimulates biphasic elevation of cytoplasmic free calcium in GH_3 cells. Further evidence that TRH mobilizes cellular and extracellular Ca^{2+}. Endocrinology 116:591–596, 1985.

134. Martin TFJ: Thyrotropin-releasing hormone rapidly activates the phosphodiester hydrolysis of polyphosphoinositides in GH_3 pituitary cells: Evidence for the role of a polyphosphoinositide-specific phospholipase C in hormone action. J Biol Chem 258:14816–14822, 1983.

135. Tan KN, Tashjian AHJ: Receptor-mediated release of plasma membrane-associated calcium and stimulation of calcium uptake by thyrotropin-releasing hormone in pituitary cells in culture. J Biol Chem 256:8994–9002, 1981.

136. Peizhi LI, Thaw CN, Sempowski GD, et al: Characterization of the calcium response to thyrotropin-releasing hormone (TRH) in cells transfected with TRH receptor complementary DNA: Importance of voltage-sensitive calcium channels. Mol Endocrinol 6:1393–1402, 1992.

137. Winikov I, Geshengorn MC: Receptor density determines secretory response patterns mediated by inositol lipid-derived second messengers. Comparison of thyrotropin-releasing hormone and carbamylcholine actions in thyroid-stimulating hormone-secreting mouse pituitary tumor cells. J Biol Chem 264:9438–9442, 1989.

138. Gershengorn MC, Rebecchi MJ, Geras E, Arevalo CO: Thyrotropin-releasing hormone (TRH) action in mouse thyrotropic tumor cells in culture: Evidence against a role for adenosine 3,5'-monophosphate as a mediator of TRH-stimulated thyrotropin release. Endocrinology 107:665–670, 1980.

139. Iriuchijimia T, Mori M: Regional dissociation of cyclic AMP and inositol phosphate formation in response to thyrotropin-releasing hormone in the rat brain. J Neurochem 52:1944–1949, 1989.

140. Hokfelt T, Elde R, Fuxe K, et al: Aminergic and peptidergic pathways in the nervous system with special reference to the hypothalamus. In Reichlin S, Baldessarini RJ, Martin JB (eds): The Hypothalamus. New York, Raven Press, 1978, pp 69–76.

141. Fukuda H, Greer MA: The effect of basal hypothalamic deafferentiation in the nictohemeral rhythm of plasma TSH. Endocrinology 97:749–754, 1975.

142. Krulich L, Giachetti A, Marchlewska KOJ, et al: On the role of the central noradrenergic and dopaminergic systems in the regulation of TSH secretion in the rat. Endocrinology 100:496–502, 1977.

143. Annunziato L, Direnzo G, Lombardi G, et al: The role of central noradrenergic neurons in the control of thyrotropin secretion in the rat. Endocrinology 100:738–743, 1977.

144. Krulich L, Mayfield MA, Steele MK, et al: Differential effects of pharmacological manipulations of central α_1- and α_2-adrenergic receptors on the secretion of thyrotropin and growth hormone in male rats. Endocrinology 110:796–801, 1982.

145. Morley JE, Brammer GL, Sharp B, et al: Neurotransmitter control of hypothalamic-pituitary-thyroid function in rats. Eur J Pharmacol 70:263–268, 1981.

146. Krulich L: Neurotransmitter control of thyrotropin secretion. Neuroendocrinology 35:139–144, 1982.

147. Mannisto PT, Ranta T: Neurotransmitter control of thyrotrophin secretion in hypothyroid rats. Acta Endocrinol 89:100–104, 1978.

148. Maeda K, Frohman LA: Release of somatostatin and thyrotropin-releasing hormone from rat hypothalamic fragments in vitro. Endocrinology 106:1837–1841, 1980.

149. Richardson SB, Nguyen T, Hollander CS: Dopamine stimulates somatostatin release from perfused hypothalamic cells. Am J Physiol 244:E560–E566, 1983.

150. Lewis BM, Dieguez C, Lewis MD, Scanlon MF: Dopamine stimulates release of thyrotrophin-releasing hormone from perfused intact rat hypothalamus via hypothalamic D_2 receptors. J Endocrinol 115:419–424, 1987.

151. Lewis BM, Dieguez C, Ham J, et al: Effects of glucose on TRH, GHRH, somatostatin and LHRH release from rat hypothalamus in vitro. J Neuroendocrinol 1:437–441, 1989.

152. Brabant G, Ranft U, Ocran K, et al: Thyrotropin—an episodically secreted hormone. Acta Endocrinol 112:315–318, 1986.

153. Brabant G, Brabant A, Ranft U, et al: Circadian and pulsatile thyrotropin secretion in euthyroid man under the influence of thyroid hormone and glucocorticoid administration. J Clin Endocrinol Metab 65:83–88, 1987.

154. Brabant G, Prank K, Ranft U, et al: Physiological regulation of circadian and pulsatile thyrotropin secretion in normal man and woman. J Clin Endocrinol Metab 70:403–409, 1990.

155. Greenspan SL, Klibanski A, Schoenfeld D, Ridgway EC: Pulsatile secretion of thyrotropin in man. J Clin Endocrinol Metab 63:661–668, 1986.

156. Rossmanith WG, Mortola JF, Laughlin GA, Yen SS: Dopaminergic control of circadian and pulsatile pituitary thyrotropin release in women. J Clin Endocrinol Metab 67:560–564, 1988.

157. Samuels MH, Veldhuis JD, Henry P, Ridgway EC: Pathophysiology of pulsatile and copulsatile release of thyroid-stimulating hormone, luteinizing hormone, follicle-stimulating hormone and α-subunit. J Clin Endocrinol Metab 71:425–432, 1990.

158. Weeke J, Laurberg P: Diurnal TSH variations in hypothyroidism. J Clin Endocrinol Metab 43:32–37, 1976.

159. Moore RY: Organization and function of a nervous system circadian oscillator. Fed Proc 42:2783–2789, 1983.

160. Sharp T, Brazell MP, Bennett GW, Marsden CA: The TRH analogue CG3509 increases in vivo catechol/ascorbate oxidation in the N. accumbens but not in the striatum of the rat. Neuropharmacology 23:617–624, 1984.

161. Lighton C, Marsden CA, Bennett GW: The effects of 5,7 dihydroxytryptamine on thyrotrophin releasing hormone in regions of the brain and spinal cord of the rat. Neuropharmacology 23:55–60, 1984.

162. Winters AJ, Eskay RL, Porter JC: Concentration and distribution of TRH and LRH in the human fetal brain. J Clin Endocrinol Metab 39:960–963, 1974.

163. Koch Y, Okon E: Localization of releasing hormones in the human brain. Int Rev Exp Pathol 19:45–62, 1979.

164. Spindel ER, Wurtman RJ, Bird ED: Increased TRH content of the basal ganglia in Huntington's disease. N Engl J Med 303:1235–1236, 1980.

165. Hokfelt T, Lundberg JM, Schultzberg M, et al: Coexistence of peptides and putative transmitters in neurons. In Costa E, Trabucchi M (eds): Neural Peptides and Neuronal Communication. New York, Raven Press, 1980, pp 1–23.

166. Johansson O, Hokfelt T, Jeffcoate SL, et al: Light and electron microscopic immunohistochemical studies on TRH in the central nervous system of the rat. In Griffiths EC, Bennett, GW (eds): Thyrotropin Releasing Hormone. New York, Raven Press, 1983, pp 19–32.

167. Emson PC, Gilbert RFT, Bennett GW, et al. The coexistence of thyrotropin releasing hormone and substance P in bulbospinal serotonergic neurones. In Griffiths EC, Bennett GW (eds): Thyrotropin Releasing Hormone. New York, Raven Press, 1983, pp 33–43.

168. Gilbert RFT, Emson PC, Hunt SP, et al: The effects of monoamine neurotoxins on peptides in the rat spinal cord. Neuroscience 7:69–87, 1982.

169. Ogawa N, Kabuto H, Hirose Y, et al: Upregulation of thyrotropin-releasing hormone receptors in rat spinal cord after co-depletion of serotonin and TRH. Regulatory Peptides 10:85–90, 1985.

170. Mori M, Prasad C, Wilber JF: Regional dissociation of histidyl-proline-diketopiperazine [cyclo-(His-Pro)] and thyrotropin-releasing hormone (TRH) in the rat brain. Brain Res 231:451–453, 1982.

171. Prasad C, Mori M, Wilber JF, et al: Distribution and metabolism of cyclo-His-Pro: A new member of the neuropeptide family. Peptides 3:393–398, 1982.

172. Prasad C, Mori M, Pierson W, et al: Development changes in the distribution of rat brain pyroglutamate aminopeptidase, a possible determinant of endogenous cyclo-His-Pro concentration. Neurochem Res 3:389–399, 1983.

173. Ogawa N, Yamawaki Y, Kuroda H, et al: Discrete regional distributions of thyrotropin-releasing hormone (TRH) receptor binding in monkey central nervous system. Brain Res 205:169–174, 1981.

174. Burt DR, Taylor RL: TRH receptor binding in CNS and pituitary. In Griffiths EC, Bennett GW (eds): Thyrotropin-Releasing Hormone. New York, Raven Press, 1983, pp 71–83.

175. Bennett GW, Edwardson JA, Holland D, et al: Release of immunoreactive luteinizing hormone-releasing hormone and thyrotropin-releasing hormone from hypothalamic synaptosomes. Nature 257:323–325, 1975.

176. Maeda K, Frohman LA: Release of somatostatin and thyrotropin releasing hormone from rat hypothalamic fragments in vitro. Endocrinology 106:1837–1842, 1980.

177. Bennett GW, Sharp T, Brazell M, Marsden CA: TRH and catecholamine neurotransmitter release in the central nervous system. In Griffiths EC, Bennett GW (eds): Thyrotropin Releasing Hormone. New York, Raven Press, 1983, pp 253–269.

178. Winokur A, Beckman AL: Effects of thyrotropin releasing hormone, norepinephrine and acetylcholine on the activity of neurons in the

hypothalamus, septum and cerebral cortex of the rat. Brain Res 150:205–209, 1978.

179. Malthe-Sorenssen D, Wood PL, Cheney DL, Costa E: Modulation of the turnover rate of acetylcholine in rat brain by intraventricular injections of thyrotropin-releasing hormone, somatostatin, neurotensin and angiotensin II. J Neurochem 31:685–691, 1978.

180. Kerwin RW, Pycock CJ: Thyrotrophin-releasing hormone stimulates release of [3H]-dopamine from slices of rat nucleus accumbens in vitro. Br J Pharmacol 67:323–325, 1979.

181. Miyamoto M, Nagawa Y: Mesolimbic involvement in the locomotor stimulant action of thyrotropin-releasing hormone (TRH) in rats. Eur J Pharmacol 44:143–152, 1977.

182. Heal DJ, Green AR: Administration of thyrotropin releasing hormone (TRH) to rat releases dopamine in n-accumbens but not n-caudatus. Neuropharmacology 18:23–31, 1979.

183. Heal DJ, Pycock CJ, Youdin MBH, Green AR: Actions of TRH and its analogues on the mesolimbic dopamine system. *In* Griffiths EC, Bennett GW (eds): Thyrotropin-Releasing Hormone. New York, Raven Press, 1983, pp 271–282.

184. Sharp T, Bennett GW, Marsden CA, Tulloch IF: A comparison of the locomotor effects induced by centrally injected TRH and TRH analogues. Regul 9:305–315, 1984.

185. Brown M, Rivier J, Vale W: Actions of bombesin, thyrotropin releasing factor, prostaglandin E$_2$ and naloxone on the thermoregulation in the rat. Life Sci 20:1681–1687, 1977.

186. Breese GR, Cott JM, Cooper BR, et al: Effects of thyrotrophin-releasing hormone (TRH) on the actions of pentobarbital and other centrally acting drugs. J Pharmacol Exp Ther 193:11–22, 1975.

187. Yarbrough GG, McGuffin-Clineschmidt JC: MK-771-induced electromyographic (EMG) activity in the rat: Comparison with thyrotropin releasing hormone (TRH) and antagonism by neurotensin. Eur J Pharmacol 60:41–46, 1979.

188. Bhargava HN: Antagonism of ketamine-induced anaesthesia and hypothermia by thyrotrophin releasing hormone and cyclo(His-Pro). Neuropharmacology 20:699–702, 1981.

189. Kalivas PW, Horita A: Involvement of the septohippocampal system in TRH antagonism of pentobarbital narcosis. *In* Griffiths EC, Bennett GW (eds): Thyrotrophin Releasing Hormone. New York, Raven Press, 1983, pp 283–290.

190. Sharp T, Tulloch IF, Bennett GW, et al: Analeptic effects of centrally injected TRH and analogues of TRH in the pentobarbitone-anaesthetized rat. Neuropharmacology 23:339–348, 1984.

191. Nemeroff CB, Bissette G, Manberg PJ, et al: Neurotensin-induced hypothermia: Evidence for an interaction with dopaminergic systems and the hypothalamic pituitary-thyroid axis. Brain Res 195:69–84, 1980.

192. Osbahr AJ, Nemeroff CB, Luttinger D, et al: Neurotensin-induced antinociception in mice: antagonism by thyrotropin-releasing hormone. J Pharmacol Exp Ther 217:645–651, 1981.

193. Hernandez DE, Nemeroff CB, Valderrama MH, Prange AJ: Neurotensin-induced antinociception and hypothermia in mice: Antagonism by TRH and structural analogs of TRH. Regul Pept 8:41–49, 1984.

194. Holaday JW, Tseng L-F, Loh HH, Li CH: Thyrotropin releasing hormone antagonizes β-endorphin hypothermia and catalepsy. Life Sci 22:1537–1543, 1978.

195. Vijayan E, McCann SM: Suppression of feeding and drinking activity in rats following intraventricular injection of thyrotropin releasing hormone (TRH). Endocrinology 100:1727–1730, 1977.

196. Morley JE, Levine AS: Thyrotropin releasing hormone (TRH) suppresses stress-induced eating. Life Sci 27:269–274, 1980.

197. Dekin MS, Richerson GB, Getting PA: Thyrotropin-releasing hormone induces rhythmic bursting in neurons of the nucleus tractus solitarius. Science 229:67–69, 1985.

198. Holaday JW, Faden AI: Thyrotropin releasing hormone: Autonomic effects upon cardiorespiratory function in endotoxic shock. Regul Pept 7:111–125, 1983.

199. Myers RD, Metcalf G, Rice JC: Identification by microinjection of TRH-sensitive sites in the cat's brain stem that mediate respiratory, temperature and other autonomic changes. Brain Res 126:105–115, 1977.

200. Hawkins EF, Beydoun SR, Haun CK, Engel WK: Analogs of thyrotrophin-releasing hormone: Hypothesis relating receptor binding to net excitation of spinal lower motor neurons. Biochem Biophys Res Commun 138:1184–1190, 1986.

201. Schmidt-Achert KM, Askansas V, Engel WK: Thyrotropin-releasing hormone enhances choline acetyltransferase and creatine kinase in cultured spinal ventral horn neurons. J Neurochem 43:586–589, 1984.

202. Lewis MD, McQueen INF, Scanlon MF: Motor neurone disease serum and β-N-methylamino-L-alanine stimulate thyrotrophin-releasing hormone production by cultured brain cells. Brain Res 537:251–255, 1990.

203. Tache Y, Vale W, Brown M: Thyrotropin-releasing hormone: Central nervous system action to stimulate gastric acid secretion. Nature 287:149–151, 1980.

204. Tache Y, Goto Y, Hamel D, Pekary A, Novin D: Mechanism underlying intracisternal TRH-induced stimulation of gastric acid secretion in rats. Regul Pept 13:21–30, 1985.

205. Kato Y, Kanno T: Thyrotropin-releasing hormone injected intracerebroventricularly in the rat stimulates exocrine pancreatic secretion via the vagus nerve. Regul Pept 7:347–356, 1983.

206. La Hann TR, Horita A: Thyrotropin-releasing hormone centrally mediated effects on gastrointestinal motor activity. J Pharmacol Exp Ther 222:66–70, 1982.

207. Prasad C, Matsui T, Williams J, Peterkofsky A: Thermoregulation in rats: opposing effects of thyrotropin-releasing hormone and its metabolite histidyl-proline-diketopiperazine. Biochem Biophys Res Comm 85:1582–1587, 1978.

208. Prasad C, Matsui T, Peterkofsky A: Antagonism of ethanol narcosis by histidyl-proline-diketopiperazine. Nature 268:142–144, 1977.

209. Yanagisawa T, Prasad C, Williams J, Peterkofsky A: Antagonism of ethanol-induced decrease in rat brain cGMP concentrations by histidyl-proline-diketopiperazine, a thyrotropin-releasing hormone metabolite. Biochem Biophys Res Comm 86:1146–1153, 1979.

210. Battaini F, Peterkofsky A: Inhibition of dopamine (DA) uptake and (Na$^+$, K$^+$)-ATPase in rat brain synaptosomes by histidyl-proline-diketopiperazine [cyclo(His-Pro)], a metabolite of thyrotropin releasing hormone (TRH). Fed Proc 39:594, 1980.

211. Leppaluoto J, Koivusalo F, Kraama R: Thyrotropin-releasing hormone factor: Distribution in neural and gastrointestinal tissues. Acta Physiol Scand 104:175–179, 1978.

212. Martino E, Lernmark A, Seo H, et al: High concentration of thyrotropin-releasing hormone in pancreatic islets. Proc Natl Acad Sci USA 75:4265–4267, 1978.

213. Morley JE, Garvin TJ, Pekary AE, Hershman JM: Thyrotropin-releasing hormone in the gastrointestinal tract. Biochem Biophys Res Commun 79:314–318, 1977.

214. Leduque P, Wolf B, Aratan-Spire S, et al: Immunocytochemical location of thyrotropin-releasing hormone (TRH) in the β-cells of adult hypothyroid rat pancreas. Regul Pept 10:281–292, 1985.

215. Engler D, Scanlon MF, Jackson IMD: Thyrotropin-releasing hormone in the systemic circulation of the neonatal rat is derived from the pancreas and other extraneural tissues. J Clin Invest 67:800–807, 1981.

216. Grasso S, Buffa R, Martino E, et al: Gastrin (G) cells are the cellular site of the gastric thyrotropin-releasing hormone in human fetuses and newborns. A chromatographic, radioimmunological and immunocytochemical study. J Clin Endocrinol Metab 74(6):1421–1426, 1992.

217. Koivusalo F, Leppaluoto J: High TRH immunoreactivity in the pancreas of fetal and neonatal rats. Life Sci 24:1655–1658, 1979.

218. Kawano H, Daikoku S, Saito S: Location of thyrotropin-releasing hormone-like immunoreactivity in rat pancreas. Endocrinology 112:951–955, 1983.

219. Wolf B, Aratan-Spire S, Czernichow P: Hypothyroidism increases pancreatic thyrotropin-releasing hormone concentrations in adult rats. Endocrinology 114:1334–1337, 1984.

220. Morley JE, Levin SR, Pehlevanian M, et al: The effects of thyrotropin-releasing hormone on the endocrine pancreas. Endocrinology 104:137–139, 1979.

221. Dolva LO, Hanssen KF, Bestad A, Frey HMM: Thyrotropin-releasing hormone inhibits the pentagastrin stimulated gastrin secretion in man: A dose response study. Clin Endocrinol 10:281–286, 1979.

222. Dolva LO, Hanssen KF, Frey HMM: Action of thyrotropin-releasing hormone on gastrointestinal function in man: Inhibition of glucose and xylose absorption from the gut. Scand J Gastroenterol 13:599–604, 1978.

223. Tonoue T, Furukawa K, Nomoto T: Transition from neurogenic to myogenic receptivity for thyrotropin-releasing hormone (TRH) in the duodenum of the neonatal rat. Endocrinology 108:723–725, 1981.

224. Vuolteenaho O, Lepp AJ, Ying SY, Samaan NA: Isolation and characterization of human thyrotropin-releasing hormone (TRH) from an endocrine pancreatic tumor. Regul Pept 31(1):33–40, 1990.

225. Pekary AE, Meyer NV, Vaillant C, Hershman JM: Thyrotropin-releasing hormone and a homologous peptide in the male rat reproductive system. Biochem Biophys Res Commun 95:993–1000, 1980.

226. Pekary AE, Sharp B, Briggs J, et al: High concentrations of p-Glu-His-Pro-NH₂ (thyrotropin-releasing hormone) occur in rat prostate. Peptides 4:915–919, 1983.
227. Pekary AE, Hershman JM, Friedman S: Human semen contains thyrotropin-releasing hormone (TRH), a TRH-homologus peptide, and TRH-binding substances. J Androl 4:399–407, 1983.
228. Rui H, Welinder BS, Purvis K, Dolva O: Thyrotrophin-releasing hormone in human ejaculate. J Endocrinol 114:329–334, 1987.
229. Thetford CR, Morrell JM, Cockle SM: TRH-related peptides in the rabbit prostate complex during development. Biochem Biophys Acta 1115:252–258, 1992.
230. Bilek R, Gkonos PJ, Tavianini MA, et al: The thyrotrophin-releasing hormone (TRH)-like peptides in rat prostate are not formed by expression of the TRH gene but are suppressed by thyroid hormone. J Endocrinol 132:177–184, 1992.
231. Pekary AE, Bhasin S, Smith V, et al: Thyroid hormone modulation of thyrotropin-releasing hormone (TRH) and TRH-Gly levels in the male rat reproductive system. J Endocrinol 114:271–277, 1987.
232. Cockle SM, Morrell JM, Smyth DG: Thyrotrophin-releasing hormone-related polypeptides in rabbit prostate and semen are different from those in the rabbit hypothalamus. J Endocrinol 120:31–36, 1989.
233. Cockle SM, Aitken A, Beg F, Smyth DG: A novel peptide, pyroglutamylglutamylproline amide, in the rabbit prostate complex, structurally related to the thyrotrophin-releasing hormone. J Biol Chem 264:7788–7791, 1989.
234. Cockle SM, Aitken A, Beg F, et al: The TRH-related peptide pyroglutamylglutamylproline amide is present in human semen. FEBS Lett 252:113–117, 1989.
235. Pekary AE, Reeve JR Jr, Smith VP, Friedman S: In-vitro production of precursor peptides for thyrotropin-releasing hormone by human semen. Int J Androl 13(3):169–179, 1990.
236. Martino E, Seo H, Lernmark A, Refetoff S: Ontogenetic patterns of thyrotropin-releasing hormone-like material in rat hypothalamus, pancreas and retina: Selective effect of light deprivation. Proc Natl Acad Sci USA 77:4345–4348, 1980.
237. Martino E, Nardi M, Vaudagna G: Thyrotropin-releasing hormone–like material in human retina. J Endocrinol Invest 3:267–271, 1980.
238. Shambaugh G III, Kubek M, Wilber JF: Thyrotropin-releasing hormone activity in the human placenta. J Clin Endocrinol Metab 48:483–486, 1979.
239. Gkonos PJ, Tavianini MA, Liu CC, Roos BA: Thyrotropin-releasing hormone gene expression in normal thyroid parafollicular cells. Mol Endocrinol 3:2101–2109, 1989.
240. Wilber JF, Spinella P: Identification of immunoreactive thyrotrophin-releasing hormone in human neoplasia. J Clin Endocrinol Metab 59:432–435, 1984.
241. Burrow GN, May PB, Spaulding SW, Donabedian RK: TRH and dopamine interactions affecting pituitary hormone secretion. J Clin Endocrinol Metab 45:65–72, 1977.
242. Yat PL, Davidson NMcD, Lidgard GP, Fyffe JA: Bromocriptine suppression of the thyrotrophin response to thyrotrophin releasing hormone. Clin Endocrinol 9:179–183, 1978.
243. Scanlon MF, Weightman DR, Shale DJ, et al: Dopamine is a physiological regulator of thyrotrophin (TSH) secretion in man. Clin Endocrinol 10:7–15, 1979.
244. Kobberling J, Darragh A, Del Pozo E: Chronic dopamine receptor stimulation using bromocriptine: Failure to modify thyroid function. Clin Endocrinol 11:367–370, 1979.
245. Sarne DH, Sobieszczyk S, Ain KB, Refetoff S: Serum thyrotropin and prolactin in the syndrome of generalized resistance to thyroid hormone: Responses to thyrotropin-releasing hormone stimulation and short term triiodothyronine suppression. J Clin Endocrin Metab 70(5):1305–1311, 1990.
246. Scanlon MF, Peters JR, Salvador J, et al: The preoperative and postoperative investigation of TSH and prolactin release in the management of patients with hyperprolactinaemia due to prolactinomas and nonfunctional pituitary tumors: Relationship to adenoma size at surgery. Clin Endocrinol 24:383–389, 1986.
247. Thorner MO: Prolactin: clinical physiology and the significance and management of hyperprolactinaemia. In Martini L, Besser GM (eds): Clinical Neuroendocrinology. London, Academic Press, 1977, pp 319–361.
248. Cobb WE, Reichlin S, Jackson IMD: Growth hormone secretory status is a determinant of the thyrotropin response to thyrotropin-releasing hormone in euthyroid patients with hypothalamic-pituitary disease. J Clin Endocrinol Metab 52:324–329, 1981.
249. Arafah BM, Brodkey JS, Kaufman B, et al: Transsphenoidal microsurgery in the treatment of acromegaly and gigantism. J Clin Endocrinol Metab 50:578–585, 1980.
250. O'Connell JE, Dominiczak AF, Isles CG, et al: A comparison of calcium pentagastrin and TRH tests in screening for medullary carcinoma of the thyroid in MEN IIA. Clin Endocrinol 32(4):417–421, 1990.
251. Ahuja S: Is thyrotropin-releasing hormone as reliable a calcitonin stimulant as pentagastrin in medullary thyroid carcinoma? Acta Endocrinol 122(5):640–642, 1990.
252. Thyrotropin and prolactin response to thyrotropin-releasing hormone in depressed and nondepressed alcoholic men. Biol Psychiatry 27(1):31–38, 1990.
253. Vanelle JM, Poirier MF, Benkelfat C, et al: Diagnostic and therapeutic value of testing stimulation of thyrotropin-stimulating hormone by thyrotropin-releasing hormone in 100 depressed patients. Acta Psych Scand 81(2):156–161, 1990.
254. Barry S, Dinan TG: Neuroendocrine challenge tests in depression: A study of growth hormone, TRH and cortisol release. J Affect Disord 18(4):229–234, 1990.
255. Prange AJ, Wilson IC, Lara OO, et al: Effects of thyrotropin-releasing hormone in depression. Lancet 2:999–1002, 1972.
256. Bartalena L, Placidi GF, Martino E, et al: Nocturnal serum thyrotropin (TSH) surge and the TSH response to TSH-releasing hormone: Dissociated behaviour in untreated depressives. J Clin Endocrinol Metab 71(3):650–655, 1990.
257. Arana GW, Zarzar MN, Baker E: The effect of diagnostic methodology on the sensitivity of the TRH stimulation test for depression: A literature review. J Biol Psychiatry 28(8):733–737, 1990.
258. Gomez S, Aez JM, Aguilar Barber AM: GH response to GH-releasing factor in dementia and its relation with TSH response to TSH-releasing factor. Recenti Prog Med (Roma) 82(10):514–516, 1991.
259. Dysken MW, Falk A, Pew B, et al: Gender differences in TRH-stimulated TSH and prolactin in primary degenerative dementia and elderly controls. J Biol Psychiatry 28(2):144–150, 1990.
260. Gold MS, Pottash ALC, Ryan N, et al: TRH-induced TSH response in unipolar, bipolar and secondary depressions: Possible utility in clinical assessment and differential diagnosis. Psychoneuroendocrinology 5:147–155, 1980.
261. Molchan SE, Lawlor BA, Hill JL, et al: The TRH stimulation test in Alzheimer's disease and major depression: Relationship to clinical and CSF measures. Biol Psychiatry 30(6):567–576, 1991.
262. Metcalf G, Dettmar PW: Is thyrotropin-releasing hormone an endogenous ergotropic substance in the brain? Lancet 1:586–589, 1981.
263. Mountjoy CQ, Weller M, Mau R, et al: A double blind crossover sequential trial of oral thyrotrophin-releasing hormone in depression. Lancet 1:958–960, 1974.
264. Evans LEJ, Hunter P, Hall R, et al: A double blind trial of intravenous thyrotropin-releasing hormone in the treatment of reactive depression. Br J Psychiatry 127:227–230, 1975.
265. Kastin AJ, Schalch DS, Ehrensing RH, Anderson MS: Improvement in mental depression with decreased thyrotropin response after administration of thyrotropin-releasing hormone. Lancet 2:740–742, 1972.
266. Engel WK, Siddique T, Nicoloff JT: Effect on weakness and spasticity in amyotrophic lateral sclerosis of thyrotropin releasing hormone. Lancet 2:73–75, 1983.
267. Modarres-Sadeghi H, Guiloff RJ: Comparative efficacy and safety of intravenous and oral administration of a TRH analogue (RX77368) in motor neuron disease. J Neurol Neurosurg Psychiatry 53(11):944–947, 1990.
268. Congia S, Tronci S, Ledda M, et al: Low doses of TRH in amyotrophic lateral sclerosis and in other neurological diseases. Italian J Neurol Sci 12(2):193–198, 1991.
269. Sobue I, Yamamoto H, Konagawa M, et al: Effect of thyrotropin-releasing hormone on ataxia of spinocerebellar degeneration. Lancet 1:418–419, 1980.
270. Wang HC, Chiu HC: Clinical manifestations and thyrotropin releasing hormone therapy in cerebellar degenerations. Chin Med J 47(3):161–168, 1991.
271. Holaday JW, D'Amato RJ, Faden AI: Thyrotrophin releasing hormone improves cardiovascular function in experimental endotoxic and hemorrhagic shock. Science 213:216–218, 1981.
272. Faden AI, Jacobs TP, Holaday JW: Thyrotropin releasing hormone improves haemorrhagic recovery after spinal trauma in cats. N Engl J Med 305:1063–1067, 1981.
273. Faden AI: Opiate antagonists and thyrotropin releasing hormone: potential role in the treatment of central nervous system injury. JAMA 252:1452–1453, 1984.

274. Holaday JW, Beraton FW: Protirelin (TRH) a potent neuromodulator with therapeutic potential. Arch Intern Med 144:1138–1140, 1984.
275. Zaloga GP, Chernow B, Zajtchuk R, et al: Diagnostic dosages of protirelin (TRH) elevate BP by noncatecholamine mechanisms. Arch Intern Med 144:1149–1152, 1984.
276. Feuerstein G, Hassen AH, Faden AI: TRH: cardiovascular and sympathetic modulation in brain nuclei of the rat. Peptides 4:617–620, 1983.
277. Nink M, Krause U, Lehnert H, et al: Thyrotropin-releasing hormone has stimulatory effects on ventilation in humans. Acta Physiol Scand 141(3):309–318, 1991.
278. Holaday JW, D'Amato RJ, Ruvio BA: Action of naloxone and TRH on the autonomic regulation of circulation. In Costa E, Trabucchi M (eds): Regulatory Peptides: Molecular Biology to Function. New York, Raven Press, 1982, pp 353–361.
279. Sergev O, Racz K, Varga I, et al: Thyrotropin-releasing hormone increases plasma atrial natriuretic peptide levels in humans. J Endocrinol Invest 13(8):649–652, 1990.
280. Possmayer F: Biochemistry of pulmonary surfactant during fetal development and in the perinatal period. In Robertson B, van Golde LMG, Batenburg JJ (eds): Pulmonary Surfactant. Amsterdam, Elsevier Science, 1984, pp 295–356.
281. Robertson B: Pathology and pathophysiology of neonatal surfactant deficiency ("respiratory distress syndrome, hyaline membrane disease"). In Robertson B, van Golde LMG, Batenburg JJ (eds): Pulmonary Surfactant. Amsterdam, Elsevier Science, 1984, pp 383–418.
282. Smith BT: Pulmonary surfactant during fetal development and neonatal adaptation: hormonal control. In Robertson B, van Golde LMG, Batenburg JJ (eds): Pulmonary Surfactant. Amsterdam, Elsevier Science, 1984, pp 383–418.
283. Roti E, Gnudi A, Braverman LE: The placental transport, synthesis and metabolism of hormones and drugs which affect thyroid function. Endocr Rev 4:131–149, 1981.
284. Thorpe-Beeston JG, Nicolaides KH, Snijders RJ, et al: Fetal thyroid-stimulating hormone response to maternal administration of thyrotropin-releasing hormone. Am J Obstet Gynecol 164:1244–1245, 1991.
285. Moya F, Mena P, Foradori A, et al: Effect of maternal administration of thyrotropin releasing hormone on the preterm fetal pituitary-thyroid axis. J Pediatr 119:966–971, 1991.
286. Morales WJ, O'Brien WF, Angel JL, et al: Fetal lung maturation: The combined use of corticosteroids and thyrotropin-releasing hormone. Obstet Gynecol 73:111–116, 1989.
287. Ballard RA, Ballard PL, Creasy RK, et al: Respiratory disease in very low birthweight infants after prenatal thyrotropin-releasing hormone and glucocorticoid. TRH Study Group. Lancet 339:510–515, 1992.

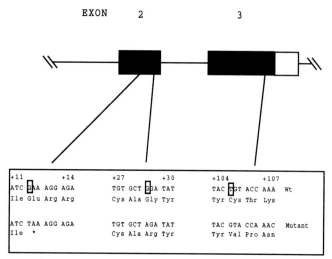

FIGURE 12–3. Point mutations of the human TSH β-subunit gene in patients with familial TSH deficiency. Three point mutations of the human TSH β-subunit gene have been described (see text). Mutations predict either a truncated TSH β-subunit or one with an amino acid change in the CAGY region.

alleles. A third kindred with a TSH-β point mutation was recently described by Rajan and co-workers.[30] This family had a frameshift deletion in codon 105 resulting in premature truncation of the TSH β-subunit. TSH was detectable at low levels in the serum, but radioactive iodine scans clearly demonstrated thyroid hypofunction in affected family members. Hypothyroidism in this family may be due either to impaired TSH secretion or secretion of TSH with reduced or absent biological activity.

Pit-1 Gene Mutations in Combined Pituitary Hormone Deficiency

In addition to its role in hormonal regulation of the prolactin and TSH β-subunit genes, Pit-1 was recently shown to be crucial for the development of certain anterior pituitary cell types in rodents: somatotrophs, lactotrophs, and thyrotrophs.[31] In humans with combined pituitary hormone deficiency (CPHD) of growth hormone, prolactin, and TSH, point mutations of the Pit-1 gene have also been identified (Fig. 12–4).[32–34] Pit-1 contains two protein domains, termed *POU-specific* and *POU-homeo*, which are both required for high-affinity Pit-1 DNA binding. In one United States patient with sporadic CPHD, a point mutation in the POU-homeo domain resulted in a Pit-1 molecule with defective transactivating function but preserved DNA binding (R271W).[33] This mutation was present on only one allele and resulted in a Pit-1 molecule that acted as a dominant inhibitor of Pit-1 action. In one Dutch and one Japanese family, DNA binding was reduced by Pit-1 gene mutations in the POU-specific domain (A158P and F172Stop).[32, 34] Since these mutations result in a Pit-1 molecule with reduced DNA-binding activity, CPHD in these families was noted only in patients with two defective alleles.

Translation of TSH Subunit Genes

TSH subunit genes are translated in the thyrotroph from separated mRNA's as precursor molecules with amino-ter-

minal extensions.[35–40] These amino-terminal extensions or leader peptides are necessary for transport of TSH subunit proteins across the membrane of the endoplasmic reticulum. During translation, the leader peptide is cleaved from precursor α- and β-subunit proteins, and high-mannose oligosaccharide chains are transferred from a dolichol phosphate carrier[41] to asparagine residues on the α- and β-subunits. The α-subunit has two glycosylation sites at amino acids 52 and 78, respectively, and the TSH β-subunit has one glycosylation site at amino acid 23. Excess α-subunit present in the rough endoplasmic reticulum (RER) begins to combine with TSH β-subunit when both subunits contain high mannose oligosaccharide chains. Subunit combination is complete in the RER, and oligosaccharide chains on TSH are processed further in the Golgi apparatus (see below).

Since α-subunit is synthesized in excess of TSH β-subunit, a small amount of free α-subunit is normally secreted from the thyrotroph. Free α-subunit, unlike α-subunit found in TSH, contains a third O-linked oligosaccharide chain at threonine 43.[42] Glycosylation at this site appears to prevent combination with the TSH β-subunit; however, the physiological significance of noncombined forms of the α-subunit is unknown.

Posttranslational Processing and Regulation

Each high-mannose oligosaccharide chain attached to TSH subunits in the RER contains 9 mannose, 3 glucose, and 2 N-acetylglucosamine residues.[43] These oligosaccharide chains are processed by glucosidases and mannosidases in the RER, yielding a "core" oligosaccharide chain of 3 mannose and 2 N-acetylglucosamine residues attached to asparagine.[44–48] In the proximal Golgi, specific glycosyltransferases attach galactose, N-acetylgalactosamine, or other residues to mannose residues of the "core" oligosaccharide chain.[49–53] Fucose residues are also added, in the RER and proximal Golgi, to the innermost N-acetylglucosamine residue attached in N-linkage to asparagine.[54–56]

In the distal Golgi, terminal sialic acid and sulfate residues are added by specific transferases to acceptor galactose or N-acetylgalactosamine sugars, respectively, on the oligosaccharide. The anterior pituitary, unlike the placenta, contains a glycosyltransferase for N-acetylgalactosamine and a sulfotransferase and thus is capable of synthesizing

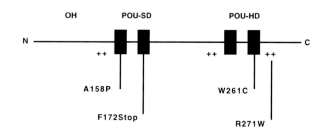

FIGURE 12–4. Mutations in the Pit-1 gene responsible for hypopituitarism. The three functional domains of Pit-1 are shown: OH, hydroxylation domain; POU-SD, POU-specific domain; and POU-HD, POU-homeo domain. Regions rich in basic amino acids are indicated by + +. Mutations of the Pit-1 molecule in mammals are shown below the functional domains. These mutations have been found in patients with CPHD, except W261C, which was found in the Snell dwarf mouse strain.

oligosaccharide chains capped by sulfate.[52] Glycoprotein hormones containing "sulfate-capped" oligosaccharide chains (FSH, LH, and TSH) have a shorter biological half-life than those capped by sialic acid residues only (CG). Differences in glycosylation structure are therefore crucial in determining the duration of action of pituitary versus placental glycoprotein hormones.

The structure of TSH oligosaccharide chains is also known to be regulated during development and by certain hormones. In a rodent model, Gyves and co-workers[57, 58] demonstrated that the complexity and number of terminal sialic acid residues on oligosaccharide chains is increased during development. Hypothyroidism has also been shown to increase the number of terminal sialic acid residues while decreasing terminal sulfate residues on both subunits of TSH.[59, 60] These changes have been shown to increase the biological half-life of TSH, prolong its duration of action, and possibly facilitate adaptation to hypothyroidism.[61] Finally, TRH can affect the glycosylation structure of TSH, but its in vitro effect appears to differ from its in vivo effects. Gesundheit and colleagues[62] demonstrated that in vitro TRH administration altered the branching of carbohydrate chains on TSH, increasing the number of biantennary forms. Taylor and co-workers[63–66] showed, however, that TRH deficiency in rodents caused by paraventricular nuclear lesions reduced the number of biantennary carbohydrate chains and that TRH administration increased the number of multiantennary carbohydrate chains to near-normal levels. The differences between these studies may relate to the in vitro (static) versus in vivo (dynamic) effects of TRH.

Regulation of TSH glycosylation produces a family of hormone isoforms with differences in in vitro and in vivo biological activities as well as in metabolic clearance rates. Some of these forms may account for decreased thyrotrophic activity in certain forms of central hypothyroidism or increased activity in certain thyrotrophic tumors (see below).

Recombinant TSH

The α and TSH-β genes have been co-transfected into Chinese hamster ovary cells resulting in the expression of heterodimeric recombinant TSH.[67] Since these cells, unlike the pituitary, have no capacity to add penultimate N-acetylgalactosamine or terminal sulfate, recombinant TSH is predominantly composed of oligosaccharide chains terminating in sialic acid. This is similar to the sialylated form of TSH that circulates in primary hypothyroidism (see above) and recombinant TSH also has a slower metabolic clearance rate compared with normal pituitary TSH. In several in vitro bioassays the activity of recombinant TSH is similar to that of pituitary TSH.[67] Currently, recombinant TSH is being employed in clinical trials to determine whether it can be used to stimulate radioiodide uptake in the diagnosis and treatment of patients with thyroid cancer (see Chapter 50).

DISORDERS OF TSH SECRETION IN HUMANS

Physiology

TSH is the major determinant of the production of iodothyronines by the thyroid gland.[68] Its daily production rate varies from 80 to 150 mIU and the plasma half-life in euthyroid subjects is 50 to 80 minutes.[69] In humans, the positive and negative modulation of TSH secretion by TRH and thyroid hormones, respectively, accounts for the principal regulatory effects on the thyrotrophic cells, whereas glucocorticoids, somatostatin, and dopamine are of pathophysiological and pharmacological importance. TSH secretion occurs in a circadian pattern characterized by a nocturnal surge that begins in the late afternoon and peaks before the onset of sleep.[70–73] Sleep withdrawal was reported to augment nightly TSH secretion, whereas sleep after a period of sleep withdrawal almost completely suppressed the circadian variation.[72] In addition, TSH appears to be secreted in a pulsatile manner with intervals of 2 to 6 hours between peaks and a nocturnal increase in the frequency and amplitude of the pulses.[74, 75] Within an individual subject the circadian TSH levels vary within 0.5 and 2 times the 24-hour mean value. The nocturnal surge in TSH is usually abolished in central hypothyroidism, thyrotoxicosis, L-T_4 suppressive therapy, and fasting.[76–79] Similarly, this nocturnal rise is diminished in states of hypercortisolism (such as Cushing's syndrome), severe nonthyroidal illness, and major depression.[79, 80] The development of the circadian rhythm begins after the first month of life[81] and persists throughout childhood and adult life.[82] However, morning TSH levels increase significantly at the age of 9 to 10 years, followed by the onset of puberty and a concomitant increase in T_3 and T_4 concentrations.[83] In healthy elderly men a decrease in pituitary responsiveness to TRH accompanied by a decrease in overall 24-hour TSH secretion has been described,[84] explaining in part the widespread prevalence of low TSH levels in older persons without hyperthyroidism.[85] In particular, the TSH response to decreased free thyroid hormone levels is inappropriately low in elderly people, indicative of an apparent resetting of the thyroid hormone feedback regulation threshold of TSH secretion.[86]

The strong negative correlation of TSH secretion with thyroid hormone serum levels was demonstrated in states of euthyroidism[87–89] and thyroid dysfunction.[87, 90–92] This feedback loop is extremely sensitive to changes in the thyroid hormone serum levels, since it has been estimated that a two-fold change in serum T_4 prompts a 100-fold change in serum TSH concentration.[93] Important interindividual differences in the slope and setpoint of the pituitary-thyroid axis are present, thereby introducing a bias if thyroid function tests are interpreted in the classical univariate manner.[94] It is important to recognize that the thyrotroph contains a high activity of type II 5'-monodeiodinase, thereby accounting for 50 to 60 per cent of the nuclear T_3 content.[95] Hence, the inhibitory effects of thyroid hormones on TSH secretion depend not only on T_3 serum levels but also on the serum T_4 concentrations and local deiodinase activity.[96] The negative feedback action of thyroid hormones on TSH synthesis and secretion occurs not only directly at the pituitary level but also by decreasing hypothalamic TRH release. The physiological importance of TRH in maintaining basal TSH secretion in humans is supported by the observation of decreased TSH concentrations and subsequent hypothyroidism in patients with hypothalamic lesions. Recent evidence suggests that the pulsatile nature of TSH secretion is regulated by TRH rather than dopamine or somatostatin.[75]

The acute administration of somatostatin or its long-acting analogue octreotide reduces basal TSH, its response to TRH, and the nocturnal peak of TSH secretion[97, 98] this effect has been exploited for the treatment of patients with TSH-producing pituitary adenomas.[99] In contrast, long-term therapy of acromegalic patients with octreotide did not alter any of the TSH pulse parameters, indicating that somatostatin is not likely to be primarily responsible for the nocturnal rise in TSH. It has been speculated that compensatory mechanisms are involved in restoring a normal TSH pulse generation during this treatment.[100, 101]

Infusion of dopamine into euthyroid subjects lowers the basal TSH and blunts the TSH response to TRH.[98] Studies with various dopamine receptor agonists suggest that the dopaminergic inhibition of basal TSH secretion and TSH pulsatility is predominantly regulated through dopamine D-2 receptors at the pituitary level, and through D-1 receptors at the hypothalamic level.[102, 103] Pharmacological amounts of glucocorticoids reduce basal TSH and blunt the response to TRH. Consequently, patients with Cushing's disease often have a suppressed TSH response to TRH, while subjects suffering from Addison's disease have elevated serum TSH levels.[71, 98, 104] Although the decrease in basal and stimulated TSH is inversely related to the serum cortisol levels under these conditions,[105] these effects occur only at supra- or infraphysiological doses and do not seem to be physiologically significant. It is nevertheless important to recognize the confounding effect of steroids or dopaminergic substances when interpreting thyroid function tests from subjects treated with one of these drugs.

Finally, the blunted TSH response to exogenous TRH in patients on chronic hemodialysis was recently shown to be restored to normal by a poorly understood mechanism after correction of the anemia by erythropoietin therapy.[106]

PATHOPHYSIOLOGY

Decreased TSH Secretion

Hyperthyroidism

In overt hyperthyroidism resulting from various etiologies (other than that resulting from inappropriate TSH secretion, described below), the serum TSH levels and the nocturnal TSH surge are invariably suppressed in the face of elevated thyroid hormone levels.[77, 87, 107] The term *subclinical hyperthyroidism* has been applied to patients with normal thyroid hormone concentrations who present with TSH levels below the reference range.[93, 108, 109] After treatment of a patient with hyperthyroidism or after discontinuing suppressive thyroid hormone therapy, the TSH levels may remain suppressed and unresponsive to TRH for several months while the thyroid hormone levels are low or normal.[110] This state of transient central hypothyroidism should be recognized and observed rather than treated prematurely with thyroid hormone replacement.

Central Hypothyroidism

While the causes of central hypothyroidism can be etiologically grouped into TRH deficiency of hypothalamic and TSH deficiency of pituitary origin, the exact site of the abnormality is often difficult to establish in a given patient.

Mass lesions (pituitary adenomas, craniopharyngiomas, meningiomas, dysgerminomas, metastases, cysts, abscesses), infiltrative lesions (tuberculosis, toxoplasmosis, syphilis, sarcoidosis, hemochromatosis, Langerhans cell histiocytosis), iatrogenic causes (surgery, radiation therapy), and idiopathic processes can cause hypothalamic and/or pituitary hypothyroidism.[111] Pituitary-specific diseases are lymphocytic hypophysitis[112] and genetic abnormalities of the TSH β-subunit or Pit-1 gene (see above).

Clinically, patients with central hypothyroidism have the signs and symptoms described for primary hypothyroidism. However, the thyroid gland is usually not palpable, and neurological manifestations of bitemporal hemianopsia, diplopia, and extraocular muscle paralysis may be present. In addition, most patients have impaired growth hormone and gonadotropin axes, whereas the adrenal axis is less frequently affected. The laboratory evaluation of patients with suspected central hypothyroidism includes a pituitary MRI scan and testing of anterior and posterior pituitary function. Specifically, in central hypothyroidism, the free T_4 levels are low, whereas the T_3 concentrations may still be normal. The basal TSH levels are undetectable in one third, normal in three fifths, and slightly elevated up to 10 mIU/L in a quarter of these patients.[113] In the latter patients it has been shown that the TSH lacks its bioactivity owing to an altered glycosylation pattern. Such patients thought to suffer from hypothalamic TRH deficiency were shown to benefit from chronic TRH administration, which was able to increase the TSH bioactivity and subsequently the circulating thyroid hormone levels in some patients.[114, 115] However, the nocturnal TSH surge is abolished in patients with secondary hypothyroidism, whereas the diurnal TSH pulsatility and pulse amplitude remain unchanged.[76, 116] TRH stimulation testing was originally thought to distinguish between central hypothyroidism of hypothalamic and pituitary origin. However, several studies have shown that the response pattern is not correlated with the site of the lesion.[113, 117, 118]

The treatment of choice is the substitution of L-T_4 after adrenal insufficiency has been excluded. However, since TSH levels as the usual end-point for titrating thyroid hormone replacement is lacking, one must rely on the clinical follow-up and if necessary on serial measurements of the parameters of thyroid hormone action, such as ankle reflex time, systolic time interval, and levels of sex hormone–binding globulin and cholesterol.[119]

Other Disorders

NONTHYROIDAL ILLNESS. With the development of the second- and third-generation assays for TSH,[87] it became apparent that 10 per cent of patients admitted to a hospital had abnormally low, but rarely suppressed (<0.01 mU/L) TSH levels.[120, 121] These abnormalities were usually normalized spontaneously within 2 to 5 days.[122] The circadian rhythmicity of TSH secretion is altered in critically ill patients. The mean 24 hours TSH level was reduced to 50 per cent of controls, reflecting a decrease in pulse amplitude. Moreover, the nocturnal TSH surge was replaced by a peak TSH levels occurring in the late afternoon.[123] It has been hypothesized that the exogenous or endogenous increase in glucocorticoids or dopamine may contribute to these alterations in TSH secretion.[87, 124]

NEUROPSYCHIATRIC DISORDERS. TRH tests were shown to be blunted in one quarter of patients with primary depression and in one quarter to one half of chronic alcoholics, whereas this was true for only 3 per cent of a healthy control population. However, disease nonspecificity and low sensitivity render this test difficult to interpret in psychiatric patients.[125] Intriguingly, decreased TSH levels were recently found to be associated with disorientation in patients with acute stroke, indicating a possible direct or indirect link of TSH secretion and cognitive functions.[126]

DRUGS. In addition to glucocorticoids and dopamine discussed earlier, diphenylhydantoin and high doses of salicylates are both capable of blunting TSH secretion.[127, 128]

Increased TSH Secretion

Primary Hypothyroidism

The most frequent cause of increased TSH levels is subclinical or overt primary hypothyroidism due to autoimmune or iatrogenic destruction of the thyroid gland. The mean 24-hour TSH pulse amplitude is increased, whereas TSH pulse frequency remains unchanged. However, the nocturnal increase of TSH is absent owing to the loss of the nocturnal increase in TSH pulse amplitude and frequency.[129] In rare instances, the thyroid gland is resistant to the action of circulating TSH, as seen for example in pseudohypoparathyroidism type I.

In overt primary hypothyroidism TSH values are invariably greater than 20 μU/ml. They may occasionally reach levels of several hundred μU/ml, but there is not a good correlation between the severity of hypothyroidism and the height of the TSH at levels greater than 50 μU/ml. TSH values greater than 20 μU/ml are diagnostic of primary hypothyroidism and there is generally no need to perform TRH stimulation tests in such patients.[87]

In certain patients with mild or "subclinical" primary hypothyroidism, in whom total and free thyroid hormone concentrations are normal or slightly low, TSH values may range between 5 and 15 μU/ml.[119] Such patients must be differentiated from certain patients with central hypothyroidism who may also have slight or modest elevations of immunoreactive TSH in the same range. In such cases a TRH test may be helpful in this differentiation. In primary hypothyroidism the TRH test shows an increased TSH response that peaks at the normal time of 20 to 30 minutes. In central hypothyroidism the TRH test may be blunted or at least not elevated. Occasionally patients with central hypothyroidism may have an exaggerated response to TRH, but such patients usually show a delayed peak of 60 minutes or longer.[113, 114]

Patients with "subclinical" primary hypothyroidism by definition have increased levels of TSH with normal levels of total and free thyroid hormones.[119] It has been demonstrated that such patients whose TSH is in the range of 5 to 12 μU/ml have no detectable metabolic impact of thyroid hormone deficiency and do not require therapy. Those whose TSH is greater than 12 μU/ml do show clear metabolic impact and may benefit from T_4 therapy.[119] However, there is no clear consensus on which patients benefit from therapy, and this is usually determined on an individual basis, sometimes as a clinical trial. Patients with mildly elevated TSH and "subclinical" hypothyroidism must be

followed at least yearly for the development of overt hypothyroidism. Moreover, such patients may be sensitive to an iodide load (e.g., secondary to a radiographic contrast study), which can rapidly precipitate overt hypothyroidism with low levels of thyroid hormone and TSH values greater than 20 μU/ml.

Following institution of thyroxine therapy for overt primary hypothyroidism, TSH levels fall to the normal range within 4 to 6 weeks. Changes in doses of thyroxine should not be made at more frequent intervals than this, and it is important to determine that a given level reflects the true steady-state value. This is particularly true of noncompliant patients who do not take therapy at prescribed doses until a few days before hormone values are determined. In such patients TSH may be elevated despite high normal or slightly elevated levels of thyroid hormones at the time blood is drawn. Such patients should have repeat determinations of TSH to ensure steady-state before further changes in thyroxine therapy are made.

Inappropriate Secretion of TSH

Patients with nonsuppressed TSH levels (>0.1 mU/L) in the presence of elevated free thyroid hormone concentrations have a syndrome of inappropriate TSH secretion, which is diagnosed after exclusion of certain conditions mimicking this syndrome. It is crucial that disorders of the binding proteins are ruled out by valid two-step assays for the measurement of free thyroid hormone levels. Furthermore, it must be ensured that the pituitary-thyroid axis of a hypothyroid patient taking thyroid hormones is in steady state at the time of testing. In a second step, the differential diagnosis of neoplastic (TSH-secreting adenoma) and nonneoplastic (syndromes of thyroid hormone resistance) causes needs to be addressed. Measurement of the free levels of the common α-subunit of the glycoprotein hormones and pituitary imaging studies should be performed. In rare cases, it may be necessary to exclude a pituitary TSH-producing microadenoma by bilateral venous petrosal sinus sampling for hormone measurements during TRH administration. In addition, TSH secretion in patients with such tumors is usually not regulated, i.e., neither stimulated by TRH nor suppressed by T_3. If a non-neoplastic cause of the inappropriate TSH secretion has been established by exclusion, generalized resistance to thyroid hormones (GRTH) and pituitary resistance to thyroid hormone (PRTH) can be differentiated on the basis of the assessment of the metabolic status of the patient and the peripheral target organs. Patients with the former condition appear clinically euthyroid and those with the latter have symptoms and signs of hyperthyroidism (see below).

TSH-Secreting Pituitary Adenomas

TSH-secreting pituitary adenomas account for less than 1 per cent of all pituitary tumors and the underlying oncogenic processes are not well understood.[130–132] Patients usually have clinical hypothyroidism and a goiter. Depending on the tumor size, headache, visual disturbances, and partial hypopituitarism may be found.[130, 131, 133] Basal TSH levels are often within the normal range,[130, 131, 133] while the pulse frequency is normal and pulse amplitude is either increased or normal.[78] To explain the clinical manifestations of hypothyroidism in such patients with inappropriately normal TSH levels, it has been demonstrated that the secreted TSH exhibits an increased bioactivity.[130, 134–136] Co-secretion of GH or PRL occurs frequently,[130, 131] while the co-secretion of TSH α- or β-subunits was detected in nearly 50 per cent of patients with acromegaly.[137] The principal treatment for TSH-secreting pituitary adenomas is surgery.[138] At the time of surgery most tumors prove to be macroadenomas, reflecting the long delays and often inappropriate therapeutic trials (antithyroid drugs, radioiodine, thyroidectomy) before the correct diagnosis is made. A quarter to half of the patients cannot be cured by surgery.[130, 131, 138] While radiotherapy is of unproved benefit in patients with residual tumor, medical therapy with the long-acting somatostatin analogue octreotide acetate has been useful.[99, 130, 138–141] However, thyroid hormone–lowering treatments should be avoided to prevent conversion of the tumor to a more aggressive form that is resistant to cure.[130, 138] These tumors may be aggressive with extensive local invasion, and there has been one report of transformation of the tumor into a pituitary carcinoma with widespread metastasis outside the central nervous system.[142]

Syndromes of Thyroid Hormone Resistance

The syndromes of thyroid hormone resistance that may present as inappropriate TSH secretion are described elsewhere in this text. These syndromes are clinically and biochemically heterogeneous, reflecting differences in the tissue distribution of the refractoriness to thyroid hormones.[143, 144] Similarly, TSH values are quite variable and may be elevated or normal but still inappropriate for the elevated levels of thyroid hormone. However, after inappropriate lowering of thyroid hormone values in such patients, TSH correlations may rise to greater than 100 μU/ml, despite residual elevation of total and free T_4.

In generalized resistance to thyroid hormone (GRTH), most tissues are refractory to T_3 and T_4. Due to the pituitary and presumably hypothalamic resistance, the setpoint of the pituitary-thyroid negative feedback axis is increased, i.e., the pituitary TSH secretion is normalized only at high circulating thyroid hormone levels. This combined tissue resistance and the subsequent compensatory rise in thyroid hormone levels are responsible for the lack of severe symptoms of hypothyroidism in affected subjects.

In apparent selective pituitary resistance to thyroid hormone (PRTH), primarily the pituitary and possibly the paraventricular nucleus of the hypothalamus (which is the site of thyrotrophin-releasing hormone synthesis) are resistant to the action of thyroid hormone. As with GRTH, the setpoint of the feedback axis is shifted to higher thyroid hormone levels; however, since the responsiveness of various peripheral tissues is preserved, these patients experience symptoms of hyperthyroidism. It has recently been demonstrated that from a pathophysiological viewpoint GRTH and PRTH may not be distinct syndromes but part of the spectrum of thyroid hormone resistance.[145, 146] Nonetheless, from a therapeutic standpoint this distinction may still be clinically useful. The extremely rare patient with selective peripheral resistance is not relevant to the syndrome of inappropriate secretion of TSH, since the secretion of TSH is per definition unaltered.

REFERENCES

1. Dracopoli NC, Rettig WJ, Whitfield GK, et al: Assignment of the gene for the β subunit of thyroid-stimulating hormone to the short arm of human chromosome 1. Proc Natl Acad Sci USA 83:1822–1826, 1986.
2. Shupnik MA, Chin WW, Habener JF, et al: Transcriptional regulation of the thyrotropin subunit genes by thyroid hormone. J Biol Chem 260:2900–2903, 1985.
3. Gurr JA, Kourides IA: Thyroid hormone regulation of thyrotropin α- and β-subunit gene transcription. DNA 4:301–307, 1985.
4. Chatterjee VKK, Lee J-K, Rentoumis A, et al: Negative regulation of the thyroid-stimulating hormone α gene by thyroid hormone: Receptor interaction adjacent to the TATA box. Proc Natl Acad Sci USA 86:9114–9118, 1989.
5. Burnside J, Darling DS, Carr FE, et al: Thyroid hormone regulation of the rat glycoprotein hormone α subunit gene promoter activity. J Biol Chem 264:6886–6891, 1989.
6. Carr FE, Burnside J, Chin WW: Thyroid hormones regulate rat thyrotropin β gene promoter activity expressed in GH₃ cells. Mol Endocrinol 3:709–716, 1989.
7. Wondisford FE, Farr EA, Radovick S, et al: Thyroid hormone inhibition of human thyrotropin β-subunit gene expression is mediated by a cis-acting element located in the first exon. J Biol Chem 264:14601–14604, 1989.
8. Wood WM, Kao MY, Gordon DF, et al: Thyroid hormone regulates the mouse thyrotropin β-subunit gene promoter in transfected primary thyrotropes. J Biol Chem 264:14840–14847, 1989.
9. Bodenner DL, Mroczynski MA, Weintraub BD, et al: A detailed functional and structural analysis of a major thyroid hormone inhibitory element in the human thyrotropin β-subunit gene. J Biol Chem 266:21666–21673, 1991.
10. Brent GA, Harney JW, Chen Y, et al: Mutations of the rat growth hormone promoter which increase and decrease response to thyroid hormone define a consensus thyroid hormone response element. Mol Endocrinol 3:1996–2004, 1989.
11. Nelson C, Albert VR, Elsholtz HP, et al: Activation of cell-specific expression of rat growth hormone and prolactin genes by a common transcription factor. Science 239:1400–1405, 1988.
12. Day RN, Maurer RA: The distal enhancer region of the rat prolactin gene contains elements conferring response to multiple hormones. Mol Endocrinol 3:3–9, 1989.
13. Shupnik MA, Rosenzweig BA, Showers MO: Interactions of thyrotropin-releasing hormone, phorbol ester, and forskolin-sensitive regions of the rat thyrotropin-β gene. Mol Endocrinol 4:829–836, 1990.
14. Steinfelder HJ, Hauser P, Nakayama Y, et al: Thyrotropin-releasing hormone regulation of human TSHB expression: Role of a pituitary-specific transcription factor (Pit-1/GHF-1) and potential interaction with a thyroid hormone-inhibitory element. Proc Natl Acad Sci USA 88:3130–3134, 1991.
15. Kapiloff MS, Farkash Y, Wegner M, et al: Variable effects of phosphorylation of Pit-1 dictated by the DNA response elements. Science 253:786–789, 1991.
16. Steinfelder HJ, Radovick S, Wondisford FE. Hormonal regulation of the thyrotropin β subunit gene by phosphorylation of the pituitary-specific transcription factor Pit-1. Proc Natl Acad Sci USA 89:5942–5945, 1992.
17. Kim MK, McClaskey JH, Bodenner DL, et al: An AP-1-like factor and the pituitary-specific factor Pit-1 are both necessary to mediate hormonal induction of human thyrotropin beta gene expression. J Biol Chem, in press.
18. Bodenner DL, McClaskey JH, Kim MK, et al: The proto-oncogenes c-fos and c-jun modulate thyroid hormone inhibition of human thyrotropin β subunit gene expression in opposite directions. Biochem Biophys Res Commun 189:1050–1056, 1992.
19. Wondisford FE, Steinfelder HJ, Nations M, et al: AP-1 antagonizes thyroid hormone receptor action on the thyrotropin β-subunit gene. J Biol Chem 268:2749–2754, 1993.
20. Perrone MH, Hinkle PM: Regulation of pituitary receptors for thyrotropin-releasing hormone by thyroid hormones. J Biol Chem 253:5168–5173, 1978.
21. Lumpkin MD, Samson WK, McCann SM: Arginine vasopressin as a thyrotropin-releasing hormone. Science 235:1070–1073, 1987.
22. Cooper DS, Klibanski A, Ridgway EC: Dopaminergic modulation of TSH and its subunits: In vivo and in vitro studies. Clin Endocrinol (Oxf) 18:265–275, 1983.

23. Scanlon WF, Weightman DR, Shale DJ, et al: Dopamine is a physiological regulator of thyrotropin (TSH) secretion in normal man. Clin Endocrinol (Oxf) 10:7–15, 1979.
24. Silver BJ, Bokar JA, Virgin JB, et al: Cyclic AMP regulation of the human glycoprotein hormone α-subunit gene is mediated by an 18-base-pair element. Proc Natl Acad Sci USA 84:2198–2202, 1987.
25. Deutsch PJ, Jameson JL, Habener JF: Cyclic AMP responsiveness of human gonadotropin-α gene transcription is directed by a repeated 10-base pair enhancer. α-promoter receptivity to the exhancer confers cell-preferential expression. J Biol Chem 262:12169–12174, 1987.
26. Hoeffler JP, Meyer TE, Yun Y, et al: Cyclic AMP-responsive DNA binding protein: structure based on a cloned placental cDNA. Science 242:1430–1433, 1988.
27. Steinfelder HJ, Radovick S, Mroczynski MA, et al: Role of a pituitary-specific transcription factor (Pit-1/GHF-1) or a closely related protein in cAMP regulation of human thyrotropin-β subunit gene expression. J Clin Invest 89:409–419, 1992.
28. Dacou-Voutetakis C, Feltquate DM, Drakopoulou M, et al: Familial hypothyroidism caused by a nonsense mutation in the thyroid-stimulating hormone β-subunit gene. Am J Hum Genet 16:998–993, 1990.
29. Hayashizaki Y, Hiraoka Y, Tatsumi K, et al: Desoxyribonucleic acid analyses of five families with familial inherited thyroid stimulating hormone deficiency. J Clin Endocrinol Metab 71:792–796, 1990.
30. Rajan SG, Kommareddi S, Nations M, et al: Familial hypothyroidism caused by a frameshift mutation in the thyrotropin beta-subunit gene: evidence for a bioinactive molecule. 66th Meeting of the American Thyroid Association, Rochester, MN, 1992, abstract 109.
31. Li S, Crenshaw EB III, Rawson EJ, et al: Dwarf locus mutants lacking three pituitary cell types result from mutations in the POU-domain gene pit-1. Nature 347:528–533, 1990.
32. Tatsumi K, Miyai K, Notomi T, et al: Cretinism with combined hormone deficiency caused by a mutation in the PIT-1 gene. Nat Genet 1:56–58, 1992.
33. Radovick S, Nations M, Du Y, et al: A mutation in the POU-homeodomain of Pit-1 responsible for combined pituitary hormone deficiency. Science 257:1115–1118, 1992.
34. Pfäffle RW, DiMattia GE, Parks JS, et al: Mutation of the POU-specific domain of Pit-1 and hypopituitarism without pituitary hypoplasia. Science 257:1118–1121, 1992.
35. Chin WW, Habener JF, Kieffer JD, Maloof F: Cell-free translation of the messenger RNA coding for the α subunit of thyroid-stimulating hormone. J Biol Chem 253:7985–7988, 1978.
36. Giudice LC, Waxdal MJ, Weintraub BD: Comparison of bovine and mouse pituitary glycoprotein hormone pre-α subunits synthesized in vitro. Proc Natl Acad Sci USA 76:4798–4802, 1979.
37. Giudice LC, Weintraub BD: Evidence for conformational differences between precursor and processed forms of thyroid-stimulating hormone β subunit. J Biol Chem 254:12679–12683, 1979.
38. Kourides IA, Vamvakopoulos NC, Maniatis GM: mRNA-directed biosynthesis of α and β subunits of thyrotropin. Processing of presubunits to glycosylated forms. J Biol Chem 254:11106–11110, 1979.
39. Kourides IA, Weintraub BD: mRNA directed biosynthesis of α subunit of thyrotropin: Translation in cell-free and whole-cell systems. Proc Natl Acad Sci USA 76:298–302, 1979.
40. Vamvakopoulos NC, Kourides IA: Identification of separate mRNAs coding for the α and β subunits of thyrotropin. Proc Natl Acad Sci USA 76:3809–3813, 1979.
41. Behrens NH, Keloir LF: Dolichol monophosphate glucose: An intermediate in glucose transfer in liver. Proc Natl Acad Sci USA 66:153–159, 1970.
42. Parsons TF, Bloomfield GA, Pierce JG: Purification of an alternate form of the α subunit of the glycoprotein hormones from bovine pituitaries and identification of its O-linked oligosaccharide. J Biol Chem 258:240–244, 1983.
43. Miura Y, Perkel VS, Magner JA: Rates of processing of the high mannose oligosaccharide units at the three glycosylation sites of mouse thyrotropin and the two sites of free α-subunits. Endocrinology 123:1296–1302, 1988.
44. Magner JA, Weintraub BD: Thyroid-stimulating hormone subunit processing and combination in microsomal subfractions of mouse pituitary tumor. J Biol Chem 257:6709–6715, 1982.
45. Magner JA, Ronin C, Weintraub BD: Carbohydrate processing of thyrotropin differs from that of free α-subunit and total glycoproteins in microsomal subfractions of mouse pituitary tumor. Endocrinology 115:1019–1030, 1984.
46. Ronin C, Stannard BS, Rosenbloom IL, et al: Glycosylation and processing of high-mannose oligosaccharides of thyroid-stimulating hormone subunits: Comparison to nonsecretory cell glycoproteins. Biochemistry 23:4503–4510, 1984.
47. Ronin C, Stannard BS, Weintraub BD: Differential processing and regulation of thyroid-stimulating hormone subunit carbohydrate chains in thyrotropic tumors and in normal and hypothyroid pituitaries. Biochemistry 24:5626–5631, 1985.
48. Magner JA, Papagiannes E: Structures of high-mannose oligosaccharides of mouse thyrotropin: differential processing of α- versus β-subunits of the heterodimer. Endocrinology 120:10–17, 1987.
49. Baenziger JU, Green ED: Pituitary glycoprotein hormone oligosaccharides: Structure, synthesis and function of the asparagine-linked oligosaccharides on lutropin, follitropin and thyrotropin. Biochem Biophys Acta 947:287–306, 1988.
50. Green ED, Baenziger JU: Asparagine-linked oligosaccharides on lutropin, follitropin, and thyrotropin. I. Structural elucidation of the sulfated and sialylated oligosaccharides on bovine, ovine, and human pituitary glycoprotein hormones. J Biol Chem 263:25–35, 1988.
51. Green ED, Baenziger JU: Asparagine-linked oligosaccharides on lutropin, follitropin, and thyrotropin. II. Distributions of sulfated and sialylated oligosaccharides on bovine, ovine, and human pituitary glycoprotein hormones. J Biol Chem 263:36–44, 1988.
52. Smith PL, Baenziger JU: A pituitary N-acetylgalactosamine transferase that specifically recognizes glycoprotein hormones. Science 242:930–933, 1988.
53. Magner JA: Assay of sulfotransfrase in subcellular fractions of hypothyroid mouse pituitary and liver tissue. Biochem Med Metab Biol 41:81–83, 1989.
54. Gesundheit N, Magner JA, Chen T, Weintraub BD: Differential sulfation and sialylation of secreted mouse thyrotropin (TSH) subunits: Regulation by TSH-releasing hormone. Endocrinology 119:455–463, 1986.
55. Magner J, Papagiannes E: Studies of double-labeled mouse thyrotropin and free α-subunits to estimate relative fucose content. Proc Soc Exp Biol Med 183:237–240, 1986.
56. Magner JA, Novak W, Papagiannes E: Subcellular localization of fucose incorporation into mouse thyrotropin and free α-subunits: studies employing subcellular fractionation and inhibitors of the intracellular translocation of proteins. Endocrinology 119:1315–1328, 1986.
57. Gyves PW, Gesundheit N, Taylor T, et al: Changes in thyrotropin (TSH) carbohydrate structure and response to TSH-releasing hormone during postnatal ontogeny: Analysis by concanavalin-A chromatography. Endocrinology 121:133–140, 1987.
58. Gyves PW, Gesundheit N, Stannard BS, et al: Alterations in the glycosylation of secreted thyrotropin during ontogenesis. Analysis of sialylated and sulfated oligosaccharides. J Biol Chem 264:6104–6110, 1989.
59. DeCherney GS, Gesundheit N, Gyves PW, et al: Alterations in the sialylation and sulfation of secreted mouse thyrotropin in primary hypothyroidism. Biochem Biophys Res Commun 159:755–762, 1989.
60. Gyves PW, Gesundheit N, Thotakura NR, et al: Changes in the sialylation and sulfation of secreted thyrotropin in congenital hypothyroidism. Proc Natl Acad Sci USA 87:3792–3796, 1990.
61. Constant RB, Weintraub BD: Differences in the metabolic clearance of pituitary and serum thyrotropin derived from euthyroid and hypothyroid rats: Effects of chemical deglycosylation of pituitary TSH. Endocrinology 119:2720–2727, 1986.
62. Gesundheit N, Fink DL, Silverman LA, et al: Effect of thyrotropin-releasing hormone on the carbohydrate structure of secreted mouse thyrotropin. Analysis by lectin affinity chromatography. J Biol Chem 262:5197–5203, 1987.
63. Taylor T, Gesundheit N, Gyves PW, et al: Hypothalamic hypothyroidism caused by lesions in rat paraventricular nuclei alters the carbohydrate structure of secreted thyrotropin. Endocrinology 122:283–290, 1988.
64. Taylor T, Gesundheit N, Weintraub BD: Effects of in vivo bolus versus continuous TRH administration on TSH secretion, biosynthesis, and glycosylation in normal and hypothyroid rats. Mol Cell Endocrinol 46:253–261, 1986.
65. Taylor T, Weintraub BD: Altered thyrotropin (TSH) carbohydrate structures in hypothalamic hypothyroidism created by paraventricular nuclear lesions are corrected by in vivo TSH-releasing hormone administration. Endocrinology 125:2198–2203, 1989.
66. Taylor T, Wondisford FE, Blaine T, et al: The paraventricular nucleus of the hypothalamus has a major role in thyroid hormone feedback regulation of thyrotropin synthesis and secretion. Endocrinology 126:317–324, 1990.
67. Thotakura NR, Desai RK, Bates LG, et al: Biological activity and metabolic clearance of a recombinant human thyrotropin produced in Chinese hamster ovary cells. Endocrinology 128:341–348, 1991.

68. Nicoloff JT, Spencer CA: Non-thyrotropin-dependent thyroid secretion. J Clin Endocrinol Metab 75:343, 1992.

69. Ridgway EC, Weintraub BD, Maloof F: Metabolic clearance and production rates of human thyrotropin. J Clin Invest 53:895–903, 1974.

70. Brabant G, Ocran K, Ranft U, Vonzurmuhlen A, et al: Physiological regulation of thyrotropin. Biochimie 71:293–301, 1989.

71. Brabant G, Brabant A, Ranft U, et al: Circadian and pulsatile thyrotropin secretion in euthyroid man under the influence of thyroid hormone and glucocorticoid administration. J Clin Endocrinol Metab 65:83–88, 1987.

72. Brabant G, Prank K, Ranft U, et al: Physiological regulation of circadian and pulsatile thyrotropin secretion in normal man and woman. J Clin Endocrinol Metab 70:403–409, 1990.

73. Toft AD: Thyrotropin: Assay, secretory physiology and testing of regulation. In Braverman LE, Utiger RD (eds): Werner and Ingbar's The Thyroid (ed 6). Philadelphia, JB Lippincott, 1991, pp 287–305.

74. Greenspan SL, Klibanski A, Schoenfeld D, et al: Pulsatile secretion of thyrotropin in man. J Clin Endocrinol Metab 63:661–668, 1986.

75. Brabant G, Prank K, Hoang-Vu C, Hesch RD, et al: Hypothalamic regulation of pulsatile thyrotropin secretion. J Clin Endocrinol Metab 72:145–150, 1991.

76. Caron PJ, Nieman LK, Rose SR, et al: Deficient nocturnal surge of thyrotropin in central hypothyroidism. J Clin Endocrinol Metab 62:960–964, 1986.

77. Bartalena L, Martino E, Falcone M, et al: Evaluation of the nocturnal serum thyrotropin (TSH) surge, as assessed by TSH ultrasensitive assay, in patients receiving long term L-thyroxine suppression therapy and in patients with various thyroid disorders. J Clin Endocrinol Metab 65:1265–1271, 1987.

78. Samuels MH, Henry P, Kleinschmidt-Demasters BK, et al: Pulsatile glycoprotein hormone secretion in glycoprotein-producing pituitary tumors. J Clin Endocrinol Metab 73:1281–1288, 1991.

79. Bartalena L, Martino E, Velluzzi F, et al: The lack of nocturnal serum thyrotropin surge in patients with nontoxic nodular goiter may predict the subsequent occurrence of hyperthyroidism. J Clin Endocrinol Metab 73:604–608, 1991.

80. Bartalena L, Martino E, Petrini L, et al: The nocturnal serum thyrotropin surge is abolished in patients with adrenocorticotropin (ACTH)-dependent or ACTH-independent Cushing's syndrome. J Clin Endocrinol Metab 72:1195–1199, 1991.

81. Mantagos S, Koulouris A, Makri M, et al: Development of thyrotropin circadian rhythm in infancy. J Clin Endocrinol Metab 74:71–74, 1992.

82. Rose SR, Nisula BC: Circadian variation of thyrotropin in childhood. J Clin Endocrinol Metab 68:1086–1090, 1989.

83. Michaud P, Foradori A, Rodriguez-Portales JA, et al: A prepubertal surge of thyrotropin precedes an increase in thyroxine and 3,5,3'-triiodothyronine in normal children. J Clin Endocrinol Metab 72:976–981, 1991.

84. Vancoevorden A, Laurent E, Decoster C, et al: Decreased basal and stimulated thyrotropin secretion in healthy elderly men. J Clin Endocrinol Metab 69:177–185, 1989.

85. Sawin CT, Geller A, Kaplan MM, et al: Low serum thyrotropin (thyroid-stimulating hormone) in older persons without hyperthyroidism. Arch Intern Med. 151:165–168, 1991.

86. Lewis GF, Alessi CA, Imperial JG, et al: Low serum free thyroxine index in ambulating elderly is due to a resetting of the threshold of thyrotropin feedback suppression. J Clin Endocrinol Metab. 73:843–849, 1991.

87. Spencer CA, Lopresti JS, Patel A, et al: Applications of a new chemiluminometric thyrotropin assay to subnormal measurement. J Clin Endocrinol Metab 70:453–460, 1990.

88. Bregengard C, Kirkegaard C, Faber J, et al: Relationships between serum thyrotropin, serum free thyroxine (T_4), and 3,5,3'-triiodothyronine (T_3) and the daily T_4 and T_3 production rates in euthyroid patients with multinodular goiter. J Clin Endocrinol Metab 65:258–261, 1987.

89. Vice PA, Clark F, Schardt W, Evered D: Studies on the control of thyrotropin secretion in normal man. Clin Endocrinol (Oxf). 5:515–529, 1976.

90. Cotton GE, Gorman CA, Mayberry WE: Suppression of thyrotropin (h-TSH) in serum of patients with myxedema of varying etiology treated with thyroid hormones. N Engl J Med 285:529–533, 1971.

91. Reichlin S, Utiger RD: Regulation of the pituitary-thyroid axis in man: Relationship of TSH concentration to concentration of free and total thyroxine in plasma. J Clin Endocrinol Metab 27:251–255, 1967.

92. Ross DS, Ardisson LJ, Meskell MJ: Measurement of thyrotropin in

93. Wehmann RE, Nisula BC: Radioimmunoassay of human thyrotropin: Analytical and clinical developments. Crit Rev Clin Lab Sci. 20:243–283, 1984.

94. Meier CA, Maisey MN, Lowry A, et al: Interindividual differences in the pituitary-thyroid axis influence the interpretation of thyroid function tests. Clin Endocrinol (Oxf) in press.

95. Silva JE, Larsen PR: Pituitary nuclear 3,5,3'-triiodothyronine and thyrotropin secretion: an explanation for the effect of thyroxine. Science 198:617–620, 1977.

96. Fish LH, Schwartz HL, Cavanaugh J, et al: Replacement dose, metabolism, and bioavailability of levothyroxine in the treatment of hypothyroidism. N Engl J Med 316:764–770, 1987.

97. Morley JE: Neuroendocrine control of thyrotropin secretion. Endocr Rev 2:396–436, 1981.

98. Hershman JM, Pekary AE: Regulation of thyrotropin secretion. In Imura H (ed): The Pituitary Gland. New York, Raven Press, 1985, pp 149–188.

99. Comi RJ, Gesundheit N, Murray L, et al: Response of thyrotropin-secreting pituitary adenomas to a long-acting somatostatin analogue. N Engl J Med 317:12–17, 1987.

100. Roelfsema F, Deboer H, Frolich M: Circadian and pulsatile thyrotropin release in treated acromegalics. J Endocrinol Invest 12:685–692, 1989.

101. Roelfsema F, Frolich M: Pulsatile thyrotropin release and thyroid function in acromegalics before and during subcutaneous octreotide infusion. J Clin Endocrinol Metab 72:77–82, 1991.

102. Boesgaard S, Hagen C, Andersen AN, et al: Effect of fenoldopam, a dopamine D-1 receptor agonist, on pituitary, gonadal and thyroid hormone secretion. Clin Endocrinol (Oxf) 30:231–239, 1989.

103. Boesgaard S, Hagen C, Hangaard J, et al: Effect of dopamine and a dopamine D-1 receptor agonist on pulsatile thyrotrophin secretion in normal women. Clin Endocrinol 32:423–431, 1990.

104. Brabant A, Brabant G, Schuermeyer T, et al: The role of glucocorticoids in the regulation of thyrotropin. Acta Endocrinol (Copenh) 121:95–100, 1989.

105. Benker G, Raida M, Olbricht T, et al: TSH secretion in Cushing's syndrome: Relation to glucocorticoid excess, diabetes, goitre, and the "sick euthyroid syndrome." Clin Endocrinol (Oxf) 33:777–786, 1990.

106. Ramirez G, Bittle PA, Sanders H, et al: Hypothalamo-hypophyseal thyroid and gonadal function before and after erythropoietin therapy in dialysis patients. J Clin Endocrinol Metab 74:517–524, 1992.

107. Roden M, Nowotny P, Vierhapper H, et al: Diagnostic relevance of suppressed basal concentrations of TSH compared with the negative TRH test in detection and exclusion of hyperthyroidism. Acta Endocrinol (Copenh) 124:136–142, 1991.

108. Caldwell G, Gow SM, Sweeting VM, et al: A new strategy for thyroid function testing. Lancet 1:1117–1119, 1985.

109. Davies PH, Franklyn JA, Daykin J, et al: The significance of TSH values measured in a sensitive assay in the follow-up of hyperthyroid patients treated with radioiodine. J Clin Endocrinol Metab 74:1189–1194, 1992.

110. Davis JRE, Black EG, Sheppard MC: Evaluation of a sensitive chemiluminescent assay for TSH in the follow-up of treated thyrotoxicosis. Clin Endocrinol (Oxf) 27:563–570, 1987.

111. Samuels MH, Ridgway EC: Central hypothyroidism. Endocrinol Metab Clin North Am 21:903–919, 1992.

112. Feigenbaum SL, Martin MC, Wilson CB, et al: Lymphocytic adenohypophysitis: A pituitary mass lesion occurring in pregnancy—proposal for medical treatment. Am J Obstet Gynecol 164:1549–1555, 1991.

113. Faglia G, Bitensky L, Pinchera A, et al: Thyrotropin secretion in patients with central hypothyroidism: Evidence for reduced biological activity of immunoreactive thyrotropin. J Clin Endocrinol Metab 48:989–996, 1979.

114. Beck-Peccoz P, Amr S, Menezes-Ferreira MM, et al: Decreased receptor binding of biologically inactive thyrotropin in central hypothyroidism. N Engl J Med 312:1085–1090, 1985.

115. Magner JA, Kane J, Chou ET: Intravenous thyrotropin (TSH)-releasing hormone releases human TSH that is structurally different from basal TSH. J Clin Endocrinol Metab 74:1306–1311, 1992.

116. Samuels MH, Lillehei K, Kleinscmidt-Demasters BK, et al: Patterns of pulsatile pituitary glycoprotein secretion in central hypothyroidism and hypogonadism. J Clin Endocrinol Metab 70:391–397, 1990.

117. Hall R, Besser GM, Ormston BJ, et al: The thyrotropin-releasing hormone test in diseases of the pituitary and hypothalamus. Lancet 1:7754, 1972.

118. Snyder PJ, Jacobs LS, Rabello MM, et al: Diagnostic value of thyrotropin-releasing hormone in pituitary and hypothalamic diseases. Am J Med 81:751–756, 1974.

119. Staub JJ, Althaus BU, Engler H, et al: Spectrum of subclinical and overt hypothyroidism—effect on thyrotropin, prolactin, and thyroid reserve, and metabolic impact on peripheral target tissues. Am J Med 92:631–642, 1992.

120. Spencer CA: Clinical utility and cost-effectiveness of sensitive thyrotropin assays in ambulatory and hospitalized patients. Mayo Clin Proc 63:1214–1222, 1988.

121. Spencer CA, Eigen A, Shen D, et al: Sensitive TSH tests: specificity limitations for screening thyroid disease in hospitalized patients. Clin Chem 33:1391–1395, 1987.

122. Nicoloff JT, Lopresti JS: Nonthyroidal illness. In Braverman LE, Utiger RD (eds): Werner and Ingbar's The Thyroid (ed 6). Philadelphia, JB Lippincott, 1991, pp 357–368.

123. Custro N, Scafidi V, Notarbartolo A: Alterations in circadian rhythm of serum thyrotropin in critically ill patients. Acta Endocrinol 127:18–22, 1992.

124. Kaptein EM, Spencer CA, Kamiel MB, et al: Prolonged dopamine administration and thyroid hormone economy in normal and critically ill subjects. J Clin Endocrinol Metab 51:387–393, 1980.

125. Loosen PT: Thyroid function in affective disorders and alcoholism. Endocrinol Metab Clin North Am 17:55–82, 1988.

126. Olsson T, Asplund K, Hagg E: Pituitary-thyroid axis, prolactin and growth hormone in patients with acute stroke. J Intern Med 228:287–290, 1990.

127. Rootwelt K, Ganes T, Johannessen SI: Effect of carbamazepine, phenytoin and phenobarbitone on serum levels of thyroid hormones and thyrotropin in humans. Scand J Lab Invest 38:731–736, 1978.

128. Dussault JH, Turcotte R, Guyda H: The effect of acetylsalicylic acid on TSH and PRL secretion after TRH stimulation in the human. J Clin Endocrinol Metab 43:232–235, 1976.

129. Adriaanse R, Brabant G, Prank K, et al: Circadian changes in pulsatile TSH release in primary hypothyroidism. Clin Endocrinol (Oxf) 37:504–510, 1992.

130. Gesundheit N, Petrick PA, Nissim M, et al: Thyrotropin-secreting pituitary adenomas: Clinical and biochemical heterogeneity. Case report and follow-up of nine patients. Ann Intern Med 111:827–835, 1989.

131. Beckers A, Abs R, Mahler C, et al: Thyrotropin-secreting pituitary adenomas: Report of seven cases. J Clin Endocrinol Metab 72:477–483, 1991.

132. Karga HJ, Alexander JM, Hedleywhyte ET, et al: Ras mutations in human pituitary tumors. J Clin Endocrinol Metab 74:914–919, 1992.

133. Gesundheit N: Thyrotropin induced hyperthyroidism. In Braverman LE, Utiger RD, (eds): Werner and Ingbar's The Thyroid (ed 6). Philadelphia, JB Lippincott, 1991, pp 682–691.

134. Beck-Peccoz P, Piscitelli G, Amr S, et al: Endocrine, biochemical, and morphological studies of a pituitary adenoma secreting growth hormone, thyrotropin (TSH), and alpha-subunit: Evidence for secretion of TSH with increased bioactivity. J Clin Endocrinol Metab 62:704–711, 1986.

135. Nissim M, Lee KO, Petrick PA, et al: A sensitive TSH bioassay based on iodide uptake in rat FRTL-5 thyroid cells: Comparison with the cyclic AMP response to human serum TSH and enzymatically deglycosylated bovine and human TSH. Endocrinology 121:1278–1287, 1987.

136. Gesundheit N, Petrick PA, Taylor T, et al: Comparison of a Pituitary TSH-Secreting Micro- versus Macroadenoma. In Medeiros-Neto G, Gaitan E (eds): Frontiers in Thyroidology. New York, Plenum, 1986, pp 259–265.

137. Assadian H, Shimatsu A, Koshiyama H, et al: Secretion of alpha and TSH-beta subunits in patients with acromegaly: an in vivo study. Acta Endocrinol (Copenh) 122:729–734, 1990.

138. McCutcheon IE, Weintraub BD, Oldfield EH: Surgical treatment of thyrotropin-secreting pituitary adenomas. J Neurosurg 73:674–683, 1990.

139. Gorden P, Comi RJ, Maton PN, et al: Somatostatin and somatostatin analogue (SMS 201–995) in treatment of hormone-secreting tumors of the pituitary and gastrointestinal tract and non-neoplastic diseases of the gut. Ann Intern Med 110:35–50, 1989.

140. Sy RA, Bernstein R, Chynn KY, et al: Reduction in size of a thyrotropin- and gonadotropin-secreting pituitary adenoma treated with octreotide acetate (somatostatin analog). J Clin Endocrinol Metab 74:690–694, 1992.

141. Chanson P, Weintraub BD, Harris AG: Treatment of TSH-secreting pituitary adenomas with octreotide: short-term and long-term effects in 52 patients; results of the International Multicenter TSH-Secreting Adenomas Study Group. Ann Intern Med, in press.

142. Mixson AJ, Friedman TC, Katz DA, et al: Thyrotropin-secreting pituitary carcinoma. J Clin Endocrinol Metab 76:529–533, 1993.

143. Usala S, Weintraub BD: Thyroid hormone resistance syndrome. Trends Endocrinol Metab 2:140–144, 1991.

144. Jameson JL: Editorial: Thyroid hormone resistance: Pathophysiology at the molecular level. J Clin Endocrinol Metab 74:708–711, 1992.

145. Geffner ME, Su F, Ross NS, et al: An arginine to histidine mutation in codon 311 of c-erbAβ gene results in a mutant thyroid hormone receptor that does not mediate a dominant negative phenotype. J Clin Invest, in press.

146. Mixson AJ, Renault JC, Weintraub BD: Identification of a novel mutation in the gene encoding the β-triiodothyronine receptor in a patient with apparent selective pituitary resistance to thyroid hormone. Clin Endocrinol 38:227–234, 1993.

13

Gonadotropin-Releasing Hormone (GnRH): Basic Physiology

DENNIS W. LINCOLN

The establishment of the amino acid sequence of GnRH in 1971 stands as one of the great landmarks of reproductive endocrinology.[1–3] This discovery confirmed beyond further question the neuroendocrine doctrine advanced by Harris and Green[4] and opened a new era in the clinical management of reproductive disorders. Twenty-one years later, the final step in the pathway was added with the publication of the amino acid sequence of the GnRH receptor of the pituitary gland.[5]

GnRH (also known as luteinizing hormone–releasing hormone, or LHRH) is produced in the hypothalamic parts of the brain and, following release to the pituitary portal blood vessels, acts on the pituitary gland to stimulate the secretion of luteinizing hormone (LH) and follicle-stimulating hormone (FSH). GnRH thereby regulates, indirectly at least, the functions of both the ovaries and the testes and their steroidal secretions. The patterns of LH and FSH secretion differ markedly, but for the most part these differences can be accounted for by changes in the pulsatile pattern of GnRH secretion and the feedback of gonadal hormones, notably estradiol and testosterone. There is no convincing evidence for the existence of a separate and specific FSH-releasing hormone, although some components of the GnRH precursor and some GnRH analogues appear to differ in the degree to which they stimulate the secretion of the two gonadotropins.[6] GnRH-like peptides and GnRH-induced effects have also been identified in the ovaries, testes, breast, placenta, sympathetic nervous system, retina, and pancreas, and the mRNA for the GnRH receptor has likewise been detected in some of these tissues. At least one other GnRH-related peptide has also been isolated from the hypothalamus of most species other than placental mammals.

This chapter focuses on mammalian GnRH and its role in the regulation of the pituitary gland.

STRUCTURE-ACTIVITY RELATIONSHIPS

Evolution of GnRH-like Peptides

Mammalian GnRH consists of a single chain of 10 amino acids and is protected at the N-terminus by cyclization of the glutamine to pyroglutamic acid and is amidated at the C-terminus (Table 13–1). Chicken GnRH-I has Arg^8 replaced by Gln^8, whereas salmon GnRH has two substitutions.[7] Collectively these three peptides could have a common lineage because one can be derived from the other by point mutations in the coding sequences. A second GnRH-related peptide has also been identified in species other than placental mammals. This second form of GnRH, typified by chicken GnRH-II, has been highly conserved and appears in cartilaginous and bony fish, amphibians, reptiles, birds, and marsupials.[8, 9] Thus most species express two distinct forms of GnRH, but only the mammalian form appears to be related to reproduction. The functions of the other GnRH-like peptides are less clear, although in some situations they act as regulatory peptides within the nervous system. The route by which these various GnRH-like peptides evolved is a matter of debate, but two families of peptides appear to have arisen about 500 million years ago, probably by gene duplication. The structure of the N- and C-terminals of all the GnRH-like peptides has been strongly conserved, suggesting that these regions are important sites of binding and receptor activation. Sequence homology, with respect to four or more amino acids, has been reported for at least 39 other proteins,[7] including the yeast α-mating factor (Table 13–1).

The pituitary GnRH receptor has likewise undergone evolutionary change such that the various forms of GnRH and GnRH analogues have markedly different potencies,

TABLE 13–1. AMINO ACID STRUCTURE OF MAMMALIAN GnRH AND RELATED PEPTIDES

1	2	3	4	5	6	7	8	9	10		
Reproductive-related GnRH peptides											
pGlu	His	Trp	Ser	Tyr	Gly	Leu	Arg	Pro	Gly-NH₂		Mammalian
—	—	—	—	—	—	—	Gln	—	—		Chicken I
—	—	—	—	—	—	Trp	Leu	—	—		Salmon
Nonreproductive GnRH peptides											
—	—	—	—	His	—	Trp	Tyr	—	—		Chicken II
—	—	Tyr	—	Leu	Glu	Trp	Lys	—	—		Lamprey
Analogues in clinical use											
—	—	—	—	—	Nal(2) D-	—	—	—	Gly aza		Nafarelin—agonist
—	—	—	—	—	Ser D-, tert. butyl	—	—	Pro-NH-CH₂-CH₃			Buserelin—agonist (nine amino acids)
Nal(2) N-Ac-D-	Phe D-pCl-	Pal(3) D-	—	Lys (Nic)	Lys D-(Nic)	—	—	Lys (iPr)	Ala D-		Antide— antagonist
Other peptides with sequence homology											
Trp	His	Trp		Leu	Gln	Trp	Lys	Pro	Gly	Gln-Pro-Met-Tyr	Yeast α-mating factor
Val	Ser	Ser	Ser	Leu	Gly	Leu	Arg	Pro	Asp		Adenovirus hexon protein

both between vertebrate groups and mammalian species. Further details are provided later in this chapter.

Enzymic Degradation

GnRH has a half-life of 5 to 7 minutes,[10] but such determinations are confounded by dilution factors and the partitioning of GnRH within different tissues of the body. Most of the GnRH released into the pituitary portal blood is removed on the first pass through the pituitary gland, either by receptor binding and internalization within gonadotropes or by enzymic degradation. Three degrading enzyme systems have been identified as active within the pituitary gland.[11] A post-proline cleaving enzyme hydrolyzes the Pro⁹-Gly¹⁰ bond, and a pyro-Glu-amino peptidase cleaves the pGlu¹-His² bond. Several enzymes cleave other parts of the peptide, but the most active of these enzymes within the pituitary gland appears to be a non–chymotrypsin-like endopeptidase that hydrolyzes the Tyr⁵-Gly⁶ bond and to a lesser extent the His²-Trp³ bond. Most metabolites of GnRH are biologically inactive. GnRH can adopt many configurations, but on the basis of conformational energy analysis,[12] the biologically active hormone is thought to contain a major fold (IIβ-bend) within the residues Tyr⁵-Gly⁶-Leu⁷-Arg.⁸ This has the effect of bringing the N- and C-terminals into close proximity.

GnRH Agonists

Many thousand derivatives of GnRH have been synthesized in an attempt to develop more potent compounds for therapeutic use. Several test systems have been used to screen these putative agonists, including LH release from isolated anterior pituitary cells, ovulation induction in pentobarbitone-blocked rats, estrus suppression, and inhibition of FSH-induced estrogen production by cultured granulosa cells.[13] The response to agonists varies markedly in these systems and, as a consequence, it is difficult to assign a single estimate of relative potency. In general terms, su-

peragonists are conformationally stabilized. They have a longer half-life and a higher receptor affinity than does the native hormone. Deletion of the terminal Gly¹⁰(des-Gly) and the addition of an ethylamide (NHEt) group to the terminal proline in position 9 potentiates the action of the peptide, possibly by blocking the action of the post-proline cleaving enzyme. An alternative stabilization of the terminal sequence involves the substitution of an aza-Gly¹⁰ group. The second major step in agonist production involved the substitution of the glycine residue in position 6 within amino acids that stabilize the β-bend and reduce enzymic degradation.[14] Thus D-Ala⁶, Pro⁹-NHEt, GnRH was produced and was found to have a potency much greater than native GnRH. Large numbers of elaborate side chains were then explored. Among the more successful substitutions were the introduction of (1) a tertiary butyl ethyl derivative of serine producing D-Ser(tert.butyl)⁶, Pro⁹-NHEt, GnRH (Table 13–1); (2) a 3(2)-naphthyl derivative of alanine producing D-Nal(2)⁶, GnRH; and (3) a benzyl derivative of histamine producing D-His(Bzl)⁶, Pro⁹-NHEt, GnRH. All three of these derivatives have potencies 100- to 200-fold greater than that of GnRH.

GnRH Antagonists

The synthesis of GnRH antagonists posed greater problems. Analogues had to be of sufficiently high affinity and persistence to displace endogenous GnRH from the pituitary receptors without evoking receptor activation and of sufficient potency to reach the pituitary gland in effective amounts after dilution and degradation within the peripheral circulation.

Deletion of the His residue in position 2 (des-His²) produced the first analogue to competitively inhibit the action of GnRH,[15] and the potency of this weakly active antagonist was then increased by incorporating those modifications in position 6 associated with the production of superagonists, namely, D-Ala⁶, D-Leu⁶, D-Phe⁶, and D-Trp⁶. The next major step was the substitution of His² with D-Phe. Indeed, D-Phe², D-Leu⁶, GnRH became the first antagonist with sufficient potency to block the ovulatory surge of LH when adminis-tered to the rat on the day of proestrus.[16] An enormous number of alternative substitutions were then investigated. A notable step was the discovery that substitutions in posi-tions 1 and 3, when coupled with the previous substitutions in positions 2 and 6, produced a range of extremely potent tetra-substituted decapeptides. Many of the most potent antagonists now contain so many aromatic amino acids that they are extremely lipophilic. As a consequence, they have to be administered in propylene glycol or as a suspension in corn oil. One approach to overcome this problem was to incorporate a hydrophilic D-amino acid in position 6 and accept the decrease in potency that was predicted. Surprisingly, the potency of several of the D-Arg[6] analogues was increased.[17] As a general rule the GnRH receptor ap-pears to tolerate a hydrophobic or hydrophilic residue in position 6 so long as it is paired with a hydrophilic (N-Ac-Pro) or hydrophobic (N-Ac-D-Nal(2)) residue in position 1, respectively. Some of the more recently derived GnRH an-tagonists have seven substitutions and express potencies 10,000 times greater than the Des-His[2] derivative discov-ered in the early 1970's (see Table 13–1).

BIOSYNTHESIS OF GnRH AND PRECURSOR PROCESSING

In 1984, Seeburg and Adelman isolated cDNA sequences from human placental tissue which encoded a GnRH pre-cursor of 92 amino acids (Fig. 13–1).[18] The first part (23 or 24 amino acids) forms a typical signal sequence and incorporates a hydrophobic center region; this probably plays a role in the processing of peptide within the rough endoplasmic reticulum and Golgi apparatus. The signal sequence abuts directly on the active hormone, and cleav-age at this site exposes the amino-terminal glutamic resi-due, which then undergoes cyclization to form the pyro-

Glu terminus of GnRH. The basic amino acids, Gly-Lys-Arg in positions 11 to 13, provide typical trypsin and carboxy-peptidase-like cleavage sites, with the glycine residue pro-viding the amino donor for C-terminal amidation.[19] The remaining 56 amino acids of the precursor, termed gona-dotropin-associated peptide (GAP), contains no sites for N-glycosylation, and no homologies are known with regard to other peptide sequences. The GnRH precursor translates into a peptide of about 10,000 daltons. A subsequent ge-nomic analysis indicates that neurons in the brain produce a peptide that is identical to the human placental precur-sor.[20] The hypogonadal mouse contains a mutation that prevents the expression of the third and fourth exons of the GnRH gene, although the full nucleotide sequence for GnRH is still present.

GnRH, once it is packaged into granules, is presumably moved by fast axonal transport to the nerve terminals in the median eminence (ME) and elsewhere for storage and subsequent degradation or release. Fast axonal transport at 1 to 3 mm/h is still a relatively slow process, and changes in the rate of biosynthesis cannot be used to compensate, other than in the long term, for changes in the rate of secretion. Large stores of GnRH are therefore maintained within the nerve terminals relative to the amounts released under physiological conditions. The hypothalamus of the sheep, for example, contains 20 to 80 ng GnRH, whereas each GnRH pulse probably contains less than 100 pg GnRH.

The cleavage of the precursor into GnRH and GAP dur-ing transport and storage should result in the co-secretion of the two peptide sequences.[21–23] This could be of great importance because GAP (and related fragments) has been reported both to inhibit the secretion of prolactin and to stimulate the secretion of LH and FSH.[24] Earlier studies had indeed provided evidence for a dopamine-free prolac-tin-inhibiting factor of about 8000 Da in those areas of the brain staining immunohistochemically for GnRH.[25] It is

```
                          TGG ATC TAA TTT GAT TGT GCA TTC ATG TGC CTT AGA


        met lys pro ile gln lys leu leu ala gly leu ile leu leu thr ser cys val glu gly cyc ser ser
        ATG AAG CCA ATT CAA AAA CTC CTA GCT GGC CTT ATT CTA CTG ACT TCG TGC GTG GAA GGC TGC TCC AGC


        1 ------------ GnRH ----------- 10  ■   ■   ■
        gln his trp ser tyr gly leu arg pro gly gly lys arg asp ala glu asn leu ile asp ser phe gln
        CAG CAC TGG TCC TAT GGA CYG CGC CCT GGA GGA AAG AGA GAT GCC GAA AAT TTG ATT GAT TCT TTC CAA
                                                          1--- GAP, FSH (LH) releasing activity ---

              ■                                          ■                                       ■
        glu ile val lys glu val gly gln leu ala glu thr gln arg phe glu cys thr thr his gln pro arg
        GAG ATA GTA AAA GAG GTT GGT CAA CTG GCA GAA ACC CAA CGC TTC GAA TGC ACC ACG CAC CAG CCA CGT
        --------13 ----------------------------------23                                         30

                    ■                                                              ■ ■
        ser pro leu arg asp leu lys gly ala leu glu ser leu ile glu glu glu thr gly gln lys lys ile
        TCT CCC CTC CGA GAC CTG AAA GGA GCT CTG GAA AGT CTG ATT GAA GAG GAA ACT GGG CAG AAG AAG ATT
                        40                                  50                              56


        TAA ATC CAT TGG GCC AGA AGG ATT GAC CAT TAC TAA CAT
```

FIGURE 13–1. Nucleotide and amino acid sequence of human prepro-GnRH. Sites of enzymic cleavage are indicated (■). Cleavage at these sites generates GnRH and a number of other peptides, collectively known as gonadotropin-associated peptides (GAP). The longest GAP, of 56 amino acids, has the potential to inhibit the release of prolactin. A shorter fragment of 23 amino acids has been reported to preferentially release FSH. (Sequence data adapted from Seeburg PH, Adelman JP: Characterization of cDNA for precursor of human luteinizing hormone releasing hormone. Nature 311:666–668, 1984.)

plausible that the pituitary gland could receive a differential signal if GAP were subject to further enzymic cleavage en route at one or more of its putative cleavage sites (Fig. 13–1). Fragments of GAP have been produced in an attempt to identify regions of biological activity. Prolactin-inhibiting activity appears to require the full GAP sequence.[26] FSH- and LH-releasing activity, on the other hand, requires only a small part of the structure. The decapeptide of GAP$_{4-13}$ contains the minimal sequence to stimulate gonadotropin secretion, with a potency about 1 per cent of GnRH.[27] There is no sequence homology between these two decapeptides. Of perhaps even more interest is the recent observation that D-Trp substitution of GAP$_{1-13}$ in position 9 produces a peptide that preferentially releases FSH, with amplification effects observed with multiple injections into the ovariectomized, estrogen-progesterone–primed rat.[6]

LOCALIZATION OF GnRH IN BRAIN

Adult Brain

Neurons that are immunoreactive for GnRH are found diffusely spread throughout the anterior parts of the hypothalamus, preoptic area, septal complex, and other parts of the forebrain, but nowhere are the cells grouped into distinct nuclei.[28] One notable species variation has been reported. Primates, including humans, have GnRH neurons located in the medial basal hypothalamus and arcuate nucleus, whereas very few have been detected in these regions in the rat and guinea pig.[29] GnRH secretion is powerfully regulated by the feedback of gonadal steroids and the central release of various neurotransmitters. However, neurons staining cytochemically for GnRH do not accumulate radioactively labeled gonadal steroids, although steroid-concentrating cells are found in very close proximity.[30] One would imagine that there must be active communication between these two cell types, and it is interesting to note that some GnRH neurons in the preoptic area engage in reciprocal synaptic connections with adjacent neural elements.[31] The neurotransmitters involved in these synaptic interconnections have not been fully characterized, but synapses containing serotonin, epinephrine, dopamine, and γ-aminobutyric acid have been identified impinging upon GnRH neurons.

Axons from GnRH neurons project to many sites within the CNS. One of the most distinct projections is from the medial preoptic area to the ME, with fibers coursing through the lateral hypothalamus or close to the third ventricle before terminating in a profuse plexus of boutons on the primary pituitary portal blood plexus. Some GnRH neurons located elsewhere in the brain also project to the pituitary portal vessels, and thus the regulation of the pituitary gland by GnRH may come under the control of more than one neural system. By contrast, not all GnRH-containing fibers project to the portal system. There is a major projection to the organum vasculosum of the lamina terminalis (OVLT) and a more diffuse projection of fibers to many regions of the brain.

The GnRH terminals of the ME are outside the blood-brain barrier (BBB), as indeed are those in the OVLT. As a consequence, the terminals of the GnRH neurons are more exposed than the cell bodies to large molecular weight hormones in the peripheral circulation. In addition, the terminals of GnRH neurons exist in much closer apposition to each other than do the cell bodies, and thus terminal interactions could be important in the organization of pulsatile secretion (see below). There is some question as to whether GnRH, once released into the portal vessels, can return across the BBB.[32] Several studies have, however, reported changes in sexual behavior following the peripheral administration of GnRH to ovariectomzied steroid-primed animals.[33] Abundant GnRH receptors have also been measured in the hippocampus and other parts of the limbic system by using the binding of [^{125}]D-Ala^6, Leu^7, Pro^9-NHEt, GnRH.[34]

Origin of GnRH Neurons

GnRH neurons originate in the olfactory placode and not in the walls of the cerebral ventricles as originally thought.[35] During early fetal development, cells staining immunoreactively for GnRH migrate through the nasal septum to enter the forebrain in association with the nervus terminalis. Subsequently, they course medially to the olfactory bulbs to enter the septum, preoptic area, and anterior hypothalamus. As a result of this unusual origin, one might expect the GnRH neurons to express features not shared with other neuroendocrine systems. Already, this discovery has provided an explanation for a number of hitherto unexplained observations. Some GnRH neurons have been reported to exhibit cilia, a feature of the olfactory epithelium.[36] Anosmia and gonadal failure are likewise linked in Kallman's syndrome. In these patients, the development of the olfactory system is severely altered, and the normal migration of GnRH neurons is arrested.[37] The major GnRH expressed by these migrating neurons appears to be identical to that found in the hypothalamus of the mature animal.

PATTERNS OF GnRH SECRETION

LH is secreted in a pulsatile pattern (Fig. 13–2), and very marked changes in LH pulse frequency and pulse amplitude have been observed in relation to puberty, the female reproductive cycle, and the time of year in seasonal breeding species.[38] A typical LH pulse increases to peak height between one blood sample and the next, and thereafter the level decays approximately in parallel with the half-life of the hormone. This indicates an abrupt and short episode of secretion, perhaps lasting no more than two to six minutes.[39] Changes in pulse frequency probably relate to changes in the pattern of GnRH secretion, as could changes in pulse amplitude, but the latter relationship is complicated by changes in the sensitivity of the pituitary gland to GnRH brought about by the feedback actions of gonadal steroids. Pulse frequency and pulse amplitude tend to be inversely related; that is, large-amplitude LH pulses are usually associated with long interpulse intervals and vice versa, although notable exceptions to this general principle do occur.

A bolus injection of GnRH or a GnRH agonist usually evokes an episode of LH secretion that commences within

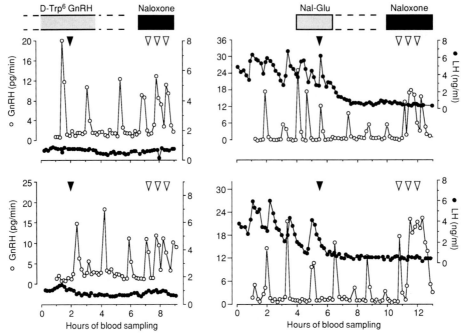

FIGURE 13–2. Effect of GnRH agonist and antagonist analogues on GnRH and LH secretion in short-term castrated rams. The effect of the administration of the D-Trp[6] agonist (0.5 mg/day intramuscularly *closed arrows, left*) to two sheep for 12 days before the simultaneous sampling of pituitary portal and jugular blood is shown in the left panel. LH levels after 12 days of agonist treatment were markedly suppressed owing to pituitary desensitization, but GnRH secretion remained pulsatile. Naloxone, the opiate antagonist, when administered in three 100-mg intravenous injections, induced an increase in GnRH pulse frequency (*open arrows*). The effect of the administration of the Nal-Glu antagonist (5 mg intramuscularly *closed arrows, right*) to two sheep on GnRH and LH secretion is shown in the right panel. Antagonist treatment caused an immediate suppression of LH secretion. The secretion of GnRH remained unaltered. Naloxone, given as above, increased mean GnRH secretion in the antagonist-treated castrated ram. (Data adapted from Caraty A, Locatelli A, Delaleu B, et al: Gonadotropin-releasing-hormone (GnRH) agonists and GnRH antagonists do not alter endogenous GnRH secretion in short-term castrated rams. Endocrinology 127:1523–1529, 1990.)

seconds and decays with a profile virtually indistinguishable from that of an endogenously evoked LH pulse. The period of GnRH secretion could therefore be much shorter than the two to six minutes estimated for LH release. Most studies of GnRH-induced LH secretion are, however, confounded by an unknown contribution from endogenous GnRH. Various approaches have been devised in an attempt to circumvent the problem. These include the pharmacological suppression of the GnRH pulse generator of the brain, the destruction of the GnRH terminals in the ME by electrolytic lesions, the transection of the pituitary stalk, and the application of active and passive immuno-neutralization of GnRH. None of these procedures eliminates the possibility of some endogenous GnRH reaching the pituitary gland, and very low levels of tonic GnRH secretion, insufficient to stimulate a measureable release of LH, could enhance the pituitary responsiveness to superimposed pulses of GnRH. Collectively, however, these studies establish beyond reasonable doubt that each LH pulse is driven by a corresponding episode of GnRH secretion from the brain. The opposite deduction does not necessarily hold. Some GnRH pulses may not release observable LH pulses. GnRH pulses may fail to elicit an effect if they have inadequate amplitude, follow too closely upon a previous pulse, or encounter a down-regulated pituitary gland.

Negative Feedback of Gonadal Steroids

The inhibition of GnRH and LH secretion by the feedback of gonadal steroids is the single most important factor governing reproduction. Castration or ovariectomy consistently results in the development of an LH profile that is characterized by large-amplitude pulses at short intervals, and the phenomenon is apparent within a few hours of surgery.[40] An increase in LH pulse amplitude and frequency has also been observed when ewes have been immunized against estradiol, androstenedione, and testosterone,[41] and similar effects have been recorded in more limited studies using rhesus monkeys.[42] Both progesterone and estradiol inhibit LH secretion when given separately, but considerable synergism is expressed when they are given together,[43] as in contraceptive pills. Testosterone expresses a similar negative feedback when given to the castrated male and appears to act without appreciable synergism with other steroid hormones.[44] Interestingly, the implantation of testosterone in the female rhesus monkey after ovariectomy has an effect similar to that of implanting estrogen and progesterone and reduces pulsatile secretion of LH from one pulse per hour to one pulse per five hours.[45] GnRH and LH secretion is, therefore, driven by a free-running GnRH pulse generator whose expression by the brain is held in check primarily by the negative feedback of gonadal hormones.

Positive Feedback of Gonadal Steroids

The neuroendocrine regulation of GnRH secretion in the female differs in two fundamental respects from that observed in the male. The pattern of steroid (and inhibin) secretion from the ovary changes dynamically during the reproductive cycle, and this modifies the suppression of the GnRH pulse generator. The time scale of these changes is related to the rate of follicle growth and the life span of the corpus luteum, and thus it can be said that the ovary determines the length of the reproductive cycle. The second difference is the expression of a positive feedback response to estrogen, which culminates in the secretion of the preovulatory LH surge.

The administration of estradiol to the female normally evokes an LH surge in the absence of high levels of progesterone. The onset of this surge commences after 12 to 36 hours, but this varies according to species. Much debate continues about the role played by the brain in the expression of positive feedback, because a wealth of evidence shows that the responsiveness of the pituitary gland to GnRH is enormously increased by estrogen, both in vivo[46] and in vitro.[47] Support for an exclusive pituitary site of action was increased by the observation that a preovulatory LH surge could be evoked in a rhesus monkey with a lesion in the medial basal hypothalamus by the simple expedient of administering a constant GnRH pulse every hour for up to 70 days.[48] On face value, this observation indicates that the hypothalamus provides no more than a permissive GnRH signal. This view has been strongly contested on the grounds that the hypothalamic lesions do not necessarily eliminate the entire endogenous GnRH signal, and constant GnRH pulse therapy has been shown to be ineffective when an impervious Teflon barrier is inserted across the pituitary stalk. However, ovulation is evoked when the pulsatile GnRH signal is replaced for 24 hours in the presence of a high estrogen titer by a low-level, continuous GnRH infusion.[49] This, in contrast to the previous study, suggests that the hypothalamus provides a specific message for the induction of the preovulatory surge. An important species difference may still underlie this controversy.

Evidence for involvement of the brain in the generation of the ovulatory LH surge is present in the LH profile because, in women, cows, rats, sheep, and monkeys, the preovulatory LH surge is composed of large-amplitude pulses that recur at short intervals. The interpulse interval is considerably shorter than that observed after ovariectomy, 8 to 10 minutes in the ewe, and indicates that the GnRH pulse generator can be driven at above the free-running rate. LH has a half-life of about 30 minutes; thus, pulses at intervals of 10 minutes or less result in a surge-like elevation in the baseline LH profile. But the situation is complicated by the fact that the half-life of LH may change at times of maximal secretion, as could the immunological to biological activity of the hormone.

Levels of GnRH in Pituitary Portal Blood

Considerable progress has now been made in a quest to resolve the controversies outlined above, based on the measurement of GnRH in the pituitary portal blood of conscious, unstressed, and unrestrained sheep. The transnasal, transsphenoidal approach for the collection of pituitary portal blood, originally devised by Clarke and Cummings,[50] has been extensively improved to allow the collection of blood from conscious, unstressed, and unrestrained animals over considerable periods of time.[51]

An excellent correlation has been observed between GnRH and LH pulses, with GnRH levels increasing in a spike-like manner between one sampling period and the next (Fig. 13–3).[51, 52] Levels of GnRH vary markedly between sheep, by two orders of magnitude in some cases. Such differences could relate to the vascular dynamics of the pituitary portal bed and the response to transection and should not be regarded as of any great significance. GnRH pulse frequency during the estrus cycle follows the pattern predicted from the measurement of circulating levels of LH, with gonadal steroids reducing pulse frequency and increasing pulse amplitude. This relationship does not apply so clearly in the nonbreeding season.[52] GnRH pulses are large and very widely spaced at this time, despite the very low circulating levels of gonadal steroids. Gonadectomy during the nonbreeding season, however, results in a massive increase in GnRH pulsatility.[53] From these results, one has to conclude that low-frequency GnRH pulsatility during the nonbreeding season relates to an enhanced

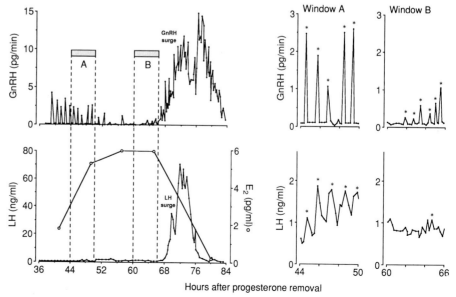

FIGURE 13–3. GnRH, LH, and estradiol profiles in simultaneous samples of portal and jugular blood of a ewe in relation to an LH surge timed by the removal of a progesterone implant. Two six-hour periods of the study are expanded on the right and rescaled to illustrate the pulsatile pattern of GnRH and LH secretion during the follicular phase. Note: The GnRH surge continued for many hours beyond the termination of the LH surge.

sensitivity of the hypothalamus to the negative feedback effects of gonadal hormones (presumably steroids).

The role of GnRH in the direct regulation of its own secretion has been challenged by the administration of GnRH agonists and antagonists in short-term castrated rams (see Fig. 13–2). Neither the D-Trp[6] agonists nor the Nal-Glu antagonist used in these studies altered GnRH pulsatility, despite reducing the level of LH secretion in both cases.[54] Thus, in the castrated ram, neither GnRH nor LH has any role in the regulation of GnRH pulsatility, thereby excluding both short- and ultrashort-loop feedback from the equation.

Recent studies,[55, 56] in contrast to some earlier publications,[57] have consistently recorded a massive increase in the portal blood level of GnRH during both estrogen-induced and spontaneous preovulatory LH surges. Both estrogen-induced and spontaneous GnRH surges exhibit a number of robust features. The surges are of very large amplitude, some are biphasic, and all continue beyond the end of the LH surge (Fig. 13–3). This apparent cessation of LH secretion, in the presence of very high levels of GnRH, could be due to down-regulation of the pituitary gland,[58] exhaustion of the readily releasable pool of LH,[58] a change in immunological characteristics of the circulating LH,[59] or the action of a putative "surge-inhibiting factor."[60] The GnRH surge has a spike-like profile, suggestive of a very high frequency pattern of GnRH secretion. However, given the relatively long sampling intervals involved, it is impossible to determine whether the GnRH surge is entirely the result of pulsatile secretion or involves a component of continuous secretion. Certainly the latter possibility cannot be excluded. A marked reduction in GnRH pulsatility is also observed in the hours preceding the preovulatory surge and appears to relate to an inhibitory action of estrogen acting at a hypothalamic level.

Based on the measurement of GnRH in pituitary portal blood, the female reproductive cycle appears to be driven by the same hypothalamic GnRH pulse generator that is present in the male. However, the cycle involves a number of sequential elements controlled by the temporal changes in the feedback of ovarian steroids, reflecting the time course of follicle and luteal development. At the start of the follicular phase, following the regression of the corpus luteum (and menstruation in women and old-world primates), the LH pulses are large and frequent, an expression of a largely unrestrained GnRH pulse generator. The amplitude of the GnRH pulses then falls as the follicular phase progresses, in response to the negative feedback of estrogen. Eventually, the increasing levels of estrogen act to elicit a massive (and pulsatile) increase in the secretion of GnRH (a GnRH surge). This, in turn, acting upon a now highly sensitized pituitary gland, elicits the preovulatory LH surge. The early luteal phase is characterized by less frequent LH pulses, related to the inhibitory actions of progesterone from the corpus luteum, acting alone or synergistically with other steroids. The mid- and late-luteal phases are characterized by prominent LH pulses. These are somewhat irregular and infrequent in their occurrence, and each is followed, in women at least, by a surge in the luteal secretion of progesterone lasting one to two hours.[61] In several situations not discussed, the pattern of GnRH secretion is further modulated by neural rather than hormonal signals, including suckling-induced lactational infertility and coitus-induced ovulation.

Two issues remain to be discussed: the nature of the hypothalamic pulse generator and the interaction of GnRH with its receptor.

GnRH PULSE GENERATION

GnRH neurons are, one assumes, electrophysiologically active, and changes in the number of action potentials transmitted to the terminals probably determine the level of hormone secretion. Electrical stimulation of the preoptic area, anterior hypothalamus, and ME readily evokes GnRH and LH release and, when appropriately timed, ovulation.[62] High rates of stimulation, simulating high rates of action potential generation, are far more efficient at releasing hormone than those rates of activity associated with the background noise of the nervous system. Thus, stimulation of the isolated mediobasal hypothalamus at 50 pulses per second releases more GnRH *per pulse* than stimulation at 10 pulses per second or less. These and other studies suggest that hormone pulses are fashioned by a relative synchronization of high-frequency electrical activity.

Recordings of the electrical activity of authenticated GnRH neurons are difficult to obtain, primarily because the cells are few in number and widely scattered. However, considerable success has been achieved using large electrodes to monitor the global activity of axons and terminals in the region of the ME of the rat[63] and rhesus monkey.[64] These "multiunit" recordings, in effect, provide a qualitative summation of electrical events in the adjacent neuropil. A massive increase in electrical activity was observed to precede each LH pulse in ovariectomized rats and monkeys, indicative of both high-frequency activation and synchronization between cells. The bursts of increased activity lasted 1 to 5 minutes in rats and preceded the rise in LH by 2 to 9 minutes.[63] Estimates of this latency are very imprecise owing to the long blood sampling intervals. The recordings from monkeys are of a similar character. Bursts of multiunit activity lasted for 8 to 16 minutes and recurred at intervals of 37 to 56 minutes.[64] More recently, using telemetric methods, the electrical activity of the ME has been tracked throughout the menstrual cycle in intact animals. The multiunit volleys recorded under these circumstances were much shorter, ranging from 3.2 minutes in the follicular phase to 4.1 minutes in the luteal phase.[65] Perhaps the most surprising discovery was the dramatic reduction in activity observed during and immediately prior to the midcycle LH surge. A similar reduction had previously been recorded in relation to the more artificial estrogen-induced LH surge.[66] This observation, consistent between animals, stands in sharp contrast to the evidence previously discussed to indicate a massive increase in GnRH secretion at this time, at least in the ewe.

The dramatic volleys of multiunit activity that have been recorded from the ME appear to reflect some aspect of the GnRH pulse generator, but whether the activity that has been recorded arises from GnRH neurons remains an open question. It is plausible that the recordings represent a neural input from elsewhere in the brain or a form of intraneural feedback. The pattern of multiunit volleys is not influenced by GnRH administration, which tends to eliminate ultrashort-loop feedback via the portal circulation. The intervolley interval is, by contrast, subject to modulation by both opioid and epinephrinergic drugs.[67, 68] The ME receives a major norepinephrine innervation from the brain stem,[69] and norepinephrine readily stimulates or augments LH secretion, presumably by stimulating GnRH secretion. Thus, the periodic activation of this norepinephrinergic input may represent the GnRH pulse generator, and electrical recordings may have been obtained from the terminals of these neurons.

GnRH neurons may be linked at a central level through interneurons or reciprocal connections. Certainly an anatomical substrate for such a system of communication has been shown to exist.[70] Indeed, one of the most remarkable observations relevant to this discussion has been the recent discovery of intrinsic pulsatile secretory activity in cultures of immortalized GnRH neurons.[71] As far as one can judge, these neurons are divorced from the neurotransmitter connections that might operate in vivo, with the exception of GnRH to GnRH connections. The door is now clearly open to the investigation of GnRH pulsatility in vitro.

GnRH-RECEPTOR INTERACTIONS

GnRH Receptor

GnRH and GnRH analogues exert their effects via membrane-bound receptors located on the pituitary gonadotropes. This coupling to the receptor and the cascade of events that follows involves hormone binding, microaggregation, internalization, release of second messengers, mobilization of calcium, and exocytosis. GnRH also stimulates the synthesis of its own receptors, the second messengers, and the gonadotropin subunits.

The cDNA for the mouse GnRH receptor has recently been sequenced using a novel combination of polymerase chain reaction (PCR) amplification and expression cloning.[5] Degenerate oligonucleotide sequences, based on transmembrane regions of the dopamine-D1 receptor, were used to amplify cDNA fragments from a mouse pituitary cDNA library. In parallel, mRNA from the transgenic αT3-1 pituitary tumor cell line was expressed in *Xenopus* oocytes. Activation of these oocytes with GnRH evokes membrane depolarization, as shown earlier in other transfection studies.[72] Antisense sequences to the PCR products were then produced, microinjected, and tested for their ability to block the expression of the αT3-1 GnRH receptor mRNA, thus allowing the identification of putative fragments of the GnRH receptor. These were sequenced and used as probes to identify full-length clones. A full-length rat GnRH receptor has since been sequenced from a rat pituitary cDNA library using homologous oligonucleotide probes derived from the mouse sequence (Fig. 13–4). The two receptors appear to be functionally identical.

The GnRH receptor consists of 327 amino acids and, as such, is one of the smallest of the 80 transmembrane receptors that have been analyzed. The external domain is relatively short and contains two putative glycosylation sites; a third site is also present on the first external loop. Where GnRH binds to the receptor is unclear. Binding could occur on either the external domain or at some point within the transmembrane channel formed by the seven transmembrane bridges, as occurs with monaminergic receptors, for example. It could be important in the context of

binding that the highly conserved aspartate of the second transmembrane domain, essential for the function of most transmembrane receptors, has been replaced with an asparagine. Six putative phosphorylation sites are present, two on each of the three cytoplasmic loops. Their role in second messenger coupling has yet to be determined. The C-terminal, located within the cell, is almost absent. This generates questions regarding the down-regulation of the GnRH receptor, because the C-terminal of other receptors has been implicated in this important phenomenon. The closest homology with other known receptors is with interleukin-8.

GnRH-like peptides express different gonadotropin-releasing activities, which suggests that differences in receptor structure may exist between not only vertebrate groups but also mammalian species.[7] Mammalian GnRH has high activity in mammals but relatively low activity in other groups. In contrast, all other forms of GnRH, with the exception of lamprey GnRH, have high potency in all groups, including mammals. Arg^8 is essential for gonadotropin release in mammals, but not in birds, reptiles, amphibians, and fish. His^5 substitution is associated with a marked reduction in activity in birds, but is without effect in mammals. Likewise, analogues differ in potency between species. It is impossible at this early stage in the analysis of the GnRH receptor to relate these differences to receptor structure.

Second Messenger Activation

The events associated with receptor binding were first visualized using a GnRH-ferritin conjugate that was visible under the electron microscope.[73] The ferritin particles were initially distributed uniformly over the gonadotrophs, with a density suggesting the existence of about 15,000 receptors per cell. Within 20 minutes the hormone receptor complexes underwent aggregation and by 30 minutes were internalized by endocytosis, presumably to be degraded by lysosomes. The time course of these events appears too slow for their involvement in the initial phase of GnRH stimulation. Furthermore, GnRH analogues retain their potency after steps have been taken to block internalization. Some degree of microaggregation, at least at the molecular level, is essential for the activation of the insulin and EGF receptors, and the same principles may apply to the GnRH receptor.[74] Bivalent antibodies to the insulin receptor express insulin-like activities because they are thought to link adjacent receptors into dimers, whereas monovalent antibodies inhibit insulin binding without promoting activation.[75] Bivalent antibodies prepared against antagonists appear to serve the same purpose and, by linking together adjacent receptors, convert antagonists into agonists.[76] The events that follow from the cross-linking of receptors are unknown. It is plausible that the inner domains of the GnRH receptor, having been drawn into close proximity, now reciprocally interact via G-proteins to catalyze the activation of the second messenger cascade. GnRH receptors are coupled to the hydrolysis of polyphosphoinositide, with the production of the two second messengers diacylglycerol and inositol triphosphate, which serve to stimulate protein phosphorylation and mobilization of calcium, respectively.[77] The receptors are not directly coupled

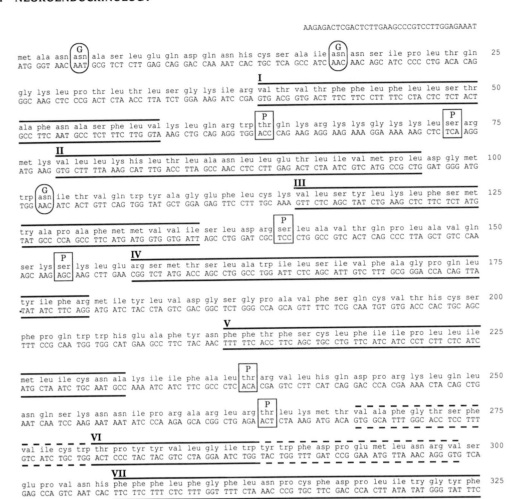

FIGURE 13–4. Nucleotide and amino acid sequence of rat GnRH receptor, as determined from a full-length pituitary cDNA clone. The putative seven transmembrane domains of the 327-amino acid receptor are illustrated by bars above and below, and numbered. The sixth transmembrane domain is difficult to place but falls somewhere between amino acids 269 and 299. Three putative glycosylation sites are present on the external domains of the receptor (G). Six putative phosphorylation sites are present, two on each of the three cytoplasmic loops (P). The rat receptor illustrated, analyzed by Dr. Karin Eidne and her team in Edinburgh, differs in only minor respects from the mouse GnRH receptor sequenced from the transgenic alpha T3-1 tumor cell line. (Data from Tsutsumi M, Zhou W, Millar RP, et al: Cloning and functional expression of a mouse gonadotropin-releasing hormone receptor. Mol Endocrinol 7:1163–1169, 1992; with permission.)

to the cAMP pathway, although a facilitatory role in gonadotropin release cannot be excluded.

Calcium, as in most secretory systems, is closely involved in LH release by exocytosis, with a mobilization of intracellular calcium determining the initial phase of GnRH stimulation and an influx of extracellular calcium determining the more sustained events associated with secretion.[66] Several attempts have been made to characterize the calcium channels involved, using isolated gonadotropes, tumor-derived cells of the gonadotrope lineage, pharmacological manipulation of the channels, the electrophysiological measurement of ion conductances, and the time-lapse visualization of intracellular free calcium. Two membrane-bound calcium channels have been identified in pituitary cells, one characterized by a fast current with rapid activation-inactivation kinetics (T-type), and a slower dihydropyridine-sensitive channel (L-type) commonly associated with second messenger activation and inactivation.[78] N-type channels, identified in other tissues, do not appear to be present. Current evidence indicates that both T- and L-type channels are involved in LH secretion. Isolated gonadotropes display the ability to generate voltage-dependent action potentials in response to depolarizing current injection,[79] but action potentials do not appear to be evoked by GnRH administration. Action potentials per se do not appear to sustain calcium entry. Thus diacylglycerol and cytosolic Ca^{2+} appear to activate protein kinase C, and this in turn, by phosphorylation,[80, 81] activates the L-type Ca^{2+} channel.

Modulation of Stimulus-Secretion Coupling

The pulsatile pattern of GnRH secretion provides an important temporal component to stimulus-secretion coupling. Gonadectomy results in an increase in GnRH receptors, but the effect can be abolished by manipulations that prevent the postcastration increase in GnRH secretion, that is, the placement of hypothalamic lesions and administration of an anti-GnRH antiserum. The response to GnRH, in terms of receptor numbers (binding sites), also depends on the pattern and dose of GnRH administered and the time at which receptor binding is measured. In the testosterone-implanted castrated rat, receptor numbers are maximal when GnRH pulses are given every 30 minutes, and a marked decline in receptor numbers is observed at shorter or longer pulse intervals.[82] Receptor numbers decline immediately following a GnRH pulse but after 30 to 60 minutes tend to rise to higher than pretreatment values. As a consequence, one GnRH pulse can augment the response to another given 30 to 60 minutes later (self-priming).[83] Evidence also indicates that pulse interval is an important factor in the differential regulation of β-LH and β-FSH gene expression.[84]

Continuous exposure of the pituitary gland to GnRH or a GnRH agonist results, after an initial stimulation, in a loss of responsiveness and virtual abolition of LH secretion (down-regulation or desensitization), and the phenomenon has been observed both in vivo[85] and in vitro.[85] This is not due to a lack of LH, because secretion can be evoked in desensitized cells by secretagogues, such as calcium ionophores and melitin. Antagonist binding does not evoke desensitization, but the phenomenon is observed if the antagonist is dimerized so as to act as an agonist.

The developing view is that voltage-dependent calcium channels (L-type), activated by protein kinase C, are involved in desensitization via a change in the ability of protein kinase C to phosphorylate the Ca^{2+} channel.[78]

FUTURE

Enormous progress has been made since the discovery of the structure of GnRH in 1971, but several major questions remain to be answered. What is the genomic structure of GnRH II, and why is this gene complex not expressed in placental mammals? How are GnRH neurons organized to produce pulsatile secretion, a phenomenon now observed in vitro? What mechanisms govern the continuous secretion of GnRH during the preovulatory surge? Why do multiunit recordings from the arcuate region of the hypothalamus fail to show increases in activity during the preovulatory GnRH surge? Are primates fundamentally different from sheep in the regulation of the GnRH surge? What species differences exist in the structure of the GnRH receptor? How are the second messenger pathways of the gonadotrope organized to differentially regulate the biosynthesis and secretion of the two gonadotropins? Can one devise peptides that selectively enhance or inhibit biosynthesis and secretion of FSH? The story is continued in Chapters 14 and 15.

REFERENCES

1. Matsuo H, Baba Y, Nair RMG, et al: Structure of the porcine LH and FSH-releasing hormone. I. The proposed amino acid sequence. Biochem Biophys Res Commun 43:1334–1339, 1971.
2. Matsuo H, Arimura A, Nair RMG, Schally AV: Synthesis of the porcine LH- and FSH-releasing hormone by the solid phase method. Biochem Biophys Res Commun 45:822–827, 1971.
3. Burgus R, Butcher M, Amoss M, et al: Primary structure of the ovine hypothalamic luteinizing hormone–releasing factor (LRF). Proc Natl Acad Sci USA 69:278–282, 1972.
4. Green JD, Harris GW: The neurovascular link between the neurohypophysis and adenohypophysis. J Endocrinol 5:136–146, 1947.
5. Tsutsumi M, Zhou W, Millar RP, et al: Cloning and functional expression of a mouse gonadotropin-releasing hormone receptor. Mol Endocrinol 7:1163–1169, 1992.
6. Yu WH, Millar RP, Milton SCF, et al: Selective FSH-releasing activity of [D-Trp^9]GAP$_{1–13}$: Comparison with gonadotropin-releasing abilities of analogs of GAP and natural LHRH's. Brain Res Bull 25:867–873, 1990.
7. Millar RP, King JA: Evolution of gonadotropin releasing hormone: Multiple usage of a peptide. News in Physiological Sciences 3:49–53, 1988.
8. King JA, Hinds LA, Mehl AE, et al: Chicken GnRH II occurs together with mammalian GnRH in a South American species of marsupial (Monodelphis domestica). Peptides 11:521–525, 1990.
9. King JA, Steneveld AA, Millar RP, et al: Gonadotropin-releasing hormone in elasmobranch (electric ray, Torpedo marmorata) brain and plasma: Chromatographic and immunological evidence for chicken GnRH II and novel molecular forms. Peptides 13:27–35, 1992.
10. Redding TW, Kastin AJ, Gonzales-Barcena D, et al: The half-life, metabolism and excretion of tritiated luteinizing hormone–releasing hormone (LH-RH) in man. J Clin Endocrinol Metab 37:626–631, 1973.
11. Horsthemke B, Knisatschek H, Rivier J, et al: Degradation of luteinizing hormone–releasing hormone and analogs by adenohypophyseal peptidases. Biochem Biophys Res Commun 100:753–759, 1981.
12. Momany FA: Conformational energy analysis of the molecule, luteinizing hormone–releasing hormone. I. Native decapeptide. J Am Chem Soc 98:2990–2995, 1976.
13. Hsueh AJW, Adashi EY, Tucker E, et al: Relative potencies of gonadotropin-releasing hormone agonists and antagonists on ovarian and pituitary functions. Endocrinology 112:689–695, 1983.
14. Fujino M, Fukuda T, Shinagawa S, et al: Synthetic analogs of luteinizing hormone–releasing hormone (LH-RH) substituted in position 6 and 10. Biochem Biophys Res Commun 60:406–413, 1974.
15. Monahan MW, Rivier J, Vale W, Guillemin R: [Gly^2]LRF and desHis^2-LRF. The synthesis, purification and characterization of two LRF analogs antagonistic to LRF. Biochem Biophys Res Commun 47:551–556, 1972.
16. Beattie CW, Corbin A, Foell TJ, et al: Anti-ovulatory/anti-pregnancy effects of [D-Phe^2]-LRH analogs administered early in the rat estrous cycle. Contraception 13:341–353, 1976.
17. Coy DH, Horvath A, Nekola MV, et al: Peptide antagonists of LH-RH: Large increases in antiovulatory activities produced by basic D-amino acids in the six position. Endocrinology 110:1445–1447, 1982.
18. Seeburg PH, Adelman JP: Characterization of cDNA for precursor of human luteinizing hormone releasing hormone. Nature 311:666–668, 1984.
19. Bradbury AF, Finnie MDA, Smyth DG: Mechanism of C-terminal amide formation by pituitary enzymes. Nature 298:686–688, 1982.
20. Adelman JP, Mason AJ, Hayflick JS, Seeburg PH: Isolation of the gene and hypothalamic cDNA for the common precursor of gonadotropin-releasing hormone and prolactin release–inhibiting factor in human and rat. Proc Natl Acad Sci USA 83:179–183, 1986.
21. Silverman AJ, Witkin JW, Millar RP: Light and electron microscopic immunocytochemical analysis of antibodies directed against GnRH and its precursor in hypothalamic neurons. J Histochem Cytochem 38:803–813, 1990.
22. Phillips HS, Nikolics K, Branton D, Seeburg PH: Immunocytochemical localization in rat brain of a prolactin release–inhibiting sequence of gonadotropin-releasing hormone prohormone. Nature 316:542–545, 1985.
23. Clarke IJ, Cummins JT, Karsch FJ, et al: GnRH-associated peptide (GAP) is cosecreted with GnRH into the hypophyseal portal blood of ovariectomized sheep. Biochem Biophys Res Commun 143:665–671, 1987.
24. Nikolics K, Mason AJ, Szonyi E, et al: A prolactin inhibiting factor within the precursor for human gonadotropin-releasing hormone. Nature 316:511–517, 1985.
25. Enjalbert A, Moos F, Carbonnel L, et al: Prolactin inhibiting activity of dopamine-free subcellular fractions from rat mediobasal hypothalamus. Neuroendocrinology 24:147–161, 1977.
26. Wormald PJ, Abrahamson MJ, Seeburg PH, et al: Prolactin-inhibiting activity of GnRH associated peptide in cultured human pituitary cells. Clin Endocrinol 30:149–155, 1989.
27. Milton RCdeL, Wormmald PJ, Brandt W, et al: The delineation of a

decapeptide gonadotropin-releasing sequence in the carboxy-terminal extension of the human gonadotropin-releasing hormone precursor. J Biol Chem 261:16990–16997, 1986.

28. King JC, Anthony ELP, Fitzgerald DM, Stopa EG: Luteinizing hormone–releasing hormone neurons in human preoptic/hypothalamus: Differential intraneuronal localization of immunoreactive forms. J Clin Endocrinol Metab 60:88–97, 1985.

29. Silverman AJ, Krey LC, Zimmerman EA: A comparative study of the luteinizing hormone releasing hormone (LHRH) neuronal networks in mammals. Biol Reprod 20:98–110, 1979.

30. Shivers BD, Harlan RE, Morrell JI, Pfaff DW: Absence of oestradiol concentration in cell nuclei of LHRH-immunoreactive neurones. Nature 304:345–347, 1983.

31. Silverman AJ, Witkin JW: Synaptic interactions of luteinizing hormone–releasing hormone (LHRH) neurons in the guinea pig preoptic area. J Histochem Cytochem 33:69–72, 1985.

32. Ermisch A, Ruhle HJ, Klauschenz E, Kretzshmar R: On the blood-brain barrier to peptides—[H-3]GnRH accumulation by 18 regions of the rat brain and by anterior pituitary. Exp Clin Endocrinol 84:112–116, 1984.

33. Moss RL: Actions of hypothalamic-hypophysiotropic hormones on the brain. Annu Rev Physiol 41:617–631, 1979.

34. Reubi JC, Maurer R: Visualization of LHRH receptors in the rat brain. Eur J Pharmacol 106:453–454, 1984.

35. Schwanzelfukuda M, Pfaff DW: Origin of luteinizing-hormone–releasing hormone neurons. Nature 338:161–164, 1989.

36. Jennes L, Stumpf WE, Sheedy ME: Ultrastructural characterization of gonadotropin-releasing hormone (GnRH)–producing neurons. J Comp Neurol 232:534–547, 1985.

37. Schwanzelfukuda M, Bick D, Pfaff DW: Luteinizing-hormone–releasing hormone (LHRH)-expressing cells do not migrate normally in an inherited hypogonadal (Kallmann) syndrome. Mol Brain Res 6:311–326, 1989.

38. Lincoln DW, Fraser HM, Lincoln GA, et al: Hypothalamic pulse generators. Recent Prog Horm Res 41:369–419, 1985.

39. Rasmussen DD, Malven PV: Characterization of cephalic arteriovenous LH differences by continuous sampling in ovariectomized ewes. Neuroendocrinology 34:415–420, 1982.

40. Lincoln GA, Short RV: Seasonal breeding: Nature's contraceptive. Recent Prog Horm Res 36:1–52, 1980.

41. Martensz ND, Scaramuzzi RJ, Van Look PFA: The plasma concentrations of luteinizing hormone and follicle-stimulating hormone during anoestrus in ewes actively immunized against oestradiol-17β, oestrone or testosterone. J Endocrinol 81:261–269, 1979.

42. Ferin M, Dyrenfurth I, Cowchock S, et al: Active immunization of 17β-estradiol and its effects upon the reproductive cycle of the rhesus monkey. Endocrinology 94:765–776, 1974.

43. Martin GB, Scaramuzzi RJ, Henstridge JD: Effects of oestradiol, progesterone and androstenedione on the pulsatile secretion of luteinizing hormone in ovariectomized ewes during spring and autumn. J Endocrinol 96:181–193, 1983.

44. Lincoln GA: Central effects of photoperiod on reproduction in the ram revealed by the use of a testosterone clamp. J Endocrinol 103:233–241, 1984.

45. Dubey AK, Plant TM: Testosterone administration to ovariectomized female rhesus monkeys (Macaca mulatta) reduces the frequency of pulsatile luteinizing hormone secretion. Biol Reprod 32:1109–1115, 1985.

46. Reeves JJ, Arimura A, Schally AV: Changes in pituitary responsiveness to luteinizing hormone–releasing hormone (LH-RH) in anestrous ewes pretreated with estradiol benzoate. Biol Reprod 4:88–92, 1971.

47. Drouin J, Lagace L, Labrie F: Estradiol-induced increase in the LH responsiveness to LH-releasing hormone LHRH in rat pituitary cells in culture. Endocrinology 99:1477–1481, 1976.

48. Knobil E: The neuroendocrine control of the menstrual cycle. Recent Prog Horm Res 36:53–88, 1980.

49. Norman RL, Gliessman P, Lindstrom SA, et al: Reinitiation of ovulatory cycles in pituitary stalk sectioned rhesus monkeys: Evidence for a specific hypothalamic message for the preovulatory release of luteinizing hormone. Endocrinology 111:1874–1882, 1982.

50. Clarke IJ, Cummins JT: The temporal relationship between gonadotrophin releasing hormone (GnRH) and luteinising hormone (LH) secretion in ovariectomised ewes. Endocrinology 111:1737–1739, 1982.

51. Caraty A, Locatelli A: Effect of time after castration on secretion of LHRH and LH in the ram. J Reprod Fertil 82:263–269, 1988.

52. Barrell GK, Moenter SM, Caraty A, Karsch FJ: Seasonal changes of gonadotropin-releasing hormone secretion in the ewe. Biol Reprod 46:1130–1135, 1992.

53. Karsch FJ, Cummings JT, Thomas GB, Clarke IJ: Steroid feedback inhibition of pulsatile secretion of gonadotropin releasing hormone in the ewe. Biol Reprod 36:1207–1218, 1987.

54. Caraty A, Locatelli A, Delaleu B, et al: Gonadotropin-releasing-hormone (GnRH) agonists and GnRH antagonists do not alter endogenous GnRH secretion in short-term castrated rams. Endocrinology 127:2523–2529, 1990.

55. Moenter SM, Caraty A, Karsch FJ: The estradiol-induced surge of gonadotropin-releasing-hormone in the ewe. Endocrinology 127:2523–2529, 1990.

56. Moenter SM, Caraty A, Locatelli A, Karsch FJ: Pattern of gonadotropin-releasing hormone (GnRH) secretion leading up to ovulation in the ewe—existence of a preovulatory GnRH surge. Endocrinology 129:1175–1182, 1991.

57. Clarke IJ: Gonadotrophin-releasing hormone secretion (GnRH) in anoestrous ewes and the induction of GnRH surges by oestrogen. J Endocrinol 117:355–360, 1988.

58. Crowder ME, Nett TM: Pituitary content of gonadotropins and receptors for gonadotropin-releasing hormone (GnRH) and hypothalamic content of GnRH during the periovulatory period of the ewe. Endocrinology 114:234–239, 1984.

59. Keel BA, Grotjan HE Jr: Luteinizing hormone microheterogeneity. In Keel BA, Grotjan HE Jr (eds): Microheterogeneity of Glycoprotein Hormones. Boca Raton, FL, CRC Press, 1989, pp 149–184.

60. Hwan J-C, Freemena ME: A physiological role of luteinizing hormone release–inhibiting factor of hypothalamic origin. Endocrinology 121:1099–1103, 1987.

61. Crowley WF Jr, Filicori M, Spratt DI, Santoro NF: The physiology of gonadotropin-releasing hormone (GnRH) secretion in men and women. Recent Prog Horm Res 41:473–526, 1985.

62. Dyer RG, Mansfield S, Yates JO: Discharge of gonadotrophin-releasing hormone from the mediobasal part of the hypothalamus: Effect of stimulation frequency and gonadal steroids. Exp Brain Res 39:453–460, 1980.

63. Kawakami M, Uemura T, Hayashi R: Electrophysiological correlates of pulsatile gonadotropin release in rats. Neuroendocrinology 35:63–67, 1982.

64. Wilson RC, Kesner JS, Kaufman J-M, et al: Central electrophysiological correlates of pulsatile luteinizing hormone secretion in the rhesus monkey. Neuroendocrinology 39:256–260, 1984.

65. O'Byrne KT, Thalabard JC, Grosser PM, et al: Radiotelemetric monitoring of hypothalamic gonadotropin-releasing hormone pulse generator activity throughout the menstrual cycle of the rhesus monkey. Endocrinology 129:1207–1214, 1991.

66. Kesner JS, Wilson RC, Kaufman J-M, et al: Unexpected responses of the hypothalamic gonadotropin-releasing hormone pulse generator to physiological estradiol inputs in the absence of the ovary. Proc Natl Acad Sci USA 84:8745–8749, 1987.

67. Kaufman J-M, Kesner JS, Wilson RC, Knobil E: Electrophysiological manifestation of luteinizing hormone–releasing hormone pulse generator activity in the rhesus monkey: Influence of α-adrenergic and dopaminergic blocking drugs. Endocrinology 116:1327–1333, 1985.

68. Nishihara M, Himura H, Kimura F: Interactions between noradrenergic and opioid peptidergic systems in controlling the electrical activity of luteinizing hormone releasing hormone pulse generation in ovariectomized rats. Neuroendocrinology 54:321–326, 1991.

69. Moore RY, Bloom FE: Central catecholamine neuron systems: Anatomy and physiology of the norepinephrine and epinephrine systems. Annu Rev Neurosci 2:113–168, 1979.

70. Leranth CS, Segura LMG, Palkovits M, et al: The LHRH containing neural network in the preoptic area of the rat. Demonstration of LHRH containing nerve terminals in synaptic contact with LHRH neurons. Brain Res 345:332–336, 1985.

71. Wetzel WC, Valenca MM, Merchenthaler I, et al: Intrinsic pulsatile secretory activity of immortalized luteinizing-hormone–releasing hormone–secreting neurons. Proc Natl Acad Sci USA 89:4149–4153, 1992.

72. Eidne KA, McNiven AI, Taylor PL, et al: Functional expression of rat pituitary gonadotrophin-releasing hormone receptors in Xenopus oocytes. J Mol Endocrinol 1:R9–12, 1988.

73. Hopkins CR, Gregory H: Topographical localization of the receptors for luteinizing hormone–releasing hormone on the surface of dissociated pituitary cells. J Cell Biol 75:528–540, 1977.

74. Conn PM, Rogers DC, Seay SG: Biphasic regulation of the GnRH receptor by receptor microaggregation and intracellular Ca²⁺ levels. Mol Pharmacol 25:51–55, 1984.

75. Jacobs S, Chang K-J, Cuatrecasas P: Antibodies to purified insulin receptor have insulin-like activity. Science 200:1283–1284, 1978.

76. Conn PM, Rogers DC, Stewart JM, et al: Conversion of a gonadotropin releasing hormone antagonist to an agonist. Nature 296:653–655, 1982.
77. Chang JP, Morgan RO, Catt KJ: Dependence of secretory responses to gonadotropin-releasing hormone on diacylglycerol metabolism. Studies with diacylglycerol lipase inhibitor, RHC 80267. J Biol Chem 263:18614–18620, 1988.
78. Izumi S, Stojilkovic SS, Iida T, et al: Role of voltage-sensitive calcium channels in $[Ca^{2+}]_i$ and secretory responses to activators of protein kinase C in pituitary gonadotrophs. Biochem Biophys Res Commun 170:359–367, 1990.
79. Mason WT, Waring DW: Electrophysiological recordings from gonadotropes: Evidence for Ca^{2+} channels mediated by gonadotropin-releasing hormone. Neuroendocrinology 42:311–322, 1986.
80. Stojilkovic SS, Chang OP, Ngo D, Catt KJ: Evidence for a role of protein kinase C in luteinizing hormone synthesis and secretion. J Biol Chem 263:17307–17311, 1988.
81. Anderson L, Hoyland J, Mason WT, Eidne KA: Characterization of the gonadotropin-releasing hormone calcium response in single αT3-1 pituitary gonadotroph cells. Mol Cell Endocrinol 86:167–175, 1992.
82. Katt JA, Duncan JA, Herbon L, et al: The frequency of gonadotropin-releasing hormone stimulation determines the number of pituitary gonadotropin-releasing hormone receptors. Endocrinology 116:2113–2115, 1985.
83. Fink G, Chiappa SA, Aiyer MS: Priming effect of luteinizing hormone releasing factor elicited by preoptic stimulation and by intravenous infusion and multiple injections of the synthetic decapeptide. J Endocrinol 69:359–372, 1976.
84. Weiss J, Jameson JL, Burrin JM, Crowley WF Jr: Divergent responses of gonadotropin subunit messenger RNAs to continuous versus pulsatile gonadotropin-releasing hormone in vitro. Mol Endocrinol 4:557–564, 1990.
85. de Koning JA, van Dieten MJ, van Rees GP: Refractoriness of the pituitary gland after continuous exposure to luteinizing hormone releasing hormone. J Endocrinol 79:311–318, 1978.
86. Smith MA, Vale W: Desensitization to gonadotropin-releasing hormone observed in superfused pituitary cells on cytodex beads. Endocrinology 108:752–759, 1981.

14

Gonadotropins

WILLIAM R. MOYLE
ROBERT K. CAMPBELL

BRIEF REVIEW OF GONADOTROPIN ACTIONS

The glycoprotein hormones that control the production of male and female gametes as well as the sex steroid hormones are termed *gonadotropins.* They are members of a family that includes the pituitary hormones follitropin (also known as FSH or follicle-stimulating hormone), lutropin (also known as LH or luteinizing hormone), and thyrotropin (also known as TSH or thyroid-stimulating hormone). In addition, the placenta of some species produces choriogonadotropin (also known as CG or chorionic gonadotropin), a hormone most closely related in structure and function to LH.

The major effects of the gonadotropins on the physiological functions of the gonads have been known for years. As its name implies, in females the principal role of FSH is to stimulate follicle maturation. While the earliest stages of follicle development occur in the absence of FSH, development of a mature follicle capable of being ovulated requires FSH stimulation. The physiological rise and fall in FSH concentration during follicular development has a key role in selecting the follicle(s) that will be ovulated at midcycle in response to LH. FSH acts on granulosa cell FSH receptors to increase the conversion of androgens to estrogens and to induce cell proliferation.[1, 2] In response to estradiol and FSH, granulosa cells become more sensitive to FSH. As a result of this positive feedback mechanism, certain follicles develop more rapidly than the others that have resumed meiosis. Once established, these "dominant" follicles continue to develop despite the decline in FSH levels during the second half of the follicular phase (see Chs. 15, 116). Follicles that have failed to become more sensitive to FSH become atretic, a process of apoptosis, or programmed cell death.[3, 3a, 4] Many follicles that would become atretic can be "rescued" if they receive additional FSH stimulation, as may happen therapeutically during ovulation induction.[5] During the later stages of follicular maturation, FSH stimulation promotes the formation of the antrum and induction of granulosa cell LH receptors.[6] This prepares the follicle for the surge of LH that causes ovulation and differentiation of the granulosa and thecal cells into a corpus luteum.

In immature males FSH is required for initiation of spermatogenesis.[7] It binds to receptors on Sertoli cells and stimulates cAMP production, androgen metabolism, and growth.[8, 9] Although FSH interacts with Sertoli cells in sexually mature males, once spermatogenesis has been initi-

ated, it can be maintained in hypophysectomized animals by pharmacological amounts of testosterone.[7] Thus, the requirement for FSH in adults has not been as clear as that during puberty. New studies have shown that immunization of male monkeys against FSH resulted in a dramatic reduction in spermatogenesis and fertility, even though plasma testosterone levels remained normal.[10–12] Infertility was reversed when the titers of the antisera declined, which indicates that FSH is needed for spermatogenesis in adults having normal Leydig cell function.

The major effects of LH are to promote ovulation and luteinization of mature Graffian follicles and to stimulate steroidogenesis in interstitial cells. The latter include the thecal cells of the follicle and the Leydig cells of the testis. Actions of LH on thecal cells are needed to produce the androgens that serve as substrates for follicular estradiol synthesis.[6, 13] Thus, LH and FSH have synergistic roles in ovarian estradiol formation. LH may also have a role in maintaining progesterone production from the corpus luteum; however, this differs widely among species. In some animals the luteotropic actions of LH are mediated by estradiol, a steroid produced in response to the actions of LH on other parts of the ovary.[14] In males, androgens produced by Leydig cells in response to LH are needed for spermatogenesis and for development of male secondary sexual characteristics.

CG is a gonadotropin produced by the placenta that is most closely related in structure and activity to LH. It has been found during pregnancy in all primates but in only a few other animals, notably the horse, donkey, and zebra.[15] In humans, hCG secretion begins about the time of implantation and reaches a maximal level before the end of the first trimester. During this time it is responsible for maintaining pregnancy by prolonging the life of the corpus luteum and for stimulating luteal progesterone synthesis. Luteal steroidogenesis remains elevated for only about one month despite the continued presence of high levels of hCG throughout pregnancy. In monkeys CG induces the corpus luteum to secrete progesterone for an even shorter time.[16] The placenta is responsible for progesterone synthesis throughout the remainder of pregnancy.

A large proportion of hCG is excreted in urine and, until recently, the urine of pregnant women has been the only practical source of the hormone. Naturally occurring β-subunit fragments of hCG have also been detected in serum and in urine. One of the more abundant of these, termed the β-*core fragment,* is an analogue of hCG β-subunit that lacks parts of the N-terminus (residues 1 to 5), C-terminus (residues 93 to 145), and residues 41 to 54 from the central portion of the β-subunit.[17] This fragment is unable to combine with the α-subunit, and its function is unknown. It has been associated with cervical carcinoma and may be useful as a tumor marker.[18, 19] Other proteins that are likely to be metabolites of hCG have also been found, but unlike the β-core fragment, these are missing only a few residues from the β-subunit near Gly47 and Val48.[20] Because these metabolites contain both α- and β-subunits, they are readily detected with most anti-hCG monoclonal antibodies and may interfere with hCG assays.[18]

Human menopausal gonadotropins (hMG) are mixtures of LH, FSH, and their metabolites isolated from the urine of menopausal women. They are found subsequent to reduced ovarian function after menopause, when plasma levels of LH and FSH become elevated. Like hCG, a high percentage of these hormones is excreted in urine. The major use of hMG has been in stimulating follicle development during ovulation induction or in ovarian hyperstimulation before in vitro fertilization,[21, 22] or GIFT.[23]

Until recently the only sources of gonadotropins were the anterior pituitary gland and urine. The genes and cDNA for both subunits of the glycoprotein hormones have now been cloned from many species and have enabled production of gonadotropins by cultured mammalian cells. This permits synthesis of large quantities of hormones and analogs. Recombinant DNA–derived hormones are in clinical trials and are expected to be available for treatment of fertility disorders within the next few years.[24]

HORMONE STRUCTURE AND FUNCTION

FSH, LH, and CG have many important current and potential clinical uses. Gonadotropins are used to induce fertility in men and women.[5, 21, 25] Measurements of gonadotropin levels are routinely employed to diagnose pregnancy and have been used to detect fetal loss prior to menses.[26] Gonadotropin measurements may also be important for diagnosing ectopic pregnancy[27] and gonadotropin-secreting tumors.[19] In some cases neutralization of hCG has been proposed as a means to disrupt tubal pregnancy[28] or as a cancer therapy.[29, 30] Immunization against gonadotropins has long been known to cause infertility, and appropriate antigenic gonadotropin analogues might be useful in contraceptive vaccines.[11, 31, 32] The rational design of new reagents that induce ovulation, stimulate spermatogenesis, and inhibit fertility, or that can be used as specific immunogens, requires detailed knowledge of the structures and functions of the hormones. Thus, understanding the relationship between the structures and functions of the gonadotropins has several potential practical applications as well as theoretical interest.

FSH, LH, and CG are structurally related glycoproteins composed of a common α-subunit and a hormone-specific β-subunit. FSH and LH have similar mechanisms of action involving binding to specific receptors and inducing the synthesis of cAMP or possibly other second messengers.[33] The subunits of the hormones can be dissociated at low pH or by agents that disrupt hydrogen bonds (e.g., urea), indicating that they are not covalently linked.[34] The confor-

mations of the subunits are altered slightly during dissociation; they can be recognized by most, but not all, monoclonal antibodies that bind to the intact hormones. Purified free subunits of the gonadotropins usually have little endocrine activity relative to that of the intact hormones in most in vitro or in vivo assays, and much of the activity of the isolated subunits appears to be due to contamination with intact hormone. One possible exception to this generalization is the ability of free α-subunit to stimulate prolactin synthesis from decidual cells.[35] When α- and β-subunits are combined, the endocrine activity of the resulting heterodimer corresponds to that of the hormone from which the β-subunit is derived. While major differences are found throughout the sequences of the β-subunits, only a small region of the β-subunit appears to control receptor-binding specificity.[36]

Glycoprotein gonadotropins have been found in all five vertebrate classes. In mammals the α-subunit is encoded by a single gene that is expressed in the anterior pituitary gland in every species and in the placenta of primates and equines.[37, 38] Some fish appear to make at least two α-subunits.[39] The highly conserved α-subunits contain 10 identically positioned cysteines that are oxidized to form five disulfide bonds (Fig. 14–1). In addition, most α-subunits contain two asparagine-linked oligosaccharides corresponding to those of the human protein at residues 52 and 78.

Differences in the primary sequences of FSH, LH, and TSH β-subunits (Fig. 14–2) are responsible for the ability of the β-subunit to confer the biological activity unique to each hormone. The LH and FSH β-subunits are each encoded by a separate gene, whereas in primates the CG β-subunits are encoded by as many as six genes that may have evolved by gene duplication.[37, 40] All six appear to be expressed in the placenta and some are alternately spliced.[41] These CG genes may also be expressed at a low level in the pituitary.[42] Preparations of hLH have been reported to contain hCG; cultured pituitary cells make small amounts of hCG, and hCG appears to be released in a pulsatile manner in normal adults. Trace amounts of hCG have also been found in the urine of menopausal women.[43] The horse has only a single gene that functions in the pituitary and placenta to make LH and CG β-subunits and the only differences between the two proteins are found in their carbohydrate moieties.[44, 44a]

The disulfide bonds are crucial for gonadotropin activity. Treatment of the gonadotropins with reducing agents disrupts the structures of both subunits and causes them to dissociate. When reduced α-subunit is oxidized, it regains its ability to combine with the β-subunit, suggesting that it also regains its tertiary structure.[34]

Several regions of the gonadotropins are thought to influence the interactions of the hormones with their receptors, but the hormone residues that make contact with the receptors have not been identified. Mutagenesis studies have suggested that lysine 91[45] of the α-subunit and aspartate 99[46] of the β-subunit have crucial roles in signal transduction and, by inference, in receptor interaction. A naturally occurring inactive analog has been identified wherein Gln54 is replaced by arginine, suggesting that this region may also interact with the receptor.[47]

Some synthetic gonadotropin fragments bind to LH and FSH receptors and a few have signal transduction activity.[48–51] The most active peptide that mimicked FSH[52, 53] contained

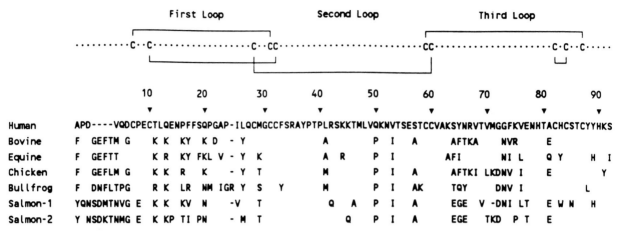

FIGURE 14–1. **Amino acid sequences of selected vertebrate glycoprotein hormone α-subunits.** This figure compares the sequences of the α-subunits from three mammals (human[135], bovine[136], equine[137]), one bird (chicken[138]), one amphibian (bullfrog[139]), and one fish (salmon[39]) to illustrate the conservation between the proteins. Sequences for reptilian α-subunits have not yet been determined. Residues identical to the human have been omitted. Lines illustrate the locations of the disulfide bonds. Numbering is the same as the human α-subunit and is that used throughout the text. The abbreviations are: A, ala; C, cys; D, asp; E, glu; F, phe; G, gly; H, his; I, ile; K, lys; L, leu; M, met; N, asn; P, pro; Q , gln; R, arg; S, ser; T, thr; V, val; W, trp; Y, tyr. The dashes (-) refer to missing residues.

residues derived from both the α- and β-subunits including Thr-Arg-Asp-Leu (hFSH β-subunit residues 34–37), Thr-Asp-Ser-Asp-Ser (hFSH β-subunit residues 92,88–91), and Ser-Arg-Ala-Tyr (hFSH α-subunit residues 34–37). This peptide stimulated rat Sertoli cell cAMP production with an ED50 of about 10^{-7} M.[52, 53] Surprisingly, residues Thr-Arg-Asp-Leu were not required for full-length hCG analogues to bind with high affinity to FSH receptors.[36] In addition, chimeras of hCG have been made that bind to FSH receptors and induce signal transduction nearly as well as FSH, even though they lack both the Thr-Arg-Asp-Leu and Asp-Ser-Asp-Ser regions (Campbell and Moyle, unpublished observations). The most active contiguous synthetic hCG fragment corresponded to the loop formed by residues between the fifth and sixth cysteines. Peptides derived from this region of the molecule bound to LH receptors and stimulated steroidogenesis at concentrations near 10^{-5} M.[51] Surprisingly, substitutions of FSH sequences within this region of hCG had no effect on its ability to bind to LH receptors or to stimulate testosterone synthesis.[36]

The residues found in active synthetic peptides have been assumed to be the parts of LH and FSH which contact the receptor. However, the synthetic peptides have very low affinities for the receptors. Further, they do not account for the activities of hormone analogues that bind to receptors with the same affinities as LH and FSH. Thus, models based on interpretations of data obtained using synthetic peptides appear to be premature. X-ray crystallographic structures of the gonadotropins and their receptors would provide the best models to explain their functions. Although both deglycosylated and desialylated hCG have been crystallized,[54, 55] no high resolution structure is yet available for any gonadotropin or its subunits.

FUNCTIONS OF THE OLIGOSACCHARIDES

N-linked (Fig. 14–3) and O-linked oligosaccharides have been found in both the α- and β-subunits (see review by Baenziger and Green[56]). The N-linked sugars appear to have roles in the clearance of the proteins from serum and in initiating signal transduction once the hormones have reached their receptors. The O-linked sugars normally found only on the C-terminus of a few β-subunits including hCG appear to extend the circulating half-lives of the hormones. While O-linked glycosylation of the α-subunit at Thr39 has also been observed, it is not found on the α-subunit isolated from LH, FSH, or hCG, and it can prevent subunit combination.[57]

The half-lives of LH and FSH are influenced by their oligosaccharides and differ depending on the hormone and the species from which it is obtained. Hormones with oligosaccharides terminating in galactose or galactosamine or that are sulfated have shortened plasma half-lives.[58, 59] They are cleared from the circulation by binding to liver parenchymal cell receptors.[56] Clearance of the sulfated hormones is controlled by a hepatic reticuloendothelial cell that recognizes *N*-acetylgalactosamine sulfate, the terminal sugar usually found on LH.[60] Owing to the more rapid clearance of sulfated hormones than sialylated hormones, the circulating half-life of a gonadotropin is largely proportional to the amount of sialic acid in the preparation being tested[58, 61] and is decreased following neuraminidase treatment.[62]

The oligosaccharides of LH and FSH are primarily terminated by sulfate and sialic acid, respectively (Fig. 14–3). Approximately 40 per cent of hLH oligosaccharides terminate in sulfate or are neutral, 25 per cent end in both sulfate and sialic acid, and 35 per cent are sialylated.[56] Bovine and ovine LH have much less sialylic acid. Comparable values for hFSH are 12 per cent, 5 per cent, and 83 per cent, respectively.[56] The higher content of sialic acid in hFSH contributes to its half-life being longer than that of LH.[56, 60] Because neither hLH nor hFSH are exclusively sulfated nor sialylated, hormone species with different half-lives are present in both pituitary LH and FSH preparations. Further, the mode of hormone clearance is complex, with much of the hormone being metabolized by the liver or excreted in urine. The half-life of plasma LH is generally considered to be 20 minutes[63] but may be shorter or longer

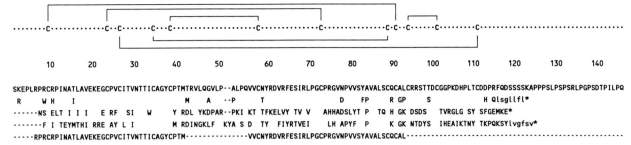

FIGURE 14–2. **Amino acid sequences of the β-subunits of the human glycoprotein hormones and the β-subunit fragment.** The sequences are aligned such that the highly conserved cysteine residues are in register and the positions of the disulfide bonds are illustrated by the horizontal lines. TSH is unique in that it has two additional amino acids between the fifth and sixth cysteines. The only known variation in the locations of the cysteines occurs in the protein from the chum salmon, in which the cysteine normally found at residue 26 is located at residue 5. This may represent a compensational pair of modifications and suggests that residue 5 and residue 26 may be near one another and residues 110 in the β subunit. Only a few of the residues besides the cysteines are conserved. These include the aspartate at residue 99, which may have a role in hormone efficacy.[46] The lower case letters at the ends of the sequences refer to residues that are not present in the secreted proteins but that may influence storage in secretion granules. The abbreviations are as in Figure 14–1 except that hCG-FRAG refers to the hCG β-fragment and "*" refers to a termination codon. The numbering system used is that for hCG β-subunit.

depending on the procedure used to measure it. A range of between 2 and 50 minutes has been reported,[58, 64] and a small fraction of LH may survive even longer.[63] The short half-life of LH is consistent with the observation that hourly LH release from the anterior pituitary during the early and midfollicular phases does not lead to an increase in plasma LH levels. Values ranging from one to four hours for the half-life of FSH have been reported.[61, 65, 66] The longer half-life of FSH accounts for much of the difficulty in observing FSH pulses at the start of the menstrual cycle when FSH levels are rising due to the hourly release of FSH into the circulation.[67]

Values for the circulating half-lives of the placental gonadotropins hCG[63, 68–70] and equine CG[15] range from 0.1 to 2 days and are greater than those of the pituitary gonadotropins. This is not surprising, since hCG and equine CG have a higher content of sialic acid due to the inability of the placenta to make sulfated glycoproteins. In addition, factors other than the composition of the N-linked oligosaccharides also contribute to the half-life of hCG. The C-terminal extension found on hCG but missing in LH contains the O-linked oligosaccharides and has long been presumed to be responsible for the longer half-life of hCG. This idea was supported by the recent observation that the protein made by fusing the C-terminus of hCG to the FSH β-subunit had a longer half-life than FSH.[71] Nonetheless, the half-life of hCG has long been known to exceed that of its α- or β-subunits by 10- to 20-fold.[70] Thus, in spite of the importance of the oligosaccharides and the C-terminal extension, other factors contribute to the stability of hCG in serum.

In addition to their involvement in the stability of the circulating hormones, the oligosaccharides have a role in signal transduction. The ability of deglycosylated LH or FSH to elicit signal transduction is proportional to its content of carbohydrate. Following deglycosylation, the efficacy of the gonadotropins is reduced in vitro[72] and gonadotropins that have been deglycosylated completely have low activity when assayed in vitro. Studies in which the glycosylation signals have been selectively removed from the human α-subunit have shown that the oligosaccharide on Asn52 is the most important for signal transduction.[73]

Those on the β-subunit do not seem to have a major role in eliciting a hormonal signal.

GONADOTROPIN SYNTHESIS

Synthesis of the gonadotropins begins with the transcription of the genes in the nucleus. Several upstream regulatory elements in the genes for each gonadotropin subunit have been identified.[38, 74–82] These mediate cyclic nucleotide, steroid, and GnRH control of gonadotropin gene transcription. In addition, elements that confer placental and pituitary regulation have also been found.[38]

Much of what is known about the early steps in the synthesis of gonadotropins is based on analogy to the synthesis of other secreted glycoproteins and has been reviewed by Baenziger and Green.[56] The mRNA for each subunit encodes a leader peptide that ensures that the α- and β-subunits will be translocated into the lumen of the endoplasmic reticulum during synthesis. During translocation high mannose oligosaccharides are transferred from a dolichol intermediate to Asn residues in the sequence Asn-X-Thr/Ser, where X is any amino acid except proline. The subunits fold in the lumen of the endoplasmic reticulum, a region of the cell known to have a high oxidizing capacity and an elevated ratio of oxidized/reduced glutathione, which facilitates disulfide bond formation.[83] The α-subunit folds rapidly and all five disulfide bonds appear to be formed within a few minutes. The β-subunit folds slowly and combines with the α-subunit in the endoplasmic reticulum.[84] The order of disulfide bond formation appears to be 34-88, 38-57, 23-72, 9-90, 93-100, and 26-110 with the last disulfide bonds forming after the α- and β-subunits have combined.[84a–c] Folding may be assisted by several heat shock proteins acting as chaperonins. The N-linked oligosaccharides also appear to contribute to efficient subunit folding and heterodimer assembly. Only a portion of the subunits appears to be assembled into mature heterodimers,[84] and both the pituitary and placenta secrete uncombined free subunits.[85, 86]

Like those of all glycoproteins, the oligosaccharides of the gonadotropins are modified during passage of the pro-

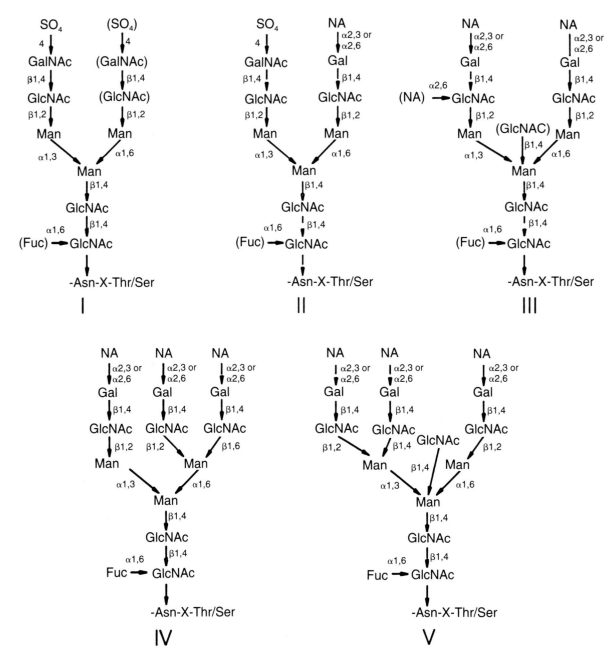

FIGURE 14–3. **Structures of the oligosaccharide of the glycoprotein hormones.** Residues in each of these structures listed in parentheses are missing in some forms of the hormones. Those forms illustrated as I or II are found predominantly in LH. FSH contains those in types II and III. hCG contains type III. Note also that the link between the sialic acid and galactose made by the placenta is primarily 2,3 whereas that made by the anterior pituitary is primarily 2,6. The abbreviations are: Glc, glucose; Man, mannose; Gal, galactose; GlcNAc, glucosamine; GalNAc, galactosamine; SA, sialic acid; Fuc, fucose. For a more complete description see the review by Baenziger and Green.[56]

teins through the endoplasmic reticulum and Golgi apparatus (Fig. 14–4). Glycosylation is completed by a process in which some sugars (primarily glucose and mannose) are trimmed and others are added (*N*-acetylglucosamine, *N*-acetylgalactosamine, and/or galactose, and sialic acid) as the protein is shuttled from the lumen of the endoplasmic reticulum through the cis-, medial-, and trans-Golgi compartments and into the trans-Golgi network, from which it is secreted or stored in granules.

The final processing of the oligosaccharides depends on one or more signals in the α- and β-subunits that determine which oligosaccharide chains are substrates for *N*-acetylgalactosamine transferase and subsequent sulfate cap-

ping.[87] This occurs at a branch point in hormone glycosylation. If *N*-acetylgalactosamine is added to the oligosaccharide chain in the medial-Golgi, it will be sulfated in the trans-Golgi. Once galactose is added in the trans-Golgi, it can no longer be sulfated and will become sialylated (Fig. 14–4). A putative recognition motif (Pro-X-Arg/Lys, where X is a hydrophobic amino acid) for pituitary *N*-acetylgalactosamine transferase has been identified in the α-subunit and the β-subunits of hCG and hLH.[88] This enzyme, found in the anterior pituitary but not the placenta, enables the pituitary to make sulfated gonadotropins. Thus, free α-subunit and hLH made by the anterior pituitary are sulfated while free α-subunit and hCG made by the placenta

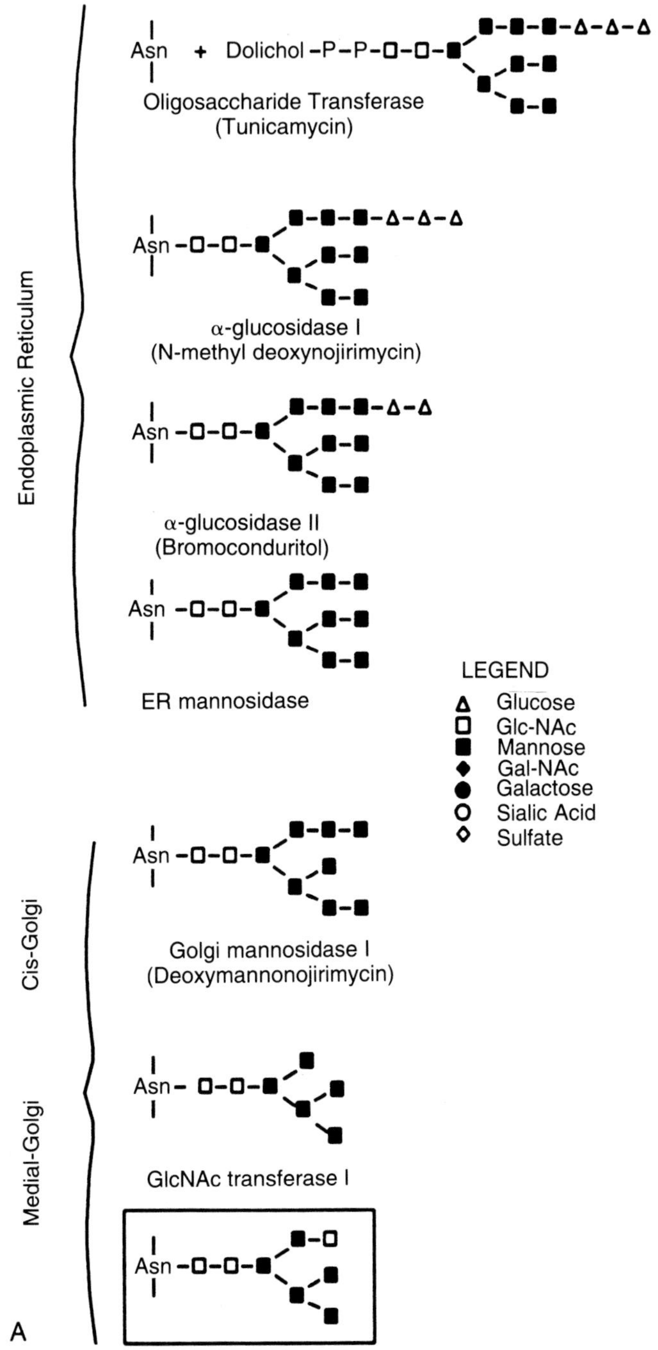

FIGURE 14–4. **Compartmentalization of hormone glycosylation.** *A,* Transfer of an oligosaccharide from dolichol to asparagine residues of the α- and β-subunits of the gonadotropins occurs as the subunits are synthesized and are transported into the lumen of the endoplasmic reticulum. While they are still in the endoplasmic reticulum, the subunits fold and combine to form the heterodimers. At least three glucoses are removed before the proteins are transferred from the endoplasmic reticulum to the *cis*-Golgi for further processing. Most glycoproteins appear to be subjected to similar oligosaccharide trimming to give the intermediate containing five mannose and three *N*-acetylglucosamine sugars (i.e., the structure illustrated in the box).

Illustration continued on following page

are not sulfated even though the α-subunit and both β-subunits contain the putative *N*-acetylgalactosamine transferase signal. Because the free α-subunit secreted from the anterior pituitary is sulfated and has a short half-life, it has been a useful tool to study pulsatile LHRH secretion.[89] Although LH and FSH are made in the same cell,[56] the oligosaccharides of both the α- and β-subunits of FSH are sialylated. When it combines with the α-subunit, the FSH β-subunit appears to obscure the Pro-Leu-Arg sequence

found in the α-subunit, thereby preventing its recognition by *N*-acetylgalactosamine transferase and subsequent sulfation.[87]

Following glycosylation, the pituitary hormones enter the regulated pathway where they are stored in secretion granules and released in response to GnRH. Although LH and FSH are made in the same cell, they are stored in different secretion granules.[56] Secretion of the gonadotropins from the anterior pituitary is highly regulated (see Ch.

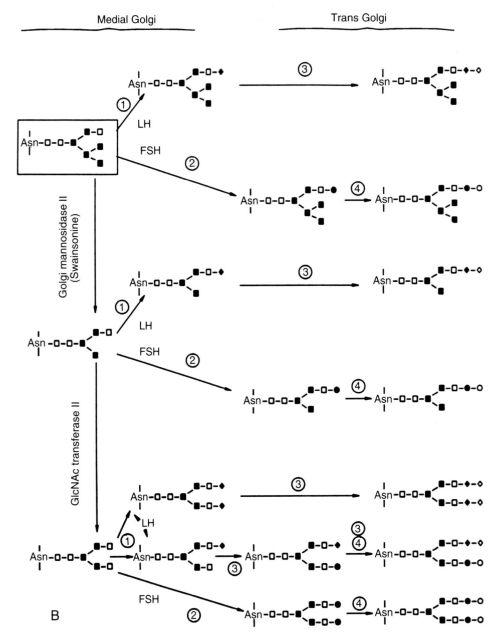

FIGURE 14–4 *Continued B,* Glycosylation of LH and FSH differ beginning in the medial-Golgi, where LH is subjected to the actions of *N*-acetylgalactosamine-transferase (enzyme 1). Sulfate is added in the trans-Golgi to oligosaccharides terminating in GalNAc by the GalNAc sulfotransferase (enzyme 3). Galactose residues are added to oligosaccharides on FSH in the trans-Golgi by galactose transferase (enzyme 2) and finally sialic acid is added by the sialyltransferase (enzyme 4).

13). In contrast to hLH and hFSH, hCG is not stored in the placenta and appears to be released as soon as it is made. Portions of the proteins that determine whether they will enter the regulated or the constitutive pathway have not been identified. Originally, the hydrophobic tail on the hLH β-subunit was thought to make the major contribution to differences in the regulation of their secretion.[90] However, in transfected cells capable of either constitutive or regulated secretion, both hLH and hCG are secreted by the regulated pathway.[91]

Some of the steps in oligosaccharide processing may not proceed to completion or are directed down a particular pathway by the order in which the sugars are removed and/or added to the oligosaccharide. For example, if *N*-acetylgalactosamine transferase acts prior to mannosidase

II, the action of mannosidase II will be blocked[56] and the oligosaccharides will contain only a single antenna. The extent and nature of the processing depends on several factors including steroids of GnRH. The unequal processing of the oligosaccharides leads to numerous hormone isoforms, which differ in size, charge, half-life, and receptor binding activity. While the majority of the oligosaccharides are biantennary, some are triantennary or bisected.[56, 92, 93] Some isoforms of the gonadotropins appear to have greater activity than others. For example, the more highly sialylated forms of hFSH are more acidic than less sialylated forms. Increased sialylation is associated with increased half-life but decreased receptor binding potency.[72, 94] Changes in the pattern of gonadotropin glycosylation might influence the biological activity of the hormones during endocrine regulation of the gonads,[95, 96] although to some extent the longer half-life of the more acidic forms compensates for their lower receptor-binding activity.[59] Nonetheless, in spite of the potential roles that hormone isoforms might have in endocrine regulation and the extensive studies designed to elucidate these roles, the physiological importance of gonadotropin isoforms has yet to be established.

GONADOTROPIN MEASUREMENT

In vivo and in vitro assays have been devised to quantify all the gonadotropins. In vivo assays are influenced by the stability of the hormones in serum as well as their ability to bind to receptors and initiate signal transduction. Thus, although they are less sensitive and more difficult to perform than most other assays, in vivo assays are useful for determining hormone potency. Bioassays for FSH are most often based on its ability to increase the weight of the ovary in hCG-stimulated immature rats.[97] In vivo bioassays of LH rely on its ability to increase testicular androgen synthesis, which results in an increase in the weight of the ventral prostate.[98] Other common in vivo assays for LH depend on its ability to promote the loss of ascorbic acid from the ovary[99] or to induce ovulation.[58]

In vitro bioassays are usually much more sensitive than in vivo bioassays. Despite the fact that in vitro assays are not influenced by hormone clearance, gonadotropins and gonadotropin analogues that are found to be active in vitro can be expected to be active in vivo, particularly if they are produced in mammalian cells known to make oligosaccharides containing sialic acid. In vitro bioassays for FSH are often based on its ability to enhance granulosa cell steroidogenesis, synthesis of plasminogen activator, or Sertoli cell cAMP accumulation.[8] The most sensitive in vitro bioassays for LH are based on its ability to induce androgen biosynthesis in isolated Leydig cells.[100] Steroidogenesis assays are sufficiently sensitive to quantify serum levels of LH and FSH. They have the disadvantage of being tedious and time-consuming and are usually not considered suitable for routine use in monitoring hormone levels.

Radioimmunoassays (RIA's) were the earliest immunoassays for gonadotropins that enabled plasma concentrations to be determined routinely.[101, 102] More recently RIA have been superseded by monoclonal antibody–based "sandwich" immunoassays.[103] Because they are not based on the competition of a ligand for an antibody, sandwich immunoassays are more sensitive than RIA. Indeed, the sensitivity of the sandwich assays permitted analysis of hCG levels before the expected menses and provided an assessment of fetal wastage during early pregnancy.[26]

While immunoassays are fast and highly sensitive, they do not necessarily monitor the biological activities of gonadotropins. Several laboratories have shown that in vitro biological assays of serum LH and FSH usually yield greater values than radioimmunoassays when pituitary hormones are employed as standards.[104, 105] The biological and immunological activity of the gonadotropins is known to vary depending on other endocrine factors, particularly steroid hormone levels and the amount of GnRH stimulation.[106–108] The reasons that unequal values are obtained in these assays are not known. Differences in the glycosylation of the

circulating and pituitary hormones could account for part of the enhanced biological activity found in serum. Another reason for the discrepancy might be that serum contains hormones and other factors that can modify the response to hormones.[8, 109] While the exact identities of these factors remain unknown, several hormones including IGF1 have been shown to influence the response to FSH.[6]

Radioligand receptor assays (RLA) have been employed to circumvent the dependence of RIA on antibodies and the difficulties of performing in vitro bioassays. These are performed similar to radioimmunoassays except that a receptor is used in place of an antibody.[110] While these have the potential ability to detect the receptor-binding region of the hormones and provide a more accurate index of biological activity, they will also detect deglycosylated hormones that may be inactive. In addition to this type of competition assay, bioassays have been devised in which hormone receptor complexes are detected using antibodies to the hormones.[111] These assays have been termed *bioimmunoradiometric assays* (bio-IRMA). The major limitation to RLA and bio-IRMA has been the availability of hormone receptors. Now that the hormone receptors have been cloned, these assays may become more widespread. In addition, by designing cell lines that express large numbers of recombinant receptors, simple sensitive bioassays that monitor binding and signal transduction are being designed.[112, 112a]

GONADOTROPIN RECEPTORS

The cloning of the receptors for LH and FSH in 1989 and 1990[113–115] was a major milestone in gonadotropin physiology. On the basis of their amino acid sequences, the receptors were recognized to be members of the G-coupled protein receptor superfamily. This had been expected since they have long been known to use cAMP as a second messenger.[116] According to their amino acid sequences, the glycoprotein hormone receptors appear to have a large extracellular N-terminus, a transmembrane domain composed of 7 hydrophobic α-helices, and a small cytoplasmic C-terminus. Support for this model comes from the abilities of antireceptor antibodies to recognize the N-terminal domain on the cell surface and the C-terminal domain within the cell.[117]

The genes for the FSH and LH receptors contain 10 and 11 exons, respectively, and the largest (i.e., exons 10 or 11) encodes a small portion of the N-terminus and the entire transmembrane domain and C-terminus.[118–120] The N-terminus of all the receptors forms the high-affinity hormone-binding site and is formed from leucine repeats of unknown function.[113] These repeats correspond to the locations of many exon/intron boundaries.[118, 119] Several alternate spliced transcripts of the LH receptor are known, including those in which portions of exon 11 are missing.[115, 118] These encode analogues lacking the transmembrane domain, and the roles of these proteins in signal transduction are unknown. If they were secreted, they would inhibit hormone action by competing with the full-length receptor for binding LH or CG. Nonetheless, while spliced variants lacking the transmembrane domain might encode soluble receptors,[121] most studies have failed to find significant amounts of these binding sites outside the cell.[122-125] Indeed, the N-terminus is nearly always retained in an intracellular compartment when attempts are made to express it without the transmembrane domain.

Due to the similarity in the gonadotropin receptors and those for the catecholamines, gonadotropin-induced signal transduction is likely to be similar to that of the catecholamines. Presumably this involves the binding of the ligand in a pocket created by the transmembrane domain, which leads to a change in its shape.[126] This results in an alteration of the transmembrane domain that enables its cytoplasmic surface to interact with G proteins. The LH receptor and FSH receptor are known to interact with G proteins; however, the locations of residues that are important for this have not been identified. By analogy to other G protein–coupled receptors, the third and possibly other cytoplasmic loops may be involved.[127] The transmembrane domain of the LH receptor has relatively low affinity for hCG,[128] an observation consistent with this model. Nonetheless, other models are also possible. Both the LH and FSH receptors have been proposed to be homodimers or possibly become part of a larger complex,[129, 130] and it is conceivable that this is needed for signal transduction. The glycoprotein hormones have also been reported to have disulfide isomerase activity.[131] It is also conceivable that the hormones might induce signal transduction by altering one or more of the disulfide bonds in the receptor.

Most LH receptors have been found in the gonads; however, they have also been detected in other tissues,[132-134] including the uterus. While their role in uterine function is unknown, they might act as receptors for hCG throughout pregnancy. This may also explain the reason that hCG is secreted at high levels throughout pregnancy.

CONCLUSIONS

The development of gonadotropin expression systems and the cloning of the hormone receptors have made major contributions to our knowledge of gonadotropin structure and function. Detailed studies of the structure and function of both the hormones and their receptors are now possible. These developments have permitted the design and initial testing of gonadotropin analogues that may have clinical utility.[36, 71] Improved bioassay systems may also be available soon.[130] New data on the structures and processing of the oligosaccharides should lead to a better understanding of hormone secretion and turnover.[56, 60, 88] Progress in crystallizing hCG has also been made and when a crystal structure is available, it may enable the design of more effective agonists and antagonists, including active peptides and hormone mimics. It may also facilitate the design of more potent immunogens that will be useful for contraception.

REFERENCES

1. Tonetta SA, DiZerega GS: Intragonadal regulation of follicular maturation. Endocr Rev 10:205–229, 1989.
2. DiZerega GS, Hodgen GD: Folliculogenesis in the primate ovarian cycle. Endocr Rev 2:27–49, 1981.
3. Tilly JL, Kowalski KI, Johnson AL, Hsueh AJ: Involvement of apoptosis in ovarian follicular atresia and postovulatory regression. Endocrinology 129:2799–2801, 1991.
3a. Tilly JL, Kowalski KI, Schomberg DW, Hseuh AJ: Apoptosis in atretic ovarian follicles is associated with selective decreases in messenger ribonucleic acid transcripts for gonadotropin receptors and cytochrome P450 aromatase. Endocrinology 131:1670–1676, 1992.
4. Raff MC: Social controls on cell survival and cell death. Nature 356:397–400, 1992.
5. Hillier SG: Ovarian manipulation with pure gonadotropins. J Endocrinol 127:1–4, 1990.
6. Hsueh AJW, Adashi EY, Jones PBC, Welsh TH Jr: Hormonal regulation of the differentiation of cultured ovarian granulosa cells. Endocr Rev 5:76–127, 1984.
7. Steinberger E: Hormonal control of mammalian spermatogenesis. Physiol Rev 51:1–22, 1971.
8. Wang C: Bioassays of follicle stimulating hormone. Endocr Rev 9:374–377, 1988.
9. Heckert LL, Griswold MD: Expression of follicle-stimulating hormone receptor mRNA in rat testes and Sertoli cells. Mol Endocrinol 5:670–677, 1991.
10. Aravindan GR, Ravindranath N, Moudgal NR: Use of DNA flowcytometry in assessing gonadotropin regulation of spermatogenesis in monkeys. In Moudgal NR, Yoshinaga K, Rao AJ, Adiga PR (eds): Perspectives in Primate Reproductive Biology. New Delhi, Wiley Eastern Limited, 1991, pp 189–199.
11. Moudgal NR, Ravindranath N, Murthy GS, et al: On the development of a male contraceptive vaccine. In Moudgal NR, Yoshinaga K, Rao AJ, Adiga PR (eds): Perspectives in Primate Reproductive Biology. New Delhi, Wiley Eastern Limited, 1991, pp 297–306.
12. Moudgal NR: The immunobiology of follicle-stimulating hormone and inhibin: Prospects for a contraceptive vaccine. Curr Opin Immunol 2:736–742, 1990.
13. Erickson GF, Magoffin DA, Dyer CA, Hofeditz C: The ovarian androgen producing cells: a review of structure/functional relationships. Endocr Rev 6:371–399, 1985.
14. Keyes PL, Wiltbank MC: Endocrine regulation of the corpus luteum. Annu Rev Physiol 50:465–482, 1988.
15. Murphy BD, Martinuk SD: Equine chorionic gonadotropin. Endocr Rev 12:27–44, 1991.
16. Hodgen GD, Itskovitz J: Recognition and maintenance of pregnancy. In Knobil E, Neill JD (eds): The Physiology of Reproduction. New York, Raven Press, 1988, pp 1995–2021.
17. Birken S, Armstrong EG, Kolks MA, et al: Structure of the human chorionic gonadotropin beta-subunit fragment from pregnancy urine. Endocrinology 123:572–583, 1988.
18. Cole LA, Hussa RO, Rao CVO: Discordant synthesis and secretion of human chorionic gonadotropin and subunits by cervical carcinoma cells. Cancer Res 41:1615–1619, 1981.
19. Hussa RO: The Clinical Marker hCG. New York, Praeger Publishers, 1987.
20. Cole LA, Kardana A, Andrade-Gordon P, et al: The heterogeneity of human chorionic gonadotropin (hCG). III. The occurrence and biological and immunological activities of nicked hCG. Endocrinology 129:1559–1567, 1991.
21. Gemzell C: Induction of ovulation with human gonadotropins. Recent Prog Horm Res 21:179–198, 1965.
22. Corsan GH, Kemmann E: The role of superovulation with menotropins in ovulatory infertility: A review. Fertil Steril 55:468–475, 1991.
23. Asch RH, Ellsworth LR, Balmaceda JP, Wong PC: Pregnancy following translaparoscopic gamete intrafallopian transfer (GIFT). Lancet 2:1034, 1984.
24. DeCherney AH, Naftolin F: Recombinant DNA-derived human luteinizing hormone: Basic science rapidly applied to clinical medicine. JAMA 259:3313–3314, 1988.
25. Haidl G, Schill WB: Guidelines for drug treatment of male infertility. Drugs 41:60–68, 1991.
26. Wilcox AJ, Weinberg CR, O'Connor JF, et al: Incidence of early loss of pregnancy. N Engl J Med 319:189–194, 1988.
27. Emancipator K, Bock JL, Burke MD: Diagnosis of ectopic pregnancy by the rate of increase of choriogonadotropin in serum: Diagnostic criteria compared. Clin Chem 36:2097–2101, 1990.
28. Frydman R, Fernandez H, Troalen F, et al: Phase I clinical trial of monoclonal anti-human chorionic gonadotropin antibody in women with an ectopic pregnancy. Fertil Steril 52:734–738, 1989.
29. Kumar S, Talwar GP, Biswas DK: Necrosis and inhibition of growth of human lung tumor by anti-α-human chorionic gonadotropin antibody. JNCI 84:42–47, 1992.
30. Acevedo HF, Raikow RB, Powell JE, Stevens VC: Effects of immunization against human choriogonadotropin on the growth of transplanted Lewis lung carcinoma and spontaneous mammary adenocarcinoma in mice. Cancer Detect Prev Suppl 1:477–486, 1987.

31. Stevens VC: Birth control vaccines and immunological approaches to the therapy of noninfectious diseases. Inf Dis Clin North Am 4:343–354, 1990.

32. Pal R, Singh O, Rao LV, Talwar GP: Bioneutralization capacity of the antibodies generated in women by the beta subunit of human chorionic gonadotropin (beta hCG) and beta hCG associated with the alpha subunit of ovine luteinizing hormone linked to carriers. Am J Reprod Immunol 22:124–126, 1990.

33. Gudermann T, Nichols C, Levy FO, et al: Ca^{2+} mobilization by the LH receptor expressed in *Xenopus* oocytes independent of 3',5'-cyclic adenosine monophosphate formation: Evidence for parallel activation of two signaling pathways. Mol Endocrinol 6:272–278, 1992.

34. Pierce JG, Parsons TF: Glycoprotein hormones: Structure and function. Ann Rev Biochem 50:465–495, 1981.

35. Blithe DL, Richards RG, Skarulis MC: Free alpha molecules from pregnancy stimulate secretion of prolactin from human decidual cells: A novel function for free alpha in pregnancy. Endocrinology 129:2257–2259, 1991.

36. Campbell RK, Dean-Emig DM, Moyle WR: Conversion of human choriogonadotropin into a follitropin by protein engineering. Proc Natl Acad Sci USA 88:760–764, 1991.

37. Fiddes JC, Talmadge K: Structure, expression, and evolution of the genes for the human glycoprotein hormones. *In* Greep RO (ed): Recent Progress in Hormone Research, Vol 40. New York, Academic Press, 1984, pp 43–78.

38. Nilson JH, Bokar JA, Clay CM, et al: Different combinations of regulatory elements may explain why placenta-specific expression of the glycoprotein hormone α-subunit gene occurs only in primates and horses. Biol Reprod 44:231–237, 1991.

39. Kitahara N, Nishizawa T, Gatanaga T, et al: Primary structure of two mRNAs encoding putative salmon alpha-subunits of pituitary glycoprotein hormone. Comp Biochem Physiol 91B:551–556, 1988.

40. Graham MY, Otani T, Boime I, et al: Cosmid mapping of the human chorionic gonadotropin beta subunit genes by field-inversion gel electrophoresis. Nucleic Acids Res 15:4437–4448, 1987.

41. Bo M, Boime I: Identification of the transcriptionally active genes of the chorionic gonadotropin β gene cluster in vivo. J Biol Chem 267:3179–3184, 1992.

42. Sawitzke AL, Griffin J, Odell WD: Purified preparations of human luteinizing hormone are contaminated with small amounts of a chorionic gonadotropin-like material. J Clin Endocrinol Metab 72:841–846, 1991.

43. Akar AH, Gervasi G, Blacker C, et al: Human chorionic gonadotrophin-like and beta-core-like materials in postmenopausal urine. J Endocrinol 125:477–484, 1990.

44. Sherman GB, Wolfe MW, Farmerie TA, et al: A single gene encodes the β-subunits of equine luteinizing hormone and chorionic gonadotropin. Mol Endocrinol 6:951–959, 1992.

44a. Smith PL, Bousfield GR, Kumar S, et al: Equine lutropin and chorionic gonadotropin bear oligosaccharides terminating with SO$_4$-4-GalNAc and Siaα2,3Gal, respectively. J Biol Chem 268:795–802, 1993.

45. Yoo J, Ji I, Ji TH: Conversion of lysine 91 to methionine or glutamic acid in human choriogonadotropin α results in the loss of cAMP inducibility. J Biol Chem 266:17741–17743, 1991.

46. Chen F, Wang Y, Puett D: Role of the invariant aspartic acid 99 of human choriogonadotropin β in receptor binding and biological activity. J Biol Chem 266:19357–19361, 1991.

47. Weiss J, Axelrod L, Whitcomb RW, et al: Hypogonadism caused by a single amino acid substitution in the β subunit of luteinizing hormone. N Engl J Med 326:179–183, 1992.

48. Salesse R, Bidart JM, Troalen F, et al: Peptide mapping of intersubunit and receptor interactions of human choriogonadotropin. Mol Cell Endocrinol 68:113–119, 1990.

49. Reed DK, Ryan RJ, McCormick DJ: Residues in the α subunit of human choriotropin that are important for interaction with the lutropin receptor. J Biol Chem 266:14251–14255, 1991.

50. Santa-Coloma TA, Crabb JW, Reichert LE Jr: A synthetic peptide encompassing two discontinuous regions of hFSH-β subunit mimics the receptor binding surface of the hormone. Mol Cell Endocrinol 78:197–204, 1991.

51. Keutmann HT: Receptor-binding regions in human glycoprotein hormones. Mol Cell Endocrinol 92:C1–C6, 1992.

52. Hage-van Noort M, Puijk WC, Plasman HH, et al: Synthetic peptides based upon a three-dimensional model for the receptor recognition site of follicle-stimulating hormone exhibit antagonistic or agonistic activity at low concentrations. Proc Natl Acad Sci USA 89:3922–3926, 1992.

53. Meloen RH, Amerongen AV, Hage van Noort ML, et al: The use of peptides to reconstruct conformational determinants; a brief review. Ann Biol Clin 49:231–242, 1991.

54. Lustbader JW, Birken S, Pileggi NF, et al: Crystallization and characterization of human chorionic gonadotropin in chemically deglycosylated and enzymatically deglycosylated states. Biochemistry 28:9239–9243, 1989.

55. Harris DC, Machin KJ, Evin GM, et al: Preliminary X-ray diffraction analysis of human chorionic gonadotropin. J Biol Chem 264:6705–6706, 1989.

56. Baenziger J, Green ED: Pituitary glycoprotein hormone oligosaccharides: structure, synthesis and function of the asparagine-linked oligosaccharides on lutropin, follitropin and thyrotropin. Biochim Biophys Acta 947:287–306, 1988.

57. Parsons TF, Pierce JG: Free alpha-like material from bovine pituitaries: Removal of its O-linked oligosaccharide permits combination with lutropin beta. J Biol Chem 259:2662–2666, 1984.

58. Baenziger JU, Kumar S, Brodbeck RM, et al: Circulatory half-life but not interaction with the lutropin/chorionic gonadotropin receptor is modulated by sulfation of bovine lutropin oligosaccharides. Proc Natl Acad Sci USA 89:334–338, 1992.

59. Smith PL, Kaetzel D, Nilson J, Baenziger JU: The sialylated oligosaccharides of recombinant bovine lutropin modulate hormone bioactivity. J Biol Chem 265:874–881, 1990.

60. Fiete D, Srivastava V, Hindsgaul O, Baenziger JU: A hepatic reticuloendothelial cell receptor specific for SO4-4GalNAc β1,4GlcNAc β1,2Manα that mediates rapid clearance of lutropin. Cell 67:1103–1110, 1991.

61. Peckham WD, Yamaji T, Dierschke DJ, Knobil E: Gonadal function and the biological and physiochemical properties of follicle-stimulating hormone. Endocrinology 92:1660–1666, 1973.

62. Morell AG, Gregoriadis G, Scheinberg IH, et al: The role of sialic acid in determining the survival of glycoproteins in the circulation. J Biol Chem 246:1461–1467, 1971.

63. Yen SSC, Llerena O, Little B, Pearson OH: Disappearance rates of endogenous luteinizing hormone and chorionic gonadotropin in man. J Clin Endocrinol Metab 28:1763–1767, 1968.

64. Veldhuis JD, Johnson ML: In vivo dynamics of luteinizing hormone secretion and clearance in man: Assessment by deconvolution mechanics. J Clin Endocrinol Metab 66:1291–1300, 1988.

65. Urban RJ, Padmanabhan V, Beitins I, Veldhuis JD: Metabolic clearance of human follicle-stimulating hormone assessed by radioimmunoassay, immunoradiometric assay, and in vitro Sertoli cell bioassay. J Clin Endocrinol Metab 73:818–823, 1991.

66. Yen SSC, Llerena LA, Pearson OH, Littell AS: Disappearance rates of endogenous follicle-stimulating hormone in serum following surgical hypophysectomy in man. J Clin Endocrinol Metab 30:325–329, 1970.

67. Hall JE, Schoenfeld DA, Martin KA, Crowley WFJ: Hypothalamic gonadotropin-releasing hormone secretion and follicle-stimulating hormone dynamics during the luteal-follicular transition. J Clin Endocrinol Metab 74:600–607, 1992.

68. Armstrong EG, Birken S, Moyle WR, Canfield RE: Immunochemistry of human chorionic gonadotropin. *In* Litwack G (ed): Biochemical Actions of Hormones, Vol 13. New York, Academic Press, 1986, pp 91–128.

69. Damewood MD, Shen W, Zacur HA, et al: Disappearance of exogenously administered human chorionic gonadotropin. Fertil Steril 52:398–400, 1989.

70. Braunstein GD, Vaitukaitis JL, Ross GT: The in vivo behavior of human chorionic gonadotropin after dissociation into subunits. Endocrinology 91:1030–1036, 1972.

71. Fares FA, Suganuma N, Nishimori K, et al: Design of a long-acting follitropin agonist by fusing the C-terminal sequence of the chorionic gonadotropin β subunit to the follitropin β subunit. Proc Natl Acad Sci USA 89:4304–4308, 1992.

72. Sairam MR, Bhargavi GN: A role for the glycosylation of the alpha-subunit in the transduction of biological signal in glycoprotein hormones. Science 229:65–67, 1985.

73. Matzuk MM, Boime I: Mutagenesis and gene transfer define site-specific roles of the gonadotropin oligosaccharides. Biol Reprod 40:48–53, 1989.

74. Keri RA, Andersen B, Kennedy GC, et al: Estradiol inhibits transcription of the human glycoprotein hormone α-subunit gene despite the absence of a high affinity binding site for estrogen receptor. Mol Endocrinol 5:725–733, 1991.

75. Chin WW, Kronenberg HM, Dee PC, et al: Nucleotide sequence of the mRNA encoding the pre-α-subunit of mouse thyrotropin. Proc Natl Acad Sci USA 78:5329–5333, 1981.

76. Gordon DF, Wood WM, Ridgway EC: Organization and nucleotide sequence of the mouse α subunit gene of the pituitary glycoprotein hormones. DNA 7:679–690, 1988.

77. Burnside J, Buckland PR, Chin WW: Isolation and characterization of the gene encoding the α-subunit of the rat pituitary glycoprotein hormones. Gene 70:67–74, 1988.

78. Fenstermaker RA, Farmerie TA, Clay CM, et al: Different combinations of regulatory elements may account for expression of the glycoprotein hormone α-subunit gene in primate and horse placenta. Mol Endocrinol 4:1480–1487, 1990.

79. Andersen B, Kennedy GC, Hamernik DL, et al: Amplification of the transcriptional signal mediated by the tandem cAMP response elements of the glycoprotein hormone α-subunit gene occurs through several distinct mechanisms. Mol Endocrinol 4:573–582, 1990.

80. Andersen B, Kennedy GC, Nilson JH: A cis-acting element located between the cAMP response elements and CCAAT box augments cell-specific expression of the glycoprotein hormone α subunit gene. J Biol Chem 265:21874–21880, 1990.

81. Kennedy GC, Andersen B, Nilson JH: The human alpha subunit glycoprotein hormone gene utilizes a unique CCAAT binding factor. J Biol Chem 265:6279–6285, 1990.

82. Kay RWH, Jameson JL: Identification of a gonadotropin-releasing hormone-responsive region in the glycoprotein hormone α-subunit promoter. Mol Endocrinol 6:1767–1773, 1992.

83. Hwang C, Sinskey AJ, Lodish HF: Oxidized redox state of glutathione in the endoplasmic reticulum. Science 257:1496–1502, 1992.

84. Peters BP, Krzesicki RF, Hartle RJ, et al: A kinetic comparison of the processing and secretion of the αβ-dimer and the uncombined α- and β-subunits of chorionic gonadotropin synthesized by human choriocarcinoma cells. J Biol Chem 259:15123–15130, 1984.

84a. Bedows E, Huth JR, Ruddon RW: Kinetics of folding and assembly of the human chorionic gonadotropin beta subunit in transfected Chinese hamster ovary cells. J Biol Chem 267:8880–8886, 1992.

84b. Huth JR, Mountjoy K, Perini F, Ruddon RW: Intracellular folding pathway of human chorionic gonadotropin beta subunit. J Biol Chem 267:8870–8879, 1992.

84c. Huth JR, Mountjoy K, Perini F, et al: Domain-dependent protein folding is indicated by the intracellular kinetics of disulfide bond formation of human chorionic gonadotropin beta subunit. J Biol Chem 267:21396–21403, 1992.

85. Edmonds M, Molitch M, Pierce JG, Odell WD: Secretion of alpha subunits of luteinizing hormone (LH) by the anterior pituitary. J Clin Endocrinol Metab 41:551–554, 1975.

86. Ruddon RW, Hartle RJ, Peters BP, et al: Biosynthesis and secretion of chorionic gonadotropin subunits by organ cultures of first trimester placenta. J Biol Chem 256:11389–11392, 1981.

87. Smith PL, Baenziger JU: Recognition by the glycoprotein hormone-specific N-acetylgalactosaminetransferase is independent of hormone native conformation. Proc Natl Acad Sci USA 87:7275–7279, 1990.

88. Smith PL, Baenziger JU: Molecular basis of recognition by the glycoprotein hormone-specific N-acetylgalactosamine-transferase. Proc Natl Acad Sci USA 89:329–333, 1992.

89. Whitcomb RW, O'Dea LS, Finkelstein JS, et al: Utility of free alpha-subunit as an alternative neuroendocrine marker of gonadotropin-releasing hormone (GnRH) stimulation of the gonadotroph in the human: Evidence from normal and GnRH-deficient men. J Clin Endocrinol Metab 70:1654–1661, 1990.

90. Matzuk MM, Spangler MM, Camel M, et al: Mutagenesis and chimeric genes define determinants in the β-subunits of human chorionic gonadotropin and lutropin for secretion and assembly. J Cell Biol 109:1429–1438, 1989.

91. Bielinska M, Rzymkiewicz D, Pixely M: Human lutropin and chorionic gonadotropin are targeted to a regulated secretory pathway in GH3 cells. 74th Annual Meeting of the Endocrine Society, San Antonio, TX, June 24–27; Abstr 1195, 1992.

91a. Bielinska M, Rzymkeiwicz D, Boime I: Human lutropin and chorionic gonadotropin are targeted to a regulated secretory pathway in GH3 cells. Mol Endocrinol, in press.

92. Lustbader J, Birken S, Pollak S, et al: Characterization of the expression products of recombinant hCG and subunits. J Biol Chem 262:14204–14212, 1987.

93. Blithe DL: N-Linked oligosaccharides on free α interfere with its ability to combine with human chorionic gonadotropin-β subunit. J Biol Chem 265:21951–21956, 1990.

94. Blum WF, Gupta D: Heterogeneity of rat FSH by chromatofocusing: Studies on serum FSH, hormone released in vitro and metabolic clearance rates of its various forms. J Endocrinol 105:29–37, 1985.

95. Veldhuis JD, Johnson ML, Dufau ML: Preferential release of bioac-

96. Padmanabhan V, Mieher CD, Borondy M, et al: Circulating bioactive follicle-stimulating hormone and less acidic follicle-stimulating hormone isoforms increase during experimental induction of puberty in the female lamb. Endocrinology 131:213–220, 1992.

97. Steelman SL, Pohley FM: Assay of follicle-stimulating hormone based on the augmentation with human chorionic gonadotropin. Endocrinology 53:604–616, 1953.

98. Greep RO, vanDyke HB, Chow BF: Use of anterior lobe of prostate gland in the assay of metakentrin. Proc Soc Exp Biol Med 46:644–649, 1941.

99. Parlow AF: A rapid bioassay method for LH and factors stimulating LH secretion. Fed Proc 17:40, 1958.

100. Veldhuis JD, Johnson ML, Dufau ML: Physiological attributes of endogenous bioactive luteinizing hormone secretory bursts in man. Am J Physiol 256:E199–E207, 1989.

101. Midgley AR Jr: Radioimmunoassay: A method for human chorionic gonadotropin and human luteinizing hormone. Endocrinology 79:10–18, 1966.

102. Midgley AR Jr: Radioimmunoassay for human follicle-stimulating hormone. J Clin Endocrinol Metab 27:295–299, 1967.

103. O'Connor JF, Schlatterer JP, Birken S, et al: Development of highly sensitive immunoassays to measure human chorionic gonadotropin, its β-subunit, and β core fragment in the urine: application to malignancies. Cancer Res 48:1361–1366, 1988.

104. Chappel SC, Ulloa Aguirre A, Coutifaris C: Biosynthesis and secretion of follicle-stimulating hormone. Endocr Rev 4:179–211, 1983.

105. Beitins IZ, Padmanabhan V: Bioactive follicle-stimulating hormone. Trends Endocrinol Metab 2:145–151, 1991.

106. Urban RJ, Veldhuis JD, Blizzard RM, Dufau ML: Attenuated release of biologically active luteinizing hormone in healthy aging men. J Clin Invest 81:1020–1029, 1988.

107. Urban RJ, Veldhuis JD, Dufau ML: Estrogen regulates the gonadotropin-releasing hormone-stimulated secretion of biologically active luteinizing hormone. J Clin Endocrinol Metab 72:660–668, 1991.

108. Urban RJ, Dahl KD, Padmanabhan V, et al: Specific regulatory actions of dihydrotestosterone and estradiol on the dynamics of FSH secretion and clearance in humans. J Androl 12:27–35, 1991.

109. Skaf R, Macdonald GJ, Sheldon RM, Moyle WR: Use of antisera to follicle-stimulating hormone (FSH) to detect non-FSH factors in human serum which modulate rat granulosa cell steroidogenesis. Endocrinology 117:106–113, 1985.

110. Schneyer AL, Sluss PM, Whitcomb RW, et al: Development of a radioligand receptor assay for measuring follitropin in serum: Application to premature ovarian failure. Clin Chem 37:508–514, 1991.

111. Moyle WR, Anderson DM, Macdonald GJ, Armstrong EG: Bioimmunoassay (BIA): a sandwich immunoassay scheme employing monoclonal antibodies and hormone receptors to quantify analytes. J Recept Res 8:419–436, 1988.

112. Kelton CA, Cheng SVY, Nugent NP, et al: The cloning of the human follicle stimulating hormone receptor and its expression in COS-7, CHO, and Y-1 cells. Mol Cell Endocrinol 89:141–151, 1992.

112a. Jia X-C, Perlas E, Su J-GJ, et al: Luminescence luteinizing hormone/choriogonadotropin (LH/CG) bioassay: measurement of serum bioactive LH/CG during early pregnancy in human and macaque. Biol Reprod, in press.

113. McFarland KC, Sprengel R, Phillips HS, et al: Lutropin-choriogonadotropin receptor: An unusual member of the G protein-coupled receptor family. Science 245:494–499, 1989.

114. Sprengel R, Braun T, Nikolics K, et al: The testicular receptor for follicle stimulating hormone: Structure and functional expression of cloned cDNA. Mol Endocrinol 4:525–530, 1990.

115. Loosfelt H, Misrahi M, Atger M, et al: Cloning and sequencing of porcine LH-hCG receptor cDNA: Variants lacking transmembrane domain. Science 245:525–528, 1989.

116. Sutherland EW, Robison GA: Role of cyclic 3'-5'AMP in responses to catecholamines and other hormones. Pharmacol Rev 18:145–161, 1966.

117. Rodriguez MC, Segaloff DL: The orientation of the lutropin/choriogonadotropin receptor in rat luteal cells as revealed by site-specific antibodies. Endocrinology 127:674–681, 1990.

118. Tsai-Morris CH, Buczko E, Wang W, et al: Structural organization of the rat luteinizing hormone (LH) receptor gene. J Biol Chem 266:11355–11359, 1991.

119. Koo YB, Ji I, Slaughter RG, Ji TH: Structure of the luteinizing hormone receptor gene and multiple exons of the coding sequence. Endocrinology 128:2297–2308, 1991.

120. Heckert LL, Daley IJ, Griswold MD: Structural organization of the follicle-stimulating hormone receptor gene. Mol Endocrinol 6:70–80, 1992.

121. Tsai Morris CH, Buczko E, Wang W, Dufau ML: Intronic nature of the rat luteinizing hormone receptor gene defines a soluble receptor subspecies with hormone binding activity. J Biol Chem 265:19385–19388, 1990.

122. Moyle WR, Bernard MP, Myers RV, et al: Leutropin/β-adrenergic receptor chimeras bind choriogonadotropin and adrenergic ligands but are not expressed at the cell surface. J Biol Chem 266:10807–10812, 1991.

123. Xie Y-B, Wang H, Segaloff DL: Extracellular domain of lutropin/choriogonadotropin receptor expressed in transfected cells binds choriogonadotropin with high affinity. J Biol Chem 265:21411–21414, 1990.

124. Ji I, Ji TH: Exons 1–10 of the rat LH receptor encode a high affinity hormone binding site and exon 11 encodes G-protein modulation and a potential second hormone binding site. Endocrinology 128:2648–2650, 1991.

125. Braun T, Schofield PR, Sprengel R: Amino-terminal leucine-rich repeats in gonadotropin receptors determine hormone selectivity. EMBO J 10:1885–1890, 1991.

126. Dixon RA, Sigal IS, Rands E, et al: Ligand binding to the beta-adrenergic receptor involves its rhodopsin-like core. Nature 326:73–77, 1987.

127. Dixon RA, Sigal IS, Candelore MR, et al: Structural features required for ligand binding to the beta-adrenergic receptor. EMBO J 6:3269–3275, 1987.

128. Ji I, Ji TH: Human choriogonadotropin binds to a lutropin receptor with essentially no N-terminal extension and stimulates cAMP synthesis. J Biol Chem 266:13076–13079, 1991.

129. Kusuda S, Dufau ML: Characterization of ovarian gonadotropin receptor. Monomer and associated form of the receptor. J Biol Chem 263:3046–3049, 1988.

130. Dattatreyamurty B, Smith RA, Vahang S-B, et al: The size of the mature membrane receptor for follicle-stimulating hormone is larger than that predicted from its cDNA. J Mol Endocrinol 9:115–121, 1992.

131. Boniface JJ, Reichert LEJ: Evidence for a novel thioredoxin-like catalytic property of gonadotropic hormones. Science 247:61–64, 1990.

132. Lei ZM, Rao ChV, Satyaswaroop PG, Day TG: The expression of hCG/LH receptors in human endometrial carcinomas. Society of Gynecologic Investigation 39th Annual Meeting, San Antonio, TX, Abstr 209, 213, 1992.

133. Lei ZM, Rao CV, Ackerman DM, Day TG: The expression of human chorionic gonadotropin/human luteinizing hormone receptors in human gestational trophoblastic neoplasms. J Clin Endocrinol Metab 74:1236–1241, 1992.

134. Reshef E, Lei ZM, Rao CV, et al: The presence of gonadotropin receptors in nonpregnant human uterus, human placenta, fetal membranes, and decidua. J Clin Endocrinol Metab 70:421–430, 1990.

135. Fiddes JC, Goodman HM: Isolation cloning and sequence analysis of the cDNA for the α-subunit of human chorionic gonadotropin. Nature 281:351–356, 1979.

136. Nilson JH, Thomason AR, Cserbak MT, et al: Nucleotide sequence of a cDNA for the common α-subunit of the bovine pituitary hormones. J Biol Chem 258:4679–4682, 1983.

137. Stewart F, Thomson JA, Leigh SEA, Warwick JM: Nucleotide (cDNA) sequence encoding the horse gonadotrophin α-subunit. J Endocrinol 115:341–346, 1987.

138. Foster DN, Galehouse D, Giordano T, et al: Nucleotide sequence of the cDNA encoding the common α subunit of the chicken pituitary glycoprotein hormones. J Mol Endocrinol 8:21–27, 1992.

139. Hayashi H, Hayashi T, Hanaoka Y: Amphibian lutropin and follitropin from the bullfrog (Rana catesbeiana): Complete amino acid sequence of the α subunit. Eur J Biochem 203:185–191, 1992.

15

Gonadotropins and the Gonad: Normal Physiology and Their Disturbances in Clinical Endocrine Diseases

JANET E. HALL
WILLIAM F. CROWLEY, Jr.

Reproductive function in men and women is crucially dependent on a precisely coordinated cascade of hormonal signals from the hypothalamus, the pituitary, and the gonads (Fig. 15–1). Pituitary secretion of the gonadotropins is initiated by the pulsatile secretion of gonadotropin-releasing hormone (GnRH) from the hypothalamus. The secreted pituitary gonadotropins functionally divide the gonads of both men and women into two components: the gametogenic compartment controlled by follicle-stimulat-ing hormone (FSH) and the steroidogenic compartment, largely dependent on luteinizing hormone (LH). Maintenance of normal reproductive function ultimately requires the collaboration of these two functionally distinct units within the gonad as well as their feedback via gonadal steroids and other peptides acting at the level of both the hypothalamus and the pituitary. This chapter focuses on the physiology and pathophysiology of the pituitary component of this system, gonadotropin synthesis, and secre-

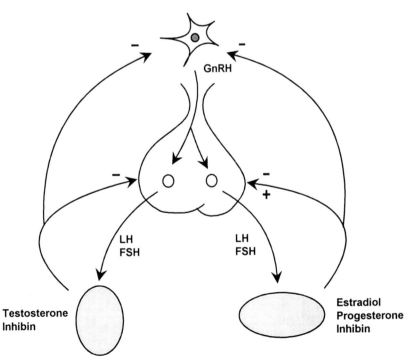

FIGURE 15–1. A diagrammatic representation of the normal reproductive axis highlighting the hormonal integration of the hypothalamus, pituitary, and gonads in the normal male *(left)* and female *(right)*. See text for detailed discussion of feedback.

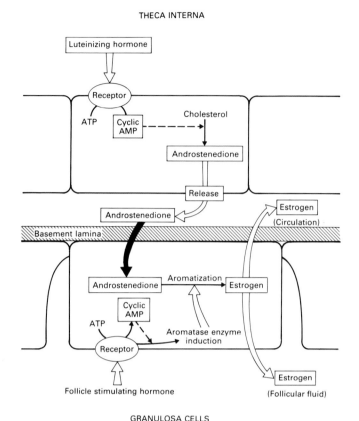

FIGURE 15-2. The two-cell conceptualization of estrogen biosynthesis in the granulosa cell from androstenedione precursors synthesized in theca cells. LH primarily controls androstenedione secretion, while FSH regulates aromatization. The precise roles of intraovarian regulators in this schema have not been clearly elucidated. (From Erickson GF: Normal ovarian function. Clin Obstet Gynecol 12:31, 1978.)

tion and its control by GnRH. An understanding of the neuroendocrine determinants of pituitary gonadotroph function provides an essential backdrop for any understanding of the clinical abnormalities of the reproductive axis in men and women. A general neuroendocrine approach to these disorders in both sexes is provided in the final sections of this chapter, while a more detailed examination of specific abnormalities is found in subsequent chapters.

THE GONADOTROPINS

The gonadotropins, LH and FSH, are members of the glycoprotein hormone family. Like the other members of this family, thyroid-stimulating hormone (TSH) and human chorionic gonadotropin (hCG), the gonadotropins are heterodimers formed from the noncovalent linkage of a common α-subunit with a unique β-subunit.[1, 2] It is only in the combination of the α-subunit and the specific β-subunit that receptor binding and functional specificity are conferred to the intact hormone. As detailed in Chapter 14, alterations in glycosylation of the protein core can result in marked heterogeneity in the forms of LH and FSH secreted from the pituitary under a variety of developmental, physiological, and pharmacological conditions. Importantly, these changes may influence clearance and/or binding of the hormones to their specific gonadal receptors

and therefore their biopotency.[3] This "microheterogeneity" may also affect the degree to which the intact hormone is recognized in various monoclonal assay systems.[4] In addition to secretion of the intact dimeric hormones, the α-subunit is secreted from both the gonadotroph and the thyrotroph in a free or uncombined form (FAS). Pulsatile secretion of FAS correlates with pulsatile LH. This and other lines of evidence indicate that the pulsatile component of FAS secretion is largely controlled by GnRH.[5]

Function of the Gonadotropins

The biological actions of LH and FSH are confined to the ovary and testis, with FSH playing a predominant role in maturation of the gonads and regulation of gametogenesis while LH regulates steroidogenesis. In the ovary, FSH stimulates the growth of the developing follicles beyond the early antral stage and is responsible for the recruitment of a cohort of follicles in each reproductive cycle.[6, 7] Estradiol synergizes with FSH both by stimulating proliferation of the granulosa cells of the ovary and by amplifying the responsiveness of the granulosa cells to FSH.[8, 9] The ultimate number of follicles that reach the preovulatory stage depends on the level of continued FSH support,[7] and hence restraint of pituitary secretion of FSH by the secretory products of the developing follicle (estradiol and possibly inhibin) is a crucial determinant of normal reproductive cycles.

In the ovary, steroidogenesis depends on the coordinated activities of the theca and the granulosa cell compartments as well as the presence of both LH and FSH (Fig. 15-2). FSH stimulates the appearance of LH receptors on both granulosa and theca cells. LH is then responsible for theca cell production of androgens from cholesterol, while FSH controls aromatization of these androgen precursors to estrogens in the granulosa cells.[10, 11] LH also plays a major role in the steroid production of the corpus luteum, which synthesizes progesterone from the cholesterol precursors that are now available to the luteinized granulosa cell owing to the invasion of new vascular channels, which appear in the ruptured follicle (now the corpus luteum) following ovulation.[12] The importance of LH in maintenance of the corpus luteum in the human was originally demonstrated in studies of the administration of LH to hypophysectomized women[13] and more recently in studies in which the addition of hCG, but not FSH, prevented luteolysis in women to whom a GnRH antagonist was administered in the luteal phase.[14]

In addition to playing a key role in ovarian steroidogenesis, a midcycle surge of LH is crucial to both ovulation and to final ovum maturation with the resumption of meiotic division, which was arrested at the diplotene stage of the first meiotic division during the second trimester in utero. The precise mechanism by which LH induces rupture of the mature follicle and extrusion of the ovum are poorly understood but are thought to involve increased synthesis of both prostaglandins and plasminogen activator within the maturing follicle.[15, 16]

In the testis, FSH is required for the development of the seminiferous tubules and for initiation of spermatogenesis at puberty,[17] although it is unclear whether it is required to sustain spermatogenesis or whether LH alone is sufficient.[18] The subsequent maintenance of spermatogenesis clearly requires high levels of intratesticular androgen that are sustained by LH secretion; receptors for both FSH and androgens are located on Sertoli cells, which surround the developing spermatogonia and spermatids in the seminiferous tubules.[19-21] It is likely that the action on spermatogenesis of both FSH and testosterone is mediated through the Sertoli cells, which contain the FSH receptors. The role of the testicular paracrine factor, PmodS, IGF, and other autocrine and paracrine factors in spermatogenesis has only recently begun to be elucidated.[22] Other actions of FSH in the testis include induction of Leydig cell maturation, enhancement of the androgen response to LH, augmentation of LH receptor number, stimulation of production of androgen binding protein, and induction of aromatase activity.[23-26]

LH interacts with its own specific high-affinity receptors, which are located only on the Leydig cells, and controls testosterone biosynthesis as evidenced by the close relationship of pulsatile testosterone secretion following pulses of LH secretion in normal men (Fig. 15-3).[27] There is an excess number of LH receptors present on the Leydig cell, and these "spare receptors" may play a key role in modulating the sensitivity of steroidogenic response to low levels of gonadotropins.[28] LH has been shown to modulate its own action by decreasing or "down-regulating" its receptor number and by postreceptor mechanisms that depend on testosterone synthesis. It is hypothesized that this is one of several intratesticular "servo-mechanisms" by which testosterone production is controlled.

Ontogeny of Gonadotropin Synthesis and Secretion

Recent studies in a number of species have detailed the development and migration of GnRH secretory neurons from epithelial cells outside the developing CNS in the olfactory placode to the median eminence, where contact is made with capillaries of the hypothalamic-pituitary portal system.[29, 30] In the human, GnRH has been detected in embryonic brain extracts as early as 4.5 weeks, GnRH neurons have been demonstrated in the fetal hypothalamus by 9 weeks, and functional connections of these neurons with the portal system are established by 16 weeks.[31] LH and

FSH are first detectable in the pituitary as early as 10 weeks and are measurable in peripheral blood by 12 weeks of gestation.[32] Low levels of gonadotropins in the pituitary and serum of anencephalic infants and the demonstration of the ability of GnRH to stimulate gonadotropin secretion and to induce LHβ mRNA synthesis in pituitary cells from second trimester fetuses support a role for GnRH in gonadotropin regulation during early fetal life.[32, 33]

An important theme of sexual dimorphism of pituitary hormone physiology begins in utero with an overall increase in pituitary content of FSH and LH and a striking preponderance of FSH over LH in female fetuses and infants up to seven years of age in comparison with males spanning a similar developmental range.[32] In addition, serum levels of both LH and FSH peak earlier in female than in male fetuses with FSH levels in females remaining well above those of males throughout gestation and into the neonatal periods.[34, 35] These variations in circulating gonadotropin levels and their ratios during gestation are consistent with the development of functioning gonadal negative feedback relatively late in fetal life. Both the male and female develop in an environment that is extraordinarily high in estrogen. Testosterone, which is crucial to the development of male external genitalia, is secreted by the testis as early as 10 weeks of gestation, and evidence of testosterone negative feedback on the pituitary has been clearly demonstrated by midgestation in the primate.[36]

Maternally derived hCG, which also binds to the LH receptor, appears to be the major determinant of testicular androgen secretion during gestation. This is most clearly demonstrated by the normal external genital development of a patient with a LHβ mutation that rendered his LH bioinactive.[37] However, abnormal gonadal development in anencephalic males by early in the third trimester[38] suggests that an additional factor, possibly FSH, is important for normal testicular development in utero. This is in contrast to the situation in the female, in whom anencephaly is associated with normal ovarian development until near term.[38] Interestingly, FSH receptors have not been demonstrated in the female gonad until the ninth month of gestation,[39] compatible with the observation that the fetal ovary does not secrete significant quantities of steroids in vivo, although it contains most of the enzymes required for de novo steroid synthesis.[40] In the absence of FSH receptors, inhibin secretion from the ovary would also not be expected to occur at this stage of development. Both α and

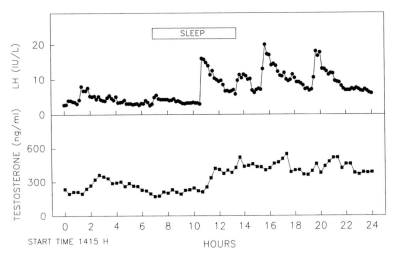

FIGURE 15-3. Serum LH and testosterone concentrations in a normal man with a slow frequency of GnRH secretion indicating the relationship of testosterone secretion to pulsatile LH secretion. (Adapted from Spratt DI et al: Neuroendocrine-gonadal axis in men: frequent sampling of LH, FSH, and testosterone. Am J Physiol 254 [Endocrinol Metab 17]:E658–66, 1988.)

β subunits of inhibin are present in the human male testis at midgestation, and secretion of α inhibin can be stimulated by HCG and FSH, while only weak staining of the inhibin subunits is present in the human ovary at a comparable time.[41] A lack of inhibin secretion by the ovary may well explain the observed increase in serum and pituitary FSH in the female fetus.

By the neonatal period, there is clear evidence of pulsatile secretion of GnRH with the predominant gonadotropin secreted in the female being FSH, while LH predominates in the male.[35] This pattern is observed both with basal and GnRH-stimulated secretion and may relate to sex differences in inhibin secretion. In childhood, pituitary gonadotropin secretion is markedly reduced.[31] The ability of the pituitary to respond to exogenous GnRH after appropriate priming throughout childhood suggests that low levels of gonadotropin secretion result from diminished hypothalamic GnRH secretion. In recent studies, sensitive serum assays have detected pulsatile gonadotropin secretion during childhood, albeit at very low levels.[42] The mechanism responsible for this quiescence of hypothalamic GnRH secretion during childhood remains an area of active investigation. In primate models, abundant GnRH mRNA is present in the hypothalamus during an equivalent developmental stage,[43] as are several modulators of its action such as endorphins. It may be that metabolizing enzymes responsible for GnRH secretion play a role in this important developmental process. Despite the long-standing hypothesis that the childhood quiescence of the hypothalamic-pituitary axis is due to a heightened sensitivity of this axis to the negative feedback of gonadal steroids, current evidence suggests that a non–sex steroid-dependent CNS factor governs the onset of puberty. Neither melatonin nor endorphins appear to be involved directly in the onset of puberty, but a role for excitatory amino acids such as N-methylaspartate has been suggested in studies in the primate.[44] In addition, several studies have inferred that a metabolic signal (which has yet to be defined) may be important in control of the onset of puberty.[45, 46]

Whatever the mechanism responsible, the onset of puberty is characterized by reactivation of hypothalamic GnRH secretion with resultant changes in both the quantity and quality of gonadotropin secretion. The earliest change in the pattern of gonadotropin secretion is an increase in pulsatile LH release associated with sleep, as initially described in the classic studies of Boyar.[47] As puberty progresses, pulsatile secretion of LH occurs throughout both the daytime and nighttime. This increase in radioimmunoassayable LH is accompanied by an even greater increase in LH bioactivity.[48] The altered sex steroid milieu that occurs during puberty similarly affects the degree of glycosylation of FSH, thus affecting its clearance and probably its bioactivity.[49] With the onset of cyclic reproductive function in adolescent females, FSH levels are increased over those of LH in the early follicular phase of each menstrual cycle.[50] Levels of both LH and FSH then become dynamically regulated in response to gonadal feedback as is discussed later, with the development of estrogen-induced positive feedback on LH representing the final developmental milestone in the hypothalamic-pituitary-ovarian axis. A similar FSH-predominant window does not appear to occur in males across pubertal development. During the period of maximal testicular growth and through the development of sperm production, both of

which are relatively early events in male sexual development, there are approximately equivalent levels of LH and FSH secreted endogenously and in response to exogenous GnRH administration.[31, 51] Whether this sexual dimorphism is related to fundamental differences in sex steroid feedback or to inhibin production is currently unclear.

With the decline in gonadal function during the menopause in women, secretion of FSH and LH is no longer restrained by gonadal feedback, and levels of both gonadotropins increase dramatically.[52] A similar hormonal pattern of elevated gonadotropins is seen with testicular failure or castration in men, although aging is generally not associated with such a dramatic decrease in gonadal function.[53] However, recent evidence suggests that there may be age-associated decreases in hypothalamic-pituitary function in men.[54]

CONTROL OF GONADOTROPIN SECRETION

The Pulsatile Nature of Gonadotropin Secretion

The intact gonadotropins and FAS are secreted in an episodic or pulsatile manner from the gonadotroph, the precise secretory pattern observed for each hormone in peripheral blood being dependent on the frequency and amplitude of hypothalamic GnRH secretion, the disappearance characteristics of the individual glycoprotein, and a frequency of blood sampling that is adequate to reflect the underlying frequency of episodic secretion (Fig. 15–4). Patterns of pulsatile gonadotropin secretion have now been documented in males and females from adolescence throughout reproductive life and into the menopause. These studies indicate that both the frequency and the amplitude of pulsatile secretion of LH, FSH, and FAS are precisely controlled.[55, 56] In addition these hormones, which are secreted from a single cell, are differentially controlled. Information about the factors that control differential gonadotropin secretion in the human has been derived from frequent sampling studies in normal men and women, from the use of the ablation-replacement model provided by GnRH-deficient subjects in whom GnRH can be replaced and experimentally varied to determine the crucial components of hypothalamic control, from the use of exogenous sex steroid administration to manipulate gonadotropin responses in the intact and GnRH-deficient model, and from the use of specific antagonists to GnRH.

GnRH Control of Gonadotropin Secretion

Hypothalamic control of pituitary function is mediated through GnRH, a decapeptide isolated and characterized in 1971 by the Nobel work of Schally and Guilleman. Although GnRH stimulates the secretion of both LH and FSH in vivo and in vitro, there are a number of physiologic and pathophysiologic situations in which the patterns of secretion of the two gonadotropins are markedly discrepant. In studies in which the GnRH receptor is blocked acutely by a pure competitive GnRH antagonist, LH levels decrease immediately by 80 to 90 per cent, while FSH

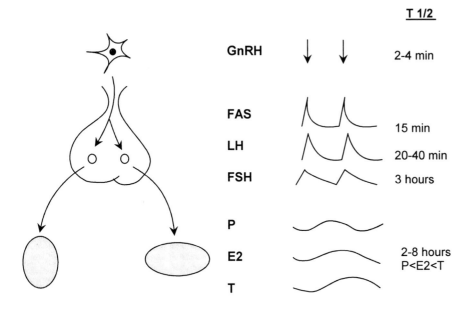

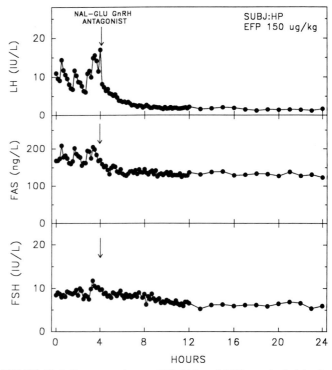

FIGURE 15–4. Diagrammatic representation of the effect of changes in hormone clearance on the characteristics of gonadotropin and sex steroid secretion in response to pulsatile secretion of GnRH.

decreases by only 40 to 60 per cent, suggesting that factors other than GnRH are responsible for the acute control of FSH secretion (Fig. 15–5).[57] These and other observations have led a number of investigators to postulate the presence of a separate, physiologically relevant hypothalamic FSH-releasing factor.[58] To date, such a hypothalamic factor has not been definitively characterized. Activin production by the gonadotroph is an excellent candidate for one such trophic hormone (see below). In addition, there is evidence that the differential secretion of LH and FSH may be accounted for by other mechanisms, including the differential effects of both GnRH pulse frequency and gonadal steroids on synthesis and secretion of the two hormones,[59] and the gonadal peptides inhibin and activin, which preferentially inhibit and stimulate FSH secretion, respectively, in in vitro studies as will be discussed below.[60–62a]

The mechanism of the generation of pulsatile secretion of GnRH is discussed in detail in Chapters 10 and 13. From the perspective of the composite integration of the reproductive axis, some generalizations are important to bear in mind. The first is that there appears to be an intrinsic circhoral frequency of endogenous GnRH secretion, which is seen most clearly in the castrate state.[63, 64] This observation strongly implies that gonadal factors have a hypothalamic site of action as will be discussed below. In addition, environmental factors including nutrition, exercises and stress in the human and other seasonal cues in a number of animal species impact upon the generation of the inherent rhythm of pulsatile GnRH secretion from the hypothalamus. The precise mechanisms by which these environmental cues are translated to alterations in the frequency or amplitude of endogenous GnRH secretion are incompletely understood, but involve several neurotransmitter systems including the adrenergic, dopaminergic, GABAergic, and opioid systems.

The Role of Pulsatile GnRH Secretion

GnRH secretion from the hypothalamus is pulsatile and is mirrored directly by the pulsatile secretion of the gonadotropins as demonstrated by the concordance of pulses of GnRH in portal blood and LH in peripheral blood in

animal models (Fig. 15–6).[65, 66] Importantly, this pulsatile mode of stimulation is an absolute requirement for normal gonadotropin synthesis and secretion. The classic studies of Knobil and colleagues,[67] in which endogenous GnRH secretion was ablated by hypothalamic lesioning in monkeys, indicated that secretion of LH and FSH could be maintained only by the pulsatile administration of exogenous GnRH, while its continuous administration resulted in a marked decrease in gonadotropin secretion. This desensitization was reversed only by the restoration of a pul-

FIGURE 15–5. Response of serum LH, FAS, and FSH to a single injection of the NAL-GLU GnRH antagonist indicating the differential response of these three glycoprotein hormones to blockade of the GnRH receptor. (From Hall JE, Crowley WF Jr: Use of GnRH antagonists as physiologic probes in the female. *In* Crowley WF Jr, Conn PM (eds): Modes of Action of GnRH and its Analogs. New York, Springer-Verlag, 1992, pp 310–321.)

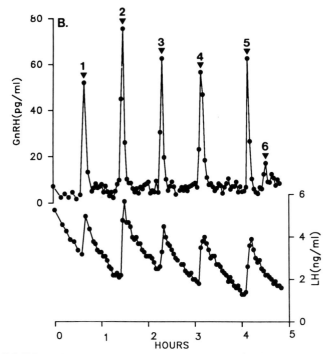

FIGURE 15–6. Portal blood GnRH and jugular LH levels in an ovariectomized ewe sampled at 2.5-min intervals. (From Clarke IJ: Exactitude in the relationship between GnRH and LH secretion. *In* Crowley WF Jr, Conn PM (eds): Modes of Action of GnRH and its Analogs. New York, Springer-Verlag, 1992, pp 179–192.)

satile mode of GnRH delivery. Subsequently, pituitary desensitization of gonadotropin secretion by continuous occupancy of the GnRH receptor has been exploited for the treatment of human disease by the use of agonist analogues of GnRH.[67a] These operate effectively as a continuous infusion when administered daily or as a depot preparation.

The Role of GnRH Pulse Frequency

The independent influence of GnRH pulse frequency on gonadotropin secretion has been investigated in patients with congenital GnRH deficiency, in whom the program of exogenous GnRH replacement can be experimentally varied.[56] Increasing the frequency of pulsatile GnRH results in an initial increase in mean LH levels but a progressive decrease in the pituitary responsiveness to each pulse of GnRH (Fig. 15–7). This decreasing pituitary responsiveness to GnRH and the observation that mean LH levels decreased at the highest frequency of GnRH stimulation indicate early desensitization of pituitary gonadotropin secretion by GnRH. Interestingly, changes in mean levels of FSH indicate that desensitization of FSH secretion by these same experiments occurs at a lower GnRH pulse frequency than for LH in this model.

There are two physiological situations in which such a frequency-mediated desensitization of gonadotropin secretion may play an important role in the human. The mechanisms underlying the onset and termination of the preovulatory LH surge have not been completely elucidated; however, the persistence of high portal vein levels of GnRH in the sheep beyond the point at which midcycle LH levels begin to decline[68] suggests that desensitization of LH secre-

tion may well play a decisive role in the termination of the midcycle surge. The second example of frequency-mediated gonadotroph desensitization may occur in a subset of patients with polycystic ovarian syndrome who have an abnormal gonadotropin profile characterized by high levels of LH in the presence of normal to low levels of FSH (Fig. 15–8),[69] a pattern reminiscent of the early phases of desensitization described earlier. These patients have been shown to have a frequency of GnRH secretion that is persistently higher than sex steroid–matched control women.[69]

Decreasing the frequency of GnRH stimulation from every 2 hours to every 8 hours is associated with pulses of LH of progressively increasing amplitude and area under the secretory curve (Fig. 15–9).[56] This series of studies was controlled for potential alterations in gonadal steroids resulting from the decreased frequency of gonadotropin stimulation and thus indicated that the frequency of GnRH alone, rather than secondary effects of sex steroid–negative feedback, are responsible for the observed amplification in LH pulse characteristics. Studies in the rat suggest that this slow luteal phase frequency of GnRH stimulation may well be important in differentially increasing the synthesis of FSH (Fig. 15–10)[59] in preparation for its subsequent preferential secretion in response to increasing GnRH stimulation during the luteal-follicular transition of the normal menstrual cycle (Fig. 15–11).[50]

Sex Steroid Modulation of Gonadotropin Secretion

The major feedback regulation of gonadotropin synthesis and secretion is mediated by the negative effects of gonadal steroids. These effects are important in both the male and female, operating either directly at the pituitary or indirectly through altering hypothalamic GnRH secretion. In addition, the normal female menstrual cycle is uniquely dependent on positive feedback for generation of the midcycle gonadotropin surge.

Estrogen and Progesterone in Women

Estrogen exerts its negative and positive feedback effects upon gonadotropin secretion at both the pituitary and the hypothalamus. The most striking evidence of its importance in the inhibition of gonadotropin secretion is the marked increase in levels of both LH and FSH that occur following removal of the ovaries and the return of these levels toward normal with estrogen replacement. While FSH is generally more sensitive to the negative feedback effects of estrogen in intact women, physiological replacement of estrogen alone in castrates does not return FSH levels to normal.[70] Studies in normal women have indicated that the pituitary response to estrogen administration is both dose- and time-dependent.[71, 72] At low levels and short durations of estrogen exposure, there is a predominantly inhibitory effect on gonadotropin secretion that is dose-dependent. During the normal menstrual cycle, it is this effect that is responsible for the decline in FSH levels from the early to the midfollicular phase, a decrease that is crucial to achieving controlled development of a single dominant follicle.[7] Higher doses and more sustained exposure to estrogen are then responsible for the positive feedback

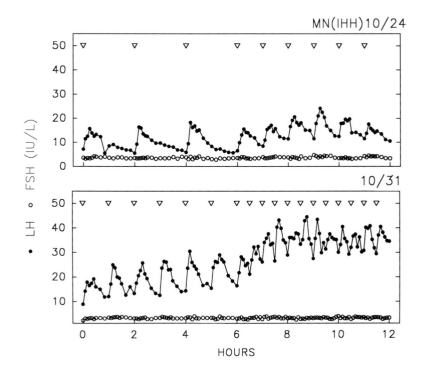

FIGURE 15–7. Acute and chronic LH (*closed circles*) and FSH (*open circles*) responses to a fixed and 'physiologic' dose of exogenous GnRH administered at the times indicated by the triangles to a GnRH-deficient man, indicating a marked increase in the LH/FSH ratio with increases in the frequency of GnRH administration. (Adapted from Spratt DI et al: Effects of increasing the frequency of low doses of gonadotropin-releasing hormone (GnRH) on gonadotropin secretion in GnRH-deficient men. J Clin Endocrinol Metab 64:1179, 1987, © The Endocrine Society.)

effects that subsequently generate the preovulatory gonadotropin surge. The observation that ovulation can be induced in GnRH-deficient women with no change in the dosage or frequency of exogenous GnRH from that required for follicular development in the early follicular phase[73, 74] suggests that, as with estrogen's negative feedback effects, the majority of estrogen-positive feedback is mediated at the level of the pituitary in the human. Estradiol induces LHβ mRNA synthesis in the rat and increases the sensitivity of LH secretion in pituitary cells to GnRH stimulation. However, the persistence of pulsatile secretion of LH throughout the normal midcycle surge in women,[75] the collapse of the surge with removal of GnRH in a GnRH-deficient woman (Crowley, personal communication), and studies in which a GnRH antagonist was used to investigate estrogen-induced positive feedback[76] all support a role for hypothalamic GnRH secretion during the midcycle.

The major effect of progesterone on gonadotropin secretion in women is mediated primarily by its effects on the frequency of hypothalamic GnRH secretion. GnRH pulse frequency decreases progressively during the luteal phase, an effect that correlates with the duration rather than the dosage of progesterone exposure.[55] Studies in which progesterone has been administered with or without estrogen suggest that this effect requires the prior presence of estrogen for its full expression,[77] possibly through induction of progesterone receptors. Several lines of evidence, including the failure to demonstrate sex steroid receptors within GnRH neurons, suggest that this effect of progesterone on GnRH pulse frequency is not exerted directly on

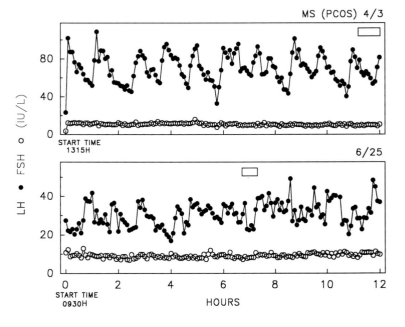

FIGURE 15–8. Pattern of serum LH and FSH secretion in a typical patient with PCOS studied on two separate occasions, indicating the increased ratio of LH to FSH and the increased amplitude and frequency of LH secretion typical of many patients with this disorder. Open bars indicate sleep.

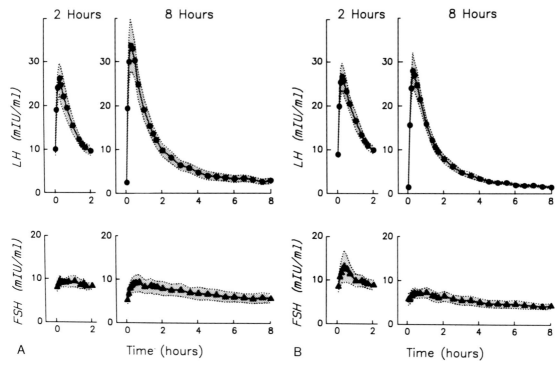

A   Time (hours)   B   Time (hours)

FIGURE 15–9. Mean ($+/-$ sem) serum LH and FSH concentrations of four GnRH-induced pulses in men with GnRH deficiency when GnRH was administered every two or eight hours (A) without testosterone replacement and (B) with testosterone replacement. (Reproduced from Finkelstein JS et al: Effects of decreasing the frequency of gonadotropin-releasing hormone stimulation on gonadotropin secretion in gonadotropin-releasing hormone-deficient men and perfused rat pituitary cells. J Clin Invest 81:1725–1733, 1988, by copyright permission of the American Society for Clinical Investigation.)

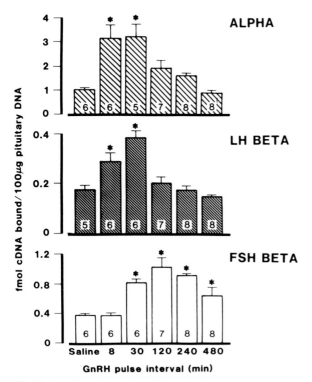

FIGURE 15–10. The effect of GnRH pulse frequency over the range indicated on expression of gonadotropin subunit mRNA expression in castrate testosterone-replaced male rats. The dose/pulse of GnRH was constant (25 ng). *$p<0.05$ vs saline. (From Dalkin AC et al: The frequency of gonadotropin-releasing-hormone stimulation differentially regulated gonadotropin subunit messenger ribonucleic acid expression. Endocrinology 125:917–924, 1989 © The Endocrine Society.)

the GnRH neurons but rather through modulation of the opioid control of the GnRH pulse generator. In GnRH-deficient women, low levels of progesterone increase LH pulse amplitude.[78] This suggests that progesterone may have an additional pituitary role in the generation of LH pulses of increased amplitude that are observed during the midcycle surge and in the early luteal phase at a time when the GnRH pulse frequency has not yet slowed.

Testosterone in Men

The site of testosterone-negative feedback in normal men was investigated by comparing the gonadotropin responses to infusions of estradiol and testosterone in normal men to those in men with GnRH deficiency in whom the dose and frequency of pulsatile GnRH replacement were experimentally fixed to physiological levels.[56] These parallel studies allowed the pituitary component of negative feedback (determined from the responses of GnRH-deficient men) to be subtracted from the total response of the normal men with intact hypothalamic-pituitary axes to arrive at the hypothalamic component of this effect. Estrogen administration decreased LH secretion similarly in the normal and GnRH-deficient men, indicating that its site of action is primarily pituitary. In contrast, testosterone has a dual site of action. It dramatically decreases the frequency of endogenous GnRH secretion in normal men similar to the effect of progesterone in women and has a mild additional negative feedback effect on mean LH levels and LH pulse amplitude in GnRH-deficient men in response to physiological doses of exogenous GnRH, suggesting both a

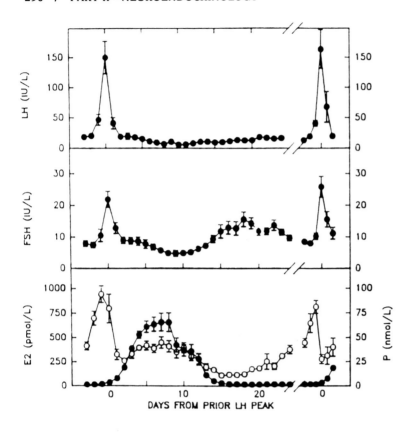

FIGURE 15–11. Mean ($+/-$ sem) of daily serum LH, FSH, E2 *(open circles)* and P *(closed circles)* levels in 12 subjects studied across the luteal follicular transition, graphed in relation to the preceding and subsequent LH surges. A slowed frequency of pulsatile GnRH secretion precedes the rise in FSH which is then correlated with an increasing frequency of pulsatile GnRH secretion. (From Hall JE et al: Hypothalamic gonadotropin-releasing hormone secretion and follicle-stimulating hormone dynamics during the luteal-follicular transition. J Clin Endocrinol Metab 74:600–607, 1992, © The Endocrine Society.)

hypothalamic and pituitary site of action. Studies in which the testosterone infusion was accompanied by administration of testolactone to reduce aromatization of testosterone to estradiol indicated that the predominant hypothalamic effect of testosterone on GnRH pulse frequency is mediated through its conversion to estradiol, but that testosterone itself has a small but direct hypothalamic effect independent of aromatization.

Gonadal Peptide Modulation of Gonadotropin Secretion

The differential secretion of LH and FSH in response to what has been proposed to be a single releasing factor has provoked a long-standing interest in the role of other gonadal regulators of pituitary function, specifically, a selective inhibitor of FSH. Although initially described in 1932, inhibin was not purified until 1985. Inhibin is a heterodimer, composed of covalently linked α and β subunits produced primarily by ovarian granulosa and testicular Sertoli cells. Its production is controlled by FSH (in conjunction with a number of other important modulators), and its main endocrine action is the selective suppression of FSH biosynthesis and secretion.[60–62] In addition, it appears to have an important intragonadal role in either a paracrine or autocrine mode. Although a number of assays for assessment of circulating levels of inhibin in the human have been developed, each has been plagued by a lack of specificity for the dimeric hormone as well as difficulty in measurement of intact inhibin in serum.[79] Thus, an understanding of the dynamic changes in inhibin and its role in human physiology has yet to be determined.

During the purification of inhibin it became apparent that another gonadal peptide, activin, a dimer composed of two of the β subunits of inhibin, could stimulate FSH secretion. This β subunit homodimer is present in a number of tissues in addition to the gonad, including pituitary and bone marrow.[62] While the physiology of activin has yet to be completely elucidated, there is increasing evidence that it may function primarily as a paracrine or autocrine growth factor especially at the pituitary level, promoting FSH biosynthesis.

Follistatin is an additional gonadal peptide that bears no structural similarity to the inhibin/activin family of peptides.[61] It is composed of a single polypeptide chain, is a potent inhibitor of FSH biosynthesis and secretion, and is synergistic with inhibin in this action, probably by serving as a binding protein for inhibin and activin with a much greater affinity for activin.

GONADOTROPINS IN THE DIAGNOSIS OF REPRODUCTIVE DISORDERS

The general principles underlying the diagnosis of disorders of the reproductive endocrine system are similar in males and females. In patients with suspected abnormalities of reproductive function, the defect may lie at the level of the hypothalamus, the pituitary, the gonad, or the outflow tract (the uterus in the female and the vas deferens in the male). A detailed history and a careful physical examination often provide many diagnostic clues and focus on laboratory testing to make the evaluation cost-effective and accurate. Once the defect has been localized to a given anatomical level, a differential diagnosis can then be generated that employs the information garnered from the history and physical examination. Key to the anatomic localization of the defect is the assessment of gonadotropin status. In general, in patients with disorders of the outflow tract, both sex steroid and gonadotropin levels will be normal. In patients with abnormalities at the gonadal level, gonadotropin levels will be elevated in the presence of low levels of gonadal steroids due to the failure of negative feedback of gonadally derived factors on gonadotropin secretion (Fig. 15–12A). Patients with either a hypothalamic or a pituitary site of disruption of the reproductive axis will have either low or normal levels of gonadotropins in the presence of low levels of sex steroids (Fig. 15–12B), the

gonadotropin levels reflecting either a disordered pattern of GnRH secretion with consequent abnormal pituitary stimulation or an abnormal gonadotrope response to pulsatile GnRH (Fig. 15–12C).

It is important to determine whether the failure of function of the reproductive axis is primary in its temporal occurrence as in the case of delayed puberty or if it follows a period of time in which any part of the reproductive axis has been functional. A primary disorder requires consider-

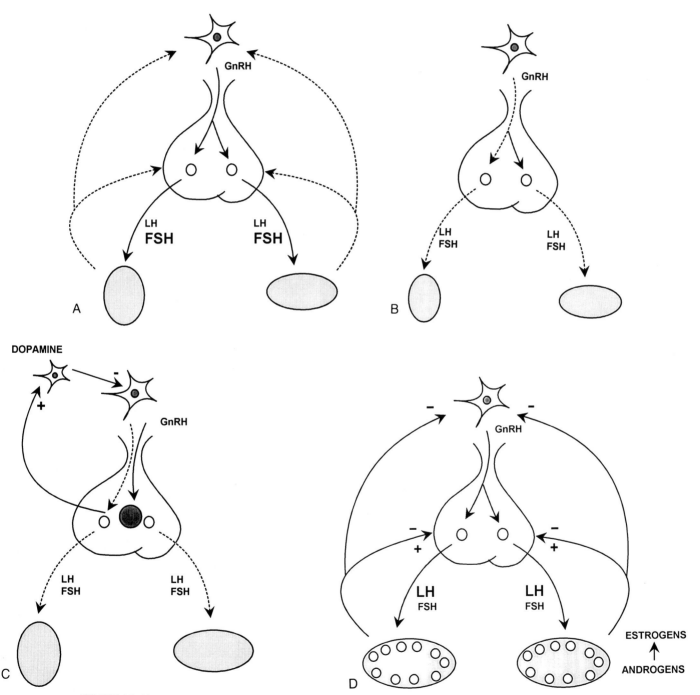

FIGURE 15–12. Diagrammatic representation of the hormonal relationships in disorders of reproductive function. *A,* Gonadal failure with absence of negative feedback restraint of gonadotropin secretion; *B,* Hypogonadotropic disorders due to hypothalamic dysfunction with abnormalities of GnRH secretion or, rarely, to failure of pituitary response to GnRH; *C,* Pituitary dysfunction with abnormalities of gonadotropin secretion occurring either directly due to a mass effect *(right)* or secondary to dopaminergic inhibition of GnRH *(left);* and *D,* Polycystic ovarian syndrome with abnormalities in hypothalamic GnRH pulse frequency, pituitary LH, and FSH dynamics and ovarian steroid secretion.

ation of a broader differential diagnosis that includes congenital abnormalities, androgen resistance syndromes, and chromosomal abnormalities. On the other hand, most processes more commonly associated with secondary hypogonadism in both males and females may also present as primary hypogonadism.

Hypergonadotropic Disorders in Women

An elevation of FSH greater than two standard deviations above the normal follicular phase range in a hypoestrogenic amenorrheic woman is virtual proof of failure of gonadal function. When this situation occurs in a women under 40 years of age, it is termed *premature ovarian failure.* In most cases LH levels will also be significantly elevated, but FSH is a more sensitive marker of gonadal deficiency. The clinical history often reveals the pathognomical finding of hot flashes causing nighttime wakening and vaginal dryness. Interestingly, the course of premature ovarian failure may be a waxing and waning one with reciprocal changes in estradiol and FSH occurring over several years and evidence of follicular development and even pregnancy in occasional hypergonadotropic patients following diagnosis.[80]

An increasing body of evidence suggests that premature ovarian failure may not be a singular entity with a single prognosis. A decrease in the initial complement of germ cells appears to underlie the ovarian failure associated with galactosemia, while an increased rate of follicular atresia during childhood appears to be the mechanism responsible for premature ovarian failure associated with abnormalities of the X chromosome such as Turner's syndrome and its variants (XO, XO/XX, XXX) and possibly also the familial syndrome resulting from an interstitial deletion of the X chromosome.[81] In such patients, menopause will occur before menarche. Premature ovarian failure is also seen in association with damage to the developing oocytes from radiation and certain chemotherapeutic agents.[82] Autoimmune mechanisms are likely to explain the development of ovarian failure in yet another subset of patients in whom lymphocytic invasion of the ovary and/or circulating

antibodies to gonadal tissue have been demonstrated.[83] Antibodies to the steroid-producing cells have been described in patients with both type I and type II polyglandular failure syndromes. Antibodies have also been identified to both the FSH receptor and the LH receptor in patients with systemic lupus erythematosus, although these have been poorly characterized. Recent data suggest that cell-mediated immune mechanisms may also play a role in the premature ovarian failure of some patients. Finally, there is a subset of patients with elevated gonadotropins in whom normal ovarian follicles are seen on biopsy. In this final subset of patients, whose condition is termed "resistant ovary syndrome," the potential etiologies include antibodies to the gonadotropin receptor, proteins that inhibit binding to the FSH and/or LH receptor, or secretion of gonadotropins that are not biologically active as may occur in patients with gonadotropin-producing pituitary tumors[84] or with structural defects in one or other of the gonadotropins.[85] In recent studies, comparison of samples in patients with premature ovarian failure in an FSH radioreceptor assay and a dimer-specific FSH immunoassay revealed a subset of patients with a high receptor to immunoassay ratio (Fig. 15–13).[86] In this subset of patients, two separate inhibitors of binding to the FSH receptor have been identified, one of which may well be a form of the α-subunit of inhibin. The use of these gonadotropin receptor assays in conjunction with immunoassays and bioassays will ultimately facilitate the classification of patients with premature ovarian failure into different subsets in which therapeutic options may differ.

Hypogonadotropic Disorders in Women

In patients with hypogonadotropic hypogonadism, the absence of cyclic gonadal function associated with gonadotropin levels that are often normal or only slightly decreased presents an apparent paradox. These patients with hypogonadotropic hypogonadism may present with either primary amenorrhea, i.e., failure to progress normally through puberty to the point of establishment of normal reproductive cycles, or with secondary amenorrhea. While

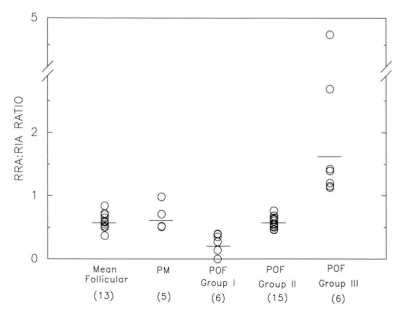

FIGURE 15–13. Radioreceptor to radioimmunoassay (RRA/RIA) ratios in patients with premature ovarian failure (POF) divided into three groups by comparison to mean follicular phase levels and to postmenopausal women (PM). (From Schneyer AL et al: Development of a radioligand receptor assay for measuring follitropin in serum: Application to premature ovarian failure. Clin Chem 37:508–514, 1991.)

this clinical presentation is most commonly seen in association with a functional hypothalamic defect, it may also occur secondary to specific neuroanatomical lesions of the hypothalamus or the pituitary.

Hypothalamic Causes

The most common group of patients in whom low levels of gonadotropins accompany hypoestrogenism, comprising two thirds to three quarters of all patients presenting with amenorrhea, are those in whom a structural neuroanatomical lesion cannot be found. The diagnosis given to such patients is "hypothalamic amenorrhea."[87] Studies in which the pattern of pulsatile secretion of LH and FSH levels in patients with hypothalamic amenorrhea has been compared to that in normal women in the early follicular phase, i.e., matched for ambient sex steroid levels, have revealed an underlying spectrum of defects of pulsatile GnRH secretion (Fig. 15–14).[51, 88, 89] The most severe form of this GnRH abnormality is characterized by a complete lack of any GnRH-induced gonadotropin secretion. This condition results in extremely low levels of LH, whereas FSH levels—which are somewhat less suppressed—are often within the normal range. This discrepancy in gona-

dotropin levels with reversal of the LH:FSH ratio is presumably caused by the differential dependence of LH versus FSH on GnRH as already discussed. This "apulsatile" group includes patients with primary amenorrhea, often in the presence of anosmia (Kallmann's syndrome), in whom the defect in GnRH secretion is congenital, and patients with anorexia nervosa,[90] in whom it is reversible with weight gain. Other abnormalities of pulsatile GnRH secretion include patterns of low amplitude, slow frequency, and nighttime augmentation—all of which are inadequate programs of GnRH secretion to sustain orderly folliculogenesis and ovulation.[51] Patients in whom amenorrhea is clinically associated with excessive exercise,[91] weight loss, stress, and acute or chronic intercurrent illness are often represented in these latter groups, attesting to the clinical consequences of environmental factors on control of the GnRH pulse generator in the human. The neuroendocrine mediators of these environmental cues may include the inhibitory influence of increased opioidergic or dopaminergic tone on the GnRH pulse generator or the effects of alterations in melatonin or CRF (see Chs. 13 and 118). This spectrum of defects in pulsatile GnRH secretion in patients with hypothalamic amenorrhea thus explains the variation in gonadotropin and estrogen levels often encountered during random diagnostic testing as well as the varying response to therapy that have long puzzled clinicians treating patients with hypothalamic amenorrhea. It also predicts a uniformly positive response to therapeutic institution of a physiological regimen of exogenous GnRH for ovulation induction in such patients.[73, 74]

Structural lesions in the hypothalamus that interfere with the normal pattern of GnRH secretion underlie the development of hypogonadotropic amenorrhea in a small subset of patients. In the majority of such cases a careful history and physical examination will specifically prompt the search for a structural neuroanatomical lesion. Such abnormalities include craniopharyngiomas that commonly present with growth retardation, visual impairment, or headache. Other tumors with a predilection for midline CNS structures, including germinomas, gliomas, meningiomas, and endodermal sinus tumors as well as rare metastatic tumors, dermoid cysts, or teratomas, may be found infrequently and are often accompanied by other localizing signs or symptoms. Langerhans histiocytosis and infiltrative disorders of the hypothalamus such as sarcoidosis and tuberculosis are usually accompanied by diabetes insipidus. Head injuries are an infrequent cause of hypogonadotropic hypogonadism. The amenorrhea associated with cranial irradiation, increasingly seen in long-term survivors of childhood malignancies, is far more likely to be of hypothalamic than of pituitary origin because of the greater sensitivity of the hypothalamus to the destructive effects of radiation.[92]

Pituitary Causes

Pituitary defects account for approximately 20 per cent of cases of amenorrhea, with the vast majority of these being prolactinomas. The presentation of headache, visual field defects, and other hormonal deficiencies, which is typical of other pituitary tumors, is rare in women with prolactinomas. Amenorrhea or galactorrhea or both are usually the earliest symptom(s) of a prolactin-secreting mi-

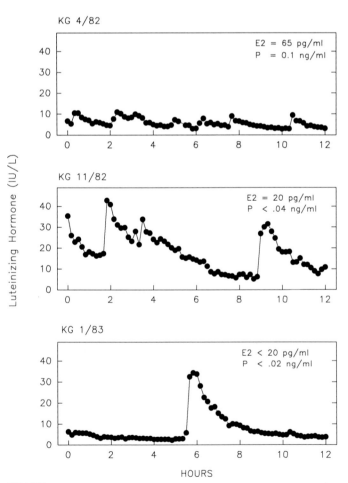

FIGURE 15–14. Serial studies in a patient with hypothalamic amenorrhea indicating the sectrum of defects of amplitude and frequency of GnRH secretion that can be seen in a single patient studied over time. (Adapted from Crowley WF Jr et al: The physiology of gonadotropin-releasing hormone (GnRH) secretion in men and women. Rec Prog Horm Res 41:473–481, 1985.)

croadenoma, although some patients also present with galactorrhea. However, their gonadotropin profile is identical to that seen in patients with hypothalamic amenorrhea. Although the anatomical defect in prolactin-secreting tumors is clearly at the level of the pituitary, the etiology of gonadotropin deficiency in this disorder is not in the inability of the pituitary to secrete gonadotropins but in the increase in dopamine turnover within the hypothalamus, which is a consequence of hyperprolactinemia and which is inhibitory to GnRH secretion (see Fig. 15–12C).[93] Thus, these patients present with a spectrum of abnormalities of pulsatile GnRH secretion and gonadotropin levels identical to that observed in patients with hypothalamic amenorrhea.

Other pituitary tumors such as those secreting GH, ACTH, or gonadotropin subunits and pituitary infarction are quite rare causes of hypothalamic amenorrhea and generally are associated with other clinical or biochemical features that help to localize the site of the defect to the pituitary. Lymphocytic hypophysitis has also been reported in association with isolated gonadotropin deficiency, primarily in the postpartum setting.[94]

Polycystic Ovarian Syndrome

Patients with polycystic ovarian syndrome (PCOS) are difficult to categorize in a schema that depends on either hypersecretion or hyposecretion of gonadotropins or reliance on neuroanatomical localization of the site of the defect, since the basic defect is unknown (see Fig. 15–12D). The clinical presentation is most typically of androgen excess (hirsutism or acne) in the presence of amenorrhea or oligoamenorrhea, generally having its onset in adolescence. Morphological and functional abnormalities of the ovary have been identified in these patients,[95, 96] but whether these abnormalities are primary or secondary to abnormal stimulation by gonadotropins, adrenal androgens, or hyperinsulinemia is as yet unresolved. High levels of LH in the presence of normal to low levels of FSH and a resultant elevation in the ratio of LH to FSH characterize the gonadotropin abnormality common to a large subset of patients with PCOS.[97] The elevation of LH has been observed using both immunoassays and bioassays, and the normal to low levels of FSH would also appear to be biologically active. An increased amplitude and frequency of pulsatile LH secretion (see Fig. 15–8)[69] has been documented as well as an increased gonadotropin responsiveness to exogenous GnRH secretion.[98] These results suggest that there are abnormalities in both hypothalamic GnRH secretion and pituitary responsiveness in PCOS, although the mechanisms responsible for these alterations remain unclear. The pattern of gonadotropin secretion may result from abnormal feedback of androgens or chronically elevated estrogen levels; however, definitive proof of this hypothesis is lacking. The similarity of the discrepant pattern of LH and FSH in association with a fast frequency of pulsatile GnRH secretion in patients with PCOS (see Fig. 15–8) to those observed in GnRH-deficient patients, in whom increasing frequencies of exogenous GnRH were administered (see Fig. 15–7), has led to the hypothesis that the abnormal pituitary responsiveness in PCOS may be due to the increased frequency of GnRH secretion, per se. This increased frequency of GnRH secretion may represent one of the intrinsic abnormalities in PCOS, as suggested by the abnormal chronobiology of LH secretion in adolescents with PCOS[99] and by the lifelong tendency of patients with PCOS to revert to an abnormal gonadotropin profile following successful ovulation induction with estrogen antagonists, exogenous gonadotropins, or exogenous pulsatile GnRH.[100]

Hypergonadotropic Disorders in Men

In men, high levels of gonadotropins—particularly FSH—almost invariably accompany testicular failure (see Fig. 15–12A). Interestingly, the gonadotropin elevations seen with gonadal failure in men are relatively modest in comparison with the changes in women, a further example of the sexual dimorphism in gonadotropin secretion already described. Clinically, patients may present with infertility secondary to defects of spermatogenesis, evidence of underandrogenization, or gynecomastia. Testicular volume is usually decreased with seminiferous tubule damage, as the seminiferous tubules account for greater than 60 per cent of testicular volume in normal men.

The most common developmental or structural testicular abnormality is Klinefelter's syndrome (XXY), which affects as many as one in 500 males and is associated with seminiferous tubule dysgenesis.[101] The classic form, which probably results from an early meiotic nondysjunction, is associated with small, firm testes, azoospermia, gynecomastia, excessive growth of the long bones, and elevated levels of FSH. Leydig cell damage is variable and thus testosterone levels and the degree of virilization may vary considerably. In general, LH levels are inversely proportional to testosterone levels. The testosterone/estradiol ratio is elevated due to increased testicular production of estrogen, resulting in a high prevalence of gynecomastia in these patients who must be monitored closely because of a 20-fold increased risk of developing breast cancer. Patients with 46 XY/XXY mosaicism and XX males show similar but more variable features of Klinefelter's syndrome.

Less common associations with hypergonadotropic hypogonadism include myotonia dystrophica and Noonan's syndrome,[102] an autosomal dominant syndrome in which a normal karyotype is associated with the somatic features found in girls with Turner's syndrome (webbed neck, short stature, cubitus valgus, shield-like chest, and various cardiovascular abnormalities). Cryptorchidism and mental retardation are common in Noonan's syndrome and LH and FSH levels are elevated in those with diminished testicular function. In rare patients, hypergonadotropic hypogonadism is the result of congenital agenesis or anorchia, in which there is no recognizable testicular tissue possibly because of testicular torsion or viral infection after the 14th week of gestation.

A number of disorders appear to preferentially damage the germinal epithelium and are therefore characterized by oligospermia or azoospermia and increased FSH levels but normal serum levels of testosterone and LH. In any of these disorders, if the testicular damage is particularly severe, Leydig cell damage may also occur with decreased testosterone and increased LH levels. The most common cause of acquired testicular failure is viral orchitis, with the mumps virus most frequently responsible. The primary damage is to the seminiferous tubules, but occasionally Leydig cell damage may result in low levels of testosterone in addition to the induced abnormalities in spermatogenesis. The position of the testis in the scrotum makes it uniquely susceptible to trauma and to temperature elevations, both of which can also result in defects in spermatogenesis. The testis is also extremely sensitive to the effects of ionizing radiation.[103] While some patients present with decreased spermatogenesis alone, Leydig cell damage from diminished testicular blood flow may also result in transient and occasionally permanent decreases in testosterone. Certain chemotherapeutic agents, anabolic steroids, alcohol, and marijuana may also result in permanent testicular damage. Rarely, testicular failure may be part of a generalized autoimmune disorder or may result from granulomatous disease or from testicular iron deposition in hemachromatosis or sickle cell anemia. Germinal cell aplasia (Sertoli cell only) is associated with failure of spermatogenesis but normal testosterone production. Its etiology is unclear, although both genetic and viral etiologies have been suggested.

While testicular damage is the most common cause of hypergonadotropic hypogonadism in men, elevations in gonadotropins may also be caused by structural abnormalities in the gonadotropin hormones or their receptors or by substances that inhibit binding of the gonadotropin hormones to their receptors. A single amino acid substitution in the β-subunit of LH, resulting in the synthesis of biologically inactive LH, has recently been described in a patient with hypergonadotropic hypogonadism.[85] In patients with gonadotropin-producing pituitary tumors, abnormal secretion of the biologically inactive α- and β-subunits may be associated with hypogonadism.[104, 105] The degree to which levels of LH and FSH are elevated will depend on the specificity of the assay for the α- and β-subunits and the intact hormone. An abnormality of the LH receptor has been suggested in a 46,XY male with primary hypogonadism by functional studies,[105a] but there have been no reports to date of gonadotropin-receptor abnormalities using molecular techniques. The cloning of the human LH and FSH receptors now makes such investigations possible. Inhibitors of LH or FSH receptor binding may occur in men as in women. Finally, abnormalities of the androgen receptor, resulting in a limited form of androgen resistance, were identified in 40 per cent of patients with idiopathic azoospermia in a study of unselected men with idiopathic infertility.[106]

Hypogonadotropic Disorders in Men

The clinical presentation in men with hypogonadotropic hypogonadism is similar to that of primary testicular damage, i.e., delayed or absent puberty or secondary evidence of hypogonadism (see Fig. 15–12B). The possibility of restoration of normal physiology including fertility makes identification of this relatively rare subset of disorders particularly important. Low testosterone levels in association with low or normal levels of gonadotropins indicate an abnormality of hypothalamic GnRH secretion or a deficient pituitary responsiveness. Unfortunately, single-bolus GnRH testing is of little value in the differentiation of hypothalamic and pituitary etiologies. In men, congenital disorders and neuroanatomical lesions of the hypothalamus or pituitary that result in hypogonadotropic hypogonadism are more common than they are in women while functional disorders of the hypothalamus occur relatively infrequently.

Hypothalamic Causes

Hypothalamic GnRH deficiency may result from any of the same neuroanatomical causes just described that affect the generation of normal GnRH pulses in women (tumors, infiltrative disorders, CNS radiation) or it can be idiopathic. Idiopathic hypogonadotropic hypogonadism (IHH) is characterized by an isolated deficiency of GnRH secretion in the absence of a structural CNS lesion.[107] The complete absence of pulsatile LH secretion combined with the ability of a pulsatile regimen of exogenous GnRH to completely reverse the gonadotropin abnormality has localized the defect in this disorder to the hypothalamus.[108] IHH is associated with anosmia in approximately 30 per cent of cases,[108] an association that was first described by Kallmann in 1944. Since the initial description, it has been recognized that other midline craniofacial defects such as cleft lip and palate, deafness, and color blindness may be present with hypogonadotropic hypogonadism or may track separately through affected families. Studies have suggested both X-linked and autosomal dominant and recessive modes of inheritance.[109, 110] In humans, the GnRH gene on chromosome 8 is normal[111, 112] in contrast to the hypogonadotropic mouse model, in which a significant deletion in the GnRH gene produces hypogonadotropic hypogonadotropism.

Recent studies in patients with the X-linked form of Kallmann's syndrome have provided evidence for a candidate gene on the short arm of the X chromosome (Xp22.3).[113] The homology of this deleted gene with N-CAM, a neural adhesion molecule,[114] strengthens the hypothesis that Kallmann's syndrome may be caused by migration arrest of GnRH neurons along their path to the hypothalamus.[115] Clinically, patients may present with microphallus and cryptorchidism at birth or with failure to progress through puberty. Occasional individuals with partial sexual maturation have been identified and may represent an acquired form of GnRH deficiency. An additional variant of hypogonadotropic hypogonadism in men is the "fertile eunuch" syndrome, in which patients have sufficient GnRH-induced gonadotropin secretion to stimulate high intratesticular testosterone levels and spermatogenesis yet inadequate testosterone levels for complete virilization. Hypogonadotropic hypogonadism can also occur as part of several other congenital syndromes discussed in Chapter 133.

In patients with protein-calorie malnutrition, Hodgkin's disease and cancer prior to chemotherapy, and in acute conditions such as myocardial infarction, head trauma, general surgery, and burns, the etiology of low levels of testosterone appears to be multifactorial.[116] Unlike in the sick euthyroid syndrome there is no evidence of interference of the binding of testosterone with its carrier protein.[117]

Pituitary Causes

Pituitary causes of hypogonadotropic hypogonadism are rare in men. Prolactin-secreting microadenomas, the most common pituitary cause of hypogonadotropin hypogonadism in women, occur infrequently in men, in whom their presentation is often late and associated with tumors of large size (see Fig. 15–12C). Nonfunctioning pituitary adenomas or those secreting either intact hormones or their subunits may result in hypogonadotropic hypogonadism because of their space-occupying effects, interference with GnRH secretion (PRL and ACTH producing tumors), or secretion of abnormal gonadotropins (LH and FSH secreting tumors; see above). Hemochromatosis and sickle cell disease can present with gonadal failure in men because of iron deposition in the pituitary, which has a predilection for the gonadotropes.[117, 118] Iron deposition may also occur at the hypothalamic and gonadal levels. Recovery of pituitary function may be possible in such patients with phlebotomy and reduction of the iron load.

CONCLUSIONS

Pituitary gonadotropin secretion is precisely controlled in normal men and women by both hypothalamic and gonadal factors. The primary level of control is via the GnRH pulse generator, which integrates a variety of environmental cues with gonadal steroid feedback. Direct feedback of gonadal steroids and peptides at the level of the pituitary provides an additional mechanism through which the precise regulation of the reproductive axis is mediated. Evaluation of gonadotropin secretion in patients presenting with hypogonadism (abnormalities of gametogenesis and/or steroidogenesis) provides the key to the diagnosis and subsequent treatment of their reproductive disorder.

REFERENCES

1. Pierce JG, Parsons TF: Glycoprotein hormones: Structure and function. Ann Rev Biochem 50:465–495, 1981.
2. Gharib SD, Wierman ME, Shupnik MA, Chin WW: Molecular biology of the pituitary gonadotropins. Endocr Rev 11:177–199, 1990.
3. Chappel SC, Ulloa-Aguirre A, Coutifaiis C: Biosynthesis and secretion of follicle-stimulating hormone. Endocr Rev 4:179–211, 1976.
4. Taylor AE, Crowley WF: Epitopic mapping of human gonadotropins. In Greenstein B (ed): Neuroendocrine Research Methods, New York, Harwood Academic, 1991, pp 955–986.
5. Whitcomb RW, O'Dea LStL, Finkelstein JS, et al: Utility of free α-subunit as an alternative neuroendocrine marker of gonadotropin-releasing hormone (GnRH) stimulation of the gonadotroph in the human: Evidence from normal and GnRH-deficient men. J Clin Endocrinol Metab 70:1654–1661, 1990.
6. Gougeon A: Dynamics of follicular growth in the human: A model from preliminary results. Human Reprod 1:81–87, 1986.
7. Hodgen GD: The dominant ovarian follicle. Fertil Steril 38:281–300, 1982.
8. Richards JS, Jonassen JA, Rolfes AI, et al: Adenosine-3′,5′-monophosphate, luteinizing hormone receptor and progesterone during granulosa cell differentiation: Effects of estradiol and follicle-stimulating hormone. Endocrinology 104:765–773, 1979.
9. Louvet JP, Vaitukaitis JL: Induction of follicle-stimulating hormone (FSH) receptors in rat ovaries by estrogen priming. Endocrinology 99:758–764, 1976.
10. Channing CP: Steroidogenesis and morphology of human ovarian cell types in tissue culture. J Endocrinol 45:297–308, 1969.
11. McNatty KP, Makris A, DeGrazia C, et al: The production of progesterone, androgens, and estrogens by granulosa cells, thecal tissue, and stromal tissue from human ovaries in vitro. J Clin Endocrinol Metab 49:687–699, 1979.
12. Koos RD: Potential relevance of angiogenic factors to ovarian physiology. Semin Reprod Endocrinol 7:29–40, 1989.
13. Vande Wiele RL, Bogumil J, Dyarenfurth I, et al: Mechanisms regulating the menstrual cycle in women. Recent Prog Horm Res 26:63–103, 1970.
14. McLachlan RI, Cohen NL, Vale WW et al: The importance of luteinizing hormone in the control of inhibin and progesterone secretion by the human corpus luteum. J Clin Endocrinol Metab 68:1078–1085, 1989.
15. Tsafriri A, Lindner HR, Zor U, Lamprecht SA: Physiological role of prostaglandins in the induction of ovulation. Prostaglandins 2:1–10, 1972.
16. Beers WH, Strickland S, Reich E: Ovarian plasminogen activator: relationship to ovulation and hormonal regulation. Cell 6:387–394, 1975.
17. Bremner WJ, Matsumoto AM, Sussman AM, Paulsen CA: Follicle-stimulating hormone and human spermatogenesis. J Clin Invest 68:1044–1052, 1981.
18. Matsumoto AM, Paulsen CA, Bremner WJ: Stimulation of sperm production by human luteinizing hormone in gonadotropin-suppressed normal men. J Clin Endocrinol Metab 55:882–887, 1984.
19. Wahlstrom T, Huhtaniemi I, Hovatta O, et al: Localization of luteinizing hormone, follicle-stimulating hormone, prolactin and their receptors in human and rat testis using immunohistochemistry and radioreceptor assay. J Clin Endocrinol Metab 57:825–830, 1983.
20. Hansson W, Weddington SC, McLean WS, et al: Regulation of seminiferous tubular function by FSH and androgen. J Reprod Fertil 44:363–375, 1975.
21. Tindall DJ, Miller DA, Means AR: Characterization of androgen receptor in Sertoli cell–enriched testis. Endocrinology 101:13–23, 1977.
22. Skinner MK: Cell-cell interactions in the testis. Endocr Rev 12:45–77, 1991.
23. Kerr JB, Sharpe RM: Follicle-stimulating hormone induction of Leydig cell maturation. Endocrinology 116:2592–2604, 1985.
24. Ketelslegers JM, Hetzel WD, Sherins RJ, et al: Developmental changes in testicular gonadotropin receptors: Plasma gonadotropins and plasma testosterone in the rat. Endocrinology 103:212–222, 1978.
25. Fritz IB, Rommerts FG, Louis BG, Dorrington JH: Regulation of FSH and dibutyryl cyclic AMP of the formation of androgen-binding protein in Sertoli cell-enriched cultures. J Reprod Fertil 46:17–24, 1976.
26. Dorrington JH, Armstrong DT: Follicle-stimulating hormone stimulates estradiol-17β synthesis in cultured Sertoli cells. Proc Natl Acad Sci USA 72:2677–2681, 1975.
27. Spratt DI, O'Dea LS, Schoenfeld D, et al: Neuroendocrine-gonadal axis in men: Frequent sampling of LH, FSH and testosterone. Am J Physiol 254:E658–E666, 1988.
28. Huhtaniemi IT, Clayton RN, Catt KJ: Gonadotropin binding and Leydig cell activation in the rat testis in vivo. Endocrinology 111:982–987, 1982.
29. Schwanzel-Fukuda M, Pfaff DW: Migration of LHRH-immunoreactive neurons from the olfactory placode rationalizes olfacto-hormonal relationships. J Steroid Biochem Molec Biol 39:565–572, 1991.
30. Gibson MJ, Charlton HM, Perlow MJ, et al: Preoptic area brain grafts in hypogonadal (hpg) female mice abolish effects of congenital hypothalamic gonadotropin-releasing hormone deficiency. Endocrinology 114:1938–1940, 1984.
31. Grumbach MM, Kaplan SL: The neuroendocrinology of human puberty: an ontogenetic perspective. In Grumbach MM, Sizonenko PC, Aubert ML (eds): Control of the Onset of Puberty. Baltimore, Williams & Wilkins, 1990, pp 1–68.
32. Kaplan SL, Grumbach MM: The ontogenesis of human foetal hormones. II Luteinizing hormone (LH) and follicle stimulating hormone (FSH). Acta Endocrinol 81:808–829, 1976.
33. Castillo RH, Matteri RL, Dumesic AD: Luteinizing hormone synthesis in cultured fetal human pituitary cells exposed to gonadotropin-releasing hormone. J Clin Endocrinol Metab 75:318–322, 1992.
34. Wierman ME, Crowley WF: Neuroendocrine control of the onset of puberty. In Falkner F, Tanner JM (eds): Human Growth, A Comprehensive Treatise (ed 2), Volume 2. New York, Plenum Press, 1986, pp 225–241.
35. Waldhauser F, Weibenbacher G, Frisch H, Pollak A: Pulsatile secretion of gonadotropins in early infancy. Eur J Pediatr 137:71–74, 1981.
36. Resko JA, Ellinwood WE: Negative feedback regulation of gonadotropin secretion by androgens in fetal rhesus macaques. Biol Reprod 33:346–352, 1985.
37. Axelrod L, Neer RM, Kliman B: Hypogonadism in a male with immunologically active, biologically inactive luteinizing hormone: An

exception to a venerable rule. J Clin Endocrinol Metab 48:279–287, 1979.

38. Baker RG, Scrimgeour JB: Development of the gonad in normal and anencephalic human fetuses. J Reprod Fertil 68:193–199, 1980.

39. Huhtaniemi IT, Yamomoto M, Ranta T, et al: Follicle-stimulating hormone receptors appear earlier in the primate fetal testis than in the ovary. J Clin Endocrinol Metab 65:1210–1214, 1987.

40. George RW, Wilson JD: Conversion of androgen to estrogen by the human fetal ovary. J Clin Endocrinol Metab 47:550–555, 1978.

41. Rabinovici J, Goldsmith PC, Roberts VJ, et al: Localization and secretion of inhibin/activin subunits in the human and subhuman primate fetal gonads. J Clin Endocrinol Metab 73:1141–1149, 1991.

42. Apter D, Cacciatore B, Alfthan H, Stenman U: Serum luteinizing hormone concentrations increase 100-fold in females from 7 years of age to adulthood, as measured by time-resolved immunofluorometric assay. J Clin Endocrinol Metab 68:53–57, 1989.

43. Wiemann JN, Clifton DK, Steiner RA: Pubertal changes in gonadotropin releasing and proopiomelanocortin gene expression in the brain of the male rat. Endocrinology 124:1760–1767, 1989.

44. Gay VL, Plant TM: N-methyl-D,L-aspartate elicits hypothalamic gonadotropin-releasing hormone release in prepubertal male Rhesus monkeys. Endocrinology 120:2289–2296, 1987.

45. Frisch RE, McArthur JW: Menstrual cycles: Fatness as a determinant of their maintenance or onset. Science 185:949–951, 1974.

46. Foster DL, Olster DH: Effect of restricted nutrition on puberty in the lamb: patterns of tonic luteinizing hormone (LH) secretion and competency of the LH surge mechanism. Endocrinology 116:375–381, 1985.

47. Boyar R, Finkelstein J, Roffwrag H, et al: Synchronization of augmented luteinizing hormone secretion with sleep during puberty. N Engl J Med 287:582–586, 1972.

48. Lucky AW, Rich BH, Rosenfield RL, et al: LH bioactivity increases more than immunoreactivity during puberty. J Pediatr 97:205–213, 1980.

49. Wide L, Wide M: Higher plasma disappearance rate in the mouse for pituitary follicle-stimulating normone of young women compared to that of men and elderly women. J Clin Endocrinol Metab 58:426–429, 1984.

50. Hall JE, Schoenfeld DA, Martin KA, Crowley WF, Jr: Hypothalamic GnRH secretion and FSH dynamics during the luteal-follicular transition. J Clin Endocrinol Metab 70:328–335, 1990.

51. Santoro N, Filicori M, Crowley WF, Jr: Hypogonadotropic disorders in men and women: diagnosis and therapy with pulsatile gonadotropin-releasing hormone. Endocr Rev 7:11–23, 1986.

52. Sherman BM, Korenman SG: Hormonal characteristics of the human menstrual cycle throughout reproductive life. J Clin Invest 55:699–706, 1975.

53. Zumoff B, Strain GW, Kearns J, et al: Age variation of the 24-hour mean plasma concentrations of androgens, estrogens and gonadotropins in normal men. J Clin Endocrinol Metab 54:534–538, 1982.

54. Vermeulen A, Kaufman JM: Role of the hypothalamo-pituitary function in the hypoandrogenism of healthy aging. J Clin Endocrinol Metab 75:704–705, 1992.

55. Crowley WF Jr, Filicori M, Spratt DI, Santoro NF: The physiology of gonadotropin-releasing hormone (GnRH) secretion in men and women. Recent Prog Hormone Res 41:473–531, 1985.

56. Crowley WF Jr, Whitcomb RW, Jameson JL, et al: Neuroendocrine control of human reproductionin the male. Recent Prog Hormone Res 47:27–67, 1991.

57. Hall JE, Whitcomb RW, Riveir JE, et al: Differential regulation of luteinizing hormone, follicle-stimulating hormone, and free α-subunit secretion from the gonadotrope by gonadotropin-releasing hormone (GnRH): Evidence from the use of two GnRH antagonists. J Clin Endocrinol Metab 70:328–335, 1990.

58. Lumpkin MD, Moltz JH, Yu WH, et al: Purification of FSH-releasing hormone: Its dissimilarity from LHRH of mammalian, avian, and piscian origin. Brain Res Bull 18:175–178, 1987.

59. Marshall JC, Dalkin AC, Haisenleder DJ, et al: Gonadotropin-releasing hormone pulses: Regulators of gonadotropin synthesis and ovulatory cycles. Recent Prog Hormone Res 47:155–187, 1991.

60. DeKretser DM, Robertson DM: The isolation and physiology of inhibin and related proteins. Biol Reprod 40:33–47, 1989.

61. Ying SY: Inhibins, activins and follistatins: Gonadal proteins modulating the secretion of follicle-stimulating hormone. Endocr Rev 9:267–293, 1988.

62. Vale W, Rivier C, Hsueh A, et al: Chemical and biological characterization of the inhibin family of protein hormones. Rec Prog Horm Res 44:1–34, 1988.

62a. Weiss J, Harris PE, Halvorson LM, Crowley WF Jr: Dynamic regulation of follicle-stimulating hormone-beta messenger ribonucleic acid levels by activin and gonadotropin-releasing hormone in perfused rat pituitary cells. Endocrinology 131:1403–1408, 1992.

63. Winters SJ, Troen P: A reexamination of pulsatile luteinizing hormone secretion in primary testicular failure. J Clin Endocrinol Metab 57:432–435, 1983.

64. Yen SS, Tsai CC, Naftolin F, et al: Pulsatile patterns of gonadotropin release in subjects with and without ovarian function. J Clin Endocrinol Metab 34:671–675, 1972.

65. Levine JE, Duffy MR: Simultaneous measurement of luteinizing hormone (LH)-releasing hormone, LH and follicle-stimulating hormone release in intact and short-term castrate rats. Endocrinology 122:2211–2221, 1988.

66. Clarke IJ: Exactitude in the relationship between GnRH and LH secretion. In Crowley WF, Jr, Conn MP (eds): Modes of Action of GnRH and its Analogs. New York, Springer-Verlag, 1992, pp 179–192.

67. Belchetz PE, Plant TM, Nakai Y, et al: Hypophysial responses to continuous and intermittent delivery of hypothalamic gonadotropin-releasing hormone. Science 202:631–633, 1978.

67a. Conn PM, Crowley WF Jr: Gonadotropin-releasing hormone and its analogues. N Engl J Med 324:93–103, 1991.

68. Moenter SM, Brand RC, Karsch FJ: Dynamics of gonadotropin-releasing hormone (GnRH) secretion during the GnRH surge: Insights into the mechanism of GnRH surge induction. Endocrinology 130:2978–2984, 1992.

69. Waldstreicher J, Santoro NF, Hall JE, et al: Hyperfunction of the hypothalamic-pituitary axis in women with polycystic ovarian disease: Indirect evidence for partial gonadotroph desensitization. J Clin Endocrinol Metab 66:165–172, 1988.

70. Geola FL, Frumar AM, Tataryn IV, et al: Biological effects of various doses of conjugated equine estrogens in postmenopausal women. J Clin Endocrinol Metab 51:620–625, 1980.

71. Yen SSC, Tsai CC: The biphasic pattern in the feedback action of ethinyl estradiol on the release of pituitary FSH and LH. J Clin Endocrinol Metab 33:882–887, 1971.

72. Keye WR Jr, Jaffe RB: Strength-duration characteristics of estrogen effects on gonadotropin response to gonadotropin-releasing hormone in women. I. Effects of varying duration of estradiol administration. J Clin Endocrinol Metab 41:1003–1008, 1975.

73. Santoro N, Wierman ME, Filicori M, et al: Intravenous administration of pulsatile gonadotropin-releasing hormone in hypothalamic amenorrhea: Effects of dosage. J Clin Endocrinol Metab 62:109–116, 1986.

74. Martin K, Santoro N, Hall J, et al: Management of ovulatory disorders with pulsatile gonadotropin-releasing hormone. J Cin Endocrinol Metab 71:1081A–G, 1990.

75. Adams JM, Hall JE, Taylor AE, Crowley WF Jr: The midcycle surge: Neuroendocrine characterization in normal women. The Endocrine Society 73rd Annual Meeting, Washington, DC, June 19–22; Abstract 856:244, 1991.

76. Kolp LA, Pavlou, Urban RJ, et al: Abrogation by a potent gonadotropin-releasing hormone antagonist of the estrogen/progesterone-stimulated surge-like release of luteinizing hormone and follicle-stimulating hormone in postmenopausal women. J Clin Endocrinol Metab 75:993–997, 1992.

77. Nippoldt TB, Reame NE, Kelch RP, Marshall JC: The roles of estradiol and progesterone in decreasing luteinizing hormone pulse frequency in the luteal phase of the menstrual cycle. J Clin Endocrinol Metab 69:67–76, 1989.

77a. Shoupe D, Montz FJ, Lobo RA: The effects of estrogen and progestin on endogenous opioid activity in oophorectomized women. J Clin Endocrinol Metab 60:178–183, 1985.

78. Couzinet B, Brailly S, Bouchard P, Schaison G: Progesterone stimulates luteinizing hormone secretion by acting directly at the pituitary. J Clin Endocrinol Metab 74:374–378, 1992.

79. Schneyer AL, Mason AJ, Burton LE, et al: Immunoreactive inhibin α-subunit in human serum: Implications for radioimmunoassay. J Clin Endocrinol Metab 70:1208–1212, 1990.

80. Rebar RW, Erickson GF, Yen SSC: Idiopathic premature ovarian failure: Clinical and endocrine characteristics. Fertil Steril 37:35–41, 1982.

81. Krauss CM, Turksoy RN, Atkins L, et al: Familial premature ovarian failure due to an interstitial deletion of the long arm of the X chromosome. N Engl J Med 317:125–131, 1987.

82. Damewood MD, Grochow LB: Prospects for fertility after chemotherapy or radiation for neoplastic disease. Fertil Steril 45:443–459, 1986.

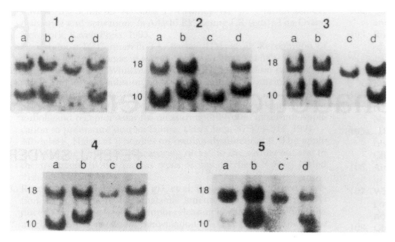

FIGURE 16–1. Demonstration of the apparent monoclonality of five pituitary adenomas. The bands represent DNA fragments of the HPRT gene from the peripheral leukocytes (lanes a and b) and pituitary adenoma cells (lanes c and d) of five women. The leukocytes of each patient show both alleles (lane a), but the adenoma cells show only one allele (lane c), supporting the hypothesis that these adenomas arose from clonal expansion of a single cell. (From Alexander JM, Biller BMK, Bikkal H, et al: Clinically nonfunctioning pituitary tumors are monoclonal in origin. J Clin Invest 86:336–340, 1990; with permission.)

gonadotroph adenomas and supranormal serum FSH concentrations lowers the FSH to normal level.[3]

PATHOPHYSIOLOGY

Secretion by gonadotroph adenomas can be characterized as inefficient, incomplete, and inconsistent. Secretion is inefficient compared with other pituitary adenomas; whereas a lactotroph adenoma 2 cm in diameter usually produces a serum prolactin concentration 100 to 1000 times normal, a gonadotroph adenoma of that size produces a serum FSH concentration no more than 10 times normal and sometimes not supranormal at all.[4] Secretion is incomplete in that secretion of both intact FSH and LH—and only them—is unusual; instead, secretion usually involves some combination of intact FSH and α, FSHβ, and LHβ subunits.[4] Secretion is inconsistent among adenomas in the relative amounts of intact FSH and LH and the subunits each secretes. These characteristics can be recognized both in vivo and in vitro and both basally and in response to stimulation.

Basal Secretion

Intact FSH and LH

Gonadotroph adenomas often produce supranormal serum concentrations of intact FSH but uncommonly of intact LH.[4, 5] This conclusion is drawn from data obtained in men because of the difficulty in interpreting basal values of gonadotropins and their subunits in women with pituitary macroadenomas. In a recent series of 38 men who had clinically nonfunctioning pituitary adenomas, most of which had in vitro evidence of gonadotroph origin, 10 had supranormal serum FSH concentrations (Fig. 16–2).[5] The degree of FSH elevation may range from minimal to 10 times the upper limit of normal. The intact FSH secreted by gonadotroph adenomas appears to be normal, or nearly normal, qualitatively. The size of the FSH is similar to that of intact FSH, and not to FSHβ or α subunits, by gel filtration.[6] The charge on the FSH molecules secreted by gonadotroph adenomas also appears to be normal, as judged by chromatofocusing patterns.[7] Biological activity of the FSH when tested in vitro is even greater than that from normal men, but biological activity has not been tested in vivo.[8]

Gonadotroph adenomas uncommonly produce supranormal serum concentrations of intact LH[9, 10] and rarely of sufficient degree to cause a supranormal serum testosterone concentration. More common than an actual elevation of intact LH is an artefactual elevation resulting from a supranormal serum α subunit concentration cross-reacting in a polyclonal assay for LH; this artefact can be circumvented by using a two-site double monoclonal assay, which has much greater specificity for the intact molecule.

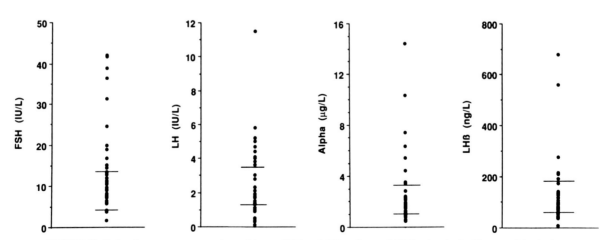

FIGURE 16–2. Basal serum concentrations of intact FSH and LH and α and LHβ subunits in 38 men with pituitary macroadenomas that were considered "clinically nonfunctioning." Eleven had elevations of FSH, 10 of LH, 8 of α subunit, and 6 of LHβ subunit. Of the 38 adenomas, 36 were studied in cell culture and 29 could be identified as gonadotroph adenomas by their secretion in culture.

Gonadotropin Subunits: α, FSHβ, and LHβ

About 15 per cent of men who have gonadotroph adenomas have supranormal basal serum concentrations of α, FSHβ, or LHβ subunits, often in combination with supranormal concentrations of another subunit or intact FSH or LH.[4, 5, 11] Occasionally, a single subunit is supranormal. When α subunit alone is supranormal, the source can be either a gonadotroph or a thyrotroph adenoma, and in vitro studies are needed to make the distinction.

Stimulated Secretion

Administration of thyroid-releasing hormone (TRH) to patients who have gonadotroph adenomas often produces an increase in the serum concentrations of intact gonadotropins and their subunits, especially the LHβ subunit.[5, 11, 12] These responses are interpretable as characteristic of gonadotroph adenomas because normal men and women show no response of intact gonadotropins and their subunits to TRH, or, in the case of intact LH and LHβ, no more than a 33 per cent increase. In a study of 16 women with pituitary macroadenomas that were clinically nonfunctioning, 11 could be identified as being of gonadotroph origin by their LHβ subunit responses to TRH; 4 had responses of LH and 3 of FSH (Fig. 16–3).[12] Of 38 men with pituitary macroadenomas that were clinically nonfunctioning, 14 had responses of LHβ, 5 of intact LH, and 4 of intact FSH.[5]

Administration of GnRH to patients who have gonadotroph adenomas results in greatly variable FSH and LH responses, from subnormal to normal, but the responses cannot be interpreted; either normal or adenomatous gonadotroph cells could be the source of the FSH or LH.

Secretion in Vitro

Gonadotroph adenomas that are recognized in vivo by supranormal basal or stimulated serum concentrations of intact gonadotropins and/or subunits usually secrete in culture relatively large amounts of the same intact hormones and subunits that they secreted in vivo. Of 11 women whose clinically nonfunctioning adenomas could be recognized to be of gonadotroph origin by their LHβ responses to TRH, 9 were established in dispersed cell culture, and all 9 secreted readily detectable amounts of LHβ.[12] In addition, gonadotroph adenomas often secrete relatively large amounts of other gonadotroph cell products in culture as well.[4, 5, 11–13] For example, some adenomas associated in vivo only with a supranormal serum basal concentration of intact FSH also secrete large amounts of LH in culture. Other adenomas associated in vivo only with a supranormal concentration of α subunit secrete intact FSH in culture, identifying them as gonadotroph adenomas. Yet other adenomas that are associated with normal basal serum concentrations of intact gonadotropins and their subunits, but a large LHβ response to TRH, secrete

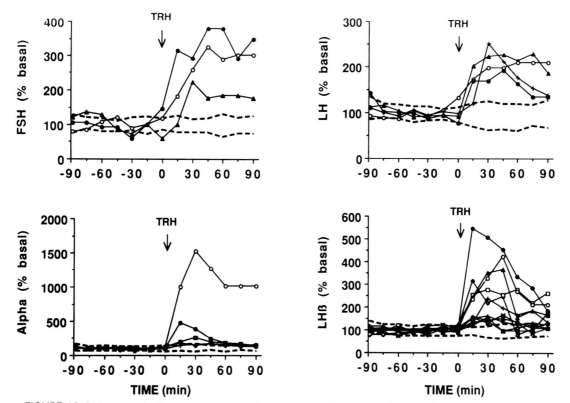

FIGURE 16–3. Increases in the serum concentrations of intact FSH, LH, α subunit, and, mostly, LHβ subunit to TRH in 16 women with adenomas that had been thought to be "nonsecreting" on the basis of basal hormone concentrations. The dashed lines show the ranges of serum concentrations in 16 age-matched healthy women. Eleven women with "nonsecreting" adenomas exhibited significant responses to TRH of LHβ subunit, four of intact LH and α subunit, and three of FSH. (From Daneshdoost L, Gennarelli TA, Bashey HM, et al: Recognition of gonadotroph adenomas in women. N Engl J Med 324:589–594, 1991; with permission.)

**TABLE 16–1. CLINICAL PRESENTATIONS OF
GONADOTROPH ADENOMAS**

Neurological Symptoms (most common)
Visual impairment
Headache
Other (e.g., diplopia, seizures, CSF rhinorrhea)
Incidental Finding
When an imaging procedure is performed because of an unrelated
    symptom
Hormonal Symptoms (least common)
Oligomenorrhea or amenorrhea in a premenopausal woman
Premature puberty when intact LH is secreted in a prepubertal boy
Symptoms of hormonal deficiencies (commonly occur but uncommonly
    are the presenting symptoms)
Large testes in men with FSH-secreting tumors

large amounts of intact FSH as well as LHβ in culture. Gonadotroph adenomas in culture respond to stimulation with both TRH and GnRH by secreting both FSH and LH.[13]

DIAGNOSIS

Clinical Presentation

Gonadotroph adenomas usually come to clinical attention when they become so large that they cause neurological symptoms (Table 16–1). They may also be detected as a coincidental finding when an imaging procedure of the head is performed for an unrelated reason. Least commonly, they may come to medical attention because of hormonal hypersecretion. The large size of gonadotroph adenomas commonly causes hormonal hyposecretion from the nonadenomatous pituitary, but these deficiencies usually do not impel the patient to seek medical attention. Gonadotroph adenomas are probably not recognized when they are microadenomas, because they are so inefficient that at that size they probably do not result in supranormal serum concentrations of intact gonadotropins or their subunits.

Impaired vision is the neurological symptom that most commonly leads a patient with a gonadotroph adenoma to seek medical attention, because suprasellar extension of the adenoma elevates and compresses the optic chiasm. Although a bitemporal visual field defect is considered the most typical abnormality, asymmetrical defects are also common. When compression becomes more severe, central visual acuity may also be impaired. The onset of the deficit is usually so gradual that patients often do not seek ophthalmological consultation for months or even years.

Other neurological symptoms that may cause a patient with a gonadotroph adenoma to seek medical attention are headaches, caused presumably by expansion of the sella; diplopia, caused by oculomotor nerve compression due to lateral extension of the adenoma; CSF rhinorrhea, caused by inferior extension of the adenoma; and the excruciating headache and diplopia caused by pituitary apoplexy.

Detection of a gonadotroph adenoma as an incidental finding when an imaging procedure of the head is performed for an unrelated reason, such as a motor vehicle accident, is the next most common presentation. The least common presentation is a consequence of hormonal hypersecretion by the adenoma. This includes oligomenor-

rhea or amenorrhea in a premenopausal woman due to excessive FSH secretion and premature puberty in a prepubertal boy due to an adenoma secreting intact LH.[14, 15] In adult men with FSH-secreting adenoma, excessively large testes may be a feature.

At the time of initial presentation due to a neurological symptom, many patients with gonadotroph adenomas, when questioned, admit to symptoms of hormonal deficiencies. Ironically, the most common pituitary hormonal deficiency is of LH, the result of compression of the normal gonadotroph cells by the adenoma and lack of secretion of a substantial amount of intact LH by the adenomatous gonadotroph cells. The result in men is a subnormal serum testosterone concentration, which produces decreased energy and libido. The result in premenopausal women is amenorrhea. Thyroid-stimulating hormone (TSH) and ACTH deficiencies, leading to thyroxine and cortisol deficiencies, may also occur.

Diagnostic Tests

The process of making the diagnosis of a gonadotroph adenoma usually proceeds from recognizing that a patient's visual abnormality or other symptom could represent an intrasellar lesion, to confirming the presence of a sellar lesion by an imaging procedure, to finding the secretory abnormalities characteristic of a gonadotroph adenoma (Table 16–2).

Tests of Vision and Imaging of the Pituitary

Neuro-ophthalmological evaluation should include a computerized test of visual fields and an assessment of visual acuity. The pituitary should be imaged, preferably by MRI (Fig. 16–4). This procedure is generally preferable to CT scanning because of its superior resolution, its ability to demonstrate the optic chiasm, and its ability to demonstrate blood and thereby recognize hemorrhage in the pituitary and distinguish an aneurysm from other lesions. MRI does not, however, show calcification in a craniopharyngioma as well as a CT scan, often does not distinguish a pituitary adenoma from other intrasellar lesions, and does not distinguish a pituitary adenoma from the nonadenomatous pituitary or one kind of pituitary adenoma from another.

Hormonal Tests

Intrasellar mass lesions detected by MRI should be evaluated further by measurement of serum concentrations of

**TABLE 16–2. HORMONAL CRITERIA FOR THE DIAGNOSIS OF
GONADOTROPH ADENOMAS* (ANY ONE OR ANY COMBINATION
OF THE FOLLOWING)**

MEN	WOMEN
Supranormal Basal Serum Concentrations of	
FSH†	FSH but not LH
α, LHβ, or FSHβ subunits	Any subunit relative to intact FSH and LH
LH and testosterone	
Supranormal Response to TRH of	
FSH	FSH
LH	LH
LHβ (most common)	LHβ (most common)

*Assuming the patient has a pituitary macroadenoma
†Assuming the patient does not have a history of primary hypogonadism

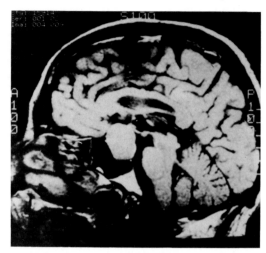

FIGURE 16–4. MRI scan showing, in a sagittal view of the head, a large gonadotroph adenoma extending superiorly to elevate the optic chiasm. Gonadotroph adenomas are often not recognized until they become this large.

pituitary hormones to determine whether the lesion is of pituitary or nonpituitary origin, and, if pituitary, the cell of origin. An adenoma of gonadotroph or thyrotroph origin should be suspected if the serum prolactin concentration is less than 100 ng/ml, the patient does not appear acromegalic, and the serum insulin-like growth factor I concentration is not supranormal, and the patient does not have Cushing's syndrome or supranormal urine cortisol excretion. Preoperative recognition that an intrasellar mass lesion is of gonadotroph origin depends on finding specific combinations of basal and stimulated concentrations of intact gonadotropins and their subunits. The combinations differ somewhat in men and women.

In a man who has a pituitary macroadenoma, elevated basal serum concentrations of intact gonadotropins and/or their subunits alone or in combination with responses of any of these to TRH are strong evidence that the adenoma is of gonadotroph origin. Elevated basal FSH is common, as are elevated basal α, FSHβ, and LHβ subunits. Patients who have elevated basal intact hormone and subunit secretion often exhibit responses of any of them to TRH.

In a woman who has a pituitary macroadenoma, basal serum concentrations of intact FSH or their subunits are usually of little diagnostic value because of the difficulty of interpreting elevated values in a woman over 50 years old, the age at which these adenomas usually present. In that situation, differentiation between the adenoma and nonadenomatous postmenopausal gonadotroph cells as the source of the elevated gonadotropins and their subunits is usually not possible. In a few situations, however, the distinction can be made, such as when intact FSH is markedly elevated but LH is not elevated at all, or when one of the gonadotropin subunits is distinctly elevated but intact FSH and LH are not elevated.[12] In a woman, therefore, the in vivo diagnosis depends on the finding of a response to TRH, of intact FSH or LH or, most commonly, of LHβ subunit.

Differential Diagnosis

Gonadotroph adenomas need to be distinguished from other kinds of pituitary adenomas, nonpituitary lesions arising within and around the sella, and long-standing primary hypogonadism. Although adenomas arising from other pituitary cells usually are recognized readily by the clinical syndromes they produce and by their secretory products, some somatotroph,[16] corticotroph,[17] and even lactotroph adenomas are clinically silent. These appear to be nonsecreting in vivo and are recognized only when studied in vitro, such as by immunospecific staining. Intrasellar and parasellar lesions of nonpituitary origin can sometimes but not always be distinguished from pituitary adenomas on the basis of their imaging characteristics, and sometimes are not recognized for what they are until they are examined histologically. Neither other pituitary adenomas nor nonpituitary lesions exhibit the hormonal abnormalities characteristic of gonadotroph adenomas. Long-standing primary hypogonadism can lead to gonadotroph cell hypertrophy and thus to pituitary enlargement, and in this way it is similar to gonadotroph adenomas, as well as in elevated serum gonadotropin concentrations. The pituitary enlargement seen with primary hypogonadism, however, is not nearly so great as that with gonadotroph adenomas at the time of presentation. In primary hypogonadism, LH as well as FSH is elevated, and neither intact gonadotropins nor their subunits respond to TRH.[6]

Clinical Utility of Diagnosing Gonadotroph Adenomas

Making the diagnosis of a gonadotroph adenoma in vivo is of value in distinguishing a pituitary rather than nonpituitary origin of a lesion and in providing a marker by which to monitor the response to treatment. Distinguishing an intrasellar lesion as of pituitary rather than nonpituitary origin is of value because it can influence treatment. If surgery is needed, for example, a pituitary lesion is almost always approached transsphenoidally, no matter how large, because it is infradural, but a meningioma is usually approached transcranially because it usually arises above the dura. Finding tumor markers characteristic of gonadotroph adenomas, such as elevated basal FSH or α or LHβ subunit concentrations, not only identifies the lesion as of gonadotroph origin but provides a means by which to follow the response to treatment. When the basal serum FSH concentration is elevated prior to surgery, for example, the decrease after surgery correlates with reduction in adenoma mass seen by imaging.[18]

THERAPY

Because gonadotroph adenomas are usually not detected until they become so large that they cause significant visual impairment, treatment usually must be directed at reducing adenoma mass and restoring vision as soon as possible. Surgery, usually transsphenoidal, is the only treatment that meets this criterion (Table 16–3). Gonadotroph adenomas are usually sensitive to radiation, which may be used to prevent regrowth if substantial adenoma tissue remains after surgery or to treat primarily if an adenoma is detected before it becomes so large as to cause neurologic symptoms. Several pharmacological treatments have been tried, but none reduces adenoma size much.

TABLE 16–3. COMPARISON OF TREATMENTS FOR GONADOTROPH ADENOMAS

TREATMENT	INDICATIONS	COMPLICATIONS
Transsphenoidal surgery	Intrasellar mass with suprasellar extension and severe visual impairment	Worsening of vision, oculomotor palsy, hematoma, CSF rhinorrhea, meningitis, seizures, diabetes insipidus, hypopituitarism
Transcranial surgery	Large, residual symptomatic extrasellar tissue following transsphenoidal surgery	Same as above, but more likely
Supervoltage radiation	Primary treatment: Intrasellar mass with only mild suprasellar extension	Transient: Fatigue, nausea, hair loss, loss of taste and smell
	Adjuvant treatment: Substantial residual adenoma tissue after surgery	Permanent: hypopituitarism
Observation	Adenoma confined to sella; patient elderly or infirm	Visual impairment
Medications (dopamine agonists, GnRH antagonists)	Experimental protocol	

Surgery

Transsphenoidal Surgery

Transsphenoidal surgery is usually the preferred treatment for gonadotroph adenomas that impair vision significantly. Seventy to 80 per cent of patients who have abnormal visual fields due to a pituitary macroadenoma do experience improvement following transsphenoidal surgery.[19, 20] Transsphenoidal surgery may also be performed because of severe headaches, diplopia, or other neurological abnormalities and elevation of the optic chiasm in the absence of visual impairment. The transsphenoidal approach is usually preferred over the transcranial as the initial procedure no matter how great the suprasellar extension, because pituitary adenomas are infradural and the risk of serious side effects is less. Serious complications of transsphenoidal surgery are uncommon but appear to be greater when the adenoma is very large, and include mortality, hemorrhage, optic and oculomotor nerve damage, CSF rhinorrhea, and meningitis. In one series the total of all serious complications due to transsphenoidal surgery by experienced neurosurgeons in 113 patients who had macroadenomas with extrasellar extension was 6 per cent.[19] Less serious complications include diabetes insipidus, which commonly occurs transiently but uncommonly occurs permanently; loss of anterior pituitary hormones; and persistent sinus symptoms. The results of surgery should be evaluated four to six weeks afterwards. Residual adenoma tissue should be evaluated by MRI and by measurement of whatever hormones or subunits were elevated before surgery. The functions of the nonadenomatous anterior pituitary should also be re-evaluated postoperatively, as should vasopressin secretion. Neuro-ophthalmological function should likewise be re-evaluated.

Other Surgery

The neurosurgeon occasionally performs transcranial surgery but usually only when extrasellar adenoma tissue that remains after transsphenoidal surgery continues to cause clinically significant neurological impairment. Neurological side effects are more likely with this approach than with the transsphenoidal. Postoperative evaluation should be performed as with transsphenoidal surgery.

Radiation

Supervoltage radiation should be used to prevent regrowth and reduce the size when a substantial amount of adenoma tissue remains after transsphenoidal surgery. If little residual adenoma remains postoperatively, radiation need not be given at that time, but only if growth becomes apparent in subsequent years. Radiation can also be used as primary treatment for gonadotroph adenomas that are large enough to warrant treatment but are not causing significant visual impairment or other neurologic symptoms.

Supervoltage radiation is administered in daily doses of 2 Gy to a total of 46 Gy. Side effects include lassitude and nausea, which last up to one to two months; diminished taste and olfaction, which may last for six months; and loss of hair at the portal sites, which may last for a year. Hypopituitarism is another side effect, sometimes beginning as soon as one month after completion of radiation, but usually not until a year or more. By 10 years afterwards, about 50 per cent of patients have a deficiency of ACTH, TSH, or LH.

Hormonal evaluation, both for excessive secretion of whichever intact gonadotropins and their subunits were secreted excessively by the adenoma prior to treatment and for deficient secretion by the nonadenomatous pituitary, should be performed 6 and 12 months after radiation and once a year thereafter. Evaluation of size by MRI should be performed one year after radiation and, if the mass is smaller, less frequently thereafter. Neuro-ophthalmological evaluation should be repeated after radiation if it was abnormal before.

Pharmacological Treatment

The extraordinary success of dopamine agonists in reducing the size of, as well as secretion by, lactotrope adenomas has prompted attempts to find a pharmacological treatment for gonadotroph adenomas. So far, however, no drug has been found that reduces adenoma size consistently and substantially.

Although dopamine does not decrease gonadotropin secretion to an appreciable degree in normal subjects, bromocriptine has been reported to reduce the secretion of intact gonadotropins and α subunit in a few patients and even to improve vision in one, but not to reduce adenoma size.[21-25] CV205-502 (quingolide) has also been reported to reduce secretion in some patients.[26]

Several agonist analogues of GnRH have been administered to patients with gonadotroph adenomas, based on the rationale that chronic administration of these agonists causes down-regulation of GnRH receptors on, and decreased secretion of FSH and LH from, normal gonadotroph cells. Administration of GnRH agonist analogues to patients with gonadotroph adenomas, however, generally produces either an agonist effect or no effect on secretion and no effect on adenoma size.[26-29]

Potent antagonist analogues of GnRH have recently been developed. Administration for one week of the GnRH antagonist, Nal-Glu GnRH, to men with gonadotroph adenomas reduced their elevated FSH concentrations to normal.[30] When Nal-Glu administration was continued for six months, however, FSH remained suppressed, but adenoma size did not decrease.[30]

REFERENCES

1. Alexander JM, Biller BMK, Bikkal H, et al: Clinically nonfunctioning pituitary tumors are monoclonal in origin. J Clin Invest 86:336–340, 1990.
2. Samaan NA, Stephans AV, Danziger J, Trujillo J: Reactive pituitary abnormalities in patients with Klinefelter's and Turner's syndromes. Arch Intern Med 139:198–201, 1979.
3. Daneshdoost L, Pavlou S, Molitch ME: Inhibition of follicle-stimulating hormone secretion from gonadotroph adenomas by repetitive administration of a gonadotropin-releasing hormone antagonist. J Clin Endocrinol Metab 71:92–97, 1990.
4. Snyder PJ: Gonadotroph cell adenomas of the pituitary. Endocr Rev 6:552–563, 1985.
5. Daneshdoost L, Gennarelli TA, Bashey HM, et al: Identification of gonadotroph adenomas in men with clinically nonfunctioning adenomas by the luteinizing hromone β-subunit response to thyrotrophin-releasing hormone. J Clin Endocrinol Metab 77:1352–1355, 1993.
6. Snyder PJ, Bashey HM, Kim SU, Chappel SC: Secretion of uncombined subunits of luteinizing hormone by gonadotroph cell adenomas. J Clin Endocrinol Metab 59:1169–1175, 1984.
7. Chappel SC, Bashey HM, Snyder PJ: Similar isoelectric profiles of FSH from gonadotroph cell adenomas and non-adenomatous pituitaries. Acta Endocrinol (Copenh) 115:311–316, 1986.
8. Galway AB, Hsueh JW, Daneshdoost L, et al: Gonadotroph adenomas in men produce biologically active follicle-stimulating hormone. J Clin Endocrinol Metab 71:907–912, 1990.
9. Snyder PJ, Sterling FH: Hypersecretion of LH and FSH by a pituitary adenoma. J Clin Endocrinol Metab 42:544–550, 1976.
10. Peterson RD, Kourides IA, Horwith M, et al: Luteinizing hormone and α-subunit-secreting pituitary tumor: Positive feedback of estrogen. J Clin Endocrinol Metab 51:692–698, 1981.
11. Katznelson L, Alexander JM, Bikkal HA, et al: Imbalanced follicle-stimulating hormone β-subunit hormone biosynthesis in human pituitary adenomas. J Clin Endocrinol Metab 74:1343–1351, 1992.
12. Daneshdoost L, Gennarelli TA, Bashey HM, et al: Recognition of gonadotroph adenomas in women. N Engl J Med 324:589–594, 1991.
13. Lamberts SWJ, Verleun T, Oosterom R, et al: The effects of bromocriptine, thyrotropin-releasing hormone, and gonadotropin-releasing hormone on hormone secretion by gonadotropin-secreting pituitary adenomas in vivo and in vitro. J Clin Endocrinol Metab 64:524–530, 1987.
14. Faggiano M, Criscuolo T, Perrone I, et al: Sexual precocity in a boy due to hypersecretion of LH and prolactin by a pituitary adenoma. Acta Endocrinol 102:167–172, 1983.
15. Ambrosi B, Basstti M, Ferrario R, et al: Precocious puberty in a boy with a PRL-, LH- and FSH-secreting pituitary tumour: Hormonal and immunocytochemical studies. Acta Endocrinol (Copenh) 122:569–576, 1990.
16. Kovacs K, Lloyd R, Horvath E, et al: Silent somatotroph adenomas of the human pituitary: A morphologic study of three cases including immunocytochemistry, electron microscopy, in vitro examination, and in situ hybridization. Am J Pathol 134:345–353, 1989.
17. Horvath E, Kovacs K, Killinger DW, et al: Silent corticotropic adenomas of the human pituitary gland. Am J Pathol 98:617–638, 1980.
18. Harris RI, Schatz NJ, Gennarelli T, et al: Follicle-stimulating hormone–secreting pituitary adenomas: Correlation of reduction of adenoma size with reduction of hormonal hypersecretion after transsphenoidal surgery. J Clin Endocrinol Metab 56:1288–1293, 1983.
19. Trautmann JC, Laws ER: Visual status after transsphenoidal surgery at the Mayo Clinic, 1971–1982. Am J Ophthalmol 96:200–208, 1983.
20. Black PM, Zervas NT, Candia G: Management of large pituitary adenomas by transsphenoidal surgery. Surg Neurol 29:443–447, 1988.
21. Berezin M, Olchovsky D, Pines A, et al: Reduction of follicle-stimulating hormone (FSH) secretion in FSH-producing pituitary adenoma by bromocriptine. J Clin Endocrinol Metab 59:1220–1222, 1984.
22. Vance ML, Ridgway EC, Thorner MO: Follicle-stimulating hormone- and α- subunit-secreting pituitary tumor treated with bromocriptine. J Clin Endocrinol Metab 61:580–584, 1985.
23. Klibanski A, Deutsch PJ, Jameson JL, et al: Luteinizing hormone-secreting pituitary tumor: Biosynthetic characterization and clinical studies. J Clin Endocrinol Metab 64:536–542, 1987.
24. Klibanski A, Shupnik MA, Bikkal HA, et al: Dopaminergic regulation of α-subunit secretion and messenger ribonucleic acid levels in α-secreting pituitary tumors. J Clin Endocrinol Metab 66:96–102, 1988.
25. Comtosis R, Bouchard J, Robert F: Hypersecretion of gonadotropins by a pituitary adenoma: Pituitary dynamic studies and treatment with bromocriptine in one patient. Fertil Steril 52:569–573, 1989.
26. Kwekkeboom DJ, Lamberts SWJ: Long-term treatment with the dopamine agonist CV 205-502 of patients with a clinically non-functioning, gonadotroph, or α-subunit secreting pituitary adenoma. Clin Endocrinol 36:171–176, 1991.
27. Roman SH, Goldstein M, Kourides IA, et al: The luteinizing hormone–releasing hormone (LHRH) agonist [D-Trp⁶-Pro⁹-NEt] LHRH increased rather than lowered LH and α-subunit levels in a patient with an LH-secreting pituitary tumor. J Clin Endocrinol Metab 58:313–319, 1984.
28. Sassolas G, Lejeune H, Trouillas J, et al: Gonadotropin-releasing hormone agonists are unsuccessful in reducing tumoral gonadotropin secretion in two patients with gonadotropin-secreting pituitary adenomas. J Clin Endocrinol Metab 67:180–185, 1988.
29. Klibanski A, Jameson JL, Biller BMK, et al: Gonadotropin and α-subunit responses to chorionic gonadotropin-releasing hormone analog administration in patients with glycoprotein hormone–secreting pituitary tumors. J Clin Endocrinol Metab 68:81–86, 1989.
30. McGrath GA, Goncalvez R, Udupa J, et al: New technique for quantitation of pituitary adenoma size: Use in evaluating treatment of gonadotroph adenomas with a GnRH antagonist. J Clin Endocrinol Metab 76:1363–1368, 1993.

17

Somatostatin

J. A. H. WASS

Somatostatin (SS; growth hormone release–inhibiting hormone, GH-RIH; somatotropin release–inhibiting factor, SRIF; growth hormone release-inhibiting factor, GRIF) has a number of different physiological roles in humans. This is suggested by its widespread distribution. It is present not only in the hypothalamus but also in extrahypothalamic areas of the brain and spinal cord. In common with a number of other peptides, it is also found in the gastrointestinal system, particularly in the D cells of the pancreas, stomach, and intestine, and in peripheral nerve fibers of the intestinal wall, as well as in peripheral nerves, the placenta, the retina, the thymus, and the adrenal medulla.

Phylogenetically, SS appeared later than insulin but earlier than glucagon and pancreatic polypeptide.[1] The evidence suggests that genes controlling production of this molecule appeared before the development of cell-to-cell and nerve-to-cell communication. Thus, it is present in early vertebrates as well as in primitive invertebrates, including protozoa (Tetrahymena pyriformis).[2] The work of Pearse has shown that it is also present in the sea squirt (Ciona intestinalis), a creature known to exist 600 million years ago.[3] Only recently, however, has SS been studied satisfactorily, and as a result of widespread interest an enormous body of literature has developed in 20 years.

ISOLATION, STRUCTURE, AND CHEMICAL SYNTHESIS

The existence of hypothalamic factors regulating anterior pituitary function via the portal system of vessels between the median eminence and the pituitary was first suggested by Green and Harris in 1974.[4] The first evidence for a hypothalamic factor inhibiting growth hormone (GH) secretion from the anterior pituitary came from the work of Krulich et al,[5] who while looking for a pituitary GH-releasing factor (GRF), discovered a fraction obtained from hypothalamic extracts which unexpectedly inhibited GH release from rat anterior pituitaries in vitro. They suggested that the secretion of GH from the pituitary is regulated by two different interacting factors, one inhibiting and the other stimulating release and both under nervous system control. During another unsuccessful search for GRF, Brazeau et al in Guillemin's laboratory isolated SS from ovine hypothalami.[6] SS was found to contain 14 amino acid residues (a tetradecapeptide) and to have a cyclic structure joined by two intramolecular disulfide bonds between the two cysteine residues (Fig. 17–1). The linear reduced sequence was synthesized by condensation and solid-phase methods and purified and was found to have the same biological activity as the cyclic form in vitro, indicating that reduction is not critical to peptide recognition by specified SS receptors. It was quickly synthesized by other groups.[7, 8] The initial concept of a peptide whose main function involves the regulation of GH has been considerably expanded,[9] and it has been shown that a family of SS-related peptides including the original peptide (now called S-14), an amino-terminal extended form (S-28), several species-specific variants, and larger forms vary in molecular size in different species from 11.5 to 15.7 kDa. In 1975 Schally and colleagues[10, 11] isolated and sequenced SS from porcine hypothalami and showed it to have the same structure as ovine SS. They also reported the presence of two larger forms that were both immunologically and biologically active and at that time were thought to represent SS precursors.

SS's in different species usually have the same structure. In mammals studied so far there are differences in the sequence of SS's obtained only in catfish and angler fish islets (Table 17–1). In the latter, it is likely that more than

H-Ala-Gly-Cys-Lys-Asn-Phe-Phe-Trp-Lys-Thr-Phe-Thr-Ser-Cys-OH

FIGURE 17–1. Amino acid sequence of cyclic somatostatin.

one gene coding for SS is present, as recombinant techniques reveal the presence of two different messages, one coding for SS I and another for SS II.[12]

MOLECULAR HETEROGENEITY

Schally et al[10, 11] found three different molecular weight forms of SS which were all biologically active. Arimura et al[13] chromatographed extracts of rat stomach and pancreas and again found both tissues to contain high molecular weight forms of SS as well as the tetradecapeptide form. In the hypothalamus, all groups have reported a 1.6-kDa form together with 3-kDa and higher molecular weight forms. Both the intermediate and high molecular weight forms do not break down during treatment with dithiothreitol, an agent that reduces disulfide bonds, indicating that they do not represent aggregates of the tetradecapeptide. Somatostatin-28 was described by Pradayrol et al.[14] This has a molecular weight of 3145 Da and contains the amino acid sequence of tetradecapeptide SS extended by 14 residues at the N-terminus. The two consecutive basic residues located just before the cleavage site which produce tetradecapeptide suggest that this may be a precursor to S-14. However, different quantities of S-28 and varying ratios of S-28 and S-14 in different tissues, together with other evidence, suggest that although it may be a precursor, it also acts as a hormone in its own right with its own somewhat different spectrum of activity in different tissues. Thus, compared with S-14, S-28 suppresses GH far longer[15]; the effects of S-28 are greater with regard to insulin but not glucagon suppression[16]; gastric acid is suppressed more effectively by S-14 than S-28. Furthermore, S-28 binds with greater affinity to pituitary receptors and acts without cleavage to S-14.[17]

In the gastrointestinal tract S-28 contributes increasingly to the total SS-like immunoreactivity from the pyloric antrum to the colon and is the predominant form in the lower gut.[18, 19] Different forms of SS occur in the circulation. Thus, gel filtration studies of rat hypophyseal portal blood has shown a major peak of tetradecapeptide SS, with a small peak of high molecular weight material.[20, 21] In peripheral venous blood the work of Penman et al[22] has shown that the major form of SS occurs in the 3.5-kDa form. The differing amounts of high molecular weight material in the brain and gut suggest different control mechanisms for processing of the prohormone in these tissues.[23, 24] Penman and Wass[25] found that CSF contains largely higher molecular weight forms.

In summary, therefore, S-14 is the principal form found. It usually has the same sequence in different species. S-14 and S-28 have overlapping but distinct bioactions and act through different receptors. In neural tissue, S-14 is present in greater quantities than S-28. There is virtually no S-28 in the stomach and duodenum, but lower down the gut S-28 is the most important molecular form, and levels of both rise after ingestion of food. It appears that the production of S-14 and S-28 is not an important biological pathway in tissues in which S-28 is present.

EFFECTS AND ACTIONS FOLLOWING EXOGENOUS ADMINISTRATION

The early work on SS focused on the effects of exogenous administration. It has been shown that SS has a broad spectrum of action other than that of GH inhibition, suggesting a biological importance beyond that of a hypothalamic-pituitary–regulating hormone.

Actions on the Pituitary Gland

Brazeau first reported the biological effects of SS in inhibiting GH release from cultured pituitary cells. It was demonstrated then to be a powerful inhibitor of GH release both in vivo and in vitro; the GH responses to all physiological and pharmacological stimuli are inhibited by SS. Thus, in humans this hormone blocks the GH responses to exercise, arginine, insulin-induced hypoglycemia, and GRF.[26–29] When SS infusions are discontinued, a rebound of GH levels occurs, suggesting that, at least in the short term, although basal hormone release is inhibited promptly, SS does not interfere with synthesis of GH.[26, 28] Suppression of GH also occurs in circumstances in

TABLE 17–1. ESTABLISHED STRUCTURES OF SOMATOSTATIN AND SOMATOSTATIN-RELATED PEPTIDES*

TYPE OF SOMATOSTATIN OR PEPTIDE															Ala	Gly	Cys	Lys	Asn	Phe	Phe	Trp	Lys	Thr	Phe	Thr	Ser	Cys
Mammalian hypothalamic																												
Catfish islet						Asp	Asn	Thr	Val	Arg	Ser	Lys	Pro	Leu	Ala	—	Met	—	Tyr	—	—	—	Ser	Ser	—	Ala	—
Angler fish islet I	Ala	Ala	Ser	Gly	Gly	Pro	Leu	Leu	Ala	Pro	Arg	Glu	Arg	Lys	—	—	—	—	—	—	—	—	—	—	—	—	—	—
Angler fish islet II	Ser	Val	Asp	Ser	Thr	Asn	Asn	Leu	Pro	Pro	Arg	Glu	Arg	Lys	—	—	—	—	—	—	Tyr	—	—	Gly	—	—	—	—
Porcine 28	Ser	Ala	Asn	Ser	Asn	Pro	Ala	Met	Ala	Pro	Arg	Glu	Arg	Lys	—	—	—	—	—	—	—	—	—	—	—	—	—	—
Rat medullary thyroid carcinoma	Ser	Ala	Asn	Ser	Asn	Pro	Ala	Met	Ala	Pro	Arg	Glu	Arg	Lys	—	—	—	—	—	—	—	—	—	—	—	—	—	—

*Sequences enclosed in the box are homologous regions of the N-extended somatostatin-28. Dashes denote homologous amino acids in somatostatin-14. (From Reichlin S: Somatostatin. N Engl J Med 309: 1495–1501, 1556–1563, 1983.)

which basal levels of circulating GH are pathologically elevated, such as in acromegaly, diabetes mellitus, Laron dwarfism, and carcinoid tumors.[26, 27, 30, 31] SS also partially inhibits thyroid-stimulating hormone (TSH) secretion basally and in response to thyrotropin-releasing hormone (TRH) in euthyroid humans and animals and in hypothyroidism.[26, 32–35]

Basal prolactin secretion is not altered in normal subjects, nor is the increase seen in prolactin after TRH- or insulin-induced hypoglycemia.[26] Basal and GnRH-stimulated levels of gonadotropins are similarly not altered by SS. Lastly, SS has no effect on basal or stress-induced release of ACTH in normal subjects and mice.[26, 36] The inhibition of elevated basal ACTH levels by SS has been reported in occasional patients with Nelson's syndrome,[37] suggesting the possibility of abnormal receptors for SS on these tumors, as SS has no effect on the raised levels of ACTH seen in Addison's disease.[38]

Actions on the Endocrine and Exocrine Pancreas

SS inhibits insulin secretion both basally and in response to oral and intravenous glucose, glucagon, and tolbutamide.[28, 31, 39, 40] This inhibition occurs by a direct action on the islet cells of the pancreas.[41, 42] Similarly, basal and stimulated glucagon responses to arginine are inhibited.[28, 31] These inhibitory effects of SS on insulin and glucagon secretion occur in insulin-dependent diabetics and acromegalics as well as in normal subjects. The effects of SS on insulin secretion occur at approximately the same concentrations of SS as those that inhibit GH secretion.[43] Long-term infusions of SS cause transient hyperglycemia 60 to 90 minutes after commencement of an infusion, but glucose then returns to normal.[44]

SS also causes a fall in basal and stimulated pancreatic polypeptide in normal subjects and in patients with maturity-onset diabetes.[45, 46] It also inhibits exocrine pancreatic function, particularly the pancreatic enzyme responses to cholecystokinin and the pancreatic bicarbonate responses to secretin.[47–49]

Actions on the Gastrointestinal Tract

Intravenous SS inhibits the secretion of a wide variety of gastrointestinal hormones.[50] Thus, both basal and stimulated gastrin levels are inhibited, as well as the elevated gastrin levels seen in patients with Zollinger-Ellison syndrome and pernicious anemia.[51, 52] Furthermore, secretory volume and both acid and pepsin output are decreased by SS. Table 17–2 shows the wide variety of peptide hormones inhibited by SS infusions, as well as the inhibitory effects on exocrine gastrointestinal function using doses of 80 to 800 μg/h. Whereas gastric acid secretion is decreased even when gastrin is administered, whether the other actions upon exocrine secretion represent direct effects of the peptide or changes secondary to the inhibition of other hormone secretion is at present unclear. SS also suppresses circulating levels of GH-releasing hormone in humans, and this is thought to be of gut or pancreatic origin.[53] It is clear, however, that SS can exert exocrine as well as endocrine

TABLE 17–2. ACTIONS OF EXOGENOUSLY ADMINISTERED SOMATOSTATIN ON ENDOCRINE AND EXOCRINE SECRETIONS

ENDOCRINE	NON-ENDOCRINE
Inhibits secretion of	Inhibition of
Pituitary	Gastric acid secretion
GH	Gastric emptying rate
TSH	Pancreatic exocrine function—
Gastrointestinal tract	volume, electrolyte, and
Gastrin	enzyme content
CCK-pancreozymin	Gallbladder contraction
Secretin	Intestinal motility
VIP	Intestinal absorption of nutrients
GIP	Splanchnic blood flow
Motilin	Liver metabolism (?)
Glicentin (enteroglucagon)	Renal water reabsorption
Pancreas	Activity of some CNS neurons
Pancreatic polypeptide	**Excitation of**
Insulin	Activity of some neurons
Glucagon	
Somatostatin	
Renin; calcitonin (?)	
PTH (?)	
Growth hormone–releasing	
hormone	

effects. Furthermore, gastrointestinal motility and blood flow decrease.[54–56] These latter findings probably explain the beneficial effects of SS in controlling severe gastrointestinal bleeding. Lastly, the peptide decreases the absorption of nutrients, including glucose, triglycerides, and amino acids.

Actions on Other Hormones

SS inhibits the release of renin after the acute and chronic administration of furosemide (frusemide) in humans.[57] No effect of SS on basal or stimulated aldosterone levels in normal subjects or isolated bovine adrenal cells[58] has been found. Some effects have been shown in thyroid cells in man, and Loos and colleagues[59] reported that it inhibits TSH-stimulated secretion of T_3 and thyroxine T_4 from human thyroid cells in vitro, but the exact physiological significance of these findings is unclear. Hargis et al[60] found SS to inhibit parathormone secretion in rats, but this has not been confirmed in humans. Again, the physiological significance of these findings is unclear.

Actions on the Nervous System

The presence of SS in regions of the brain outside the hypothalamus suggests that it may be a neurotransmitter or modulator in the nervous system. Direct actions of SS on the nervous system have been demonstrated, and there have been reports of both excitatory and inhibitory effects. Thus SS has been reported to depress the activity of neurons in the cerebral and cerebellar cortex and in the hypothalamus in the rat.[61] A potent excitatory effect of SS on some nervous system neurons has been reported by Dodd and Kelly.[62] SS has been shown to act directly within the rat brain to affect glucose regulation.[63] It also shows partial binding to opiate receptors in the rat brain[64] and produces analgesic and other opiate-like effects when administered centrally.[65] No behavioral effects of infusions have been reported in a number of clinical studies.[26, 28, 30, 31]

MECHANISM OF ACTION, STRUCTURAL REQUIREMENTS, AND ANALOGUES

The effect of SS is rapid in onset and brief in duration. Following this there is a rebound in secretion, suggesting that it acts on secretory and not synthetic processes, possibly by depression of exocytosis.[66] SS does not appear to require protein synthesis for its action, and cyclohexamide, an inhibitor of protein synthesis, does not prevent the inhibition of GH secretion by SS in vitro.[67]

The four amino acid residues in positions 7 to 10 at the β-turn are most important for receptor binding.[68, 69] SS receptors have been demonstrated by competitive-binding assays on anterior pituitary cells secreting GH, TSH, and prolactin, in the brain in the highest concentrations in the cerebral cortex, thalamus, hypothalamus, and striatum,[17] and in the exocrine pancreas and adrenal cortex. Srikant and Patel[17] have suggested that brain and pituitary SS receptors are different, with a greater proportion of S-14 receptors in the brain and a greater proportion of S-28 cells in the pituitary, and that the ratio of receptor density to endogenous SS content is higher in the cortex than in the hypothalamus. SS receptors have also been shown to exist on pancreatic islet cells secreting insulin, glucagon, and SS[70, 71] and on gastric cells.

In the rat, work on pancreatic acinar plasma membranes has suggested that the receptors are glycoproteins of approximately 90 kDa, but characterization is not yet complete.[72]

SS acts by first binding to receptors or plasma membranes of pituitary cells or those of pancreatic islets or neurons. There are at least two classes of receptor. Receptor binding leads to activation of one or more membrane-bound guanine-binding proteins, which in turn lower cAMP and intracellular free Ca^{2+} concentration.

There is no clear picture of the postreceptor mechanism of the effects of SS intracellularly, but it may have actions at several sites. SS has been reported to lower cyclic $3',5'$-AMP levels in the pituitary and the pancreatic islets as well as in rat gastric glands.[73–75]

Cyclic AMP–independent mechanisms exist, and SS reduces membrane permeability by calcium; its inhibition of insulin and glucagon secretion by pancreatic islets can be overcome by increasing the concentration of calcium ions in the medium.[76, 77] Blocking the outward flux of potassium interferes with the effects of SS on insulin,[78] suggesting that one effect of SS is to cause increased permeability of the cell membrane.

Little is known about the mode of action of SS in the nervous system. It has been shown to influence the uptake and release of calcium ions by synaptosomes.[79] In view of the crucial role of calcium ions in nerve terminal depolarization, as well as in hormone secretion, it has been speculated that SS may exert its action as both a neurotransmitter and a hormone by affecting calcium transport through the nerve cell and endocrine cell membrane, respectively.[80]

Depolarization by exposure to high K^+ stimulates SS release in dispersed fetal rat cerebral cortical cells. The effect is Na^+ and Ca^{2+} dependent. The release is inhibited by GABA (γ-aminobutyric acid), histamine, and benzodiazepines and stimulated by potassium, the GABA antagonist pictrotoxin, acetylcholine, vasoactive intestinal peptide, dopamine, and norepinephrine.[81]

Structural Requirements for Somatostatin Bioactivity

Both linear and cyclic forms of SS have bioactivity in vitro.[6] The amino-terminus is not required for activity. Analogues that cannot form a covalent cyclic structure because of the cysteine residues are either substituted by alanine or, in cases where the sulfhydryl groups have been alkylated, exhibit greatly reduced but still significant bioactivity. This suggests that the disulfide bond is probably necessary for interaction with the receptor.[82–84] Although the disulfide bond is important, the size of the ring is not critical. The amino acid residues seen in positions 7 to 10 appear to be essential, and in general the length of action can be increased by substituting tryptophan in position 8. Thus, analogues of SS have been synthesized which are more potent, longer acting, and more specific than the native peptide. Some inhibit insulin more effectively than glucagon and vice versa,[85, 86] and it has been found that increased GH suppression can be obtained.[87, 88] Inhibition of gastrin secretion appears to involve unique structural requirements. Because of these variations, differences in the structural requirements of SS receptors on the α and β cells of the gastrointestinal tract and pituitary cells seem possible.

MEASUREMENT

BIOASSAY. Because of the broad spectrum of biological action of SS, a number of bioassays for the peptide have been developed which depend on suppression of GH, insulin, or glucagon secretion.[32, 77, 83] They are useful for measuring biological potency of synthetic SS preparations, analogues, and heterogeneous molecular forms. They are used for measuring SS content of tissue extracts, but measurement of blood is limited by the presence of other hormones and biologically active peptides that interfere with these biological responses.

RADIOIMMUNOASSAY. The first radioimmunoassay of SS was reported by Arimura et al.[89, 90] For measurement of SS in tissues, most laboratories have in the past used nonextracted radioimmunoassays. There are large discrepancies between the estimates of SS tissue content by different laboratories, even when tissues from the same species are compared (Table 17–3). The differences may be due to a number of factors, including the use of different antibodies differently affected by the presence of SS-binding protein in tissues, different methods of storage and extraction of tissues, and different degrees of purity of synthetic SS preparations used as standards for the assays.[91]

The radioimmunoassay of SS in blood presents several problems. Endogenous SS is rapidly degraded in the presence of plasma, and this is also true for the iodinated SS tracer. Because of this and the fact that SS binds to a high molecular weight plasma protein, it is now generally agreed that in order to be measured accurately SS must first be extracted from plasma by one of a variety of methods.[91] Using extraction, basal circulating SS levels are usually below 100 pg/ml (Table 17–4). Levels are much higher in patients with tumors secreting SS, ranging up to 25,000 ng/ml. These assays have established that some nonpancreatic tumors secrete the peptide, and abnormal secretion

TABLE 17–3. SOMATOSTATIN LEVELS IN DIFFERENT LOCATIONS IN RAT AND HUMAN

LOCATION	SPECIES	LEVEL (ng/mg wet wt of tissue)	REFERENCE
Hypothalamus	Rat	2.12	Brownstein et al., 1975[90]
Hypothalamus	Rat	1.11	Kronheim et al., 1976[121]
Hypothalamus	Rat	2.3	Patel and Reichlin, 1978[183]
Pancreas	Rat	0.14	Arimura et al., 1975[184]
Pancreas	Rat	0.34	Vale et al., 1976[185]
Pancreas	Rat	0.033	McIntosh et al., 1978[186]
Pancreas	Human	0.25	McIntosh et al., 1978[186]
Stomach (fundus)	Rat	0.46	Arimura et al., 1975[184]
	Rat	0.046	McIntosh et al., 1978[186]
Stomach (fundus)	Human	0.60	Chayvialle et al., 1978[187]
Stomach (fundus)	Human	0.29	McIntosh et al., 1978[186]
Stomach (antrum)	Rat	0.43	Arimura et al., 1975[184]
Stomach (antrum)	Rat	0.050	McIntosh et al., 1978[186]
Stomach (antrum)	Human	1.68	Chayvialle et al., 1978[187]
Stomach (antrum)	Human	0.46	McIntosh et al., 1978[186]
Duodenum	Rat	0.025	Arimura et al., 1975[184]
Duodenum	Rat	0.15	Patel and Reichlin, 1978[183]
Duodenum	Human	1.35	Chayvialle et al., 1978[187]

has been demonstrated in lung and thyroid tumors (see below).[22]

ANATOMICAL LOCALIZATION

The peptide is widely but not universally distributed and displays specific and selective functions that differ according to its location. SS-containing neurons are found in the parts of the hypothalamus regulating the anterior pituitary, the posterior pituitary, the extrahypothalamic brain, and the brain stem and spinal cord.

The Nervous System

HYPOTHALAMUS. The distribution of immunoreactive SS was first studied immunocytochemically in the guinea pig brain.[92] Many cells terminate in the external layers of the median eminence around the capillary loops of the hypophyseal portal vessels, and the principal source of these tuberoinfundibular fibers is the anterior periventricular re-

TABLE 17–4. PUBLISHED NORMAL RANGES FOR PERIPHERAL PLASMA SOMATOSTATIN LEVELS IN DIFFERENT SPECIES

SPECIES	SOMATOSTATIN RANGE (pg/ml)*	REFERENCES
Human	174 ± 9 (92%) 1000 ± 41 (8%)	Kronheim et al., 1978[128]
Human	88 ± 8	Krejs et al., 1979[188]
Human	80 ± 25†	Lundqvist et al., 1979[189]
Human	675 ± 95‡	Pipeleers et al., 1979[190]
Human	11.9 ± 1.6	Saito et al., 1980[191]
Rat	10.5 ± 2.6	Arimura et al., 1978[192]
Pig	138 ± 20	Gustavsson and Lundqvist, 1978[193]
Dog	119.7 ± 7.6	Schusdziarra et al., 1977[194]
Dog	<10	Arimura et al., 1978[195]
Dog	28.5 ± 8.4	Chayvialle et al., 1978[196]

*Values quoted are the mean of the normal range plus or minus one standard error of the mean, except for†, for which values are quoted as the mean plus one standard deviation, and‡, for which the limits of the range are not given.

gion of the hypothalamus just under the ependymal lining.[93] Some axons of SS cell bodies in the hypothalamic periventricular area lead to the median eminence and terminate there, near portal capillaries. Others project either to hypothalamic nuclei, which are part of the limbic system,[94] or to the brain stem and spinal cord.[95] SS is also present in nerve endings in the suprachiasmatic nuclei, a part of the brain thought to generate circadian rhythms.

CEREBRAL CORTEX. The highest concentration of SS in the rat and human brain is found in the median eminence and arcuate nucleus, but it is also present in high concentrations in other hypothalamic nuclei as well as throughout the extrahypothalamic brain, especially in the preoptic area of the cerebral cortex and in the spinal cord.[90, 96] None of the cerebral hemisphere SS comes from the hypothalamus. Anatomical studies show that SS in the extrahypothalamic brain is present mainly in short interconnecting neurons; thus, it has a local regulatory role in this part of the nervous system. In the deeper layers of the cortex SS-containing neurons extend from the spinal cord.

Studies on subcellular preparations of both hypothalamic and extrahypothalamic areas of the rat brain and indeed all SS neuronal systems that have been studied in detail have shown that SS is localized in the synaptosome fraction in secreting granules in nerve endings, thus suggesting its role as a neurotransmitter.[97, 98] When hypothalamic cells of fetal rats in cell culture are exposed to electrolyte or neurotransmitter changes, they make and release SS.[99] A wide variety of neurotransmitters and neuropeptides affect SS release (Table 17–5). Ultrastructural and immunocytochemical studies have shown that brain SS is present in neurosecretory granules larger than those storing acetylcholine and epinephrine.[100] Ontogenetically, SS is first detectable at 16 weeks near the third ventricle in the human brain.[101]

In CSF, SS is detected in levels of 46 to 112 pg/ml.[102] Patients with acromegaly have normal concentrations,[102, 103] but clearly this does not necessarily mean that hypothalamic secretion is unchanged, as the hypothalamus is not the only source of SS in the CSF.

PERIPHERAL NERVOUS SYSTEM. Many sensory neurons contain SS.[104] The fibers of cell bodies located in spinal

TABLE 17–5. SUMMARY OF PANCREATIC ISLET CELL REGULATORY FACTORS*

SUBSTRATES	SOMATOSTATIN	INSULIN	GLUCAGON
Glucose	↑	↑	↓
Amino acids	↑	↑	↑
Neurotransmitters			
Acetylcholine (muscarinic receptors)	↑	↑	↑
α_1-Adrenergic	↓		
α_2-Adrenergic	↓	↓	↑
β-Adrenergic (NE,E)	↑	↑	↑
Dopamine	↓		
GABA	↓	↔	
Neuropeptides			
Somatostatin	↓	↓	↓
Insulin	↓ ?	?	?
Glucagon	↑	?	?
Pancreatic polypeptide	?	?	?
VIP	↑	↑	↑
Secretin	↑		
Substance P	↑	↓↑	↑
Cholecystokinin	↑	↑	↑
Gastrin	↑		
Bombesin	↔	↑	↑
Neurotensin	↑	↑↓	↑
Endorphins	↓	↑↓	↑
Prostaglandin E, cyclic nucleotides	↑	↑↓	↑

Data are derived from McCann et al[197] and Reichlin.[198]
* ↑ = Increase; ↓ = decrease; ↔ = no change; ↓↑ = conflicting reports.
NE = Norepinephrine; E = epinephrine; VIP = vasoactive intestinal polypeptide.

sensory ganglia terminate in the dorsal part of the spinal cord, intermingling there with other sensory nerve endings.

SS also coexists with catecholamines in some sympathetic neurons, suggesting dual cell control.[104] How this dual control is effected is at present uncertain; other interneuronal connections may alter expression, for example, of the SS gene. In the parasympathetic tract, accumulation of SS proximal to a ligature can be demonstrated in the vagus nerves of rats and other species, thus demonstrating axonal transport. This external transport is blocked by colchicine, which disrupts microtubules.[105] SS is also present in the human retina.[106] It is thus clear that SS fibers projecting centrally from the periphery subserve a wide variety of sensory functions.

The Gastrointestinal Tract

All laboratories have found high concentrations of SS in the stomach, pancreas, and intestine, particularly in the visceral autonomic nervous system and the endocrine cells of the gut.[107, 108] Large amounts are detectable in the gastric antrum, duodenum, and pancreas, and smaller amounts may be found in the remainder of the gut. SS is also detected in the lumen of the stomach and duodenum. SS is first detectable in the pancreas at the age of eight weeks.[109] Although the concentration of SS in the gastrointestinal tract is considerably lower than that in the median eminence, the total amount of SS is much greater than in the hypothalamus. Immunocytochemically SS has been shown

to be localized in the D cells of the pancreas and in the mucosa of the gastrointestinal tract from the fundus of the stomach to the colon. SS cells occur with greatest frequency in the gastric fundus and antrum and the duodenal mucosa.[107, 110] D cells are situated in the lower third of the crypts and possess long cytoplasmic processes that reach along the basal membranes to the basal pole of neighboring glands,[109] thus providing a paracrine means of affecting the secretion of other endocrine cells in the gut (e.g., gastrin). They also possess microvilli that come into contact with the lumen, presumably providing the means whereby changes in the gut contents are sensed by the D cell and alter SS secretion. Secretion can occur in either direction, into the lumen of the gut or into the circulation.

The gut is innervated by both extrinsic and intrinsic SS-containing neurons, and the latter are located in both the submucosal and myenteric plexuses. Lastly, SS cells have been found in the salivary gland of the monkey,[111] and the flow of saliva and amylase content are decreased by it. SS is present in saliva.

Other Locations

SS-staining cells have been reported in the parafollicular ("C") cells of humans, together with calcitonin, and the peptide is synthesized by some medullary carcinoma cells.[112] It is not clear whether SS inhibits calcitonin secretion. SS can also occur in catecholamine-secreting cells of the human adrenal medulla and in the cytotrophoblastic layer of human placental villi.[113–116]

BIOSYNTHESIS, PROCESSING, AND TRANSPORT

It is now well established that SS-14 and SS-28 are synthesized as part of a large precursor, pre-prosomatostatin, which is about eight times larger than SS itself.[117] The mature hormones arise as a result of post-translational cleavage. Genetic recombinant techniques have elucidated the sequence of pre-prosomatostatin using cloned cDNA's generated from a number of species, including fish pancreatic islets,[12] a rat medullary carcinoma,[118] and a human somatostatinoma.[119] Rat and human pre-prosomatostatin are virtually identical in amino acid sequence, differing in only 4 of 116 residues, 2 in the signal peptide and 2 in the propeptide. Angler fish and catfish both have two SS precursors and have little homology to the mammalian precursors. The overall organization of pre-prosomatostatin consists of a hydrophobic signal peptide of amino acids followed by a pre-region of 90 to 100 residues. The mature hormones SS-14 and SS-28 are located at the carboxyl-terminus of the pre-region, and the latter is preceded by pairs of basic amino acids: Arg-Ly. The rat gene was sequenced in 1984,[120] and to date there is no evidence for a separate gene for SS-14 and SS-28.

The pre-hormone is synthesized in the endoplasmic reticulum of neurons and epithelial cells and translocated to the Golgi system, guided by the leader sequence, which is then cleaved off the prohormone, a precursor of amino acids.[121, 122] Some prohormone is further processed within the secretory granules to form SS-14 and SS-28. Differences in the relative proportions of the various forms of SS in different tumors presumably reflect differences in post-translational processing and are cell-specific or organ-specific. This is important because of the differences in function of the varying molecular forms. At present the mechanisms of control of intracellular post-translational processing are poorly understood, but tissue-specific container or silencer regions may occur in the gene concerned. After packaging of hormone into granules, granules move from the cell body of neurons to neuronal processes by axoplasmic flow.

METABOLISM

SS circulates bound to a binding protein.[123] In vivo studies of the time course of inhibition of hormone release have suggested that SS has a short biological half-life. Thus the half-life of exogenously administered SS has been calculated by radioimmunoassay to vary from 1.1 to 3.0 minutes in humans.[124] The half-life is longer in patients with renal failure and probably also in those with hepatic failure.[125] These data therefore suggest that both the kidney and the liver may be important sites of SS metabolism. However, other tissues may be important, and peptidases that cleave SS have been reported in rat brain.[126, 127] The circulation may be another site of SS metabolism, as it is known that SS-degrading enzymes occur in plasma.[128] In the circulation SS is rapidly converted to des-ala^1-SS.[129]

PHYSIOLOGICAL ROLE

SS almost certainly has a number of different physiological roles over and above what the name implies. With regard to the pituitary, it acts as a neurohormone, secreted by nerve cells into the blood. In the nervous system it is a neurotransmitter or neuromodulator. Outside the brain, it can either act on cells by paracrine means (e.g., in the pancreas or gut) or act as a true hormone (e.g., on the pancreas or gastrointestinal tract after circulating in the blood). It can influence its own secretion (an autocrine function) and it may affect the gut after it is secreted into the lumen (a "lumone").

Pituitary Regulation

GROWTH HORMONE. Because of its properties in inhibiting both basal and stimulated release of GH, SS has a physiological role acting via the hypophyseal portal system in regulating GH from the anterior pituitary. Evidence for this comes from a number of different studies. Active and passive immunization of dogs with SS antiserum increases basal GH levels, and it prevents the inhibition of GH secretion following stress.[130, 131] Active immunization against SS in rats increases basal GH levels and diminishes episodic bursts of GH secretion.[131, 132]

It has been demonstrated in rats that the level of SS in the hypophyseal portal blood is considerably higher than that in the jugular vein, and an inverse relationship has been found between hypophyseal portal SS and plasma GH[133–135]; portal SS levels rise prior to GH troughs in rats,

so that intermittent secretion appears to be an important regulator of GH pulses. Intraventricular GH increases the level of SS in hypophyseal portal blood and suppresses GH secretion.[136] In vitro studies in rats have shown that GH has an inhibiting effect on its own action by affecting SS cell bodies in the periventricular region of the hypothalamus. Furthermore, somatomedin-C causes an increase of SS in hypothalamic tissue.[137] In addition, lesions of the medial preoptic area of the hypothalamus in rats increase the pulses of secretion of GH, both in frequency and in amplitude.

Several neurotransmitters, including acetylcholine, epinephrine, and dopamine, modify SS secretion, and the effects of these on GH are probably accounted for in part by their effect on SS secretion itself.

TSH. SS inhibits the release of thyrotropin from isolated pituitary cells and reduces TRH-induced TSH release in man. In hypothyroidism, basal TSH levels are reduced. The role of SS in the control of TSH secretion is suggested by the fact that hypothyroid rats have increased brain, pancreatic, and gut SS levels, which can be normalized by the administration of T$_4$.[138, 139] Furthermore, SS antibody potentiates the TSH response to TRH in man but not in sheep.[140, 141] It seems clear, therefore, that TSH secretion is regulated both by TRH positively and by SS and thyroid hormone negatively. SS has no physiological effects on other anterior pituitary hormones.

Neurotransmitter Function

The presence of SS in the extrahypothalamic brain and spinal cord suggests a role in the regulation of the nervous system, independent of any action in modulating GH and thyrotropin secretion. The presence of SS receptors further supports the neurotransmitter role of SS. Lastly, a demonstration that SS is released from rat brain tissue in vitro in response to membrane depolarization gives further support to the concept that SS has an important, if unclear, physiological role in the nervous system.

Somatostatin in Neurological Disease

Inaccessibility of tissue and ethical difficulties in obtaining CSF create problems in studying SS in human brain disease. Intrahypocampal injections of cysteamine in rats deplete SS and cause a decrease in memory and locomotion, but whether these effects are reversible by SS is unclear at present. There are now several reports of markedly reduced concentrations of SS in the brains of patients with Alzheimer's disease,[142, 143] together with a decrease in SS-binding sites. Acetylcholine and possibly CRF are similarly involved, but other neurotransmitter systems, including dopaminergic, noradrenergic, and serotoninergic systems are well maintained in Alzheimer's disease. The role of SS in normal brain function in man is unclear at present, as low concentrations are found in some patients who apparently function normally.

Recent studies suggest that various central tumors, including glioma, meningioma, and neuroma, do not immunostain or secrete SS.[144] One hypothalamic hamartoma associated with precocious puberty has been reported to contain SS.[145]

Pathological increases in CSF SS have been reported in patients with various structural diseases of the CNS; these probably represent nerve cell damage.[103] Patients with multiple sclerosis in relapse may have lower levels of SS in the CSF,[146] but this has not yet been confirmed. In unipolar depression, SS levels in the CSF are reduced[147, 148] and may return to normal on recovery. The importance of these findings is not yet clear. Manic patients do not have altered levels of CSF SS.

Pancreas

SS is important in insulin and glucagon regulation but less so in the control of pancreatic polypeptide secretion. The localization of SS in the D cells of the pancreatic islets bears a close relation to those cells secreting glucagon and insulin (α and β cells). This, together with the observed effects of intravenous SS in inhibiting secretion of insulin, glucagon, and indeed SS itself, has led to the suggestion that SS plays a local paracrine regulatory role in the pancreas.[149] The treatment of isolated rat pancreatic islets in vitro with SS antiserum has been shown to increase insulin and glucagon release.[150, 151] That this is a paracrine action is further suggested by the fact that neutralization of circulating SS with antiserum effects no changes in plasma insulin or glucagon levels.[152–154] These effects have been confirmed in humans,[155] because SS responses to various stimuli, including insulin-induced hypoglycemia and food ingestion, bear no relationship to the circulating insulin or glucagon responses seen after these stimuli. Similarly, neither exogenously administered glucagon nor intravenous insulin has a regulating effect on SS.[156] Patel has found SS receptors on α and β cells as well as on D cells.[157]

How these actions relate to physiological mechanisms is not known. With glucagon, there seems to be a negative feedback system as glucagon stimulates SS in vitro and SS in turn inhibits glucagon. However, the situation with insulin is unclear, because its administration has little effect on SS release, although deficiency does induce SS secretion. The α cell is more transient than the β cell, accounting for the mild hyperglycemia seen in patients receiving SS long term.

Somatostatin in Pancreatic Diseases

DIABETES MELLITUS. No clear role for SS has emerged in the pathogenesis or manifestations of diabetes mellitus. There is no evidence that diabetes in man is caused by excess SS release.

SOMATOSTATINOMA. The somatostatinoma syndrome was first recognized in 1979.[158] SS-secreting tumors are associated with some of the biological effects seen after exogenous administration of the peptide (Table 17–6). These tumors are rare; as of 1981 only seven had been reported; there are now approximately 25 cases of pancreatic somatostatinoma in the literature. Most originate in the pancreas, and most are malignant. The patients usually show diabetes mellitus due to suppression of insulin and glucagon secretion, but hyperglycemia is mild and may require only dietary management; other signs of suppression include GH responses to provocative stimuli, malabsorption from the gut with steatorrhea, and in some patients gall-

stones, probably related to cholecystokinin suppression and cholestasis, and hypochlorhydria. Circulating SS levels are considerably elevated.[158] SS is seldom the sole hormone involved, and coexistant hypersecretion of other peptide hormones can cause hypoglycemia, flushing, Cushing's syndrome, and diarrhea. These make for considerable variability in symptoms, and recognition is difficult. Many patients with somatostatinoma present with liver metastases of the islet cell tumor with symptoms that in retrospect have been present for many years.

Gastrointestinal somatostatinomas also occur mainly in the duodenal wall and ampulla of Vater. SS is released much less commonly than with pancreatic somatostatinoma, so the syndrome is not often present. They present with intestinal or biliary obstruction. Histologically they are psammomatous tumors. Somatostatinoma of the papilla of Vater has been described in association with neurofibromatosis type I.

Gastrointestinal Tract

SS affects a very wide variety of physiological gut actions (see Table 17–2), including the inhibition of endocrine and exocrine function, decreased absorption and motor activity, and decreased mesenteric blood flow. The effect of SS on the gut may be paracrine, truly endocrine as has been shown for lipid digestion,[159] or through luminal secretion.[160]

Experiments in a number of species, primarily in dogs and subsequently in humans, have shown that food, particularly oral protein and fat, causes a rise in circulating SS levels.[155, 161–163] Several groups of workers have measured SS levels in the hepatic portal vein in a number of different species and have found that they are higher than simultaneously collected peripheral samples. Thus most of the measured circulating SS arises from the gastrointestinal tract. If SS is infused at rates that produce postprandial concentrations, there is a decrease in insulin and glucagon responses to feeding. Immunocytochemical studies have shown that SS in gastric cells localized in the lower part of the antral mucosa bears a close anatomical relationship to the gastrin-secreting cells and parietal cells. Because the intravenous administration of SS inhibits both gastric acid and gastrin secretion, it is highly likely that SS is acting in a paracrine role in this regard. It may be that intraluminal SS is acting in a paracrine manner. Support for these paracrine actions comes from reports that vagal stimulation releases SS into the gastric antral lumen of cats and that

TABLE 17–6. FEATURES OF PANCREATIC SOMATOSTATINOMA

Hyperglycemia
Cholelithiasis
Steatorrhea
Hypochlorhydria
Diarrhea
Abdominal pain
Weight loss
Anemia
Elevated plasma and tissue somatostatin
Histologically malignant
May be associated with ACTH, calcitonin, secretion

intragastric instillation of SS in healthy human subjects and dogs reduces basal acid secretion.[164, 165]

Cholinergic mechanisms have an important inhibitory effect on SS release, as has been shown in dogs and humans.[166] The important question is whether the rise in circulating SS seen postprandially has any physiological significance. Recent studies have shown that when SS is infused in postprandial concentrations physiological levels may influence GH and insulin secretion[167]; nevertheless, postprandial changes in SS and GH bear no functional relationship. SS therefore seems to have an important role in the gut, controlling by a variety of means the rate at which nutrients enter the circulation.[164]

Endogenous Somatostatin and Gastrointestinal Disease

No evidence exists to suggest that abnormalities of SS secretion underlie any gastrointestinal disease. Clearly, excessive acid secretion or gastrin secretion may result from gut SS deficiency, but no changes in SS of the gastric antrum or differential counts of gastrin (G) or D cells have been found in patients with peptic ulceration.

CLINICAL USES OF SOMATOSTATIN

Native Somatostatin

The major limitation in the clinical use of this compound is its short half-life of less than three minutes in the circulation. It is not absorbed orally and therefore has to be given parenterally.

SS has been used as an investigative tool in the hormonal regulation of metabolism and has been used in an attempt to treat brittle diabetes mellitus, secreting pancreatic tumors, upper gastrointestinal bleeding, pancreatitis, and acromegaly.

NORMAL SUBJECTS. When SS is infused into normal subjects, insulin, glucagon, and GH are suppressed, resulting in a lowering of blood glucose, particularly because of glucagon suppression. If the infusion continues, blood glucose then rises because of continued suppression of insulin secretion.

DIABETES MELLITUS. When SS is infused into patients with Type I diabetes, a lowering of blood glucose and a marked diminution of hyperglycemia and ketosis occur after insulin withdrawal. These reactions are not completely prevented, however, leading Gerich to suggest that glucagon is an important component of diabetic acidosis.[168] SS has also been given to improve the control of brittle diabetes by reducing the degree of change in blood glucose, but no consistent effects are seen; it is at present unclear how useful this treatment is in practical terms.

In Type II diabetes, metabolic control is worsened by SS infusions, largely because of loss of residual insulin secretion. The hypoglycemic action of insulin is enhanced by SS administration, presumably because of loss of glucagon counterregulation.

PANCREATIC TUMORS. Pancreatic tumors, including secreting gastrinomas, insulinomas, glucagonomas, and VIPomas, have been treated by parenteral administration of SS, but its short duration of action has confined its use to brief periods only. Nesidioblastosis, which causes neonatal and infantile hyperinsulinemia and hypoglycemia because of a pancreatic disorder characterized by hyperfunctioning islets, has also been managed with SS prior to total pancreatectomy.

UPPER GASTROINTESTINAL BLEEDING. Because of its effect of reducing acid and gastrin secretion as well as decreasing mesenteric blood flow, SS can be useful in controlling acute upper gastrointestinal bleeding. In a controlled trial by Kayasseh et al,[169] when SS was given as an intravenous bolus of 250 μg followed by administration of 250 μg/h, it controlled bleeding due to gastric ulcer and stress gastritis, usually within a few hours, and was superior to cimetidine. It may also be useful in the treatment of upper gastrointestinal bleeding due to esophageal varices,[170] lowering hepatic wedge pressure by 20 per cent. It is not superior to vasopressin in the control rate but has markedly fewer side effects.[171]

ACUTE PANCREATITIS. Acute pancreatitis may also be successfully treated with SS.[172] Pancreatic fistulae may respond to SS, presumably owing to the actions of the peptide in inhibiting exocrine pancreatic secretion.

ACROMEGALY. Patients with acromegaly respond to SS infusions with a suppression of GH and improvement in glucose tolerance.[31] Again, the short-term effect of native SS has precluded long-term trials.

Side Effects

Intravenous administration of SS has no serious adverse effects. Normal subjects may experience a transient increase in blood pressure and pulse. Occasionally with high-dose infusions dizziness, sweating, nausea, and passage of bulky steatorrheic stools may be encountered. The need for intravenous administration of the peptide, its short duration of action, and the postinfection hypersecretion of hormones greatly diminished initial enthusiasm for clinical use of native SS and led to the development of longer-acting analogues.

Somatostatin Analogues

The potential for developing analogues with a different spectrum of effects that are resistant to degradation and therefore have a longer half-life and might be effective orally has stimulated a great deal of research. One such analogue has been developed in Switzerland[173] and is now licensed in the treatment of carcinoid tumors, VIPoma, and acromegaly. Its structure is shown in Figure 17–2. It is an octapeptide variant of SS (octreotide) with a half-life of approximately 110 minutes in the peripheral circulation. It inhibits the secretion of GH 45 times, glucagon 11 times, and insulin 1.3 times more actively than native SS. No rebound secretion occurs.

CARCINOID TUMORS. Carcinoid tumors may contain SS

Somatostatin octapeptide (201–995)

H-(D)Phe-Cys-Phe-(D)Trp-Lys-Thr-Cys-Thr-ol,acetate

FIGURE 17–2. Amino acid sequence of the somatostatin octapeptide, octreotide (SS 201–995).

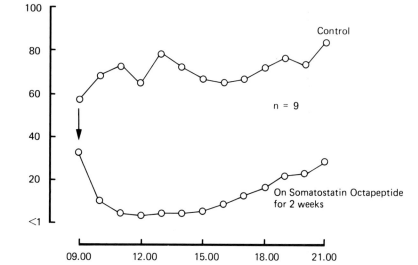

FIGURE 17–3. Long-term treatment with the somatostatin octapeptide, octreotide, 100 μg subcutaneously twice daily, in 9 patients with acromegaly: the effect on mean serum growth hormone. A dose was given as indicated by the arrow.

receptors. In these patients systemic treatment with octreotide may improve diarrhea and flushing attacks. Kvols et al[174] have shown that octreotide causes frequent symptomatic and biochemical responses. To date no antitumor effects of octreotide against carcinoids have been demonstrated. Prediction of the subsequent response to octreotide may be obtained with scanning using octreotide labeled with radioactive iodine or indium.[175, 176]

PANCREATIC TUMORS. A number of VIP-secreting tumors have been studied, and a dramatic improvement in diarrhea as well as a reduction in circulating VIP levels have occurred with long-term treatment.[177] The response to octreotide depends on the presence of SS receptors. The duration of the response is variable. Eventually in those malignant tumors there is escape. Octreotide does not control tumor growth and so should be used as symptomatic treatment in addition to other approaches aimed at debulking the tumor or giving cytotoxic therapy. Other pancreatic tumors secreting glucagon, gastrin, GRF, and insulin may respond to octreotide.

ACROMEGALY. The octapeptide analogue of SS (octreotide) has now been used in the treatment of many patients with acromegaly and appears to have a valuable place in therapy[178–180] (Fig. 17–3). It appears possible to control GH secretion in the long term with subcutaneous administration of 100 μg three times a day, and control of GH levels is often better than that obtained with dopamine agonists such as bromocriptine. Responses to octreotide correlate with the number of somatostatin receptors present in the tumor subsequently obtained at transsphenoidal operation.[181] The addition of bromocriptine to SS does not further suppress GH levels in the patients so far studied. Carbohydrate tolerance does not worsen and may improve in some patients, presumably related to GH suppression. At the commencement of treatment, a decrease in pituitary tumor size is seen in about half the acromegalic patients treated,[179] but this is less marked than that observed during bromocriptine therapy of prolactin-secreting tumors. Occasional patients experience diarrhea or colicky abdominal pain, and steatorrhea may be seen, presumably because of inhibition of pancreatic exocrine secretion. These effects settle with time on treatment. Gallstones develop in pa-

tients on octreotide owing to suppression of cholecystokinin release and increased bile cholesterol. They are rarely a problem clinically. Octreotide is the most effective long-term means of controlling acromegaly by medical treatment.

TSH-OMAS. Inhibition of hormone release and tumor shrinkage have also been reported during therapy with octreotide in TSH-secreting pituitary tumors.[182]

GUT DISEASE. Because of its effect on gastrointestinal motility and blood flow and pancreatic exocrine function, octreotide has also been used in the treatment of diarrhea associated with ileostomy, radiation damage, diabetic neuropathy, and AIDS. It has also been used in the treatment of bleeding esophageal varices and peptic ulcer and also to inhibit pancreatic secretion in pancreatic fistulae. It is not yet licensed for these uses.

SUMMARY

SS with its widespread distribution has a number of different but important physiological roles. Analogues of SS are of potential importance therapeutically as well as in controlling hormone-secreting tumors. SS may also be effective in control of symptoms due to peptic ulceration and bleeding esophageal varices.

The effects of SS on behavior are unknown in humans, although numerous effects have been described in animals. Not only has the physiology of this compound been elucidated in a wide variety of studies, but new insights have been gained into molecular evolution. Because of its widespread and diverse actions, it appears to have a number of important clinical uses that are in the process of being evaluated.

REFERENCES

1. Falkmer S: Immunocytochemical studies of the evolution of islet hormones. J Histochem Cytochem 27:1281–1282, 1979.
2. Berelowitz M, LeRoith D, Von Schenk H, et al: Somatostatin-like immunoreactivity and biological activity is present in *Tetrahymena pyriformis*, a ciliated protozoan. Endocrinology 110:1939–1944, 1982.

3. Pearce AGE: The phylogeny of the common peptides. Proc R Soc Lond 210:61–62, 1980.
4. Green JD, Harris GW: The neurovascular link between the neurohypophysis and adenohypophysis. J Endocrinol 5:136–145, 1947.
5. Krulich L, Dhariwal APS, McCann SM: Stimulatory and inhibitory effects of purified hypothalamic extracts on growth hormone release from rat pituitary in vitro. Endocrinology 83:783–790, 1968.
6. Brazeau P, Vale W, Burgus R, et al: Hypothalamic polypeptide that inhibits the secretion of immunoreactive pituitary growth hormone. Science 178:77–79, 1973.
7. Coy DH, Coy EJ, Arimura A, Schally AV: Solid phase synthesis of growth hormone release inhibiting factor. Biochem Biophys Res Commun 54:1267–1273, 1973.
8. Yamashiro D, Li CH: Synthesis of a peptide with full somatostatin activity. Biochem Biophys Res Commun 54:882–888, 1973.
9. Reichlin S: Somatostatin. N Engl J Med 309:1495–1501, 1556–1563, 1983.
10. Schally AV, Dupont A, Arimura A, et al: Isolation of porcine GH release inhibiting hormone (GH-RIH): The existence of 3 forms of GH-RIH. Fed Proc 34:584, 1975.
11. Schally AV, Dupont A, Arimura A, Redding TW: Isolation and structure of somatostatin from porcine hypothalami. Biochemistry 15:509–514, 1976.
12. Hobart P, Crawford R, Shen LP, et al: Cloning and sequence analysis of cDNAs encoding two distinct somatostatin and precursors found in the endocrine pancreas of angler-fish. Nature 288:137–141, 1980.
13. Arimura A, Sato H, Dupont A, et al: Somatostatin: Abundance of immunoreactive hormone in rat stomach and pancreas. Science 189:1007–1009, 1975.
14. Praydayrol L, Jörnvall H, Mutt V, Ribet A: N-terminally extended somatostatin: The primary structure of somatostatin-28. FEBS Lett 109:55–58, 1980.
15. Rodriguez-Arnao MD, Gomez-Pan A, Rainbow SJ, et al: Aspects of prosomatostatin on growth hormone and prolactin response to arginine in man: Comparison with somatostatin. Lancet 1:353–356, 1981.
16. Brown M, Rivier J, Vale W: Biological activity of somatostatin and somatostatin analogs on inhibition of arginine-induced insulin and glucagon release in the rat. Endocrinology 98:336–343, 1976.
17. Srikant CB, Patel YC: Somatostatin receptors: Identification and characterization in rat brain membranes. Proc Natl Acad Sci USA 78:3930–3934, 1981.
18. Descos F, de Parseau L, Olive C, Chayvialle JA: Somatostatin-like immunoreactivity in human gastrointestinal mucosa. 2nd International Symposium on Somatostatin, Athens, 1–3 June 1981, Abst 31.
19. Penman E, Wass JAH, Butler MG, et al: Distribution and characterisation of immunoreactive somatostatin in human gastrointestinal tract. Regul Pept 7:53–65, 1983.
20. Chihara K, Arimura A, Schally AV: Immunoreactive somatostatin in rat hypophyseal portal blood: Effects of anesthetics. Endocrinology 104:1434–1441, 1979.
21. Gillioz P, Giraud P, Conte-Devaux B, et al: Immunoreactive somatostatin in rat hypophyseal portal blood. Endocrinology 104:1407–1410, 1979.
22. Penman E, Lowry PJ, Wass JAH, et al: Molecular forms of somatostatin in normal subjects and in patients with pancreatic somatostatinoma. Clin Endocrinol 12:611–620, 1980.
23. Patel YC: A high molecular weight form of somatostatin-28 (1–12) like immunoreactive substance within somatostatin-14, immunoreactivity in the rat pancreas: Evidence that somatostatin-14 synthesis can occur independently of somatostatin-28. J Clin Invest 72:2137–2143, 1983.
24. Zingg HH, Patel YC: Processing of somatostatin-28 to somatostatin-14 by rat hypothalamic synaptosomal membranes. Life Sci 33:1241–1247, 1983.
25. Penman E, Wass JAH: Radioimmunoassay of somatostatin: Methodological problems and physiological investigations. In Bizollom CA (ed): Physiological Peptides and New Trends in Radioimmunology. Proceedings of the 5th International Symposium on Radioimmunology, Lyon, France, 9–11 April, 1981. Amsterdam, Elsevier 1981, pp 3–18.
26. Hall R, Schally AV, Evered D, et al: Action of growth hormone release inhibitory hormone in healthy men and in acromegaly. Lancet 2:581–584, 1973.
27. Prange Hansen A, Ørskov H, Seyer-Hansen K, Lundbaek K: Some actions of growth hormone release inhibiting factor. Br Med J 3:523–524, 1973.
28. Mortimer CH, Carr D, Lind T, et al: Effects of growth hormone

29. release inhibiting hormone on circulating glucagon, insulin and growth hormone in normal, diabetic, acromegalic and hypopituitary patients. Lancet 1:697–701, 1974.
29. Wehrenberg WB, Ling N, Böhlen P, et al: Physiological roles of somatocrinin and somatostatin in the regulation of growth hormone secretion. Biochem Biophys Res Commun 109:562–567, 1982.
30. Besser GM, Mortimer CH, McNeilly AS, et al: Long term infusion of growth hormone release inhibiting hormone in acromegaly: Effects on pituitary and pancreatic hormones. Br Med J 4:620–627, 1974.
31. Besser GM, Mortimer CH, Carr D, et al: Growth hormone release inhibiting hormone in acromegaly. Br Med J 1:352–355, 1974.
32. Vale W, Rivier C, Brazeau P, Guillemin R: Effects of somatostatin on the secretion of thyrotropin and prolactin. Endocrinology 95:968–977, 1975.
33. Weeke J, Hansen AP, Lundbaek K: The inhibition by somatostatin of the thyrotropin response to thyrotropin releasing hormone in normal subjects. Scand J Clin Lab Invest 33:101–103, 1974.
34. Weeke J, Hansen AP, Lundbaek K: Inhibition by somatostatin of basal levels of serum thyrotropin (TSH) in normal men. J Clin Endocrinol Metab 41:168–171, 1975.
35. Lucke C, Höffken B, von zur Mühlen A: The effect of somatostatin on TSH levels in patients with primary hypothyroidism. J Clin Endocrinol Metab 41:1082–1084, 1975.
36. Richardson UI, Schonbrunn A: Inhibition of adrenocorticotropin secretion by somatostatin in pituitary cells in culture. Endocrinology 108:281–290, 1981.
37. Tyrrell JB, Lorenzi M, Gerich JE, Forsham PH: Inhibition by somatostatin of ACTH secretion in Nelson's syndrome. J Clin Endocrinol Metab 40:1125–1127, 1975.
38. Oki S, Nakai Y, Nako K, Imura H: Plasma B endorphin responses to somatostatin, thyrotropin-releasing hormone, or vasopressin in Nelson's syndrome. J Clin Endocrinol Metab 50:194–197, 1980.
39. Alberti KGMM, Christensen SE, Iversen J, et al: Inhibition of insulin secretion by somatostatin. Lancet 2:1229–1301, 1973.
40. Gerich JE, Lorenzi M, Schneider V, Forsham PH: Effects of somatostatin on plasma glucose and insulin responses to glucagon and tolbutamide in man. J Clin Endocrinol Metab 39:1057, 1974.
41. Iversen J: Inhibition of pancreatic glucagon release by somatostatin in vitro. Scand J Clin Lab Invest 33:125–129, 1974.
42. Curry DL, Bennet LL: Reversal of somatostatin inhibition of insulin secretion by calcium. Biochem Biophys Res Commun 60:1015–1019, 1974.
43. Brown M, Rivier J, Vale W: Biological activity of somatostatin and somatostatin analogs on inhibition of arginine-induced insulin and glucagon release in the rat. Endocrinology 98:336–343, 1976.
44. Rizza R, Verdonk C, Miles J, et al: Somatostatin does not cause sustained fasting hyperglycaemia in man. Horm Metab Res 11:643–644, 1979.
45. Adrian TE, Bloom SR, Besterman HS, Bryant MG: PP-physiology and pathology. In Bloom SR (ed): Gut Hormones. New York, Churchill Livingstone, 1978, pp 254–260.
46. Floyd JC, Fajans SS, Pek S: Physiological regulation of plasma levels of P.P. in man. In Bloom SR (ed): Gut Hormones. New York, Churchill Livingstone, 1978, pp 247–253.
47. Boden G, Sivitz MC, Owen OE, et al: Somatostatin suppresses secretin and pancreatic exocrine secretion. Science 190:163–164, 1975.
48. Dollinger HC, Raptis S, Pfeiffer EF: Effects of somatostatin on exocrine and endocrine pancreatic function stimulated by intestinal hormones in man. Horm Metab Res 8:74–78, 1976.
49. Konturek SJ, Tasler J, Obtulowicz W, et al: Effect of growth hormone release inhibiting tissue on hormones stimulating exocrine pancreatic secretion. J Clin Invest 58:1–6, 1976.
50. Arnold R, Linkisch BG: Somatostatin and the gastrointestinal tract. Clin Gastroenterol 9:733–753, 1980.
51. Bloom SR, Mortimer CH, Thorner MO, et al: Inhibition of gastrin and gastric acid secretion by growth hormone release inhibiting hormone. Lancet 2:1106–1109, 1974.
52. Raptis S, Dollinger HC, von Berger L, et al: Effects of somatostatin on gastric secretion and gastrin release in man. Digestion 13:15–26, 1975.
53. Sopwith AM, Penny ES, Besser GM, Rees LH: Secretion of circulating immunoreactive human growth hormone releasing factor is inhibited by somatostatin. J Endocrinol 108(Suppl):Abst 260, 1986.
54. Bloom SR, Ralphs DN, Besser GM, et al: Effect of somatostatin on motilin levels and gastric emptying. Gut 16:834, 1975.
55. Wahren J, Felig P: Influence of somatostatin on carbohydrate disposal and absorption in diabetes mellitus. Lancet 2:1213–1215, 1976.
56. Konturek SJ, Krol R, Pawlik W, et al: Pharmacology of somatostatin.

In Bloom SR (ed): Gut Hormones. New York, Churchill Livingstone, 1978, pp 457–462.

57. Gomez-Pan A, Snow MH, Piercy DA, et al: Actions of growth hormone release inhibiting hormone (somatostatin) on the renin aldosterone system. J Clin Endocrinol Metab 43:240–243, 1976.

58. Diel F, Holz J, Bethge N: Failure of somatostatin and B endorphin to affect bovine adrenal cortex cells in vitro. Horm Metab Res 13:95–98, 1981.

59. Loos U, Kampshoff H, Birk J, Rothenbuckner G: Secretion of T3 and T4 by isolated human thyroid cells and its inhibition by somatostatin. Proceedings of the Vth International Congress of Endocrinology, Hamburg, 1976. Abst 646.

60. Hargis GK, Williams GA, Reynolds WA, et al: Effect of somatostatin on parathyroid hormone and calcitonin secretion. Endocrinology 102:745–750, 1978.

61. Renaud LP, Martin JB, Brazeau P: Depressant action of TRH, LHRH and somatostatin on activity of central neurons. Nature 255:233–235, 1975.

62. Dodd J, Kelly JS: Is somatostatin an excitatory transmitter in the hippocampus? Nature 273:674–675, 1978.

63. Brown M, Rivier J, Vale W: Somatostatin: Central nervous system actions on glucoregulation. Endocrinology 104:1709–1715, 1979.

64. Terenius L: Somatostatin and ACTH are peptides with partial antagonist-like selectivity for opiate receptors. Eur J Pharmacol 38:211–213, 1976.

65. Rezek M, Havlicek V, Leybin L, et al: Opiate-like naloxone-reversible actions of somatostatin given intracerebrally. Can J Physiol Pharmacol 56:227–231, 1978.

66. Kraicer J, Spence JW: Release of growth hormone from purified somatotrophs: Use of high K^+ and the ionophore A23187 to elucidate interrelations among Ca^{++}, adenosine $3',5'$-monophosphate, and somatostatin. Endocrinology 108:651–657, 1981.

67. Vale W, Brazeau P, Rivier C, et al: Somatostatin. Recent Prog Horm Res 31:365–397, 1975.

68. Veber DF, Holly FW, Nutt RF, et al: Highly active cyclic and bicyclic somatostatin analogues of reduced ring size. Nature 280:512–514, 1979.

69. Veber DF, Freidinger RM, Schwenk-Perlow D, et al: A potent cyclic hexapeptide analogue of somatostatin. Nature 292:55–58, 1981.

70. Mehler PS, Sussman AL, Maman A, et al: Role of insulin secretagogs in the regulation of somatostatin binding by isolated rat islets. J Clin Invest 66:1334–1338, 1980.

71. Reyl F, Silve C, Lewin MJM: Somatostatin receptors on isolated gastric cells. *In* Rosselen G, Fromageot P, Bonfils S (eds): Hormone Receptors in Digestion and Nutrition. Amsterdam, Elsevier, 1979, pp 391–400.

72. Williams JA, Susini CS: Structural characterisation of pancreatic somatostatin receptors. International Conference on Somatostatin, Washington, May 6–8, 1986, Abst 12.

73. Borgeat P, Labrie F, Drouin J, Belanger A: Inhibition of adenosine $3',5'$ monophosphate accumulation in anterior pituitary gland in vitro by growth hormone release inhibiting hormone. Biochem Biophys Res Commun 56:1052–1059, 1974.

74. Efendic S, Grill V, Luft R: Inhibition by somatostatin of glucose induced $3',5'$-monophosphate (cyclic AMP) accumulation and insulin release in isolated pancreatic islets of the rat. FEBS Lett 55:131–133, 1975.

75. Gespach C, Dupont C, Bataille D, Rosseling G: Selective inhibition by somatostatin of cyclic AMP production in rat gastric glands. FEBS Lett 114:247–252, 1980.

76. Curry DL, Bennett LL, Li CH: Direct inhibition of insulin secretion by synthetic somatostatin. Biochem Biophys Res Commun 58:885–889, 1974.

77. Bhathera SJ, Perrino PV, Voyles NR, et al: Reversal of somatostatin inhibition of insulin and glucagon secretion. Diabetes 25:1031–1040, 1976.

78. Pace CS, Tarvin JT: Somatostatin: Mechanism of action in pancreatic islet B cells. Diabetes 30:836–842, 1981.

79. Tan AT, Tsang D, Renaud LP, Martin JB: Effect of somatostatin on calcium transport in guinea pig cortex synaptosomes. Brain Res 123:193–196, 1977.

80. Luft R, Efendic S, Hökfelt T: Somatostatin: Both hormone and neurotransmitter? Diabetologia 14:1–13, 1978.

81. Reichlin S: Somatostatin: Regulation of secretion and synthesis. J Endocrinol 108(Suppl): Abst 2, 1986.

82. Sarantakis D, Teichman J, Fenichel R, Lien E: Des-Ala¹-Gly²-His⁴˒⁵D Trp⁸-somatostatin: A glucagon specific and long acting somatostatin analog. FEBS Lett 92:153–155, 1978.

83. Rivier J, Brazeau P, Vale W, Guillemin R: Somatostatin analogs: Relative importance of the disulphide bridge and of the Ala-Gly side chain for biological activity. J Med Chem 18:123–126, 1975.

84. Vale W, Rivier J, Brown M: Regulatory peptides of the hypothalamus. Annu Rev Physiol 39:473–527, 1977.

85. Brown M, Vale W, Rivier J: Insulin selective somatostatin (SS) analogs. Diabetes 26(Suppl 1):29, 1977.

86. Brown M, Rivier J, Vale W: Somatostatin-28: Selective action on the pancreatic B cell and brain. Endocrinology 108:2391–2393, 1981.

87. Veber DF, Holly FW, Nutt RF, et al: Highly active cyclic and bicyclic somatostatin analogues of reduced ring size. Nature 280:512–514, 1979.

88. Voyles NR, Bhathera SJ, Recant L, et al: Selective inhibition of glucagon and insulin secretion by somatostatin analogs. Proc Soc Exp Biol Med 160:76–79, 1979.

89. Arimura A, Sato H, Coy DH, Schally AV: Radioimmunoassay for GH-release inhibiting hormone. Proc Soc Exp Biol Med 148:784–789, 1975.

90. Brownstein M, Arimura A, Sato H, et al: The regional distribution of somatostatin in the rat brain. Endocrinology 96:1456–1461, 1975.

91. Penman E, Wass JAH, Lund A, et al: Development and validation of the specific radioimmunoassay for somatostatin in human plasma. Ann Clin Biochem 16:15–25, 1979.

92. Hökfelt T, Efendic S, Johansson O, et al: Immunohistochemical localization of somatostatin (growth hormone release-inhibiting factor) in the guinea pig brain. Brain Res 80:165–169, 1974.

93. Alpert C, Brawer JR, Patel YC, Reichlin S: Somatostatinergic neurons in anterior hypothalamus: Immunohistochemical localization. Endocrinology 98:255–258, 1976.

94. Bennett-Clarke C, Romagnano MA, Joseph SA: Distribution of somatostatin in the rat brain: Telencephalon and diencephalon. Brain Res 188:473–486, 1980.

95. Krisch B: Somatostatin-immunoreactive fiber projections into the brain stem and the spinal cord of the rat. Cell Tissue Res 217:531–552, 1981.

96. Emson PC, Rossor M, Lee CM: Original distribution and chromatographic behaviour of somatostatin in human brain. Neurosci Lett 22:319–324, 1981.

97. Leading Article: Brain peptides—new synaptic messages? Lancet 2:895–896, 1980.

98. Berelowitz M, Hudson A, Pimstone B, et al: Subcellular localization of growth hormone release inhibiting hormone in rat hypothalamus, cerebral cortex, striatum and thalamus. J Neurochem 31:751–753, 1978.

99. Delfs J, Robbins R, Connolly JL, et al: Somatostatin production by rat cerebral neurones in dissociated cell cultures. Nature 283:676–677, 1980.

100. Pelletier G, Dube O, Puvaini R: Somatostatin electron microscope immunohistochemical localisation in secretory neurons of rat hypothalamus. Science 196:1469–1470, 1977.

101. Chayvialle JA, Paulin J, Dubois PM, et al: Ontogeny of somatostatin in the human gastrointestinal tract, endocrine pancreas and hypothalamus. Acta Endocrinol 94:1–10, 1980.

102. Wass JAH, Penman E, Medbak S, et al: CSF and plasma somatostatin levels in acromegaly. Clin Endocrinol 13:235–241, 1980.

103. Patel YC, Rao K, Reichlin S: Somatostatin in human cerebrospinal fluid. N Engl J Med 296:529–533, 1977.

104. Hökfelt T, Johansson O, Ljungdahl A, et al: Peptidergic neurons. Nature 284:515–521, 1980.

105. Gilbert RFT, Emson PC, Fahrenkiug J, et al: External transport of neuropeptides in the cervical vagus nerve of the rat. J Neurochem 34:108–113, 1980.

106. Rorstad OP, Brownstein MJ, Martin JB: Immunoreactive and biologically active somatostatin-like material in rat retina. Proc Natl Acad Sci USA 76:3019–3023, 1979.

107. Polak JM, Pearse AGE, Grimelius L, et al: Growth hormone release inhibiting hormone in gastrointestinal and pancreatic D cells. Lancet 1:1220–1222, 1975.

108. Orci L, Baetens D, Dubois MP, Rufener C: Evidence for the D-cell of the pancreas secreting somatostatin. Horm Metab Res 7:400–402, 1975.

109. Larsson LI, Goltermann N, de Magistris L, et al: Somatostatin cell processes as pathways for paracrine secretion. Science 205:1393–1395, 1979.

110. Dubois MP: Immunoreactive somatostatin is present in discrete cells of the endocrine pancreas. Proc Natl Acad Sci USA 72:1340–1343, 1975.

111. Girod C, Dubois MP, Durand N: Immunocytochemical evidence for

the presence of somatostatin-like immunoreactivity in scattered cells of the duct system of the submandibular glands in the monkey, *Macaca irus*. Histochemistry 69:137–143, 1980.

112. Sundler F, Alumets J, Hakanson R, et al: Somatostatin immunoreactive cells in medullary carcinoma of the thyroid. Am J Pathol 88:381–386, 1977.

113. Hökfelt T, Fuxe K, Goldstein M: Applications of immunohistochemistry to studies on monoamine cell systems with special reference to nervous tissues. Ann NY Acad Sci 254:407–432, 1975.

114. Parsons JA, Erlandsen SL, Hegre OD, et al: Central peripheral localization of somatostatin, immunochemical studies. J Histochem Cytochem 24:872–882, 1976.

115. Lundberg JM, Hamberger B, Schultzberg M, et al: Enkephalin and somatostatin-like immunoreactivities in human adrenal medulla and pheochromocytoma. Proc Natl Acad Sci USA 76:4079–4083, 1979.

116. Kumasaka T, Nishi N, Yaoi Y, et al: Demonstration of immunostatin-like substance in villi and decidua in early pregnancy. Am J Obstet Gynecol 134:39–44, 1979.

117. Shields D: In vitro biosynthesis of fish islet pre-somatostatin: Evidence of processing and segregation of a high molecular weight precursor. Proc Natl Acad Sci USA 76:4074, 1980.

118. Goodman RH, Jacobs JW, Dee PC, Habener JF: Somatostatin-28 encoded in a cloned cDNA obtained from a rat medullary thyrocarcinoma. J Biol Chem 257:1156–1159, 1982.

119. Shan LP, Pictet RL, Rutter WJ: Human somatostatin 1: Sequence of the cDNA. Proc Natl Acad Sci USA 79:4575–4579, 1982.

120. Montminy MR, Goodman RH, Horovitch SJ, Habener JF: Primary structure of the gene encoding rat pre-pro-somatostatin. Proc Natl Acad Sci USA 81:3337–3340, 1984.

121. Kronheim S, Berelowitz M, Pimstone BL: A radioimmunoassay for growth hormone release–inhibiting hormone: Method and quantitative tissue distribution. Clin Endocrinol 5:619–630, 1976.

122. Goodman RH, Montminy MR, Lowe MJ, Habener JF: Biosynthesis of rat pre-pro-somatostatin. *In* Patel YC, Tannenbaum GS (eds): Somatostatin. New York, Plenum Publishing, 1985, pp 31–47.

123. Kronheim S, Sheppard MC, Shapiro B, Pimstone BL: Ultra centrifugation evidence for a somatostatin binding protein in serum. Biochim Biophys Acta 586:568–573, 1979.

124. Sheppard M, Shapiro B, Pimstone B, et al: Metabolic clearance and plasma half-disappearance time of exogenous somatostatin in man. J Clin Endocrinol Metab 48:50–53, 1979.

125. Kastin AJ, Arimura A, Gonzalez-Barcena D, et al: Dynamics of injected somatostatin in blood of patients with hepatic failure and acromegaly. Peptides 1:257–259, 1980.

126. Marks N, Stern F: Inactivation of somatostatin (GH-RIH) and its analogs by crude and partially purified rat brain extracts. FEBS Lett 55:220–224, 1975.

127. Griffiths EC, Jeffcoate SL, Holland DT: Inactivation of somatostatin by peptidases in different areas of the rat brain. Acta Endocrinol 85:1–10, 1977.

128. Kronheim S, Berelowitz M, Pimstone BL: The characterization of somatostatin-like immunoreactivity in human serum. Diabetes 27:523–529, 1978.

129. Mark F, Schenkel L, Petrach B, et al: Rapid conversion of somatostatin to active metabolites in human plasma. FEBS Lett 127:22–24, 1981.

130. Schusdziarra V, Rouiller D, Arimura A, Unger RH: Antisomatostatin serum increases levels of hormones from the pituitary and gut, but not from the pancreas. Endocrinology 103:1956–1959, 1978.

131. Steiner RA, Stewart JK, Barber J, et al: Somatostatin: A physiological role in the regulation of growth hormone secretion in the adolescent male baboon. Endocrinology 102:1587–1594, 1978.

132. Arimura A, Smith WD, Schally AV: Blockade of stress-induced decrease in blood GH by anti-somatostatin serum in rats. Endocrinology 98:540–543, 1976.

133. Molitch ME, Hlivyak LE: Growth hormone shortlived feedback: Anatomic specificity of growth hormone stimulation of hypothalamic somatostatin concentration. Horm Metabol Res 12:559–560, 1980.

134. Chihara K: Stimulation by rat growth hormone of somatostatin release into hypophyseal portal blood in the rat. Program of the 61st Meeting of the Endocrine Society, Anaheim, 1979, Abst 290.

135. Gillioz P, Giraud P, Cont-Devolx B, et al: Immunoreactive somatostatin in rat hypophyseal portal blood. Endocrinology 104:1407–1410, 1979.

136. Chihara K, Minamitani N, Kaji H, et al: Intraventricularly injected growth hormone stimulates somatostatin release into rat hypophyseal portal blood. Endocrinology 109:2279–2281, 1981.

137. Berelowitz M, Szabo M, Frohman LA, et al: Somatomedin C mediates

growth hormone negative feedback by effects on both the hypothalamus and the pituitary. Science 212:1279–1281, 1981.

138. Berelowitz M, Pimstone B, Shapiro B, et al: Tissue growth hormone release in inhibiting hormone-like immunoreactivity in experimental hypothyroidism and hypopituitarism. Clin Endocrinol 9:185–191, 1978.

139. Berelowitz M, Maeda K, Harris SL, Frohman LA: Manipulation of growth hormone (GH) and thyrotropin (TSH) homeostasis in vivo provides evidence of a hypophysiotropic role for hypothalamic somatostatin (SRIF). Program of the VIth International Congress of Endocrinology, Melbourne, 1980, Abst 78.

140. Morley JE: Neuroendocrine control of thyrotropin secretion. Endocr Rev 2:396–436, 1981.

141. Varner MA, Davis SL, Reeves JJ: Temporal serum concentrations of growth hormone, thyrotropin, insulin, and glucagon in sheep immunized against somatostatin. Endocrinology 106:1027–1032, 1980.

142. Davies P, Katzman R, Terry RD: Reduced somatostatin-like immunoactivity in cerebral cortex from cases of Alzheimer's disease and Alzheimer senile dementia. Nature 288:279–280, 1980.

143. Rossor MN, Emsen PC, Mountjoy CQ, et al: Reduced amounts of immunoreactive somatostatin in the temporal cortex in senile dementia of Alzheimer type. Neurosci Lett 20:373–377, 1980.

144. Davidson K, Penny E, McLoughlin L, et al: Peptide hormones in primary and secondary tumours of the central nervous system. J Endocrinol 104(Suppl):65, 1985.

145. Hockman HI, Judge DM, Reichlin S: Precocious puberty and hypothalamic hamartoma. Pediatrics 67:236–244, 1981.

146. Sorensen KV, Christensen SE, Dupont E, et al: Low somatostatin content in cerebrospinal fluid in multiple sclerosis. Acta Neurol Scand 61:186–191, 1980.

147. Gerner RH, Yamada T: Altered neuropeptide concentrations in cerebrospinal fluid or psychiatric patients. Brain Res 238:298–302, 1982.

148. Rubinow DR, Gold PW, Post RM, et al: CSF somatostatin in affective illness. Arch Gen Psychiatry 40:409–412, 1983.

149. Unger RH, Orci L: Possible roles of the pancreatic D-cell in the normal and diabetic states. Diabetes 26:241–244, 1977.

150. Barden N, Lavoie M, Dupont A, et al: Stimulation of glucagon release by addition of antisomatostatin serum to islets of Langerhans in vitro. Endocrinology 101:635–638, 1977.

151. Taniguchi H, Utsumi M, Hasegawa M, et al: Physiological role of somatostatin: Insulin release from rat islets treated by somatostatin antiserum. Diabetes 26:700–702, 1977.

152. Schusdziarra V, Zyznar E, Rouiller D, et al: Splanchnic somatostatin: A hormonal regulator of nutrient homeostasis. Science 207:530–532, 1980.

153. Itoh M, Mandarino L, Gerich JE: Antisomatostatin gamma globulin augments secretion of both insulin and glucagon in vitro: Evidence for a physiologic role for endogenous somatostatin in the regulation of pancreatic A- and B-cell function. Diabetes 29:693–696, 1980.

154. Schatz H, Kullek U: Studies on the local (paracrine) actions of glucagon, somatostatin and insulin in isolated islets of rat pancreas. FEBS Lett 122:207–210, 1980.

155. Wass JAH, Penman E, Dryburgh J, et al: Circulating somatostatin after food and glucose in man. Clin Endocrinol 12:569–574, 1980.

156. Webb S, Levy I, Wass JAH, et al: Studies on the mechanisms of somatostatin release after insulin induced hypoglycemia in man. Clin Endocrinol 21:667–675, 1984.

157. Patel YC, Amherd TM, Orchy L: Quantitative electron microscopic autoradiography of insulin, glucagon and somatostatin-binding sites on islets. Science 217:1155–1156, 1982.

158. Wright J, Abolfathi A, Penman E, Marks V: Pancreatic somatostatinoma presenting with hypoglycemia. Clin Endocrinol 12:603–608, 1980.

159. Schusdziarra V: Somatostatin—a regulatory modulator connecting nutrient entry and metabolism. Horm Metab Res 12:563–576, 1980.

160. Uvnäs-Wallensten K, Efendic S, Luft R: Vagal release of somatostatin into the antral lumen of cats. Acta Physiol Scand 99:126–128, 1977.

161. Schusdziarra V, Harris V, Arimura A, Unger RH: Evidence for a role of splanchnic somatostatin in the homeostasis of ingested nutrients. Endocrinology 104:1705–1708, 1979.

162. Penman E, Wass JAH, Medbak S, et al: Response of circulating immunoreactive somatostatin to nutritional stimuli in normal subjects. Gastroenterology 81:692–699, 1981.

163. Lucey MR, Fairclough PD, Wass JAH, et al: Response of circulating somatostatin, insulin, gastrin and GIP, to intraduodenal infusion of nutrients in normal man. Clin Endocrinol 21:209–217, 1984.

164. Schusdziarra V, Rouiller D, Harris V, Unger RH: Release of gastric somatostatin-like immunoreactivity during acidification of the duodenal bulb. Gastroenterology 76:950–953, 1979.

165. Johansson C, Wisen O, Kolberg B, et al: Effects of intragastrically administered somatostatin on basal and pentagastrin stimulated gastric acid secretion in man. Acta Physiol Scand 104:232–234, 1978.

166. Wass JAH: Somatostatin and its physiology in man in health and disease. *In* Besser GM, Martini L (eds): Clinical Neuroendocrinology. New York, Academic Press, 1982, pp 359–395.

167. Skamene A, Patel YC: Infusion of graded concentrations of somatostatin in man: Pharmacokinetics and differential inhibitory effects on pituitary and islet hormones. Clin Endocrinol 20:555–564, 1984.

168. Gerich JE: Somatostatin and diabetes. Am J Med 70:619–626, 1981.

169. Kayasseh L, Gyr K, Keller U, et al: Somatostatin and cimetidine in peptic ulcer—haemorrhage. Lancet 1:844–848, 1980.

170. Jenkins SA, Baxter JN, Corbett W, et al: A prospective randomised controlled clinical trial comparing somatostatin and vasopressin in controlling acute variceal haemorrhage. Br Med J 290:275–278, 1985.

171. Kravetz D, Bosch J, Teres J, et al: Comparison of intravenous somatostatin and vasopressin infusions in treatment of acute variceal haemorrhage. Hepatology 4:442–446, 1984.

172. Usadel KH, Luschner U, Uberla KK: Treatment of acute pancreatitis with somatostatin: A multicenter double blind trial. N Engl J Med 303:999–1000, 1980.

173. Bauer W, Briner U, Dopfner W, et al: SMS 201–995: A very potent selective octapeptide analog of somatostatin with prolonged action. Life Sci 31:1133–1140, 1982.

174. Kvols LK, Moertel CG, O'Connell MJ, et al: Treatment of malignant carcinoid syndrome. Evaluation of a long-acting somatostatin analogue. N Engl J Med 351:663–666, 1986.

175. Krenning EP, Breeman WAP, Kooij PPM, et al: Localisation of endocrine-related tumours with radioiodinated analogue of somatostatin. Lancet 1:242–244, 1989.

176. Ur E, Bomanji J, Mather SJ, et al: Localisation of carcinoid tumours and insulinomas using radiolabelled somatostatin analogues: ^{123}I-TOCT and ^{111}In-DOCT. Clin Endocrinol 38:501–506, 1993.

177. Kraenglin ME, Ch'ng JLL, Wood SM, et al: Long-term treatment of a VIP with somatostatin analogue resulting in remission of symptoms and possible shrinkage of metastases. Gastroenterology 88:185–187, 1985.

178. Plewe G, Beyer J, Krause U, et al: Long acting and a selective suppression of growth hormone secretion by somatostatin analog SMS 201–995 in acromegaly. Lancet 2:782–784, 1984.

179. Lamberts SWJ, Uitterlinden P, Verschoor L, et al: Long term treatment of acromegaly with somatostatin analog SMS 201–995. N Engl J Med 313:1576–1580, 1985.

180. Wass JAH, Lytras N, Besser GM: Somatostatin octapeptide (SMS 201–995) in the medical treatment of acromegaly. Scand J Gastroenterol 21(Suppl 119):136–140, 1986.

181. Reubi JC, Landolt AM: The growth hormone responses to octreotide in acromegaly correlate with adenoma somatostatin receptor status. J Clin Endocrinol Metab 68:844–850, 1989.

182. Guillausseau PJ, Chanson P, Timsit J, et al: Visual improvement with SMS 201–995 in patient with a thyrotropin-secreting pituitary adenoma. N Engl J Med 317:53–54, 1987.

183. Patel YC, Reichlin S: Somatostatin in hypothalamus, extra hypothalamic brain and peripheral tissues of the rat. Endocrinology 102:523–530, 1978.

184. Arimura A, Sato H, Dupont A, et al: Somatostatin: Abundance of immunoreactive hormone in rat stomach and pancreas. Science 189:1007–1009, 1975.

185. Vale W, Ling N, Rivier J, et al: Anatomic and phylogenetic distribution of somatostatin. Metabolism 25(Suppl 1):1491–1494, 1976.

186. McIntosh C, Arnold R, Bothe E, et al: Gastrointestinal somatostatin: Extraction and radioimmunoassay in different species. Gut 19:655–663, 1978.

187. Chayvialle JAP, Descos F, Bernard C, et al: Somatostatin in mucosa of stomach and duodenum in gastroduodenal disease. Gastroenterology 75:13–19, 1978.

188. Krejs GJ, Orci L, Conlon JM, et al: Somatostatinoma syndrome: Biochemical, morphologic and clinical features. N Engl J Med 301:285–292, 1979.

189. Lundqvist G, Gustavsson S, Hällgren R: Plasma levels of somatostatin-like immunoreactivity independent of kidney function. Clin Endocrinol 10:489–492, 1979.

190. Pipeleers D, Somers G, Gepts W, et al: Plasma pancreatic hormone levels in a case of somatostatinoma: Diagnostic and therapeutic implications. J Clin Endocrinol Metab 49:572–579, 1979.

191. Saito H, Ogawa T, Ishmaru K, et al: Plasma somatostatin in normal and diseased states. Program of the VIth International Congress of Endocrinology, Melbourne, 1980, Abst 75.

192. Arimura A, Lundqvist G, Rothman J, et al: Radioimmunoassay of somatostatin. Metabolism 27(Suppl 1):1139–1144, 1978.

193. Gustavsson S, Lundqvist G: Participation of antral somatostatin in the local regulation of gastrin release. Acta Endocrinol 88:329–346, 1978.

194. Schusdziarra V, Dobbs RE, Harris V, Unger RH: Immunoreactive somatostatin levels in plasma of normal and alloxan diabetic dogs. FEBS Lett 81:69–72, 1977.

195. Arimura A, Itoh Z, Aizawa I, Rothman J: Radioimmunoassay for plasma somatostatin and its application in studying somatostatin release from dog stomach. Program of the 60th Meeting of the Endocrine Society, Miami, 1978, Abst 155.

196. Chayvialle JA, Miyata M, Rayford PL, Thompson JC: Effect of food ingestion on vasoactive intestinal peptide and somatostatin plasma levels in control and antrectomised dogs. Scand J Gastroenterol 13(Suppl 49):37, 1978.

197. McCann SM, Krulich L, Negro-Vilar A, et al: Regulation and function of pan-hevin (somatostatin). Adv Biochem Psychopharmacol 22:131–143, 1980.

198. Reichlin S: Somatostatin. *In* Krieger DT, Brownstein N, Martin JB (eds): Brain Peptide. New York, John Wiley & Sons, 1982, pp 712–752.

18

Growth Hormone–Releasing Hormone: Basic Physiology and Clinical Implications

MICHAEL J. CRONIN
MICHAEL O. THORNER

BASIC PHYSIOLOGY

History

Growth hormone–releasing hormone (GHRH), the last of the originally proposed hypophysiotropic factors, was identified structurally in 1982. A generation earlier, Reichlin had proposed the existence of a GHRH because selective hypothalamic lesions yielded a growth hormone deficiency and growth failure.[1, 2] Although many groups attempted to isolate GHRH, success was achieved first via GHRH-producing abdominal tumors rather than from the traditional physiological source of the hypothalamus. In 1973 it was first reported that extracts of various human tumors enhance GH release.[3] Eight cases of presumed ectopic GHRH-secreting tumors were described,[4-13] and a partial purification of GHRH from an extrapituitary tumor was reported in 1980.[14] In October 1980 we studied in Charlottesville a patient with acromegaly and Turner's syndrome whose acromegaly was due to somatotroph hyperplasia rather than a pituitary adenoma,[15] a diagnosis that became evident after acromegaly persisted despite transsphenoidal surgery. Therefore, we sought a source for ectopic GHRH secretion and found a 5-cm tumor in the pancreas. It was from this tumor that two different teams[16-18] isolated a 40-amino acid peptide designated growth hormone–releasing factor GHRH(1-40)OH. Simultaneously, the Guillemin laboratory sequenced three GHRH peptides from a tumor obtained in Lyon, France[19, 20]: GHRH(1-44)-NH$_2$, GHRH(1-40)OH, and GHRH(1-37)OH. The amino acid sequences were identical for all three factors, with the extensions indicating the possibility of processing before release. The biological activity resided in residues 1 to 29, and the sequence demonstrated that this was a member of the glucagon/secretin family of peptides. There were no disulfide bonds and no evidence of glycosylation of this peptide factor. These GHRH's eventually fulfilled the requirements of a hypophysiotropic GHRH. This chapter provides a limited summary of basic and clinical GHRH research.

Molecular and Cellular Biology

SEQUENCE. Using knowledge of the GHRH's isolated from the tumors, the first hypothalamic GHRH was identified in the rat.[21, 22] This peptide contained 43 amino acids with a free acidic group and differed from that in the human by 15 substitutions or deletions. The alterations included a substitution of tyrosine for histidine at position 1, which is more typical of the glucagon/secretin family. The human, porcine, caprine, bovine, and murine hypothalamic GHRH's have also been identified.[23-26] Their sequences and the percentage identities relative to human are listed in Table 18–1. Both GHRH(1-44)NH$_2$ and GHRH(1-40)OH can be found in the human hypothalamus[21, 23, 26, 27] and in the pituitary of acromegalics,[28] as well as in mice transgenic for human GHRH.[29] GHRH can be made synthetically[17, 30] and recombinantly in *E. coli*.[31] Peptidic analogues of increased potency[32, 33] and a GHRH antagonist[34, 35] were developed from the GHRH scaffold.

GENE. Messenger RNA (mRNA) extracted from two different tumors allowed cDNA probes to be constructed and the single-copy GHRH gene to be identified[36, 37] on human chromosome 20. This includes five exons,[18, 38] the third of which encodes the biologically active 1 to 31 sequence. Much like in the human, the rat[39] and mouse[40] GHRH genes span about 10 kilobases of genomic DNA that contain five exons encoding the active hormone and its precursor.

TISSUE DISTRIBUTION. In the human and a number of species GHRH immunoreactivity is present in the basal hypothalamus, appropriate anatomically for release into the pituitary portal vessels.[27, 41-50] GHRH cell bodies directing processes to the median eminence originate from both the perifornical nucleus[47] and the arcuate (rat) or infundibular (human) nucleus.[26, 43-45, 47, 51, 52] GHRH perikarya are also found in the ventromedial nucleus,[41, 46, 47] a region that can induce increased GH release upon electrical stimulation.[13] There is a reciprocal innervation between GHRH and somatostatin neurons in the rat hypothalamus,[53] providing the potential for direct communication between the

TABLE 18–1. GROWTH HORMONE–RELEASING HORMONE SEQUENCES

		PER CENT IDENTITY				
		1	2	3	4	5
1. Human	YADAIFTNSY RKVLGQLSAR KLLQDIMSRQ QGESNQERGA RARL	–				
2. Porcine	YADAIFTNSY RKVLGQLSAR KLLQDIMSRQ QGERNQEQGA RVRL	93	–			
3. Bovine*	YADAIFTNSY RKVLGQLSAR KLLQDIMNRQ QGERNQEQGA KVRL	88	95	–		
4. Ovine	YADAIFTNSY RKILGQLSAR KLLQDIMNRQ QGERNQEQGA KVRL	86	93	97	–	
5. Murine	HVDAIFTTNY RKLLSQLYAR KVIQDIMNKQ QGERIQEQRA RL	60	65	65	65	–
6. Rat	HADAIFTSSY RRILGQLYAR KLLHEIMNRQ QGERNQEQRS RFN	67	72	72	74	65

*Bovine and caprine sequences are identical.

major stimulatory and inhibitory neurons governing GH release. This relationship may participate in the ultradian oscillation of hypothalamic GHRH and somatostatin mRNA's.[54] A number of other brain regions outside of the hypothalamus contain immunoreactive GHRH.[45–47, 49, 55] The ontogeny of GHRH neurons suggests that they appear in the human fetus between 18 and 29 weeks of gestation[43, 44] and in the rat on embryonic day 18, reaching adult levels by postnatal day 30.[56]

Outside the central nervous system, GHRH mRNA and immunoreactivity appears in a number of cell types and tissues in humans and rodents. In general, its function remains to be established outside the GH axis. mRNA for GHRH is found in leukocytes,[57–59] testis,[60, 61] ovary,[62] and placenta.[61, 63–65] Immunoactive or bioactive GHRH content or release is measured in the anterior pituitary,[66] adrenal medulla,[67] leukocytes,[57, 58] placenta,[63, 68, 69] testis,[50, 60] ovary,[62] pancreas,[70, 71] and gastrointestinal tract.[71–73] Initial studies in the somatotroph found immunoreactive GHRH in secretory granules and the nuclei of somatotrophs,[74] whereas more recent data indicate internalization into another intracellular compartment.[75] It remains to be established whether this is a degradative or signaling process. Human tumors can also express,[28] and pituitary adenomas release,[66] immunoreactive GHRH.

GHRH Neuron and Target Cell Activity

RECEPTOR AND DISTRIBUTION. In 1992 three groups achieved the molecular cloning of anterior pituitary receptors for GHRH in human, rat, and mouse.[76–78] The isolated cDNAs encoded a 423-amino acid protein that has seven putative transmembrane domains characteristic of G protein–coupled receptors (Fig. 18–1). The rat and human sequences are 82 per cent identical.[77] The sequences predict ten extracellular cysteines that are conserved in the rat, mouse, and human GHRH receptors (GHRH-R) and also in secretin and VIP receptors. Six of these ten are conserved in all reported members of this receptor family; seven of the ten are in the N-terminal domain. These residues may stabilize an extracellular hormone-binding domain.[77]

Rat cDNA clones revealed a 41-amino acid insert at amino acid 325. However, analysis of rat pituitary mRNA by polymerase chain reaction (PCR) revealed only evidence of the shorter form.[77] In mouse there is evidence of alternate splicing coding for both an extended form and for a receptor devoid in the first transmembrane domain. Interestingly, this latter cDNA codes for a receptor that appears to be biologically active.[78]

The human GHRH receptor is a member of the secretin

GHRH Receptor

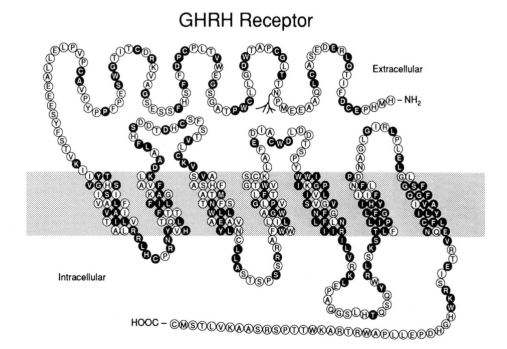

FIGURE 18–1. Cartoon representation of deduced sequence of GHRH receptor. Shaded amino acids are conserved in related receptors. (From Gaylinn BD, Harrison JK, Zysk JR et al: Molecular cloning and expression of a human anterior pituitary receptor for GHRH. Mol Endocrinol 7:77–84, 1993.)

family of G protein–coupled receptors, having 47, 42, 35, and 28 per cent identity with receptors for VIP, secretin, calcitonin, and parathyroid hormone, respectively,[76] and similar homology was found for the rat sequence.[77] Transient expression of this cDNA in COS cells induced saturable, high-affinity GHRH-specific binding and also stimulated the accumulation of intracellular cAMP in response to physiological concentrations of GHRH. A specific GHRH antagonist blocked both binding and second-messenger response. Northern analysis indicated that GHRH-receptor mRNA was most abundant in extracts of pituitary and was not detected in other tissues.[76–78] Two transcripts of approximately 2.5 and 4 kilobases (Kb) were identified in rat pituitary, 2.0 and 2.1 Kb in mouse, and 3.5 Kb in ovine pituitary.[76–78] Further, in mouse it has been shown that the receptor is expressed in a spatial and temporal pattern corresponding to GH gene expression.[78] In the mouse, the first evidence of Pit-1 (a pituitary-specific transcription factor) expression occurred at embryonic day 14.5, while transcripts encoding the cloned receptor first appeared on embryonic day 16.5. The receptor apparently is not expressed in the pituitary of dw/dw mice, which are deficient in functional Pit-1 gene expression. Thus it appears that GHRH-R is dependent on Pit-1, and a deficiency of Pit-1 leads to lack of GHRH-R gene expression and thus of somatotroph development.

These data are consonant with earlier data that demonstrated cross-linking of ^{125}I-GHRH analogue to sheep pituitary membranes, revealing high-affinity binding sites with an apparent molecular weight of 55 kDa. However, after deglycosylation and taking into account the mass of the coupled GHRH analogue, the MW of the native ovine receptor protein was estimated at 42 kDa,[79, 80] in agreement with the prediction from the human cDNA sequence of 45 kDa, assuming cleavage of a signal peptide.[76] The deglycosylation studies, as well as the structure predicted from the cDNA, suggest that the receptor has one N-linked glycosylation site at amino acid 50. Further, the binding characteristics of the natural receptor and the cloned receptor are largely in agreement with a single high-affinity site with a K_d of 0.2 nM.

Various radiolabeled forms of GHRH bind to membranes of the pituitary, thymus, and spleen. The dissociation constants estimated in these studies vary widely from 41 pM[81] to 590 nM.[82] No binding was measurable in three nonfunctional pituitary adenomas, while there was consistent GHRH binding to five acromegalic adenomas, with dissociation constants averaging 0.3 nM.[83]

INTRACELLULAR SIGNALING. Hypothalamic GHRH is released in vitro by interleukin-1 and is inhibited by somatostatin,[84] perhaps by direct innervation by somatostatin neurons.[85] Likewise, cAMP analogues and calcium stimulate GHRH release from cultured hypothalamus, while protein kinase C modulates these effectors.[86] Indirect studies in vivo suggest that alpha$_2$-adrenergic and opioid agonists' stimulation of GH release is also via GHRH.[87]

At the somatotroph, GHRH activates many of the classical signaling systems, including calmodulin, calcium mobilization, cAMP, and phospholipid pathways, indicating a significant commitment of the GH cell to respond to GHRH. As with many secretory cells, GHRH-accelerated GH release requires both calcium[88–92] and calmodulin.[89, 93] Intracellular calcium is elevated within seconds of a GHRH stimulus, both in pituitary cells[94–96] and in thymocytes.[97]

cAMP Metabolism. Native GHRH derived from the Charlottesville tumor is an excellent stimulus for cAMP accumulation and GH release; somatostatin blocks these responses.[98, 99] Once synthetic GHRH became available, the effects of native GHRH were confirmed and extended.[88–90, 92, 98, 100–108] Glucocorticoid pretreatment enhances both the potency and efficacy of GHRH in driving cAMP accumulation and GH release[109]; this steroid is necessary for GHRH-induced cAMP accumulation after several days in culture. Adenylate cyclase activity in membranes of normal rat pituitary or human acromegalic tumors[110] is enhanced by GHRH in a guanine nucleotide-[93, 111] and calmodulin-[93] sensitive manner. Pertussis toxin enhances GHRH-initiated cAMP accumulation and GH release.[98, 101, 105] The spontaneous reduction in GHRH-stimulated cAMP levels that occurs over time can be blocked by cycloheximide,[98] while the stimulatory ability of GHRH is potentiated by protein kinase C activation.[104, 105, 108, 112] This indicates that another receptor system that stimulates C kinase may directly enhance the productivity of the GHRH-R–coupling protein–adenylate cyclase complex[113, 114]; a candidate for this is growth hormone–releasing peptide (GHRP).[112]

Phospholipids. GHRH increases phosphatidylinositol labeling[115] as well as free arachidonate levels[116] in the pituitary, although no effect of GHRH on polyphosphoinositide hydrolysis has been reported.[117] Several metabolic pathways involving phospholipid metabolism may be activated by or may modulate GHRH activity.[95, 103] cAMP metabolism can be dissociated from GH release after GHRH with some phospholipid metabolic enzyme inhibitors, indicating that they can act distal to the cAMP system to evoke exocytosis.[103]

GH mRNA AND RELEASE DYNAMICS IN CULTURE. GHRH stimulates the level or transcription rate of GH mRNA,[118, 119] the release of newly synthesized GH[120] and total GH (stored plus released),[121] as well as the proliferation of somatotrophs in vitro.[122] The GHRH effect on the somatotroph varies according to the anatomical location of the somatotroph within the pituitary,[123] and the GH-releasing effect is further enhanced by glucocorticoids,[30, 109, 124] possibly through increased GHRH binding.[81] Like glucocorticoids, T$_3$[124] and GH-releasing peptide[112] can amplify GHRH-stimulated GH secretion. In contrast, IGF-I[30] and somatostatin[106, 124] are noncompetitive inhibitors of GHRH-accelerated GH release in vitro.

Accelerated GH release occurs immediately after exposure to GHRH[98, 100, 125–128] and remains elevated for the duration of the GHRH pulse,[98, 100, 125, 127, 128] albeit at declining rates of release after about 10 minutes.[12, 100, 121, 125, 128–130] This spontaneous decline could occur without GH content depletion[12] and could be blocked by cycloheximide, suggesting the participation of a rapidly turning-over inhibitory protein.[98] The reciprocal interaction of GHRH and somatostatin, suggested neuroanatomically[53] and in pituitary portal blood measurements,[131, 132] results in a greater mass of GH release per GHRH pulse. This has been demonstrated in perfusion culture.[133]

Picomolar to nanomolar concentrations of GHRH that probably are present in pituitary portal blood[131, 132] regulate a graded GH response from the somatotroph.[17, 20, 21, 30, 99] Reports exist that GHRH stimulates modest prolactin release at low GHRH concentrations in vitro[134, 135] and the secretion of an unidentified pituitary protein.[136] As GHRH can interact with vasoactive intestinal peptide (VIP) receptors (VIP is a prolactin secretagogue) in intestinal epithelium[137] and GH$_3$ cells,[138] it is possible that pharmacological or pathological levels of GHRH can activate this and other receptor types.

Animal Studies

GHRH EFFECTS ON THE GH AXIS. After the first demonstration in vivo of GHRH-enhanced GH release in anesthetized rats,[139, 140] routine responses to GHRH were then achieved by passive immunization against somatostatin[141–143] or rat GHRH.[141, 142] It was apparent soon thereafter that GHRH could enhance GH secretion in every vertebrate tested, from monkey[144] to bovine[145–150] to chicken.[151] In heifers and swine, GHRH(1-44)OH and GHRH(1-29)OH were equipotent.[152]

GHRH is necessary for endogenous pulsatile GH secretion and optimal statural growth in the rat because anti-GHRH antibody treatment eliminated and slowed these processes, respectively.[141, 153] Conversely, GHRH administered over several days to weeks enhances body or organ growth and function in experimental animals.[154–157] This is particularly striking in mice transgenic for GHRH.[158, 159] Pulses of GHRH are measured in pituitary portal plasma of unanesthetized sheep with peak values of 25 to 40 pg/ml, and a period of 71 minutes.[132] Degradation of GHRH in the circulation is primarily through dipeptidylpeptidase IV.[40]

During development, basal GH responses to exogenous GHRH decrease from postnatal days 1 to 28 in the rhesus monkey[160]; passive immunization against GHRH shows that endogenous GHRH is an active secretagogue up to day 9.[161] In the rat GHRH injections do not increase GH levels at postnatal day 2,[162] whereas there are stimulatory responses of similar magnitude measured at postnatal days 10, 30, and 75 as well as at 14 months.[163] Likewise, 5 days of GHRH injections elevate GH biosynthesis in rat pituitaries at postnatal day 10.[164] During suckling and weaning, lambs are equally responsive to GHRH-induced GH release.[165] Interestingly, passive immunization of pregnant rats against GHRH results in larger fetuses, perhaps due to the higher insulin-like growth factor content of fetal tissues.[166]

There are significant changes in GHRH status during aging as well. In the hypothalamus there is a reduction in GHRH gene expression and content[167] as well as a decrease in GHRH binding to pituitary in 18-month-old rats.[168] This may contribute to the diminished pituitary response to GHRH in aged male rats[169–172] and men.[73, 173]

The GHRH system is also strongly gender-dependent. Hypothalamic GHRH mRNA level is greater in male than female rat,[174, 175] is reduced by orchidectomy and increased by testosterone treatment in intact[176] or castrated[177] male rats; estradiol has no effect on hypothalamic GHRH mRNA.[175, 176] The ability of GHRH to elicit a GH response in vivo varies during the rat estrous cycle,[178] is of greater magnitude in the male than female,[163, 179] and is strongly sex steroid–dependent.[179] Somatotrophs from male rats likewise have a greater cAMP and GH response to GHRH than those from female rats when studied in static[102] or perfusion[179] cultures. Furthermore, the intact and castrated male rat treated with testosterone yields the most GHRH

responsive somatotrophs,[179] as does direct testosterone treatment of cultured somatotrophs.[180] Gender differences can be measured at the level of the single somatotroph using the hemolytic plaque assay[181]; testosterone (administered in vivo) increases secretory capacity and recruits a subpopulation of somatotrophs, while estradiol has the opposite effects.[182]

In addition to feedback effects of sex steroids, free fatty acids[183] and GH itself[184] reduce the in vivo release of GH in response to GHRH. GH treatment can either restore immunoreactive GHRH levels in the hypothalamus after hypophysectomy[185] or decrease hypothalamic GHRH content in intact rats.[186] Likewise, T$_4$ replacement can recover hypothalamic immunoreactive GHRH levels reduced by thyroidectomy in rats,[187] and both T$_3$ and cortisol can protect against the reduction in GHRH-stimulated GH release in hypothyroid[188] or adrenalectomized rats,[189, 190] respectively. Indeed, evidence now supports an effect of glucocorticoids at the level of the GHRH neuron in vivo.[191]

Months of excess GHRH exposure in transgenic mice is associated with increased pituitary mass and mammosomatotroph hyperplasia[158, 159] that eventually results in adenoma formation after 12 months.[192, 193] This is reminiscent of the clinical findings in patients with ectopic GHRH secretion. What was surprising was the rapidity of this effect: GHRH infusions were capable of inducing enlargement of the anterior pituitary within days in intact normal rats.[194] The dosage range of this acute effect has yet to be defined, and this observation does not address the potential replacement value of GHRH in deficiency states. In pituitary allograft studies in orchidectomized hamsters, exogenous GHRH maintains somatotroph size without affecting the percentage of GH cells.[195]

GHRH EFFECTS ON FUNCTIONS OUTSIDE THE GH AXIS. GHRH can increase gastrin release,[196] as well as secretion of insulin, glucagon, and somatostatin.[197–199] In the brain, GHRH coexists with tyrosine hydroxylase[85] and can enhance its activity[200] as well as that of choline acetyltransferase,[201] while inhibiting thyrotropin-releasing hormone secretion from the rat hypothalamus.[202] GHRH influences eating behavior,[121, 203–206] and circulating GHRH is increased by feeding in humans.[207] Most of these activities, including the control of GH status, suggest that GHRH acts as a nutrient partitioning hormone in regulating body composition.

CLINICAL IMPLICATIONS

A significant amount of literature has appeared since GHRH became available for clinical use in late 1982. The development of the peptide as a diagnostic and therapeutic agent continues. There is reason to believe that GHRH will prove useful in both diagnosis and therapy. The evidence for this prediction will be presented within the context of three areas of potential clinical application: the measurement of GHRH levels in tissues and body fluids (basally or in response to pharmacological stimuli), the administration of GHRH as a test of pituitary function, and the administration of GHRH to enhance GH secretion and to induce growth.

Measurement of GHRH Levels

INTRODUCTION. Following the synthesis of GHRH, radio-immunoassays (RIA's) to measure the peptide were developed rapidly and are now being utilized to document concentrations of the releasing hormone in tissues and body fluids. Initially it was hoped that GHRH in the peripheral circulation would be principally of hypothalamic origin and its measurement would thus serve as an index of hypothalamic secretion. However, it is clear that most circulating GHRH is not of hypothalamic origin but instead comes from the gut.[208, 209] Further, the RIA would ideally measure intact biologically active hormone. However, GHRH(1-44)NH$_2$ has a very short half-life in the circulation of 6.8 min and the metabolite GHRH(3-44)NH$_2$ appears within one minute of an intravenous injection of GHRH(1-44)NH$_2$.[210] GHRH is cleaved by a dipeptidylaminopeptidase IV in the circulation. The biological activity of GHRH(3-44)NH$_2$ is $<10^{-3}$ that of GHRH(1-44)NH$_2$.[211] Unfortunately most RIA's measure GHRH(1-44)NH$_2$ and GHRH(3-44)NH$_2$ with equal efficiency and therefore do not reflect biological activity in the circulation. Most assays are directed to the midportion of the GHRH molecule and therefore do not distinguish between different circulating forms. Using assays to the N- and C-terminal portions of the molecule and gel filtration and ion exchange chromatography, three forms of GHRH have been identified in pooled normal plasma—the major portion being GHRH(1-40)OH and two minor peaks coinciding with GHRH(1-44)NH$_2$ and GHRH(1-37)OH.[212] With the same assay used, most GHRH in both human hypothalamus and pheochromocytomas was in the form of GHRH(1-44)NH$_2$, with only a minor portion as GHRH(1-40)OH. In two pancreatic islet tumors that secreted ectopic GHRH, the major portion of GHRH was in the form of GHRH(1-40)OH and also contained a small peak of GHRH(1-37)OH; the smallest peak was GHRH(1-44)NH$_2$.

Unstimulated plasma levels of GHRH appear to be within the range of 10 to 70 pg/ml in normal adults,[209, 213, 214] with no apparent difference between the sexes.[213] Similar values (11 to 54 pg/ml) have been reported in the cerebrospinal fluid (CSF) of children and adults of both sexes with no known endocrine disease.[215] Although peripheral levels of GHRH are not elevated in the maternal circulation, they are increased in cord blood, as are levels of growth hormone.[213] Levels of cord blood GHRH were 78.3 ± 8.4 pg/ml at 40 weeks of gestation, while levels of 27 ± 2.6 pg/ml were observed at 38 weeks.[216] There is a marked increase in circulating concentrations of GHRH just before the GH surge observed in the initial slow-wave stage of sleep.[213] Plasma GHRH levels were measured in 180 normal children, 93 boys and 87 girls between ages of 8 and 18.[217] GHRH levels were five times higher at midpuberty in girls (159 ± 28.5 pg/ml) versus prepubertal levels of 30.3 ± 4.3 pg/ml. In midpubertal boys GHRH levels (101.4 ± 11.5 pg/ml) were twice those in prepubertal boys (48.1 ± 5.2 pg/ml). These results suggest that a rise of GHRH levels at puberty may be responsible for the increase in GH secretion at that time. In normal adults, plasma GHRH levels rise two- to three-fold within 40 to 80 minutes after administration of 500 mg L-dopa.[213, 218] Moreover, since GH levels rise 120 minutes after L-dopa, GHRH has been implicated as the mediator of L-dopa–associated GH release.[218, 219] Other factors that increase circulating immunoreactive-GHRH levels in normal subjects include insulin-induced hypoglycemia,[220, 221] late phase after oral glucose load,[221] sauna bath (in young but not old men),[222] and a mixed meal.[208]

In addition to the studies performed in normal subjects, serum or CSF levels of GHRH have now been documented in several clinical disorders.

GHRH Levels in Acromegaly. There has been intense interest in defining the frequency of ectopic GHRH production and establishing it as a cause of acromegaly. Two extensive studies have addressed these issues. In a study of 80 patients with acromegaly, 76 had GHRH levels in the normal range.[209] Of the four with elevated levels, one was known to harbor a GHRH-secreting tumor. Extensive evaluation of the other three failed to determine a source for the GHRH. In a second study, 3 of 177 patients with acromegaly exhibited elevated serum levels of GHRH.[214] In all cases, the GHRH levels were markedly elevated (i.e., in the nanogram per milliliter range), and the patients were previously known to have GHRH-secreting tumors. Thus, although apparently rare, ectopic secretion of GHRH must be considered as a possible cause of acromegaly, and measurement of peripheral GHRH seems prudent as a part of the evaluation. Since it is known that the release of ectopic hormones may be intermittent and since only 300 pg/ml of GHRH is necessary to stimulate GH release in normal subjects, a single normal or modestly elevated GHRH determination may not exclude ectopic GHRH-associated acromegaly.

The subject of GHRH-producing tumors has been extensively reviewed.[223] GHRH-producing tumors associated with acromegaly are rare. In that review 30 tumors were accepted as definitive. Unique features of the patients with acromegaly who harbored tumors secreting GHRH were: young age, female preponderance, foregut derivation and benign biological behavior of the tumors, small secretory granules in the tumors, and frequent association with MEN type 1 syndrome. The pancreas and lung are common primary sites. GHRH-containing tumors unassociated with acromegaly include those of gut and thymus, small cell carcinoma of lung, and medullary carcinoma of thyroid. Several tumors are plurihormonal. In contrast to somatotroph adenoma seen in patients with classical acromegaly, the hypophyseal lesion represents somatotroph hyperplasia in acromegalic patients with GHRH-producing tumor. This finding indicates that GHRH not only increases somatotroph secretory activity but also causes somatotroph proliferation. Studies of GHRH-producing tumors are of fundamental importance to obtain insight into endocrine activity of pituitary somatotrophs and the pathogenesis of GH-secreting pituitary adenomas associated with acromegaly; the importance of GHRH in the etiology of acromegaly is still unresolved. To address whether GHRH can produce tumors, transgenic mice expressing the human GHRH gene have been developed. These animals, exposed to excessive quantities of GHRH throughout development and life, developed mammosomatotroph or somatotroph adenomas.[192, 193] The significance of these observations to the human disease is unclear. The relationship between GHRH-secreting tumors and MEN type 1 syndrome is controversial; further studies are required to elucidate whether they represent two distinct entities or whether GHRH-producing tumors accompanied by acromegaly are only "forme fruste" manifestations of MEN type 1 syndrome. Several cases of acromegaly due to ectopic GHRH secretion associated with MEN type 1 syndrome have been described.[224–227]

In a study to determine whether small cell carcinoma of the lung is associated with elevated circulating IR-GHRH, IR-GHRH was measured in plasma from 28 patients with non–small cell lung cancer, 44 patients with small cell carcinoma of the lung, 10 patients with nonmalignant lung disease, and 37 normal subjects. The mean circulating GHRH levels (pg/ml) were small cell carcinoma of lung, 49.4 ± 9.4; non–small cell carcinoma of lung, 23.9 ± 8.8; nonmalignant disease, 12.7 ± 5.5; and the controls, 16.3 ± 2.1. No patients had clinical acromegaly and GH levels were $<5\ \mu g/L$ in all but five subjects with small cell carcinoma and one subject with non–small cell carcinoma.

Eutopic GHRH Secretion. Occasionally hypothalamic gangliocytomas may be associated with acromegaly. Immunocytochemical staining of such tumors for GHRH has been described. It has been suggested that these tumors should be considered as an unusual cause of acromegaly.[228] On occasion these tumors are intrasellar; in such cases, the observation that somatotrophs are in close anatomical association with neurons suggests that GHRH not only stimulates GH secretion but may also cause adenoma formation. A more recent report described a case of an intrasellar gangliocytoma with somatotroph adenoma. The gangliocytoma was strongly positive for gastrin and weakly positive for GHRH. Since gastrin administered intracerebroventricularly increases GH secretion, it has been suggested that gastrin release may act in a paracrine manner on gangliocytoma to enhance GHRH secretion and thus cause somatotroph adenoma.[229]

GHRH Levels in Growth Hormone–Deficient Children. Many reports concerning serum and CSF concentrations of GHRH in children with various forms of growth deficiency have appeared. Of 22 children with the diagnosis of constitutional short stature (defined as two to three SD below the predicted mean height for age, peak levels of GH in excess of $10\ \mu g/L$ during at least one provocation test, and bone age approximating chronological age), basal GHRH levels (8 to 148 pg/ml) were no different from those noted in normal children.[230] In addition, in five of nine children, GHRH levels rose two-fold 15 minutes after administration of L-dopa (500 mg PO). In another study of 16 children with idiopathic delayed puberty, the peak serum GHRH concentration following L-dopa was 41 ± 10 pg/ml, and this compared with 96 ± 25 pg/ml in children with constitutional short stature.[231] Similarly, in patients with hypothalamic hypopituitarism there was no increase in circulating GHRH levels after L-dopa, which contrasts with responses in normal subjects.[218, 219] These patients with hypothalamic hypopituitarism do respond to exogenous GHRH administration. Insulin-induced hypoglycemia increased circulating GHRH levels in normal subjects but not in six patients with isolated GH-deficiency.[221] In 10 children with short stature, GHRH levels increased at 15 minutes after hypoglycemia from 10 ± 0.5 to 17.1 ± 3.1 pg/ml.[220] There was no increase in GHRH after arginine, even though hypoglycemia alone or arginine alone increased GH concentrations.

However, in contrast to children with constitutional short stature, five children with GH deficiency associated with hypothalamic germinomas were reported to have undetectable amounts of GHRH in the CSF.[215] In addition, children with idiopathic GH deficiency have GHRH present in the CSF but at concentrations lower than those in normal children (15.1 ± 1.0 versus 29.3 ± 2.0 pg/ml; mean + SEM).

Other Disorders. Patients with cirrhosis of the liver and those with renal failure apparently have plasma GHRH levels within the normal range.[213] Patients with Type 1 diabetes mellitus have normal basal GHRH levels but blunted circulating GHRH responses to a mixed meal.[232]

Administration of GHRH as a Diagnostic Procedure

Before the availability of GHRH, testing of GH reserve utilized procedures dependent on effects mediated by the hypothalamus. Thus, the administration of arginine or L-dopa and insulin-induced hypoglycemia are assumed to elicit a hypothalamic signal that, having impinged upon the somatotrophs, resulted in GH release. Obviously, a defect at either the hypothalamic or pituitary level would be expected to produce an abnormal response. The availability of GHRH for clinical testing has now provided the potential to separate hypothalamic from pituitary disease.

Numerous studies have now demonstrated that GHRH selectively stimulates the release of GH in the human. In Tables 18–2, 18–3, and 18–4 are shown serum GH concentrations in healthy men, women, and children after several doses of GHRH(1-40)OH or GHRH(1-44)NH$_2$ and GHRH(1-29)NH$_2$ given intravenously.[73, 233–243] GHRH stimulates the release of GH within 5 minutes, and peak levels are achieved between 30 and 60 minutes. Except for a slight decrease in blood pressure noted by one group,[235] vital signs are said to be unaffected by GHRH. Dose-response relationships between GHRH and GH release have been documented in young adult men and women.[236, 237] The dose of GHRH(1-44)NH$_2$ required for half-maximal GH secretion is $0.4\ \mu g/kg$ in men and $0.2\ \mu g/kg$ in women. However, maximal GHRH-stimulated GH release does not appear to differ between young men and women or during several phases of the menstrual cycle[237, 240] (Tables 18–2 and 18–3).

Although the number of reports of GHRH-stimulated GH release in normal children is small, the number of subjects studied is relatively large. As shown in Table 18–4, the effect of GHRH on GH release has been defined both in normal children with short stature[241] and in boys and girls at several developmental stages.[242] In the latter study, 45 girls and 40 boys were investigated. The stage of puberty for each child was determined by evaluation of breast development or testicular size. No difference in GHRH-stimulated GH secretion was found for girls among the pubertal stages or in comparison with normal adult women. In boys, a slight decrease in responsivity was seen at midpuberty, but overall no differences were found between girls and boys. There is one report of greater GH response in tall pubertal girls compared with boys.[243] Therefore, GH responses to GHRH appear consistent between children and young adults. It is also of interest that estrogen priming of the GH response is observed in response to hypoglycemia but not to GHRH. This suggests that estrogen does not affect the pituitary response to GHRH[244, 245] and may

TABLE 18–2. GH RESPONSES IN NORMAL MEN TO BOLUS IV INJECTIONS OF GHRH

	GHRH	DOSE (μg/kg)	NORMAL MEN (No.)	MEAN PEAK (μg/L ± SEM)
Thorner et al[233]	1–40	1.0	6	20.4 ± 6.5
Wood et al[234]	1–44	10 μg dose	8	7.8 ± 3.0
		30 μg dose		11.9 ± 2.8
		100 μg dose		15.9 ± 2.1
Rosenthal et al[235]	1–44	0.5	5	26.6 ± 10.6*
		5.0	6	24.3 ± 4.5*
		10.0	5	26.6 ± 6.0*
Shibasaki et al[73]	1–44	100 μg dose	8 (20's)	29.6 ± 7.2
			7 (30's)	30.2 ± 10.0
			5 (40's)	9.7 ± 2.3
			5 (50's)	10.9 ± 2.4
			5 (60's)	8.4 ± 2.2
			7 (70's)	8.1 ± 2.8
Vance et al[236]	1–40	0.1	6	11.4 ± 2.8*
		0.3	6	14.6 ± 1.7*
		1.0	6	17.0 ± 3.0*
		3.3	6	14.5 ± 8.4*
		10.0	5	15.6 ± 6.2*
Gelato et al[237]	1–44	0.01	6	4†
		0.1	7	11†
		1.0	8	34†
		10.0	6	36†
				MEAN (RANGE)
Sassolas et al[238]	1–44	0 μg dose	10	1.5 (0.5–7.2)
		75 μg dose	10	21.4 (10.3–29.0)
		150 μg dose	10	27.8 (7.7–54.9)
		300 μg dose	10	20.8 (5.4–36.3)
		600 μg dose	10	23.0 (10.7–48.7)
Lang et al[239]	1–44	1.0	29 (18–30 yr)	8.7 ± 5.711*
			10 (31–60 yr)	5.7 ± 3.9*
			7 (51–70 yr)	4.9 ± 2.5*
			13 (71–95 yr)	2.7 ± 1.9*

*Increment in GH. †Estimated from Figure 2, Gelato et al.[237]

enhance endogenous hypothalamic GHRH secretion or inhibit somatostatin secretion.

The question of an effect of the aging process on GHRH-stimulated GH release is less clear. Indeed, this issue has been addressed by several groups with conflicting results. GH secretion in response to GHRH has been reported to be markedly diminished in older versus younger men[73] and to be unaltered by aging.[173] However, a word of caution should be introduced with regard to the interpretation of these and similar studies. In a study of 116 normal women

TABLE 18–3. GH RESPONSES IN NORMAL WOMEN TO BOLUS IV INJECTIONS OF GHRH

	GHRH	DOSE (μg/kg)	NORMAL WOMEN No.	NORMAL WOMEN Phase of Cycle	MEAN PEAK (μg/L ± SEM)
Gelato et al[237]	1–44	0.01	6	Midfollicular	4*†
		0.1	6	Midfollicular	16*†
		1.0	5	Midfollicular	36*†
		10.0	5	Midfollicular	33*†
		1.0	8	Midluteal	42.5 ± 6.0
Evans et al[240]	1–40	3.3	10	Early follicular	34.9 ± 8.3
		3.3	10	Late follicular	25.2 ± 6.8
		3.3	10	Luteal	32.7 ± 12.8
Lang et al[239]	1–44	1.0	21	(18–30 yr)‡	13.3 ± 9.4*
			10	(31–50 yr)‡	14.6 ± 12.7*
			7	(51–70 yr)	5.5 ± 5.0*
			19	(71–95 yr)	1.8 ± 2.0*

*Increment in GH. †Estimated from Figure 2, Gelato.[237] ‡19 studied at follicular phase and 12 at luteal phase, Lang et al.[239]

and men, a greater GH increase in response to GHRH was observed in premenopausal women compared with age-matched men, and an age-dependent decrease in GHRH-stimulated GH secretion was observed in both men and women.[239]

There is general agreement that the variability among individuals to GHRH-stimulated GH release is remarkable. Such variability makes it difficult or impossible to detect subtle differences in responsivity among various groups and may limit the usefulness of GHRH as a diagnostic tool. Indeed, all physicians considering the use of GHRH within clinical settings need to be fully aware of these concerns and require that properly obtained data on normal reference groups (e.g., with regard to age, sexual development, nutritional status, body weight, GH assay used) be available for comparison of results in patients under investigation. In contrast to the large variability between subjects, repeated studies separated by at least one week of normal men demonstrated relatively small within-subject variability when challenged with 100 or 200 μg GHRH(1-44)NH₂.[246]

The potential use of GHRH analogues as diagnostic agents is beginning to receive attention. On the basis of the observation that amidated GHRH(1-29)NH₂ is biologically active in vitro, this agent has now been tested in humans.[247] When given intravenously as a 200-μg bolus to normal subjects, GHRH(1-29)NH₂ stimulated GH release to the same degree as an equivalent dose of GHRH(1-40)OH. Similarly, Nleu²⁷GHRH(1-29)NH₂ stimulated GH secretion in normal men.[248] Many GHRH analogues have

TABLE 18–4. GH RESPONSES IN NORMAL CHILDREN TO BOLUS IV INJECTIONS OF GHRH

	GHRH	DOSE (μg/kg)	NO.		MEAN PEAK (μg/L ± SEM)
Chihara et al[241]	1–44	1.0	13	8.2–14.6 yr	18.5 ± 2.5
				TANNER STAGE	**MEAN CHANGE (μg/L ± SEM)**
Gelato et al[242]	1–44	1.0	45 girls	I	30 ± 7
				II	29 ± 10
				III	23 ± 5
				IV	27 ± 7
				V	26 ± 8
				TESTICULAR SIZE (cc)	
	1–44	1.0	40 boys	< 5	32 ± 5
				5–12	30 ± 17
				13–20	18 ± 4
				> 20	33 ± 8
					MEAN PEAK (μg/L ± SEM)
Smals et al[243]	1–44	100 μg dose	10 tall adolescent girls		34 ± 4
			8 tall adolescent boys		19 ± 3

been synthesized and some have been tested in humans. The major problem is that these compounds are rapidly degraded, and even though analogues have been designed to be resistant to metabolism, none with clinically significant prolonged GH stimulatory activity in humans has been described.[249, 250] Further, the problem of lower subcutaneous bioavailability when compared with the intravenous route has not been overcome in humans. Because these shortened peptides with simpler structures are less expensive to synthesize, the use of such GHRH analogues will almost certainly become an attractive alternative to the utilization of native peptide.

Hypopituitarism. Both adults and children with hypopituitarism have been challenged with GHRH. Table 18–5 lists several studies in hypopituitary adult men.[234, 247, 251–254] Of eight men with various hypothalamic-pituitary disorders tested with both GHRH(1-44)NH₂ and insulin-induced hypoglycemia, GH release (which was similar after both testing methods) was impaired when compared with results in normal men.[234] In patients who had previously undergone

TABLE 18–5. GH RESPONSES IN HYPOPITUITARY PATIENTS TO BOLUS IV INJECTIONS OF GHRH

	GHRH	DOSE	NO.	RESULTS
Wood et al[234]	1–44	100 μg	8	All impaired responses; comparable to responses to insulin-induced hypoglycemia
Grossman et al[247]	1–40	200 μg	6	5 had no response to hypoglycemia; greater response to GHRH (1–40) and GHRH (1–29); all 6 responded
	1–29	200 μg		
Borges et al[251]	1–40	10 μg/kg	12	All impaired; 8 had no response; 4 had increase of GH by ≥1.5 μg/L
Hashimoto et al[252]		1.0 μg/kg	16 nonfunctioning pituitary tumors • 9 chromophobe adenoma • 3 craniopharyngioma • 2 Rathke's cleft cyst • 1 intrasellar cyst • 1 tuberculum sella meningioma	>70% had impaired response before and after surgery
				MEAN PEAK GH (μg/L ± SEM)
Gelato et al[253]	1–44	1 μg/kg	9 Hand-Schüller-Christian disease	9 of 9 responded 6.4 ± 2.1
			9 IGHD	5 of 9 responded 1.3 ± 0.2
			8 normal young	35 ± 8
			Comment: with priming (1 μg/kg) qd for 5 days responses increased: HSCD	5.1 ± 2.5 to 12 ± 6.8
			IGHD	1.4 ± 0.2 to 2.9 ± 0.6
Crosnier et al[254]	1–44	2 μg/kg	19 prepubertal children—cranial irradiation (24 Gy) for ALL or LS	Impaired in 16/19 16.7 ± 2.5
			14 prepubertal children—constitutional short stature	52.6 ± 8.5

ALL, Acute lymphoblastic leukemia; LS, lymphosarcoma.

external pituitary irradiation for prolactinomas,[247] the responses to GHRH(1-40)OH or GHRH(1-29)NH$_2$ and to insulin-induced hypoglycemia were dissociated: the GH response to hypoglycemia was clearly diminished and the response to GHRH was substantially higher. These results suggest that GH deficiency seen after cranial irradiation is more likely due to hypothalamic damage (with the subsequent failure to secrete GHRH) rather than to a pituitary defect. When 12 adult males who had presented in childhood with short stature were tested with 10 μg/kg GHRH(1-40)OH, GH release was, in contrast to that in normal men, diminished in 66 per cent.[251] In addition, the mean GHRH-stimulated GH level of those who did respond was less than that of normal men. In follow-up to this study, adult patients who had presented in childhood with idiopathic GH deficiency were given 10 μg/kg GHRH(1-40)OH before and after five days of treatment with 0.33 μg/kg GHRH(1-40)OH administered IV every three hours.[255] In response to the initial GHRH bolus, the mean maximal GH level achieved was the same as the response to a control injection of diluent for GHRH. After five days of treatment, the mean maximal GH level reached in response to GHRH was higher than in response to the control substance. These results suggest that potentially functional somatotrophs are present in the pituitaries of at least some patients with idiopathic GH hormone deficiency but that such cells may require priming (perhaps in a manner analogous to that for gonadotrophs in patients with Kallmann's syndrome) by the appropriate hypothalamic factor prior to demonstrating normal responsivity. These results are encouraging within the context of the potential of GHRH as a therapeutic agent in GH deficiency.

Children with Short Stature. A number of studies have focused on GHRH-stimulated GH release in children with short stature[244, 256-267] (Table 18–6). To date, the results have generally been consistent: Children who have short stature but no GH deficiency by conventional criteria respond to GHRH in a manner similar to that seen in young adults. However, in children with GH deficiency documented by conventional means, GHRH-stimulated GH release is variable. Of 27 GH-deficient children, 16 failed to respond to GHRH(1-44)NH$_2$ with a rise in GH of greater than 5μg/L.[256] When children with short stature were divided into GH-sufficient, deficient, and partially deficient groups and challenged with GHRH(1-44)NH$_2$, the GH-sufficient group released an amount of GH similar to that of normal young adults.[257] Of the 20 subjects in the deficient group, 17 exhibited a rise in GH of at least 1 μg/L, with peak levels at least twice those of baseline. Children with partial GH deficiency demonstrated GHRH-stimulated GH release to levels intermediate between the intact and deficient groups.

The effect of GHRH(1-40)OH in children with short stature of several etiologies, including constitutional delay, intrauterine growth retardation, organic hypopituitarism, and idiopathic GH deficiency, has been reported.[258] In addition to being listed in Table 18–6, the results of this study are shown diagrammatically in Figure 18–2. In each group,

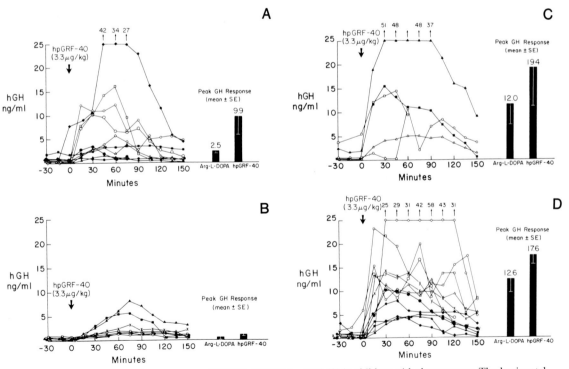

FIGURE 18–2. GH release in response to GHRH(1-40)OH (hpGRF-40) in children with short stature. The horizontal axis is time (min) before and after the IV injection of GHRH, 3.3 μg/kg as a bolus dose. The vertical axis is GH concentration (ng/ml or μg/L). Each set of symbols represents an individual patient. *A,* Idiopathic GH deficiency (IGHD); *B,* Organic hypopituitarism; *C,* Intrauterine growth retardation (IUGR); *D,* Constitutional delay (CD) and/or familial short stature. Bars at the lower right of each panel are the mean ±SE of the peak responses to the arginine/L-dopa and to human pancreatic tumor growth hormone–releasing hormone 40 in children with short stature. (From Rogol AD, Blizzard RM, Johanson AJ, et al: Growth hormone release in response to human pancreatic tumor GHRH-40 in children with short stature. J Clin Endocrinol Metab 59:580–586, © by the Endocrine Society, 1984.)

TABLE 18–6. GH RESPONSES IN CHILDREN WITH SHORT STATURE TO BOLUS IV INJECTIONS OF GHRH

	GHRH	DOSE	NO.	RESULTS
Takano et al[256]	1–44	1–2 μg/kg	28 normal GH (by conventional criteria)	All equivalent responses to adult responses
			27 GHD	16/27 no response; 11 were >5 μg/L
				MEAN PEAK GH (μg/L ± SEM)
Schriock et al[257]	1–44	5 μg/kg	20 GHD	17 responded (5.1 ± 1.2)
			6 partial GHD	6 responded (13.1 ± 1.8)
			GH sufficient	6 responded (27.2 ± 3.5)
Rogol et al[258]	1–40	3.3 μg/kg	10 idiopathic GHD	9.9 ± 3.9
			7 organic hypopituitarism	3.4 ± 1.0
			5 intrauterine growth retardation	19.4 ± 8.1
			18 constitutional delay of growth or familial short stature	17.6 ± 1.9
				RANGE (μg/L) (NO. RESPONDED)
Laron et al[259]	1–44	1 μg/kg	7 idiopathic GHD	0.5–22 [4/7]
			1 MPHD	2.2 [1/1]
			3 constitutional short stature	18–100 [3/3]
				MEAN PEAK GH (μg/L ± SEM)
Pintor et al[260]	1–40	1 μg/kg	4 normal prepubertal males	41.7 ± 3
			6 constitutional growth delay, males	13.1 ± 2
				PEAK GH (μg/L)
Lannering et al[261]	1–40	2 μg/kg	19 treated with CNS radiation for tumors of eye, brain, epipharynx	3 nonresponders (<7, range 2.5–5)
				13 of 16 responded (>7, range 10–43)
			Comment: response to GHRH inversely correlated with time elapsed since radiotherapy.	
Cappa et al[262]	1–40	1 μg/kg	20 normal short	~35 ± 5
			12 prepubertal girls	34.2 ± 5.6
			12 Turner's syndrome	7/12 were >10
				5/12 were <10
			• 7 with 45 X,O	5/7 poor response
			• 5 mosaicism and/or 46 X,iX	All normal response
Bozzola et al[263]	1–44	2 μg/kg	17 GHD	8/17 responded (>10)
			6 partial GHD	4/6 responded (>10)
			7 prepubertal short normal	6/7 responded (>10)
Reiter et al[264]		0.5 μg/kg	Constitutional short stature	39.2 ± 5.1
			17 Turner's syndrome	17 ± 3.6
Ranke et al[265]	1–29	1 μg/kg	131 children	
			• 38 controls	45.3
			• 18 constitutional delay	28.0
			• 10 IUGR	67.2
			• 8 dysmorphic short stature	85.9
			• 8 Turner's syndrome	25.8
			• 45 IGHD/19 IGHD/26 MPHD	5.1
Chatelain et al[244]	1–44	2 μg/kg	394 prepubertal	
			• 210 constitutional short stature (>10 μg/L)	22.9 ± 2.4
			• 73 partial GHD (>5–<10 μg/L)	14.6 ± 3.2
			• 111 severe GHD (<5 μg/L)	8.4 ± 1.6
Takano et al[267]	1–44	1 μg/kg if <18 yr 100 μg if ≥18 yr	141 short normal	39.5 ± 2.2
			• 73 IGHD (severe)	7.2 ± 0.9
			• 30 mild IGHD	27.2 ± 3.7
			• 29 secondary GHD	5.2 ± 0.8
			• 3 primary hypothyroidism	9.7 ± 4.4
			• 21 Turner's syndrome	25.1 ± 2.8
			• 25 other diseases	323 ± 4.8
				AUC (μg/L/h)
Sartorio et al[266]	1–44	1 μg/kg	17 prepubertal (Tanner II–III)	
			• 9 short normal (below 5th percentile but GV ≥ 5 cm/yr)	788 ± 244
			• 8 normal (GV > 10th percentile)	984 ± 242

MPHD, Multiple pituitary hormone deficiencies; IUGR, intrauterine growth retardation.

the GH response to GHRH exceeded that seen after administration of arginine and L-dopa. Children with organic hypopituitarism, all of whom had hypothalamic tumors previously treated by surgery and/or irradiation, responded least well to GHRH. Those with constitutional delay or intrauterine growth retardation responded best, with GH levels overlapping those seen in young adults. Children with idiopathic GH deficiency had quite variable degrees of GHRH-stimulated GH release, ranging from essentially no response to responses considered normal for young adults. In another study, four of seven children with isolated GH deficiency, one with multiple anterior pituitary deficiencies, and three with constitutional short stature, responded to GHRH(1-44)NH2.[259] In each case the response to the releasing hormone was greater than that to insulin-induced hypoglycemia.

In addition, an investigation examining children with constitutional delay as the cause of short stature compared GHRH-stimulated GH release in six such prepubertal males with that seen in four normal prepubertal males.[260] Compared with normal children, those with constitutional growth delay demonstrated only a slight increase in GH within 15 minutes after administration of GHRH but achieved higher levels 40 to 120 minutes after injection.

Two studies have addressed the GH response to GHRH in children who received cranial radiation for CNS tumors. Both studies demonstrated that GH secretion was impaired in the majority of such children, either when studied over a 24-hour period or in response to conventional pharmacological stimuli. The longer the duration after the radiation therapy, the higher the percentage of children with GH deficiency.[254, 261] In both studies the GH response to GHRH for the group of children was impaired, but because the characteristics of the 24-hour GH profile did not correlate with the response to GHRH, the authors of one paper argued that GHRH should not be used as a test of GH reserve.[261]

Children with Turner's syndrome have short stature of unknown etiology. Five of seven such patients had impaired responses to GHRH (range of peak GH, $\mu g/L$) of 5 to 18 in 45 XO Turner girls, 16 to 29 in mosaic Turner girls, and 17 to 53 in control girls.[262] These data suggest that one of many factors giving rise to short stature in girls with Turner's syndrome may be reduced GH response to GHRH, which may reflect hypothalamic GHRH deficiency, since all children respond to GHRH. In another study the GH response to GHRH was also found to be impaired in girls with Turner's syndrome, but these authors considered that this was due, at least in part, to the increase in adipose tissue in girls with Turner's syndrome compared with the controls, in addition to their higher IGF-I concentrations.[245]

In a further study, 17 GH-deficient children (GH peak after two conventional tests and sleep $<5 \mu g/L$), six partially GH-deficient children (peak 5 to 10 $\mu g/L$), and seven prepubertal short normal children (peak $>10 \mu g/L$) were tested with GHRH.[263] In the control subjects the response to GHRH ranged from 10 to 100 $\mu g/L$. Thus, these authors defined a "normal" response as $>10 \mu g/L$. Eight of 17 GH-deficient children had responses $>10 \mu g/L$, as did four of six partially GH-deficient children and six of seven normal short children. These authors concluded that the test was useful in identifying those patients with normal GHRH responses who had impaired responses to pharmacological tests or sleep. They suggested that these patients have a hypothalamic defect. In another large study 131 children were evaluated.[265] The normal range (defined as mean $\pm$ 2SD) was from 11.8 to 172.4 $\mu g/L$. Thus 10 $\mu g/L$ was defined as a normal response. GH deficiency previously had been defined as a peak response to arginine or insulin of $<7 \mu g/L$, and partial GHD as 7 to 10 $\mu g/L$. Of 86 children without GH deficiency, only three did not reach 10 $\mu g/L$ in response to GHRH. Two were obese and one had Turner's syndrome and thus presumably had increased adiposity. Of the 45 GH-deficient children, 34 had peak responses to GHRH below 10 $\mu g/L$ (i.e., 75 per cent of the patients). Although there was no significant relationship between the maximal GH response to GHRH and those to insulin and arginine, there was a weak relationship between the maximal GH response to GHRH and during deep sleep (r = 0.35, P $<$ 0.05). These authors concluded that in children with obesity the test may be subnormal in the absence of GH deficiency. However, in a normal-weight child suspected of having GH deficiency, a GHRH test should be performed. Although 25 per cent of such children may have a response greater than 10 $\mu g/L$, a response below 10 $\mu g/L$ establishes GH deficiency, particularly when taken together with the serum IGF-I level.

The largest study published to date tested 574 prepubertal children suspected of having disorders of growth.[244] Of these, 394 were evaluable; of the 179 who were excluded, 81 were above pubertal stage 1, 17 did not have growth failure, 59 did not have valid reference data, seven had inappropriate chronological age, nine had insufficient endocrine data, and six were excluded for miscellaneous reasons. On the basis of conventional tests, the 394 children were subdivided into three groups: (1) constitutional short stature (GH peak $>10 \mu g/L$, n = 210), (2) partial GH deficiency (GH peak >5 to $<10 \mu g/L$, n = 73), and (3) severe GH deficiency (peak GH $<5 \mu g/L$, n = 111). In those children being treated with GH, it was discontinued at least 15 days before the GHRH test. The mean peak GH responses to GHRH in the three groups were 22.0 $\pm$ 2.4, 14.6 $\pm$ 3.2, and 8.4 $\pm$ 1.6 $\mu g/L$, respectively. Thus, there was a graded reduction in the response depending on the degree of GH deficiency. There was overlap between the groups. However, if a peak of at least 10 $\mu g/L$ is taken as normal, then 90 per cent of the constitutionally short children had a normal response while 61 per cent of the severely GH deficient and 24 per cent of the partially GH-deficient children had a subnormal response. These authors concluded that most children with severe GH deficiency had a subnormal response to GHRH, while only 10 per cent of the constitutional short stature children had a subnormal response. However, they remark that this degree of false-positive result is comparable with other tests of GH reserve. Further, from the published data it is not possible to determine whether this 10 per cent sample of the constitutional short stature children with "subnormal" responses contained children with obesity, since obesity is known to blunt the GH response to GHRH.

GHRH tests in 322 short Japanese children and young adults were reported. The subjects consisted of 141 normal short children, 73 with severe GH deficiency (peak GH to standard pharmacological tests $<5 \mu g/L$), 30 with partial GH deficiency (GH peak >5 to $<7 \mu g/L$), 29 patients with secondary GH deficiency (due to structural hypothalamic lesions and peak GH $<8 \mu g/L$), 3 with primary hypothyroidism, 21 with Turner's syndrome, and 25 with other diseases.[267] Mean responses are shown in Table 18–6 and follow a similar pattern as that observed in the other studies just described.

In this and other studies in GH-deficient subjects, but not in normal subjects, there was a significant negative correlation between peak GH response to GHRH and chronological age or bone age.[244, 257, 265] In this study several values were taken to see which peak GH level would be a good discriminator for GH deficiency. If a peak GH in response to GHRH of $>15 \mu g/L$ was taken as normal, 87.9 per cent of normal short children had a "normal" response, while only 9.6 per cent of severely GH deficient subjects and 63.2 per cent of partially GH deficient subjects had "normal" responses. If $>10 \mu g/L$ were taken as the cut-off, 95 per cent, 21.9 per cent and 80 per cent had normal responses, respectively. Similarly, 13.8 per cent of secondarily GH deficient subjects had normal responses. Thus the GHRH test may be useful as a screening test, with the caveat that as with other tests of GH reserve there are false-positive and -negative results.

In order to determine whether there is a more subtle abnormality in the regulation of GH secretion in children with constitutional growth delay, two consecutive bolus injections of GHRH were administered intravenously 120 minutes apart in normal children and children with constitutional delay.[266] In contrast to the response in adults, in whom there is refractoriness to the second dose of GHRH, in both normal children and children with constitutional growth delay there was only attenuation in the response to the second dose. However, in response to the first or second dose of GHRH, there was no difference between normal and constitutional delay groups. Considered as a group, these studies imply that GH deficiency rarely results from an absence of functional somatotrophs but rather derives from hypothalamic disease. Moreover, an absent or diminished response to GHRH does not necessarily imply pituitary disease, as somatotrophs that have presumably remained dormant in the absence of hypothalamic stimulation may require priming in order to demonstrate normal responsivity. Using a strict criterion for the GHRH test of a peak GH of <10 μg/L in nonobese short children, there can be a degree of certainty that the child is GH deficient. If the response is >10 μg/L, the child may still suffer from GH deficiency.

Acromegaly. GHRH receptors in pituitary adenoma cell membranes from five patients with acromegaly were characterized using ^{125}I [His^1,Nleu^{27}]GHRH(1-29)NH$_2$ as ligand.[83] The specific binding of ^{125}I [His^1,Nleu^{27}]GHRH(1-29)NH$_2$ to the membranes was saturable; Scatchard analysis of the data revealed an apparent single class of high-affinity GHRH receptors; the mean dissociation constant was 0.3 $\pm$ 0.07 nmol/L and the mean maximal binding capacity was 26.7 $\pm$ 7.0 fmol/mg protein. In three nonfunctioning pituitary adenomas, GHRH receptors were not detected. There was no correlation between the in vivo plasma GH response to 100 μg GHRH intravenous bolus in four of the acromegalic patients and the characteristics of the tumor GHRH receptors.

Several studies have been performed in which patients with acromegaly have been tested with GHRH[234, 268–271] (Table 18–7). Of 29 patients with acromegaly, all responded to GHRH(1-40)OH with the exception of four patients who had previously received external pituitary irradiation.[269]

There was significant variability in responsiveness, a finding also noted by others.[268] This investigation did not, however, confirm the findings of a study in which a relationship was described between suppression of GH levels (by $\sim$ 20 per cent) with oral glucose and the response to GHRH(1-44)NH$_2$.[234] Of interest are observations that acromegalic patients who respond to bromocriptine have poorer responses to GHRH than do patients who are bromocriptine-unresponsive.[270] Similarly, no relationship between GHRH- and TRH-stimulated GH release has been documented.

Whether GHRH will prove useful in defining the pathophysiological mechanism(s) responsible for acromegaly remains to be determined. In three preliminary reports, GHRH failed to stimulate GH release in patients with the ectopic GHRH syndrome.[272–274] That pituitary tumors do respond with GH secretion to natural or synthetic GHRH has been documented both in vivo (GHRH-stimulated GH release diminishes after transsphenoidal resection of pituitary tumors[269]) and in vitro.[110, 275–278]

Experimental and Other Pathophysiological Settings.

Glucocorticoids. In rats glucocorticoids potentiate GHRH action and enhance spontaneous GH secretion. In normal humans there is a biphasic effect of pharmacological doses of glucocorticoids. When normal men were treated with a single intravenous bolus of 4 mg dexamethasone and 3 hours later were challenged with a bolus injection of GHRH, the peak GH response to GHRH increased from 9.9 $\pm$ 2 μg/L to 29.2 $\pm$ 5.7 μg/L. When the dexamethasone dose was increased to 8 mg intravenously 12 hours before GHRH bolus, the peak GH response to GHRH was attenuated to 3 $\pm$ 1.1 μg/L. These results suggest an acute stimulatory response followed by a later inhibitory effect.[279] The effect of dexamethasone on GH response to GHRH has been studied in acromegaly.[280] Six acromegalic patients were studied before and after two days of dexamethasone (9 mg/day). Blood glucose was increased and insulin-like growth factor-I (IGF-I) was decreased by dexamethasone. GH response to GHRH was decreased by dexamethasone. In contrast, culture of adenomas from three of these patients demonstrated that 50 nM dexamethasone for two days augmented GH release basally and in response to GHRH (100 pM to 1 nM). These results indicate that the potentiating action of two days of treatment with dexamethasone in vitro is overcome in vivo by some extrapituitary action, probably in the CNS. This is considered to be mediated by enhanced somatostatin secretion because the

TABLE 18–7. GH RESPONSES IN ACROMEGALIC PATIENTS TO BOLUS IV INJECTIONS OF GHRH

	GHRH	DOSE		NO.	RESULTS
Wood et al[234]	1–44	100 μg	6	2 untreated	3 normal increment
				4 untreated (^{99}Y or external) irradiation	3 "exaggerated"
Shibasaki et al[268]	1–44	100 μg	10	5 untreated	3 exaggerated (4-fold increase)
				5 treated by surgery but not cured	5 "normal" (2-fold increase)
Gelato et al[269]	1–40	1.3 μg/kg	29	8 untreated	2 with $<$2-fold increase
				21 previously treated	25/29 increase
					4 no response (all previously irradiated)
Chiodini et al[270]	1–44	100 μg	35		22/35 $>$100% increase from basal
					MEAN PEAK GH (μg/L$\pm$SEM)
Smals et al[271]	1–44	100 μg	31	27 untreated	175 $\pm$ 49 highly variable responses (maximum
				4 previously treated, not cured	change 1–999)

effect may be overcome by pyridostigmine.[281] Other evidence suggesting that high levels of glucocorticoids inhibit GH secretion in humans comes from studies in patients with Cushing's syndrome, in whom the GH response to GHRH is attenuated.[282]

Hypoglycemia and Hyperglycemia. Under normal circumstances in humans, hypo- and hyperglycemia are associated with enhanced and suppressed levels of circulating GH, respectively—observations that are used clinically to document abnormalities in the hypothalamic-pituitary axis. Thus the failure of stimulation of GH release in response to insulin-induced hypoglycemia is considered to reflect hypothalamic and/or pituitary dysfunction. In addition, failure of glucose to suppress serum GH levels in a patient with suspected acromegaly is considered a diagnostic finding. With the availability of GHRH, there has been interest in the effects of hypo- or hyperglycemia on GHRH-stimulated GH release. After insulin-induced hypoglycemia, which alone prompts the release of GH, exogenous GHRH fails to stimulate further GH release.[283] These results are compatible with the hypothesis that hypoglycemia elicits endogenous GHRH release, which, via desensitization, renders the somatotrophs unresponsive to a further challenge with exogenous GHRH. Alternatively, enhanced somatostatin secretion, resulting from the increase in circulating GH levels in response to hypoglycemia, may attenuate the response to GHRH.

When GHRH is administered to normal subjects with pharmacologically induced hyperglycemia, GH secretion is markedly attenuated.[284, 285] These data are consistent with the hypothesis that hyperglycemia stimulates hypothalamic somatostatin release, which then inhibits GHRH-stimulated GH release. However, within this context, the findings that neither well- nor poorly controlled patients with diabetes mellitus demonstrate abnormalities in GHRH-stimulated GH release are of interest.[285, 286] There are other studies suggesting that the GH response to GHRH may be enhanced in Type I diabetics. These data, coupled with the clinical observation that diabetic individuals may have increased levels of circulating GH, are consistent with an abnormality of glucose-mediated GH suppression in this disorder. In a study of poorly controlled Type I diabetics, the effects of insulin and hyperglycemia on the GH response to GHRH were studied. The GH response to GHRH in poorly controlled diabetics (with hyperglycemia 16.8 mM) in the absence of insulin was similar to that seen in normal subjects who were euglycemic. When insulin was infused in the same subjects (insulin clamp) to produce combined hyperinsulinemia (528 ± 90 pM) and hyperglycemia (16.5 ± 1.98 mM), the GHRH-induced GH rise was markedly exaggerated (65 ± 11 versus 20 ± 4 μg/L without insulin infusion). This enhancement of GHRH-stimulated GH release by insulin was strikingly attenuated in five well-controlled diabetics studied under similar conditions of hyperinsulinemia and hyperglycemia. In normal subjects acute hyperinsulinemia tended to reduce the GH response to GHRH.[287]

Obesity. It has long been held that GH secretion in obese subjects is reduced. The effect of obesity on GHRH-stimulated GH release was compared (1) with GH release associated with insulin-induced hypoglycemia and (2) in response to GHRH(1-40)OH in both nonobese control subjects and obese patients.[288] In addition, the obese subjects were tested both before and after gastrointestinal surgery. Compared with nonobese controls, GHRH-stimulated GH secretion was markedly diminished in the preoperative obese patients and was somewhat greater (although not normal) after gastric bypass surgery. The response to GHRH correlates with both the percentage above ideal body weight and the response to insulin. These results suggest that, in obesity, impaired GH release in response to insulin-induced hypoglycemia is mediated at the pituitary level by diminished effectiveness of GHRH. That this defect is reversed with weight reduction implies that this abnormality is a consequence of obesity rather than a cause.

Combined Hypothalamic Hormone Test. The potential of combining several hypothalamic hormones as a test for anterior pituitary function has been explored by assessing the effects of corticotropin-releasing factor (CRF) (1 μg/kg), gonadotropin-releasing hormone (GnRH) (100 μg), GHRH (1 μg/kg), and thyrotropin-releasing hormone (TRH) (200 μg) given simultaneously.[289] Studies in normal young men revealed neither synergism nor inhibition of anterior pituitary hormone release in response to the administration of combined hypothalamic hormones when compared with the responses when the releasing hormones were given individually. These studies were extended to compare the stimulated hormone release in men with that in normal young women in the early follicular phase of the menstrual cycle. The results are summarized in Table 18–8. Except for a slightly higher luteinizing hormone response in men and a slightly higher prolactin response in women, no significant male versus female differences were detected. In addition, these data suggest that an acceptable amount of clinically useful information can be obtained by assaying a basal and two or three postinfusion samples, depending on the specific hormones in question (Table 18–9). The utility of this procedure in the clinical assessment of patients with hypothalamic and/or pituitary disease remains to be demonstrated.

Administration of GHRH as a Therapeutic Agent

Many studies have now examined the potential of GHRH as an agent to increase growth velocity in children. The initial study made use of the observation that in growing children, five to nine discrete pulses of GH are detected

TABLE 18–8. EFFECTS OF HYPOTHALAMIC RELEASING HORMONES ON IR-HORMONE LEVELS

	MEN	WOMEN
IR-ACTH (pg/ml)	40 ± 7.6	40 ± 6.6
IR-cortisol (μg/dl)	9.5 ± 1.0	9.8 ± 1.2
IR-FSH (mIU/ml)	2.7 ± 0.6	3.0 ± 0.2
IR-LH (mIU/ml)	21 ± 2.6	13.9 ± 1.9
IR-TSH (μU/ml)	12 ± 1.2	15 ± 2.1
IR-PRL (ng/ml)	46 ± 5.0	92 ± 15
IR-GH (ng/ml)	23 ± 7.1	55 ± 20

Maximum increments (mean $\pm$ SEM) in plasma or serum IR-hormone levels in 14 men and 12 women after receiving the combination of all four hypothalamic releasing hormones. (From Sheldon WR Jr, DeBold CR, Evans WS, et al: Rapid sequential intravenous administration of four hypothalamic releasing hormones as a combined anterior pituitary function test in normal subjects. J Clin Endocrinol Metab 60:623–630, © by the Endocrine Society, 1985.)

TABLE 18–9. RECOMMENDED SCHEDULE FOR ASSAYING PLASMA HORMONE LEVELS DURING COMBINED ANTERIOR PITUITARY FUNCTION TEST

PLASMA/SERUM HORMONE ASSAYED	TIME AFTER INFUSION (Min)							TOTAL ASSAYS
	0	10	15	30	45	60	90	
IR-ACTH	X	X			X	X		4
IR-cortisol	X				X	X		3
IR-FSH	X				X	X		3
IR-LH	X		X	X				3
IR-TSH	X		X	X				3
IR-PRL	X	X	X					3
IR-GH	X				X	X	X	4
Total Assays	7	2	3	2	4	4	1	23

From Sheldon WR Jr, DeBold CR, Evans WS, et al: Rapid sequential intravenous administration of four hypothalamic releasing hormones as a combined anterior pituitary function test in normal subjects. J Clin Endocrinol Metab 60:623–630, © by the Endocrine Society, 1985.

every 24 hours. Thus, GHRH(1-40)OH was administered subcutaneously (via a miniature peristaltic pump) every three hours to two children with organic hypopituitarism.[290] The regimen of three hourly doses of 1 or 3 μg/kg GHRH was continued for six months. Within the first week of treatment, both children exhibited evidence of enhanced GH secretion, including enhanced nitrogen retention and increased urinary calcium excretion. GH secretion was increased after pulses with GHRH during the entire six-month period and linear growth was accelerated. One child grew at a rate of 7.1 cm/year during therapy, compared with 4.6 cm/year before therapy. The second child grew 13.7 cm/year during therapy, compared with 2.1 cm/year before administration of GHRH(1-40)OH.

Subsequently there have been more than a dozen reports on the use of GHRH to accelerate growth in children. All investigators have administered GHRH by the subcutaneous route; the procedure includes administration by pump every 3 hours over 24 hours or every 3 hours overnight only or continuously; by twice-daily injection; or by once-daily injection. The results of these studies are summarized below. A number of circumstances exist that make the discussion problematic. The groups of children who were treated are not homogeneous. Thus the children's diagnoses varied from GH deficiency and short stature to normal variant short stature without GH deficiency. The GHRH preparations used were different: GHRH(1-40)OH,

GHRH(1-44)NH₂, GHRH(1-29)NH₂. The regimens varied and the criteria for response differed.

The majority of GH-deficient children with short stature and growth failure have a disorder of hypothalamic regulation of the anterior pituitary rather than a defect of the somatotroph. In these children single injections of GHRH may stimulate GH secretion. In our multicenter study of treatment of 24 children with GHRH(1-40)OH, growth was accelerated over six months in 88 per cent of patients. The three children who did not respond received GHRH administered by pump overnight only (with the lowest average dose of 6 to 8 μg/kg/day) and therefore received only half the dose given to children treated by pump throughout the 24-hour period.[291]

In Table 18–10 are shown the results of GHRH administration by pump treatment.[291, 293] All groups demonstrated an acceleration in growth velocity in 71 to 100 per cent of patients. The growth rate on GHRH therapy varied from 6.2 to 10 cm/year over the first six months and was maintained in patients for up to five years.[291, 294] Growth velocity appears to be related to the total daily dosage,[291] although the significance of the frequency and mode of administration (continuous compared with intermittent therapy) has not been established. The rationale for administering GHRH continuously came from observations in normal young men in whom GHRH was administered by continuous intravenous infusion over 24 hours or over 14 days. These studies, as well as measurement of GHRH and GH levels every 20 minutes for 24 hours in an acromegalic man who harbored a GHRH-secreting metastatic carcinoid tumor, suggested that continuous GHRH might enhance pulsatile GH secretion. Eight children with partial GH deficiency were treated with continuous GHRH(1-29)NH₂ and Nleu²⁷GHRH(1-29)NH₂ administered subcutaneously.[293] The growth velocity in five patients who completed one year of treatment increased from (cm/year) 4.6 ± 0.3 to 7.0 ± 1.4 at one year. Their 24-hour GH profiles, which were repeated at three-month intervals, demonstrated sustained augmented pulsatile GH secretion during treatment. After treatment ceased growth velocity returned to pretreatment growth velocity.

In Table 18–11 are shown the results of twice-daily GHRH administration.[291, 295–299] In doses varying from 2 to 20 μg/kg, growth velocity was accelerated in 16 to 100 per cent of patients. The results of twice-daily administration are quite variable. In one study only two of seven patients

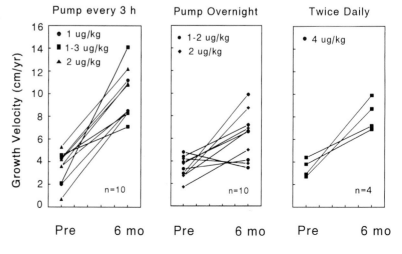

FIGURE 18–3. The effect of three different regimens of GHRH(1-40)OH therapy on growth velocity (cm/year). (From Thorner MO, Rogol AD, Blizzard RM et al: Acceleration of growth rate in GH-deficient children treated with human growth hormone–releasing hormone. Pediatr Res 24:145–151, 1988.)

TABLE 18–10. CHILDREN TREATED WITH SUBCUTANEOUS GHRH BY PUMP TO ACCELERATE GROWTH

REFERENCE	NO. OF CHILDREN	DIAGNOSIS* (Peak GH μg/L)	GHRH	DOSE (μg/kg)	TOTAL DOSAGE (μg/day)†	GROWTH VELOCITY (Mean ± SEM)		% RESPONDERS	COMMENTS
						Pre	During		
Thorner et al[291]	10	GHD (<10)	1–40	1–3 q 3h	200–600	3.5 ± 1.4 (±SD)	10.0 ± 2.2 (6 mo)	100%	Ab 11/20
	10	GHD (<10)	1–40	1–2 q 3h overnight only	100–200	3.4 ± 1.0	6.2 ± 2.1 (6 mo)	80%	
Low et al[292]	7	GHD (<2)	1–44	1–2 q 3h	200–400	2.7 ± 0.2	8.4 ± 2.5 (2 mo) 5.4 ± 0.7 (12 mo)	71%	Ab–none
Brain et al[293]	5 (12 mo) 3 (3–6 mo)	Partial GHD (<10)	1–29	Continuous	2150	4.6 ± 0.3 (±SD)	7.0 ± 1.4 (12 mo) (similar GV in 3 at 3–6 mo)	100%	Ab–all

*Peak GH response to standard pharmacological tests. †Assumes 25 kg child.

with GH deficiency responded with accelerated growth.[298] In two other studies only about half the patients responded with accelerated growth; in one of the studies the children had been pretreated with GH. Those children with the poorest response to GH also had the poorer responses to GHRH.[295] The most impressive results were achieved in a multicenter study using GHRH(1-44)NH$_2$ in 20 GH-deficient children. In that study 100 per cent of the children responded with accelerated growth velocity. In addition, none developed antibodies to GHRH. The pretreatment, 6-month, and 12-month growth velocities (cm/year) were 3.6 ± 1.1, 8.6 ± 2.5, and 8.1 ± 1.5, respectively.[299]

In Table 18–12 are shown the results with once-daily GHRH injections.[300-304] Again the responses varied, ranging from 0 to 83 per cent of children demonstrating accelerated growth velocity. The dosage varied from 1.6 to 23 μg/kg/dose. The poorest results were seen in older children who had previously been treated with GH.[302] The best results were observed when five of six GH-deficient children responded with accelerated growth velocity during treatment with 10 μg/kg/dose GHRH(1-44)NH$_2$. The optimal growth velocity was observed in the first nine months of therapy.[300]

The total amount of GHRH administered per day varied greatly from one report to the next. Those patients treated with three hourly doses of GHRH delivered by pump re-

ceived 100 to 600 μg/day. In contrast, the patients who received the continuous GHRH delivered by pump received 2150 μg/day. The subjects who received the twice- or once-daily injections received 200 to 1000 and 190 to 450 μg/day, respectively. There are no predictors for excellent responses: clearly a critical dose needs to be exceeded, but there is no clear dose-response relationship across these studies. It appears that at least 200 μg/day is required. The pretreatment or intratreatment GH response to an intravenous bolus of GHRH and pretreatment IGF-I level were not helpful in predicting response.[265, 291, 305]

Routes of Administration. Because GHRH has been shown to stimulate growth in the human, numerous questions arise regarding potential routes and timing of administration of GHRH as well as the possibilities for the use of peptide fragments or analogues. Assuming chronic use, intravenous infusion of peptide would be highly impractical. Moreover, if GHRH is required several times per day, intranasal administration might prove more acceptable than subcutaneous injection. With regard to routes of administration, data have been presented that detail the response to GHRH given intranasally versus subcutaneously or intravenously.[306, 307]

Intranasal Administration of GHRH. Intranasal GHRH(1-40)OH stimulated GH release in normal young adult men. However, 300-fold higher doses were required to effect the

TABLE 18–11. CHILDREN TREATED WITH SUBCUTANEOUS GHRH BY TWICE-DAILY INJECTIONS

REFERENCE	NUMBER OF CHILDREN	DIAGNOSIS* (μg/L)	GHRH	DOSE (μg/kg)	TOTAL DOSAGE (μg/day)†	GROWTH VELOCITY (Mean ± SD)		% RESPONDERS	COMMENTS
						Pre	During		
Ross et al[295]	18	GHD (<3.5) (including 10 IGHD, 4 MPHD, 3 cranial irradiation, 1 septo-optic dysplasia)	1–29	≤ 25‡	500–1000	R-1.7 ± 1.2 after 3 mo NR-3.4 ± 1.6	7.2 ± 2.5 (6 mo) 3.0 ± 1.2 (6 mo)	44	Ab 14/17
Takano et al[296]	4	2 IGHD (<7) 2 germinoma	1–44	50–100 μg dose	100–200	#1 3.5 #2 3.1 #3 2.0 #4 1.0	8.2 (6 mo) 3.8 (#1 and 3) 9.8 0.8	50	Ab 2/4
Thorner et al[291]	4	GHD (<10)	1–40	4	200	3.2 ± 1.8	7.9 ± 2.4 (6 mo)	100	Ab 1/4
Smith and Brook[297]	8	GHD (8.5) some MPHD	1–29	4–8	200–400		5.1 ± 0.3 (4 μg) 5.9 ± 0.4 (8 μg) (mean—9 mo)	63	Ab not done
Butenandt and Staudt[298]	7	GHD (<3)	1–29	4–6	200–300	3.0 (1.9–3.8)	4.0 (0.5–8.2) (6–15 mo)	29	7/7 responded to subsequent GH; Ab not done
Duck et al[299]	20	GHD (<10)	1–44	10–20[a]	500–1000	3.6 ± 1.1	8.6 ± 2.5 (6 mo) 8.1 ± 1.5 (12 mo)	100	Ab–none

*Peak GH to standard pharmacological tests; † assumes 25-kg child; ‡250 μg dose if wt <20 kg (n = 8) or 500 μg dose if wt >20 kg (n = 10); [a]16 subjects, 10 μg dose for 1 yr; 4 subjects, 10 μg for 6 mo and 20 μg for 6 mo.

TABLE 18–12. CHILDREN TREATED WITH SUBCUTANEOUS GHRH BY ONCE-DAILY INJECTION

REFERENCE	NO. OF CHILDREN	DIAGNOSIS* (<μg/L)	GHRH	DOSAGE (μg/kg)	TOTAL DOSE (μg/day)†	GROWTH VELOCITY (Mean ± SEM)		% RESPONDERS	COMMENTS
						Pre	During		
Rochiccioli et al[300]	6	Partial GHD (<11)	1–44	10 μg/kg	250	4.2 ± 1.1 (±SD)	10 ± 3.3 (6 mo) 8.6 ± 1.8 (12 mo)	83 (at 12 mo)	Reduced GV at 9–12 mo; Ab 1/6
Bozzola et al[301]	25	10 GHD (<5) 15 partial GHD (<10)	1–44	1.6–18 μg/kg	40–450	3.5 ± 0.2 3.7 ± 0.2	7.3 ± 0.4 (6 mo)‡ 4.1 ± 0.3	40 (at 6 mo) 32 (at 12 mo)	Responders Nonresponders Ab-6/25
Romer et al[302]	11 9	GHD (<5) GHD (<3)	1–44 1–44	10 μg/kg "(3 × a week)	250	3.3 (n = 20)	2.6 (6 mo) 3.0 (for all 20)	0	Older children 19/21 pretreated with GH 2/20 >2 cm/yr
GEMS[303]	111	GHD (<10)	1–44	1.3–23.1 kg	30–300	≤ −2 SDS 3.8 ± 0.1	>2 cm/yr (6 mo) 6 ± 0.2	50 increased GV	Ab 13.5% 42% had catch-up
Wit et al[304]§	5 6	GHD (<10)	1–44	7.5 μg/kg 15 μg/kg	190 380	2.5 2.7	4.6 (3 mo) 7.0 (3 mo)	40 >2 cm/yr 50	"Insuff response" 10 pretreated with GH; Ab–none

Subsequent GH treatment (2 IU-4X/wk): at 3 mo average growth velocity similar for those on higher dose of GHRH; 3 had better response on GHRH.
*Peak GH to standard pharmacological tests.
†Assumes 25 kg child.
‡NOTE: After withdrawal of GHRH, responders GV decreased from 7.3 ± 0.4 to 5.1 ± 1.7; treated with GH (0.6 U/kg for 6 mo):
GEMS - GHRH European Multicenter Study, Lievre et al, 1992.
§3 mo study—10/12 pretreated with GH

release of amounts of GH similar to those stimulated by GHRH given intravenously. Of interest, 30-fold more GHRH is required when given subcutaneously than intravenously. The probable reason for these results is that plasma levels of immunoreactive GHRH after intravenous administration of GHRH(1-40)OH are 60- and 500-fold higher than those achieved after administration of the same dose subcutaneously and intranasally, respectively.[306] Therefore, although encouraging in the sense that intranasal administration of GHRH is a viable option, the amounts that would be required make the intranasal administration of native peptide economically unfeasible. However, if subsequent studies were to demonstrate that less expensive forms of GHRH can be utilized, intranasal administration may emerge as a viable option. Similar results were obtained with GHRH(1-29)NH$_2$. However, in longer-term studies nasal irritation was observed, and growth velocity results were poor.

Frequency of GHRH Administration. The possibility that GHRH or its analogues can be given subcutaneously less frequently than in the original studies is under active investigation. It is remarkable that some studies have demonstrated good responses with once- or twice-daily injections.[291, 299, 300] This may be explained by the fact that GHRH may only be required to stimulate GH synthesis and pulsatile GH may be regulated by intermittent somatostatin withdrawal. Further, it should be remembered that the profile of GH concentrations achieved during GH therapy is far from physiological, with one pharmacological peak achieved after each injection, which spans about 12 hours. The need for a pulsatile pattern of GH to sustain growth has not been established in humans, although intuitively this seems logical since that is the profile of normal GH secretion in growing children.

Prospects for the Future. In studies in normal men, continuous administration of GHRH by intravenous infusion over 14 days appears to augment pulsatile GH secretion associated with an increase in IGF-I. Similarly, the results of accelerated growth and augmentation of endogenous pulsatile GH secretion in children treated with continuous

subcutaneous GHRH suggests that a sustained release preparation may achieve these objectives. Thus, the prospect exists for either the development of a delayed-release preparation of GHRH or the use of a long-acting analogue. These observations are of particular importance, since it appears that GHRH does not lead to desensitization as does GnRH. GHRH may therefore hold promise as an effective stimulator of GH secretion in children and adults and, in the former, is likely to lead to accelerated linear growth. The cloning of the receptor for GHRH offers the prospect of wide-scale screening of nonpeptide compounds for GHRH agonist activity. This may open a horizon in the search for new methods to enhance endogenous GH secretion.

Over the last few years a synthetic peptide, growth hormone–releasing peptide (GHRP), has been shown to be an effective secretagogue of GH in multiple species[308–311] and in humans.[312, 313] GHRP acts through non-GHRH and nonsomatostatin receptors. Its in vivo activity is far greater than its in vitro effects on GH release from the pituitary. Thus, it has been proposed that it acts both at the hypothalamus and the pituitary. At the hypothalamus it may increase endogenous GHRH release, or release a hitherto unidentified GH releasing factor, or antagonize the effects of somatostatin. Further, at the pituitary it acts directly to functionally antagonize the effects of somatostatin as well as augmenting GHRH effects. A nonpeptide mimetic of this compound has been developed.[314] Obviously, a compound with oral bioactivity that mimics the effects of GHRP theoretically has a major role in therapy to enhance GH secretion.

REFERENCES

1. Reichlin S: Growth and the hypothalamus. Endocrinology 67:760–773, 1960.
2. Reichlin S: Growth hormone content of pituitaries from rats with hypothalamic lesions. Endocrinology 69:225–230, 1961.

3. Beck C, Larkins RG, Martin TJ, et al: Stimulation of growth hormone release from superfused rat pituitary by extracts of hypothalamus and of human lung tumours. J Endocrinol 59:325–333, 1973.

4. Southern AL: Functioning metastatic bronchial carcinoid with elevated levels of serum and cerebrospinal fluid serotonin and pituitary adenoma. J Clin Endocrinol Metab 20:298–305, 1960.

5. Weiss L, Ingram M: Adenomatoid bronchial tumors: A consideration of the carcinoid tumors and the salivary tumors of the bronchial tree. Cancer 14:161–178, 1961.

6. Buse J, Buse MG, Roberts WJ: Eosinophilic adenoma of the pituitary and carcinoid tumors of the rectosigmoid area. J Clin Endocrinol Metab 21:735–738, 1961.

7. Dabek JT: Bronchial carcinoid tumor with acromegaly in two patients. J Clin Endocrinol Metab 38:329–333, 1974.

8. Sonksen PH, Ayres AB, Braimbridge M, et al: Acromegaly caused by pulmonary carcinoid tumours. Clin Endocrinol (Oxf) 5:503–513, 1976.

9. Ballard HS, Frame B, Hartsock RJ: Familial multiple endocrine adenoma-peptic ulcer complex. Medicine 43:481–516, 1964.

10. Caplan RH, Koob L, Abellera RM, et al: Cure of acromegaly by operative removal of an islet cell tumor of the pancreas. Am J Med 64:874–882, 1978.

11. Shalet SM, Beardwell CG, MacFarlane IA, et al: Acromegaly due to production of a growth hormone releasing factor by a bronchial carcinoid tumor. Clin Endocrinol (Oxf) 10:61–67, 1979.

12. Zafar MS, Mellinger RC, Fine G, et al: Acromegaly associated with a bronchial carcinoid tumor: evidence for ectopic production of growth hormone-releasing activity. J Clin Endocrinol Metab 48:66–71, 1979.

13. Leveston SA, McKeel DW, Jr., Buckley PJ, et al: Acromegaly and Cushing's syndrome associated with a foregut carcinoid tumor. J Clin Endocrinol Metab 53:682–689, 1981.

14. Frohman LA, Szabo M, Berelowitz M, et al: Partial purification and characterization of a peptide with growth hormone–releasing activity from extrapituitary tumors in patients with acromegaly. J Clin Invest 65:43–54, 1980.

15. Thorner MO, Perryman RL, Cronin MJ, et al: Somatotroph hyperplasia. Successful treatment of acromegaly by removal of a pancreatic islet tumor secreting a growth hormone–releasing factor. J Clin Invest 70:965–977, 1982.

16. Spiess J, Rivier J, Thorner M, et al: Sequence analysis of a growth hormone releasing factor from a human pancreatic islet tumor. Biochemistry 21:6037–6040, 1982.

17. Rivier J, Spiess J, Thorner M, et al: Characterization of a growth hormone–releasing factor from a human pancreatic islet tumour. Nature 300:276–278, 1982.

18. Esch FS, Bohlen P, Ling NC, et al: Characterization of a 40 residue peptide from a human pancreatic tumor with growth hormone releasing activity. Biochem Biophys Res Commun 109:152–158, 1982.

19. Sassolas G, Chayvialle JA, Partensky C, et al: Acromegaly, clinical expression of the production of growth hormone releasing factor in pancreatic tumors. Ann Endocrinol (Paris) 44:347–354, 1983.

20. Guillemin R, Brazeau P, Bohlen P, et al: Growth hormone–releasing factor from a human pancreatic tumor that caused acromegaly. Science 218:585–587, 1982.

21. Rivier J, Spiess J, Vale W: Human and rat hypothalamic growth hormone releasing factor (GRF). In Hubry VJ, Rich DH (eds): Peptides: Structure and Function. Rockford, IL, Pierce Chemical Co., 1983, pp 853–856.

22. Spiess J, Rivier J, Vale W: Characterization of rat hypothalamic growth hormone–releasing factor. Nature 303:532–535, 1983.

23. Bohlen P, Brazeau P, Bloch B, et al: Human hypothalamic growth hormone releasing factor (GRF): Evidence for two forms identical to tumor derived GRF-44-NH2 and GRF-40. Biochem Biophys Res Commun 114:930–936, 1983.

24. Bohlen P, Esch F, Brazeau P, et al: Isolation and characterization of the porcine hypothalamic growth hormone releasing factor. Biochem Biophys Res Commun 116:726–734, 1983.

25. Esch F, Bohlen P, Ling N, et al: Isolation and characterization of the bovine hypothalamic growth hormone releasing factor. Biochem Biophys Res Commun 117:772–779, 1983.

26. Ling N, Esch F, Bohlen P, et al: Isolation, primary structure, and synthesis of human hypothalamic somatocrinin: growth hormone–releasing factor. Proc Natl Acad Sci USA 81:4302–4306, 1984.

27. Lin HD, Bollinger J, Ling N, et al: Immunoreactive growth hormone–releasing factor in human stalk median eminence. J Clin Endocrinol Metab 58:1197–1199, 1984.

28. Asa SL, Kovacs K, Thorner MO, et al: Immunohistological localiza-
tion of growth hormone–releasing hormone in human tumors. J Clin Endocrinol Metab 60:423–427, 1985.

29. Brar AK, Downs TR, Heimer EP, et al: Biosynthesis of human growth hormone–releasing hormone (hGRH) in the pituitary of hGRH transgenic mice. Endocrinology 129:3274–3280, 1991.

30. Brazeau P, Ling N, Bohlen P, et al: Growth hormone releasing factor, somatocrinin, releases pituitary growth hormone in vitro. Proc Natl Acad Sci USA 79:7909–7913, 1982.

31. Engels JW, Glauder J, Mullner H, et al: Enzymatic amidation of recombinant (Leu27) growth hormone releasing hormone-Gly45. Protein Eng 1:195–199, 1987.

32. Kovacs M, Gulyas J, Bajusz S, et al: An evaluation of intravenous, subcutaneous, and in vitro activity of new agmatine analogs of growth hormone–releasing hormone hGH-RH (1-29)NH2. Life Sci 42:27–35, 1988.

33. Bokser L, Zarandi M, Schally AV: Evaluation of in vivo biological activity of new agmatine analogs of growth hormone–releasing hormone (GH-RH). Life Sci 46:999–1005, 1990.

34. Coy DH, Murphy WA, Sueiras-Diaz J, et al: Structure-activity studies on the N-terminal region of growth hormone releasing factor. J Med Chem 28:181–185, 1985.

35. Robberecht P, Coy DH, Waelbroeck M, et al: Structural requirements for the activation of rat anterior pituitary adenylate cyclase by growth hormone–releasing factor (GRF): discovery of (N-Ac-Tyr1, D-Arg2)-GRF(1-29)- NH2 as a GRF antagonist on membranes. Endocrinology 117:1759–1764, 1985.

36. Mayo KE, Vale W, Rivier J, et al: Expression-cloning and sequence of a cDNA encoding human growth hormone-releasing factor. Nature 306:86–88, 1983.

37. Gubler U, Monahan JJ, Lomedico PT, et al: Cloning and sequence analysis of cDNA for the precursor of human growth hormone-releasing factor, somatocrinin. Proc Natl Acad Sci USA 80:4311–4314, 1983.

38. Mayo KE, Cerelli GM, Rosenfeld MG, et al: Characterization of cDNA and genomic clones encoding the precursor to rat hypothalamic growth hormone–releasing factor. Nature 314:464–467, 1985.

39. Mayo KE, Cerelli GM, Lebo RV, et al: Gene encoding human growth hormone-releasing factor precursor: Structure, sequence, and chromosomal assignment. Proc Natl Acad Sci USA 82:63–67, 1985.

40. Frohman MA, Downs TR, Chomczynski P, et al: Cloning and characterization of mouse growth hormone-releasing hormone (GRH) complementary DNA: Increased GRH messenger RNA levels in the growth hormone-deficient lit/lit mouse. Mol Endocrinol 3:1529–1536, 1989.

41. Bloch B, Brazeau P, Bloom F, et al: Topographical study of the neurons containing hpGRF immunoreactivity in monkey hypothalamus. Neurosci Lett 37:23–28, 1983.

42. Bloch B, Brazeau P, Ling N, et al: Immunohistochemical detection of growth hormone-releasing factor in brain. Nature 301:607–608, 1983.

43. Bloch B, Gaillard RC, Brazeau P: Topographical and ontogenetic study of the neurons producing growth hormone releasing factor in human hypothalamus. Regul Pept 8:21–31, 1984.

44. Bresson JL, Clavequin MC, Fellman D, et al: Ontogeny of the neuroglandular system revealed with hpGRF antibodies in human hypothalamus. Neuroendocrinology 39:68–73, 1984.

45. Bugnon C, Gouget A, Fellman D, et al: Immunocytochemical demonstration of a novel peptidergic neurone system in the cat brain with an anti-growth hormone–releasing factor serum. Neurosci Lett 38:131–137, 1983.

46. Jacobowitz DM, Schulte H, Chrousos GP, et al: Localization of GRF-like immunoreactive neurons in the rat brain. Peptides 4:521–524, 1983.

47. Merchenthaler I, Vigh S, Schally AV, et al: Immunocytochemical localization of growth hormone-releasing factor in the rat hypothalamus. Endocrinology 114:1082–1085, 1984.

48. Sawchenko PE, Swanson LW, Rivier J, et al: The distribution of growth hormone–releasing factor (GRF) immunoreactivity in the central nervous system of the rat: an immunohistochemical study using antisera directed against rat hypothalamic GRF. J Comp Neurol 237:100–115, 1985.

49. VandePol CJ, Leidy JW, Jr., Finger TE, et al: Immunohistochemical localization of GRF-containing neurons in rat brain. Neuroendocrinology 42:143–147, 1986.

50. Tsargarakis S, Ge F, Besser GM, et al: Similar high molecular weight forms of growth hormone–releasing hormone are found in rat brain and testis. Life Sci 49:1627–1634, 1991.

51. Leidy JW, Robbins RJ: Regional distribution of human growth hor-

mone–releasing hormone in the human hypothalamus by radioim-munoassay. J Clin Endocrinol Metab 62:372–378, 1986.

52. Horvath S, Palkovits M: Synaptic interconnections among growth hormone releasing hormone (GHRH) containing neurons in the arcuate nucleus of the rat hypothalamus. Neuroendocrinology 48:471–476, 1988.

53. Horvath S, Palkovits M, Gorcs T, et al: Electron microscopic immu-nocytochemical evidence for the existence of bidirectional synaptic connections between growth hormone releasing hormone and so-matostatin neurons in the hypothalamus of the rat. Brain Res 481:8–15, 1989.

54. Zeitler P, Tannenbaum GS, Clifton DK, et al: Ultradian oscillations in somatostatin and growth hormone–releasing hormone mRNAs in the brains of adult male rats. Proc Natl Acad Sci USA 88:8920–8924, 1991.

55. Bruhn TO, Anthony EL, Wu P, et al: GRF immunoreactive neurons in the paraventricular nucleus of the rat: An immunohistochemical study with monoclonal and polyclonal antibodies. Brain Res 424:290–298, 1987.

56. Ishikawa K, Katakami H, Jansson JO, et al: Ontogenesis of growth hormone–releasing hormone neurons in the rat hypothalamus. Neu-roendocrinology 43:537–542, 1986.

57. Weigent DA, Blalock JE: Immunoreactive growth hormone releasing hormone in rat leukocytes. J Neuroimmunol 29:1–13, 1990.

58. Stephanou A, Knight RA, Lightman SL: Production of a growth hormone–releasing hormone-like peptide and its mRNA by human lymphocytes. Neuroendocrinology 53:628–633, 1991.

59. Weigent DA, Riley JE, Galin FS, et al: Detection of growth hormone and growth hormone-releasing hormone–related messenger RNA in rat leukocytes by the polymerase chain reaction. Proc Soc Exp Biol Med 198:643–648, 1991.

60. Berry SA, Pescovitz OH: Identification of a rat GHRH-like substance and its messenger RNA in rat testis. Endocrinology 123:661–663, 1988.

61. Suhr ST, Rahal JO, Mayo KE: Mouse growth hormone–releasing hormone: Precursor structure and expression in brain and placenta. Mol Endocrinol 3:1693–1700, 1989.

62. Bagnato A, Moretti C, Ohnishi J, et al: Expression of the growth hormone-releasing hormone gene and its peptide product in the rat ovary. Endocrinology 130:1097–1102, 1992.

63. Margioris AN, Brockmann G, Bohler HCJ, et al: Expression and localization of growth hormone releasing hormone messenger ribo-nucleic acid in rat placenta: In vitro secretion and regulation of its peptide product. Endocrinology 126:151–158, 1990.

64. Gonzalez-Crespo S, Boronat A: Expression of the rat growth hor-mone–releasing hormone gene in placenta is directed by an alter-native promoter. Proc Natl Acad Sci USA 88:8749–8753, 1991.

65. Pescovitz OH, Johnson NB, Berry SA: Ontogeny of growth hormone releasing hormone and insulin-like growth factors-I and -II messen-ger RNA in rat placenta. Pediatr Res 29:510–516, 1991.

66. Joubert D, Benlot C, Lagoguey A, et al: Normal and growth hormone (GH)–secreting adenomatous human pituitaries release somato-statin and GH-releasing hormone. J Clin Endocrinol Metab 68:572–577, 1989.

67. Nicholson WE, DeCherney GS, Jackson RV, et al: Pituitary and hy-pothalamic hormones in normal and neoplastic adrenal medullae: Biologically active corticotropin-releasing hormone and corticotro-pin. Regul Pept 18:173–188, 1987.

68. Tanaka Y, Saito S, Nambo O, et al: Study on human pancreatic growth hormone releasing factor-like substance in human placenta. 7th Internatl Congr Endocrinol, Quebec, Canada (Abst 2335):1984.

69. Meigan G, Sasaki A, Yoshinaga K: Immunoreactive growth hormone releasing hormone in rat placenta. Endocrinology 123:1098–1102, 1988.

70. Shibasaki T, Kiyosawa Y, Masuda A, et al: Distribution of growth hormone–releasing hormone-like immunoreactivity in human tissue extracts. J Clin Endocrinol Metab 59:263–268, 1984.

71. Bosman FT, Van Assche C, Kruseman ACN, et al: Growth hormone releasing factor immunoreactivity in the human and rat gastrointes-tinal tract and pancreas. J Histochem Cytochem 32:1139–1144, 1984.

72. Christofides ND, Stephanou A, Suzuki H, et al: Distribution of im-munoreactive growth hormone-releasing hormone in the human brain and intestine and its production by tumors. J Clin Endocrinol Metab 59:747–751, 1984.

73. Shibasaki T, Shizume K, Nakahara M, et al: Age-related changes in plasma growth hormone response to growth hormone-releasing fac-tor in man. J Clin Endocrinol Metab 58(1):212–214, 1984.

74. Morel G, Mesguich P, Dubois MP, et al: Ultrastructural evidence for

75. Mentlein R, Buchholz C, Krisch B: Binding and internalization of gold-conjugated somatostatin and growth hormone–releasing hor-mone in cultured rat somatotropes. Cell Tissue Res 258:309–317, 1989.

76. Gaylinn BD, Harrison JK, Zysk JR, et al: Molecular cloning and expression of a human anterior pituitary receptor for growth hor-mone-releasing hormone. Mol Endocrinol 7:77–84, 1993.

77. Mayo KE: Molecular cloning and expression of a pituitary-specific receptor for growth hormone-releasing hormone. Mol Endocrinol 6:1734–1744, 1992.

78. Lin C, Lin SC, Chang CP, et al: Pit-1–dependent expression of the receptor for growth hormone releasing factor mediates pituitary cell growth. Nature 360:765–769, 1992.

79. Gaylinn BD, Lyons CE, Jr: Characterization of the receptor for growth hormone releasing factor from ovine pituitary membranes. 73rd Annual Meeting of the Endocrine Society, p 423, 1991, Abst.

80. Gaylinn BD, Lyons CE, Jr: Photoaffinity cross-linking of a receptor for growth hormone releasing factor from ovine pituitary mem-branes. 74th Annual Meeting of the Endocrine Society, 1992, Abstr.

81. Seifert H, Perrin M, Rivier J, et al: Binding sites for growth hormone releasing factor on rat anterior pituitary cells. Nature 313:487–489, 1985.

82. Abribat T, Boulanger L, Gaudreau P: Characterization of human growth hormone-releasing factor (1-44) amide binding to rat pitui-tary: Evidence for high and low affinity classes of sites. Brain Res 528:291–299, 1990.

83. Ikuyama S, Natori S, Nawata H, et al: Characterization of growth hormone–releasing hormone receptors in pituitary adenomas from patients with acromegaly. J Clin Endocrinol Metab 66:1265–1271, 1988.

84. Honegger J, Spagnoli A, D'Urso R, et al: Interleukin-1 beta modu-lates the acute release of growth hormone-releasing hormone and somatostatin from rat hypothalamus in vitro, whereas tumor necrosis factor and interleukin-6 have no effect. Endocrinology 129:1275–1282, 1991.

85. Horvath S, Mezey E, Palkovits M: Partial coexistence of growth hor-mone–releasing hormone and tyrosine hydroxylase in paraventricu-lar neurons in rats. Peptides 10:791–795, 1989.

86. Cugini CD, Jr., Millard WJ, Leidy JW, Jr: Signal transduction systems in growth hormone-releasing hormone and somatostatin release from perifused rat hypothalamic fragments. Endocrinology 129:1355–1362, 1991.

87. Miki N, Ono M, Shizume K: Evidence that opiatergic and alpha-adrenergic mechanisms stimulate rat growth hormone release via growth hormone–releasing factor (GRF). Endocrinology 114:1950–1952, 1984.

88. Bilezikjian LM, Vale WW: Stimulation of adenosine 3′,5′-monophos-phate production by growth hormone–releasing factor and its inhi-bition by somatostatin in anterior pituitary cells in vitro. Endocrinol-ogy 113:1726–1731, 1983.

89. Mougin C, Brazeau P, Ling N, et al: Roles of cyclic AMP and calcium in the mechanism of the release of growth hormone by somatocri-nin. CR Acad Sci (Paris) 299:83–88, 1984.

90. Brazeau P, Ling N, Esch F, et al: Somatocrinin (growth hormone releasing factor) in vitro bioactivity: Ca^{++} involvement, cAMP-me-diated action and additivity of effect with PGE2. Biochem Biophys Res Commun 109:588–594, 1982.

91. Beck-Peccoz P, Volpi A, Maggioni AP, et al: Evidence for an inhibi-tion of thyroid hormone effects during chronic treatment with amio-darone. Horm Metab Res 18:411–414, 1986.

92. Hart GR, Ray KP, Wallis M: Mechanisms involved in the effects of TRH on GHRH-stimulated growth hormone release from ovine and bovine pituitary cells. Mol Cell Endocrinol 56:53–61, 1988.

93. Schettini G, Cronin MJ, Hewlett EL, et al: Human pancreatic tumor growth hormone-releasing factor stimulates anterior pituitary adenyl-ate cyclase activity, adenosine 3′,5′-monophosphate accumulation, and growth hormone release in a calmodulin-dependent manner. Endocrinology 115:1308–1314, 1984.

94. Holl RW, Thorner MO, Leong DA: Intracellular calcium concentra-tion and growth hormone secretion in individual somatotropes: Ef-fects of growth hormone–releasing factor and somatostatin. Endocri-nology 122:2927–2932, 1988.

95. Snyder GD, Yadagiri P, Falck JR: Effect of epoxyeicosatrienoic acids on growth hormone release from somatotrophs. Am J Physiol 256:E221–E226, 1989.

96. Rawlings SR, Hoyland J, Mason WT: Calcium homeostasis in bovine somatotrophs: Calcium oscillations and calcium regulation by growth hormone-releasing hormone and somatostatin. Cell Calcium 12:403–414, 1991.

97. Guarcello V, Weigent DA, Blalock JE: Growth hormone releasing hormone receptors on thymocytes and splenocytes from rats. Cell Immunol 136:291–302, 1991.

98. Cronin MJ, Hewlett EL, Evans WS, et al: Human pancreatic tumor growth hormone (GH)–releasing factor and cyclic adenosine 3',5'-monophosphate evoke GH release from anterior pituitary cells: The effects of pertussis toxin, cholera toxin, forskolin, and cycloheximide. Endocrinology 114:904–913, 1984.

99. Cronin MJ, Rogol AD, Dabney LG, et al: Selective growth hormone and cyclic AMP stimulating activity is present in human pancreatic islet cell tumor. J Clin Endocrinol Metab 55:381–383, 1982.

100. Cronin MJ, Rogol AD, MacLeod RM, et al: Biological activity of a growth hormone–releasing factor secreted by a human tumor. Am J Physiol 244:E346–E353, 1983.

101. Cronin MJ, Rogol AD: Sex differences in the cyclic adenosine 3',5'-monophosphate and growth hormone response to growth hormone-releasing factor in vitro. Biol Reprod 31:984–988, 1984.

102. Cronin MJ, Rogol AD, Myers GA, et al: Pertussis toxin blocks the somatostatin-induced inhibition of growth hormone release and adenosine 3',5'-monophosphate accumulation. Endocrinology 113:209–215, 1983.

103. Cronin MJ, MacLeod RM, Canonico PL: Modification of basal and GRF-stimulated cyclic AMP levels and growth hormone release by phospholipid metabolic enzyme inhibitors. Neuroendocrinology 40:332–338, 1985.

104. Cronin MJ, Canonico PL: Tumor promoters enhance basal and growth hormone releasing factor stimulated cyclic AMP levels in anterior pituitary cells. Biochem Biophys Res Commun 129:404–410, 1985.

105. Cronin MJ, Summers ST, Sortino MA, et al: Protein kinase C enhances growth hormone releasing factor (1-40)–stimulated cyclic AMP levels in anterior pituitary. Actions of somatostatin and pertussis toxin. J Biol Chem 261:13932–13935, 1986.

106. Arimura A, Culler MD, Turkelson CM, et al: In vitro pituitary hormone releasing activity of 40 residue human pancreatic tumor growth hormone releasing factor. Peptides 4:107–110, 1983.

107. Culler MD, Kenjo T, Obara N, et al: Stimulation of pituitary cAMP accumulation by human pancreatic GH-releasing factor-(1-44). Am J Physiol 247:E609–E615, 1984.

108. Ray KP, Wallis M: Regulation of growth hormone secretion and cyclic AMP metabolism in ovine pituitary cells: Interactions involved in activation induced by growth hormone-releasing hormone and phorbol esters. Mol Cell Endocrinol 58:243–252, 1988.

109. Michel D, Lefevre G, Labrie F: Dexamethasone is a potent stimulator of growth hormone–releasing factor-induced cyclic AMP accumulation in the adenohypophysis. Life Sci 35:597–602, 1984.

110. Spada A, Vallar L, Giannattasio G: Presence of an adenylate cyclase dually regulated by somatostatin and human pancreatic growth hormone (GH)–releasing factor in GH-secreting cells. Endocrinology 115:1203–1209, 1984.

111. Labrie F, Gagne B, Lefevre G: Growth hormone–releasing factor stimulates adenylate cyclase activity in the anterior pituitary gland. Life Sci 33:2229–2233, 1983.

112. Cheng K, Chan WW, Barreto A Jr, et al: The synergistic effects of His-D-Trp-Ala-Trp-D-Phe-Lys-NH2 on growth hormone (GH)–releasing factor-stimulated GH release and intracellualr adenosine 3',5'-monophosphate accumulation in rat primary pituitary cell culture. Endocrinology 124:2791–2798, 1989.

113. Summers ST, Cronin MJ: Phorbol esters induce two distinct changes in GH3 pituitary cell adenylate cyclase activity. Arch Biochem Biophys 262:12–18, 1988.

114. Summers ST, Cronin MJ: Phorbol esters enhance basal and stimulated adenylate cyclase activity in a pituitary cell line. Biochem Biophys Res Commun 135:276–281, 1986.

115. Canonico PL, Cronin MJ, Thorner MO, et al: Human pancreatic GRF stimulates phosphatidylinositol labeling in cultured anterior pituitary cells. Am J Physiol 245:E587–E590, 1983.

116. Canonico PL, Speciale C, Sortino MA, et al: Growth hormone releasing factor (GRF) increases free arachidonate levels in the pituitary: A role for lipoxygenase products. Life Sci 38:267–272, 1986.

117. Dobson PRM, Merritt JE, Baird JG, et al: The effect of growth hormone releasing factor on cyclic AMP accumulation and phosphatidylinositol breakdown. 5th Internatl Conf Cyclic Nucleotides Protein Phosphorylation 101, 1983.

118. Barinaga M, Yamamoto G, Rivier C, et al: Transcriptional regulation of growth hormone gene expression by growth hormone–releasing factor. Nature 306:84–85, 1983.

119. Barinaga M, Bilezikjian LM, Vale WW, et al: Independent effects of growth hormone releasing factor on growth hormone release and gene transcription. Nature 314:279–281, 1985.

120. Stachura ME, Tyler JM, Farmer PK: Fractional reduction of somatostatin concentration interacted with rat growth hormone releasing hormone to titrate the magnitude of pulsatile growth hormone and prolactin release in perifusion. Neuroendocrinology 48:500–506, 1988.

121. Dieguez C, Foord SM, Shewring G, et al: The effects of long term growth hormone releasing factor (GRF 1-40) administration on growth hormone secretion and synthesis in vitro. Biochem Biophys Res Commun 121:111–117, 1984.

122. Billestrup N, Swanson LW, Vale W: Growth hormone–releasing factor stimulates proliferation of somatotrophs in vitro. Proc Natl Acad Sci USA 83:6854–6857, 1986.

123. Perez FM, Hymer WC: A new tissue-slicing method for the study of function and position of somatotrophs contained within the male rat pituitary gland. Endocrinology 127:1877–1886, 1990.

124. Vale W, Vaughan J, Yamamoto G, et al: Effects of synthetic human pancreatic (tumor) GH releasing factor and somatostatin, triiodothyronine and dexamethasone on GH secretion in vitro. Endocrinology 112:1553–1555, 1983.

125. Borges JL, Uskavitch DR, Kaiser DL, et al: Human pancreatic growth hormone–releasing factor 40 (hpGRF-40) allows stimulation of GH release by TRH. Endocrinology 113:1519–1521, 1983.

126. Almeida OF, Schulte HM, Rittmaster RS, et al: Potency and specificity of a growth hormone-releasing factor in a primate and in vitro. J Clin Endocrinol Metab 58:309–312, 1984.

127. Vigh S, Schally AV: Interaction between hypothalamic peptides in a superfused pituitary cell system. Peptides 5 Suppl 1:241–247, 1984.

128. Badger TM, Millard WJ, McCormick GF, et al: The effects of growth hormone (GH)-releasing peptide on GH secretion in perifused pituitary cells of adult male rats. Endocrinology 115:1432–1438, 1984.

129. Ceda GP, Hoffman AR: Growth hormone–releasing factor desensitization in rat anterior pituitary cells in vitro. Endocrinology 116:1334–1340, 1985.

130. Gelato MC, Rittmaster RS, Pescovitz OH, et al: Growth hormone responses to continuous infusions of growth hormone–releasing hormone. J Clin Endocrinol Metab 61:223–228, 1985.

131. Plotsky PM, Vale W: Patterns of growth hormone–releasing factor and somatostatin secretion into the hypophysial-portal circulation in the rat. Science 230:461–463, 1985.

132. Frohman LA, Downs TR, Clarke IJ, et al: Measurement of growth hormone-releasiing hormone and somatostatin in hypothalamic-portal plasma of unanesthetized sheep. Spontaneous secretion and response to insulin-induced hypoglycemia. J Clin Invest 86(1):17–24, 1990.

133. Weiss J, Cronin MJ, Thorner MO: Periodic interactions of GH-releasing factor and somatostatin can augment GH release in vitro. Am J Physiol 253:E508–E514, 1987.

134. Law GJ, Ray KP, Wallis M: Effects of growth hormone–releasing factor, somatostatin and dopamine on growth hormone and prolactin secretion from cultured ovine pituitary cells. FEBS Lett 166:189–193, 1984.

135. Stachura ME, Tyler JM, Farmer PK: Human pancreatic growth hormone–releasing factor 44 differentially stimulates release of stored and newly synthesized rat growth hormone in vitro. Endocrinology 116:698–706, 1985.

136. Tachibana K, Marquardt H, Yokoya S, et al: Growth hormone–releasing hormone stimulates and somatostatin inhibits the release of a novel protein by cultured rat pituitary cells. Mol Endocrinol 2:973–978, 1988.

137. Bergstrom RW, Hansen KL, Clare CN, et al: Hypogonadotropic hypogonadism and anosmia (Kallmann's syndrome) associated with a marker chromosome. J Androl 8:55–60, 1987.

138. Zeytin F, Brazeau P: GRF (somatocrinin) stimulates release of neurotensin, calcitonin and cAMP by a rat C cell line. Biochem Biophys Res Commun 123:497–506, 1984.

139. Wehrenberg WB, Ling N, Bohlen P, et al: Physiological roles of somatocrinin and somatostatin in the regulation of growth hormone secretion. Biochem Biophys Res Commun 109:562–567, 1982.

140. Wehrenberg WB, Ling N, Brazeau P, et al: Somatocrinin, growth hormone releasing factor, stimulates secretion of growth hormone in anesthetized rats. Biochem Biophys Res Commun 109:382–387, 1982.

141. Wehrenberg WB, Bloch B, Phillips BJ: Antibodies to growth hormone–releasing factor inhibit somatic growth. Endocrinology 115:1218–1220, 1984.
142. Wehrenberg WB, Brazeau P, Luben R, et al: Inhibition of the pulsatile secretion of growth hormone by monoclonal antibodies to the hypothalamic growth hormone releasing factor (GRF). Endocrinology 111:2147–2148, 1982.
143. Tannenbaum GS, Ling N: The interrelationship of growth hormone (GH)–releasing factor and somatostatin in generation of the ultradian rhythm of GH secretion. Endocrinology 115:1952–1957, 1984.
144. Koritnik DR, Cronin MJ, Orth DN, et al: Pituitary response to intravenous hypothalamic releasing peptides in cynomolgus monkeys treated with contraceptive steroids. J Clin Endocrinol Metab 65:37–45, 1987.
145. Johke T, Hodate K, Ohashi S, et al: Growth hormone response to human pancreatic growth hormone releasing factor in cattle. Endocrinol Jpn 31:55–61, 1984.
146. Hodate K, Johke T, Kawabata A, et al: Effect of synthetic growth hormone releasing factor from a human pancreatic tumor on bovine and caprine growth hormone secretion. Jpn J Zootech Sci 55:66–68, 1983.
147. Moseley WM, Krabill LF, Friedman AR, et al: Administration of synthetic human pancreatic growth hormone-releasing factor for five days sustains raised serum concentrations of growth hormone in steers. J Endocrinol 104:433–439, 1985.
148. Moseley WM, Krabill LF, Friedman AR, et al: Growth hormone response of steers injected with synthetic human pancreatic growth hormone-releasing factors. J Anim Sci 58:430–435, 1984.
149. Enright WJ, Olsen RF, Moseley WM, et al: Growth hormone releasing factor induced release of growth hormone in lactating cows. J Dairy Sci 67(Suppl 1):161, 1984.
150. Enright WJ, Zinn SA, Chapin LT, et al: Growth hormone (GH) release in bull calves after injections or infusion of growth hormone releasing factor. J Anim Sci 59(Suppl 1):193, 1984.
151. Leung FC, Taylor JE: In vivo and in vitro stimulation of growth hormone release in chickens by synthetic human pancreatic growth hormone releasing factor (hpGRFs). Endocrinology 113:1913–1915, 1983.
152. Peticlerc D, Pelletier G, Lapierre H, et al: Dose response of two synthetic human growth hormone–releasing factors on growth hormone release in heifers and pigs. J Anim Sci 65:996–1005, 1987.
153. Cella SG, Locatelli V, Mennini T, et al: Deprivation of growth hormone–releasing hormone early in the rat's neonatal life permanently affects somatotropic function. Endocrinology 127:1625–1634, 1990.
154. Thorner MO, Cronin MJ: Growth hormone–releasing factor: Clinical and basic studies. In Mueller EE, MacLeod RM, Frohman LA (eds): Neuroendocrine Perspectives. Amsterdam, Elsevier, 1985, pp 95–144.
155. Ling N, Zeytin F, Bohlen P, et al: Growth hormone releasing factors (Review). Annu Rev Biochem 54:403–423, 1985.
156. Enright WJ, Chapin LT, Moseley WM, et al: Growth hormone–releasing factor stimulates milk production and sustains growth hormone release in Holstein cows. J Dairy Sci 69:344–351, 1986.
157. Clark RG, Robinson IC: Growth induced by pulsatile infusion of an amidated fragment of human growth hormone releasing factor in normal and GHRF-deficient rats. Nature 314:281–283, 1985.
158. Mayo KE, Hammer RE, Swanson LW, et al: Dramatic pituitary hyperplasia in transgenic mice expressing a human growth hormone–releasing factor gene. Mol Endocrinol 2:606–612, 1988.
159. Stefaneanu L, Kovacs K, Horvath E, et al: Adenohypophysial changes in mice transgenic for human growth hormone–releasing factor: A histological, immunocytochemical, and electron microscopic investigation. Endocrinology 125:2710–2718, 1989.
160. Wheeler MD, Wehrenberg WW, Styne DM: Growth hormone regulation by growth hormone-releasing hormone in infant rhesus monkeys. Biol Neonate 60:19–28, 1991.
161. Wheeler MD, Styne DM: Longitudinal changes in growth hormone response to growth hormone–releasing hormone in neonatal rhesus monkeys. Pediatr Res 28:15–18, 1990.
162. Acs Z, Lonart G, Makara GB: Role of hypothalamic factors (growth hormone–releasing hormone and gamma-aminobutyric acid) in the regulation of growth hormone secretion in the neonatal and adult rat. Neuroendocrinology 52:156–160, 1990.
163. Ge F, Tsagarakis S, Rees LH, et al: Relationship between growth hormone-releasing hormone and somatostatin in the rat: Effects of age and sex on content and in-vitro release from hypothalamic explants. J Endocrinol 123:53–58, 1989.
164. Cozzi MG, Zanini A, Locatelli V, et al: Growth hormone-releasing hormone and clonidine stimulate biosynthesis of growth hormone in neonatal pituitaries. Biochem Biophys Res Commun 138:1223–1230, 1986.
165. Barenton B, Duclos M, Diaz J, et al: Characteristics of growth hormone response to the administration of growth hormone–releasing hormone (GRF) in the lamb. Reprod Nutr Dev 27:491–500, 1987.
166. Spatola E, Pescovitz OH, Marsh K, et al: Interaction of growth hormone–releasing hormone with the insulin-like growth factors during prenatal development in the rat. Endocrinology 129:1193–1200, 1991.
167. Colonna VD, Zoli M, Cocci D, et al: Reduced growth hormone releasing factor (GHRF)–like immunoreactivity and GHRF gene expression in the hypothalamus of aged rats. Peptides (Brief Comm) 10:705–708, 1989.
168. Abribat T, Deslauriers N, Brazeau P, et al: Alterations of pituitary growth hormone-releasing factor binding sites in aging rats. Endocrinology 128:633–635, 1991.
169. Sonntag WE, Hylka VW, Meites J: Impaired ability of old male rats to secrete growth hormone in vivo but not in vitro in response to hpGRF(1-44). Endocrinology 113:2305–2307, 1983.
170. Sonntag WE, Gough MA: Growth hormone releasing hormone induced release of growth hormone in aging male rats: Dependence on pharmacological manipulation and endogenous somatostatin release. Neuroendocrinology 47:482–488, 1988.
171. Ceda GP, Valenti G, Butturini U, et al: Diminished pituitary responsiveness to growth hormone-releasing factor in aging male rats. Endocrinology 118:2109–2114, 1986.
172. Lang I, Kurz R, Geyer G, et al: The influence of age on human pancreatic growth hormone releasing hormone stimulated growth hormone secretion. Horm Metab Res 20:574–578, 1988.
173. Pavlov EP, Harman SM, Merriam GR, et al: Responses of growth hormone (GH) and somatomedin C to GH-releasing hormone in healthy aging men. J Clin Endocrinol Metab 62:595–600, 1986.
174. Argente J, Chowen JA, Zeitler P, et al: Sexual dimorphism of growth hormone–releasing hormone and somatostatin gene expression in the hypothalamus of the rat during development. Endocrinology 128:2369–2375, 1991.
175. Maiter D, Koenig JI, Kaplan LM: Sexually dimorphic expression of the growth hormone–releasing hormone gene is not mediated by circulating gonadal hormones in the adult rat. Endocrinology 128:1709–1716, 1991.
176. Zeitler P, Argente J, Chowen-Breede JA, et al: Growth hormone releasing hormone messenger ribonucleic acid in the hypothalamus of the adult male rat is increased by testosterone. Endocrinology 127:362–368, 1990.
177. Zeitler P, Vician L, Chowen-Breede JA, et al: Regulation of somatostatin and growth hormone-releasing hormone gene expression in the rat brain. Metabolism 39:46–49, 1990.
178. Aguilar I, Pinilla L: Ovarian role in the modulation of pituitary responsiveness to growth hormone–releasing hormone in rats. Neuroendocrinology 54:286–290, 1991.
179. Evans WS, Krieg RJ, Limber ER, et al: Effects of in vivo gonadal hormone environment on in vitro hGRF-40–stimulated GH release. Am J Physiol 249:E276–E280, 1985.
180. Hertz P, Silbermann M, Even L, et al: Effects of sex steroids on the response of cultured rat pituitary cells to growth hormone–releasing hormone and somatostatin. Endocrinology 125:581–585, 1989.
181. Leong DA, Lau SK, Sinha YN, et al: Enumeration of lactotropes and somatotropes among male and female pituitary cells in culture: Evidence in favor of a mammosomatotrope subpopulation in the rat. Endocrinology 116:1371–1378, 1985.
182. Ho KY, Thorner MO, Krieg RJ, Jr, et al: Effects of gonadal steroids on somatotroph function in the rat: Analysis by the reverse hemolytic plaque assay. Endocrinology 123:1405–1411, 1988.
183. Alvarez CV, Mallo F, Burguera B, et al: Evidence for a direct pituitary inhibition by free fatty acids of in vivo growth hormone responses to growth hormone–releasing hormone in the rat. Neuroendocrinology 53:185–189, 1991.
184. Grings EE, Scarborough R, Schally AV, et al: Response to a growth hormone-releasing hormone analog in heifers treated with recombinant growth hormone. Domest Anim Endocrinol 5:47–53, 1988.
185. Ganzetti I, De Gennaro V, Redaelli M, et al: Effect of hypophysectomy and growth hormone replacement on hypothalamic GHRH. Peptides 7:1011–1014, 1986.
186. Maiter DM, Gabriel SM, Koenig JI, et al: Sexual differentiation of growth hormone feedback effects on hypothalamic growth hormone–releasing hormone and somatostatin. Neuroendocrinology 51:174–180, 1990.

187. Katakami H, Downs TR, Frohman LA: Decreased hypothalamic growth hormone–releasing hormone content and pituitary responsiveness in hypothyroidism. J Clin Invest 77:1704–1711, 1986.

188. Edwards CA, Dieguez C, Scanlon MF: Effects of hypothyroidism, triiodothyronine and glucocorticoids on growth hormone responses to growth hormone–releasing hormone and His-D-Trp-Ala-Trp-D-Phe-Lys-NH2. J Endocrinol 121:31–36, 1989.

189. Wehrenberg WB, Baird A, Ling N: Potent interaction between glucocorticoids and growth hormone–releasing factor in vivo. Science 221:556–558, 1983.

190. Wehrenberg WB, Baird A, Klepper R, et al: Interactions between growth hormone–releasing hormone and glucocorticoids in male rats. Regul Pept 25:147–155, 1989.

191. Miell J, Corder R, Miell PJ, et al: Effects of glucocorticoid treatment and acute passive immunization with growth hormone–releasing hormone and somatostatin antibodies on endogenous and stimulated growth hormone secretion in the male rat. J Endocrinol 131:75–86, 1991.

192. Asa SL, Kovacs K, Stefaneanu L, et al: Pituitary mammosomatotroph adenomas develop in old mice transgenic for growth hormone–releasing hormone. Proc Soc Exp Biol Med 193:232–235, 1990.

193. Asa SL: The role of hypothalamic hormones in the pathogenesis of pituitary adenomas. Pathol Res Pract 187:581–583, 1991.

194. Cronin MJ, Burnier J, Clark RG: Growth hormone releasing hormone infusion in normal rats enlarges the pituitary within days. J Endocrinol Invest 14(1):34, 1991.

195. Horacek MJ, Campbell GT, Blake CA: Effects of growth hormone–releasing hormone on somatotrophs in anterior pituitary gland allografts in hypophysectomized, orchidectomized hamsters. Cell Tissue Res 253:287–290, 1988.

196. Accary JP, Dubrasquet M, Lehy T, et al: Growth hormone releasing hormone stimulates the release of gastrin in rat. Peptides 7 Suppl 1:241–243, 1986.

197. Hermansen K, Kappelgaard AM: Characterization of growth hormone releasing hormone stimulation of the endocrine pancreas: Studies with alpha- and beta-adrenergic and cholinergic antagonists. Acta Endocrinol (Copenh) 114:589–594, 1987.

198. Bailey CJ, Wilkes LC, Flatt PR, et al: Effects of growth hormone–releasing hormone on the secretion of islet hormones and on glucose homeostasis in lean and genetically obese-diabetic (ob/ob) mice and normal rats. J Endocrinol 123:19–24, 1989.

199. Green IC, Southern C, Ray K: Mechanism of action of growth hormone–releasing hormone in stimulating insulin secretion in vitro from isolated rat islets and dispersed islet cells. Horm Res 33:199–204, 1990.

200. Kentroti S, Vernadakis A: Growth hormone–releasing hormone influences neuronal expression in the developing chick brain. I. Catecholaminergic neurons. Brain Res 49:275–280, 1989.

201. Kentroti S, Vernadakis A: Growth hormone–releasing hormone and somatostatin influence neuronal expression in developing chick brain. II. Cholinergic neurons. Brain Res 51:297–303, 1990.

202. Mitsuma T, Nogimori T, Hirooka Y: Effects of growth hormone–releasing hormone and corticotropin-releasing hormone on the release of thyrotropin-releasing hormone from the rat hypothalamus in vitro. Exp Clin Endocrinol 90:365–368, 1987.

203. Imaki T, Shibasaki T, Hotta M, et al: The satiety effect of growth hormone-releasing factor in rats. Brain Res 340:186–188, 1985.

204. Dickson PR, Vaccarino FJ: Characterization of feeding behavior induced by central injection of GRF. Am J Physiol 259:651–657, 1990.

205. Vaccarino FJ, Bloom FE, Rivier J, et al: Stimulation of food intake in rats by centrally administered hypothalamic growth hormone–releasing factor. Nature 314:167–168, 1985.

206. Ruckebusch Y, Malbert CH: Stimulation and inhibition of food intake in sheep by centrally administered hypothalamic releasing factors. Life Sci 38:929–934, 1986.

207. Penny ES, Sopwith AM, Patience RL, et al: Characterization by high-performance liquid chromatography of circulating growth hormone–releasing factors in normal subjects. J Endocrinol 111:507–511, 1986.

208. Rosskamp R, Becker M, Haverkamp F, et al: Plasma levels of growth hormone-releasing hormone and somatostatin in response to a mixed meal and during sleep in children. Acta Endocrinol (Copenh) 116:549–554, 1987.

209. Penny ES, Penman E, Price J, et al: Circulating growth hormone releasing factor concentrations in normal subjects and patients with acromegaly. Br Med J (Clin Res) 289:453–455, 1984.

210. Frohman LA, Downs TR, Williams TC, et al: Rapid enzymatic degradation of growth hormone–releasing hormone by plasma in vitro

and in vivo to a biologically inactive product cleaved at the NH2 terminus. J Clin Invest 78:906–913, 1986.

211. Frohman LA, Downs TR, Williams TC, et al: Rapid enzymatic degradation of growth hormone-releasing hormone by plasma in vitro and in vivo to a biologically inactive product cleaved at the NH2 terminus. J Clin Endocrinol Metab 78:906–913, 1986.

212. Sasaki A, Sato S, Yumita S, et al: Multiple forms of immunoreactive growth hormone-releasing hormone in human plasma, hypothalamus, and tumor tissues. J Clin Endocrinol Metab 68:180–185, 1989.

213. Saito H, Saito S, Yamazaki R, et al: Clinical value of radioimmunoassay of plasma growth hormone–releasing factor (letter). Lancet 2:401–402, 1984.

214. Thorner MO, Frohman LA, Leong DA, et al: Extrahypothalamic growth-hormone-releasing factor (GRF) secretion is a rare cause of acromegaly: Plasma GRF levels in 177 acromegalic patients. J Clin Endocrinol Metab 59:846–849, 1984.

215. Kashio Y, Chihara K, Kaji H, et al: Presence of growth hormone–releasing factor-like immunoreactivity in human cerebrospinal fluid. J Clin Endocrinol Metab 60:396–398, 1985.

216. Argente J, Acquafredda A, Cavallo L, et al: Growth hormone-releasing hormone. Studies in cord blood from term human newborns. Biol Neonate 52:264–267, 1987.

217. Argente J, Evain-Brion D, Munoz-Villa A, et al: Relationship of plasma growth hormone–releasing hormone levels to pubertal changes. J Clin Endocrinol Metab 63:680–682, 1986.

218. Mitsuhashi S, Yamasaki R, Miyazaki S, et al: Effect of oral administration of L-dopa on the plasma levels of growth hormone-releasing hormone (GHRH) in normal subjects and patients with various endocrine and metabolic diseases. Nippon Naibunpi Gakkai Zasshi 63:934–946, 1987.

219. Chihara K, Kashio Y, Kita T, et al: L-dopa stimulates release of hypothalamic growth hormone–releasing hormone in humans. J Clin Endocrinol Metab 62:466–473, 1986.

220. Rosskamp R, Becker M, Tegeler A, et al: Effect of insulin-induced hypoglycemia on circulating levels of plasma growth hormone–releasing hormone and somatostatin in children. Horm Res 27:121–125, 1987.

221. Kashio Y, Chihara K, Kita T, et al: Effect of oral glucose administration on plasma growth hormone–releasing hormone (GHRH)-like immunoreactivity levels in normal subjects and patients with idiopathic GH deficiency: Evidence that GHRH is released not only from the hypothalamus but also from extrahypothalamic tissue. J Clin Endocrinol Metab 64:92–97, 1987.

222. Leppaluoto J, Tapanainen P, Knip M: Heat exposure elevates plasma immunoreactive growth hormone–releasing hormone levels in man. J Clin Endocrinol Metab 65:1035–1038, 1987.

223. Sano T, Asa SL, Kovacs K: Growth hormone–releasing hormone-producing tumors: Clinical, biochemical, and morphological manifestations (Review). Endocr Rev 9:357–373, 1988.

224. Sano T, Yamasaki R, Saito H, et al: Growth hormone–releasing hormone (GHRH)-secreting pancreatic tumor in a patient with multiple endocrine neoplasia type I. Am J Surg Pathol 11:810–819, 1987.

225. Asa SL, Singer W, Kovacs K, et al: Pancreatic endocrine tumour producing growth hormone–releasing hormone associated with multiple endocrine neoplasia type I syndrome. Acta Endocrinol 115:331–337, 1987.

226. Ramsay JA, Kovacs K, Asa SL, et al: Reversible sellar enlargement due to growth hormone–releasing hormone production by pancreatic endocrine tumors in an acromegalic patient with multiple endocrine neoplasia type I syndrome. Cancer 62:445–450, 1988.

227. Yamasaki R, Saito H, Sano T, et al: Ectopic growth hormone-releasing hormone (GHRH) syndrome in a case with multiple endocrine neoplasia type I. Endocrinol Jpn 35:97–109, 1988.

228. Asa SL, Scheithauer BW, Bilbao JM, et al: A case for hypothalamic acromegaly: a clinicopathological study of six patients with hypothalamic gangliocytomas producing growth hormone–releasing factor. J Clin Endocrinol Metab 58:796–803, 1984.

229. Bevan JS, Asa SL, Rossi ML, et al: Intrasellar gangliocytoma containing gastrin and growth hormone-releasing hormone associated with a growth hormone–secreting pituitary adenoma (see comments). Clin Endocrinol (Oxf) 30:213–224, 1989.

230. Donnadieu M, Evain-Brion D, Tonon MC, et al: Variations of plasma growth hormone (GH)–releasing factor levels during GH stimulation tests in children. J Clin Endocrinol Metab 60:1132–1134, 1985.

231. Argente J, Evain-Brion D, Donnadieu M, et al: Impaired response of growth hormone-releasing hormone (GHRH) measured in plasma after L-dopa stimulation in patients with idiopathic delayed puberty. Acta Paediatr Scand 76:266–270, 1987.

232. Foot AB, Davidson K, Edge JA, et al: The growth hormone releasing hormone (GHRH) response to a mixed meal is blunted in young adults with insulin-dependent diabetes mellitus whereas the somatostatin response is normal. Clin Endocrinol (Oxf) 32:177–183, 1990.

233. Thorner MO, Rivier J, Spiess J, et al: Human pancreatic growth hormone–releasing factor selectively stimulates growth hormone secretion in man. Lancet 1:24–28, 1983.

234. Wood SM, Ch'ng JL, Adams EF, et al: Abnormalities of growth hormone release in response to human pancreatic growth hormone releasing factor (GRF [1-44]) in acromegaly and hypopituitarism. Br Med J (Clin Res) 286:1687–1691, 1983.

235. Rosenthal SM, Schriock EA, Kaplan SL, et al: Synthetic human pancreas growth hormone-releasing factor (hpGRF1–44-NH2) stimulates growth hormone secretion in normal men. J Clin Endocrinol Metab 57:677–679, 1983.

236. Vance ML, Borges JL, Kaiser DL, et al: Human pancreatic tumor growth hormone-releasing factor: Dose-response relationships in normal man. J Clin Endocrinol Metab 58:838–844, 1984.

237. Gelato MC, Pescovitz OH, Cassorla F, et al: Dose-response relationships for the effects of growth hormone–releasing factor-(1-44)-NH2 in young adult men and women. J Clin Endocrinol Metab 59:197–201, 1984.

238. Sassolas G, Chatelain P, Cohen R, et al: Effects of human pancreatic tumor growth hormone-releasing hormone (hpGRH1-44-NH2) on immunoreactive and bioactive plasma growth hormone in normal young men. J Clin Endocrinol Metab 59:705–709, 1984.

239. Lang I, Schernthaner G, Pietschmann P, et al: Effects of sex and age on growth hormone response to growth hormone-releasing hormone in healthy individuals. J Clin Endocrinol Metab 65:535–540, 1987.

240. Evans WS, Borges JL, Vance ML, et al: Effects of human pancreatic growth hormone–releasing factor-40 on serum growth hormone, prolactin, luteinizing hormone, follicle–stimulating hormone, and somatomedin-C concentrations in normal women throughout the menstrual cycle. J Clin Endocrinol Metab 59:1006–1010, 1984.

241. Chihara K, Kashio Y, Abe H, et al: Idiopathic growth hormone (GH) deficiency, and GH deficiency secondary to hypothalamic germinoma: Effect of single and repeated administration of human GH-releasing factor (hGRF) on plasma GH level and endogenous hGRF-like immunoreactivity level in cerebrospinal fluid. J Clin Endocrinol Metab 60:269–278, 1985.

242. Gelato MC, Malozowski S, Nicoletti M, et al: Responses to growth hormone-releasing hormone (GHRH) during development and puberty in normal boys and girls. Symposium on recent developments in the study of growth factors: GRF and Somatomedin. Paris, 1985.

243. Smals AE, Pieters GF, Smals AG, et al: Sex difference in growth hormone response to growth hormone–releasing hormone between pubertal tall girls and boys. Acta Endocrinol 116:161–164, 1987.

244. Chatelain P, Alamercery Y, Blanchard J, et al: Growth hormone (GH) response to a single intravenous injection of synthetic GH-releasing hormone in prepubertal children with growth failure. J Clin Endocrinol Metab 65:387–394, 1987.

245. Ross RJ, Grossman A, Davies PS, et al: Stilboestrol pretreatment of children with short stature does not affect the growth hormone response to growth hormone–releasing hormone. Clin Endocrinol (Oxf) 27:155–161, 1987.

246. Hotta M, Shibasaki T, Masuda A, et al: The inter- and intra-subject variabilities of plasma GH response to human growth hormone–releasing hormone (1-44) NH2 in men. Endocrinol Jpn 32:673–680, 1985.

247. Grossman A, Lytras N, Savage MO, et al: Growth hormone releasing factor: Comparison of two analogues and demonstration of hypothalamic defect in growth hormone release after radiotherapy. Br Med J (Clin Res) 288:1785–1787, 1984.

248. Vance ML, Evans WS, Kaiser DL, et al: The effect of intravenous, subcutaneous, and intranasal GH-RH analog, [Nle27]GHRH(1-29)-NH2, on growth hormone secretion in normal men: Dose-response relationships. Clin Pharmacol Ther 40:627–633, 1986.

249. Aitman TJ, Rafferty B, Coy D, et al: Bioactivity of growth hormone releasing hormone (1-29) analogues after SC injection in man. Peptides 10:1–4, 1989.

250. Barron JL, Coy DH, Millar RP: Growth hormone responses to growth hormone-releasing hormone (1-29)-NH2 and a D-Ala2 analog in normal men. Peptides 6:575–577, 1985.

251. Borges JL, Blizzard RM, Gelato MC, et al: Effects of human pancreatic tumour growth hormone releasing factor on growth hormone and somatomedin C levels in patients with idiopathic growth hormone deficiency. Lancet 2:119–124, 1983.

252. Hashimoto K, Makino S, Hirasawa R, et al: Combined anterior pituitary function test using CRH, GRH, LH-RH, TRH and vasopressin in patients with non-functioning pituitary tumors. Acta Med Okayama 44:141–147, 1990.

253. Gelato MC, Oldfield E, Loriaux DL, et al: Pulsatile growth hormone secretion in patients with acromegaly and normal men: The effects of growth hormone–releasing hormone infusion. J Clin Endocrinol Metab 71:585–590, 1990.

254. Crosnier H, Brauner R, Rappaport R: Growth hormone response to growth hormone-releasing hormone as an index of growth hormone secretory dysfunction after prophylactic cranial irradiation for acute lymphoblastic leukemia. Acta Paediatr Scand 77:681–687, 1988.

255. Borges JL, Blizzard RM, Evans WS, et al: Stimulation of growth hormone (GH) and somatomedin C in idiopathic GH-deficient subjects by intermittent pulsatile administration of synthetic human pancreatic tumor GH-releasing factor. J Clin Endocrinol Metab 59:1–6, 1984.

256. Takano K, Hizuka N, Shizume K, et al: Plasma growth hormone (GH) response to GH-releasing factor in normal children with short stature and patients with pituitary dwarfism. J Clin Endocrinol Metab 58:236–241, 1984.

257. Schriock EA, Lustig RH, Rosenthal SM, et al: Effect of growth hormone (GH)-releasing hormone (GRH) on plasma GH in relation to magnitude and duration of GH deficiency in 26 children and adults with isolated GH deficiency or multiple pituitary hormone deficiencies: Evidence for hypothalamic GRH deficiency. J Clin Endocrinol Metab 58:1043–1049, 1984.

258. Rogol AD, Blizzard RM, Johanson AJ, et al: Growth hormone release in response to human pancreatic tumor growth hormone–releasing hormone-40 in children with short stature. J Clin Endocrinol Metab 59:580–586, 1984.

259. Laron Z, Keret R, Bauman B, et al: Differential diagnosis between hypothalamic and pituitary hGH deficiency with the aid of synthetic GH-RH 1-44. Clin Endocrinol (Oxf) 21:9–12, 1984.

260. Pintor C, Puggioni R, Fanni V, et al: Growth-hormone releasing factor and clonidine in children with constitutional growth delay. Evidence for defective pituitary growth hormone reserve. J Endocrinol Invest 7:253–256, 1984.

261. Lannering B, Albertsson Wikland K: Growth hormone release in children after cranial irradiation. Horm Res 27:13–22, 1987.

262. Cappa M, Loche S, Borrelli P, et al: Growth hormone response to growth hormone releasing hormone 1-40 in Turner's syndrome. Horm Res 27:1–6, 1987.

263. Bozzola M, Tato L, Cisternino M, et al: Synthetic growth hormone-releasing hormone (GHRH 1-44) in the differential diagnosis between hypothalamic and pituitary GH deficiency. J Endocrinol Invest 9:503–506, 1986.

264. Reiter JC, Craen M, van Vliet G: Decreased growth hormone response to growth hormone-releasing hormone in Turner's syndrome: Relation to body weight and adiposity. Acta Endocrinol (Copenh) 125:38–42, 1991.

265. Ranke MB, Gruhler M, Rosskamp R, et al: Testing with growth hormone-releasing factor (GRF[1-29]NH2) and somatomedin C measurements for the evaluation of growth hormone deficiency. Eur J Pediatr 145:485–492, 1986.

266. Sartorio A, Spada A, Conti A, et al: Effect of two consecutive administrations of GHRH in children with constitutional growth delay. Eur J Pediatr 149:678–679, 1990.

267. Takano K, Shizume K, Imura H, et al: Plasma growth hormone (GH) response to GH-releasing factor (SM-8144) in children of short stature and patients with GH deficiency. Endocrinol Jpn 34:117–128, 1987.

268. Shibasaki T, Shizume K, Masuda A, et al: Plasma growth hormone response to growth hormone–releasing factor in acromegalic patients. J Clin Endocrinol Metab 58:215–217, 1984.

269. Gelato MC, Merriam GR, Vance ML, et al: Effects of growth hormone–releasing factor on growth hormone secretion in acromegaly. J Clin Endocrinol Metab 60:251–257, 1985.

270. Chiodini PG, Liuzzi A, Dallabonzana D, et al: Changes in growth hormone (GH) secretion induced by human pancreatic GH releasing hormone-44 in acromegaly: A comparison with thyrotropin-releasing hormone and bromocriptine. J Clin Endocrinol Metab 60:48–52, 1985.

271. Smals AE, Pieters GF, Smals AG, et al: The higher the growth hormone response to growth hormone releasing hormone the lower the response to bromocriptine and thyrotrophin releasing hormone in acromegaly. Clin Endocrinol (Oxf) 27:43–47, 1987.

272. Losa M, Schopohl J, Stalla GK, et al: Growth hormone releasing

factor test in acromegaly: Comparison with other dynamic tests. Clin Endocrinol (Oxf) 23:99–109, 1985.

273. Lytras N, Grossman A, Wass JAH, et al: Growth hormone-releasing hormone test in patients with hypothalamic disease, Cushing's syndrome and acromegaly. 7th Internatl Congr Endocrinol, Quebec, Canada, Abstract 1444:1984.

274. Schulte HM, Benker G, Windeck R, et al: Failure to respond to growth hormone releasing hormone (GHRH) in acromegaly due to a GHRH secreting pancreatic tumor: dynamics of multiple endocrine testing. J Clin Endocrinol Metab 61:585–587, 1985.

275. Webb CB, Thominet JL, Frohman LA: Ectopic growth hormone releasing factor stimulates growth hormone release from human somatotroph adenomas in vitro. J Clin Endocrinol Metab 56:417–419, 1983.

276. Adams EF, Winslow CL, Mashiter K: Pancreatic growth hormone releasing factor stimulates growth hormone secretion by pituitary cells (letter). Lancet 1:1100–1101, 1983.

277. Daniels M, Turner SJ, Cook DB, et al: Effect of GRF 1-44, somatostatin and cycloheximide on GH secretion from human somatotropinomas in culture. 7th Internatl Congr Endocrinol, Quebec, Canada, Abstract 678:1984.

278. Lamberts SW, Verleun T, Oosterom R: The interrelationship between the effects of somatostatin and human pancreatic growth hormone–releasing factor on growth hormone release by cultured pituitary tumor cells from patients with acromegaly. J Clin Endocrinol Metab 58:250–254, 1984.

279. Casanueva FF, Burguera B, Tome MA, et al: Depending on the time of administration, dexamethasone potentiates or blocks growth hormone–releasing hormone–induced growth hormone release in man. Neuroendocrinology 47:46–49, 1988.

280. Nakagawa K, Akikawa K, Matsubara M, et al: Effect of dexamethasone on growth hormone (GH) response to growth. J Clin Endocrinol Metab 60:306–310, 1985.

281. Giustina A, Girelli A, Doga M, et al: Pyridostigmine blocks the inhibitory effect of glucocorticoids on growth hormone–releasing hormone stimulated growth hormone secretion in normal man. J Clin Endocrinol Metab 71:580–584, 1990.

282. Hotta M, Shibasaki T, Masuda A, et al: Effect of human growth hormone–releasing hormone on GH secretion in Cushing's syndrome and non-endocrine disease patients treated with glucocorticoids. Life Sci 42:979–984, 1988.

283. Shibasaki T, Hotta M, Masuda A, et al: Plasma GH responses to GHRH and insulin-induced hypoglycemia in man. J Clin Endocrinol Metab 60:1265–1267, 1985.

284. Sharp PS, Foley K, Chahal P, et al: The effect of plasma glucose on the growth hormone response to human pancreatic growth hormone releasing factor in normal subjects. Clin Endocrinol (Oxf) 20:497–501, 1984.

285. Press M, Tamborlane WV, Thorner MO, et al: Pituitary response to growth hormone–releasing factor in diabetes. Failure of glucose-mediated suppression. Diabetes 33:804–806, 1984.

286. Giampietro O, Ferdeghini M, Miccoli R, et al: Effect of growth hormone-releasing hormone and clonidine on growth hormone release in type 1 diabetic patients. Horm Metab Res 19:636–641, 1987.

287. Press M, Caprio S, Tamborlane WV, et al: Pituitary response to growth hormone releasing hormone in insulin-independent diabetes: Abnormal responses to insulin and hyperglycemia. Diabetes 41:17–21, 1992.

288. Williams T, Berelowitz M, Joffe SN, et al: Impaired growth hormone responses to growth hormone–releasing factor in obesity. A pituitary defect reversed with weight reduction. N Engl J Med 311:1403–1407, 1984.

289. Sheldon WR, Jr., DeBold CR, Evans WS, et al: Rapid sequential intravenous administration of four hypothalamic releasing hormones as a combined anterior pituitary function test in normal subjects. J Clin Endocrinol Metab 60:623–630, 1985.

290. Thorner MO, Reschke J, Chitwood J, et al: Acceleration of growth in two children treated with human growth hormone–releasing factor. N Engl J Med 312:4–9, 1985.

291. Thorner MO, Rogol AD, Blizzard RM, et al: Acceleration of growth rate in growth hormone-deficient children treated with human growth hormone–releasing hormone. Pediatr Res 24:145–151, 1988.

292. Low LCK, Wang C, Cheung PT, et al: Long term pulsatile growth hormone (GH)-releasing hormone therapy in children with GH deficiency. J Clin Endocrinol Metab 66:611–617, 1988.

293. Brain CE, Hindmarsh PC, Brook CG: Continuous subcutaneous

GHRH(1-29)NH2 promotes growth over 1 year in short, slowly growing children. Clin Endocrinol (Oxf) 32:153–163, 1990.

294. Low LCK: The therapeutic use of growth hormone–releasing hormone. J Pediatr Endocrinol 6:15–20, 1993.

295. Ross RJ, Rodda C, Tsagarakis S, et al: Treatment of growth-hormone deficiency with growth hormone–releasing hormone. Lancet 1:5–8, 1987.

296. Takano K, Hizuka N, Asakawa K, et al: Human growth hormone-releasing hormone (hGH-RH; hGRF) treatment of four patients with GH deficiency. Endocrinol Jpn 35:775–781, 1988.

297. Smith PJ, Brook CG: Growth hormone releasing hormone or growth hormone treatment in growth hormone insufficiency? Arch Dis Child 63:629–634, 1988.

298. Butenandt O, Staudt B: Comparison of growth hormone releasing hormone therapy and growth hormone therapy in growth hormone deficiency. Eur J Pediatr 148:393–395, 1989.

299. Duck SC, Schwarz HP, Costin G, et al: Subcutaneous growth hormone-releasing hormone therapy in growth hormone–deficient children: First year of therapy. J Clin Endocrinol Metab 75:1115–1120, 1992.

300. Rochiccioli PE, Tauber MT, Coude FX, et al: Results of 1-year growth hormone (GH)-releasing hormone (1-44) treatment on growth, somatomedin C, and 24-hour GH secretion in six children with partial GH deficiency. J Clin Endocrinol Metab 65:268–274, 1987.

301. Bozzola M, Biscaldi I, Cisternino M, et al: Long term growth hormone (GH)-releasing hormone and biosynthetic Gh therapy in GH-deficient children: Comparison of therapeutic effectiveness. J Endocrinol Invest 13:236–239, 1990.

302. Romer TE, Rymkiewicz-Kluczynska B, Olivier M, et al: Growth hormone–releasing hormone reverses secondary somatotroph unresponsiveness. J Clin Endocrinol Metab 72:503–506, 1991.

303. Lievre M, Chatelain P, van Vliet G, et al: Treatment with growth hormone–releasing hormone (GHRH) 1-44 in children with idiopathic growth hormone deficiency: A randomized double-blind dose-effect study. Fundam Clin Pharmacol 6:359–366, 1992.

304. Wit JM, Otten BJ, Waelkens JJ, et al: Short-term effect on growth of two doses of GRF 1-44 in children with growth hormone deficiency: Comparison with growth induced by methionyl-GH administration. Horm Res 27:181–189, 1987.

305. Smith PJ, Brook CG: The place of intravenous GHRH 1-40 studies in the therapy of growth hormone–deficient children with GHRH. Clin Endocrinol (Oxf) 27:97–105, 1987.

306. Evans WS, Borges JL, Kaiser DL, et al: Intranasal administration of human pancreatic tumor GH-releasing factor 40 stimulates GH release in normal men. J Clin Endocrinol Metab 57:1081–1083, 1983.

307. Evans WS, Vance ML, Kaiser DL, et al: Effects of intravenous, subcutaneous, and intranasal administration of growth hormone (GH)-releasing hormone 40 on serum GH concentrations in normal men. J Clin Endocrinol Metab 61:846–850, 1985.

308. Bowers CY, Momany FA, Reynolds GA, et al: On the in vitro and in vivo activity of a new synthetic hexapeptide that acts on the pituitary to specifically release growth hormone. Endocrinology 114:1537–1545, 1984.

309. Croom WJ, Leonard ES, Baker PK, et al: The effects of synthetic growth hormone releasing hexapeptide BI 679 on serum growth hormone levels and production in lactating dairy cattle. J Dairy Sci 67:109, 1984.

310. Malozowski S, Hao EH, Ren SG, et al: Growth hormone (GH) responses to the hexapeptide GH-releasing peptide and GH-releasing hormone (GHRH) in the Cynomolgus macaque: Evidence for non-GHRH-mediated responses. J Clin Endocrinol Metab 73:314–317, 1991.

311. Clark RG, Carlsson LMS, Trojnar J, et al: The effects of a growth hormone–releasing peptide and growth hormone–releasing factor in conscious and anaesthetized rats. J Neuroendocrinol 1:249–255, 1989.

312. Bowers CY, Reynolds GA, Durham D, et al: Growth hormone (GH)-releasing peptide stimulates GH release in normal men and acts synergistically with GH-releasing hormone. J Clin Endocrinol Metab 70:975–982, 1990.

313. Hartman ML, Farello G, Pezzoli SS, et al: Oral administration of growth hormone (GH)-releasing peptide (GHRP) stimulates GH secretion in normal men. J Clin Endocrinol Metab 74:1378–1384, 1992.

314. Smith RG, Cheng K, Schoen WR, et al: A non-peptidyl growth hormone secretagogue. Science 260:1640–1643, 1993.

19

Growth Hormone, Insulin-Like Growth Factors, and Acromegaly

WILLIAM H. DAUGHADAY

GROWTH HORMONE (GH)

Structure of GH-Related Peptides

Human growth hormone (hGH) is a single-chain peptide of 191 amino acids with two intramolecular S−S bonds which is devoid of carbohydrate substituents (Fig. 19–1). About 10 per cent of the hGH in the pituitary has a molecular weight of 20 kDa rather than 22 kDa. This smaller variant GH is missing amino acid residues 32 to 46 of the 22-kDa form.[1] As discussed later, this variant arises from aberrant processing of GH mRNA precursor. Pituitary extracts and serum contain even smaller concentrations of other GH peptides.[2] A "big" GH, twice the size of hGH, represents an interchain disulfide dimer rather than a precursor form of the hormone. Even larger nondissociable aggregates of hGH, "big-big" GH, are described. GH derivatives have been isolated in which there is enzymatic cleavage of the large peptide loop between amino acids 139 and 140. In some assay systems such molecules have enhanced growth-promoting activity and decreased diabetogenic activity. However, little evidence indicates that these two-chain molecules contribute significantly to GH action in vivo. Deamidation of the GH molecule gives rise to additional heterogeneity of electrophoretic migration.

The human placenta secretes a unique GH (GH-V) that differs from pituitary GH in 13 of its 191 amino acids.[3, 4] In addition, this GH is present in a 25-kDa glycated form.[5]

Supported by grant (2P01HD20805) of the National Institutes of Child Health and Human Development.

The concentration of GH-V in serum rises progressively during pregnancy.[6, 7]

GH is related structurally to human chorionic somatomammotropin (hCS), a peptide secreted in large amounts by the placenta. hCS, like hGH, contains 191 amino acids, of which 161 are in positions identical to those present in hGH.[8] The positions of the intramolecular S−S bonds are comparable in hGH and hCS. All of these structural similarities indicate a relatively recent evolutionary derivation from a common precursor molecule. Because hCS is closer to hGH in primary structure than to other mammalian CS's, a simple derivation of hCS from a common mammalian CS precursor is impossible (Fig. 19–2). Either primate CS arose by a new duplication of the primate GH gene, or there has been interchange of large portions of the primate GH gene with a pre-existing CS-type gene. Despite these molecular similarities, hCS has only 0.1 per cent the growth-promoting potency of hGH.

Prolactin (PRL) is a more distant member of the growth hormone family. It has 199 amino acids and an additional S−S intramolecular bond. Only 16 per cent of the amino acids of PRL are in positions identical to those of hGH.

The GH Gene

Members of the hGH gene family are present as a linear array on the long arm of chromosome 17 (Fig. 19–3).[9, 10] The gene for pituitary GH (GH-N) is followed in the 3′ direction by a pseudogene with similarities to the genes for CS. Next in sequence is the first of two genes for CS-A, followed by the gene for the placental variant GH (GH-V), and finally the second CS gene (CS-B). Both CS genes are expressed in the placenta, and the translation products

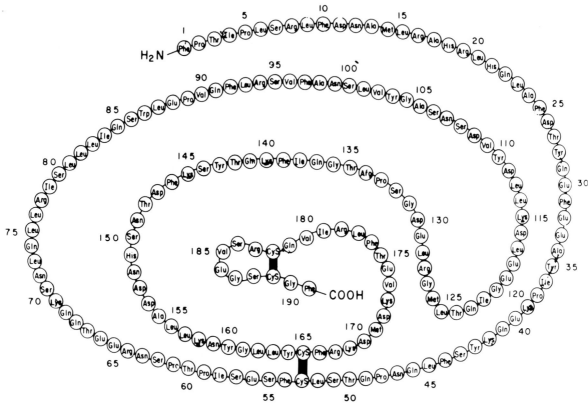

FIGURE 19–1. **Covalent structure of hGH.** (Reprinted with permission from Chawla RK, Parks JS, Rudman D: Structural variants of human growth hormone: Biochemical, genetic and clinical aspects. Ann Rev Med 34:519–547, 1983. Copyright 1983 by Annual Reviews Inc.)

differ at only one amino acid position in the signal peptide. The individual genes of the GH family share a similar basic structure of five introns separated by four exons (Fig. 19–3). Alternative splicing of intron 3 of the GH-N gene oc-

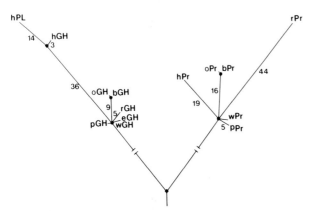

FIGURE 19–2. **Evolutionary tree for the growth hormone–prolactin family.** Branch lengths are accepted point mutations per 100 residues. GH, growth hormone; bGH, bovine (ox) GH; oGH, ovine (sheep) GH; pGH, porcine (pig) GH; eGH, equine (horse) GH; rGH, rat GH; wGH, sei whale GH; hGH, human GH; hPL, human placental lactogen; Pr, prolactin; bPR, bovine Pr; oPr, ovine Pr; pPr, porcine Pr; rPr, rat Pr; wPr, fin whale prolactin; hPr, human prolactin. Solid circles are points of divergence of one or more species. Branch lengths leading to oGH, eGH, wGH, pGH, oPH, oPr, bPr, and wPr are 1.0, 0.3, 3.4, 0, 1.8, 1.0, 0, and 3.4, respectively. (Reprinted with permission from Wallis M: The molecular evolution of pituitary growth hormone, prolactin and placental lactogen. A protein family showing variable rates of evolution. J Mol Evol 17:10–18, 1981. Copyright Springer-Verlag, 1981.)

curs in about 10 per cent of the primary transcripts and gives rise to 20-kDa GH. Although the GH-V gene has a similar intron 3 structure, alternative splicing at this site rarely if ever occurs.

The expression of the GH-N gene is limited almost exclusively to the somatotrope cells of the anterior pituitary, but recently low levels of expression of the GH-N gene have been recognized in monocytes.[11] The restricted expression of the GH gene in somatotroph cells is determined by two promoter sites just 5′ to a TATA box.[12] A specific transcription factor, GHF-1 (sometimes called Pit-1), is expressed in the differentiation of somatotroph cells and permits low levels of expression of the GH-N gene. GHF-1 is a member of a family of homeodomain transcription factors found in organisms as remote as *Drosophila* and yeast. Occupancy of two sites of the GH promoter by GHF-1 allows synergistic interaction with a number of secondary activator sites, including those for the glucocorticoid receptor and the cAMP-induced transcription factor that mediates the action of the GH-releasing factor (GRF). In rodents the thyroid hormone response element is a major determinant of GH gene expression, and hypothyroidism in this species results in virtual disappearance of GH mRNA and peptide from the pituitary.

Little is known about the regulation of expression of the genes of the GH family in the placenta. Rat Pit-1 binds only to a single distal site of the hGH-V gene and a single proximal site of the hCS-B gene.[13] Other differences in the transcription-regulating factors of the placenta must exist.

Repetitive, highly homologous nucleotide sequences in the different members of the GH gene family increase the

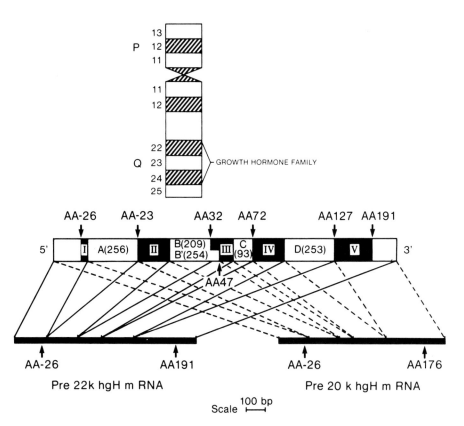

FIGURE 19–3. *Top*, Representative of the pattern of chromosome 17 under standard staining techniques. The dark and light bands are given numbers outward from the centromere to facilitate identification. The GH gene family is located on the long arm, designated q, somewhere within the region of bands 22 to 24. *Bottom*, Theoretical representation of the hGH gene and the mRNA from it. The hGH gene contains three introns: intron A between amino acids (AA) 24 and 25, intron B between AA 31 and 32, and intron C between AA 71 and 72. These are excised when the gene is transcribed into the mRNA for the 22-kDa hGH. Also shown is the alternative splicing transcribed into the mRNA of 20-kDa hGH. (Reprinted with permission from Chawla RK, Parks JS, Rudman D: Structural variants of human growth hormone: Biochemical, genetic and clinical aspects. Ann Rev Med 34:519–547, 1983. Copyright 1983 by Annual Reviews Inc.)

risk of unequal recombination with subsequent gene deletion. Homozygous deletions of the GH gene occur in some cases of severe isolated GH deficiency.[14] Such individuals are very short and lack immunodetectable GH in their serum. Many such children make an initial excellent growth response when treated with hGH but subsequently develop high titers of GH antibodies and cease to respond to GH treatment.

Unequal recombination has also led to large deletions with loss of the CS-A, GH-V, and CS-B genes.[15] When this large deletion is homozygous in the fetal genome, the maternal serum lacks both of these placental hormones. The fact that fetal development proceeds normally and delivery is uncomplicated indicates that these hormones are not essential for fetal survival. More detailed studies might detect metabolic deviations in the mother or fetus from the lack of these hormones.

Regulation of GH Secretion

For a more complete discussion, see Chapters 17 and 18.

Hypophysiotropic Hormone Regulation

The secretion of GH is regulated by the balance between a GH-releasing hormone (GRH), also known as somatocrinin, and a GH release–inhibitory factor, somatostatin (SS). The complete GRH peptide has 44 amino acids, but forms lacking the terminal 4 and 7 amino acids have been isolated and are active. The N-terminal domain of the GRH molecule contains the active site, because nearly complete biological activity is retained by the 29-N terminal amino

acids. GRH-containing cells are located primarily in the arcuate nucleus of the hypothalamus, with axonic processes terminating in the median eminence (ME). GRH acts selectively on the somatotroph cells to secrete GH by a cAMP-mediated mechanism. It also stimulates GH mRNA translation and transcription after more prolonged exposure to somatotroph cells.

SS was originally recognized in hypothalamic extracts by its ability to inhibit GH secretion by isolated rat pituitaries. The predominant form of SS in the hypothalamus has 14 amino acids. SS neuron cell bodies are concentrated in the anterior periventricular region of the hypothalamus close to the ependymal lining. Axons from these neurons lead to the ME. Although these SS tracts are most important in regulating GH secretion, other SS cells are found throughout the CNS and gastrointestinal tract, including pancreatic islets. In many of these locations the principal SS has 28 amino acids. The somatotroph cell has a single type of high-affinity SS receptor. SS is capable of blocking GH secretion provoked by a wide variety of secretagogues.

Both GRH and SS are involved in the negative feedback induced by GH on its own secretion. Intraventricular injection of small quantities of GH inhibits pulsatile GH secretion in the rat, an effect that appears to be mediated by stimulating SS secretion. GH can also stimulate SS production by hypothalamic fragments in vitro.

GH inhibits its own secretion by a second pathway. Insulin-like growth factor I (IGF I) is a GH-dependent peptide that mediates many of the growth-promoting actions of GH. IGF I alone or in combination with IGF II can act directly on the hypothalamus to promote the secretion of SS and, in primary cultures of rat pituitaries, can inhibit the ability of GRH to stimulate GH secretion.

Neurotransmitter Substances

For more complete coverage, see Chapters 8 and 18 and for diagnostic tests see Chapter 31.

Many stimuli of GH secretion, including exercise, hypoglycemia, arginine, and L-dopa, act through an α-adrenergic mechanism and are inhibited by the α-adrenergic receptor blocker phentolamine and potentiated by the β-blocker propranolol. L-Dopa is first converted to dopamine and subsequently to norepinephrine. The efficacy of phentolamine in blocking L-dopa action suggests that dopamine itself has little importance compared with norepinephrine in promoting GH secretion. Clonidine, a central α-agonist, is also a potent stimulus for GH secretion. Serotonin may also be important in regulating GH secretion. Impairment of serotonin synthesis by p-chlorophenylalanine suppresses GH secretion in the rat, and administration of 5-OH tryptophan, a serotonin precursor, can increase GH secretion.

Other neurotransmitters and neuromodulators such as cholecystokinin, vasoinhibitory peptide, opioid peptides, and acetylcholine can also modify GH secretion. These various factors appear to affect the secretion of SS and GRH rather than acting directly on somatotroph cells.

Physiological Secretion

GH secretion by the fetal pituitary is established by the end of the first trimester, and levels of GH in fetal serum thereafter are markedly elevated.[16] GH concentrations are high in cord serum and in serum of premature compared with full-term infants. The high concentrations of GH in fetal serum have been attributed to a delay in maturation of the SS system of somatotroph regulation.

GH secretion is characterized by brief surges followed by secretory inactivity. Under basal conditions, serum GH concentration of normal adults is less than 1 μg/L.[17] The surges of secretion occur at three- to five-hour intervals, with the greatest surge in young individuals occurring 60 to 90 minutes after the onset of deep sleep (Fig. 19–4). Sleep deprivation aborts or greatly reduces the expected GH surge.

The episodic pattern of GH secretion makes the estimation of mean GH concentration of a patient impossible with a single blood specimen. Investigators have resorted to continuous sampling or intermittent sampling at frequent intervals to estimate mean GH concentration. The results of one such study in boys before and during puberty and in young men is shown in Table 19–1.[18] A modest rise in pulse amplitude and mean GH concentration occurs in late puberty. Studies of older men have established a progressive fall in mean GH concentration. Similar studies of mean GH concentration in women have shown a small but statistically significant higher concentration than in men of the same age. Because of differences in the sensitivity and specificity of various radioimmunoassays, results from different studies may differ.

Estimates can be made of total daily GH secretion of boys going through puberty and of young men. These are based on older measurements of the volume of distribution of injected GH (80 ml/kg) and the metabolic clearance rate of GH (30 ml/kg/min).[19] In prepubertal boys the

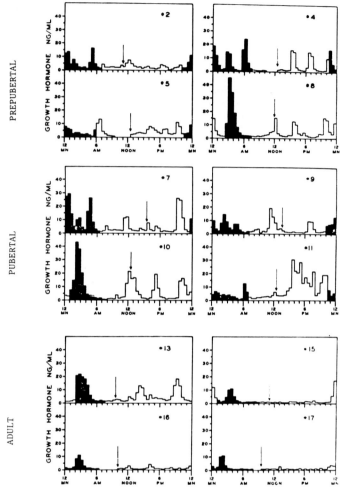

FIGURE 19–4. Circadian pattern of serum GH concentrations. The top four patterns were obtained in studies on prepubertal children; the center four patterns were from pubertal children; and the bottom four patterns were from adult subjects. Samples obtained during sleep are shown in solid black. (Reprinted with permission from Plotnick LP, Thompson RC, Kowarski A, et al: Circadian variation of integrated concentration of growth hormone in children and adults. J Clin Endocrinol Metab 40:240–247, 1975. Copyright by the Endocrine Society.)

estimated GH secretory rate is about 30 μg/kg/24 h, rises to 60 μg/kg/24 h during late puberty, and subsequently falls to about 20 μg/kg/24 h in young adults. For a 70-kg young man, this predicts a pituitary secretion of GH of about 1.2 mg/day. Although these calculations are based on a number of assumptions, they do provide an approximation of the daily secretion.

GH secretion is modified by several nutrients. Acute hypoglycemia regularly provokes GH secretion 30 to 45 minutes after the glucose nadir. In some experiments with normal subjects, lowering fasting plasma glucose by 10 to 15 mg/dl may suffice to provoke GH secretion. Despite the regular GH response to hypoglycemia, the insulin antagonism of a GH peak is delayed for several hours. Thus, GH is less important than glucagon and catecholamines in counteracting the acute effects of hypoglycemia. In slowly developing hypoglycemia, adrenergic arousal and increased GH secretion may not occur. Glucose administration inhibits the GH responses to physical and psychological stress as well as to L-dopa and certain other

TABLE 19–1. CHARACTERISTICS OF GH SECRETION IN CHILDREN AT VARIOUS STAGES OF PUBERTY AND YOUNG ADULTS

	Pre-	Early	Late	Post	Adult
Age (years)	9.0 ± 0.3	11.5 ± 0.2	14.4 ± 0.2	16.4 ± 0.4	23.0 ± 0.6
24-hour GH concentration (μg/L)	6.7 ± 1.0	4.7 ± 0.7	$13.8 \pm 2.4*$	4.4 ± 0.9	3.9 ± 0.5
GH pulse amplitude (μg/L)	14.4 ± 1.3	12.8 ± 1.3	$22.4 \pm 2.8*$	14.7 ± 3.9	10.3 ± 1.3
GH pulse per 24 hours	$8.8 \pm 0.7*$	7.0 ± 0.5	$7.8 \pm 0.6*$	6.6 ± 0.6	6.1 ± 0.5
GH secretion (μg/kg/24 h)†	29	20	60	19	17

Data from Martha PM Jr, Gorman KM, Blizzard RM, et al: Endogenous growth hormone secretion and clearance rates in normal boys, as determined by deconvolutional analysis: Relationship to age, pubertal status, and body mass. J Clin Endocrinol Metab 74:336, 1992, © by the Endocrine Society.
*Values that are statistically greater than unmarked values.
†Estimated GH secretion based on volume of distribution and metabolic clearance rate of GH (Owens et al[19]).

pharmacological stimuli. Glucose administration does not abort the sleep-related GH surge.

GH secretion is stimulated by a high-protein meal and by the oral or intravenous administration of several amino acids, most notably arginine and leucine.[20] The intravenous administration of arginine in a dose of 0.5 g/kg over 30 minutes provides a useful clinical provocative test of GH secretion. GH secretion can also be modulated by fatty acids. Conditions that raise serum free fatty acids inhibit GH secretion, and conditions that lower serum free fatty acids potentiate GH secretion. Obese patients have suppressed spontaneous and induced GH secretory peaks. It is not known to what extent alterations in plasma free fatty acids contribute to this GH suppression in obese patients.

GH Receptors

Progress in understanding the action of primate GH lagged behind that of the GH's of the principal large farm animals. GH prepared from such species was fully potent in stimulating the growth of laboratory animals but was virtually inactive when injected into humans and other primates. This was attributed to impurities present in early nonprimate GH preparations or to the development of immune resistance. The critical observations of Knobil and Greep[21] established the restricted species specificity of primate GH responsiveness. In a series of beautiful experiments, they established that both monkey and beef GH were fully active in laboratory rats, but only monkey GH was potent in affecting carbohydrate and protein metabolism of monkeys. This clearly established a restricted specificity of the primate response mechanism. At that time the concept of hormone receptors was rudimentary and the authors speculated that "effector sites for growth hormone action are more selective in primates than they are in the rat in terms of the time-honored lock and key concept."

The next major advance in our understanding of the human GH receptor (GH-R) resulted from studies of membrane binding made possible by labeling GH with radioactive iodine. It was found that membranes prepared from human liver[22] and human lymphoid (IM-9) cells[23] had many specific binding sites for labeled hGH. This binding was inhibitable by unlabeled hGH, but not by GH's of nonprimate species. In contrast, membranes from rat livers specifically bound labeled hGH equally to bovine GH and rat GH. It was evident from these studies that modifications of both the lock and key have occurred in primate evolution, but evolution of the lock (receptor) was critical in determining primate GH specificity.

Primary Structure

Despite the restricted binding specificity of the human GH-R cited above, the primary structure of the GH-R differs little from that of nonprimate species.[24] The cloning of the GH-R cDNA was accomplished by screening rabbit and human liver cDNA libraries using an oligonucleotide probe synthesized from the known N-terminal amino acid sequence of the isolated rabbit GH-R and binding protein. Both rabbit and human cDNA receptor clones contain an open reading frame specifying a 638-amino acid protein. After a signal peptide of 18 amino acids, there are 620 amino acids in the mature molecule with a formula weight of 70 kDa. The rabbit and human GH-R proteins have 84 per cent amino acid identity. Both proteins consist of an extracellular domain of 247 amino acids, a transmembrane domain of 24 amino acids, and an intracellular domain of 397 amino acids. The extracellular domain contains five possible glycosylation sites, and glycosylation of these sites in the mature molecule increases apparent size of electrophoretic gels from 95 kDa to about 130 kDa.

The intracellular domain of the human GH-R has no recognizable protein phosphokinase sequences, but there are reports of an associated protein tyrosine kinase (in the cell membrane), which is activated by ligand occupancy of the extracellular GH-binding site of the receptor.[25] The GH-R in the cell membrane may also be closely associated with ubiquitin, a protein involved in the degradation of other cellular proteins. This association may account for the short half-life of the GH-R on the cell membrane, which in rat liver is estimated to be less than one hour.

The binding site for GH on the human GH-R has been identified by systematically substituting alanine residues for charged residues in the extracellular domain of the GH-R by site-directed mutagenesis of the cDNA and expression in *Escherichia coli*.[26] Figure 19–5 shows that the critical residues for GH binding lie at the tips of seven strands of an immunoglobulin-like portion of the GH-R.[27] The basis of specificity of the human GH-R for hGH is not clarified by this analysis. Of the 29 amino acids recognized as critical for GH binding by the human GH-R, the bovine GH-R has 19 identical residues, 2 positions are deleted, and only 8 positions are nonidentical. Moreover, these 8 amino acids are not unique for the human GH-R but are found in other mammalian GH's. The basis of the specificity of the human GH-R must reside in subtle changes of the GH-R molecule.

Two regions of the GH molecule which react with the GH-R have been defined by alanine substitution of charged amino acids. The loci of substitution which markedly decrease binding of the isoform to the GH-R are scattered over much of the primary amino acid sequence. When these sites are shown on a representation of structure of the GH molecule derived from x-ray crystallography, the active site is discretely localized on the surface of the molecule (Fig. 19–6).

In addition to the primary site on the GH molecule that reacts with the receptor, a second site binds to the receptor. In experiments with recombinantly synthesized fragments of the GH-R representing the extracellular domain, two molecules of this extracellular receptor domain reacted with a single GH molecule.[27, 28] Site one has the highest affinity for hGH and binds first. When the first site is occupied, a second site is exposed for binding by a second GH-R. This site, as deduced from mutagenesis results, occupies a separate aspect of the GH molecule (Fig. 19–6). These observations suggest that dimerization of two GH-R's may be required for full biological activity of GH. Although dimerization of other receptors is well known, this is the first example of dimerization induced by a single hormonal ligand.

hGH differs from nonprimate GH's in having high affinity for the prolactin receptor and possessing high lactogenic potency. The affinity for the prolactin receptor, but not for the GH-R, is zinc dependent.[29, 30] Zinc ion induces dimerization of GH, which is the active ligand for the prolactin receptor. Zinc binding, dimer formation, and affinity for the prolactin receptor were all reduced by substituting Ala for His[18], His[21], and Glu[174] of the hGH molecule.

The amino acid sequence of placental GH (GH-V) differs from hGH in only 13 residues. It has full affinity for GH receptors but has much reduced affinity for the PRL receptors.[31] This may be explained in part by the substitu-

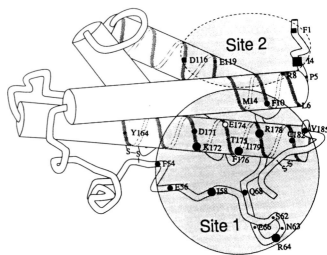

FIGURE 19–6. **Probable location of two sites reactive with the GH-R projected on a model of the GH structure.** The cylinders represent four predominantly helical domains. Alanine substitutions in hGH that disrupt binding of hGHbp at either site 1 or site 2 are generally delineated by the large shaded circles. Residues for which alanine mutants reduce site 2 binding by two- to four-fold, four- to ten-fold, 10- to 50-fold, and more than 50-fold are shown by graduated squares (■, ■, ■, and ■, respectively). Residues marked by the symbols •, ●, ●, and ○ represent sites where Ala mutations in site 1 of hGH cause reductions of two- to four-fold, four- to ten-fold, greater than 10-fold, or a four-fold increase in binding affinity for the hGHbp, respectively, using the MAb 5 immunoprecipitation assay. (Reprinted from Cunningham BC, Ultsch M, de Vos AM, et al: Dimerization of the extracellular domain of the human growth hormone receptor: Crystal structure of the complex. Science 254:821–825, with permission of the American Association for the Advancement of Science.)

tion of Arg for His[18] and Tyr for His[21]. These substitutions greatly reduce the ability of GH-V to form dimers.

The GH-R and the PRL receptor are both members of a large superfamily of cytokine receptors.[32] Other members of this superfamily include receptors for interleukin (IL)-2, IL-3, IL-4, IL-6, IL-7, erythropoietin, and granulocyte/monocyte colony stimulating factor. The structural features of the superfamily are indicated in Figure 19–7. All are glycosylated single-chain proteins with an amino-terminal extracellular domain with four conserved cysteine residues. An exception is the IL-7 receptor, which has only two cysteines. All but the GH-R have a Trp-Ser-X-Trp-Ser sequence near the transmembrane domain whose significance is not yet known.

Regulation

The distribution of GH-R's has been studied most completely in the rat by radioligand binding and by detection of receptor mRNA. Evidence for receptors has been found in many tissues, with the highest concentrations of rat GH-R mRNA in liver, heart, kidney, intestine, and muscle.[38] Marked changes in the concentration of GH-R's occur during development. Rat liver receptor concentrations are very low at birth, but receptor number increases progressively during the first 10 weeks of life.

Direct measurements of GH-R number or mRNA during human development are scanty, but indirect evidence of a similar pattern is provided by measurement of serum GH-binding protein (GH-BP).[39–41] Cord serum from premature infants has very little GH-BP. This is increased at birth and

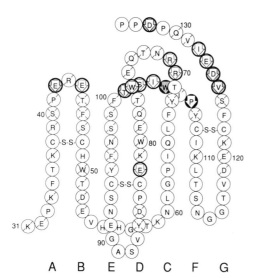

FIGURE 19–5. **Probable location of the GH-binding site of the GH-R in the cysteine-rich part of the extracellular domain.** Residues in the hGHbp causing a two-fold or greater effect upon binding to hGH mapped upon an immunoglobulin-like folding diagram predicted for the cysteine-rich domain. Seven antiparallel β-strands (A-G) compose a β-sandwich by folding the G strand around the back until it hydrogen binds to the A strand. Residues causing less than a two-fold reduction (Ⓚ), a two- to four-fold reduction (Ⓡ), a four- to ten-fold reduction (Ⓖ), a 10- to 100-fold reduction (Ⓕ), and greater than 100-fold reduction (Ⓦ) in binding are indicated. Residues that gave low expression yields are indicated by (Ⓕ). (Reprinted with permission from Bass SH, Mulkerrin MG, Wells JA: A systematic mutational analysis of hormone-binding determinants in the human growth hormone receptor. Proc Natl Acad Sci USA 88:4498, 1991.)

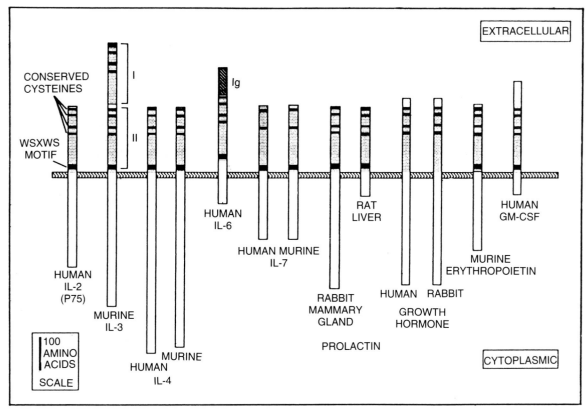

FIGURE 19–7. **The hematopoietin receptor superfamily.** Schematic representations of the structures of all the known members of the family are shown. Horizontal bars represent conserved cysteine residues. The black boxes represent the conserved Trp-Ser-X-Trp-Ser (WSXWS) motif. The stippled areas show the stretch of ~210 amino acids within which the receptor homologies are contained. The immunoglobulin-like domain at the N-terminus of the IL-6 receptor is also indicated. (Reprinted with permission from Casman D, Lyman SD, Idzerda RL, et al: A new cytokine receptor superfamily. Trends Biochem Sci 15:265–270, 1990.)

rises progressively during childhood to reach adult levels at about 20 years (Fig. 19–8). The developmental pattern of the GH-R concentration correlates well with the known GH independence of fetal growth. The rise in the hepatic GH-R concentration coincides with the progressive increase of serum IGF I concentration during the period of childhood growth. The limiting determinant of hepatic IGF I synthesis and secretion may not be the GH concentration per se, but the presence of hepatic GH-R's. The

widespread tissue distribution of GH-R's indicates that GH effects are not restricted to liver.

In the hepatocyte, only a small fraction of the total receptor concentration is found in the plasma membrane, and the remainder is present in Golgi and endoplasmic membranes. Hepatic GH-R's have a rapid turnover, and the intracellular receptors are at various stages of post-translational processing and in transit to the cell membrane. The turnover of GH-R's is probably acutely in-

FIGURE 19–8. **Measurements of GH-binding protein (GHBP) in premature and term cord-serum and sera from children and adults of various ages.** Binding is compared with reference serum from a young adult woman. (Reprinted with permission from Daughaday WH, Trivedi B, Andrews BA: The ontogeny of serum GH binding protein in man: A possible indicator of hepatic GH receptor development. J Clin Endocrinol Metab 65:1072–1074, 1987. © by the Endocrine Society, 1987.)

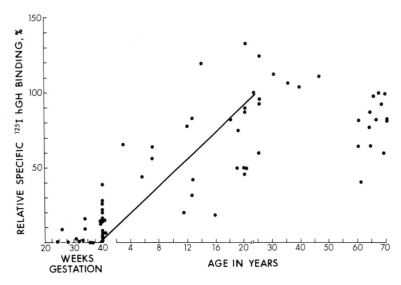

creased by a bolus injection of GH, leading to a transient down-regulation of GH-R number. More prolonged exposure to GH has usually resulted in an increase in hepatic GH-R concentration in experimental animals. The concentration of hepatic GH-R's in hypophysectomized rats is reduced and rises with GH treatment. In rats and rabbits pregnancy leads to a marked increase in hepatic GH-R's. In humans, the increase in serum GH in acromegaly and GH-V in pregnancy results in little change in serum GH-BP. In experimental diabetes and malnutrition, hepatic GH-R's are reduced. Insulin treatment of diabetic rats promptly restores GH-R number to normal.

GH-Binding Protein (GH-BP)

It was first recognized that rabbit serum contains a specific GH-BP[33] and later established that the rabbit GH-BP consists of the extracellular domain of the GH-R. Human GH-BP is a single-chain glycoprotein with a molecular weight of about 60 kDa.[34, 35] It has three disulfide bridges forming small loops. The hGH-BP binds hGH with high affinity (3 to 9 $\times$ 10^8 L/mol) and with specificity for primate GH. Human prolactin has approximately 10 per cent of the affinity of hGH for GH-BP, and hCS has about 0.1 per cent of the affinity of hGH.

Normal adult plasma GH-BP has a binding capacity of 59 $\pm$ 2 nmol/L, and 25 to 35 per cent of plasma GH is bound by GH-BP at physiological GH concentrations. Considerable evidence exists that GH-BP inhibits access of the hormone to tissue receptors. The importance of this role in total GH disappearance kinetics is not clear. Binding of GH by GH-BP is reversible, which permits transfer of GH to GH-R's of tissues. The $T_{1/2}$ of hGH after bolus injection or stopping sustained infusions of GH is about 20 to 30 minutes, which is not very different from that of other nonglycosylated peptide hormones of this size.

Although the identity of structure of GH-BP and the extracellular domain of the GH-R is clearly established, the mechanism of formation of GH-BP remains uncertain. Rats and mice have similar GH-BP's in their serum that arise from truncated GH-R mRNA's lacking a hydrophobic transmembrane domain.[36] A similar truncated form of the GH-R mRNA has not been found in human liver. Some insight into the process of GH-BP release is provided by IM-9 human lymphoid cells.[37] These cells, rich in GH-R's, can be induced to shed their surface GH-R's very rapidly after exposure to reducing agents such as iodoacetamide and N-ethylmaleimide. The shedding of GH-BP by these cells appears to result from activation of a plasma membrane–associated endopeptidase.

The source of plasma GH-BP is not known with certainty, but because liver has by far the highest concentration of GH-R's, it is generally held that it is the major contributor to plasma GH-BP. In general, there has been a good correlation between the concentration of membrane-bound GH-R's and the concentration of plasma GH-BP in a number of species. In humans, the concentration of GH-R's in ethically accessible tissues is too low for accurate measurement, but serum GH-BP can be reliably estimated by a number of methods of separating bound from unbound [^{125}I]hGH, including conventional gel filtration, fast protein liquid exclusion chomatography, and immunoprecipi-

tation. Clinical investigators have used these methods as indirect indices of GH-R changes in normal and abnormal growth, as discussed below.

GH-Receptor Signal Transduction

After GH is bound to specific sites on the extracellular domain of the GH-R, a conformational change results, which transmits a signal across the plasma membrane and activates the cytoplasmic domain to initiate intracellular biochemical processes. Despite considerable research, little is known about how these processes work. The cytoplasmic domain of the GH-R lacks the recognizable tyrosine kinase motifs present in the insulin and IGF I receptors. It has been observed, however, that tyrosines in the cytoplasmic domain of the GH-R of several cell types are rapidly phosphorylated after exposure to GH.[42] Moreover, GH-R's that have been isolated by immunoprecipitation have an associated tyrosine kinase molecule. Therefore, an attractive hypothesis is that the activated GH-R in turn activates an associated tyrosine kinase, which results in tyrosine phosphorylation of the receptor and perhaps other key compounds. The significance of the phosphorylation of the GH-R itself is equally murky because it apparently lacks intrinsic kinase activity.

Activation of protein kinase C occurs early in several cell types after exposure to GH. In mouse preadipocytes this leads to expression of the c-fos, and c-jun and jun-B oncogenes in fetal mouse calvarial osteoblasts.[43, 44] Information about the participation of phospholipase C in mediating early actions of GH is unclear. Within minutes after the exposure of mouse osteoblasts diacyl glycerol[43] accumulates, and basal lateral membranes of canine renal proximal tubular cells treated with GH have a prompt increase in the release of both diacylglycerol and inositol triphosphate.[45] In contrast, insulin induction of phospholipase C reportedly is blocked by prior GH treatment in adipose tissue of ob/ob mice.[46]

Direct Actions of GH

The effects of GH on tissues are exerted both directly and by the mediation of IGF's. Most of the effects of GH on the liver are direct because after fetal life the liver is rich in GH-R's and has a few Type 1 IGF-R's. After GH administration there is the early increase in synthesis of 8 to 10 proteins. Among the proteins destined for export are IGF I, α_2 microglobulin,[47] and the serine protease inhibitors Spi 2.1 and Spi 2.3.[48] A nuclear transcription factor induced by GH regulates the increased expression of the Spi 2.1 gene. Ornithine decarboxylase is a cytosolic protein whose gene expression is increased markedly by GH. This enzyme is responsible for polyamine synthesis, which may regulate aspects of cell proliferation.

GH affects gene expression in many cell types. The increased expression of c-fos in the mouse osteoblasts mentioned above is of interest because it reaches a maximum within 30 minutes.[44] In contrast, the increase in expression of the IGF I gene in the same cell was significant only after 6 hours and reached a maximum at 48 hours. In the rat hepatocyte, the increase in expression of the P-450$_{15\beta}$, IGF

I, and GH-R genes is greatly augmented by the simultaneous presence of GH, insulin, IGF I, and T_3.[49] The regulation of GH gene expression appears complex and requires considerable study.

We now recognize that many nonhepatic tissues have GH-R's that mediate direct rapid metabolic actions such as the promotion of glucose and amino acid transport in muscle and fat and the stimulation of lipolysis in fat and muscle. GH also stimulates IGF I gene expression in a number of extrahepatic tissues. Local production of IGF I can contribute to cell multiplication and differentiated functions by autocrine/paracrine actions. Distinguishing between direct and indirect actions of GH in these tissues is difficult and in experimental systems usually requires the demonstration that the GH effect is not blocked by antibodies raised against IGF I or the Type 1 IGF-R.

The overall actions of GH are most clearly recognized after the administration of GH to GH-deficient children. There is a prompt resumption of skeletal, muscular, and visceral growth. This is reflected in a prompt stimulation of protein anabolism with a diversion of amino acids from oxidation to protein synthesis, which leads to a markedly positive nitrogen balance. Concomitant with these changes is a promotion of lipolysis in adipose tissue and in muscle. This action of GH leads to a loss of subcutaneous fat in young children with GH deficiency, who tend to have a cherubic plumpness before treatment. At the same time there are changes in glucose metabolism with a decrease in the sensitivity to insulin, which leads to an increase in the insulin response to glucose ingestion. These changes may be mediated in part by an increase in free fatty acids in serum and in muscle. If there is an inherited or acquired limitation of insulin secretion, impaired glucose tolerance and diabetes may result.

GH exerts effects on mineral metabolism. Associated with protein anabolism, there is retention of intracellular potassium, magnesium, and phosphate. Sodium is retained without significant changes in aldosterone secretion. Hypercalciuria without hypercalcemia occurs during the early weeks of GH administration. Because this is associated with increase in intestinal absorption of calcium, positive calcium balance is maintained. GH administration has several effects on the kidney. It promotes 1-hydroxylation of 25-hydroxyvitamin D, increases glomerular filtration, and increases the reabsorption of phosphate by the proximal renal tubule. GH increases the synthesis of extracellular matrix. This can be documented by measuring the rise in urinary hydroxyproline. In GH excess there is accumulation of hyaluronate and chondroitin sulfate sufficient to be recognized as facial and acral puffiness. This brief synopsis does not exhaust the biological effects of GH. Additional effects of GH in humans on bone, heart, liver, intestine, and other organs have been documented.

Disorders of GH Receptors

Patients with the Laron syndrome have the clinical features of severe GH deficiency, but circulating GH is markedly elevated and serum levels of IGF I are markedly reduced.[50] These patients fail to respond to administered GH. Many of these patients come from consanguineous parents and have affected siblings, indicative of a recessive

mode of inheritance. Most cases of the Laron syndrome have occurred in Asiatic Jews, but a clustering of cases has recently been recognized in an inbred population in Ecuador.[51] In two affected subjects, defective [^{125}I]hGH binding was demonstrated in membranes obtained by liver biopsy.[52] The condition now is readily diagnosed by showing that the level of serum GH-BP is markedly decreased or absent.[53, 54]

A number of molecular defects have been recognized in the GH-R gene of patients with the Laron syndrome. These include deletions of exons 3, 5, and 6, which code for the extracellular domain of the GH-R,[55] and two nonsense mutations that lead to premature termination of the intracellular domain of the GH-R.[56] In one family, a mutation resulted in substitution of phenylalanine by serine in position 96 of the GH-R.[56] Although phenylalanine in this position is conserved in many receptors of the cytokine family, it does not affect the ability of this receptor to bind hGH. Recent transfection studies have explained this apparent contradiction.[57] COS-7 monkey kidney cells, which lack GH-R's, were transfected with normal GH-R cDNA. The transfected cells expressed GH-R's on their plasma membrane. When, however, cDNA of the [Ser^{96}]GH-R mutant was transfected into COS-7 cells, there was no GH-R on plasma membrane, but intracellular GH-R was increased by immunofluorescence and membranes recovered from lysosomal vesicles contained GH-R's. These results suggest that the mutant GH-R's fail to follow the correct intracellular transport pathway.

A more subtle abnormality of the GH-R occurs in African pygmies, an ethnic group whose adult stature reaches only 132 to 146 cm.[41] The adults have normal GH secretion but reduced serum concentrations of IGF I. Figure 19–9 shows the progressive rise in serum GH-BP in children with normal stature. In pygmies, however, the progressive rise does not occur. Serum GH-BP levels in young pygmies were not remarkably low but failed to rise as childhood progressed.

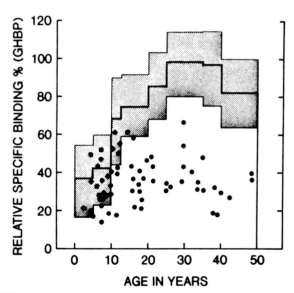

FIGURE 19–9. **Measurement of relative GH-binding protein (GHBP) activity** in normal children and African pygmies as a function of age. (Reprinted from Merimee TJ, Bauman G, Daughaday WH: Growth hormone–binding protein: II. Studies in pygmies and normal statured subjects. J Clin Endocrinol Metab 71:1183–1188, © by the Endocrine Society, 1990.)

These results suggest that the GH-R is normal, but its developmental regulation is impaired. This accounts for failure of serum IGF I to have the expected pubertal rise and the fact that growth deficit increases as childhood progresses.

INSULIN-LIKE GROWTH FACTORS (IGF's)

Many of the growth-promoting actions of GH are not exerted directly but rather through the intermediate actions of peptides called somatomedins. This was first recognized because cartilage from a hypophysectomized rat had a marked anabolic response (recognized as the incorporation of [35S]-sulfate into chondroitin sulfate) when GH is given in vivo.[58] When GH was added to cartilage explants in vitro, with or without hypophysectomized rat serum, little anabolic response occurred. When, however, sera from normal rats and GH-treated hypophysectomized rats were added in vitro, a marked stimulation of sulfate uptake occurred. The anabolic agent was present in peptide fractions of plasma extracts. These experiments suggested an endocrine pathway of somatomedin action. Subsequent research has established that somatomedins can be produced in many tissues and can also act in an autocrine/paracrine mode. This is discussed more fully below.

IGF Structure

As the result of extensive extraction and purification efforts, Rinderknecht and Humbel in 1978 isolated two peptides from human plasma with insulin-like and somatomedin-like actions.[59, 60] Because the primary amino sequence of these two peptides resembles proinsulin, the peptides were identified as insulin-like growth factor I and II (IGF I and IGF II), and the structural domains of the peptide were named according to the convention for proinsulin (Fig. 19–10). Human IGF I is a single-chain, basic peptide with 70 amino acids, and IGF II is a slightly acidic peptide of 67 amino acids. The domain homologous to the C-peptide of proinsulin is much shorter in the IGF's and consists of only 12 amino acids, which remain in the fully processed peptides. The IGF's have carboxyl extension (D domain) of 8 amino acids for IGF I and 6 amino acids for IGF II. The structures of IGF I and IGF II are highly conserved in mammals and birds. In the case of IGF I, this has also been extended to amphibians (*Xenopus*) and teleosts (salmon) (for a review see ref. 61).

The primary translation product of IGF I mRNA includes a signal peptide of 48 amino acids and one of two possible carboxyl extensions (Fig. 19–11). Both E domains have a common sequence of 16 amino acids. The IGF IA prohormone contains an additional 19 amino acids and the IGF IIB contains an additional 61 nonhomologous amino acids.

The primary translation product of human IGF II includes a 24-amino acid signal peptide and an 89-amino acid E domain. A variant form of IGF II arising from alternative splicing of exon 8 results in substitution of Arg-Leu-Pro-Gly for serine 29. This variant may compose as much as 15 per cent of the circulating IGF II.[62]

IGF Genes and mRNA's

The human IGF I gene occupies 80 kilobases (Kb) with six exons and is found on chromosome 12. The coding sequences for the mature peptide are found on exons 3 and 4. Alternative splicing of exons 5 and 6 give rise to prepro IGF IA and IGF IB, respectively. Because two alternative initiation sites in the gene are present on exons 1 and 2, mRNA species of 7.6 Kb, 1.1 Kb, and 1.3 Kb are found in different proportions in various tissues.

The IGF II gene is found on chromosome 11 in close

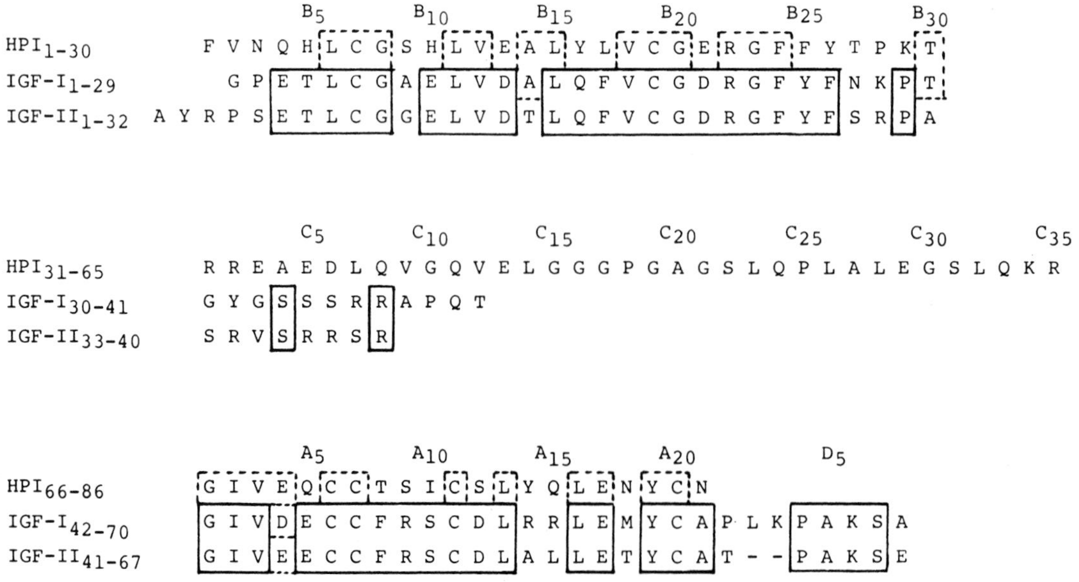

FIGURE 19–10. **Comparison of the primary structures of human proinsulin (HPI), IGF I, and IGF II.** The portion of the molecules related to insulin B chain is shown on the top, the proinsulin C-peptide is shown in the middle. The identities between IGF I and II are enclosed in solid boxes. Identities between proinsulin and one or both IGF's are enclosed in the broken line. (Reprinted with permission from Rinderknecht E, Humbel RE: Primary structure of human insulin-like growth factor II. FEBS Lett 89:283–286, 1978. Copyright Elsevier.)

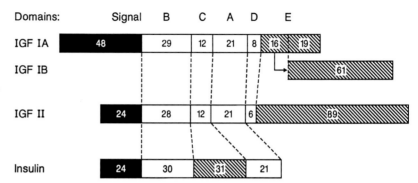

FIGURE 19–11. Comparison of the amino acid number in the separate domains of the pre-pro forms of IGF IA, IGF IB, IGF II, and insulin.

proximity to the insulin gene and contains nine exons. Because there are four alternate promoters and two polyadenylation sites, a great variety of sizes of IGF II mRNA's (6.0, 5.3, 5.0, 4.8, 2.2, and 1.8 Kb) have been recognized which have tissue- and age-specific expression. It is not known if these mRNA's are all translated. For reviews, see references 61 and 63.

Both IGF I and IGF II mRNA species are expressed in many tissues of human fetuses of 16 to 20 weeks' gestation (Fig. 19–12).[64] The concentration of IGF II mRNA is much higher than that of IGF I mRNA in liver, intestine, adrenal, skin, kidney, and pancreas. The concentration of IGF I mRNA in fetal rat liver is lower than in most other tissues, whereas in the adult liver, it is much higher. In the rat, expression of the IGF II gene is primarily a fetal phenomenon, and soon after birth the level of mRNA falls and is virtually undetectable in most adult rat tissues except the choroid plexus. In the adult human the IGF II gene continues to be expressed in the liver in high concentrations and in other tissues in lower concentrations. The concentration of IGF I and IGF II peptides in human fetal tissues does not accurately reflect the concentration of mRNA observed.[65] This may mean that there is variable translation of the different mRNA species.

IGF-Binding Proteins

IGF's circulate in association with multiple specific binding proteins (IGFBP).[66] Four principal IGFBP's are present in human plasma (Table 19–2). About three quarters of the IGF I and II of human plasma are present as a ternary complex of 150 kDa consisting of IGF peptide bound to a 53-kDa glycosylated binding protein (IGFBP-3) and a second glycosylated, acid labile subunit of 85 kDa[67] (Fig. 19–13). The concentration of IGFBP-3 is GH dependent and approximates that of IGF I plus IGF II. Once IGFBP-3 binds to IGF I or II, an allosteric change occurs in IGFBP-3 so that it becomes reactive with an acid labile protein, the α subunit. As the α subunit is always present in excess, the reaction is driven toward complex formation. It is likely that IGF I and IGF II dissociate from IGFBP-3 only after IGFBP-3 dissociates from the α subunit. The ternary complex provides a circulating reserve pool of IGF's which is not directly available to tissues. Evidence suggests that the half-time of disappearance of the ternary complex from the circulation may be as long as 12 hours. The sources of plasma IGFBP-3 and α subunit are not known with certainty, although the liver is probably a major contributor. Because the concentration of IGFBP-3 is regulated primar-

ily by IGF availability, its measurement in the plasma provides an indirect indication of the GH status of the subject which may be diagnostic in pituitary dwarfism.

IGFBP-2 is a nonglycosylated BP of 33 kDa which is present in serum in the second highest concentration and is

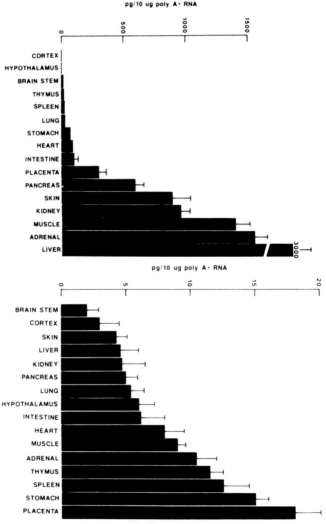

FIGURE 19–12. **Abundance of IGF IA mRNA** (*above*) **and IGF II mRNA** (*below*) in various tissues from 16- to 20-week human fetuses. Measurements were made by densitometry of dot blots. (Reprinted from Han VKM, Lund PK, Lee DC, D'Ercole AJ: Expression of somatomedin/insulin-like growth factor messenger ribonucleic acid in the human fetus: Identification, characterization, and tissue distribution. J Clin Endocrinol Metab 66:422–429, © by the Endocrine Society, 1988.)

of the Type I receptor. Multiple phosphorylations of the β chain greatly activate the intrinsic tyrosine kinase activity. Insulin receptor substrate-1 (IRS-1) is phosphorylated rapidly and may be an important intracellular mediator of both insulin and IGF I action.[86] A number of incompletely characterized intracellular proteins are rapidly phosphorylated, leading to separate response mechanisms by largely unknown pathways.

The Type II IGF-R is a bifunctional molecule that consists of a single chain whose amino acid sequence predicts a molecular weight of 270,000.[87] The extracellular portion of this receptor is large and contains 15 repeated homologous segments. A transmembrane domain is followed by a relatively short intracellular domain. The extracellular portion of the Type II receptor has a binding site for IGF II and multiple sites for mannose-6-phosphate containing glycoproteins. The Type II IGF-R has high affinity for IGF II, much reduced affinity for IGF I, and virtually no affinity for insulin. The mannose-6-phosphate sites have an important intracellular role in directing certain hydrolytic enzymes to lysozymes. The intracellular signal transduction system of the Type II receptor appears to differ from that of the Type I receptor. In a reconstituted system, the Type II receptor was coupled with G-protein activation.[88]

The internalization of the Type II receptor, particularly when occupied by IGF II, is extremely rapid, and one postulated role of the receptor is to promote IGF II degradation. The importance of the Type II receptor in mediating cell responses appears to be limited. There are reports that IGF II stimulates glycogen synthesis in a hepatoma cell line[89] and calcium flux and thymidine uptake in mouse fibroblasts through this receptor[90] and promotes motility of rhabdomyosarcoma cells.[91]

Actions of IGF

Endocrine and Autocrine/Paracrine

The hypothesis that GH acts indirectly on cartilage by the mediation of a hormonal factor was based on the observation that GH added to cartilage segments of hypophysectomized rats does not significantly stimulate mitosis and matrix formation. The relative inactivity of GH has been confirmed with embryo-chick cartilage, porcine cartilage, rabbit cartilage, and human cartilage. These observations suggest that GH acts on an extraskeletal target, presumably the liver, to increase IGF I synthesis and release. IGF I reaches the skeletal target via the circulation and acts as an endocrine factor.

In conflict with this view, much evidence now indicates that GH does have direct actions on growth cartilage (for a review, see ref. 92). Local exposure of the epiphyseal growth cartilage to GH by local infusion or by unilateral femoral artery infusion increases the ipsilateral growth of cartilage. This effect of GH is mediated by IGF I because it can be blocked by antiserum directed against IGF I.[93] It is also known that growth cartilage contains GH-R's, and GH in vivo and in vitro results in an increase in cartilage IGF I gene expression and IGF I release, which acts locally in an autocrine/paracrine mode.

These two opposing views of IGF I action have provoked controversy. In the author's opinion, both modes of IGF I action are required for full restitution of cartilage growth in the hypophysectomized animal.[94] The direct action of GH on growth cartilage is real but small in magnitude and must be supplemented by IGF I reaching the cartilage from the circulation. A unique GH requirement for the clonal expansion and differentiation of primary cultures of prechondrocytes isolated from rat tibial epiphyseal plates has been proposed (Fig. 19–16).[95]

Cellular Effects

The past 35 years has seen extensive study of the effects of somatomedins on isolated tissues and cell lines. A great variety of normal cell types of ectodermal, endodermal, and mesenchymal origin require high concentrations of insulin for thymidine uptake and propagation. In most cases insulin can be replaced by IGF I in more physiological concentrations. Many neoplastic cells depend on IGF I

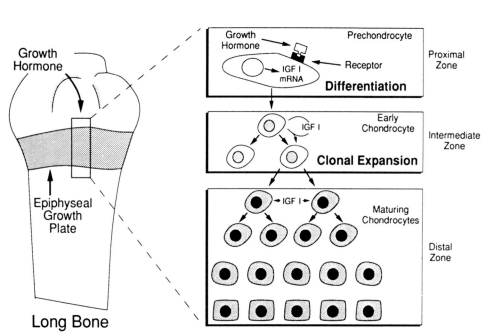

FIGURE 19–16. The proposed sequential dependence of GH for proliferation and differentiation of prechondrocytes and the subsequent IGF I dependence of early chondrocytes and maturing chondrocytes. (Modified from Isaksson OGP, Isgaard J, Nilsson A, et al: Direct action of growth hormone. *In* Bercu BB (ed): Basic and Clinical Aspects of Growth Hormone. New York, Plenum, 1988, pp 199–211.)

for propagation in vitro,[81] but other tumor cell lines exhibit insulin and IGF-independent growth but no longer grow in the presence of IGF I or IGF I receptor antibodies. This is evidence that these cells are producing their own IGF's, which act in an autocrine/paracrine manner. In other cases the mitogenic action of another hormone is mediated by inducing the local synthesis of IGF's. For example, TSH stimulation of thyroid (FRTL-5) cell proliferation is greatly augmented by local production of IGF II.[96]

Despite the abundant evidence that IGF's stimulate mitogenesis in many cell types, including fibroblasts, preadipocytes, and premyocytes,[97–99] it may not be able to stimulate mitogenesis without the prior action of a competence factor such as platelet-derived growth factor or fibroblast growth factor. GH may have such an initiation action on prechondrocytes.[84]

IGF's can promote the differentiation of several cell types by stimulating the synthesis of specific proteins. They promote expression of the myogenin gene in differentiating myoblasts,[100] the synthesis and secretion of collagen and chondroitin sulfate in chondrocytes, and the elongation and synthesis of delta crystallin in chick embryo lens epithelial cells.[101]

IGF I can also synergize with other hormones. Granulosa cells of the rat ovary cannot divide. When exposed to IGF I alone, they show little increase in progesterone and estrogen synthesis. A limited response follows exposure to FSH, but when IGF I and FSH are both added to cultures of granulosa cells, a marked increase in progesterone and estrogen synthesis results.[102]

The above responses to IGF's require time to develop. IGF's also have rapid metabolic effects in fibroblasts such as stimulation of the uptake of the model amino acid, α-aminoisobutyric acid, and glucose. Acute metabolic effects are also induced in myocytes and adipocytes.

In Vivo Effects of IGF I

ACUTE EFFECTS. Studies of the in vivo effects of IGF I and IGF II were retarded by the limited supply of the peptides isolated from human plasma. The number of experiments that could be done and their duration were greatly restricted. This situation has now changed owing to advances in molecular biology, which have permitted studies of the excessive secretion of IGF I in transgenic mice and the production of recombinant IGF I and IGF II.

Hypoglycemia followed the bolus intravenous injection of 13 nmol/kg of IGF I in human volunteers, but in this study IGF I had one thirteenth the potency of insulin.[103] In another study human volunteers who received subcutaneous injections of 15.6 nmol/kg also experienced hypoglycemia.[104] When normal volunteers received a continuous infusion of IGF I given at rates of 0.91, 1.82, and 2.73 nmol/kg/h, plasma glucose levels were maintained but serum insulin and C-peptide concentrations fell.[105] This may reflect an inhibitory action of IGF I on insulin secretion. GH secretion was also inhibited by negative feedback on the hypothalamus.

Despite the similarity of actions of IGF I and insulin on glucose metabolism, important differences exist. Both insulin and IGF I stimulate peripheral utilization of glucose, but in both rats[106] and dogs[107] IGF I has little or no ability to inhibit hepatic glucose release. This is consistent with

the differences in receptor population of the two peptides. The liver is richly endowed with insulin receptors but has few IGF I receptors. Human volunteers receiving IGF I infusions during a glucose clamp demonstrated inhibition of hepatic glucose release, probably as a result of inhibition of glucagon secretion.[108] The hypoglycemic action of IGF I is mediated by the Type 1 IGF-R rather than cross-over binding to the insulin receptor. These observations suggest that IGF I may be of clinical use in the control of hyperglycemia in insulin-resistant patients. Preliminary results are encouraging in the treatment of three patients with acanthosis nigricans and insulin resistance[109] and in one insulin-resistant patient with the Mendenhall syndrome.[110]

In addition to these effects on glucose metabolism, other metabolic changes were found in young volunteers receiving 9.8 nmol/kg and 11.6 nmol/kg of IGF I as a bolus.[111] Little change occurred in plasma free fatty acids after IGF I, but a 70 per cent fall occurred after insulin. This difference in response is again attributable to the paucity of IGF I receptors in human adipose tissue. IGF I suppressed plasma leucine concentration without increasing leucine oxidation. The nonoxidative leucine disappearance was also unchanged, which suggested to the investigators that IGF I was inhibiting body protein breakdown.

The few studies of IGF II effects in vivo have shown that it exhibited the same general effects as IGF I, but its potency was reduced.

EFFECTS ON GROWTH. The ability of IGF I to stimulate skeletal growth was first established by implanting osmopumps in hypophysectomized rats, which delivered 100 or 200 μg/day of plasma-derived IGF I.[112] After 10 days there was an increase in the width of the tibial epiphyseal cartilage plate.

The growth-promoting effects of IGF I have also been observed in mice transgenic for the human IGF I gene. In one study the IGF I transgene was expressed in the liver and many other tissues.[113] After six months body weight increased about 40 per cent in male and 80 per cent in female transgenic mice over that of appropriate control mice. The relative increase in the weights of brain, spleen, and pancreas exceeded the overall increase in weight. Despite these positive results, no increase in skeletal growth was noted.

A much more convincing demonstration of the growth-promoting effects of IGF I transgene was found in mice made hyposomatotropic by diphtheria toxin selectively targeted to the somatotrope cells.[114] When the hIGF I gene was introduced in such mice, the serum IGF I was raised from the very low levels characteristic of the hyposomatotropism to levels that were 60 per cent greater than in normal control mice. Gain of both body weight and skeletal size of the transgenic mice was observed. Again in these animals there was a disproportionate gain in brain weight. It is clear from these animal studies that IGF I can restore growth in the absence of GH.

Long-term clinical studies with IGF I are in progress. IGF I administration has little role in the treatment of hypopituitary dwarfism unless high levels of antibodies to hGH are present. IGF I should be effective for those patients who have GH resistance attributable to abnormal GH receptors (Laron syndrome). A patient with the Laron syndrome has already been shown to have appropriate acute metabolic responses to IGF I administration,[115] and there has been a preliminary announcement that IGF I can stimulate growth in patients with the Laron syndrome.[116] IGF I in a dose of 150 μg/kg given as a single daily subcutaneous injection to five children with Laron syndrome for three to five months resulted in very significant increases in growth velocity. These studies indicate that GH action on prechondrocytes is not required for IGF I promotion of sustained skeletal growth.

HYPERSOMATOTROPISM

Increased secretion of GH occurs physiologically during normal development, in compensation for conditions associated with resistance to GH action, and in primary hypersecretion of GH and GRF.

Physiological

Physiological hypersecretion of GH is present in both the human fetus and the mother in pregnancy. Beginning late in the first trimester, fetal serum GH rises to levels that in adults would lead to acromegaly, yet fetal growth does not depend on GH until the very last weeks of gestation. Fetal GH reaches a peak of about 100 μg/L (5 nmol/L) by the end of the second trimester and thereafter falls progressively to term.[16] This fetal GH hypersecretion may be attributable in part to a delay in maturation of the hypothalamic regulation of somatotrope secretion. Also, the low levels of IGF I in fetal serum may not effectively inhibit GH secretion.

Hypersecretion of GH occurs also in the mother beginning early in pregnancy but arises from the placenta by the expression of the GH variant gene (discussed above). The levels reached late in pregnancy are about 20 to 30 μg/L by radioimmunoassay and even higher by specific radioreceptor assay.[6, 7] Placental secretion of GH shuts off pituitary GH secretion. By most assays, serum IGF I concentrations are elevated but usually not to the degree found in acromegaly.[7] Subtle changes indicative of facial and acral growth may be observed in pregnant women.

Puberty is another period of physiological increase of GH secretion. Although quantitation is difficult, mean serum GH levels in puberty may double with a similar rise in serum IGF I (see Table 19–1).[18] Sex hormones contribute to the marked acceleration of growth that occurs at puberty. If this degree of elevation of GH and IGF I did not abate, pathological growth would result. The hormonal changes in puberty make it difficult to distinguish normal from pathological growth at this age.

A compensatory increase in GH secretion commonly occurs in a number of conditions of GH resistance. The most dramatic example exists in the Laron syndrome, a condition associated with defective GH-R's.[117] Serum GH levels in this condition are markedly elevated and fluctuate wildly, particularly in children. The ability of the liver to respond to GH with IGF I synthesis depends on normal nutrition. Increased GH secretion often is found in cirrhosis, malnutrition, uncontrolled diabetes, and some wasting diseases. Despite elevations of GH, serum IGF I levels are usually reduced, and confusion with primary GH excess seldom arises.

In primary hypersomatotropism the normal negative feedback mechanisms of IGF I and GH acting on the hypothalamic-pituitary unit are upset but may not be absent. Many acromegalics respond to arginine and glucose with increased secretion of GH by mechanisms that must include hypophysiotropic hormones. In clinical acromegaly serum GH measurements may vary considerably from hour to hour, and the mean of multiple samples is required to establish the degree of elevation. Administration of 75 g of glucose by mouth lowers normal serum GH to less than 2 μg/L and prevents misinterpreting physiological surges of GH secretion as pathological. It should be remembered that many GH radioimmunoassays are not specific for active GH at this level, and two-site immunoassays are preferable.[17] The mean GH levels of patients with clinical acromegaly vary from barely elevated (around 5 μg/L) to more than 500 μg/L with a median level of about 30 μg/L.

The measurement of serum IGF I is very useful in the evaluation of patients whose mean GH concentration is minimally elevated because serum IGF I concentrations appear to be a function of the logarithm of the GH concentration (Fig. 19–15).[75] In adults a rise in serum IGF I is evident when the mean serum GH increases above 4 to 5 μg/L. Figure 19–15 also indicates that the increases in serum IGF I reach a maximum with serum GH levels of 60 to 100 μg/L.

In the past there was great interest in studying the GH secretory responses of patients with acromegaly to the administration of thyrotropin-releasing hormone (TRH), gonadotropin-releasing hormone, L-dopa, and glucose.[118] These responses indicate alterations in secretory regulation but are inconsistent and of little diagnostic importance. The persistence of an abnormal response to TRH after transsphenoidal adenomectomy suggests an incomplete operation and increased likelihood of recurrence. The practical usefulness of TRH and other provocative testing is not generally accepted.

Pituitary and Extrapituitary Causes

GH-secreting pituitary tumors account for the vast majority of cases of acromegaly. Although macroadenomas were present in about 90 per cent of the cases from surgical clinics in the past, patients are now diagnosed earlier in their disease and microadenomas now represent an increasing fraction of cases, 33 per cent in one series.[119] There is a tendency for microadenomas to be found in the lateral wings of the adenohypophysis. Many macroadenomas are locally invasive, but true carcinomas are very rarely found.

GH-secreting adenomas have been classified on the basis of immunostaining of their secretory granules, cytological characteristics, and in vitro secretion of hormones.[120] Somatotroph adenomas contain GH granules with no immunohistochemical evidence of other hormones. Plurihormonal adenomas contain granules with immunohistochemical evidence of other pituitary hormones in addition to GH. PRL is the most common companion of GH. If both GH and PRL immunoreactivity reside within the same tumor cell, it is called a mammosomatotroph adenoma. In mixed somatotroph-lactotroph adenomas, GH and PRL are found in separate cells. Relatively undifferentiated, poorly granulated tumors with both GH and PRL immunoactivity are called acidophil stem cell adenomas. Infrequently, immunocytological evidence of thyrotropin and gonadotropins may be detected in GH-secreting tumors or in medium conditioned by such tumors maintained in primary culture. Rarely, pituitary tumors that can secrete GH exist outside the sella in the sphenoid sinus and parapharyngeal tissue.

Clonality and Mutations in Somatotroph Adenomas

Many have speculated that pituitary adenomas might arise from hyperplasia resulting from prolonged stimulation by hypophysiotropic releasing factors. Against such a mechanism commonly occurring in acromegaly is the finding that somatotroph cells in the normal pituitary remnant appear to be suppressed and successful adenomectomy restores normal function. Strong evidence exists from X-chromosome inactivation analysis that pituitary tumors arise from clonal expansion of a single mutant cell line.[121, 122] Restriction length polymorphisms are known for two genes on the X-chromosome specifying hypoxanthine phosphoribosyl transferase and phosphoglycerate kinase. X-chromosome analysis is possible when normal cells are heterozygous for one or both of the polymorphic genes. Genes that occur on the inactive X-chromosome are methylated, which makes them resistant to methylation-sensitive enzymes. It is therefore possible to distinguish whether one or both X-chromosome alleles are expressed in a tumor. This analysis has now been conducted in 22 pituitary tumors, including tumors from three patients with acromegaly. The great majority of these tumors had monoclonal expansion. In the few cases in which both X-chromosomal alleles were found active in pituitary adenomas, infiltration of the tumor with normal cells was evident histologically.

One type of mutation may explain the clonal growth of many somatotroph adenomas. When GRF binds to its receptor on normal somatotroph cells, it increases cAMP by activating the GTP binding complex (Gs). This response to GRF occurs normally in about 60 per cent of somatotroph adenomas. In the remainder there is constitutive activation of cAMP so that no further increase in cAMP or stimulation of GH secretion occurs after exposure to GRF.[123] Because cAMP mediates somatotroph proliferation as well as promoting GH secretion, its constitutive increase gives the mutant cells a growth advantage that could explain adenoma formation. Two sites of mutation of the Gs α peptide have been recognized in pituitary adenomas. In one arginine-201 is replaced with either cysteine or histidine and in the other glutamine-227 is replaced with arginine.

The McCune-Albright syndrome is a condition manifested by polyostotic fibrous dysplasia, café-au-lait pigmented nevi, and endocrine abnormalities. Autonomous hypersecretion of ovary, adrenal, thyroid, and pituitary occur. Hyperplastic or adenomatous tissues from these affected glands have shown Gs α mutations similar to those found in acromegaly.[124] It is likely that these endocrine tissues and also many nonendocrine tissues are a mosaic of normal and Gs mutant cells.

Multiple endocrine neoplasia type 1 (MEN 1) syndrome is an autosomal dominant disease in which pancreatic, parathyroid, and pituitary adenomas can develop. The gene associated with this condition has been located on chromosome 11 at q13.[125, 126] The normal gene's action is that of tumor suppressor, the mutant forms of the gene found in MEN 1 adenomas are inactive, and the development of adenomas occurs with loss of heterozygosity. If the normal gene is lost in a clone of glandular cells, an adenoma is likely to develop.

Ectopic GH Secretion

GH immunoactivity has been found in many different nonendocrine tumors, but questions of specificity of the immune reaction have been raised. Melmed et al[127] have presented convincing evidence that a mesenteric pancreatic islet cell tumor was responsible for acromegaly. This tumor had high GH concentration, and there was a high arteriovenous gradient of GH across the tumor. Removal of the tumor lowered serum GH and IGF I levels to normal. The tumor expressed GH mRNA and released GH in primary culture.

GRF-Producing Tumors

A small minority of the cases of acromegaly (less than 1 per cent) are the result of the hypersecretion of GRF by tumors.[128, 129] There are now seven well-documented cases of gangliocytomas associated with acromegaly. In five cases the tumors were located in the sella turcica. The other two were suprasellar. GRF has been demonstrated in such tumors immunohistochemically.

More than 50 cases of extrasellar tumors producing GRF have been described, with unequivocal demonstration of ectopic GRF in 39.[127] Pulmonary and gastrointestinal carcinoids are the most common tumors, and next in frequency are islet cell tumors of the pancreas. Single cases of bronchial adenoma, pheochromocytoma, and paraganglioma have been found to secrete GRF. The pituitaries of patients with ectopic GRF-secreting tumor may be either hyperplastic or adenomatous. In some cases the diagnosis of adenoma was made, but the distinction between adenomatous hyperplasia and adenomas is indistinct.

The clinical presentation of most cases of GRF hypersecretion does not differ from other cases of acromegaly, and the diagnosis was suspected only after it was found that the pituitary was hyperplastic rather than containing a somatotroph adenoma. Many of these cases had persistent hypersomatotropism after transsphenoidal operation. A minority of patients with islet tumors or carcinoids had evidence of secretion of other peptide hormones such as ACTH, parathyroid-related peptide, and gastrin. Immunohistological staining for GH was present in one carcinoid also secreting GRF.[130] Diarrhea and other features of the carcinoid syndrome may be present with the acromegaly.

If suspected, the diagnosis of ectopic GRF-mediated acromegaly can be confirmed by radioimmunoassay. Plasma levels of 300 ng/L up to 50 mg/L have been reported.[131] The assay, however, is technically demanding and not widely available. Because ectopic GRF syndrome is such a rare condition, routine radioimmunoassay screening of acromegalic patients is not cost effective.

Manifestations of GH Excess (Table 19–3)

SKIN AND CONNECTIVE TISSUE. The stimulation of connective tissue growth occurs throughout the body, but it is

TABLE 19–3. MANIFESTATIONS OF HYPERSOMATOTROPISM

	Recognition Class
I. Skin and connective tissue growth	
1. Soft tissue swelling	
Facial	+ + +
Acral	+ + +
2. Excess sweating	+
3. Hirsutism	
4. Laryngeal thickening (deep voice)	+ +
II. Skeletal and articular changes	
1. Gigantism (with childhood onset)	+ +
2. Costal growth (barrel chest)	+
3. Mandibular growth (prognathism)	+ +
4. Calvarial growth	
Frontal bossing	+
Frontal sinus	+
5. Vertebral bony overgrowth	
6. Phalangeal bony overgrowth	
7. Articular cartilage growth	
Widening joint space	
Accelerated osteoarthritis	
III. Visceral growth	
1. Cardiac (ventricular and septal thickening)	
2. Hepatic	
3. Renal	
4. Pulmonary	
5. Thyroid	
IV. Changes in metabolism	
1. Insulin resistance	
Hyperinsulinemia	
Impaired glucose tolerance	+
Diabetes mellitus	+
2. Increase in 1,25-dihydroxycholecalciferol	
3. Hypercalciuria (renal lithiasis)	
V. Associated endocrine abnormalities	
1. Hyperprolactinemia (galactorrhea)	+
2. FSH, LH	
Women: menstrual irregularity, amenorrhea	
Men: impotence	
3. TSH	
Hypersecretion—very rare	
Hyposecretion—uncommon	
4. ACTH	
Hypersecretion—very rare	
Hyposecretion—uncommon	
5. Vasopressin	
Hyposecretion—uncommon	
VI. Neuromuscular manifestations	
1. Headache	+ + +
2. Visual field loss	+ +
3. Sleep apnea	+ +
4. Peripheral nerves	
Entrapments (carpal tunnel)	+ +
Hypertrophic neuropathy	
5. Myopathy	

most evident in dermal and subdermal tissues and recognized clinically as facial puffiness and acromegaly. These changes occur early and are the key to early recognition of the disease. They may be recognized as a boggy feeling of the handshake or an increase in heel pad thickness. The increase in shoe size and glove size is largely the result of soft tissue swelling. The tongue, soft palate, uvula, and pharyngeal tissues are also affected by this process and can cause sleep apnea, a complication common in acromegaly.[132] Laryngeal thickening gives rise to the characteristic deep voice of the acromegalic patient.

The skin itself is affected by GH excess with increase in its appendages. Women complain of excess growth of coarse facial hair. Sweat and sebaceous gland hypertrophy result in excessive ill-smelling sweat. In advanced cases, deep facial and scalp furrowing occurs.

During the early years of acromegaly soft tissue swelling regresses rapidly after successful treatment. This reflects the relatively short half-life of hyaluronic acid and chondroitin sulfate. As the duration of acromegaly extends, the reversibility of soft tissue swelling becomes progressively less owing to increased collagen deposition.

SKELETAL AND ARTICULAR GROWTH. When GH excess occurs in childhood, there is an acceleration of linear growth which, if untreated, results in gigantism (Figs. 19–17 and 19–18).[133, 134] In the most striking examples of gigantism, accelerated growth begins in infancy and is often associated with stigmata of the McCune-Albright osteodystrophy such as café-au-lait spots, polyostotic fibrous dysplasia, and other endocrinopathies. Many children with gigantism fail to enter puberty or experience incomplete pubertal development. This results in the persistence of skeletal cartilage growth plates and further extends the period of skeletal growth, with development of eunuchoid body proportions (Fig. 19–18).

Pituitary gigantism is a rare disorder, but the increased monitoring of growth of children with appropriate growth charts should permit recognition early in the course of the condition. Normal children after the age of three usually follow the same growth channel until puberty. Any sustained increase in growth velocity of otherwise healthy children without evidence of premature pubertal changes should arouse suspicion. Also, consideration of GH excess

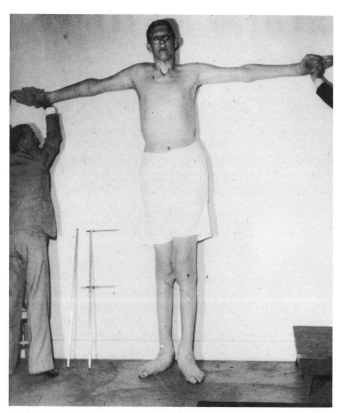

FIGURE 19–17. The "Alton giant" at age 20 years shortly before his death. Obvious are the eunuchoid body proportions and the deformity of his feet due to Charcot-type bony destruction and distal muscular atrophy secondary to severe neuropathy.

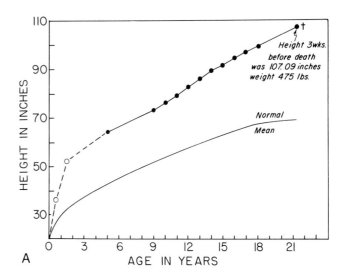

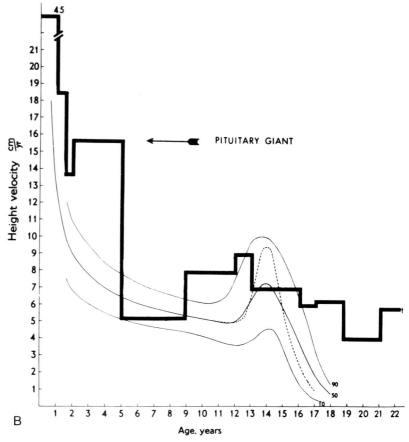

FIGURE 19–18. *A*, Growth attainment curve of the "Alton giant," showing that most of the increment over normal was acquired during the first three years of life. *B*, Growth velocity curve of the "Alton giant," which shows the remarkable increase in growth velocity which occurred before the age of four years. Also, note that there was little pubertal increase in growth velocity and that growth continued beyond age 21 years. (Reprinted with permission from Daughaday WH: Extreme gigantism. N Engl J Med 297:1267, 1977.)

is warranted for children more than 2 SD's above the calculated midparental height.

Few conditions induce the degree of skeletal growth present in gigantism. Conditions such as Marfan's syndrome, neurofibromatosis, and sex chromosome redundancy, which may be associated with tall stature, have characteristic features that should not cause diagnostic confusion.

The condition of "cerebral gigantism" needs to be distinguished from pituitary gigantism.[135, 136] These children, unlike those with GH excess, are large at birth and have accelerated infantile growth. Heads, hands, and feet are disproportionately large. Mental and motor development is often impaired. Bone age is advanced, and growth velocity declines in childhood so that eventual height may not be increased. Despite intensive study, no endocrine abnormalities in these children have been found that could account for their early growth. Measurements of serum GH levels and IGF I levels are normal.

When hypersomatotropism begins in adulthood (acromegaly), there is no increase in height because of fusion of the epiphyses (Fig. 19–19). The ribs, however, may continue to grow in length because of cartilage proliferation at the costochondral junctions. This growth leads to the barrel chest of untreated acromegalics. The mandible also can increase in length with GH excess. Here the prolifera-

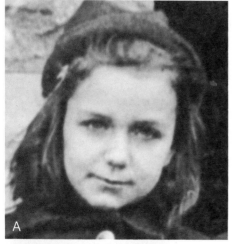

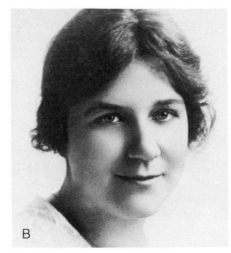

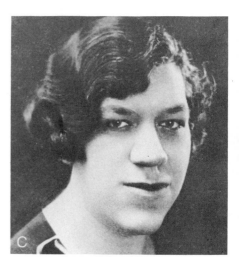

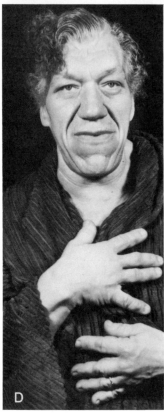

FIGURE 19-19. Photographic record of the progression of acromegaly. *A*, Facial features of the patient at age 9 years. *B*, At the age of 16 years there is a suggestion of soft tissue swelling and mandibular prominence. *C*, At the age of 33 years the nasal soft tissue swelling and prognathism are clearly evident. *D*, At the age of 52 years the thickening of the skin is markedly increased and prognathism has progressed. The patient died soon after this photograph from congestive heart failure. (Reprinted with permission from Clinical Pathological Conferences. Am J Med 20:133, 1956.)

tion of cartilage occurs at the temporomandibular articulation, which results in the development of prognathism in many acromegalics. Alert dentists can recognize this change. There is also increased spacing of the teeth in acromegaly of long duration, but this cannot be due to growth arising from the cartilage at the articulation. It is likely that the enlarged tongue promotes jaw remodeling by exerting persistent lateral pressure.

GH excess stimulates periosteal growth, which results in thickening of the calvarium. This is recognized clinically by the prominent brow associated with enlargement of the frontal sinuses. Distal tufting of the phalanges is recognized radiologically. Vertebrae are increased by ossification on their anterior surface, which may bridge the disc space. Articular cartilage growth is stimulated by GH excess. This leads to widening of the joint spaces, altered joint mechanisms, and degenerative arthritis.

VISCERAL GROWTH. The major viscera are enlarged in acromegaly, but this usually is not recognized by physical examination. There is thickening of the cardiac ventricular wall and interventricular septum. These changes, combined with an increased prevalence of hypertension, contribute to the excess mortality of untreated acromegaly. The liver is increased in weight at autopsy, and functional studies in life have documented increased blood flow and biliary transport. The kidneys are also increased in weight with large glomeruli, and glomerular filtration rate and renal plasma flow are increased. Thyromegaly is recognized in about 20 per cent of patients even in the absence of disturbed thyroid function. Lung volumes are increased in many acromegalic patients, and intrathoracic airway obstruction is demonstrated in 25 per cent of patients.[137]

CHANGES IN METABOLISM. GH excess induces insulin resistance. Early in the disease there is hyperinsulinism without hyperglycemia, but later, impaired glucose tolerance develops in 30 to 40 per cent of patients and overt diabetes in 10 to 20 per cent.[138] Retinopathy and nephropathy can occur in acromegaly with diabetes, but whether it is more or less common than in uncomplicated diabetes is disputed. Hypertriglyceridemia occurs in 19 to 44 per cent of acromegalic patients.[139] Hepatic triglyceride lipase and lipoprotein lipase activities are reduced in acromegaly.

In acromegaly there is an increase in calcium absorption from the gut attributable to an increase in serum 1,25-dihydroxycholecalciferol.[140, 141] Serum 25-hydroxycholecalciferol levels tend to be low, which suggests increases in 1α-hydroxylase activity. Serum calcium is normal and urine calcium increased. There is a 6 to 12 per cent prevalence of urolithiasis. Serum phosphorus is increased owing to a direct effect of GH on phosphorus transport in the proximal tubule. Despite increased bone calcium turnover, increased bone density is found early in the disease, but if hypogonadism develops early and is severe, osteoporosis occurs. Kyphosis due to spinal osteoporosis was present in three of eight patients with gigantism examined in later life.[142]

DISTURBED PITUITARY FUNCTION. As previously discussed, somatomammotropic adenomas contain both GH and PRL. Serum PRL is increased in 15 to 40 per cent of patients with acromegaly. About 20 per cent of women with acromegaly have galactorrhea, but its occurrence is not necessarily associated with hyperprolactinemia because human GH has high intrinsic lactogenic activity.

Gonadal function is often disturbed in acromegaly. Menstrual abnormalities occur in about 75 per cent of women, and clinical or laboratory evidence of hypogonadism, often with impotence, is present in 25 to 50 per cent of men. These changes reflect decreased gonadotropin secretion, which can have various causes, including direct effects of the pituitary tumors on portal blood flow and destruction of normal pituitary cells. In some cases these gonadal changes are due to functional suppression of gonadotropin secretion by elevated serum PRL or the lactogenic action of excess GH.

Goiter is found in about 30 per cent of acromegalic patients, but in most cases, thyroid function is normal. The frequency of hyperthyroidism is less than 10 per cent. Most of these cases represent toxic nodular goiter. Hyperthyroidism attributable to excess secretion of TSH has been reported.[143]

Hypoadrenocorticism in acromegaly is very rare and occurs only with the most aggressive tumors. There have been few documented cases of hyperadrenocorticism in acromegalic patients. In one unusual case, ACTH hypersecretion was attributed to corticotropic hyperplasia in the nonadenomatous portion of the pituitary.[144]

NEUROLOGICAL MANIFESTATIONS. Headaches are prominent complaints in more than half the patients with acromegaly and have been attributed to stretching of the dural coverings of the sella. The possibility that they could have a hormonal basis is suggested by the very rapid relief of headache which often occurs with octreotide therapy. An equally likely explanation of this finding is that relief results from a reduction of tumor size. Even a very slight reduction in tumor size, which might not be detectable by imaging, would reduce tension within the restricted confines of the sella turcica.

Pressure on the optic chiasm with visual field defects remains the most common parasellar complication in acromegaly but is now found in only about 20 per cent of patients. Involvement of other cranial nerves, obstructive hydrocephalus, and symptomatic hypothalamic involvement are fortunately rare. About 5 per cent of patients complain of excessive sleepiness, but when sleep studies are performed, as many as 60 per cent have sleep apnea.[132] Although this could be attributable to upper airway obstruction in two thirds of the cases, in the remaining one third, a central mechanism was suspected.

Peripheral neuropathy is an important complication of acromegaly. Entrapment syndromes, especially in the carpal tunnel, are particularly common.[145, 146] Its presence is recognized in almost 50 per cent of acromegaly with careful clinical examination and confirmatory electrophysiological studies. Remission often follows successful treatment of the acromegaly.

A more diffuse hypertrophic neuropathy occurs with long-standing hypersomatotropism, particularly in gigantism.[133, 146] This is associated with paresthesia and sensory defects in a stocking-glove distribution and the presence of enlarged cordlike peripheral nerves. In severe examples of this condition, which occur in gigantism, motor weakness is present. Cases have been reported with neuropathic (Charcot) bone necrosis of the feet.[133]

A mild proximal myopathy is commonly found in acromegaly.[146] Hypertrophy of Type 1 fibers and atrophy of Type 2 fibers have been reported. Mild enzyme elevations and electromyographic changes occur.

Prognosis

Untreated acromegaly decreases life expectancy.[147–149] Acromegaly carries an increased risk for development of diabetes with its attendant complications. Between 25 and 35 per cent of patients develop hypertension, and death from cardiovascular and cerebrovascular disease causes a three-fold increase in risk. Acromegalic patients are also at increased risk of dying of respiratory disease, but the exact reason for this has not been established.

There has been much speculation about the role of GH in the induction of malignancies and the possible role of GH in increasing the rate of growth of established malignancies.[150] Experimental data exist for such an association. Long-term administration of GH to hypophysectomized rats led to lymphosarcomas in 40 per cent, adrenal neoplasms in 67 per cent, adrenomedullary carcinomas in 20 per cent, solid ovarian tumors in 13 per cent, and breast tumors.[151]

Information about the prevalence of malignant tumors in acromegalic patients is incomplete. The number of patients followed up is comparatively small, and the information about treatment and its success is fragmented. Nevertheless, two follow-up studies suggested that malignant tumors are more common as a cause of death than expected.[147, 149]

More suggestive evidence links acromegaly with an increased risk of colon polyps and cancer. In one report, the prevalence of colon polyps was reported to be 53 per cent.[152] An association of colon polyps with more than three skin tags (acrochordons) has been reported. In another report, the prevalence of colon cancer was 6.9 per cent in acromegalic patients, particularly among those with a family history of colon cancer.[153] Ezzat and Melmed[150] suggested that the risk factors for colon polyps are (1) patient older than 50, (2) acromegaly for more than 10 years, and (3) more than three skin tags. On the basis of present information, these authors recommend full colonoscopy for acromegalic patients over 50 years of age every three to five years.

Treatment

An occasional patient with obvious features of gigantism or acromegaly is encountered with normal or low levels of serum GH and IGF I. In most cases this is the result of hemorrhagic infarction of a pituitary adenoma. Some of these patients recall an episode of sudden, severe retroorbital headache that lasted for several days. The frequency with which these spontaneous remissions occur is not known, but it is not rare. Obviously, no further treatment of such patients is required other than replacement of hormonal deficits.

Surgery

Patients with persistent hypersomatotropism should be treated regardless of whether continued increase in acromegalic features is occurring. Surgery remains the first-line therapy for this condition.[154, 155] In most cases a pituitary adenoma can be approached transsphenoidally, a procedure associated with low morbidity and mortality. The transfrontal approach is required only for macroadenomas with extensions that cannot be reached transsphenoidally. The success of the procedure in restoring serum GH to normal is largely determined by the size of the tumor and whether or not it has invaded parasellar structures. Cure can be anticipated with microadenomas but seldom is achieved with giant adenomas or with cavernous sinus invasion.

Recurrence of hypersomatotropism is rare if the serum GH postoperatively is less than 2 μg/L after oral glucose. With serum GH above 5 μg/L, a slow rise in serum GH levels can be anticipated without additional therapy. Reoperation can be considered for patients with circumscribed residual tumor demonstrable by MRI.

Removal of a microadenoma rarely impairs, and may improve, pituitary function. Various degrees of hypopituitarism may result from more extensive adenomectomy. This most frequently involves gonadotropin function. Adrenal and thyroid functions are generally maintained postoperatively. Diabetes insipidus developed in only 2.6 per cent of the cases in one series.[155] Postoperative complications of transsphenoidal surgery with experienced surgeons occur in less than 7 per cent of the cases[154] and include postoperative rhinorrhea, vascular damage, and localized meningitis. Mortality with this procedure has been about 1 per cent.[154]

Radiation Therapy

Various modalities of radiation therapy have been used in the treatment of acromegaly.[156, 157] These include the local implantation of yttrium pellets, proton beam radiation, and super-voltage x-ray therapy. The latter has been improved by discrete focusing on the pituitary tumor (stereotactic radiation therapy). All these methods have been shown to lower serum GH, but the response to therapy may be delayed for two years and longer. Even after 10 years, as many as 10 to 15 per cent of patients treated with x-ray remain hypersomatotropic. Among radiation-treated patients, 15 to 50 per cent develop one or more deficiencies of normal pituitary function. Hypothalamic damage may result from treatment of tumors with significant suprasellar extension. Rarely, damage to the optic nerve occurs. These complications of radiation therapy are less likely to occur with lower doses of radiation.

Radiation therapy at present is used primarily for patients who have residual hypersomatotropism after transsphenoidal adenomectomy, patients who are not candidates for surgery because of medical contraindications, and patients whose vascular or bony abnormalities would make the transsphenoidal approach hazardous.

Medical Therapy

Large doses of estrogens can lower serum IGF I levels of acromegalic patients,[158] but sustained clinical benefit has never been established. Interest in medical treatment of acromegaly has increased greatly with the development of more specific therapeutic agents.

DOPAMINERGIC AGENTS. When L-dopa is given to normal individuals, an acute stimulation of GH secretion results. This is attributable largely to formation of dopamine and norepinephrine in the hypothalamus with inhibition of somatostatin secretion.[159] An opposite response is seen in most patients with GH-secreting tumors given dopamine or dopaminergic agents. More than half of the patients have a fall in serum GH. In vitro studies have confirmed that dopamine can act directly on somatotroph tumors to inhibit GH release.[159]

The structures of dopaminergic agonists, which are effective after oral administration and have sufficient duration of action to be clinically useful, are shown in Figure 19–20. Bromocriptine and pergolide are available in the United States but have not yet been approved by the FDA for the treatment of acromegaly. Only bromocriptine has been approved for the treatment of prolactinomas. Bromocriptine must be given every 8 to 12 hours, whereas pergolide often can be given once a day. Slowly absorbed parental preparations of bromocriptine are under study with sustained therapeutic effects for weeks. Lisuride and cabergoline are dopaminergic agents that also have much prolonged action. These agents have been used primarily in prolactinomas by European investigators.

Jaffe and Barkan[160] have summarized the reports of 549 patients treated with bromocriptine. The dose of bromocriptine (7.5 to 80 mg/day) required in acromegaly is larger than that needed in patients with prolactinomas, but it is unlikely that much is gained in the treatment of acromegaly by increasing the dose above 20 to 30 mg. GH levels less than 10 μg/L were achieved in 53 per cent and less

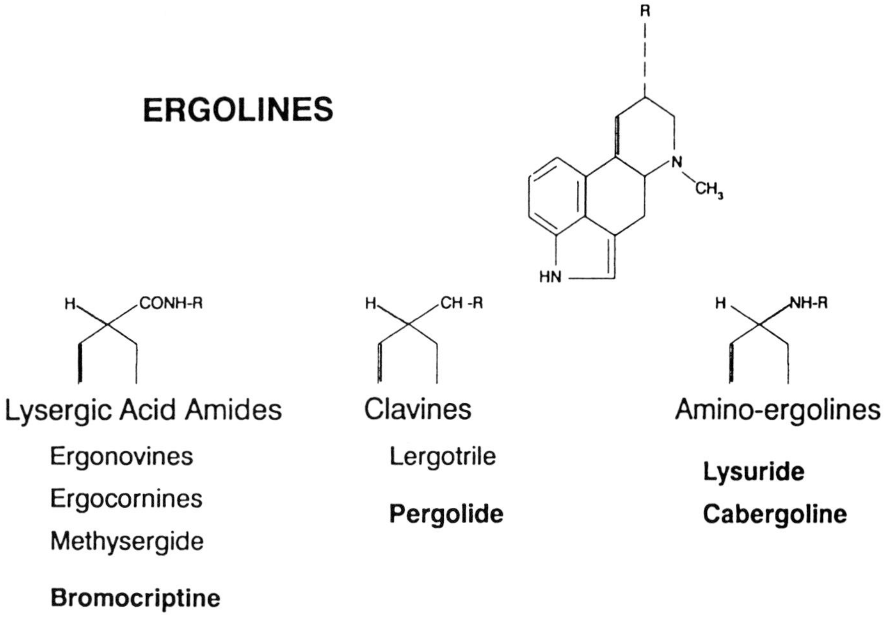

ERGOLINES

FIGURE 19–20. Structure of classes of the dopaminergic agents that have been developed. Compounds in bold type have been shown to exhibit clinical efficacy in reducing prolactin (PRL) and/or GH levels. (Reprinted with permission from Frohman LA: Therapeutic options in acromegaly. J Clin Endocrinol Metab 72:1175, 1991. © by the Endocrine Society, 1991.)

Lysergic Acid Amides
Ergonovines
Ergocornines
Methysergide
Bromocriptine

Clavines
Lergotrile
Pergolide

Amino-ergolines
Lysuride
Cabergoline

than 5 μg/L in 20 per cent. Measurement of serum IGF I is a more rigorous criterion of response than serum GH, and normal levels of IGF I were achieved in only 10 per cent of 116 cases. A decrease in tumor size with modern imaging occurred in 29 per cent of cases and was most likely to occur in patients with elevated PRL levels. Therapeutic effectiveness may be increased when bromocriptine is combined with octreotide.[161]

Side effects, including nausea, vomiting, nasal stuffiness, and hypotension, may occur early in treatment with bromocriptine. These are minimized by starting treatment with 1.25 or 2.5 mg at night and slowly increasing the dose as tolerated. It must be taken in the middle of a meal. More severe CNS symptoms of insomnia, sedation, confusion, paranoia, hallucinations, and nightmares may be encountered with the highest doses reported.

Bromocriptine therapy is most useful for patients with slightly elevated serum GH and IGF I concentrations after surgical or radiation treatment. Although substantial lowering of serum GH occurs with bromocriptine in patients with more severe hypersomatotropism, serum IGF I usually remains elevated and clinical response is minimal.

SOMATOSTATIN ANALOGUES. The intravenous administration of SS lowers serum GH concentrations in most patients and decreases GH secretion of somatotrope adenoma cells in culture. The short half-life of SS in the circulation of only a few minutes, precludes the use of the natural 14-amino acid hormone in therapy. This has prompted pharmaceutical research into prolonging the action of SS by molecular modification. The result of this effort was the synthesis of octreotide. This agent retains a truncated form of the S–S bonded loop of SS but has the substitution of two D-amino acids that greatly reduce susceptibility to peptidase cleavage. When octreotide is given by subcutaneous injection to normal subjects, a marked suppression of serum GH occurs for six to eight hours without a subsequent rebound hypersecretion that occurs with the native hormone.

There has now been extensive experience with this agent in treating patients with acromegaly.[162] Therapy is usually

started with 50 μg given subcutaneously every eight hours. The dose is increased, as required, up to 100 μg three times daily. Little further improvement is observed with higher subcutaneous doses but may occur when octreotide is given by continuous subcutaneous injection by pump or by the addition of bromocriptine. Serum GH and IGF I levels are lowered in 80 to 90 per cent of patients. Normalization of serum GH (mean < 3.3 μg/L) was achieved in 8 of 27 patients in one series.[163]

Tumor size decreases in about half the patients but is generally much less dramatic than occurs with bromocriptine treatment of prolactinomas. Shrinkage is not the result of tumor cell death but is due to loss of cytoplasmic volume with increase in lysosomes.[164] In short-term in vitro studies, SS action does not decrease GH mRNA.[165]

In experimental animals and probably also in humans, octreotide has a more profound effect in inhibiting GH secretion than insulin secretion. During octreotide treatment the response of insulin to a glucose challenge is blunted, but the long-term effects on glucose metabolism of octreotide treatment of acromegalic patients are usually slight because the drug also removes the insulin resistance of GH excess and inhibits the secretion of glucagon.

SS and octreotide also have effects on gastrointestinal motor activity, blood flow, and glandular secretion. Nevertheless, the gastrointestinal symptoms of octreotide treatment have been comparatively mild.[166] Nausea and cramps occur early in treatment. Mild steatorrhea is common. Gastritis related to *Heliobacter pylori* with impaired vitamin B_{12} absorption has been reported. Octreotide inhibits biliary flow and gallbladder contraction, which results in new gallstone formation in up to 10 per cent of patients with acromegaly within two years of treatment.[166, 167]

Practical considerations make octreotide treatment undesirable as a first-line treatment of acromegaly. Many patients find the requirement of three daily subcutaneous injections for an indefinite period onerous. The present price of the drug raises the cost of a year's treatment to nearly $10,000. If oral anticholilithogenic treatment is also required, the cost of therapy is higher. Despite the extensive experience with the drug in the United States and abroad, it has not yet received FDA approval and for this reason, there may not be insurance coverage. For these reasons, octreotide in the United States is indicated only for patients not responding fully to surgical or radiation treatment.

REFERENCES

1. Lewis UJ: Variants of growth hormone and prolactin and their post-translational modifications. Annu Rev Physiol 46:33, 1984.
2. Baumann G: Growth hormone heterogeneity: Genes, isohormones, variants and binding proteins. Endocrine Rev 1992, 12:424, 1991.
3. Miller WL, Eberhardt NL: Structure and evolution of the growth hormone gene family. Endocrine Rev 4:97, 1983.
4. Frankenne F, Rentier-Delrue F, Scippo ML, et al: Expression of the growth hormone variant gene in human placenta. J Clin Endocrinol Metab 64:635, 1987.
5. Ray J, Jones BK, Liebhaber SA, et al: Glycosylated human growth hormone variant. Endocrinology 125:566, 1989.
6. Hennen G, Frankenne F, Closset J, et al: A human placental GH: Increasing levels during second half of pregnancy with pituitary GH suppression as revealed by monoclonal antibody radioimmunoassays. Int J Fertil 30:27, 1985.
7. Daughaday WH, Trivedi B, Winn HN, et al: Hypersomatotropism in pregnant women as measured by a human liver radioreceptor assay. J Clin Endocrinol Metab 70:215, 1990.
8. Wallis M: The molecular evolution of pituitary growth hormone prolactin and placental lactogen: A protein family showing variable rates of evolution. J Mol Evol 17:10, 1981.
9. Seeburg PH: The human growth hormone gene family: Nucleotide sequences show recent divergence and predict a new polypeptide hormone. DNA 1:239, 1982.
10. Chen EY, Liao Y-C, Smith DH, et al: The human growth hormone locus: Nucleotide sequence, biology, and evolution. Genomics 4:479, 1989.
11. Weigent DA, Baxter JB, Wear WE, et al: Production of immunoreactive growth by mononuclear leukocytes. FASEB J 2:2812, 1988.
12. Karin M, Castrillo J-L, Theill LE: Growth hormone gene regulation: A paradigm for cell-type-specific gene activation. Trends Genet 6:92, 1990.
13. Nickel BE, Nachtigal MW, Bock ME, et al: Differential binding of rat pituitary–specific nuclear factors to the 5′-flanking region of pituitary and placental members of the human growth hormone gene family. Mol Cell Biochem 106:181, 1991.
14. Vnencak-Jones CL, Phillips JA III, Chen EY, et al: Molecular basis of human growth hormone gene deletions. Proc Natl Acad Sci USA 85:5615, 1988.
15. Wurzel JM, Parks JS, Herd JE, et al: Gene deletion is responsible for absence of immunoassayable human chorionic somatomammotropin. DNA 1:251, 1982.
16. Gluckman PD, Grumbach MM, Kaplan SL: The neuroendocrine regulation and function of growth hormone and prolactin in the mammalian fetus. Endocrine Rev 2:363, 1981.
17. Imura H, Shimatsu A, Hattori N, et al: Ultrasensitive assays in evaluation of growth hormone disorders. In Melmed S, Robbins RJ (eds): Current Issues in Endocrinology and Metabolism. Boston, Blackwell Publishing, 1991, p 261.
18. Martha PM Jr, Gorman KM, Blizzard RM, et al: Endogenous growth hormone secretion and clearance rates in normal boys, as determined by deconvolutional analysis: Relationship to age, pubertal status, and body mass. J Clin Endocrinol Metab 74:336, 1992.
19. Owens D, Srivastava MC, Tompkins CV, et al: Studies of the metabolic clearance rate, apparent distribution space and plasma half-disappearance time of unlabelled human growth hormone in normal subjects and patients with liver disease, renal disease, thyroid disease and diabetes mellitus. Europ J Clin Invest 3:284, 1973.
20. Bratusch-Marrain P, Waldhausl W: The influence of amino acids and somatostatin on prolactin and growth hormone release in man. Acta Endocrinol 90:403, 1979.
21. Knobil E, Greep RO: The physiology of growth hormone with particular reference to its action in the Rhesus monkey and the ''species specificity'' problem. Rec Progr Hormone Res 15:1, 1959.
22. Carr D, Friesen HG: Growth hormone and insulin binding to human liver. J Clin Endocrinol Metab 42:484, 1972.
23. Lesniak MA, Roth J, Gorden P, et al: Binding of ^{125}I-human growth hormone to specific receptors in human cultured lymphocytes. J Biol Chem 249:1661, 1974.
24. Leung DW, Spencer SA, Cachianes G, et al: Growth hormone receptor and serum binding protein: Purification, cloning and expression. Nature 330:537, 1987.
25. Stred SE, Stubbart JR, Argetsinger LS, et al: Demonstration of growth hormone (GH) receptor associated tyrosine kinase activity in multiple GH-responsive cell types. Endocrinology 127:2506, 1990.
26. Bass SH, Mulkerrin MG, Wells JA: A systematic mutational analysis of hormone-binding determinants in the human growth hormone receptor. Proc Natl Acad Sci USA 88:4498, 1991.
27. Cunningham BC, Ultsch M, de Vos AM, et al: Dimerization of the extracellular domain of the human growth hormone receptor by a single molecule. Science 254:821, 1991.
28. de Vos AM, Ultsch M, Kosiakoff AA: Human growth hormone and extracellular domain of its receptor: Crystal structure of the complex. Science 255:306, 1992.
29. Cunningham BC, Bass S, Fuh G, et al: Zinc mediation of the binding of human growth hormone to the human prolactin receptor. Science 250:1709, 1990.
30. Cunningham BC, Mulkerrin MG, Wells JA: Dimerization of human growth hormone by zinc. Science 253:545, 1991.
31. Ray J, Okamura H, Kelly PA, et al: Human growth hormone-variant demonstrates a receptor binding profile distinct from that of normal pituitary hormone. J Biol Chem 265:7929, 1990.
32. Kelly PA, Djiane J, Postel-Vinay M-C, et al: The prolactin/growth hormone receptor family. Endocr Rev 12:235, 1991.
33. Ymer SI, Herington AC: Evidence for the specific binding of growth hormone to a receptor-like protein in rabbit serum. Mol Cell Endocrinol 41:153, 1985.
34. Baumann G, Stolar MW, Amburn K, et al: A specific growth hormone–binding protein in human plasma: Initial characterization. J Clin Endocrinol Metab 62:134, 1986.
35. Herington AC, Ymer S, Stevenson J: Identification and characterization of specific binding proteins for growth hormone in normal human sera. J Clin Invest 77:1817, 1986.
36. Smith WC, Linzer DI, Talamantes F: Detection of two growth hormone receptor mRNAs and primary translation products in the mouse. Proc Natl Acad Sci USA 85:9576, 1988.
37. Trivedi B, Daughaday WH: Release of growth hormone binding protein from IM-9 lymphocytes by endopeptidase is dependent on sulfydryl group inactivation. Endocrinology 123:2201, 1988.
38. Mathews LS, Enberg B, Norstedt G: Regulation of rat growth hormone receptor gene expression. J Biol Chem 264:9905, 1989.
39. Daughaday WH, Trivedi B, Andrews BA: The ontogeny of serum GH binding protein in man: A possible indicator of hepatic GH receptor development. J Clin Endocrinol Metab 65:1072, 1987.
40. Silbergeld A, Lazar L, Erster LB, et al: Serum growth hormone binding protein activity in healthy neonates, children and young adults: Correlation with age, height and weight. Clin Endocrinol 31:295, 1989.
41. Merimee TJ, Baumann G, Daughaday W: Growth hormone-binding protein: II. Studies in pygmies and normal statured subjects. J Clin Endocrinol Metab 71:1183, 1990.
42. Carter-Su C, Stubbart JR, Wang X, et al: Phosphorylation of highly purified growth hormone receptors by a growth hormone receptor-associated tyrosine kinase. J Biol Chem 264:18644, 1989.
43. Doglio A, Dani C, Grimaldi P, et al: Growth hormone stimulates c-fos gene expression by means of a protein kinase C without increasing inositol lipid turnover. Proc Natl Acad Sci USA 86:1148, 1989.
44. Slootweg MC, de Groot RP, Herrmann-Erlee MPM, et al: Growth hormone induces expression of c-jun and jun B oncogenes and employs a protein kinase C signal transduction pathway for the induction of c-fos oncogene expression. J Mol Endocrinol 6:179, 1991.
45. Rogers S, Hammerman MR: Growth hormone activates phospholipase C in proximal tubular basolateral membranes from canine kidney. Proc Natl Acad Sci USA 86:1148, 1989.
46. Roupas P, Chou SY, Towns RJ, et al: Growth hormone inhibits activation of phosphatidylinositol phospholipase C in adipose plasma membranes: Evidence for growth hormone-induced change in G protein function. Proc Natl Acad Sci USA 88:1691, 1991.
47. Lynch KR, Dolan KP, Nakhasi HL, et al: The role of growth hormone in α2μ globulin synthesis: A reexamination. Cell 28:185, 1982.
48. Yoon J-B, Berry SA, Seelig S, et al: An inducible nuclear factor binds to a growth hormone-regulated gene. J Biol Chem 265:19947, 1990.

49. Tollet P, Enberg B, Mode A: Growth hormone (GH) regulation of cytochrome P-450 IIX12, insulin-like growth factor-I (IGF-I), and GH receptor messenger RNA expression in primary rat hepatocytes: A hormonal interplay with insulin, IGF-I and thyroid hormone. Mol Endocrinol 4:1934, 1990.

50. Laron Z: Laron-type dwarfism (hereditary somatomedin deficiency). Adv Int Med Ped 51:117, 1984.

51. Rosenbloom AL, Aguirre JG, Rosenfeld RG, et al: The little women of Loja: Growth hormone–receptor deficiency in an inbred population of southern Ecuador. N Engl J Med 323:1367, 1990.

52. Eshet R, Laron Z, Pertzelan S, et al: Defect of human growth hormone receptors in the liver of two patients with Laron-type dwarfism. Israel J Med Sci 20:8, 1984.

53. Daughaday WH, Trivedi B: Absence of serum growth hormone binding protein in patients with growth hormone receptor deficiency (Laron dwarfism). Proc Natl Acad Sci USA 84:4736, 1987.

54. Baumann G, Shaw MA, Winter RJ: Absence of the plasma growth hormone–binding protein in Laron-type dwarfism. J Clin Endocrinol Metab 65:814, 1987.

55. Godowski PJ, Leung DW, Meacham LR, et al: Characterization of the human growth hormone receptor gene and demonstration of a partial deletion in two patients with Laron-type dwarfism. Proc Natl Acad Sci USA 86:8083, 1989.

56. Amselem S, Duquesnoy P, Attree O, et al: Laron dwarfism and mutations of the growth hormone–receptor gene. N Engl J Med 321:989, 1989.

57. Duquesnoy P, Sobrier ML, Amselem SS, et al: Defective membrane expression of human growth hormone (GH) receptor causes Laron-type GH insensitivity syndrome. Proc Natl Acad Sci USA 88:10272, 1991.

58. Salmon WD Jr, Daughaday WH: A hormonally controlled serum factor which stimulates sulfate incorporation by cartilage in vitro. J Lab Clin Med 49:825, 1957.

59. Rinderknecht E, Humbel RE: The amino acid sequence of human insulin-like growth factor I and its structural homology with proinsulin. J Biol Chem 253:2769, 1978.

60. Rinderknecht E, Humbel RE: Primary structure of human insulin-like growth factor II. FEBS Lett 89:283, 1978.

61. Rotwein P: Structure, evolution, expression and regulation of insulin-like growth factors I and II. Growth Factors 5:3, 1991.

62. Hampton B, Burgess WH, Marshak DR, et al: Purification and characterization of an insulin-like growth factor II variant from human plasma. J Biol Chem 32:19155, 1989.

63. Daughaday WH, Rotwein P: Insulin-like growth factors I and II. Peptide, messenger ribonucleic acid and gene structures, serum, and tissue concentrations. Endocr Rev 10:68, 1989.

64. Han VKM, Lund PK, Lee DC, et al: Expression of somatomedin/insulin-like growth factor messenger ribonucleic acids in the human fetus: Identification, characterization, and tissue distribution. J Clin Endocrinol Metab 66:422, 1988.

65. Hill DJ: Relative abundance and molecular size of immunoreactive insulin-like growth factors I and II in human fetal tissues. Early Hum Dev 21:49, 1990.

66. Clemmons DR: Insulin-like growth factor binding proteins. Trends Endocrinol Metab 1:412, 1990.

67. Baxter RC: Insulin-like growth factor (IGF) binding proteins: The role of serum IGF-BPs in regulating IGF availability. Acta Paediatr Scand 372:107, 1991.

68. Lewitt MS, Baxter RC: At the cutting edge, insulin-like growth factor-binding protein-1: A role in glucose counterregulation? Mol Cell Endocrinol 79:C147, 1991.

69. Shimasaki S, Shimonaka M, Zhang H-P, et al: Isolation and molecular characterization of three novel insulin-like growth factor binding proteins (IGFBP-4, 5 and 6). In Spencer EM (ed): Modern Concepts of Insulin-Like Growth Factors. New York, Elsevier, 1991, pp 343–358.

70. Elgin RC, Busby WH, Clemmons DR: An insulin-like growth factor binding–protein enhances the biologic response to IGF-I. Proc Natl Acad Sci USA 84:3254, 1987.

71. Kortleve DJ, Groffen CAH, Schuller A, et al: The evolution of the insulin-like growth factor binding protein family. In Spencer EM (ed): Modern Concepts of Insulin-Like Growth Factors. New York, Elsevier, 1991, pp 311–328.

72. Silbergeld A, Litwin A, Bruchis S, et al: Insulin-like growth factor I (IGF-I) in healthy children, adolescents and adults as determined by a radioimmunoassay specific for the synthetic 53-70 peptide region. Clin Endocrinol 25:67, 1986.

73. Rosenfeld RG, Wilson DM, Lee PDK, et al: Insulin-like growth factors I and II in evaluation of growth retardation. J Pediatr 109:428, 1986.

74. Rosenfeld RG, Kemp SF, Hintz RL: Constancy of somatomedin response to growth hormone treatment of hypopituitary dwarfism, and lack of correlation with growth rate. J Clin Endocrinol Metab 53:611, 1981.

75. Barkan AL, Beitins IZ, Kelch RP: Plasma insulin-like growth factor-I/somatomedin-C in acromegaly: Correlation with the degree of growth hormone hypersecretion. J Clin Endocrinol Metab 67:69, 1988.

76. Clemmons DR, Klibanski A, Underwood LE, et al: Reduction of plasma immunoreactive somatomedin-C during fasting in humans. J Clin Endocrinol Metab 53:1247, 1981.

77. Grant D, Hambley J, Becker D, et al: Reduced sulphation factor in undernourished children. Arch Dis Child 48:596, 1973.

78. Underwood LE, Thissen J-P, Moats-Staats BM, et al: Nutritional regulation of IGF-I and postnatal growth. In Spencer EM (ed): Modern Concepts of Insulin-Like Growth Factors. New York, Elsevier, 1991, pp 37–48.

79. Isley WH, Underwood LE, Clemmons DR: Dietary components that regulate serum somatomedin-C concentrations in humans. J Clin Invest 71:175, 1983.

80. Wu J-C, Daughaday WH, Lee S-D, et al: Radioimmunoassay of serum IGF-I and IGF-II in patients with chronic liver diseases and hepatocellular carcinoma with or without hypoglycemia. J Lab Clin Med 112:589, 1988.

81. Daughaday WH, Deuel TF: Tumor secretion of growth factors. Endocrinol Metab Clin North Am 20:539–563, 1991.

82. Daughaday WH, Kapadia M: Significance of abnormal serum binding of insulin-like growth factor II in the development of hypoglycemia in patients with non–islet-cell tumors. Proc Natl Acad Sci USA 86:6778, 1989.

83. Baxter RC, Daughaday WH: Impaired formation of the ternary insulin-like growth factor binding protein complex in patients with hypoglycemia due to non–islet cell tumors. J Clin Endocrinol Metab 73:696, 1991.

84. Neely EK, Beukers MW, Oh Y, et al: Insulin-like growth factor receptors. Acta Paediatr Scand 372:116, 1991.

85. Jacobs S, Maxham CP: Hybrid IGF-I receptors. In Spencer EM (ed): Modern Concepts of Insulin-Like Growth Factors. New York, Elsevier, 1991, pp 431–438.

86. Shoelson SE, Chatterjee S, Chaudhuri M, et al: YMXM motifs of IRS-1 define substrate specificity of the insulin receptor kinase. Proc Natl Acad Sci USA 89:2027, 1992.

87. Morgan DO, Edman JC, Standring DN, et al: Insulin-like growth factor 2 receptor as a multifunctional binding protein. Nature (London) 329:301, 1987.

88. Nishimoto I, Kojima I, Ohkuni Y, et al: Insulin-like growth factor-II increases cytoplasmic free calcium in competent balb/c3T3 cells treated with epidermal growth factor. Biochem Biophys Res Commun 142:275, 1987.

89. Hari J, Pierce SB, Morgan DO, et al: The receptor for insulin-like growth factor II mediates an insulin-like response. EMBO J 6:3367, 1987.

90. Kojima I, Nishimoto I, Iiri T, et al: Evidence that type II insulin-like growth factor receptor is coupled to calcium gating system. Biochem Biophys Res Commun 154:9, 1988.

91. El-Badry OM, Minniti C, Kohn EC, et al: Insulin-like growth factor II acts as an autocrine growth and mobility factor in human rhabdomyosarcoma tumors. Cell Growth Differentiation 1:325, 1990.

92. Lindahl A, Isgaard J, Isaksson O: Growth and differentiation. Bailliere's Clin Endocrinol Metab 5:671, 1991.

93. Schlechter NL, Russell SM, Spencer EM, et al: Evidence to suggest that the direct growth promoting effects of growth hormone on cartilage in vivo are mediated by local production of somatomedin. Proc Natl Acad Sci USA 83:2932, 1986.

94. Daughaday WH: A personal history of the origin of the somatomedin hypothesis and recent challenges to its validity. Perspect Biol Med 32:194, 1989.

95. Lindahl A, Nilsson A, Isaksson OGP: Effects of growth hormone and insulin-like growth factor-I on colony formation of rabbit epiphyseal chondrocytes at different stages of maturation. J Endocrinol 115:263, 1987.

96. Maciel RMB, Moses AC, Villone G, et al: Demonstration of the production and physiological role of insulin-like growth factor II in rat thyroid follicular cells in culture. J Clin Invest 82:1546, 1988.

97. Morikawa M, Nixon T, Green H: Growth hormone and the adipose conversion of 3T3 cells. Cell 29:783, 1982.

98. Nixon BT, Green H: Growth hormone promotes the differentiation of myoblasts and preadipocytes generated by azacytadine treatment of 10T1-2 cells. Proc Natl Acad Sci USA 81:3429, 1984.

99. Zizulak KM, Green H: The generation of insulin-like growth factor-I sensitive cells by growth hormone action. Science 233:551, 1986.

100. Florini JR, Ewton DZ, Roof SL: Insulin-like growth factor-I stimulates terminal myogenic differentiation by induction of myogenin gene expression. Mol Endocrinol 5:718, 1991.

101. Beede DC, Silver MH, Belcher KS, et al: Lentropin, a protein that controls lens fiber formation, is related functionally and immunologically to the insulin-like growth factors. Proc Natl Acad Sci USA 84:2327, 1987.

102. Adashi EY, Resnich CE, D'Ercole AJ, et al: Insulin-like growth factors as intraovarian regulators of granulosa cell growth and function. Endocrine Rev 6:400, 1985.

103. Guler HP, Zapf J, Froesch ER: Short-term metabolic effects of recombinant human insulin-like factor I in healthy adults. N Engl J Med 317:137, 1987.

104. Takano K, Hizuka N, Asakawa K, et al: Effects of s.c. administration of recombinant human insulin-like growth factor I (IGF-I) on normal human subjects. Endocrinol Jpn 37:309, 1990.

105. Guler H-P, Schmidt C, Zapf J, et al: Effects of recombinant insulin-like growth factor I on insulin secretion and renal function in normal human subjects. Proc Natl Acad Sci USA 86:2868, 1989.

106. Jacob R, Barrett E, Plewe G, et al: Acute effects of insulin-like growth factor I on glucose and amino acid metabolism in the awake fasted rat. Comparison with insulin. J Clin Invest 83:1717, 1989.

107. Moxley RT II, Arner P, Moss A, et al: Acute effects of insulin-like growth factor I and insulin on glucose metabolism in vivo. Am J Physiol 259:E561, 1990.

108. Sherwin RS: Metabolic effects of insulin-like growth factor I in humans: Comparison to insulin. Program 74th Annual Meeting, The Endocrine Society, 1992, p 42.

109. Schoenle EJ, Zenobi PD, Torresani T, et al: Recombinant human insulin-like growth factor I (rhIGF-I) reduces hyperglycemia in patients with extreme insulin resistance. Diabetalogia 34:675, 1991.

110. Quin JD, Fisher BM, Paterson KR, et al: Acute response to recombinant insulin-like growth factor I in a patient with Mendenhall's syndrome. N Engl J Med 323:1425, 1990.

111. Elahi D, McAloon-Dyke M, Fukagawa NK, et al: Hemodynamic and metabolic responses to human insulin-like growth factor I (IGF-I) in men. In Spencer EM (ed): Modern Concepts of Insulin-Like Growth Factors. New York, Elsevier, 1991, pp 219–224.

112. Schoenle E, Zapf J, Humbel RE, et al: Insulin-like growth factor I stimulates growth in hypophysectomized rats. Nature 296:252, 1982.

113. Mathews LS, Hammer RE, Behringer RR, et al: Growth enhancement of transgenic mice expressing human insulin-like growth factor I. Endocrinology 123:2827, 1988.

114. Behringer RR, Lewin TM, Quaife CJ, et al: Expression of insulin-like growth factor I stimulates normal somatic growth in growth hormone–deficient transgenic mice. Endocrinology 127:1033, 1990.

115. Walker JL, Ginalska-Malinowska M, Romer TE, et al: Effects of the infusion of insulin-like growth factor I in a child with growth hormone insensitivity syndrome (Laron dwarfism). N Engl J Med 324:1483, 1991.

116. Laron Z, Klipper-Aurbach Y, Klinger B: Effects of insulin-like growth factor on linear growth, head circumference, and body fat in patients with Laron-type dwarfism. Lancet 339:1258, 1992.

117. Laron Z: Laron-type dwarfism (hereditary somatomedin deficiency): A review. Ergebnisse der Innern Medizin und Kinderheilkunde. Adv Intern Med Pediatr 51:117, 1984.

118. Chang-DeMoranville BM, Jackson IMD: Diagnosis and endocrine testing in acromegaly. Endocrinol Metab Clin North Am 21:649, 1992.

119. Fahlbusch R, Honegger J, Buchfelder M: Surgical management of acromegaly. Endocrinol Metab Clin North Am 21:669, 1992.

120. Asa SL, Kovacs K: Pituitary pathology in acromegaly. Endocrinol Metab Clin North Am 21:553, 1992.

121. Alexander JM, Biller BMK, Zervas NT, et al: Clinically nonfunctioning pituitary tumors are monoclonal in origin. J Clin Invest 86:336, 1990.

122. Herman V, Fagin J, Gonsky R, et al: Clonal origin of pituitary adenomas. J Clin Endocrinol Metab 71:1427, 1990.

123. Spada A, Arosio M, Bochicchio D, et al: Clinical, biochemical and morphological correlates in patients bearing growth hormone–secreting pituitary tumors with or without constitutively active adenylyl cyclase. J Clin Endocrinol Metab 71:1421, 1990.

124. Weinstein LS, Shenker A, Gejman PV, et al: Activating mutations of the stimulatory G protein in the McCune-Albright syndrome. N Engl J Med 325:1688, 1991.

125. Bystrom C, Larsson C, Blomberg C, et al: Localization of the MEN 1 gene to a small region within chromosome 11q13 deletion mapping in tumors. Proc Natl Acad Sci USA 87:1968, 1990.

126. Bale AE, Norton JA, Wong EL, et al: Allelic loss on chromosome 11 in hereditary and sporadic tumors related to familial multiple endocrine neoplasia type 1. Cancer Res 51:1154, 1991.

127. Melmed S, Ezrin C, Kovacs K, et al: Acromegaly due to secretion of growth hormone by an ectopic pancreatic islet-cell tumor. N Engl J Med 312:9, 1985.

128. Kovacs K: Growth hormone–releasing hormone–producing tumors: Clinical, biochemical, and morphological manifestations. Endocr Rev 9:357, 1987.

129. Faglia G, Arosio M, Bazzoni N: Ectopic acromegaly. Endocrinol Metab Clin North Am 21:575, 1992.

130. Leveston SA, McKeel DW Jr, Buckley PJ, et al: Acromegaly and Cushing's syndrome associated with a foregut carcinoid tumor. J Clin Endocrinol Metab 52:682, 1981.

131. Frohman LA, Downs TR: Ectopic GRH syndromes. In Robbins RJ, Melmed S (eds): A Century of Scientific and Clinical Progress. New York, Plenum Publishing, 1987, p 115.

132. Grunstein RR, Ho KY, Sullivan CE: Sleep apnea in acromegaly. Ann Intern Med 115:527, 1991.

133. Daughaday WH: Pituitary gigantism. Endocrinol Metab Clin North Am 21:633, 1992.

134. Daughaday WH: Extreme gigantism. N Engl J Med 297:1267, 1977.

135. Sotos JF, Dodge PR, Muirhead D, et al: Cerebral gigantism in childhood. N Engl J Med 271:109, 1964.

136. Hook EB, Reynolds JW: Cerebral gigantism: Endocrinological and clinical observations of six patients including a congenital giant, concordant monozygotic twins and a child who achieved adult gigantic size. J Pediatr 70:900, 1967.

137. Trotman-Dickenson B, Weetman AP, Hughes JMB: Upper airflow obstruction and pulmonary function in acromegaly: Relationship to disease activity. Q J Med 79:527, 1991.

138. Nabarra JDN: Acromegaly. Clin Endocrinol 26:481, 1987.

139. Takeda R, Tatami R, Ueda K, et al: The incidence and pathogenesis of hyperlipidaemia in 16 consecutive acromegalic patients. Acta Endocrinol 100:358, 1982.

140. Eskildsen PC, Lund B, Sorensen OH, et al: Acromegaly and vitamin D metabolism: Effect of bromocriptine treatment. J Clin Endocrinol Metab 49:484, 1979.

141. Takamoto S, Tsuchiya H, Onishi T, et al: Changes in calcium homeostasis in acromegaly treated by pituitary adenomectomy. J Clin Endocrinol Metab 61:71, 1985.

142. Whitehead EM, Shalet SM, Davies D, et al: Pituitary gigantism: A disabling condition. Clin Endocrinol 17:271, 1982.

143. Carlson HE, Linfood JA, Braunstein GD, et al: Hyperthyroidism and acromegaly due to a thyrotropin- and growth hormone–secreting pituitary tumor. Lack of hormonal response to bromocriptine. Am J Med 74:915, 1983.

144. Ludmerer K, Kissane JM (eds): Clinicopathologic conference: Multiple pituitary hormonal abnormalities in a 60-year old man. Am J Med 83:1111, 1987.

145. O'Duffy JD, Randall RV, MacCarty CS: Median neuropathy (carpal-tunnel syndrome) in acromegaly. A sign of endocrine over-activity. Ann Intern Med 78:379, 1973.

146. Pickett JBE III, Layzer RB, Levin SR, et al: Neuromuscular complications of acromegaly. Neurology 25:638, 1975.

147. Wright AD, Hill DM, Lowy C, et al: Mortality in acromegaly. Q J Med 39:1, 1970.

148. Alexander L, Appleton D, Hall R, et al: Epidemiology of acromegaly in the Newcastle region. Clin Endocrinol (Oxf) 12:71, 1980.

149. Bengtsson BA, Eden S, Ernest I, et al: Epidemiology and long-term survival in acromegaly. Acta Med Scand 223:327, 1988.

150. Ezzat S, Melmed S: Are patients with acromegaly at increased risk for neoplasia. J Clin Endocrinol Metab 72:245, 1991.

151. Moon HD, Simpson ME, Li CH, et al: Neoplasms in rats treated with pituitary growth hormone I. Pulmonary and lymphatic tissues. Cancer Res 10:297, 1950.

152. Klein I, Parveen G, Gavoeler JS, et al: Colonic polyps in patients with acromegaly. Ann Intern Med 97:27, 1982.

153. Brunner JE, Johnson CC, Zafar S, et al: Colon cancer and polyps in acromegaly: Increased risk associated with family history of colon cancer. Clin Endocrol (Oxf) 32:65, 1990.

154. Fahlbusch R, Honegger J, Buchfelder M: Surgical management of acromegaly. Endocrinol Metab Clin North Am 21:669, 1992.

155. Ross DA, Wilson CB: Results of transsphenoidal microsurgery for growth hormone–secreting pituitary adenoma in a series of 214 patients. J Neurosurg 68:854, 1988.

156. Eastman RC, Gorden P, Glatstein E, et al: Radiation therapy of acromegaly. Endocrinol Metab Clin North Am 21:693, 1992.

157. Littley MD, Shalet SM, Beardwell CG: Radiation and the hypothalamic pituitary axis. *In* Gutin PH, Leibel SA, Sheline GE (eds): Radiation Injury to the Nervous System. New York, Raven Press, 1991, p 303.

158. Clemmons DR, Underwood LE, Ridgway EG, et al: Estradiol treatment of acromegaly: Reduction of immunoreactive somatomedin-C and improvement of metabolic status. Am J Med 69:571, 1980.

159. Adams EF, Ghuttacharji SC, Halliwell CL, et al: Effect of pancreatic growth hormone releasing factors on GH secretion by human somatotrophic pituitary tumours in cell culture. Clin Endocrinol 21:709–718, 1984.

160. Jaffe CA, Barkan AL: Treatment of acromegaly with dopamine agonists. Endocrinol Metab Clin North Am 21:713–735, 1992.

161. Chiodini PG, Cozzi R, Dallabonzana D, et al: Medical treatment of acromegaly with SMS 201-995, a somatostatin analog: A comparison with bromocriptine. J Clin Endocrinol Metab 64:447–453, 1987.

162. Lamberts SWJ, Reubi J-C, Krenning EP: Somatostatin analogs in the treatment of acromegaly. Endocrinol Metab Clin North Am 21:737, 1992.

163. Lamberts SWJ, Uitterlinden P, Schuijff PC, et al: Therapy of acromegaly with Sandostatin: The predictive value of an acute test, the value of serum somatomedin-C measurements in dose adjustment and the definition of a biochemical "cure." Clin Endocrinol 29:411, 1988.

164. Asa SL, Felix I, Singer W, et al: Effects of somatostatin on human pituitary somatotroph adenomas: An in vitro functional and morphologic study. Program of the Endocrine Soc 1990 (abstract 93).

165. Hofland LJ, Velkeniers B, van Koetsveld PM, et al: The relationship between growth hormone (GH) messenger ribonucleic acid levels and hormone release from individual cells derived from human GH–secreting pituitary adenomas. Clin Endocrinol 34:5, 1991.

166. Plockinger U, Dienermann D, Quabbe H-J: Gastrointestinal side-effects of octreotide during long term treatment of acromegaly. J Clin Endocrinol Metab 71:1658, 1990.

167. Ho KY, Weissberger AJ, Marbach P, et al: Therapeutic efficacy of the somstostatin analog SMS 201-995 (octreotide) in acromegaly. Effects of dose and frequency and long-term safety. Ann Intern Med 112:173, 1990.

20

Growth Hormone Insufficiency: Clinical Features, Diagnosis, and Therapy

MICHAEL B. RANKE

The existence of a pituitary hormone responsible for the regulation of growth has been recognized for many years.[1, 2] The first isolated growth hormone (GH), which was bovine, was found to be ineffective in humans[3, 4] owing to the structural difference between primate and nonprimate growth hormone.[5] It was only after GH was isolated from human cadaver pituitaries that the treatment of growth hormone deficiency (GHD) became possible.[6, 7] But the limited availability of extracted GH posed a problem in itself, which was overcome when, through modern gene technology, methionyl human GH (met-hGH)[8] and authentic recombinant GH (r-hGH)[9] were produced. As a result of the dramatic increase in therapeutical possibilities, a wide range of disorders linked with impaired GH secretion can now be defined, as can their pathogenetic level. The discoveries of the effect of the somatomedin mediators on growth and of their complex regulatory system have further increased our understanding of the pathogenesis of such disorders. Thus, it is now accepted that GHD occurs in a spectrum of disorders in which the clinical and auxological pictures are relatively identical.

ETIOLOGY OF GROWTH HORMONE DEFICIENCY

Growth hormone deficiency comprises a spectrum of etiologically and pathogenetically different disorders. A gene defect causing the inability to synthesize GH,[10, 11] i.e., GH deficiency in the true sense, must be considered separately, as the border between normal GH secretion and that in insufficient GH secretion is quite blurred. In gen-

eral, the term *GH insufficiency* (GHI) is preferable to GHD in referring to patients with impaired GH secretion. Here the term GHD will be reserved only to describe abnormal growth arising from a gene deletion or the absence of the pituitary gland. An attempt to classify the different disorders according to common criteria is at present not relevant, as our knowledge is still too limited.[12]

The most frequent form of GHD is the idiopathic growth hormone deficiency or insufficiency (IGHD/IGHI), which occurs either isolated or combined with other pituitary hormonal deficiencies, e.g., multiple pituitary hormone deficiency (MPHD). The incidence of IGHD is yet unknown and may vary from nation to nation; some population surveys have led to estimates of an incidence of between 1:5000 and 1:10,000.[13, 14] It has also been widely observed that more males suffer from IGHD than do females, the ratio being approximately 2:1. Until recently investigators could not determine any definite etiological factors in this group of disorders. It has been suggested, however, that head trauma at birth leads to hypothalamic or pituitary damage.[15, 13] Interestingly, the number of breech deliveries is relatively high in this group.[16] On the other hand, a high percentage of children with IGHI were delivered by cesarean section, an obstetrical measure taken to help reduce neonatal trauma, especially in cases of breech presentation. Thus, it remains an enigma as to whether functional and anatomical lesions in the pituitary and hypothalamic area cause irregularities at birth, such as breech presentation, or whether these abnormalities result from such anomalies. These lesions were also observed more frequently in patients with assumed IGHD when modern imaging techniques were used.[17, 18] The fact that the mothers of patients with IGHD are relatively shorter than their fathers may indicate that the risk of perinatal trauma in normal-sized newborns[19] is higher. Short stature in parents of children with isolated IGHD may also point to a genetic link between the affected children and their parents.

In some forms of isolated GHD, heredity is a determining factor.[20] The autosomal recessive form of GHD, for instance, is caused by the deletion of the hGH-1 gene (type IA).[10, 21] Whether growth-attenuating antibodies to exogenous GH are formed or not clearly depends on the molecular basis of the defect.[22, 23] In the autosomal dominant form (type IB), the hGH-1 gene is not defective, which explains why residual GH is secreted. There have been reports of an autosomal dominant form (type II)[24]; also, a fourth variation, possibly an X-linked recessive form associated with hypogammaglobulinemia (type III), is known to exist.[25] It can be assumed that further defects of the genes that regulate the synthesis and/or secretion of GH will be discovered in the future.

In the group of patients whose disorders are characterized by a disturbed pattern of GH secretion and cannot be diagnosed by using conventional criteria (see later), the underlying cause is unknown. The majority of congenital or acquired forms of GHI caused by functional or anatomical lesions are sometimes linked with other hormonal deficiencies of the pituitary gland or hypothalamus. It is difficult to answer the question as to whether the isolated form of idiopathic GHD occurs more frequently than does the multiple GHD form, as the results of various series have been so dissimilar.[26] A selection bias may account for this, as also may the timing and extent of testing for additional deficiencies. Thus figures on the occurrence of IGHD vary.

Many congenital central malformations, such as those of septo-optical dysplasia (synonymous with the de Morsier syndrome),[27] empty sella syndrome,[28] and solitary central maxillary incisor syndrome,[29] are associated with midline defects and cleft palate.[30] Among the defined syndromes, there are several in which congenital GHI is a major disorder.[20] In general, GHI may occur in specific syndromes causing short stature or increasing its severity. Prenatal infections such as rubella may also cause hypothalamic or pituitary damage.[31]

Acquired forms of GHD can result from tumors in or around the hypothalamus or pituitary gland (e.g., craniopharyngeoma and dysgerminoma). The former is reported to occur more frequently, and GHI can be diagnosed either at the time of presentation or after surgery and/or radiotherapy.[32] Of cranial tumors distant from the hypothalamus and pituitary area, medulloblastomas are the most common. Damage to this area is invariably caused by high-dose cranial irradiation, a therapeutical measure needed in about 70 per cent of these cases.[33, 34] In fact, recent advances in medical treatment are also the reason why many children with tumors outside the cranium (e.g., leukemia, lymphoma) suffer from GHI, since cranial irradiation is now part of many standard treatment regimens and will damage the hypothalamus and pituitary area.[35] Other causes of acquired GHD/GHI, such as head injury, CNS infection, hydrocephalus, granulomatous disease, Langerhans' histiocytosis (histiocytosis X), deposition of hemosiderin, and vascular anomalies, are rare. A fascinating thought, which may soon steer the course of research in this field, is that an autoimmune process at the level of the hypothalamus and pituitary area may actually cause GHI.[36]

CLINICAL FEATURES

The clinical appearance of children with GHI varies from patient to patient, as does the degree to which GH secretion is impaired. Severe cases of GHI, however, allow an immediate clinical diagnosis, as the clinical picture is characteristic: the body proportions are normal; the forehead is prominent and the bridge of the nose sunken; the cranium, hands, and feet are particularly small; a marked increase in the amount of subcutaneous fat along the trunk is present; in whites the skin is so pallid that the subcutaneous veins show up; the hair is thin but not sparse; nail growth is slow; and the child has a high-pitched voice (Fig. 20–1). As a rule dental eruption is retarded, and permanent teeth are irregularly positioned. The delay in bone maturity usually matches the degree of growth retardation (Fig. 20–2). Although the onset of puberty is delayed in cases of isolated GHD, it generally keeps pace with bone age.[37] In congenital GHI affecting male children, microphallus is sometimes an additional anomaly.

During the neonatal period, prolonged icterus and hypoglycemia may be signs of GHI, but it is the auxology that is the bedrock of diagnosis. The degree of height deviation from the normal is a determining factor with respect to the age at which the diagnosis is made (Fig. 20–3). Interestingly, in children who presented with short stature and in whom idiopathic GHI was found, height at time of diagnosis was less than the height at diagnosis of children whose short stature was due to GHD or GHI associated with an organic lesion.[38] It has been suggested that sex and race can affect the timing of diagnosis.[39] Because it takes a normally tall child a long time to fall beyond the 3rd percentile—particularly if the target height is high—height in itself is not the best parameter in diagnosing abnormal

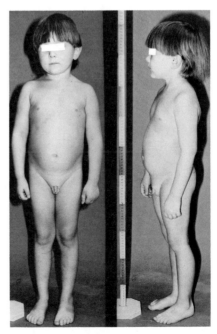

FIGURE 20–1. Clinical appearance of an 11-year-old boy with isolated IGHI (height = 102 cm.)

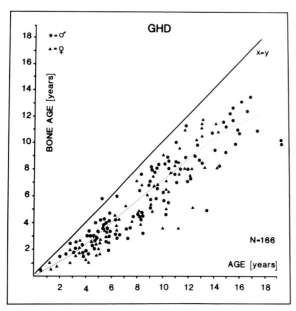

FIGURE 20–2. Bone age at diagnosis in children with IGHI.

growth. Growth velocity, on the other hand, will outline a continuous decrease in height velocity up to or well below the 25th percentile in a child with GHD. The determination of height velocity takes the two distant height measurements into consideration, with their error measurement, and, in addition, the error of height velocity depends on the time interval of the measurements.

$$\frac{\text{SD of error of measurement}}{1.41 \times \text{duration of interval/yr}} = \text{SD error of height velocity}$$

It remains controversial whether the prenatal or perinatal onset of GHD/GHI influences neonatal size or early postnatal growth. It used to be thought that GH was unim-

portant in prenatal growth.[40] Some reports have shown that a high proportion of children with IGHD are small at birth[15, 41] and that height velocity sinks rapidly immediately after. Thus the degree of impaired growth reflecting the extent of GH insufficiency and the careful eye of the medical examiner are crucial to the timely diagnosis of growth problems.

It is well known that in children with GHI more subcutaneous fat is measurable by caliper.[42] However, probably as a result of compensatory reduction in muscle mass, the weight-for-height ratio tends to be normal during the prepubertal period. A detailed account of alterations in body composition using modern techniques is thus needed in children with GHD/GHI.[43]

BIOCHEMICAL DIAGNOSIS

While the diagnosis of the complete absence of GH production (e.g., GHD type IA) is straightforward, it is hard to pinpoint insufficient GH secretion in this rare condition. The difficulty lies in proving that the amount of GH secreted in a slowly growing child does not suffice to maintain growth within normal limits. The modalities formerly used to diagnose GHD/GHI were developed on the basis of available possibilities and empirically deduced conventions. According to conventional criteria, the diagnosis of GHI is established only if the clinical and auxological criteria are compatible and if the GH levels do not exceed a limit set in standard stimulation tests. It is accepted practice that two tests are done. However, this method of defining "classical" GHI/GHD should be challenged in the light of recent developments, the most important of which will be covered later in this chapter.

In the evaluation of GH testing, it should be remembered that secondary factors also influence GH secretion. Hypercortisolism, for instance, as well as hypothyroidism and obesity, impair GH secretion. Hypothyroidism is signif-

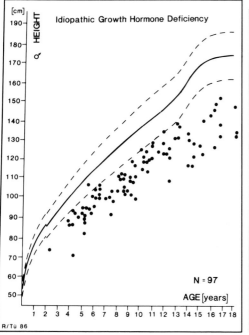

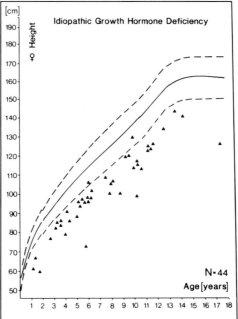

FIGURE 20–3. Height at diagnosis in children with IGHI compared to normal ranges.

icant in the case of a short, obese child, because one noticeable indication of GHI is the aforementioned thickness of subcutaneous fat. Emotional factors, such as those known to impair GH secretion in anorexia nervosa, may also affect test results. The question of whether GH secretion is primarily diminished in Crohn's disease is currently being discussed.

DETERMINATION OF GROWTH HORMONE

GH circulating in body fluids is composed of a mixture of peptides,[44] the major component—about 90 per cent—being a polypeptide of 191 amino acids with a molecular weight of 22,000 (the "22 k" form). It is the product of the hGH-1 gene, which is located on the long arm of chromosome 17 along with other members of the hGH and human chorionic somatomammotropin (hCS) family.[45] Through alternate splicing, a smaller hGH (the "20 k" form) is produced from the hGH-1 gene. Constituents of the different forms of GH circulating in the body vary, as does their biological potency.[46, 47] GH in blood is measured using immunoassays using monoclonal or polyclonal antibodies that potentially recognize different epitopes of the growth hormones.[48] Without an external internationally accepted quality control of tests, it is fruitless to compare results from various laboratories; the new international standard, IRP WHO 80/505 r-hGH, has a potency of 3.3 IU/mg r-hGH, in sharp contrast to the earlier IRP 66/217, which is equivalent to 2 IU/mg Pit-hGH. This indicates that a general cut-off level that merely divides GHI patients from non-GHI patients is also questionable from the perspective of GH measurements. Receptor assays and bioassays for GH do exist but have not found their way into standard diagnostic procedures in clinical practice.[49]

GROWTH HORMONE SECRETION AND STIMULATION TESTS

GH secretion in the pituitary gland can be provoked by physiological stimuli such as sleep, exercise, and specific components in food, as well as by pharmacological stimuli such as clonidine, L-dopa, and insulin (as a means of inducing hypoglycemia). The mechanisms by which various stimuli transmit their message to the pituitary gland are complex (Fig. 20–4). In the hypothalamus, different substances bind to various receptors in the neurotransmitter network, following which GH release is either positively or negatively affected. Thus a combination of GHRH and somatostatin (growth hormone release–inhibiting hormone, GHRIH) is directly or indirectly released at the hypothalamic level. It is now known that agonists of the α- and β-receptor, as well as the dopaminergic and serotoninergic agonists, stimulate GH release, whereas their respective antagonists inhibit it. Moreover, further neurotransmitter systems are involved in the regulation of GH secretion.[50, 51]

Since a standardized exercise plan can provoke the secretion of GH, it is often used to screen outpatients.[52] The disadvantage of this method is that it often yields "false-positive" results. The most widely used pharmaceutical substances in the standardized stimulation of GH are

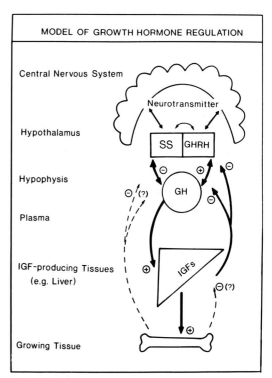

FIGURE 20–4. Model of growth hormone regulation.

the amino acids arginine-HCl and ornithine, clonidine, L-dopa, and (despite the potential risk of hypoglycemia) insulin.[53, 54] Since these substances act in different ways, a combination of tests might be useful in pinpointing the mechanisms underlying impaired GH secretion. The therapeutical consequences of such an approach have not yet been adopted into routine medical practice.

The potency of each testing procedure in provoking a certain degree of GH release differs. Clonidine is probably the most potent drug for this purpose. As a rule, the highest GH level observed in a test is considered as the response. Since all these pharmacological tests tend to provoke GH secretion insufficiently (the "false-positive" response can be as high as 25 per cent), it has become common practice to base the diagnosis of GHD/GHI on the results of at least two tests. A predefined cut-off level for all of these tests is questionable, as mentioned earlier. Responsiveness to the various agents differs according to age, sex, and stage of development, and normal values cannot be established. This unresolved issue of setting "normal" values also casts doubt on the principally justified approach in which "priming" with sex steroids is done before a test.[55] The best that can be said in defense of using the widely accepted cut-off level of 10 μg/L = 20 mIU/L is that just a few patients in need of GH will be deprived of therapy. Cut-off levels of 10 mIU/L and 14 mIU/L, respectively, formerly were part of the definition of "total" GHD, and levels between 10 and 20 mIU/L were considered to indicate "partial" GHD. In various national studies, different cut-off levels were fixed to define impaired GH secretion.[56] It might be best to reserve the term "total," however, for cases of gene deletion or the absence of the pituitary gland.

GROWTH HORMONE–RELEASING HORMONE TESTING

Both naturally occurring GHRH-40 and GHRH-44 are the result of alternate splicing from the same gene.[57] Their molecules, shortened to 37 N-terminal residues and GHRH (1-29) amide, are equally potent, on a molar basis, in provoking GH release from the pituitary somatotrophs. The highest amount of GH release can be induced by an intravenous injection of 1 µg/kg BW of these peptides. In cases in which the source of GHI is the pituitary gland, the GH release induced by GHRH does not exceed 10 µg/L of GH, and GH responsiveness tends to be delayed. Although the test has a high sensitivity in cases of GHD/GHI diagnosed through standard stimulation tests, its specificity is low.[58] Therefore, this test is mainly used to differentiate between GHI originating in the pituitary gland (impaired response to GHRH) from that originating in the hypothalamus (response to GHRH). The latter, however, can be definitely established only after longer exposure to GHRH indicates that "dormant" somatotrophs can be stimulated into actively secreting GH. The modalities of such priming have not yet been standardized. It is now accepted that most cases of GHI formerly classified as being of pituitary origin were, in fact, hypothalamic cases.

SPONTANEOUS GROWTH HORMONE SECRETION

Measurements of spontaneous GH secretion taken over time reflect the status of GH secretion and its relationship to growth better than do measurements arising from pharmacological stimuli.[59, 60] In some cases of GHI, "normal" GH levels are reached in standard tests, and low amounts of GH are secreted spontaneously.[59, 61] Nevertheless, although spontaneous GH secretion may be considered as the "gold standard" in defining GHI, many problems limit its usefulness as a diagnostic tool.[60] Many questions remain open, e.g., whether integrated versus discrete sampling should be conducted, what the correct sampling intervals should be, and what constitutes the optimal duration of sampling in order to achieve the most accurate results; at the same time, there is the challenge of making testing as inexpensive and convenient as possible. A complex analysis of data is needed if discrete sampling is done.[62] It is not absolutely clear which of the parameters characterizing a secretion profile (e.g., area under the curve [AUC], sum of peak heights, and frequency of peaks) is best associated with the growth process. A limited number of reference values have been established using different methods,[60] but the relatively high intraindividual reproducibility of less than 30 per cent (as in standard tests) makes the evaluation of spontaneous GH secretion a research tool rather than an established method in clinical endocrinology. If the total amount of GH secreted were the major determining factor of growth[63] rather than the complex pattern, it would suffice to use less-demanding sampling techniques to determine spontaneous GH secretion.[64]

URINARY GROWTH HORMONE

Although only minimal amounts of GH are excreted in urine in comparison to the total amount secreted, there seems to be a good correlation between these parameters.[65] Ultrasensitive assays have recently been developed that enable even minute amounts of GH in urine to be measured.[66, 67] Since urine—particularly early morning urine—can easily and repeatedly be obtained, a good picture of the GH secretory status of a child can be delineated through long-term measurements. Provided that the factors influencing GH excretion at the renal level are excluded, the measurement of urinary GH might become another possibility in screening for GHD/GHI.

INSULIN-LIKE GROWTH FACTORS

Since the somatomedin hypothesis[68] was put forward, there has been heated discussion of whether the growth-promoting effect is a direct consequence of GH or whether it occurs indirectly through a somatomedin or other insulin-like growth factors (IGF's). Moreover, it is still a point of debate as to whether IGF activity is mediated by the endocrine system or whether it is channeled through the paracrine and autocrine route. The "dual effector theory of GH action" (regardless of whether it is proved or disproved) incorporates both these diverging views,[65] and the recent success of the latest attempt in treating Laron-type dwarfism, in which IGF-I is applied systemically, indicates that IGF's probably are an integral part of the endocrine system. What we do know, however, is that the blood levels of both IGF-I and its major binding protein (IGFBP-3) are highly correlated with the total amount of GH secreted.[70] Indeed, both factors have been proved to be highly sensitive and specific in confirming GHD/GHI that has been diagnosed by conventional criteria.[70, 71] Although the nutritional status and liver or kidney function are known to influence the IGF-I and IGFBP-3 levels in blood, it can be taken for granted that impaired GH secretion is highly unlikely if test results show normal levels of these variables (Fig. 20–5).[72] IGF measurements are now crucial in correctly establishing bioactive GH,[73] as either normal or high levels of GH measured in these cases invariably confound the diagnosis. A strong case could actually be made to place IGF-I and IGFBP-3 measurements at the top of an algorithm grading the different stages in dealing with sus-

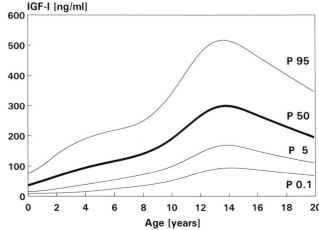

FIGURE 20–5. Normal age-dependent levels (RIA) of IGF-I and IGFBP-3.

pected GHI or GHD (Table 20–1), because when these parameters are normal, it is highly improbable that the patient has GHD or GHI. One method of establishing or ruling out syndromes involving GH insensitivity is a short-term test of the GH-dependent IGF-I and IGFBP-3 levels. Such testing would further extend the diagnostic possibilities, but, unfortunately, this has not yet been standardized.[72]

TREATMENT OF GROWTH HORMONE DEFICIENCY

The aim of treatment in children with GHD must be to ensure normal height during childhood and in adult life. Besides accomplishing this, the treatment method should

be convenient for the patient and treatment risks and costs should be minimal. A discussion of the factors possibly influencing the growth response—route, frequency, and timing of GH administration as well as dosage and the pharmaceutical product itself—follows. Other aspects of treatment, such as the first year, treatment during the prepubertal stage as well as during puberty, and substitution therapy in which other hormones are used are also considered briefly.

Route of Growth Hormone Administration

Until the end of the 1970's, the intramuscular route was used in injecting GH. This was probably not only a result of traditional practice[7] but also because of apprehensions concerning lipoatrophy and the increase in antibodies.[74] In comparing the subcutaneous and the intramuscular routes, it appears that the former is characterized by slower rates of appearance and disappearance[75] as well as by lower figures for maximum values, which in turn are probably caused by increases in local degradation.[76] Since the fear of side effects is unfounded in using the subcutaneous route and also since the growth response per dose injected is similar,[77] the subcutaneous injection offered a good solution—it causes less pain, can even be given by a lay person, and above all it is safe—it is the standard route of application.

Frequency and Timing

In animal experiments, improved results were achieved when daily injections were tested against twice- or thrice-weekly injections.[78] Daily doses of GH are intrinsically important in the treatment of children, as they provide by far the best regimen for its most effective use.[79–81] Further studies will show whether two subcutaneous injections per day are more advantageous or not. Caution is recommended in increasing daily subcutaneous injections, however, as GH levels might not reach physiological nadirs, thus jeopardizing the safety of treatment. The animal experiments, on the other hand, showed that continuous subcutaneous infusion of one daily dose of GH produced better results.[82] GH products causing the protracted release of GH at the site of the injection have been tested successfully in children.[83] Even though pulsatile GH secretion clearly offers the most physiologically effective alternative in using GH to promote growth and enhance other metabolic effects, growth rates in children correlated best with integrated levels of GH secreted over a certain period of time.[84] Moreover, IGF-I and IGFBP-3 are highly significant in terms of the total daily GH secretion.[85] Thus, pharmaceutical products that release GH slowly may well be an effective alternative in the future.

There have been no longitudinal investigations conducted on whether GH should be injected in the morning or in the evening. There were no differences observed in some short-term metabolic responses.[86, 87] Recent tests, however, have shown that evening injections interfere to a lesser extent with the normal metabolic homeostasis.[88] It can thus be concluded that the common practice of giving evening injections may not only be convenient but also physiologically sound.

TABLE 20–1. A THEORETICAL ALGORITHM FOR THE BIOCHEMICAL DIAGNOSIS OF GHD/GHI DISORDERS

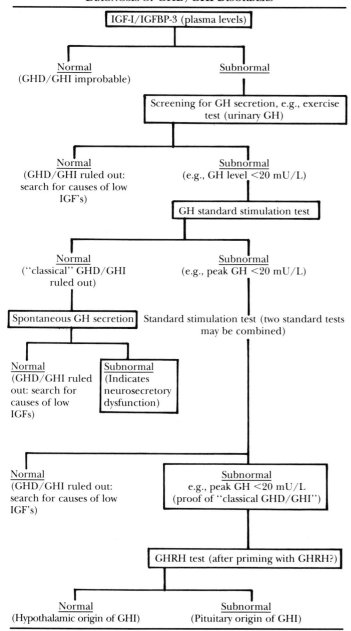

Dosage

The positive relationship between the logarithm of a total weekly GH dose and growth velocity in treating GHD is indisputable.[89, 90] The correct dosage of GH to achieve optimal childhood and adult height in the most efficient manner in substitution therapy, however, is still a matter of concern. Even though it has been shown that current dosage of GH influences growth during the first two years of treatment in IGHD,[80–92] the optimal dose for each individual is a complex problem, as the auxology always varies. It is taken for granted that, during the prepubertal stage in patients with IGHD, a weekly dose of 0.5 IU/kg BW ($\cong 14$ IU/m^2 BS) is adequate. My colleagues and I prefer to calculate dosage by basing it on the body surface area. There is, however, a simple transformation between the recently reported dose/m^2 and dose/kg, i.e., dose/m^2 = 27 $\times$ dose/kg.[93] During puberty, when spontaneous GH secretion increases by a factor of about two, an equivalent increase in the GH dose may be recommended, although the empirical basis for this needs verification.[94] The relationship between growth and therapeutic variables in GHI may differ as a result of any treatment for malignancies.[95]

Side Effects

Although GH therapy in GHD is aimed at substitution, side effects sometimes occur. The cause may lie in the product itself, in the mode of application, or in the disposition of the treated subject. Unfortunately, no detailed data are available on the incidence of adverse events (acute and late) related to GH therapy. Even in studies in which the reporting of an adverse event is mandatory, it is difficult to judge whether the information is complete.[96] One of the undesirable side effects of GH supplements is the formation of antibodies.

Antibody Formation

The variability in the formation of antibodies against injected hGH depends on the type of material injected,[97] the site of the injection (with the subcutaneous route probably allowing easier antibody formation[74]), and the patient's susceptibility. Formerly, when rather impure products based on extracted GH[98] were available and also during the transitional period during which meth-hGH[99] was used, antibody formation was often an impediment in therapy. A change occurred, however, with r-hGH.[100] The appearance of growth-attenuating antibodies is now very rare, except when there is a GH gene deletion.[11] Interestingly, GH antibodies, if directed to the appropriate epitopes of the molecule, may even enhance the effects of GH.[101]

One irreversible side effect of single lots of pituitary GH is the sporadic occurrence of the fatal Creutzfeldt-Jakob disease,[102] which results from improper effacement of the infecting agent during the production process. Not surprisingly, this led to the withdrawal of Pit-hGH for treatment in humans. The duration of incubation is unclear, and there have been cases in which it lasted for as long as 13 years after the cessation of therapy. Little data exist on the incidence of this disease, although in the United Kingdom

it is now estimated that approximately 1 in 200 patients who were treated with pituitary GH were affected. Local side effects (i.e., at the site of GH injection) such as pain, lipoatrophy, and hypertrophy are relatively rare. Slipped capital femoral epiphysis, although also a rare event, has long been described as being associated with GH treatment.[103] The phenomenon can be explained by the instability present in this mechanically exposed area, when rapid growth is induced, as, for instance, during GH treatment. Similarly, a commonly reported but yet unexplained symptom, "pain in the knee," may also have an pathophysiological basis. Whether or not GH substitution therapy induces malignant diseases looms as a big question: there are concerns that leukemias, particularly, may result from such therapy or that tumors may be induced or reappear and that an existing malignancy may worsen. One can allay these fears by stating that no convincing evidence exists showing that malignancies are caused or worsened by GH substitution therapy.[104–106] It must be added, however, that this knowledge has not been drawn from data from a large series. Therefore, the indication for GH substitution needs careful evaluation whenever an increased risk of malignancy is present (e.g., GHD caused by malignancy, GHD associated with disorders that would place the patient at risk per se).

TREATMENT OF ASSOCIATED HYPOTHALAMIC-PITUITARY DEFICIENCIES

IGHD often occurs together with other deficiencies of the hypothalamus and pituitary gland (e.g., MPHD). The ratio of isolated deficiencies versus multiple deficiencies in IGHD varies in different reports[26] and depends on the sample investigated and the diagnostic tools applied. While deficiencies of TSH, ACTH, and gonadotropins have a bearing on growth development in GHI, it remains uncertain whether this holds true for deficiencies of prolactin and adrenal androgens. Secondary hypothyroidism requires substitution with T$_4$ (approximately 100 μg/m^2 BS d), and an ACTH deficiency, in which the risk of hypoglycemia is inherent, must always be substituted with cortisol. Doses lower than those given to patients suffering from hypocortisolism should be considered for children with GHI, since glucocorticoid treatment can inhibit growth. A total daily dose of about 10 (15) mg/m^2 BS can be recommended here.

It is a complex matter to use sex steroids as substitutes in gonadotropin deficiency. It is, on the one hand, known that patients with delayed spontaneous puberty or no signs of puberty at all tend to have a better growth prognosis.[107–110] On the other hand, the development of secondary sex characteristics is, psychologically, of utmost consequence in adolescents. Thus, the timing of gender-specific sex steroid (testosterone and estrogens) use should be appropriate, i.e., in girls, not later than 12 years of age; in boys, 14 years, and dosages must be low enough to avoid advancement of bone age. Dosages of GH should also be prescribed according to the developmental state of the child. A detailed discussion of the induction of puberty is beyond the scope of this article; nevertheless, it should be kept in mind that the major factor determining adult height is the height reached at the start of spontaneous or induced puberty.[109] Thus, GH substitution should be started as early as possible, and an appropriate prepubertal treatment regimen is mandatory if normal height is to be achieved in patients.

ALTERNATIVE TREATMENT

Growth Hormone–Releasing Hormone

Since idiopathic GHD or GHI in most patients originates in the hypothalamus, it follows logically that the "dormant" pituitary should be stimulated with exogenous GHRH. Various GHRH products and modes of application (such as constant infusion or frequent subcutaneous injections) have been investigated.[111–113] The resulting growth rates were not encouraging, as they were lower than those achieved when GH treatment was given; the reason for this may be suboptimal therapy. If there is no basic objection to a therapy in which GHRH possibly causes an overstimulation of the somatocytes, it may be only a matter of time before appropriate modes of application (e.g., depot preparations, intranasal sprays or drops) make this a suitable alternative to GH.

Neurotransmitters

Another possibility of treating certain cases of GHD and GHI is by stimulating endogenous GH production by means of neurotransmitters.[114] Clonidine is a likely choice, as it enhances endogenous GHRH, possibly in combination with physostigmin, which in turn diminishes the endogenous tone of somatostatin.[115] At present, no evidence of the effectiveness of this approach is available.

IGF-I

After the recombinant DNA technique made the production of IGF-I possible,[116] it was used to promote growth in GH insensitivity syndromes such as Laron-type dwarfism.[117] IGF-I may potentially be used alone or in combination with GH to promote growth in GHD, particularly in cases in which diabetes mellitus poses a risk. The clinical use of IGF-I is still experimental.

CONCLUSIONS

The final height reached in patients treated for GHD and GHI is ultimately the most important consideration. Outcome is related to several issues: the timing of GH therapy beginning so that therapy is optimized, treatment modalities and duration, and the substitution of other hormonal deficiencies if required. In the past, GH therapy was governed by the limited availability of pituitary GH. The long-term results reported are at best a reflection of the inadequacies of therapy resulting from the prevailing circumstances and limited knowledge.[107, 108, 110, 118, 119] Usually patients with IGHD who were put on GH at about 10 years of age and who were then treated with weekly doses of about 12 IU/m², given 2 to 3 times weekly, reached only the third growth percentile of the normal population.[107, 109] The late start of treatment[120] as well as the dosages of GH used at that time now appear to be incongruous. Intermittent treatment was found to be less beneficial.[121] This issue must, however, be reconsidered today. Patients who additionally have a gonadotropin deficiency usually have a better outcome than those who entered puberty spontaneously.[107] The reason this happens is not yet absolutely clear. We have observed that final height correlates well with height at the start of puberty, and that, as a rule, nothing is gained during spontaneous or induced puberty.[109] We suggested, therefore, that height normalization was a battle that had to be won before puberty. Bourguignon found that the total gain in height during puberty appeared to match the bone age at the onset of puberty in males with IGHD.[122] The dosage of GH, however, also appears to determine growth in puberty.[93, 109] Thus, on the basis of historical data, it is difficult to reach a conclusion on what actually determines optimal growth. Recently, in an attempt to optimize treatment, we developed prediction models by considering the auxological parameters and treatment modalities over the first two years of GH substitution in prepubertal children with IGHD.[92] Our analysis showed that the response to GH over a certain period of time leads to changes in responsiveness to GH. The aim of such a complex analysis, in which longitudinal data are sought and for which a large number of patients is required, is to find a means of using growth hormone so that height can be normalized during childhood and adult life according to the individual needs of each patient and that the least expensive therapy with the least risk to the patient can be evolved.

REFERENCES

1. Cushing H: Pituitary Body and its Disorders. Philadelphia, JB Lippincott, 1912.
2. Evans HM, Long JA: The effect of anterior lobe administered intraperitoneally upon growth, maturity, and oestrus cycles of the rat. Anatomical Record 21:62 (Abstract), 1921.
3. Li HC: The chemistry of human pituitary hormone: 1956–1966. *In* Pecile A, Mueller EE (eds): Growth Hormone. Amsterdam, Excerpta Medica, 1968, pp 3–28.
4. Wallis M: The molecular evolution of pituitary hormones. Biological Review 50:35, 1975.
5. Bennet LL, Weinberger H, Escamilla R: Failure of hypophyseal growth hormone to produce nitrogen storage in a girl with hypophyseal dwarfism. J Clin Endocrinol 10:492–499, 1950.
6. Raben M: Preparation of growth hormone from pituitaries of man and monkey. Science 125:883, 1957.
7. Raben M: Treatment of a pituitary dwarf with human growth hormone. Clin Endocr Metab 18:901–903, 1958.
8. Frykluund LM, Bierich JR, Ranke MB: Recombinant human growth hormone. Clin Endocrinol Metab 15:511–536, 1986.
9. Bennett WF, Chloupek R, Harris R, Canova-Davis, et al: Characterization of natural-sequence recombinant human growth hormone. *In* Mueller E, Cocchi D, Locatelli V (eds): Advances in Growth Hormone and Growth Factor Research. Rome, Pythagoras Press, 1989, pp 29–50.
10. Braga S, Phillips JA, Joss E, et al: Familial growth hormone deficiency resulting from a 7.6 kb deletion within the growth hormone gene cluster. Am J Med Genet 25:443–452, 1986.
11. Illig R, Prader A, Ferrandez A, Zachmann M: Hereditary prenatal growth hormone deficiency with increased tendency to growth hormone antibody formation ("A-type" of isolated growth hormone deficiency). Acta Paediatr Scand (Suppl) 60:607, 1971.
12. Ranke MB: The Kabi Pharmacia International Growth Study: Aetiol-

ogy classification list with comments. Acta Paediatr Scand (Suppl) 379:87–92, 1991.

13. Rona RJ, Tanner JM: Aetiology of idiopathic growth hormone deficiency in England and Wales. Arch Dis Childh 52:197–208, 1977.

14. Vimpani G, Vimpani A, Lidgard G, Cameron N, Farquhar J: Prevalence of severe growth hormone deficiency. Br Med 2:427–430, 1977.

15. Bierich JR: On the aetiology of hypopituitary dwarfism. *In* Pecile A, Mueller EE (eds): Growth and Growth Hormone. Amsterdam, Excerpta Medica, 1972, pp 408–413.

16. Albertsson-Wikland K, Niklasson A, Karlberg P: Birth data for patients who later develop growth hormone deficiency: Preliminary analysis of a national register. Acta Paediatr Scand (Suppl) 370:115–120, 1990.

17. Stanhope R, Hindmarsh P, Kendall B, et al: High resolution scanning of the pituitary gland in growth disorders. Acta Paediatr Scand 75:779–786, 1986.

18. Scotti G, Triulzi F, Chiumello G, et al: New imaging techniques in endocrinology: Magnetic resonance of the pituitary gland and sella turcica. Acta Paediatr Scand (Suppl) 356:5–14, 1989.

19. The International Board of Kabi International Growth Study: Parental height of children with idiopathic growth hormone deficiency: Analysis from the Kabi International Growth Study. Acta Paediatr Scand (Suppl) 356:178–180, 1989.

20. Rimoin DL, Graham JM, Jr: Syndromes associated with growth deficiency. Acta Paed Scand (Suppl) 349:3–10, 1989.

21. Poskitt EME, Rayner PHW: Isolated growth hormone deficiency. Two families with autosomal dominant inheritance. Arch Dis Childh 49:55–59, 1974.

22. Mullis PE, Akinci A, Kanaka Ch, et al: Prevalence of human growth hormone-1 gene deletions among patients with isolated growth hormone deficiency from different populations. Pediatr Res 31:532–534, 1992.

23. Parks JS, Meacham LR, McKean MC, et al: Growth hormone (GH) gene deletion is the most common cause of severe GH deficiency among Oriental Jewish children. Pediatr Res 25:90A (Abstr), 1989.

24. Phillips JA III: Genetic disorders: Differentiating growth disorders. Hosp Practice 20:85–114, 1985.

25. Phelen PD, Connelly J, Martin FIR, et al: X-linked recessive hypopituitarism. *In* Birth Defects, Original Article Series, Vol VII: 6. New York, Alan R. Liss, 1971, pp 24–27.

26. Ranke MB: Stunted growth with more or less normal appearance. II. Hypothalamic-pituitary dwarfism: therapeutic problems. Eur J Pediatr 139:218–221, 1982.

27. De Morsier G: Etudes sur les dysraphies cranio-encephaliques. 20.III Agenesie du septum pellucidum avec malformation du tractus optique. La dysplasia septo-optique. Schweiz Arch Neurol Psychiatr 77:267–292, 1956.

28. Sipponen P, Simila S, Collan Y, et al: Familial syndrome with panhypopituitarism, hypoplasia of the hypophysis, and poorly developed sella turcica. Arch Dis Child 53:664, 1978.

29. Rappaport EB, Ulstrom RA, Gorlin RJ, et al: Solitary maxillary incisor and short stature. J Pediatr 91:924–928, 1977.

30. Laron Z, Taube E, Kaplan I: Pituitary growth hormone insufficiency associated with cleft lip and palate. An embryonal developmental defect. Helv Pediatr Acta 24:576–581, 1969.

31. Preece MA, Kearney PJ, Marshall WC: Growth hormone deficiency in congenital rubella. Lancet II:842, 1977.

32. Lyen KR, Grant DB: Endocrine function, morbidity and mortality after surgery for craniopharyngioma. Arch Dis Child 57:837–841, 1982.

33. Lannering B, Marky I, Mellander L, Albertsson-Wikland K: Growth hormone secretion and response to growth hormone therapy after treatment for brain tumour. Acta Paediatr Scand (Suppl) 343:146–151, 1988.

34. Shalet SM, Clayton PE, Price DA: Growth impairment following treatment for childhood brain tumours. Acta Paediatr Scand 343:137–145, 1988.

35. Shalet SM, Clayton PE, Price DA: Growth and pituitary function in children treated for brain tumours or acute lymphoblastic leukemia. Horm Res 30:53–61, 1988.

36. Bottazzo GF, McIntosh C, Stanford W, et al: Growth hormone cell antibodies and partial growth hormone deficiency in a girl with Turner's syndrome. Clin Endocrinol 12:1–9, 1980.

37. Tanner JM, Whitehouse RH: A note on the bone age at which patients with ''isolated'' growth hormone deficiency enter puberty. J Clin Endocrinol Metab 41:788–790, 1975.

38. Vandershueren-Lodeweyckx M (on behalf of the Executive Scientific Committee of KIGS): Who is treated with growth hormone today? Acta Paediatr Scand (Suppl) 370:107–113, 1990.

39. August GP, Lippe BM, Blethen SL, et al: Growth hormone treatment in the United States: Demographic and diagnostic features of 2331 children. J Pediatr 116:899–903, 1990.

40. Sizonenko PC, Hubert ML: Pre- and perinatal endocrinology. *In* Falkner F, Tanner JM (eds): Human Growth, Vol 1. London, Baillier-Tindall, 1978, pp 549–592.

41. Chatelain P: Dramatic early post-natal growth failure in children with early onset growth hormone deficiency. Acta Paediatr Scand (Suppl) 379:100–102, 1991.

42. Tanner JM, Hughes PCR, Whitehouse RH: Comparative rapidity of response of height, limb muscle and limb fat to treatment with human growth hormone in patients with and without growth hormone deficiency. Acta Endocrinologica 84:681–691, 1977.

43. Parra A, Argote RM, Garcia G, et al: Body composition in hypopituitary dwarfs before and during human growth hormone therapy. Metabolism 28:851–857, 1979.

44. Chawla RK, Parks JS, Rudman D: Structural variants of human growth hormone: Biochemical, genetic, and clinical aspects. Ann Rev Med 34:519–547, 1983.

45. George DL, Phillips JA III, Francke U, Seeburg PH: The genes for growth hormone and chorionic somatomammotropin are on the long arm of human chromosome 17 in the region q21-gter. Hum Gen 57:138–141, 1981.

46. Rudman D, Chawla RK, Kutner MH: Heterogeneity of growth hormone in nocturnal serum of children. Pediatr Res 19:981–985, 1985.

47. Baumann G, Winter RJ, Shaw M: Circulating molecular variants of growth hormone in childhood. Pediatr Res 22:21–22, 1987.

48. Chatelain P, Boullat B, Cohen R, et al: Assay of growth hormone levels in human plasma using commercial kits: Analysis of some factors influencing the results. Acta Paediatr Scand (Suppl) 370:56–62, 1990.

49. Friesen HG: Receptor assay for growth hormone. Acta Paediatr Scand (Suppl) 370:87–91, 1990.

50. Mueller EE: Neural control of somatotropic function. Physiol Rev 67(3):962–1053, 1987.

51. Camanni F, Ghigo E, Mazza E, et al: Aspects of neurotransmitter control of GH secretion: Basic and clinical studies. *In* Mueller EE, Cocchi D, Locatelli V (eds): Advances in Growth Hormone and Growth Factor Research. Rome, Pythagoras Press, 1989, pp 263–281.

52. Lacey KA, Hewison A, Parkin JM: Exercise as a screen test for growth hormone deficiency in children. Arch Dis Child 48:508–512, 1973.

53. Ranke MB, Haber P: Growth hormone stimulation tests. *In* Ranke MB (ed): Functional Endocrinology Diagnostics in Children and Adolescents. Mannheim, J&J Verlag, 1992, pp 61–75.

54. Frasier SD: A review of growth hormone stimulation tests in children. Pediatrics 54:929–937, 1974.

55. Illig R, Bucher H: Testosterone priming of growth hormone release. *In* Laron Z, Butenandt O (eds): Evaluation of GHJ Secretion (Pediatric and Adolescent Endocrinology), Vol 12. Basel, Karger, 1983, pp 75–85.

56. Raiti S: Statistical aspects of hGH therapy for hypopituitarism. *In* Laron Z, Butenandt O, Raiti O (eds): Clinical Use of Growth Hormone. Basel, Karger, 1987, pp 1–12.

57. Mayo KE: Structure and expression of growth hormone–releasing hormone (GHRH) genes. *In* Mueller EE, Cocchi D, Locatelli V (eds): Advances in Growth Hormone and Growth Factor Research. Rome, Pythagoras Press, 1989, pp 219–226.

58. Ranke MB, Gruhler M, Rosskamp R, et al: Testing with growth hormone–releasing factor (GRG (1-29) NH2) and somatomedin C measurements for the evaluation of growth hormone deficiency. Eur J Pediatr 145:485–492, 1986.

59. Bercu BB, Shulman D, Root AW, Spiliotis BE: Growth hormone (GH) provocative testing frequently does not reflect endogenous GH secretion. J Clin Endocrinol Metab 63:709–716, 1986.

60. Albertsson-Wikland K, Rosberg S: Methods of evaluating spontaneous growth hormone secretion. *In* Ranke MB (ed): Functional Endocrinologic Diagnostics in Children and Adolescents. Mannheim, J&J Verlag, 1992, pp 76–101.

61. Albertsson-Wikland K, Rosberg S: Analyses of 24-hour growth hormone (GH) profiles in children. J Clin Endocrinol Metab 67:493–500, 1988.

62. Veldhuis JD, Faria A, Vance ML, et al: Contemporary tools for the analysis of episodic growth hormone secretion and clearance in vivo. Acta Paediatr Scand (Suppl) 347:63–82, 1988.

63. Hindmarsh P, Smith PJ, Brook CGD, Mathews DR: The relationship between height velocity and growth hormone secretion in short prepubertal children. Clin Endocrinol 27:581–597, 1987.

64. Zadik Z, Chalew SA, Raiti S, Kowarski AA: Do short children secrete insufficient growth hormone? Pediatrics 76:335–360, 1985.

65. Green H, Morikawa M, Nixon T: A dual effector theory of growth hormone action. Differentiation 29:195–198, 1985.

66. Sukegawa I, Hizuka N, Takano K, et al: Urinary growth hormone measurements for evaluating endogenous growth hormone secretion. J Clin Endocrinol Metabol 66:1119–1123, 1988.

67. Girard J, Celniker A, Price A, et al: Urinary measurement of growth hormone secretion. Acta Paediatr Scand (Suppl) 366:149–154, 1990.

68. Sukegawa I, Hizuka N, Takano K, et al: Measurement of nocturnal urinary growth hormone values. Acta Endocrinol (Copenh) 121:290–296, 1989.

69. Salmon WD, Jr, Daughaday WH: A hormonally controlled serum factor which stimulates sulfate incorporation by cartilage in vitro. J Lab Med 49:825–836, 1957.

70. Blum WF: Insulin-like growth factors and their binding proteins. In Ranke MB (ed): Functional Endocrinologic Diagnostics in Children and Adolescents. Mannheim, J&J Verlag, 1992, pp 102–118.

71. Blum WF, Ranke MB, Kietzmann K, et al: A specific radioimmunoassay for growth hormone (GH)–dependent somatomedin-binding protein: its use for diagnosis of GH deficiency. J Clin Endocrinol Metab 70:1292–1298, 1990.

72. Ranke MB, Blum WF, Bierich JR: Clinical relevance of serum measurements of insulin-like growth factors and somatomedin binding protein. Acta Paediatr Scand (Suppl) 347:114–126, 1988.

73. Kowarski AA, Schneider J, Ben Galim E: Growth failure with normal serum RIA-GH and low somatomedin activity: Somatomedin restoration and growth acceleration after exogenous GH. J Clin Endocrinol Metab 47:461–466, 1978.

74. Underwood LE, Voina SJ, Van Wyk JJ: Restoration of growth by growth hormone (Roos) in hypopituitary dwarfs immunized by other human growth hormone preparations. J Clin Endocrinol Metab 38:288–297, 1974.

75. Russo L, Moore WV: A comparison of subcutaneous and intramuscular administration of human growth hormone in the therapy of growth hormone deficiency. J Clin Endocrinol Metab 55:1003–1006, 1982.

76. Joergensen JOL: Human growth hormone replacement therapy: Pharmacological and clinical aspects. Endocr Rev 12:189–207, 1991.

77. Wilson DM, Baker B, Hintz RL, Rosenfeld RG: Subcutaneous versus intramuscular growth hormone therapy: Growth and acute somatomedin response. Pediatrics 76:361, 1985.

78. Jansson JO, Albertsson-Wikland K, Eden S, Thorngren KG, et al: Effect of the frequency of growth hormone administration on longitudinal bone growth and body weight in hypophysectomized rats. Acta Physiol Scand 114:261–265, 1982.

79. Kastrup KW, Christiansen JS, Koch Andersen J, Oerskov H: Increased growth rate following transfer to daily sc administration from three weekly im injections of hGH in growth hormone deficient children. Acta Endocrinol (Copenh) 104:148–152, 1983.

80. Ranke MB, Guilbaud O: Growth response in pre-pubertal children with idiopathic growth hormone deficiency during first year of treatment with human growth hormone. Analysis of the Kabi International Growth Study. Acta Paediatr Scand (Suppl) 370:1220–1230, 1990.

81. Albertsson-Wikland K, Westphal O, Westgreen U: Daily subcutaneous administration of human growth hormone in growth hormone deficient children. Acta Paediatr Scand 75:89–97, 1986.

82. Cotes PM, Bartlett WA, Gaines Das RE, Flecknell P, et al: Dose regimes of human growth hormone: Effects of continuous infusion and of a gelatine vehicle on growth in rats and rate of absorption in rabbits. J Endocrinol 87: 303–312, 1980.

83. Lippe B, Frasier SD, Kaplan SA: Use of growth hormone gel. Arch Dis Childh 54:609–613, 1979.

84. Albertsson-Wikland K, Rosberg S, Libre E, et al: Growth hormone secretory rates in children as estimated by deconvolution analyses of 24 h plasma concentration profiles. Am J Physiol 257:E809–E814, 1989.

85. Blum WF, Ranke MB: Use of insulin-like growth factor binding protein 3 for the evaluation of growth disorders. Horm Res (Suppl) 34:31–37, 1990.

86. Rudman D, Freides D, Patterson JH, Gibbas DL: Diurnal variation in the responsiveness of human subjects to human growth hormone. J Clin Invest 52:912, 1973.

87. Matusik MC, Furnaletto RW, Meyer WJ: Chronobiologic considerations in human growth hormone therapy. J Pediatr 103:543–547, 1983.

88. Joergensen JOL, Moeller N, Lauritzen T, Alberti KGMM, et al: Evening versus morning injections of growth hormone (GH) in GH-deficient patients: Effects of 24-hour pattern of circulating hormones and metabolites. J Clin Endocrinol Metab 70:207–214, 1990.

89. Frasier SD, Costin G, Lippe MB, et al: A dose response curve for hGH. J Clin Endocrinol Metab 52:1213–1217, 1981.

90. Preece MA, Tanner JM, Whitehouse RH, Cameron N: Dose dependence of growth response to hGH in GH deficiency. J Clin Endocrinol Metab 42:466–483, 1976.

91. Bundak R, Hindmarsh PC, Smith PJ, Brook CGD: Long-term auxological effects of human growth hormone. J Pediatr 112:875–890, 1988.

92. Ranke MB, Guilbaud O: Growth response in pre-pubertal children with idiopathic growth hormone deficiency during the first two years of treatment with human growth hormone. Analysis of the Kabi International Growth Study. Acta Paediatr Scand (Suppl) 379:109–115, 1991.

93. Preece MA: New insights from a large international collaborative growth study. Acta Paediatr Scand (Suppl) 370:103–104, 1990.

94. Price DA: Puberty in children with idiopathic growth hormone deficiency on growth hormone treatment: Preliminary analysis of the data from the Kabi Pharmacia International Growth Study. Acta Paediatr Scand (Suppl) 379:117–124, 1991.

95. Price DA, Ranke MB, Guilbaud O: Growth response in the first year of growth hormone treatment in pre-pubertal children with organic growth hormone deficiency: A comparison with idiopathic growth hormone deficiency. Acta Paediatr Scand (Suppl) 370:131–137, 1990.

96. Ranke MB: Adverse events (AE) reported during growth hormone therapy. Results of the Kabi International Growth Study (KIGS). Biannual Report 6:13–16, 1991.

97. Chalkley SR, Tanner JM: Incidence and effects on growth of antibodies to human growth hormone. Arch Dis Child 46:160–166, 1971.

98. Moore WV, Leppert P: The role of aggregated human growth hormone (hGH) in development of antibodies to hGH. J Clin Endocrinol Metab 51:691–697, 1980.

99. Bierich JR: Treatment of pituitary dwarfism with biosynthetic growth hormone. Acta Paediatr Scand (Suppl) 325:13–18, 1986.

100. Takano K, Shizume K, Hizuka N, Okuno A, et al: Treatment of pituitary dwarfism with authentic recombinant human growth hormone (SM-9500). Endocrinol Jpn 34:291–297, 1987.

101. Holder AT, Aston R, Preece MA, Ivanyi J: Potentiation of the somatogenic and lactogenic activity of human growth hormone with monoclonal antibodies. J Endocrinol 110:381–388, 1986.

102. Brown P, Gajdusek DC, Gibbs CJ, Jr, Asher DM: Potential epidemic of Creutzfeldt-Jakob disease from human growth hormone therapy. N Engl J Med 313:728–731, 1985.

103. Rappaport EB, Fife D: Slipped capital femoral epiphysis in growth hormone deficient patients. Am J Dis Child 139:396–399, 1985.

104. Stahnke N, Zeisel HJ: Growth hormone therapy and leukaemia. Eur J Pediatr 148:591–596, 1989.

105. Arslanian SA, Becker DJ, Lee PA, et al: Growth hormone therapy and tumour recurrence. Am J Dis Child 139:347–350, 1985.

106. Clayton PE, Shalet SM, Gattemaneni HR, Price DA: Does growth hormone cause relapse of brain tumour? Lancet 1:711–713, 1987.

107. Burns EC, Tanner JM, Preece MA, Cameron N: Final height and pubertal development in 55 children with idiopathic growth hormone deficiency, treated for between 2 and 15 years with human growth hormone. Eur J Pediatr 137:155–164, 1981.

108. Ranke MB, Weber J, Bierich JR: Long-term response to human growth hormone in 36 children with idiopathic growth hormone deficiency. Eur J Pediatr 132:221–238, 1979.

109. Ranke MB, Butenandt O: Idiopathic growth hormone deficiency: final height to treatment with growth hormone and effects of puberty and sex steroids. In Frisch H, Laron Z (eds): Induction of Puberty in Hypopituitarism. Ares-Serono Symposium, Vol 16, pp 85–102, Rome, 1988.

110. Hibi I, Tanaka T, Tanae A: Final height of patients with idiopathic GH deficiency after long-term GH treatment. Acta Endocrinol (Copenh) 120:409–415, 1989.

111. Rochicchioli PE, Tauber M, Coude F, et al: Results of 1-year growth hormone (GH)–releasing hormone (1-44) treatment on growth, somatomedin C, and 24-hour GH secretion in six children with partial GH deficiency. J Clin Endocrinol Metab 63:1100–1105, 1986.

112. Smith PJ, Brook CGD, Rivier J, et al: Nocturnal pulsatile growth hormone–releasing hormone treatment in growth hormone deficiency. Clin Endocrinol (Oxf) 25:35–44, 1986.

113. Thorner MO, Reschke J, Chitwood J, et al: Acceleration of growth in two children treated with growth hormone releasing factor, N Engl J Med 312:4–9, 1985.

114. Pintor C, Loche S, Puggioni R, Cella SG, et al: Growth hormone deficiency states: approach by CNS-acting compounds. In Mueller E,

Cocchi C, Locatelli V (eds): Advances in Growth Hormone and Growth Factor Research. Rome, Pythagoras Press, 1989, pp 375–387.

115. Ghigo E, Mazza E, Imperiale E, et al: The enhancement of the cholinergic tone by pyridostigmine promotes both basal and growth hormone (GH)–releasing hormone–induced GH secretion in children of short stature. J Clin Endocrinol Metab 65:452–456, 1987.

116. Skottner A, Clark RG, Robinson ICAF, Fryklund I: Recombinant human insulin-like growth factor: Testing the somatomedin hypothesis in hypophysectomized rats. J Endocrinol 112:123–132, 1987.

117. Laron Z, Anin S, Klipper-Aurbach Y, Klinger B: Effects of insulin-like growth factor on linear growth, head circumference, and body fat in patients with Laron-type dwarfism. Lancet 339:1258–1261, 1992.

118. Zuppinger K, Joss EE, Rotten A, et al: Endresultate bei hypophysaerem Kleinwuchs nach Wachstumhormontherapie. Schweiz Rundschau Medizin Praxis 34:1197–1204, 1990.

119. Job JC, Chaussain JL, Garnier PE, et al: Dose response relationship in the treatment of hypopituitary children with hGH: A retrospective study. Acta Paediatr Scand (Suppl) 337:93–105, 1987.

120. Tanner JM: Toward complete success in the treatment of growth hormone deficiency: A plea for earlier ascertainment. Health Trends 7:61–65, 1975.

121. Preece MA, Tanner JM: Results of intermittent treatment of growth hormone deficiency with growth hormone. J Clin Endocrinol Metab 45:159–170, 1977.

122. Bourguignon JP, Vandenwegh M, Vanderschueren-Lodeweyckx M, et al: Pubertal growth and final height in hypopituitary boys: A minor role of bone age at onset of puberty. J Clin Endocrinol Metab 63:376–382, 1982.

21

Corticotropin-Releasing Hormone: Basic Physiology and Clinical Applications

ASHLEY GROSSMAN

In 1948 Geoffrey Harris proposed that the hypothalamus acts as the key mediator between the central nervous system (CNS) and the pituitary gland, effecting a wide range of adaptive responses to both physical and psychological stimuli.[1] It was shown that adrenal corticosteroid secretion was regulated by a pituitary hormone, adrenocorticotropin (ACTH), and then Saffran and Schally[2] and Guillemin and Rosenberg[3] demonstrated the presence in hypothalamic extracts of humoral factors capable of stimulating the secretion of ACTH from the pituitary gland in vitro. Evidence increasingly suggested that one significant ACTH secretogogue was arginine vasopressin (AVP). However, there remained another elusive yet important stimulator of ACTH release in hypothalamic extracts that led to the relative disregard of AVP and the continued search for a dominant corticotropin-releasing hormone.

A number of methodological problems meant that more than a quarter-century elapsed between the postulation and the conclusive isolation, sequencing, and synthesis of the 41-amino acid *corticotropin-releasing hormone* (CRH; previously termed CRF, CRF-41, or CRH-41).[4] While this does indeed appear to be the principal ACTH-releasing hormone, it should be recognized that CRH remains only one part of the stimulatory complex to ACTH release. Vasopressin was an important component of the original ACTH-releasing factors, but there may be other ACTH-releasing hormones yet to be identified. Certain cytokines may have direct pituitary effects, while in some species catecholamines may act directly on the pituitary. Evidence is also increasing in favor of an inhibitory agent to corticotroph ACTH release. Thus, in many circumstances CRH

appears to set the basal permissive tone of the hypothalamic-pituitary-adrenal (HPA) axis, while changes in other factors mediate responses to specific dynamic stimuli.

ANATOMY AND PHYSIOLOGY

Localization of Corticotropin-Releasing Hormone

There are several major systems of CRH neurons. The best characterized of these is the paraventricular nucleus–median eminence (PVN-ME) pathway, which is responsible for the majority of the ACTH regulatory activity associated with CRH. The axons from these neurons curve around the mediobasal hypothalamus to terminate medially in the median eminence, and high concentrations of CRH can be measured in hypophyseal portal blood.[5] These neurons appear from about the 12th week of life in the human fetal hypothalamus.[6] Many of the parvicellular PVN CRH-containing neurons also contain vasopressin, although this appears to be a plastic property insofar as the proportion of each changes according to the corticosteroid milieu. Thus, adrenalectomy increases the proportion of CRH neurons that co-store and presumably co-secrete vasopressin.[7] Lesser amounts of CRH are found in other hypothalamic nuclei, such as the supraoptic and arcuate nuclei, in the limbic system (particularly the amygdala and the nucleus of the stria terminalis), and as scattered interneurons within the cerebral cortex. There is particularly intense immunopositive staining for CRH in several hippocampal fields, and it has also been located in the cerebellar cortex, inferior olive, and in fibers tracking down to the locus ceruleus.[8] In addition, CRH immunoreactivity has been localized to a number of peripheral sites, including the lungs, liver, thymus, gastrointestinal tract, pancreas (in "glucagon" cells), adrenal medulla, and testis, but the role played by CRH at these sites is unclear. The primate placenta is particularly rich in CRH immunoreactivity, and its presence there has been the object of considerable study. CRH has been identified in cells of the immune system, where its presence has been taken as further evidence in favor of an endocrine-immune axis. Finally, CRH has also been demonstrated in a number of tumors, and its secretion from an ectopic source may give rise to Cushing's syndrome.

Corticotropin-Releasing Hormone Gene

The CRH gene has been isolated from a variety of species and shows considerable interspecies homology. The rat and human sequences share 94 per cent nucleotide homology, while the ovine sequence shares approximately 80 per cent of its bases with each of these. In humans, the gene is located on chromosome 8.[9] Tissue-specific expression of the rat CRH gene has been reported[10] and closely parallels its immunohistochemical distribution; there is also a reasonably close parallel between CRH and its presumptive receptor, occasional discrepancies now being explicable in terms of the distribution of the CRH-binding protein. As far as the gene product is concerned, the rat and human peptides are identical, whereas the ovine molecule varies by only seven aminoacid substitutions (Fig. 21–1).

Corticotropin-Releasing Hormone Actions

CRH is the most significant secretogogue for ACTH from the pituitary gland. Its stimulatory action causes a

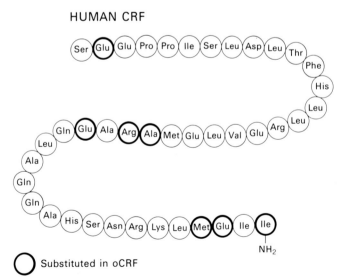

HUMAN CRF

○ Substituted in oCRF

FIGURE 21–1. The structure of human and rat CRH, which is identical. Ovine CRH differs from the human/rat peptide by 7 amino acid substitutions.

dose-related increase in the synthesis and secretion of ACTH: this effect is brought about by the binding of the peptide to specific cell membrane receptors on corticotrophs. In addition to the pituitary, CRH receptors are also present in most areas of the cerebral cortex, limbic system, and brain stem known to contain CRH neurons.[11] Most studies have agreed that there is only one class of receptor; this is coupled to guanyl nucleotide (G) proteins and adenylate cyclase. Activation induces a rise in intracellular cAMP, transmembrane Ca^{2+} flux, ACTH secretion, and pro-opiomelanocortin (POMC) synthesis.[12] These characteristics suggest that the receptor is part of the family of transmembrane-spanning G protein–linked receptors, although attempts to clone the receptor assuming this have so far proved unsuccessful. Virtually all evidence suggests that ACTH is secreted in parallel with other POMC cleavage products, although the functions of these other peptides (if any) remain controversial (see Ch. 22). Recent data indicate that as the concentration of CRH increases there is a dose-responsive increase in ACTH output from individual corticotrophs; by contrast, vasopressin appears to cause an all-or-none response from corticotrophs of varying threshold sensitivities that are progressively recruited.[13] Vasopressin also differs from CRH in that its receptor is linked to the phospholipase C/phosphatidylinositol pathway and does not cause changes in ACTH synthesis.

Regulation of Corticotropin-Releasing Hormone: Physiology

The regulation of the HPA axis is achieved by the combined activities of a multiplicity of neuronal pathways that project onto both the PVN and the median eminence, working in concert with a variety of circulating factors, particularly the glucocorticoids. Significant among the extrahypothalamic neuronal inputs are relays via the stria terminalis from limbic structures that include the amygdala and the hippocampus (predominantly stimulatory and inhibitory, respectively).[14] Ascending visceral sensory information (stimulatory) is relayed via noradrenergic fibers from the nucleus tractus solitarius and the ventrolateral medulla, with a small input from the locus ceruleus. The PVN is also served by a wealth of fibers connecting it to all the other hypothalamic nuclei. Studies of hypothalamic mRNA levels by in situ hybridization show rises following adrenalectomy[15] and insulin-induced hypoglycemia[16] and falls following prolonged administration of dexamethasone. Other areas of the brain expressing CRH mRNA are unaffected by such maneuvers, confirming that they belong to physiologically distinct systems.

The feedback effects of glucocorticoids onto the HPA axis are exerted at multiple levels and in a variety of time frames. Rapid-onset inhibition at the level of the pituitary is associated with suppression of CRH-stimulated, but not basal, ACTH secretion. This effect occurs within minutes and may be mediated by a membrane-dependent process.[17] Slow-onset feedback at the level of the corticotroph occurs over several hours or days and involves suppression of basal and stimulated ACTH. This inhibition involves nuclear-mediated long-term changes. The possible involvement of peptide intermediaries in the medium-term feedback effects (particularly lipocortin/annexin[18]) remain intriguing but unsubstantiated.

Parallel phenomena can be seen at the level of the PVN where the concentration of glucocorticoid receptors is high, particularly in cells containing immunoreactive CRH.[19] Glucocorticoid receptors are also found in high concentrations in the CA1 and CA2 regions of the dorsal hippocampus,[20] and there is evidence to suggest a role for these in HPA axis inhibition through effects on CRH.[21] Thus feedback effects of corticosteroids act at several levels of the control of CRH to inhibit both release and synthesis and modify stress-induced responses. Furthermore, recent data suggest that a separate class of steroids synthesized by astrocytes, the neurosteroids,[23] may also regulate CRH release by interacting allosterically with the γ-aminobutyric acid receptor (and possibly other receptors). Since this class includes dehydroepiandrosterone sulfate, one of the adrenocortical "androgens" that may paradoxically increase CRH release, steroid feedback effects may be even more complex than previously recognized.

The secretion of glucocorticoids is vital in maintaining the body's homeostasis under stress: it is the end point of a neuroendocrine cascade of events generated in the CNS in reaction to a variety of physical and emotional stressful stimuli. A vast body of animal data converge on the concept that HPA axis activation occurs in response to stress, whether these be primarily hemodynamic (hemorrhage, hypotension), metabolic (hypoglycemia) or psychological (immobility, pain, and the like). Recent work on CRH and AVP, whether in portal blood measurements or changes in peptide or mRNA levels, has shown that the relative changes in the proportion of the two peptides are stressor- and intensity-specific and are also contingent on the corticosteroid milieu. Thus mild hypoglycemia may increase both AVP and CRH, whereas CRH alone is recruited principally at more severe hypoglycemic changes.[24] Nevertheless, immunoneutralization and CRH-antagonist studies have demonstrated that a basal-permissive secretion of CRH is necessary for any activation of the HA axis to occur. The presence of CRH is apparently obligatory for a normal ACTH secretory response to most stimuli, with CRH acting either in a dynamic manner to drive ACTH secretion or permissively to determine the set point for the expression of the other intrinsically weaker ACTH secretogogues.[25] Most stressors must intercept this process to prevent rapid feedback negating the induced activation. Indeed, there is evidence that a priming effect of repeated stress precisely equals the attenuating effect of steroid feedback inhibition, such that the corticosteroid response is preserved.[26]

In the human, much of the extensive early data on HPA axis activation may be summarized in the following terms: such activation will occur in response to physical stressors, as in animal studies (hypoglycemia, acute exercise, hypotension) and also in response to psychological or emotional stressors that are severe and, most importantly, for which the person has no clear coping strategy.[27] Some of these situations have been investigated in terms of hypothalamic mediators; thus, acute exercise probably involves activation of hypothalamic AVP, whereas hypoglycemia probably involves both AVP and CRH.[28] Circumstantial evidence suggests that emotional stress and long-term training in professional athletes results in persistent central CRH activation.

In addition to its role in ACTH regulation, there is increasing evidence that CRH may act as the central executive regulator of the response to stress. Central administration off the peptide suppresses the gonadal and growth axes[29] (by suppression of gonadotropin-releasing hormone and stimulation of somatostatin, respectively), increases sympathetic outflow with the expected metabolic and cardiovascular consequences,[30] and results in a behavioral pattern of increased arousal accompanied by inhibition of feeding and sexual activity.[31] These observations are compatible with the view that activation of CRH within the hypothalamus can concurrently activate and coordinate the metabolic, circulatory, and behavioral responses that are adaptive in stressful situations. In the human, the evidence is of necessity much more indirect. Nevertheless, most studies of behavioral disorders associated with apparent stress have shown increases in cerebrospinal fluid (CSF) CRH concentrations, compatible with increased HPA activity.

Regulation of Corticotropin-Releasing Hormone

Specific Regulators of CRH Secretion

ACETYLCHOLINE. Early animal studies implicated a central stimulatory effect of acetylcholine on ACTH secretion, with peripherally administered anticholinesterase agents increasing corticosterone secretion, while subsequent studies demonstrated similar changes following intracerebroventricular injections or median eminence implantation of cholinergic agonists.[32] In vitro studies measuring bioassayable corticotropin-releasing activity from incubated rat hypothalami have consistently shown stimulation following administration of acetylcholine. Further studies measuring CRH by radioimmunoassay (RIA) indicated that at least part of the increased corticotropin-releasing bioactivity following acetylcholine treatment is due to elevation of CRH.[33, 34] While both in vivo and in vitro studies uniformly demonstrated a stimulatory role for acetylcholine on CRH secretion, uncertainties still exist about the species of cholinergic receptor involved. Most evidence suggests the predominant involvement of the muscarinic receptor in the control of CRH. In the human, reports showing a cholinergic stimulation of the HPA have mostly been discounted, such changes as do occur being attributed to nonspecific side effects of the drugs used.[35, 36]

CATECHOLAMINES. There is good evidence for a rich catecholaminergic innervation of this part of the brain; the majority of the catecholaminergic afferents projecting onto the hypothalamus arise in the ventrolateral medulla (A1 cell group) and dorsolateral medulla (nucleus tractus solitarius, A2 cell group[37]), while a few also arise from the locus ceruleus (A6 cell group). Epinephrine-synthesizing neurons located in the ventrolateral medulla (C1 cell group) and the dorsal vagal complex (C3 cell group) also project to the hypothalamus. The bulk of the neuronal endings in close proximity to the CRH neurons are PNMT-positive and thus presumably epinephrine-secreting. While an anatomical link between the central catecholaminergic system and CRH has clearly been established, inferences from various studies regarding the nature (inhibitory or facilitatory) of these afferents have been the subject of considerable controversy over many years.[38] However, there is little disagreement from in vitro studies that the major catecholaminergic influence on CRH release is *facilitatory,* although some controversy still exists in regard to the receptors involved in mediating this stimulatory effect, with evidence in favor of both α- and β-adrenoceptors.[39, 40] Human studies have also shown that the HPA can be stimulated by methoxamine and that this α-adrenergic pathway is involved in food-stimulated[41] ACTH release but not in circadian rhythmicity[42]—probably both CRH and AVP are involved in this process. Drugs that are active at α2-adrenoceptors generally inhibit pituitary-adrenal activity in the human, and it has been assumed that this occurs via presynaptic inhibition of a stimulatory noradrenergic pathway. However, there is recent evidence that hypothalamic atriopeptin, which may be a physiological inhibitor of ACTH release,[43] is specifically activated by α2-adrenoceptors,[44] and thus the situation is currently unclear.

SEROTONIN. Serotonin is widely distributed in the brain, with the highest concentrations found in the hypothalamus and the brain stem. Ascending serotoninergic fibers from the midline raphe nuclei, which contain the bulk of serotonin-positive cell bodies, innervate a variety of hypothalamic areas, including the PVN. CRH is stimulated by serotonin, as demonstrated using both acute hypothalamic explants[45] and long-term hypothalamic cultures.[46] However, the physiological significance of serotonin inputs in regulating CRH secretion in relation to stress and circadian periodicity remains unclear. Furthermore, while there are scattered reports favoring a stimulatory role for serotonin in the human, the poor specificity of putative serotonin antagonists has complicated understanding of their physiological role. The development of newer drugs with closely delimited affinities for specific serotoninergic receptor subtypes will be of great help.

GABA. Several studies have suggested an important role for GABA in the control of ACTH secretion through an action within the hypothalamus. Early in vivo studies demonstrated that GABA and GABA-agonist drugs inhibit, while GABA antagonists augment, stress-induced adrenocortical activation.[47] Furthermore, administration of GABA antagonists stimulates the HPA axis under basal conditions. In vitro, studies measuring both bioassayable corticotropin-releasing activity and CRH by RIA have reproducibly shown inhibition of stimulated release by GABA and GABA agonists.[48] This interaction is potentiated by benzodiazepines.[49] Anatomical evidence indicates the presence of a rich GABA-ergic innervation of CRH neurons which consists of a dense network of GABA-ergic fibers closely surrounding the PVN, and GABA may also be co-stored and co-released from CRH neurons acting on presynaptic receptors in the median eminence. Therefore, all current animal data point to the existence of an important interaction between GABA and CRH secretion. Human studies, which are few, have generally shown either no or only mildly inhibitory effects of GABA-enhancing drugs, such as sodium valproate.[50] Benzodiazepines may also inhibit the HPA axis in the human, probably by activating the GABA receptor at an allosteric site, but do not affect the pituitary-adrenal response to CRH.

ENDOGENOUS OPIOIDS. The role of opioids in the regulation of the HPA axis has been the subject of considerable controversy and dispute. In humans, pharmacological studies have consistently shown that opioids inhibit ACTH secretion while high doses (about 0.1 mg/kg) of the opiate antagonist naloxone stimulate ACTH release, suggesting that there is a tonic opioid–mediated inhibitory influence on the HPA axis.[51] The effects of naloxone appear to be mediated via an adrenergic pathway,[52] and as they are additive to a maximal dose of CRH are probably contingent on vasopressin; this would suggest that naloxone cannot be used as a simple alternative to CRH in the assessment of the HPA in humans. In rodents, however, chronic administration of the opiate alkaloid morphine inhibits adrenocortical responses to stress, and acute administration of naloxone stimulates the secretion of ACTH, while acute administration of morphine *increases* both ACTH and corticosterone secretion.[53]

More recent in vitro studies have shown that opioid peptides and morphine consistently inhibited CRH secretion stimulated by either neurotransmitters or depolarising agents.[54] These data are in good agreement with the growing body of evidence for an inhibitory modulatory role of opioids in CRH secretion. It is of note, however, that only peptides active at μ- and κ-, but not δ-receptors, are capable of inhibiting CRH secretion.[55] This may indicate the endogenous ligands involved in the negative regulation of CRH. One possibility is that the dynorphins, which are co-stored with CRH and preferentially activate κ-receptors,[56] are important endogenous regulators. Alternatively, cleavage products of proenkephalin such as adrenorphin, which is particularly active at both μ- and κ-receptors, could represent an alternative endogenous mediator for the inhibitory actions of opioids. There is also evidence that hypothalamic metenkephalin varies in parallel with CRH in response to certain stressors.[57] In summary, therefore, opioids predominantly stimulate the HPA axis in the rat and inhibit it in the human. In both species the principal site of action is probably the hypothalamus; the effects of naloxone in the human are unlikely to be mediated by CRH.

OTHER NEUROPEPTIDES. CRH neurons in the PVN are at the exact center of a complex interaction with a variety of peptides in this nucleus. Although not all of these substances have been investigated in relation to their effects on CRH secretion, there is evidence that at least some of them could, under specified circumstances, modulate CRH neurons. Of some interest are the opposing effects of angiotensin II and atrial natriuretic peptide (ANP) on CRH secretion. ANP counteracts angiotensin II–induced adrenal stimulation of aldosterone secretion in the periphery and, as shown by more recent data, angiotensin II stimulates while ANP's inhibit CRH secretion from the hypothalamus.[58-60] It is therefore likely that these peptides, stimulated under conditions of deranged water homeostasis, may manipulate the HPA centrally in a similar manner to their peripheral effects. Another interesting interaction is the stimulatory effect of NPY on CRH secretion[61] in view of the fact that this peptide is often related to catecholamine action, and catecholamines have pronounced effects on CRH secretion. Substance P, somatostatin, and the potent vasodilator nitric oxide also inhibit CRH directly.[62-64] Human studies have shown inconsistently inhibitory effects of oxytocin and somatostatin on the HPA, but these peptides probably do not significantly inhibit the ACTH response to CRH. There is some evidence that the atriopeptins can, under certain circumstances, directly inhibit the release of pituitary ACTH: two reports in the human have produced inconsistent results.[65, 66]

CYTOKINES. Over the last few years there has been an increasing body of evidence in favor of a two-way communication between the immune and the neuroendocrine systems, particularly in relation to the HPA axis. Thus several substances released from immune cells during the immune response, now known as cytokines, have been reported to modify ACTH secretion. Besedovsky et al.[67] reported that intravenous interleukin-1 (IL-1) acutely stimulated ACTH and glucocorticoid secretion in the rat. Although it has been suggested that subacute effects of interleukins may be mediated directly at the pituitary level,[68] most studies have demonstrated a more substantial role for a central site of action of IL-1. IL-6 is also able to stimulate CRH release from the rat hypothalamus in vitro,[69] and there are reports of direct effects of IL-2 and TNF.[70] The responses to both IL-1 and IL-6 are blocked by specific antagonists of the enzyme cyclo-oxygenase, suggesting that prostaglandin or prostacyclin intermediaries are involved. Furthermore, IL-1, IL-6, and lipopolysaccharide (LPS) directly stimulate hypothalamic prostaglandin E_2 (PGE_2) release, while both PGE_2 and LPS increase the secretion of hypothalamic IL-1.[71, 72] Thus, it is possible that stimulation of CRH by circulating IL-1 occurs by increasing hypothalamic PGE_2, possibly in or near the organum vasculosum of the lamina terminalis,[73] which in turn releases hypothalamic IL-1. This may also apply to IL-6. LPS may thereby activate the HPA by inducing a feedforward self-regenerating response, leading to explosive bursts of activity (Fig. 21–2).

There are few data on specific HPA responses to cytokines in the human, reports of increased HPA activity following IL-2 administration probably being a result of the nonspecific side effects. However, early studies on the responses to pyrogen probably represent the sequelae of endogenous IL-1 and IL-6 activation; these demonstrated extremely high ACTH levels in response to such stimula-

tion.[74] This degree of responsiveness almost certainly reflects activation of both CRH and AVP, although direct pituitary effects are also possible. The current knowledge regarding neuromodulation of CRH release is summarized in Figure 21–3.

CLINICAL ASPECTS

Studies in Normal Subjects

Physiology

CRH has been synthesized by solid-phase techniques and administered by bolus or continuous intravenous infusion to normal volunteers in many studies. In the earliest published study, it was demonstrated that 100 μg ovine CRH (oCRH), given as an acute bolus injection, leads to a rapid rise in plasma ACTH peaking at around 10 minutes, followed by a more gradual rise in serum cortisol, peaking at 45 to 60 minutes. No side effects were observed other than transient facial flushing.[75] No change was seen in serum prolactin, GH, TSH, LH, or FSH. It therefore appeared that oCRH was a safe, sensitive, and specific test of the readily releasable pool of ACTH in the corticotroph. Subsequent studies have confirmed that oCRH-41 acutely stimulates the secretion of ACTH and cortisol. Serum 11-deoxycortisol, the immediate precursor of cortisol, is also elevated, as is corticosterone. There is also a small but significant rise in aldosterone after 200 μg oCRH.[76] This is consistent with the known mild stimulatory effects of ACTH on mineralocorticoid pathways. Detailed dose-response studies have demonstrated a threshold dose of 0.01 to 0.03 μg/kg,[77] with most observers reporting a maximally effective dose of approximately 1 μg/kg. Further increases in ACTH above this dose are probably a consequence of the hypotensive effects of oCRH. Other pituitary hormones respond little or not at all to oCRH in normal subjects, nor do plasma catecholamines alter. There does not appear to be any age or sex difference in responsiveness to oCRH in adults, and CRH responsiveness does not vary with age from early childhood through to late adult life.[78] CRH may cause small changes in adrenal androgens such as dehydroepiandrosterone sulfate that are less pronounced prepubertally and in the elderly.

The side effects associated with oCRH have caused some uncertainty in the past. At a dose of 100 μg or 1 μ/kg, which have come to be most used in clinical testing, most investigators have reported little or no change in pulse rate or blood pressure, although facial flushing is common. This is usually transient but can be prolonged and is more common and more sustained at higher doses. However, in one study it was noted that three of 60 patients suffered "absences" after 200 μg of oCRH, and one had junctional cardiac dysrhythmia followed by cardiac arrest. No serious side effects were observed in 140 subjects given 1 μg/kg.[79] It would seem likely that CRH causes peripheral vasodilatation and possibly mild hypotension at all doses but that these are rarely a problem at or below a total dose of 100 μg. In several hundred normal subjects and patients investigated over the past ten years, we have observed symptomatic hypotension after oCRH only in patients with adrenocorticoid insufficiency whose replacement therapy was inadequate or withheld. It is possible that the more severe

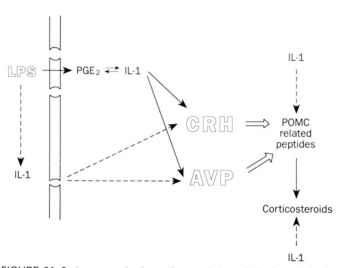

FIGURE 21–2. A suggested scheme for regulation of the hypothalamic-pituitary-adrenal axis by lipopolysaccharide (LPS) and interleukin-1 induced by endotoxemia. LPS may enter the CNS where the blood-brain barrier is deficient and thereby induce local release of prostaglandin E_2 (PGE_2). This may in turn induce a positive feedback release of hypothalamic interleukin-1 (IL-1) and hence the release of CRH. IL-1 either locally or from the circulation can also release AVP, which will synergize with CRH in activation of the pituitary-adrenal axis. IL-1 may also directly affect the pituitary and adrenal.

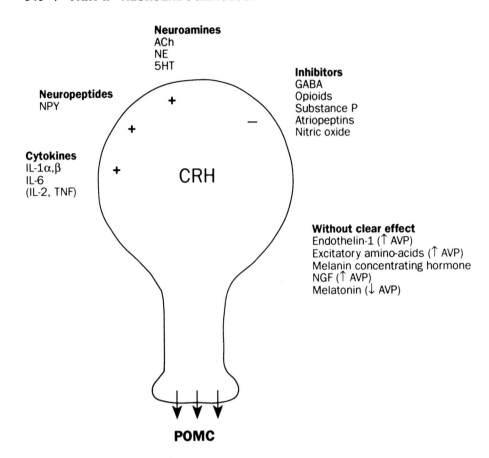

Neuroamines
ACh
NE
5HT

Neuropeptides
NPY

Cytokines
IL-1α,β
IL-6
(IL-2, TNF)

Inhibitors
GABA
Opioids
Substance P
Atriopeptins
Nitric oxide

CRH

Without clear effect
Endothelin-1 (↑ AVP)
Excitatory amino-acids (↑ AVP)
Melanin concentrating hormone
NGF (↑ AVP)
Melatonin (↓ AVP)

POMC

FIGURE 21–3. Summary of the neurotransmitter regulation of CRH. These data, produced from a composite of in vivo and in vitro studies, do not necessarily imply that the relevant receptors are directly on the CRH neuron. Many agents that activate the pituitary-adrenal axis may be without effect on CRH itself and may act via AVP.

reactions previously reported were due to impurities in the preparation of oCRH.

Experience with human CRH is much more limited, but the few published reports indicate that peak ACTH and cortisol responses to hCRH are similar to those after oCRH, although they may be slightly less, but the duration of the hormonal changes is much diminished.[80] Detailed half-life studies have provided some explanation for these differences. Intravenous injection of oCRH produces a rapid rise in the plasma level of oCRH, followed by a gradual fall consisting of two, or possibly three, phases. The initial half-life of between 6 and 12 minutes probably reflects distribution into a volume representing the plasma space.[81] The second half-life of 46 to 73 minutes is likely to represent metabolic clearance and is considerably in excess of the reported half-lives of the shorter-acting hypothalamic peptides TRH and GnRH. It is likely that the prolonged effect of injected oCRH is secondary to this delayed clearance, which appears to be constant throughout the day.

It has also been noted that the infusion of oCRH may be followed by a polyphasic response in plasma ACTH and serum cortisol, in that an initial rise in hormone levels is followed by a fall and subsequent delayed secondary rise. In view of the prolonged half-life of oCRH, it is most probable that the secondary suppression in pituitary-adrenal activity is due to exhaustion of the readily releasable pool of the corticotroph. Further accumulation of readily releasable ACTH consequent to oCRH activity then produces the secondary rise. However, hCRH has a much more rapid clearance in humans. In a detailed study of the pharmacokinetics of CRH,[82] it was found that the metabolic half-life of hCRH in the human was significantly less than that of

oCRH; in the sheep, the half-lives of the two peptides were similar and comparable to that of oCRH in humans. Since the sheep has no CRH-binding protein (CRH-BP; see below), and oCRH does not bind to the human CRH-BP, this suggests that the uniquely short half-life of hCRH in the human is a function of CRH-BP specifically "addressing" it for rapid metabolism. Clinically, this may not be particularly important if the discriminatory power of hCRH between normal and pathological states is equivalent to oCRH, and this appears to be the case, as discussed later.

The administration of CRH is associated with a rise in other ACTH-related peptides, including β-endorphin, as well as the recently demonstrated N-terminal peptide derived from pro-opiomelanocortin, pro-γ-MSH. It therefore appears that there is mobilization and release of all the normal cleavage products of pro-opiomelanocortin.[83, 84]

The response to oCRH is also determined by the level of circulating corticosteroids. Pretreatment with dexamethasone blocks the pituitary-adrenal response to oCRH, while the higher the basal cortisol, the lower the incremental response to oCRH. Thus the incremental response to oCRH late in the afternoon or at night is more easily seen than in the morning. For this reason, some authorities recommend that CRH testing be carried out in the late afternoon, when the low basal HPA activity enhances apparent CRH responsiveness.[85] High doses of oCRH also blunt subsequent circadian increases in pituitary-adrenal activity, while continuous infusions lead to little or no response to subsequent bolus injections. (These studies also demonstrated a lack of down-regulation to CRH.[86]) Thus corticosteroid feedback acts, at least in part, at the pituitary level in humans and blocks or attenuates the response to exogenous CRH.

It is also possible to administer oCRH by the subcutaneous and intranasal routes. In a study of 10 normal men, subcutaneous oCRH was found to be approximately equipotent to intravenous oCRH, whereas intranasal oCRH was only 1 per cent as effective.[87] In terms of the therapeutic use of CRH, the subcutaneous route for oCRH is feasible for long-term administration.

Potentiation of Corticotropin-Releasing Hormone

It has been noted that, even at quite high doses, the response to oCRH is less than that following insulin-induced hypoglycemia in both normal subjects and patients with a history of hypothalamic-pituitary disease. One possibility is that the prolonged and continuous stimulation of the corticotroph in this situation is less effective than the pulsatile release of endogenous CRH induced by hypoglycemia and other stressors. However, as has been previously discussed, it is more likely that there are other ACTH-releasing factors that are required to potentiate the action of CRH, particularly vasopressin. This has been directly demonstrated by the administration of vasopressin together with CRH; a vasopressin dose that is poorly stimulatory alone is able to greatly potentiate the ACTH-releasing activity of oCRH in normal subjects.[88] As noted earlier, evidence from animal studies suggests that while CRH activates a cAMP-mediated series of events, vasopressin acts through a quite separate cAMP-independent pathway involving phospholipase C and the phospatidylinositol pathway. The enhancement of endogenous vasopressin release by hypertonic saline infusion is also able to potentiate the effect of CRH on the release of ACTH.[89] In the rat, there is additional evidence for the direct stimulation of the corticotroph by angiotensin, circulating catecholamines at high concentrations, and a potentiation of the action of CRH by gastrin-releasing peptide (GRP). However, in humans, increases in circulating angiotensin do not appear to enhance the effectiveness of CRH, and infusions of epinephrine are also without effect.[90] GRP has been extracted from several endocrine tumors in humans, and in one patient high circulating levels of tumor-derived GRP were found in association with pituitary-dependent Cushing's syndrome.[91]

The massive adrenocortical response to endogenous pyrogen administration also suggests that vasopressin and/or other factors are released in this situation over and above endogenous CRH. Responsiveness to CRH is blunted by opiate alkaloids and peptides, but there are discrepant reports on the effects of somatostatin, oxytocin, and atriopeptin. While there is a suggestion that CRH responsiveness may be diminished in massive obesity, this has not been confirmed in more recent reports. Finally, it may be noted that CRH can be combined with other hypothalamic investigative peptides such as GnRH, TRH, and GHRH: in the main, there is no evidence for any important interactions between these agents.[92]

Disorders of the Hypothalamic-Pituitary-Adrenal Axis

Patients who demonstrate cortisol deficiency secondary to dysfunction above the level of the adrenal glands may have a functional defect at the level of the pituitary, in the hypothalamus, or in their connections. The standard test of adrenocortical reserve, insulin-induced hypoglycemia, assesses the whole hypothalamic-pituitary axis, so that a lesion along these pathways cannot be precisely located. Numerous studies have been published demonstrating that patients with hypothalamic lesions show maintained, or even enhanced, ACTH responses to CRH, whereas in those with primary pituitary pathology there is little or no response.[93] As this finding occurs in patients who may have long-standing abnormalities, it further implies that endogenous CRH is not required for the maintenance of the corticotroph's secretory capacity. Because of the rapid onset of adrenal atrophy, cortisol responses to CRH in either group of patients are usually quite poor. It therefore appears that a standard test with CRH may discriminate between pituitary and hypothalamic pathology, although modern imaging techniques make the test superfluous in most instances.

Isolated ACTH Deficiency

The syndrome of isolated ACTH deficiency has been considered to be of varied etiology, so it is not surprising that the responses of these patients to oCRH have been heterogenous. Of the reported patients with isolated ACTH deficiency who have received CRH, all but one failed to respond with a rise in ACTH, suggesting primary corticotroph failure[94]; the single responder had a delayed rise in plasma ACTH that was still increasing at the end of the test.[95] It is likely that she had an acquired deficiency in either the synthesis of endogenous CRH or its access to the pituitary.

Primary Adrenal Failure

In primary adrenal failure, the elevated basal levels of plasma ACTH respond excessively to CRH. In one study of eight patients basal plasma ACTH rose from a mean level of 1494 pg/ml to a peak of 2601 pg/ml 10 minutes after 100 µg CRH. There was a highly significant correlation between basal plasma ACTH and the incremental response to CRH.[96] This enhanced response is likely to be a consequence of the hypertrophy or hyperplasia of the corticotrophs. It is possible that a discrepancy between the ACTH and cortisol responses to CRH may indicate early adrenal failure, or minor enzyme abnormalities, in cases in which exogenous pharmacological doses of ACTH do not reveal any adrenal pathology.

Cushing's Syndrome

CRH has come to play an increasingly significant role in the biochemical work-up in the diagnosis and differential diagnosis of Cushing's syndrome; indeed, this is probably its most important use in clinical practice. The test usually involves the administration of 1 µg/kg or 100 µg of human or ovine CRH, given intravenously at 9 A.M., 4 P.M., or 5 P.M., with determination of cortisol and ACTH levels at 15-minute intervals for two hours thereafter. While patients with pituitary-dependent disease usually show exaggerated ACTH responses, those with an ectopic source of the hormone are distinguished by their flat responses. However, the predictive value of the CRH test in distinguishing between ectopic and eutopic disease remains a matter of some debate. Early reports demonstrated that patients with pituitary-dependent Cushing's syndrome respond to CRH with a rise in ACTH and cortisol, and that little or no response is seen shortly after transsphenoidal selective adenomectomy; this suggested that the tumor cells themselves were responsive to CRH, but not the suppressed normal cells.[97] Nevertheless, this differentiation is not absolute, and some patients with histologically proven pituitary disease have clearly shown "normal" or even absent responses.[98] It should be noted that a high level of plasma cortisol greatly attenuates the response to CRH in normal subjects. It appears that the responsiveness of the hyperplastic/adenomatous corticotrophs to CRH in Cushing's disease is a reflection of their insensitivity to steroidal feedback, as also revealed by the dexamethasone suppression test. In general, when basal plasma ACTH and cortisol are normal in Cushing's disease, a peak ACTH or cortisol response to CRH beyond the level in normal subjects is seen in approximately 80 per cent of patients, and is thus extremely useful in differentiating Cushing's disease from simple obesity and depressive illness.

In terms of the differential diagnosis between pituitary-dependent Cushing's syndrome and occult ectopic ACTH syndrome, the clinical value of CRH has been difficult to assess because different centers have utilized different protocols, types of CRH, and definitions of responsiveness. In spite of this, there is only a single published report in which a patient with a proved ectopic source of ACTH responded to a CRH with a rise in serum cortisol. We published the results of a patient with an apparent occult ectopic ACTH syndrome who responded to oCRH, but he was subsequently shown to harbor a pituitary ACTH-secreting tumor. However, we have since seen a patient with a histologically proved bronchial carcinoid who did indeed respond, while intermittent or periodic secretors of tumoral ACTH further complicate interpretation. On the other hand, some 20 per cent of patients with pituitary-dependent Cushing's disease also show a poor or absent response. Thus, a patient with a high-normal serum cortisol who does not appear to respond to CRH may simply be stressed or may have Cushing's syndrome due to either a pituitary or ectopic source of ACTH or CRH. This obviously limits the usefulness of the CRH test. Nevertheless, in the patient with ACTH-dependent Cushing's syndrome and no obvious source for the ACTH, an exaggerated response to CRH suggests Cushing's disease, whereas a completely absent response favors ectopic secretion of ACTH (or CRH).

Combining the results from the CRH test with those of the low- and high-dose dexamethasone suppressive tests has considerably increased the ability to diagnose the source of ACTH secretion in ACTH-dependent Cushing's syndrome. Hermus et al.[99] in a meta-analysis of 83 patients with Cushing's disease showed that, of these, 90 per cent had a cortisol rise in response to CRH. This suggests that responsiveness to CRH almost always excludes the ectopic ACTH syndrome, while the absence of any response coupled with failure of suppression with high-dose dexamethasone administration is highly suggestive of an ectopic source. Nevertheless, assuming that a pituitary source of ACTH is 10 times more common than an ectopic source as a cause of Cushing's syndrome, this analysis suggests that a

patient who *neither* responds to CRH *nor* suppresses with high-dose dexamethasone still has an almost 30 per cent probability of having pituitary-dependent disease. In general, a significant rise in serum cortisol (peak level 20 per cent greater than mean basal) makes the diagnosis of the ectopic ACTH syndrome extremely improbable.

In order to further improve diagnostic reliability, several centers have looked at ACTH levels in venous samples obtained simultaneously from both inferior petrosal sinuses after stimulation with human or ovine CRH. Many relatively small series have been published following the original description of the technique. In the largest series to date, involving nearly 300 cases, Oldfield et al.[100] showed that while basal samples of ACTH with an inferior petrosal sinus:peripheral plasma ratio greater than 2.0 identified 205 out of 215 patients with Cushing's disease (sensitivity 95.3 per cent) with no false positives (specificity 100 per cent), a peak ACTH:peripheral plasma ratio greater than 3.0 after oCRH stimulation identified all 203 patients who received CRH (sensitivity 100 per cent) with no false positives (specificity 100 per cent) (Fig. 21–4).

Analysis of our own data suggests that CRH certainly improves the diagnostic accuracy of interior petrosal sinus catheters in differentiating central from peripheral sources of ACTH, although it is still less than 100 per cent. Most other reports concur that in expert radiological hands the technique is extremely powerful, while lacking absolute precision. We have also found that human CRH, which is commercially available in Europe, is as good as or better

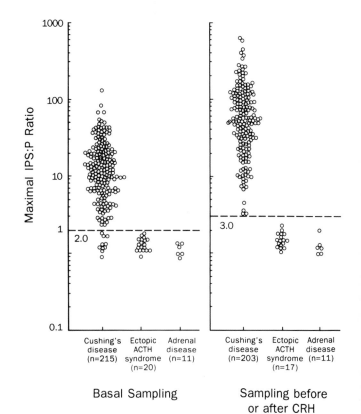

FIGURE 21–4. The maximal ratio of ACTH in plasma from one inferior petrosal sinus to the concentration in the peripheral blood (IPS:P) in patients with Cushing's syndrome. (Data from Oldfield EH, et al: Petrosal sinus sampling with and without CRH for the differential diagnosis of Cushing's syndrome. N Engl J Med 325:897–905, 1991.)

than the ovine molecule in clinical practice. In terms of tumor lateralization, most evidence suggests that this is accurate in only around 70 per cent of patients. This finding should not be particularly surprising, as tumors 2 to 6 mm in diameter in a fossa measuring 10 mm may not be clearly lateralized, and it is an unwarranted assumption that the venous drainage is uniform. A tumor measuring half the size of the normal pituitary with an aberrant venous drainage will clearly be falsely localized on a petrosal catheter. Nevertheless, it may be useful to provide the neurosurgeon with any information in regard to lateralization so that a generous hemihypophysectomy can be performed on the suggested side if no tumor is clearly visible. It should also be stressed that the petrosal catheter technique is of absolutely no value in the actual diagnosis of Cushing's syndrome, i.e., to differentiate Cushing's syndrome from normality or depressive illness.

With regard to postoperative CRH tests, the data are not yet available to indicate that they have a clear role in predicting the likelihood of recurrence. In our experience, a series of postoperative basal cortisols that remain <50 nmol/L are the best indication of cure; levels above this necessitate further therapeutic intervention.[101] In patients with Nelson's syndrome, there is usually a delayed but exaggerated response to CRH.[102]

Patients with Cushing's syndrome due to adrenal adenomas, carcinomas, or micronodular hyperplasia have low or undetectable basal levels of ACTH. These have failed to respond to CRH in most studies, although in patients with mild disease the "normal" pituitary may not be fully suppressed and thus may show a small response.

Several authors have recently suggested that, while AVP alone has no diagnostic advantage over CRH in the investigation of Cushing's syndrome, by combining a low dose of AVP with the CRH the false-negative rate for Cushing's disease may be largely eliminated. However, in view of the added complexity of this procedure, plus the inherent vasopressor activity of AVP, it is not recommended that this be introduced into routine clinical practice.

Depression

As noted later, there is substantial evidence in favor of abnormalities of the HPA in patients with depressive illness, compatible with the notion that there may be overdrive of endogenous hypothalamic CRH in many. The standard CRH test will show a normal rise in serum cortisol, but the ACTH response is often significantly attenuated in such patients, albeit usually still within the normal range.[103, 104] Clinically, this pattern is quite different from that seen in Cushing's disease, and the test may thereby be of clinical use, although it is more often used in a research setting. Patients with anorexia nervosa and panic disorder may show responses similar to those of depressed patients,[105] while in schizophrenia the responses are reported to be normal.

Acromegaly

In two studies of the effects of CRH in acromegaly, one reported that one patient (of eight) apparently responded to CRH with a paradoxical rise in serum GH, although this was still within the normal range. In the second study, two of six patients were said to have responded paradoxically, although no control infusion was given, so that spontaneous fluctuations in serum GH may have accounted for these responses.

Localization of Corticotropin-Releasing Hormone in Humans

Using immunocytochemical techniques, CRH immunoreactivity has been found in the human hypothalamus, where it is localized to the parvocellular neurons in the anterior part of the paraventricular nucleus. Axon terminals containing CRH were found to run down to abut on the portal vessels in the islands of von Greving, the functional counterpart of the zona externa in humans, but were also seen in the vicinity of the zona intermedia.[106] The more recent introduction of immunoassays specifically directed against CRH has confirmed the presence of CRH in the hypothalamus and posterior pituitary but has also located CRH in the cortex, thalamus, cerebellum, pons, medulla, and spinal cord. It has been suggested that hypothalamic CRH neurons act as central coordinators of stress hormone responses, and local activation of these neurons will inhibit GnRH release and stimulate the sympatho-adrenomedullary axis. CRH was localized to the adrenal, whereas lesser concentrations were found in the lung, liver, stomach, duodenum, and pancreas. These extra-adrenal sources of CRH appear to be identical to CRH on high-performance liquid chromatography. However, Nieuwenhuyzen-Kruseman and colleagues found CRH immunoreactivity in the mucosal cells of the gastric antrum that was not identical to hypothalamic CRH; a third form of CRH has been found within the somatotrophs of the anterior pituitary.[107] The discovery of a CRH-like peptide in the gut may be of physiological importance, because administering CRH leads to a rise in circulating pancreatic polypeptide in normal humans[108]; CRH also causes a fall in blood pressure thought to principally be the result of splanchnic vasodilatation. No change in any other gut or pancreatic peptides has been noted. CRH decreases gastric acid secretion in the dog, but this appears to be a central action rather than a paracrine effect.

Detectable CRH has also been isolated in various sites in pathological conditions, including tumors. CRH immunoreactivity is present in low but detectable concentrations in human CSF. The level was lower in patients with Cushing's disease, in those on corticosteroid treatment, and in patients with Sheehan's syndrome; high-normal levels were seen in three patients with Nelson's syndrome and one with Addison's disease.[109] The authors suggest that these results demonstrate that corticosteroids suppress hypothalamic, and hence CSF, CRH concentrations. High levels of CRH have also been reported in the CSF of patients with depressive illness and anorexia nervosa (see later).

CRH Levels in Normal Subjects

Plasma levels of CRH of approximately 3 to 4 pmol/L appear to be derived from both hypothalamic and extrahypothalamic sources and are thus not physiologically representative of various states of HPA activation. Thus, there is poor evidence for circadian variation in plasma CRH levels, and most studies report nonsuppression with administration of exogenous glucocorticoid and no increases after metyrapone. Nevertheless, during extreme stress such as severe hypoglycemia some, but not all, studies have reported a small rise in circulating CRH, suggesting that there may be a hypothalamic component to its plasma level.[110] CSF levels of CRH appear to be higher in neonates but fall off rapidly, reaching adult levels within 24 months.[111]

Corticotropin-Releasing Hormone Levels in Pregnancy

The placenta is an important source of CRH, both peptide and mRNA, although this appears to be true only in primates. Most of the CRH is of the same molecular weight as hypothalamic CRH, although higher molecular weight forms are also present, and it has been shown to be biologically active. Evidence exists that this CRH may be secreted and may influence the release of placental ACTH. Factors regulating the secretion of placental CRH are broadly similar to those active on the hypothalamus, with stimulation by norepinephrine and IL-1, for example, but glucocorticoids are stimulatory rather than inhibitory.[112] Placental CRH is also secreted into the circulation: in the first trimester of pregnancy, plasma CRH levels are low and do not differ from those of nonpregnant women, but levels begin to rise in the second trimester and reach a peak at term (about 250 to 300 pmol/L), declining rapidly within 24 hours after parturition.[113] Similar changes are found in CRH levels in amniotic fluid.

Studies of CRH levels in maternal and umbilical cord blood samples have been shown to be elevated in a number of pathological conditions in pregnancy, including twin pregnancy, hypertension of pregnancy (pre-eclampsia, but not chronic hypertension), and intrauterine growth retardation.[114] However, there remains considerable disagreement as to the precise cell of origin of CRH in the feto-placental unit. Thus CRH immunoreactivity has been localized to the syncytiocytotrophoblast and intermediate trophoblast in the placenta, the epithelium and subepithelial cells of the amnion, and the amniotic epithelium of the umbilical cord. CRH may modify the release of other placental peptides and synergizes with oxytocin to increase gestational myometrial activity.[115] This pattern of distribution indicates that CRH plays a paracrine role in interactions within and between the placenta, fetal membranes, and decidua, that it may be associated with the maturation of the fetal HPA axis, and that it may be instrumental in the physiology of labor. Recent reports suggest that fetal CRH may have an important signaling role in the initiation of labor in some species. However, pregnancy-associated CRH can be fully understood only in relation to the CRH-binding protein (see later).

CRH-Binding Protein

Although maternal plasma CRH concentrations in the later phases of pregnancy approach those of hypothalamic portal blood, there is only a moderate increase in maternal

plasma ACTH with advancing gestation, and even in the terminal stages of pregnancy levels remain within the range of nonpregnant individuals. It has now been demonstrated that a 38-kDa peptide-binding glycoprotein is present in human plasma, inactivating CRH and thus preventing pituitary-adrenal stimulation.[116] This binding protein has recently been cloned and partially sequenced,[117] and is clearly quite different from the CRH receptor insofar as it binds only rat and human CRH and not ovine CRH, whereas the rat and human respond both in vivo and in vitro to both forms. Both rat and human recombinant CRH-BP have been shown to inhibit CRH binding to a CRH antibody and to block CRH-induced ACTH release by corticotrophs in vitro. Saphier et al. have shown that the half-life of hCRH is specifically shortened in the human, whereas both hCRH and oCRH have a relatively long half-life in the sheep, which lacks a CRH-BP.[117a] These findings suggest that CRH-BP enhances the clearance of human CRH.

Although the role of CRH-BP remains unclear, it is possible that CRH-BP protects the body from the effects of the high CRH levels seen in pregnancy. It will be recalled that only primate placenta synthesizes CRH, and only in the human does circulating CRH progressively increase during gestation. This in turn suggests that placental CRH plays a unique human role in pregnancy. However, the slow time course of the association of CRH with CRH-BP (about 5 to 8 minutes) still allows rapid hypothalamic pulses of CRH to stimulate pituitary ACTH release at first pass. There is some evidence that CRH may, under certain circumstances, stimulate monocytes to release an ACTH-like moiety, and thus excessive free levels may require sequestration. Recent data suggest that there may be a marked fall in CRH-BP levels in the final weeks of pregnancy[118] (Fig. 21–5), and it has also been shown that infused human

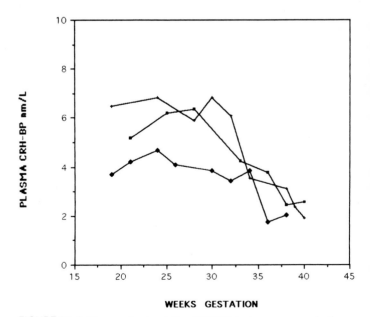

FIGURE 21–5. Changes in circulating CRH-BP during pregnancy in three sequentially sampled women. In the 3rd trimester circulating CRH-BP falls markedly; together with the rise in total CRH, this fall produces a marked rise in the free level of CRH. This may be associated with changes in myometrial activity. (Data from Linton EA, et al: CRH-BP: Plasma levels decrease during the 3rd trimester of normal human pregnancy. J Clin Endocrinol Metab 76: 260–262, 1992.)

CRH leads to a fall in available CRH-BP[119] (Fig. 21–6). Thus free levels of CRH may increase more rapidly than previously had been suspected in the final stages of pregnancy, further emphasizing the possibility that placental CRH is intimately involved in parturition.

CRH-BP has been located immunohistochemically in rat brain in a specific distribution suggesting that it may play a functional role, possibly by inactivating local CRH.[120] Some preliminary evidence indicates that it may help to explain some of the apparent discrepancies between the distribution of CRH and CRH "receptors." Finally, the fact that CRH-BP has a much greater affinity for a peptide such as sauvagine rather than CRH itself has prompted the speculation that the endogenous ligand for the binding protein may be other than CRH. This intriguing suggestion awaits further study.

Ectopic Corticotropin-Releasing Hormone

Tumors that are able to secrete CRH ectopically have been increasingly described since the first report of a prostatic tumor that had metastasized to the hypothalamus. Other examples include bronchial carcinoids, nephroblastomas, pheochromocytomas, medullary carcinomas of the thyroid, and islet cell tumors. However, such tumors usually also co-secrete ACTH, and it is often difficult to know whether to ascribe any associated Cushing's syndrome to the CRH or ACTH hypersecretion. The biochemical and radiological characteristics of such tumors are essentially those of the ectopic ACTH syndrome, with a failure to respond to high-dose dexamethasone and a "flat" response to exogenous CRH (see earlier). Nevertheless, under some circumstances the CRH can serve as a tumor marker to assess the course of the disease and its response to therapy.

Corticotropin-Releasing Hormone and Major Depression

Maintained hypersecretion of cortisol and ACTH have consistently been demonstrated in a proportion of patients with major depression, usually around 40 to 70 per cent. It has been suggested that this heightened pituitary-adrenal activity is a consequence of excessive CRH drive, and this hypothesis is compatible with the majority of abnormalities of the HPA described in depressive illness. Various groups have shown raised levels of immunoreactive CRH in the CSF of depressed subjects, although not all studies have been equally conclusive, and one recent study utilizing sequential CSF sampling unexpectedly reported lower CSF CRH levels in this group of patients.[121] CSF CRH levels have also been reported to be elevated in anorexia nervosa, reduced in dementia of the Alzheimer's type, and are probably normal in schizophrenia.

Studies looking at hormonal responses to a bolus intravenous dose of ovine or human CRH have shown characteristic attenuated ACTH but normal cortisol responses, consistent with endogenous CRH overdrive in the face of functionally robust negative feedback. Continuous 24-hour infusions of CRH in normal subjects have resulted in a modest hypercortisolemia that shared some of the features of that found in major depression, including the preservation of circadian rhythms in cortisol and ACTH secretion and a blunted ACTH response to a further bolus dose of CRH. When negative feedback inhibition is reduced by administering metyrapone, an 11β-hydroxylase inhibitor, hypercortisolemic patients with depressive illness show exaggerated rises in ACTH as compared with normocortisolemic controls,[122] similar to responses shown by normal subjects infused with CRH over 48 hours.[123] Nevertheless, it remains unclear whether these biological markers reflect primary derangements in neural mechanisms that modulate HPA axis activity or whether they exist purely as stress-related epiphenomena. It was noted earlier that CRH produces behavioral and neuroendocrine changes characteristic of severe stress, many of which are also seen in major depression. It has therefore been proposed that activation of CRH, both hypothalamic and possibly extrahypothalamic, plays a crucial role in many of the central and peripheral manifestations of depressive illness. Further studies in this area should clarify whether changes in hypothalamic CRH are truly of pathogenetic significance in depression.

Corticotropin-Releasing Hormone: Appetite and Arthritis

Two other areas under detailed scrutiny currently are the involvement of CRH in appetite control and in inflam-

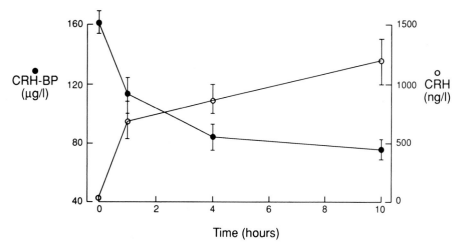

FIGURE 21–6. Changes in circulating CRH-BP following the infusion of a high dose of human CRH in a group of six normal subjects. Note the marked fall in circulating CRH-BP, probably due to sequestration and metabolism after binding to the infused CRH. (Data from Ur E, et al: Continuous human corticotrophin-releasing hormone infusion in normal subjects inhibits circulating corticotrophin-releasing hormone binding protein. J Endocrinol 132:50, 1992.)

matory arthritis. Central administration of CRH results in reduced appetite, and there is evidence for disruption of the regulation of hypothalamic CRH in the genetically obese Zucker rat.[124] Such animals may show weight loss following adrenalectomy, an effect independent of peripheral effects of circulating corticosteroids. Further studies on the involvement of CRH in other forms of obesity, its relationship to other satiety factors such as CCK, and the precise regulatory pathways are under way. In clinical practice it has been suggested that the efficacy of serotonin-uptake inhibitors, such as dexfenfluramine, in decreasing appetite is contingent upon stimulation of endogenous CRH by serotonin.

A surprising recent finding has been that the arthritis-prone Lewis rat may be rendered normal by corticosteroid administration, and such rats may be shown to have a defect in the releasability of central CRH.[125] However, the interpretation of these data is complicated by the fact that in normal rats with induced inflammatory arthritis the principal activator, the HPA, is not CRH, which may even be suppressed.[126] It is therefore difficult to be certain that changes in the regulation of CRH in the Lewis rat are relevant to the pathogenesis of the arthritis. Discordant data in the human suggest that patients with rheumatoid arthritis may have elevated basal pituitary-adrenal activity but an inherently less reactive pituitary-adrenal axis. While such work in the human is fraught with methodological problems, these findings do suggest a whole new area of pathogenetic and possibly therapeutic significance.

ACKNOWLEDGMENTS: I am very grateful to Drs. Peter Trainer, Stylianos Tsagarakis and Ehud Ur for their assistance in preparing this chapter, and to Miss Valerie Taylor and Mrs. Elzbieta Marcar for secretarial help.

REFERENCES

1. Harris GW: Neural control of the pituitary gland. Physiol Rev 28:139–179, 1948.
2. Saffran M, Schally AV: Release of corticotrophin by anterior pituitary tissue in vitro. Can J Biochem 33:408–415, 1955.
3. Guillemin R, Rosenberg B: Humoral hypothalamic control of the anterior pituitary: Study with combined tissue cultures. Endocrinology 57:599–607, 1955.
4. Vale W, Spiess J, Rivier C, Rivier J: Characterization of a 41-residue ovine hypothalamic peptide that stimulates secretion of corticotropin and β-endorphin. Science 213:1394–1397, 1981.
5. Plotsky P: Pathways to the secretion of adrenocorticotrophin: A view from the portal. J Neuroendocrinol 3:1–9, 1991.
6. Ackland JF, Ratter SJ, Bourne GL, Rees LH: Corticotropin-releasing factor-like immunoreactivity and bioactivity of human fetal and adult hypothalami. J Endocrinol 108:171, 1986.
7. Whitnall MH: Distribution of pro-vasopressin expressing and pro-vasopressin deficient CRH neurons in the paraventricular hypothalamic nucleus of colchicine-treated normal and adrenalectomized rats. J Comp Neurol 275:13–28, 1988.
8. Powers RE, DeSouza EB, Walker LC, et al: Corticotropin-releasing factor as a transmitter in the human olivocerebellar pathway. Brain Res 415:347, 1987.
9. Arbiser JL, Morton CC, Bruns GA, Majzoub JA: Human corticotropin releasing hormone gene is located on the long arm of chromosome 8. Cytogenet Cell Genet 47:113–116, 1988.
10. Thompson RC, Seasholtz AF, Douglass JO, Herbert E: The rat corticotropin-releasing hormone gene. Ann NY Acad Sci 512:1–11, 1987.
11. Aguilera G, Millan M, Hauger RL, Catt KJ: Corticotropin-releasing factor receptors: Distribution and regulation in brain, pituitary, and peripheral tissues. Ann NY Acad Sci 512:48–66, 1987.
12. Insel TR, Battaglia G, Fairbanks DW, De Souza EB: The ontogeny of brain receptors for corticotropin-releasing factor and the development of their functional association with adenylate cyclase. J Neurosci 8:4151–4158, 1988.
13. Leong DA, Canny BJ, Jia L-G: New modes of secretion from individual corticotrope studies. Abstract S-6.3 presented at Ninth International Congress of Endocrinology. Nice, France (Aug 30th–Sept 5th), 1992.
14. Sawchenko PE, Imaki T, Potter E, et al: The functional neuroanatomy of corticotropin-releasing factor. CIBA Foundation Symposium 177. Chichester, Wiley, 1993, pp 5–29.
15. Swanson LW, Simmons DM: Differential steroid hormone and neural influences on peptide MRNA levels in CRH cells of the paraventricular nucleus: A hybridization histochemical study in the rat. J Comp Neurol 285:413–435, 1989.
16. Suda T, Tozawa F, Yamada M: Insulin-induced hypoglycaemia increases corticotropin-releasing factor messenger ribonucleic acid levels in rat hypothalamus. Endocrinology 123:1371–1375, 1988.
17. Orchinik M, Murray TF, Morre FL: A corticosteroid receptor in neuronal membranes. Science 252:1848–1851, 1991.
18. Loxley, HD, Cowell A-M, Flower RJ, Buckingham JC: Effects of lipocortin 1 and dexamethosone on the secretion of corticotropin-releasing factors in the rat: In vitro and in vivo studies. J Neuroendocrinol 5:51–62, 1993.
19. Fuxe K, Wikstrom AC, Okret S et al: Mapping of the glucosotricoid receptor immunoreactive neurons in the rat tel- and diencephalon using a monoclonal antibody against rat liver glucocorticoid receptor. Endocrinology 117:1803–1812, 1985.
20. Seckl J, Dickson KL, Fink G: Central 5, 7-dihydroxytryptamine lesions decrease hippocampal glucocorticoid and mineralocorticoid receptor messenger ribonucleic acid expression. J Neuroendocrinol 2:911–916, 1990.
21. Kovacs K, Kiss JZ, Makara GB: Glucocorticoid implants around the hypothalamic paraventricular nucleus prevent the increase of corticotropin-releasing factor and arginine vasopressin immunostaining induced by adrenalectomy. Neuroendocrinology 44:229–234, 1986.
22. De Kloet ER: Brain corticosteroid receptor balance and homeostatic control. Front Neuroendocrinol 12:95–164, 1991.
23. Baulieu E-E, Robel P: Neurosteroids: A new brain function? J Steroid Biochem Molec Biol 37:395–403, 1990.
24. Berkenbosch F, De Goeij CE, Tilders FJH: Hypoglycemia enhances turnover of corticotropin-releasing factor and of vasopressin in the zona externa of the rat median eminence. Endocrinology 125:28–34, 1989.
25. Plotsky PM, Bruhn TO, Vale W: Hypophysiotopic regulation of adrenocorticotropin secretion in response to insulin-induced hypoglycemia. Endocrinology 117:323, 1985.
26. Walker C-D, Dallman MF: Neonatal facilitation of stress-induced adrenocorticotropin secretion by prior stress: Evidence for increased central drive to the pituitary. Endocrinology 132:1101–1107, 1993.
27. Mason JW: A review of psychoendocrine research on the pituitary-adrenal cortical system. Psychosom Med 30:576–607, 1968.
28. Howlett TA, Grossman A, McLoughlin L, et al: The effect of ovine corticotrophin-releasing factor on the hormone response to insulin-induced hypoglycemia. Clin Endocrinol 30:185–190, 1989.
29. Ono N, Lumpkin MD, Samson WK, et al: Intrahypothalamic action of corticotropin-releasing factor (CRF) to inhibit growth hormone and LH release in the rat. Life Sci 35:117, 1984.
30. Brown MR, Fisher LA, Spiess J, et al: Corticotropin releasing factor: Actions on the sympathetic nervous system and metabolism. Endocrinology 111:928, 1982.
31. Sutton RE, Koob GE, Le Moal M, et al: Corticotrophin releasing factor produces behavioural activation in rats. Nature 297:331, 1982.
32. Krieger HP, Krieger DT: Chemical stimulation of the brain: Effect on adrenal corticoid release. Am J Physiol 218: 1632, 1970.
33. Calogero AE, Gallucci WT, Bernardini R, et al: Effect of cholinergic agonists and antagonists on rat hypothalamic corticotropin-releasing hormone secretion in vitro. Neuroendocrinology 47:303, 1988.
34. Tsagarakis S, Holly JMP, Rees LH, et al: Grossman A: Acetylcholine and norepinephrine stimulate the release of corticotropin releasing factor-41 from the rat hypothalamus in vitro. Endocrinology 123: 1962, 1988.
35. Lewis DA, Sherman BM, Kathol RG: Analysis of the specificity of physostigime stimulation of adrenocorticotropin in man. J Clin Endocrinol Metab 58:570–573, 1984.
36. Freeman E, Touzel R, Grossman A, et al: Pyridostigmine, an acetylcholinesterase inhibitor, stimulates growth hormone release, but has no effect on basal TSH or ACTH levels, or on the TSH response to TRH. J Neuroendocrinol 2:429–432, 1990.

37. Sawchenko PE, Swanson LW: The organisation of noradrenergic pathways from the brainstem to the paraventricular and supraoptic nuclei in the rat. Brain Res Rev 4:275, 1982.

38. Al-Damluiji S: Review: Adrenergic mechanisms in the control of corticotropin secretion. J Endocrinol 119:5, 1988.

39. Calogero AE, Galluci WT, Chrousos GP, Gold PW: Catecholamine effect upon rat hypothalamus corticotropin-releasing hormone secretion in vitro. J Clin Invest 82: 839, 1988.

40. Hillhouse EW, Milton NGF: Effect of noradrenaline and gamma-aminobutyric acid on the secretion of corticotropin-releasing factor-41 and arginine vasopressin from the rat hypothalamus in vitro. J Endocrinol 122:719, 1989.

41. Al Damluji S, Iveson T, Thomas JM, Pendlebury DJ, Rees LH, Besser GM: Food induced cortisol secretion is mediated by central alpha-1 adrenoceptor modulation of pituitary ACTH secretion. Clin Endocrinol (Oxf) 26:629–636, 1987.

42. Al-Damluji S, Cunnah D, Perry L, et al: The effect of alpha-adrenergic manipulation on the 24 hour pattern of cortisol secretion in man. Clin Endocrinol (Oxf) 1987.

43. Antoni FA, Dayanithi G: Secretion of ACTH by periperfused isolated rat anterior pituitary cells: Pulse of secretogogue enhance the secretory response and modify the effect of atriopeptin. J Endocrinol 125:365–373, 1990.

44. Huang W, Lee D, Yang Z, et al: Plasticity of adrenoceptor responsiveness on irANP secretion and pro-ANP MRNA expression in hypothalamic neuron cultures: Modulation by dexamethasone. Endocrinology 131:1562–1564, 1992.

45. Tsagarakis S, Navarra P, Rees LH, et al: Morphine directly modulates stimulated CRH-41 release from the rat hypothalamus in vitro. Endocrinology 124:2330, 1989.

46. Calogero AE, Bernardini R, Margioris AN, et al: Effects of serotonergic agonists and antagonists on corticotropin-releasing hormone secretion by explanted rat hypothalami. Peptides 10:189, 1989.

47. Makara JB, Stard E: Effect of gamma-aminobutyric acid (GABA) and GABA antagonist drugs on ACTH release. Neuroendocrinology 16:178, 1974.

48. Tsagarakis S, Rees LH, Besser GM, Grossman A: GABA modulation of CRH-41 secretion from the rat hypothalamus in vitro. J Endocrinol 2:221, 1990.

49. Calogero AE, Galluci WT, Chrousos GP, Gold PW: Interaction between GABAergic neurotransmission and rat hypothalamic corticotropin-releasing hormone secretion in vitro. Brain Res 463:28, 1988.

50. Abraham RR, Dornhorst A, Wynn V, et al: Corticotrophin, cortisol, prolactin and growth hormone responses to insulin-induced hypoglycaemia in normal subjects given sodium valproate. Clin Endocrinol (Oxf) 22:639–644, 1985.

51. McMurray RG, Newbould E, Bouloux P, et al: High-dose naloxone modifies cardiovascular and neuroendocrine function in ambulant subjects. Psychoneuroendocrinology 16:447–455, 1991.

52. Grossman A, Besser GM: Opiates control ACTH through a noradrenergic mechanism. Clin Endocrinol (Oxf) 17:287–290, 1982.

53. Jezova D, Vigas M, Jurcoticova J: ACTH and cortisone response to naloxone and morphine in normal, hypophysectomized and dexamethasone rats. Life Sci 31:307–312, 1982.

54. Plotsky PM: Opioid inhibition of immunoreactive corticotropin-releasing factor secretion into hypophysialportal circulation of rats. Regul Pept 15:235, 1986.

55. Tsagarakis S, Rees LH, Besser GM, Grossman A: Opiate receptor subtype regulation of CRF-41 release from rat hypothalamus in vitro. Neuroendocrinology 51:599, 1990.

56. Roth KA, Weber E, Barchas JD, Chang D, Chang JK: Immunoreactive dynorphin (1–8) and corticotropin-releasing factor in subpopulation of hypothalamic neurons. Science 219:189, 1983.

57. Lightman SL, Young S: Changes in hypothalamic preproenkephalin A MRNA following stress and opiate withdrawal. Nature 238:263, 1987.

58. Takao T, Hashimoto K, Ota Z: Effect of atrial natriuretic peptide on acetylcholine-induced release of corticotropin-releasing factor from rat hypothalamus in vitro. Life Sci 42:1199, 1988.

59. Ibanez-Santos J, Tsagarakis S, Rees LH, Besser GM, Grossman A: Atrial natriuretic peptides inhibit the release of CRF-41 from the rat hypothalamus in vitro. J Endocrinol 126:223, 1990.

60. Plotsky PM, Sutton SW, Bruhn TO, Ferguson AV: Analysis of the role of angiotensin II in mediation of adrenocorticotropin secretion. Endocrinology 122:538, 1988.

61. Tsagarakis S, Rees LH, Besser GM, Grossman A: Neuropeptide Y stimulates CRF-41 release from the rat hypothalamus in vitro. Brain Res 502:167, 1989.

62. Faria M, Navarra P, Tsagarakis S, et al: Inhibition of CRH-41 release by substance p, but not substance k, from the rat hypothalamus in vitro. Brain Research 538:76–78, 1990.

63. Brown MR, Rivier C, Vale W: Central nervous system regulation of adrenocorticotrophin secretion: Role of somatostatins. Endocrinology 114:1546–1549, 1984.

64. Costa A, Trainer P, Besser GM, Grossman A: Nitric oxide inhibits the induced release of corticotrophin releasing hormone from the rat hypothalamus in vitro. Brain Res 605:187–192, 1993.

65. Ur E, Faria M, Tsagarakis S, et al: Atrial natriuretic peptide in physiological doses does not inhibit the ACTH or cortisol response to corticotrophin releasing hormone-41 in normal human subjects. J Endocrinol 131:163–167.

66. Kellner M, Wiedemann K, Holsboer F: Atrial natriuretic factor inhibits the CRH-stimulated secretion of ACTH and cortisol in man. Life Sci 50:1835–1842, 1992.

67. Besedovsky A, Del Rey A, Sorkin E, Dinarello CA: Immunoregulatory feedback between interleukin-1 and glucocorticoid hormones. Science 233:652, 1986.

68. Kehrer P, Turnhill D, Dayer J-M, et al: Human recombinant interleukin-1β and -α, but not recombinant tumour necrosis factor-α, stimulate ACTH release from rat anterior pituitary cells in vitro in a prostaglandin E$_2$ and cAMP independent manner. Neuroendocrinology 48:160–166, 1988.

69. Navarra P, Tsagarakis S, Faria MS, et al: Interleukins-1 and -6 stimulate the release of corticotrophin releasing hormone-41 from rat hypothalamus in vitro via the eicosanoid cyclo-oxygenase pathway. Endocrinology 128:37–44, 1991.

70. Bernardini R, Kamilaris TC, Calogero AE, et al: Interactions between tumor necrosis factor-α, hypothalamic corticotropin-releasing hormone, and adrenocorticotropin secretion in the rat. Endocrinology 126:2876–2881.

71. Navarra A, Pozzoli G, Brunetti L, et al: Interleukins-1β and -6 specifically increase the release of prostaglandin E2 from rat hypothalamic explants in vitro. Neuroendocrinology 56:61–68, 1992.

72. Navarra P, Pozzoli G, Becherucci C, et al: Prostaglandin E$_2$ and bacterial lipopolysaccharide stimulate bioactive interleukin-a release by rat hypothalamic explants. Neuroendocrinology 57:257–261, 1993.

73. Katsuura G, Gottschall PE, Dahl RR, Arimura A: Adrenocorticotropin release induced by intracerebroventricular injection of recombinant human interleukin-1 in rats: Possible involvement of prostaglandins. Endocrinology 122:1773, 1988.

74. Staub JJ, Jenkins JS, Ratcliffe JG, Landon J: Comparison of corticotropin and corticosteroid response to lysine vasopressin, insulin, and pyrogen in man. Br Med J 1:267–269, 1973.

75. Grossman A, Kruseman ACN, Perry L, et al: A new hypothalamic hormone, CRF, specifically stimulates the release of adrenocorticotrophin and cortisol in man. Lancet 1:921–922, 1982.

76. Conaglen JV, Donald RA, Espiner EA, et al: The effect of ovine corticotropin-releasing factor on catecholamine, vasopressin and aldosterone secretion in normal man. J Clin Endocrinol Metab 58:463, 1984.

77. Orth DN, Jackson RV, DeCherney GS, et al: Effect of synthetic ovine corticotropin-releasing factor: Dose response of plasma adrenocorticotropin and cortisol. J Clin Invest 71:587, 1983.

78. Pavlov EP, Harman SM, Chrousos GP, et al: Responses of plasma adrenocorticotropin, cortisol and dehydroepiandrosterone to ovine corticotropin-releasing hormone in healthy aging men. J Clin Endocrinol Metab 62:767–776, 1986.

79. Schulte HM, Chrousos GP, Chatterji DC, et al: Safety of corticotrophin-releasing hormone. Lancet 1:1222, 1983.

80. Schurmeyer TH, Avggerinos PC, Gold PW, et al: Human corticotropin-releasing factor in man: Pharmacokinetic properties and dose-response of plasma adrenocorticotropin and cortisol secretion. J Clin Endocrinol Metab 59:1103.

81. Nicholson WE, DeCherney GS, Jackson RV, et al: Plasma distribution, disappearance half-time, metabolic clearance rate, and degradation of synthetic ovine corticotropin-releasing factor in man. J Clin Endocrinol Metab 57:1263, 1983.

82. Saphier PW, Faria M, Grossman A, et al: A comparison of the clearance of ovine and human corticotrophin-releasing hormone (CRH) in man and sheep: A possible role for CRH-binding protein. J Endocrinol 133:487–495, 1992.

83. Jackson RV, DeCherney GS, Jackson RV, et al: Synthetic ovine corticotrophin-releasing hormone: Simultaneous release of proopiolipomelanocortin peptides in man. J Clin Endocrinol Metab 58:740, 1984.

84. McLoughlin L, Tomlin S, Grossman A, et al: CRF-41 stimulates the release of β-lipotrophin and β-endorphin in normal human subjects. Neuroendocrinology 38:282, 1984.

85. DeCherney GS, DeBold CR, Jackson RV, et al: Diurnal variation in the response of plasma adrenocorticotropin and cortisol to intravenous ovine corticotropin-releasing hormone. J Clin Endocrinol Metab 61:273, 1985.

86. Schulte HM, Chrousos GP, Gold PW, et al: Continuous administration of synthetic ovine corticotropin-releasing factor in man. Physiological and pathophysiological implications. J Clin Invest 75:1781, 1985.

87. DeBold CR, Sheldon WR, DeCherney GS, et al: Effect of subcutaneous and intranasal administration of ovine corticotropin-releasing hormone in man: Comparison with intravenous administration. J Clin Endocrinol Metab 58:836–840, 1985.

88. DeBold CR, Sheldon WR, DeCherney GS, et al: Arginine vasopressin potentiates adrenocorticotropin release induced by ovine corticotropin-releasing factor. J Clin Invest 73:1087, 1984.

89. Milsom SR, Conaglen JV, Donald RA, et al: Augmentation of the response to CRF in man: Relative contribution of endogenous angiotensin and vasopressin. Clin Endocrinol 22:623–630, 1985.

90. Al-Damluji S, Cunnah D, Grossman A, et al: Effect of adrenaline on basal and ovine corticotropin releasing factor stimulated ACTH secretion in man. J Endocrinol 112:145–150, 1987.

91. Howlett TA, Price J, Hale AC, et al: Pituitary ACTH-dependent Cushing's Syndrome due to ectopic production of a bombesin-like peptide by a medullary carcinoma of the thyroid. Clin Endocrinol 22:91–101, 1985.

92. Sheldon Jr WR, DeBold CR, Evans WS, et al: Rapid sequential intravenous administration of four hypothalamic releasing hormones as a combined anterior pituitary function test in normal subjects. J Clin Endocrinol Metab 60:623, 1985.

93. Schulte HM, Chrousos GP, Avgerinos P, et al: The corticotropin-releasing hormone stimulation test: A possible aid in the evaluation of patients with adrenal insufficiency. J Clin Endocrinol Metab 58:1064, 1984.

94. Gordon D, Beastall GH, Thomson C, Thomson JA: ACTH deficiency: Hypothalamic or pituitary in origin? Scott Med J 32:49, 1987.

95. Lytras N, Grossman A, Perry L, et al: Corticotropin releasing factor: Responses in normal subjects and patients with disorders of the hypothalamus and pituitary. Clin Endocrinol (Oxf) 20:71, 1984.

96. Hermus ARMM, Pieters GFFM, Pesman GJ, et al: ACTH and cortisol responses to ovine corticotropin-releasing factor in patients with primary and secondary adrenal failure. Clin Endocrinol (Oxf) 22:761–769, 1985.

97. Avgerinos PC, Chrousos GP, Nieman LK, et al: The corticotropin-releasing hormone test in the postoperative evaluation of patients with Cushing's syndrome. J Clin Endocrinol Metab 65:906, 1987.

98. Trainer PJ, Grossman A: The diagnosis and differential diagnosis of Cushing's syndrome. Clin Endocrinol 34:317–330, 1991.

99. Hermus AR, Pieters GF, Benraad TJ, et al: The CRH test and the high-dose dexamethasone test in the differential diagnosis of Cushing's Syndrome. In Casanueva FF, Diguez C (eds): Recent Advances in Basic and Clinical Neuroendocrinology. Amsterdam, Elsevier, 1990, pp 351–354.

100. Oldfield EH, Doppman JL, Nieman LK: Petrosal sinus sampling with and without corticotropin-releasing hormone for the differential diagnosis of Cushing's syndrome. N Engl J Med 325:897–905, 1991.

101. Trainer PJ, Lawrie HS, Verhelst J, et al: Transsphenoidal resection in Cushing's disease: Undetectable serum cortisol as the definition of successful treatment. Clin Endocrinol (Oxf) 38:73–79, 1993.

102. Oldfield EH, Schulte HM, Chrousos GP, et al: Corticotropin-releasing hormone (CRH) stimulation in Nelson's syndrome: response of adrenocorticotropin secretion to pulse injection and continuous infusion of CRH. J Clin Endocrinol Metab 62:1020, 1986.

103. Gold PW, Loriaux DL, Roy A, et al: Responses to corticotrophin-releasing hormone in the pathophysiology of hypercortisolism in depression and Cushing's disease. N Engl J Med 314:1329–1335, 1986.

104. Holsboer F, Van Bardeleben U, Buller R, et al: Stimulation response to corticotropin-releasing hormone (CRH) in patients with depression, alcoholism and panic disorder. Horm Metab Res 16:80–88, 1987.

105. Roy-Byrne PP, Uhde TW, Post RM, et al: The corticotropin-releasing hormone stimulation test in patients with panic disorder. Am J Psychiatry 143:896–899, 1986.

106. Ohtani H, Mouri T, Sasaki A, Sasano N: Immunoelectron microscopic study of corticotropin-releasing factor in the human hypothalamus and pituitary gland. Neuroendocrinology 45:104, 1987.

107. Nieuwenhuyzen-Kruseman AC, Linton EA, Ackland J, et al: Heterogeneous immunocytochemical reactives of oCRF-41-like material in the human hypothalamus, pituitary, and gastrointestinal tract. Neuroendocrinology 38:212–216, 1984.

108. Lytras N, Grossman A, Rees LM, et al: Corticotrophin releasing factor: Effects on circulating gut and pancreatic peptides in man. Clin Endocrinol (Oxf) 20:725–728, 1984.

109. Tomori N, Suda T, Tozawa F, et al: Immunoreactive corticotrophin-releasing factor concentrations in cerebrospinal fluid from patients with hypothalamic-pituitary-adrenal disorders. J Clin Endocrinol Metab 57:1305–1307, 1983.

110. Suda T, Tomori N, Yajima F, et al: Immunoreactive corticotrophin-releasing factor in human plasma. J Clin Invest 76:2026, 1985.

111. Hedner JT, Lundell KH, Bissette G, O'Connor L, Nemeroff CB: Cerebrospinal fluid concentrations of neurotensin and corticotropin-releasing factor in pediatric patients. Biol Neoate 55:260, 1989.

112. Robinson BG, Emanuel RL, Frim DM, Majzoub JA: Glucocorticoid stimulates expression of corticotropin-releasing hormone gene in human placenta. Proc Natl Acad Sci USA 85:5244, 2988.

113. Petraglia F, Giardino L, Coukos G, et al: Corticotropin-releasing factor and parturition: Plasma and amniotic fluid levels and placental binding sites. Obstet Gynecol 75:784–770, 1991.

114. Wolfe CDA, Patel SP, Linton EA, et al: Plasma CRH in abnormal pregnancy. Br J Obstet Gynaecol 95:1003–1006, 1988.

115. Quattero HPW, Fry CH: Placental corticotropin releasing hormone may modulate human parturition. Placenta 10:439–443, 1989.

116. Orth DN, Mount CD: Specific high affinity binding protein for human CRH in normal human plasma. Biochem Biophys Res Commun 143:411–417, 1987.

117. Potter E, Behan DP, Fischer WH, Linton EA, Lowry PJ, Vale WW: Cloning and characterisation of the cDNA for human and rat corticotropin-releasing factor binding-proteins. Nature 349:423–426, 1991.

117a. Saphier PW, Faria M, Grossman A, et al.: A comparison of the clearance of ovine and human corticotropin-releasing hormone (CRH) in man and sheep: A possible role for CRH-binding protein. J Endocrinol 133:487–495, 1992.

118. Linton, EA, Perkins AV, Woods RJ, et al: Corticotropin releasing hormone-binding protein (CRH-BP): Plasma levels decrease during the third trimester of normal human pregnancy. J Clin Endocrinol Metab 76:260–262, 1992.

119. Ur E, Woods R, Grossman A, et al: Continuous human corticotropin-releasing hormone infusion in normal subjects inhibits circulating corticotropin-releasing hormone-binding protein. J Endocrinol 132 (Abstract), 1992.

120. Potter E, Behan DP, Linton EA, et al: The central distribution of a corticotropin-releasing factor (CRF)-binding protein predicts multiple sites and modes of interaction with CRF. Proc Nat Acad Sci USA: 4192–4196, 1992.

121. Geracioti Jr TC, Orth DN, Ekhator NN, et al: Serial cerebrospinal fluid corticotropin-releasing hormone concentrations in healthy and depressed humans. J Clin Endocrinol Metab 74:1325, 1992.

122. Ur E, Dinan T, O'Keane V, et al: The effect of metyrapone on the pituitary-adrenal axis in depression: Relation to dexamethasone suppressor status. Neuroendocrinology 56:533–538, 1992.

123. Ur E, Capstick C, McLoughlin L, et al: Continuous administration of human corticotropin-releasing hormone in the absence of glucocorticoid feedback in man. J Endocrinol 131 (Suppl): P18 (Abstract), 1991.

124. Plotsky PM, Thrivikraman KV, Watts AG, Hauger RL: Hypothalamic-pituitary-adrenal axis function in the Zucker obese rat. Endocrinology 130:1931–1941, 1992.

125. Sternberg EM, Young III WS, Bernardini R, et al: A central nervous system defect in biosynthesis of corticotropin-releasing hormone is associated with susceptibility to streptococcal cell wall-induced arthritis in Lewis rats. Proc Natl Acad Sci USA 86:4771–4775, 1989.

126. Harbuz MS, Rees RG, Eckland D, et al: Paradoxical responses of hypothalamic corticotropin-releasing factor (CRF) messenger ribonucleic acid (mRNA) and CRF-41 peptide and adenohypophysial proopiomelanocortin mRNA during chronic inflammatory stress. Endocrinology 130:1394–1400, 1992.

Adrenocorticotropic Hormone

HIROO IMURA

Adrenocorticotropic hormone (ACTH) is a peptide hormone that is secreted from the anterior lobe of the pituitary gland and stimulates the adrenal cortex to secrete glucocorticoids, mineralocorticoids, and adrenal androgens. Secretion of ACTH is regulated by the CNS and serum levels of glucocorticoids. The precursor of ACTH is a large molecule called pro-opiomelanocortin (POMC), and several bioactive peptides are derived from this precursor molecule. Over the last 15 years, the primary structure of POMC has been determined by molecular cloning, and extensive studies have been made on molecular biology and processing of POMC and regulation of secretion of ACTH and related peptides.

HISTORY

The pioneering work by Smith (1930) demonstrated that ACTH is a factor separate from other pituitary hormones which maintains the weight of the adrenal cortex. Introduction of the oxycellulose method to purify ACTH significantly accelerated the purification and determination of the primary structure of ACTH by Bell[1] (1954) and some other groups. The pituitary was found also to contain substances that enhance the darkening of frog skin, and two melanocyte-stimulating hormones, α-MSH and β-MSH, were purified by Lerner and Lee[2] (1955) and some other investigators. In 1964, Li[3] isolated a 91-amino acid peptide from sheep pituitary and named it β-lipotropin (β-LPH) owing to its lipolytic activity. Following the discovery of opioid peptides, enkephalins, from the brain in 1975, three peptides having opioid activity were isolated from the pituitary gland and named α-, β-, and γ-endorphin.[4, 5] β-LPH contains the structure of β-MSH and endorphins, and ACTH contains the structure of α-MSH in their molecules. That all these peptides are derived from the common pre-

cursor was demonstrated by Eipper and Mains[6] using biosynthetic labeling of POMC. Secretion of ACTH from the anterior pituitary is enhanced by a hypothalamic hormone, corticotropin-releasing hormone (CRH). This was first demonstrated by Saffran and Schally, and Guillemin and Rosenberg (1955), and its primary structure was determined in 1981 by Vale et al.[7]

PRECURSOR OF ACTH AND ITS GENE

Pro-opiomelanocortin (POMC)

Peptide hormones are generally synthesized in endocrine cells as precursor forms, which are susequently processed to mature hormones. The existence of a big molecule with ACTH-like immunoreactivity was first demonstrated in plasma and pituitary or tumor tissues by using gel filtration combined with radioimmunoassay.[8] Later studies using mouse ACTH-producing pituitary tumor cells, AtT-20 cells,[9] and human ectopic ACTH-producing tumor cells[10] demonstrated that ACTH is biosynthesized as a large molecule of approximately 31 kDa. In vitro translation product of mRNA encoding the precursor of ACTH also had a molecular weight of approximately 35 kDa.[11] Because ACTH has a molecular weight of only 4.5 kDa, the question was what other peptides exist in the remaining portion of the precursor molecule.

Using a pulse-chase technique and anti-ACTH and anti–β-endorphin antisera, Eipper and Mains[6] showed that both ACTH and β-endorphin are derived from the common precursor through intermediate forms in AtT-20 cells. Nakanishi et al[12] and Roberts and Herbert[13] demonstrated that the in vitro translation product of mRNA coding for the precursor of ACTH is immunoprecipitated by both anti-ACTH and anti–β-endorphin antisera. These results indicated that ACTH and β-endorphin/β-LPH are derived from the common precursor.

To elucidate the primary structure of the ACTH/β-LPH precursor, Nakanishi et al.[14] cloned DNA complementary to mRNA (cDNA) encoding the precursor that was purified from bovine neurointermediate pituitary. The amino acid sequence of the precursor deduced from the nucleotide sequence of cDNA has shown that the bovine precursor consists of 265 amino acids, including a signal peptide of 26 amino acids (Fig. 22–1). The protein sequence of β-LPH, of which the C-terminal portion corresponds to β-endorphin, is located at the C-terminal portion of the precursor. The N-terminus of β-LPH is connected by paired basic amino acid residues, Lys-Arg, with ACTH. There are again paired basic amino acids, Lys-Arg, at the N-terminus of ACTH, which are connected with a previously unknown N-terminal portion. There is a sequence of Met-X-His-Phe-Arg-Trp in this N-terminal portion, which is named γ-MSH because of its sequence homology with α- and β-MSH.

The N-terminus of the precursor is considered to be Trp because partial amino acid sequencing of the N-terminal peptide isolated from human and rat pituitary and AtT-20 cells all have Trp residue at the N-terminus. Human N-terminal peptide consists of 76 amino acids.[15] Between the N-terminal peptide and ACTH is a peptide sequence flanked by paired basic amino acids that is called joining peptide or hinge peptide. Because this precursor can produce multiple hormones, the name pro-opiomelanocortin was proposed and has been extensively used.

The primary structures of human, porcine, rat, mouse, frog, and salmon POMC have been deduced from nucleotide sequences of cloned cDNA or genes. Figure 22–1 compares amino acid sequences of bovine, human, mouse, and pig POMC deduced from nucleotide sequences. There are three highly conserved regions: the N-terminal peptide (aligned position 27-106), the ACTH region (aligned position 144-182), and the β-MSH/β-endorphin region (aligned position 230-278).[16] Three MSH peptide sequences and their corresponding nucleotide sequences (ATG-GAG-CAC-TTC-TGG-GAC) are very highly conserved between mammalian and frog species and within the three MSH regions of a single species. This suggests that POMC arose as a result of two tandem gene duplication events. Salmon POMC is exceptional in that it lacks the γ-MSH region, although it has both α-MSH and β-MSH sequences. There are two hypervariable regions in POMC: the joining peptide region and the N-terminal portion of β-LPH. As shown in Figure 22–1, all peptides have several paired basic amino acid residues, which are considered to be processing sites. N- or O-glycosylation sites occur in the N-terminal peptide region in all POMC molecules.

Structure of the POMC Gene

The structural organization of the POMC gene has been studied in human, bovine, porcine, and mouse genes.[16] The rat POMC gene has also been partially cloned. The human POMC gene is composed of 7665 base pairs (bp) and has the following organization: exon 1 (86 bp)—intron A (3708 bp)—exon 2 (152 bp)—intron B (2886 bp)—exon 3 (833 bp).[17] The first exon encodes the 5'-noncoding region. The second exon encodes the 5'-noncoding sequence, signal peptide, and the N-terminal portion of POMC. Most of the sequence of POMC, including three MSH regions, is encoded in exon 3 (Fig. 22–2). The structural organizations of POMC genes of other species are very similar. For example, the position of the intron B is between Leu[44] and Ala[45] in all species.[16] Mouse and pig genomes have two copies of POMC-related sequences. In the mouse, one copy is certainly a pseudogene because it has a termination codon. This pseudogene appears to be generated by a reverse-transcriptase mechanism.

The POMC gene has also similarities with the preproen-

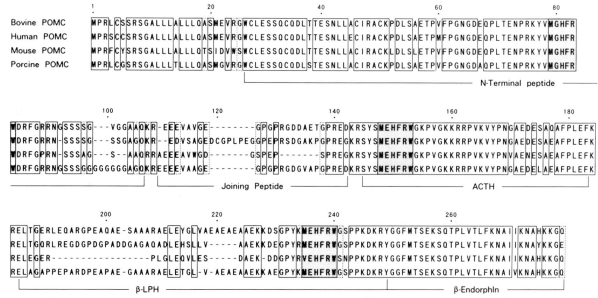

FIGURE 22–1. Amino acid sequences of bovine, human, murine, and porcine POMC deduced from nucleotide sequences of cloned cDNA's. One-letter amino acid notation is used. Sets of identical residues are enclosed by solid lines and sets of residues considered to be the favored amino acid substitution are enclosed by dotted lines. Shaded areas show three MSH sequences.

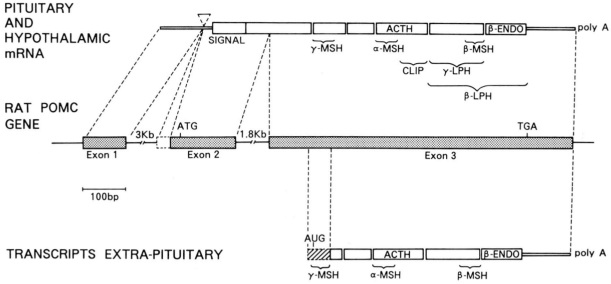

FIGURE 22–2. Organization of rat POMC gene and pituitary or hypothalamic mRNA and extrapituitary transcript. Alternative splicing at the 3' portion of intron A gives rise to a longer mRNA in the hypothalamus. Similar alternative splicing can occur in human ectopic ACTH-producing tumors. Extrapituitary tissues contain mRNA shorter than POMC mRNA in the pituitary. This is a product of aberrant transcription beginning in the γ-MSH portion of exon 3, with several different transcription starting sites *(dotted line)*. (From Drouin J, Sun YL, Nemer M: Regulatory elements of the pro-opiomelanocortin gene. Pituitary specificity and glucocorticoid repression. TEM 2:219–225, 1990.)

kephalin A and preproenkephalin B (prodynorphin) genes.[16] The preproenkephalin A gene has also three exons, and most of the protein-coding sequence resides in exon 3. The preproenkephalin B gene consists of four exons, having an additional exon in the 5'-region, and most parts of the precursor protein are encoded in exon 4. The translation initiation site exists in a very similar position—exon 2 in the POMC and preproenkephalin A genes and exon 3 in the preproenkephalin B gene. These similarities suggest that these three genes have evolved by an analogous mechanism.

Expression of the POMC Gene

Expression of the POMC gene has been studied by Northern blotting and in situ hybridization. POMC mRNA is most abundantly detected in corticotrophs of the anterior pituitary and melanotrophs of the intermediate pituitary.[18] Although much less in amount, POMC mRNA could be detected in the hypothalamus, especially in the arcuate nucleus.[18] Very low levels of POMC mRNA have been identified in many extracranial tissues, such as the testes, ovaries, placenta, adrenal medulla, and leukocytes. POMC mRNA expressed in the normal pituitary or hypothalamus has a size of approximately 1100 nucleotides. On the other hand, mRNA in extracranial tissues has a size approximately 300 nucleotides shorter than that of the pituitary,[19] but in ectopic ACTH-producing tumors, it is approximately 200 nucleotides longer than that of the pituitary mRNA.[20, 21] The shorter mRNA was studied by several groups and was found to be aberrant translation products of the POMC gene.[19] As shown in Figure 22–2, multiple translation initiation sites occur in the 5'-region of exon 3. It is still not known whether or not this short mRNA is

translated into peptides. Even if translated, the peptide is not secreted because of the lack of signal peptide.

Ectopic ACTH-producing tumors and the hypothalamus sometimes contain larger POMC mRNA.[20, 22] Jeannotte et al[22] reported a long poly-A tail in POMC mRNA extracted from the hypothalamus. There is also a site of alternative splicing at the 5' end of exon 2, which may increase the size of mRNA for about 50 nucleotides. Another possibility is an altered initiation site of translation.

Regulation of Expression of the POMC Gene

The POMC gene is abundantly expressed only in a limited number of cell types, such as pituitary corticotrophs and melanotrophs and the neuronal cells of the arcuate nucleus. This suggests the presence of a mechanism responsible for tissue-specific expression of the gene. To study the mechanism, two major approaches have been used: introduction of the POMC gene or its 5'-flanking region with a reporter gene into cultured cells or into mouse oocytes.

A fragment of the POMC gene including a large 5'-flanking region was transfected into the AtT-20 cells, mouse fibroblast L cells, and rat glial C6 cells, together with the neomycin-resistant gene.[23] In the transformed AtT-20 cells, the introduced human POMC gene was transcribed correctly and the transcript was spliced faithfully. On the other hand, most of the transcripts of the human POMC gene were not correctly initiated in L cells or C6 cells, and the levels of mRNA were low. This suggests the presence of tissue-specific translation factors in pituitary corticotrophs or repressors in extrapituitary tissues. To study the DNA element responsible for tissue-specific expression of the POMC gene, deletion experiments were performed. These studies suggest that two DNA sequences, -480 to -323 and -166 to -34, seem to be important.[24] DNA mobility-shift binding assay and the footprint method provided evidence for a nuclear factor that binds the -478 to -320 DNA fragment of the 5′-flanking region of the POMC gene. More recent studies using in vitro footprinting and replacement mutagenesis have shown that at least nine regulatory elements are required for full activities and have suggested that several translation factors, including proteins of SP-1 and COUP families, are involved.[24]

The in vivo specificity of POMC 5′-flanking sequences was assessed in transgenic mice bearing a POMC-neochimeric gene.[25] The pattern of transgene expression mimicked very closely the expression of endogenous POMC; that is, the transgene expression was high in the pituitary but was not observed in other tissues except for the testis. In the latter case, the expression of the transgene was not observed in all transgenic mice. It was demonstrated that no more than 760 bp of the POMC gene were required to direct cell-specific transgene expression in both corticotrophs and melanotrophs.

Expression of the POMC gene is regulated by several factors. CRH, which is an important stimulator of ACTH secretion, also enhances POMC gene expression in corticotrophs both in vivo and in vitro. The effects of CRH on melanotrophs are somewhat different. Acute stimulation by CRH increased peptide secretion in vivo and gene expression in vitro. Chronic CRH injection, however, suppressed the gene expression in about 30 per cent of control animals. This is in contrast to the effect of chronic CRH administration on corticotrophs, which induced a significant increase of POMC gene expression.

CRH is considered to act through the activation of adenylate cyclase to stimulate ACTH secretion. Forskolin, a direct stimulator of adenylate cyclase, and 8-bromo-cAMP, an analogue of cAMP, also enhance POMC gene expression in both anterior or intermediate pituitary cells in vitro,[26] suggesting a common pathway in the release of ACTH and expression of the POMC gene. Using a DNA deletion method and chloramphenicol acetyltransferase (CAT) as a reporter gene, the 5′-flanking sequence of the rat POMC gene between -320 and -133 bp was reported to confer both CRH and forskolin responsiveness. However, this region contains no consensus sequence known as the cAMP-responsive elements (CRE's). In the human POMC gene, the region between -417 and -97 bp from the translation initiation site was demonstrated to be involved in the regulation by cAMP.[27] This region was shown to confer cAMP responsiveness when placed upstream of a heterogeneous viral promoter. The DNA elements responsible for cAMP responsiveness, CRE's, consist of core octamer motifs, 5′-TGACGTCA-3′.[27] Around -340 and -320 bp upstream from the translational start site of the human POMC gene, there are two regions with 75 per cent homologies to CRE.

ACTH secretion from corticotrophs is stimulated by certain factors other than CRH, such as vasopressin and catecholamines. These factors have no clear-cut effects on POMC gene expression, although phorbol ester, a direct stimulator of C kinase, was reported to enhance POMC gene expression. Expression of the POMC gene in the intermediate lobe is inhibited by dopamine and enhanced by haloperidol, a dopamine antagonist,[28] suggesting an inhibitory control of dopamine on the intermediate lobe.

Another factor involved in the regulation of the POMC gene in the intermediate lobe is γ-aminobutyric acid (GABA) because GABA-ergic agents are implicated in the negative influence on the POMC gene expression.

Glucocorticoids are well-known inhibitors of ACTH secretion. In animal experiments, adrenalectomy increases and glucocorticoids decrease POMC mRNA levels in the anterior pituitary.[29] This inhibitory effect of glucocorticoids is explained partly by a direct effect on corticotrophs because glucocorticoids inhibit POMC mRNA levels in cultured pituitary or AtT-20 cells. Glucocorticoids also inhibit pituitary POMC mRNA levels through the brain, acting at or above the level of the hypothalamus. Hypothalamic CRH mRNA levels were reported to increase after adrenalectomy and decrease after glucocorticoid treatment.

The effects of glucocorticoids on the POMC gene in the neurointermediate lobe are different from those on the anterior pituitary. In intact animals, glucocorticoids have essentially no effects on POMC mRNA levels in the intermediate lobe. This can be explained by the absence of glucocorticoid receptors in the intermediate lobe under physiological conditions. The glucocorticoid receptors may be expressed in melanotrophs in culture. Concordant with this observation, glucocorticoids inhibit POMC gene expression in cultured melanotrophs.

In vitro effects of glucocorticoids have been studied extensively in AtT-20 cells. Detection of the POMC primary transcript by using a specific probe or the nuclear run-off assay has provided evidence that glucocorticoids act mainly at the level of translation and that antagonistic interaction with CRH is present at this level. The DNA element responsible for the negative regulation by glucocorticoids has not yet been identified. The stimulatory effects of glucocorticoids on gene translation are mediated by a glucocorticoid-responsive element (GRE). However, the 5′-flanking region of the POMC gene does not have a GRE. To localize the DNA fragment responsible for negative regulation, Gagner and Drouin[30] performed deletion studies and found that deletion of a fragment (-38 to -138) abolished glucocorticoid repression. Using a mutagenesis technique, they found also that a double point mutation at -70 and -71 of the upstream fragment also abolished the glucocorticoid repression. They hypothesized that proteins of COUP family bind a DNA fragment around -63 bp and that glucocorticoid receptors may interfere with the function of COUP, one of the translation factors for POMC gene expression. More recent study disclosed, however, that not only the -77 to -51 region but also the -480 to -320 region is required for glucocorticoid repression. If this is the case, the mechanism of glucocorticoid-induced repression of the gene is complex.

ACTH secretion is enhanced by a variety of stresses, such as pain, infection, and electrical shock. These stresses increase POMC mRNA levels of the pituitary. Such increases can be explained by an increase in hypothalamic CRH release. It has been observed, however, that cytokines, such as interleukin-1 (IL-1) and IL-2, increase the POMC mRNA content of AtT-20 cells.[31] This suggests an additional direct action of cytokines on pituitary corticotrophs. Bacterial lipopolysaccharides enhance also the production of cytokines in the pituitary, which may act to enhance POMC gene expression. Growth factors may also be included in the category of cytokines and are produced in the pituitary or brain. Among them, activin, a gene from the family including transforming growth factor β, was reported to inhibit expression of the POMC gene.[32] Physiological significance of this observation must await further clarification.

PROCESSING OF PRECURSOR

Translation of the POMC mRNA gives rise to pre-POMC, which has a signal peptide at the N-terminus. This precursor undergoes a series of co- and post-translational modifications. The first step of co-translational events is the cleavage of the N-terminal signal sequence, which is considered to play an important role in the binding and entrance of the peptide into the endoplasmic reticulum.[33] Another co-translational event is N-glycosylation at the Asn residue in the sequence of Asn-X-Ser in the γ-MSH region.[33] N-glycosylation may occur to some extent in the corticotropin-like intermediate lobe polypeptide (CLIP) sequence of mouse POMC. Another type of post-translational processing that occurs in the Golgi apparatus is phosphorylation at a Ser[31] residue in the C-terminal region of the ACTH molecule. This is thought to occur while POMC is an intact molecule.[38] There is also evidence that POMC may contain sulfate, which is thought to be linked covalently with the oligosaccharide moiety or to be sulfation of the tyrosine moiety.

The major step of post-translational processing of POMC is the endopeptidase cleavage that takes place within secretory granules.[33] The endopeptidase cleavage of POMC varies in different tissues. Following the endopeptidase cleavage, the exopeptidase cleavage is thought to remove basic amino acids from the carboxy-terminus. Other modifications of POMC include α-amidation and N-acetylation. Pituitary secretory granules have been reported to contain α-amidation activity.[34] α-MSH is the major POMC-derived peptide amidated at the C-terminus, although other fragments may also be amidated. N-acetylation occurs in both β-endorphin and α-MSH in the intermediate lobe and also, although to a lesser extent, in the anterior lobe or other tissues. The occurrence of pyroglutamic acid at the N-terminus of β-lipotropin and joining peptide has also been reported.[35]

Processing in the Anterior Pituitary

In corticotrophs of the anterior pituitary, the endopeptidase cleavage occurs at specific paired basic amino acid residues, Lys-Arg and Arg-Arg. Other pairs of basic amino acids—Arg-Lys, Lys-Lys, and Lys-Lys-Arg-Arg—are not cleaved in corticotrophs. It is still not known why Lys-Arg residues in the sequence of Lys-Lys-Arg-Arg of the ACTH molecule are not cleaved. It is not due to the conformation of the ACTH molecule but to processing enzymes because this portion is cleaved in melanotrophs. Thus, the major endoproducts in the anterior pituitary are the N-terminal peptide (1-76 in human), the joining peptide, ACTH and β-LPH, although β-LPH is further processed to β-endorphin to a certain extent (Fig. 22–3).[36, 37] β-MSH is not produced in human pituitary postpartum and the previously isolated human β-MSH (1-22) was an artefactual product.[38] There are some other minor products. Either C-terminally and/or N-terminally truncated forms of ACTH have been isolated: ACTH 1-37, ACTH 1-38, ACTH 7-39, ACTH 7-38, and ACTH 7-31. C-terminally truncated forms of β-endorphin– or α-MSH–like peptides are N-acetylated. N-acetylation products are also very scarce in human pituitary. Further processing of ACTH to α-MSH and CLIP occurs to a very limited extent in rat anterior pituitary.

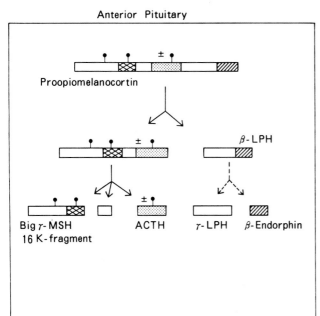

Anterior Pituitary

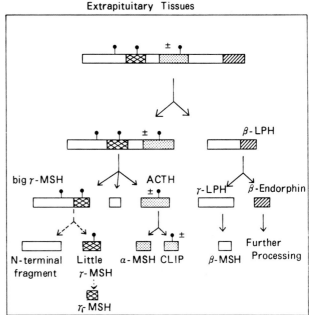

Neurointermediate Pituitary
Extrapituitary Tissues

FIGURE 22–3. Diagrammatic representation of the processing of POMC in the anterior pituitary *(left)* and neurointermediate pituitary *(right)*. Processing in other tissues is more or less similar to that in the neurointermediate lobe, although there are considerable tissue-to-tissue differences (see text). Connected filled circles indicate putative glycosylation sites.

Processing in the Intermediate Lobe

Processing of ACTH into α-MSH and CLIP occurs quite extensively in the intermediate lobe, by the process of endo- and exopeptidase cleavage, acetylation, and amidation. β-LPH is also cleaved into β-endorphin or its C-terminally truncated forms and these β-endorphin–like peptides are N-terminally acetylated to a large extent.[36] N-terminal peptide is partly cleaved at the Arg-Lys portion, thus producing γ-MSH. This processing occurs when POMC lacks an o-linked sugar chain. Several small molecular forms of γ-MSH have been isolated. The smallest form has Lys at the N-terminus and Phe-NH2 at the C-terminus. Thus, α-MSH, CLIP, and N-acetyl β-endorphin are the principal products of the intermediate lobe (Fig. 22–3).[37]

Processing in the CNS and Extracranial Tissues

Processing of POMC in the brain is somewhat similar to that in the intermediate lobe, although there are some differences. ACTH is cleaved in the brain to a large extent, but α-MSH–like peptide produced is not N-terminally acetylated, consistent with low α-N-acetyltransferase activity in hypothalamic extracts. CLIP may have several molecular forms by further processing. Unlike the intermediate lobe, β-endorphin is N-acetylated to only a limited extent and C-terminally truncated forms are scanty; thus β-endorphin 1-31 is the principal form in the hypothalamus. N-terminal peptide is also processed to small molecular forms of γ-MSH.

Processing of POMC in extracranial and extrapituitary tissues is more or less similar to that in the intermediate lobe, although certain tissue-to-tissue differences exist. In the thyroid, N-acetylated β-endorphin is predominant with a small amount of ACTH.[39] In the pancreas, ACTH and N-acetylated β-endorphins are identified.[39] The gastrointestinal tract contains β-endorphin rather than β-LPH and also ACTH-like immunoreactivity eluted at the position of ACTH 1-39,[37] whereas γ-MSH is in a large molecular form, the N-terminal peptide. In the adrenal medulla, most of immunoreactive β-endorphin is β-endorphin 1-31 and not β-LPH.[39] ACTH and deacetylated α-MSH are also found. Human placenta contains ACTH, β-LPH, β-endorphin, and N-terminal peptide.[37] Immunoreactive β-endorphin was detectable throughout the male reproductive tract, being the highest in the testis, and was reported to be compatible with β-endorphin 1-31.[39] More recent study has shown, however, that N-acetylated α-endorphin and γ-endorphin are the major molecular species, with a small amount of N-acetyl β-endorphin. The female reproductive tract also contains β-endorphin, which is co-eluted with β-endorphin 1-31. ACTH 1-39 is also present, although large molecular forms of ACTH are predominant.

Recent studies have shown that POMC-derived peptides are produced in macrophages and lymphocytes. β-endorphin–like immunoreactivity corresponds to β-endorphin 1-31 with some other molecular species,[39] whereas the principal form of immunoreactive ACTH was reported to be ACTH 1-25.

Processing of POMC in Human ACTH-Producing Tumors

Processing of POMC in pituitary adenomas in Cushing's disease is essentially the same as that in normal corticotrophs, although there are minor differences.[40] The major proportion of immunoreactive ACTH corresponds to ACTH 1-39. Further processing of ACTH may occur in the adenoma because concomitant secretion of ACTH and α-MSH has been reported.[41] Processing of β-LPH to β-endorphin is a little more accelerated; therefore, the peak of β-endorphin is almost comparable to that of β-LPH on gel filtration chromatography.[40] Partial processing of the N-terminal peptide to γ-MSH–like peptide could also occur in Cushing's adenomas. Lamberts et al.[42] have proposed that there are two types in Cushing's adenoma—an anterior lobe type and an intermediate lobe type. This hypothesis has not yet been confirmed by others, and it is still not known whether the processing of POMC differs between the two types.

Processing of POMC in ectopic ACTH-producing tumors varies considerably from tumor to tumor. As first reported by Yalow and Berson,[8] big ACTH, the precursor or intermediate form, is usually more abundant than in the normal pituitary, and some tumors have only big ACTH compatible with the precursor form.[20] On the other hand, further processing of ACTH to α-MSH–like peptide and CLIP can occur in some tumors.[20] The processing of β-LPH to β-endorphin also varies considerably, and multiple molecular forms were observed. N-terminal peptide is also heterogeneous on gel filtration, suggesting the processing to γ-MSH. Furthermore, glycosylation of the N-terminal peptide seems also to be altered in some cases, because the binding to a lectin column was reported to be decreased.[43] The limited processing of the precursor and the accelerated processing of ACTH, β-LPH, and N-terminal peptide resemble the processing in the neonatal pituitary.

Characteristics of Processing of Prepropeptide in Corticotrophs

To elucidate the capacity of corticotrophs to process various prepropeptides, cDNA's encoding peptide precursors were introduced into AtT-20 cells and the peptides produced were analyzed. These studies have shown that most peptide precursors transfected into AtT-20 cells are cleaved into small molecular forms at paired basic amino acid residues, Lys-Arg or Arg-Arg. This indicates that the cleaving enzymes act on both endogenous and exogenous precursor molecules.

The site-directed mutagenesis has been introduced to study the peptide sequence for faithful processing.[44] Neuropeptide Y has a single paired basic amino acid cleavage site, Lys-Arg. This portion was mutated to Arg-Arg, Arg-Lys, or Lys-Lys, and the mutants were transfected into AtT-20 cells; the Lys-Arg and Arg-Arg sites were easily cleaved, whereas the cleavage of Arg-Lys was slow and limited and that of Lys-Lys was very poor. Disruption of N- or O-glycosylation sites in the N-terminal portion does not affect the processing, but the change of Arg-Lys to Arg-Arg before the γ-MSH portion induces almost complete cleavage at this site. These results suggest that the glycosylation does not much affect the processing and that the amino acid sequence is important as a processing signal.[44]

Processing Enzymes

The processing of POMC requires one or more endo-peptidases, exopeptidases, α-amidating enzymes, and acetyltransferases to produce mature hormones.[45] Recent studies have succeeded in purifying or cloning at least some of these enzymes. As to the endopeptidase, it is still not clear how many enzymes are involved in the processing of POMC. Purification of such enzymes was very difficult, but a breakthrough was brought about by the discovery of yeast endopeptidase, KEX-2. This is a Ca^{2+}-dependent serine protease with a bacterial subtilisin-like catalytic domain which is involved in the processing of pro-α-factor. The KEX-2 protease expressed in mammalian cells was demonstrated to cleave co-expressed POMC. Based on this observation, several mammalian homologues of KEX-2 have been cloned. One is PC-2, a subtilisin-like protein identified in human insulinoma cells by homology to KEX-2. Another is PC-1 (called PC-3 by some investigators) cloned from AtT-20 cells.[46] Pituitary corticotrophs express high levels of PC-1 mRNA with little PC-2, whereas both PC-1 and PC-2 genes are highly expressed in the intermediate lobe.[47] It has been shown also that glucocorticoids, thyroid hormone, and dopamine are involved in the expression of PC-1 and PC-2 genes.[47] Both PC-1 and PC-2 were demonstrated to accurately cleave the Lys-Arg or Arg-Arg portion of POMC when both genes were co-expressed and are thought to be major endopeptidases for POMC processing. Another endoprotease that is potentially involved in peptide processing is furin, a protein that is encoded by the upstream region of the c-fos/fps proto-oncogene and that has homology with KEX-2. The furin gene is expressed widely in all tissues and is possibly involved in constitutive secretory pathways.

Carboxypeptidase E (EC 3.4,17.10) is an exopeptidase that removes a Lys or Arg residue at the C-terminus of small peptides. It is encoded in a single gene, and the protein synthesized has a molecular weight of 55 kDa. This enzyme is expressed almost constantly in many tissues, but in corticotrophs it is co-secreted with ACTH and related peptides in response to secretagogues.

α-Amidation of peptides is catalyzed by peptidyl-glycine α-amidating monoxygenase (EC 1, 14, 17, 3), which is encoded by a single complex gene and has multiple molecular forms as a result of alternative splicings. Some of the molecular forms have a transmembrane domain. When expressed in AtT-20 cells, significantly enhanced enzyme activity was observed.

CHEMISTRY, BIOLOGICAL ACTIVITY, AND STRUCTURE-FUNCTION RELATIONSHIPS OF POMC-DERIVED PEPTIDES

ACTH

ACTH is a single-chain polypeptide consisting of 39 amino acids, and only one or two amino acids are substituted between 25 and 33 amino acids in mammals (Fig. 22–4). In birds, amphibians, and fishes, several amino acid substitutions are seen between 13 and 24 amino acids and at the N-terminal end.[48] However, the sequence between 2

A

```
         1              5            10            15            20
H-Ser-Tyr-Ser-Met-Glu-His-Phe-Arg-Trp-Gly-Lys-Pro-Val-Gly-Lys-Lys-Arg-Arg-Pro-Val-

              25            30            35
Lys-Val-Tyr-Pro-Asn-Gly-Ala-Glu-Asp-Glu-Ser-Ala-Glu-Ala-Phe-Pro-Leu-Glu-Phe-OH
```

B

FIGURE 22–4. Amino acid sequence of human ACTH (A) and amino acid sequences of mammalian, avian, amphibian, and fish ACTH (B). In B, one-letter amino acid notation is used.

	1	10	20	30	39
Human :	SYSMEHFRWG	KPVGKKRRPV	KVYPNGAE-DE	SAE-AFPLEF	
Bovine :	· · · · · · · · · ·	· · · · · · · · · ·	· · · · · · · · – ·	· · Q - · · · · · ·	
Ovine :	· · · · · · · · · ·	· · · · · · · · · ·	· · · · D · · · · – ·	· · Q - · · · · · ·	
Porcine :	· · · · · · · · · ·	· · · · · · · · · ·	· · · · · · · · · – ·	L · · · · · · · · ·	
Rat :	· · · · · · · · · ·	· · · · · · · · · ·	· · · · · V · - N ·	· · · · · · · · · ·	
Turkey :	· · · · · · · · ·	· · · · RRK · · I	· · · · · · SV-BZ	ZQA-SY · V · ·	
Ostrich :	· · · · · · · · · ·	· · · · R · · · · I	· · · · · VQ-E ·	TS - - G · · · · ·	
Chicken :	· · · · · · · · · ·	· · · · R · · · · I	· · · · · VQ-E ·	· · · · -SY · M · ·	
Xenopus	A · · · · · · · · ·	· · · · R · · · · I	· · · · · · V · -E ·	· · · -SY · M · L	
Dogfish :	· · · · · · · · ·	· · M · R · · ·	· · · · · SF-· · ·	· V · -NMGP · L	
Salmon	· · · · · · · · ·	· · I · H · · · · I	· · · ASSL · GGD	· S · GT · · · QA	

α-MSH

and 12 amino acids is identical throughout the species, suggesting the importance of this portion for biological activity.

The major biological activity of ACTH is to stimulate secretion of adrenal steroids. Glucocorticoid (cortisol in man and corticosterone in rats) secretion is regulated principally by ACTH, although some other substances modulate the action of ACTH. Among them, corticostatin, a group of neutrophil peptides, has recently been shown to compete with ACTH at the receptor level. ACTH also enhances secretion of adrenal androgens, but other factors may regulate secretion of androgens. Acute injection of ACTH causes a rise of plasma aldosterone. However, the renin-angiotensin system is a more important determinant of aldosterone secretion in ambulant men, and chronic ACTH excess does not result in increased aldosterone secretion because of suppression of the renin-angiotensin system. The mechanism of action of ACTH is discussed in Chapter 93. Beside the steroidogenic action, ACTH has melanocyte-stimulating activity in frogs, enhances lipolysis in rats and rabbits, accelerates the acquisition of conditioning in rats, induces stretching or yawning in rats, and induces hypoglycemia and hyperinsulinemia in rats. These extra-adrenal actions are not evident in humans except that ACTH increases skin pigmentation. Because α- and β-MSH do not exist in humans, the major pigmentary hormone in humans is thought to be ACTH.

The steroidogenic activity of ACTH resides in the N-terminal portion because synthetic ACTH 1-24 and ACTH 1-23 have almost full activity. Studies using a variety of synthetic peptide preparations have revealed that ACTH 1-13 has little steroidogenic activity, which increases with an extension of the C-terminal end of the peptide, reaching the full activity at ACTH 1-23. Further extension of the C-terminal sequence toward ACTH 1-39 gives stability to ACTH when incubated in plasma in vitro, suggesting the protective action from proteolytic cleavage. It has been proposed that steroidogenic activity of ACTH resides in the 6 to 10 amino acid residues (His-Phe-Arg-Trp-Gly) and that four basic amino acid residues, Lys-Lys-Arg-Arg (15-18), are the binding site for ACTH receptor. The His-Phe-Arg-Trp portion is also essential for melanocyte-stimulating activity or other extrapituitary actions of ACTH.

MSH

α-MSH consists of 13 amino acids and is derived from ACTH by proteolysis, N-terminal acetylation, and C-terminal amidation. That is, α-MSH is an N-acetyl ACTH 1-13 amide. The amino acid sequence of α-MSH is identical in mammals but somewhat different in fish at the N- and C-termini (Fig. 22–4). α-MSH is produced in melanotrophs of the intermediate lobe of the pituitary in most mammals.

In the adult human pituitary, however, the intermediate lobe is not present. Scattered intermedia-type cells are present in the anterior lobe adjacent to the posterior lobe. α-MSH–like immunoreactivity is present in the anterior lobe in man, but which cells contain immunoreactive α-MSH is still controversial; some reports claim them to be intermedia-type cells, whereas others identify them as normal anterior pituitary cells. The human pituitary has weak N-acetylating activity. Therefore, most immunoreactive α-MSH in the human pituitary appears not to be the N-acetylated form. Human brain contains immunoreactive α-MSH, but its N-terminus is not acetylated.

Studies using synthetic peptide have shown that the minimum peptide for melanocyte-stimulating activity is His-Phe-Arg-Trp. CLIP first isolated from pig and rat intermediate pituitaries consists of the 18-39 portion of ACTH and is possibly produced by the cleavage of ACTH as a by-product of α-MSH. It has no clear-cut biological function.

β-MSH has been isolated from mammalian and non-mammalian pituitary. It is an 18-amino acid peptide in most species. Human β-MSH was originally reported to consist of 22 amino acids, but later studies have shown that β-MSH is not present in vivo and is an artefact produced during the process of extraction.[38] Circulating immunoreactive β-MSH in man is β-LPH or γ-LPH, detected by cross-reactivity with anti–β-MSH antisera.

β-LPH and β-Endorphin

β-LPH is a peptide originally isolated from sheep pituitary.[3] Sheep β-LPH consists of 91 amino acids and its C-terminal 31-amino acid sequence corresponds to β-endorphin. The N-terminal portion, 1-58 in sheep, was also isolated from pituitary gland and is called γ-LPH. This suggests that β-LPH is cleaved to give rise to β-endorphin and γ-LPH. The C-terminal 18 amino acids of γ-LPH (41-58 in sheep) correspond to the sequence of β-MSH. The primary structure of β-LPH has been elucidated in several species by either peptide sequencing or gene cloning. These studies have revealed that the N-terminal portion of β-LPH shows considerable species differences and that the portions of β-endorphin and β-MSH are well conserved.

β-endorphin is a 31-amino acid peptide in mammals and the N-terminal five amino acids are identical to the sequence of methionine enkephalin (met-enkephalin).[4] Several C-terminally truncated forms of β-endorphin have been isolated from the brain or pituitary. They are α-endorphin (β-endorphin 1-16), γ-endorphin (β-endorphin 1-17), and δ-endorphin (β-endorphin 1-27). N-terminally acetylated forms of β- and δ-endorphins have also been isolated from the pituitary.

β-LPH has weak lipolytic and opiate-like activities. Using synthetic peptides, it has been shown that the lipolytic activity of β-LPH resides in the 48-58 region, which corresponds to the sequence of β-MSH. On the other hand, opiate-like activity is present in the C-terminal portion, which coincides with β-endorphin.

β-endorphin has potent opiate-like analgesic and spasmolytic activity. It also affects feeding, sexual behavior, and learning and modulates neuroendocrine function when administered into the cerebral ventricle or the brain.[49] Analgesic activity resides in the N-terminal sequence of β-endorphin, which corresponds to met-enkephalin. However, there are differences in receptor selectivity between met-enkephalin and β-endorphin. Met-enkephalin binds preferentially to δ-receptors, whereas β-endorphin binds μ and δ receptors. Such differences in receptor selectivity cause some differences in biological activity between the two opioid peptides.

N-Terminal and Joining Peptide

A glycosylated peptide with 76 amino acids was isolated from the human pituitary.[15] This peptide has Trp at the N-terminus and the γ-MSH sequence in the C-terminal portion. N-glycosylation occurs at Asn[65] and O-glycosylation at Thr.[45] There are two disulfide bridges, linking Cys 2-8 and Cys 20-24. This peptide was reported to release aldosterone from isolated cells of human aldosterone-producing adenoma[50] and to potentiate the steroidogenic action of ACTH 1-24 on the rat adrenal cortex.[51]

N-terminal peptide can be further processed into a small peptide, γ-MSH, in the intermediate lobe or brain. Three γ-MSH preparations, γ$_1$-, γ$_2$-, and γ$_3$-MSH, were synthesized and shown to have weak steroidogenic, melanotropic, and behavioral actions.[52]

The joining peptide was also isolated from human pituitary,[53] and three different forms were identified. The proposal that the joining peptide has adrenal androgen-stimulating activity has not been supported by subsequent studies.

REGULATION OF SECRETION OF ACTH AND RELATED PEPTIDES

Regulation of secretion of ACTH and POMC-derived peptides has been studied extensively by measuring plasma levels of these peptides in humans and animals. In vitro studies using pituitary cells have been performed also. These studies have shown that secretion of ACTH and related peptides from the anterior pituitary is regulated by the CNS via humoral factors such as CRH and vasopressin. On the other hand, secretion of ACTH, α-MSH, and β-endorphin from the intermediate lobe of rats is regulated by nerves, and dopamine, norepinephrine, and GABA are involved as neurotransmitters.

Many studies have shown that all POMC-derived peptides, ACTH, β-LPH, β-endorphin, and N-terminal peptide (or γ-MSH–like immunoreactivity) are concomitantly secreted from the anterior pituitary,[52, 54, 55] although some studies reported discordant secretion. Such discordance in secretion of POMC-derived peptides may be partly explained by different processing of POMC under certain conditions, although exact reasons are still unknown. Parallel secretion of ACTH and related peptides observed in most instances suggests that POMC-derived peptides are packed in the same granules and secreted concomitantly by the process of exocytosis.

CRH, Vasopressin, and Other Hypothalamic Factors

CRH, which is produced in parvocellular neurons of the paraventricular nucleus and secreted from the median eminence into pituitary portal vessels, is a major regulator of ACTH secretion. It acts through CRH receptors on corticotrophs and stimulates adenylate cyclase activity. CRH not only stimulates ACTH secretion very rapidly but also enhances biosynthesis of ACTH. Chemistry and physiology of CRH are discussed in detail in Chapter 21.

Arginine vasopressin is another important factor that is produced in parvocellular neurons of the paraventricular nucleus and secreted into pituitary portal vessels from the median eminence. It acts through vasopressin receptors on corticotrophs and stimulates ACTH release, probably by activating phosphatidyl inositol turnover. Although CRH is of prime importance in regulating ACTH secretion, vasopressin synergistically acts with CRH to augment ACTH secretion. Other hypothalamic factors that are possibly involved in regulating ACTH secretion are epinephrine, oxytocin, and angiotensin II, but their contribution is, if any, minimal.[56]

The physiological significance of CRH was demonstrated by an increase of CRH levels in pituitary portal blood in response to stress, such as hemorrhagic shock.[56] Vasopressin and epinephrine contents were also increased. There was a positive correlation between the magnitude of hemorrhage and an increase of CRH. Furthermore, passive immunization with anti-CRH antisera blunted plasma ACTH response to ether stress to 15 per cent of the control value in rats.[57] This suggests that most of the ACTH response to stress is mediated by CRH. The remaining portion can be ascribed to other factors, especially vasopressin, although the completeness of immunoneutralization must be carefully evaluated. The contribution of CRH or other factors to ACTH secretion may vary under different conditions of stress. In insulin-induced hypoglycemia, participation of vasopressin and catecholamines is regarded as more important than in other stresses, although CRH is obligatory in these also.

Intravenous injection of ovine or human CRH causes an increase of plasma ACTH and cortisol levels,[58] although the former is a little more potent than the latter. Therefore, a CRH test can be used to evaluate the reserve of corticotrophs. If vasopressin is given along with CRH, exaggerated responses of plasma ACTH to CRH are observed, suggesting synergistic action in humans (Fig. 22–5). Although vasopressin alone has weak ACTH-secreting activity in normal subjects, it is a potent secretagogue for ACTH in most patients with an ACTH-secreting pituitary adenoma of Cushing's disease.

Neurotransmitters and ACTH Secretion

Putative neurotransmitters or neuromodulators influence ACTH secretion, probably by modulating the release of CRH or other hypothalamic factors. It has been shown that cholinergic agents, norepinephrine, serotonin, histamine, and GABA affect ACTH secretion. The role of norepinephrine in regulating ACTH secretion has been controversial, but recent studies using small amounts of norepinephrine have shown that norepinephrine plays a stimulatory role in CRH release acting through α$_1$-receptors.[59, 60] However, activation of α$_2$-receptors localized on presynaptic membrane rather inhibits firing rates of neurons. Cholinergic agents and serotonin stimulate CRH release and are possibly involved in circadian rhythm and stress responses of the hypothalamic-pituitary-adrenal (HPA) axis.[61] More recently, the involvement of histamine and the excitatory amino acid N-methyl-D-aspartate is suggested, especially in the acute activation of the HPA axis.[62, 63] On the other hand, GABA may act as a transmitter of inhibitory interneurons.

Peptidergic neurons may also be involved in ACTH secretion. Opioid peptides, such as β-endorphin, enkephalin, and its potent analogue, DAMME(D-ala²-mephe⁴met-enkephalin-(0)-ol), inhibit ACTH secretion in humans and animals, possibly acting either directly or indirectly in CRH neurons.[64, 65] The opioid antagonist naloxone increases plasma ACTH and cortisol levels, suggesting that endogenous opioid peptides have tonic inhibitory effects on ACTH secretion.

Several other neuropeptides were also reported to affect ACTH secretion. Angiotensin II, gastrin-releasing peptide, neuropeptide Y, and thyrotropin-releasing hormone stimulate ACTH secretion when administered centrally. Possible mediation of CRH in this stimulatory action is suggested. Cholecystokinin stimulates ACTH secretion even when administered by a systemic route, although CRH may be involved in cholecystokinin action. On the other hand, atrial natriuretic peptide, galanin, vasopressin, and substance P were reported to inhibit ACTH secretion when given centrally. The physiological significance of these peptides, their sites of action, and their interactions with classic transmitters in regulating CRH release remain to be elucidated.

Glucocorticoid Effects on ACTH Secretion

The negative feedback effect of glucocorticoids on ACTH secretion is a complex mechanism involving both the brain and the pituitary. Glucocorticoids act directly on corticotrophs but act also on the hypothalamus or other parts of the brain to alter CRH secretion. There are two types of feedback inhibition—rapid, occurring within minutes, and delayed, occurring after two or more hours. The inhibition between 30 minutes and two hours is sometimes called intermediate or slow-type feedback.[66] The delayed mechanism can be explained by the glucocorticoid inhibition of POMC gene expression in corticotrophs, as discussed above. There is an antagonistic interaction between CRH and glucocorticoids in regulation POMC gene expression. Glucocorticoids also decrease prepro-CRH mRNA levels in the hypothalamus acting directly on the hypothalamus or indirectly through other brain areas. The rapid feedback mechanism also exerts its effect on corticotrophs and the brain, probably through nongenomic mechanisms. The effect appears between 10 and 30 minutes when glucocorticoids are added to corticotrophs in vitro. The site of action of glucocorticoids in the brain is controversial. CRH occurs in neurons of the hypothalamus, but evidence suggests that the hippocampus or other brain areas may also be involved.[67] Implantation of glucocorticoids into the dorsal hippocampus was shown to inhibit adrenalectomy-induced ACTH secretion.

There are two types of glucocorticoid receptors, type I and type II. Relative steroid-binding affinity of type I receptors is corticosterone > aldosterone > dexamethasone, whereas that of type II receptors is dexamethasone > corticosterone > aldosterone. Type II receptors are expressed in the paraventricular nucleus, several other hypothalamic nuclei, the limbic system, and the brain stem, whereas type I receptors are confined to the limbic system and brain stem nuclei. Which type of receptor is more important in the negative feedback is still not completely elucidated. It may be different in discrete brain regions and the pituitary

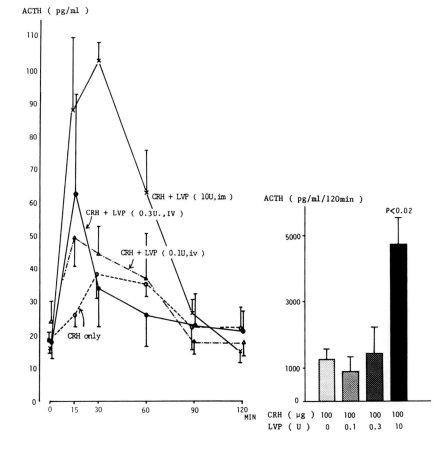

FIGURE 22–5. Plasma ACTH responses to 100 μg human CRH alone or in combination with 0.1 to 10 μU of lysine vasopressin (LVP) in normal subjects. CRH was given intravenously and LVP intramuscularly.

because the rank order of ACTH-inhibiting activity of corticosterone and dexamethasone varies under different experimental conditions.

Glucocorticoids inhibit ACTH secretion in humans. There seem to be at least two sites of the action, the pituitary and the brain. Glucocorticoid pretreatment inhibits CRH-induced ACTH secretion, suggesting that glucocorticoids exert rapid feedback effects on the pituitary. On the other hand, glucocorticoids lower plasma CRH levels, suggesting site(s) of action in the brain, although the plasma CRH level is not a sensitive and accurate index of hypothalamic CRH secretion. Exogenous administration of 2.5 mg or more of prednisolone causes suppression of ACTH secretion. Larger doses of prednisolone or other glucocorticoids (such as dexamethasone) are required to demonstrate significant suppression of ACTH secretion in Cushing's disease. Therefore, a low-dose dexamethasone suppression test has been used extensively in the diagnosis of Cushing's syndrome.

Long-term glucocorticoid administration or endogenous glucocorticoid hypersecretion induces profound inhibition of the HPA axis with marked adrenal atrophy. After steroid withdrawal or ablation of tumors, patients sustain low levels of plasma ACTH and cortisol. The duration of low hormone levels varies in relation to the duration and extent of glucocorticoid excess. In Cushing's syndrome, it may last 6 to 12 months. During the recovery period, ACTH secretion increases first, followed by an increase of cortisol secretion.[68]

Circadian Rhythmicity and Basal Secretion

Plasma levels of ACTH, other POMC-derived peptides, and cortisol show considerable parallel fluctuation during a day. In humans they start to rise during the later sleep period around 3 A.M., reach the peak around 8 A.M., and then decrease, remaining low in the late evening.[69] Shifts in the ACTH and cortisol secretory cycle are observed in night workers. In "free-run" experiments performed by eliminating all external stimuli, an endogenous circadian rhythm slightly longer than 24 hours is observed. Therefore, the sleep/wake cycle or social activity becomes a synchronizer of the intrinsic circadian rhythm. The circadian rhythm of ACTH secretion is well-established in humans from the age of three and persists throughout life. Even adrenalectomized patients or patients with primary adrenal failure show the circadian rhythm of plasma ACTH, but patients with Cushing's disease or Cushing's syndrome do not demonstrate significant periodicity. Some patients with lesions of the hypothalamus or the limbic system show disruption of the rhythm. Circadian rhythm of plasma ACTH and corticosterone in rats is opposite to that of man, and high levels are observed before the dark period. The suprachiasmatic nucleus is thought to be the major brain area involved in the circadian periodicity.

Frequent blood sampling with measurement of plasma ACTH and cortisol discloses a burst-like mode of hormone secretion. Such pulsatile secretion of ACTH is seen in humans and animals. Pulses of ACTH occur at average intervals of 15 to 20 minutes in rats, sheep, and rhesus monkey. In humans previous reports gave discordant values owing to different sampling paradigms, but recent studies by

Veldhuis et al.[70] disclosed a mean interburst interval of 39 minutes and a half-duration of bursts of 19 minutes. The amplitude modulation, but not the frequency of bursts, gives rise to the circadian changes of the hormones. Plasma β-endorphin and cortisol levels exhibit a synchrony with ACTH.

The origin of pulses is still not completely understood. A pulse generator in the hypothalamus seems to regulate pulsatile secretion of CRH. However, neutralization of endogenous CRH by anti-CRH antisera in rats does not abolish the high-frequency pulses, although it inhibits the amplitude of the pulses.[71] This suggests the presence of periodicity independent of CRH, either of hypothalamic or pituitary origin. Whether "basal" secretion of ACTH occurs besides bursts is not completely clear. Evidence suggests, however, that ACTH is secreted only by a burst-like mode without constant basal secretion.[70]

Stress

Both physical and psychological stresses, such as pain, hemorrhage, hypoglycemia, ether anesthesia, immobilization, forced exercise, noise, and fear induce rapid release of ACTH, overriding feedback and circadian control.[56] The pathway by which CRH neurons are finally activated to release CRH varies by the type of stress, but the final common pathway seems to be the median eminence, where CRH, vasopressin, and epinephrine are secreted. Among the hormones secreted into pituitary portal vessels, CRH plays a predominant role in hemorrhagic stress.[56] In hypoglycemia, however, vasopressin or epinephrine seems more important than in hemorrhage, suggesting some differences in hypothalamic hormones under different stress conditions.

The magnitude of plasma ACTH responses to stress varies at different times of the day in both humans and rats. This may not be due to varied negative feedback effect of plasma glucocorticoid levels but possibly to the effect of circadian rhythmicity.

Effect of Cytokines

Microbial infection or tissue damage is known to activate the HPA axis, and bacterial pyrogen can be used to test the integrity of this axis. Besedovsky et al.[72] first reported that systemic administration of IL-1 into mice caused a prompt rise of plasma ACTH, reaching the peak within 30 minutes. Thereafter, IL-1α, IL-1β, IL-2, IL-6, and tumor necrosis factor α were found to increase plasma ACTH, although IL-2 elicited a sluggish increase.[73] The action of cytokines (except for IL-2) is thought to be mediated by CRH because anti-CRH antisera abolish plasma ACTH responses and because CRH concentrations in pituitary portal blood increase in response to cytokines. How cytokines in circulating blood reach the brain to stimulate CRH release is still unknown. They may act on the organum vasculosum of the lamina terminalis,[74] where the blood-brain barrier is weak, or they may act directly on CRH neurons at the median eminence or other sites of the hypothalamus. Cytokines also increase hypothalamic prepro-CRH mRNA levels. Cytokines may act directly on the pituitary cortico-

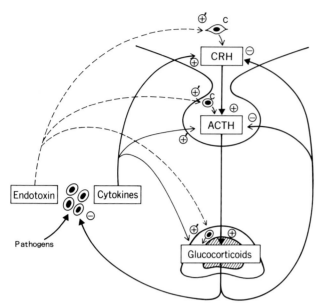

FIGURE 22–6. Interactions between the immune and neuroendocrine system. Cytokines produced in inflammatory foci act on the hypothalamic-pituitary-adrenal (HPA) axis at three different levels (solid line). Bacterial lipopolysaccharides act on the brain pituitary and adrenal to stimulate local production of cytokines (dashed line), which may also act to activate the HPA axis. Glucocorticoids thus produced inhibit the pituitary-adrenal axis through a long-loop feedback mechanism and possibly suppress cytokine production in inflammatory foci. (From Imura H, Fukata J, Mori T: Cytokines and endocrine function: An interaction between the immune and neuroendocrine systems. Clin Endocrinol 35:107–115, 1991.)

trophs, although the action is weak and slow. Direct stimulating effect of cytokines on the adrenal cortex is also seen but requires a latent period of more than 12 hours. Thus, rapid effects of cytokines are mediated by CRH release, but slow effects may be exerted at levels of the hypothalamus, pituitary, and adrenal.

More recently, lipopolysaccharide has been reported to produce IL-1α, IL-1β, tumor necrosis factor α, and IL-6 in the hypothalamus, pituitary, and adrenal, probably by enhancing the gene expression, because a latent period of more than one hour is required. Although the role of cytokines produced locally is not clear, they may act as local regulators in a way similar to that of cytokines given by a systemic route. Thus, the effect of inflammation on the HPA axis is complex and differs according to the duration of inflammation. Glucocorticoids produced by the activation of this axis possibly inhibit cytokine production in inflammatory foci, because the addition of glucocorticoids inhibits the production of cytokines by macrophages and lymphocytes in vitro. Thus, a negative feedback mechanism overriding the immune and endocrine systems may operate during inflammation (Fig. 22–6).

REFERENCES

1. Bell PH: Purification and structure of β-corticotropin. J Am Chem Soc 76:5565–5567, 1954.
2. Lerner AB, Lee TH: Isolation of homogenous melanocyte stimulating hormone from hog pituitaries. J Am Chem Soc 77:1066–1077, 1955.
3. Li CH: Lipotropin, a new active peptide from pituitary glands. Nature 201:924, 1964.
4. Li CH, Chung D, Doneen BA: Isolation, characterisation and opiate

activity of β-endorphin from human pituitary glands. Biochem Biophys Res Commun 72:1542–1547, 1976.
5. Guillemin R, Ling N, Lazarus L, et al: The endorphins, novel peptides of brain and hypophysial origin, with opiate-like activity: Biochemical and biological studies. Ann NY Acad Sci 297:131–157, 1977.
6. Eipper BA, Mains RE: Analysis of the common precursor to corticotropin and endorphin. J Biol Chem 253:5732–5744, 1978.
7. Vale W, Spiess J, Rivier C, Rivier J: Characterisation of a 41-residue ovine hypothalamic peptide that stimulates secretion of corticotropin and β-endorphin. Science 213:1394–1397, 1981.
8. Yalow RS, Berson SA: Size heterogeneity of immunoreactive human ACTH in plasma and in extracts of pituitary gland and ACTH-producing thymoma. Biochem Biophys Res Commun 43:439–445, 1971.
9. Eipper BA, Mains RE: High molecular weight forms of adrenocorticotropin in the mouse pituitary and in a mouse pituitary tumor cell line. Biochemistry 14:3836–3844, 1975.
10. Hirata Y, Yamamoto H, Matsukura S, Imura H: In vitro release and biosynthesis of tumor ACTH in ectopic ACTH producing tumors. J Clin Endocrinol Metab 41:106–114, 1975.
11. Nakanishi S, Taii S, Hirata Y, et al: A large product of cell free translation of messenger RNA coding for corticotropin. Proc Natl Acad Sci USA 73:4319–4323, 1976.
12. Nakanishi S, Inoue A, Taii S, Numa S: Cell-free translation product containing corticotropin and β-endorphin encoded by messenger RNA from anterior lobe and intermediate lobe of bovine pituitary. FEBS Lett 84:105–109, 1977.
13. Roberts JL, Herbert E: Characterisation of a common precursor to corticotropin and β-endorphin: Cell-free synthesis of the precursor and identification of corticotropin peptides in the molecule. Proc Natl Acad Sci USA 74:4826–4830, 1977.
14. Nakanishi S, Inoue A, Kita T, et al: Nucleotide sequence of cloned cDNA for bovine corticotropin-β-lipotropin precursor. Nature 278:423–427, 1979.
15. Seidah NG, Chretien M: Complete amino acid sequence of a human pituitary glycopeptide: An important maturation product of proopiomelanocortin. Proc Natl Acad Sci USA 78:4236–4240, 1981.
16. Numa S, Imura H: ACTH and related peptides: Gene structure and biosynthesis. In Imura H (ed): The Pituitary Gland. New York, Raven Press, 1985, pp 83–102.
17. Takahashi H, Teranishi Y, Nakanishi S, Numa S: Isolation and structural organisation of the human corticotropin-beta-lipotropin precursor gene. FEBS Lett 135:97–110, 1981.
18. Lundblad JR, Roberts JL: Regulation of proopiomelanocortin gene expression in pituitary. Endocr Rev 9:135–158, 1988.
19. Jingami H, Nakanishi S, Imura H, Numa S: Tissue distribution of messenger RNAs coding for opioid peptide precursors and related RNA. Eur J Biochem 142:441–447, 1984.
20. Imura H, Matsukura S, Nakai Y, et al: Clinical and biochemical features of ectopic hormone-producing tumors: Possible mechanism of hormone production. In Bresciani F, King RJB, Lippman ME, et al (eds): Progress in Cancer Research and Therapy. New York, Raven Press, 1984, pp 569–583.
21. de Bold CR, Menefee JK, Nicholson WE, Orth DN: Proopiomelanocortin gene is expressed in many normal human tissues and in tumors not associated with ectopic adrenocorticotropin syndrome. Mol Endocrinol 2:862–870, 1988.
22. Jeannotte L, Burbach JPH, Drouin J: Unusual POMC ribonucleic acids in extrapituitary tissues: Intronless transcripts in testes and long poly A tails in hypothalamus. Mol Endocrinol 1:749–757, 1987.
23. Usui T, Nakai Y, Tsukada T, et al: Expression of the human proopiomelanocortin gene introduced into a rat glial cell line. J Mol Endocrinol 4:169–175, 1990.
24. Therrien M, Drouin J: Pituitary pro-opiomelanocortin gene expression requires synergistic interactions of several regulatory elements. Mol Cell Biol 11:3492–3503, 1991.
25. Tremblay Y, Tretjakoff I, Peterson A, et al: Pituitary-specific expression and glucocorticoid regulation of a pro-opiomelanocortin (POMC) fusion gene in transgenic mice. Proc Natl Acad Sci USA 85:8890–8894, 1988.
26. Roberts JL, Lundblad JR, Eberwine JH, et al: Hormonal regulation of POMC gene expression in pituitary. Ann NY Acad Sci 512:275–285, 1987.
27. Usui T, Nakai Y, Tsukada T, et al: Cyclic AMP–responsive region of the human proopiomelanocortin (POMC) gene. Mol Cell Endocrinol 62:141–146, 1989.
28. Hollt V, Haarmann I, Seizinger BR, Herz A: Chronic haloperidol treatment increases the level of in vitro translatable messenger ribonucleic acid coding for the β-endorphin/adrenocorticotropin precur-

sor proopiomelanocortin in the pars intermedia of the rat pituitary. Endocrinology 110:1885–1891, 1982.

29. Drouin J, Sun YL, Nemer M: Regulatory elements of the proopiomelanocortin gene. Pituitary specificity and glucocorticoid repression. TEM 2:219–225, 1990.

30. Gagner J-P, Drouin J: Opposite regulation of pro-opiomelanocortin gene transcription by glucocorticoids and CRH. Mol Cell Endocrinol 40:25–32, 1985.

31. Fukata J, Usui T, Naitoh Y, et al: Effects of recombinant human interleukin-1α, -1β, 2 and 6 on ACTH synthesis and release in the mouse pituitary tumor cell line AtT-20. J Endocrinol 122:33–39, 1989.

32. Bilezikjian LM, Blount AL, Campen CA, et al: Activin A inhibits proopiomelanocortin messenger RNA and adrenocorticotropin secretion of AtT 20 cells. Mol Endocrinol 5:1389–1395, 1991.

33. Mains RE, Eipper BA: The tissue-specific processing of proACTH/endorphin. TEM 1:388–394, 1990.

34. Bradbury AF, Finnie MDA, Smyth DG: Mechanisms of C-terminal amide formation by pituitary enzymes. Nature 298:686–688, 1982.

35. Bennett HPJ, Bateman A, Solomon S: Examination of the heterogeneity of the joining peptide and the amino-terminal fragment of β-lipotropin of bovine POMC. In Proceedings of the 71st Annual Meeting of the Endocrine Society, Seattle, WA, 1989, p 261 (Abstract 955).

36. Eipper BA, Mains RE: Structure and biosynthesis of proadrenocorticotropin/endorphin and related peptides. Endocr Rev 1:1–27, 1980.

37. Imura H, Nakai Y, Nakao Y, et al: Biosynthesis and distribution of opioid peptides. J Endocrinol Invest 6:139–149, 1983.

38. Scott AP, Lowry PJ: Adrenocorticotrophic and melanocyte-stimulating peptides in the human pituitary. Biochem J 139:593–602, 1974.

39. Smith AI, Funder JW: Proopiomelanocortin processing in the pituitary, central nervous system and peripheral tissues. Endocr Rev 9:159–179, 1988.

40. Imura H, Nakai Y, Nakao K, et al: Adrenocorticotropic hormone and related peptides in human tissue. In Block PM et al (eds): Secretory Tumors of the Pituitary Gland. New York, Raven Press, 1984, pp 227–243.

41. McLouglin L, Rees LH: The relevance of pro-opiomelanocortin (POMC) processing pattern in Cushing's syndrome. In Lüdecke DK, Chrousos GP, Tolis G (eds): ACTH, Cushing's Syndrome and Other Hypercortisolemic States. New York, Raven Press, 1990, pp 115–121.

42. Lambers SW, de Lange SA, Stefanko SZ: Adrenocortioctropin-secreting pituitary adenomas originate from the anterior or the intermediate lobe in Cushing's disease: Differences in the regulation of hormone secretion. J Clin Endorcinol Metab 54:286–291, 1982.

43. Tanaka I, Nakai Y, Nakao K, et al: γ-Melanotropin-like immunoreactivity in bovine and human pituitaries, ACTH-producing pituitary adenoma and ectopic ATCH-producing tumors. Evidence for an abnormality in glycosylation in ectopic ACTH-producing tumours. Clin Endocrinol 15:353–361, 1981.

44. Noel G, Keutmann HT, Mains RE: Investigation of the structural requirements for peptide precursor processing in AtT 20 cells using site-directed mutagenesis of proadrenocorticotropin/endorphin. Mol Endocrinol 5:404–413, 1991.

45. Mains RE, Dickerson IM, May V, et al: Cellular and molecular aspects of peptide hormone biosynthesis. Frontiers Neuroendocrinol 11:52–89, 1990.

46. Thomas L, Leduc R, Thorne BA, et al: Kex 2-like endopeptidase PC2 and PC3 accurately cleave a model prohormone in mammalian cells: Evidence for a common core of neuroendocrine processing enzymes. Proc Natl Acad Sci USA 88:5297–5301, 1991.

47. Day R, Schater MK-H, Watson SJ, et al: Distribution and regulation of the prohormone convertase PC1 and PC2 in rat pituitary. Mol Endocrinol 6:485–497, 1992.

48. Hayashi H, Imai K, Imai K: Characterization of chicken ACTH and α-MSH: the primary sequence of chicken ACTH is more similar to xenopus ACTH than to other avian ACTH. Gen Comp Endocrinol 82:434–443, 1991.

49. Loh HH, Ross DH (eds): Neurochemical Mechanisms of Opiates and Endorphins. New York, Raven Press, 1979, pp 1–563.

50. Seidah NG, Rochemont J, Hamelin J, et al: Primary structure of the major human pituitary pro-opiomelanocortin NH₂-terminal glycopeptide: Evidence for an aldosterone-stimulating activity. J Biol Chem 256:7977–7984, 1981.

51. Pedersen RC, Brownie AC, Ling NC: Pro-adrenocorticotropin/endorphin-derived peptides: Coordinate action on adrenal steroidogenesis. Science 208:1044–1046, 1980.

52. Imura H: ACTH, β-endorphin and related peptides. In Cumming IA, Funder JW, Mendelsohn FAO (eds): Endocrinology. Canberra, Australian Academy of Science, 1980, pp 58–65.

53. Seidah NG, Rochemont J, Hamelin J, et al: The missing fragment of the pro-sequence of human pro-opiomelanocortin: Sequence and evidence for C-terminal amidation. Biochem Biophys Res Commun 102:710–716, 1981.

54. Chan JS, Seidah NH, Chrétien M: Measurement of N-terminal (1-76) of human proopiomelanocortin in human plasma: Correlation with adrenocorticotropin. J Clin Endocrinol Metab 56:791–796, 1983.

55. Jefficoate WJ, Rees LH, Lowry PJ, Besser GM: A specific radioimmunoassay for human β-lipotrophin. J Clin Endocrinol Metab 47:160–167, 1978.

56. Plotzky PM: Hypophysiotropic regulation of stress-induced ACTH secretion. Adv Exp Med Biol 245:65–81, 1988.

57. Rivier C, Rivier J, Vale W: Inhibition of adrenocorticotropin secretion in the rat by immunoneutralization of corticotropin-releasing factor. Science 218:377–379, 1982.

58. Orth DN: Corticotropin-releasing hormone in humans. Endocr Rev 13:164–191, 1992.

59. Al-Damluji S: Adrenergic mechanisms in the control of corticotropin. J Endocinol 119:5–14, 1988.

60. Plotzky PM, Cunningham ET Jr, Widmaier EP: Catecholaminergic modulation of corticotropin-releasing factor and ACTH secretion. Endocr Rev 10:437–458, 1989.

61. Krieger DT, Krieger HP: Chemical stimulation of the brain: Effect of adrenal corticoid release. Am J Physiol 218:1632–1641, 1970.

62. Knigge U, Bach FW, Matzen S, et al: Effect of histamine on the secretion of proopiomelanocortin derived peptides in the rats. Acta Endocrinol 119:312–319, 1988.

63. Farah JM Jr, Rao TS, Mick SJ, et al: N-methyl-D-aspartate treatment increases circulating adrenocorticotropin and luteinizing hormone in the rat. Endocrinology 128:1875–1880, 1991.

64. Stubbs WA, Delitala G, Besser GM, et al: Hormonal and metabolic responses to an enkephalin analogue in normal man. Lancet 2:1225–1227, 1978.

65. Buckingham JC, Cooper TA: Influence of opioid substances on hypothalamo-pituitary-adrenocortical activity in the rat. In Delitala G, Motta M, Serio M (eds): Opioid Modulation of Endocrine Function. New York, Raven Press, 1984, pp 81–87.

66. Keller-Wood ME, Dallman MF: Corticosteroid inhibition of ACTH secretion. Endocr Rev 5:1–24, 1984.

67. Jacobson L, Sapolsky R: The role of the hippocampus in feedback regulation of the hypothalamic-pituitary-adrenocortical axis. Endocr Rev 12:118–134, 1991.

68. Graber AL, Ney RL, Nicholson WE, et al: Natural history of pituitary-adrenal recovery following long-term suppression with corticosteroids. J Clin Endocrinol Metab 25:11–16, 1965.

69. Krieger DT: Regulation of circadian periodicity of plasma ACTH levels. In Krieger DT, Ganong WF (eds): ACTH and Related Peptides: Structure, Regulation and Action. New York, New York Academy of Science, 1977, pp 561–567.

70. Veldhuis JD, Iranmanesh A, Johnson ML, Lizarralde G: Amplitude, but not frequency, modulation of adrenocorticotropin secretory bursts gives rise to the nyctohemeral rhythm of the corticotropic axis in man. J Clin Endocrinol Metab 71:451–463, 1990.

71. Carnes M, Lent SJ, Goodman B, et al: Effects of immunoneutralization of corticotropin-releasing hormone on ultradian rhythm of plasma adrenocorticotropin. Endocrinology 126:1904–1913, 1990.

72. Besedovsky H, Ray D, Sorkin A, Dinarello CA: Immunoregulatory feedback between interleukin 1 and glucocorticoid hormones. Science 233:651–654, 1986.

73. Imura H, Fukata J, Mori T: Cytokines and endocrine function: An interaction between the immune and neuroendocrine systems. Clin Endocrinol 35:107–115, 1991.

74. Katsuura G, Arimura A, Koves K, Gottschall PE: Involvement of organum vasculosum of lamina terminalis and preoptic area in interleukin 1β-induced ACTH release. Am J Physiol 258:E163–E171, 1990.

23

Prolactin: Basic Physiology

NANCY E. COOKE

HISTORICAL PERSPECTIVE

Among the hormones of the anterior pituitary, prolactin (PRL), with more than 85 functions documented among various vertebrate species, is by far the most versatile.[1] PRL was first discovered in 1928, based upon its ability to cause lactation in pseudopregnant rabbits.[2] Anterior pituitary extracts were subsequently shown to stimulate the pigeon crop sac to form "crop milk," a secretion used by brooding pigeons to feed their young.[3] This biological phenomenon became the classic assay for PRL bioactivity.[4] The hormone was first purified from sheep pituitaries and named prolactin in 1932,[5] but it was not until 1971 that human PRL was purified and verified to be distinct from human growth hormone (GH).[6, 7] In the early 1980's the cDNA and gene for human PRL were cloned and sequenced, and the PRL gene was defined as a member of a multigene family that includes the GH and chorionic somatomammotropin (CS) genes.[8, 9] The suckling-induced release of PRL, a universal response in mammals, has emerged as a classic experimental model for the study of neuroendocrine interactions.[10] In the late 1980's, the cloning and characterization of Pit-1 as a tissue-specific transactivator of PRL gene transcription enhanced understanding of pituitary cell development and PRL gene regulation.[11] The cloning of several forms of the PRL receptor within the past few years has led to the recognition that this receptor is a member of a large family of hematopoietic cytokine receptors. The diversity of the PRL receptor isoforms and the structural overlap with the receptors in this family may partially explain PRL's bewildering array of biological actions.[12] PRL's role in immunoregulation has been confirmed in the last few years[13] and should prove to be an important area for future research.

GENOMIC ORGANIZATION AND HETEROGENEITY

The PRL-GH Gene Family

The concept that PRL, GH, and CS are evolutionarily related polypeptide hormone genes was first proposed based upon comparison of their amino acid sequences.[14] The hypothesis was strengthened when it was found that GH and PRL shared an even higher degree of nucleotide than amino acid sequence identity[15] and that both genes contained five exons with four introns interrupting homologous positions in the coding sequence.[9] Despite their evolutionary similarity, the GH and PRL genes have been dispersed to chromosomes 17 and 6, respectively.[16] Recent studies on the PRL/GH gene family in fish have provided new information on the family's evolution. The rainbow trout GH gene contains an additional intron in exon 5, and the coding segments of the gene lack the internally homologous exonic regions noted in the rat and human gene sequences.[17] This has forced a re-evaluation of the previous hypothesis that the ancestral progenitor of this gene family arose by multiple duplications of a small primordial subexonic gene to generate five exons. An additional member of the PRL/GH gene family has recently been detected in the genome of certain fish. Because the sequence of this protein is 24 per cent identical to both fish GH and PRL, it was named somatolactin. Although the five-exon structure is maintained, the somatolactin gene, at 16 kilobases (kb) in length, is now the largest gene in the family (Fig. 23–1). These findings have led to the hypothesis that somatolactin is the direct descendant of the ancestral gene common to both GH and PRL.[18] The existence of a somatolactin gene in mammals has not been reported.

Multiple PRL-Related Genes

In humans the GH gene is a member of a gene cluster containing five closely related genes: pituitary GH itself, and four placentally expressed genes—GH-variant and CS-A, -B, and -L.[19] At present it appears that the more distantly related human PRL gene is encoded as a single gene in the human genome. This is in clear contrast to the situation in rats, mice, hamsters, and cattle in which a family of structurally related, PRL-like genes are found in the genome and are expressed in the placenta during gestation. In further contrast to humans, there appears to be only a single GH gene in these species. There are at least eight or nine rodent PRL-related genes. These genes can be divided into two classes: those that bind to PRL receptors, referred to as lactogens, and those that do not, the nonlactogens.[20] The receptors for the latter group have not yet been identified. Among the rat lactogens are placental lactogen-I (PL-I) and PL-II, which were first detected by a lactogen radioreceptor assay from midgestation or late placental extracts, respectively. A developmental switch occurs within a single placental cell type between the expression of these two genes, PL-I declining as PL-II expression begins. The level of PL-II in maternal serum correlates with the number of conceptuses, is stimulated by the fetus, and is inhibited

by the pituitary, probably by GH.[20] PL-I and PL-II have been cloned.[20] Some of their characteristics are summarized in Table 23–1. Recently a third placental lactogen, PL-I variant (PL-Iv), was detected by cross-reaction with anti-PL-I antibodies and by cross-hybridization to a PL-I cDNA.[21]

PRL-like protein A (PLP-A) and PLP-B were discovered during the cloning of rat PL-II, and each was then independently characterized.[22, 23] Both molecules are present in maternal circulation at high levels.[24] PLP-C was discovered as a contaminant of PLP-A.[25] PLP-A and possibly PLP-B and PLP-C do not bind to the PRL receptor and thus are not lactogens. The rat decidua has long been recognized to generate a factor, decidual luteotropin (LTH), that prolongs corpus luteum function. In contrast to the PLP's, LTH binds to lactogen receptors and is recognized by antiserum to PRL.[26] The structure of LTH, anticipated to be a member of the PRL family, is not yet known. Several characteristics of LTH have suggested that it may be PLP-B[27] or, more likely, the newly characterized decidual PRL-related protein (dPRP) (Table 23–1).[28] Along with prolactin, PL-I, PL-Iv, PL-II, PLP-A, PLP-B, PLP-C, and dPRP have been localized to chromosome 17 in the rat. PLP-A, PLP-B, PLP-C, and PL-Iv have not been detected in the mouse and may be unique to the rat.[20]

Each of the rat PRP's is expressed at a specific time during pregnancy, suggesting that each is required for specific functions (Fig. 23–2). Initially, maternal pituitary PRL secretion is activated by the copulatory stimulus, initiating the nocturnal and diurnal PRL surges. By day six of gestation, PL-I, decidual LTH, and PLP-B are secreted. Pituitary PRL production declines by about day 11, at which time it is replaced by placental PL-II, PLP-A, PLP-B, PLP-C, and PL-Iv secretion. The pattern of dPRP is not yet known. Fetal pituitary PRL secretion is detectable by day 17, and maternal pituitary PRL secretion returns just before partu-

CHUM SALMON SOMATOLACTIN

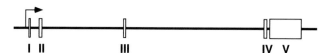

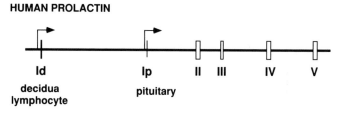

FIGURE 23–1. **Structures of the related chum salmon somatolactin, human PRL, and hGH genes.** Exons are indicated by rectangles and are numbered; introns and flanking regions are indicated by the line. The fifth exon of somatolactin includes a long 3′-nontranslated region. All three genes are drawn approximately to the scale in kilobase pairs (kb) shown at the bottom of the figure. Note that the human PRL gene contains a promoter and exon 1 utilized in decidua and lymphocytes (ld) and a different promoter and exon 1 utilized in the pituitary (lp). The arrowheads indicate location of promoters and direction of transcription. The somatolactin gene with about 24 per cent identity to fish GH and PRL genes may be the common ancestor to both.

HUMAN GROWTH HORMONE

TABLE 23–1. THE PROLACTIN FAMILY IN RATS AND MICE

| | Functional Characteristics | | | | Structural Characteristics | | |
Hormone	Similarity to Prolactin*	MW (kDa)	#Cys	Glycoprotein	Prolactin Receptor Binding	Homologue in Mouse	Homologue in Rat
Prolactin	100%	25	6	No	Yes	Yes	Yes
Placental lactogen-I	38%	30;36–40	8	Yes	Yes	Yes	Yes
Placental lactogen-II	47%	25	4	No	Yes	Yes	Yes
PRL-like protein-A	39%	29;33	5	Yes	No	No	Yes
PRL-like protein-B	39%	30	4	Yes	?	No	Yes
PRL-like protein-C	34%	25;29	7	Yes	?	No	Yes
Placental lactogen-Iv	43%	29;33	5	Yes	Weak	No	Yes
Luteotropin	?	29	?	Yes	Yes	?	Yes
Decidual PRL-related protein	37%	29	6	Yes	?	?	Yes
Proliferin 1/proliferin 2†	37%	22	6	Yes	No	Yes	No
PRL-related protein (proliferin-related)	39%	38–45	5	Yes	No	Yes	No

*Includes conservative amino acid substitutions.

†Proliferin 1 and 2 differ by four amino acids.

Adapted from Soares MJ, Faria TN, Roby KF, Deb S: Pregnancy and the prolactin family of hormones: Coordination of anterior pituitary, uterine, and placental expression. Endocr Rev 12:402–423, 1991; © The Endocrine Society.

rition.[20] Proposed roles for the gestational PRL-related molecules include preparation of the mammary gland for lactation, nutrient transport to the fetus, growth and differentiation of the endometrium, interactions with the immune system, placental ion/water transfer, and fetal growth and development.[20] They may also participate in the maintenance of the corpus luteum, perhaps via inhibition of ovarian proteases[29] and regulation of aromatase.[30] These cells contact only the maternal blood supply and hence are suited for secretion into this vascular bed. Only PL-II is detected in the giant cells of the placental labyrinth and is in direct contact with the fetal blood supply, suggesting that only PL-II may play a direct role in the rat fetus.

The mouse genome contains PL-I and PL-II genes, and in addition there may be up to four additional PLP's, termed proliferins (PLF's). These are apparently found only in the mouse.[31] Three of these PLF's, PLF-1, PLF-2, and PRP, have been characterized (Table 23–1). PLF-1 was initially detected as a cell-cyle immediate early gene in synchronized cultured fibroblasts.[32] Subsequently PLF-2 was found to be a glycoprotein secreted from the midgestation mouse placenta.[33] PLF-2 is synthesized in trophoblastic giant cells of the placenta and is secreted into the serum and amniotic fluid of pregnant mice with levels reflecting the number of conceptuses.[34] Mouse PRP is secreted by the basal zone of the mouse placenta, and the protein is detectable in maternal serum throughout the last half of gestation.[35] In searching for a PLF receptor, it was unexpectedly found that PLF binds to the mannose 6-phosphate receptor present in fetal liver and maternal placental membranes but was inactive in binding to PRL or GH receptors. The mannose 6-phosphate receptor is involved in targeting enzymes to lysosomes. Therefore, one or more of the PLF's may be a lysosomal protein or may be degraded or processed in the lysosome.[36] It was noted that PLF was synthesized in multipotential 10T1/2 cells but not in differentiated myoblasts and that transfection of PLF-1 (but not PLF-2, the predominant form) into myoblasts results in cells that are no longer myogenic. Of note, addition of purified PLF-1 protein to the media surrounding the cells does not similarly repress myogenesis. These data suggest that the action of PLF-1 is not mediated by a cell surface receptor but via an intracellular route.[37] The concept of an intracellular action for PRL has also been reported in lymphocyte proliferation,[13] but a clear understanding of the mechanism has yet to emerge (see Immune Regulation).

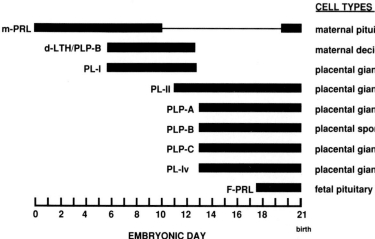

CELL TYPES

m-PRL — maternal pituitary lactotrope
d-LTH/PLP-B — maternal decidual cell
PL-I — placental giant cell
PL-II — placental giant cell
PLP-A — placental giant cell/spongiotrophoblast
PLP-B — placental spongiotrophoblast
PLP-C — placental giant cell/spongiotrophoblast
PL-Iv — placental giant cell/spongiotrophoblast
F-PRL — fetal pituitary lactotrope

EMBRYONIC DAY
0 2 4 6 8 10 12 14 16 18 21
birth

FIGURE 23–2. **The developmental stage- and cell-specific expression of the rat PRL gene family.** Abbreviations are as follows: mPRL, maternal pituitary PRL; d-LTH, decidual luteotropin; F-PRL, fetal pituitary PRL. The scale refers to the duration of gestation in the rat. (Adapted from Soares MJ, Faria TN, Roby KF, Deb S: Pregnancy and the prolactin family of hormones: Coordination of anterior pituitary, uterine, and placental expression. Endocr Rev 12:402–423, 1991; © The Endocrine Society.)

Microheterogeneity of PRL Isoforms

PRL and most of the PRP's have been detected in more than one form. This structural diversity is generated by both post-transcriptional and post-translational modifications. Many of the PRL's are glycosylated (Table 23–1). Human pituitary PRL (Fig. 23–3) also has been detected in a diversity of protein isoforms, including a glycosylated hormone. It was recently discovered that the rat PRL gene can be alternatively spliced so that exon 4 is excluded. Such an alternatively spliced product would maintain an open reading frame and predicts a protein with a molecular weight of 15.9 kDa instead of the usual 23 kDa. This protein has not yet been identified.[38] In humans there are two alternatively used promoters and first exons in the PRL gene, both spliced to the single exon 2. The more 5' or upstream promoter and exon 1 are active and expressed in the maternal decidua and lymphocytes, whereas the more 3' promoter is active in the anterior pituitary (see Fig. 23–1). Because exon 1 in both cases encodes only the 5' non-translated region, this alternative processing of the PRL transcript does not result in any structural changes in the protein (see Decidual Prolactin and Immune Regulation).[39]

Human PRL consists of 199 amino acid residues (Fig. 23–3) and migrates on reducing gels at an apparent molecular size of 23 kDa. A cleaved, two-chain form of pituitary PRL has been detected in serum and pituitary preparations of rodents and man. This isohormone is the product of specific enzymatic cleavage in the large disulfide loop by an acid protease, resulting in 8- and 16-kDa chains held together with a single disulfide bond.[40] Data on the 16-kDa cleaved form of PRL must be interpreted with care, because the 16-kDa protein can be generated as an in vitro artefact in acidic conditions.[41] Despite this, evidence suggests that 16-kDa PRL is a physiologically significant isoform. Cleaved PRL appears to be generated by contact with its target tissues, specifically prostate, mammary gland, and liver. Because cleavage is maximal at pH 3.4 to 5.5, the pH range within coated vesicles and lysosomes, it has been postulated that the cleaved products might be produced secondary to normal intracellular processing.[42] Mammary glands from lactating rats produce more cleaved PRL than kidney or liver from the same rats. The ability of the mammary gland to produce cleaved PRL in different physiological states is as follows: pregnant > cycling > lactating, suggesting that the generation of cleaved forms of PRL has physiological specificity.[43] It appears that a distinct isoreceptor exists in some tissues for 16-kDa PRL. Although 16-kDa PRL binds to the same liver PRL receptors to which 23-kDa PRL binds, it is only 6.5 per cent as active as the full-length molecule. In contrast, 16-kDa PRL is 30 times more potent than intact hormone in binding to kidney microsomal membranes, the organ with highest affinity for the 16-kDa form (Fig. 23–4). The receptors for the 16-kDa form are present in brain and liver as well. Although 16-kDa PRL has biological effects via the standard PRL receptor as a mitogen on mammary epithelium, in the pigeon crop sac, in the Nb2 bioassay, and in casein biosynthesis (see Methods of Detection),[42] its activities are always lower than those of intact PRL. Therefore it was a significant finding that reduced 16-kDa PRL, both recombinant and enzymatically cleaved, but not intact PRL, inhibited fibroblast growth factor-stimulated growth of cultured bovine capillary endothelial cells in a dose-dependent fashion through the specific 16-kDa receptor.[44] These data resulted in the hypothesis that the 16-kDa form is an angiolytic factor of potential therapeutic significance in the treatment of tumor growth. Therefore the 16-kDa receptor appears to transduce a growth-inhibitory effect following 16-kDa binding, whereas the standard PRL receptor transmits a growth-stimulating effect. The 16-kDa PRL has reduced detectability in some radioimmunoassays (RIA's) and may account for previous reports of high bioassay:RIA ratios of PRL in some sera, tissues, and incubation media.

A glycosylated form of PRL, migrating at 25 kDa, has been isolated from human, ovine, porcine, turkey, and mouse pituitaries.[45] In humans, the asparagine at residue 31 (Fig. 23–3) contains the carbohydrate moiety. Two distinct glycoslyated forms of this modified human PRL have been identified.[46] Glycosylated PRL represents 13 to 25 per cent of PRL in the human pituitary gland, circulates in the sera of men and women, and has been detected in amniotic fluid. In receptor binding assays, glycosylated ovine PRL has 20 per cent of the potency of the nonglycosylated form, only 24 per cent activity in the Nb2 bioassay, and 80

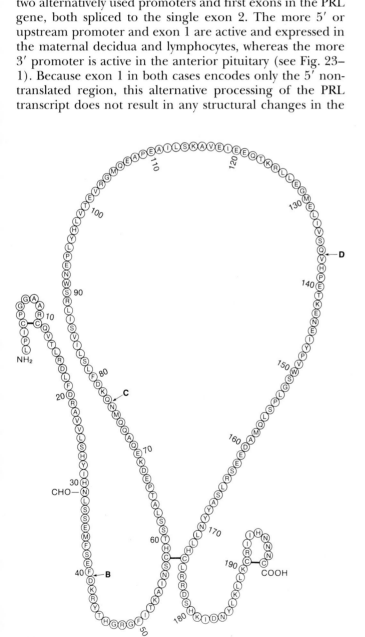

FIGURE 23–3. The human PRL molecule. The human PRL amino acid sequence[15] is displayed in the single-letter amino acid code. The lettered arrows indicate the points at which the coding region of the PRL gene is interrupted by introns. Intron A, located in the signal peptide, is not shown in this diagram, which depicts only the mature protein. The N-linked glycosylation site at residue 31, asparagine, is indicated by CHO.

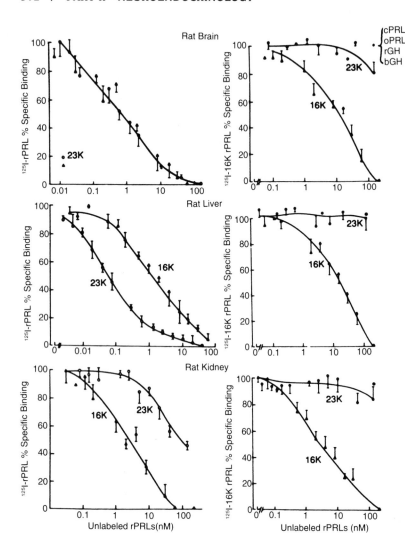

FIGURE 23–4. **A unique receptor for the 16-kDa fragment of PRL in rat tissues.** The displacement binding curves of iodinated 23-kDa rat PRL or its 16-kDa fragment are shown for brain, liver, and kidney. (Reproduced from Clapp C, Sears PS, Nicoll CS: Binding studies with intact rat prolactin and a 16K fragment of the hormone. Endocrinology 125:1054–1059, 1989; © The Endocrine Society.)

per cent activity in casein production.[47] The differential release of the various glycosylated forms of PRL in physiologically relevant states seems to reflect preferential secretion of unmodified, newly synthesized PRL.[48] Phosphorylated and deamidated forms of PRL have also been reported.[49] The phosphorylated forms may inhibit cell division in the rat pituitary-derived GH3 cell line, whereas the dephosphorylated form may act as an autocrine growth factor in these cells.[50] A 21-kDa PRL has been detected in the pituitaries and sera of rodents and man. The concentration of this form is altered by PRL secretagogues.[51] It has been postulated that 21-kDa PRL may be the translation product of an alternatively spliced PRL transcript, similar to the 20-kDa alternatively spliced form of hGH.[52] Finally, a human Burkitt lymphoma cell line secretes an immunologically detectable 29-kDa PLP (PLP 29) that appears essential to the growth of the cell line in serum-free media; however, this cell also secretes GH.[53a] This could represent a post-translational modification or be the product of a human PRL-related gene.

Fractionation of human serum by Sephadex G-100 chromatography resolves PRL into three immunoreactive peaks: 23 kDa, 48- to 56-kDa, and 150-kDa forms. Some reports have suggested that the 48- to 56-kDa form is a dimer of PRL, that can be converted to 23-kDa PRL with reducing agents. The origin of 150-kDa PRL is less clear; it

may represent heterogeneous or homogeneous aggregates of PRL. 150-kDa PRL demonstrates decreased receptor binding and biological activity, as well as decreased serum clearance. These facts may explain the clinical syndrome of sustained hyperprolactinemia of the 150-kDa form with minimal symptoms, that is, normal menses and minimal galactorrhea.[54] Serum from the infant of one such pregnant patient also demonstrated increased levels of 150-kDa PRL, suggesting that genetic factors may influence the presence of this form because this large molecule is unlikely to pass from mother to fetus via the circulatory system.[55] High molecular weight forms of PL-II in rodents and CS in humans have been attributed to heterodimers formed with α_2-macroglobulin. Whether PRL also exists in such complexes remains unknown. It cannot be assumed that the standard RIA accurately detects all of the PRL isohormones present in sera or tissue extracts. These findings suggest that PRL is only one in a family of related proteins and may itself represent a prohormone form that is further activated by post-translational processing. Differences in the structural features of the various PRL isoforms may result in differences in their biological activities. These variants may each possess unique bioactivities that, when combined in different ratios, may be responsible for the many known actions of PRL. Additionally, the production of some of these variants may be controlled by independent mechanisms, explaining the perplexing complexity of PRL regulation.

GENOMIC REGULATION

Regulation of Tissue-Specific PRL Gene Expression

The driving force behind cell and organ differentiation is the temporal and cell-specific expression of certain highly regulated genes. Therefore a major problem in molecular biology has been to understand what determines an individual gene's cell-specific expression. The cell-specific regulation of the PRL and GH genes has emerged as a model system for such studies. The differentiated anterior pituitary lactotroph and somatotroph are defined by a high-level expression of the PRL and GH gene, respectively. Tissue-specific nuclear proteins known as transactivators are responsible for the transcriptional activation of genes such as PRL that define a differentiated phenotype. These transactivators act in a combinatorial fashion to both activate and restrict the expression of the given gene, often by binding directly to DNA sequences upstream from the gene (cis elements). In the case of PRL, expression is activated in the pituitary lactotroph but restricted from the somatotroph. This regulation occurs by the interaction of the tissue-specific transactivators with discrete DNA segments, promoters, and enhancers associated with the gene.

The Structure and Regulation of the PRL Gene Promoter

The rat PRL promoter contains a cluster of four pituitary transactivator binding sites just upstream of the TATAAA element, called the proximal element. A cluster of four more binding sites over 1 kb further upstream and adjacent to an estrogen receptor binding site is known as the distal element. The normal expression of the PRL gene depends on an interaction between these distal and proximal elements. Because a subpopulation of pituitary cells simultaneously expresses both PRL and GH, a common transcription factor likely activates both GH and PRL genes, and two similar binding sites were detected upstream of the GH gene. Each of the eight protected elements in the PRL promoter and the two identified in the GH promoter were noted to contain an AT-rich DNA sequence motif with the consensus nucleotide sequence A(T/A)(T/A)TATNCAT. Each region of the promoter containing this motif was bound by a protein specific to pituitary cell nuclei.[56]

Properties of Pit-1

The nuclear protein that binds to each of the proximal and distal elements was purified 4000-fold by DNA-affinity chromatography from GC cells using a multimer of the DNA-binding motif as the affinity reagent. The purified transacting factor was named Pit-1.[57] Properties of Pit-1 were shared with GHF-1, a transacting factor purified by binding to cis elements of the hGH gene.[58] Antisense Pit-1 oligonucleotides decrease both GH and PRL expression and proliferation in pituitary cell lines, and it is now gen-

erally accepted that the independently discovered Pit-1 and GHF-1 are identical.[59]

Rat Pit-1/GHF-1 mRNA is expressed in both lactotrophs and somatotrophs. When transfected into fibroblasts, Pit-1 selectively activates expression from the PRL and GH gene promoters. When transfected into a lactotroph cell line, Pit-1 activates PRL, but not GH gene expression, suggesting that a restrictive mechanism is responsible for excluding GH expression from lactotrophs.[57] A globally restrictive mechanism has been demonstrated by the fusion of non–hormone-secreting cell lines with PRL- and GH-secreting GH3 cells. Such fusions result in the extinction of Pit-1 gene expression, with subsequent loss of both PRL and GH expression from the fused GH3 cells.[60, 61] Although Pit-1 is essential for the expression of PRL and GH, it must act in concert with a variety of additional factors to establish the full cellular phenotype.

Pit-1 was found to contain a conserved stretch of about 155 amino acids with homology to a family of eukaryotic transcription factors. This homology unit is called the POU domain (for pit-1, oct-1, and unc-86, the original homologous transcription factors) and it is made up of two subdomains, the POU-specific domain and the POU-homeobox domain.[62] The homeobox domain contains a helix-turn-helix region described in all homeodomains and is required and sufficient for low-affinity DNA binding. The POU-specific domain is necessary for high-affinity binding (up to a 1000-fold increase) and accurate recognition of the Pit-1 cis elements and mediates DNA-dependent protein-protein interaction between two Pit-1 molecules, necessary for efficient transcriptional activation of the PRL gene.[57]

Ontogeny of Pit-1 Expression

The earliest expression of Pit-1 in the pituitary correlates with the appearance of distinct pituitary cell types. Pit-1 transcripts are first detectable on rat embryonic day 11 in the neural tube, and the Pit-1 protein is first detected in the rat pituitary on embryonic days 15 to 16, before the coactivation of PRL and GH genes by about embryonic days 16 to 17. This timing is consistent with the model that Pit-1 triggers the initial transcriptional activation of both hormone genes. However, Pit-1 transcripts are detected in all pituitary cell types, but Pit-1 protein is detected in somatotrophs, lactotrophs, and thyrotrophs only (Fig. 23–5). Pit-1's role in the thyrotroph is still somewhat unclear. Although GH gene expression reaches its maximum by embryonic days 19 to 20, the PRL gene exhibits a gradual increase to full levels at days 10 to 15 after birth. This suggests that additional transactivators are necessary for the PRL gene to achieve full expression. It has been suggested that synergism between Pit-1 and the estrogen receptor which binds to an element (ERE) located adjacent to the distal enhancer element may be responsible for the post-birth increase in PRL gene expression.[63] Somatotroph and lactotroph lineage ablation studies in transgenic mice[64, 65] and reverse hemolytic plaque assay studies of isolated pituitary cells (see Mammosomatotrophs) are consistent with the notion that most, if not all, lactotrophs are derived from a presomatotroph lineage and that this transition may be regulated by estrogen. Finally, Pit-1 has been found to autoregulate its own gene expression, which

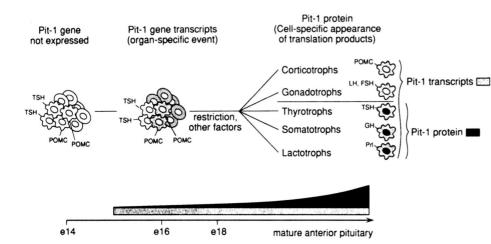

FIGURE 23–5. **Ontogeny of Pit-1 mRNA and protein expression in the various cell types of the developing rat pituitary.** The scale represents rat embryonic days (e). (From Simmons DM, Voss JW, Ingraham HA, et al: Pituitary cell phenotypes involve cell-specific pit-1 mRNA translation and synergistic interactions with other classes of transcription factors. Genes Dev 4:695–711, 1990.)

should result in the maintenance of the pituitary phenotype. The embryonic appearance of Pit-1 probably represents one of the last steps in the pathway leading to formation of fully determined lactotrophs and somatotrophs. At present, little is known about the preceding steps in the regulatory cascade, although a transactivator named pituitary transcription factor (PTF) that may induce Pit-1 expression during development has been identified.[66]

Pit-1 Mutations

A mutation of Pit-1 would be predicted to abolish GH and PRL expression and result in a dwarf phenotype. There are three genetically dwarf mouse strains, the allelic Snell and Jackson strains (*dw*) and the nonallelic Ames dwarf mouse (*df*). In the *dw* mutation, the pituitary is hypoplastic, with no evidence of lactotrophs, somatotrophs, or thyrotrophs, and no immunologically detectable PRL, GH, or thyroid-stimulating hormone (TSH). Administration of exogenous hormones reverses much of the phenotype, with the exception of the hypocellularity of the pituitary.[67] Analyses of the Pit-1 gene in these dwarf mice revealed that the Snell mouse has a point mutation in the POU-homeodomain that abolishes Pit-1 binding to DNA. Similarly, the Jackson mouse Pit-1 gene contains a 4-kb insertion, disrupting its function.[68] The Ames dwarf mouse pituitary does not express Pit-1, but the Pit-1 gene is intact and the *df* mutation has been assigned to a unique chromosome 11 locus not associated with the Pit-1 gene.[69] These results suggest that the products of the *df* locus might be involved in the regulation of Pit-1. It is not yet known whether the *df* locus gene and PTF are identical.

Recently Pit-1 mutations have been discovered in three human kindreds exhibiting pituitary dwarfism. In the first report, the proband presented with cretinism and was subsequently found to be deficient in GH and PRL synthesis as well. A nonsense mutation was found at codon 172 that eliminated the POU-homeodomain.[70] A point mutation in the POU-specific domain of Pit-1 was found in a Dutch family with dwarf siblings demonstrating combined TSH, GH, and PRL deficiency. This mutation reduced the binding affinity of Pit-1 and abolished activation of both GH and PRL in transfection assays but did not result in pituitary hypoplasia.[71] In the third report, a point mutation in only one of the two Pit-1 alleles resulted in a dominant inhibition of Pit-1 action in the pituitary.[71a] These cases may

represent the first recognized instances of genetic diseases resulting from mutations in transcription factor genes.

Hormone-Mediated Regulation of the PRL Gene

The transcription of the PRL gene is known to be regulated by a variety of different hormones and growth factors: estradiol, thyroid-releasing hormone (TRH), dopamine, glucocorticoids, transforming growth factor-β, and epidermal growth factor (EGF). Many of these hormones use intracellular second messengers such as cAMP, calcium, or diacylglycerol. In addition to mediating pituitary-specific expression, the PRL promoter also contains *cis* elements that respond to hormonal signals or second-messenger cascades. Study of the DNA sequences and *trans*-acting factors through which these effects are mediated has become a major area of research.

Steroid Hormones

Steroid hormones have both positive and negative effects on PRL gene transcription. These effects are mediated either through direct binding of the steroid hormone receptor to promoter regions or through interaction with another transcription factor that binds directly to the promoter. Injections of estrogen into rats result in a rapid increase in PRL gene transcription, confirmed by transcriptional run-on assays in GH4 cells in which a 4.5-fold increase in transcription is seen. This estrogen-response element (ERE), located near PRL's distal enhancer, is unusual in that it is nonpalindromic, suggesting that interaction between the estrogen receptor and another transcription factor may be necessary for the estrogen responsiveness of the PRL gene.[72] The ERE and Pit-1 binding sites appear to interact because cotransfection of Pit-1 and the estrogen receptor into a cell line lacking endogenous estrogen receptors results in an estrogen-mediated boost in PRL transcription by 8- to 15-fold, whereas estrogen receptor alone had no effect.[63] Pit-1 and the estrogen receptor appear to act in concert to activate the distal enhancer element, and an interaction between the proteins has been suggested.[73] Glucocorticoids normally induce a negative transcriptional effect on the PRL promoter and a negative glucocorticoid regulatory element has been localized in the PRL promoter.[74]

Thyroid hormone influences PRL transcription. Whether transcription is induced or inhibited depends upon the pituitary cell line studied.[75] The 5'-flanking region of the rat PRL gene contains both a distal positive and a proximal negative thyroid response element. The thyroid receptor does not bind directly to the proximal element, suggesting that protein-protein interactions mediate the negative effect. The receptor can bind directly to the distal stimulatory element, however.[76]

Dopamine

A variety of other hormonal stimuli act indirectly on the PRL gene via intracellular second-messenger systems. Dopamine mediates its negative effect on PRL gene transcription via decreases in intracellular cAMP. The cAMP-responsive element has been mapped to the region between −127 and +73 in the rat PRL gene.[77] A single Pit-1 binding site linked to the PRL TATAA box was able to confer partial dopamine responsiveness to a reporter gene.[78] This has raised the possibility that the cAMP effect may be partially indirect, mediated through a cAMP-response element in the promoter of the Pit-1 gene itself.[66]

Others

TRH and EGF rapidly stimulate PRL gene transcription via increases in intracellular calcium.[79] A TRH response element as well as a calcium response element (CaRE) have been mapped to the first Pit-1 binding site of the rat PRL proximal promoter region, suggesting that the TRH and calcium effect is mediated by Pit-1.[80] Furthermore, the distal PRL promoter region also directs a TRH and calcium response. Calcium can stimulate multiple signaling pathways. The use of pharmacological calcium channel agonists has implicated the movement of calcium through "L" type channels in the transcriptional response of both proximal and distal PRL promoter elements. Protein kinase C is apparently not involved.[81] It is interesting that TRH is known to activate protein kinase C in pituitary cell lines, and that this activation has been implicated in the regulation of PRL *secretion* from these cells by TRH. Thus the apparent absence of this enzyme from the pathway of action of TRH on PRL gene expression implies a divergence of the actions of TRH on PRL secretion and gene expression before the level of protein kinase C activity.[80]

EGF, cAMP, and tissue plasminogen activator, each of which activates a specific protein kinase, also transcriptionally regulate the PRL gene and the regulation is mediated via Pit-1 binding sites. It has been proposed that these Pit-1–mediated interactions might occur via phosphorylation of the Pit-1 protein. In fact, phosphorylation of Pit-1 has been shown to modulate its conformation, increasing binding at some promoter sites and decreasing it at others.[11] Virtually every hormonal regulator of PRL gene transcription except estrogen has been demonstrated to exert its action through a Pit-1 *cis* element. Whether these effects are mediated through the transcriptional regulation of *pit-1* levels, Pit-1 structure, or protein-protein interactions involving Pit-1 remains to be determined.

BIOSYNTHESIS

Methods of Detection

The most common means of measuring PRL is by standard RIA. A less specific but overlapping approach is the PRL radioreceptor assay, which detects all "lactogenic" hormones, including hGH and CS.[82] Recent progress in cloning and characterizing the lactogen family of receptors (see Receptors) will likely render this assay too nonspecific, and it may soon be replaced by individual radioreceptor assays. A number of assays directly detect PRL bioactivity. The original bioassay is the pigeon crop sac assay in which systemic or local injection of PRL induces proliferation of the mucosal epithelium of the crop sac. Another bioassay detects secretory changes in mouse mammary tissue explants in response to added PRL. The most commonly used PRL bioassay is based on the mitogenic effect of PRL on the Nb2 lymphoma cell line.[83] Cell division in this cell line, which depends upon PRL for proliferation, is easily quantitated by counting cells after a 72-hour incubation with various concentrations of PRL. None of these bioassays is specific in that they detect any lactogen. The Nb2 assay is the most sensitive; it detects PRL concentrations as low as 0.4 ng/ml.

Two techniques have been developed to quantify hormone secretion from individual cells. The cell immunoblot assay requires the transfer of cells cultured on coverslips to a nylon membrane, followed by immunostaining. In this approach, stored hormone is quantitated.[84] With the reverse hemolytic plaque assay (RHPA), PRL or any hormone secreted from individual living cells is visualized microscopically after incubation of the cells with hormone-specific antiserum followed by detection using protein A–coated ovine erythrocytes and complement. Clear zones of hemolysis, proportional to the amount of hormone secreted, form around the hormone-secreting cell (Fig. 23–6).[85] This technique can also be used to detect more than one secreted hormone by using two different antisera, added sequentially along with fresh erythrocytes and complement. This is referred to as the sequential RHPA and has been used to detect the GH- and PRL-secreting mammosomatotroph cell.

Pituitary PRL

Mammosomatotrophs

The capacity of the pituitary to synthesize hormones predates histological differentiation of the pituitary cells into lactotrophs (PRL-secreting cells) and somatotrophs (GH-secreting cells). In all species studied, GH secretion predates PRL secretion. Studies in neonatal rats using the sequential RHPA for PRL and GH have indicated that of every 100 acidophils present, 62.5 release GH only, 1.7 release PRL only, but 35.8 release both hormones (mammosomatotrophs).[86] In humans the numbers are similar.[86] Furthermore, cells containing only PRL could not be detected until about 23 weeks of age.[87] This has led to the hypothesis that somatotrophs give rise to lactotrophs by way of a mammosomatotroph intermediate cell. Studies in transgenic mice support this hypothesis.[64, 65] When the herpes simplex virus thymidine kinase gene is expressed in

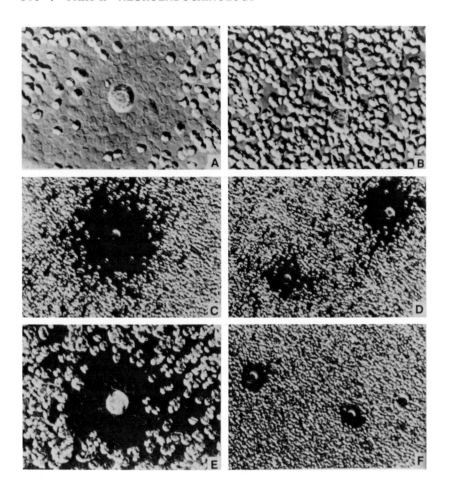

FIGURE 23–6. **Reverse hemolytic plaque assay.** *A,* A high-power magnification of a single pituitary cell that secretes PRL. This cell is surrounded by sheep erythrocytes that are lysed by the interaction of anti-PRL IgG and secreted PRL on the erythrocytes when complement is added. *B,* A pituitary cell not secreting PRL is surrounded by intact erythrocytes. *C* and *D,* Lower magnification views of PRL-secreting pituitary cells. *E* and *F,* High and low magnifications, respectively, of cells secreting GH. Antibodies and sheep red blood cells can be applied sequentially to document cells secreting both hormones (not shown here). (From Leong DA, Lau SK, Sinha YN, et al: Enumeration of lactotropes and somatotropes among male and female pituitary cells in culture: Evidence in favor of a mammosomatotrope subpopulation in the rat. Endocrinology 116:1371–1378, 1985; © The Endocrine Society.)

a dividing cell, the exposure of that cell to the synthetic nucleoside FIAU (1-(2-deoxy-2-fluoro-δ-β-arabinofuranosyl)-5-iodouracil) results in cell death. When transgenic mice are generated that carry the thymidine kinase gene transcriptionally controlled by the GH promoter, these mice develop dwarfism, loss of both somatotrophs and lactotrophs in their pituitaries, and markedly decreased GH and PRL secretion. In contrast, mice carrying the thymidine kinase gene driven by the PRL promoter and exposed to FIAU have normal pituitaries. Because the toxicity of FIAU in these transgenic mice depends upon cell division, it is concluded that lactotrophs are post-mitotic, terminally differentiated cells derived from a stem-cell mammosomatotroph. It is extrapolated from these data that the stem mammosomatotroph persists in the adult animal and is capable of repopulating the pituitaries of the FIAU-treated animals with mature GH- and PRL-producing cells.[65]

Data have accumulated supporting the concept that GH- and PRL-secreting cells present in the adult animal may be interconvertible. This has been suggested by the observation of marked increases in dual-secreting mammosomatotrophs in male rat pituitaries exposed to estrogen associated with a commensurate decrease in GH-secreting cells. Also chronic treatment with gonadotropin-releasing hormone (GnRH) increases PRL-secreting cells with a reciprocal decrease in GH cells. Whether this reciprocal shift in phenotype is due to interconversion between cell types or differential cell death and mitosis of the stem cell is not clear. Regardless of the mechanism, some hormones that increase PRL secretion may function, at least in part, as lactotroph recruitment factors.

Storage and Secretion

Pituitary preprolactin, like all secreted proteins, is synthesized and its signal peptide is removed on the membrane-bound ribosomes of the rough endoplasmic reticulum. From there the processed PRL is transported to the Golgi, where it is glycosylated to a variable extent and packaged into secretory granules. PRL is concentrated in the secretory granules, along with the storage proteins chromogranin and the secretogranin. At this point the PRL becomes electron dense, suggesting that it is in the form of insoluble aggregates. These secretory granules go through a maturation process during which they enlarge in size, develop a regular shape, become even more dense, and migrate to the periphery of the cell prior to release.[88] The mechanisms underlying the formation of these granules have not been determined. PRL was originally thought to be secreted by two pathways, the regulated secretory granule pathway described above and a constitutive pathway, characterized by lack of secretory granule formation and rapid transport to the cell surface. The constitutive pathway was considered to be the bulk flow default pathway, whereas the secretory granule pathway was considered to be the pathway responding to secretagogues.[89] New evidence suggests that lactotrophs may in fact secrete granule-stored hormone to a significant extent even in the basal state in the absence of secretagogues.[90]

Decidual PRL

In addition to its major site of synthesis in the pituitary, human PRL is also synthesized in the decidua basalis of the pregnant uterus,[91] the decidualized endometrium of the nongravid uterus during days 22 to 28 of the normal menstrual cycle,[92] and the myometrium.[93] PRL is present in amniotic fluid at levels 100-fold higher than in maternal or fetal blood. Amniotic fluid PRL levels peak at midgestation and decrease during the third trimester, while maternal pituitary PRL levels are still rising. PRL produced by the decidual cell appears to be 50 per cent glycosylated, whereas that produced by the pituitary is only 10 per cent glycosylated. The PRL found in the amniotic fluid is heavily glycosylated.[94] Taken together, these findings suggest that the source of amniotic fluid PRL is the decidua. This transport from decidua to amniotic fluid appears to depend upon the cellular adhesion between the maternal decidua and the fetal chorion layers of the placenta in vivo.[95]

At present, only a single type of PRL appears to be synthesized by the human decidua. The coding region of a PRL cDNA clone isolated from the human decidua is identical to pituitary PRL.[96] However, the mRNA for decidual PRL is approximately 150 nucleotides larger than pituitary PRL mRNA. This discrepancy is explained by the existence of a previously unrecognized 5'-noncoding exon, located approximately 8 kb upstream of the originally reported first noncoding exon (see Fig. 23–1). The presence of this upstream exon is found in PRL mRNA expressed in the decidua and in lymphocytes[97] but not when PRL is expressed in the pituitary. This reflects the specific activation of a tissue-specific alternative 5' promoter in decidua/lymphocytes.[39] The existence of two alternatively utilized promoters, the more 5' active in decidua and lymphocytes and the more 3' active in pituitary, results in a totally different transcriptional regulatory profile of PRL gene expression in these tissues. The IM-9-P3 B-lymphoblastoid cell line has been used as a model to study the gene regulation of the decidual/lymphocyte form of the PRL gene. Dexamethasone has been found to negatively regulate PRL secretion by decreasing mRNA stability in these cells. In addition, in these cells PRL apparently has no effect on its own secretion and does not serve as an autocrine growth factor,[98] although autocrine regulation in pituitary-derived GH3 cells has been reported.[50]

In clear distinction to the pituitary, PRL in the decidua and endometrium is not stored in secretory granules. Consistent with this difference, the secretory regulation of decidual PRL is also quite different from that of the pituitary.[99] Studies on isolated decidual cells indicate that modulators of pituitary PRL secretion such as dopamine, bromocriptine, and TRH are ineffective in the decidua. Induction of endometrial PRL synthesis depends upon progesterone-induced decidualization. Once decidualized, these cells continue to secrete PRL in the absence of progesterone. Estradiol depresses the stimulation caused by progesterone.[100] Decidual explants incubated with media conditioned by human placental explants were noted specifically to release more PRL than controls.[101] The factor in the conditioned media responsible for this release, *decidual prolactin-releasing factor,* has been purified as a 23.5-kDa protein and shown to stimulate both the synthesis and release of decidual PRL at a concentration of about 3 nM.[102] A *decidual prolactin-inhibiting factor* has also been partially purified. It prevents PRL release in response to the decidual PRL-releasing factor.[103] Lipocortin-I, present in decidual homogenates, can inhibit the basal and decidual PRL-releasing factor–stimulated synthesis and release of decidual

but not pituitary PRL in a autocrine/paracrine fashion.[104] Arachidonic acid also inhibits decidual PRL release.[103] Insulin growth factor 1 (IGF-1), insulin, endothelin, and relaxin all stimulate the dose-dependent release of decidual PRL through their respective receptors.[105] It appears that a novel feedback regulation between fetal membranes, placenta, and decidua coordinates the synthesis and release of decidual PRL (Fig. 23–7).

PRL in Body Fluids

Cerebrospinal Fluid

In addition to serum and amniotic fluid, PRL immunoreactivity has been detected in several other body fluids. PRL has been detected in the CSF,[106] as is the case with all of the adenohypophyseal hormones. Considerable evidence supports the presence of PRL in the brain: immunocytochemical, RIA, and bioassay data, as well as evidence for PRL gene expression in both hypothalamic and extrahypothalamic brain. PRL in brain appears to be largely concentrated in nerve endings, suggesting a trans-synaptic function.[107] After hypophysectomy or bromocriptine treatment, PRL immunoreactivity in the CNS remains constant,[108] consistent with independent forms of gene regulation. PRL-binding sites and PRL receptor mRNA have been identified in the brain and in some peripheral neurons.[109] In fact, a role in behavior modification for CNS PRL is suggested by experiments in which microinfusions in the midbrain increase lordosis and maternal behavior in the nulliparous rat.[110] In some studies CSF PRL levels reflect serum levels with serum-to-CSF ratios ranging from 3 to 10.[111] Some serum PRL enters the CSF via a receptor-mediated mechanism located at the choroid plexus.[112] PRL may also gain direct access from the pituitary to the CSF via retrograde flow through the hypothalamic-hypophyseal portal system.[113] Whether any endogenous brain PRL enters the CSF remains unknown.

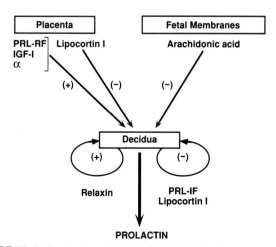

FIGURE 23–7. **Regulation of human decidual PRL release by paracrine and autocrine placental factors.** PRL-RF refers to PRL-releasing factor and PRL-IF to PRL-inhibiting factor isolated from placenta and decidua, respectively. (Adapted from Handwerger S, Markoff E, Richards R: 3. Regulation of the synthesis and release of decidual prolactin by placental and autocrine/paracrine factors. Placenta 12:121–130, 1991.)

Milk

PRL is secreted into breast milk at levels that appear to represent average circulating PRL concentrations.[114] At present the physiological significance of milk PRL is unclear. In nursing human mothers, serum levels rise over the first three to five postpartum days, reaching 157 ng/ml, then fall with continued nursing to about 24 ng/ml by day 13 postpartum, suggesting a role for milk PRL in the early neonatal period.[115] In lactating animals, iodinated PRL injected intravenously appears in the breast milk and is subsequently transferred to lysosomes or across the transepithelial pathway to the plasma of suckling pups via intestinal epithelia PRL receptors. Significant quantities of PRL are potentially transferred in this manner.[116]

Semen

PRL is present in human semen at levels about 1.6-fold higher than those in serum. Because levels fall about 50 per cent in the second week after vasectomy, it was postulated that both the seminal vesicles and the testicular-epididymal unit secrete PRL into the seminal pool.[117] PRL is known to have biological effects on the male reproductive tract; in the testis it increases the number of luteinizing hormone (LH) receptors and enhances testosterone synthesis and secretion, whereas in the prostate and seminal vesicles it increases organ weight and enhances uptake of testosterone. The data suggest that PRL originates in the cells of the male reproductive tract, but the possibility remains that PRL may be concentrated across the blood-testis barrier.

Ovarian Follicular Fluid

PRL is present in ovarian follicular fluid. Although the follicular fluid levels of follicle-stimulating hormone (FSH) and LH parallel serum levels, PRL levels there are higher, suggesting either an active transport mechanism or local synthesis. PRL is maximal in the early follicular phase and falls during the late follicular phase. The levels appear to be inversely related to follicular fluid volumes and correlate with maturational changes in the preovulatory human follicle.[118] The immunoreactive follicular fluid PRL is also bioactive in the Nb2 assay.[119] In the rat, in which PRL is luteotropic, PRL enhances progesterone production in granulosa cells isolated from preovulatory rat follicles.[120] It has also been reported to inhibit estrogen secretion in immature follicles and androgen secretion from theca/interstitial cells.[121] Whether local follicular fluid PRL is responsible for these actions is not known.

REGULATION OF SECRETION

Physiological Observations

Normal Circadian Secretion

Like all anterior pituitary hormones, PRL is secreted episodically, with a distinctive 24-hour pattern. In normal human subjects, there are about 14 pulses of PRL secretion in 24 hours, approximately one each 95 minutes.[122] Superimposed upon this pattern is a bimodal 24-hour pattern of secretion, with a major nocturnal peak beginning after sleep onset and peaking in midsleep. Minimal levels (the smallest spikes) occur around noon, followed by a lesser peak of secretion in the evening.[122, 123] The enhancement of secretion during the night is due to increases in the amplitude of each pulse, unaccompanied by an increase in pulse frequency.[124] PRL secretion remains pulsatile in patients with prolactinomas, whereas circadian variation is abolished. Furthermore, rat anterior pituitaries transplanted under the pituitary capsule of hypophysectomized rats release PRL in pulses of 8- to 10-minute intervals. Because hypothalamic connections have been severed, this short periodicity appears to be intrinsic to the lactotroph.[125] These data from both human and rat studies support the concept that these short pulses are not controlled by the hypothalamus but arise within the gland.[126]

Secretion During the Menstrual Cycle, Pregnancy, and Lactation

Serum PRL levels are generally higher in women than in men. This reflects the effects of estrogen. The daytime peak of PRL secretion is more pronounced during the luteal than follicular phase of the menstrual cycle.[127] During pregnancy, maternal serum PRL levels begin to rise during the first trimester and increase steadily throughout pregnancy, resulting in about a 10-fold increase by term, presumably due to the high levels of estrogen during pregnancy.[128] In contrast to maternal serum levels, the levels of PRL in amniotic fluid peak at 17 to 25 weeks of gestation, then decline to a lower plateau at 36 weeks.[129] Serum PRL levels fall during labor by about 50 per cent, reaching a nadir about two hours prior to delivery. After delivery, serum PRL levels rise markedly, peaking about two hours postpartum and then falling again six hours later.[130] The postpartum period is characterized by physiological hyperprolactinemia, which progressively drops toward normal nulliparous levels over a period of four weeks despite continued suckling.[131] Whether lactational hyperprolactinemia plays a direct role in postpartum anovulation and infertility remains controversial.[132] Periods of suckling are immediately followed by PRL secretory activity separated by intervals of secretory quiescence (Fig. 23–8). This pattern continues for twice the duration of the suckling period.[133] In most nonpregnant women and some men, nipple stimulation causes a similar rapid rise in PRL levels.[134]

Stress

In 1960, stress was found to initiate lactation in estrogen-primed virgin rats.[135] Since then, human PRL secretion has been shown to increase after many types of stress, including general anesthesia, surgery, exercise, and insulin-induced hypoglycemia. In each case the stress causes a significantly greater PRL increase in women than in men. Following general surgery, levels as high as five-fold over basal have been reported.[136] It has been postulated that the stress-induced increase in PRL is partially mediated by the opiate peptides, particularly β-endorphin.[137] Neuronal histamine and arginine vasopressin have been implicated as mediators in other studies,[138] whereas melanocyte-stimulating hormone (MSH) has been implicated as an inhibitor of stress-induced increases in PRL.[139] The dual control by

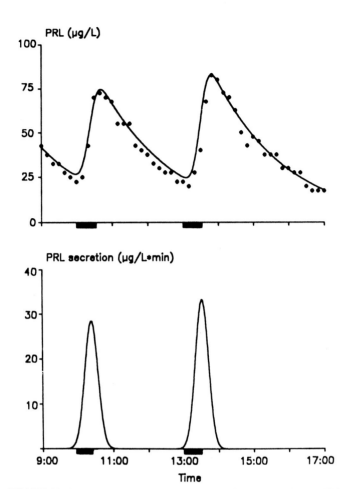

FIGURE 23–8. **PRL suckling response in a lactating woman.** Serum PRL levels are shown in the top panel. The suckling intervals are indicated by the black bars along the abscissa. The lower graph shows the PRL secretory profile using the mathematical deconvolution model. (Adapted from Kremer JAM, Borm G, Schellekens LA, et al: Pulsatile secretion of luteinizing hormone and prolactin in lactating and nonlactating women and the response to naltrexone. J Clin Endocrinol Metab 72:294–300, 1991; © The Endocrine Society.)

β-endorphin and MSH, two products of the pro-opiomelanocortin precursor, suggests that the processing of these two peptides must be physiologically regulated.

Endocrine Regulation

Estrogen

Estrogen regulates the secretion of PRL in many different species. Initial observations in the rat indicated that long-term estrogen treatment results in hyperplasia and hypertrophy of the acidophils of the pituitary.[140] Oophorectomy reduces the size and number of lactotrophs, effects that are reversed within four days by treatment with estrogen.[141] Surveys of human pituitaries at autopsy have demonstrated that estrogen increases the number of PRL-secreting cells.[142] In line with this, it has long been known that high estrogen levels induce prolactinomas in certain strains of rats.[143] The concept that an uncommitted mammosomatotroph could be converted to a lactotroph under the influence of estrogen was first proposed in 1974.[144] This has been studied more recently using the RHPA to monitor

changes in the ratio of PRL- and GH-secreting cells during pregnancy through lactation. Estrogen-mediated increments in the lactotroph population at the expense of mammosomatotrophs were found at three physiological time points: the transitions from virgin to midgestation, from delivery to early lactation and again in late lactation.[145] A direct study in which male rat pituitary cells were exposed to estradiol for six days revealed a marked increase in the proportion of mammosomatotrophs and a commensurate decrease in somatotrophs.[146] Estrogen has such a major impact on PRL expression in the neonate that it has been proposed as the controlling factor in the ontogeny of the lactotrophs. Thus it appears that somatotrophs and lactotrophs are interconvertible via the dual-secreting mammosomatotroph and that this interconversion is significantly influenced by estrogen.

Estrogen can also increase the level of PRL gene expression within an existing lactotroph. Primary pituitary cell cultures incubated with physiological levels of estradiol demonstrate an increase in preprolactin mRNA after one day, followed by a two- to three-fold increase in PRL secretion after two days.[147] Estrogen stimulates induction of PRL mRNA in vivo: 2.3-fold and 5.4-fold in males and immature females, respectively, after six days of estradiol injection.[148] Subsequently it was demonstrated that estrogen stimulates transcription from the PRL gene both in vivo and in vitro, within 30 minutes of a single injection of estradiol.[149] Using a short-acting estrogen, 16α-estradiol, the kinetics of PRL mRNA accumulation were shown to be biphasic. The first phase, which lasts for two hours, is independent of new protein synthesis. This is considered to be the estrogen receptor–mediated stimulation of gene transcription. The second phase, which starts three hours after stimulation and continues for several days, was shown to depend on new protein synthesis. The cellular mechanism of this second level of control is unclear but is postulated to be mediated through the effect of estrogen on the hypothalamus.[150]

Estrogen modulates the responsiveness of the pituitary gland to hypothalamic factors that control PRL production: two specific examples of this are a decrease in responsiveness to dopamine, a PRL-inhibiting factor, and an increase in responsiveness to TRH, a stimulatory factor. The mechanisms involved include decreasing the number of dopamine receptors and increasing the number of TRH receptors,[151] as well as a direct suppression by estrogen of dopamine secretion.[152] Estrogens exert a powerful effect on the tuberoinfundibular neuron; activity is two to three times greater in female than in male rats, and dopamine concentrations in pituitary stalk blood are concomitantly higher in the female rat.[153]

Some of the direct actions of estradiol on lactotroph proliferation may be mediated by a locally synthesized growth factor, galanin. This was first suggested when galanin was isolated from an estrogen-induced pituitary cDNA library.[154] Galanin also stimulates lactotroph proliferation and PRL secretion in the rat via a hypothalamic effect.[155] The actions of estrogen on the pituitary may also be modulated by one of estrogen's metabolites that has the opposite effect on PRL release. The pituitaries of rats and humans have the enzyme necessary for the conversion of estrogen into this metabolite, 2-hydroxyestrogen, which is capable of suppressing PRL secretion.[156] Thus the overall regulation of PRL by estrogen uses at least four distinct mechanisms: PRL gene regulation, lactotroph differentiation, neuroendocrine modulation, and perhaps the local and inhibitory effects just mentioned. The many in vivo correlations between estrogen and PRL levels indicate that estrogen is one of the most important regulators of PRL secretion.

Insulin

Physiological doses of insulin stimulate PRL expression in GH3 cells; PRL mRNA levels increase 3- to 10-fold and secretion is accelerated. This effect is specific because GH levels are not altered.[157] This effect is also detectable in primary pituitary cells[158] and in decidua.[105] The direct mitogenic effect of PRL on the islet β-cell and its proposed role in the maintenance of normal glucose levels during pregnancy suggest a feedback loop on the islets.[159] This further suggests that insulin regulation of PRL is likely to be physiologically important. The physiological significance of these findings is unclear at present.

Neuroendocrine Regulation

Several examples of the neuroendocrine control of PRL secretion have been discussed above: the sleep-related, stress, and suckling-induced surges of PRL. The suckling stimulus represents a neuroendocrine reflex and is a popular experimental model; the magnitude of the PRL response is closely coupled to the intensity of the stimulus.[160] An example of a highly complex neuroendocrine reflex unique to PRL is the release of PRL in response to stimulation of the uterine cervix in the rat. Either artificial cervical stimulation or normal mating results in a twice-daily surge of PRL release, peaking at about three-fold over baseline. This twice-daily pattern continues for up to 13 days after the stimulus and in the absence of fertilization induces a state known as pseudopregnancy.[161] Although the exact molecular mechanisms controlling these responses are incompletely understood at present, a variety of PRL-releasing factor and PRL-inhibitory factors have been discovered that may be of importance. The neuroendocrine regulation of PRL secretion is a complex subject that can be addressed only briefly here. The interested reader is referred to several recent comprehensive reviews for greater detail.[10, 153, 162, 163]

PRL-Inhibiting Factors (PIF's)

DOPAMINE. The connections between the median eminence (ME) and the anterior pituitary are critical to the maintenance of physiological control over PRL secretion. PRL synthesis, unlike that of other adenohypophyseal hormones, continues after pituitary stalk section, after transplantation of the pituitary of the renal capsule, and after transfer of the pituitary or its cells into culture.[164] Therefore the hypothalamus exerts a predominantly negative control over spontaneous pituitary PRL secretion. Dopamine, a catecholamine present in the ME and the hypophyseal portal blood at levels sufficient to inhibit PRL release,[165] acts as the major physiological PIF via a direct action on the pituitary. If dopamine or its agonists are administered intravenously to humans, PRL levels fall in

normal individuals as well as in most patients with hyperprolactinemia.[166] Although other PIF's have been identified, current evidence supports dopamine as the physiologically significant PIF.

The CNS contains several dopaminergic pathways that differ in distribution and function. Of these, the tuberoinfundibular-dopaminergic (TIDA) system is the one that primarily regulates PRL secretion. The cell bodies of these neurons are located in the arcuate nucleus of the medial basal hypothalamus (Fig. 23–9B), and their terminals project to the ME and pituitary stalk.[165] In some areas of the rat ME the dopamine terminals constitute up to 35 per cent of all terminals, making this one of the most dense projections of a single system in the mammalian brain, suggesting that these terminals subserve particularly important functions.[167] Because there are no direct neural connections to the anterior lobe, dopamine secreted by these terminals is transported to the anterior lobe via the long hypophyseal portal vessels.[168] Dopamine is also present in the posterior lobe of the pituitary in high concentrations, and this source of dopamine appears to play a role in inhibiting PRL secretion.[169] Posterior pituitary dopamine can reach the anterior pituitary lactotrophs via the short portal vessels. Posterior lobectomy elevates basal PRL secretion and abolishes the suckling-induced rise in PRL (Fig. 23–9A).[162] Therefore, dopamine transported via the long portal vessels from the ME and via short portal vessels from the posterior lobe seems quantitatively sufficient to account for the inhibition of spontaneous PRL release.

Dopamine has a series of specific isoreceptors, but only the D2 receptor subtype is present on anterior pituitary cells.[170] The number of D2 receptors is up-regulated by decreases in the level of dopamine reaching the anterior pituitary and appears to be down-regulated by estrogen to a lesser extent.[171] The cytoplasmic domain of the D2 receptor is linked to adenylate cyclase, and dopamine binding at nanomolar concentrations results in decreased adenylate cyclase activity and decreased cAMP accumulation within minutes.[172] Reciprocally, withdrawal of dopamine results in a rapid, significant rise in intracellular cAMP.[163] Lactotrophs, much like neurosecretory cells, exhibit action potentials with an important calcium component. PRL, like a neurotransmitter, is secreted by exocytosis, suggesting a link between the action potential and hormone secretion.[173] Dopamine reduces the action potential discharge from lactotrophs and reduces calcium fluxes across the cell membrane, resulting in decreased intracellular calcium and decreased hormone secretion.[174] Dopamine may also attenuate phosphoinositide levels in the pituitary.[175] Therefore, dopamine mediates its effects through multiple signal transduction pathways.

SHORT FEEDBACK LOOP. PRL secretion cannot be regulated via a traditional long-loop feedback through the peripheral circulation because it is not generally considered to produce a target organ hormone (however, see Synlactin Hypothesis). Instead PRL serves as its own inhibiting factor via an autoregulatory, pituitary-to-hypothalamus, short-loop feedback. PRL binds to PRL receptors in the ME,[176] resulting in increased dopamine synthesis and turnover, which in turn suppress PRL secretion by the pituitary. Elevation of PRL by tumors or pharmacological agents[177] is accompanied by an increase in dopamine, whereas hypophysectomy leads to a decrease in dopamine that can be restored to normal by PRL injections. PRL has also been

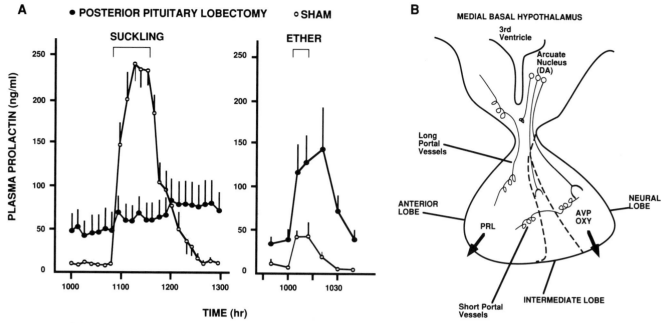

FIGURE 23–9. **The posterior pituitary elaborates a potent PRL-releasing factor.** *A,* Abolishment of the suckling-induced rise in PRL following posterior pituitary lobectomy in the rat. In contrast, the anterior pituitary PRL-secreting response is maintained after the surgery. *B,* Representation of some of the neural and vascular connections within the hypothalamopituitary complex. The role of a PRL-releasing factor from the posterior pituitary/neural lobe has been postulated. It could reach the anterior pituitary via the short portal vessels. (Adapted from Ben-Jonathan N, Arbogast LA, Hyde JF: Neuroendocrine regulation of prolactin release. Progr Neurobiol 33:399–447, 1989. Copyright 1989, Pergamon Press Ltd.)

shown to exert an autoregulatory role on its own secretion at the lactotroph level in vitro, but the physiological significance of this is unclear.[178]

Miscellaneous Factors. An attempt to purify nondopaminergic PRL-inhibiting activity from the hypothalamus resulted in the purification of GABA.[179] GABA receptors are present in the anterior pituitary,[180] GABA is present in the hypophyseal portal system,[181] and GABA inhibits PRL in vitro. However, GABA's potency is 100-fold lower than dopamine's, bringing into question the importance of its physiological role.

The existence of a peptide PIF has been predicted based upon the partial purification of such a factor from the sheep ME.[182] A candidate to fulfill this role is the 56-amino acid peptide encoded by the carboxyl-terminal portion of rat and human pro-GnRH. In the original reports, this GnRH-associated peptide (GAP) inhibits PRL secretion in primary pituitary cultures at a potency comparable to that of dopamine. Antibodies developed after immunization of rabbits with GAP cause uniform elevations in PRL levels.[183] GAP inhibits PRL release in rats in a variety of physiological conditions in which prolactin is elevated, such as stress and lactation.[184] The situation is somewhat different in sheep; although GAP is secreted into the hypophyseal portal blood, it does not affect PRL release.[185] In vitro GAP inhibits PRL release, but recent studies suggest its potency is much less than originally described.[186] Therefore it remains controversial whether GAP is the elusive peptide PIF. Other PIF's include somatostatin, which is active only in the presence of estrogen,[187] and α-MSH.[188] The physiological importance of these PIF's remains to be determined.

PRL-Releasing Factors (PRF's)

The existence of the suckling and copulomimetic induction of acute PRL release, the stress response, and the proestrus PRL surge all argue for the existence of PRF's. Loss of tonic inhibition of PRL release by dissociation of dopamine from its receptor is the most parsimonious explanation. However, it cannot explain all observations, and the dissociation of dopamine from its receptor is likely to work in conjunction with PRF's, not alone.[163]

TRH. The tripeptide TRH was the first identified PRF. TRH induces PRL release by a direct action on the pituitary gland, and the TRH regulation of PRL gene transcription was discussed above. In humans, TRH administered intravenously causes PRL secretion, even at the lowest doses capable of inducing a TSH response.[189] Although levels of TRH in hypophyseal portal blood have been reported to increase in parallel with PRL in several studies,[190] more recent contradictory reports have appeared.[191] TRH is a PRF, but its role in the physiologically important PRL surges remains elusive.

Vasoactive Intestinal Peptide (VIP). VIP was first isolated from intestinal extracts but has subsequently been shown to be present in many sites including hypophyseal portal blood at levels 19-fold over peripheral levels.[192] VIP and its cosynthesized peptide, peptide-histidine-isoleucine (PHI), stimulate PRL release from isolated pituitary glands.[193] VIP and PHI act through a shared binding site to increase PRL mRNA levels, perhaps secondary to the induction of cAMP. Antisera to VIP block basal and stress-induced PRL secretion and alter the profile of the suckling-induced rise.[194] The action of VIP is sluggish, and, unlike TRH, an escape from dopamine inhibition does not increase its effect.[163] The level at which VIP is active remains controversial; some report activity at nanomolar concentrations, others at micromolar—again leaving confusion regarding its physiological significance.

SEROTONIN. Serotonin or its precursor 5-hydroxytryptamine (5-HT) stimulates PRL release in vivo but not in vitro. Two mechanisms have been proposed: reduction in the activity of the TIDA neurons, or stimulation of the release of PRF(s).[162] It has been difficult to distinguish between these possibilities based on current experimental results. 5-HT administration decreases dopamine synthesis in the ME with an associated rise in serum PRL,[195] but paradoxically serotonin still stimulates PRL release when dopamine is infused at high levels.[196]

ADDITIONAL PRF'S. The posterior pituitary was concluded to contain a PRF based upon the observation that posterior pituitary lobectomy abolishes the suckling-induced rise in PRL (Fig. 23–9A) and the nocturnal surge of PRL in early pregnancy without altering basal secretion.[197] Furthermore, extracts from the posterior lobe stimulate PRL release.[162] It has been postulated that this PRF is oxytocin[198] or the 39-amino acid glycopeptide that arises from the carboxyl terminus of the vasopressin-neurophysin precursor,[199] but these conflicting claims remain to be resolved. A large list of additional putative PRF's has been reported in recent years. Among these are β-endorphin, met- and leu-enkephalin, dynorphin, α- and β-neoendorphin, bombesin, substance P, neurotensin, histamine, melatonin, bradykinin, epidermal growth factor, fibroblast growth factor, tumor necrosis factor-α, α-subunit of LH, gastrin, acetylcholine, and others.[160, 161]

Paracrine and Autocrine Regulation

Data supporting cell-to-cell interactions in the regulation of PRL secretion have been accumulating. Initially it was shown that GnRH stimulates PRL release, but only if lactotrophs are co-cultured with gonadotrophs.[200] The mediator for this effect may be angiotensin II because angiotensin II is localized in the gonadotroph and is released in response to GnRH, and high-affinity angiotensin II binding sites have been detected on the lactotroph.[201] Angiotensin II stimulates PRL secretion in vivo, and in vitro angiotensin II is an extremely potent PRF, effective at 1 nM levels.[202] Pituitary folliculostellate cells inhibit PRL secretion when co-cultured with lactotrophs. The identity of the mediator is unknown.[203] Recent data have implicated VIP, which is also located in the anterior pituitary, perhaps in both lactotroph and folliculostellate cells,[204] as an autocrine or paracrine regulator of PRL release because antisera or antagonists to VIP inhibit basal PRL release in dispersed pituitary cells.[205] This effect may be additive to the effect of hypothalamic VIP. Another potential autocrine regulatory factor, galanin, was discussed in the Estrogen section (above). The intrinsic pulsatility of PRL release, thought to originate within the pituitary gland, has been hypothesized to arise as a result of such paracrine or autocrine influences.[153]

PRL ACTIONS

Receptors

The first step in PRL's action is binding to a specific plasma membrane receptor. Specific lactogen receptors have been identified by binding studies in a wide variety of tissues: mammary gland, liver, kidney, adrenals, ovaries, uterus, placenta, testis, prostate, seminal vesicles, hypothalamus, choroid plexus, pancreatic islets, lymphoid tissues, brain, intestine, peripheral blood mononuclear cells, and others. This list includes tissues that are known targets for PRL action and some that are not.[206] The multitude of tissues that bind PRL correlates with the profusion of biological activities attributed to PRL. The PRL receptor has been localized not only to the plasma membrane but also to endosomes, Golgi apparatus, and lysosomes. Furthermore a soluble, highly specific lactogen-binding protein with binding characteristics similar to those of the membrane-bound receptor has been detected in liver, kidney, and mammary gland cytosol.[207] The receptors for PRL and GH are among the few receptors for which the mechanism of postreceptor signal transduction remains unknown. The recent cloning and structural analysis of the PRL and GH receptors should facilitate studies to critically probe their mechanisms.[12]

Receptor Structure

The PRL receptor was initially cloned from rat liver. Analysis of the predicted receptor amino acid structure indicated that it was made up of an extracellular domain of 210 residues, including five cysteines, a transmembrane hydrophobic domain of 24 residues, and a short cytoplasmic domain of 51 residues. Localized regions of high sequence conservation compared with the cloned GH receptor were noted, leading to the conclusion that the PRL and GH receptors, like their respective ligands, constitute a multigene family.[208] This conclusion was solidified by the finding that both receptors are encoded within the same region of chromosome 5 in man and chromosome 15 in mouse.[209] This contrasts with the finding that GH and PRL have been dispersed to separate chromosomes and prompted the suggestion that the divergence of the ligands may have driven the divergence of the receptors. Subsequently, both hormone receptors were shown to belong to a superfamily of hematopoietic receptors that includes the receptors for a large number of cytokines: granulocyte colony-stimulating factor, erythropoietin, granulocyte-macrophage colony-stimulating factor, interferon, IL-2 through IL-7, and gp 130, which share structural similarities in their binding domains but not in their cytoplasmic domains (Fig. 23–10).[210] The relative positions of the four extracellular cysteines are conserved. Also conserved is the primary structure of a subregion within the extracellular region adjacent to the membrane that retains homology to a portion of the cell adhesion molecule fibronectin (Fig. 23–10, FBN). Recent data suggest that a hematopoietic receptor gene lacking its binding domain may be an oncogene (Fig. 23–10, v-mpl),[211] as may be the related erythropoietin receptor when it is constitutively activated by a point muta-

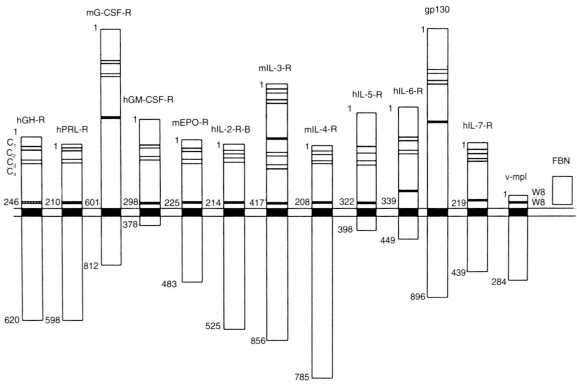

FIGURE 23–10. The members of the hematopoietic-cytokine receptor family that includes the receptors for PRL and GH. Selected amino acids of each receptor are numbered. Homologous regions reside in the extracellular domains, marked at the amino-terminal end by the pairs of cysteines (C1-C4, indicated by thin lines). A common WSXWS motif is indicated by the thick line. The transmembrane regions are in black. (Adapted from Kelly PA, Djiane J, Postel-Vinay M-C, Edery M: The prolactin/growth hormone receptor family. Endocr Rev 12:235–251, 1991; © The Endocrine Society, 1991.)

tion.[212] Whether the related PRL and GH receptors share postreceptor binding activation mechanisms with the hematopoietic receptor family or can be mutated into functional oncogenes is not currently known.

Additional isoforms of the PRL receptor have been cloned subsequent to the initial isolation of the rat liver cDNA. The rabbit mammary gland receptor cDNA predicted a receptor composed of 592 amino acids rather than 291. The difference between the liver and mammary PRL receptors is in the length of their cytoplasmic domains. The long rabbit mammary form is more comparable to the GH receptor, which contains 620 residues. It contains additional segments of sequence similarity to the GH receptor within its cytoplasmic region, although no consensus sequences known to be involved in signal transduction have been found. A human PRL receptor, cloned from the hepatoma cell line HepG2, was found to contain a long cytoplasmic domain.[213] So far, only long receptor forms have been identified in rabbit and human. These data suggested that the two types of intracellular domain might mediate different biological actions.

In contrast to the single form of PRL receptor in humans, the rat PRL receptor family contains considerable complexity. In rat ovary and liver, a long form of receptor with extracellular and transmembrane domains identical to the short form, but with a 357-residue intracellular domain, was cloned.[214] The rat PRL receptor gene contains at least 11 exons, and the eleventh exon appears to encode the short form of the cytoplasmic region, whereas the tenth

exon encodes the long form of the cytoplasmic domain.[12] A short ovarian receptor form was cloned that contains only the extracellular domain and a 20-amino acid unique carboxyl-terminal extension, suggesting that it might be a soluble PRL-binding protein.[215] That such a soluble PRL-binding protein may be ubiquitous is suggested by the finding that a PRL-binding protein has been immunoprecipitated by a monoclonal antibody against the PRL receptor from rabbit breast milk.[216] The rat Nb2 lymphoma cell line was found to encode a 393-residue receptor that lacks amino acids 323 through 520 of the cytoplasmic domain of the long form of the rat receptor. This receptor displays a 3.3-fold higher affinity for PRL than the long form and is the product of a mutated PRL receptor gene lacking the codons for these amino acids.[217] Not all of the receptor isoforms have been characterized yet, and from the data so far it appears that significant species specificity will emerge. These data strongly suggest that complex alternative splicing of the rodent PRL receptor gene transcript occurs. The physiological role of the PRL receptor isoforms is unclear but should prove to be very interesting.

Receptor Regulation

PRL receptor levels are differentially regulated depending upon the tissue that is studied. The liver contains the highest concentration of PRL receptors, although their function is unclear. PRL has long been considered to upregulate its own receptor, although it has been suggested that this effect may reflect induction of serum PRL anti-bodies in some experiments[218] and uncovering of cryptic receptor sites in others.[219] During development, PRL receptor mRNA is not detectable by Northern analysis until about 21 days of age. There is an increase at 40 days, corresponding to puberty; then levels stabilize. However, PRL-binding sites continue to increase in the liver after 40 days, whereas mRNA levels are stable, suggesting that regulation of receptor levels is both transcriptional and post-transcriptional during development. Similarly, estrogen injections increase receptor levels by action at both transcriptional and post-transcriptional levels in vivo.[220] The regulation of receptor mRNA levels was studied in rat liver and mammary gland during pregnancy and lactation. In liver, there is a marked increase in all transcripts at day 19 of pregnancy, followed by a fall to very low levels at the onset of lactation. In the breast, levels increase on day 21 of gestation and continue to increase throughout lactation, indicating differential receptor gene regulation in the breast, perhaps uniquely induced by the decline of progesterone at the end of pregnancy.[221] The short form of the receptor was noted to predominate in rat mammary gland (70 per cent) as in liver. The two receptors have been compared for their relative abilities to stimulate milk protein gene transcription by co-transfecting either receptor with a chloramphenicol acetyl transferase (CAT) reporter gene under the transcriptional control of the milk protein β-lactoglobulin gene promoter. Only the long form of the receptor was able to stimulate CAT activity in the presence of PRL in serum-free medium, establishing that the long form of the receptor is specifically involved in milk protein gene transcription.[222] The mutant Nb2 cell form of the receptor is reported to stimulate reporter gene transcription as well.[12] The short form of the receptor was noted to be more similar to receptors that act as transporters, such as the transferrin receptor and the LDL receptor.[222] Furthermore, PRL has been detected in a number of bodily fluids, including milk, as noted previously. Therefore it has been postulated that the short form of the receptor may serve to internalize PRL into certain cell types, whereas the long form may be critical to the transcriptional activation of PRL-responsive genes.

Human GH, but not nonprimate GH's, binds with high affinity to the PRL receptor. The detailed study of the binding of hGH to its receptors has provided a number of conclusions that may be applicable to all of the members of this receptor supergene family. The binding affinity of hGH to the extracellular domain of the PRL receptor increases 8000-fold with the addition of zinc. This is due to the co-chelation of a single zinc molecule by three amino acid residues in hGH and one residue in the PRL receptor. Substitutions of these three residues in subprimate GH's and the hGH variant with nonchelating amino acids[223] explain their decreased affinity for the PRL receptor.[224] Zinc is also required for CS to bind to the PRL receptor, but not for PRL itself to bind. The disulfide bonding pattern of the extracellular domain of the GH receptor involves the sequential pairwise association of its six extracellular domain cysteines. Mutational analysis of the hGH-binding domain of the GH receptor demonstrates that ligand binding depends on the spatial association of several discontinuous regions.[225] A single GH molecule forms a 1:2 complex with the extracellular domain of two GH receptors via a two-step sequential binding reaction. Remarkably the same region of the receptor binds to two distinct domains of GH.[226] The dimerization of the receptor that results has been demonstrated to be necessary for signal transduction to occur. This was further demonstrated by the finding that certain monoclonal antibodies against the receptor act as agonists, whereas their monovalent fragments, unable to promote dimerization, act as antagonists (Fig. 23–11).[227] Earlier data demonstrated that certain bivalent anti-PRL receptor antibodies mediate an increased synthesis of β-casein in primed mammary glands in vitro and in vivo. Monovalent antibodies do not mediate a biological effect,[228] strongly suggesting that the PRL receptor also requires dimerization for at least some of its activities. These detailed studies of the hGH receptor may foreshadow similar conclusions for the related PRL receptor. For example, mutational analysis of the PRL receptor confirms that its extracellular cysteines are necessary for ligand binding. Deletion of 55 of the 57 intracellular amino acids of the short receptor isoform increases ligand-binding affinity by five-fold and decreases the rate of receptor internalization.[229]

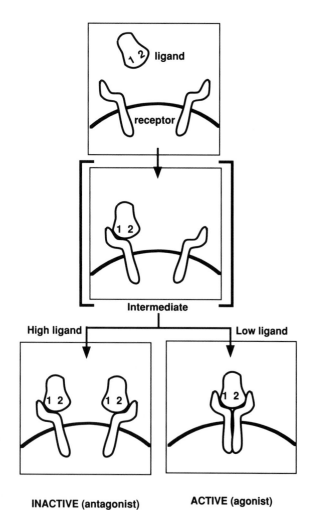

FIGURE 23–11. **The two-step binding and dimerization model based on studies of the GH receptor.** The ligand binds to the first receptor molecule, then to the second, resulting in the active, dimerized receptor. In the presence of excess ligand, the receptor does not dimerize and is not activated. (Reproduced from Fuh G, Cunningham BC, Fukunaga R, et al: Rational design of potent antagonists to the human growth hormone receptor. Science 256:1677–1680, 1992. Copyright 1992 by the AAAS.)

Signal Transduction

Because PRL has such a diversity of effects and receptor isoforms, it seems unlikely that a single mode of signal transduction suffices for all of its bioactivities. The earliest postreceptor binding events in the rat Nb2 lymphoma cell line appear to include the activation of Na^+/H^+ exchange via a plasma membrane antiporter. This was based on the finding that PRL-induced mitogenesis in this cell line is blocked by amiloride, an inhibitor of the antiporter.[230] G proteins may modulate PRL action in Nb2 cells based upon the responses to cholera toxin and pertussis toxin.[231] The Nb2 PRL receptor was shown to be associated with G proteins by chemical cross-linking. Both G_i and G_s proteins have been detected immunologically in Nb2 cells, and hGH acting at the PRL receptor has been shown to enhance pertussis toxin–stimulated ADP-ribosylation of G_i in the Nb2 cell membranes.[232] These data strongly suggest that the PRL receptor may mediate its signal through G proteins in the Nb2 cell, although perhaps not through adenylate cyclase activation.[233] It is unclear at this time whether the PRL receptor is phosphorylated, although rapid stimulation of tyrosine kinase activity is detected after PRL binding to Nb2 cells, resulting in the phosphorylation of several cellular proteins. The sizes of these phosphorylated substrates suggest that the PRL receptor itself is not phosphorylated.[234] The early transcriptional activation of several growth-related genes has been identified in PRL-stimulated Nb2 cells. These include c-myc, actin, interferon-regulatory factor 1, ornithine decarboxylase, and a heat shock protein 70 homologue.[235] How these genes orchestrate the proliferative response is unknown.

Synlactin Hypothesis

It has long been known that PRL as well as GH can stimulate the secretion of bioactive somatomedins from liver in vivo and in vitro. The PRL- and GH-induced somatomedins differ in that those stimulated by GH enhance linear bone growth.[236] A factor has been identified that is secreted in response to PRL from the livers of rats, mice, pigeons, fish, and turtles—representatives of the five major vertebrate classes—that augments the mitogenic effects of PRL in the pigeon crop sac assay.[237] Direct delivery of PRL to the liver in vivo via the hepatic portal vein of hypophysectomized rats has shown that this hepatic response to PRL is physiologically important in PRL's mammotropic but not its galactopoietic actions.[238] A similar factor has been reported in human serum that enhances PRL-stimulated mitogenesis in the Nb2 lymphoma bioassay.[239] In each case the factor increases PRL's activity in the respective bioassay. Because of this synergizing effect with PRL, the factor has been named synlactin.[237] It is postulated that synlactin may be identical to the PRL-induced somatomedin because the hormones of the IGF family such as proinsulin, relaxin, and somatomedin C are slightly synergistic with PRL in the crop sac bioassay.[240] Recently the action of ovine PRL in stimulating hepatic IGF-I was confirmed. Following an intraperitoneal injection of ovine PRL to hypophysectomized rats, a 15-fold increase in IGF-I gene expression could be detected. These rats demonstrated a small but significant weight gain over the 10-day period of administration.

These experiments indicate that PRL has intrinsic somatogenic activity in the rat, although it was not determined whether this effect was exerted via binding to the PRL receptor.[241] Taken together, these results suggest that this IGF-I and synlactin might be identical.

Recently it was demonstrated that mouse PRL induces a novel mouse IGF-binding protein in mammary epithelial cells significantly more efficiently than does mouse GH itself. IGF-I demonstrated an additive effect on the expression of this 29-kDa IGF-binding protein, and it was postulated that this lactogen-induced IGF-binding protein may mediate the effects of IGF's on lactogen-dependent growth and development of the mammary gland during gestation.[242] There are IGF-I receptors on mammary gland membranes, and IGF-I has been demonstrated to enhance PRL-induced lactogenesis in the rabbit[243] as well as mammary cell mitogenesis in vitro.[244] It remains unclear whether IGF-I itself is produced locally in the breast.

Reproductive Actions

Unique among hormones of the adenohypophysis, PRL did not specialize early in vertebrate evolution. Instead, it is used by different species to control a wide variety of functions, many of which are species specific. From comparative studies, osmoregulation, growth, and development may be the most fundamental actions of the hormone. In adult humans, PRL's role is incompletely delineated but seems to be involved primarily with reproductive functions.

Male

PRL receptors are present in the Leydig cells of the testis, the prostate, and seminal vesicles of the rat, suggesting a direct, local role in male reproduction. PRL increases and maintains the concentration of LH receptors on the Leydig cell membrane, increasing the sensitivity of the testis to LH stimulation and therefore helping to sustain testosterone levels.[245] PRL potentiates the effects of androgens on the growth and secretory activity of male accessory glands in the rodent, as well as displaying androgen-independent, direct effects.[246] PRL in seminal fluid stimulates glucose and fructose utilization and influences sperm motility and fertilizing capacity.[247] PRL also affects male reproduction indirectly. Elevated PRL levels may inhibit copulatory behavior in male rats, causing them to take longer to ejaculate than control males owing to slower pacing of copulation.[248] A decrease in the frequency of erections has also been noted.[249] The effects of increased PRL levels is postulated to be secondary to dopamine depletion in subregions of the hypothalamus.[250] Evidence remains circumstantial for a role of endogenous PRL, although it has been reported that PRL is released in male rats after exposure to an estrous female, even in the absence of copulation.[251] However, disorders that produce chronically elevated levels of PRL in men result in a decrease in libido and potency and in some cases hypogonadism. These symptoms are reversible when PRL levels are lowered but usually not reversible with testosterone treatment alone.[252]

Female

OVARY. The role that PRL plays in ovarian function is complex, differing among species and within each species during various stages of reproductive function. The frequent development of amenorrhea in women with hyperprolactinemia demonstrates the critical role of PRL in human ovarian function. In contrast, hypoprolactinemia does not appear to interfere with cyclicity. There is a preovulatory PRL surge in rodents and ruminants but not in primates. This appears to be due to the rising titer of estrogen at this time and appears to require the posterior pituitary.[253] PRL receptors are present in the luteinized rat ovary. PRL has an important role in maintaining the corpus luteum in the rat, but not in humans, during early pregnancy. This includes the stimulation of luteal cell growth and progesterone secretion by the corpus luteum. PRL does this by maintaining appropriate numbers of LH receptors on the developing corpus luteum, thereby enhancing its steroidogenic response to LH.[254] PRL downregulates annexin production in the corpus luteum, and annexins (or lipocortins) inhibit phospholipase A2, an important enzyme in prostaglandin synthesis, and prostaglandin in turn decreases progesterone biosynthesis in the ovary.[255]

In women, an optimal window of PRL levels appears to be necessary for normal corpus luteum function. For example, lactation impairs follicular development in all mammals. Paradoxically, high PRL levels suppress progesterone synthesis by the ovary and decrease induction of aromatase, resulting in decreased estrogen production.[256] Such a bell-shaped response curve is characteristic of many of PRL's actions and is reminiscent of the antagonistic properties of high levels of GH in preventing receptor dimerization and action (Fig. 23–11). These effects could result in direct inhibition of ovarian function, but hyperprolactinemia also acts centrally on the hypothalamus to decrease the frequency and amplitude of LH pulses, possibly at the level of the GnRH pulse generator.[257]

BREAST. PRL is essential to the initiation and maintenance of lactation, as originally demonstrated by the fact that hypophysectomy in rodents inhibits lactation and results in reduced mammary cell number.[258] Contrary to the original concept that PRL was responsible for both actions, it is now becoming clear that the mammary mitogenic effect is due to GH, not PRL. This was demonstrated in primates when selective inhibition of PRL with ergot drugs did not adversely affect full mammary development. However, both rat GH (nonlactogenic) and hGH were demonstrated to be 10- to 20-fold more potent mammary mitogens, acting perhaps through a putative mammary gland IGF-I.[259] When nursing rhesus mothers were treated with GH, their neonatal offspring had significantly greater body weight gain than controls, and it was concluded that this was due to increased mammary gland development, the mammotropic rather than the galactopoietic actions of GH.[260] In fact, precocious mammary gland development and lactogenesis have been noted in transgenic mice expressing GH locally in the mammary gland in the absence of pregnancy.[261] This suggests that the local expression or internalization of a lactogen and/or somatogen may be critical to mammary development and lactogenesis.

PRL specifically induces milk protein synthesis in mammary explants and cultured breast cells by binding to its receptors on the mammary epithelial cell.[262] Only the long form of the PRL receptor can activate transcription of milk protein genes. A 20-fold increase in the number of PRL receptors occurs at parturition, indicating that the breast becomes more sensitive to PRL at that time.[263] PRL- and GH-binding proteins have been detected in milk.[216] That these hormones in milk may remain bioactive after transfer to the neonate has been suggested by the finding of PRL receptors in neonatal gut and the stimulation of neonatal pituitary lactotrophs by a 6000-Da milk peptide.[264, 265] There is extensive turnover of phospholipids in the breast during lactation, reflecting the exocrine nature of the mammary gland and the fact that a major component of breast milk is triglycerides surrounded by apical plasma membrane. PRL, in conjunction with insulin and cortisone, increases the rate of fatty acid synthesis, maintains the activity of breast lipoprotein lipase, and stimulates phospholipid biosynthesis in mouse mammary explants.[263, 266] PRL mediates certain immune events in the breast. It appears to enhance the specific migration of IgA lymphoblasts from the gut-associated lymphatic tissue to the mammary gland during pregnancy. Progeny of these cells produce IgA antibodies, which are then transported across the mammary epithelium into milk.[267]

Osmoregulation

One of the most basic functions of PRL throughout the animal kingdom is its role in osmoregulation. During the migration of fish from salt to fresh water, pituitary PRL serves the critical role of adapting the gills and kidneys to conserve salt and maintain mineral homeostasis. Additional targets for the osmoregulatory effects of PRL in fish and tetrapods include the gut, urinary bladder, and skin.[1] In mammals the role of PRL in osmoregulation is less clear-cut. Early PRL preparations were contaminated with vasopressin, making experiments using these preparations difficult to interpret.

Evidence for renal synthesis of PRL and the presence of PRL receptors in the human kidney suggest a local role in fluid and electrolyte balance. PRL binds to the proximal tubules of the kidney[268] and has been detected in the cytoplasm of proximal tubular epithelium. Studies in response to PRL infusion via kidney micropuncture in the rat have reported a decrease in water, sodium, and potassium excretion without renal hemodynamic changes. No alteration of proximal tubular reabsorption could be detected, suggesting that the principal site of PRL action may be distal to this point.[269] The sodium-conserving effect of PRL is exaggerated in the dehydrated state.[270] PRL may also modulate the chloride ion content of human sweat,[271] and alter the action of mineralocorticoids on the kidney by interacting with the renin-angiotensin system. Angiotensin II receptors are present on pituitary lactotrophs, and angiotensin II stimulates PRL release from cultured rat pituitary cells, suggesting the presence of a feedback loop.

A role for PRL in amniotic fluid osmoregulation has been proposed. This is based upon studies in which fetal placental membranes were stretched across diffusion chambers. PRL could decrease diffusion of water from the fetal to the maternal side of the membranes, but only when PRL was added to the fetal side. This effect was blocked by an antibody to PRL and could not be mimicked by GH or human CS.[272] Such a decrease in amniotic fluid diffusion would prevent dehydration of the fetus at times when amniotic fluid is hypotonic. Because the first action of PRL in fetal life may be osmoregulation, and osmoregulation is a main function of PRL in lower species, it has been proposed that during the development of individual higher vertebrates, the actions of PRL may "recapitulate its phylogeny."[273]

The osmoregulatory effects of PRL in the rat are also exerted on the intestinal mucosa. PRL administration stimulates absorption of fluid and monovalent and divalent ions by the rat small intestine.[274] The increase in intestinal calcium absorption that occurs in the pregnant rat does not depend on vitamin D and may instead be a response to the elevated PRL levels of gestation. Vitamin D–deficient, hypocalcemic rats, when injected with PRL in vivo, increase their serum calcium by eight hours. Examination of calcium transport across everted gut sacs indicates an increase in calcium transport within four hours of PRL injection, peaking at eight hours.[275] One of the main effects of PRL on ionic fluxes in the mammal may be this effect on calcium retention.

Immune Regulation

Involvement of pituitary hormones in immune regulation was first proposed as early as 1930, when hypophysectomy was noted to cause thymic involution in rats. This effect was reversed by implantation of GH3 cells secreting GH and PRL.[276] Hypophysectomized rats display an impaired immune response; they do not develop contact sensitivity to dinitrochlorbenzene, and they do not form antibodies appropriately in response to injected sheep red blood cells. In addition, DNA synthesis in their lymphocytes is profoundly decreased. Daily treatment with either GH or PRL restores immunological competence and promotes DNA synthesis and growth of lymphoid tissue.[277] Blocking pituitary PRL release with bromocriptine reduces lymphoctye reactivity in the in vitro graft-versus-host reaction[278] and inhibits macrophage interaction, T-cell proliferation, and cytokine production in rodents.[279] In animal models of disease states, bromocriptine administration suppresses the postpartum exacerbation of collagen-induced arthritis,[280] autoimmune uveitis,[281] and systemic lupus erythematosus.[282] In addition, PRL levels have been noted to increase just before transplantation rejection episodes.[283] Cyclosporine A, an immunosuppressive agent used to limit transplant rejection, may function by blocking PRL action and by antagonizing its normal functions on the immune system.[284] It has therefore been concluded that PRL stimulates humoral and cell-mediated immunity and that lymphocytes are an important target for PRL in vivo. The elevated PRL levels of pregnancy and lactation have also been reported to suppress immunity, as has hyperprolactinemia in situations other than pregnancy.[285]

The mechanism of action of PRL on the immune system has been studied in vitro. It is known that the Nb2 lymphoma cell possesses PRL receptors and responds to PRL with cell division. Recently it was demonstrated that normal lymphocytes also proliferate in response to PRL and that PRL induces the expression of the IL-2 receptor, DNA synthesis, and IL-2 production in the splenic lymphoctyes of ovariectomized but not estrogen-treated rats.[286] Addition of antibody against PRL to cultured lymphocytes prevents their proliferation in response to a series of mitogens.[287]

Secretion of PRL-like immunoreactive proteins from murine lymphocytes has been reported,[288] as well as secretion by the blast cells of a patient with acute leukemia.[289] A Burkitt lymphoma cell line, sfRamos, appears to secrete a 29-kDa PRL-related protein, which the cell line is dependent upon for serum-free proliferation.[53] Synthesis of PRL by normal lymphoid cells was recently confirmed. It was found that PRL mRNA could be detected in primary human mononuclear cells and that these transcripts originate from the alternative upstream promoter and exon also utilized in the decidua (see Fig. 23–1, exon Id). In the same study, PRL protein was detected by metabolic labeling of the mononuclear cells. In addition, PRL receptor transcripts were found to be ubiquitously present in B cells, T cells, and monocytes. It was suggested from these data that PRL has an autocrine/paracrine effect on immune cell function (Fig. 23–12). PRL could not be detected in rat mononuclear cells, suggesting that the expression of PRL in immune cells may be a species-specific phenomenon.[97] In the murine T-cell line, L-2, IL-2 stimulation results in the translocation of PRL from the culture media to the nucleus and the translocation of PRL receptor to the nuclear periphery, whereas anti-PRL antiserum results in a dose-dependent decrease in L-2 proliferation. This was interpreted as indicating that nuclear PRL is necessary for cell cycle progression.[290] Perhaps uptake from the media occurs in species that do not express PRL endogenously in their lymphocytes. To test this hypothesis, the Nb2 cell line was transfected with a chimeric PRL construct lacking its own signal peptide sequence but containing the DNA sequences directing the nuclear localization of SV40 large T antigen. In this transfected cell line PRL could be detected only in the nucleus. This cell line proliferated continuously in response to IL-2 stimulation in the presence of antiserum to PRL, whereas controls transfected with the PRL gene plus its signal peptide did not. It was concluded that nuclear PRL is necessary for IL-2 stimulated proliferation of rat Nb2 cells and that PRL can function without binding to its cell surface receptor.[13] In the L-2 cell line, it has been proposed that PRL may be a necessary complement to IL-2 for cell cycle progression into S phase.[291] It appears clear that PRL modulates immune function, but the full spectrum of its activity remains to be elucidated.

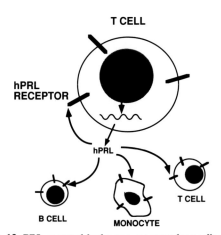

FIGURE 23–12. **PRL secreted by human mononuclear cells may have an autocrine/paracrine role in the function of immune cells.** (From Pellegrini I, Lebrun J-J, Ali S, Kelly PA: Expression of prolactin and its receptor in human lymphoid cells. Mol Endocrinol 6:1023–1031, 1992; © The Endocrine Society, 1992.)

REFERENCES

1. Nicoll CS: Physiological actions of prolactin. *In* Knobil E, Sawyer WH (eds): Handbook of Physiology, section 7: Endocrinology, Vol IV, part 2, pp 253–292. Washington, DC, American Physiological Society, 1974.

2. Stricker P, Grueter R: Action du lobe anterieur de l'hypophyse sur la montee laiteuse. Compt Rend Soc Biol (Paris) 99:1978–1980, 1928.

3. Riddle O, Braucher PF: Studies on the physiology of reproduction in birds. XXX. Control of the special secretion of the crop-gland in pigeons by anterior pituitary hormone. Am J Physiol 97:617–627, 1931.

4. Riddle O, Bates RW, Dykshorn SW: The preparation, identification and assay of prolactin—a hormone of the anterior pituitary. Am J Physiol 105:191–206, 1933.

5. Riddle O, Bates RW, Dykshorn SW: A new hormone of the anterior pituitary. Proc Soc Exp Biol Med 29:1212–1215, 1932.

6. Lewis UJ, Singh RNP, Seavey BK: Human prolactin: Isolation and some properties. Biochem Biophys Res Commun 44:1169–1176, 1971.

7. Hwang P, Guyda H, Friesen H: Purification of human prolactin. J Biol Chem 247:1955–1958, 1972.

8. Cooke NE, Coit D, Weiner RI, et al: Structure of cloned DNA complementary to rat prolactin messenger RNA. J Biol Chem 255:6502–6510, 1980.

9. Cooke NE, Baxter JD: Structural analysis of the prolactin gene suggests a separate origin for its 5'-end. Nature 297:603–606, 1982.

10. Leong DA, Frawley LS, Neill JD: Neuroendocrine control of prolactin secretion. Annu Rev Physiol 45:109–127, 1983.

11. Rosenfeld MG: POU-domain transcription factors: Pou-er-ful developmental regulators. Genes Dev 5:897–907, 1991.

12. Kelly PA, Djiane J, Postel-Vinay M-C, Edery M: The prolactin/growth hormone receptor family. Endocr Rev 12:235–251, 1991.

13. Clevenger CV, Altmann SW, Prystowsky MB: Requirement of nuclear prolactin for interleukin-2 stimulated proliferation of T lymphocytes. Science 253:77–79, 1991.

14. Niall HD, Hogan ML, Sauer R, et al: Sequences of pituitary and placental lactogenic and growth hormone: Evolution from a primordial peptide by gene reduplication. Proc Natl Acad Sci USA 68:866–869, 1971.

15. Cooke NE, Coit D, Shine J, et al: Human prolactin: cDNA structural analysis and evolutionary comparisons. J Biol Chem 256:4007–4016, 1981.

16. Owerbach D, Rutter WJ, Cooke NE, et al: The prolactin gene is located on chromosome 6 in humans. Science 212:815–816, 1981.

17. Agellon LB, Davies SL, Chen TT, Powers DA: Structure of a fish (rainbow trout) growth hormone gene and its evolutionary implications. Proc Natl Acad Sci USA 85:5136–5140, 1988.

18. Takayama Y, Rand-Weaver M, Kawauchi H, Ono M: Gene structure of chum salmon somatolactin, a presumed pituitary hormone of the growth hormone/prolactin family. Mol Endocrinol 5:778–786, 1991.

19. Cooke NE, Jones BK, Urbanek M, et al: Placental expression and function of the human growth hormone gene cluster. *In* Soares MJ, Handwerger S, Talamantes F (eds): Trophoblast Cells: Pathways for Maternal-Embryonic Communication. New York, Springer-Verlag, 1993.

20. Soares MJ, Faria TN, Roby KF, Deb S: Pregnancy and the prolactin family of hormones: Coordination of anterior pituitary, uterine, and placental expression. Endocr Rev 12:402–423, 1991.

21. Deb S, Faria TN, Roby KF, et al: Identification and characterization of a new member of the prolactin family: Placental lactogen-I variant. J Biol Chem 266:1605–1610, 1991.

22. Duckworth ML, Peden LM, Friesen HG: Isolation of a novel prolactin-like cDNA clone from developing rat placenta. J Biol Chem 261:10879–10884, 1986.

23. Duckworth ML, Peden LM, Friesen HG: A third prolactin-like cDNA clone from developing rat placenta: Complementary deoxyribonucleic acid sequence and partial structure of the gene. Mol Endocrinol 2:912–920, 1988.

24. Ogilvie S, Duckworth ML, Larkin LH, et al: De novo synthesis and secretion of prolactin-like protein-B by rat placental explants. Endocrinology 126:2561–2566, 1990.

25. Deb S, Roby KF, Faria TN, et al: Identification and immunochemical characterization of a major placental secretory protein related to the prolactin–growth hormone family, prolactin-like protein-C. Endocrinology 128:3066–3072, 1991.

26. Jayatilak PG, Glaser LA, Basuray R, et al: Identification and characterization of a prolactin-like hormone produced by the rat decidual tissue. Proc Natl Acad Sci USA 82:217–221, 1985.

27. Croze F, Kennedy TG, Schroedter IC, Friesen HG: Expression of rat prolactin-like protein B in deciduoma of pseudopregnant rat and in decidua during early pregnancy. Endocrinology 127:2665–2674, 1990.

28. Ogilvie S, Buhn WC, Olsen JA, Shiverick KT: Identification of a novel family of growth hormone–related proteins secreted by rat placenta. Endocrinology 126:3271–3273, 1990.

29. Gaddy-Kurten D, Hickey GJ, Fey GH, et al: Hormonal regulation and tissue-specific localization of α_2-macroglobulin in rat ovarian follicles and corpora lutea. Endocrinology 125:2985–2995, 1989.

30. Krawnow JS, Hickey GJ, Richards JS: Regulation of aromatase mRNA and estradiol biosynthesis in rat ovarian granulosa and luteal cells by prolactin. Mol Endocrinol 4:13–21, 1990.

31. Wilder EL, Linzer DIH: Expression of multiple proliferin genes in mouse cells. Mol Cell Biol 6:3283–3286, 1986.

32. Linzer DIH, Nathans D: Growth-related changes in specific mRNAs of cultured mouse cells. Proc Natl Acad Sci USA 80:4271–4275, 1983.

33. Linzer DIH, Lee S-J, Ogren L, et al: Identification of proliferin mRNA and protein in mouse placenta. Proc Natl Acad Sci USA 82:4356–4359, 1985.

34. Lee S-J, Talamantes F, Wilder E, et al: Trophoblastic giant cells of the mouse placenta as the site of proliferin synthesis. Endocrinology 122:1761–1768, 1988.

35. Colosi P, Swiergiel JJ, Wilder EL, et al: Characterization of proliferin-related protein. Mol Endocrinol 2:579–586, 1988.

36. Lee S-J, Nathans D: Proliferin secreted by cultured cells binds to mannose 6-phosphate receptors. J Biol Chem 263:3521–3527, 1988.

37. Wilder EL, Linzer DIH: Participation of multiple factors, including proliferin, in the inhibition of myogenic differentiation. Mol Cell Biol 9:430–441, 1989.

38. Emanuele NV, Jurgens JK, Halloran MM, et al: The rat prolactin gene is expressed in brain tissue: Detection of normal and alternatively spliced prolactin messenger RNA. Mol Endocrinol 6:35–42, 1992.

39. DiMattia GE, Gellersen B, Duckworth ML, Friesen HG: Human prolactin gene expression: The use of an alternative noncoding exon in decidua and the IM-9-P3 lymphoblast cell line. J Biol Chem 265:16412–16421, 1990.

40. Mittra I: A novel "cleaved" prolactin in the rat pituitary. II, In vivo mammary mitogenic activity of its N-terminal 16K moiety. Biochem Biophys Res Commun 95:1760–1767, 1980.

41. Casabiell X, Robertson MC, Friesen HG, Casanueva FF: Cleaved prolactin and its 16K fragment are generated by an acid protease. Endocrinology 125:1967–1972, 1989.

42. Clapp C: Analysis of the proteolytic cleavage of prolactin by the mammary gland and liver of the rat: Characterization of the cleaved and 16K forms. Endocrinology 121:2055–2064, 1987.

43. Baldocchi RA, Tan L, Nicoll CS: Processing of rat prolactin by rat tissue explants and serum in vitro. Endocrinology 130:1653–1659, 1992.

44. Clapp C, Weiner RI: A specific, high affinity, saturable binding site for the 16-kilodalton fragment of prolactin on capillary endothelial cells. Endocrinology 130:1380–1386, 1992.

45. Lewis UJ, Singh RNP, Sinha YN, Vanderlaan WP: Glycosylated human prolactin. Endocrinology 116:359–363, 1985.

46. Lewis UJ, Singh RNP, Lewis LJ: Two forms of glycosylated human prolactin have different pigeon crop sac–stimulating activities. Endocrinology 124:1558–1563, 1989.

47. Markoff E, Sigel MB, Lacour N, et al: Glycosylation selectively alters the biological activity of prolactin. Endocrinology 123:1303–1306, 1988.

48. Liu JH, Lee DW, Markoff E: Differential release of prolactin variants in postpartum and early follicular phase women. J Clin Endocrinol Metab 71:605–610, 1990.

49. Oetting WS, Tuazon PT, Traugh JA, Walker AM: Phosphorylation of prolactin. J Biol Chem 261:1649–1652, 1986.

50. Krown KA, Wang Y-F, Ho TWC, et al: Prolactin isoform 2 as an autocrine growth factor for GH3 cells. Endocrinology 131:595–602, 1992.

51. Sinha YN, Jacobsen BP: Structural and immunologic evidence for a small molecular weight ("21K") variant of prolactin. Endocrinology 123:1364–1370, 1988.

52. Estes PA, Cooke NE, Liebhaber SA: A native RNA secondary structure controls alternative splice-site selection and generates two growth hormone isoforms. J Biol Chem 267:14902–14908, 1992.

53. Baglia LA, Cruz D, Shaw JE: An Epstein-Barr virus-negative Burkitt lymphoma cell line (sfRamos) secretes a prolactin-like protein during continuous growth in serum-free medium. Endocrinology 128:2266–2272, 1991.

53a. Lytras A, Quan N, Vrontakis ME, et al: Growth hormone expression in human Burkitt lymphoma serum-free Ramas cell line. Endocrinology 132:620–628, 1993.

54. Andersen AN, Pedersen H, Djursing H, et al: Bioactivity of prolactin in a woman with an excess of large molecular size prolactin, persistent hyperprolactinemia and spontaneous conception. Fertil Steril 38:625–628, 1982.

55. Jackson RD, Wortsman J, Malarkey WB: Persistence of large molecular weight prolactin secretion during pregnancy in women with macroprolactinemia and its presence in fetal cord blood. J Clin Endocrinol Metab 68:1046–1050, 1989.

56. Nelson C, Albert VR, Elsholtz HP, et al: Activation of cell-specific expression of rat growth hormone and prolactin genes by a common transcription factor. Science 239:1400–1405, 1988.

57. Ingraham HA, Chen R, Mangalam HJ, et al: A tissue-specific transcription factor containing a homeodomain specifies a pituitary phenotype. Cell 55:519–529, 1988.

58. Bodner M, Castrillo J-L, Theill LE, et al: The pituitary-specific transcription factor GHF-1 is a homeobox-containing protein. Cell 55:505–518, 1988.

59. Castrillo J-L, Theill LE, Karin M: Function of the homeodomain protein GHF1 in pituitary cell proliferation. Science 253:197–199, 1991.

60. Supowit SC, Ramsey T, Thompson EB: Extinction of prolactin gene expression in somatic cell hybrids is correlated with the repression of the pituitary-specific trans-activator GHF-1/Pit-1. Mol Endocrinol 6:786–792, 1992.

61. Triputti P, Guerin SL, Moore DD: Two mechanisms for the extinction of gene expression in hybrid cell lines. Science 241:1205–1207, 1988.

62. Herr W, Sturm RA, Clerc RG, et al: The POU-domain: Large conserved region in the mammalian Pit-1, oct-2, oct-2, and Caenorhabditis elegans unc-86 gene products. Genes Dev 2:1513–1516, 1988.

63. Simmons DM, Voos JW, Ingraham HA, et al: Pituitary cell phenotypes involve cell-specific Pit-1 mRNA translation and synergistic interactions with other classes of transcription factors. Genes Dev 4:695–711, 1990.

64. Behringer RR, Mathews LS, Palmiter RD, Brinster RL: Dwarf mice produced by genetic ablation of growth hormone-expressing cells. Genes Dev 2:453–460, 1988.

65. Borelli E, Heyman RA, Arias C, et al: Transgenic mice with inducible dwarfism. Nature 339:538–541, 1989.

66. McCormick A, Brady H, Fukushima J, Karin M: The pituitary-specific regulatory gene GHF1 contains a minimal cell type-specific promoter centered around its TATA box. Genes Dev 4:1490–1503, 1991.

67. Camper SA, Saunders TL, Katz RW, Reeves RH: The Pit-1 transcription factor gene is a candidate for the murine Snell dwarf mutation. Genomics 8:586–590, 1990.

68. Li S, Crenshaw EB, Rawson EJ, et al: Dwarf locus mutants lacking three pituitary cell types result from mutations in the POU-domain gene Pit-1. Nature 347:528–533, 1990.

69. Buckwalter MS, Katz RW, Camper SA: Localization of the panhypopituitary dwarf mutation (df) on mouse chromosome 11 in an intersubspecific backcross. Genomics 10:515–526, 1991.

70. Tatsumi K, Kiyoshi M, Notomi T, et al: Cretinism with combined hormone deficiency caused by a mutation in the Pit-1 gene. Nature Genetics 1:56–58, 1992.

71. Pfäffle RW, Di Mattia GE, Parks JS, et al: Mutation of the POU-specific domain of Pit-1 and hypopituitarism without pituitary hypoplasia. Science 257:1118–1121, 1992.

71a. Radovick S, Nations M, Du Y, et al: A mutation in the homeodomain of Pit-1 responsible for combined pituitary hormone deficiency. Science 257:1115–1118, 1992.

72. Waterman ML, Adler S, Nelson C, et al: A single domain of the estrogen receptor confers deoxyribonucleic acid binding and transcriptional activation of the rat prolactin gene. Mol Endocrinol 2:14–21, 1988.

73. Day RN, Koike S, Kakai M, et al: Both Pit-1 and the estrogen receptor are required for estrogen responsiveness of the rat prolactin gene. Mol Endocrinol 4:1964–1971, 1990.

74. Camper SA, Yao YAS, Rottman FAM: Hormonal regulation of the bovine prolactin promoter in rat pituitary tumor cells. J Biol Chem 260:12246–12251, 1985.

75. Stanley F: Transcriptional regulation of prolactin gene expression by

76. Day RN, Maurer RA: Thyroid hormone–responsive elements of the prolactin gene: Evidence for both positive and negative regulation. Mol Endocrinol 3:931–938, 1989.

77. Keech CA, Gutierrez-Hartmann A: Analysis of rat prolactin promoter sequences that mediate pituitary-specific and 3′,5′-cyclic adenosine monophosphate–regulated gene expression in vivo. Mol Endocrinol 3:832–839, 1989.

78. Elsholtz HP, Lew AM, Albert PR, Sundmark VC: Inhibitory control of prolactin and Pit-1 gene promoter by dopamine. J Biol Chem 34:22919–22925, 1991.

79. White BA, Bancroft FC: Epidermal growth factor and thyrotropin-releasing hormone interact synergistically with calcium to regulate prolactin mRNA levels. J Biol Chem 258:4618–4622, 1983.

80. Yan G-Z, Bancroft C: Mediation by calcium of thyrotropin-releasing hormone action on the prolactin promoter via transcription factor Pit-1. Mol Endocrinol 5:1488–1497, 1991.

81. Day RN, Maurer RA: Pituitary calcium channel modulation and regulation of prolactin gene expression. Mol Endocrinol 4:736–742, 1990.

82. Shiu RPC, Kelly PA, Friesen HG: Radioreceptor assay for prolactin and other lactogenic hormones. Science 180:968–971, 1973.

83. Tanaka T, Shiu RPC, Gout PW, et al: A new sensitive and specific bioassay for lactogenic hormones: Measurement of prolactin and growth hormone in human serum. J Clin Endocrinol Metab 51:1058–1063, 1980.

84. Kendall ME, Hymer WC: Cell blotting: A new approach to quantify hormone secretion from individual rat pituitary cells. Endocrinology 121:2260–2262, 1987.

85. Frawley LS, Neill JD: Detection of hormone release from individual cells in mixed populations using a reverse hemolytic plaque assay. Endocrinology 112:1135–1137, 1983.

86. Mulcahey JJ, Jaffe RB: Detection of a potential progenitor cell in the human fetal pituitary that secretes both growth hormone and prolactin. J Clin Endocrinol Metab 66:24–32, 1988.

87. Asa SL, Kovacs K, Horvath E, et al: Human fetal adenohypophysis: Electron microscopic and ultrastructural immunocytochemical analysis. Neuroendocrinology 48:423–431, 1988.

88. Farquhar MG, Reid JJ, Daniell LW: Intracellular transport and packaging of prolactin: A quantitative electron microscope autoradiographic study of mammotrophs dissociated from rat pituitaries. Endocrinol 102:296–311, 1978.

89. Burgess TL, Kelly RB: Constitutive and regulated secretion of proteins. Annu Rev Cell Biol 3:243–293, 1987.

90. Hinkel PM, Scammel JG, Shanshala ED II: Prolactin and secretogranin-II, a marker for the regulated pathway, are secreted in parallel by pituitary GH4C1 cells. Endocrinology 130:3503–3511, 1992.

91. Clements J, Whitfield P, Cooke NE, et al: Expression of the prolactin gene in human decidua-chorion. Endocrinology 112:1133–1134, 1983.

92. Maslar IA, Riddick DH: Prolactin production by human endometrium during the normal menstrual cycle. Am J Obstet Gynecol 135:751–754, 1979.

93. Gellersen B, Bonhoff A, Hunt N, Bohnet HG: Decidual-type prolactin expression by the human myometrium. Endocrinology 129:158–168, 1991.

94. Lee DW, Markoff E: Synthesis and release of glycosylated prolactin by human decidua in vitro. J Clin Endocrinol Metab 62:990–993, 1986.

95. McCoshen JA, Tagger OY, Wodzicki A, Tyson JE: Choriodecidual adhesion promotes decidual prolactin transport by human fetal membranes. Am J Physiol 243:R552–R557, 1982.

96. Takahashi H, Nabeshima Y, Nabeshima YI, et al: Molecular cloning and nucleotide sequence of DNA complementary to human decidual prolactin mRNA. J Biochem 95:1491–1499, 1984.

97. Pellegrini I, Lebrun J-J, Ali S, Kelly PA: Expression of prolactin and its receptor in human lymphoid cells. Mol Endocrinol 6:1023–1031, 1992.

98. Gellersen B, DiMattia GE, Friesen HG, Bohnet HG: Regulation of prolactin secretion in the human B-lymphoblastoid cell line IM-9-P3 by dexamethasone but not other regulators of pituitary prolactin secretion. Endocrinology 125:2853–2861, 1989.

99. Handwerger S, Wilson S, Conn PM: Different subcellular storage sites for decidual-and pituitary-derived prolactin: Possible explanation for differences in regulation. Mol Cell Endocrinol 37:83–87, 1984.

100. Huang JR, Tseng L, Bischof P, Jänne OA: Regulation of prolactin

production by progestin, estrogen, and relaxin in human endometrial stromal cells. Endocrinology 121:2011–2017, 1987.

101. Handwerger S, Barry S, Markoff E, et al: Stimulation of the synthesis and release of decidual prolactin by a placental polypeptide. Endocrinology 112:1370–1374, 1983.

102. Golander A, Richards R, Thrailkill K, et al: Decidual prolactin (PRL)-releasing factors stimulates the synthesis of PRL from human decidual cells. Endocrinology 123:335–339, 1988.

103. Handwerger S, Markoff E, Richards R: Regulation of the synthesis and release of decidual prolactin by placental and autocrine/paracrine factors. Placenta 12:121–130, 1991.

104. Pihoker C, Feeney RJ, Su J-L, Handwerger S: Lipocortin-I inhibits the synthesis and release of prolactin from human decidual cells: Evidence for autocrine/paracrine regulation by lipocortin-I. Endocrinology 128:1123–1128, 1991.

105. Thrailkill KM, Golander A, Underwood LE, et al: Insulin stimulates the synthesis and release of prolactin from human decidual cells. Endocrinology 124:3010–3014, 1989.

106. DeVito WJ: Immunoreactive prolactin in the hypothalamus and cerebrospinal fluid of male and female rats. Neuroendocrinology 50:182–186, 1989.

107. Emmanuele NV, Jurgens JK, Halloran MM, et al: The rat prolactin gene is expressed in brain tissue: Detection of normal and alternatively spliced prolactin messenger RNA. Mol Endocrinol 6:35–42, 1992.

108. DeVito WJ: Distribution of immunoreactive prolactin in the male and female rat brain: Effect of hypophysectomy and intraventricular administration of colchicine. Neuroendocrinology 48:39–44, 1988.

109. Shiu S, Koos RD, Wise PM: Detection of prolactin receptor (PRL-R) mRNA in the rat hypothalamus and pituitary gland. Endocrinology 130:1747–1749, 1992.

110. Bridges RS, Numan M, Ronsheim PM, et al: Central prolactin infusions stimulate maternal behavior in steroid-treated nulliparous female rats. Proc Natl Acad Sci USA 87:8003–8007, 1990.

111. Lenhard L, Deftos LJ: Adenohypophyseal hormones in the CSF. Neuroendocrinology 34:303–304, 1982.

112. Mangurian LP, Walsh RJ, Posner BI: Prolactin enhancement of its own uptake at the choroid plexus. Endocrinology 131:698–702, 1992.

113. Assies J, Schellekens APM, Touber JL: Protein hormones in cerebrospinal fluid: Evidence for retrograde transport of prolactin from the pituitary to the brain in man. Clin Endocrinol 8:487–491, 1978.

114. Ostrom DM: A review of the hormone prolactin during lactation. Prog Food Nutr Sci 14:1–43, 1990.

115. Taketani Y, Mizuno M: Studies on prolactin in human milk. Endocrinology 32:837–844, 1985.

116. Whitworth N, Grosvenor CE: Transfer of milk prolactin to the plasma of neonatal rats by intestinal absorption. J Endocrinol 79:191–199, 1978.

117. Rui H, Torjesen PA, Jacobsen H, Purvis K: Testicular and glandular contributions to the prolactin pool in human semen. Arch Androl 15:129–136, 1985.

118. Seibel MM, Smith D, Dlugi AM, Levesque L: Periovulatory follicular fluid hormone levels in spontaneous human cycles. J Clin Endocrinol Metab 68:1073–1077, 1989.

119. Subramanian MC, Sacco AG, Moghissi KS, et al: Prolactin size heterogeneity in human follicular fluid: A preliminary study. Int J Fertil 36:367–371, 1991.

120. Crisp TM: Hormone requirements for early maintenance of rat granulosa cell cultures. Endocrinology 101:1286–1297, 1977.

121. Margoffin DA, Erickson GP: Prolactin inhibition of luteinizing hormone stimulated androgen synthesis in ovarian interstitial cells cultured in defined medium: Mechanisms of action. Endocrinology 111:2001–2007, 1982.

122. Van Cauter E, L'Hermite M, Copinschi G, et al: Quantitative analysis of spontaneous variations of plasma prolactin in normal man. Am J Physiol 241:E355–E363, 1981.

123. Sassin JF, Frantz AG, Kapen S, Weitzman ED: The nocturnal rise of human prolactin is dependent on sleep. J Clin Endocrinol Metab 37:436–440, 1973.

124. Veldhuis JD, Johnson ML: Operating characteristics of the hypothalamo-pituitary-gonadal axis in men: Circadian, ultradian, and pulsatile release of prolactin and its temporal coupling with luteinizing hormone. J Clin Endocrinol Metab 67:116–123, 1988.

125. Shin SH, Reifel CS: Adenohypophysis has an inherent property for pulsatile prolactin secretion. Neuroendocrinology 32:139–144, 1981.

126. Samuels MH, Kleinschmidt-Demasters B, Lillehei K, Ridgway EC: Pulsatile prolactin secretion in hyperprolactinemia due to presumed pituitary stalk interruption. J Clin Endocrinol Metab 73:1289–1293, 1991.

127. Tennekoon KH, Lenton EA: Early evening prolactin rise in women with regular cycles. J Reprod Fertil 73:523–527, 1985.

128. Rigg LA, Lein A, Yen SSC: Pattern of increase in circulating prolactin levels during human gestation. Am J Obstet Gynecol 129:454–456, 1977.

129. Kletzky OA, Rossman F, Bertolli SI, et al: Dynamics of human chorionic gonadotropin, prolactin, and growth hormone in serum and amniotic fluid throughout normal human pregnancy. Am J Obstet Gynecol 151:878–884, 1985.

130. Rigg LA, Yen SSC: Multiphasic prolactin secretion during parturition in human subjects. Am J Obstet Gynecol 128:215–218, 1977.

131. Battin DA, Marrs RP, Fleiss PM, Mishell DR: Effect of suckling on serum prolactin, luteinizing hormone, follicle-stimulating hormone, and estradiol during prolonged lactation. Obstet Gynecol 65:785–788, 1985.

132. McNeilly A: Suckling and the control of gonadotropin secretion. In Knobil E, Neill JD (eds): The Physiology of Reproduction, Vol 2. New York, Raven Press, 1988, pp 2337–2339.

133. Kremer JAM, Borm G, Schellekens LA, et al: Pulsatile secretion of luteinizing hormone and prolactin in lactating and nonlactating women and the response to naltrexone. J Clin Endocrinol Metab 72:294–300, 1991.

134. Kolodny RC, Jacobs LS, Daughaday WH: Mammary stimulation causes prolactin secretion in non-lactating women. Nature 238:284–286, 1972.

135. Nicoll CS, Talwalker PK, Meites J: Initiation of lactation in rats by nonspecific stresses. Am J Physiol 5:1103–1106, 1960.

136. Noel GL, Suh HK, Stone JG, Frantz AG: Human prolactin and growth hormone release during surgery and other conditions of stress. J Clin Endocrinol Metab 35:840–851, 1972.

137. Pontiroli AE, Baio G, Stella L, et al: Effects of naloxone on prolactin, luteinizing hormone, and cortisol responses to surgical stress in humans. J Clin Endocrinol Metab 55:378–380, 1982.

138. Kjaer A, Knigge U, Olsen L, et al: Mediation of the stress-induced prolactin release by hypothalamic histaminergic neurons and the possible involvement of vasopressin in this response. Endocrinology 128:103–110, 1991.

139. Khorram O, Bedran de Castro JC, McCann SM: Physiological role of α-melanocyte–stimulating hormone in modulating the secretion of prolactin and luteinizing hormone in the female rat. Proc Natl Acad Sci USA 81:8004–8008, 1984.

140. Pasteels JL: Recherches morphologiques et experimentales sur la secretion de prolactine. Arch Biol Liege 74:439–453, 1963.

141. Osamura RY, Komatsu N, Izumi S, et al: Ultrastructural localization of prolactin in the rat anterior pituitary glands by preembedding peroxidase-labeled antibody method. J Histochem Cytochem 30:919–925, 1992.

142. Asa SL, Penz G, Kovacs K, Ezrin C: Prolactin cells in the human pituitary: A quantitative immunocytochemical analysis of human pituitaries taken at autopsy. Arch Pathol Lab Med 106:360–363, 1982.

143. Franks S: Regulation of prolactin secretion by oestrogens: Physiological and pathological significance. Clin Sci 65:457–462, 1983.

144. Strattman IE, Ezrin C, Sellers EA: Estrogen-induced transformation of somatotrophs into mammotrophs in the rat. Cell Tissue Res 152:229–238, 1974.

145. Frawley LS, Boockfor FR: Mammosomatotropes: Presence and functions in normal and neoplastic pituitary tissue. Endocr Rev 12:337–355, 1991.

146. Boockfor FR, Hoeffler JP, Frawley LS: Estradiol induces a shift in cultured cells that release prolactin or growth hormone. Am J Physiol 250:E103–E105, 1986.

147. Stone RT, Maurer RA, Gorski J: Effect of estradiol-17β on preprolactin messenger ribonucleic acid activity in the rat pituitary gland. Biochem 16:4915–4921, 1977.

148. Ryan R, Shupnik MA, Gorski J: Effect of estrogen on preprolactin messenger ribonucleic acid sequences. Biochemistry 18:2044–2048, 1979.

149. Maurer RA: Estradiol regulates the transcription of the prolactin gene. J Biol Chem 257:2133–2135, 1982.

150. Shull JD, Gorski J: The hormonal regulation of prolactin gene expression: An examination of mechanisms controlling prolactin synthesis and the possible relationship of estrogen to these mechanisms. Vitamins Hormones 43:197–249, 1986.

151. Raymond V, Beaulieu M, Labrie F, Boissier J: Potent antidopaminergic activity of estradiol at the pituitary level on prolactin release. Science 200:1173–1175, 1978.

152. Cramer OM, Parker CR, Porter JC: Estrogen inhibition of dopamine release into hypophysial portal blood. Endocrinology 104:419–422, 1979.
153. Lamberts SWJ, MacLeod RM: Regulation of prolactin secretion at the level of the lactotroph. Physiol Rev 70:279–318, 1990.
154. Vrontakis ME, Peden LM, Duckworth ML, Friesen HG: Isolation and characterization of a complementary DNA (galanin) clone from estrogen-induced pituitary tumor messenger RNA. J Biol Chem 262:16755–16758, 1987.
155. Nordstrom O, Melander T, Hökfelt T, et al: Evidence for an inhibitory effect of the peptide galanin on dopamine release from the rat median eminence. Neurosci Lett 72:21–26, 1987.
156. Fishman J, Tulchinsky D: Suppression of prolactin secretion in normal young women by 2-hydroxyestrone. Science 210:74, 1980.
157. Stanley F: Stimulation of prolactin gene expression by insulin. J Biol Chem 263:13444–13448, 1988.
158. Prager D, Yamashita S, Melmed S: Insulin regulates prolactin secretion and messenger ribonucleic acid levels in pituitary cells. Endocrinology 122:2946–2952, 1988.
159. Brelje TC, Sorenson RL: Role of prolactin versus growth hormone on islet B-cell proliferation in vitro: Implications for pregnancy. Endocrinology 128:45–57, 1991.
160. Neill JD: Prolactin secretion and its control. In Knobil E, Neill JD (eds): The Physiology of Reproduction. New York, Raven Press, 1988, pp 1379–1390.
161. Gunnett JW, Freeman ME: The mating-induced released of prolactin: A unique neuroendocrine response. Endocr Rev 4:44–61, 1983.
162. Ben-Jonathan N, Arbogast LA, Hyde JF: Neuroendocrine regulation of prolactin release. Prog Neurobiol 33:399–447, 1989.
163. Martinez de la Escalera G, Weiner RI: Dissociation of dopamine from its receptor as a signal in the pleiotropic hypothalamic regulation of prolactin secretion. Endocr Rev 13:241–255, 1992.
164. Everett J: Luteotrophic function of autografts of the rat hypophysis. Endocrinology 54:685–690, 1954.
165. Ben-Jonathan N, Oliver C, Winer HJ, et al: Dopamine in hypophysial portal plasma of the rat during the estrous cycle and throughout pregnancy. Endocrinology 100:452–458, 1977.
166. LeBlanc H, Lachelin GCL, Abu-Fadil S, Yen SSC: Effects of dopamine infusion on pituitary hormone secretion in humans. J Clin Endocrinol Metab 43:668–674, 1976.
167. Brownstein MJ, Palkovits M, Saavedra JM, Kizer JS: Distribution of hypothalamic hormones and neurotransmitters within the diencephalon. Front Neuroendocrinol 4:1–24, 1976.
168. Baertschi AJ: Portal vascular route from hypophysial stalk/neural lobe to adenohypophysis. Am J Physiol 239:R463–R469, 1980.
169. Peters LL, Hoefer MT, Ben-Jonathan N: The posterior pituitary: Regulation of anterior pituitary prolactin secretion. Science 213:659–661, 1981.
170. Creese I, Sibley DR, Leff SE: Agonist interactions with dopamine receptors. Focus on radioligand-binding studies. Fed Proc 43:2779–2784, 1984.
171. Pasqualini C, Lenoir V, El Abed A, Kerdelhue B: Anterior pituitary dopamine receptors during the rat estrous cycle. Neuroendocrinology 38:39–44, 1984.
172. Swennen L, Denef C: Physiological concentrations of dopamine decrease adenosine 3′5′-monophosphate levels in cultured rat anterior pituitary cells and enriched populations of lactotrophs: Evidence for a causal relationship to inhibition of prolactin release. Endocrinology 111:398–405, 1982.
173. Kidokoro Y: Spontaneous calcium action potentials in a clonal pituitary cell line and their relationship to prolactin secretion. Nature 258:741–742, 1975.
174. Drouva S, Rerat E, Bihoreau C, et al: Dihydropyridine-sensitive calcium channel activity related to prolactin, growth hormone, and luteinizing hormone release from anterior pituitary cells in culture: Interactions with somatostatin, dopamine, and estrogens. Endocrinology 123:2762–2773, 1988.
175. Jarvis WD, Judd AM, MacLeod RM: Attenuation of anterior pituitary phosphoinositide phosphorylase activity by the D2 dopamine receptor. Endocrinology 123:2793–2799, 1988.
176. Walsh RJ, Posner BI, Kopriwa BM, Brawer JR: Prolactin binding sites in rat brain. Science 201:1041–1043, 1978.
177. Gudelsky GA, Porter JC: Release of dopamine from tuberoinfundibular neurons into pituitary stalk blood after prolactin or haloperidol administration. Endocrinology 106:526–529, 1980.
178. Bentley AM, Wallis M: In vitro evidence for the autoregulation of prolactin secretion at the level of the pituitary gland in the rat. J Endocrinol 115:13–18, 1987.

179. Schally AV, Redding TW, Arimura A, et al: Isolation of γ-aminobutyric acid from pig hypothalami and demonstration of its prolactin-release inhibiting (PIF) activity in vivo and in vitro. Endocrinology 100:681–691, 1977.
180. Grandison L, Guidotti A: γ-Aminobutyric acid receptor function in rat anterior pituitary: Evidence for control of prolactin secretion. Endocrinology 105:754–759, 1979.
181. Mulchahey JJ, Neill JD: γ-Aminobutyric acid (GABA) levels in hypophyseal stalk plasma of rats. Life Sci 31:453–456, 1982.
182. Mizunuma H, Khorram O, McCann SM: Purification of a non-dopaminergic and non-GABAergic prolactin release-inhibiting factor (PIF) in sheep stalk-median eminence. Proc Soc Exp Biol Med 178:113–120, 1985.
183. Nikolics K, Mason AJ, Szonyi E, et al: A prolactin-inhibiting factor within the precursor for human gonadotropin-releasing hormone. Nature 316:511–517, 1985.
184. Yu WH, Seeburg PH, Nikolics K, McCann SM: Gonadotropin-releasing hormone–associated peptide exerts a prolactin-inhibiting and weak gonadotropin-releasing activity in vivo. Endocrinology 123:390–395, 1988.
185. Thomas GB, Cummins JT, Boughton BW, et al: Gonadotropin-releasing hormone associated peptide (GAP) and putative processed GAP peptides do not release luteinizing hormone or follicle-stimulating hormone or inhibit prolactin secretion in the sheep. Neuroendocrinology 48:342–350, 1988.
186. Wormald PJ, Abrahamson MJ, Seeburg PH, et al: Prolactin-inhibiting activity of GnRH associated peptide in cultured human pituitary cells. Clin Endocrinol 30:149–155, 1989.
187. Lamberts SWJ, Zuyderwijk JJ, Den Holder F, et al: Studies on the conditions of the effects of somatostatin on adrenocorticotropin, prolactin and thyrotropin release by cultured rat pituitary cells. Neuroendorinology 50:44–50, 1989.
188. Wardlow SL, Smeal MM, Markowitz CE: Antagonism of β-endorphin-induced prolactin release by α-melanocyte-stimulating hormone and corticotropin-like intermediate lobe peptide. Endocrinology 119:112–118, 1986.
189. Noel GL, Dimond RC, Wartofsky L, et al: Studies of prolactin and TSH secretion by continuous infusion of small amounts of thyrotropin releasing hormone (TRH). J Clin Endocrinol Metab 39:6–17, 1974.
190. Fink G, Koch Y, Ben Aroya N: Release of thyrotropin releasing hormones into hypophysial portal blood is high relative to other neuropeptides and may be related to prolactin secretion. Brain Res 243:186–189, 1982.
191. Sheward WJ, Fraser HM, Fink G: Effect of immunoneutralization of thyrotropin-releasing hormone on the release of thyrotropin and prolactin during suckling or in response to electrical stimulation of the hypothalamus in the anaesthetized rat. J Endocrinol 106:113–119, 1985.
192. Said SI, Porter JC: Vasoactive intestinal polypeptide: Release into hypophyseal portal blood. Life Sci 24:227–230, 1979.
193. Werner SK, Hulting A-L, Hökfelt T, et al: Effect of the peptide PHI-27 on prolactin release in vitro. Neuroendocrinology 37:476–478, 1983.
194. Nagy G, Mulchahey JJ, Neill JD: Autocrine control of prolactin secretion by vasoactive intestinal peptide. Endocrinology 122:364–366, 1988.
195. Johnston CA, Negro-Vilar A: Maturation of the prolactin and proopiomelanocortin-derived peptide responses to ether stress and morphine: Neurochemical analysis. Endocrinology 118:797–804, 1988.
196. Pilotte NS, Porter JC: Dopamine in hypophysial portal plasma and prolactin in systemic plasma of rats treated with 5-hydroxytryptamine. Endocrinology 108:2137–2141, 1981.
197. Averill RLW, Grattan DR, Norris SK: Posterior pituitary lobectomy chronically attenuates the nocturnal surge of prolactin in early pregnancy. Endocrinology 128:705–709, 1991.
198. Mori M, Vigh S, Miyata A, et al: Oxytocin is the major prolactin releasing factor in the posterior pituitary. Endocrinology 126:1009–1013, 1991.
199. Nagy G, Mulchahey JJ, Smyth DG, Neill JD: The glycopeptide moiety of vasopressin-neurophysin precursor is neurohypophysial prolactin releasing factor. Biochem Biophys Res Commun 151:524–529, 1988.
200. Denef C, Andries M: Evidence for paracrine interaction between gonadotrophs and lactotrophs in pituitary cell aggregates. Endocrinology 112:813–822, 1983.
201. Deschepper CF, Crumrine DA, Ganong WF: Evidence that the gonadotrophs are the likely site of production of angiotensin II in the anterior pituitary of the rat. Endocrinology 119:36–43, 1986.

202. Steele MK, Negro-Vilar A, McCann SM: Effect of angiotensin II on in vivo and in vitro release of anterior pituitary hormones in the female rat. Endocrinology 109:893–899, 1981.

203. Baes M, Allaerto W, Denef C: Evidence for functional communication between folliculostellate cells and hormone-secreting cells in perifused anterior pituitary cell aggregates. Endocrinology 120:685–691, 1987.

204. Lam KSL, Lechan RM, Minamitani N, et al: Vasoactive intestinal peptide in the anterior pituitary is increased in hypothyroidism. Endocrinology 124:1077–1084, 1989.

205. Nagy G, Mulchahey JJ, Neill JD: Autocrine control of prolactin secretion by vasoactive intestinal peptide. Endocrinology 122:364–366, 1988.

206. Kelly PA, Djiane J, Katoh M, et al: The interaction of prolactin with its receptors in target tissues and its mechanism of action. Recent Prog Horm Res 40:379–439, 1984.

207. Ymer SI, Stevenson JL, Herington AC: Differences in the developmental patterns of somatotrophic and lactogenic receptors in rabbit liver cytosol. Endocrinology 125:516–523, 1989.

208. Boutin JM, Jolicoeur C, Okamura H, et al: Cloning and expression of the rat prolactin receptor, a member of the growth hormone/prolactin receptor gene family. Cell 53:69–77, 1988.

209. Barton DE, Foellmer BE, Wood WI, Francke U: Chromosome mapping of the growth hormone receptor gene in man and mouse. Cytogenet Cell Genet 50:137–141, 1989.

210. Bazan JF: Structural design and molecular evolution of a cytokine receptor superfamily. Proc Natl Acad Sci USA 87:6934–6938, 1990.

211. Souryi M, Vignon I, Penciolelli J-F, et al: A putative truncated cytokine receptor gene transduced by the myeloproliferative leukemia virus immortalizes hematopoietic progenitors. Cell 63:1137–1147, 1990.

212. Longmore GD, Lodish HF: An activating mutation in the murine erythropoietin receptor induces erythroleukemia in mice: A cytokine receptor superfamily oncogene. Cell 67:1089–1102, 1991.

213. Boutin J-M, Edery M, Shirota M, et al: Identification of a cDNA encoding a long form of prolactin receptor in human hepatoma and breast cancer cells. Mol Endocrinol 3:1455–1461, 1989.

214. Shirota M, Banville D, Ali S, et al: Expression of two forms of prolactin receptor in rat ovary and liver. Mol Endocrinol 4:1136–1143, 1990.

215. Zhang R, Buczko E, Tsai-Morris C-H, et al: Isolation and characterization of two novel rat ovarian lactogen receptor cDNA species. Biochem Biophys Res Commun 168:415–422, 1990.

216. Postel-Vinay M-C, Belair L, Kayser C, et al: Identification of prolactin and growth hormone binding proteins in rabbit milk. Proc Natl Acad Sci USA 88:6687–6690, 1991.

217. Ali S, Pellegrini I, Kelly PA: A prolactin-dependent immune cell line (Nb2) expresses a mutant form of prolactin receptor. J Biol Chem 266:20110–20117, 1991.

218. Hughes JP, Elsholtz HP, Friesen HG: Up-regulation of lactogenic receptors—an immunological artifact? Endocrinology 111:702–704, 1982.

219. Dave JR, Witorsch RF: Prolactin increases lipid fluidity and prolactin binding of rat prostatic membranes. Am J Physiol 248:E687–E693, 1985.

220. Jolicoeur C, Boutin J-M, Okamura H, et al: Multiple regulation of prolactin receptor gene expression in rat liver. Mol Endocrinol 3:895–900, 1989.

221. Jahn GA, Edery M, Belair L, et al: Prolactin receptor gene expression in rat mammary gland and liver during pregnancy and lactation. Endocrinology 128:2976–2984, 1991.

222. Lesueur L, Edery M, Ali S, et al: Comparison of long and short forms of the prolactin receptor on prolactin-induced milk protein gene transcription. Proc Natl Acad Sci USA 88:824–828, 1991.

223. Ray J, Okamura H, Kelly PA, et al: Human growth hormone–variant demonstrates a receptor binding profile distinct from that of the normal pituitary growth hormone. J Biol Chem 265:7939–7944, 1990.

224. Cunningham BC, Bass S, Fuh G, Wells JA: Zinc mediation of the binding of human growth hormone to the human prolactin receptor. Science 250:1709–1712, 1990.

225. Bass SH, Mulkerrin MG, Wells JA: A systematic mutational analysis of hormone-binding determinant in the human growth hormone receptor. Proc Natl Acad Sci USA 88:4498–4502, 1991.

226. de Vos AM, Ultsch M, Kossiakoff AA: Human growth hormone and extracellular domain of its receptor: Crystal structure of the complex. Science 255:306–312, 1992.

227. Fuh G, Cunningham BC, Fukunaga R, et al: Rational design of potent antagonists to the human growth hormone receptor. Science 256:1677–1680, 1992.

228. Elberg G, Kelly PA, Djiane J, et al: Mitogenic and binding properties of monoclonal antibodies to the prolactin receptor in Nb2 rat lymphoma cells: Selective enhancement by anti-mouse IgG. J Biol Chem 265:14770–14776, 1990.

229. Rozakis-Adcock M, Kelly PA: Mutational analysis of the ligand-binding domain of the prolactin receptor. J Biol Chem 266:16472–16477, 1991.

230. Too CKL, Walker A, Murphy PR, et al: Identification of amiloride-sensitive Na$^+$/H$^+$ exchange in rat NB2 node lymphoma cells. Stimulation by 12-O-tetradecanoyl-phorbol-13-acetate. Endocrinology 121:1503–1511, 1987.

231. Larsen JL, Dufau ML: Modulation of prolactin-stimulated Nb2 lymphoma cell mitogenesis by cholera toxin and pertussis toxin. Endocrinology 123:438–444, 1988.

232. Larsen JL: Human hormone enhances pertussis toxin–stimulated ADP-ribosylation of G$_i$ in Nb2 cell membrane. J Biol Chem 267:10583–10587, 1992.

233. Kornberg LJ, Liberti JP: Nb2 cell mitogenesis: Effect of lactogens on cAMP and protein phosphorylation. Biochim Biophys Acta 1011:205–211, 1989.

234. Rillema JA, Campbell GS, Lawson DM, Carter-Su C: Evidence for a rapid stimulation of tyrosine kinase activity in Nb2 rat lymphoma cells. Endocrinology 131:973–975, 1992.

235. Yu-Lee L-Y, Hrachovy JA, Stevens AM, Schwarz LA: Interferon-regulatory factor 1 is an immediate-early gene under transcriptional regulation by prolactin in Nb2 T cells. Mol Cell Biol 10:3087–3094, 1990.

236. Francis MJO, Hill DJ: Prolactin-stimulated production of somatomedin by rat liver. Nature 285:167–168, 1975.

237. Delidow BC, Hebert N, Steiny S, Nicoll CS: Secretion of prolactin-synergizing activity (Synlactin) by the liver of ectothermic vertebrates in vitro. J Exp Zool 238:147–153, 1986.

238. English DE, Russell SM, Katz LS, Nicoll CS: Evidence for a role of the liver in the mammotrophic action of prolactin. Endocrinology 128:1505–1510, 1991.

239. McNeilly AS, Friesen HG: Presence of a nonlactogenic factor in human serum which synergistically enhances prolactin-stimulated growth of Nb2 rat lymphoma cells in vitro. J Clin Endocrinol Metab 61:408–411, 1985.

240. Anderson TR, Pitts DS, Nicoll CS: Prolactin's mitogenic action on the pigeon crop-sac mucosal epithelium involves direct and indirect mechanisms. Gen Comp Endocrinol 54:236–246, 1984.

241. Murphy LJ, Tachibana K, Friesen HG: Stimulation of hepatic insulin-like growth factor-I gene expression by ovine prolactin: Evidence for intrinsic somatogenic activity in the rat. Endocrinology 122:2027–2033, 1988.

242. Fielder PJ, Thordarson G, English A, et al: Expression of a lactogen-dependent insulin-like growth factor–binding protein in cultured mouse mammary epithelial cells. Endocrinology 131:261–267, 1992.

243. Duclos M, Houdebine L-M, Djiane J: Comparison of insulin-like growth factor I and insulin effects on prolactin-induced lactogenesis in the rabbit mammary gland in vitro. Mol Cell Endocrinol 65:129–134, 1989.

244. Deeks S, Richards J, Nandi S: Maintenance of normal rat mammary epithelial cells by insulin and insulin-like growth factor I. Exp Cell Res 174:448–460, 1988.

245. Aragona C, Bohnet HG, Friesen HG: Localization of prolactin binding in prostate and testis: The role of serum prolactin concentration on the testicular LH receptor. Acta Endocrinol 84:402–409, 1977.

246. Nevalainen MT, Valve EM, Mäkelä SI, et al: Estrogen and prolactin regulation of rat dorsal and lateral prostate in organ culture. Endocrinology 129:612–622, 1991.

247. Bartke A: Role of prolactin in reproduction in male mammals. Fed Proc 39:2577–2581, 1980.

248. Doherty PC, Bartke A, Smith MS: Hyperprolactinemia and male sexual behavior: Effects of steroid replacement with estrogen plus dihydrotestosterone. Physiol Behav 35:99–104, 1985.

249. Doherty PC, Baum MJ, Todd RB: Effects of chronic hyperprolactinemia on sexual arousal and erectile function in male rats. Neuroendocrinology 42:368–375, 1986

250. Kalra PS, Simpkins JW, Luttge WG, Kalra SP: Effects of male sex behavior and preoptic dopamine neurons of hyperprolactinemia induced by MtTW15 pituitary tumors. Endocrinology 113:2065–2071, 1983.

251. Kamel F, Wright WW, Mock EF, Frankel AI: The influence of mating and related stimuli on plasma levels of luteinizing hormone, follicle

stimulating hormone, prolactin, and testosterone in the male rat. Endocrinology 101:421–429, 1977.

252. Drago F: Prolactin and sexual behavior: A review. Neurosci Biobehav Rev 8:433–439, 1984.
253. Murai I, Reichlin S, Ben-Jonathan N: The peak phase of the proestrus prolactin surge is blocked by either posterior pituitary lobectomy or antisera to vasoactive intestinal peptide. Endocrinology 124:1050–1055, 1989.
254. Richards JS, Williams JL: Luteal cell receptor content for prolactin (PRL) and luteinizing hormone (LH). Regulation by LH and PRL. Endocrinology 99:1571–1581, 1976.
255. Albarracin CT, Gibori G: Prolactin action on luteal protein expression in the corpus luteum. Endocrinology 129:1821–1830, 1991.
256. Dorington J, Gore-Langton RE: Prolactin inhibits oestrogen synthesis in the ovary. Nature 290:600–602, 1981.
257. Cohen-Becker IR, Selmanoff M, Wise PM: Hyperprolactinemia alters the frequency and amplitude of pulsatile luteinizing hormone secretion in the ovariectomized rat. Neuroendocrinology 42:328–333, 1986.
258. Selye H, Collip JB, Thomson DL: Effect of hypophysectomy upon pregnancy and lactation in mice. Proc Soc Exp Biol Med 31:82–83, 1933.
259. Kleinberg DL, Ruan W, Catanese V, et al: Non-lactogenic effects of growth hormone on growth and insulin-like growth factor-I messenger ribonucleic acid of rat mammary gland. Endocrinology 126:3274–3275, 1990.
260. Wilson ME, Gordon TP, Chikazawa K, et al: Effects of growth hormone on neonatal growth in nursing rhesus monkeys. J Clin Endocrinol Metab 72:1302–1307, 1991.
261. Bchini O, Andres AC, Schubaur B, et al: Precocious mammary gland development and milk protein synthesis in transgenic mice ubiquitously expressing human growth hormone. Endocrinology 128:539–546, 1991.
262. Rosen JM, Matuski RJ, Richards DA, et al: Multihormonal regulation of casein gene expression at the transcriptional and posttranscriptional levels in the mammary gland. Rec Prog Horm Res 36:157–193, 1980.
263. Shiu RPC, Friesen HG: Mechanism of action of prolactin in the control of mammary gland function. Annu Rev Physiol 42:83–96, 1980.
264. Dusanter-Fourt I, Belair L, Gespach C, Djiane J: Expression of prolactin (PRL) receptor gene and PRL-binding sites in rabbit intestinal epithelial cells. Endocrinology 130:2877–2882, 1992.
265. Porter TE, Frawley SL: Stimulation of prolactin cell differentiation in vitro by a milk-borne peptide. Endocrinology 129:2707–2713, 1991.
266. Rillema FA, Foley KA, Etindi RN: Temporal sequence of prolactin actions on phospholipid biosynthesis in mouse mammary gland explants. Endocrinology 116:511–515, 1985.
267. Weisz-Carrington P, Roux ME, McWilliams M, et al: Hormonal induction of the secretory immune system in the mammary gland. Proc Natl Acad Sci USA 75:2928–2932, 1978.
268. Mountjoy K, Cowden EA, Dobbie JW, Ratcliffe JG: Prolactin receptors in kidney. J Endocrinol 87:47–54, 1980.
269. Stier CT, Cowden EA, Friesen HG, Allison MEM: Prolactin and the rat kidney: A clearance and micropuncture study. Endocrinology 115:362–367, 1984.
270. Horrobin DF: Prolactin as a regulator of fluid and electrolyte metabolism in mammals. Fed Proc 39:2567–2570, 1980.
271. Robertson MY, Boyajian MJ, Patterson K, Robertson WVB: Modulation of the chloride concentration of human sweat by prolactin. Endocrinology 119:2439–2444, 1986.
272. Tyson JE: The evolutionary role of prolactin in mammalian osmoregulation: Effects on fetoplacental hydromineral transport. Semin Perinatol 6:216–228, 1982.
273. Nicoll CS: Ontogeny and evolution of prolactin's functions. Fed Proc 39:2563–2566, 1980.
274. Mainoya JR, Bern HA, Regan JW: Influence of ovine prolactin on transport of fluid and sodium chloride by the mammalian intestine and gallbladder. J Endocrinol 63:311–317, 1974.
275. Pahuja DN, DeLuca HF: Stimulation of intestinal calcium transport and bone calcium mobilization by prolactin in vitamin D–deficient rats. Science 214:1038–1039, 1981.
276. Kelley KW, Brief S, Westly HJ, et al: GH3 pituitary adenoma cells can reverse thymic aging in mice. Proc Natl Acad Sci USA 83:5663–5667, 1986.
277. Berczi I, Nagy E, de Toledo AM, et al: Pituitary hormones regulate c-myc and DNA synthesis in lymphoid tissue. J Immunol 146:2201–2206, 1991.
278. Hiestand PC, Meckler P, Nordmann R, et al: Prolactin as a modulator of lymphocyte responsiveness provides a possible mechanism for cyclosporine. Proc Natl Acad Sci USA 83:2599–2603, 1986.
279. Bernton E, Meltzer MS, Holaday J: Suppression of macrophage activation and T-lymphocyte function in hypoprolactinemic mice. Science 239:401–404, 1988.
280. White A, Williams RO: Bromocriptine suppresses postpartum exacerbation of collagen-induced arthritis. Arthritis Rheum 31:927–928, 1988.
281. Palestine AG, Muellenberg-Coulombre CG, Kim MK, et al: Bromocriptine and low dose cyclosporine in the treatment of experimental autoimmune uveitis in the rat. J Clin Invest 79:1078–1081, 1987.
282. McMurray R, Keisler D, Kanuckel K, et al: Prolactin influences autoimmune disease activity in the female B/W mouse. J Immunol 147:3780–3787, 1991.
283. Carrier M, Russell DH, Wild JC, et al: Prolactin as a marker of rejection in human heart transplantation. Transplant Proc 19:3442–3443, 1987.
284. Russell DH, Kibler R, Matrisian L, et al: Prolactin receptors on human T and B lymphocytes: Antagonism of prolactin binding by cyclosporin. J Immunol 134:3027–3031, 1985.
285. Vidaller A, Llorente L, Larrea F, et al: T-cell dysregulation in patients with hyperprolactinemia: Effect of bromocriptine therapy. Clin Immunol Immunopathol 38:337–343, 1986.
286. Viselli SM, Stanek EM, Mukherjee P, et al: Prolactin-induced mitogenesis of lymphocytes from ovariectomized rats. Endocrinology 129:983–990, 1991.
287. Hartman D, Holoday J, Bernton E: Inhibition of lymphocyte proliferation by antibodies to prolactin. FASEB J 3:2194–2202, 1989.
288. Montgomery DW, LeFevre JA, Ulrich ED, et al: Identification of prolactin-like proteins synthesized by normal murine lymphocytes. Endocrinology 127:2601–2603, 1990.
289. Hatfill SJ, Kirby R, Hanley M, et al: Hyperprolactinemia in acute leukemia and indication of ectopic expression of human prolactin in blast cells of a patient of subtype M4. Leuk Res 14:57–62, 1990.
290. Clevenger CV, Russell DH, Appasamy PM, Prystowsky MB: Regulation of interleukin 2–driven T-lymphocyte proliferation by prolactin. Proc Natl Acad Sci USA 87:6460–6464, 1990.
291. Clevenger CV, Sillman AL, Hanley-Hyde J, Prystowsky MB: Requirement for prolactin during cell cycle regulated gene expression in cloned T-lymphocytes. Endocrinology 130:3216–3222, 1992.

24

Prolactin: Hyperprolactinemic Syndromes and Management

MARY LEE VANCE
MICHAEL O. THORNER

NATURAL HISTORY OF
HYPERPROLACTINEMIA

HYPERPROLACTINEMIA: CLINICAL
PRESENTATION

ANATOMIC EVALUATION OF THE
PITUITARY GLAND

BIOCHEMICAL EVALUATION

PREGNANCY AND
HYPERPROLACTINEMIA

TREATMENT OF HYPERPROLACTINEMIA

Hyperprolactinemia is the most common hypothalamic-pituitary disorder encountered in clinical endocrinology. The causes of pathological hyperprolactinemia are diverse, and treatment depends upon identification of the precise cause. Pathological hyperprolactinemia is defined as a consistently elevated serum prolactin level (greater than 20 ng/ml) in the absence of pregnancy or postpartum lactation. Because prolactin is secreted in a pulsatile fashion, several determinations should be obtained, such as three samples on different mornings, to correctly establish the diagnosis of hyperprolactinemia.

Causes of hyperprolactinemia are listed in Table 24–1. Any process that interferes with dopamine synthesis, its transport to the pituitary, or its action at the lactotrope dopamine receptors may produce hyperprolactinemia. Hypothalamic lesions that cause elevated serum prolactin levels include tumors, infiltrative disease, and cranial irradiation. Pituitary diseases, other than prolactin-secreting tumors, include acromegaly, Cushing's disease, pituitary stalk section, the empty sella syndrome, and other "nonfunctioning" tumors, which may effectively produce a stalk section by pressure, interrupting the portal capillary blood flow. A careful history of drug ingestion may obviate further investigations. Numerous drugs that interfere with dopamine synthesis or dopaminergic inhibition of prolactin secretion cause hyperprolactinemia that is reversible with discontinuation of the drug. The more commonly prescribed drugs include neuroleptics, some antidepressants, estrogens (oral contraceptives), some antihypertensives, and the dopamine receptor blockers, metoclopramide and domperidone. Although basal prolactin levels are usually normal in primary hypothyroidism, in some patients both basal and stimulated (after thyrotropin-releasing hormone [TRH] administration) prolactin levels are elevated[1]; both basal and stimulated levels are lowered by appropriate thyroid hormone replacement, but this takes longer than thy-

roid-stimulating hormone (TSH) to decrease to normal.[1, 2] Hyperprolactinemia occurs in 20 to 75 per cent of men and women with chronic renal failure; it is not altered by hemodialysis but is normalized by successful transplantation.[3–7] The precise mechanism for hyperprolactinemia in

TABLE 24–1. ETIOLOGIES OF PATHOLOGICAL HYPERPROLACTINEMIA

1. Hypothalamic Disease
   A. Tumor (e.g., craniopharyngioma, third ventricle cyst, glioma, hamartoma, metastatic)
   B. Infiltrative disease (e.g., sarcoidosis, giant cell granuloma, tuberculosis, eosinophilic granuloma)
   C. Pseudotumor cerebri
   D. Cranial radiation
2. Pituitary Disease
   A. Prolactinoma (microadenoma, macroadenoma)
   B. Acromegaly
   C. Cushing's disease
   D. Glycoprotein-producing tumor (LH, FSH, TSH, α-subunit)
   E. Other tumors (metastatic, intrasellar germinoma, meningioma, nonsecretory pituitary tumor)
   F. Pituitary stalk section (trauma)
   G. Empty sella
   H. Infiltrative disease (lymphocytic hypophysitis, giant cell granuloma, sarcoidosis)
3. Drugs
   A. Neuroleptics (perphenazine, fluphenazine, thorazine, promazine, trifluoperazine, haloperidol, chlorpromazine)
   B. Dopamine receptor blockers (metoclopramide, sulpiride, domperidone)
   C. Antidepressants (amoxapine, imipramine, amitriptyline)
   D. Antihypertensives (α-methyldopa, reserpine, verapamil)
   E. Estrogens
   F. Opiates
   G. Cimetidine (intravenous)
4. Primary Hypothyroidism
5. Chronic Renal Failure
6. Cirrhosis
7. Neurogenic (spinal cord lesions, chest wall lesions, breast stimulation)
8. Stress (physical, psychological)
9. Idiopathic

Data from refs. 108–118.

This work is supported in part by US Public Health Service Grants DK 32632 and RR 00847.

chronic renal failure is not known. Although estrogens are known to stimulate the lactotroph with consequent secretion of prolactin, there does not appear to be an association between the use of oral contraceptives and the development of a pituitary tumor[8, 9] or the use of conjugated estrogens and hyperprolactinemia. The polycystic ovarian syndrome is associated primarily with the hypersecretion of androgens by the adrenal glands, the ovaries, or both. Some women with mild hyperandrogenemia also have hyperprolactinemia, and some evidence suggests that elevated prolactin levels may alter adrenal function, particularly the production of dehydroepiandrosterone sulfate (DHEAS), which decreases following treatment of the hyperprolactinemia.[10]

Once drugs are excluded as a cause of hyperprolactinemia, the most common cause of this disorder is a pituitary tumor, either a macroadenoma (greater than 10 mm in diameter) or a microadenoma (less than 10 mm in diameter). The precise prevalence of prolactinomas is not known. The reported occurrence of microadenomas varies between 23 and 27 per cent.[11, 12] In one study of 120 unselected autopsy specimens, a microadenoma was present in 27 per cent of the pituitary glands examined. There was no antemortem evidence of pituitary disease and no predilection for gender. Forty per cent of these microadenomas were positive for prolactin with the immunoperoxidase stain.[12] The prevalence of macroadenomas is not known, but in clinical practice these occur much less frequently than do microadenomas. A higher proportion of prolactinomas in men and in postmenopausal women than in women of reproductive age appears to be macroadenomas at diagnosis. This is likely related to the duration of disease, the gradual development of symptoms, and, in postmenopausal women, the lack of menses as a marker of gonadal function. In contrast, women of reproductive age usually seek medical attention promptly because of a change in menstrual cycles and are more likely to have a small tumor at diagnosis. In one study of 682 patients with infertility, hyperprolactinemia was present in 23 per cent of women with secondary amenorrhea, 8 per cent with oligomenorrhea, and 3 per cent with unexplained infertility. Three per cent of men with oligospermia and infertility had hyperprolactinemia.[13] Although this represents a select group of patients, this study indicates that the prevalence of hyperprolactinemia is significant in otherwise healthy adults.

NATURAL HISTORY OF HYPERPROLACTINEMIA

The cause of hyperprolactinemia is identifiable in the majority of patients. However, despite careful evaluation, including pituitary imaging studies, the cause may not be apparent in some patients. These patients are then given the diagnosis of idiopathic hyperprolactinemia. The obvious concern in these patients and in patients with moderate hyperprolactinemia (less than 200 ng/ml) and a radiographically identifiable microadenoma is the risk of progression of disease and development of a large tumor. From the information available, the risk of progression to an identifiable tumor appears small, on the order of 3 to 7 per cent, in patients evaluated by serial polytomography and/or CT scans.[14–17] When serum prolactin levels are used

as an indication of disease activity, a substantial number of patients have either no change or a decrease in serum prolactin over time. In 41 patients with idiopathic hyperprolactinemia followed for up to 12 years (mean 5.5 years), 83 per cent had either no change or a decrease in prolactin and in 34 per cent the prolactin level fell to normal. Seven of the 41 (17 per cent) had a greater than 50 per cent increase in serum prolactin. The initial prolactin concentration was important in that none of the patients who had an initial value of greater than 60 ng/dl had a decrease in serum prolactin to normal, whereas 67 per cent of patients with an initial level of less than 40 ng/dl had a decrease to normal. Only one patient in this series developed evidence of a pituitary tumor; this patient had an initial serum prolactin of 150 ng/ml.[17] A prospective study of 30 untreated hyperprolactinemic women followed for three to seven years (mean 5.2 years) revealed that 35 per cent had improvement in clinical symptoms; serum prolactin decreased to normal in six and menses became normal in six. Six women had an increase in prolactin of greater than 50 per cent of baseline during the study. Changes in pituitary size, assessed by either hypocycloidal polytomography or CT scan in 27 women, included a return to normal in 4 of 13 (15 per cent) with an abnormal initial study, tumor progression in 2 (8 per cent), and no change in 7 (26 per cent). Four of 14 women (29 per cent) with a normal study at entry developed radiographic evidence of a pituitary tumor; however, none developed a macroadenoma or pituitary insufficiency.[18]

The most consistent effect of chronic hyperprolactinemia is gonadal dysfunction. As noted, it appears that only a minority of patients with hyperprolactinemia develop a large pituitary tumor, but this must be a consideration in all patients. Only recently has another potential complication of long-standing hyperprolactinemia been recognized, that is, an effect on bone density in both men and women. Of 14 hyperprolactinemic-amenorrheic women, bone mineral content was measured by direct photon absorptiometry of the radius and compared with 16 age-matched normal women and 19 postmenopausal women who had no history of osteoporosis or estrogen replacement therapy. The duration of amenorrhea ranged from less than 1 year to 18 years; the median was 3 years. Serum prolactin values ranged from 22 to 99 ng/ml. Serum estradiol levels ranged from undetectable (less than 20 pg/ml) to 90 pg/ml; 43 per cent of hyperprolactinemic women had estradiol levels comparable to those of postmenopausal women. The serum estradiol level did not correlate with duration of amenorrhea or serum prolactin level. The hyperprolactinemic-amenorrheic women had a significant reduction in bone density compared with age-matched normal controls, and the patients with undetectable serum estradiol concentrations had significantly decreased bone density compared with age-matched controls and with patients with estradiol levels above 20 pg/ml. The patients with undetectable estradiol concentrations also had significantly lower bone density than did the postmenopausal women between the ages of 48 and 69 years. No significant correlation between serum prolactin and bone density was demonstrated.[19] The relationship between serum prolactin levels and bone density was also investigated by Schlechte et al.[20] in a study of amenorrheic women with and without hyperprolactinemia and compared with a group of women with histologically proven prolactin-secreting adenomas who were cured two to five years after surgery, that is, had normal menses and normal serum prolactin levels. An additional group of healthy volunteers was also studied. Bone mineral content was significantly reduced in both groups of women with hyperprolactinemia, those who had a normal postoperative prolactin as well as those who remained hyperprolactinemic after surgery. Regardless of the surgical outcome, the women with prolactin-secreting tumors had significantly decreased bone density that was not related to serum estradiol, androgen, or gonadotropin concentrations. It is well known that premature menopause and attendant hypoestrogenemia are associated with accelerated bone loss in women.

This study suggests that hyperprolactinemia itself may play some role in the promotion of bone loss. Men with chronic hyperprolactinemia and attendant hypogonadism also have decreased bone density compared with age-matched normal men. The decreases occurred in both forearm and vertebral bones and were not related to the absolute prolactin or testosterone concentrations.[21] Reversal of hyperprolactinemia and restoration of gonadal function resulted in a significant increase in radial bone density and a slight increase in vertebral bone density; men who remained hypogonadal despite suppression of prolactin did not exhibit any increase in bone density.[22] Although the decision to treat hyperprolactinemia in the absence of a demonstrable tumor is subject to discussion, the foregoing studies are supportive of the opinion that patients with hyperprolactinemia should receive definitive therapy to lower the prolactin level to normal, to promote return of gonadal function, to halt progression of osteopenia, and possibly to reverse the process.

HYPERPROLACTINEMIA: CLINICAL PRESENTATION

The usual clinical manifestations of hyperprolactinemia are those of gonadal dysfunction, or, with a large tumor, symptoms related to a mass may predominate, such as headaches, visual field disturbances, ophthalmoplegia, and diminished visual acuity. These patients are often seen initially by physicians of diverse specialties. It is not uncommon for a patient to be first evaluated by a neurologist, ophthalmologist, gynecologist, urologist, psychiatrist, or pediatrician. Women of reproductive age are most often seen by the gynecologist because of menstrual irregularities, amenorrhea, galactorrhea, or infertility. The incidence of galactorrhea in women with hyperprolactinemia varies among reports, occurring in 30 to 80 per cent.[23, 24] Conversely, galactorrhea may occur in the presence of normal serum prolactin levels, as demonstrated in 76 women with galactorrhea and normal menses; prolactin was normal in 86 per cent of this group.[25] That hyperprolactinemia frequently causes amenorrhea, oligomenorrhea, and infertility is well described. A less well-defined role of prolactin in female infertility is that of transient preovulatory increases in prolactin. In 48 women with regular menstrual periods and idiopathic infertility, 94 per cent had a preovulatory elevation in serum prolactin levels ranging from 27 to 70 ng/ml over one to three days, which coincided with the preovulatory estradiol peak. In this uncontrolled study,

the increase in prolactin was suppressed with bromocriptine therapy, and 40 per cent of women became pregnant within one to three months of treatment.[26] Another frequent cause of infertility is the polycystic ovarian syndrome. Mild hyperprolactinemia may play a role in a subgroup of women with this disorder. The prevalence of hyperprolactinemia in women with polycystic ovarian syndrome has been reported as 13 to 41 per cent. A more precise prevalence of 17 per cent was observed in 150 women with polycystic ovarian syndrome when multiple serum prolactin determinations were made. Comparison of the hyperprolactinemic and normoprolactinemic women revealed a significantly greater elevation of the serum testosterone in the hyperprolactinemic group.[27] Hyperprolactinemia is also associated with sexual dysfunction in women. This has been most fully characterized in hyperprolactinemic women undergoing hemodialysis for chronic renal failure; 50 to 80 per cent reported decreased libido and frequency of sexual activity,[7, 28] which improved during treatment with bromocriptine.[7] Other psychological disturbances, including hostility, depression, and anxiety, appear to occur more often in women with hyperprolactinemic amenorrhea than in women with normoprolactinemic amenorrhea and women with normal cycles.[29]

Men with hyperprolactinemia usually have some gonadal dysfunction that may initially be considered psychogenic in origin. In 136 men seeking treatment for diminished libido and impotence, 8.1 per cent had hyperprolactinemia.[30] However, in men with documented prolactin-secreting tumors the incidence of impotence was 91 per cent and likely reflects sample bias and/or a more advanced stage of disease.[31] Although most men have diminished libido and/or impotence, only a minority actually report abnormal sexual function. However, after correction of hyperprolactinemia, these men invariably report improvement in libido and potency.[32] From 14 per cent to approximately 33 per cent of men with hyperprolactinemia have galactorrhea; its presence may depend on the vigor with which it is sought.[10, 31] As a likely reflection of the duration of disease prior to diagnosis, a higher proportion of hyperprolactinemic men and postmenopausal women present with visual field defects than do premenopausal women. In one group of 22 men with prolactinomas, 41 per cent had visual impairment.[31] Infertility may also prompt men to seek medical attention. In one survey of 171 infertile men, 7 (4 per cent) had hyperprolactinemia that was reversible with bromocriptine treatment.[33]

Headaches occur commonly in patients with pituitary tumors, particularly macroadenomas. Additionally, there appears to be an increased occurrence of headaches in women with hyperprolactinemia and presumed microadenomas. Fifty-eight per cent of women with hyperprolactinemia and normal radiological evaluation had more than one severe headache per week, compared with 27 per cent of a control group. There was no correlation between the serum prolactin level and the frequency or severity of these headaches, and the precise relationship between an elevated serum prolactin level in the setting of normal radiological studies and headaches is unclear.[34]

Hyperprolactinemia may also cause delayed or arrested puberty and, rarely, precocious puberty. Galactorrhea, infantile genitalia, and short stature have also been observed in these patients.[35–37]

ANATOMIC EVALUATION OF THE PITUITARY GLAND

When clinical and/or biochemical findings are suggestive of hypothalamic-pituitary disease, the anatomy of the pituitary gland and hypothalamus must be defined to determine if a mass or infiltrative lesion is present. With the advent of MR imaging and high-resolution CT scanning, the anatomy of the pituitary gland and surrounding sella turcica is more precisely visualized than with a plain radiograph of the skull or hypocycloidal polytomography. MRI and CT are noninvasive methods to directly visualize the hypothalamic-pituitary region and have replaced the skull radiograph, cerebral arteriography, and pneumoencephalography as initial studies. Comparison of hypocycloidal polytomography with high-resolution CT scanning demonstrated that only 83 per cent of 12 patients with surgically proven microadenomas had abnormal polytomograms.[38] Another study comparing roentgenographic anatomy and histopathology in 205 autopsy specimens demonstrated that 30 per cent of specimens had abnormal radiographic findings that did not correlate with histopathological findings. Abnormalities of the sella such as asymmetry of the floor or minor cortical changes may be normal variations without pathological significance.[39] The definition of normal pituitary anatomy has undergone changes with the introduction of the high-resolution CT and MR scans. Of 107 women with no evidence of pituitary or hypothalamic disease, contrast-enhanced high-resolution direct coronal CT scanning demonstrated that the height of a normal gland may be up to 9 mm, that the upward surface may be convex, and that the larger glands and a convex contour occur in younger women.[40] Swartz et al.[41] studied 50 healthy female volunteers between the ages of 18 and 35 who had no pituitary disease and found that 44 per cent had upwardly convex intrasellar contents, gland density was variable, and 36 per cent had focal defects. These observations are important in considering the diagnosis of a microadenoma. Further complexity of this subject is illustrated by a study of 51 patients who underwent surgery for presumed prolactin-secreting microadenomas; only 39 per cent had documented adenomas at surgery, and of this group only 85 per cent had abnormal CT findings. Conversely, 66 per cent of patients with hyperprolactinemia and no microadenoma at surgery had abnormal CT findings. In this series, only focal lesions of the gland were determined to be significant in the identification of microadenomas.[42]

Currently, the most accurate method of defining pituitary anatomy is the MR scan with gadolinium diethylenetriaminopentaacetic acid (Gd-DTPA) enhancement. The second most accurate study is a high-resolution CT scan with direct coronal sections or reformatted sections in coronal and sagittal planes. Contiguous images, with 1.5-mm collimation through the pituitary gland, is the most precise way to image the gland with CT. Intravenous contrast as a rapid intravenous bolus followed by a drip infusion should be administered to assess gland homogeneity and the presence or absence of focal lesions. MR imaging is superior to CT because it allows visualization of the optic chiasm and cavernous sinus regions, thus defining the superior and lateral borders of a mass, optic chiasm compression, stalk deviation, or cavernous sinus invasion. Gland size on MR imaging correlates with both CT and autopsy studies; normal gland height ranges from 3 to 9 mm. On MR scan, approximately 75 per cent of the pituitary is the anterior portion, which is usually isointense with brain white matter on most sequences; gland heterogeneity may occur in normal subjects. The posterior pituitary is identifiable by a high signal intensity, which probably reflects lipid-containing substances within vasopressin-containing neurons. The optic chiasm lies directly above the pituitary fossa in 80 per cent of subjects, and the pituitary stalk is posterior to the chiasm. The cavernous sinus is lateral to and isointense with the pituitary; cranial nerves III, IV, VI, the V_1 and V_2 divisions of V, and the internal carotid artery are located in the cavernous sinus. The cranial nerves are lower in signal intensity than the pituitary, and the carotid artery has very low signal intensity (signal void, black), reflecting blood flow. Incidental hemorrhage is occasionally present, and a partially empty sella is observed frequently in normal subjects.[43]

Both CT (if performed properly) and MR techniques are approximately equivalent in identifying a large pituitary mass. However, MR imaging is superior in defining a tumor's full extent and relationship to surrounding structures and is more accurate in identifying small lesions (Fig. 24-1). In patients with surgically proven microadenomas, the MR scan correctly identified the lesion and its location in 100 per cent, whereas accurate identification by CT

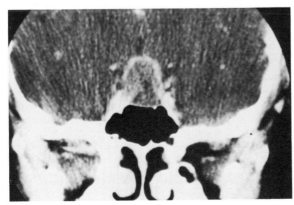
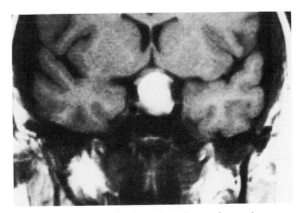

FIGURE 24–1. Coronal CT (*left*) and MR (*right*) scan of a 15-year-old girl with primary amenorrhea and a cystic macroprolactinoma (serum prolactin 350 µg/L).

occurred in only 50 per cent.[44] Although superior, the MR image may not identify all small lesions as demonstrated by a study of patients with Cushing's disease; only 83 per cent of surgically proven tumors were visualized on MR images.[45] A microadenoma on MR imaging is usually round and hypointense with the normal gland on T1-weighted images; lesions are best demonstrated with coronal images and have a higher signal than normal gland on T2-weighted images. Pituitary stalk (infundibulum) deviation to the side opposite the tumor may be a helpful indicator of tumor location. Macroadenomas tend to have signal characteristics similar to those of the normal gland and cystic or hemorrhagic areas may be present.[43]

Hemorrhage has a characteristic appearance on the MR image and depends on the age of the hemorrhage and disruption of the blood-brain barrier. An acute hemorrhage, less than one week old, consists of deoxyhemoglobin and is isointense with the gland on T1-weighted images and has low signal intensity on T2-weighted images. A subacute hemorrhage, one to four weeks in age, contains methemoglobin, which forms from the periphery to the center and appears as high signal on both T1- and T2-weighted images. A hemorrhage older than four weeks appears as a homogeneous high signal on both T1 and T2 images; hemosiderin appears as a ring around the hemorrhage.[46]

BIOCHEMICAL EVALUATION

While the diagnosis of hyperprolactinemia may be made with a single serum sample if the concentration is sufficiently elevated, this hormone is secreted in a pulsatile fashion and levels vary throughout a 24-hour period. Although a single elevated morning level may be adequate to diagnose excess prolactin secretion, a potential problem is a mildly elevated level—20 to 40 ng/ml—which may reflect a peak determination or may be a result of stress. For these reasons, it is prudent to obtain several samples before making the diagnosis of pathological hyperprolactinemia. This can easily be achieved by obtaining a single sample on three separate days or three sequential samples from an indwelling venous catheter every 30 minutes when the patient is sufficiently relaxed. Once the diagnosis of hyperprolactinemia is established, the numerous causes should be considered before proceeding to more elaborate testing. After pregnancy, hypothyroidism, and drugs are eliminated as possible causes, the search for hypothalamic or pituitary disease is necessary. As mentioned in the section on radiographic evaluation, MR imaging or high-resolution CT scanning with intravenous contrast administration characterizes hypothalamic and pituitary anatomy. Despite these technological advancements, imaging studies may not always demonstrate a tumor. For this reason, numerous dynamic tests have been proposed to differentiate hypothalamic from pituitary disease and to determine if a pituitary tumor is present. The most widely used test is administration of TRH with measurement of the prolactin response. Other agents such as the dopamine receptor antagonist sulpiride, the dopamine-releasing agent nomifensine, the histamine-2 receptor blocker cimetidine, and D-amphetamine, an inhibitor of dopamine uptake, have also been used. As a general rule, a majority of patients with a prolactin-secreting tumor have a diminished prolactin response

to intravenous TRH, but this observation is not a consistent finding and this test should not be used to diagnose or exclude a tumor. Additionally, this test is not specific to distinguish between hypothalamic and pituitary diseases. In a review of several series, totaling more than 600 hyperprolactinemic patients, only 11 per cent had a normal increase in prolactin of greater than 100 per cent over the basal level. However, a blunted prolactin response to TRH is not specific for a pituitary disease, as was demonstrated in a study of 49 patients with hyperprolactinemia; 82 per cent of patients with a prolactinoma had a blunted response and 64 per cent with suprasellar tumors (nonprolactinomas) also had a blunted prolactin response to TRH.[47] Sulpiride, nomifensine, cimetidine, and D-amphetamine have also been used in an attempt to distinguish the cause of hyperprolactinemia.[48–50] The response to these agents is no more specific and thus of little practical use in a diagnostic evaluation.

Serum prolactin levels have been measured in patients with a variety of intracranial diseases, including patients with pituitary tumors. Prolactin levels were measured in 205 patients with a spectrum of disorders, including intracranial aneurysm, craniopharyngioma, stroke, head trauma, seizures, headaches, suspected pituitary tumor, and third ventricle tumor. Five clinical entities were associated with an elevation of serum prolactin, including craniopharyngioma, meningioma, ectopic pinealoma, third ventricle tumor, and aneurysm; additionally, one patient taking amitriptyline also had an elevated serum prolactin level. Prolactin levels were less than 100 ng/ml in these patients, compared with patients with a documented pituitary tumor who had elevations ranging from 30 to 22,000 ng/ml. Fourteen patients were suspected of having a pituitary tumor; six had an elevated prolactin level of 30 to 200 ng/ml. In the entire group of 205 patients, 63 had elevated prolactin levels and 46 of these had tumors verified by biopsy; thus, 73 per cent of these hyperprolactinemic patients had definite evidence of a pituitary adenoma. Of particular note in this study was the age distribution at the time of diagnosis of patients with surgically documented pituitary adenomas. The majority of women were between 15 and 44 years of age, whereas the majority of men ranged in age from 45 to 74 years.[51] This supports the clinical impression that men more often present later in the course of disease than do women. Caution should be exercised in presuming that a macroadenoma is a prolactinoma if the serum prolactin is only moderately elevated. This is exemplified by a report of two women with macroadenomas in whom the initial prolactin level was less than 100 ng/ml; bromocriptine effectively suppressed prolactin to normal, but there was no reduction in tumor size. Pathological examination of the tumors with immunoperoxidase staining demonstrated no prolactin-secreting cells in one, and only 10 per cent of the cells contained prolactin in the other.[52] As a general guide, most patients with macroprolactinomas have a serum prolactin of greater than 200 ng/ml.

PREGNANCY AND HYPERPROLACTINEMIA

Once a woman has received effective treatment for hyperprolactinemia, fertility is usually re-established. After the serum prolactin level has been suppressed and there is a return of regular cyclic menses, the chances of achieving pregnancy are theoretically and practically the same as those of a normal woman of the same age. Hyperprolactinemic women with documented pituitary tumors treated with bromocriptine had a pregnancy rate of 37.5 to 81 per cent.[53–56] Of 200 women treated with transsphenoidal surgery, 90 desired pregnancy and 78 became pregnant (87 per cent). However, 37 of these (47 per cent) required postoperative bromocriptine, radiation therapy, or a combination of the two prior to conception.[57]

The management of women with prolactinomas during pregnancy remains controversial, although there is general agreement that these patients should be followed very closely for development of symptoms of pituitary expansion, such as headache, visual field defects, and ophthalmoplegia. Because the volume of the normal pituitary gland increases by approximately 70 per cent during normal pregnancy,[58] expansion in women harboring a microadenoma or macroadenoma is of particular concern. From the available information, pregnant women with microadenomas appear to have a very low risk for development of complications related to pituitary expansion, perhaps less than 1 per cent. The precise risk in women with macroadenomas is difficult to determine but is probably less than 25 per cent. These estimates are based on two published series of retrospective studies. Magyar and Marshall[59] reported the results of a survey of 45 obstetricians on the outcome of 91 pregnancies in 73 women with previously untreated pituitary tumors. Sixty-five of the women had either an abnormal plain radiograph of the sella turcica or abnormal sellar tomograms prior to pregnancy; there was no estimation of tumor size. Twenty-three per cent of these 73 women had headaches during pregnancy, and 25 per cent developed visual field abnormalities; 61 per cent remained asymptomatic. Treatment included surgery or radiation therapy either during or after pregnancy in 22 of the 73; two were treated during pregnancy with dexamethasone and one with bromocriptine. Seven women developed visual field abnormalities and received no therapy during pregnancy; none of these had permanent sequelae after delivery. Surgical complications included diabetes insipidus in five, which was transient in three; one had postoperative anosmia; and one had a persistent visual field defect. Gemzell and Wang[53] reported the results of 91 pregnancies in 85 women with previously untreated microadenomas; 1.1 per cent of these patients developed headaches and visual field abnormalities during pregnancy. Forty-six per cent of women with previously untreated macroadenomas had 46 pregnancies; headaches and visual field abnormalities occurred in 25 per cent. However, the incidence of these symptoms during 70 pregnancies in 67 women with previously treated pituitary tumors was 2.8 per cent; these women received either surgery or radiation therapy or both prior to conception. There was no predilection for time with regard to development of complications; they occurred with equal frequency during the first, second, and third trimesters. Women who developed complications during pregnancy either were treated with surgery, yttrium-90 implantation, corticosteroids, or bromocriptine or were observed. There were no permanent sequelae related to the tumor in any of the women. In a discussion of pregnancy and hyperprolactinemia, Molitch[60] reviewed the literature of complications

during pregnancy. Of 246 women with previously untreated microadenomas, 1.6 per cent had symptoms of tumor enlargement, and 4.5 per cent had asymptomatic enlargement demonstrated radiographically. In 45 women with untreated macroadenomas, 15.5 per cent had symptomatic tumor enlargement and 8.9 per cent had asymptomatic enlargement. In an additional group of 46 women with macroadenomas who received prior treatment with irradiation or surgery, only 4.3 per cent had symptomatic tumor enlargement and none had asymptomatic enlargement. Samaan and colleagues[61] described 18 women with hyperprolactinemia and no evidence of pituitary tumor on polytomography or CT scan who became pregnant while taking bromocriptine; there were no complications during pregnancy. Rjosk and colleagues[62] reported no complications during 65 pregnancies in 81 women. Only 2 of 13 women who received transsphenoidal surgery had a normal postoperative serum prolactin level; 11 were treated with bromocriptine prior to pregnancy. Regardless of measures taken prior to pregnancy, there is no guarantee that prepregnancy radiation or surgery will prevent complications secondary to pituitary expansion during pregnancy as evidenced by ophthalmologic complications despite prior pituitary irradiation, but this is a very rare event because properly planned radiation therapy is safe and highly effective in preventing this complication.[63, 64] The development of significant pituitary expansion and complications may be managed expectantly, medically with a dopamine agonist, or surgically with transsphenoidal surgery. That the dopamine agonist bromocriptine promotes rapid suppression of prolactin and a decrease in pituitary size is well-documented; moreover, it does not appear to interfere with pregnancy.[65–67]

TREATMENT OF HYPERPROLACTINEMIA

The goals of any therapy for hyperprolactinemia are straightforward. These include suppression of excessive hormone secretion, reduction in the mass of any demonstrable tumor, restoration to normal of any disturbance of vision and/or cranial nerve function, preservation or restoration of other anterior pituitary function, and prevention of recurrence or progression of disease. Currently, there are several choices for therapy, including observation, surgical resection (that is, transsphenoidal microsurgery), pituitary radiation, and medical treatment with a dopamine agonist. Any therapeutic decision should be based upon these goals, clinical features, results and risks of treatment, and patient preference. The long-term consequences of persistent hyperprolactinemia include gonadal dysfunction with resultant infertility and the potential for development of large tumors with adverse effects on the visual system, as well as adverse effects on bone density. Although the precise risk of development of a large pituitary tumor is not known, it must be presumed that only a minority of patients will have a progressive increase in tumor size.[14–17]

Prior to the advent of medical treatment for hyperprolactinemia, therapy usually consisted of surgical resection and/or pituitary irradiation. From the limited information available on prolactin-secreting adenomas, it is apparent that only a minority of patients treated with pituitary irradiation achieve a normal serum prolactin level within a short time span. Additionally, achievement of a normal serum prolactin level with radiation therapy appears to occur most readily in patients with relatively lower pretreatment levels. In 28 patients reported by Sheline and colleagues,[68] only 8 had normal serum prolactin levels 2 to 10 years (mean 4.2 years) following radiation therapy. Antunes et al.[69] followed six patients with prolactinomas for 13 to 72 months (mean 32 months) who were treated with radiation therapy and found that serum prolactin levels were reduced by 94 per cent for the group; however, no patient achieved a normal serum prolactin concentration. Nabarro[70] reported that in 15 patients treated with radiation therapy, 3 of 14 had reduction of prolactin to normal within 21 to 33 months, and an additional patient had a normal prolactin 6 years after radiation therapy. In another study of 6 patients with prolactinomas who were treated with surgery prior to radiation therapy and followed for 6 to 84 months (mean 39 months), prolactin levels fell by 75 per cent; however, none of the patients achieved a normal serum prolactin level.[31] It is apparent from these reports that although pituitary radiation does not produce a rapid reduction in serum prolactin, it does appear effective in preventing progression of disease over the long term. An alternative is dopamine agonist medical therapy in conjunction with pituitary radiation. Grossman and colleagues studied the effects of radiation therapy in 36 women with small prolactinomas who were treated with 4500 rads (4.5 Gy) and then given a dopamine agonist—bromocriptine, lisuride, or pergolide. Twenty-eight were later evaluated when dopamine agonist therapy was withdrawn; 25 had a decrease in serum prolactin and 8 had a normal serum prolactin two to eight years after radiation therapy. No patient had tumor expansion, even during pregnancy, at which time the dopamine agonist therapy was discontinued. The fertility rate in the women treated with combination radiation therapy and a dopamine agonist was 73 per cent of those who desired fertility, and the apparent ovulation rate was 94 per cent. That the beneficial effect on gonadal function was more likely related to the dopamine agonist than to radiation therapy is suggested by the observation that 92 per cent of the women who successfully conceived did so within four months of treatment.[64]

Transsphenoidal resection of prolactinomas has been performed in a large number of patients at various centers. Surgical success depends on two important factors: the size of the tumor and the experience of the neurosurgeon. In reports from centers in which this procedure is performed frequently, a normal postoperative serum prolactin level is achieved in 60 to 80 per cent of patients with microadenomas (less than 10 mm in diameter) and ranges from 0 to 40 per cent of those with macroadenomas (more than 10 mm in diameter).[69, 71–75] As exemplified in a report by Hardy,[75] there is a good correlation between the size of the pituitary tumor, the preoperative serum prolactin concentration, and the operative cure rate, that is, normal postoperative serum prolactin. Of 266 women who underwent transsphenoidal surgery, 14 had a preoperative prolactin level of 20 to 250 ng/ml, and 86 per cent of these had a normal postoperative prolactin. When the preoperative prolactin level was between 251 and 500 ng/ml, the postoperative cure rate was 48 per cent, and when the preoperative prolactin level was greater than 1000 ng/ml, only 6 per cent had a normal serum prolactin level following

transsphenoidal surgery. Similar results were obtained in 55 men with prolactinomas. Of 100 patients who underwent transsphenoidal surgery at the Mayo Clinic, 54 of the 84 women had a microadenoma. Of the 32 with a preoperative serum prolactin of less than 100 ng/ml, 88 per cent had a normal postoperative serum prolactin level. Only 50 per cent of patients with a microadenoma and preoperative prolactin level of greater than 100 ng/ml had a successful result. Of 10 women with a diffuse noninvasive macroadenoma, 50 per cent had a surgical cure, whereas only 25 per cent of the 20 women with an invasive adenoma were cured. All of the 16 men had a macroadenoma; 43 per cent with a diffuse adenoma had a normal postoperative prolactin level and 19 per cent with an invasive adenoma had a successful outcome. Operative complications included cerebrospinal rhinorrhea in one patient and transient diabetes insipidus in nine patients; there were no operative deaths.[74] In another series from the Mayo Clinic, assessment of the risks and benefits of transsphenoidal surgery following unsuccessful prior therapy was carried out in 158 patients. In this heterogeneous group of patients, 35 per cent of patients with pituitary hypersecretion had a successful surgical result, 59 per cent of patients with visual disturbance had an improvement in vision, and 74 per cent had successful repair of CSF rhinorrhea. Fifty of the 158 patients (32 per cent) experienced new complications following transsphenoidal surgery, including four deaths, stroke or vascular injury, hemorrhage, visual loss, meningitis, CSF rhinorrhea, cranial nerve palsy, permanent diabetes insipidus, hypopituitarism, and nasal septal perforation. It is clear from these results that the surgical risks for a patient who has received prior therapy, particularly previous surgery, are significantly greater than for a previously untreated patient undergoing the same procedure.[76] Although surgery affords the opportunity for rapid decompression of a prolactinoma and potential cure, the incidence of recurrent hyperprolactinemia and tumor regrowth must be considered. Serri and colleagues[77] reported the long-term follow-up of 44 patients treated with transsphenoidal microsurgery. Twenty-eight patients with microadenomas had a normal serum prolactin level following surgery (85 per cent); hyperprolactinemia recurred in 50 per cent after 4 ± 1.3 years. Sixteen patients had macroadenomas, and five of these had a normal serum prolactin level following surgery; hyperprolactinemia recurred in four of five (80 per cent) 2.5 ± 1.6 years following surgery. In another study of late recurrence of tumor, Rodman and colleagues[78] reported a 17 per cent recurrence after 50 ± 3 months in women who underwent successful surgery for a microadenoma. In women with a macroadenoma and a normal serum prolactin following transsphenoidal resection, 20 per cent developed recurrent hyperprolactinemia.[78] As mentioned, the highest rate of surgical cure occurs in patients with a microadenoma and a preoperative prolactin level of less than 250 ng/ml. However, even these patients have a significant risk of recurrence of disease.

The introduction of specific dopamine agonists into clinical medicine, beginning in 1971, afforded a new therapeutic approach for patients with hyperprolactinemia and prolactinomas. Bromocriptine, 2-Br-α-ergocryptine mesylate, is a semisynthetic ergot alkaloid that was specifically developed as an inhibitor of prolactin secretion and is the prototype for other dopamine agonist preparations. Although bromocriptine is the only dopamine agonist currently approved for use in the United States, other compounds such as lisuride and pergolide are available in other countries. Newer compounds undergoing evaluation include a long-acting ergot-derivative, cabergoline, and a nonergot compound, quinagolide (CV 205-502). Bromocriptine directly stimulates neuronal and pituitary cell membrane dopamine receptors[79–81] and competes with specific binding of ^{3}H-dopamine to dopamine receptors of isolated bovine pituitary membranes.[81] This specific dopamine receptor agonist inhibits prolactin secretion both in vitro[82, 83] and in vivo.[84] Following a single oral dose of bromocriptine, serum prolactin remains suppressed for up to 14 hours,[85] after which time no drug remains detectable in the circulation.[86] The most common side effects of bromocriptine and other dopamine agonists are nausea and orthostatic hypotension, which usually occur upon initiation of therapy. These side effects may be prevented or minimized by initially administering a low dose at bedtime in the middle of food. The dose is then gradually increased over days or weeks to that which achieves a therapeutic response, the drug being always taken during a meal. Other less commonly encountered side effects of dopamine agonists include headache, fatigue, abdominal cramps, nasal congestion, and constipation.[32] Hallucinations have also been reported to occur with these drugs. A review of 600 patients treated with either bromocriptine or lisuride noted that eight developed psychosis during drug therapy. The symptoms included auditory hallucinations, delusions, and appreciable mood changes, and all symptoms abated when treatment was stopped. Although this adverse reaction occurred in only 1.3 per cent of this group of patients, both physicians and patients should be aware of this possibility.[87] Additionally, symptoms of nausea and abdominal pain may be exacerbated by concomitant ingestion of alcohol, and patients should be cautioned of this potential interaction.[88] Bromocriptine has been administered by the vaginal route to normal and hyperprolactinemic women. In normal women, vaginal administration produced higher bromocriptine serum concentrations than did an equivalent oral dose (2.5 mg); serum prolactin concentrations declined to less than 90 per cent of baseline values.[89, 90] Fifteen hyperprolactinemic women were treated for four weeks with a single daily vaginal bromocriptine dose (2.5 mg); serum prolactin decreased to normal in 13 (87 per cent). Side effects included one episode of mild nausea and two cases of transient constipation. Retrospective comparison with oral bromocriptine therapy suggested that the vaginal route of administration produced much fewer gastrointestinal side effects.[91]

Although the dopamine agonists usually suppress serum prolactin, there is a spectrum of responsiveness. A single oral dose of 2.5 mg of bromocriptine suppressed serum prolactin by 47 to 96 per cent, and this effect lasted for at least nine hours. Chronic treatment with 2.5 mg of bromocriptine three times daily resulted in further lowering of serum prolactin levels[92, 93] (Fig. 24–2). Numerous investigators have reported the effectiveness of bromocriptine and other dopamine agonists in decreasing serum prolactin levels, in abolishing galactorrhea, in restoring gonadal function, and in causing a decrease in tumor size. In a review of 13 reported series on the effectiveness of bromocriptine in 286 hyperprolactinemic women, between 64 and 100 per cent of patients had suppression of prolactin to normal, 64 to 100 per cent had improvement in galactorrhea, 57 to 100 per cent had return of menses, and 57 to 100 per cent had documented ovulation.[32] After six months of therapy, more than 80 per cent of women have return of normal menstrual cycles.[93] Although most women have improvement or cessation of galactorrhea, this may persist despite lowering of prolactin levels to normal.

The response to dopamine agonist therapy in patients with macroadenomas is similar to that in patients with microadenomas who have substantially lower pretreatment serum prolactin levels. However, although dopamine agonists are effective in decreasing serum prolactin levels and the size of a large pituitary tumor, achievement of normal serum prolactin concentrations usually requires a longer treatment time than in patients with microadenomas. This probably reflects tumor mass rather than unresponsiveness to dopamine receptor stimulation. This is perhaps best exemplified by two reports of long-term follow-up of patients with macroadenomas treated with either bromocriptine or lisuride. In a prospective study of 27 patients with macroadenomas who received bromocriptine for 12 to 15 months as primary therapy (no other treatment), 67 per cent had a decrease in serum prolactin to normal and 100 per cent had a decrease in tumor size. Nine of 10 patients with visual field defects had improvement in these abnormalities.[94] In another study of 38 patients treated with bromocriptine or lisuride for 30 to 88 months (mean 57 ± 14 months), 79 per cent had suppression of prolactin to normal and 76 per cent had a decrease in tumor size.[95] Numerous other studies have been done of patients with macroadenomas treated with bromocriptine or lisuride and, as a general rule, from 50 to 100 per cent of patients have suppression of prolactin to normal. Again, this may depend on the length of treatment.[32, 94, 95] It should be emphasized that although some patients may not have a reduction in

FIGURE 24–2. Mean (± SEM) serum prolactin levels in seven women with hyperprolactinemia after an initial oral dose of 2.5 mg of bromocriptine and after three and six months of treatment with 2.5 mg three times daily. Marked suppression of prolactin occurs with the first dose and is maintained during chronic treatment. (From Thorner MO, McNeilly AS, Hagan C, Besser GM: Long-term treatment of galactorrhea and hypogonadism with bromocriptine. BMJ 2:419–422, 1974.)

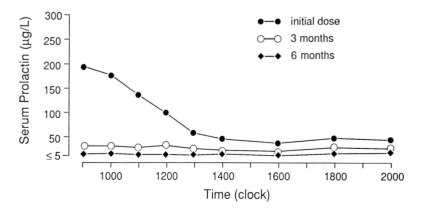

serum prolactin to normal during dopamine agonist therapy, a majority have a substantial reduction in serum prolactin levels. Of particular note is the finding that most patients with macroadenomas have a reduction of serum prolactin prior to any radiographically detectable change in tumor size.[94] The standard dose of bromocriptine is 2.5 mg three times daily, and the usual dose of lisuride is 0.2 mg three times daily; however, some patients may require up to 20 mg of bromocriptine/d or 0.8 mg of lisuride daily. The precise dose may not remain constant, as exemplified by the patients reported by Liuzzi and colleagues.[95] These investigators reduced the dose of either bromocriptine or lisuride in 30 patients with macroadenomas who had achieved normal serum prolactin levels during medical therapy. Twenty-one of the 30 patients had continued suppression of serum prolactin, and there was no change in tumor size when they took lower doses of bromocriptine or lisuride for 6 to 52 months.

Newer dopamine agonist drugs include a long-acting compound, cabergoline, which can be administered once or twice weekly. This ergoline derivative reduced serum prolactin concentrations to normal in 22 of 30 hyperprolactinemic women (73 per cent) after 1 to 36 weeks of therapy (mean 6 weeks). Five of seven patients had at least 50 per cent reduction in tumor size after one year of therapy. Side effects occurred in 13 and were similar to those with bromocriptine (nausea, hypotension, headache, gastric pain, dizziness, weakness) but disappeared in 10 women.[96] In another group of 11 hyperprolactinemic women with a demonstrable pituitary tumor, prolactin was suppressed to normal in all patients, and all had evidence of a decrease in tumor size. No side effects occurred in these women.[97] CV 205-502 (quinagolide), a nonergot compound that stimulates the D_2 receptor, is undergoing clinical evaluation for treatment of hyperprolactinemia. This compound is administered once daily, and its effect on reducing prolactin and tumor size is similar to that of other dopamine agonists[98–101] (Figs. 24–3 and 24–4). In some patients, CV 205-502 produces fewer side effects than the ergot derivatives; of 22 hyperprolactinemic women treated for six months with either CV 205-502 or bromocriptine (double-blind study), four patients receiving bromocriptine discontinued treatment because of side effects but

none of the women in the CV 205-502 group stopped treatment. Serum prolactin decreased to normal in 8 of 11 CV 205-502–treated women and in 2 of 9 bromocriptine-treated women.[101] A long-acting depot injectable bromocriptine preparation that can be administered repeatedly appears to suppress prolactin concentrations for up to 28 days. Serum prolactin was substantially reduced in 6 women with a microadenoma and in 8 men and women with a macroadenoma; prolactin decreased to normal in 9 of 14 patients (64 per cent) after six months. Mild nausea and vomiting occurred in 2 patients, and 4 had symptomatic postural hypotension within the first 24 hours after the injection.[102]

As noted, an alternate modality of therapy is the combination of pituitary radiation and a dopamine agonist, with intermittent withdrawal of medical treatment to determine the effectiveness of pituitary irradiation. Grossman and colleagues[64] noted that 26 of 27 women with prolactinomas treated with megavoltage radiation therapy and either bromocriptine, lisuride, or pergolide had a decrease in serum prolactin levels when medical therapy was withdrawn 1 to 11 years after radiation therapy (mean 4.2 years); serum prolactin levels became normal in 8 of these patients. This combined approach appears beneficial over the long term; however, these patients require monitoring for the potential development of hypopituitarism, which does not occur with dopamine agonist therapy alone. Dopamine agonist therapy must be considered chronic therapy because withdrawal of the drug usually results in return of hyperprolactinemia and tumor expansion with the risk of visual compromise.[9, 37, 95, 103] In this context, dopamine therapy must be considered "replacement" treatment for a functional dopamine deficiency.

Although most patients have a satisfactory biochemical and clinical response to dopamine agonist therapy, there have been isolated reports of a few patients in whom progression of disease has occurred during bromocriptine therapy.[104–106] This occurrence serves to emphasize the need for close monitoring of all patients with a pituitary tumor.

Because dopamine agonists are used to treat infertility secondary to hyperprolactinemia, the question of potential teratogenicity during pregnancy is important. This has

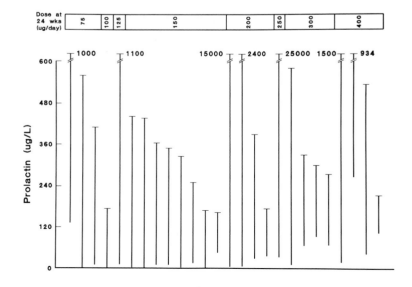

FIGURE 24–3. Serum prolactin concentrations in 26 patients with a prolactin-secreting macroadenoma before and after 24 weeks of CV 205-502 therapy (normal serum prolactin is < 20 μg/L). (From Vance ML, Lipper M, Klibanski A, et al: Treatment of prolactin-secreting pituitary macroadenomas with the long-acting non-ergot dopamine agonist CV 205-502. Ann Intern Med 112:668–673, 1990.)

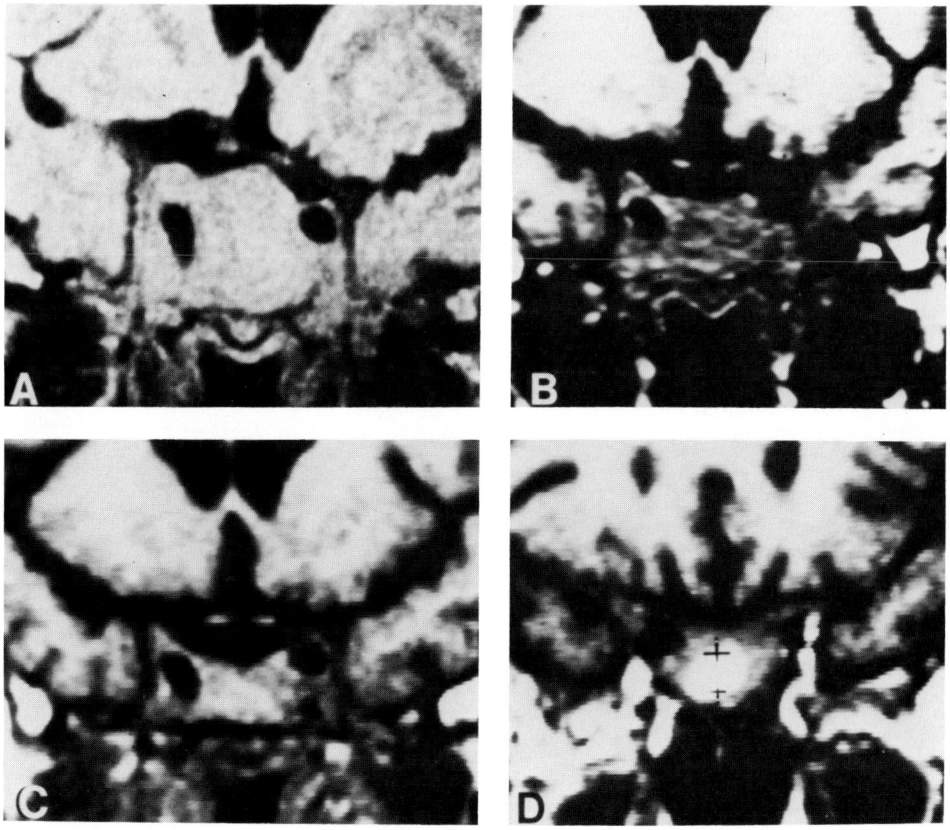

FIGURE 24-4. Coronal MR scans in a man with a prolactin-secreting pituitary macroadenoma before (A) and after 8 (B) and 24 (C) weeks of treatment with CV 205-502. Note an area of spontaneous hemorrhage in the tumor, which did not produce pituitary insufficiency (D). Serum prolactin decreased from 15,000 to 11 μg/L after 12 weeks of treatment. (From Vance ML, Lipper M, Klibanski A, et al: Treatment of prolactin-secreting pituitary macroadenomas with the long-acting non-ergot dopamine agonist CV 205-502. Ann Intern Med 112:668–673, 1990.)

been studied in 1410 pregnancies in 1335 women who received bromocriptine. There was no associated increased risk to the fetus; the mean duration of bromocriptine ingestion after conception for 1278 pregnancies was 21 days; 9 women took the drug throughout pregnancy and 4 took the drug late in pregnancy. Spontaneous abortion occurred in 11.1 per cent, compared with a 10 to 15 per cent rate in the normal population. Multiple births occurred in 1.8 per cent of women who took bromocriptine. The incidence of congenital abnormalities detected at birth was 3.5 per cent; 1 per cent of these were life threatening or required surgery, and the remaining 2.5 per cent were minor abnormalities. This incidence of congenital abnormalities is comparable to that in the normal population. The duration of fetal exposure to bromocriptine was 30.6 days (mean) for the group with congenital abnormalities and 30.5 days (mean) in the group with normal children. The calculated dose of bromocriptine ingested by the mothers was not different.[108] Although these data suggest no increased risk of spontaneous abortions or congenital abnormalities associated with exposure to bromocriptine, continuous surveillance of this group of children is required to exclude any late-appearing effects of the drug.

As outlined in this chapter, the diagnosis and treatment of patients with hyperprolactinemia are relatively straightforward. The wide availability of the prolactin radioimmunoassays and immunoradiometric assays allows for prompt recognition of hyperprolactinemia as the cause of a multiplicity of clinical presentations, the most common of which is gonadal dysfunction. Serum prolactin determinations in conjunction with an MR or high-resolution CT scan of the pituitary afford the opportunity to assess both secretory activity and anatomy of the gland, both of which

should be delineated prior to institution of therapy. The choice of therapy should be made on the basis of goals outlined earlier, and careful follow-up is mandatory for these patients.

REFERENCES

1. Edwards CRW, Forsyth IA, Besser GM: Amenorrhea, galactorrhoea and primary hypothyroidism with high circulating levels of prolactin. Br Med J 111:462–464, 1971.
2. Refetoff S, Fang VS, Rappaport B, Friesen HG: Interrelationships in the regulation of TSH and prolactin secretion in man: Effect of L-dopa, TRH, and thyroid hormone in various combinations. J Clin Endocrinol Metab 38:450–457, 1974.
3. Chirito E, Bonda A, Friesen HG: Prolactin in renal failure (abstract). Clin Res 20:423, 1972.
4. Nagel TC, Freinkel N, Bell RH, et al: Gynecomastia, prolactin, and other peptide hormones in patients undergoing chronic hemodialysis. J Clin Endocrinol Metab 36:428–432, 1973.
5. Olgaard K, Hagen C, McNeilly AS: Pituitary hormones in women with chronic renal failure: The effect of chronic haemo- and peritoneal dialysis. Acta Endocrinol 80:237–246, 1975.
6. Hagen C, Olgaard K, McNeilly AS, Fisher R: Prolactin and the pituitary-gonadal axis in male uremic patients on regular dialysis. Acta Endocrinol 82:29–38, 1976.
7. Weizman R, Weizman A, Levi J, et al: Sexual dysfunction associated with hyperprolactinemia in males and females undergoing hemodialysis. Psychosom Med 45:259–269, 1983.
8. Coulam CB, Annegers JF, Abboud CF, et al: Pituitary adenoma and contraceptives: A case-control study. Fertil Steril 31:25–28, 1979.
9. Hull MGR, Bromham DR, Savage PE, et al: Post-pill amenorrhea: A causal study. Fertil Steril 36:472–476, 1981.
10. Thorner MO, Edwards CRW, Hanker JP, et al: Prolactin and gonadotropin interaction in the male. In Troen P, Nankin H (eds): The Testis in Normal and Infertile Men. New York, Raven Press, 1977, pp 351–366.
11. Costello RT: Subclinical adenoma of the pituitary gland. Am J Pathol 12:205–216, 1936.

12. Burrow GN, Wortzman G, Rewcastle NB, et al: Microadenomas of the pituitary and abnormal sellar tomograms in an unselected autopsy series. N Engl J Med 304:156–158, 1980.

13. Pepperell RJ: Prolactin and reproduction. Fertil Steril 35:267–274, 1981.

14. March CM, Kletzky OA, Davajan V, et al: Longitudinal evaluations of patients with untreated prolactin-secreting pituitary adenomas. Am J Obstet Gynecol 139:835–844, 1981.

15. Von Werder K, Fahlbusch R, Rjosk HK: Macroprolactinoms: Clinical and therapeutic aspects. In Tolis G, Sterfanis C, Monatokalakis T, and Labine F (eds): Prolactin and Prolactinomas. New York, Raven Press, 1983, pp 415–429.

16. Koppelman MCS, Jaffe MJ, Rieth KG, et al: Hyperprolactinemia, amenorrhea, and galactorrhea: A retrospective assessment of twenty-five cases. Ann Intern Med 100:115–121, 1984.

17. Martin TL, Kim M, Malarkey WB: The natural history of idiopathic hyperprolactinemia. J Clin Endocrinol Metab 60:855–858, 1985.

18. Schlechte J, Dolan K, Sherman B, et al: The natural history of untreated hyperprolactinemia: A prospective analysis. J Clin Endocrinol Metab 68:412–418, 1989.

19. Klibanski A, Neer RM, Beitins IZ, et al: Decreased bone density in hyperprolactinemic women. N Engl J Med 303:1511–1514, 1980.

20. Schlechte JA, Sherman B, Martin R: Bone density in amenorrheic women with and without hyperprolactinemia. J Clin Endocrinol Metab 56:1120–1123, 1983.

21. Greenspan SL, Neer RM, Reigway EC, Klibanski A: Osteoporosis in men with hyperprolactinemic hypogonadism. Ann Intern Med 104:777–782, 1986.

22. Greenspan SL, Oppenhiem DS, Klibanski A: Importance of gonadal steroids to bone mass in men with hyperprolactinemic hypogonadism. Ann Intern Med 110:526–531, 1989.

23. Franks S, Nabarro JDN, Jacobs HS: Prevalence and presentation of hyperprolactinemia in patients with "functionless" pituitary tumours. Lancet 1:778–780, 1977.

24. Thorner MO, Besser GM: Bromocriptine treatment of hyperprolactinemic hypogonadism. Acta Endocrinol 88(Suppl 216):131–146, 1978.

25. Kleinberg DL, Noel GL, Frantz AG: Galactorrhea: A study of 235 cases, including 48 with pituitary tumors. N Engl J Med 296:589–600, 1977.

26. Ben-David M, Schenker JG: Transient hyperprolactinemia: A correctable cause of idiopathic female infertility. J Clin Endocrinol Metab 57:442–444, 1983.

27. Luciano AA, Chapler FK, Sherman BM: Hyperprolactinemia in polycystic ovary syndrome. Fertil Steril 41:719–725, 1984.

28. Mastrogiacomo L, DeBesi L, Serafini E, et al: Hyperprolactinemia and sexual disturbances among uremic women on hemodialysis. Nephron 37:195–199, 1984.

29. Fava M, Fava GA, Kellner R, et al: Psychosomatic aspects of hyperprolactinemia. Psychother Psychosom 40:257–262, 1983.

30. Schwartz MF, Baumann JE, Masters WH: Hyperprolactinemia and sexual disorders in men. Biol Psychiatry 17:861–876, 1982.

31. Carter JN, Tyson JE, Tolis C, et al: Prolactin-secreting tumors and hypogonadism in 22 men. N Engl J Med 299:847–852, 1978.

32. Vance ML, Evans WS, Thorner MO: Drugs five years later: Bromocriptine. Ann Intern Med 100:78–91, 1984.

33. Segal S, Yaffe H, Laufer N, Ben-David M: Male hyperprolactinemia effects on fertility. Fertil Steril 32:556–561, 1979.

34. Kemmann E, Jones JR: Hyperprolactinemia and headaches. Am J Obstet Gynecol 145:668–671, 1983.

35. Slonim AE, Glick AD, Island DP, Kasselberg AG: Hyperprolactinemia associated with advanced puberty in a male. J Pediatr 101:236–239, 1982.

36. Patton ML, Wooif PD: Hyperprolactinemia and delayed puberty: A report of three cases and their responses to therapy. Pediatrics 71:572–575, 1983.

37. Thorner MO, Perryman RL, Rogol AD, et al: Rapid changes of prolactinoma volume after withdrawal and reinstitution of bromocriptine. J Clin Endocrinol Metab 53:480–483, 1981.

38. Cusisk JF, Haughton VM, Hagen TC: Radiological assessment of intrasellar prolactin-secreting tumors. Neurosurgery 6:376–379, 1980.

39. Muhr C, Bergstrom K, Grimelius L, Larson SG: A parallel study of roentgen anatomy of the sella turcica and the histopathology of the pituitary gland in 205 autopsy specimens. Neuroradiology 21:55–65, 1981.

40. Wolpert SM, Molitch ME, Goldman JA, Wood JB: Size, shape, and appearance of the normal female pituitary gland. AJR 143:377–381, 1984.

41. Swartz JD, Russell KB, Basile BA, et al: High-resolution computed tomographic appearance of the intrasellar contents in women of childbearing age. Radiology 147:115–117, 1983.

42. Davis PC, Hoffmann JC, Tindall JT, Braun IF: Prolactin-secreting pituitary microadenomas: Inaccuracy of high resolution CT imaging. AJNR 5:721–726, 1984.

43. Chakers DW, Curtin A, Ford G: Magnetic resonance imaging of pituitary and parasellar abnormalities. Radiol Clin North Am 27:265–281, 1989.

44. Kulkarni MV, Lee KF, McArdle CB, et al: 1.5-T MR imaging of pituitary microadenomas: Technical considerations and CT correlation. AJNR 9:5–11, 1988.

45. Dwyer AJ, Frank JA, Doppman JL, et al: Pituitary adenoma in patients with Cushing's disease: Initial experience with Gd-DTPA-enhanced MR imaging. Radiology 163:421–426, 1987.

46. Gomori JM, Grossman RI, Zimmerman RA, Bilaniuk CT: Intracranial hemorrhage: Imaging by high-field MRI. Radiology 157:87–93, 1985.

47. Klijn JGM, Lamberts SWJ, DeJong FH, Birkenhager JC: The value of the thyrotropin-releasing hormone test in patients with prolactin-secreting pituitary tumors and suprasellar non-pituitary tumors. Fertil Steril 35:155–161, 1981.

48. Ferrari C, Rampini P, Benco R, et al: Functional characterization of hypothalamic hyperprolactinemia. J Clin Endocrinol Metab 55:897–901, 1982.

49. Iodice M, Lombardi G, Tommaselli A, et al: Agreement of prolactin response to cimetidine and nomifensine in patients with prolactin-secreting tumors and idiopathic hyperprolactinemia. Neuroendocrinology 35:333–335, 1982.

50. DeLeo V, Cella SG, Carmanni F, et al: Prolactin-lowering effect of amphetamine in normoprolactinemic subjects and in physiological and pathological hyperprolactinemia. Horm Metab Res 15:439–443, 1983.

51. Balagura S, Frantz AG, Housepain EM, Carmel PW: The specificity of serum prolactin as a diagnostic indicator of pituitary adenoma. J Neurosurg 51:42–46, 1979.

52. Boulanger CM, Mashak CA, Chang RJ: Lack of tumor reduction in hyperprolactinemic women with extrasellar macroadenomas treated with bromocriptine. Fertil Steril 44:532–535, 1985.

53. Gemzell C, Wang CF: Outcome of pregnancy in women with pituitary adenoma. Fertil Steril 31:363–372, 1979.

54. Skrabanek P, McDonald D, Meagher D, et al: Clinical course and outcome of thirty-five pregnancies in infertile hyperprolactinemic women. Fertil Steril 33:391–395, 1980.

55. Nillius SJ, Bergh KT, Larson SG: Pituitary tumors and pregnancy. In Jedynak CP, Peillon F (eds): Pituitary Adenomas. New York, Asclepious Publishers, 1980, pp 103–111.

56. Wollesen F, Andersen T, Karle A: Size reduction of extrasellar pituitary tumors during bromocriptine treatment: Quantitation of the effect on different types of tumors. Ann Intern Med 96:281–286, 1982.

57. Laws ER Jr, Fode NC, Randall RV, et al: Pregnancy following transsphenoidal resection of prolactin-secreting pituitary tumors. J Neurosurg 58:685–688, 1983.

58. Erdheim J, Stumme E: Uber die Schwangerschaftsveranderung der Hypophyse. Beitr Pathol Anat 46:1, 1909.

59. Magyar DM, Marshall JR: Pituitary tumors and pregnancy. Am J Obstet Gynecol 132:739–751, 1978.

60. Molitch ME: Pregnancy and the hyperprolactinemic woman. N Engl J Med 312:1364–1370, 1985.

61. Samaan NA, Leavens ME, Sacca R, et al: The effects of pregnancy on patients with hyperprolactinemia. Am J Obstet Gynecol 148:466–473, 1984.

62. Rjosk HK, Fahlbusch R, Von Werder K: Influence of pregnancies on prolactinomas. Acta Endocrinol 100:337–346, 1982.

63. Lamberts SWJ, Klijn JGM, de Lange SA, et al: The incidence of complications during pregnancy after treatment of hyperprolactinemia with bromocriptine in patients with radiologically evident pituitary tumors. Fertil Steril 31:614–619, 1979.

64. Grossman A, Cohen BL, Charlesworth M, et al: Treatment of prolactinomas with megavoltage radiotherapy. Br Med J 288:1105–1109, 1984.

65. Canales ES, Garcia IC, Ruiz JE, Zarate A: Bromocriptine as prophylactic therapy in prolactinoma during pregnancy. Fertil Steril 36:524–526, 1981.

66. Van Roon E, Van der Vijver JCM, Gerretsen G, et al: Rapid regression of a suprasellar extending prolactinoma after bromocriptine treatment during pregnancy. Fertil Steril 36:173–177, 1981.

67. Konopka P, Raymond JP, Merceron RE, Seneze J: Continuous admin-

istration of bromocriptine in the prevention of neurological complications in pregnant women with prolactinomas. Am J Obstet Gynecol 146:935–938, 1983.

68. Sheline GE, Grossman A, Jones AE, Besser GM: Radiation therapy for prolactinomas. *In* Black PM, Zervas NT, Ridgway EC, Martin JB (eds): Secretory Tumors of the Pituitary Gland. New York, Raven Press, 1984, pp 93–108.

69. Antunes JL, Housepain EM, Frantz AG, et al: Prolactin-secreting pituitary tumors. Ann Neurol 2:148–153, 1977.

70. Nabarro JDN: Pituitary prolactinomas. Clin Endocrinol 17:129–155, 1982.

71. Chang RJ, Keye WR, Young JR, et al: Detection, evaluation, and treatment of pituitary microadenomas with galactorrhea and amenorrhea. Am J Obstet Gynecol 128:356–363, 1977.

72. Tindall GT, McLanahan CS, Christy JH: Transsphenoidal microsurgery for pituitary tumors associated with hyperprolactinemia. J Neurosurg 48:849–860, 1978.

73. Post KD, Biller BJ, Adelman LS, et al: Selective transsphenoidal adenomectomy in women with galactorrhea-amenorrhea. JAMA 242:158–162, 1979.

74. Randall RV, Laws ER, Abboud CF, et al: Transsphenoidal microsurgical treatment of prolactin-producing pituitary adenomas: Results in 100 patients. Mayo Clin Proc 58:108–121, 1983.

75. Hardy J: Transsphenoidal microsurgery of prolactinomas. *In* Black PM, Zervas NT, Ridgway EC, Martin JB (eds): Secretory Tumors of the Pituitary Gland. New York, Raven Press, 1984, pp 73–81.

76. Laws ER, Fode NC, Redmond MJ: Transsphenoidal surgery following unsuccessful prior therapy: An assessment of benefits and risks in 158 patients. J Neurosurg 63:823–829, 1985.

77. Serri O, Rasio E, Beauregard H, et al: Recurrence of hyperprolactinemia after selective transsphenoidal adenomectomy in women with prolactinoma. N Engl J Med 309:280–283, 1983.

78. Rodman EF, Molitch ME, Post KD, et al: Long-term follow-up of transsphenoidal selective adenomectomy for prolactinoma. JAMA 252:921–924, 1984.

79. Hokfelt T, Fuxe K: On the morphology and the neuroendocrine role of the hypothalamic catecholamine neuron. *In* Knigge KM, Scott DR, Weidl A (eds): Brain-Endocrine Interaction. Basel, Karger, 1972, pp 181–223.

80. Corrodi H, Fuxe K, Hokfelt T, et al: Effect of ergot drugs on central catecholamine neurons: Evidence for a stimulation of central dopamine neurons. J Pharm Pharmacol 25:409–412, 1973.

81. Calabro MA, MacLeod RM: Binding of dopamine to bovine anterior pituitary membranes. J Clin Endocrinol 40:363–366, 1974.

82. Pasteels JL, Dangery A, Freotte M, Ectors F: Inhibition de la secretion de prolactine par l'eregocornine et al 2-Br-alpha-ergocryptin: Action directe sur l'hypophyse en culture. Ann Endocrinol 32:188–192, 1975.

83. Yeo T, Thorner MO, Jones A, et al: The effects of dopamine, bromocriptine, lergotrile, and metoclopramide on prolactin release from continuously perfused columns of isolated rat pituitary cells. Clin Endocrinol 10:123–130, 1979.

84. Fluckinger E, Doepfner W, Marko M, Nieder W: Effects of ergot alkaloids on the hypothalamic-pituitary axis. Postgrad Med 52 (Suppl 1):57–61, 1976.

85. Muller EE, Panerai AE, Cocchi D, Mantegazza P: Endocrine profile of ergot alkaloids. Life Sci 21:1545–1558, 1977.

86. Schran HF, Bhuta SI, Schwarz HJ, Thorner MO: The pharmacokinetics of bromocriptine in man. *In* Goldstein M, Calne DB, Lieberman A, Thorner MO (eds): Ergot Compounds and Brain Function: Neuroendocrine and Neuropsychiatric Aspects. New York, Raven Press, 1980, pp 125–139.

87. Turner TH, Cookson JC, Wass JAH, et al: Psychotic reactions during treatment of pituitary tumours with dopamine agonists. Br Med J 289:1101–1103, 1984.

88. Ayres J, Maisey MN: Alcohol increases bromocriptine's side effects. N Engl J Med 302:806, 1980.

89. Vermesh M, Fossum FT, Kletzky OA: Vaginal bromocriptine: Pharmacology and effect on serum prolactin in normal women. Obstet Gynceol 72:693–698, 1988.

90. Katz E, Weiss BE, Hassell A, et al: Increased circulating levels of bromocriptine after vaginal compared with oral administration. Fertil Steril 55:882–884, 1991.

91. Kletzky OA, Vermesh M: Effectiveness of vaginal bromocriptine in treating women with hyperprolactinemia. Fertil Steril 51:269–272, 1989.

92. Thorner MO, Schran HF, Evans WS, et al: A broad spectrum of prolactin suppression by bromocriptine in hyperprolactinemic women: A study of serum prolactin and bromocriptine levels after acute and chronic administration of bromocriptine. J Clin Endocrinol Metab 50:1026–1033, 1980.

93. Thorner MO, McNeilly AS, Hagan C, Besser GM: Long-term treatment of galactorrhea and hypogonadism and bromocriptine. Br Med J 2:419–422, 1974.

94. Molitch ME, Elton RL, Blackwell RE, et al: Bromocriptine as primary therapy for prolactin-secreting macroadenomas: Results of a prospective multicenter study. J Clin Endocrinol Metab 60:698–705, 1985.

95. Liuzzi A, Dallabonzana D, Oppizzi G, et al: Low doses of dopamine agonists in the long-term treatment of macroprolactinomas. N Engl J Med 313:656–659, 1985.

96. Ciccarelli E, Guisti M, Miola C, et al: Effectiveness and tolerability of long term treatment with cabergoline, a new long-lasting ergoline derivative, in hyperprolactinemic patients. J Clin Endocrinol Metab 69:725–728, 1989.

97. Melis GB, Bambacciani M, Paoletti AM, et al: Reduction in the size of prolactin-producing pituitary tumor after cabergoline administration. Fertil Steril 52:412–415, 1989.

98. Vance ML, Cragun JR, Reimnitz E, et al: CV 205-502 treatment of hyperprolactinemia. J Clin Endocrinol Metab 68:336–339, 1989.

99. Vance ML, Lipper M, Klibanski A, et al: Treatment of prolactin-secreting pituitary macroadenomas with the long-acting non-ergot dopamine agonist CV 205-502. Ann Intern Med 112:668–673, 1990.

100. Newman CB, Hurley AM, Kleinberg DL: Effect of CV 205-502 in hyperprolactinaemic patients intolerant of bromocriptine. Clin Endocrinol 31:391–400, 1989.

101. Homburg R, West C, Browness J, Jacobs HS: A double-blind study comparing a new non-ergot, long-acting dopamine agonist, CV 205-502, with bromocriptine in women with hyperprolactinemia. Clin Endocrinol 32:565–571, 1990.

102. Ciccarelli E, Miola C, Avataneo T, et al: Long-term treatment with a new repeatable injectable form of bromocriptine, Parlodel LR, in patients with tumorous hyperprolactinemia. Fertil Steril 52:930–935, 1989.

103. Von Werder K, Fahlbusch R, Landgraf R, et al: Treatment of patients with prolactinomas. J Endocrinol Invest 1:47–58, 1978.

104. Martin NA, Hales M, Wilson CB: Cerebellar metastasis from a prolactinoma during treatment with bromocriptine. J Neurosurg 55:615–619, 1981.

105. Crosignani PG, Mattei A, Ferrari C, Giovanelli MA: Enlargement of a prolactin-secreting pituitary macroadenoma during bromocriptine. Br J Obstet Gynaecol 89:169–170, 1982.

106. Breidahl HD, Topliss DJ, Pike JW: Failure of bromocriptine to maintain reduction in size of a macroprolactinoma. Br Med J 287:451–452, 1983.

107. Turkalj I, Braun P, Krupp P: Surveillance of bromocriptine in pregnancy. JAMA 247:1589–1591, 1982.

108. Molitch ME, Reichlin S: Hyperprolactinemia. DM 28:1–58, 1982.

109. Lundberg PO, Osterman PO, Wide L: Serum prolactin in patients with hypothalamic and pituitary disorders. J Neurosurg 55:194–199, 1981.

110. Goldman M, Rabin A: Case report: Hyperprolactinemia in patient with pseudotumor cerebri. J Med Soc NJ 81:501–502, 1984.

111. Gharib H, Frey HM, Laws ER, et al: Coexistent primary empty sella syndrome and hyperprolactinemia. Arch Intern Med 143:1383–1386, 1983.

112. Marcovitz S, Guyda HJ, Finlayson MH, et al: Intrasellar germinoma associated with hyperprolactinemia. Surg Neurol 22:387–396, 1984.

113. Shen DY, Guay AT, Silverman ML, et al: Primary intrasellar germinoma presenting with secondary amenorrhea and hyperprolactinemia. Neurosurgery 15:417–420, 1984.

114. Braunstein GD, Hassen G, Kamdar V, Nelson JC: Anterior pituitary hormone levels in the cerebrospinal fluid of patients with pituitary and parasellar tumors. Fertil Steril 36:164–172, 1981.

115. Turkington RW: Prolactin secretion in patients treated with various drugs. Arch Intern Med 130:349–354, 1972.

116. Cooper DS, Gelenberg AJ, Wojcik JC, et al: The effect of amoxapine and imipramine on serum prolactin levels. Arch Intern Med 141:1023–1025, 1981.

117. Gluskin LE, Strasberg B, Shaah JH: Verapamil-induced hyperprolactinemia and galactorrhea. Ann Intern Med 95:66–67, 1981.

118. Fearrington EL, Rand CH, Rose JD: Hyperprolactinemia-galactorrhea induced by verapamil. Am J Cardiol 51:1466–1467, 1983.

25

Vasopressin and Its Neurophysin

PETER H. BAYLIS

SYNTHESIS AND METABOLISM

Vasopressin, the antidiuretic hormone of most vertebrates, is the major determinant of renal water excretion and therefore plays a central role in the maintenance of water balance.

Background

In 1895 Oliver and Schäfer[1] reported potent hypertensive effects of fresh pituitary gland extracts injected intravenously into mammals; the pressor activity was subsequently shown to reside solely in the neurohypophysis.[2] The renal effects of posterior pituitary extracts were described later by Schäfer.[3] Profound polyuria caused by mechanical injury to dog pituitaries was reversed by injection of pituitary extracts. The efficacy of pituitary extracts in the treatment of patients suffering from diabetes insipidus is attributed to two independent workers within weeks of each other.[4, 5]

The chemical structure of arginine vasopressin (AVP), found in most mammals (Table 25–1), was elucidated in du Vigneaud's laboratory and synthesized within a few months of its discovery.[6] It is a nonapeptide, molecular weight 1084 Da, and a strongly basic molecule (isoelectric point pH 10.9).[7] Lysine vasopressin is the antidiuretic hormone of the pig family. Biological activity is readily destroyed by oxidation or reduction of the disulfide bond.[8] Nonmammalian species have a variety of nonapeptides related closely to vasopressin and oxytocin (Table 25–1). Single nucleotide changes account for most of the amino acid substitutions, which tend to occur at positions 3, 4, and 8. Thus, considerable structural uniformity is conserved, which has led to the hypothesis that a single ancestral gene evolved along two evolutionary lines, one being vasotocin-vasopressin and the other isotocin-mesotocin-oxytocin.[9] More recent evidence, however, indicates that multiple genes may encode numerous vasopressin-like hormones.[10]

Molecular Biology

AVP is derived from a large 145-amino acid precursor molecule comprising a signal peptide, AVP, AVP-specific neurophysin, and a glycosylated moiety[11] (Fig. 25–1). Se-

TABLE 25–1. AMINO ACID SEQUENCES OF ARGININE VASOPRESSIN AND RELATED NEUROHYPOPHYSIAL NONAPEPTIDES

	1 2 3 4	5	6 7 8 9	Distribution
Arginine vasopressin:	Cys-Tyr-Phe-Glu$(NH)_2$-Asp(NH_2)-Cys-Pro-Arg-Gly(NH_2)			Most mammals
Lysine vasopressin:	Phe Glu(NH_2)		Lys	Pig family
Arginine vasotocin:	Ile Glu(NH_2)		Arg	Nonmammalian vertebrates
Oxytocin:	Ile Glu(NH_2)		Leu	Mammals, birds
Mesotocin:	Ile Glu(NH_2)		Ile	Reptiles
Isotocin:	Ile Ser		Ile	Fish
Glumitocin:	Ile Ser		Glu(NH_2)	Fish
Valitocin:	Ile Glue(NH_2)		Val	Fish
Aspartocin:	Ile Asp(NH_2)		Leu	Fish

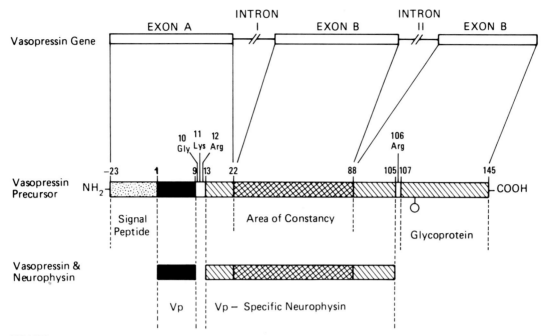

FIGURE 25–1. **Vasopressin gene, vasopressin precursor molecule, and AVP with its specific neurophysin.** Three exons code for the precursor molecule, which comprises a signal protein, AVP hormone, AVP-specific neurophysin, a glycoprotein moiety, coupled by amino acids. (Adapted from Land H, Schütz G, Schmale H, Richter D: Nucleotide vasopressin-neurophysin II precursor. Nature 295:299–303, 1982.)

quence analysis of the genes encoding the AVP precursor molecule and recombinent DNA techniques have confirmed the structure of the AVP-neurophysin complex.[11] The gene for this complex is located in chromosome 20, linked closely to the oxytocin gene and separated by only 11 kb of sequence.[12] The gene has three exons encoding the AVP-neurophysin complex, which are separated by two introns (Fig. 25–1). In all species analyzed at the DNA level so far, the part of neurophysin moiety is very highly conserved.

Studies on the regulation of mammalian AVP gene suggest a close correlation with the expression of oxytocin in some animals. Not only does osmotic salt loading cause dramatic accumulation of AVP mRNA in the neurohypophysis[13] and up-regulation of the AVP gene but it also concomitantly increases oxytocin gene transcription.[14] Conversely, lactation triggers transcription of both oxytocin and vasopressin genes.[15] In rats, AVP and oxytocin genes are expressed in separate groups of hypothalamic neurons, each specific for either vasopressin or oxytocin. Because the same stimulus can promote identical expression of AVP and oxytocin genes, a cell-specific mechanism is suspected to exist that allows activation of only one or the other of the genes in the hypothalamic neurons.

Expression of the AVP gene has been observed in extrahypothalamic tissues, such as adrenal gland, gonads, cerebellum, and probably the pituicytes of the posterior pituitary gland.[16]

Studies in lower vertebrates (e.g., teleost fish) suggest that at least two genes encode the vasotocin precursor, the counterpart of the mammalian AVP precursor.[16] A second AVP gene would be convenient to explain the observation that the Brattleboro rat (genetically deficient in hypothalamic AVP) has normal concentrations of AVP in peripheral tissues.[17] It is well recognized that the Brattleboro rat has a single nucleotide deletion in the portion of the hypothalamic gene encoding the AVP-specific neurophysin, which causes a frame shift in the translation product, leading to intracellular degradation of the mutant AVP precursor.[18]

Biosynthesis and Metabolism

Synthesis of the AVP precursor occurs principally in the hypothalamic neurons of the supraoptic and paraventricular nuclei. As the precursor complex migrates along the neuronal axons at a rate of about 2 mm/h, it undergoes specific cleavage, and the products that include AVP are stored as neurosecretory granules in the posterior pituitary.[19] Release of AVP from the neural lobe is associated with an increase in the rate of phasic firing of electrical impulses.[20] Exocytosis of AVP is calcium dependent. Only a percentage of the peptides are ever released, as some AVP-containing neurosecretory granules migrate from the nerve endings as a result of an aging process and their contents become unavailable for release.[21]

AVP and its specific neurophysin are co-secreted into the systemic circulation in equimolar quantities.[22] Apart from acting as a transport protein for AVP in the neuronal axons, neurophysin appears to serve no other biological function. The half-life of AVP in the blood volume is about 5 to 15 minutes.[23] After release from the neurohypophysis, AVP circulates unbound to proteins in the blood[23] but does bind to platelet receptors, causing platelet-rich AVP plasma concentrations to be about five-fold higher than platelet-depleted plasma.[24]

At least four main sites of enzymatic cleavage have been identified on the AVP molecule.[23] During pregnancy and the immediate postpartum period an extremely active cysteine aminopeptidase or vasopressinase (E.C.3.4.11.3) of placental syncytiotrophoblastic origin degrades AVP rapidly.[23]

NEUROANATOMY

The posterior lobe of the pituitary gland is an extension of the forebrain. Vasopressor activities from the neurohypophysis have been detected as early as the tenth week of gestation[25] in humans. At birth the weight of the whole pituitary gland is approximately 100 mg, and it attains an adult human weight of about 600 mg, 20 per cent of which is the posterior lobe.[26]

Figure 25–2 shows the neuroanatomical relationships of the posterior pituitary in humans. The major site of AVP synthesis is in the magnocellular neurons of the supraoptic and paraventricular nuclei; additional magnocellular neurons containing AVP are found in and near the hypothalamus. Smaller neurons (parvocellular) synthesizing AVP are present in the suprachiasmatic and paraventricular nuclei.[27] Three major vasopressinergic neuronal projections arise from the supraoptic and paraventricular nuclei. The principal pathway originates mainly from the supraoptic nucleus and travels to the posterior lobe; another important pathway terminates in the zona externa of the median eminence, these fibers arising from the medial parvocellular paraventricular nucleus.[27] Extrahypothalamic vasopressinergic neurons project to the forebrain, brain stem, and spinal cord, most of which originate from the paraventricular nucleus.[28, 29] Complex neuronal interconnections exist between paraventricular and supraoptic nuclei, and the brain stem nuclei, the nucleus of tractus solitarius, and the locus coeruleus, via dorsal and ventral ascending noradrenergic bundles.

Release of AVP is controlled and modulated by a series of sensory influences. Osmotic regulation is mediated by putative osmoreceptors, anatomically distinct from the supraoptic and paraventricular nuclei. They are located in the anterior circumventricular structures, probably in the organum vasculosum of the lamina terminalis, the subfornical organ, or the AV3V region.[30, 31] The appreciation of thirst, although a cortical function, depends upon osmotically sensitive nuclei situated in the anterior or lateral hypothalamus and the integrity of neuronal pathways projecting to the ventromedial nucleus.[30, 31] It is probable that osmoreceptors for thirst are distinct from AVP osmoreceptors. Baroregulatory influences on vasopressin-synthesizing neurons arise from peripheral high- and low-pressure receptors located in the arch of the aorta, the carotid vessels, the atria of the heart, and the great veins within the thorax.[32] Afferent fibers in the vagus and glossopharyngeal nerves terminate in the brain stem nuclei, sensory information then being passed to the AVP neurons in the hypothalamus.

CONTROL OF SECRETION

Neurotransmitters

Two major classes of substances, the biogenic amines and peptides, act as neurotransmitters that regulate the secretion of AVP.[33] Catecholamines certainly influence AVP secretion. Dopamine is the most abundant amine to be found in the neurohypophysis, together with both D-1 and D-2 receptors. Although evidence indicates that dopamine may act as an inhibitory neurotransmitter in the posterior pituitary, it is a potent stimulant of AVP from rat hypothalami.[34] Dopamine appears to be involved in the release of AVP after nausea and/or emesis,[33] but data conflict on whether cerebral dopamine stimulates or inhibits osmoregulated AVP secretion.[34, 35] Norepinephrine has been found in the supraoptic and paraventricular nuclei by histochemical and immunocytochemical techniques.[36] Central norepinephrine fibers stimulate AVP release via α_1 receptors.[37] Comprehensive studies by Schrier and col-

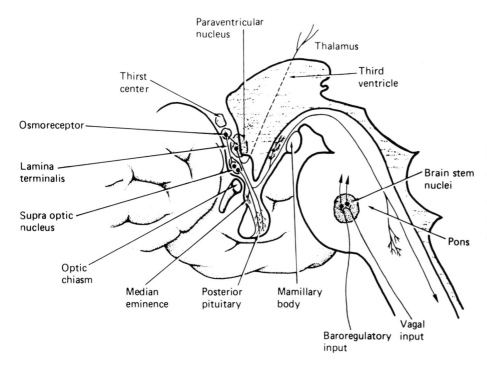

FIGURE 25–2. Schematic representation of hypothalamus, posterior pituitary, and surrounding structures. Major neuronal tracts arise from the supraoptic and paraventricular nuclei, which pass to the posterior lobe of the pituitary, the median eminence, the brain stem and spinal cord, and the forebrain. Afferent fibers to these nuclei originate from the osmoreceptors and baroreceptors, the latter passing via brain stem nuclei.

leagues[38] provide clear evidence for hemodynamic roles for α- and β-adrenergic agonists, causing inhibition and stimulation of neurohypophysial AVP, respectively.

Acetylcholine is also present in both supraoptic and paraventricular nuclei. Although data that acetylcholine stimulates basal and enhances osmoregulated AVP secretion are unequivocal, controversy remains about whether its action is mediated by the muscarinic or nicotinic receptors.[33]

The peptide angiotensin II enhances osmotically stimulated AVP secretion from the posterior pituitary when administered by peripheral infusion or intracerebroventricular injection. Its site of action is the organum vasculosum of the lamina terminalis, a putative site for the osmoreceptor.[39]

Rat studies suggest that atrial natriuretic peptide inhibits AVP secretion[40] by acting on the subfornical organ, but in humans there is little evidence that circulating physiological concentrations influence osmoregulated AVP release.[41] Recent work indicates that brain natriuretic peptide inhibits the activity of the supraoptic neurons and those in the AV3V region of the anterior hypothalamus.[42]

Opioid peptides also influence AVP secretion. Leu-enkephalin is present in the supraoptic and paraventricular nuclei and in the nerve terminals containing AVP in the neurohypophysis.[43] The consensus of opinion is that the enkephalins and β-endorphin inhibit AVP secretion; probably via a κ opioid receptor.[44]

Many other substances have been implicated in the neurotransmitter control of AVP (steroids, prostaglandins, serotonin, γ-aminobutyric acid), but their physiological significance remains to be determined.[33]

Osmoregulation

After a series of elegant studies on dogs, Verney[45] in 1947 first proposed the concept that secretion of AVP is regulated by the osmolality of body water. He concluded that intracranial osmoreceptors very sensitive to changes in blood sodium concentration and other solutes control AVP release. Initial confirmation of Verney's proposals came from bioassay techniques,[46] but recent studies[47–49] from a variety of laboratories have clearly demonstrated the exquisitely sensitive relationship between plasma osmolality and AVP concentrations. In healthy adults, the infusion of concentrated saline (855 mmol/L) to steadily increase plasma osmolality (pOs) results in progressive rises in peripheral plasma AVP concentrations (pAVP). Although pulsatile release of AVP can be detected in the internal jugular vein, no evidence exists of minute-to-minute fluctuation in AVP concentration in peripheral veins.[50] A direct correlation exists between the two variables (Fig. 25–3), which is defined by the function, pAVP = 0.43 (pOs − 284), r = +0.96, P < 0.001. The abscissal intercept, 284 mosmol/kg, indicates the plasma osmolality at which plasma AVP starts to increase, thus providing a measure of the set of the osmoreceptor mechanism or the osmotic threshold for AVP release. Whether AVP secretion can be completely suppressed remains unclear,[51] but using a cytochemical method to measure plasma AVP, AVP secretion could not be switched off by hypotonicity.[52] Nevertheless, the concept of a threshold of AVP release remains a pragmatic means

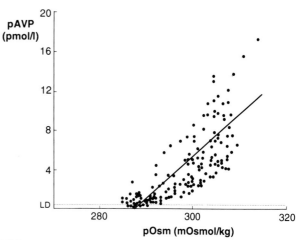

FIGURE 25–3. **Relationship between plasma osmolality and plasma AVP.** Increases in plasma AVP in response to hypertonicity induced by infusion of 855 mmol/L saline in a group of healthy adults. The mean regression line (—) is defined by pAVP = 0.43 (pOs − 284); r = +0.96; P < 0.001. LD represents the limit of detection of the assay, 0.3 pmol/L. (Adapted from Thompson CJ: Polyuric states in man. *In* Baylis PH (ed): Water and Salt Homeostasis in Health and Disease. London, Bailliere Tindall, 1989, pp 473–497.)

to characterize osmoregulatory function and analyze disorders of osmoregulation.[49] The slope of the regression line reflects sensitivity or gain of the osmoreceptor/AVP–releasing unit. Estimates of osmoreceptor gain and threshold for AVP release obtained by indirect methods of assessing AVP concentrations by measuring urine osmolality correspond well to the above values.[53] Fast rates of hypertonic saline infusion result in exaggerated AVP responses,[47] thereby giving a curvilinear relationship between pAVP and pOs. Complete disconnection of AVP-secreting neurons from their osmoreceptors appears to cause persistent low-grade AVP release, resulting in plasma AVP values about 1.0 pmol/L.[54] Thus, AVP secretion is increased from this "basal" rate by stimulation of facilitatory osmoreceptor cells but is decreased to minimal values by activation of inhibitory cells.

Despite considerable variations in osmoreceptor sensitivity and threshold for AVP release between individuals, these constants remain unchanged within an individual tested over a short period of time.[55] Recent studies have shown that the constants for slope and threshold are similar in monozygotic twins, suggesting a genetic determinant for the set of the osmoregulatory system.[56] Pregnancy causes a lowering of the threshold for AVP secretion without alteration of the gain of the osmoreceptor in both rats[57] and humans,[58] which accounts for the hypo-osmolality of pregnancy. In the luteal phase of the normal human ovulatory menstrual cycle, a small but significant fall in plasma osmolality occurs as a result of lowering of thresholds for thirst and vasopressin release.[59]

The response of the osmoreceptor to solutes other than sodium chloride is variable. In the presence of insulin, moderate hyperglycemia fails to stimulate AVP secretion,[60] but insulinopenic rats do release AVP with severe hyperglycemia.[61] Furthermore, urea has about one third the stimulatory effect on AVP release of sodium chloride,[60] and alcohol suppresses AVP secretion.[62] As plasma AVP rises, antidiuresis and urinary concentration increase. At plasma concentrations of immunoreactive AVP of 0.5 pmol/L or

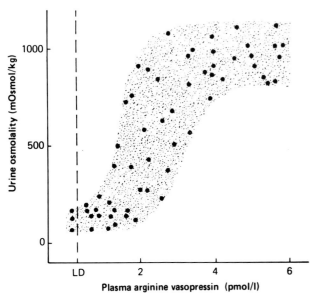

FIGURE 25–4. **Relationship between plasma AVP and urine osmolality during water load and fluid restriction in a group of healthy adults.** Maximum urine concentration is achieved by plasma AVP values greater than 4 pmol/L. LD represents the limit of detection of the assay, 0.3 pmol/L. (From Baylis PH, Robertson GL: Physiological control of vasopressin secretion. *In* Baylis PH, Padfield PL (eds): The Posterior Pituitary: Hormone Secretion in Health and Disease. New York, Marcel Dekker, 1985, pp 119–139.)

less, maximum diuresis occurs (Fig. 25–4). In response to rising plasma osmolality from 284 mosmol/kg (osmotic threshold for AVP release), plasma AVP concentration rises progressively to achieve increases in urinary concentration. Because plasma osmolality exceeds, on average, 295 mosm/kg when plasma AVP attains about 4 pmol/L, maximum antidiuresis is attained. Greater hyperosmolality, although releasing more AVP, fails to conserve any more renal water, exposing the body to potentially severe dehydration. This is avoided in healthy individuals by the stimulation of thirst to promote drinking.[47, 63] The intake of fluid results in lowering of plasma osmolality to levels at which renal water excretion can again be regulated by changes in AVP secretion, that is, less than 295 mosmol/kg. Drinking to quench osmotically stimulated AVP release does not return an individual's response back down the osmoregulatory line (see Fig. 25–3), but a precipitous fall occurs in plasma AVP, suggesting a rapid total inhibition of AVP secretion.[64] An oropharyngeal reflex is probably responsible for this observation. If fluid volumes greater than those demanded by thirst are consumed, then AVP secretion is suppressed to very low levels (< 0.3 pmol/L), at which stage the kidney is capable of excreting 15 to 20 L of urine in 24 hours. Only ingestion of fluid volumes in excess of this results in further lowering of plasma osmolality in healthy adults. The osmoregulatory system for thirst and AVP secretion maintains plasma osmolality within the narrow limits of about 284 to 295 mosmol/kg.

Baroregulation

Blood volume and pressure are widely recognized to influence AVP secretion. Early work in sheep suggested that reductions of at least 10 per cent were necessary to increase

antidiuretic activity.[65] In humans, falls in arterial blood pressure of the order of 5 to 10 per cent are necessary to increase significantly circulating immunoreactive AVP concentrations (Fig. 25–5).[66] In contrast to the simple linear correlation between plasma osmolality and plasma AVP, the pressure-AVP relationship is exponential. Changes in blood volume are mediated by low pressure receptors in the left atrium and great veins within the chest, whereas arterial blood pressure regulation is mediated by baroreceptors situated in the arch of the aorta and the carotid walls.[67] Recent evidence suggests that ventricular receptors may also be involved in baroregulation.[68]

Baroregulation of AVP does not operate in isolation, as responses are modified by neurohumoral influences. Atrial natriuretic peptides appear to inhibit AVP responses, whereas norepinephrine augments responses.[69] Similarly, an interrelationship exists between osmoregulatory and baroregulatory AVP secretion, such that as hypovolemia develops the AVP osmoregulatory line is shifted to the left of normal.[70, 71] Thus, under conditions of moderate hypovolemia, osmoregulation is preserved around a lower setpoint of plasma osmolality. As hypovolemia becomes more severe, very high plasma AVP values are attained which override the osmoregulatory system.

Other Regulatory Mechanisms

Nausea and emesis are potent stimuli to AVP secretion. In primates, circulating AVP values in excess of 500 pmol/L have been recorded,[72, 73] which are independent of osmotic and hemodynamic input. Traction on the intestines during surgery, for example, is a similar powerful

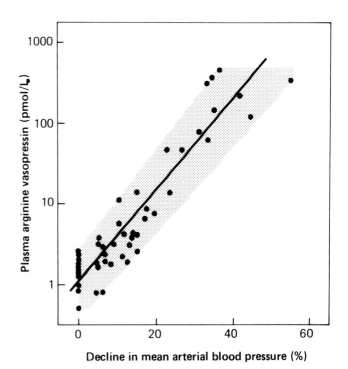

FIGURE 25–5. Relationship of plasma AVP to the percentage decline in mean arterial blood pressure (MABP) induced by infusion of increasing doses of trimethaphan in a healthy man. The regression line is defined by log (pAVP) = 0.06 (MABP + 0.67), r = +0.98, $P < 0.001$, n = 48. (From Baylis PH: Posterior pituitary function in health and disease. Clin Endocrinol Metab 12:747–770, 1983.)

nonosmotic stimulus to AVP release.[74] Both phenomena probably contribute to the high plasma AVP values observed after gastrointestinal surgery and cause hyponatremia if excess fluid is administered in the postoperative period.

Neuroglucopenia is another independent stimulus to AVP secretion, but plasma values attained are only moderate, up to about 6 pmol/L.[75] Whether AVP is a true stress hormone remains controversial.

THIRST

For many decades a "thirst center" has been postulated,[45] but only in the last few years has it been located to the anterior hypothalamic structures, the organum vasculosum of the lamina terminalis, the AV3V region, or the subfornical organ.[76] Whether they are sodium sensors or respond to osmotic change is not clear.[77] Little doubt exists, however, that thirst is an extremely powerful sensation that drives the seeking and drinking of water.

A major experimental obstacle has been quantitation of thirst sensation, but recent work in humans using visual analogue scales has overcome the problem to an extent. In contrast to previous concepts, it is now apparent that a simple linear correlation exists between thirst and plasma osmolality, and small changes in blood tonicity are readily appreciated by thirst.[63] A function defining the relationship between thirst (Th) and plasma osmolality can be derived: Th = 0.39 (pOsm − 285), r = +0.95, P < 0.001. The abscissal intercept, 285 mosmol/kg, represents the osmotic threshold for thirst perception (Fig. 25–6), which is statistically no different from the threshold for AVP release. Despite wide individual variations in the value of the thirst osmotic threshold, it remains remarkably consistent within individuals.[55] Indeed, the functional characteristics of the osmoregulatory lines for AVP release and thirst are very similar. Drinking causes a dramatic fall in osmotically stimulated thirst analogue scores identical to AVP.[64]

In addition, thirst can be stimulated by extracellular volume depletion. Underfilling of the low-pressure thoracic circulation leads to drinking in animals,[78] an effect probably mediated by the left atrium via the vagus nerve. Angiotensin II is a powerful dipsogen that is present in the anterior circumventricular organs but may also act as a peripheral agent, having been generated in the circulation from renin released by an underperfused kidney.[79, 80]

ACTIONS OF VASOPRESSIN

The effects of AVP are mediated by two major classes of receptor (Table 25–2).[81] The V_1 receptor is coupled to phospholipase C and thus increases the turnover of the inositol phosphates and allows the influx of Ca^{2+} to raise intracellular Ca^{2+} concentrations. This receptor is subdivided into V_{1a} and V_{1b} because the binding properties of the pituitary corticotrope (V_{1b}) to a variety of vasopressin agonists and antagonists differ from those of other V_1 receptor tissues. The rat V_{1a} arginine vasopressin receptor has recently been cloned in hepatocytes and has seven transmembrane domains.[82] The V_2 receptor is coupled via the regulatory G proteins to adenylate cyclase and is found principally in the kidney.[83] Both the human and the rat V_2 receptors have been cloned.[84, 85] The gene, located on the long arm of the X chromosome, encodes a 370-amino acid protein with transmembrane topography characteristic of G protein–coupled receptors.

Renal Effects

Two well-recognized sites of action of AVP have been located in the mammalian kidney, the collecting tubule, and the medullary thick ascending limb of Henle's loop. AVP may also act on other parts of the nephron, including the glomerulus.

Its effect on the collecting tubule to concentrate urine depends upon a solute gradient across the tubular cells, which arises from a hypertonic renal interstitium and hypotonic luminal fluid in the tubule.[86, 87] The hypertonic interstitium results from the active transport of solute from the loops of Henle, which act as a countercurrent multiplier. The vasa recta following the course of the loops function as the countercurrent exchanger. Consequently, a small solute gradient is created between ascending and descending limbs of Henle's loop, which allows the formation of a progressively more concentrated interstitium from the corticomedullary junction to the papilla. In the presence of AVP, the water permeability of the collecting tubules that pass through the hypertonic interstitium is increased. This allows water to move along the gradient from lumen to renal medulla, resulting in urinary concentration.[87]

The increase in water permeability is mediated by a complicated cascade of intracellular events, starting with activation of adenylate cyclase to increase intracellular cAMP. Stimulation of a cAMP-dependent protein kinase rearranges the intracellular microfilaments and microtubules in response to AVP, but the precise nature and sequence

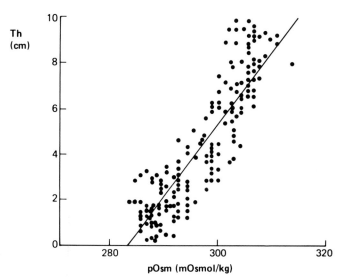

FIGURE 25–6. **Relationship between thirst (Th) and plasma osmolality during a hypertonic saline (855 mmol/L) infusion in a group of healthy adults.** The mean regression line (—) is defined by Th = 0.39 (pOsm − 285), r = +0.95, P < 0.001. (Adapted from Thompson CJ: Polyuric states in man. *In* Baylis PH: Water and Salt Homeostasis in Health and Disease. London, Bailliere Tindall, 1989, pp 473–497.)

TABLE 25–2. CLASSIFICATION OF ARGININE VASOPRESSIN RECEPTORS

V_{1a} receptor
  Coupled to phospholipase C
  Increased turnover of inositol phosphates
  Increased influx of Ca^{2+}
  Sites: vascular smooth muscle
         liver
         platelets
         cerebrum
V_{1b} receptor
  Intracellular effects similar to V_{1a} receptor
  AVP analogue binding profiles different from V_{1a} receptor
  Site: pituitary corticotroph
V_2 receptor
  Coupled to adenylate cyclase
  Generation of cAMP
  Sites: renal collecting tubule
         renal medullary thick ascending limb of Henle's loop

of these events are obscure. The final step involves the insertion of aggregates of water-conducting particles into the luminal membrane of the collecting tubule[88] (Fig. 25–7). These aggregates arise from cytoplasmic tubular structures that fuse with the luminal membrane.

In addition to AVP-sensitive water channels in the terminal collecting duct, there is a distinct AVP-regulated urea transporter in the distal collecting tubule of the mammalian kidney.[89] By cycling urea into the renal interstitium, urea is conserved to contribute to the osmotic gradient essential for the water channels.

The other major renal site of AVP action is the medullary thick ascending limb of Henle's loop, which possesses, in some species, an AVP-sensitive adenylate cyclase.[90, 91] Clear evidence exists that sodium can be actively transported into the renal interstitium following AVP stimulation of the thick ascending limb.[92] The effect of AVP on this part of the nephron assists the generation of a hypertonic interstitial renal medulla and increases the osmotic gradient across the collecting tubules, resulting in augmentation of its antidiuretic action.

Cardiovascular Effects

Although AVP is a potent pressor agent, plasma concentrations required to increase arterial blood pressure in healthy individuals are many times higher than those observed under normal basal conditions.[93] Nevertheless, AVP can produce considerable constriction of numerous regional arteries and arterioles (e.g., splanchnic, renal, hepatic) at nearly physiological plasma concentrations (10 pmol/L).[94] Using specific V_{1a} antagonists, the importance of endogenous AVP in maintaining blood pressure in mild volume depletion has emerged.[95, 96] The pressor effect of AVP varies according to the vascular bed, and differential pressor effects on intrarenal vessels account for the shunting of blood from the medulla to the cortex under the influence of AVP.[97] Cardiac output and oxygen consumption are reduced by AVP through a variety of mechanisms.[98]

However, little evidence indicates that AVP plays a substantial role in the development of essential hypertension in humans, although it may be important in the cause and maintenance of hypertension in some animal models (e.g., deoxycorticosterone-salt hypertension).[99]

Effect on the Pituitary

Corticotropin-releasing factor (CRF) and AVP are the main secretagogues for corticotropin release from the anterior pituitary. They act synergistically. AVP, synthesized in the parvocellular part of the paraventricular nucleus, is released from the median eminence into the portal blood to supply the anterior pituitary gland. The corticotroph expresses a large number of V_{1b} receptors.[100]

Adrenalectomy in the rat results in elevated CRF and AVP in the paraventricular neurons, where the two peptides are co-localized within the same cell.[101] Administration of corticosterone reverses the effect of adrenalectomy. Recent studies indicate that these steroid manipulations regulate AVP mRNA.[102] Regulation of corticotropin secretion by AVP is physiologically important. AVP does not influence the secretion of other anterior pituitary hormones. Miscellaneous effects of AVP are given in Table 25–3.

POLYURIC SYNDROMES

Classification

Diabetes insipidus or polyuria can be defined by the excretion of copious urine, in excess of 3 L/24 hours. One of three pathogenetic mechanisms may be responsible for polyuria.[112] The first is a deficiency, usually not absolute, of AVP and is called hypothalamic diabetes insipidus (HDI). The second mechanism is a partial or total renal resistance to the antidiuretic action of AVP, termed nephrogenic di-

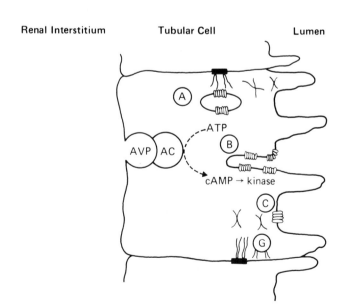

FIGURE 25–7. Schematic view of an AVP-sensitive collecting tubule, depicting the binding of AVP to the contraluminal surface and activating adenyl cyclase (AC) to generate cAMP from ATP and subsequently to phosphorylate protein kinases. A: cytoplasmic tubule containing water-conducting particles; B: fusion and particle delivery to luminal membrane; C: particle aggregates in luminal membrane. The function of G, the large granule, is unknown. (From Hays RM: Alteration of luminal membrane structure by antidiuretic hormone. Am J Physiol 245:C289–C296, 1983.)

TABLE 25–3. MISCELLANEOUS EFFECTS OF ARGININE VASOPRESSIN

Action	Receptor	Reference
Clotting factors		
Factor VIII released from hepatocytes	V_2	100
von Willebrand factor, released from vascular endothelium	V_2	101, 102
Liver		
Glycogen phosphorylase A activated	V_{1a}	103, 104
Brain		
Central blood pressure control	V_{1a}	105
Central temperature control	V_{1a}	105
Animal behavior stimulated	V_{1a}	106
? Retrieval of information	V_{1a}	107
? Function of CSF AVP		108

abetes insipidus (NDI). NDI has many causes, from the severe congenital form to the acquired types that may be reversible if they are due to metabolic disturbances (diabetes mellitus, hypercalcemia). Excessive inappropriate drinking, termed primary polydipsia or dipsogenic diabetes insipidus, is the third cause of polyuria. Table 25–4 gives a classification of conditions leading to polyuria.[112]

Hypothalamic Diabetes Insipidus

HDI is a disorder of urinary concentration resulting from impaired osmoregulated AVP secretion. It is also known as neurogenic, central, or cranial diabetes insipidus. Most patients have detectable plasma AVP concentrations that are inappropriately low with respect to the concomitant plasma osmolalities. Persistent polyuria leads to hypertonic dehydration, and patients maintain water balance through an intact thirst mechanism.

It is an uncommon disorder, with an estimated preva-

TABLE 25–4. CLASSIFICATION OF POLYURIA

A. Hypothalamic diabetes insipidus
  Primary: Idiopathic
               Hereditary (dominant or recessive)
               DIDMOAD (Wolfram) syndrome
               Autoimmune
  Secondary: Head injury
               Post cranial surgery
               Tumors (craniopharyngioma, pinealoma, dysgerminoma, pituitary macroadenoma, hypothalamic metastases)
               Granulomata (sarcoidosis, histiocytosis)
               Infections (meningitis, encephalitis)
               Vascular (infarction, aneurysms, sickle cell anemia)
               Pregnancy (associated with vasopressinase)
B. Nephrogenic diabetes insipidus
  Primary: Hereditary (sex-linked recessive)
               Idiopathic
  Secondary: Chronic renal disease (polycystic kidneys, obstructive uropathy)
               Metabolic disease (hypercalcemia, hypokalemia)
               Drug-induced (lithium, demeclocycline)
               Osmotic diuresis (glucose, mannitol)
               Systemic disorders (amyloidosis, myelomatosis)
               Pregnancy
C. Primary Polydipsia:
               Idiopathic
               Associated with psychosis
               Hypothalamic disease (sarcoidosis)
               Drug-induced (anticholinergic, tricyclic antidepressants)

lence of 1:25,000 and equal gender distribution. Destruction of at least 80 per cent of hypothalamic neurons synthesizing AVP is necessary before symptoms of polyuria and polydipsia become manifest.

Cause

The majority of causes of HDI are secondary to disease acquired during life (see Table 25–4). Blotner's review[113] in 1958 suggested that the most common form of HDI, accounting for 45 per cent of cases, was idiopathic, but recent surveys indicate that the current figure is lower (30 per cent).[114] Some patients have circulating antibodies to hypothalamic AVP-secreting neurons, a manifestation possibly of an autoimmune process.[115] The presence of plasma AVP antibodies in untreated patients is exceedingly rare.[116] Occasionally, a "triple-phase response" to trauma of the pituitary stalk has been observed.[117] Immediately after the insult transient polyuria occurs for a few days, followed by a period of continual antidiuresis lasting up to one week, after which permanent HDI ensues. Pituitary tumors that compress or invade the posterior lobe rarely cause HDI, although metastatic deposits in the hypothalamus, often from carcinoma of the breast or bronchus, result in HDI. In childhood, tumors affecting the hypothalamus (e.g., craniopharyngioma, dysgerminoma) account for up to 50 per cent of all cases of HDI. Sheehan's syndrome remains an uncommon cause of HDI, but maximal urine-concentrating ability appears to be impaired in some patients, implying a minimal defect in osmoregulated AVP release.[118] Very rarely diabetes insipidus occurs in pregnancy, which may in some instances be due to increased activity of circulating vasopressinase,[119] the aminopeptidase of placental origin. The hypothalamic form of pregnancy-associated diabetes insipidus must be differentiated from the transient nephrogenic type occasionally seen in pregnancy.[120]

A number of familial varieties of HDI have been described, inherited as either a dominant or a recessive trait. Genetic studies on one family with dominant inheritance show a single nucleotide substitution in the second exon, resulting in an amino acid change in the AVP-neurophysin moiety.[121] Another type of familial HDI can be associated with diabetes mellitus, optic atrophy, nerve deafness, and abnormalities of the renal tract, the DIDMOAD syndrome.[122]

Investigation

Because no clinical features definitely identify the cause of polyuria in a particular patient, diagnosis must rest on the results of investigations. Direct measurement of plasma AVP during osmotic stimulation establishes the diagnosis of HDI, but reliable methods to measure AVP are not always readily available. Consequently, indirect methods of assessing antidiuretic activity during a period of fluid deprivation are commonly used.

Having established that the patient is polyuric (24-hour urine volume greater than 3 L), a fluid deprivation test can be performed, with subsequent assessment of renal concentrating ability in response to exogenous AVP. Although a variety of tests have been described,[66, 123, 124] a common protocol is given in Chapter 31. Patients with severe HDI can be distinguished by their low urine osmolality (<300 mOsm/kg), high plasma osmolality (>295 mOsm/kg) after dehydration, and urine concentration to greater than 750 mOsm/kg following administration of desmopressin (DDAVP). Severe NDI can be identified by failure to increase urine osmolality above 300 mOsm/kg after dehydration and desmopressin. Unfortunately, many patients have partial defects, and mild forms of HDI and NDI and primary polydipsia cannot always be differentiated by this type of test.[125] Prolonged periods of fluid deprivation have been advocated to improve diagnosis,[124] as have the infusions of hypertonic saline to raise plasma osmolality quickly.[126]

Difficulties in establishing a diagnosis arise with fluid deprivation tests because prolonged polyuria from any cause leads to partial resistance to the antidiuretic action of AVP, probably owing to reduction in tonicity of the renal medullary interstitium.[127] Accurate diagnosis of HDI can be made, however, by direct measurement of plasma AVP concentration during infusion of hypertonic saline[125, 128] (Fig. 25–8A). Patients with HDI are identified by the subnormal or undetectable plasma AVP concentrations with respect to plasma osmolalities that fall to the right of the normal distribution. Primary polydipsia and NDI patients have plasma AVP responses that fall into the normal range, but distinction between these two diagnoses can be made by relating plasma AVP concentration to urine osmolality after a short period of dehydration. NDI is characterized by inappropriately high plasma AVP values for the concomitant urine osmolality, whereas primary polydipsia patients show an appropriate relationship (Fig. 25–8B).

As accurate AVP assays may not be readily available, an alternative approach to diagnosis can be made by instituting a careful therapeutic trial of DDAVP, preferably in hospital. Administration of 10 µg of DDAVP intranasally once daily for two to four weeks causes progressive dilutional hyponatremia in primary polydipsia. Patients with NDI remain unaffected whereas those with HDI experience an improvement in thirst and polyuria.

Treatment

With severe HDI profound polyuria is a great inconvenience and may lead to bladder distention, hydroureter, hydronephrosis, and secondary NDI. The treatment of choice for these patients is DDAVP, a synthetic, long-acting vasopressin analogue that possesses minimal pressor activity and twice the antidiuretic potency of AVP.[129] It is often administered as an intranasal spray (5 to 40 µg daily) or parenterally, but there is considerable individual variation in the dose required to control symptoms.[129] An oral preparation of DDAVP is now available; patients require 100 to 600 µg daily in divided doses to control polyuria. To avoid the potential complication of dilutional hyponatremia, DDAVP should be withdrawn at regular intervals to allow patients to become polyuric. If DDAVP is too potent, then lysine vasopressin can be prescribed, which acts for up to four hours but has the disadvantage of possessing considerable pressor activity. Pitressin tannate in oil for intramuscular administration or pitressin snuff is poorly tolerated and has been replaced by DDAVP.

Patients with mild forms of HDI, who have low circulating AVP concentrations, can also be treated with a variety of oral agents. Chlorpropamide (250 to 500 mg daily) has been the most frequently used agent and appears to potentiate the antidiuretic action of circulating AVP,[130] reducing urine output by 50 per cent, but troublesome side effects of hypoglycemia and hyponatremia do occur. Thiazides, carbamazepine, clofibrate, and tolbutamide cause an antidiuresis in some patients with HDI but are generally less effective than chlorpropamide.

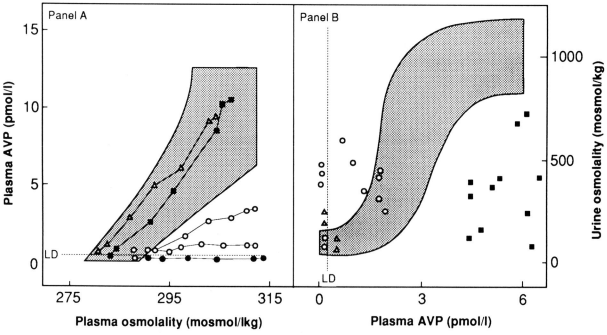

FIGURE 25–8. **Results of dynamic tests in patients with polyuria.** *(Panel A)* Plasma osmolality and plasma AVP responses to hypertonic saline (855 mmol/L) infusion. *(Panel B)* Plasma AVP and urine osmolality responses to a period of fluid restriction. The stippled area defines the normal response; circles, patients with HDI; squares, NDI; triangles, primary polydipsia. LD is the limit of detection of the assay, 0.3 pmol/L.

TABLE 25–5. CLASSIFICATION OF HYPOTONIC HYPONATREMIA

CLINICAL FLUID ASSESSMENT	HYPOVOLEMIA		EUVOLEMIA	HYPERVOLEMIA	
Extracellular sodium	Na ($\downarrow\downarrow$)		Na ($\rightarrow$)	Na ($\uparrow$)	
Total body water	H_2O ($\downarrow$)		H_2O ($\uparrow$)	H_2O ($\uparrow\uparrow$)	
Common causes	Renal losses	Extrarenal losses	SIADH	Cardiac failure	Renal failure
	Diuretics	Vomiting	Hypothyroidism	Cirrhosis	
	Mineralocorticoid deficiency	Diarrhea	"Sick cell" syndrome	Nephrotic syndrome	
	Salt-losing nephritis	Burns	Glucocorticoid deficiency		
Urinary sodium concentration (mmol/L)	>20	<10	>20	<10	>20

*Adapted from Berl T, Anderson RJ, McDonald KM, Schrier RW: Clinical disorders of water metabolism. Kidney Int 10:117–132, 1976.

Nephrogenic Diabetes Insipidus

The causes of NDI, renal resistance to the antidiuretic action of AVP, are given in Table 25–4. The rare yet severe sex-linked form presents usually in the first year of life.[131] The abnormal gene has been localized to the Xq28 region of the long arm of the X chromosome,[132] which probably accounts for the abnormalities of the V_2 receptor.[133] Various metabolic disorders including hypokalemia, hypercalcemia, and prolonged polyuria itself can produce acquired NDI, which is often reversible with correction of the underlying cause. Lithium is a common cause of NDI which may not be reversible.[134] Diagnosis is confirmed by recording inappropriately low urine osmolality with respect to the circulating plasma AVP concentration after a period of controlled fluid restriction (Fig. 25–8).

Other than removal of the underlying cause and ensuring adequate hydration, specific therapy for diabetes insipidus is difficult. Thiazide diuretics in conjunction with salt restriction, prostaglandin synthetase inhibitors such as indomethocin, and very high dose DDAVP, singly or in combination, are useful but rarely reduce urine volumes by more than 50 per cent.[131, 135]

Primary Polydipsia

Primary polydipsia is a syndrome characterized by excessive fluid intake and polyuria. It is often observed in psychotic patients, who may be motivated by irrational beliefs rather than genuine thirst (Table 25–4). Rarely, structural abnormalities such as hypothalamic sarcoidosis may cause primary polydipsia. Recent work using visual analogue scales to assess thirst has identified a group of patients with lowered osmotic thirst thresholds (see Fig. 25–6) but normal osmoregulated AVP secretion and renal function.[136] Confirmation of the diagnosis of primary polydipsia is obtained by observing normal osmoregulated AVP secretion and renal function (Fig. 25–8). Reduction of fluid intake is the only rational treatment.

HYPOTONIC SYNDROMES

Hyponatremia

Hyponatremia, defined as a serum sodium level less than 130 mmol/L, is a common electrolyte disorder, occurring in about 15 per cent of hospitalized patients.[137] A pragmatic classification is given in Table 25–5. Clinical assessment identifies the extracellular volume status of most patients, although problems can arise in distinguishing mild forms of hypervolemia and hypovolemia from euvolemia. Pseudohyponatremia due to excessive concentrations of blood glucose, proteins, or lipids is excluded because plasma is not hypotonic. Clinical features of hyponatremia (Table 25–6) may develop as serum sodium falls below 115 mmol/L or if there is a very rapid decrease in serum sodium.[138, 139] Otherwise patients remain asymptomatic. Values of serum sodium around 100 mmol/L are life-threatening. Most hyponatremic patients have detectable or elevated plasma AVP concentrations and their urine osmolality tends to be higher than plasma osmolality,[140, 141] so that neither is diagnostic of the syndrome of inappropriate antidiuresis (SIAD). Measurement of urinary sodium concentration aids classification (see Table 25–5).

Syndrome of Inappropriate Antidiuresis

Inappropriate antidiuretic hormone secretion was proposed many years ago to account for serum hypochloremia observed in tuberculosis,[142] but it re-emerged as a syndrome associated with a variety of conditions described and defined by Bartter and Schwartz[143] (Table 25–7). Support for the hypothesis of inappropriate antidiuretic hormone secretion came from early studies on healthy adults given exogenous vasopressin and oral fluids to produce dilutional hyponatremia.[144] Recent studies have confirmed a variety of abnormalities of AVP secretion in the syndrome.[145]

TABLE 25–6. CLINICAL FEATURES OF HYPOTONIC HYPONATREMIA

Anorexia	Muscle cramps	Headache
Nausea	Myoclonus	Confusion
Vomiting	Abdominal ileus	Convulsions
Fatigue	Ataxia	Coma and death

TABLE 25–7. CARDINAL FEATURES OF THE SYNDROME OF INAPPROPRIATE ANTIDIURETIC HORMONE SECRETION

Hyponatremia with appropriately low plasma osmolality
Urine osmolality greater than plasma osmolality
Excessive renal sodium excretion
Absence of hypotension, hypovolemia, and edema-forming states
Normal renal and adrenal function

Cause

Many conditions associated with dilutional hyponatremia have been reported in which the cause has been attributed to SIAD (Table 25–8).

Small cell carcinoma of the bronchus is probably the most common neoplastic cause of SIAD. AVP has been demonstrated in tumor extracts, suggesting that the tumor was the source of AVP, and evidence that tumorous tissue can synthesize AVP has come from studies on in vitro biosynthesis of AVP.[146] However, not all patients with SIAD associated with neoplastic disease have ectopic AVP production because abnormal excessive AVP secretion from the posterior pituitary has been demonstrated.[147] Studies have suggested that abnormal forms of AVP are secreted by some tumors and that others synthesize AVP ectopically but SIAD does not result.

Pathophysiology

The basic abnormality in most cases of SIAD is a failure to maximally suppress AVP secretion as plasma osmolality falls below the theoretical osmotic threshold for AVP release. Thus, AVP continues to circulate at concentrations that are inappropriately high in relation to the hypo-osmolality of body fluids, although the absolute AVP values may not be particularly elevated. For reasons not well understood, patients continue to drink and this, combined with a degree of persistent antidiuresis due to circulating AVP, leads to dilutional hyponatremia.[148] Investigation of osmoregulated AVP secretion in a large group of patients, all of whom fulfilled the criteria laid down by Bartter and Schwartz and who had a variety of underlying disorders, revealed four distinct patterns of AVP release[147] (Fig. 25–9).

The first pattern (Type A, Fig. 25–9) is characterized by wide fluctuations in plasma AVP concentration which occur at random and bear no relationship to changes in plasma osmolality. Such erratic release could be accounted

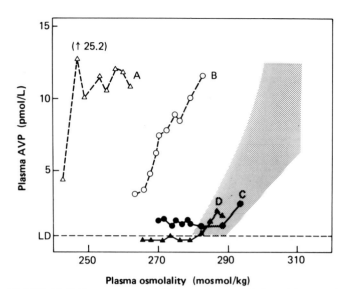

FIGURE 25–9. **Four patterns of AVP response to infusion of hypertonic saline** in a group of hyponatremic patients with the syndrome of inappropriate antidiuretic hormone secretion. A: erratic release; B: reset osmostat; C: AVP leak; D: normal osmoregulated AVP release. (Adapted from Zerbe R, Stropes L, Robertson GL: Vasopressin function in the syndrome of inappropriate antidiuresis. Ann Rev Med 31:315–327, 1980.)

for by ectopic secretion from neoplastic tissue, but similar patterns occur in non-neoplastic disease, suggesting a lesion in the posterior pituitary or any of its regulatory afferent neurons. Type A accounts for about 35 per cent of patients with SIAD.

A second group, accounting for one third of patients, demonstrates resetting of the osmostat to the left of normal (Type B). In these patients, plasma AVP is responsive to changes in plasma osmolality, but the threshold for AVP release and thirst is subnormal. Such patients are still able to osmoregulate water excretion, retaining the ability to dilute and concentrate urine, but around a plasma osmolality that is lower than normal. Again, this pattern of AVP release is observed in both neoplastic and non-neoplastic disease. Because similar shifts to the left of normal are observed in hypovolemia and hypotension, one cause is suspected to be a lesion in the afferent baroregulatory pathways.

In some cases, AVP secretion cannot be entirely suppressed and the hormone "leaks out" at low plasma osmolality (Type C). However, increasing plasma osmolality results in a normal plasma AVP response. The last group (Type D), accounting for less than 10 per cent of patients, has entirely normal osmoregulated AVP secretion; nevertheless, the patients fulfill the criteria of Bartter and Schwartz, fail to excrete a water load, and cannot maximally dilute urine. It is not known whether this abnormality is due to increased renal sensitivity to extremely low concentrations of AVP or to another antidiuretic factor.

Treatment

Patients with SIAD who have plasma sodium concentrations greater than 125 mmol/L rarely have significant symptoms from hyponatremia itself and may not require specific treatment to raise plasma sodium. With more severe degrees of hyponatremia, some form of therapy may be required.

TABLE 25–8. SOME CAUSES OF THE SYNDROME OF INAPPROPRIATE ANTIDIURETIC HORMONE SECRETION

Neoplastic Disease	Chest Disorders
Carcinoma (bronchus, duodenum, pancreas, bladder, ureter, prostate)	Pneumonia
	Tuberculosis
	Empyema
Thymoma	Cystic fibrosis
Mesothelioma	Pneumothorax
Lymphoma, leukemia	Asthma
Ewing's sarcoma	**Drugs**
Carcinoid	Vasopressin and analogues
Bronchial adenoma	Oxytocin
CNS Disorders	Chlorpropamide
Head injury	Clofibrate
Brain abscess or tumor	Vincristine, vinblastine, cisplatin
Meningitis, encephalitis	
Guillain-Barré syndrome	Thiazides
Cerebral hemorrhage	Phenothiazides
Cavernous sinus thrombosis	Monoamine oxidase inhibitors
Hydrocephalus	**Miscellaneous**
Cerebellar and cerebral atrophy	Idiopathic
	Psychosis, delirium tremens
Shy-Drager syndrome	
Porphyria	
Peripheral neuropathy	
Epilepsy	

Adequate treatment directed toward the underlying cause of SIAD is the most appropriate, but if this fails and the patient requires therapy for life-threatening or symptomatic chronic hyponatremia, total fluid intake should be restricted to 500 ml/24 hours, aiming to raise serum sodium slowly no higher than 130 mmol/L.[49, 149] Because fluid restriction can be distressing, particularly when prolonged, additional drug therapy is advocated to manage chronic hyponatremia. The antidiuretic action of AVP can be blocked by demeclocycline (600 to 1200 mg daily) or the less reliable and more toxic lithium carbonate (600 to 1800 mg daily).[150] The NDI induced by these drugs may take up to six weeks to develop fully. Specific antagonists to the V_2 receptor have been synthesized. Although their efficacy has been confirmed in animals, they have failed to fulfill their potential in humans.[151] Drugs to suppress neurohypophysial AVP secretion (e.g., phenytoin) have met with limited success.[152] An alternative therapeutic approach is the administration of oral furosemide (40 to 80 mg daily) together with salt supplementation (3 g daily).[153] If the serum sodium is exceedingly low (100 mmol/L), hypertonic saline can be infused very slowly to raise serum sodium no more rapidly than 0.5 mmol/L/h to attain about 130 mmol/L final concentration.

Severe hyponatremia and its treatment are associated with high mortality and morbidity. Rapid correction of chronic low serum sodium (<115 mmol/L) by any method can cause central pontine and extrapontine myelinolysis or osmotic demyelination syndrome,[154] in which the patient develops brain edema, seizures, and coma and risks death, often two to four days after correction of the hyponatremia. Recent studies have confirmed that both the rate and magnitude of the increase in serum sodium during correction are risk factors for the development of demyelinating lesions in chronically hyponatremic rats.[155]

THIRST DEFICIENCY SYNDROMES

Defects in osmoregulated thirst are extremely uncommon. They lead to a chronic inadequate intake of fluid which, in the majority of cases, causes profound hypernatremia.[156, 157] These disorders are referred to as hypodipsic or adipsic hypernatremia. Not infrequently an associated disturbance of osmoregulated AVP release is present.

Cause

Thirst deficiency syndromes develop as a result of a variety of pathological processes involving the putative thirst osmoreceptor cells in the anterior circumventricular organs of the hypothalamus or their neuronal connections. Table 25–9 lists the specific diseases recognized to cause hypodipsic or adipsic hypernatremia.[156] Tumors due to either neoplastic conditions or granulomatous diseases account for the majority.

Pathophysiology

With the development of visual analogue scales to estimate thirst and precise AVP assays, it is now possible to

TABLE 25–9. CAUSES OF THIRST DEFICIENCY SYNDROMES

Neoplastic (50%)	Granulomatous (20%)
Primary: Craniopharyngioma	Histiocytosis
Pinealoma	Sarcoidosis
Meningioma	**Miscellaneous (15%)**
Pituitary tumor	Hydrocephalus
Secondary: Bronchial	Ventricular cyst
carcinoma	Trauma
Breast carcinoma	Idiopathic
Vascular (15%)	
Internal carotid ligation	
Anterior communicating artery aneurysm	
Intrahypothalamic hemorrhage	

Adapted from Robertson GL, Aycinena P, Zerbe RL: Neurogenic disorders of osmoregulation. Am J Med 72:339–353, 1982.

classify these syndromes into different pathogenetic entities.

Resetting of the osmotic thresholds for thirst and AVP release to the right of normal (see Figs. 25–3 and 25–6) accounts for patients with "essential" hypernatremia.[158] These patients have persistent hypernatremia but are still able to dilute and concentrate urine and appreciate thirst but do so around a higher plasma osmolality set point.[49, 154]

Complete destruction of the osmoreceptors leads to total adipsia and, interestingly, a persistently low level of AVP secretion that fails to respond to osmotic stimuli. There are, however, normal AVP responses to nonosmotic stimuli. Severe hypernatremia ensues, as these patients never experience thirst and, if left to themselves, do not drink. Because of persistent minimal non-osmoregulated AVP secretion, hyponatremia can develop if patients are given large fluid loads, as hypo-osmolality does not suppress AVP release.[157]

A third type of defect was described recently in which there is normal osmoregulated AVP secretion but total absence of osmoregulated thirst.[159] This clinical observation supports the concept of two populations of osmoreceptor cells, one serving AVP pathways and the other thirst appreciation.

Treatment

The cornerstone of management of patients with thirst deficiency syndromes is adequate fluid intake if the underlying cause cannot be treated. Hypodipsic patients rarely develop life-threatening hypernatremia because thirst develops when plasma osmolality rises sufficiently. Fluid intake then returns serum sodium toward normal.

Adipsia with absent osmoregulated AVP secretion presents a major management problem, and these patients run the risk of profound hypernatremia. One therapeutic approach is the administration of oral fluid, the volume of which is based on the previous day's body weight change. Frequent intermittent checks of serum sodium are essential to avoid extreme fluctuations in serum sodium. Nevertheless, wide swings from hypernatremia to hyponatremia can still occur.[49] This form of adipsia is indeed life-threatening.

107. Spruce BA, McCulloch AJ, Burd J, et al: The effect of vasopressin infusion on glucose metabolism in man. Clin Endocrinol 22:463–468, 1985.
108. Pittman QJ, Landgraf R: Vasopressin in thermoregulation and blood pressure control. *In* Jard S, Jamison R (eds): Vasopressin. Montrouge, France, John Libbey, 1991, pp 177–184.
109. Ferris CF, Singer EA, Meenan DM, Albers HE: Inhibition of vasopressin-stimulated flank marking behaviour by V₁-receptor antagonists. Eur J Pharmacol 154:153–159, 1988.
110. Sargal A, Keith AB, Wright C, Edwardson JA: Failure of vasopressin to enhance memory in a passive avoidance task in rats. Neuroscience Lett 28:87–92, 1982.
111. Schwartz WJ, Coleman RJ, Reppert SM: A daily vasopressin rhythm in rat cerebrospinal fluid. Brain Res 263:105–112, 1983.
112. Thompson CJ: Polyuric states in man. *In* Baylis PH (ed): Water and Salt Homeostasis in Health and Disease. London, Baillière Tindall, 1989, pp 473–497.
113. Blotner H: Primary or idiopathic diabetes insipidus: A system disease. Metabolism 7:191–206, 1958.
114. Moses AM, Notman DD: Diabetes insipidus and syndrome of inappropriate antidiuretic hormone secretion (SIADH). Adv Intern Med 27:73–110, 1982.
115. Scherbaum WA, Bottazzo GF: Autoantibodies to vasopressin cells in idiopathic diabetes insipidus: Evidence for an autoimmune variant. Lancet 1:897–901, 1983.
116. Vokes TJ, Gaskill MB, Robertson GL: Antibodies to vasopressin in patients with diabetes insipidus. Ann Intern Med 108:190–195, 1988.
117. Hollinshead WH: The interphase of diabetes insipidus. Proc Mayo Clinic 39:95–100, 1964.
118. Jialal I, Desai K, Rajput MC: An assessment of posterior pituitary function in patients with Sheehan's syndrome. Clin Endocrinol 27:91–95, 1987.
119. Baylis PH, Thompson CJ, Burd JM, et al: Recurrent pregnancy-induced polyuria and thirst due to hypothalamic diabetes insipidus: An investigation into possible mechanisms responsible for polyuria. Clin Endocrinol 24:459–466, 1986.
120. Barron WM, Cohen LH, Ulland LA, et al: Transient vasopressin-resistant diabetes insipidus of pregnancy. N Engl J Med 310:442–444, 1984.
121. Ito M, Mori Y, Oiso Y, Saito H: A single base substitution in the coding region for neurophysin II associated with familial central diabetes insipidus. J Clin Invest 87:725–728, 1991.
122. Cremers CWRJ, Wijdeveld PGAB, Pinckers AJLG: Juvenile diabetes mellitus, optic atrophy, hearing loss, diabetes insipidus, atonia of the urinary tract and bladder, and other abnormalities (Wolfram syndrome). Acta Paediatr Scand (Suppl) 264:1–16, 1977.
123. Dashe AM, Cramm RE, Crist CA, et al: A water deprivation test for the differential diagnosis of polyuria. JAMA 185:699–703, 1963.
124. Miller M, Dalakos T, Moses AM, et al: DHP: Recognition of partial defects in antidiuretic hormone secretion. Ann Intern Med 73:721–729, 1970.
125. Zerbe RL, Robertson GL: A comparison of plasma vasopressin measurements with a standard indirect test in the differential diagnosis of polyuria. N Engl J Med 305:1539–1546, 1981.
126. Moses AM, Streeten DHP: Differentiation of polyuric states by measurement of responses to changes in plasma osmolality induced by hypertonic saline infusion. Am J Med 42:368–377, 1967.
127. Robertson GL: Diagnosis of diabetes insipidus. *In* Czernichow P, Robinson AG (eds): Diabetes Insipidus in Man. Frontiers of Hormone Research, Vol 13. Basel, Karger, 1985, pp 176–189.
128. Baylis PH, Robertson GL: Vasopressin response to hypertonic saline infusion to assess posterior pituitary function. J R Soc Med 73:255–260, 1980.
129. Cobb WE, Spare S, Reichlin S: Neurogenic diabetes insipidus: Management with DDAVP (1-desamino-8-D arginine vasopressin). Ann Intern Med 88:183–188, 1978.
130. Miller M, Moses AM: Potentiation of vasopressin action by chlorpropamide in vivo. Endocrinology 86:1024–1027, 1970.
131. Niaudet P, Dechaux M, Trivinc C, et al: Nephrogenic diabetes insipidus: Clinical and pathophysiological aspects. Adv Nephrol 13:247–260, 1984.
132. Kambouris M, Dlouhy SR, Trofatter JA, et al: Localisation of the gene for X-linked nephrogenic diabetes insipidus to Xq28. Am J Med Genet 29:239–246, 1988.
133. Moses AM, Miller JL, Levine MA: Two distinct pathophysiological mechanisms in congenital nephrogenic diabetes insipidus. J Clin Endocrinol Metab 66:1259–1264, 1988.
134. Simon NM, Garber E, Arieff AL: Persistent nephrogenic diabetes insipidus after lithium carbonate. Ann Intern Med 86:446–447, 1977.
135. Niaudet P, Dechaux M, Leroy D, Boyer M: Nephrogenic diabetes insipidus in children. *In* Czernichow P, Robinson AG (eds): Diabetes Insipidus in Man. Frontiers of Hormone Research, Vol 13. Basel, Karger, 1985, pp 224–231.
136. Robertson G, Aycinena P, Vokes T, Weiss N: Dipsogenic diabetes insipidus: A variant of primary polydipsia caused by abnormal osmoregulation of thirst. *In* Yoshida S, Share L (eds): Recent Progress in Posterior Pituitary Hormones 1988. Amsterdam, Elsevier Science Publishers BV, 1988, pp 411–418.
137. Flear CTG, Gill GV, Burn J: Hyponatremia: Mechanisms and management. Lancet 2:26–31, 1981.
138. Berl T, Anderson RJ, McDonald KM, Schrier RW: Clinical disorders of water metabolism. Kidney Int 10:117–132, 1976.
139. Arieff AL, Flach F, Massry SG: Neurological manifestations and morbidity of hyponatremia, correlation with brain, water and electrolytes. Medicine 55:121–129, 1976.
140. Anderson RJ, Chung H-M, Kluge R, Schrier RW: Hyponatremia: A prospective analysis of its epidemiology and the pathogenetic role of vasopressin. Ann Intern Med 102:164–168, 1985.
141. Gross PA, Pehrisch H, Rascher W, et al: Pathogenesis of clinical hyponatremia: Observations of vasopressin and fluid intake in 100 hyponatremic medical patients. Eur J Clin Invest 17:123–129, 1987.
142. Winkler AW, Crankshaw OF: Chloride depletion in conditions other than Addison's disease. J Clin Invest 17:1–6, 1938.
143. Bartter FC, Schwartz WB: The syndrome of inappropriate secretion of antidiuretic hormone. Am J Med 42:790–806, 1967.
144. Leaf A, Bartter FC, Sautos RF, Wrong O: Evidence in man that urinary electrolyte loss induced by pitressin is a function of water retention. J Clin Invest 32:868–878, 1952.
145. Verbalis JG: Hyponatremia. *In* Baylis PH (ed): Water and Salt Homeostasis in Health and Disease. London, Baillière Tindall, 1989, pp 499–530.
146. Carney DN, Gazdar AF, Oie HK, et al: The in vitro growth and characterization of small cell lung cancer. *In* Greco FA (ed): Biology and Management of Lung Cancer. Boston, Martinus Nijhoff, 1983, pp 1–24.
147. Zerbe R, Stropes L, Robertson GL: Vasopressin function in the syndrome of inappropriate antidiuresis. Ann Rev Med 31:315–327, 1980.
148. Rolls B: Thirst in human hypo- and hypernatremic states. *In* Jard S, Jamison R (eds): Vasopressin. Montrouge, France, John Libbey, 1991, pp 549–556.
149. Kovacs L, Robertson GL: Disorders of water balance—hyponatremia and hypernatremia. Clin Endocrinol Metab 6:107–127, 1992.
150. Forrest JN Jr, Cox M, Hong C, et al: Superiority of demeclocycline over lithium in the treatment of chronic syndrome of inappropriate secretion of antidiuretic hormone. N Engl J Med 298:173–177, 1978.
151. Kinter LB, Ilson BE, Caltabianol S, et al: Antidiuretic hormone antagonism in humans: Are there predictors? *In* Jard S, Jamison R (eds): Vasopressin. Montrouge, France, John Libbey, 1991, pp 321–329.
152. Tanay A, Yust I, Peresecenschi G, et al: Longterm treatment of the syndrome of inappropriate antidiuretic hormone secretion with phenytoin. Ann Intern Med 90:50–52, 1979.
153. Decaux G, Waterlot Y, Gennette F, et al: Inappropriate secretion of antidiuretic hormone treated with furosemide. Br Med J 285:89–90, 1982.
154. Sterns RH, Riggs J, Schochet SS: Osmotic demyelination syndrome following correction of hyponatremia. N Engl J Med 314:1535–1542, 1986.
155. Verbalis JG, Martinez AJ: Determinants of brain myelinolysis following correction of chronic hyponatremia in rats. *In* Jard S, Jamison R (eds): Vasopressin. Montrouge, France, John Libbey, 1991, pp 539–547.
156. Robertson GL, Aycinena P, Zerbe RL: Neurogenic disorders of osmoregulation. Am J Med 72:339–353, 1982.
157. Robertson GL: Abnormalities of thirst regulation. Kidney Int 25:460–469, 1984.
158. de Rubertis FR, Michelis MF, Beck N, et al: "Essential hypernatremia" due to ineffective osmotic and intact volume regulation of vasopressin secretion. J Clin Invest 50:97–111, 1971.
159. Hammond DN, Moll GW, Robertson GL, Chelmicka-Schorr E: Hypodipsic hypernatremia with normal osmoregulation of vasopressin. N Engl J Med 315:433–436, 1986.
160. Land H, Schütz G, Schmale H, Richter D: Nucleotide vasopressin-neurophysin II precursor. Nature 295:299–303, 1982.
161. Baylis PH, Robertson GL: Physiological control of vasopressin secretion. *In* Baylis PH, Padfield PL (eds): The Posterior Pituitary: Hormone Secretion in Health and Disease. New York, Marcel Dekker, 1985, pp 119–139.

26

Oxytocin

BRIAN T. PICKERING

The first description of what later came to be recognized as an action of oxytocin was almost an aside by Henry Dale,[1] who mentioned that an intravenous injection of an extract of ox pituitary into a cat caused the animal's uterus to contract. Dale went on to explore more thoroughly this property of what he showed to be associated with the posterior lobe of the gland and, although he wrote, "It does not seem justifiable . . . to draw . . . the conclusion that the principle acting on the plain muscle of the uterus is different from that which acts on the arteries," the uterotonic action of oxytocin had been discovered.[2] Within a year or two, Ott and Scott[3] had shown that posterior pituitary extracts increase milk flow in lactating goats and thus, by 1910, the two principal actions of oxytocin—on milk letdown and on uterine activity—had been established.

It is interesting to note that as well as establishing the action of neurohypophysial extracts on the promotion of milk flow, Ott and Scott[4] also reported that "the corpus luteum, pineal body and thymus increased the quantity of milk fourfold in five minutes." These findings appear to have been completely overlooked, and it was some 70 years later before ovarian oxytocin was rediscovered[5] and, indeed, that the corpus luteum was found to synthesize the hormone.[6, 7] Similarly, there has been much interest recently in oxytocin produced by the thymus and its role in immunological responses.[8] Most of this chapter is devoted to pituitary oxytocin, but a mention of gonadal oxytocin is made at the end.

Although crude posterior pituitary extract had been used by Blair Bell[9] to assist labor, the clinical use of its biological actions became easier when it was purified into its constituent hormones. In spite of Dale's belief in a single active principle, it was in his laboratory that the first steps in separating oxytocin from vasopressin were taken.[9, 10] By the end of the 1920's, separate preparations of oxytocin and vasopressin were available commercially,[12] so that it became possible to use oxytocin clinically to assist labor without the undesirable vasopressor actions of accompanying vasopressin.

Even though the separation of oxytocin from vasopressin in the laboratory had been clearly demonstrated, arguments continued about the possible existence of a single parent molecule in the animal. Such arguments received support from the isolation of an apparently homogeneous protein—"the Van Dyke protein"—that showed all of the activities associated with the posterior pituitary gland.[13] The solution to this paradox came with the discovery[14] of neurophysin, a protein—or family of proteins—that formed an ionic complex with the hormones. It was this complex that constituted the "Van Dyke protein." Moreover, with the elucidation of the structures of oxytocin and vasopressin (Fig. 26–1), it became clear that the overlap of biological activity, which had contributed to the argument for a single pluripotent hormone, resulted from the great homology in the sequence of amino acids in the two peptides (see ref. 15). Thus, oxytocin was shown to be an independent hormone and, in the following pages, its biosynthesis and physiology are discussed and reference is given to some of its clinical applications.

CELLS OF ORIGIN AND BIOSYNTHESIS OF OXYTOCIN

From Neurosecretion to Peptidergic Neurons

The oxytocin stored in and released from the posterior pituitary gland is produced in neurons whose cell bodies are located in the supraoptic and paraventricular nuclei of

CyS. Tyr. Ile. Gln. Asn. CyS. Pro. Leu. Gly(NH$_2$)
Oxytocin

CyS. Tyr. Phe. Gln. Asn. CyS. Pro. Arg. Gly(NH$_2$)
Arginine Vasopressin

FIGURE 26–1. The neurohypophysial hormones.

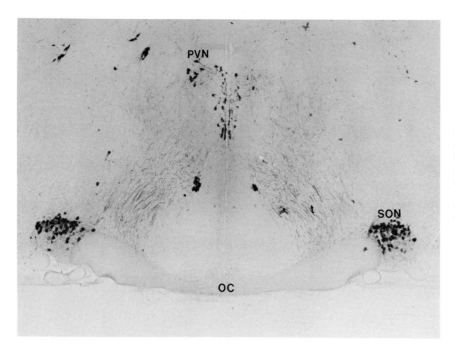

FIGURE 26–2. **Location of the neurons that produce the neurohypophysial hormones in the hypothalamus.** Section of rat hypothalamus stained immunocytochemically for oxytocin-neurophysin (by peroxidase-antiperoxidase method). SON, supraoptic nucleus; PVN, rostral end of paraventricular nucleus; t, fibers from PVN coursing down to join hypothalamic-neurohypophysial tract; OC, optic chiasm.

the hypothalamus (Fig. 26–2). Because of their size, these cells are often referred to as magnocellular neurons.

These days, the concept of active peptides being synthesized in neurons is not difficult to accept, but this has not always been so. Because the posterior pituitary is composed largely of nerve fibers and cells recognized as modified astroglia (pituicytes), it was naturally assumed that the posterior pituitary hormones would be secreted by the latter.[16] Although the idea that some neurons might be secretory—neurosecretion, enunciated by Scharrer[17]—provided an alternative hypothesis, it was not widely explored; even when Bargmann[18] provided definitive evidence for the hypothalamic-neurohypophysial system being neurosecretory, it was some time before it was generally accepted.

Examination with the electron microscope[19] showed the axons in the neurohypophysis to have many dilatations filled with secretory granules (Fig. 26–3) which, on preparation in the centrifuge, proved to contain the hormones and the neurophysins.[20–23]

With the development of immunocytochemical techniques for the localization of peptide-containing cells in tissues, it soon became apparent that oxytocin and vasopressin are far from unique as neuropeptides and that peptidergic neurons have a major role to play in the functioning of the nervous system (e.g., see ref. 24). Thus, although the concept of neurosecretion has been expanded almost beyond its definition, it has given birth to the peptidergic neuron, and oxytocin has played a significant role in this development.[25]

Separate Oxytocin and Vasopressin Cells

Immunocytochemical techniques clearly differentiate oxytocin-containing neurons from those making vasopressin,[26] and there is very little doubt that, at least in the hypothalamus, the hormones are synthesized in separate cells.[27, 28] Early studies[29, 30] suggested that each hypothalamic nucleus elaborated a separate peptide, the supraop-

tic (SON) synthesizing vasopressin and the paraventricular (PVN) oxytocin, but this has not been substantiated: Each nucleus makes both hormones.[28, 31, 32] There is some differential distribution within the nuclei, with more oxytocin cells in the rostral part and more vasopressin cells in the caudal part of both the SON and PVN in the rat.[33] It has been customary to refer to the SON and PVN as if the

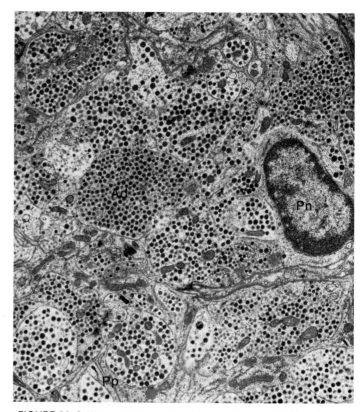

FIGURE 26–3. **Electron micrograph of the rat posterior pituitary** showing the axonal dilatations (Ad) filled with secretory granules and invested with pituicyte processes (Pp). A pituicyte nucleus (Pn) is also shown ($\times$ 15,000).

oxytocin-producing cells of the hypothalamus are confined to these anatomical entities, but a three-dimensional reconstruction by Fisher et al[34] showed this to be true for less than half of the cells, with the rest being in "accessory nuclei" (see also ref. 35).

Oxytocin-Neurophysin

Soon after Acher and his co-workers[14] showed that the Van Dyke protein was in fact a complex between the hormones and an "inert" protein, which they named neurophysin, the latter was found to be a family of related proteins rich in cystine and consisting of 93 to 95 amino acid residues. The reported size of this family has fluctuated over the years, largely because it was not recognized initially that the posterior pituitary is rich in proteases active in weakly acidic solutions. It now seems certain that there are two primary neurophysins in each species, one associated with oxytocin and one with vasopressin.[36, 37] A great deal of structural homology exists among the neurophysins, with the sequence of 65 amino acids from 10 to 74 showing very few substitutions. What variations do occur between different neurophysins are restricted to the amino- and carboxy-terminal sequences. Moreover, even in the variable amino-terminal region, some functional conservation occurs such that, in the limited number of species that have been examined, homology exists among the neurophysins associated with vasopressin and among those related to oxytocin which is greater than the homology between the two neurophysins in a given species. This has led Acher and his colleagues[38] to describe two groups of neurophysins, MSEL neurophysins and VLDV neurophysins, using the single letter code to designate the residues in positions 2, 3, 6, and 7 (M, methionine; S, serine; E, glutamic acid; L, leucine; V, valine, D, aspartic acid). Where a specific association has been demonstrated, MSEL neurophysins are associated with vasopressin and VLDV neurophysins with oxytocin. However, because the Acher nomenclature is not precisely correct in all species, it seems more appropriate to refer to a vasopressin-neurophysin and an oxytocin-neurophysin.

Although it will become obvious later on, it is perhaps worth stressing that oxytocin-neurophysin is a molecule that is associated with oxytocin in the cell. It does not show greater affinity for oxytocin than for vasopressin during the formation of complexes in the test tube: Both neurophysins bind both hormones.

The Common Hormone-Neurophysin Precursor: The Pathway to Oxytocin

In the mid-1960's, Sachs and his colleagues[39] showed that vasopressin is synthesized by way of a larger protein precursor (see Chapter 25) and, not unexpectedly, oxytocin was shown to be made in a similar way.[40] One possibility entertained by Sachs was that vasopressin and neurophysin shared a common precursor, and this suggestion became more acceptable when it was realized that a separate neurophysin is associated with each hormone. Moreover, observation of parallel synthesis of each hormone and its neurophysin strengthened the common-precursor hypoth-

esis,[41] which was vindicated by the isolation of the molecules by Russell et al.[42] Purification of the messenger RNA from bovine hypothalami, preparation of complementary DNA, and amplification in a bacterial system allowed a German group to elucidate the amino acid sequence of the oxytocin-neurophysin precursor,[43, 44] which is represented in Figure 26–4.

Even as long ago as the mid-1950's, Vogt[45] concluded that, if primary synthesis of oxytocin occurs in the hypothalamus, the molecule must undergo some chemical modification on its journey to the posterior pituitary gland to account for the higher oxytocic relative to vasopressor activity in the gland compared with the hypothalamus. Studies on the rate of transport of oxytocin and its neurophysin along the axons of the hypothalamic-neurohypophysial tract[40, 41] supported the idea that the common precursor is packaged into granules in the neuronal perikarya in the hypothalamus and processed into the secretory products as the granule moves along the axon toward the terminals in the posterior pituitary. These ideas have now been fully substantiated by the isolation of the appropriate components from different parts of the tract.[46, 47] Once they are packaged, processing of the precursor commences and continues to completion. The necessary enzymes are present within the granule,[48] and processing does not depend on the environment through which the granule moves because it continues normally when transport is switched off with colchicine.[49]

Formation of oxytocin from its precursor (Fig. 26–4) entails cleavage of the primary polypeptide chain and amidation of what becomes the terminal glycine residue in the hormone. The −Gly.Lys.Arg− sequence, which separates the oxytocin and neurophysin sequences, is the cryptic message for both of these events. Proteolytic cleavage sites in polypeptide precursors that yield secretory products are most frequently identified by pairs of basic amino acid residues,[50] and it is now being appreciated that a glycine residue usually acts as the nitrogen donor in the formation of peptides with terminal amides.[51]

We know very little about the precise mechanism by which the secretory granules are transported along the axons. Radioactive oxytocin can be isolated from the neural lobe of the pituitary gland about 1.5 hours after an intracerebral injection of $[^{35}S]$cysteine[52, 53] so that the granules move along the axons with a velocity of approximately 50 mm/day. This puts oxytocin granules into the group of rapidly transported substances referred to as class II by Baitinger and colleagues.[54] Like other components of this group, the oxytocin granules are arrested by vinca alkaloids such as colchicine,[53–56] suggesting that microtubules may be involved in their transport. However, although much has been written about intra-axonal transport of polypeptides,[59] the nature of the interaction of granule and microtubule is still unknown.

As discussed below, hormone release requires the fusion of the secretory granule with the axonal membrane, and the dilatations referred to above and shown in Figure 26–3 are the storage sites. The pituitary contains large

signal-OXYTOCIN-**Gly.Lys.Arg**-neurophysin-His

FIGURE 26–4. The oxytocin precursor.

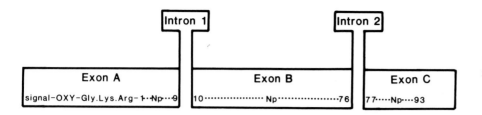

FIGURE 26–5. A representation of the oxytocin gene.

The Oxytocin Gene

Nucleotide sequences have been determined for both bovine[60] and rat[61] oxytocin genes. As shown in Figure 26–5, the gene consists of three exons separated by two introns. (Exons contain nucleotide sequences that are transcribed into mRNA, whereas the nucleotide sequences of introns are not transcribed but are spliced out in the formation of mRNA.) It is interesting that the highly conserved part of the amino acid sequence of neurophysin (residues 10 to 74), referred to above, represents almost the whole exon B, with the variable parts of the molecule being coded for by exons A and C.

The oxytocins and vasopressin genes are structurally closely linked: In humans they are both located on chromosome 20 and are separated by less than 8 kb.[62] A similar situation exists in the rat, in which it has been established that the genes are present on the same chromosome (11 kb apart) but on different DNA strands such that they are transcribed in opposite directions.[63]

ROLE OF OXYTOCIN IN LACTATION

The Milk-Ejection Reflex

Of all of the known biological actions of oxytocin, the milk-ejection activity is probably the one that has the soundest physiological footing. Originally described by Ott and Scott[3] as an action on milk secretion, the ability of oxytocin to bring about an increase in milk flow is now known to result from the contraction of myoepithelial cells. These contractile cells form a meshlike arrangement around the alveoli in the mammary glands,[64] and their contraction under the influence of oxytocin squeezes milk out of the alveoli into the ducts. The milk-ejection reflex is a classic neuroendocrine reflex arc (see reviews in refs. 65 and 66). Stimulation of the nipple by the sucking infant leads to a release of oxytocin from the maternal pituitary.

Activity of Hypothalamic Neurons During Milk Ejection

In most animals, milk ejection does not occur under anesthesia, but, fortunately, the rat is an exception and continues to express the reflex under surgical anesthesia, so that it is possible to record the electrical activity of the neurons producing oxytocin while the rat continues to suckle her young. Such experiments have shown a burst of electrical activity in the neurons some 10 to 12 seconds before the rise of intramammary pressure which delivers the milk to the young,[67] and implantation of microwire recording electrodes have enabled Summerlee and Lincoln[68] to demonstrate the same phenomenon in unanesthetized lactating rats. Thus the reflex arc can be illustrated as shown in Figure 26–6: Stimulation of the nipple allows activation of the oxytocin neuron in SON and PVN, resulting in a release of oxytocin into the circulation from the terminals in the posterior pituitary.

Afferent Pathways and Patterns of Oxytocin Release

With regard to the afferent limb of this reflex arc, it is not appropriate to delineate here the neuroanatomical pathways by which information is conveyed from the nipples to the hypothalamus, but rather the reader is directed to reviews in which these are considered.[66, 69] However, some comments must be made about input to the system. The reflex is not a simple one: Stimulation of the nipple does not lead inevitably to activation of the oxytocin neuron and release of the hormone. Rather, a central gating mechanism determines whether the stimulus gets through. This rather complex process involves a number of central controls modulating the primary information and resulting in the recruitment of most if not all of the oxytocin-producing magnocellular neurons,[66, 69, 70] so that only a brief mention of some of its consequences is made here. When an anesthetized lactating rat is maintained with 10 to 12 pups attached to her nipples, milk ejections, preceded by bursts of activity in hypothalamic neurons, occur at 5- to 10-minute intervals throughout the period of the experiment. That this periodic effect requires afferent input from the nipples is clear from the fact that it does not occur in the absence of suckling pups. Moreover, it requires a threshold level of stimulus because application of six or fewer sucking pups to the nipples of a mother rat does not stimulate milk ejection even after considerable time, whereas addition of a seventh baby immediately elicits oxytocin release and a normal milk-ejection pattern. On the other hand, when a full complement of young are first put to the nipples, a long latent period occurs before the onset of the first burst of action potentials and consequent milk ejection. The first burst is very small, increasing over the next two to three responses.

The study of an anesthetized rat with its young constantly sucking is not as artificial as it may first appear. The conscious rat spends a total of about 18 hours per day with its young attached to the nipples. During this period, each pup sucks briefly about every 20 seconds, and there is no

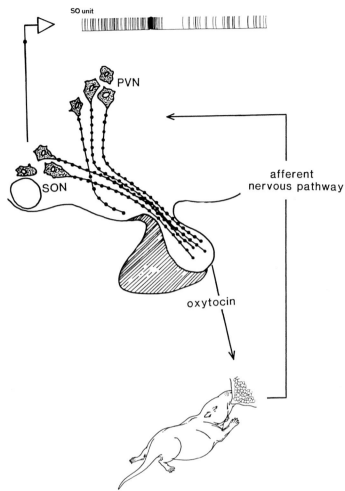

FIGURE 26–6. **The milk-ejection reflex arc.** The upper part of the figure shows the electrical activity of a neuron in the supraoptic nucleus recorded during a milk ejection.

Release of Oxytocin

The primary action that initiates the release of hormone from the nerve terminals is the influx of calcium ions resulting from membrane depolarization consequent to the arrival of action potentials (for reviews, see refs. 69 and 77). Thus, calcium provides the link for "stimulus-secretion coupling."[78, 79] The exact mechanism of calcium's action is not known, but it results in the movement of secretory granules to the limiting membranes of the terminals, where they fuse to release their contents by exocytosis. A direct relationship does not exist between the number of action potentials that arrive at the nerve terminals and hormone release. The same number of potentials is more effective in bringing about oxytocin release when delivered as high-frequency bursts than as a low-frequency train. Maximal release seems to occur at a frequency of 30 to 50 Hz—the frequency seen during the suckling-related bursts illustrated in Figure 26–6.[69]

Synchronization of activity appears to occur in all the oxytocin neurons of the SON during the burst of electrical activity that precedes milk ejection (see Fig. 26–6) and results in hormone release. The mechanism for this synchronization is still unknown, but one suggestion is that it occurs by electronic coupling (e.g., through gap junctions). Interestingly, morphological studies have shown a great increase of membrane apposition in neurons within the nuclei under conditions in which oxytocin release is enhanced, such as lactation.[80-82]

During the past decade, attention was once again focused on the pituicyte as a component in hormone release. In the past there have been numerous reports of changes in pituicyte morphology in relation to different levels of hormone release, but proposals for the explanation of such changes have usually proved incorrect.[83] The pituicyte has long cell processes that wrap around the hormone-containing nerve terminals (see Fig. 26–3), but the work of Tweedle and his colleagues[84] has shown that stimuli for oxytocin release (parturition, suckling) result in a decrease in the extent to which the axons are invested by pituicytes. Thus it seems that the pituicytes may shield the release areas from the extracellular environment in the resting state but move away during hormone release to allow it to be dissipated.

Pharmacological studies have implicated a number of neurotransmitters in the release of oxytocin (for review, see refs. 69 and 85), although the transmitter at the final synapse with the oxytocin cell is still unknown. Acetylcholine, dopamine, and norepinephrine have all been shown to affect hormone release, although the effects of each appear complex. For example, norepinephrine appears to operate through two apparently opposing mechanisms: A stimulating effect is obtained through α-receptors, whereas β-agonists inhibit oxytocin release. The latter effect may be the result of a presynaptic inhibition at the terminals releasing oxytocin in the posterior pituitary because intracerebroventricular injection of isoproterenol (a β-agonist) has no effect on the periodic bursts of electrical activity in the oxytocin neurons of the lactating rat but switches off milk ejection even though the mammary gland remains sensitive.[86]

synchronization among the litter except for a short time every 5 to 10 minutes when a milk ejection is occurring.[71] Both in the anesthetized and in the conscious nursing rat, oxytocin release and hence provision of milk occur only when the EEG recorded from the mother's cerebral cortex shows synchronized, large-amplitude, slow waves like those seen when the animal is asleep. Any stimulus leading to arousal blocks the milk-ejection reflex.[72]

Suckling behavior and hence oxytocin release vary greatly from species to species,[65, 69, 73] and it appears that there are variations in the operation of the central gate such that the reflex is tailored to the needs of the species in relation to its habitat and way of life. In contrast to the rat, which nurses for most of the day, the rabbit suckles her young for a short period (about 5 minutes) once a day. An intermediate situation exists in the pig, in which the sow suckles for 5 to 15 minutes every 45 to 60 minutes, and a single milk ejection occurs during each suckling period. Moreover, whereas milk ejection is associated with sleeplike behavior in the rat, quite the reverse is true for pig and rabbit, in which oxytocin release seems to be associated with an EEG pattern of arousal.[74-76]

The Role of Opioids in the Regulation of Oxytocin Release

Intracerebroventricular injection of morphine leads to a cessation of milk ejection in the rat without affecting the electrical activity of the oxytocin neurons, suggesting an inhibition of hormone release effected at the nerve terminals,[87] and this is supported by the action being present in the neural lobe in vitro.[87] A great deal of immunocyto-chemical evidence exists for the presence of opioid peptides in the posterior pituitary,[88, 90] so that there is every possibility for this inhibitory effect to be of physiological significance. On the other hand, some investigators maintain that the opioid peptides found in the posterior pituitary are present in neurons that are separate from hormone-containing ones and, moreover, that these fibers innervate the pituicytes.[92] Certainly, pituicytes express receptors for opiates[93] and, as mentioned above, pituicytes have been suggested to play a role in oxytocin release.

There is now no doubt that opioids do have an important role to play in the control of oxytocin release, in relation to both milk let-down and parturition (see below).[66] Opioid action is not confined to the axon terminals but indicates inhibition of the electrical activity of the neurons.[66] Our understanding of the central effects of opioids in the oxytocin system has been improved greatly by the model introduced by Russell and his colleagues in which rats are made morphine-tolerant by a regimen of chronic drug administration.[94] Using this paradigm, these authors conclude that the magnocellular neurons are subject to an inhibitory opioid tone, but whether this applies to morphine-naïve as well as morphine-tolerant rats still must be determined.[66, 95] Certainly, naloxone potentiates the release of oxytocin brought about by the injection of cholecystokinin, but this is not accompanied by an increase in electrical activity of the neurons.[96]

OXYTOCIN AND PARTURITION

Stimulation of the uterus to contract was the first action of oxytocin to be discovered,[1] yet controversy still exists about whether this activity has physiological relevance, particularly for the human.

There is no doubt that, were it released, oxytocin could play a major role in parturition. The number of oxytocin receptors in the myometrium of the rat increases some 40-fold in the hours preceding the onset of labor,[97, 98] and the electrical stimulation of the pituitary stalk in rabbits toward the end of gestation promotes "normal" delivery within minutes.[99] Thus there is little doubt that a mechanism to bring about oxytocin release at term *could* initiate as well as promote parturition. Available evidence, however, substantially opposes such a simple mechanism.[100]

Attempts to gather data relevant to the release of oxytocin at parturition have been frustrated by a number of problems: the pulsatile nature of oxytocin release,[101, 102] the short half-life of oxytocin in blood,[103] and the presence in human blood (but not that of usual experimental animals) of a pregnancy-related degradative enzyme, oxytocinase.[104] Moreover, the stimulation of oxytocin release by distention of the cervix, the Ferguson reflex,[105] makes it more difficult to differentiate between a rise in oxytocin concentration that might initiate parturition and one that results from the commencement of labor.

The majority of studies have shown an increase in circulating oxytocin in association with labor (for review, see ref. 100). One problem is to establish whether the uterine contractions have resulted from oxytocin release or have initiated it as a response to distention of the birth canal. In other words, does oxytocin release merely facilitate labor, or does it play a part in the initiation of parturition? There may not be a straightforward answer to this question, and what applies to one species may not apply to another.

It now seems generally accepted that parturition in sheep is initiated by the release of cortisol from the fetal adrenal gland.[106] Once labor is underway, distention of the canal may lead to an increase in oxytocin release from the mother's pituitary,[107, 108] and this facilitates labor. Moreover, even in this species, maternal oxytocin release could be an earlier event, stimulated as a consequence of fetal prostaglandin $F_{2\alpha}$ secretion, and there is evidence of oxytocin levels increasing throughout pregnancy to reach a peak at term, perhaps arising from increased frequency of pulses of release.[102]

In the rat, the build-up of pituitary hormones[109] and neurophysins[110] during gestation and their precipitous fall at parturition suggest that oxytocin release is associated with labor. Moreover, putative oxytocin neurons, recorded in the conscious rat during labor, showed high-frequency bursts of activity just prior to the delivery of a fetus or placenta,[111] suggesting the release of a pulse of oxytocin. Again, there is no way of assessing whether the release of the hormones initiates or is stimulated by parturition. However, the large increase in the number of oxytocin receptors in the myometrium in the hours before birth[97] has been taken as an indicator that the resultant increase in sensitivity to oxytocin allows the hormone to trigger parturition.

In the human, too, an enormous increase (100- to 200-fold) occurs in the myometrial oxytocin receptors during pregnancy.[111] This results in the human myometrium becoming extremely sensitive to oxytocin such that the levels of hormone detected at the commencement of labor could be sufficient to initiate the process.[100] However, the increase in uterine receptors is not confined to the myometrium but is also seen in the uterine decidua. This tissue responds to oxytocin in vitro by the release of prostaglandin $F_{2\alpha}$,[111, 113] a substance that probably plays an important role in the progress of labor.[100] Thus, as Fuchs and Fuchs[100] point out, the human uterus at term is perfectly primed to respond to a small increase in oxytocin, both by contracting and by prostaglandin releasing $F_{2\alpha}$, which itself brings about contractions.

Chard et al.[114] first demonstrated that oxytocin is released by the human fetus during labor and suggested that this fetal oxytocin may play a role in the initiation of labor. Other workers have also reported oxytocin release by the human fetus,[100, 115, 116] and similar data have been obtained for the rat fetus.[117] Moreover, although injection of oxytocin antibody into pregnant rats had no effect on the timing of parturition,[118] injection into the fetuses in utero caused a mean delay of 18 hours in its onset.[117]

Clearly, it is not unreasonable to suggest that the arrival of this fetal oxytocin at the primed uterus initiates contractions. Labor then develops by a complex interplay involving uterine prostaglandin $F_{2\alpha}$ and, perhaps, also maternal oxytocin.[100]

It is of course reasonable to suggest that onset of parturition is timed by the removal of an inhibition. This could be inhibition of muscular contraction or of oxytocin release. Relaxin is a hormone that has long been held to have a role in the inhibition of uterine tone,[119] and circulating levels of this rise during the latter part of gestation and fall at term.[120] Summerlee and his colleagues[121] showed that relaxin also had central effects inhibiting oxytocin release and suggested that this inhibition was mediated by opioids.[122] Thus, a decrease in relaxin at term would simultaneously remove an inhibition of oxytocin release and of uterine sensitivity. On the other hand, Way and Leng[123] have evidence that relaxin increases the release of oxytocin in the rat and that this effect is independent of opioids. Clearly, much remains to be learned about the complex interactions of all of these peptides.

Clinical Uses of Oxytocin

Oxytocin has been used to assist labor almost since its initial discovery[9, 124] and has also been used to relieve breast engorgement (for recent review, see ref. 125).

OXYTOCIN AS A NEUROPEPTIDE TRANSMITTER

Oxytocin nerve terminals are not confined to the median eminence and posterior pituitary gland but are located throughout the CNS, even reaching the lower spinal cord.[126–128] The presence of these extrahypothalamic pathways raises the possibility that, besides its hormonal action, oxytocin may act as a neurotransmitter or neuromodulator in neuron-neuron interactions. Certainly, oxytocin applied iontophoretically to hippocampal neurons, a region of the brain where oxytocin has been localized,[128–130] increases their firing pattern and does so by affecting receptors that show pharmacological similarities to those of the uterus.[131, 132]

The physiological role(s) of oxytocin within the CNS is still obscure. Certainly, the peptide does have behavioral effects related to the retention of information,[133] although these may be due to a metabolite of oxytocin rather than to the peptide itself.[134]

GONADAL OXYTOCIN

The Ovary

As mentioned earlier, it is interesting that, although Ott and Scott[4] showed clearly that the corpus luteum contains an oxytocin-like substance, very little attention was paid to this for the next 70 years. It was the juxtaposition of two laboratories, one isolating relaxin from ovine corpora lutea and the other working on the biochemistry of oxytocin, which led to the identification of a uterus-stimulating substance in the ovary as oxytocin.[5]

The hormone is synthesized in the large luteal cells,[135, 136] along with a neurophysin, by a pathway very similar to that

in the hypothalamus[6]; indeed, the ovarian oxytocin gene is almost identical to the hypothalamic one.[7]

In the cow, a waxing and waning of luteal oxytocin occurs, with maximum concentrations of the hormone toward the middle part of the life of the corpus luteum.[137] The physiological role of luteal oxytocin is still obscure,[138–140] but it does seem to be secreted because the blood draining from the ovary of a sheep in the luteal phase of its cycle has a higher concentration of oxytocin than the blood entering through the ovarian artery.[141] A great deal of evidence links oxytocin with luteolysis (for review, see refs. 138 and 139); for example, immunization against the hormone prolongs the luteal phase,[142, 143] and injection of a prostaglandin analogue (a known luteolysin) leads to massive release of oxytocin from the ovary.[141] However, no direct relationship exists between oxytocin content and progesterone secretion, because luteal oxytocin falls off quite normally when the animal becomes pregnant, even though the corpus luteum is maintained and continues to secrete progesterone.[137]

High concentrations (micrograms per gram) of luteal oxytocin have been found only in ruminants: sheep,[5] cow,[144] and goat (Homeida and Cooke, cited in ref. 139). The corpora lutea of other species do have luteal oxytocin but in smaller (nanograms per gram) amounts: human,[145–147] monkey,[148] pig,[149] and guinea pig (Swann and Smith, unpublished observations). Oxytocin is contained within granules much like those seen in the neurohypophysis.[150] Such granules have been described in luteal cells in the past but associated with progesterone.[151]

Interestingly, although the ovarian oxytocin gene is switched on at the time of ovulation,[152] oxytocin does not build up until several days later,[137] suggesting an initial build-up of precursor and subsequent delay in post-translational processing. Such a suggestion is supported by immocytochemical evidence.[153]

The Testis

The synthesis of oxytocin by the ovary and the observation that the neurohypophysial hormones influence androgen production by testis cells in vitro[154] raised the question of the presence of oxytocin in the male gonad. Both immunoreactive oxytocin and neurophysin have been measured in testicular extracts from rat and human.[155] Immunocytochemical studies[156, 157] (Fig. 26–7) suggest that the oxytocin resides in the Leydig cells. Indeed such cells, in vitro, synthesize oxytocin, and the synthesis is enhanced by luteinizing hormone.[158]

The physiological function of testicular oxytocin is still unclear, although evidence is mounting that it has a role as an intragonadal hormone.[140, 159] Certainly, the mobility of seminiferous tubules is enhanced by low levels of oxytocin[160] and while tubules removed from untreated animals are spontaneously active, those taken from animals manipulated to be devoid of testicular oxytocin are quiescent.[140] Thus, oxytocin may play a part in moving the seminiferous tubule contents along the lumen or may agitate the seminiferous epithelium to facilitate the movement of the developing germ cell toward the lumen.[140]

Neurohypophysial hormones have long been known to influence steroidogenesis in the testis,[154] although there

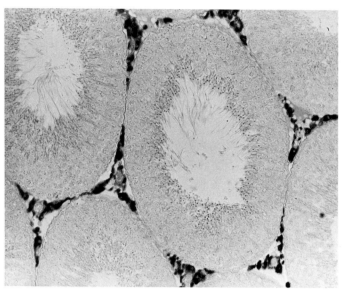

FIGURE 26–7. Oxytocin in the testis. A section of a rat testis stained immunocytochemically for oxytocin. Note that the stain is confined to the interstitial tissue.

have been conflicting reports about whether they were inhibiting or stimulating. The apparent paradox is explained by the finding that in rats chronically treated with oxytocin implants in the testis, a fall in testosterone with a concomitant rise in dihydrotestosterone[161] occurs. Thus it may be that oxytocin plays a paracrine role in the testis, perhaps providing local signaling of the stage of the spermatogenic cycle in different parts of the testis.[156, 162]

THE OXYTOCIN RECEPTOR

The cloning of a cDNA corresponding to the human oxytocin receptor and its expression to give a 388-amino acid receptor protein[163] has opened another door in oxytocin research. It is now possible to ask questions about the pathophysiology of the hormone by considering the expression of the receptor gene as well as that for the production of liquid.

REFERENCES

1. Dale HH: On some physiological actions of ergot. J Physiol Lond 34:163–206, 1906.
2. Dale HH: The action of extracts of the pituitary body. Biochem J 4:427–447, 1909.
3. Ott I, Scott JC: The action of infundibulin upon the mammary secretion. Proc Soc exp Biol NY 8:48–49, 1910.
4. Ott I, Scott JC: The galactagogue action of the thymus and corpus luteum. Proc Soc Exp Biol 8:49, 1910.
5. Wathes DC, Swann RW: Is oxytocin an ovarian hormone? Nature 297:225–227, 1982.
6. Swann RW, O'Shaughnessy PJ, Birkett SD, et al: Biosynthesis of oxytocin in the corpus luteum. FEBS Lett 174:262–266, 1984.
7. Ivell R, Richter D: The gene for the hypothalamic peptide hormone oxytocin is highly expressed in the bovine corpus luteum: Biosynthesis, structure and sequence analysis. EMBO J 3:2351–2354, 1984.
8. Greenen V, Legros J-J, Franchimont P, et al: The thymus as a neuroendocrine organ. Synthesis of vasopressin and oxytocin in human thymic epithelium. Ann NY Acad Sci 496:56–66, 1987.
9. Blair Bell W: The pituitary body and the therapeutic value of the infundibular extract in shock, uterine atony and intestinal paresis. Br Med J 2:1609–1613, 1909.
10. Dudley HW: Some observations on the active principles of the pituitary gland. J Pharm Exp Therap 14:295–312, 1919.
11. Dudley HW: On the active principles of the pituitary gland. J Pharm Exp Therap 21:103–122, 1923.
12. Kamm O, Aldrich TB, Grote IW, et al: The active principles of the posterior lobe of the pituitary gland. J Am Chem Soc 50:573–601, 1928.
13. van Dyke HB, Chow BF, Greep RO, Rothen A: Isolation of a protein from the pars neuralis of the ox pituitary with constant oxytocic pressor and diuresis-inhibiting activities. J Pharmacol Exp Ther 74:190–209, 1942.
14. Acher R, Manoussos G, Olivry G: Sur les relations, entre l'ocytocine et la vasopressine d'une part et la protéine de van Dyke d'autre part. Biochim Biophys Acta 16:155–156, 1955.
15. Du Vigneaud V: Hormones of the posterior pituitary gland: Oxytocin and vasopressin. Harvey Lectures 51:1–26, 1956.
16. Bucy PC: The pars nervosa of the bovine hypophysis. J Comp Neurol 50:505–519, 1930.
17. Scharrer E: Die Lichtempfindlicheit blinder Elritzen (Untersuchungen uber das Zwischenhirn der Fische I). Z Vgl Physiol 7:1–38, 1928.
18. Bargmann W: Uber die neurosekretorische Verknupfung von Hypothalamus und Neurohypophyse. Z Zellforsch Mikrosk Anat 34:610–634, 1949.
19. Palay SL: The fine structure of the neurohypophysis. In Waelsch H (ed): Ultrastructure and Cellular Chemistry of Neural Tissue. New York, Hoeber, 1957, pp 31–49.
20. Weinstein H, Malamed S, Sachs H: Isolation of vasopressin-containing granules from the neurohypophysis of the dog. Biochim Biophys Acta 50:385–386, 1961.
21. Barer R, Heller H, Lederis K: The isolation, identification and properties of the hormonal granules of the neurohypophysis. Proc R Soc B 158:388–416, 1963.
22. LaBella FS, Reiffenstein RJ, Beaulieu G: Subcellular fractionation of bovine posterior pituitary glands by centrifugation. Arch Biochem Biophys 100:399–408, 1963.
23. Ginsburg M, Ireland M: The role of neurophysin in the transport and release of neurohypophysial hormones. J Endocrinol 35:289–298, 1966.
24. Krieger DT, Brownstein MJ, Martin JB (eds): Brain Peptides. New York, Wiley, 1983.
25. Pickering BT: The neurosecretory neurone in the 1980s. In Farner DS, Lederis K (eds): Neurosecretion: Molecules, Cells, Systems. New York, Plenum, 1981, pp 417–433.
26. Aspeslagh MR, Vandesande F, Dierickx K: Electron microscopic immunocytochemical demonstration of separate neurophysin-vasopressinergic and neurophysin-oxytocinergic nerve fibres in the neural lobe of the rat hypophysis. Cell Tissue Res 171:31–37, 1976.
27. Morris JF, Sokol HW, Valtin H: One neuron–one hormone? Recent evidence from Brattleboro rats. In Moses AM, Share L (eds): Neurohypophysis. Basel, Karger, 1977, pp 58–66.
28. Dierickx F, Vandesande F, Goossens N: The one neuron–one hormone hypothesis and the hypothalamic magnocellular neurosecretory system of the vertebrates. In Vincent JD, Kordon C (eds): Cell Biology of Hypothalamic Neurosecretion. Paris, CNRS, 1978, pp 391–398.
29. Olivecrona H: Paraventricular nucleus and pituitary gland. Acta Physiol Scand 40:1–178, 1957.
30. Nibblelinck DW: Paraventricular nuclei, neurohypophysis and parturition. Am J Physiol 200:1229–1232, 1961.
31. Sokol HW: Evidence for oxytocin synthesis after electrolytic destruction of the paraventricular nucleus in rats with hereditary hypothalamic diabetes insipidus. Neuroendocrinology 6:90–97, 1970.
32. Burford GD, Dyball REJ, Moss RL, Pickering BT: Synthesis of both neurohypophysial hormones in both the paraventricular and supraoptic nuclei of the rat. J Anat 117:261–296, 1974.
33. Swaab DF, Pool CW, Nijveldt F: Immunofluorescence of vasopressin and oxytocin in the rat hypothalamo-neurohypophysial system. J Neural Transm 36:195–215, 1975.
34. Fisher AWF, Price PG, Burford GD, Lederis K: A 3-dimensional reconstruction of the hypothalamo-neurohypophysial system of the rat. Cell Tissue Res 204:343–354, 1979.
35. Rhodes CH, Morrell JI, Pfaff DW: Immunobiochemical analysis of magnocellular elements in rat hypothalamus: Distribution and numbers of cells containing neurophysin, oxytocin and vasopressin. J Comp Neurol 198:45–64, 1981.
36. Pickering BT, Jones CW: The neurophysins. In Li CH (ed): Hor-

monal Proteins and Peptides, Vol 5. New York, Academic Press, 1978, pp 103–158.

37. Breslow E: Chemistry and biology of the neurophysins. Ann Rev Biochem 48:251–274, 1979.
38. Chauvet M-T, Chauvet J, Acher R: Phylogeny of neurophysins: Partial amino acid sequence of a sheep neurophysin. FEBS Lett 52:212–215, 1975.
39. Sachs H, Fawcett P, Takabatake Y, Portanova R: Biosynthesis and release of vasopressin and neurophysin. Rec Prog Horm Res 25:447–491, 1969.
40. Pickering BT, Jones CW, Burford GD: Biosynthesis and intraneuronal transport of neurosecretory products in the hypothalamo-neurohypophysial system. In Wolstenholme GEW, Birch J (eds): Neurohypophysial Hormones (Ciba Study Grp 39). London, Livingstone, Churchill, 1971, pp 58–74.
41. Pickering BT, Jones CW, Burford GD, et al: The role of neurophysin proteins: Suggestions from the study of their transport and turnover. Ann NY Acad Sci 248:15–35, 1975.
42. Russell JT, Brownstein MJ, Gainer H: Biosynthesis of vasopressin, oxytocin, and neurophysins: Isolation and characterization of two common precursors (propressophysin and prooxyphysin). Endocrinology 107:1880–1891, 1980.
43. Schmale H, Richer D: In vitro biosynthesis and processing and composite common precursors containing amino acid sequences identified immunologically as neurophysin I/oxytocin and as neurophysin II/arginine vasopressin. FEBS Lett 121:358–362, 1980.
44. Land H, Grez M, Ruppert S, et al: Deduced amino acid sequence from the bovine oxytocin-neurophysin I precursor cDNA. Nature 303:342–344, 1983.
45. Vogt M: Vasopressor, antidiuretic, and oxytocic activities of extracts of the dog's hypothalamus. Br J Pharmacol 8:193–196, 1953.
46. Brownstein MJ, Russell JT, Gainer H: Synthesis transport, and release of posterior pituitary hormones. Science NY 207:373–378, 1980.
47. Swann RW, Gonzalez CB, Birkett SD, Pickering BT: Harbingers and hormones: Inter-relationships of rat neurohypophysial hormone precursors in vivo. In Cross BA, Leng G (eds): The Neurohypophysis: Structure, Function and Control. Progress in Brain Research, Vol 60. Amsterdam, Elsevier, 1983, pp 235–239.
48. North WG, Morris JF, LaRochelle TF, Valtin H: Enzymatic interconversions of neurophysins. Endocrinology 101:110–118, 1977.
49. Birkett SD, Swann RW, Gonzalez CB, Pickering BT: Analysis of the neurohypophysial components accumulating in the supraoptic nucleus of the rat after injection of colchicine. Arch Biochem Biophys 225:430–435, 1983.
50. Steiner DF, Quinn PS, Chan SJ, et al: Processing mechanisms in the biosynthesis of proteins. Ann NY Acad Sci 343:1–16, 1980.
51. Bradbury AF, Finnie MDA, Smyth DG: Mechanism of C-terminal amide formation by pituitary enzymes. Nature 298:686–688, 1982.
52. Jones CW, Pickering BT: Rapid transport of neurohypophysial hormones in the hypothalamo-neurohypophysial tract. J Physiol Lond 208:73–74P, 1970.
53. Jones CW, Pickering BT: Intra-axonal transport and turnover of neurohypophysial hormones in the rat. J Physiol Lond 227:553–564, 1972.
54. Baitinger C, Levine J, Lorenz T, et al: Characteristics of axonally transported proteins. In Weiss DG (ed): Axoplasmic Transport. Berlin, Springer-Verlag, 1982, pp 110–120.
55. Norstrom A, Hansson HA, Sjostrand J: Effects of colchicine on axonal transport and ultrastructure of the hypothalamo-neurohypophysial system of the rat. Z Zellforsch Mikrosk Anat 113:271–293, 1971.
56. Flament-Durand J, Dustin P: Studies on the transport of secretory granules in the magnocellular hypothalamic neurons. Z Zellforsch Mikrosk Anat 130:440–454, 1972.
57. Hindeland-Gertner C, Stoeckel ME, Porte A, Stutinsky F: Colchicine effects on neurosecretory neurones and other hypothalamic and hypophysial cells, with special reference to changes in the cytoplasmic membranes. Cell Tissue Res 170:17–41, 1976.
58. Parish DC, Rodriguez EM, Birkett SD, Pickering BT: Effects of small doses of colchicine on the components of the hypothalamo-neurohypophysial system of the rat. Cell Tissue Res 220:809–827, 1981.
59. Weiss DG, (ed): Axoplasmic Transport. Berlin, Springer-Verlag, 1982.
60. Ruppert S, Scherer G, Schutz G: Recent gene conversion involving bovine vasopressin and oxytocin precursor genes suggested by nucleotide sequence. Nature 308:554–557, 1984.
61. Ivell R, Richter D: Structure and comparison of the oxytocin and vasopressin genes from rat. Proc Natl Acad Sci USA 81:2006–2010, 1984.
62. Sausville E, Carney D, Battey J: The human vasopressin gene is linked to the oxytocin gene and is selectively expressed in a cultured lung cancer cell. J Biol Chem 260:10236–10241, 1985.
63. Mohr E, Schmitz E, Richter D: A single rat genomic DNA fragment encodes both the oxytocin and vasopressin genes separated by 11 kilobases and oriented in opposite transcriptional directions. Biochimie 70:649–654, 1988.
64. Richardson KC: Contractile tissues in the mammary gland, with special reference to myoepithelium in the goat. Proc R Soc B 136:30–45, 1949.
65. Lincoln DW, Paisley AC: Neuroendocrine control of milk ejection. J Reprod Fertil 65:571–586, 1982.
66. Crowley WR, Armstrong WE: Neurochemical regulation of oxytocin secretion in lactation. Endocr Rev 13:33–65, 1992.
67. Wakerley JB, Lincoln DW: The milk-ejection reflex of the rat: A 20- to 40-fold acceleration of the firing of paraventricular neurones during oxytocin release. J Endocrinol 57:477–493, 1973.
68. Summerlee AJS, Lincoln DW: Electrophysiological recordings from oxytocinergic neurones during suckling in the unanaesthetised lactating rat. J Endocrinol 90:255–265, 1981.
69. Poulain DA, Wakerley JB: Electrophysiology of hypothalamic magnocellular neurones secreting oxytocin and vasopressin. Neuroscience 7:773–808, 1982.
70. Wakerley JB, Ingram CD: Synchronisation of hypothalamic oxytocin neurones: Possible coordinating mechanisms. News in Physiological Sciences 8:129–133, 1993.
71. Wakerley JB, Drewett RF: Pattern of suckling in the infant rat during spontaneous milk-ejection. Physiol Behav 15:277–281, 1975.
72. Lincoln DW, Hentzen K, Hin T, et al: Sleep: A prerequisite for reflex milk ejection in the rat. Exp Brain Res 38:151–162, 1980.
73. Bisset GW: Milk ejection. In Knobil EL, Sawyer WH (eds): Handbook of Physiology (Sect. 7) Endocrinology, Vol IV, pt 1. Washington, DC, American Physiological Society 1974, pp 493–520.
74. Ellendorff F, Forsling ML, Poulain DA: The milk-ejection reflex in the pig. J Physiol Lond 333:577–594, 1982.
75. Neve HA, Paisley AC, Summerlee AJS: Arousal: A pre-requisite for suckling in the conscious rabbit? Physiol Behav 28:213–217, 1982.
76. Paisley AC, Summerlee AJS: Suckling and arousal in the rabbit: Activity of neurones in the cerebral cortex. Physiol Behav 31:471–475, 1983.
77. Pickering BT, Swann RW: Secretion in the posterior pituitary gland. In Cantin M (ed): Cell Biology of the Secretory Process. Basel, Karger, 1984, pp 247–275.
78. Douglas WW: Involvement of calcium in exocytosis and the exocytosis-vesiculation sequence. Biochem Soc Symp 39:1–28, 1974.
79. Rubin RP: Stimulus-secretion coupling. In Cantin M (ed): Cell Biology of the Secretory Process. Basel, Karger, 1984, pp 52–72.
80. Theodosis DT, Poulain DA, Vincent J-D: Possible morphological basis for synchronisation of neuronal firing in the rat supraoptic nucleus during lactation. Neuroscience 6:919–929, 1981.
81. Hatton GI, Tweedle CD: Magnocellular neuropeptidergic neurons in hypothalamus: Increases in membrane apposition and number of specialized synapses from pregnancy to lactation. Brain Res Bull 8:197–204, 1982.
82. Theodosis DT, Poulain DA: Evidence that oxytocin-secreting neurones are involved in the ultrastructural reorganisation of the rat supraoptic nucleus apparent at lactation. Cell Tissue Res 235:217–219, 1984.
83. Morris JF, Nordmann JJ, Dyball REJ: Structure-function correlation in mammalian neurosecretion. Int Rev Exp Path 18:1–95, 1978.
84. Tweedle CD: Ultrastructural manifestations of increased hormone release in the neurohypophysis. In Cross BA, Leng G (eds): The Neurohypophysis: Structure, Function and Control. Amsterdam, Elsevier, 1983, pp 259–272.
85. Clarke G, Merrick LP: Electrophysiological studies of the magnocellular neurons. Curr Topics Neuroendocr 4:17–59, 1985.
86. Moos F, Richard P: Double contrôle noradrénergique de la libération d'ocytocine pendant le réflexe d'éjection de lait chez la rate. CR Hebd Seanc Acad Sci Paris 290:1261–1264, 1980.
87. Clarke G, Wood P, Merrick L, Lincoln DW: Opiate inhibition of peptide release from the neurohumoral terminals of hypothalamic neurones. Nature 282:746–748, 1979.
88. Rossier J, Battenberg E, Pittman Q, et al: Hypothalamic enkephalin neurones may regulate the neurohypophysis. Nature 277:653–655, 1979.
89. Martin R, Voigt KH: Enkephalins co-exist with oxytocin and vasopressin in nerve terminals of rat neurohypophysis. Nature 289:502–504, 1981.

90. Geis R, Weber E, Martin R, Voigt KH: Hypothalamo-posterior pituitary system in Brattleboro rats: Immunoreactive levels of leucine-enkephalin, dynorphin (1–17), dynorphin (1–8) and α-neo-endorphin. Life Sci 31:1809–1812, 1982.

91. Martin R, Geis R, Holl R, et al: Co-existence of unrelated peptides in oxytocin and vasopressin terminals of rat neurohypophysis: Immunoreactive methionine⁵-enkephalin–, leucine⁵-enkephalin– and cholecystokinin-like substances. Neuroscience 8:213–227, 1983.

92. van Leeuwen FW, Pool CW, Sluiter AA: Enkaphalin immunoreactivity in synaptoid elements on glial cells in the rat neural lobe. Neuroscience 8:229–241, 1983.

93. Lightman SL, Ninkovic M, Hunt SP, Iversen LL: Evidence for opiate receptors on pituicytes. Nature 305:235–237, 1983.

94. Bicknell RJ, Leng G, Lincoln DW, Russell JA: Naloxone excites oxytocin neurones in the supraoptic nucleus of lactating rats after chronic morphine treatment. J Physiol (Lond) 396:297–317, 1988.

95. Leng G, Russell JA: Opioids, oxytocin and parturition. In Dyer RA, Bicknell RJ (eds): Brain Opioid Systems in Reproduction. Oxford, Oxford University Press, pp 231–256, 1989.

96. Leng G, Dyball REJ, Way SA: Naloxone potentiates the release of oxytocin induced by systemic administration of cholecystokinin without enhancing the electrical activity of supraoptic neurones. Exp Brain Res 88:321–325, 1992.

97. Soloff MS, Alexandrova M, Fernstrom MJ: Oxytocin receptors triggers for parturition and lactation? Science NY 204:1313–1315, 1979.

98. McCracken JA: Hormone receptor control of prostaglandin F 2α secretion by the ovine uterus. Adv Prost Thromb Res 8:1329–1344, 1980.

99. Lincoln DW: Labour in the rabbit: Effect of electrical stimulation applied to the infundibulum and median eminence. J Endocrinol 50:607–618, 1971.

100. Fuchs AR, Fuchs F: Endocrinology of human parturition: A review. Br J Obstet Gynecol 91:948–967, 1984.

101. Gibbens GLD, Chard T: Observations of maternal oxytocin release during human labor and the effect of intravenous alcohol administration. Am J Obstet Gynecol 126:243–246, 1976.

102. Mitchell MD, Kraemer DL, Brennecke SP, Webb R: Pulsatile release of oxytocin during the estrous cycle, pregnancy and parturition in sheep. Biol Reprod 27:1169–1173, 1982.

103. Ginsburg M, Smith MW: The fate of oxytocin in male and female rats. Br J Pharmac Chemother 14:327–333, 1959.

104. Page EW: The value of plasma pitocinase determinations. Am J Obstet Gynecol 52:1014–1021, 1946.

105. Ferguson JKW: Study of motility of intact uterus at term. Surg Gynecol Obstet 73:359–366, 1941.

106. Thornburn GD, Challis JRG, Robinson JS: Endocrine control of parturition. In Wynn RM (ed): Biology of the Uterus. New York, Plenum, 1977, pp 653–732.

107. Flint APF, Forsling ML, Mitchell MD, Turnbull AC: Temporal relationship between changes in oxytocin and prostaglandin F levels in response to vaginal distension in the pregnant and puerpural ewe. J Reprod Fertil 43:551–554, 1975.

108. Roberts JS, Share L: Inhibition by progesterone of oxytocin secretion during vaginal stimulation. Endocrinology 87:812–815, 1970.

109. Fuchs AR, Saito S: Pituitary oxytocin and vasopressin content of pregnant and parturient rats before, during and after parturition. Endocrinology 88:574–578, 1971.

110. Nicholson HD, Pickering BT: Changes in rat neural lobe neurophysin during pregnancy and lactation. J Endocrinol 72:60–61P, 1977.

111. Summerlee AJS: Extracellular recordings from oxytocin neurones during the expulsive phase of birth in unanaesthetised rats. J Physiol 321:1–9, 1981.

112. Fuchs AR, Fuchs R, Husslein P, et al: Oxytocin receptors and human parturition: A dual role for oxytocin in the initiation of labour. Science NY 215:1396, 1982.

113. Roberts JS, McCracken JA, Gavagen JE, Soloff MS: Oxytocin-stimulated release of prostaglandin F 2α from ovine endometrium in vitro: Correlation with estrous cycle and oxytocin-receptor binding. Endocrinology 99:1107–1114, 1976.

114. Chard T, Boyd NRH, Forsling ML, et al: The development of a radioimmunoassay for oxytocin: The extraction of oxytocin from plasma, and its measurement during parturition in human and goat blood. J Endocrinol 48:223–234, 1970.

115. Dawood MY, Wang CF, Gupta R, Fuchs F: Fetal contribution to oxytocin in human labor. Obstet Gynecol 52:205–209, 1978.

116. Sellers SM, Hodgson HT, Mountford LA, et al: Is oxytocin involved in parturition? Br J Obstet Gynaecol 88:725–729, 1981.

117. Schriefer JA, Lewis PR, Miller JW: Role of fetal oxytocin in parturition in the rat. Biol Reprod 27:362–368, 1982.

118. Kumaresan P, Kagan A, Glick SM: Oxytocin antibody and lactation and parturition in rats. Nature 230:468–469, 1971.

119. Weiss G: Relaxin. Ann Rev Physiol 46:43–52, 1984.

120. Sherwood OD, Crnekovic VE, Gordon WL, Rutherford JE: Radioimmunoassay of relaxin throughout pregnancy and during parturition in the rat. Endocrinology 107:691–698, 1980.

121. Summerlee AJS, O'Byrne KT, Paisley AC, et al: Relaxin affects central control of oxytocin release. Nature 309:372–374, 1984.

122. Jones SA, Summerlee AJS: Relaxin acts centrally to inhibit oxytocin release: An effect that is reversed by naloxone. J Endocrinol 111:99–102, 1986.

123. Way SA, Leng G: Relaxin increases the firing rate of supraoptic neurones and increases oxytocin secretion in the rat. J Endocrinol 132:149–158, 1992.

124. Theobald GW, Graham A, Campbell J, et al: The use of postpituitary extract in physiological amounts in obstetrics. Br Med J 2:123–127, 1948.

125. Petrie RH: The pharmacology and use of oxytocin. Clin Perinatol 8:35–47, 1981.

126. Swanson LW: Immunohistochemical evidence for a neurophysin-containing autonomic pathway arising in the paraventricular nucleus of the hypothalamus. Brain Res 128:346–353, 1977.

127. Swanson LW, McKellar S: The distribution of oxytocin- and neurophysin-stained fibers in the spinal cord of the rat and monkey. J Comp Neurol 188:87–106, 1979.

128. Sofroniew MV, Weindl A: Central nervous system distribution of vasopressin, oxytocin and neurophysin. In Martinez JL Jr, Jensen RA, Messing RB, et al: (eds): Endogenous Peptides and Learning and Memory Processes. New York, Academic Press, 1981, pp 327–369.

129. Buijs RM: Intra- and extrahypothalamic vasopressin and oxytocin pathways in the rat. Pathways to the limbic system. Cell Tissue Res 192:423–435, 1978.

130. Buijs RM: Vasopressin and oxytocin—their role in neurotransmission. Pharmacol Ther 22:127–141, 1983.

131. Muhlethaler M, Dreifuss JJ, Gahwiler BH: Vasopressin excites hippocampal neurones. Nature 296:749–751, 1982.

132. Muhlethaler M, Sawyer WH, Manning MM, Dreifuss JJ: Characterization of a uterine-type oxytocin receptor in the rat hippocampus. Proc Natl Acad Sci USA 80:6713–6717, 1983.

133. de Wied D, Gispen WH: Behavioral effects of peptides. In Gainer H (ed): Peptides in Neurobiology. New York, Plenum Press, 1977, pp 397–448.

134. Burbach JPH, Bohus B, Kovacs GL, et al: Oxytocin is a precursor of potent behaviourally active neuropeptides. Eur J Pharmacol 94:125–131, 1983.

135. Watkins WB: Immunohistochemical localization of neurophysin and oxytocin in the sheep corpora lutea. Neuropeptides 4:51–54, 1983.

136. Guldenaar SEF, Wathes DC, Pickering BT: Immunocytochemical evidence for the presence of oxytocin and neurophysin in the large cells of the bovine corpus luteum. Cell Tissue Res 237:349–352, 1984.

137. Wathes DC, Swann RW, Pickering BT: Variations in oxytocin, vasopressin and neurophysin concentrations in the bovine ovary during the oestrous cycle and pregnancy. J Reprod Fertil 71:551–557, 1984.

138. Wathes DC: Possible actions of gonadal oxytocin and vasopressin. J Reprod Fertil 71:315–345, 1984.

139. Wathes DC, Swann RW, Porter DG, Pickering BT: Oxytocin as an ovarian hormone. Curr Topics Neuroendocrinol 6:129–152, 1986.

140. Pickering BT, Ayad VJ, Birkett SD, et al: Neurohypophysial hormones in the gonads: Are they real and do they have a function? Reprod Fertil Dev 2:245–262, 1990.

141. Flint APF, Sheldrick EL: Ovarian secretion of oxytocin is stimulated by prostaglandin. Nature 297:587–588, 1982.

142. Sheldrick EL, Mitchell MD, Flint AP: Delayed luteal regression in ewes immunized against oxytocin. J Reprod Fertil 59:37–42, 1980.

143. Schams D, Prokopp S, Barth D: The effect of active and passive immunization against oxytocin on ovarian cyclicity in ewes. Acta Enocrinol (Copenh) 103:337–344, 1983.

144. Wathes DC, Swann RW, Birkett SD, et al: Characterization of oxytocin, vasopressin, and neurophysin from the bovine corpus luteum. Endocrinology 113:693–698, 1983.

145. Wathes DC, Swann RW, Pickering BT, et al: Neurohypophysial hormones in the human ovary. Lancet 2:410–412, 1982.

146. Khan-Dawood FS, Dawood MY: Human ovaries contain immunoreactive oxytocin. J Clin Endocrinol Metab 57:1129–1132, 1983.

147. Schaeffer JM, Liu J, Hsueh AJW, Yen SSC: Presence of oxytocin and arginine vasopressin in human ovary, oviduct, and follicular fluid. J Clin Endocrinol Metab 59:970–973, 1984.

148. Khan-Dawood FS, Marut EL, Dawood MY: Oxytocin in the corpus

luteum of the cynomolgus monkey (*Macaca fascicularis*). Endocrinology 115:570–574, 1984.

149. Pitzel L, Welp K, Holtz W, Konig A: Neurohypophysial hormones in the corpus luteum of the pig. Neuroendocrinol Lett 6:1–5, 1984.

150. Theodosis DT, Wooding FBP, Sheldrick EL, Flint APF: Ultrastructural localisation of oxytocin and neurophysin in the ovine corpus luteum. Cell Tiss Res 243:129–135, 1986.

151. Gemmell RT, Stacy BD, Thorburn GD: Ultrastructural study of secretory granules in the corpus luteum of the sheep during the estrous cycle. Biol Reprod 11:447–462, 1974.

152. Ivell R, Brackett KH, Fields MJ, Richter D: Ovulation triggers oxytocin gene expression in the bovine ovary. FEBS Lett 190:263–267, 1985.

153. Wathes DC, Guildenaar SEF, Swann RW, et al: A combined radioimmunoassay and immunocytochemical study of ovarian oxytocin production in the periovulatory period in the ewe. J Reprod Fertil 78:167–183, 1986.

154. Adashi EY, Hsueh AJW: Direct inhibition of testicular androgen biosynthesis revealing antigonadal activity of neurohypophysial hormones. Nature 293:650–652, 1981.

155. Nicholson HD, Swann RW, Burford GD, et al: Identification of oxytocin and vasopressin in the testis and in adrenal tissue. Regul Pept 8:141–146, 1984.

156. Guldenaar SEF, Pickering BT: The localization of gonadal oxytocin by immunocytochemistry. J Anat 139:736–737, 1984.

157. Guldenaar SEF, Pickering BT: Immunocytochemical evidence for the presence of oxytocin in rat testis. Cell Tissue Res 240:485–487, 1985

158. Nicholson HD, Hardy MP: Lutenising hormone differentially regulates the secretion of testicular oxytocin and testosterone by purified adult rat Leydig cells *in vitro*. Endocrinology 130:671–677, 1992.

159. Nicholson HD, Pickering BT: Oxytocin, a male intragonadal hormone. Regul Pept 45:253–256, 1993.

160. Worley RTS, Nicholson HD, Pickering BT: Testicular oxytocin: An initiator of seminiferous tubule movement. *In* Saez JM (ed): Proceedings of the Workshop of the European Study Group. Molecular and Cellular Endocrinology of the Testis. Paris, INSERM, 1985, pp 205–212.

161. Nicholson HD, Guldenaar SEF, Boer GJ, Pickering BT: Testicular oxytocin: Effects of intratesticular oxytocin in the rat. J Endocrinol 130:231–238, 1991.

162. Pickering BT, Birkett SD, Guldenaar SEF, et al: Oxytocin in the testis: What, where and why? Ann NY Acad Sci 564:198–209, 1989.

163. Kimura T, Tanizawa O, Mori K, et al: Structure and expression of a human oxytocin receptor. Nature 356:526–529, 1992.

27

The Pineal Gland: Basic Physiology and Clinical Implications

JOSEPHINE ARENDT

STRUCTURE AND BIOCHEMISTRY OF THE PINEAL GLAND

Structure

The pineal gland (epiphysis cerebri) is a small, unpaired central structure, essentially an appendage of the brain. Great variation in size and position is seen even within species.[1] In humans the pineal weighs around 100 to 150 mg. It assumes a shape resembling a pine cone (hence pineal) and, again owing to its shape, has been referred to as the "penis of the brain."

The mammalian pineal is a secretory organ, whereas in fish and amphibians it is directly photoreceptive and in reptiles and birds it has a mixed photoreceptor and secretory function.[2] The extracranial parietal (parapineal, frontal) organ found in some lower vertebrates has been referred to as the "third eye."[1, 2] The principal cellular component is the pinealocyte, and elements of its photoreceptive evolutionary history remain in both structure and function.[1-3] In some species, including humans, calcified lumps are frequently present in pineal tissue after puberty, although this appears not to be associated with a decline in metabolic activity.[4-6] The gland is richly vascularized. Its principal innervation is sympathetic, arising from the superior cervical ganglion.[7] In addition, there is good evi-

dence for parasympathetic, commissural, and peptidergic innervation.[8] Its primary function in all species studied to date is to transduce information concerning light-dark cycles to body physiology, particularly for the organization of body rhythms. This information is encoded in the secretion patterns of the major pineal hormone melatonin, 5-methoxy-N-acetyltryptamine.[9]

Synthesis and Metabolism of Melatonin

Melatonin is synthesized within the pineal from tryptophan via the pathway shown in Figure 27–1.[10, 11] Most synthetic activity occurs during the dark phase, with a major increase in the activity of serotonin–N-acetyltransferase (NAT). The rhythm of production is endogenous, being generated in the suprachiasmatic nucleus (SCN), the major central rhythm-generating system or "clock."[11] It is synchronized to 24 hours primarily by the light-dark cycle acting via the retina and the retinohypothalamic projection to the SCN. Melatonin is also synthesized in the retina, the harderian gland, and probably the gut, but these structures contribute little to circulating concentrations in mammals.

Melatonin is metabolized primarily within the liver by 6-hydroxylation, followed by sulfate and/or glucuronide con-

432

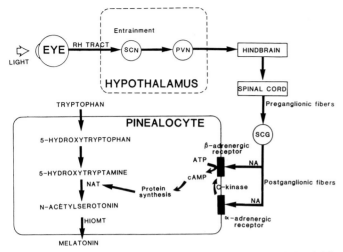

FIGURE 27–1. Control of melatonin synthesis in the pineal gland. The rhythm of secretion is generated in the suprachiasmatic nucleus (SCN) and entrained by the light-dark cycle. RH, retinohypothalamic; PVN, paraventricular nucleus; SCG, superior cervical ganglion; NA, norepinephrine; NAT, 5-hydroxytryptamine(serotonin)-N-acetyltransferase; HIOMT, hydroxyindole-O-methyltransferase.

jugation.[12] A number of minor metabolites are also formed through ring-splitting, cyclization of the side chain, or demethylation (see ref. 13 for bibliography). In humans and rodents exogenous oral or intravenous melatonin has a short metabolic half-life (20 to 60 minutes, depending on author and species), with a large hepatic first-pass effect and a biphasic elimination pattern. In ruminants longer half-lives are seen after oral administration.[14–17]

Other Pineal Factors

Although the pineal contains and synthesizes a multitude of other indoles together with biologically active peptides (for reviews, see refs. 18 and 19), they have not yet been attributed important physiological functions. Most effects of pinealectomy can be reversed by melatonin in physiological concentrations; hence, it is difficult to consider other compounds as major pineal hormones.

Neural Control of Melatonin Synthesis

Pineal denervation, or ganglionectomy, abolishes the rhythmic synthesis of melatonin and the light-dark control of its production. Norepinephrine is clearly the major transmitter, acting via β_1-adrenoceptors with potentiation by α_1 stimulation, but the role of neural serotonin is probably not negligible. There is a day-night variation in pineal norepinephrine, with highest values at night, approximately 180 degrees out of phase with the pineal serotonin rhythm. cAMP acts as a second messenger and stimulates NAT activity through a mechanism that involves both transcription and translation, although whether synthesis of new NAT molecules occurs is not yet clear (Fig. 27–1). β-Adrenergic receptor binding sites in the rat pineal vary over a 24-hour period, the lowest number being found toward the end of the dark phase, increasing shortly after lights on.[10, 11, 20, 21]

Other Control Mechanisms

The pineal contains very large numbers of other neuroreceptors and hormone receptors, but evaluation of their physiological importance is in its infancy.[22] Receptors have been detected in the pineal for a number of steroid hormones[23] and prostaglandins,[24] and administration of these can undoubtedly affect pineal metabolic activity.[23, 24] The significance of these relationships in vivo is not clear.

The pineal, the retina, and the SCN together form the basic structures perceiving and transducing nonvisual effects of light. Melatonin provides a closed loop to this system.

PHYSIOLOGY OF THE PINEAL

Light-Dark Control of Melatonin Synthesis

A Darkness Hormone

In virtually all species studied to date, whether nocturnal or diurnal, melatonin is synthesized and secreted during the dark phase of the day. Remarkably, even the unicellular alga *Gonyaulax* appears to produce melatonin during the dark phase.[25] Melatonin production is clearly a highly evolutionary conserved phenomenon. In most vertebrates the rhythm is endogenous, that is, internally generated. It persists in the absence of time cues, in general assuming a period deviating slightly from 24 hours, and is thus a true circadian rhythm.[6, 26]

In some lower vertebrates and birds the circadian rhythm of pineal melatonin production is clearly generated within the pineal itself.[27, 28] In mammals the pineal is not a self-sustaining rhythm generator. This role is taken over by the SCN.[27, 29] Lesions of the SCN lead to a loss of the vast majority of circadian rhythms such as locomotor activity, sleep, behavior, hormones including melatonin, and urinary constituents. Circadian rhythms are entrained (synchronized) to the 24-hour day primarily by light-dark cycles. Factors (zeitgebers) other than light-dark cycles which are involved in entrainment include behavioral imposition such as forced activity and rest, social and nutritional (rhythmic feeding) cues, temperature variations, knowledge of clock time, certain drugs, and melatonin itself.

Melatonin Secretion in Relation to Daylength

In most species melatonin secretion is related to the length of the night: The longer the night, the longer the duration of secretion.[30] This has been particularly well demonstrated in sheep, in which melatonin rises within a few minutes of lights off and in photoperiods of more than around 14 hours of light does not decline until lights on. In such photoperiods, light serves to entrain the rhythm and to suppress secretion at the beginning and/or the end of the dark phase (Fig. 27–2).

The most consistent observation in humans is that melatonin profiles show a phase change from winter to summer, with earlier secretion in summer than in winter (see ref. 13 for references). However, if humans are kept strictly in darkness for 14 hours per day for a period of two months,

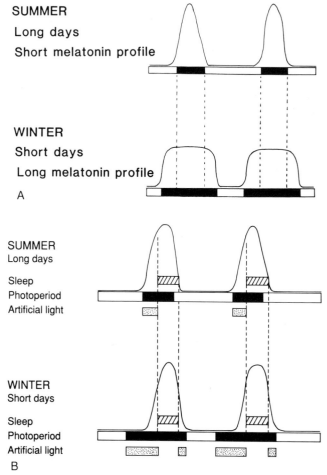

SUMMER
Long days
Short melatonin profile

WINTER
Short days
Long melatonin profile
A

SUMMER
Long days

Sleep
Photoperiod
Artificial light

WINTER
Short days

Sleep
Photoperiod
Artificial light
B

FIGURE 27–2. **Diagrammatic representation of melatonin secretion in relation to daylength.** *A,* The change in duration with length of the natural dark phase acts as a seasonal time cue in photoperiodic species. *B,* Social behavior and artificial lighting in humans lead to minimal change in duration but phase advances in summer. If a long or short dark phase is imposed, the pattern reverts to that shown in *A.*

the melatonin secretion pattern expands to cover almost the entire dark period and concomitantly, in extended periods of 14 hours of light, the rhythm contracts to less than 10 hours, with accompanying changes in body temperature and sleep.[31]

Light Suppression of Melatonin Secretion

Even a brief exposure to light of sufficient intensity at night rapidly suppresses melatonin production.[32] In general, the most effective light is in the green band (540 nm), corresponding to the rhodopsin absorption spectrum in both rodents and humans.[33] The amount of light required to suppress melatonin secretion during the night varies from species to species, with time of night, and with previous light exposure.[33] In humans Lewy et al. observed that 2500 lux (domestic light is around 300 to 500 lux) is required to completely suppress melatonin at night.[34]

This observation has been of very considerable importance, not only for an understanding of the control of human melatonin secretion but also for a general appreciation of the role of light in human physiology, in particular its importance in the control of human rhythms and in the

treatment of winter depression (seasonal affective disorder—SAD[35]).

Entrainment of the Melatonin Rhythm

A single daily light pulse of suitable intensity and duration in otherwise constant darkness is sufficient to phase shift and to synchronize the melatonin rhythm to 24 hours in animals.[35] Phase shifting and entrainment have been demonstrated in humans with suitable intensity and duration of light treatment.[13, 36, 37] However, the relative contribution of light to the entrainment of melatonin in a normal environment remains to be fully determined. Studies in Antarctica suggest that a structured social routine in a dim light environment suffices to synchronize melatonin to 24 hours.[13] However, many blind people living in a normal social environment show desynchronized melatonin and other circadian rhythms.[36]

Role in Photoperiodic Seasonal Functions

Photoperiodism

Most species show seasonal variations in their physiology and behavior, even humans. The reproductive cycle is timed so that environmental conditions are propitious for the growth of the young, and variations in behavior, pelage (coat growth and color), appetite, body weight, and fat are such that survival in ambient temperature conditions is optimized and camouflage protects against predators. When seasonal functions are primarily timed by daylength, species are referred to as photoperiodic.[39] Photoperiod is often critical for the timing of pubertal development.[40] In general, puberty is reached only during the adult mating season. It is now clear that in photoperiodic mammals and marsupials, an intact innervated pineal gland is essential for the perception of photoperiodic change.[17, 41–43] Most information derives from studies on reproductive function in hamsters and sheep.

Role of Melatonin

Pinealectomy removes the vast majority of circulating melatonin in rodents, primates, and ungulates.[42] It was therefore the first pineal hormone to be investigated as a pineal photoneuroendocrine transducer. It is possible to administer melatonin by daily infusion or feeding so as to generate at will circulating profiles with a duration characteristic of particular photoperiods in the intact or pinealectomized animal.[17, 42–45] In this way it has become clear that a particular melatonin duration is the necessary and sufficient condition for the induction of a given seasonal response and is equipotent with a particular photoperiod. Long-duration melatonin is equivalent to short days and short-duration melatonin is equivalent to long days (Fig. 27–2). The interpretation of the signal, as with daylength, depends on the physiology (for example, long- or short-day breeder) of the species in question. In sheep there is good evidence that long days or short-duration melatonin can time the whole seasonal cycle, at least of reproduction, acting as a seasonal zeitgeber for a presumed endogenous annual rhythm.[45] Animals become refractory to a specific duration of melatonin as they do to a particular photoperiod. For example, a period of long days (or a long-day melatonin signal) is required before a short-day melatonin signal advances the reproductive cycle in sheep.[45]

Puberty

Photoperiod via melatonin secretion determines the timing of puberty in some species, provided that a sufficient degree of physical maturity has been reached.[40] Interestingly, photoperiod perception by the fetus is present before birth in rodents and ungulates and ensures a rate of development appropriate to environmental conditions.[46] Melatonin crosses the placenta in a number of species, and injections to the mother can dictate postnatal reproductive development.

The laboratory rat is only marginally photoperiodic. Nevertheless, injections of melatonin during the late light phase or during a small window in the late dark phase, specifically during the period of pubertal development, delay reproductive maturity in both males and females.[47] Full sexual maturity is eventually achieved; thus the system is not permanently compromised. Moreover in vitro melatonin inhibits gonadotropin-releasing hormone (GnRH)–induced luteinizing hormone (LH) release by cultured rat pituitary glands from prepubertal animals.[48] These observations constitute the main evidence for a possible causal role of melatonin in the pubertal development of humans.

Nonreproductive Seasonal Functions

The pineal gland via melatonin secretion probably plays a role in all photoperiod-dependent functions in mammals. Evidence exists to substantiate this statement with respect to behavior, body weight, coat constitution and color (for example, the white winter coat of some polar species), prolactin variations, antler growth, thyroid activity, appetite, thermoregulation, delayed implantation, embryonic diapause, and hibernation.[17, 28, 41–43, 49] Partly because the ability to control reproduction is of applied interest in commercially important domestic species such as sheep, this aspect has received more attention than others. The winter coat of animals such as mink, arctic foxes, and cashmere goats also has commercial significance and can be manipulated by photoperiod and melatonin administration. Implanted melatonin induces short-day effects, and a number of commercial preparations of melatonin have been developed to this end.

Role of the Pineal Gland and Melatonin in Circadian Rhythms

Nonmammalian Vertebrates

There is an extensive literature on the importance of the pineal (and also the retina) to the control of circadian rhythms in lower vertebrates. Melatonin is produced rhythmically by both the pineal and the retina in many lower vertebrates and probably serves as the common humoral signal for circadian organization.[27]

Role of the Pineal in Mammalian Circadian Rhythms

Until quite recently opinion was that the pineal did not have a role in the mammalian circadian system. However, as early as 1970 Quay[50] reported that when rats are subjected to forced phase shifts of the light-dark cycle, pinealectomy increases the rate of re-entrainment; very recently Cassone[51] has shown that pinealectomy of hamsters in constant light leads to a major disruption of the circadian system. In parallel, a substantial body of work implicates melatonin in circadian thermoregulation (see ref. 49 for a review). Many such effects may involve the thyroid gland.[52]

Effects of Timed Administration of Melatonin

BEHAVIOR, HORMONES, AND TEMPERATURE. In rats, daily melatonin injections synchronize free-running activity and temperature rhythms in constant darkness and partially or completely synchronize disrupted activity rhythms in constant light.[27, 53] A phase response curve to single injections of melatonin can be demonstrated with small phase advances of at most one hour during the late subjective day.[53] Timed administration hastens adaptation of activity and melatonin production to forced phase shift and can change the direction of re-entrainment.[53, 54] Disagreement continues concerning the entrainment of adult hamsters; however, fetal hamsters can be entrained by maternal injections of melatonin at 24-hour intervals at specific circadian phases.[55] The physiological significance of these observations remains ambiguous, however, because the effective dose may be supraphysiological.

GESTATION. In the rat, gestation length depends on the ambient light-dark cycle. Small advances or delays of parturition can be induced by daylengths shorter or longer than 24 hours, and the effect can partially be mimicked by timed melatonin administration.[56]

ESTROUS CYCLE. As the pineal is involved in circadian timing, the presumption must be that it is concerned with the timing of the LH surge and indeed with general estrous timing. Melatonin administered into the lateral ventricles (albeit in very large amounts) during the "critical period" on the day of proestrus was able to block ovulation in rats. Of greater physiological relevance perhaps is evidence that in rats, timed melatonin administration can mimic the effects of extending the light-dark cycle on the timing of the LH surge. Observations of the melatonin rhythm itself show a decreased amplitude during proestrus in rodents but with conflicting reports in other species (see refs. 13, 41, and 57 for reviews).

AGING. A consistent observation in pineal research is the decline in amplitude of the melatonin rhythm in old age. Pinealectomy accelerates the aging process, and there is some evidence that daily melatonin administration in mice increases life span. Two hypotheses have been put forward to explain these insubstantial but interesting observations. One proposes that melatonin enhances immune responses via an opiatergic mechanism. The other considers that appropriately timed daily melatonin administration optimizes circadian relationships, especially of phase, and increases circadian amplitude (see ref. 58 for references).

IN VITRO PHASE SHIFTS. The metabolic activity of the rodent SCN in vivo and the electrical activity of various in

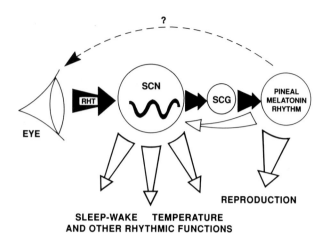

FIGURE 27–3. **A model for closed-loop feedback of melatonin within the circadian system.** Rhythm generation in the suprachiasmatic nucleus can be modulated in phase and amplitude by melatonin, with a possible influence also on retinal light processing.

vitro SCN preparations can be modified by melatonin; it inhibits 2-deoxyglucose uptake into the nuclei in late subjective day with no effect at other times and inhibits electrical activity also during late subjective day.[27] By far the most convincing evidence is the phase-advancing effect of melatonin on the circadian rhythm of electrical activity in cultured SCN.[59] The effect was large, acute, and time-dependent, with shifts of up to several hours being observed. Thus melatonin acts directly on a central biological clock to change its phase.

RETINAL RHYTHMS. There is good evidence for circadian rhythms in several retinal functions such as visual sensitivity and some photomechanical processes.[60, 61] In a limited number of studies to date, the dark-induced reactions can be induced by melatonin and the light effects by dopamine.

SUMMARY. The interrelationships of the SCN, the retina, and the pineal have been integrated into a model, originally for the avian circadian system, modified by Steinlechner[61] for mammals with further modifications here (Fig. 27–3). It is reasonable to conclude that in adult mammals melatonin serves to modulate circadian phase and strengthen coupling. In fetal and neonatal mammals it helps to program the circadian system and to determine the timing of developmental stages, especially puberty.

THE PINEAL IN HUMAN PHYSIOLOGY AND PATHOLOGY

Clearly the importance of the pineal in humans depends on the importance of light in human physiology. It is reasonable to assume that the pineal conveys information concerning light-dark cycles for the organization of seasonal and circadian rhythms in humans as in animals. Pinealectomy in humans removes virtually all plasma melatonin.[62] Other consequences of the operation consist of diffuse neurological problems that do not add up to a consistent functional effect as yet and may be more related to nonspecific effects of operation.

Human Melatonin Production

Basic Characteristics

MECHANISMS. Early work demonstrated the presence of hydroxyindole-O-methyltransferase activity in tissue from postmortem pineals. The melatonin content of human pineals is related to the time of death with, as expected, higher values at night. Pathological or traumatic denervation of the pineal abolishes the plasma melatonin rhythm. β-Adrenergic antagonists suppress melatonin production, and increased availability of norepinephrine and serotonin are stimulatory (see reviews in refs. 13, 63, and 64). There is thus good evidence that the neural and biochemical pathways known to control pineal function in rats are similar in humans.

MELATONIN AND aMT6s PRODUCTION. In a "normal" environment, melatonin is secreted during the night in healthy humans as in all other species. The average maximum levels attained in plasma in adults are of the order of 60 to 70 pg/ml when measured with high-specificity assays. Mean maximum concentrations of 6-sulfatoxymelatonin (aMT6s) attain 80 to 100 pg/ml (in different mammalian species there is a relatively narrow range of circulating concentrations, although birds have more). Minimum concentrations of both compounds are often below the limit of detection of radioimmunoassay in plasma and are usually below 10 pg/ml. The peak concentrations of melatonin in plasma normally occur between 0200 and 0400 hours. The onset of secretion is usually around 2100 to 2200 hours and the offset at 0700 to 0900 hours in adults in temperate zones. The appearance and peak levels of aMT6s in plasma are delayed by 1 to 2 hours and the morning decline by 3 to 4 hours (Fig. 27–4).[13] In urine 70 to 80 per cent of aMT6s appears in the overnight sample

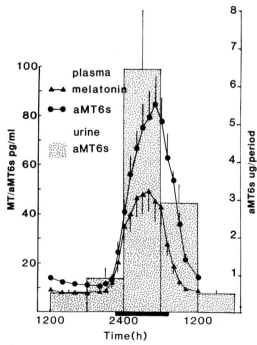

FIGURE 27–4. Plasma melatonin (MT) and 6-sulfatoxymelatonin (aMT6s) concentrations in young adults (N = 22) together with urinary excretion of aMT6s over 24 hours. S.I. Units: 100 pg/ml = 0.43 nM/L. (From Arendt J: Melatonin. Clin Endocrinol 29:205–229, 1988.)

(2400 to 0800 hours), and it is low but rarely undetectable in the afternoon and early evening. Secretion is probably pulsatile, but through tissue diffusion and metabolism this is damped in the peripheral circulation.[13]

The rhythm is endogenous, with a period usually greater than 24 hours.[37, 65] Possibly the most striking characteristic of the normal human melatonin rhythm is its reproducibility from day to day and from week to week in normal individuals, rather like an hormonal fingerprint.[13] In spite of intra-individual stability, there is very large variability in amplitude of the rhythm between subjects. A small number of apparently normal individuals have no detectable melatonin in plasma at all times of day.[66]

ASSOCIATION WITH TEMPERATURE. Many associations of melatonin with temperature exist in humans. The most striking is the reciprocal relationship in circadian profiles, where the temperature nadir correlates closely with the peak of melatonin. The ovulatory rise in temperature during the menstrual cycle is associated with a reported decline in amplitude of melatonin, but the decline in melatonin is not a consistent observation. There is a possible causal relationship, as exogenous melatonin can acutely depress body temperature in humans.[49]

ASSOCIATION WITH SLEEP. There are obvious correlations between melatonin production at night and sleep, and again some specific causal relationships may exist. However, sleep deprivation does not abolish the melatonin rhythm and in dim light does not affect secretion.[67] During sleep deprivation self-rated fatigue exhibits a circadian rhythm that is closely correlated with plasma melatonin.[67] Many studies have attempted to relate sleep stages to detailed melatonin profiles, but no striking associations have emerged.

OTHER ASSOCIATIONS. Obviously any variable with a marked circadian rhythm shows correlations with melatonin, if necessary displaced in time. Examples include cortisol, prolactin, thyroid-stimulating hormone, aspects of the immune system, and many others.[13, 63]

The relationships of stress, exercise, and some other nonpharmacological interventions in modification of melatonin production are controversial and do not appear to play a major role in humans. Insufficient data are available to make further judgments.

Development, Puberty, and Aging

Shortly after birth very little melatonin or aMT6s is detectable in body fluids. The melatonin rhythm appears around 6 to 8 weeks of life.[68] Whether in specific individuals this corresponds to the organization and synchronization of other circadian variables such as sleep remains a question of very considerable interest. If melatonin serves to set circadian phase in humans as it does in rodents, it is quite possible that breast-fed babies absorbing maternal melatonin develop circadian organization before bottle-fed babies.

The plasma concentration of melatonin increases rapidly thereafter and reaches a lifetime peak on average at 3 to 5 years old.[69] The increment is much greater at night. Subsequently a steady decrease is seen, reaching mean adult concentrations in mid to late teens with the major decline occurring before puberty (Fig. 27–5). Values remain relatively unchanged until 35 to 40 years, and a final decline

in amplitude then takes place until very low levels are seen in old age.[68, 68a, 69] Reports of differences in secretion in adults with gender, height, or body weight are not consistent. However, the measured plasma concentrations of melatonin in children are probably related to body weight.[13]

The decline in plasma melatonin in early life in no way proves that it is involved in human pubertal development. The effects of photoperiod on human puberty are entirely unknown, although circumstantial evidence for a role of light exists. For example, blind subjects may have abnormally timed pubertal development, and there may be seasonal influences on the timing of menarche.[70] Studies in precocious and delayed puberty have not yet proved very rewarding. Although lower melatonin has been reported in precocious puberty compared with age-matched controls,[71, 72] it may be more related to skeletal age. Ovarian suppression with a GnRH analogue in precocious girls is not accompanied by changes in melatonin secretion.[73] However, reports of increased melatonin in delayed puberty exist,[71, 74] and in one case report induction of sexual development with estrogen was associated with a very rapid decline of melatonin metabolite excretion.[74]

Menstrual Cycle

Some of the very earliest reports on human melatonin described low preovulatory concentrations in the morning prior to ovulation and suggested that low melatonin was

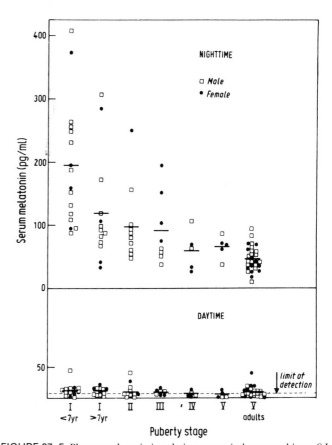

FIGURE 27–5. Plasma melatonin in relation to age in human subjects. S.I. Units: 100 pg/ml = 0.43 nM/L. (From Waldhauser F, Frisch H, Waldhauser M, et al: Fall in nocturnal serum melatonin during prepuberty and pubescence. Lancet 1:362–365, 1984.)

facilitatory to the preovulatory LH peak.[13] This is an inconsistent observation, however, and the most recent work indicates that neither the amplitude nor the phase of melatonin is altered in the course of the normal cycle.[57, 75]

It is difficult to eliminate altogether a possible function of melatonin in the human cycle, given the presence of circadian and seasonal effects in human reproduction.[13, 70] More direct evidence is given by the amplification of LH pulses in early follicular phase by pharmacological amounts of oral melatonin at 0800 hours.[76] High-amplitude, low-frequency pulses characterize anestrus, that is, reproductive involution in long days in sheep.[43] The results of this study partially support the contention that large doses of melatonin suitably administered can inhibit human reproductive activity. In primary hypothalamic amenorrhea the amplitude of melatonin secretion is increased, but this is a correlative and not necessarily a causal association.[57, 75]

Chronic administration of huge (300 mg) daily doses of melatonin to cycling women significantly suppresses plasma LH but not estradiol after four months of treatment. The combination of these large daily doses of melatonin and suboptimal norethisterone (as a synthetic progestin minipill) inhibits ovulation in women and in the absence of side effects may prove to be clinically useful.[77] In the author's opinion, low, timed doses of melatonin used to reinforce circadian organization are likely to improve fertility in humans.

Pathology

Pineal Hyperplasia and Hypoplasia

A number of reports of variations in postmortem pineal weight as a function of cause of death have been summarized by Tapp.[5] Of the most interesting, hypoplasia of the pineal in association with retinal disease may be causally interrelated. Tapp has reported that pineals in patients dying of carcinoma of the breast or melanoma are heavier than those from patients with other cancers. Very large pineals (1 g) have been described in a rare genetic syndrome with insulin resistance.[78] Sudden infant death syndrome (SIDS) is associated with small pineals and decreased melatonin production.[79, 80] SIDS deaths usually occur at night and may be associated with abnormalities of sleep. If melatonin helps to coordinate circadian organization in the developing infant, its underproduction may contribute to the disorder.

Pineal Tumors

Tumors of the pineal region in children are frequently associated with abnormal pubertal development.[81] The original hypothesis to explain precocious puberty in boys with pineal tumors was that the tumors destroyed the capacity of the pineal to inhibit sexual development. In fact much evidence suggests that precocity is due to the production of human chorionic gonadotrophin (β-hCG) by germ cell tumors of the pineal.[82, 83] This relationship has nevertheless stimulated much work on the possible role of the pineal through the secretion of melatonin as a means of timing human puberty.

Pineal tumors are heterogeneous and may arise from germ cells (teratomas, germinomas, choriocarcinomas, endodermal sinus tumors, mixed germ cell tumors), pineal parenchymal cells (pineoblastoma and pineocytoma), and the supporting stroma (gliomas).[7] All are rare (less than 1 per cent of intracranial space-occupying lesions) and tend to occur below 20 years of age with the exception of parenchymal cell tumors, which occur equally in adults and children. Germinomas respond well to radiation therapy, whereas primary surgery is more frequently the treatment of choice in other types. Tumor markers in CSF, α-fetoprotein, and β-hCG, together with CSF cytology and imaging (CT or MRI) aid in differential diagnosis. The most common symptoms are secondary to hydrocephalus (headache, vomiting, and drowsiness) together with the triad of visual problems, diabetes insipidus, and reproductive abnormalities.[84] Germinomas and teratomas occur predominantly in males. Both precocious and delayed puberty have been associated with pineal tumors. Precocious puberty is more commonly associated with teratoma. Cohen and co-workers[83] have recently reviewed the occurrence of precocious puberty in parallel with β-hCG–secreting pineal tumors. As β-hCG is identical to β-LH, they conclude that pubertal development can be directly attributed to ectopic β-hCG production in many cases. Moreover, the predominance in boys may be explained on the basis that LH alone can stimulate testosterone production, whereas in girls both LH and FSH are required for ovarian follicular development and estrogen production.

There is no consistent information on overproduction or underproduction of melatonin with specific types of tumor. However, pinealectomy removes circulating melatonin,[62] and radiation therapy appears to greatly suppress melatonin. At present long-term evaluation of patients after surgery is under way in a number of centers.

Other Solid Tumors

The relationship of the pineal and melatonin to cancer is a subject that arouses much interest following early work suggesting that the pineal contains oncostatic activity. Cohen and co-workers[85] proposed in 1978 that human breast cancer is a melatonin-deficient disease. Since that time many clinical studies have been performed to assess melatonin secretion in cancer patients. Low levels may be associated at least with (stage-dependent) breast and prostatic cancer[86, 87]; however, not all studies are consistent. A number of broad studies that have included various oncological conditions report significant differences, both increases and decreases, in plasma melatonin between types of cancer and control populations. At present these are uninterpretable.

General Pathology

Many clinical attempts have been made to relate circulating melatonin to endocrine and other pathology. The results on the whole are difficult to interpret and inconsistent (see refs. 13, 63, and 88 for reviews). Liver disease such as cirrhosis, which impairs metabolic function, leads to higher than normal plasma concentrations of melatonin.[63] Drugs that stimulate or suppress hydroxylation and conjugation mechanisms or that compete for metabolic pathways can be expected to affect circulating melatonin. Surprisingly, little evidence exists for a disturbance of melatonin secretion in major sleep disorders such as narcolepsy and Klein-Levine syndrome,[89] and in delayed sleep phase insomnia only a small delay in the rhythm is found.[90]

Psychiatry

Abnormalities of circadian function have been postulated in depression and mania. Melatonin is arguably the best index of biological clock function; only bright light "masks" the expression of the endogenous rhythm,[26] and it has been extensively used in psychiatry and in other fields to assess biological clock status. There is evidence for a decline in amplitude of the melatonin rhythm in depression associated with an increase in cortisol, and possibly an increase in mania, although not all studies are consistent.[64]

There is little evidence for abnormal timing of melatonin, although Lewy et al have reported exceptionally delayed melatonin rhythms in winter in patients with SAD compared with the small delay seen in normals.[91] This observation remains to be confirmed but is of considerable interest. The treatment originally proposed for SAD patients was the creation of an artificial summer daylength using three hours of bright full-spectrum light (Vitalite, 2500 lux) morning and evening.[35] The "melatonin hypothesis" predicted that such light treatment would shorten the duration of melatonin secretion, thus generating a summer daylength signal by analogy with animal work. The light treatment appears to be efficient, but it does not appear to work through melatonin. Bipolar (manic-depressive) patients are more sensitive to light suppression of melatonin than are normals. This observation may prove to be of both diagnostic and therapeutic importance.[64]

Most pharmacological antidepressant treatments stimulate melatonin secretion, acting through increased availability of the precursors tryptophan and serotonin and the major pineal neurotransmitter norepinephrine, or by direct action on serotonin and catecholamine receptors.[64] There may be a link between an increase in melatonin production and efficacy of treatment, and this possibility merits exploration.

EFFECTS OF MELATONIN IN HUMANS

Therapeutic Potential and Significance to Health

A very large number of people would benefit from the ability to manipulate rhythms at will. Circadian rhythm disturbance is associated (among other things) with shift work, jet lag, blindness, insomnia, and old age. A search for a general chronobiotic—a compound able rapidly to shift the biological clock in all its manifestations—occupies much scientific time and effort. To date bright light is the only treatment that in suitable intensity and duration is able to do this. A number of pharmaceutical products and steroid hormones have been shown to shift aspects of the circadian system in animals, usually the activity-rest cycle. The possible use of melatonin in this area has become evident.

Early Work

Enormous doses of up to 6.6 g (the daily production of about 200,000 people!) in the daytime had no beneficial effects on parkinsonism, Huntington's chorea, depression (which was worsened), and schizophrenia. Skin pigmentation was not affected; human pigment cells do not resemble amphibian melanophores in pigment migration phenomena. Small decreases in plasma LH and FSH were observed.[92] Large amounts of melatonin such as these may produce headache, abdominal cramps, and somnolence.

Much lower (2 mg intranasally, 10 to 240 mg orally or intravenously) but still pharmacological doses of melatonin can induce transient sleepiness or sleep but cannot maintain sleep as efficiently as conventional hypnotics.[13, 65] A brief decline in visual reaction time, accompanied by an increase in fatigue ratings but with no effect on memory, has been reported.[93] Acute oral doses of melatonin stimulate prolactin secretion.[94] This may relate to the ability of melatonin in pharmacological amounts to inhibit some dopaminergic functions. The pharmacological properties of melatonin in animals include sedation, hypothermia, anxiolysis, muscle hypotonia, decrease in locomotor activity with a rebound increase on increasing the dose, slight analgesia, slight protection against electroconvulsive shock, and very low toxicity.[95]

Timed Administration

Daily feeding of low-dose (2 to 5 mg) melatonin in the late afternoon advanced the timing of evening self-rated fatigue, the endogenous melatonin rhythm (Fig. 27–6), and the morning decline of prolactin compared with placebo. There were no significant effects on self-rated mood, or on LH, FSH, testosterone, cortisol, growth hormone, or thyroxine. No deleterious effects were reported by the subjects.[13, 65] Thus in low doses melatonin has some chronobiotic effects in humans, but it showed no significant reproductive effects and indeed the dose is well below that needed to influence human reproduction as a combined contraceptive.[77] Recently Lewy et al. described a human phase response curve to melatonin, using endogenous melatonin as a marker rhythm, with advances in the late light phase and small delays in the early morning.[96]

Jet Lag and Shift Work

Melatonin treatment timed to induce phase advances and delays has been used in the alleviation of jet lag in both real life and simulation conditions. Field studies show that self-rated jet lag can be reduced on average by 50 per cent with appropriately timed treatment both westward and eastward.[13] The improvement is greater with larger numbers of time zones.[97] The subjective impressions are reinforced by improved latency and quality of sleep, greater daytime alertness, and more rapid resynchronization of melatonin and cortisol rhythms. Comparable simulation studies have shown a marked increase in the rate of reentrainment of both hormonal and electrolyte rhythms and an immediate effect of lowering body temperature which persists as more rapid re-entrainment.[98] Neither the dose nor the timing of melatonin administration has been fully optimized. A minority (less than 10 per cent) of subjects feel worse after melatonin.[99] In these cases the individ-

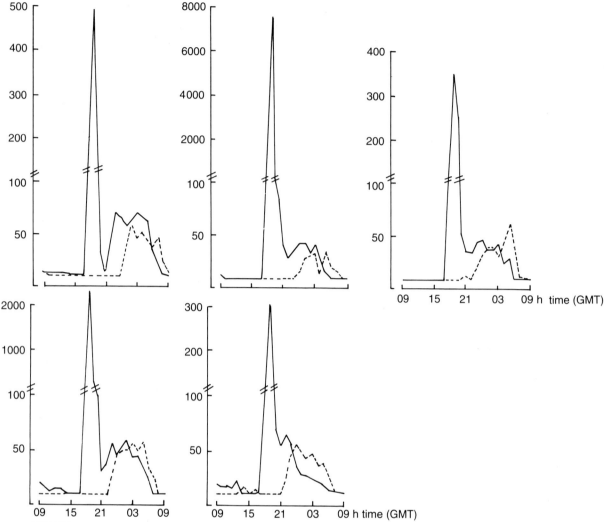

FIGURE 27-6. Administration of melatonin (2 mg) daily at 1700 h to human volunteers provokes a phase advance of the endogenous melatonin rhythm (solid line) compared with placebo (dashed line). Plasma melatonin profiles from individual subjects are shown in which the exogenous contribution to plasma concentrations, with a peak at 1800 h, is clearly distinguished from the succeeding endogenous night-time rise. This phase advance is accompanied by earlier sleepiness or sleep. (From Evered D, Clark S (eds): Photoperiodism, melatonin and the pineal. Ciba Foundation Symposium 117. London, Pitman, 1985.)

ual circadian status is probably a major determinant of response in that undesirable changes in direction of entrainment may occur with inappropriate timing of treatment. Moreover, unpredictable exposure to bright light can theoretically act in opposition to the desired result.

Very little work has been published on the use of melatonin in shift work, although exposure to bright light during the night is clearly beneficial to night shift workers.[100] Preliminary work suggests improved sleep and increased daytime alertness in night shift workers receiving melatonin at the desired bedtime during a night shift week compared with placebo and baseline conditions.[100a] Performance needs to be carefully evaluated during treatment.

Blindness

Only a small number of studies have been reported, but in the author's experience about one third of blind subjects reporting sleep problems derive benefit from melatonin ingestion (5 mg) at desired bedtime. The major effect

is a stabilization of sleep onset.[101] Whether other circadian variables are entrained in these circumstances remains controversial.

Delayed Sleep Phase Insomnia

Patients with delayed sleep phase insomnia cannot sleep at the socially acceptable time of night and delay sleep onset until the early hours of the morning, sleeping through much of the day. This condition has been successfully treated with bright light in the early morning to induce phase advances of the clock. In others evening melatonin (5 mg at 2200 hours) also advances sleep time significantly.[90] Judicious, timed application of both melatonin and bright light as time cues may well be the treatment of choice for rhythm disturbances.

Cancer

There is good evidence for photoperiod dependency and/or melatonin responsiveness of the initiation and evolution of certain cancers, particularly hormone-dependent cancers, in animals. Oncostatic effects are reported on some human cell lines, and in general the pineal and melatonin have antitumor activity.[102] In dimethylbenzanthracene-induced mammary tumors in rats, pinealectomy greatly increased the incidence of induced tumor growth, and daily melatonin administration in the late light phase greatly decreased incidence.[103] Not all reports show positive results, however. Melatonin when appropriately administered has generally stimulatory effects on aspects of the immune system, and positive effects on cancer may be a consequence.[102, 104] One interpretation of this phenomenon is that melatonin acts as an antistress hormone on the brain opioid system, with consequent up-regulation of the immune system.[104] Very recent evidence suggests that it may also act as a free-radical scavenger.[104a]

SITES AND MECHANISM OF ACTION OF MELATONIN

Target Sites

The actions of melatonin are multiple and must derive essentially from modification of events in the CNS. However, peripheral actions are not excluded. Obvious potential target sites in mammals, from the foregoing discussion, are the retina, the SCN and other central neuroendocrine control systems, and the pituitary gland. Lesions of the SCN and the anterior hypothalamic area can block photoperiodic and/or circadian effects of melatonin in some rodents, but with a degree of disparity between laboratories.[105] Implants of melatonin in the hypothalamus suppress LH release in rats.[57] Implants or infusion of melatonin in the hypothalamus mimics or blocks photoperiodic responses in several species.[105] In prepubertal rats melatonin inhibits GnRH-induced LH release in pituitary cultures at concentrations comparable to those circulating in the blood.[48] There is evidence that melatonin influences GnRH secretion from the hypothalamus in co-cultures of median eminence and pars tuberalis.[106]

Uptake and Binding Studies

Early work using low specific activity radiolabeled melatonin served to focus attention on the brain as a site of uptake and binding of melatonin.[107, 108] The development of 2-^{125}I iodomelatonin as a high specific activity ligand has permitted the identification of high-affinity (Kd 25 to 175 pM), saturable, specific, and reversible melatonin binding to cell membranes in the CNS, initially in the SCN[109] and the pars tuberalis of the pituitary.[110]

Species variation of melatonin-binding sites in the brain is of course apparent, but in rodents the SCN, the pars tuberalis, the PVN, the paraventricular nucleus of the thalamus, the habenula, the ventromedial nucleus, the preoptic area, the amygdala, and the area postrema have all shown labeling.[105, 110, 111] In ungulates binding is found in the pars tuberalis, rarely in the SCN, in septal and preoptic areas, in the inner and outer molecular layers of the hippocampus and the stratum lacunosum, in the entorhinal cortex, in the subiculum, and in apical interpeduncular nucleus.[110, 111] The SCN shows clear binding in human post-

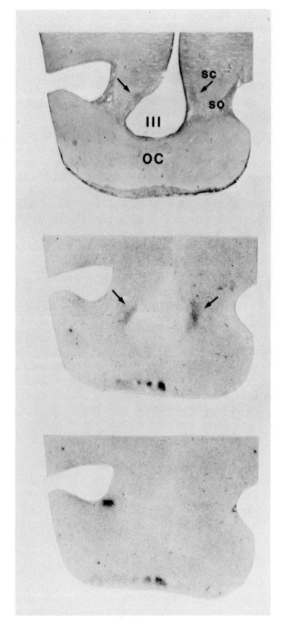

FIGURE 27–7. Localization of specific ^{125}I-iodomelatonin binding in the human suprachiasmatic nucleus (SCN) by in vitro autoradiography. *Upper panel*, 60-μm section of hypothalamus stained with cresyl violet to show location of the SCN. *Middle panel*, On an adjacent 20-μm section ^{125}I-iodomelatonin binding over the SCN was apparent as dark densities *(arrows)* by autoradiography. SCN binding was eliminated when melatonin (1 μg) was added to the incubation solution *(lower panel, autoradiograph)*. OC, optic chiasm; SC, suprachiasmatic nucleus; SO, supraoptic nucleus. (From Weaver DR, Rivkees SA, Carlson LL, Reppert SM: Localization of melatonin receptors in mammalian brain. *In* Klein DC, Moore RY, Reppert SM: Suprachiasmatic Nucleus: The Mind's Clock; New York, Oxford University Press, 1991, pp 289–308.

mortem tissue (Fig. 27–7).[112] Some of these sites (anterior hypothalamus, preoptic area, SCN) represent potential targets for the effects of melatonin on seasonal and circadian rhythms. The most consistent (but not universal) binding site between species is the pars tuberalis, but the function is currently unknown. The rise of the pars tuberalis as a primary candidate for a melatonin target tissue has stimulated work on function. Gonadotrophs constitute part of the cell population. In vitro co-culture with median eminence from the rat suggests that melatonin-provoked LH release from the pars tuberalis inhibits GnRH release from the median eminence.[106] Most of the ovine pars tuberalis, however, is constituted of agranular unidentified cells which, according to Morgan,[113] are largely responsible for melatonin-induced effects. He has proposed that they secrete an entirely new hormone that subsequently mediates the physiological effects of melatonin—an exciting prospect. Much more extensive binding can be seen in the brains of birds and lower vertebrates, especially in retino-recipient areas.[111]

There are changes in detectable binding with age; for example, in fetal rats the first appearance of binding is in the pituitary: pars distalis and pars tuberalis with SCN labeling appearing in later gestation. Pars distalis binding is absent in adult rats but persists after birth in the neonate.[114] This suggests that binding may indeed underlie function, as melatonin inhibits GnRH induced pituitary LH release in prepuberty but not in adulthood.

In parallel with these brain studies, Krause and Dubocovich have demonstrated a functional melatonin receptor initially in rabbit and chicken retina (inhibition of calcium-dependent dopamine release) which is localized in the inner plexiform layer containing dopamine amacrine cells in rabbits, in the outer and inner segments in mice, and possibly in the pigmented layer in some mammals.[61, 116]

High- and Low-Affinity Binding Sites

A range of low nanomolar to low picomolar binding to membranes has been reported by some authors using ^{125}I-melatonin,[115, 116] although more recently the existence of different classes of sites has been disputed.[117] In most mammals melatonin is thought to be secreted primarily into the blood, subsequently entering the brain, and blood concentrations are in the picomolar to femtomolar range. For such concentrations to be physiologically relevant, receptor affinity should be in this range. Melatonin, however, has many effects if administered in quantities so as to generate nanomolar concentrations or above. They may or may not be related to endogenous effects. They are nevertheless of interest, and some are exploitable therapeutically. Binding sites have been shown to vary systematically with physiological status.[116, 117a]

Melatonin Receptor Pharmacology

White and co-workers have demonstrated that melatonin-induced pigment aggregation in amphibian melanophores is a pertussis toxin–sensitive system and that melatonin inhibits forskolin-activated cAMP formation.[118] Inhibition of cAMP production may be a general feature of melatonin receptors. Intensive investigation of the properties of the pars tuberalis binding site has revealed that physiological doses of melatonin inhibit forskolin-activated cAMP production in vitro in a time- and dose-related manner.[110] There is other good evidence that the binding sites are coupled to G proteins. GTP analogues, which interfere with the regeneration of G_i-coupled receptors, decrease the affinity and sometimes the capacity of ^{125}I-melatonin binding in reptiles, birds, and mammals.[111]

Melatonin Antagonists and Agonists

The 6- and 2-substituted halogenated melatonins are good agonists both in vivo and in vitro.[110, 117] Presumably in both cases but particularly in the 6-substituted molecule there is protection against metabolic degradation and hence a lower dose requirement for the induction of a given effect. A series of agonists have recently been developed from napthalene derivatives. They show a range of affinity for the pars tuberalis melatonin receptor, some being of much higher affinity than melatonin.[119] The most interesting have similar effects to melatonin on rhythm physiology in rodents. Only two antagonists have been reported to date, but neither has proved to be consistently useful.[115, 116]

SUMMARY

To date the evidence indicates that ^{125}I-melatonin binding sites are genuine receptors, although by no means have all binding sites been investigated. So far, however, there is no conclusive direct link to a physiological response such as onset or offset of seasonal reproductive activity. It is hoped that such a link will emerge in the very near future.

REFERENCES

1. Vollrath L: The Pineal Organ. Heidelberg, Springer-Verlag, 1981.
2. Collin JP: Differentiation and regression of the cells of the sensory line in the epiphysis cerebri. In Wolstenholme GEW, Knight J (eds): The Pineal Gland. Edinburgh, Churchill Livingstone, 1972, pp 79–125.
3. Korf H-W, Moller M, Gery I, et al: Immunocytochemical demonstration of retinal S antigen in the pineal organ of four mammalian species. Cell Tissue Res 239:81–85, 1985.
4. Welsh MG: Pineal calcification: Structural and functional aspects. Pineal Res Rev 3:41–68, 1985.
5. Tapp E: The histology and pathology of the human pineal gland. Prog Brain Res 52:481–500, 1979.
6. Bojkowski C, Arendt J: Factors influencing urinary 6-sulphatoxymelatonin, a major melatonin metabolite, in normal human subjects. Clin Endocrinol 33:435–444, 1990.
7. Kappers JA: Innervation of the epiphysis cerebri in the albino rat. Anat Record 136:220–221, 1960.
8. Moller M, Korf H-W: The innervation of the mammalian pineal gland with special reference to central pinealopetal projections. Pineal Res Rev 2:41–86, 1984.
9. Lerner AB, Case JD, Takahashi Y, et al: Isolation of melatonin, pineal factor that lightens melanocytes. J Am Chem Soc 80:2587, 1958.
10. Axelrod J: The pineal gland: A neurochemical transducer. Science 184:1341–1348, 1974.
11. Klein DC: Photoneural regulation of the mammalian pineal gland. In Evered D, Clark S (eds): Photoperiodism, melatonin and the pineal. Ciba Foundation Symposium 117. London, Pitman, 1985, pp 38–56.
12. Kveder S, McIsaac WM: The metabolism of melatonin (N-acetyl-5-methoxytryptamine) and 5-methoxytryptamine. J Biol Chem 236:3214–3220, 1961.
13. Arendt J: Melatonin. Clin Endocrinol 29:205–229, 1988.
14. Vakkuri O, Leppaluoto J, Kauppila A: Oral administration and distribution of melatonin in human serum, saliva and urine. Life Sci 37:489–495, 1985.
15. Mallo C, Zaidan R, Galy G, et al: Pharmacokinetics of melatonin in man after intravenous infusion and bolus injection. Eur J Clin Pharmacol 38:297–301, 1990.
16. Lane EA, Moss HB: Pharmacokinetics of melatonin in man: First pass hepatic metabolism. J Clin Endocrinol Metab 61:1214–1216, 1985.
17. Tamarkin K, Baird CJ, Almeida OFX: Melatonin: A coordinating signal for mammalian reproduction. Science 227:714–720, 1985.

18. Pevet P: The 5-methoxyindoles different from melatonin: Their effects on the sexual axis. *In* Axelrod J, Fraschini F, Velo GP (eds): The Pineal Gland and its Endocrine Role. New York, Plenum, 1983, pp 331–348.

19. Pevet P: Physiological role of neuropeptides in the mammalian pineal gland. Adv Pineal Res 6:275–282, 1991.

20. Sugden D, Weller JL, Klein DC, et al: α-Adrenergic potentiation of β-adrenergic stimulation of rat pineal N-acetyltransferase: Studies using citazoline and fluorine analogs of norepinephrine. Biochem Pharmacol 33:3947–3950, 1984.

21. Zatz M: Sensitivity and cyclic nucleotides in the rat pineal gland. J Neural Trans (Suppl 13):97–114, 1978.

22. Ebadi M, Govitrapong P: Orphan transmitters and their receptor sites in the pineal gland. Pineal Res Rev 4:1–54, 1986.

23. Cardinali DP, Vacas MI: Feedback control of pineal function by reproductive hormones—a neuroendocrine paradigm. J Neural Trans (Suppl 13):175–201, 1978.

24. Cardinali DP, Ritta MN: Role of prostaglandins in neuroendocrine junctions: Studies in the pineal gland and the hypothalamus. Neuroendocrinology 36:152–160, 1983.

25. Poggeler B, Balzer I, Hardeland R, Lerchl A: Pineal hormone melatonin oscillates also in the dinoflagellate *Gonyaulax polyedra*. Naturwissenschaften 78:268–269, 1991.

26. Wever RA: Characteristics of circadian rhythms in human functions. *In* Wurtman RJ, Waldhauser RJ (eds): Melatonin in Humans. J Neural Trans (Suppl 21):323–374, 1986.

27. Cassone VM: Effects of melatonin on vertebrate circadian systems. Trends Neurosci 13:457–463, 1990.

28. Binkley S: The Pineal: Endocrine and Nonendocrine Function. Englewood Cliffs, NJ, Prentice Hall, 1988.

29. Rusak B, Zucker I: Neural regulation of circadian rhythms. Physiol Rev 59:449–526, 1979.

30. Arendt J: Mammalian pineal rhythms. Pineal Res Rev 3:161–213, 1985.

31. Wehr TA: The durations of human melatonin secretion and sleep respond to changes in daylength (photoperiod). J Clin Endocrinol Metab 73:1276–1280, 1991.

32. Illnerova H: Entrainment of mammalian circadian rhythms in melatonin production by light. Pineal Res Rev 6:173–217, 1988.

33. Reiter RJ: Action spectra, dose-response relationships and temporal aspects of light's effects on the pineal gland. *In* Wurtman RJ, Baum MJ, Potts JR Jr (eds): The Medical and Biological Effects of Light. Ann NY Acad Sci 453:215–230, 1985.

34. Lewy AJ, Wehr TA, Goodwin FK, et al: Light suppresses melatonin secretion in humans. Science 210:1267–1269, 1980.

35. Rosenthal NE, Sack DA, Gillin JC, et al: Seasonal affective disorder. A description of the syndrome and preliminary findings with light therapy. Arch Gen Psychiatry 41:72–79, 1984.

36. Shanahan TL, Czeisler CA: Light exposure induces equivalent phase shifts of the endogenous circadian rhythms of circulating plasma melatonin and core body temperature in man. J Clin Endocrinol Metab 73:227–235, 1991.

37. Wever RA: Characteristics of circadian rhythms in human functions. *In* Wurtman RJ, Waldhauser F (eds): Melatonin in Humans. J Neural Trans (Suppl 21):323–374, 1986.

38. Lewy AJ, Newsome DA: Different types of melatonin circadian secretory rhythms in some blind subjects. J Clin Endocrinol Metab 56:1103–1107, 1983.

39. Hoffman K: Photoperiodism in vertebrates. *In* Aschoff J (ed): Handbook of Behavioural Neurobiology. (Suppl 4). 1981, pp 449–473.

40. Ebling FJP, Foster DL: Pineal melatonin rhythms and the timing of puberty in mammals. Experientia 45:946–955, 1989.

41. Reiter RJ: The pineal and its hormones in the control of reproduction in mammals. Endocr Rev 1:109–131, 1980.

42. Arendt J: Role of the pineal gland and melatonin in seasonal reproductive function in mammals. Oxford Rev Reprod Biol 8:266–320, 1986.

43. Evered D, Clark S (eds): Photoperiodism, melatonin and the pineal. Ciba Foundation Symposium 117. London, Pitman, 1985.

44. Carter DS, Goldman BD: Antigonadal effects of timed melatonin infusion in pinealectomised male Djungarian hamsters *(Phodopus sungorus sungorus);* Duration is the critical parameter. Endocrinology 113:1261–1267, 1983.

45. Karsch FJ, Malpaux B, Wayne NL, Robinson JE: Characteristics of the melatonin signal that provide the photoperiodic code for timing seasonal reproduction in the ewe. Reprod Nutr Develop 28:459–472, 1988.

46. Weaver DR, Reppert SM: Maternal melatonin communicates day-

length to the fetus in Djungarian hamsters. Endocrinology 119:2861–2863, 1986.

47. Rivest RW, Aubert ML, Lang U, Sizonenko PC: Puberty in the rat: Modulation by melatonin and light. Neural Trans (Suppl 21):81–108, 1986.

48. Martin JE, Klein DC: Melatonin inhibition of neonatal pituitary response to luteinising hormone–releasing factor. Science 191:301–302, 1975.

49. Badia P, Myers B, Murphy P: Melatonin and thermoregulation. *In* Reiter RJ, Yu HS (eds): Melatonin: Biosynthesis, Physiological Effects, and Clinical Applications. Boca Raton, FL, CRC Press, 1992.

50. Quay WB: Precocious entrainment and associated characteristics of activity patterns following pinealectomy and reversal of photoperiod. Physiol Behav 5:1281–1290, 1970.

51. Cassone V: The pineal gland influences rat circadian activity rhythms in constant light. J Biol Rhythms 7:27–40, 1992.

52. Vriend J: Evidence for pineal gland modulation of the neuroendocrine-thyroid axis. Neuroendocrinology 36:68–78, 1983.

53. Armstrong SM: Melatonin and circadian control in mammals. Experientia 45:932–939, 1989.

54. Illnerova H: *In* Klein DC, Moore RY, Reppert SM (eds): Suprachiasmatic Nucleus, The Minds Clock. Oxford, Oxford University Press, 1991, pp 197–219.

55. Davis FC, Mannion J: Entrainment of hamster pup circadian rhythms by prenatal melatonin injections. Am J Physiol 255:R439–R448, 1988.

56. Bosc MJ: Time of parturition in rats after melatonin administration or change of photoperiod. J Reprod Fertil 80:563–568, 1987.

57. Brzezinski A, Wurtman RJ: The pineal gland: Its possible roles in human reproduction. Obstet Gynecol Survey 43:197–207, 1988.

58. Armstrong SM, Redman J: Melatonin: A chronobiotic with anti-aging properties. Med Hypotheses 34:300–309, 1991.

59. McArthur AJ, Gillette MU, Prosser RA: Melatonin directly resets the rat suprachiasmatic circadian clock in vitro. Brain Res 565:158–161, 1991.

60. Rémé CE, Wirz-Justice A, Terman M: The visual imput stage of the mammalian circadian pacemaking system: 1. Is there a clock in the mammalian eye? J Biol Rhythms 6:5–29, 1991.

61. Steinlechner S: In search of a physiological role for retinal melatonin. Adv Pineal Res (Suppl 5):123–128, 1991.

62. Neuwelt EA, Mickey B, Lewy AJ: The importance of melatonin and tumour markers in pineal tumours. *In* Wurtman RJ, Waldhauser F (eds): Melatonin in Humans. J Neural Trans (Suppl 21):397–413, 1986.

63. Vaughan GM: Melatonin in humans. Pineal Res Rev 2:141–201, 1984.

64. Arendt J: Melatonin—a new probe in psychiatric investigation. Br J Psychiatry 155:585–590, 1989.

65. Arendt J, Bojkowski C, Folkard S, et al: Some effects of melatonin and the control of its secretion in man. *In* Evered D, Clark S (eds): Photoperiodism, melatonin and the pineal. Ciba Foundation Symposium 117. London, Pitman, 1985, pp 266–283.

66. Arendt J: Mammalian pineal rhythms. Pineal Res Rev 3:161–213, 1985.

67. Akerstedt T, Froberg JE, Friberg W, Wetterberg L: Melatonin excretion, body temperature and subjective arousal during 64 hours of sleep deprivation. Psychoneuroendocrinology 4:219, 1979.

68. Das Gupta D, Riedel L, Frick JH, et al: Circulating melatonin in children: In relation to puberty, endocrine disorders, functional tests and racial origin. Neuroendocrinol Lett 5:63–78, 1983.

68a. Iguchi M, Kato K, Ibayashi M: Age dependent reduction in serum melatonin concentration in healthy human subjects. J Clin Endocrinol Metab 55:27–29, 1982.

69. Waldhauser F, Frisch H, Waldhauser M, et al: Fall in nocturnal serum melatonin during prepuberty and pubescence. Lancet 1:362–365, 1984.

70. Parkes AS: Patterns of Sexuality and Reproduction. Oxford, Oxford University Press, 1976.

71. Attanasio A, Borrelli P, Marini R, et al: Serum melatonin in children with early and delayed puberty. Neuroendocrinol Lett 5:387, 1983.

72. Waldhauser F, Boepple P, Schemper M, Crowley WF: Serum melatonin in central precocious puberty is lower than in age matched prepubertal children. J Clin Endocrinol Metab 73:793–796, 1991.

73. Berga SL, Jones KL, Kaufmann S, Yen SSC: Nocturnal melatonin levels are unaltered by ovarian suppression in girls with central precocious puberty. Fertil Steril 52:937–941, 1989.

74. Arendt J, Labib MH, Bojkowski C, et al: Rapid decrease in melatonin production during treatment of delayed puberty with oestradiol in a case of craniopharyngioma. Lancet 1:1326, 1989.

75. Berga SL, Mortola JF, Yen SSC: Amplification of nocturnal melatonin

secretion in women with functional hypothalamic amenorrhea. J Clin Endocrinol Metab 66:242–244, 1988.

76. Cagnacci A, Elliot JA, Yen SSC: Amplification of pulsatile LH secretion by exogenous melatonin in women. J Clin Endocrinol Metab 73:210–212, 1991.

77. Voordow BCG, Euser R, Verdonk RER, et al: Melatonin and melatonin-progestin combinations alter pituitary-ovarian function in women and can inhibit ovulation. J Clin Endocrinol Metab 74:108–117, 1992.

78. West RJ, Leonard JV: Familial insulin resistance with pineal hyperplasia: Metabolic studies and effect of hypophysectomy. Arch Dis Child 55:619–621, 1980.

79. Sparks DL, Hunsaker JC III: The pineal gland in sudden infant death syndrome: Preliminary observations. J Pineal Res 5:111–118, 1988.

80. Sturner WQ, Lynch HJ, Deng MH, Wurtman RJ: Melatonin levels in the sudden infant death syndrome. Forensic Sci Intern 45:171–180, 1990.

81. Axelrod L: Endocrine dysfunction in patients with tumours of the pineal region. In Schmidek HH (ed): Pineal Tumours. New York, Masson Publishing, 1977, pp 61–77.

82. Wass JAL, Jones AE, Rees LH, Besser GM: hCGβ producing pineal choriocarcinoma. Clin Endocrinol 17:423–431, 1982.

83. Cohen AR, Wilson JA, Sadeghi-Nejad A: Gonadotrophin-secreting pineal teratoma causing precocious puberty. Neurosurgery 28:597–602, 1991.

84. Horowitz MB: Central nervous system germinomas, a review. Arch Neurol 48:652–657, 1991.

85. Cohen M, Lippman M, Chabner B: Role of pineal gland in aetiology and treatment of breast cancer. Lancet 2:814–816, 1978.

86. Tamarkin L, Danforth D, Lichter A, et al: Decreased nocturnal plasma melatonin peak in patients with estrogen receptor positive breast cancer. Science 216:1003–1005, 1982.

87. Bartsch C, Bartsch H, Fluchter SH, et al: Evidence for modulation of melatonin secretion in men with benign and malignant tumours of the prostate: Relationship with the pituitary hormones. J Pineal Res 2:121–132, 1985.

88. Gupta D, Attanasio A: Pathophysiology of pineal function in health and disease in children. Pineal Res Rev 6:261–300, 1988.

89. Thompson C, Obrecht R, Franey C, et al: Neuroendocrine rhythms in a patient with the Kleine-Levin syndrome. Br J Psychiatry 147:440–443, 1985.

90. Dahlitz M, Alvarez B, Vignau J, et al: Delayed sleep phase syndrome response to melatonin. Lancet 1:1121–1124, 1991.

91. Lewy AJ, Sack RL, Miller LS, Hoban TM: Anti-depressant and circadian phase-shifting effects of light. Science 235:352–354, 1987.

92. Lerner AB, Nordlund JJ: Melatonin: Clinical Pharmacology. J Neural Trans (Suppl 13):339–347, 1978.

93. Lieberman HR, Waldhauser F, Garfield G, et al: Effects of melatonin on human mood and performance. Brain Res 323:201–207, 1984.

94. Waldhauser F, Steger H, Vorkapic P: Melatonin secretion in man and the influence of exogenous melatonin on some physiological and behavioural variables. Adv Pineal Res 2:207–223, 1987.

95. Sugden D: Psychopharmacological effects of melatonin in mouse and rat. J Pharmacol Exp Therap 227:587–591, 1983.

96. Lewy AJ, Ahmed S, Jackson JML, Sack RL: Melatonin shifts human circadian rhythms according to a phase-response curve. Chronobiol Int 9:380–392, 1993.

97. Nickelsen T, Lang A, Bergau L: The effect of 6-, 9- and 11-hour time shifts on circadian rhythms: Adaptation of sleep parameters and hormonal patterns following the intake of melatonin or placebo. Adv Pineal Res 5:303–306, 1991.

98. Samel A, Wegman HM, Vejvoda M, Maas H: Influence of melatonin treatment on human circadian rhythmicity before and after a simulated 9 hour time shift. J Biol Rhythms 6:235–248, 1991.

99. Skene DJ, Aldhous M, Arendt J: Melatonin, jet-lag and the sleep-wake cycle. In Horne J (ed): Sleep '88, Proceedings of the European Sleep Congress, Jerusalem, 1988. Basel, Karger, 1989, pp 39–41.

100. Czeisler CA, Johnson PJ, Duffy JF, et al: Exposure to bright light and darkness to treat physiologic maladaptation to night-work. N Engl J Med 322:1253–1259, 1990.

100a. Folkard S, Arendt J, Clark M: Can melatonin improve shiftworkers' tolerance of the night shift? Some preliminary findings. Chronobiol Int, in press.

101. Arendt J, Aldhous M: Synchronisation of a disturbed sleep-wake cycle in a blind man by melatonin treatment. Lancet 2:772–773, 1988.

102. Karasek M, Fraschini F: Is there a role for the pineal gland in neoplastic growth? In Fraschini F, Reiter RJ (eds): Role of melatonin and pineal peptides in neuroimmunomodulation. New York, Plenum Press, 1991, pp 243–251.

103. Tamarkin L, Cohen M, Roselle D, et al: Melatonin inhibition and pinealectomy enhancement of 7,12-dimethylbenz(a)anthracene–induced mammary tumours in the rat. Cancer Res 41:4432–4436, 1981.

104. Maestroni GJM, Conti A, Pierpaoli W: Melatonin, stress and the immune system. Pineal Res Rev 7:268, 1989.

104a. Reiter RJ, Poeggler B, Tan D-X, Chen L-D, Manchester LC, Guerrero JM: Antioxidant capacity of melatonin: a novel action not requiring a receptor. Neuroendocrinol Lett 15:103–116, 1993.

105. Hastings MH, Maywood ES, Ebling FJP, et al: Sites and mechanism of action of melatonin in the photoperiodic control of reproduction. Adv Pineal Res 5:147–157, 1991.

106. Nakazawa K, Marubayashi U, McCann SM: Mediation of the short-loop feedback of luteinising hormone (LH) on LH-releasing hormone release by melatonin-induced inhibition of LH release from the pars tuberalis. Proc Natl Acad Sci USA 88:7576–7579, 1991.

107. Cardinali DP, Hyyppa MT, Wurtman RJ: Fate of intracisternally injected melatonin in the rat brain. Neuroendocrinology 12:30–40, 1973.

108. Cardinali DP, Vacas MI, Boyer EE: Specific binding of melatonin in bovine brain. Endocrinology 105:437–441, 1979.

109. Vanecek J, Pavlik A, Illnerova H: Hypothalamic melatonin receptor sites revealed by autoradiography. Brain Res 453:359–362, 1987.

110. Morgan PJ, Williams LM: Central melatonin receptors; implications for a mode of action. Experientia 45:955–965, 1989.

111. Weaver DR, Rivkees SA, Carlson LL, Reppert SM: Localisation of melatonin receptors in mammalian brain. In Klein DC, Moore RY, Reppert SM: Suprachiasmatic Nucleus: The Mind's Clock. New York, Oxford University Press, 1991, pp 289–308.

112. Reppert SM, Weaver DR, Rivkees SA, et al: Putative melatonin receptors in a human biological clock. Science 242:78–81, 1988.

113. Morgan PJ, King TP, Lawson W, et al: Ultrastructure of melatonin responsive cells in the ovine pars tuberalis. Cell Tissue Res 263:529–534, 1991.

114. Williams LM, Martinoli MG, Titchener LT, Pelletier G: The ontogeny of central melatonin binding sites in the rat. Endocrinology 128:2083–2090, 1991.

115. Zisapel N, Oaknin S, Anis Y, Nir I: Melatonin receptors in discrete areas of the rat and Syrian hamster brain: Modulation by melatonin, pinealectomy, testosterone and the photoperiod. Adv Pineal Res 5:175–181, 1991.

116. Krause DN, Dubocovich ML: Regulatory sites in the melatonin system of mammals. Trends Neurosci 13:464–470, 1990.

117. Sugden D, Chong NWS: Pharmacological identity of 2-(125-I)iodomelatonin binding sites in chicken brain and sheep pars tuberalis. Brain Res 539:151–154, 1991.

117a. Skene DJ, Masson-Pevet M, Pevet P: Seasonal changes in melatonin binding sites in the pars tuberalis of male European hamsters and the effect of testosterone manipulation. Endocrinology 132:1682–1686, 1993.

118. White BH, Sekura RD, Rollag MD: Pertussis toxin blocks melatonin-induced aggregation in Xenopus dermal melanophores. J Comp Physiol B 157:153–159, 1987.

119. Yous S, Antrieux J, Howell HE, et al: Novel napthalenic ligands with a high affinity for the melatonin receptor. J Med Chem 35:1484–1486, 1992.

28

Hypothalamus and Hormone-Regulated Behaviors

D. W. PFAFF
A. H. LAUBER

Hypothalamic neurons, because of complex synaptic connectivity, hormone receptors, and a rich array of neuropeptides, are in a unique position to integrate neuroendocrine control of pituitary and autonomic functions with behavior. Hormone-regulated actions have offered some of the clearest opportunities to understand how the brain controls behavior. This process has been greatly facilitated by molecular reagents and techniques of molecular biology. Thus, molecular studies of hypothalamic neurons have added a new dimension to the analysis of hormonal effects on the brain, and, correspondingly, specific steroid-regulated behaviors. Cell groups within the hypothalamus and limbic system contain the highest concentrations of receptors for gonadal steroids of anywhere in the brain. Indeed, these cells confer hormonal responsiveness to other regions of the central nervous system, some of which are concerned with higher cognitive and motivational functions; others are implicated in control of reflexes and movement. Generally, hypothalamic neurons do not "produce" particular behavioral responses in the manner of an upper-level command motor neuron. Instead, hypothalamic cells have permissive effects, thereby facilitating or promoting sequences of behaviors, while contributing, most importantly, hormonal regulation.

The purpose of this chapter is to provide a general overview of hypothalamic and hormone contributions to three hormone-regulated responses: male and female reproductive behaviors and maternal behavior. Presented here are discussions of (1) contrasts in the cell groups implicated in these differing behaviors; (2) the neural circuitry and molecular mechanisms that control lordosis, the primary female-typical reproductive behavior in quadrupeds; and (3) how synergies implicit in transcription factor binding upstream of hormone-regulated genes can help to encode

biological signals properly for specific hypothalamically controlled hormone-regulated behaviors.

DIFFERENT HYPOTHALAMIC CELL GROUPS FACILITATE DIFFERENT BEHAVIORS

Complexes of different behaviors and autonomic responses are controlled by different portions of the hypothalamus and preoptic area. Moreover, hypothalamic brain regions are not committed solely to regulation of any one particular function. This is exemplified best, perhaps, by the classic studies of Hess and colleagues, who discovered that parasympathetic autonomic responses are facilitated most easily from preoptic tissue and cells anterior to the preoptic area in the basal forebrain. Parasympathetic responses include decreased heart rate and respiration, pupillary constriction, increased digestion, and other functions common to an organism in a relaxed environment. In contrast, cell groups in the posterior hypothalamus promoted sympathetic autonomic responses such as increased blood pressure, respiration, and other faculties necessary for "flight"-type responses. As mentioned later, male reproductive responses appear more dependent on preoptic functions, whereas female-typical reproductive behavior depends most exquisitely on cells in the ventromedial hypothalamic nucleus. Whenever hypothalamic control of behavior is evaluated, it is important to consider that autonomic regulation contributes to various aspects of behaviors facilitated by the hypothalamus.

The full range of data on male reproductive behavior has been reviewed most extensively by Sachs and Meisel,[1]

445

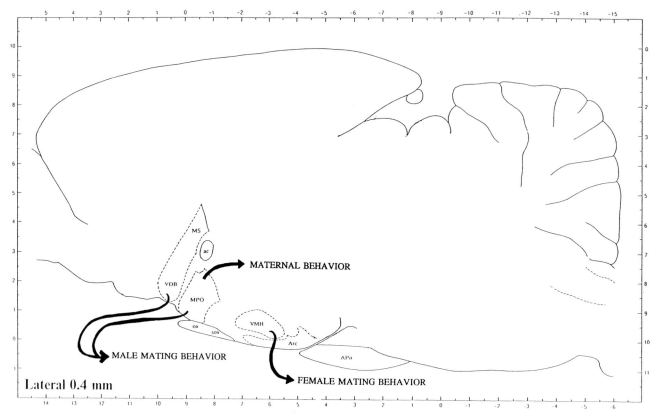

FIGURE 28–1. Different cell groups in the hypothalamus are primarily responsible for facilitating different steroid-regulated behaviors. The schematic drawing summarizes three major bodies of data deriving from physiological, anatomical, and behavioral studies. Ventromedial hypothalamic (VMH) neurons clearly support estrogenic and progestin facilitation of lordosis behavior. Important axonal trajectories are through a periventricular route and through a route sweeping laterally and dorsally across the medial forebrain bundle on a curved trajectory to the midbrain central gray. Large lesions of the medial preoptic area (MPO), especially those which extend forward into the ventral limb of the diagonal band of Broca (VDB), abolish male-typical mating behavior. Effective lesions tend to be medial, wiping out the medial preoptic nucleus proper. Cells more dorsally and laterally placed in the preoptic area appear most important for maternal behavior in rats, with the most important anatomical connections going laterally and then projecting down the medial forebrain bundle. (Schematic drawing uses plate [Lateral 0.4 mm] from Paxinos G, Watson C: The Rat Brain in Stereotaxic Coordinates, 2nd ed. San Diego, Academic Press, 1993; author's information superimposed.)

and this brief account derives from their conclusions. Male-typical reproductive behavior in the rat is dependent, in part, on cellular regulation at the level of the preoptic area. This area has a relatively high concentration of receptors for estrogen and testosterone, adding hormonal control to regulation of the behavior. The hormone-stimulated male requires olfactory cues denoting the presence of an estrous female. Then, chasing, mounting, intromission, and, eventually, ejaculation will occur.

Neural control over the concatenation of male behaviors is complex. The most constant and generalizable result is that lesions of the medial preoptic area, especially when relatively large, eliminate male copulation.[2, 3] When destruction is smaller, the results are more variable and deficits are less severe. Across species there is a tendency for preoptic tissue to display the neuroendocrine characteristics required for the normal control of male reproductive function.[4] Even beyond the preoptic area, tissue in the limbic forebrain has proved more essential for male reproductive behavior than that for females. For example, Giantonio et al.[5] found that destruction of the corticomedial amygdala could reduce male reproductive behavior. Finally, it is not surprising that removal of olfactory systems can reduce male reproductive behavior under circum-

stances in which, and in species for which, chemosensory inputs are crucial for finding the female and arousing the male. Notably, some effects of chemosensory inputs from the female may not be mediated by the olfactory epithelium and olfactory bulb (projecting through the lateral olfactory tract) but rather by the vomeronasal organ projecting through the vomeronasal nerve to the accessory olfactory bulb whose axons, in turn, follow a more medial projectory to the medial amygdala. Even the nervus terminalis, projecting from the nasal septum to the basal forebrain, might be important because some of its cell bodies contain gonadotropin-releasing hormone (GnRH) (reviewed in ref. 6). All of these findings are different for male and for female reproductive behavior, making it clear that controls for the two sorts of behaviors are different neurally as well as hormonally (Fig. 28–1).

Parental behavior is even more complex because of the large numbers of coordinated responses required and because of the marked effects of experience. Its neural and hormonal control has been reviewed extensively by Numan,[7] on whose chapter this brief summary depends. In dramatic contrast to male copulatory behavior, the main olfactory bulb and vomeronasal nerves as well as the amygdala actually inhibit maternal behavior in virgin rats.[8] Damage to the medial preoptic area of the rat will disrupt maternal behavior. An extensive series of knife cut experiments designed to damage axonal connections of the medial preoptic area in different directions revealed that only the lateral-going connections were crucial for maternal behavior in the rat and that, among those, the dorsolateral connections were most important.[9–11] Several components of this complex chain of behavioral responses (e.g., retrieving of the pups, nest building, and nursing) all can be reduced by preoptic damage. Whether or not individual preoptic neurons important for male sex behavior are also crucial for parental behavior remains to be determined, although it seems unlikely. The most effective lesions for male copulatory behavior often are ventral and medial to the more dorsolateral placements most intimately tied to parental behavior. In whatever way that question is answered, preoptic projections to the ventral tegmental area are crucial for maternal behavior.[12] Even with the conclusion that a dorsolateral preoptic area to medial forebrain bundle to midbrain tegmentum pathway is important for maternal behavior, the manner of termination and more caudal projections in the midbrain remains an open question.

Hormone Binding in Cell Nucleus

While a generation of neurobiological experiments used techniques that destroyed parts of nerve cells to demonstrate those neuronal groups crucial for particular hormone-regulated behaviors, a complementary approach used hormone-binding techniques to pinpoint where sex steroids might facilitate such behaviors. With respect to endocrine mechanisms that might be important for all vertebrates, it is especially noteworthy that there exist preoptic and hypothalamic neuronal groups that, in every case studied, have neurons with nuclear receptors for sex steroids. These include medial preoptic neurons, bed nucleus of the stria terminalis, anterior hypothalamus, ventromedial nucleus of the hypothalamus, arcuate nucleus of the hypothalamus, and ventral premammillary nucleus. Moreover, limbic forebrain structures that project to the hypothalamus—such as those in the medial and cortical nuclei of the amygdala and the lateral nucleus of the septum—always can be found to have sex steroid hormone receptors (reviewed in ref. 13). Incidentally, it is not always the case that androgen receptors exclusively, for example, are important for male reproductive behavior. Aromatization of testosterone to estradiol comprises part of the control over male reproductive behavior in the adult. Likewise, masculinization of the neonatal brain by androgenic hormones also can depend on aromatization. Thus, among androgen, estrogen, and progestin receptors, all may contribute with various strengths and weights to female reproductive behavior, masculine behavior, and parental behavior.

Orderliness of the Organization of Neural Output Pathways

Given that female-typical copulatory reflexes depend most strongly on the ventromedial hypothalamic nucleus,

the question arises of how the separate groups of cells mentioned in the foregoing paragraphs project to influence behavior control mechanisms in the brain stem. Compared with neuroanatomical regions and systems famous for their point-to-point connectivity—the visual system is a prototype of precise mapping from stimulus to retina to thalamus to cortex—neuronal groups in the hypothalamus and limbic forebrain were reputed to be more of a mixed character: less straightforward anatomically and more multifunctional. Thus it came as a surprise that the first generation of studies using modern autoradiographic neuroanatomical techniques suggested an organization of fiber systems descending through the hypothalamus and the medial forebrain bundle.[14] This theoretical suggestion followed a detailed analysis of projections from the preoptic area, anterior hypothalamus, periventricular nucleus, and ventromedial nucleus of the hypothalamus. According to this scheme, it seems clear that more medially placed neurons have axons that tend to descend medially, while axons of more lateral neurons run more laterally (Fig. 28–2). Extending this concept, the bed nucleus of the stria terminalis borders on the preoptic area dorsally, and its projections are, with few exceptions, similar to the preoptic area but with axons running in a position generally *dorsal* to that of medial preoptic area axons. From these and other data the idea of an orderly medial-lateral arrangement of descending axons in the hypothalamus and medial forebrain bundle can be extended to include the notion that axons from dorsally located neurons tend to run in a relatively dorsal position. None of these neuroanatomical tendencies applies with a point-to-point determinacy reminiscent of the visual system. However, it is apparent that descending axons in and around the medial forebrain bundle, heading for the midbrain to exert behavior and autonomic controls, tend to be ordered along medial-lateral and dorsal-ventral "gradients."

The neuroanatomical data are strong enough to suggest further that efferents descending from the anterior hypothalamus, preoptic area, and basal forebrain run in a spatial arrangement that resembles laminar flow (Fig. 28–2B). That is, the relative anterior-posterior levels of the neurons whose axon is in question determines the position that the axon will take in descending through the hypothalamus and medial forebrain bundle.[14] Axons of the most anterior neurons in this system, in the basal forebrain, enter the medial forebrain bundle as far laterally as possible, wrapping around the projections from more posterior cell groups. Conversely, axons of progressively more posterior neurons "lie into" the medial forebrain bundle, in positions medial to the axons just mentioned, from more anterior sources.

The system thus encompassed by this tendency toward anatomical orderliness includes the hypothalamus and medial forebrain bundle. Within this system, axons descending from the ventromedial hypothalamic neurons important for female reproductive behavior can either follow a periventricular route or a completely separate route that crosses the medial forebrain bundle (see below). In contrast, axons necessary for controlling brain stem mechanisms important for male reproductive behavior and parental behavior travel through the medial forebrain bundle itself.

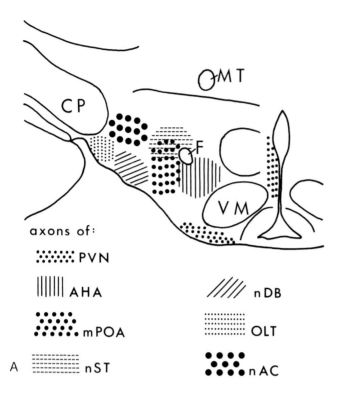

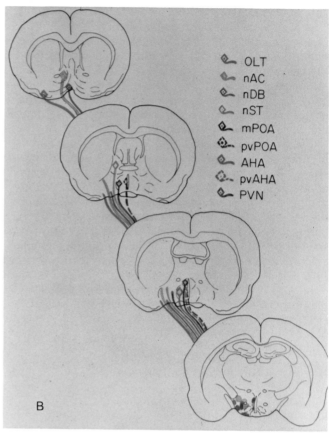

FIGURE 28–2. *A*, Schematic illustration of the relative positions of axons descending from paraventricular nucleus (PVN), anterior hypothalamic (AHA), medial preoptic area (mPOA), bed nucleus of the stria terminalis (nST), nuclei of the diagonal band (nDB), nucleus accumbens (nAC), and olfactory tubercle (OLT) neurons in the hypothalamus and MFB at the level of the ventromedial nucleus. *B*, Schematic illustration of the "laminar flow" of axons descending from the paraventricular nucleus (PVN), anterior hypothalamus (AHA), medial preoptic area (mPOA), bed nucleus of the stria terminalis (nST), nuclei of the diagonal band (nDA), nucleus accumbens (nAC), and olfactory tubercle (OLT) through the medial basal forebrain, hypothalamus, and medial MFB. Projections from more anterior cell groups appear to "wrap around" those from more posterior cell groups in hypothalamus and basal forebrain. Orderliness of descending projections from hypothalamus and basal forebrain through the MFB apparently is greater than appreciated in the older neuroanatomical literature. (From Pfaff DW, Conrad LCA: Hypothalamic neuroanatomy: Steroid hormone binding and patterns of axonal projections. In Bourne G (ed): International Review of Cytology, Vol 54. New York, Academic Press, 1978, pp 245–265.)

NEURAL CIRCUIT FOR A HYPOTHALAMICALLY CONTROLLED MAMMALIAN BEHAVIOR

The relative simplicity of the primary female typical reproductive behaviors in rodents, combined with their strong controls by estradiol and progesterone, allowed a focused series of investigations on hormone action in the hypothalamus and on lordosis mechanisms that permitted elucidation of the first circuit known for a mammalian behavior. The anatomical and chemical properties of sex hormone receptors in the medial hypothalamus and preoptic area have been reviewed.[15, 16]

Following the flow of neural activity through the cell groups responsible for lordosis behavior all the way from application of the stimulus by the male to muscular contraction by the female, showed that it is possible to explain the neural circuitry responsible for initiating lordosis.[17] Stimuli triggering the behavior are cutaneous, and action potentials deriving from these stimuli enter the dorsal horn of the spinal cord over lumbar and sacral dorsal routes. Females with the spinal cord isolated from higher neural centers do not perform lordosis; therefore, supraspinal facilitation must be required. Ascending fibers participating in the obligatory supraspinal loop travel through the anterolateral columns of the spinal cord and terminate in the medullary reticular formation, the lateral vestibular nucleus, and in and around the midbrain central gray. Notably, in the medullary reticular formation, virtually all the reticulospinal neurons that respond to behaviorally adequate sensory stimulation also receive a convergent input from a higher behaviorally relevant center, the midbrain central gray.

Estrogen acts on cells of the ventromedial nucleus of the hypothalamus to prepare the system in such a way that the female rat will engage in lordosis behavior when an appropriate stimulus is present. In a nonhormonally prepared state, the female will not show lordosis. However, when estrogen is present, followed by progesterone, the female will hop and dart in the presence of a male rat. If the male is interested, he will follow and eventually mount her. Stimulation of the female's flanks and perineum by the male will elicit raising of the head with concomitant spinal dorsiflexion, characteristic of the lordosis reflex. This allows

the male adequate access for copulation. The lordosis reflex itself is exquisitely dependent upon estrogen. Progesterone facilitates estrogen action by inducing the hop and dart response and potentiates deepening of the spinal dorsiflexion. In the absence of previous estrogen stimulation progesterone is completely ineffectual. How it is that progesterone facilitates estrogen action is unknown but involves the production of proteins facilitated by the presence of both hormones.

Maximal lordosis behavior requires estrogenic stimulation of cells within the ventromedial nucleus of the hypothalamus and to some extent upon cells within the preoptic area. As will become evident later, estrogen and progestin receptors (ER and PR) are present within certain hypothalamic and preoptic cells, altering protein synthesis. Estrogen also induces increased firing of previously silent neurons within the ventromedial nucleus presumably leading to the increased deposition of hormone-facilitated products through stimulus-secretion coupling. The preoptic area is inhibitory for lordosis, and here estrogen appears to quiet cells, leading to a "disinhibition" of the neural circuit mediating the lordosis reflex. Altered gene expression dependent on sex hormone administration is mentioned later.

Ventromedial hypothalamic effects on lordosis behavior operate over a relatively long time course—minutes to hours. Axons from ventromedial hypothalamic neurons can reach the midbrain either of two ways: a periventricular route or a sweeping lateral route (crossing the medial forebrain bundle on the way to the lateral midbrain before turning back in toward the midbrain central gray). Combinations of bilateral knife cuts prove the necessity of connections between the ventromedial hypothalamus and midbrain central gray.[18] Hypothalamic effects on midbrain neurons are such that the electrical excitability of behaviorally relevant dorsal midbrain neurons is elevated, and, in turn, these midbrain neurons facilitate lordosis behavior with a fast time course (measured in seconds). The entire circuit is illustrated in Figure 28–3.

A behaviorally important action of midbrain central gray cells seems to be to facilitate the actions of lower medullary reticulospinal neurons. These neurons act synergistically with lateral vestibulospinal neurons functioning, respectively, through reticulospinal and vestibulospinal mechanisms. These two descending pathways control motor neurons for axial muscles. They branch at different vertebral levels and act bilaterally—all of these properties making them particularly suitable for upper-level motor control of lordosis behavior. The gradual "warming up" of medullary reticulospinal electrophysiological effects on deep back muscles—increased amplitude of responses with repeated electrical stimulation—indicates that this system works most effectively with a chronic excitatory drive. This is also concordant with the long time course of hormonally facilitated excitatory drives from the hypothalamus mediated through midbrain central gray neurons.

Medullary reticulospinal and lateral vestibulospinal tracts help to prepare lumbar spinal circuits for lordosis initiation. They increase the responsiveness of deep back muscles to subsequent stimuli coming in from the pudendal nerve. While there are monosynaptic connections from reticulospinal and vestibulospinal axons to the motoneurons for deep back muscles, the descending influences responsible for facilitating lumbar spinal lordosis circuitry may

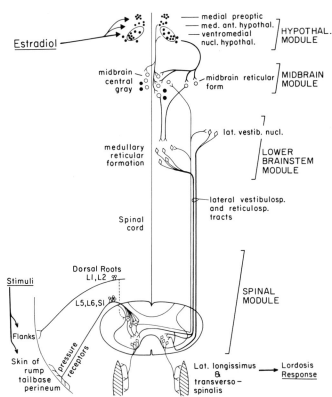

FIGURE 28–3. Summary diagram of neural circuit for activating lordosis behavior. Entire circuit is shown, from somatosensory stimuli required for activating the behavior, through the ascending pathways up to midbrain, and including ventromedial hypothalamus, where estradiol and progesterone act to facilitate the behavior. Descending pathways from hypothalamus to midbrain, to medullary reticular formation, and in turn to lumbar spinal cord are also shown. Contraction of the deep back muscles lateral longissimus and transversospinalis causes the behavior. All stimuli, neural pathways, hormone actions, and responses are bilateral, and are shown here on one side for convenience of illustration. (From Pfaff DW: Estrogens and Brain Function. New York, Springer-Verlag, 1980.)

also operate through interneurons documented at lumbar levels. Finally, excitation of the motor neurons for the deep back muscles lateral longissimus and transversospinalis causes the contractions of those muscles, which in turn execute the vertebral dorsiflexion of lordosis. In this manner, hormonal inputs to hypothalamic neurons provide an "enabling" or "permissive" influence on a complex circuit that allows the female to respond to mounting by the male in a manner required for fertilization.

PRINCIPLES OF HYPOTHALAMIC CONTROL AND CIRCUIT OPERATION

In the broadest terms, our very knowledge of the female reproductive behavior circuit, its survival as a body of fact and concept over more than 10 years, and the ability of neuroendocrinologists to add detail to this paradigm proves that it is possible to achieve a detailed cellular explanation for a mammalian behavior. That is, at least four fundamental questions can be asked about hypothalamic control of behavior. First, what causes a particular behavioral response to occur? Second, given that this behavior can occur, what regulates its amplitude? Third, as this response is occurring, what prevents other responses? Fourth, as Sherrington asked in 1906, what executes the transition from one behavioral response to another? The circuitry known for the hypothalamic control over female reproductive behavior and the cellular analyses provided, importantly, for its control by estradiol and progesterone answer the first and second questions in considerable detail.

Modular Nature of Neural Control

The circuitry for lordosis behavior clearly is arranged according to modules represented by different levels of neuraxis (Fig. 28–3), which also correspond neatly to embryologically recognized subdivisions of the central nervous system.[16] The spinal cord module receives behaviorally relevant somatosensory input, filters that input within each spinal cord segment, receives descending facilitatory signals from the reticulospinal and vestibulospinal systems, and generates the motor neuronal output for the deep back muscles which execute lordosis. The lower brain stem module integrates postural adaptations across spinal segments. The midbrain module serves as a receiving zone for hypothalamic and preoptic inputs, notably borne by endocrinologically important neuropeptides. It appears to serve as a transmission zone integrating hypothalamic signals, which have a very slow time course typical of endocrine mechanisms, with faster changing electrophysiological signaling systems typical of the rest of the nervous system. Hierarchically, it facilitates reticulospinal cells and enables the medullary reticulospinal system to synergize with lateral vestibulospinal mechanisms in control of the lumbar spinal cord. The hypothalamic module adds the most important endocrine control component to the behavioral mechanism. Steroid hormone binding, and the molecular and electrophysiological effects of estrogens and progesterone on medial hypothalamic and preoptic neurons, account for the strong steroid hormone dependence of the neural circuit and the behavior as a whole.

While the main force of mechanisms from the spinal cord through the hypothalamic module account for the generation of the behavior, the net contribution of cell groups in the forebrain module (such as the septum and the olfactory bulb) is to inhibit the behavior.

Principles of Sensory Operations

SUMMATION. Among sensory neurons mediating information relevant to lordosis behavior, stimulus information *converges* from neuron to neuron. Indeed, this convergence is the neural mechanism by which behavioral summation—the ability of stimuli applied over space and time to add in order to trigger the behavioral response—can occur.

SELECTIVE DISTRIBUTION. As sensory information travels from the primary receptors into the circuitry for lordosis behavior, not all sensory information is transferred. In some cases there is a loss of precision—receptive fields on the skin become larger. In the extreme case, there is an absence of responsivity—for example, few medial hypothalamic cells respond immediately to lordosis-eliciting stimuli. It appears that only the amount and form of sensory information required to manage the behavior is passed on.[17]

Hypothalamic Neuroendocrine Mechanisms

Conservation of endocrine mechanisms manifested in the effects of steroid hormones on target tissues is an obvious feature of hypothalamic mechanisms when compared with peripheral tissues. For example, estrogen and progestin receptors in the brain seem to be of the same chemical form as in the periphery. Similar discontinuous schedules of estrogen administration are sufficient to initiate certain endocrine-dependent events both in uterine and hypothalamic cells. In both peripheral tissues and hypothalamic cells, synthesis of ribosomal RNA is increased after estrogen treatment and rates of synthesis for certain proteins are altered. In specific ventromedial hypothalamic neurons, some aspects of the ultrastructural and chemical responses to estrogen look like the "growth" responses obvious in the uterus.

Synchronization of reproductive behavior with the gametogenic preparations for reproduction as well as appropriate environmental conditions is a clear principle of operation. The very actions of estrogen and progesterone operating through hypothalamic neurons render behavioral responses appropriate to ovarian cycles. The promotion of reproductive behavior by GnRH[19, 20] similarly helps to guarantee that pituitary output and reproductive behavior will be timed adaptively with respect to each other.

Amplification of steroid hormone effects on nerve cells leading toward reproductive behavior occurs in at least three ways. First, early estrogen-stimulated events set the stage for later hormone-dependent events to occur in the manner of a cascade.[16] Moreover, progesterone actions on the medial hypothalamus amplify the effects of estrogen on lordosis. At the neural circuitry level the high degree of interconnectedness[21] gives multiple opportunities for effects of hormones on different neuronal groups to add or multiply. At the behavioral level it is clear, in the entire chain of courtship and copulatory behavioral responses, that early hormone-dependent responses in the signaling between females and males set the stage for later hormone-dependent copulatory responses to occur.

Principles of Motor System Operations

The *hierarchial* nature of the motor pathways responsible for executing lordosis behavior appears from the following arrangement: dorsal midbrain neurons, notably in the central gray, facilitate cells in the lower brain stem module—particularly reticulospinal cells in the ventral-medial-caudal medullary reticular formation. In turn, lateral vestibulospinal and reticulospinal cells cooperate to facilitate motor neurons in their response to behaviorally relevant somatosensory input at the lumbar spinal cord level.

The *economy* of use of neural circuitry in achieving biologically adapative motor control is revealed by the fact that specificity has not been built into this system where it has not been required. Large lesions of reticulospinal systems and large transections of descending axons are required for significant behavior losses. These facts suggest an upper limit on specificity with which these descending systems could control lordosis behavior. Moreover, terminations of these descending axons occur over a wide range of spinal cord levels, often bilaterally, again indicating a massive descending facilitatory effect. Indeed, such a widespread effect fits the requirements for lordosis behavior control, in which the dorsiflexion response occurs over the entire vertebral column, bilaterally.

Once activated by hypothalamic and brain stem mechanisms, the lordosis behavior response has a *ballistic* quality. In fact, the small number of muscle spindles in the bulk of the deep back muscles equipped with fast twitch fibers and the very weakness of monosynaptic stretch reflexes suggest a lack of fine control over the precise degree of contraction. Biologically, since this behavioral response does not have a "target" in the manner of a guided limb response, it appears that once activated the deep back muscles contract with the maximum force available during lordosis as needed to support the weight of the male.

MOLECULAR MECHANISMS IN THE HYPOTHALAMUS

Understanding neural mechanisms subserving lordosis behavior has been predicated upon identification of neuroanatomical circuitry illuminating the neurons and projections required. The gonadal steroid hormone receptors are themselves transcription factors and thereby regulate gene expression. Asking questions of how hormones prepare the system and which genes are implicated has been possible in view of the previously elucidated physiological details.

Over a large series of studies dealing with steroid hormone effects on hypothalamic neurons, it is clear that even for an individual sex steroid hormone such as estradiol, when dealing with a well-defined hormonal effect on a simple vertebrate behavior such as lordosis, we are not dealing with a one hormone–one gene–one behavior system. In fact, early responses to estrogen by cells in the ventromedial hypothalamus appear to prepare the way for later responses. At the very least, we have elaboration of ribosomal RNA in response to estrogen, as well as activation of the progesterone receptor gene, enhanced α-1 adrenergic responses, heightened muscarinic responsivity, increased transcription of the preproenkephalin gene, activation of oxytocin and its receptors, and, importantly, effects on the GnRH system (reviewed in ref. 16). All of these molecular responses can be tied to female reproductive behavior and thus can be considered to be part of the molecular mechanism of the behavior as a whole.

The lordosis reflex is a prominent example of the modulatory effects of estrogen on brain function. This reproductive behavior is displayed by female rats and other rodents in response to male mounting, which stimulates somatosensory receptors within the female's flanks. Lordosis can be elicited late into the proestrus phase of the characteristic four-day estrous cycle or approximately 24 hours following sequential estrogen and progesterone treatment of ovariectomized rats. The amount of lordosis exhibited is quantifiable, and levels displayed by ovariectomized rats are related in a dose-responsive manner to the amount of estrogen administered.[22, 23] The well-elaborated estrogen dependence, neural circuitry, sex specificity, and requirement for a genomic mode of steroid action (see later) make the lordosis reflex a sensitive and quantifiable

physiological indicator of estrogen efficacy and an excellent system for studying effects of estrogen on the nervous system.

Mechanisms of estrogen action have been studied extensively since the discovery of high-affinity estrogen binding approximately 30 years ago. Molecular mechanisms of steroid hormone action have become better elucidated since the cloning of the ER and other members of the steroid hormone receptor superfamily.[24, 25] The ER is a ligand-activated transcription factor, localized within the cellular nucleus. Upon binding hormone, the protein enhances, or in some cases represses, gene expression, regulating concentrations and activities of other proteins necessary for cell survival and neural communication. As with other nuclear transcription factors, the ER is modular in structure, consisting of separate domains dedicated to binding ligand, or binding to DNA, along with regions that participate in the transactivation of target genes. Ligand binding to the ER initiates formation of receptor dimers that bind regions of chromatin-containing specific DNA sequences, known as estrogen response elements (ERE). The canonical ERE consists of the sequence GGTCANNNTGACC and is found in the upstream regulatory region of the *Xenopus* vitellogenin A2 gene. Other imperfect ERE's have been identified, sometimes consisting of multiple half sites (e.g., TGACC) such as in the chicken ovalbumin gene. More usually a dyad sequence of inverted repeats separated by three intervening nucleotides, which resembles the consensus ERE, is thought to facilitate binding of the ER dimer. The DNA-bound hormone-activated receptor associates with, and stabilizes, other proteins comprising the transcriptional complex. In concert, these proteins regulate gene expression.[24, 26, 27]

One of the best examples of a protein regulated by estrogen is the progestin receptor. Induction of PR has been used widely as an index of estrogen efficacy in many target tissues. Although the precise mechanisms governing PR concentrations are unknown, it is clear that estrogen regulates transcription of the PR gene,[28–30] presumably altering levels of the PR transcript available for translation. The precise location of the ERE(s) has not been confirmed completely, although putative sequences have been found upstream of the PR start site in the human PR gene[31] as well as within the coding region of the rabbit PR.[30] The additional possibilities of estrogen affecting message stabilization or translation or both of the PR mRNA have not been excluded. The PR also acts as a transcription factor, recognizing a sequence of DNA separate from that of an ERE. PR-regulated genes are not as well identified as those regulated by ER. Genes possesing both an ERE and a PR response element within regulatory regions may be regulated by both hormones. Estrogen regulates levels of PR, making more receptor available for enhancement of target gene expression. Interactions among ER, PR, and other transcription factors appear highly likely. Thus, synergistic actions of steroid hormones may well be mediated at the genome.

The molecular mechanisms by which estrogen modulates neuronal function are not completely understood. While estrogen induces cell proliferation in uterus, breast, and breast cancer cells, this is not a mode of action in the brain. Adult neurons are terminally differentiated cells and do not undergo the G1-S transition and replication. Directly analogous to other target tissues, however, estrogen does enhance gene expression and regulates concentrations of proteins such as the neurochemicals and receptors that ultimately mediate hormonal effects in the brain.[15]

In most instances in which estrogen acts through genomic mechanisms estrogen requires hours to yield effects. Certainly this is the case for regulation of the lordosis reflex. The behavior cannot be elicited until approximately 18 hours following exogenous hormone treatment. Indeed, the long time course of activation is consistent with the genomic actions of estrogen that are required for regulation of reproductive behavior. Early studies showed that RNA and protein synthesis inhibitors administered to ovariectomized rats just before estrogen block the ability of the hormone to induce lordosis behavior. Concomitantly, estrogen induction of PR also is obviated by synthesis blockers, demonstrating that PR concentrations in the hypothalamus are regulated via the genomic effects of estrogen.[32]

The precise effects of estrogen on brain function depend on the timing of hormone exposure. During development, estrogen guides differentiation of the brain and peripheral tissues in accordance with genetic sex. This can be shown by use of antiestrogens or, more recently, synthetic DNA that is "antisense" to ER messenger RNA (mRNA).[33] Thus, gonadal steroids present during early development permanently alter neuroanatomical organization as well as peripheral physiology and thereby determine the organism's future responses to hormones.

The rat model of sexual differentiation has revealed clearly direct relations between prenatal and perinatal hormonal milieus and the pattern of hormone secretion and steroid-dependent reproductive behaviors driven by estrogen in adulthood.[34] Early castration and replacement studies demonstrated that, for the most part, the male phenotype develops in the presence of testosterone (and estrogen), while the female phenotype depends on the relative absence of gonadal steroids in prenatal and perinatal life. The ramifications of early steroidal actions are evident morphologically in the adult brain even at the light microscopic levels. For example, there is a large nucleus present in the preoptic area of adult males (the sexually dimorphic nucleus) that is barely apparent in females.[35, 36] Even patterns of dendritic branching and synaptic spine density in the adult preoptic area are determined by hormonal exposure during crucial periods of development.[37, 38] Early sexual differentiation contributes to the many sex-specific responses activated by the gonadal steroids secreted in adulthood. Sex differences in estrogen regulation of luteinizing hormone, growth hormone-releasing factor,[39] as well as levels of PR[40, 44] and female reproductive behavior, are well-documented.

Sex-specific elicitation of female reproductive behavior is illustrative of differences in estrogen efficacy, presumably reflecting an entire sequence of events mediated by the hormone. Male rats rarely display the lordosis reflex, whereas females do so readily under proper hormonal stimulation. However, male rats can display estrogen-facilitated lordosis under some hormonal circumstances, demonstrating that the neural connections subserving lordosis are intact but are activated only under highly controlled conditions (see ref. 41 for review). The mechanisms underlying differential ability to display estrogen-facilitated lordosis behavior could be due, in part, to differences in neuroanatomical connections that mediate the behavior.[42] However, sex-related differences in estrogen action have

extensive precedents and are implicated in differential propensity toward display of the behavior.

The most parsimonious explanation for sex differences in estrogen action would be differential levels of ER available to mediate hormone action. Indeed, males have fewer ER's than females in cells in periventricular preoptic layers, medial preoptic area, and ventromedial nucleus (VMN) of the hypothalamus.[43, 44] Males also have lower levels of soluble PR in these brain regions than are observed in females.[40] Lower PR levels may be ascribed, in part, to less ER available to induce the protein. In addition, less ER is associated with hypothalamic chromatin from genetic males and females treated neonatally with androgens than occurs in phenotypical females.[45, 46] These findings are consistent with differential propensities toward display of estrogen-induced lordosis behavior. Thus, lower levels of nuclear and chromatin-associated ER may suggest less estrogen-mediated gene expression, representing one substrate for differential estrogen efficacy between males and females.

Estrogen Regulates ER and PR Messenger RNA Levels in the Hypothalamus

To ascertain if sex differences in hormone-regulated gene expression correlate with differential estrogen-dependent protein and behavioral responsivity, mRNAs for ER, PR, and proenkephalin, known to be regulated by estrogen, were chosen for study. The precise manner in which estrogen regulates levels of the ER message is not known, especially in the brain, in which levels of the protein, and mRNA, are quite low and therefore are difficult to study. In situ hybridization was chosen and modified for ultimate sensitivity in order to detect and quantify relative levels of ER mRNA in rat hypothalamus.

Estrogen down-regulates ER mRNA as a function of exogenous estrogen dose in the ventromedial and arcuate nuclei of ovariectomized females.[47] Moreover, levels of the ER mRNA remain depressed in the continued presence of the hormone.[48] Gonadectomized male and female rats were implanted with indwelling Silastic capsules containing estrogen (or cholesterol control) for two weeks to ensure that the systems were at steady state. The results showed that under the basal, gonadectomized conditions there is significantly less ER mRNA in the ventromedial and arcuate nuclei of males as compared with females. Estrogen treatment significantly reduced ER mRNA levels in the female brain, but the effect was not robust in males (Fig. 28–4).[48] These studies showed that there are sex differences in relative ER mRNA levels in hypothalamic nuclei implicated in the neural regulation of gonadal function and reproductive behavior. Indeed, these data suggest that differences in relative ER mRNA levels may be a substrate for lower levels of the ER protein and less estrogen efficacy in male hypothalamic nuclei. The functional significance of estrogen-induced down-regulation of ER mRNA in brain and other tissues is not yet known.

Differences in estrogen-regulated PR gene expression were evaluated according to the hypothesis that sex differences in PR mRNA levels might be a substrate for the differential protein concentrations.[43] Rats were gonadectomized and treated with estrogen or testosterone or left

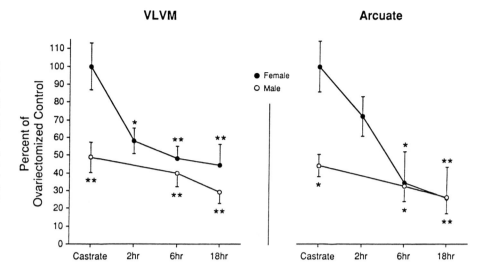

FIGURE 28–4. ER mRNA levels for male and female VLVM and arcuate hypothalamic neurons plotted as percentage of OVX control. Values reflect the mean (and SEM) for n = 4–6 rats per condition. Quantitation of grains over cells was per *Materials and Methods*.*, *P*<0.05 compared to OVX controls; **, *P*<0.01 compared to OVX controls. (From Lauber AH, Mobbs CV, Muramatsu M, Pfaff DW: Estrogen receptor mRNA expression in the rat hypothalamus as a function of genetic sex and estrogen dose. Endocrinology 129:3180–3186, 1991, © by the Endocrine Society.)

intact. Relative levels of PR mRNA were assessed in various hypothalamic nuclei using quantitative in situ hybridization. The results of these experiments are summarized in Figure 28–5. Clearly, estrogen increased relative PR mRNA levels in the VMN and arcuate nucleus of the female rats. As expected, there was no significant effect of estrogen on PR mRNA levels in female dorsomedial hypothalamic or amygdaloid nuclei, consistent with receptor levels.[49, 50] Interestingly, there were no apparent differences in basal PR mRNA levels between males and females in any brain region investigated.[51]

Estrogen failed to regulate PR message levels in the ventromedial or arcuate nuclei of males. Moreover, testosterone treatment had no apparent effect on PR mRNA levels in males. However, it was most interesting to note that levels of PR message in the ventromedial and arcuate nuclei of *intact* males were indistinguishable from levels in estrogen-stimulated females. This outcome necessitates the speculation that chronic stimulation in the male brain by testicular products may support PR message levels in males.

Taken together, these findings indicate that the sex difference in regulation of PR message levels is due to estrogen-related factors and not to mechanisms driving constitutive gene expression, because basal levels were similar between males and females. The functional importance of increased PR messenger RNA synthesis is revealed by antisense DNA experiments: Antisense to PR mRNA, when delivered to ventromedial hypothalamus, reduced female reproductive behaviors.[52] This line of experimentation overall has proved for the first time the effect of a specific transcription factor (PR) on a particular behavior.

Estrogen Regulates Levels of the Proenkephalin Message

Evidence suggests that endogenous opiates have a regulatory function in reproductive systems, especially pertaining to regulation of ovulation. The specific role of enkephalin in these systems has been elusive. Enkephalin might be implicated in regulation of lordosis behavior through delta opiate receptors, but its precise role is still under investigation. It is clear, however, that levels of this neuropeptide are under estrogenic regulation.

DuPont et al.[53] found that levels of the enkephalin neuropeptide fluctuate in accordance with the estrous cycle, peaking at proestrus when estrogen levels are highest. There are high amounts of its precursor mRNA in the ventrolateral portion of the ventromedial hypothalamus nucleus.[54] This is especially pertinent since this is the predominant nucleus controlling estrogen-regulated lordosis behavior, and this nucleus has some of the highest ER concentrations of any brain region.

Romano et al.[55] determined that estrogen stimulated a three-fold induction of proenkephalin mRNA levels in the ventrolateral ventromedial hypothalamic nucleus in hormone-treated ovariectomized rats. Further, the mRNA levels are enhanced within one hour of estrogen treatment and fall rapidly following removal of the estrogen capsule, but they can be sustained if progesterone is administered just following estrogen withdrawal.[54]

Gonadal hormone stimulation of proenkephalin message levels appears to be sex-specific, as neither estrogen nor testosterone enhances message levels in the male hypothalamus.[56] To determine if the sex difference in estrogen-regulated proenkephalin levels results from perinatal brain sexual differentiation, neonatal female rats were androgenized with exogenous testosterone and evaluated for display of lordosis and estrogen regulation of proenkephalin mRNA levels in adulthood. Female rats given testosterone immediately following birth become "defeminized" and, like genetic males, did not cycle and did not readily display lordosis in response to estrogen stimulation at maturity. The defeminized rats showed responses to estrogen that were intermediate between normal males and females. In this case, androgenized females displayed lordosis only under some conditions and estrogen induced only a modest increase in proenkephalin mRNA in the ventromedial hypothalamic nucleus. These data suggested that at least part of the sex difference in estrogen induction of proenkephalin message may be determined by hormonal events occurring during development.

The full range of factors controlling proenkephalin mRNA transcription may be revealed by in vivo promoter

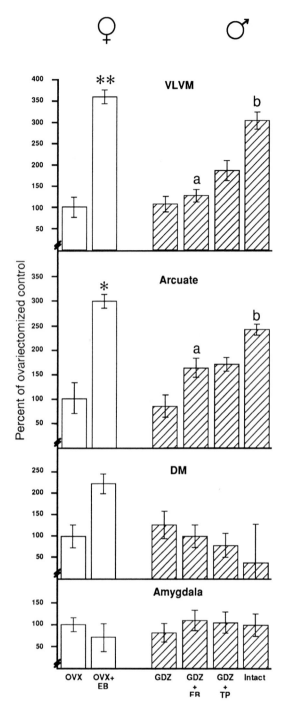

FIGURE 28–5. Mean numbers of grains per cell (± SEM) expressed as per cent of OVX control for VLVMN, DMN, arcuate and amygdaloid nuclei across sex and hormonal conditions are shown. Data show hybridization for progesterone receptor mRNA. Values which differed significantly as determined by one-way ANOVA followed by post-hoc analyses are indicated. **$P<0.01$, compared to OVX female. There was no difference between GDZ male and OVX female (Dunnett two-tailed test). *$P<0.05$ compared to OVX female. There was no difference between GDZ male and OVX female (Dunnett two-tailed t-test). [a]$P<0.05$ compared to EB female (post-hoc two-tailed t-test); [b]$P<0.05$ compared to OVX female (post-hoc two-tailed t-test). (From Lauber AH, Romano GJ, Pfaff DW: Sex difference in estradiol regulation of progestin receptor mRNA in rat mediobasal hypothalamus as demonstrated by in situ hybridization. Neuroendocrinology 53:608–613, 1991.)

analysis in the brain,[57] using a herpes-based defective neurotropic viral vector.[58] For example, using this viral vector it was seen that 2.7 kilobases (Kb) of the rat proenkephalin promoter (driving the reporter gene β-galactosidase) is sufficient for brain region–specific expression in the adult rat brain.[57]

Further studies have been conducted to assess relations between estrogen-regulated proenkephalin mRNA levels in conjunction with lordosis behavior. Ovariectomized rats were implanted with estrogen capsules of various doses and evaluated two weeks later for display of lordosis. The amount of proenkephalin mRNA was then measured in the ventromedial nuclei of the same animals. The data showed that relative levels of estrogen-stimulated proenkephalin message increased in a monotonic manner in accordance with estrogen concentration[23] (Fig. 28–6A). Further, the dose-response curves between proenkephalin and lordosis were nearly identical (Fig. 28–6B).

The parallels between estrogen induction of lordosis and proenkephalin mRNA levels are strongly suggestive of a role for enkephalin in behavior. Axons of enkephalin-containing neurons in the ventromedial nucleus project to midbrain central gray neurons,[59] and these cells may comprise part of the lordosis circuitry (see earlier discussion).

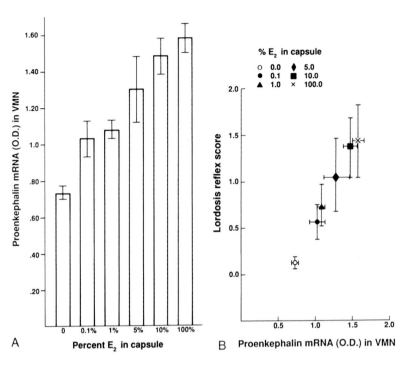

FIGURE 28–6. *A*, Effect of estradiol concentration on level of preproenkephalin mRNA in VMN. These data show the mean (and SEM) normalized O.D. values for preproenkephalin mRNA in VMN across estradiol conditions. The effect of estradiol is significant statistically (see text). The means represent values from the 5–8 animals per estradiol dose. *B*, Relationship between lordosis quotient (LQ) and preproenkephalin mRNA level in VMN across estradiol concentrations. Means (and SEM's) for LQ are plotted against preproenkephalin mRNA level in VMN at the 6 concentrations of estradiol. The systematic relationship between the two measures is clear. (From Lauber AH, Romano GJ, Mobbs CV, et al: Estradiol induction of proenkephalin messenger RNA in hypothalamus: Dose-response and relation to reproductive behavior in the female rat. Mol Brain Res 8:47–54, 1990.)

ROLES OF HYPOTHALAMIC GENE PRODUCTS WITH RESPECT TO REPRODUCTIVE BEHAVIORS

How do individual gene products expressed in hypothalamic neurons facilitate specific behaviors? Clearly these do not merely propel particular hormone-dependent reflexes all by themselves—that is the role taken by neurotransmitters in the spinal cord. Instead, the question must be formulated to see how hypothalamic gene products modulate the timing or intensity of reproductive behaviors such that their biological adaptiveness is maximized.

An obvious case is that of GnRH. This decapeptide can facilitate mating behavior[19, 20] as well as cause LH and FSH release from gonadotrophs in the anterior pituitary. It is evident that a consequence of its dual role would be to help synchronize behavioral responsiveness with ovulation. In fact, structure-function relations have been analyzed and local sites of GnRH application documented for positive behavioral effects in the female in extenso (reviewed in ref. 60). Still obscure is the functional importance of the unusual origin of GnRH neurons in the fetal olfactory placode.[61] Migrating along a scaffolding formed by neural cell adhesion molecule, GnRH neurons move from the olfactory epithelium, across the nasal septum, along the bottom of the brain to end up in the preoptic area, basal forebrain, and, in some species, anterior hypothalamus.[62] It could be that the olfactory placode origin of GnRH neurons merely speaks of the phylogenetic history of this system or that it rationalizes olfactohormonal relationships that are strong in many species. For behavioral controls, however, it is evident from work with hypophysectomized animals[20] that the deposition of this decapeptide within the central nervous system can facilitate lordosis responding. Acting as a neuromodulator, GnRH can facilitate responses to classical transmitters,[63] and based on the local application studies reviewed by Moss and Dudley,[64] these neuromodulatory actions may occur in the preoptic area, hypothalamus, or midbrain central gray.

The hypothalamic peptide oxytocin presents a subtler example. This peptide is estrogen-regulated and necessary for uterine contractions accompanying parturition and milk letdown necessary for lactation. It is entirely logical that oxytocin can facilitate maternal behavior, but it turns out that for maximum behavioral effectiveness, the assays must be conducted under conditions of mild stress.[65] Oxytocin may subserve only a limited role in facilitation of rat maternal behavior. Across a range of behavioral studies on the pharmacological actions of oxytocin, it appears that secretion of oxytocin at specific points in the central nervous system may safeguard biologically adaptive instinctive responses: It may protect them from disruption caused by mild stress.[66] With respect to female reproductive behavior, it is interesting that estrogen can induce oxytocin receptors in the ventromedial hypothalamus[67] and that oxytocin applied in that same region of the hypothalamus can facilitate reproductive behavior.[68]

The peptide product of the preproenkephalin gene (discussed earlier) presents another example of an apparent neuromodulation that, at the behavioral level, is likely to act indirectly. That is, enkephalin, acting through delta receptors can facilitate female reproductive behavior[69, 70] even though opioid peptides working through μ receptors tend to interfere with various reproductive functions. In these experiments the δ agonist was put in the lateral ventricles. During subsequent experiments designed to explicate the exact hypothalamic and limbic site of action of enkephalin (Brown et al., unpublished observations), it has become clear that one major mode of action might be to allow reproductive behavior by depressing rejection behaviors—those behaviors that are so antagonistic to the male that reproduction could not occur. In fact the very rapidity of estrogenic action on preproenkephalin mRNA suggests that the peptide product of this gene might be important for social behaviors early in a chain of events that leads ultimately to reproduction. Thus, if an opioid peptide such as enkephalin can work against those antagonistic behaviors that would prevent social contact leading to reproduction, a clear molecular mechanism would be tied to a subtle indirect behavioral step in the service of female typical behavior that allows insemination.

HYPOTHALAMIC COORDINATION OF HORMONAL AND ENVIRONMENTAL CONTROLS ON REPRODUCTIVE BEHAVIOR

Hypothalamic control over reproductive behavior by steroid hormones has permitted some of the most penetrating analyses of the biological mechanisms for behavior during the past 30 years. Nevertheless, hypothalamic regulation of reproduction cannot rely upon the steroids alone. What are the obvious biological requirements for the adaptive timing of reproduction? We emphasize here only those clear requirements that involve the CNS and assume that gametogenesis and implantation will be well managed by peripheral mechanisms. Obviously the sperm and egg need to achieve contact, thus requiring reproductive behavior. Assuming that circulating hormones are driving this behavior in order to coordinate central neural mechanisms with peripheral preparations for reproduction, nerve cells executing reproductive behavior must in addition receive inputs about the existence of the mating partner. Other permissive influences that help to guarantee the success of reproduction include adequate nutrition, adequate water and salt supplies, appropriate temperature and daylength, appropriate time of day, the existence of nesting material, and the absence of stress.

How are these biological requirements signaled to the hypothalamic "decision makers" for reproductive behavior? Of course, extrahypothalamic circuitry and standard synaptic signaling within the hypothalamus could be part of the arrangement. It is also striking, however, that transcription factors that depend upon synaptic input in hypothalamic neurons—in addition to the nuclear hormone receptors themselves—may be important. Taking examples from the liver,[71] we note that even in liver cells a combination of several liver-specific transcription factors may be required to bind to the promoters of the genes for liver-specific products. Likewise, for genes expressed in hypothalamic neurons, we may expect that, even for those promoters that contain classical steroid hormone response elements, other transcription factors binding to the promoter might signal the existence of permissive synaptic inputs. For example, the complex of proteins that bind to the κ-β sequences upstream of the preproenkephalin promoter provide an obvious opportunity for neural integration at the molecular level (Grandison et al., unpublished observations). As a broad view of biologically important molecular mechanisms in the hypothalamus, therefore, we envision that the combinatorial logic and the opportunities for synergies among transcription factors binding to hormone-responsive genes might provide opportunities for signaling those combinations of events that render the hypothalamic control of reproduction appropriate to environmental conditions.

REFERENCES

1. Sachs BD, Meisel RL: The physiology of male sexual behavior. *In* Knobil E, Neill JD (eds): The Physiology of Reproduction. New York, Raven Press, 1988, pp 1393–1486.

2. Heimer L, Larsson K: Drastic changes in the mating behavior of male rats following lesions in the junction of diencephalon and mesencephalon. Experientia 20:460–461, 1964.

3. Hart BL, Leedy MG: Neurological bases of sexual behavior: A comparative analysis. *In* Adler N, Pfaff D, Goy RW (eds): Handbook of Behavioral Neurobiology, Vol 7. New York, Plenum, 1985.

4. Kelley DB, Pfaff DW: Generalizations from comparative studies on neuroanatomical and endocrine mechanisms of sexual behavior. *In* Hutchison J (ed): Biological Determinants of Sexual Behavior. Chichester, England, Wiley, 1978, pp 225–254.

5. Giantonio GW, Lund NL, Gerall AA: Effect of diencephalic and rhinencephalic lesions on the male rat's sexual behavior. J Comp Physiol Psychol 73:38–46, 1970.

6. Schwanzel-Fukuda M, Jorgenson K, Bergen H, et al: Biology of normal LHRH neurons during and after their migration from olfactory placode. Endocr Rev 13:623–633, 1992.

7. Numan M: Maternal behavior. *In* Knobil E, Neill JD (eds): The Physiology of Reproduction (ed 3). New York, Raven Press, 1993.

8. Fleming A, Vaccarino F, Tambosso L, Chee P: Vomeronasal and olfactory system modulation of maternal behavior in the rat. Science 203:372–374, 1979.

9. Numan M, Callahan EC: The connections of the medial preoptic region and maternal behavior in the rat. Physiol Behav 25:653–665, 1980.

10. Terkel J, Bridges RS, Sawyer CH: Effects of transecting lateral neural connections of the medial preoptic area on maternal behavior in the rat: Nest building, pup retrieval and prolactin secretion. Brain Res 169:369–380, 1979.

11. Numan M, McSparren J, Numan MJ: Dorsolateral connections of the medial preoptic and maternal behavior in rats. Behav Neurosci 104:964–979, 1990.

12. Numan M, Smith HG: Maternal behavior in rats: Evidence for the involvement of preoptic projections to the ventral tegmental area. Behav Neurosci 98:712–727, 1984.

13. Morrell JI, Pfaff DW: A neuroendocrine approach to brain function: Localization of sex steroid concentrating cells in vertebrate brains. Am Zool 18:447–460, 1978.

14. Pfaff DW, Conrad LCA: Hypothalamic neuroanatomy: Steroid hormone binding and patterns of axonal projections. *In* Bourne G (ed): International Review of Cytology, Vol 54. New York, Academic Press, 1978, pp 245–265.

15. Lauber A, Pfaff DW: Estrogen regulation of mRNAs in the brain and relationship to lordosis behavior. Curr Top Neuroendocr 10:115–147, 1990.

16. Pfaff DW, Schwartz-Giblin S, McCarthy MM, Kow L-M: Cellular and molecular mechanisms of female reproductive behaviors. *In* Knobil E and Neill JD (eds): The Physiology of Reproduction (ed 2). New York, Raven Press, 1993.

17. Pfaff DW: Estrogens and Brain Function. New York, Springer-Verlag, 1980.

18. Hennessey AC, Camak L, Gordon F, Edwards DA: Connections between the pontine central gray and the ventromedial hypothalamus are essential for lordosis in female rats. Behav Neurosci 104:477–488, 1990.

19. Moss RL, McCann SM: Action of luteinizing hormone-releasing factor (LRF) in the initiation of lordosis behavior in the estrone-primed ovariectomized female rat. Neuroendocrinology 17:309–318, 1975.

20. Pfaff DW: Luteinizing hormone releasing factor (LRF) potentiates lordosis behavior in hypophysectomized ovariectomized female rats. Science 182:1148–1149, 1973.

21. Cottingham SL, Pfaff DW: Interconnectedness of steroid hormone–binding neurons: Existence and implications. Curr Top Neuroendocr 7:223–249, 1986.

22. Whalen RE: Estrogen-progesterone induction of mating in female rats. Horm Behav 5:157–162, 1974.

23. Lauber AH, Romano GJ, Mobbs CV, et al: Estradiol induction of proenkephalin messenger RNA in hypothalamus: Dose-response and relation to reproductive behavior in the female rat. Mol Brain Res 8:47–54, 1990.

24. Green S, Chambon P: The oestrogen receptor: From perception to mechanism. *In* Parker MG (ed): Nuclear Hormone Receptors. New York, Academic Press, 1991, pp 15–39.

25. Evans RM: The steroid and thyroid hormone receptor superfamily. Science 240:889–896, 1988.

26. Carson-Jurica MA, Schrader WT, O'Malley BW: Steroid receptor family: Structure and functions. Endocr Rev 11:201–220, 1990.

27. Bagchi MK, Tsai MJ, O'Malley BW, Tsai SY: Analysis of the mechanism of steroid hormone receptor dependent gene activation in cell-free systems. Endocr Rev 13:525–535, 1992.

28. Nardulli AM, Greene GL, O'Malley BW, Katzenellenbogen BS: Regulation of progesterone receptor messenger ribonucleic acid and protein levels in MCF-7 cells by estradiol: Analysis of estrogen's effect on progesterone receptor synthesis and degradation. Endocrinology 122:935–944, 1988.

29. Misrahi M, Loosfelt H, Atger M, et al: Organization of the entire rabbit progesterone receptor mRNA and of the promoter and 5′ flanking region of the gene. Nucl Acids Res 16:5459–5472, 1988.

30. Savouret JF, Bailly A, Misrahi M, et al: Characterization of the hormone responsive element involved in the regulation of the progesterone receptor gene. EMBO 10:1875–1883, 1991.

31. Kastner P, Krust A, Turcotte B, et al: Two distinct estrogen-regulated promoters generate transcripts encoding the two functionally different human progesterone receptor forms A and B. EMBO 9:1603–1614, 1990.

32. Parsons B, Pfaff DW: Progesterone receptors in CNS correlated with reproductive behavior. Curr Top Neuroendocr 5:103–140, 1985.

33. McCarthy MM, et al: Endocrinology, in press.

34. Whalen RE: Sexual differentiation: Methods, models and mechanisms. In Friedman MF, Richart RM, Van de Wiele RL (eds): Sex Differences in Behavior. New York, John Wiley & Sons, 1974, pp 467–480.

35. Gorski RA, Gordon JH, Shryne JE, Southam AM: Evidence for a morphological sex difference within the medial preoptic area of the rat brain. Brain Res 148:333, 1978.

36. Arai K, Akira M, Nishizuka M: Gonadal steroid control of synaptogenesis in the neuroendocrine brain. In Leung PCK, Armstrong DR, Ruf KB, et al (eds): Endocrinology and Physiology of Reproduction. New York, Plenum, 1987, pp 13–21.

37. Raisman G, Field PM: Sexual dimorphism in the neuropil of the preoptic area of the rat and its dependence on neonatal androgen. Brain Res 54:1, 1973.

38. Arai Y: Synaptic sexual differentiation of the neuroendocrine brain. In Ochiai K (ed): Endocrine Correlates of Reproduction. Berlin, Springer-Verlag, 1984, pp 29–40.

39. Painson JC, Thorner MO, Krieg J, Tannanbaum GS: Short term adult exposure to estradiol feminizes the male pattern of spontaneous and growth hormone–releasing factor-stimulated growth hormone secretion in the rat. Endocrinology 130:511–519, 1992.

40. Brown TJ, Clark AS, MacLusky NJ: Regional sex differences in progestin receptor induction in the rat hypothalamus: Effects of various doses of estradiol benzoate. J Neurosci 7:2529–2536, 1987.

41. Blaustein JD, Olster DH: Gonadal steroid hormone receptors and social behaviors. In Balthazart J (ed): Molecular and Cellular Basis of Social Behavior in Vertebrates. Advances in Comparative and Environmental Physiology, Vol 3. Berlin, Springer-Verlag, 1989, pp 31–104.

42. Yamanouchi K, Arai Y: Presence of a neural mechanism for the expression of female sexual behaviors in the male rat brain. Neuroendocrinology 40:393–397, 1985.

43. Brown TJ, Hochberg RB, Zielinski JE, MacLusky NJ: Regional sex differences in cell nuclear estrogen binding capacity in the rat hypothalamus and preoptic area. Endocrinology 123:1761–1770, 1988.

44. Brown TJ, MacLusky NJ, Shanabrough M, Naftolin F: Comparison of age and sex-related changes in cell nuclear estrogen–binding capacity and progestin receptor induction in the rat brain. Endocrinology 126:2865–2872, 1990.

45. Whalen RE, Olsen KL: Chromatin binding of estradiol in the hypothalamus and cortex of male and female rats. Brain Res 152:121–131, 1978.

46. Olsen KL, Whalen RE: Sexual differentiation of the brain: Effects on mating behavior and 3H-estradiol binding by hypothalamic chromatin rats. Biol Reprod 22:1068–1072, 1980.

47. Lauber AH, Romano GJ, Mobbs CV, Pfaff DW: Estradiol regulation of estrogen receptor mRNA in rat mediobasal hypothalamus: An in situ hybridization study. J Neuroendocr 2:605–611, 1990.

48. Lauber AH, Mobbs CV, Muramatsu M, Pfaff DW: Estrogen receptor mRNA expression in the rat hypothalamus as a function of genetic sex and estrogen dose. Endocrinology 129:3180–3186, 1991.

49. Parsons B, Rainbow TC, Pfaff DW, McEwen BS: Progestin receptor levels in rat hypothalamic and limbic nuclei. J Neurosci 2:1446–1452, 1982.

50. Romano GJ, Krust A, Pfaff DW: Expression and estrogen regulation of progesterone receptor mRNA in neurons of the mediobasal hypothalamus: An in situ hybridization study. Mol Endocr 3:1295–1300, 1989.

51. Lauber AH, Romano GJ, Pfaff DW: Sex difference in estradiol regulation of progestin receptor mRNA in rat mediobasal hypothalamus as demonstrated by in situ hybridization. Neuroendocrinology 53:608–613, 1991.

52. Ogawa et al., submitted, 1993.

53. DuPont A, Bardin N, Cusan L, et al: β-endorphin and metenkephalins: Their distribution, modulation by estrogens and haloperidol and role in neuroendocrine control. Fed Proc 39:2544–2550, 1980.

54. Romano GJ, Mobbs CV, Howells RD, Pfaff DW: Estrogen regulation of proenkephalin gene expression in the ventromedial hypothalamus of the rat: Temporal qualities and synergy with progesterone. Mol Brain Res 5:51–58, 1989.

55. Romano GJ, Harlan RE, Shivers BD, et al: Estrogen increases proenkephalin messenger ribonucleic acid levels in the ventromedial hypothalamus of the rat. Mol Endocr 2:1320–1328, 1988.

56. Romano GJ, Mobbs CV, Lauber AH, et al: Differential regulation of proenkephalin gene expression by estrogen in the ventromedial hypothalamus of male and female rats: Implications for the molecular basis of a sexually differentiated behavior. Brain Res 536:63–68, 1990.

57. Kaplitt MG, Lipworth L, Rabkin SD, Pfaff DW: In vivo analysis of the rat preproenkephalin promoter using an HSV defective viral vector. Soc Neurosci Abstr 18:588 (#254.5), 1992.

58. Kaplitt MG, Pfaus JG, Kleopoulos SP, et al: Expression of a functional foreign gene in adult mammalian brain following in vivo transfer via a herpes simplex virus type 1 defective viral vector. Mol Cell Neurosci 2:320–330, 1991.

59. Yamano M, Inagaki S, Kito S, et al: Enkephalinergic projection from the ventromedial hypothalamic nucleus to the midbrain central gray matter in the rat: An immunocytochemical analysis. Brain Res 398:337–344, 1986.

60. Moss RL, Dudley CA, Gosnell BA: Behavior and the hypothalamus. In DeGroot LJ (ed): Endocrinology (ed 2). Philadelphia, W. B. Saunders Company, 1989, pp 254–263.

61. Schwanzel-Fukuda M, Pfaff DW: Origin of luteinizing hormone-releasing hormone neurons. Nature 338:161–164, 1989.

62. Schwanzel-Fukuda M, Abraham S, Crossin KL, et al: Immunocytochemical demonstration of neural cell adhesion molecule along the migration route of luteinizing hormone-releasing hormone neurons in mice. J Comp Neurol 321:1–18, 1992.

63. Pan J-T, Kow L-M, Kendall DA, et al: Electrophysiological test of an amphiphilic β-structure in LHRH action. Mol Cell Endocr 48:161–166, 1986.

64. Moss RL, Dudley CA: Luteinizing hormone-releasing hormone (LHRH): A role in extrapituitary function. In Barker JL, Smith TG (eds): The Role of Peptides in Neuronal Function. New York, Marcel Dekker, 1980, pp 456–478.

65. Fahrbach SE, Morrell JI, Pfaff DW: Effect of varying the duration of pre-test cage habituation on oxytocin induction of short-latency maternal behavior. Physiol Behav 37:135–139, 1986.

66. McCarthy MM, Chung SK, Ogawa S, et al: Behavioral effects of oxytocin: Is there a unifying principle? In Jard S, Jamison R (eds): Vasopressin. Collogue INSERM, John Libbey Eurotext Ltd, 1991, pp 195–212.

67. DeKloet ER, Voorhees DAM, Boschma Y, Elands J: Estradiol modulates density of putative "oxytocin receptors" in discrete rat brain regions. Neuroendocrinology 44:415–421, 1986.

68. Schumacher M, Coirini H, Pfaff DW, McEwen BS: Behavioral effects of progesterone associated with rapid modulation of oxytocin receptors. Science 250:691–694, 1990.

69. Pfaus JG, Gorzalka BB: Selective activation of opioid receptors differentially affects lordosis behavior in female rats. Peptides 8:309–317, 1987.

70. Pfaus JG, Pfaff DW: μ-, δ-, and k-opioid receptor agonists selectively modulate sexual behaviors in the female rat: Differential dependence on progesterone. Horm Behav 26:457–473, 1992.

71. Xanthopoulos KG, Mirkovitch J, Becker T, et al: Cell-specific transcriptional control of the mouse DNA binding protein mC/EBP. PNAS 86:4117–4121, 1989.

29

Tumor Mass Effects of Lesions in the Hypothalamus and Pituitary

SHLOMO MELMED

Both neoplastic and non-neoplastic sellar masses may arise from regions within and adjacent to the hypothalamus and pituitary. They manifest either as a result of their local pressure effects on surrounding vital structures or as a result of distant metabolic or hormonal derangements. Rarely, sellar masses may be the presenting feature of a previously undiagnosed systemic disorder.

This chapter outlines the natural history and local and metabolic sequelae of mass lesions arising in the parasellar region; the characteristics of the specific lesions causing these sequelae are described. Although the functional anatomy of the hypothalamic regions has been well demarcated (see Ch. 8), the relatively close contiguity of these vital centers results in manifestations of distant metabolic derangements that are not necessarily dependent on the nature, or even the exact localization, of the parasellar mass lesion. In fact, similar hypothalamic "syndromes" may be caused by a large number of different pathological processes, all of which arise in the general parasellar region.[1-3] Consequently, the natural history and long-term prognosis of a hypothalamic mass is important in managing the specific lesion, whose exact microanatomical localization in and of itself may not necessarily be clinically precise.

Natural History of a Pituitary or Parasellar Mass

Prior to the advent of sensitive pituitary imaging techniques, a wide spectrum of clinical sequelae were evident from the effects of an enlarging mass arising from within the pituitary or its adjacent structures (Table 29–1). Although it is today relatively uncommon for such a mass to be invasive at the time of diagnosis, the relative subtlety of clinical features may delay the anatomical imaging of such a mass.

Most pituitary and hypothalamic masses are benign neoplasms, with the very rare occurrence of a true primary malignancy with proved distant metastases. Nevertheless, these benign lesions may be aggressively invasive locally into contiguous structures resulting in clinical features that depend on the anatomical location of the impinging mass. Hemorrhage and infarction, which may often be coincidental, may occur in these masses, especially during pregnancy, when the normal pituitary and its surrounding soft tissue structures are edematous and swollen. Diabetes mellitus and hypertension have also been associated with pituitary infarction. Hemorrhage and infarction of the pituitary and hypothalamus are true endocrine emergencies. Acute pituitary failure may lead to hypoglycemia, hypothermia, hypotension, apoplexy, and death.

Clearly, many pituitary masses undergo silent infarction as evidenced by histological proof of old infarct tissue in patients with otherwise normal pituitary function. Large infarcts may lead to development of a partial or totally empty pituitary sella. Most of these patients exhibit normal pituitary reserve, implying that the surrounding rim of pituitary tissue is fully functional. Large cysts associated with the hypothalamic-pituitary unit will also give the radiological appearance of an empty sella. Rarely, functional pituitary adenomas may arise within the remnant pituitary tissue, and these tumors, although their presence is indicated by classical endocrine hyperactivity, may not be visible by sensitive magnetic resonance imaging (MRI) (i.e., <2 mm in diameter). Acute or chronic infection with abscess formation may be an extremely rare occurrence in the pituitary or hypothalamic mass. Finally, many of these mass lesions present with clinically evident hormonal derangements caused by hormone hypersecretion or, more commonly, by failure of pituitary trophic hormone reserve.

TABLE 29–1. COMPLICATIONS OF A PITUITARY OR PARASELLAR MASS

Local invasion
Malignant transformation
Hemorrhage
Infarction
Empty sella
Infection (abscess)
Hormonal derangement

Pituitary hormone hyposecretion may be due to the direct pressure effects of the expanding mass on the anterior pituitary hormone–secreting cells. Alternatively, parasellar pressure effects may directly attenuate synthesis or secretion of hypothalamic hormones, with resultant pituitary failure. In contrast, a not uncommon association of hypothalamic masses is overproduction of a specific hypothalamic hormone with resultant hyperfunctioning of a specific hypothalamic-pituitary-target hormone axis.

The important diagnostic dilemma facing the clinician is to effectively distinguish an adenoma arising from the anterior pituitary gland from other parasellar masses. The compelling reason for this diagnosis is the fact that the management and prognosis of true anterior pituitary neoplasms differ so markedly from those of other nonpituitary masses. Most masses arising from within the sella are benign hormonally functional or nonfunctional adenomas, with relatively good prognosis after appropriate therapy. Their invasiveness is relatively limited and only rarely will local vital structures be compromised. In contrast, parasellar masses arising from structures contiguous with the pituitary are often malignant or invasive and usually portend a less favorable prognosis.

LOCAL MASS EFFECTS OF AN ENLARGING SELLAR MASS

The anatomical location of the pituitary sella results in several possible local functional derangements caused by a mass in the midline region of the base of the brain. The intrasellar mass may invade either soft tissue or bony surrounding structures. Because of its anatomical location, the dorsal roof of the sella presents the least resistance to expansion from within the confines of the bony sella. Nevertheless, both suprasellar and parasellar invasion inexorably occurs with an enlarging mass, with resultant clinical manifestations (Table 29–2).

GENERAL EFFECTS. Headaches are common features of intrasellar tumors, even without demonstratable suprasellar extension. Because of the confined nature of the pituitary gland within the sella, small changes in the intrasellar pressure presumably caused by a microadenoma are sufficient to increase pressure and stretching of the dural plate with resultant headache. Complaints of headache do not appear to correlate with the size of the adenoma or the presence of suprasellar extension.[4] In fact, relatively minor distortions of the sellar diaphragm or dural impingement are accompanied by persistent headache. Furthermore, successful medical management of small functional pituitary tumors with bromocriptine or octreotide is often accompanied by a remarkable disappearance of headache.

OPTIC TRACT. Pressure on the optic chiasm as a result of upward compression may result in visual defects ranging from small field defects to blindness.[5] The advent and refinement of sensitive pituitary imaging techniques during the past decade have resulted in earlier diagnosis of parasellar masses than previously feasible. Therefore, the incidence of optic tract compression by a large mass is certainly diminishing. Nevertheless, through 1972, 40 per cent of 1000 patients with pituitary tumors had either bitemporal hemianopsia or superior bitemporal defects.[5] One third of patients had evidence of blindness, scotomas, or other visual disturbances.[5]

Reproducible assessment of visual fields using perimetry techniques should be performed on all patients with an intra- or extrapituitary mass lesion. Loss of red perception appears to be an early sign of optic tract pressure, and red colored visual signals should preferably be utilized.[6] Anterior frontal mass lesions may cause unilateral visual loss, while chiasmic or posterior pressure by the mass will usually result in bilateral defects. Classically, elevation and distortion of the optic chiasm results in bitemporal hemianopsia, while dorsal chiasmic compression also results in field cuts. Homonymous hemianopsias may result from tumor or vascular pressure on the regions of the optic tract lying anterior to the chiasm. Transient visual disorders, asymmetrical deficits, or enlargement of the blind spot may all indicate the presence of a parasellar mass. If the mass causes an internal hydrocephalus by obstructing CSF flow, secondary visual disturbances and papilledema may ensue.

PITUITARY STALK. Compression of the stalk by an expanding intrasellar or parasellar mass may result in pituitary failure caused by encroachment of the portal vessels that normally provide pituitary access to the hypothalamic hormones. Stalk compression usually leads to hyperprolactinemia and failure of the other pituitary trophic hormones.

CAVERNOUS SINUS. Lateral invasion of pituitary lesions or ventrolateral encroachment by parasellar or hypothalamic masses may impinge upon the cavernous sinus and its neural contents. This invasion may lead to lesions of the third, fourth, and sixth cranial nerves as well as the ophthalmic and maxillary branches of the fifth cranial nerve. Varying degrees of diplopia, ptosis, ophthalmoplegia, and decreased facial sensation occur, depending on the extent of the neural involvement by the cavernous sinus mass.

SPHENOID SINUS. Dorsal extension into the sphenoid sinus implies that the parasellar mass has already eroded the bony sellar floor. Although no vital structures are located in the sinus, aggressive tumors may invade the roof of the palate and cause severe nasopharyngeal obstruction, infection, and even CSF leakage.

TABLE 29–2. LOCAL NEUROLOGICAL EFFECTS OF AN IMPINGING PITUITARY OR HYPOTHALAMIC MASS

IMPACTED STRUCTURE	CLINICAL EFFECT
Optic tract	Loss of red perception, bitemporal hemianopsia, superior or bitemporal field defect, scotoma, blindness
Hypothalamus	Temperature dysregulation, appetite disorders, obesity, thirst disorders, diabetes insipidus, sleep disorders, behavioral dysfunction, autonomic nervous system dysfunction
Cavernous sinus	Ptosis, diplopia, ophthalmoplegia, facial numbness
Temporal lobe	Uncinate seizures
Frontal lobe	Personality disorder, anosmia
Central	Headache, hydrocephalus, psychosis, dementia, laughing seizures

BRAIN. Both the temporal and frontal brain lobes may be invaded by the expanding parasellar mass. Uncinate seizures, personality disorders, and anosmia may result from localized tumor involvement.

METABOLIC SEQUELAE OF HYPOTHALAMIC LESIONS

In addition to the anatomical lesions caused by the expanding mass just described, direct hypothalamic involvement of the encroaching mass may lead to important non-endocrine sequelae[7] (Table 29–3). Clinical features associated with hypothalamic masses depend to a large extent on the site of the lesion rather than the nature of the pathological process. The enlarging hypothalamic mass, regardless of its etiology, will usually result in local pressure effects, including headaches and recurrent vomiting with or without associated extrapyramidal or pyramidal tract involvement. Common metabolic clinical sequelae, which occur in about one third of these patients, include precocious puberty or hypogonadism, diabetes insipidus, sleep disturbances, dysthermia, and appetite disorders (Table 29–3). Because of the very close microanatomic contiguity of several highly specialized hypothalamic cells, precise site-function effects of an expanding mass are rarely documented. Most patients therefore exhibit a spectrum of metabolic sequelae that occur regardless of the etiology or site of the pathological process.

Temperature Dysregulation

Both peripheral and central inputs control body temperature.[8] Receptors on the skin and several internal organs sense temperature changes, while central temperature-sensitive neurons are found in the anterior hypothalamic nuclei. The latter neurons transduce temperature changes to subserve changes in body temperature, cardiovascular function, and hormonal regulation. Body temperature is maintained within narrow limits, and the hypothalamus oversees a net balance of heat generated by metabolic activity and by external sources, with heat lost to the environment. Although injection of a number of neuropeptides has been shown to result in increased or decreased body heat, none has been determined as the mediator of body temperature control.

Table 29–3. METABOLIC SEQUELAE OF HYPOTHALAMIC MASS LESIONS

Temperature dysregulation	Sleep disorders
Hyperthermia	Reversal of sleep-wake cycle
Hypothermia	Akinetic mutism
Appetite disorders	Somnolence and coma
Obesity	Behavioral dysfunction
Hyperphagia	Hyperkinesis
Anorexia and emaciation	Rage
Aphagia	Autonomic dysfunction
Thirst disorders	Cardiac arrhythmias
Adipsia	Loss of sphincter control
Compulsive drinking	Cardiac failure
Hypernatremia	

Adapted from Martin JB, Reichlin S: Clinical Approach to Hypothalamic Pituitary Disease in Clinical Neuroendocrinology. Philadelphia, F.A. Davis, 1987.

HYPERTHERMIA. Lesions involving the anterior hypothalamus and its preoptic area cause paradoxical vasoconstriction, tachycardia, and hyperthermia. Chronic hyperthermia typically is associated with cold clammy skin and few of the classical physical signs of fever. This disorder may often be transient, lasting for only a few days, or may be sporadic.[9] Acute hyperthermia, presumably due to loss of heat-dissipating mechanisms in the face of ongoing heat generation, is usually due to a hypothalamic hemorrhagic insult. The malignant hyperthermia syndrome occurs postoperatively in patients harboring a skeletal muscle defect leading to hypersensitivity to muscle relaxants or neuroleptics.[10] Although hypothalamic dysregulation is probably not a major determinant of its etiology, an impairment of hypothalamic heat dissipation mechanisms has been implicated in some patients. Prolonged and sustained hyperthermia is probably not associated with hypothalamic disease. Poikilothermia, in which body temperature parallels that of the environment, is occasionally associated with the presence of hypothalamic mass lesions.

HYPOTHERMIA. Central disorders of thermoregulation leading to hypothermia occur after damage to the posterior hypothalamic nuclei by neoplastic, infectious, vascular, or granulomatous processes. Metabolic disturbances, especially hypoglycemia, and consumption of alcohol and barbiturates may lead to intracellular glucopenia and hypothermia.[11] Defective central thermoregulation may also occur with aging and in patients with anorexia nervosa. These conditions may cause either an altered set-point of normal temperature or impaired heat production. The *periodic hypothermia syndrome* may present with episodic attacks of icy coldness with rectal temperatures below 30°C, accompanying sweating, vasodilation, vomiting, and bradycardia.[12] Most of these patients have been shown to have agenesis of the corpus callosum, and rarely the syndrome is accompanied by signs of diabetes insipidus and growth hormone deficiency.

Appetite Disorders

The metabolic balance of food intake with heat and energy output is controlled by the hypothalamus.[13] Several hormones including insulin, cholecystokinin, glucagon, thyrotropin-releasing hormone, and other pancreatic peptides have been proposed as satiety factors. The precise endocrine regulation of food intake, however, remains elusive. Although compulsive eating is a recognized clinical entity associated with several nonspecific brain disorders, true hyperphagia has been well documented with hypothalamic lesions.[14]

HYPERPHAGIA AND OBESITY. Unopposed eating has been associated with lesions of the ventromedial hypothalamus leading to unopposed activity of a feeding "nucleus." Cells in this region also may have a "glucostat" function, further contributing to the metabolic control exerted by the hypothalamus. Hypothalamic damage is commonly associated with hypogonadism, hyperphagia, and resultant obesity.[15] Antisocial rage behavior and inappropriate aggression often accompany hypothalamic obesity. Although hypothalamic hypogonadism probably due to defective gonadotropin-releasing hormone (GnRH) synthesis is often associated with hyperphagia and obesity, the two conditions may occur independently of each other. Diabetes insipidus may also be frequently encountered with hyperphagia, probably attesting to involvement of the hypothalamic median eminence by the causative mass lesion leading to loss of antidiuretic hormone (ADH)-producing neural bodies.[16] The common causes of hypothalamic obesity include solid tumors (especially craniopharyngiomas), trauma or surgical damage, and inflammatory disorders. Associated gonadal failure and diabetes insipidus occur in about half of all patients.[16]

ANOREXIA AND APHAGIA. Lesions of the hypothalamus may in fact also lead to increasing anorexia, aphagia, and even death by inanition.[17] In the *diencephalic syndrome of infancy,* usually caused by a hypothalamic glioma, progressive emaciation and growth failure occur despite apparently normal food intake. Although these infants are alert and often euphoric, increasing intracranial pressure and almost total loss of body fat result in early death[18] (Table 29–4).

Thirst Disorders

Regulation of water intake is mediated by central osmoreceptors situated in the preoptic areas of the hypothalamus.[19] Lesions of the hypothalamus, including craniopharyngiomas, granulomas, germinomas, optic nerve gliomas, and large cysts, may lead to impaired thirst regulation with resultant marked perturbations in serum sodium levels.[20] The *cerebral salt retention syndrome* consists of hypodipsia and hypernatremia associated with normal extracellular fluid volume, normal blood pressure, and intact renal function.[21] These patients appear to respond to administered ADH with an increase in urine osmolarity, suggesting that partial diabetes insipidus may also be a component of the syndrome. Serum sodium levels may rise to over 160 mEq/L, with resultant weakness, muscle cramps, and irritability leading to eventual coma. Clinically, many of these patients also exhibit signs of concomitant pituitary failure or obesity or both.[22]

Sleep Disorders

The hypothalamus plays a central mediating role in regulating the rhythm of the sleep cycle. Classically, hypotha-

TABLE 29–4. CLINICAL FEATURES OF DIENCEPHALIC SYNDROME OF INFANCY

Emaciation
Endocrine dysfunction
Alertness and hyperkinesis
Vomiting
Euphoria
Pallor
Nystagmus and optic atrophy
Hydrocephalus
Tremor and sweating
Large hands/feet
Large genitalia
Polyuria
Papilledema

Adapted from Burr IM, Slonim AE, Danisk RK et al: Diencephalic syndrome revisited. J Pediatr 88:439–444, 1976.

lamic inflammatory processes and slow-growing masses are associated with increased somnolence. About a quarter of patients with hypothalamic tumors exhibit some degree of increased drowsiness, often associated with obesity.[23] Posterior hypothalamic lesions leading to somnolence are also associated with hypothermia and emotional irritability.[24] In contrast, hyposomnia or insomnia are relatively infrequently encountered in patients harboring hypothalamic lesions. Disruption of the night-day sleep cycle with nocturnal hyposomnia and daytime drowsiness has been documented in patients with cystic hypothalamic lesions.[25]

Behavioral Dysfunction

Although central behavioral control is highly complex, with supratentorial, limbic, and hypothalamic components, the hypothalamus functions to integrate appropriate emotional expression. Rage, aggression, labile emotions, and destructive antisocial behavior are hallmarks of the wide spectrum of behavioral disorders, associated especially with lesions impinging on the ventromedial nuclei of the hypothalamus.[26] Rarely a functional hypersexual activity has been reported,[27] with compulsive masturbation, hyperphagia, and hallucinations. However, most sexual dysfunction associated with hypothalamic disease is hypogonadal. Laughing seizures, diencephalic epilepsy, and classical epileptic seizures are rarely encountered and may occur in children with hypothalamic hamartomas or tumors impinging on the floor of the third ventricle.

Autonomic Dysfunction

Sympathetic nervous system activation, associated with elevated epinephrine and norepinephrine levels, hypercortisolemia, and vagal activation may result from lesions involving central hypothalamic nuclear bodies.[27] Signs of autonomic dysfunction include reduced threshold for cardiac arrhythmias, hypertension, gastric erosions and hemorrhage, and rarely acute pulmonary edema.

Functional Hypothalamic Syndromes

These conditions are not associated with specific hypothalamic or pituitary mass lesions but are clearly caused by deranged hypothalamic function or regulatory disorder.

LAURENCE-MOON-BARDET-BIEDL SYNDROME. This autosomal recessive syndrome consists of obesity, pigmentary retinopathy, mental retardation, and hypogonadism. Most of these patients also have an extra digit. Decreased visual acuity and progressive night blindness culminate in blindness in most afflicted individuals before the age of 30.[28]

SEPTO-OPTIC PITUITARY DYSPLASIA. Dysgenesis of the septum pellucidum or corpus callosum may lead to hypothalamic dysfunction and pituitary failure; the syndrome consists of cleft palate, ear deformities, syndactyly, hypertelorism, optic atrophy, micropenis, and anosmia. These children typically have short stature because of growth hormone deficiency, diabetes insipidus, and less commonly thyroid dysfunction.[29]

PRADER-WILLI SYNDROME. This relatively common syndrome, occurring in about 1:25,000 live births, is associated with a defect on chromosome 15. It consists of hyperphagia, obesity, short stature, mental retardation, and hypogonadism.[30] Neonatal muscle hypotonia is a common early sign and is often associated with prematurity or low birth weight. Varied somatic abnormalities, including cranial structure defects, hypertelorism, micrognathism, clinodactyly, palate defects, and small hands and feet may occur.[14] Morbid obesity, mental retardation, and hypogonadism invariably are present. Because the pituitary responses to dynamic testing are usually intact, hypothalamic dysfunction has been implicated in the pathogenesis of the pituitary failure.

PARASELLAR MASSES (Table 29–5)

RATHKE'S CYST. During early embryogenesis, the anterior and intermediate lobes of the pituitary gland arise from Rathke's pouch. If the pouch fails to obliterate, cystic remnants remain at the interface between the anterior and posterior pituitary lobes. These small cysts (<5 mm) are found in about 20 per cent of pituitary glands at autopsy.[31] Occasionally a pituitary adenoma may also contain small cleft cysts.[32] The imaging of these cysts on MRI reveals hyperdense or hypodense masses on either T1 or T2 images. CT scan reveals the presence of homogenous hypodense areas that may allow differentiation from pituitary adenomas.[33] Other sellar cysts include arachnoid, epidermoid, and dermoid cysts. Although these lesions are seen mainly in the cerebellopontine angle, they may also occur in the suprasellar region. Clinical features of compression include internal hydrocephalus visual disturbances and rarely growth hormone or ACTH deficiency.[34, 35] Rarely, a squamous cell carcinoma may develop in the cyst.[36]

TABLE 29–5. PITUITARY AND NONPITUITARY SELLAR MASSES

Cysts
  Rathke's
  Arachnoid
  Epidermoid
  Dermoid
Tumors
  Hormone-secreting or nonfunctional pituitary
    adenoma
  Granular cell tumor
  Craniopharyngioma
  Chordoma
  Meningioma
  Sarcomas
  Glioma
  Schwannoma
  Germ cell tumor
  Vascular tumor
  Solid or hematological metastases
Malformation and hamartomas
  Ectopic pituitary, neurohypophyseal, or salivary tissue
  Hypothalamic hamartoma
  Gangliocytoma
Miscellaneous lesions
  Aneurysms
  Lymphocytic hypophysitis
  Infections
  Sarcoidosis
  Giant cell granuloma
  Langerhan's histiocytosis

GRANULAR CELL TUMORS. Pituitary choristomas, or schwannomas, usually present only after the age of 20 and are probably acquired lesions.[37, 38] Their abundant cytoplasmic granules do not contain any of the known pituitary hormones, nor are these tumors associated with endocrine syndromes. However, several pituitary adenomas have been coincidentally associated with these tumors.

CHORDOMAS. These midline tumors arise from remnants of the notochord, are slow growing and locally invasive, and may metastasize.[39–41] Most arise from the vertebrae while about one third involve the clivus region. Characteristically, they contain a mucin-rich matrix that allows for histological diagnosis by fine-needle aspiration. On imaging, the tissue mass is associated with osteolytic bony erosion and calcification. Nasopharyngeal obstruction may rarely occur, in addition to the more commonly encountered headaches and asymmetrical visual disturbances. After surgical excision, local invasion and recurrence commonly occur, with mean patient survival of about five years. Rarely, chordomas become sarcomatous, with an aggressive natural history.

CRANIOPHARYNGIOMAS. This common parasellar tumor constitutes about 3 per cent of all intracranial tumors and up to 10 per cent of childhood brain tumors.[42] Although the tumor may present at any age, it is commonly diagnosed during childhood and adolescence. The mass may arise from embryonic squamous remnants of Rathke's pouch extending dorsally toward the diencephalon. These tumors may be large (>10 cm in diameter) and invade the third ventricle and associated brain structures. About two thirds arise from within the sella, while the remaining tumors arise from cell rests situated in the parasellar region. The cystic mass is usually filled with cholesterol-rich viscous fluid, and calcification may be present. Histology shows these tumors as comprising two cell populations: lining the cyst is a squamous epithelium containing islands characterized by columnar cells; a mixed inflammatory reaction may also occur with calcification. Although craniopharyngiomas may be quite large and may obstruct CSF flow, they rarely undergo malignant transformation.[43] Interestingly, cyst fluid contains immunoreactive hCG, which may actually leak into the CSF. Features of increased intracranial pressure, including headache, projectile vomiting, papilledema, and somnolence are usually encountered in children. Only about one third of patients are over 40 years of age, and they commonly present with asymmetrical visual field damage.

On imaging, most children and about half of all adults have a characteristic flocculent or convex calcification pattern of the tumor. Rarely, however, pituitary adenomas, other parasellar tumors, and even vascular lesions may be calcified.

The endocrine manifestations of craniopharyngioma usually result from partial or complete pituitary deficiency. Growth hormone deficiency, with resultant short stature and diabetes insipidus, and gonadal failure are common. Compression of the pituitary stalk or damage to the dopaminergic neurons in the hypothalamus results in hyperprolactinemia. This latter feature is especially important in the differential diagnosis of prolactinoma. The management of these common latter adenomas differs markedly from that of a craniopharyngioma, and careful imaging techniques may not easily distinguish the two lesions.[44] Certainly, a highly asymmetrical mass (especially with preferential posterior or dorsal extension) that does not shrink on bromocriptine therapy should arouse suspicion of craniopharyngioma. The hyperprolactinemia associated with a craniopharyngioma will also respond quite effectively to bromocriptine. This favorable biochemical response to the dopamine agonist therefore does not rule out the presence of a craniopharyngioma. Thus, craniopharyngioma may mimic a prolactinoma in terms of intrapituitary imaging, presence of hyperprolactinemia, and biochemical response to bromocriptine.

The treatment of these lesions is radical surgery, radiotherapy, or a combination of these modalities. In selected centers, stereotactic irradiation of the mass has been performed with some success. Nevertheless, regardless of which form of therapy is chosen, the ablation of the mass invariably results in anterior and/or posterior pituitary hormone deficits. Postoperative recurrence may occur in about a fifth of patients who undergo radical surgical excision,[47] while no appreciable difference is noted in the outcome in those who undergo a subtotal surgical excision followed by radiotherapy.[45, 46] The presence of pure papillary squamous cellular elements may portend a higher surgical recurrence rate.[47] The long-term effects of childhood irradiation for these tumors are considered elsewhere (Ch. 32).

MENINGIOMAS. Meningiomas account for about one quarter of all intracranial tumors.[48] These tumors arise from arachnoid and meningioendothelial cells, and those occurring in the sellar and parasellar region account for only about one fifth of all meningiomas.[49] They are usually well circumscribed and do not achieve the size of craniopharyngiomas. Suprasellar meningiomas may invade the pituitary ventrally, while intrasellar tumor origins are extremely rare. Several patients with functional pituitary adenomas have also been described who harbored coincidental parasellar meningiomas.[50] These tumors are not hormonally active and they usually present with local mass effects including headache and visual disturbances. Diagnosis by imaging is difficult because the differential radiological diagnosis of a suprasellar meningioma with ventral extension from a pituitary adenoma with dorsal extension may be difficult. Improved MRI techniques have been used in attempts to distinguish the borders of meningiomas from adenomas, but the radiological diagnosis remains difficult.[51] Because of their rich vascularization, these tumors pose an increased intraoperative risk that results in a higher surgical mortality rate than usually encountered for pituitary tumor resection.[52]

GLIOMAS. Optic gliomas and low-grade astrocytomas present with optic atrophy, papilledema, visual loss, and pituitary failure in children; in adults they may be more aggressively invasive. Most of these tumors actually arise from within the optic chiasm or optic tracts, and less than one third are intraorbital.[53, 54] Von Recklinghausen's disease is present in about one third of all patients with these tumors. Occasionally, these tumors may actually accompany growth retardation and delayed or precocious puberty,[55] and some may be malignant.[56] Mass effects include visual field disturbances, diencephalic syndrome, diabetes insipidus, and hydrocephalus.[57] Gliomas arising within the pituitary sella are exceedingly rare, and if present may be associated with hyperprolactinemia and should be considered as an uncommon mimicker of a prolactin-secreting pituitary adenoma. The important distinguishing features include the young age of these patients (80 per cent <10 years old), relatively intact pituitary function, gross visual disturbances, and imaging localization of the mass.

HYPOTHALAMIC MASSES. Hypothalamic hamartomas are benign tumors composed of a mixture of neurons, astrocytes, and oligodenrocytes. These cell types are organized in varying degrees of differentiation, and they may express peptides released from the hypothalamus. Most commonly these tumors occur before the age of two years and have been shown to express GnRH with associated precocious puberty.[58] In those tumors in which GnRH immunoreactivity could not be demonstrated, a hypothalamic dysfunction was postulated as causing the precocious puberty because injection of GnRH results in a pubertal gonadotrophin response.[59] Most of these patients have psychomotor delay and seizures. Curiously, these tumors may also be associated with laughing seizures, emotional lability, and rage.[60–62] The Pallister-Hall syndrome consists of a hypothalamic hamartoblastoma; abnormalities of the craniofacial area, heart, kidneys, and lungs; imperforate anus; and hypopituitarism.[63, 64] Although surgical excision was usually advocated for hamartomas, long-acting GnRH analogues have effectively been used to down-regulate gonadotropin secretion and control precocious puberty. The hypothalamic hamartomas are slow-growing tumors and are rarely invasive. In contrast, gangliocytomas arising in the hypothalamic or intrasellar area do grow progressively. These tumors may be associated with pituitary tumors, and ganglion cells present with the pituitary adenoma may stain positively for hormones released from the hypothalamus. Although MRI distinction may be difficult,[65] when these tumors occur in association with concurrent pituitary adenomas, it has been tempting to speculate that the hypothalamic hormone expressed by the tumor is implicated in the pathogenesis of the pituitary adenoma. In fact, besides GnRH, these tumors have been shown to express growth hormone–releasing hormone (GHRH)[66–71] and corticotropin-releasing hormone (CRH)[72–73] and to be associated with acromegaly and Cushing's syndrome, respectively.

Suprasellar germ cell tumors may be histologically indistinguishable from germinomas, teratomas, embryonal carcinomas, and choriocarcinomas.[74–78] Some of these tumors express immunoreactive β-human chorionic gonadotropin, human placental lactogen, or other placental peptides. These tumors may present with precocious puberty in addition to diabetes insipidus and visual field abnormalities. Thirst disorders, with associated hypernatremia, emaciation, or even obesity, may also occur. Suppressed growth hormone secretion with growth delay is found in over 95 per cent of these patients. After biopsy diagnosis, high-dose radiotherapy has proved to be a very effective therapy, with about 70 per cent long-term survival.

Hypothalamic astrocytomas (gliomas), often arising in the anterior hypothalamus and associated with hypophagia of infancy, are rare tumors that may be malignant.

SECONDARY METASTASES TO THE PITUITARY REGION

Pituitary metastases occur quite commonly and are found in up to 3.5 per cent of cancer patients[79–82] (Table

TABLE 29–6. NEOPLASTIC SOURCE OF PITUITARY METASTASES IN 238 PATIENTS

PRIMARY NEOPLASM	PERCENTAGE OF PATIENTS
Breast	47
Lung	19
Gastrointestinal tract	6
Prostate	6
Leukemia	3
Pancreas	3
Unknown origin	2
Nasopharynx	<2
Melanoma	<2
Thyroid	<2
Plasmacytoma	<2
Endometrium	<1
Renal	<1
Ovary	<1
Liver	<1
Penis	<1

*Included is data from references 79–82.

29–6). The posterior pituitary is the preferred site for blood-borne metastatic spread. This may be explained by the vascular supply to the posterior pituitary; blood flows into it directly from the systemic circulation via the internal carotid arteries. The predominant blood supply to the anterior pituitary, in contrast, is by way of the hypothalamic portal system. The common primary carcinomas that metastasize to the pituitary include those of the lung, gastrointestinal tract, and breast. Up to one quarter of patients with metastatic breast cancer have pituitary metastases. Interestingly, symptomatic pituitary metastases may be the presenting sign of previously undiscovered malignancy and even of malignancy of unknown origin. Although anterior pituitary failure is rare, an isolated metastatic deposit in the pituitary stalk without involvement of the anterior lobe may also present with pituitary failure (Table 29–7). Metastases to the posterior pituitary lobe are far more common. About 15 per cent of patients with diabetes insipidus harbor metastases from extrapituitary sources. Unfortunately, imaging of the pituitary mass does not distinguish these deposits from a pituitary adenoma unless extensive bony erosion is present. In fact, metastatic pituitary lesions may masquerade as a pituitary adenoma. In several instances the diagnosis of pituitary metastasis will be made only by histological study of the specimen removed at transsphenoidal surgery.

Acute lymphoblastic leukemia may be associated with periglandular pituitary infiltrates with minimal pituitary dysfunction. Rarely, SIADH has been reported in this condition. Primary lymphoma may also involve the hypothalamus and pituitary stalk, and these patients may present with resultant hypopituitarism. Isolated patients with soli-

TABLE 29–7. PRESENTING CLINICAL FEATURES IN PATIENTS WITH PITUITARY METASTASIS

	PERCENTAGE
Diabetes insipidus	70
Visual disturbances	20
Cranial nerve palsy	15
Anterior pituitary failure	15

tary pituitary plasmacytomas have been reported who do not develop classical multiple myeloma. Rarely, Langerhans' histiocytosis (histiocytosis X) lesions may be confined to the hypothalamic pituitary axis. These patients usually have diabetes insipidus and occasionally hyperprolactinemia caused by destruction of the hypothalamic portal tract.

Miscellaneous Parasellar Masses

Aneurysms arising from within or adjacent to the parasellar vasculature may mimic a pituitary adenoma. Preoperative or intraoperative rupture are potentially catastrophic complications, underlying the absolute need for early diagnosis. The differentiating features from other pituitary masses may be subtle, including eye pain, very intense headaches, and relatively sudden onset of cranial nerve palsies. Although CT and MRI techniques are now able to distinguish blood and hemorrhage from solid tumor or tissue, a highly vascular meningioma may be confused with an aneurysm.

Other rare parasellar masses include granulomata and those of sarcoidosis, tuberculosis, and Langerhans' histiocytosis (histiocytosis X). Fungal infection, especially in immunocompromised hosts, may also be localized to the parasellar region. Usually these conditions present as diabetes insipidus, with or without anterior pituitary dysfunction, and hyperprolactinemia. Gonadal dysfunction may be an early peripheral sign in adults.

REFERENCES

1. Lechan RM: Neuroendocrinology of pituitary hormone regulation. Endocrinol Metab Clin 16:475–501, 1987.
2. Bruesch SR: Anatomy of the human hypothalamus. In Givens JR, Kitabchi AE, Robertson JT (eds): The Hypothalamus. Chicago, Year Book Medical Publishers, 1984, pp 1–16.
3. Garnica AD, Netzloff ML, Rosenbloom AL: Clinical manifestations of hypothalamic tumors. Ann Clin Lab Sci 10:474–485, 1980.
4. Melmed S, Braunstein GD: Growth hormone and prolactin-secreting pituitary tumors. Ann Intern Med 105:238–253, 1986.
5. Hollenhorst RW, Younge BR: Ocular manifestations produced by adenomas of the pituitary gland: analysis of 1000 cases. In Kohler PO, Ross GT (eds): Diagnosis and Treatment of Pituitary Tumors. Amsterdam, Excerpta Medica, 1973, pp 53–64.
6. Melan O: Neuro-ophthalmologic features of pituitary tumors. Endocrinol Metab Clin North Am 16:585–608, 1987.
7. Carmel PW: Vegetative dysfunctions of the hypothalamus. Acta Neurochirurgica 75:113–121, 1985.
8. Marques PR, Illner P, Williams DD: Hypothalamic control of endocrine thermogenesis. Am J Physiol 241:E420, 1981.
9. Bauer HG: Endocrine and other clinical manifestations of hypothalamic disease. J Clin Endocrinol Metab 14:13–31, 1954.
10. Guze BH, Baxter LR Jr: Neuroleptic malignant syndrome. N Engl J Med 313:163–166, 1985.
11. Fox RH, Davis TW, Marsh FP, Urich H: Hypothermia in a young man with an anterior hypothalamic lesion. Lancet 2:185–188, 1970.
12. Mooradian AD, Morley GK, McGeachie R, et al: Spontaneous periodic hypothermia. Neurology 34:79–82, 1984.
13. Newman MM, Halmi KA: The endocrinology of anorexia nervosa and bulimia nervosa. Neurol Clin 6:195–212, 1988.
14. Bray GA, Gallagher TJ Jr: Manifestations of hypothalamic obesity in man: A comprehensive investigation of eight patients and a review of the literature. Medicine 54:301–330, 1975.
15. Mecklenberg RS, Loriaux DL, Thompson RH, et al: Hypothalamic dysfunction in patients with anorexia. Medicine 53:147–159, 1974.
16. Lewin K, Mattingly D, Millis RR: Anorexia nervosa associated with hypothalamic tumor. Br Med J 2:629–630, 1972.

17. Russell A: A diencephalic syndrome of emaciation in infancy and childhood. Arch Dis Child 26:274, 1951.
18. Burr IM, Slonim AE, Danish RK, et al: Diencephalic syndrome revisited. J Pediatr 88:439–444, 1976.
19. Scherbaum WA, Wass KAJ, Besser GM, et al: Autoimmune cranial diabetes insipidus: Its association with other endocrine diseases and with histiocytosis X. Clin Endocrinol 25:411–420, 1986.
20. Weitzman RE, Kleeman CR: The clinical physiology of water metabolism. West J Med 132:16–38, 1980.
21. DeRubertis FR, Michelis MF, Davis BB: "Essential" hypernatremia. Report of three cases and review of the literature. Arch Intern Med 134:889–895, 1974.
22. Hayek A, Peake GT: Hypothalamic adipsia without demonstrable structural lesion. Pediatrics 70:275–278, 1982.
23. Plum F, VanUitert R: Nonendocrine diseases and disorders of the hypothalamus. In Reichlin S, Baldessarini RJ, Martin JB (eds): The Hypothalamus. New York: Raven Press, 1978, pp 415–573.
24. Jennings MT, Gelman R, Hochberg F: Intracranial germ-cell tumors: Natural history and pathogenesis. J Neurosurg 63:155–167, 1985.
25. Imura H, Kato Y, Nakai Y: Endocrine aspects of tumors arising from suprasellar, third ventricular regions. Prog Exp Tumor Res 30:313–324, 1987.
26. Reeves AG, Plum F: Hyperphagia, rage, and dementia accompanying a ventromedial hypothalamic neoplasm. Arch Neurol 20:616–624, 1969.
27. Haugh RM, Markesbery WR: Hypothalamic astrocytoma. Syndrome of hyperphagia, obesity, and disturbances of behavior and endocrine and autonomic function. Arch Neurol 40:560–563, 1983.
28. DuRivage SK, Winter RJ, Brouillette RT, et al: Idiopathic hypothalamic dysfunction and impaired control of breathing. Pediatrics 75:896–898, 1985.
29. Arslanian SA, Rothfus WE, Foley TP Jr, Becker DJ: Hormonal metabolic, and neuroradiologic abnormalities associated with septo-optic dysplasia. Acta Endocrinol 107:282–288, 1984.
30. Jeffcoate WJ, Laurance BM, Edwards CRW, Besser GM: Endocrine function in the Prader-Willi syndrome. Clin Endocrinol 12:81, 1980.
31. Barrow DL, Spector RH, Takei Y, Tindall GT: Symptomatic Rathke's cleft cysts located entirely in the suprasellar region: Review of diagnosis, management and pathogenesis. Neurosurgery 16:766–772, 1985.
32. Nishio S, Mizuno J, Barrow DL, et al: Pituitary tumors composed of adenohypophysial adenoma and Rathke's cleft cyst elements: A clinicopathological study. Neurosurgery 21:371–377, 1987.
33. Kucharczyk W, Peck WW, Kelly WM, et al: Rathke cleft cysts: CT, MR imaging and pathologic features. Radiology 165:491–495, 1987.
34. Baskin DS, Wilson CB: Transsphenoidal treatment of non-neoplastic intrasellar cysts. Report of 38 cases. J Neurosurg 60:8–13, 1984.
35. Yamakawa K, Shitara N, Genka S, et al: Clinical course and surgical prognosis of 33 cases of intracranial epidermoid tumors. Neurosurgery 24:568–573, 1989.
36. Lewis AJ, Cooper PW, Kassel EE, Schwartz ML: Squamous cell carcinoma arising in a suprasellar epidermoid cyst. Case report. J Neurosurg 59:538–541, 1983.
37. Schlachter LB, Tindall GT, Pearl GS: Granular cell tumor of the pituitary gland associated with diabetes insipidus. Neurosurgery 6:418–421, 1980.
38. Morrison JG, Gray GF, Dao AH, Adkins RB: Granular cell tumors. Am Surgeon 53:156–160, 1987.
39. Perzin KH, Pushparaj N: Nonepithelial tumors of the nasal cavity, paranasal sinuses, and nasopharynx. A clinicopathological study. XIV: Chordomas. Cancer 57:784–796, 1986.
40. Meyer JE, Oot RF, Lindfors KK: CT appearance of clival chordomas. J Comput Assist Tomogr 10:34–36, 1986.
41. Volpe R, Mazabraud A: A clinicopathologic review of 25 cases of chordoma (a pleomorphic and metastasizing neoplasm). Am J Surg Pathol 7:161–170, 1983.
42. Petito CK, DeGirolami U, Earle KM: Craniopharyngiomas: A clinical and pathological review. Cancer 37:1944–1952, 1976.
43. Harris PE, Perry L, Chard T, et al: Immunoreactive human chorionic gonadotrophin from the cyst fluid and CSF of patients with craniopharyngioma. Clin Endocrinol 29:503–508, 1988.
44. Pigeau I, Sigal R, Halimi P, et al: MRI features of craniopharyngiomas at 1.5 tesla. J Neuroradiol 15:276–287, 1988.
45. Yasargil MG, Curcic M, Kis M, et al: Total removal of craniopharyngiomas. Approaches and long term-results in 144 patients. J Neurosurg 73:3–11, 1990.
46. Wen BC, Hussey DH, Staples J, et al: A comparison of the roles of surgery and radiation therapy in the management of craniopharyngiomas. Int J Radiat Oncol Biol Phys 16:17–24, 1989.
47. Adamson TE, Wiestler OD, Kleihues P, Yasargil MG: Correlation of clinical and pathological features in surgically treated craniopharyngiomas. J Neurosurg 73:12–17, 1990.
48. Rohringer M, Sutherland GR, Louw DF, Sima AAF: Incidence and clinicopathological features of meningioma. J Neurosurg 71:665–672, 1989.
49. Grisoli F, Vincentelli F, Raybaud C, et al: Intrasellar meningioma. Surg Neurol 20:36–41, 1983.
50. Yamada K, Hatayama T, Ohta M, et al: Coincidental pituitary adenoma and parasellar meningioma: case report. Neurosurgery 19:267–270, 1986.
51. Michael AS, Paige ML: MR imaging of intrasellar meningiomas simulating pituitary adenomas. J Comput Assist Tomogr 12:944–946, 1988.
52. Andrews BT, Wilson CB: Suprasellar meningiomas: The effect of tumor location on postoperative visual outcome. J Neurosurg 69:523–528, 1988.
53. Alvord EC, Lofton S: Gliomas of the optic nerve or chiasm. Outcome by patients age, tumor site, and treatment. J Neurosurg 68:85–98, 1988.
54. Rush JA, Younge BR, Campbell RJ, MacCarty CS: Optic glioma. Long-term follow-up of 85 histopathologically verified cases. Ophthalmology 89:1213–1219, 1982.
55. Flickinger JC, Torres C, Deutsch M: Management of low-grade gliomas of optic nerve and chiasm. Cancer 61:635–642, 1988.
56. Rudd A, Rees JE, Kennedy P, et al: Malignant optic nerve gliomas in adults. J Clin Neuroophthalmol 5:238–243, 1985.
57. Albers GW, Hoyt WF, Forno LS, Shratter LA: Treatment response in malignant optic glioma of adulthood. Neurology 38:1071–1074, 1988.
58. Judge DM, Kulin HE, Page R, et al: Hypothalamic hamartoma. A source of luteinizing-hormone releasing factor in precocious puberty. N Eng J Med 296:7–10, 1977.
59. Hirsch-Pescovitz O, Comite F, Hench K, et al: The NIH experience with precocious puberty: diagnostic subgroups and response to short-term luteinizing hormone releasing hormone analogue therapy. J Pediatr 108:47–54, 1986.
60. Curatolo P, Cusmai R, Finocchi G, Boscherini B: Gelactic epilepsy and true precocious puberty due to hypothalamic hamartoma. Dev Med Child Neurol 26:509–514, 1984.
60a. Nishio S, Fujiwara S, Aiko Y, et al: Hypothalamic hamartoma. Report of two cases. J Neurosurg 70:640–645, 1989.
61. Berkovic SF, Andermann F, Melanson D, et al: Hypothalamic hamartomas and ictal laughter: Evolution of a characteristic epileptic syndrome and diagnostic value of magnetic resonance imaging. Ann Neurol 23:429–239, 1989.
62. Breningstall GN: Gelactic seizures, precocious puberty and hypothalamic hamartoma. Neurology 35:1180–1183, 1985.
63. Iafolla K, Fratkin JD, Spiegel PK, et al: Case report and delineation of the congenital hypothalamic hamartoblastoma syndrome (Pallister-Hall syndrome). Am J Med Genet 33:489–499, 1989.
64. Hall JG, Pallister PD, Clarren SK, et al: Congenital hypothalamic hamartoblastoma, hypopituitarism, imperforate anus, and postaxial polydactyly—a new syndrome. Part I. Clinical, causal, and pathogenetic considerations. Am J Med Genet 7:47–74, 1980.
65. Hubbard AM, Egelhoff JC: MR imaging of large hypothalamic hamartomas in two infants. Am J Neuroradiol 10:1277, 1989.
66. Bevan JS, Asa SL, Rossi ML, et al: Intrasellar gangliocytoma containing gastrin and growth hormone-releasing hormone associated with a growth hormone-secreting pituitary adenoma. Clin Endocrinol 30:213–224, 1989.
67. Markin RS, Leibrock LG, Huseman CA, McComb RD: Hypothalamic hamartoma: A report of two cases. Pediatr Neurosci 13:19–26, 1987.
68. Asa SL, Scheithauer BW, Bilbao JM, et al: A case for hypothalamic acromegaly: A clinicopathological study of six patients with hypothalamic gangliocytomas producing growth hormone-releasing factor. J Clin Endocrinol Metab 58:796–803, 1984.
69. Kamel OW, Horoupian DS, Silverberg GD: Mixed gangliocytoma-adenoma: A distinct neuroendocrine tumor of the pituitary fossa. Hum Pathol 20:1198–1203, 1989.
70. Li JY, Racadot O, Kujas M, et al: Immunocytochemistry of four mixed pituitary adenomas and intrasellar gangliocytomas associated with different clinical syndromes: Acromegaly, amenorrhea-galactorrhea, Cushing's disease and isolated tumoral syndrome. Acta Neuropathol 77:320–328, 1989.
71. Yamada S, Stefaneanu L, Kovacs K, et al: Intrasellar gangliocytoma with multiple immunoreactivities. Endocr Pathol 1:58–63, 1990.
72. Pelletier G, Desy L, Cote J, et al: Light microscope immunohistochemical localization of growth hormone-releasing factor (GRF) in the human hypothalamus. Cell Tiss Res 245:461–464, 1986.

73. Asa SL, Kovacs K, Tindall GT, et al: Cushing's disease associated with an intrasellar gangliocytoma producing corticotrophin-releasing factor. Ann Intern Med 101:789–793, 1984.
74. Jennings MT, Gelman R, Hochberg F: Intracranial germ cell tumors: Natural history and pathogenesis. J Neurosurg 63:155–167, 1985.
75. Marsden HB, Birch JM, Swindell R: Germ cell tumours of childhood: a review of 137 cases. J Clin Pathol 34:879–883, 1981.
76. Furukawa F, Haebara H, Hamashima Y: Primary intracranial choriocarcinoma arising from the pituitary fossa. Report of an autopsy case with literature review. Acta Pathol Jpn 36:773–781, 1986.
77. Poon W, Ng HK, Wong K, South JR: Primary intrasellar germinoma presenting with cavernous sinus syndrome. Surg Neurol 30:402–405, 1988.
78. Kageyama N, Kobayashi T, Kida Y, et al: Intracranial germinal tumors. Prog Exp Tumor Res 30:255–2267, 1987.
79. Post KD, McCormick PC, Kandji AD, Hays AP: Metastatic carcinoma to pituitary adenoma: report of two cases. Surg Neurol 30:286–292, 1988.
80. Duchen LW: Metastatic carcinoma in the pituitary gland and hypothalamus. J Pathol Bacteriol 91:247–355, 1966.
81. Hagerstrand I, Schoneback J: Metastases to the pituitary gland. Acta Pathol Microbiol Scand 75:64–70, 1969.
82. Max MB, Deck MDF, Rottenberg DA: Pituitary metastasis: incidence in cancer patients and clinical differentiation from pituitary adenoma. Neurology 31:998–1002, 1981.

30

Radiographic Evaluation of the Pituitary and Anterior Hypothalamus

ROBERT J. WITTE
LEIGHTON P. MARK
DAVID L. DANIELS
VICTOR M. HAUGHTON

Methods for imaging the pituitary gland and hypothalamus have continued to improve. CT provided the first imaging technique that directly visualized the pituitary gland.[1-6] MR imaging subsequently provided a noninvasive imaging technique without imaging radiation which demonstrates the contents of the pituitary gland and hypothalamus with even better contrast resolution.[7-10] Because of CT and MR imaging, radiography, conventional tomography, angiography, venography, and pneumoencephalography have become obsolete in the evaluation of the sella. Both CT and MR imaging are effective means for detecting intrasellar and hypothalamic processes. CT is particularly effective in demonstrating the osseous structure of the sella and calcification within sellar lesions. MR imaging is accurate in demonstrating the soft tissue contents of the pituitary fossa and is sensitive for detecting tissue with paramagnetic qualities such as deoxyhemoglobin, methemoglobin, and melanin. MR imaging also provides an angiographic capability useful for demonstrating the cavernous carotid arteries. The purpose of this chapter is to describe CT and MR imaging of the pituitary fossa and to discuss the detection and differential diagnosis of intrasellar processes. Conventional techniques that have limited applications are mentioned only briefly.

Radiography

Some sellar abnormalities are discovered incidentally by means of skull radiography. With frontal and lateral radiographs obtained with a small focal spot (0.3 mm), low kilovoltage (60 to 65 kVp), high-resolution film-screen combinations, and fine collimation, the dimensions and morphology of the sella can be determined accurately. Normally the sella is less than 17 mm in length (tuberculum sellae to dorsum sellae) and less than 14 mm in depth (vertical distance between anteroposterior diameter and sellar floor). Tumors, cysts, and empty sella, which cause enlargement of the sella, are not effectively distinguished by radiography.

Tomography

Complex motion (hypocycloidal or spiral) tomography effectively shows the osseous structure of the sella. Typically 1-mm thick sections, 1 mm apart are obtained in a coronal projection. The indirect signs of an intrasellar process are changes in the shape of the sella and erosion of the sella. However, tomography has been replaced by CT and MR imaging, which are more specific in diagnosing intrasellar processes.

Cavernous Sinus Venography

Prior to the introduction of CT and MR imaging, the cavernous sinuses were opacified via a frontal or jugular vein injection to detect radiographically the invasion of the cavernous sinuses by pituitary adenoma.

Computed Tomography

Effective CT scanning of the pituitary fossa requires a spatial resolution of less than 1 mm, contrast resolution of less than 1 per cent, a gantry tilting to at least 20 degrees from vertical, a modified head holder that permits the patient to lie comfortably with the neck extended maximally, slice thicknesses as narrow as 1.5 mm, and scan speeds of 5 seconds or less. Modern scanners with fine matrices, closely spaced detectors, and large-capacity data acquisition systems provide these capabilities. A reconstruction algorithm such as targeting, zoom reconstruction, and three-dimensional reformatting can be effectively used in imaging the sella.

Coronal plane images provide the most efficient diagnosis of processes affecting the infundibulum, hypothalamus, cavernous sinuses, and pituitary gland.[11, 12] Coronal images are obtained directly by positioning the patient so that the gantry is perpendicular to the sellar floor or by using a three-dimensional program to reformat thin coronal sections obtained from direct axial images (Figs. 30–1 and 30–2). The best spatial resolution in the sella is provided by the direct coronal images.

Except for patients in whom it is contraindicated, intravenous contrast medium is used routinely in evaluation of the pituitary gland and anterior hypothalamus. The pituitary gland and infundibulum, because they lack a blood-brain barrier, are demonstrated more effectively after the injection of the intravenous contrast medium. The venous spaces and carotid artery in the cavernous sinuses increase conspicuously in density after administration of the intravenous contrast medium. For effective imaging of the normal pituitary gland and cavernous sinuses and for detection of pituitary adenomas, a dose of contrast medium containing 30 to 40 g of iodine is administered. Contrast between the normal pituitary gland and pituitary adenoma is maximized by injecting the contrast medium rapidly and minimizing the time between injection and imaging. One effective technique is to administer 250 ml of 30 per cent meglumine iothalamate or diatrizoate within seven minutes and then infuse an additional 50 ml at a slower rate while the scanning is taking place. Common side effects of the contrast medium include nausea, vomiting, and a feeling of warmth. Approximately one patient in 15,000 develops bronchospasm or hypotension, which may be life threatening if not effectively treated. In patients with a history of serious allergic reaction to contrast media, premedication with corticosteroids and antihistamines and preparation for emergency resuscitation are warranted prior to injecting the contrast medium. When the intravenous contrast medium is omitted, CT may still effectively demonstrate large pituitary adenomas.

The CT examination usually consists of six contiguous coronal 1.5-mm thick images obtained through the sella. If the sella is enlarged, a larger number of coronal images

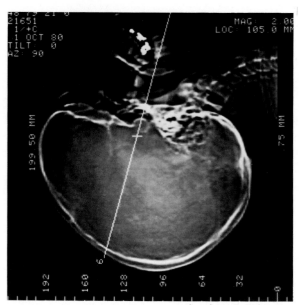

FIGURE 30–1. **Lateral localizer CT image.** The white cursor line through the pituitary fossa indicates the optimal angle to obtain direct coronal images of the sella. (From Daniels DL: The sella and juxta-sellar region. *In* Williams AL, Haughton VM: Cranial Computed Tomography: A Comprehensive Text. St. Louis, CV Mosby Company, 1985.)

may be needed. The kilovoltage, milliamperage, and reconstruction algorithm are chosen to maximize resolution.

Dynamic CT scanning has been used to study pituitary adenomas and the vascular structures related to the pituitary gland.[13–15] For dynamic scanning the scanner is programmed to obtain a series of images at a chosen level. A bolus of contrast medium (for example, 30 ml of 60 per cent iodinated agent) is injected intravenously, and images are acquired at about one per second starting five seconds after the injection. This sequence of images shows the rapid wash-in and wash-out of contrast medium in vascular structures.

Intrathecal contrast medium once had a role in the evaluation of a suspected empty sella but is no longer used.

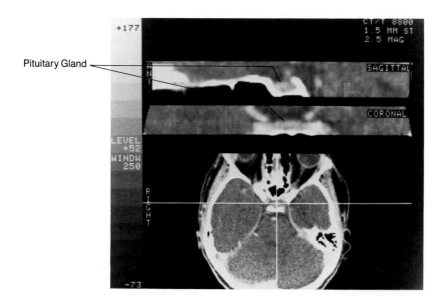

FIGURE 30–2. **Sagittal and coronal images reformatted from axial CT images.** The normal pituitary gland has a nearly straight upper contour in both reformatted views. (From Daniels DL: The sella and juxta-sellar region. *In* Williams AL, Haughton VM: Cranial Computed Tomography: A Comprehensive Text. St. Louis, CV Mosby Company, 1985.)

Angiography

Carotid angiography to demonstrate the relationship of the intracavernous carotid arteries to an intrasellar abnormality has been replaced by MR imaging and CT. Magnification and high-resolution angiography may still be used effectively in studying the neovascularity of some tumors. In particular, the faint homogeneous late blush of a pituitary adenoma can be distinguished from the earlier denser blush and palisade of vessels associated with meningioma. For angiography biplane or single plane 2× magnification, high-speed film changer, small focal spot radiographic tube, digital imaging capability, and power injection are indicated.

Magnetic Resonance Imaging

MR imaging has replaced CT as the primary modality for imaging the pituitary fossa.[16-18] The sensitivity of MR imaging and CT to microadenomas and to other disease in the pituitary fossa is comparable. With MR imaging the serious risks associated with an intravenous iodinated contrast medium are avoided. MR imaging, because of its multiplanar capabilities, obviates the need for hyperextension of the head, which may be uncomfortable for some patients. Although MR imaging usually costs more than CT, it avoids exposure of patients to ionizing radiation. Contrast medium such as gadopentetate, gadodiamide, or gadoteridol, 0.1 mmol/kg, is injected intravenously in a dose of 0.1 mmol/kg. Side effects from these contrast media are rare. No serious complications directly related to the contrast medium have been reported in an experience of several million injections. Bronchospasm, which has occurred in patients receiving the contrast medium, is questionably related to the contrast. In patients with severe claustrophobia or with a contraindication to MR imaging (cardiac pacemaker, other implanted device with electrical conductors, or aneurysm clips that are not MR safe) or to the contrast medium, CT represents an effective alternative to MR imaging.

Imagers of various field strengths produce sufficiently high resolution images to evaluate the pituitary gland and its anatomical relationships effectively. The MR study is usually a combination of T1- and possibly T2-weighted images in sagittal and coronal planes. Typically a T1-weighted spin-echo series with TR of 300 to 500 msec and TE of 15 to 20 msec is obtained in sagittal projection with 3-mm slice thickness, 256 × 256 matrix, 2 NEX, and 20 to 24 cm field of view. Coronal T1-weighted images are obtained with 3-mm slice thickness and with techniques to optimize spatial resolution. A T2-weighted sequence in coronal projection may be useful to characterize abnormalities detected on the T1-weighted images. In particular, deoxyhemoglobin, hemosiderin, and the fluid contents of a cyst may have characteristic appearances on T2-weighted images. For the T2-weighted sequence, the coronal projection, 3-mm slice thickness, TR of 2500 to 4000 msec, and TE of 80 to 120 msec are appropriate. Fast spin-echo, gradient-echo, steady-state, and three-dimensional acquisitions are being evaluated for studying the pituitary fossa. A single three-dimensional acquisition provides data from which coronal, sagittal, or axial images can be analyzed. Phase contrast, time-of-flight, two-dimensional, and three-dimensional MR angiographic techniques are also being evaluated in the larger blood vessels near the pituitary fossa. These techniques provide excellent visualization of the carotid arteries and their major branches.

For dynamic MR imaging of the sella, a technique has also been developed. For this technique images are usually acquired in a coronal plane at one-second intervals. The contrast medium is injected intravenously as a bolus, with images obtained over a period of approximately two minutes after injection.

NORMAL ANATOMY

The osseous landmarks of the pituitary fossa—that is, the tuberculum sellae, lamina dura, dorsum sellae, planum sphenoidale, and chiasmatic sulcus—have a characteristic high density on CT images and low signal intensity on MR images.[19-31] Air in the sphenoid sinus just below the floor of the sella has no signal on either CT or MR imaging. The CSF in the chiasmatic cistern above the pituitary gland contrasts in both CT and MR images with the pituitary gland. The contents of the pituitary fossa include the anterior and posterior lobes of the pituitary gland and the pars intermedia. A small amount of fat in paramidline locations and small venous channels that connect the sphenoid sinuses are also present in the sella. In CT images the pituitary gland appears relatively homogeneous. Sometimes the posterior lobe appears less homogeneous than the anterior lobe. CT may demonstrate the fat within the pituitary fossa. The intercavernous veins and a small tuft of capillaries within the gland may be visualized, especially when the dynamic techniques are used. In MR imaging the gland may be homogeneous or inhomogeneous. Within the posterior lobe of normal individuals a region of high signal intensity may be identified, which appears to be related to phospholipid structures in vacuoles in the neurohypophysis. This region of high signal intensity is absent in diabetes insipidus and in some normals. In cases of transected infundibulum, the region of high signal intensity may be found in the residual stalk or inferior hypothalamus.

In CT and MR images the pituitary gland normally has a flat or slightly concave upper surface (Figs. 30–3 to 30–5). In adolescents and pregnant or menstruating women the gland may be mildly convex. The height of the gland is 2 to 9 mm in women and is usually smaller in men.[16-22] In MR or CT studies the gland shows nearly homogeneous contrast enhancement. After intravenous administration of a paramagnetic contrast medium, the signal intensity of the pituitary gland increases markedly and nearly homogeneously to nearly the same degree as the cavernous sinuses (Fig. 30–6). The carotid arteries within the cavernous sinus, however, do not enhance in MR imaging owing to time-of-flight effects. In CT, the gland enhances with iodinated contrast medium so that it is at or slightly below the density of the enhanced cavernous sinuses. Both the carotid arteries and the venous channels in the cavernous sinuses enhance with the CT contrast medium. The cranial nerves in the cavernous sinuses which do not enhance to the same degree may be resolved as filling defects in a contrast-enhanced study.

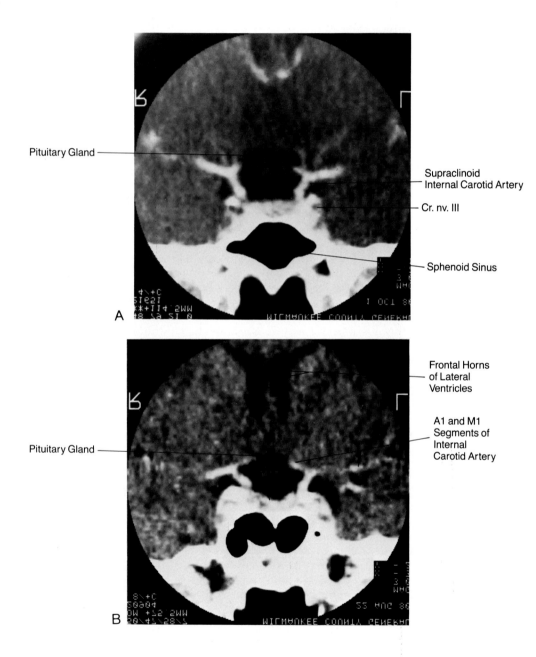

Pituitary Gland

Supraclinoid
Internal Carotid Artery

Cr. nv. III

Sphenoid Sinus

A

Frontal Horns
of Lateral
Ventricles

A1 and M1
Segments of
Internal
Carotid Artery

Pituitary Gland

B

FIGURE 30–3. **Direct coronal images of the normal sella, after the intravenous injection of iodinated contrast medium.** The upper surface of the pituitary gland is normally flat (A) or slightly concave (B). The gland enhances slightly less intensely and homogeneously than the cavernous sinuses and carotid arteries. (From Daniels DL: The sella and juxta-sellar region. *In* Williams AL, Haughton VM: Cranial Computed Tomography: A Comprehensive Text. St. Louis, CV Mosby Company, 1985.)

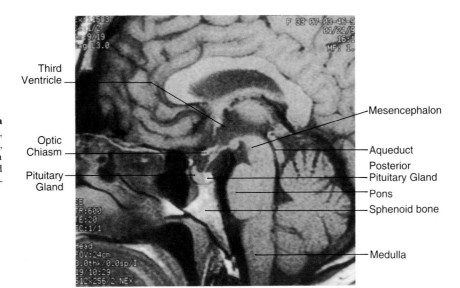

FIGURE 30-4. **Normal appearance of the sella in a sagittal T1-weighted MR image.** The pituitary gland, optic chiasm, third ventricle, aqueduct, mesencephalon, pons, and medulla have been labeled. Note the high signal intensity in bone marrow within the sphenoid bone. High signal intensity is also evident in the posterior lobe of the pituitary gland.

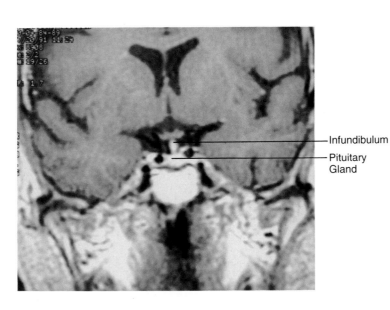

FIGURE 30-5. **Coronal T1-weighted MR image after intravenous contrast medium.** The brain and optic chiasm do not show contrast enhancement. Marked enhancement is noted, however, in the infundibulum and the pituitary gland. The carotid arteries are evident as a region of very low or negligible signal intensity. The upper surface of the pituitary gland is concave.

FIGURE 30-6. **Coronal CT images demonstrating the small midline capillary tuft below the surface of the pituitary gland.** This image is from the arterial phase of a coronal dynamic CT scanning sequence. (From Daniels DL: The sella and juxta-sellar region. *In* Williams AL, Haughton VM: Cranial Computed Tomography: A Comprehensive Text. St. Louis, CV Mosby Company, 1985.)

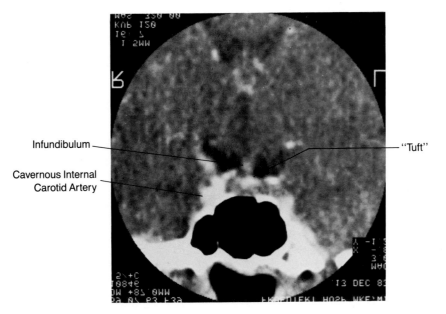

The pituitary stalk, tuber cinereum, and optic chiasm are conspicuous landmarks in CT and MR images.[26-28] With the exception of the pituitary stalk and median eminence, these structures do not enhance with the intravenous contrast media. In CT these structures have a higher density than the adjacent chiasmatic cistern. In MR imaging, the contrast between these structures and CSF depends on the pulse sequence used. In coronal sections the normally symmetrical optic chiasm can be identified. Posterior to the optic chiasm, the inverted triangular shape of the tuber cinereum is found. The infundibulum, which connects the pituitary gland and the tuber cinereum, lies in the midline or often just slightly off the midline.

In coronal CT or MR images the cavernous sinuses have a nearly triangular shape (Figs. 30–7 and 30–8). In CT without the administration of contrast medium the cavernous sinuses are isodense with the brain and uniform in density.[29-31] After intravenous contrast medium, the density of the cavernous sinuses increases to the same degree as that of the carotid artery. Filling defects visible on the enhanced CT images represent the location of the cranial nerves. Superior and lateral to the carotid artery, the oculomotor nerve (cranial nerve III) is often identified. Portions of the first and second division of the fifth cranial nerve are often identified in the cavernous sinus, and the third portion can be identified in locating the foramen ovale. The fourth and sixth nerves, which lie in close proximity to the first division of the fifth nerve in the cavernous sinus, are not readily identified. The density of the cavernous sinus on enhanced images normally exceeds that of the adjacent pituitary gland. In MR images, the cavernous sinus also enhances with intravenous contrast medium so that the cranial nerves and the carotid artery, which has negligible signal, may be distinguished.

PITUITARY ADENOMA

The most common intrasellar tumor is a pituitary adenoma.[32-34] For discussions of imaging, pituitary adenomas are usually divided into macroadenomas (a maximal diameter greater than 1 cm) and microadenomas (Figs. 30–9 and 30–10). The enlargement of the pituitary fossa, invasion of the sphenoid sinus, and displacement of the cavernous sinuses resulting from macroadenomas are readily identified on CT and MR images (Figs. 30–11 and 30–12). On unenhanced CT images, macroadenomas have a density slightly less than that of the normal pituitary gland or cavernous sinuses.[35] The upward enlargement of the tumor appears as a mass with a curvilinear margin effacing the chiasmatic cistern. Inferior extension results in a mass in the sphenoid sinus. Neoplasm in the cavernous sinuses usually enhances slightly less intensely than the normal portions of the cavernous sinus. Necrosis and cyst formation within adenomas produce regions of diminished density and diminished attenuation within the tumor (Fig. 30–13).[36-38] Small flecks of calcification in the tumor capsule are unusual findings in pituitary adenomas. Displacement, irregularity, thinning, and sloping of the sellar floor may also be demonstrated by CT in patients with pituitary adenomas.

MR imaging without contrast enhancement shows pituitary adenomas as a tissue mass that has slightly lower signal intensity on T1-weighted images and often slightly greater signal intensity on T2-weighted images than does a normal pituitary gland.[7-10] The encroachment of the tumor on the sphenoid sinus and chiasmatic cistern is recognized by displacement of air and CSF, respectively.[39] Involvement of the cavernous sinus is recognized by displacement laterally of the flow voids within the carotid arteries. With contrast enhancement the pituitary adenomas increase markedly in signal intensity but usually to a lesser degree than the cavernous sinuses. Low-intensity regions within the tumor usually represent necrosis or cyst formation (see Figs. 30–12 and 30–13). Hemorrhage within a pituitary adenoma produces a characteristic high signal intensity on unenhanced T1-weighted images. Other paramagnetic substances within pituitary adenomas may also account for regions of increased signal intensity on T1-weighted images. Therefore, MR is particularly effective in diagnosing hemorrhage into pituitary tumors in cases of pituitary apoplexy. MR is less effective than CT in demonstrating calcifications within

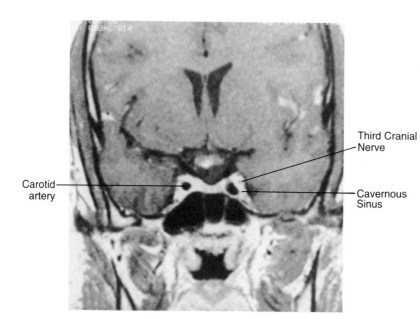

Carotid artery

Third Cranial Nerve

Cavernous Sinus

FIGURE 30–7. **Coronal contrast-enhanced MR image demonstrating the normal cavernous sinuses.** The carotid arteries, which appear as a signal void, are prominent landmarks. Small filling defects in the cavernous sinuses indicate the location of cranial nerves. The pituitary gland has slightly less signal intensity than the normal cavernous sinuses.

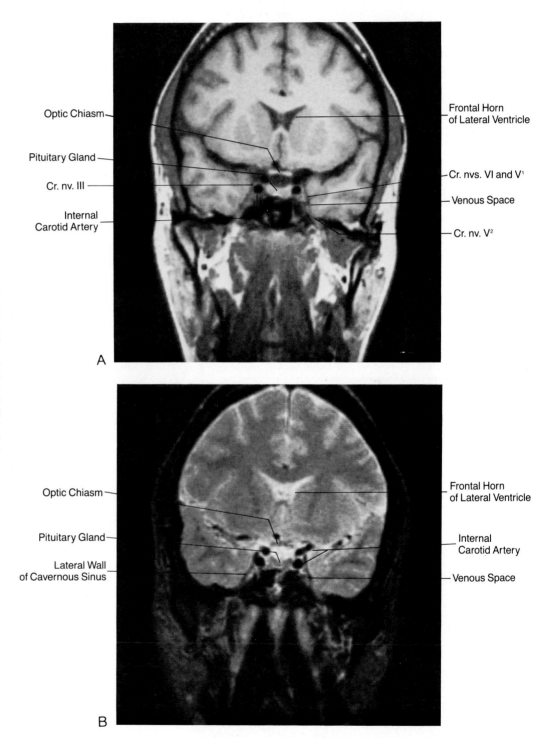

FIGURE 30–8. **The normal pituitary gland in normal MR images.** The pituitary gland contrasts with low signal intensity of the CSF in T1-weighted images (*A*) and the high signal intensity of CSF in T2-weighted images (*B*). In both images flowing blood in the internal carotid artery has a low signal intensity. (From Daniels DL: The sella and juxta-sellar region. *In* Williams AL, Haughton VM: Cranial Computed Tomography: A Comprehensive Text. St. Louis, CV Mosby Company, 1985.)

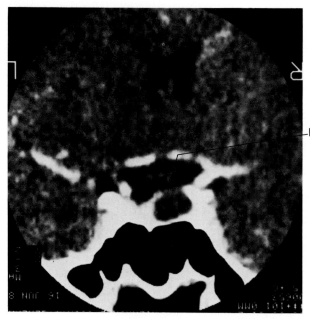

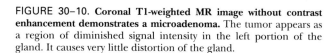

FIGURE 30-9. **Coronal enhanced CT image showing a microadenoma** in a patient with elevated prolactin. The prolactinoma appears as a low-density region in a mildly enlarged pituitary gland.

FIGURE 30-10. **Coronal T1-weighted MR image without contrast enhancement demonstrates a microadenoma.** The tumor appears as a region of diminished signal intensity in the left portion of the gland. It causes very little distortion of the gland.

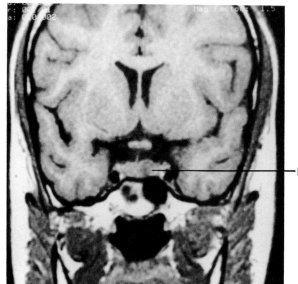

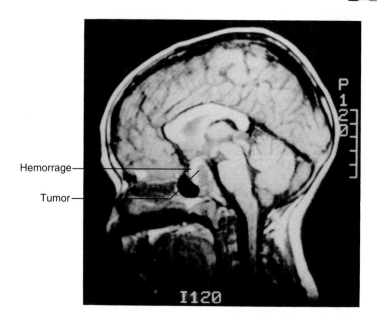

FIGURE 30-11. **Sagittal MR image showing a large pituitary adenoma** that fills the pituitary fossa and obliterates the chiasmatic cistern. Note the rim of high signal intensity indicating hemorrhage in the tumor in this patient with pituitary apoplexy.

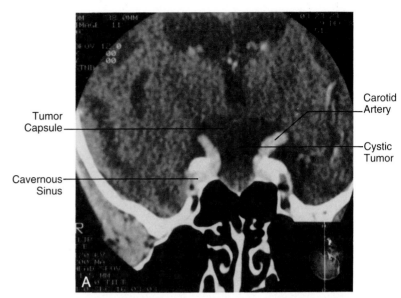

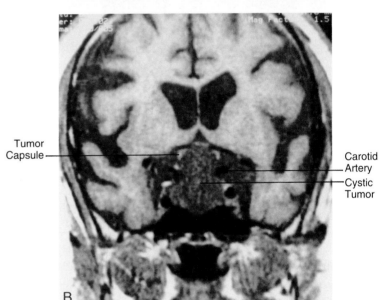

FIGURE 30–12. **A cystic pituitary adenoma shown on a coronal CT (*A*) and MR image (*B*).** In the CT study the margin of the capsule of the tumor is barely visible in the chiasmatic cistern. The cystic tumor is differentiated from an empty sella by the absence of a pituitary stalk visible in the sella. The carotid arteries and cavernous sinuses appear normal. In the T1-weighted MR image, the capsule is somewhat better defined, and the tumor has a slightly different signal from CSF.

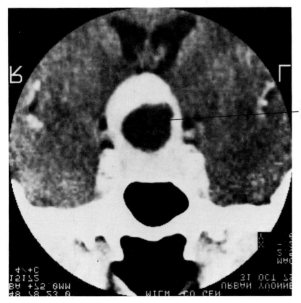

FIGURE 30–13. **Coronal CT image of a partially necrotic pituitary adenoma** that extends into the chiasmatic cistern.

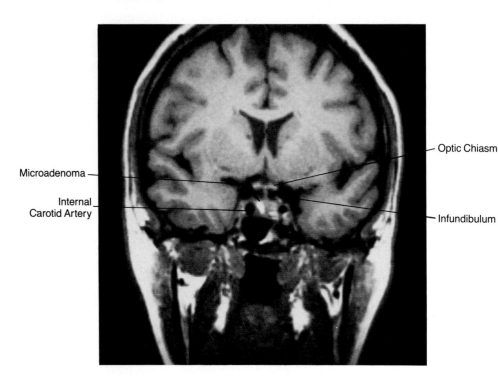

Microadenoma

Internal Carotid Artery

Optic Chiasm

Infundibulum

FIGURE 30-14. A T1-weighted image shows a prolactin-secreting microadenoma containing high signal intensity presumed to be secondary to bromocriptine treatment. The gland does not appear enlarged. (From Daniels DL, Pojunas KW, Pesch P, Haughton VM: Magnetic Resonance Imaging of the Sella and Juxta-Sellar Region. General Electric Company, 1984.)

pituitary adenomas. The most common pituitary microadenoma, a prolactin-secreting adenoma, is detected efficiently with either CT or MR imaging. Adenomas as small as 3 mm have been detected. These tumors appear as a region of diminished enhancement within the pituitary gland in either a CT or an MR image (see Figs. 30–9 and 30–10). In approximately 75 per cent of prolactinomas, the upper surface of the gland is abnormally convex and the height of the gland is greater than 9 mm. An incidental cyst within the pituitary gland may have a similar appearance to a small adenoma. In MR images the prolactin-secreting microadenomas typically have a lower signal intensity on T1-weighted images and higher signal intensity on T2-weighted images, but some variation is observed, possibly as the result of hemorrhage or other paramagnetic substances in the tumor (Fig. 30–14).

In ACTH- and hGH-secreting microadenomas CT and MR imaging are less sensitive and less specific (Figs. 30–15 and 30–16). About 50 per cent of these tumors have an abnormally convex upper gland surface and an abnormal height. A focal region of diminished enhancement within the gland is less easily identified in these tumors than in the prolactin-secreting adenomas. Some of the hGH- and ACTH-secreting pituitary adenomas are associated with normal-appearing pituitary glands on CT or MR imaging.

DIFFERENTIAL DIAGNOSIS

Meningioma

Meningiomas that arise from the surface of the diaphragma sellae, the cavernous sinus, or rarely from within

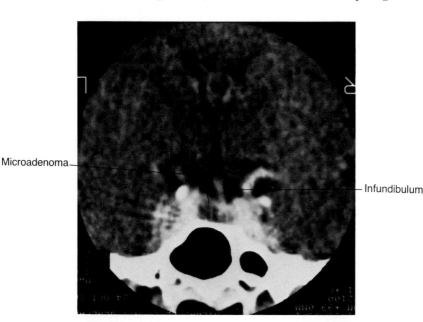

Microadenoma

Infundibulum

FIGURE 30–15. Coronal CT image showing an ACTH-secreting adenoma. The tumor appears as a low-density region in a slightly enlarged gland. The infundibulum is displaced contralaterally.

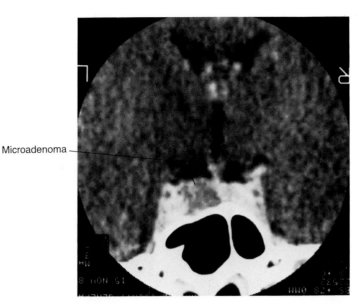

FIGURE 30–16. Enhanced coronal CT image demonstrating an hGH-secreting adenoma. The microadenoma appears as a region of diminished enhancement within the mildly expanded pituitary gland.

the pituitary fossa, are less common than pituitary adenomas. Like pituitary adenomas, they may have a homogeneous density or signal intensity before contrast enhancement. They also enhance markedly with intravenous contrast medium (Fig. 30–17). The focal calcifications often contained within the tumor appear as focal zones of hyperdensity in CT images and, if they are detected by MR imaging, as focal zones of diminished signal intensity. Hyperostotic bone adjacent to the meningioma in the tuberculum sellae and anterior or posterior clinoid processes may be demonstrated effectively by CT and less effectively by MR imaging.[40] Spread of tumor along the petroclinoid

ligament or dura is more characteristic of meningioma than of pituitary adenoma. Necrotic and cystic areas within meningioma are rarer in meningiomas than in adenomas. Meningiomas can usually be differentiated from pituitary adenomas by MR imaging and CT by identifying its anatomic relationship to the planum sphenoidale, tuberculum sellae, or dorsum sellae rather than to the pituitary fossa. Rare intrasellar meningiomas are difficult to distinguish radiographically from intrasellar adenomas.

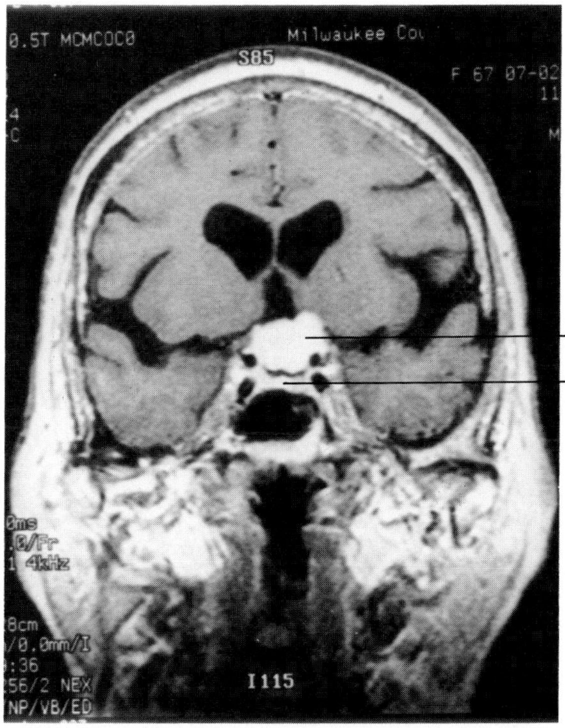

Craniopharyngioma

Although they are uncommon tumors of the chiasmatic region, craniopharyngiomas in many cases have characteristic radiographic findings that allow them to be differentiated from meningiomas or adenomas. They occur at any age but have peaks of incidence in the second and fifth decades of life. Their symptoms depend on the relationship of the tumor to the pituitary gland, hypothalamus, and optic chiasm. The discrete cysts and dense globular calcifications that characterize many craniopharyngiomas are usually evident in CT images (Fig. 30–18).[35] In MR images the cystic regions may have variable signal intensity due to varying amounts of blood, cholesterol, and protein within the cyst. Because they invade the chiasmatic cistern and/or the hypothalamus, these tumors are readily detected by CT and MR imaging. The solid portions of the tumor enhance markedly with contrast medium. Rare craniopharyngiomas that homogeneously enhance without evident calcification or cyst formation are difficult to distinguish radiographically from adenomas.

Metastases

Tumors of the nasopharynx, lung, breast, kidney, or gastrointestinal tract may metastasize to the hypothalamus or sella, producing diabetes insipidus or hypopituitarism. Metastatic tumors enhance modestly and homogeneously after intravenous contrast medium administration (Fig. 30–19).[31] Calcification and cyst formation are rare in these

FIGURE 30–17. Coronal T1-weighted contrast-enhanced MR image demonstrating a suprasellar meningioma. The tumor shows marked contrast enhancement. A thin line of low signal intensity, probably representing the diaphragma sellae, separates the tumor from the pituitary gland.

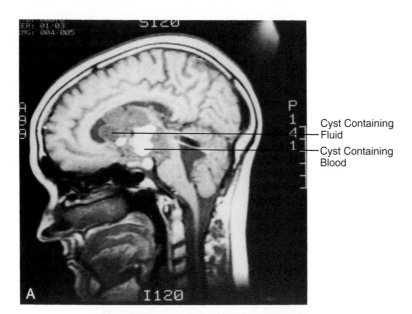

Cyst Containing Fluid

Cyst Containing Blood

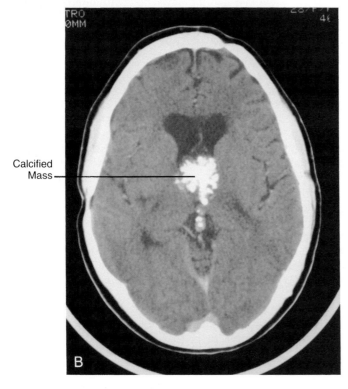

Calcified Mass

FIGURE 30–18. **Sagittal T1-weighted MR image (*A*) and axial CT image without intravenous contrast (*B*) demonstrate a craniopharyngioma.** In the MR image the lobulated mass in the suprasellar region distorts the third and lateral ventricles and contains a mixture of high and low signal intensity. The low signal intensity regions represent cysts. In the CT image, the foci of increased density represent calcification.

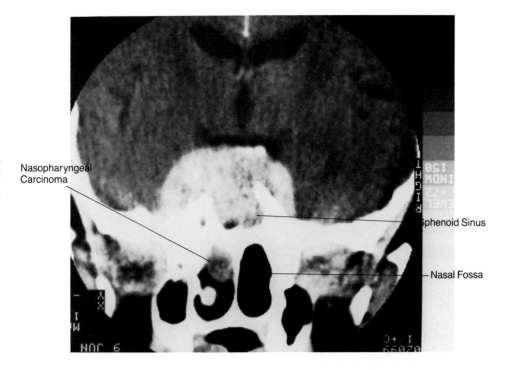

FIGURE 30–19. **Coronal CT contrast-enhanced image demonstrating a nasopharyngeal carcinoma** that erodes the sellar floor and fills the sphenoid sinus. The tumor enhances homogeneously.

Nasopharyngeal Carcinoma

Sphenoid Sinus

Nasal Fossa

metastases. The characteristic feature of these metastases is bone destruction, which CT or MR imaging may show.

Aneurysm

Rarely, an aneurysm (Fig. 30–20) may mimic an intrasellar or parasellar mass. In an unenhanced CT image, an intrasellar aneurysm appears slightly denser than cerebral tissue or if a large clot is present substantially denser than cerebral tissue. With intravenous contrast medium it may enhance homogeneously and with the same intensity as normal carotid arteries if no clot is present. When clot is present, the enhancement may be confined to the periphery of the clot. In MR imaging, flowing blood within the aneurysm usually has a characteristic signal void. The presence of clot or turbulent flow within the aneurysm may create a variety of different patterns. The lumen of the aneurysm does not enhance in MR imaging because of time-of-flight effects unless clot is present. Conventional or digital angiography must be used to document or exclude an aneurysm in questionable cases.

Lymphoid Hypophysitis

Lymphoid hypophysitis causes an enlarged and homogeneously enhancing pituitary gland.[41–43] It presents in a postpartum woman who has thyrotoxicosis or hyperpituitarism. In CT images lymphoid hypophysitis resembles a solid pituitary tumor with suprasellar extension. Enlargement of the sella, cystic changes, inhomogeneity of the gland, and calcification are uncommon (Fig. 30–21). The diagnosis of lymphoid hypophysitis should be suggested when an enlarged pituitary gland is seen post partum. Regression either spontaneously or after hormone replacement is characteristic of lymphoid hypophysitis.

Empty Sella

Empty sella is usually an incidental finding. It is usually due to incompetence of the diaphragma sellae, through which the chiasmatic cistern communicates with the pituitary fossa. Some empty sellae may result from regression of a pituitary tumor and some from a congenitally incomplete diaphragma sellae. Empty sellae are more common in women than in men. Both CT and MR imaging effectively show enlargement of the pituitary fossa and displacement of the remaining pituitary gland into the inferior portion of the fossa. An important sign of empty sella is a pituitary stalk that extends from the infundibulum through the empty sella to the residual pituitary gland (Fig. 30–22). Without identification of the infundibulum, an intrasellar cyst cannot be excluded.[44]

Hypothalamic Glioma

Hypothalamic gliomas, which usually are astrocytomas on histologic examination, usually produce symptoms of hypothalamic dysfunction in children and young adults.[45] In infants they typically produce a syndrome of hyperactivity and failure to thrive in spite of adequate caloric intake. In adults, malignant astrocytomas are more common. CT (Fig. 30–23) or MR imaging shows the hypothalamic glioma as a lobulated mass with increased signal intensity on T2-weighted images. Cystic or necrotic areas may be present. With intravenous contrast medium these tumors usually enhance on CT or MR imaging. Because they are in a suprachiasmatic location, they are not usually confused with pituitary adenomas.

Chiasmal Gliomas

Chiasmal gliomas occur most often in adolescent girls or patients with neurofibromatosis and produce visual loss

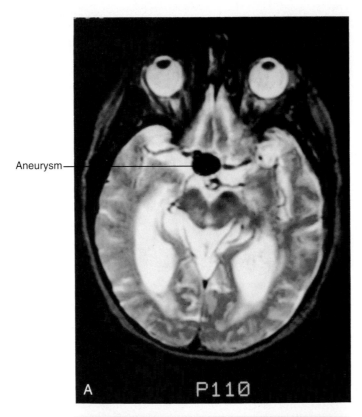

Aneurysm—

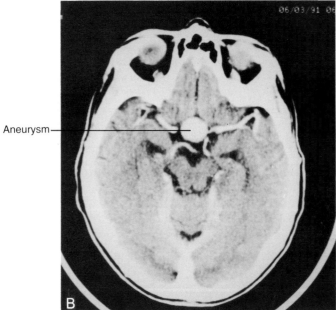

Aneurysm—

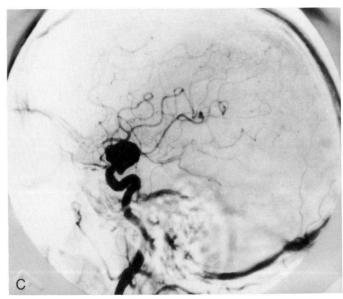

FIGURE 30–20. **Axial MR** (*A*) **and CT** (*B*) **and lateral angiogram** (*C*) **of a suprasellar aneurysm.** Notice that in the MR image, the aneurysm has a characteristic signal void. In CT, the aneurysm enhances to the same degree as the adjacent middle cerebral and basilar arteries.

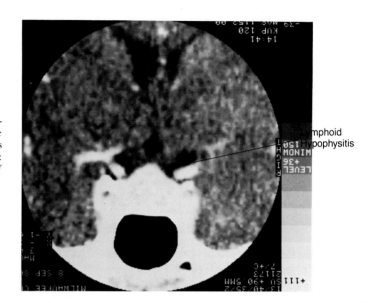

FIGURE 30–21. **Coronal CT contrast-enhanced image demonstrating lymphoid hypophysitis.** In this woman, who is three weeks post partum, the pituitary gland is enlarged and homogeneously enhancing. (From Daniels DL: The sella and juxta-sellar region. *In* Williams AL, Haughton VM: Cranial Computed Tomography: A Comprehensive Text. St. Louis, CV Mosby Company, 1985.)

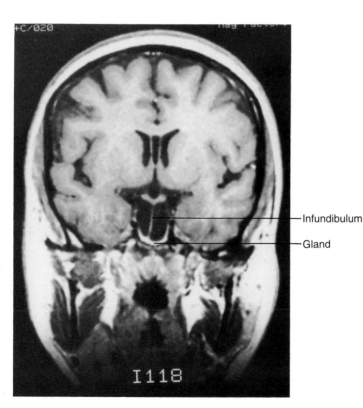

FIGURE 30–22. **Coronal MR image with intravenous contrast medium demonstrating an empty sella.** Note that the infundibulum and pituitary gland are enhanced. The identification of the infundibulum connecting the pituitary gland directly with the hypothalamus excludes a cystic tumor.

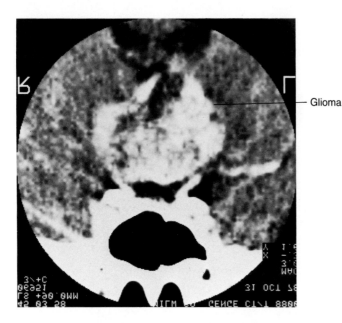

— Glioma

FIGURE 30–23. **Enhanced coronal CT image demonstrating a hypothalamic glioma.** This mass presented with prolactinemia and amenorrhea. (From Daniels DL: The sella and juxta-sellar region. *In* Williams AL, Haughton VM: Cranial Computed Tomography: A Comprehensive Text. St. Louis, CV Mosby Company, 1985.)

and optic atrophy.[32, 45] MR imaging and CT show the enlarged optic chiasm or optic nerve effectively because of its contrast with the surrounding CSF. In CT images the mass is usually isodense with brain. In MR images the mass is homogeneous and nearly isointense with brain. With intravenous contrast medium little enhancement of optic gliomas is noted in MR imaging or CT. In CT, slight hyperintensity may be noted if calcification is present (Fig. 30–24).[23] The optic tracts are often hyperintense in cases of aggressive chiasmal gliomas. These tumors are usually distinguished easily from other suprasellar masses because they are confined to the optic chiasm.

Hamartoma of the Tuber Cinereum

Hamartomas of the tuber cinereum contain cells similar to those normally found in the hypothalamus.[46] Hamartomas are usually found in children with precocious puberty, seizures, or behavior disorders, and intellectual deterioration.[43] They may secrete hypophysiotropic hormones. The usual appearance of a hamartoma of the hypothalamus in CT or MR imaging is a pedunculated soft tissue mass at the posterior hypothalamus. In CT it may be isodense with respect to the adjacent brain and usually nonenhancing. In MR imaging it may also be isointense with brain or may be hyperintense in T1-weighted images (Fig. 30–25).

Infundibular Tumors

Tumors of the infundibulum include metastases, glioma, and lymphoma.[33, 47–49] Other conditions that cause enlargement of the infundibulum include histiocytosis X and sarcoid. Patients with these tumors often present with diabetes insipidus and variable degrees of hypopituitarism. Either CT or MR imaging shows the enlarged infundibulum. The normal upper limit for the diameter of the infundibulum is 4.5 mm. Often tumor causes the infundibulum to lose its fusiform shape and become conical. Contrast enhancement is typical in these lesions, which are not usually mistaken for a pituitary adenoma.

Germinal Cell Tumors

Germinal cell tumors such as teratomas, teratocarcinomas, and germinomas (atypical teratomas) occasionally involve the suprasellar region.[50] Suprasellar germ cell tumors have a variable appearance in MR imaging and CT (Figs. 30–26 and 30–27). The germinomas and teratocarcinomas that spread via CSF pathways characteristically appear as linear or nodular enhancing regions on the surface of the brain. Suprasellar germ cell tumors may appear similar to glial tumors. The suprasellar location of germinal tumors distinguishes these from adenomas.

Epidermoid and Dermoid Cysts

Intrasellar dermoid cysts that contain dermis with hair, calcium, or fat or epidermoids that contain squamous epithelium have been reported.[51] On CT images, these tumors often have a density of CSF (5 to 15 HU) (Fig. 30–28). Fat and calcium in the dermoid may be distinguished in the mass as low (-40 HU) and high (>100 HU) densities, respectively. Intrathecal contrast agent may be required to define the margins of purely cystic tumors. In MR imaging, dermoid and epidermoid tumors appear as cysts with signal intensities consistent with a mixture of fluid, strands of tissue, calcium, or fat.

Arachnoid Cyst

The rare suprasellar arachnoid cysts often present with visual impairment and endocrine dysfunction or hydrocephalus.[52] They may also occur in adults who present with hypopituitarism and/or visual defects. Arachnoid cysts have a density in CT and signal intensity in MR imaging similar to that of CSF. Enhancement with intravenous contrast medium does not occur. They commonly displace the infundibulum and hypothalamus. An enhancing rim or dense globular calcification is more consistent with a cystic glioma or craniopharyngioma, respectively, than with an arachnoid cyst.

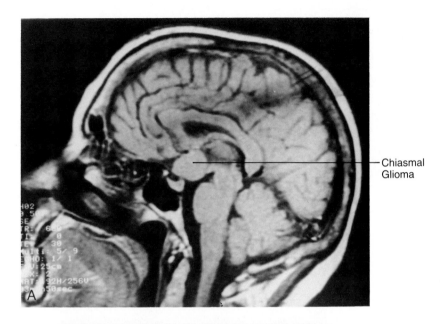

Chiasmal
Glioma

FIGURE 30–24. Sagittal (*A*) and coronal (*B*) MR images demonstrating a chiasmal glioma. Note that the mass enlarges the optic chiasm. On the contrast-enhanced coronal image (*B*), it fails to enhance, unlike the adjacent pituitary gland and cavernous sinuses.

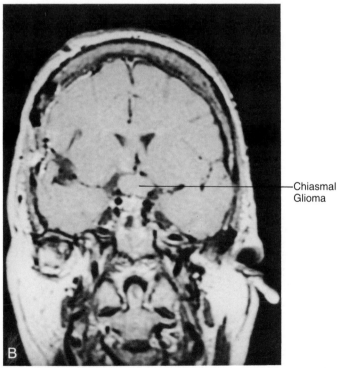

Chiasmal
Glioma

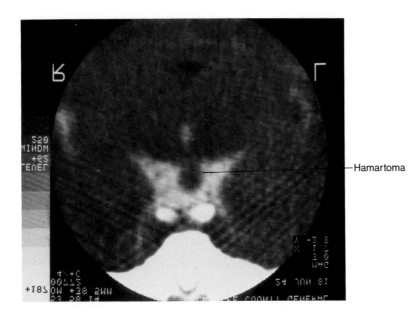

FIGURE 30–25. **Coronal CT with intrathecal enhancement demonstrating a rare hamartoma of the tuber cinereum.** (From Daniels DL: The sella and juxta-sellar region. *In* Williams AL, Haughton VM: Cranial Computed Tomography: A Comprehensive Text. St. Louis, CV Mosby Company, 1985.)

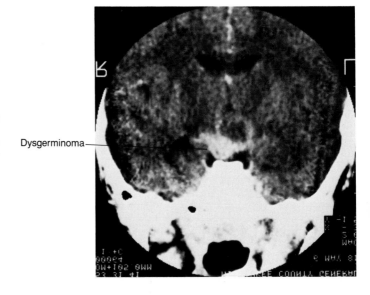

FIGURE 30–26. **Coronal enhanced CT demonstrating a hypothalamic dysgerminoma.** The tumor enhances inhomogeneously and enlarges the hypothalamus. (From Daniels DL: The sella and juxta-sellar region. *In* Williams AL, Haughton VM: Cranial Computed Tomography: A Comprehensive Text. St. Louis, CV Mosby Company, 1985.)

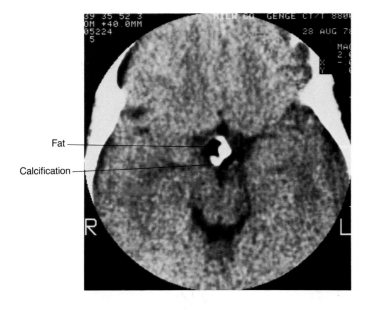

FIGURE 30–27. **Axial CT image without intravenous contrast medium showing a suprasellar teratoma.** Fat produces the characteristic low density on the MR image and calcium the characteristic high density. (From Daniels DL: The sella and juxta-sellar region. *In* Williams AL, Haughton VM: Cranial Computed Tomography: A Comprehensive Text. St. Louis, CV Mosby Company, 1985.)

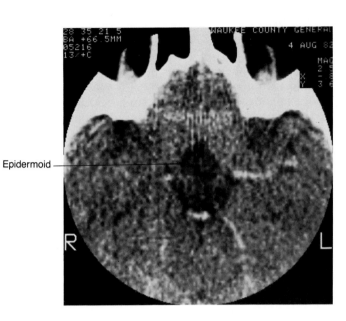

FIGURE 30–28. **Axial CT image showing a suprasellar epidermoid.** The tumor has signal intensity comparable to CSF and shows no contrast enhancement. (From Daniels DL: The sella and juxta-sellar region. *In* Williams AL, Haughton VM: Cranial Computed Tomography: A Comprehensive Text. St. Louis, CV Mosby Company, 1985.)

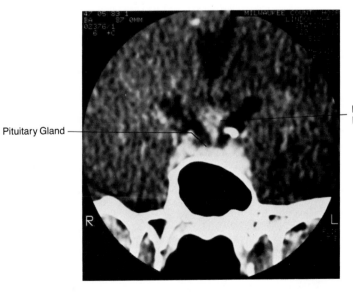

FIGURE 30–29. **Coronal CT-enhanced image showing a sarcoid granuloma in the infundibulum.** The tumor causes the abnormal cone shape of the infundibulum. (From Daniels DL: The sella and juxta-sellar region. *In* Williams AL, Haughton VM: Cranial Computed Tomography: A Comprehensive Text. St. Louis, CV Mosby Company, 1985.)

Granulomatous Disease of the Hypothalamus

Sarcoidosis, eosinophilic granuloma, or histiocytosis X may involve the hypothalamus or infundibulum (Fig. 30–29). Involvement appears in MR imaging as enlargement of the infundibulum or a coating of abnormal tissue along the pial surface of the hypothalamus, brain stem, and optic chiasm. The enlargement of the infundibulum may be detected on T1- or T2-weighted images. The abnormal tissue coating the base of the brain is detected most effectively on MR images obtained after administration of intravenous contrast medium. The radiologic differential diagnosis includes leptomeningeal carcinomatosis, basal meningitis, tuberculous meningitis, and cryptococcal meningitis.

REFERENCES

1. Reich NE, Zelch JV, et al: Computed tomography in the detection of juxtasellar lesions. Radiology 118:333–335, 1976.
2. Gyldensted C, Karle A: Computed tomography of infra- and juxtasellar lesions. A radiological study of 108 cases. Neuroradiology 14:5–13, 1977.
3. Belloni G, Baciocco A, Burelli P, et al: The value of CT for the diagnosis of pituitary microadenomas in children. Neuroradiology 15:179–181, 1978.
4. Wolpert SM, Pool KD, Biller BJ, et al: The value of computed tomography in evaluating patients with prolactinomas. Radiology 131:117–119, 1979.
5. Gardeur D, Naidich TP, Metzger J: CT analysis of intrasellar pituitary adenomas with emphasis on patterns of contrast enhancement. Neuroradiology 20:241–247, 1981.
6. Daniels DL: The sella and juxtasellar region. In Williams AL, Haughton VM (eds): Cranial Computed Tomography: A Comprehensive Text. St. Louis, CV Mosby, 1985.
7. Macpherson P, Hadley DM, Teasdale G, et al: Pituitary microadenomas: Does gadolinium enhance their demonstration? Neuroradiology 31:293–298, 1991.
8. Stadnik TW, Stevenaert P, Beckers A, et al: Pituitary microadenomas: Diagnosis with two and three dimensional MR imaging at 1.5T before and after gadolinium. Radiology 176:419–423, 1990.
9. Mike Y, Matsuo M, Nishizawa S, et al: Pituitary adenomas and normal pituitary tissue: Enhancement patterns on gadopentetate enhanced MR imaging. Radiology 177:35–41, 1990.
10. Sakamoto Y, Takahashi M, Korogi Y, et al: Normal and abnormal pituitary glands. Gadopentetate enhanced MR imaging. Radiology 178:441–448, 1991.
11. Earnest FIV, McCullough EC, Frank DA: Fact or artifact: An analysis of artifact in high-resolution computed tomographic scanning of the sella. Radiology 140:109–114, 1981.
12. Taylor S: High resolution computed tomography of the sella. Radiol Clin North Am 20:207–236, 1982.
13. Cohen WA, Pinto RS, Kricheff II, et al: Dynamic CT scanning for visualization of the parasellar carotid arteries. AJNR 3:185–189, 1982.
14. Pinto RS, Cohen WA, Kricheff II, et al: Giant intracranial aneurysms: Rapid sequential computed tomography. AJNR 3:495–499, 1982.
15. Wing SD, Anderson RE, Osborn AG: Dynamic cranial computed tomography: Preliminary results. AJNR 1:135–139, 1980.
16. Mark L, Pech P, Daniels D, et al: The pituitary fossa: A correlative anatomic and MR study. Radiology 153:453–457, 1984.
17. Pojunas K, Daniels D, Williams A, Haughton V: MRI of prolactin-secreting microadenomas. AJNR 7:209–213, 1986.
18. Daniels DL, Pojunas KW, Pech P, Haughton VM: Magnetic resonance imaging of the sella and juxtasellar region. General Electric Company, 1984.
19. Wolpert SM, Molitch ME, Goldman JA, et al: Size, shape and appearance of the normal female pituitary gland. AJNR 5:263–267, 1984.
20. Gardeur D, Metzger J: Pathologic sellaire. Paris, Ellipses, 1982, p 10.
21. Swartz JD, Russell KB, Basile BA, et al: High resolution computed tomographic appearance of the intrasellar contents in women of child-bearing age. Radiology 147:115–117, 1983.
22. Syvertsen A, Haughton VM, Williams AL, et al: The computed tomographic appearance of the normal pituitary gland and pituitary microadenomas. Radiology 133:385–391, 1979.
23. Roppolo HMN, Latchaw RE: Normal pituitary gland. 2. Microscopic anatomy—CT correlation. AJNR 4:937–944, 1983.
24. Roppolo HMN, Latchaw RE, Meyer JD, et al: Normal pituitary gland. 1. Macroscopic anatomy—CT correlation. AJNR 4:927–935, 1983.
25. Bonneville JF, Cattin F, Moussa-Bacha K, et al: Dynamic computed tomography of the pituitary gland: The "tuft sign." Radiology 149:145–148, 1983.
26. Peyster RG, Hoover ED, Adler LP: CT of the normal pituitary stalk. AJNR 5:45–47, 1984.
27. Daniels DL, Haughton VM, Williams AL, et al: Computed tomography of the optic chiasm. Radiology 137:123–127, 1980.
28. Daniels DL, Herfkins R, Gager WE, et al: Magnetic resonance imaging of the optic nerves and chiasm. Radiology 152:79–83, 1984.
29. Kline LB, Acker JD, Post MJD, et al: The cavernous sinus: A computed tomographic study. AJNR 2:229–305, 1981.
30. Umansky F, Nathan H: The lateral wall of the cavernous sinus with special reference to the nerves related to it. J Neurosurg 56:228–234, 1982.
31. Daniels DL, Pech P, Mark L, et al: Magnetic resonance imaging of the cavernous sinus. AJNR 6:187–192, 1985.
32. Merritt HH: A Textbook of Neurology. Philadelphia, Lea & Febiger, 1969, pp 243–254, 269–279, 281–282.
33. Chason JL: Nervous system and skeletal muscle. In Anderson WAD (ed): Pathology. St. Louis, CV Mosby, 1971, pp 1403–1428, 1796–1799, 1838–1842.
34. Post MJD, David NJ, Glasen JS, et al: Pituitary apoplexy: Diagnosis by computed tomography. Radiology 134:665–670, 1980.
35. Daniels DL, Williams AL, Thornton RS, et al: Differential diagnosis of intrasellar tumors by computed tomography. Radiology 141:697–701, 1981.
36. Critin CM, Davis DO: Computed tomography in the evaluation of pituitary adenomas. Invest Radiol 12:27–35, 1977.
37. Hemminghytt S, Kalkhoff RK, Daniels DL, et al: Computed tomographic study of hormone-secreting microadenomas. Radiology 146:65–69, 1983.
38. Russell EJ, George AE, Kricheff II, et al: Atypical computed tomographic features of intracranial meningioma: Radiological-pathological correlation in a series of 131 consecutive cases. Radiology 135:673–682, 1980.
39. Bilaniuk LT, Zimmerman RA, Wehrli FW, et al: Magnetic resonance imaging of pituitary lesions using 1.0 to 1.5 T field strength. Radiology 153:415–418, 1984.
40. Lee KL: The diagnostic value of hyperostosis in midline subfrontal meningioma. Radiology 119:121–130, 1976.
41. Hungerford GD, Biggs J, Levine JH, et al: Lymphoid adenohypophysitis with radiologic and clinical findings resembling a pituitary tumor. AJNR 3:444–446, 1982.
42. Quencer RM: Lymphocytic adenohypophysitis: Autoimmune disorder of the pituitary gland. AJNR 1:343–345, 1980.
43. Zeller JR, Cerletty JM, Rabinovitch RA, et al: Spontaneous regression of a post-partum pituitary mass demonstrated by computed tomography. Arch Intern Med 142:373–374, 1982.
44. Haughton VM, Rosenbaum AE, Williams AL, et al: Recognizing the empty sella by CT: The infundibulum sign. AJNR 1:527–529, 1980.
45. Miller JH, Pena AM, Segall HD: Radiological investigation of sellar region masses in children. Radiology 134:81–87, 1980.
46. Shu-Ren L, Bryson MM, Goblen RP, et al: Radiologic findings of hamartomas of the tuber cinereum and hypothalamus. Radiology 127:697–703, 1978.
47. Manelfe C, Lonvey JP: Computed tomography in diabetes insipidus. J Comput Assist Tomogr 3:309–316, 1979.
48. Peyster RG, Hoover ED: CT of the abnormal pituitary stalk. AJNR 5:49–52, 1984.
49. Brooks BS, Gammal TE, Hungerford GD, et al: Radiologic evaluation of neurosarcoidosis: Role of computed tomography. AJNR 3:513–521, 1982.
50. Futrell NN, Osborn AG, Chason BD: Pineal region tumors: Computed tomographic-pathologic spectrum. AJNR 2:415–420, 1981.
51. Paul LW, John H: The Essentials of Roentgen Interpretation. Hagerstown, MD, Harper and Row, 1972, pp 366–372, 375.
52. Armstrong EA, Harwood-Nash DCF, Hoffman H, et al: Benign suprasellar cysts: The CT approach. AJNR 4:163–166, 1983.

31

Tests of Pituitary Function

JOHN A. H. WASS
MICHAEL BESSER

It is increasingly rare to see undiagnosed, long-standing, or severe endocrine syndromes. Endocrine diagnosis depends more and more on laboratory tests. Thus, the aim of every endocrinologist should be to make an early diagnosis before symptoms develop. Increasing emphasis, therefore, has been put on dynamic pituitary function tests, which establish states of endocrine deficiency or excess.

Collection, Transport, and Storage of Samples

Appropriate collection, transport, and storage are clearly essential if reliable measurements of hormone concentrations in biological fluids are to be made, but comparatively little information is available on these topics despite their obvious importance. Before collection, the laboratory to which samples will be sent should be consulted to determine specific requirements; often special forms and containers for transporting specimens are needed. Particular attention should be paid to the exact time and conditions of the sample, e.g., fasting, stress, sleep, or posture. Furthermore, essential clinical details and drugs being taken at the time of blood sampling should be noted. A large number of drugs may affect anterior pituitary hormone secretion (for example, centrally acting drugs may affect prolactin; concurrent steroid or estrogen therapy affects glucocorticoid, thyroid, or androgenic hormone measurements; and anticonvulsants may alter thyroid function tests). Serum or plasma samples should, if possible, be transported to the laboratory within a few hours. They can usually be sent on ice, as most peptide and steroid hormones are stable in plasma at 0° to 4°C for many hours. It has been shown that transport at ambient temperature does not alter levels of thyroid-stimulating hormone (TSH), luteinizing hormone (LH), follicle-stimulating hormone (FSH), and probably growth hormone (GH) and prolactin.[1] Samples for ACTH need to be taken rapidly, centrifuged immediately, and the plasma separated and put straight onto Dry Ice or into a freezer because of the rapid degradation of this peptide by circulating peptidases. Prior to assay, samples should be stored at $-20°C$.

This chapter deals with pituitary function tests, discussing in turn those used for each of the individual hormones

to delineate first deficient and then excess secretion. Each laboratory department develops its own detailed test procedures and normal ranges based upon different assay reagents and standards. The systems described are based predominantly on those currently in use in the Department of Endocrinology at St. Bartholomew's Hospital, London.

HYPOPITUITARISM

Hypopituitarism is encountered frequently in clinical endocrine practice. If progressive pituitary hormone deficiency occurs, there is usually a characteristic order of loss, with GH deficiency occurring first, closely followed by LH. Prolactin deficiency is rare. FSH, TSH, and ACTH deficiencies usually occur much later. Antidiuretic hormone (ADH) deficiency usually implies a primary hypothalamic disturbance, as it is virtually unknown in patients with anterior pituitary tumors not exposed to surgery.

Anterior Pituitary Deficiency

Growth Hormone Deficiency

GH deficiency may occur as a result of either anterior pituitary failure or failure of hypothalamic GH-releasing hormone (GRH) secretion.

BASAL TESTS. Secretion of GH in normal subjects is below levels detectable by routine radioimmunoassay (RIA) but sometimes just detectable by the more sensitive double antibody immunoradiometric assays (IRMA) basally (<0.5 ng/ml, 1 mU/L) for most of the day. Episodic bursts of GH occur with greater frequency at night, especially during EEG stages III and IV of sleep, although occasional bursts of secretion are seen during the day, approximately every four hours. For this reason it is not possible to differentiate hypopituitarism from normal by the measurement of basal samples of GH because low levels may be seen in both states. Measurement of GH secretion rates has been achieved by the use of continuous sampling,[2] but this is too time consuming and expensive for routine diagnostic use.

Insulin-like Growth Factor I (IGF-I). IGF I measurements may aid in the diagnosis of GH deficiency. The IGF's are a family of peptide growth factors, some of which are GH-

TABLE 31–1. BIOCHEMISTRY AND RESPONSES TO TREATMENT IN VARIOUS CAUSES OF SHORT STATURE

CAUSE	SERUM GH		SERUM IGF I		
	Basal	*Stimulated*	*Basal*	*On GH Therapy*	*Response to GH Treatment*
Isolated GH deficiency	↓	↓	↓	N	Growth
Hypopituitarism	↓	↓	↓	N	Growth
Constitutional short stature	N	N	N (↓)	N	Growth
Laron's syndrome	↑	↑	↓	↓	No growth
Pygmy	N	N	↓	↓	

dependent. Most importantly, IGF-I is GH-dependent. Until recently, assays of the IGF's have been unreliable, but now the reliability of these assays has improved because of improved biochemical knowledge of their structures and plasma-binding proteins.[3, 4] IGF-I assays may assist in the classification of a number of short stature syndromes, including GH deficiency, normal variant short stature, the Laron syndrome, and the pygmy (Table 31–1).

DYNAMIC TESTS.[4a] Dynamic tests designed to stimulate secretion of GH and therefore to test for GH deficiency include sleep and exercise studies, insulin-induced hypoglycemia, stimulation with the amino acid arginine, and the use of drugs including L-dopa, clonidine, and propranolol, together with other hormones, e.g., GRF, thyrotropin-releasing hormone (TRH), and glucagon (Table 31–2). Propranolol is sometimes given together with another stimulation procedure such as arginine, as it enhances GH secretion. A number of conditions and drugs may affect the GH responses to stimulatory tests, and these are shown in Table 31–3.

PHYSIOLOGICAL TESTS. For physiological assessment, GH levels can be sampled during the onset of slow-wave sleep (EEG stages III and IV), occurring 30 to 90 minutes after sleep commences, as this is the time when maximal GH release occurs, accounting for the majority of the 24-hour GH release. Clearly the patient needs to be admitted to hospital and the study performed ideally during the second night because the initial night's sleep may not be accompanied by a normal EEG pattern. No drugs should be taken. As this procedure needs admission to hospital, currently it is not used widely. GH levels should rise above 15

TABLE 31–2. TESTS OF GROWTH HORMONE SECRETION

A. Physiological stimuli
    Sleep
    Exercise
B. Pharmacological stimuli
    Insulin-induced hypoglycemia
    Arginine
    Drug stimuli
        L-Dopa
        Clonidine
        Propranolol
    Hormone stimuli
        GRH
        TRH
        Glucagon

TABLE 31–3. CONDITIONS AND DRUGS KNOWN TO AFFECT GH RESPONSES TO STIMULATORY TESTS

INCREASED	DECREASED
Conditions	
Stress	Old age
Fasting	Obesity
Malnutrition	Delayed puberty
Anorexia nervosa	Hypothyroidism
Renal failure	Cushing's syndrome
Hepatic cirrhosis	Endogenous depression
Carcinoid syndrome	Emotional deprivation
Diabetes (poorly controlled)	
Laron's syndrome	
Drugs	
Propranolol	
α-Methyldopa	Corticosteroids
Estrogen	Chlorpromazine
Opiates	L-Dopa
	Phentolamine
	Cyproheptadine
	Methyldopa
	Ethanol
	Cannabinoids

mU/L (7.5 ng/ml). Sleep-induced GH release correlates well with that seen after insulin-induced hypoglycemia.[5]

Exercise is also a profound stimulus to GH release. Clearly it should not be undertaken in patients with coronary artery insufficiency or exercise-induced asthma. It can be performed using a bicycle ergometer, and the work load should be sufficient to achieve a pulse of 180 beats per minute. Samples should be taken basally, after 10 minutes exercise, and 10 and 30 minutes after stopping. GH levels should rise above 20 mU/L (10 ng/ml).

PHARMACOLOGICAL TESTS. Some workers have doubted the useful relationship of the GH references to dynamic pharmacological tests and the physiological GH secretory profiles. However, most believe that the relationships generally hold good, and they have been accepted as practical and valid over many years of use.

Insulin-Induced Hypoglycemia (Insulin Tolerance Test, ITT). This is the standard test for GH deficiency.[6–9] Provided that it is carefully monitored, it is safe and we have encountered no serious side effects with this test in regular use over a period of nearly 28 years.

Background. Hypoglycemia and neuroglycopenic stress are profound stimuli to the release of GH, and areas of the hypothalamus, particularly laterally, are sensitive to falls in blood glucose. Intravenous insulin is used to provide a reproducible and standardized hypoglycemic stimulus. Adequate hypoglycemia occurs when the blood glucose falls to less than 2.2 mmol/L (40 mg/dl) associated with signs of neuroglycopenia, including tachycardia and sweating, which lasts between 10 and 20 minutes. Hypoglycemia simultaneously stimulates ACTH/cortisol and prolactin secretion (see subsequent sections) as well as catecholamines, and these may be simultaneously measured. Insulin hypoglycemia tests the whole hypothalamic-pituitary axis. In a patient with panhypopituitarism, it can be used to demonstrate GH, ACTH (cortisol), and prolactin deficiency.

Preparation and Contraindications (Table 31–4). Before the test day, a plasma cortisol measurement should be taken between 7 and 9 A.M. and shown to be normal, as basal hypocortisolemia is a contraindication to testing ow-

TABLE 31–4. CONTRAINDICATIONS TO PERFORMING THE INSULIN TOLERANCE TEST (ITT)

1. Severe uncorrected hypopituitarism (basal cortisol <100 nmol/L [3.6 μg/dl])
2. Ischemic heart disease
3. Cardiac conduction disorder
4. Epilepsy, drop attacks

ing to the danger of inducing severe and prolonged hypoglycemia in such a patient. Glycogen stores will be low and the glucose therefore fails to rise in response to the release of counter-regulatory hormone release (e.g., catecholamines and glucagon). Thyroxine in serum should also be normal, as hypothyroidism impairs both GH and ACTH secretion. An ECG should be taken, as both myocardial ischemia and cardiac conduction disorders are contraindications to this test because they can both be exacerbated by hypoglycemia and catecholamine release. The test should never be performed on known epileptics, as hypoglycemia may induce a seizure.

The test should be performed in the morning after an overnight fast (water allowed) with the subject at rest on a bed or couch. It may be performed on an outpatient basis. Regular medical surveillance is necessary throughout. The subject should be asked about the symptoms of neuroglycopenia and should be seen to sweat, and the timing of these events should be noted. Fifty per cent dextrose and hydrocortisone should be readily available for use in an emergency.

Procedure. The patient is weighed. (1) Insert a reliable cannula at a convenient time prior to 8:30 A.M. and keep it patent with heparinized saline (1 ml of 10,000 U/ml heparin in 10 ml saline). (2) After 30 minutes draw blood for glucose, GH, and cortisol. Note time. (3) Give insulin intravenously via the cannula, ensuring that it is all washed into the vein. The dose of insulin is usually 0.1 to 0.15 U/kg (see next). (4) After withdrawing dead-space heparinized saline and discarding, blood is withdrawn as mentioned for glucose, serum GH, and cortisol at 30, 60, and 90 minutes after the insulin injection. (5) If there is no clinical evidence of hypoglycemia at 45 minutes (i.e., no sweating or tachycardia), the total insulin dose may be repeated and blood sampling repeated as mentioned. (6) After the 90-minute blood sample is taken, the patient should drink 25 g glucose and eat a carbohydrate-based breakfast.

It is useful to have a glucose meter available for the immediate measurement of the blood glucose level even though such bedside analyses are not as accurate as laboratory measurements of low blood sugar levels. This is advisable to assess whether adequate hypoglycemia has been achieved. Neutral, purified, or human insulin is used. The usual dose is 0.15 U/kg. Larger doses (0.2 to 0.3 U/kg are used only in patients with insulin resistance, e.g., Cushing's syndrome or acromegaly). This is not the case in hypopituitary patients. In children under the age of eight years, 0.1 U/kg is usually given; the test is rarely performed in children under the age of five years. It is very rarely necessary to terminate the test prematurely, but this is indicated in severe or prolonged sweating (more than 20 minutes) or in the presence of impending or actual loss of consciousness or seizures. If necessary, give 20 ml 50 per cent dextrose intravenously followed by a drip of 5 per cent dextrose. Sampling should be continued until the end of the test in these circumstances, because an adequate stress stimulus would have been achieved before the glucose was given.

Normal Responses. The GH level should certainly rise above 20 mU/L (10 ng/ml), but a number of factors shown in Table 31–3 may alter the responses. Levels between 10 and 20 mU/L (5 and 10 ng/ml) are equivocal. Occasionally, just before or in early puberty, the increase in serum GH is borderline in children whose growth subsequently appears normal. In such cases, especially when the bone age is 10 years or more, the test should be repeated after priming with stilbestrol, 1 mg twice daily for 48 hours, or intramuscular testosterone, 100 mg five days before.

There are a number of second-line tests of GH reserve:

Arginine Test.[10-13] *Background.* Several amino acids cause GH release, including arginine, histidine, lysine, phenylalanine, leucine, valine, methionine, and threonine. These may be given as a complexed protein meal or beef extract,[13] but the arginine test is more reproducible and reliable.

Procedure. The arginine test should be performed in the morning after an overnight fast. The patient is weighed. Two forearm venous cannulae are inserted before 9 A.M. After 30 minutes the arginine is given as an intravenous infusion of 10 per cent solution in saline in a dose of 0.5 g/kg body weight (to a maximum of 30 g) over a period of 30 minutes through one of the cannulas. The subject should be recumbent throughout the test, during which samples for GH are taken through the other intravenous cannula at 30-minute intervals for two hours. There are no side effects.

Normal Responses. GH should rise to at least 15 mU/L (7.5 ng/ml), and peak values are usually seen around 60 minutes after commencing the test. Occasionally normal subjects do not respond. Peripubertal patients can be pretreated with stilbestrol or testosterone (as described earlier). Women and children respond more consistently and have a greater rise than men. The GH response to arginine is not influenced by a number of conditions that inhibit the response to hypoglycemia, including treatment with steroids.

L-Dopa.[14] Dopaminergic mechanisms are important for GH release, and L-dopa (10 mg/kg, or 500 mg in an adult) in normal subjects stimulates GH release. Peak GH levels are seen 60 to 120 minutes after the drug is administered, but there is a failure rate of 25 to 40 per cent in normal adults; this may be reduced to 2 to 10 per cent by the prior administration of propranolol (0.75 mg/kg up to a maximum of 40 mg), which potentiates the GH response to L-dopa. A major disadvantage is the induction by L-dopa of nausea and vomiting in up to 40 per cent of subjects. Patients should fast prior to the test.

Clonidine. Clonidine, an α-adrenoceptor agonist, has been observed to stimulate GH release. The usual dose is 0.15 mg/m² orally or as an intravenous dose of 0.2 μg/kg body weight given over a period of 10 minutes. Release of GH occurs between 60 and 90 minutes following ingestion or 60 minutes after the intravenous dose. All subjects experience a fall of systolic blood pressure of 20 to 25 mm Hg, and this may persist for one to three hours. The drug may also cause drowsiness. The locus and mechanism of action are not known, nor is the relationship to physiological GH secretion. More data on its reliability exist in children and adolescents than in adults.

Glucagon.[18, 19] *Background.* Glucagon stimulates the release of insulin and subsequently GH and ACTH in normal subjects. The peak GH response occurs later than that after insulin-induced hypoglycemia, between 120 and 180 minutes following injection. Evidence suggests that GH response follows the rapid drop in blood glucose which is seen after the initial rise induced by glucagon. However, a high failure rate is seen in GH responses to glucagon in normal adult subjects, as high as 40 per cent if it is given intramuscularly or intravenously. This can be reduced to 10 to 15 per cent by the prior administration of propranolol and by subcutaneous administration of glucagon. This test is routinely used in patients who cannot be tested with insulin, especially children. Estrogen or testosterone priming may be used as for the insulin test. It is not reliable in patients with diabetes mellitus.

Procedure. The test is performed after an overnight fast with the subject at rest. An indwelling forearm venous cannula is inserted before 9 A.M. After 30 minutes, two basal samples are taken and then a dose of 1 mg of glucagon is given subcutaneously. In children 0.5 mg may be used, and for adults weighing more than 90 kg, 1.5 mg is administered. Sampling for blood glucose, GH, and cortisol continues at 30-minute intervals for 240 minutes.

Side effects may be noted, and some patients are nauseated and vomit during the second half of the test. Normally a GH level of greater than 20 mU/L (10 ng/ml) should be achieved. Glucagon usually stimulates ACTH release. Therefore, it may be used simultaneously to test ACTH reserve. Rarely, normal subjects fail to show a GH or cortisol rise, and the test is unreliable in diabetes mellitus.

Growth-Releasing Factor (GRF) Test. *Background.* Administration of GRF tests the readily releasable pool of GH in the pituitary gland. Because it acts directly on the pituitary, not the whole hypothalamic-pituitary axis, it cannot alone establish a diagnosis of hypopituitarism. It does, however, distinguish between a hypothalamic and a pituitary deficit in a patient with established deficiency of GH. GRF occurs mainly as a 1-40 peptide, but it has been shown that the biological activity resides in the first 29 amino acid residues. Thus, the GH-releasing activity of synthetic GRF (1-29) NH$_2$ in normal subjects is identical to that seen with GRF (1-40).[20] GRF testing may be important because a number of patients (for example, after radiation therapy or surgery) with apparent GH deficiency are in fact GRF deficient owing to defective synthesis of GRF or its delivery to the pituitary. A rise in serum GH after GRF in a patient who has an absent GH rise after insulin-induced hypoglycemia suggests hypothalamic deficiency of GRF. There are no contraindications to the administration of GRF. Although priming with estrogen enhances the GH response to hypoglycemia and L-dopa, this is not seen with GRF testing,[21] suggesting that the priming effect works at a hypothalamic, not a pituitary, level.

Procedure. After an overnight fast a cannula is inserted. Two basal samples are taken and GRF, 100 μg or 1.5 μg/kg in a child, is administered as a bolus over two minutes. Samples are taken for serum GH at 15-minute intervals for 120 minutes. Transient facial flushing, lasting up to five minutes, occurs in most subjects. Normally a rise greater than 10 mU/L (5 ng/ml) is seen.

Gonadotropin Deficiency

In contrast to the stimulatory tests necessary for the diagnosis of GH deficiency, the diagnosis of gonadotropin deficiency can be made largely by measuring basal serum LH and FSH and gonadal steroids—testosterone in men and estradiol in women—simultaneously. This gives information as to whether the hypothalamus or pituitary is at fault or the hypogonadism is due to primary gonadal failure. Thus, for example, with high gonadotropins and a low estradiol or testosterone, the hypogonadism is of gonadal origin, whereas with low or normal gonadotropins and a low estradiol or testosterone level, the hypogonadism is caused by a disturbance of hypothalamic or pituitary function. Further tests are needed to decide whether the hypothalamus or the pituitary is malfunctioning.

In women who have menstrual cycles, basal gonadotropins and estradiol are measured in the follicular phase of the cycle and the adequacy of ovulation is assessed with serial progesterone measurements in the luteal phase of the cycle (e.g., days 18 to 25). Serial ovarian ultrasound studies may also be performed to establish normal follicular and corpus luteum development. In men, basal serum testosterone and LH/FSH levels are measured at 9 A.M.

DYNAMIC TESTS. The various tests assess different aspects of the hypothalamic-pituitary-gonadal axis. Thus the clomiphene test assesses hypothalamic function, and gonadotropin-releasing hormone (GnRH) directly stimulates pituitary gonadotropin secretion. Gonadotropins themselves stimulate the gonads. For the latter test, either human menopausal urinary gonadotropin in women (hMG, e.g., Pergonal; containing both LH and FSH activity), or human chorionic gonadotropin (hCG) in men (containing predominantly LH activity) is generally used.

Clomiphene Test. *Background.* Clomiphene can be used to test the integrity of the negative feedback system, which involves the gonad and the hypothalamic-pituitary axis. Clomiphene combines weak estrogenic with antiestrogen effects. Its main action is to compete for the estradiol receptors of the hypothalamus and the pituitary; the hypothalamic blockade of estrogen action leads it to cause an elevation of both LH and FSH. This effect takes two to four days to begin to appear. Clomiphene therefore tests whether the GnRH secretory reserve is normal. It has direct estrogenic effects on the liver, so it also increases circulating levels of sex hormone and other binding globulins. Total circulating concentrations of sex hormones rise, especially testosterone, but those of free non–protein-bound hormones do not, unless LH/FSH levels also rise.

Contraindications. The use of clomiphene should be avoided in patients with liver disease and those with a recent history of depression. Thus, patients should be warned that sometimes this drug induces depression, particularly in men, and may cause flickering at the periphery of the visual fields. Both of these side effects disappear rapidly after cessation of the drug.

Procedure. Clomiphene is usually administered in a dosage of 3 mg/kg/day up to a maximum of 200 mg/day for 7 days. LH and FSH are measured on days 0, 4, 7, and 10. In women, if it is desired, subsequent ovulation and corpus luteum function can be assessed by measuring LH and FSH levels between days 10 and 14 to see whether a rise in gonadotropins occurs around the expected time of the ovulatory peak. In these circumstances, progesterone is measured between days 14 and 28; usually a single value of serum progesterone obtained on day 21 suffices to demonstrate the presence or absence of apparent ovulation.

Normal Responses. In both sexes the gonadotropins double by day 10. In Kallmann's syndrome (isolated GnRH deficiency) and in other hypothalamic diseases, sometimes after pituitary irradiation and in weight-related amenorrhea, no gonadotropin rise is seen. In prepubertal patients gonadotropins actually decrease during clomiphene administration. As weight is regained or puberty progresses, clomiphene responsiveness becomes apparent. Adequate corpus luteum function is usually presumed if the day 21 serum progesterone level exceeds 30 nmol/L (10 µg/L).

GnRH Test. Synthetic GnRH stimulates the pituitary gonadotrophs directly to release their readily releasable pool of LH and FSH. It does not totally deplete the pituitary of its hormone. There are no contraindications to the administration of GnRH.

Procedure. No preparation is needed, and the patient need not fast. Basally serum estradiol or testosterone should be measured after an intravenous cannula has been inserted. Blood samples are withdrawn for LH and FSH before and at 20 and 60 minutes after intravenous GnRH (100 µg). Normally serum LH levels rise rapidly after the bolus, reaching maximal levels at 20 minutes and falling by 60 minutes. FSH may rise more slowly and peak at 60 minutes, but in adults LH responses normally exceed FSH. The responses vary with gender and reproductive status. In females they vary considerably between stages of the menstrual cycle, being lowest in the early follicular phase. If the patient is cycling it is conventional to assess the LH and FSH response to GnRH during the middle of the follicular phase. In prepubertal children baseline gonadotropin levels are lower and responses to GnRH are less than those of adults. In the early stages of puberty FSH responses are greater than those of LH, but as puberty progresses LH peak values overtake those of FSH.

The GnRH test is a valuable tool in investigating the physiology and pathophysiology of the human hypothalamic-pituitary axis. However, it has limited value in establishing a diagnosis of LH/FSH deficiency or, in an established case, in helping to determine the level of the lesion. Thus gonadotropin deficiency is established when serum LH/FSH levels are not elevated in patients with low circulating basal gonadal steroids. Because the gonadotroph remains intact and contains releasable hormone, often in the presence of a pituitary tumor producing hypopituitarism by pituitary stalk compression, and virtually always with hypothalamic or stalk lesions, the GnRH test cannot distinguish between these levels of lesion. Thus normal, impaired, or excessive responses may be seen in both pituitary and hypothalamic causes of hypopituitarism. Absent LH/FSH responses are usually characteristic of a destroyed pituitary, but these can also be seen in prepubertal patients with long-standing hypothalamic lesions (e.g., craniopharyngioma) and in Kallmann's syndrome, if the gonadotroph has not been exposed to sufficient endogenous GnRH to promote LH/FSH synthesis. However, in the typical less severe cases of Kallmann's syndrome, basal LH/FSH levels are low but show a significant although often subnormal rise after GnRH.

Gonadotropin Stimulation Test. The gonads may be tested in women by administering hMG (Pergonal), which contains both LH and FSH activity. Three ampules (each containing 75 units of LH and FSH activity) may be given intramuscularly daily for three days, and serum testosterone or estradiol is measured before and 24 hours after the last dose. The response is impaired if the basal value is low and does not rise at least three-fold. In men, hCG is used; 2000 units given intramuscularly daily for three days should result in a tripling of low basal testosterone levels or a rise to levels outside the normal basal range.

Prolactin Deficiency

Prolactin deficiency is very rare except in Sheehan's syndrome (postpartum pituitary necrosis), anorexia nervosa, and total pituitary infarction. It has no human clinical sequelae except in causing failure of lactation in Sheehan's syndrome. TRH normally stimulates prolactin release. If it is necessary to assess prolactin reserve, a standard TRH test may be performed. As well as TSH (see next section), prolactin levels may be measured. Metoclopramide and domperidone, because of their actions as dopamine receptor antagonists, also cause prolactin secretion; this has been used as a research tool when prolactin deficiency is suspected but is not used in routine clinical practice.

Thyroid-Stimulating Hormone Deficiency

BASAL TESTS. These are usually enough to assess TSH reserve. Thus, T_4 and TSH measured simultaneously usually indicate whether the low serum T_4 is due to a central cause (hypothalamic or pituitary) if the TSH is not elevated, or the presence of primary thyroid disease when the serum TSH is elevated. No additional purpose is served by measuring T_3 in these circumstances. Very rarely the T_4 is low with a normal TSH in patients with thyroid-binding globulin (TBG) deficiency. In such cases a low thyroid hormone–binding test is seen and the diagnosis may be confirmed by direct TBG measurement. See also Chapter 39 for a full discussion of thyroid function tests.

DYNAMIC TESTS. *Thyrotropin-Releasing Hormone (TRH) Test.*[23, 24] Synthetic TRH may be given intravenously in a dose of 200 µg in 2 ml. It has been used as a test of hypothalamic-pituitary function and as a test for autonomy of thyroid function, but this has largely been superseded by sensitive TSH assays. Usually when given to patients with pituitary or hypothalamic disturbances, it is used to assess the readily releasable pool of pituitary TSH, but occasionally prolactin, as already mentioned, and GH (see later) may also be measured.

Procedure. No specific preparation is required. The patient need not fast, and the test should be performed in the morning because there is a greater TSH response to TRH in the evening than the morning. After insertion of an intravenous cannula, samples are withdrawn basally for serum TSH and for T_4 and T_3 if indicated. Following this, 200 µg of TRH is injected rapidly and TSH is measured at 20 (peak TSH level) and 60 minutes (to detect a delayed TSH rise). Rarely, mild and transient nausea occurs, flushing may be seen, and a perineal constricting feeling associated with a desire to micturate is noticed in about 70 per cent of subjects. These are immediate and always transient side effects, probably related to stimulation of smooth muscle in the gastrointestinal and genitourinary tracts. Very rarely TRH induces pituitary hemorrhage, giving a severe persistent headache associated with signs of pituitary expansion.[25]

In normal subjects TSH levels rise rapidly, reaching a maximum at 20 minutes and falling significantly by 60 minutes. Women have a slightly greater response because of circulating estrogens, and the response is blunted with increasing age in men. In central (i.e., pituitary/hypothalamic) hypothyroidism, the TSH response is usually reduced. It is only rarely absent. A value at 60 minutes greater than at 20 minutes suggests a hypothalamic lesion but is far from totally reliable. TSH responses may be normal in the presence of a pituitary tumor despite unequivocal secondary hypothyroidism. The TRH test therefore fails to diagnose the level of the lesion with any certainty.

The TRH test has also been used in the detection of thyroid autonomy when there is no serum TSH rise after TRH. Any rise in TSH after TRH excludes complete thyroid autonomy. A number of conditions, hormones, and drugs blunt the TSH response to TRH; these are shown in Table 31–5. Thus, a rise in TSH after TRH excludes hyperthyroidism; the absence of such a rise, however, does not necessarily indicate a diagnosis of thyrotoxicosis (Table 31–5). The newly developed sensitive TSH assays have largely obviated the TRH test in thyroid disease because subnormal levels can be differentiated from the normal range. In primary hypothyroidism the TSH response to TRH is exaggerated and prolonged. However, in primary hypothyroidism, basal TSH is elevated, thus obviating the TRH test.

ACTH Deficiency

Dynamic tests are needed to diagnose ACTH deficiency unless it is severe. In these circumstances the early morning cortisol is persistently low, less than 100 nmol/L (4 μg/dl). The whole hypothalamic-pituitary-adrenal axis may be tested using either insulin-induced hypoglycemia or glucagon. Intravenous corticotropin-releasing hormone (CRH) may be used to distinguish between hypothalamic CRH and primary pituitary ACTH deficiency. Exogenous ACTH is used to test the adrenal reserve.

DYNAMIC TESTS. *Insulin Tolerance Test.* The insulin tolerance test has been described on p. 488. If significant hypoglycemia is produced and the ACTH reserve is normal, the cortisol should rise above 550 nmol/L (20 μg/dl). Failure of this to occur in a patient with hypothalamic or pituitary disease, when the plasma cortisol response to exogenous ACTH is normal, suggests an impaired reserve of ACTH secretion.

Glucagon Test. The glucagon test is used if there are contraindications to insulin-induced hypoglycemia, for example epilepsy or ischemic heart disease. Similarly, glucagon should cause a rise in serum cortisol to above 550 nmol/L (20 μg/ml). However, this test, as with GH secretion, is less reliable than the insulin tolerance test and stimulates ACTH secretion in only 70 per cent of subjects with a normal ACTH reserve.

CRH Test. CRH stimulates ACTH secretion and is selective in its action. CRH tests are used in the diagnosis of isolated ACTH deficiencies and in the differential diagnosis of pituitary and ectopic ACTH secretion. There are no contraindications to its administration.

CRH is given intravenously, and blood samples for cortisol and ACTH are drawn at 15-minute intervals for 120 minutes. Normally a rise in ACTH and cortisol occurs.[26] Facial flushing is experienced as with other hypothalamic peptides but is transient. The CRH test has eliminated the need for the vasopressin test (vasopressin may act as a CRH), which often causes unpleasant side effects such as pallor, abdominal pain, and diarrhea.

ACTH Stimulation Tests. These are used for the demonstration of a normal adrenocortical reserve. Low plasma corticosteroids that do not rise after exogenous ACTH administration confirm disease of the adrenal cortex itself. If this persists after prolonged ACTH administration, primary adrenocortical failure is indicated rather than secondary adrenocortical atrophy due to impaired pituitary ACTH secretion, resulting either from prolonged corticosteroid therapy or from ACTH deficiency due to hypothalamic-pituitary disease.

Short ACTH Stimulation Test. Synthetic ACTH (1-24) is generally employed (tetracosactrin, Synacthen, or Cortrosyn). A dose of 250 μg is given intramuscularly, and plasma cortisol is measured at 0, 30, and 60 minutes. The test should be carried out at 9 A.M., and there is no contraindication.

A normal increment is 200 nmol/L (7 μg/dl) and poststimulation levels should exceed 550 nmol/L (20 μg/dl). Very rarely, patients with mild primary adrenal failure and elevated ACTH levels have a normal response to the short tetracosactrin test because the dose conventionally used is 1000 times the physiologically maximum effective dose. There are no side effects.

Long ACTH Stimulation Test. This test should be carried out in patients who have failed to respond to the short test. A depot preparation of 1 mg synthetic ACTH (1-24) (depot tetracosactrin, Synacthen depot, Cortrosyn depot) can be injected intramuscularly and has a duration of action of between 24 and 48 hours. Two procedures are available: (a) 1 mg depot tetracosactrin is injected by deep intramuscular injection at 9 A.M., and blood is sampled for cortisol before and at 1, 4, 6, 8, and 24 hours after injection. Normally, plasma cortisol levels peak by eight hours. In secondary adrenocortical atrophy there is a delayed rise in corticosteroids, and values remain low for the first four hours. This is followed by a rise that reaches a peak at 24 hours. In primary adrenocortical failure corticosteroid values remain low throughout. Alternatively, (b) in cases of very suppressed adrenal glands, 1 mg of depot tetracosactrin can be given daily intramuscularly for three days fol-

TABLE 31–5. CONDITIONS AND DRUGS ALTERING THE TSH RESPONSES TO TRH

INCREASED	DECREASED
Primary hypothyroidism	Thyroxine
Estrogen therapy	Triiodothyronine therapy
Excess antithyroid therapy	Glucocorticoids—prolonged
Hyperprolactinemia	Cushing's syndrome
	Growth hormone
	Somatostatin
	L-Dopa
	Ophthalmic Graves' disease
	Graves' disease/euthyroid early on treatment
	Autonomous thyroid adenoma
	Multinodular goiter
	Hypopituitarism
	Acromegaly

lowed on the fourth day by a short ACTH stimulation test. A clear rise in plasma cortisol to above 550 nmol/L (20 µg/dl) excludes adrenal atrophy. It is important to note that a normal short or long tetracosactrin test does not exclude ACTH deficiency.

A flow diagram for the diagnosis of adrenal insufficiency is shown in Figure 31–1.

Posterior Pituitary Deficiency

Polyuria, defined as the passage of more than 2 L of urine per day in an adult, when persistent may be due to central cranial diabetes insipidus with deficiency of ADH, nephrogenic diabetes insipidus in which there is resistance to the renal action of ADH, or to an excessive intake of water, primary polydipsia. In assessing posterior pituitary function, it is important to note that cortisol deficiency may decrease the glomerular filtration rate to such an extent that symptomatic diabetes insipidus is obscured unless, if present, this is adequately treated. It is therefore essential to evaluate fully the anterior pituitary function in patients with potential ACTH deficiency and to give replacement, if necessary, with corticosteroids prior to assessing posterior pituitary function. Similarly, patients should be euthyroid. In the presence of low cortisol or thyroid hormone levels, patients often cannot excrete excess water normally.

DYNAMIC TESTS. *Water Deprivation.* In the assessment of ADH deficiency two tests are used. The eight-hour water deprivation test (modified from Dashe et al.[28]) and in equivocal cases the prolonged water deprivation test (modified from Miller et al.[29]). Water deprivation is the most physiological way of testing posterior pituitary function. The essential step is to see whether the patient can concentrate urine in response to a rise in plasma osmolality. Water deprivation can, however, be dangerous, particularly if a large amount of fluid is lost through polyuria, as severe dehydration and electrolyte disturbances can occur. Patients have to be carefully supervised, therefore, on account of this and also to avoid surreptitious water drinking. The test aims at differentiating between central cranial diabetes insipidus, nephrogenic diabetes insipidus, and primary polydipsia. There are no contraindications.

Procedure. Patients need not fast, but before the test, which is started in the morning, they are encouraged to drink water only so that they are well hydrated. Tea, coffee, alcohol, and smoking, all of which may modify ADH secretion, are not allowed from midnight before the test. Clearly, if the patient is on a vasopressin preparation, this should be omitted the night prior to the test. The patient empties the bladder at a set time in the morning after a light breakfast and is then weighed. An intravenous cannula is inserted, and no water is allowed for eight hours. Consideration should be given to stopping the test if more than 3 per cent of the initial body weight is lost, as this may mark excessive dehydration. The patient should therefore be weighed before beginning the test and after four, six, seven, and eight hours. Five urine samples over an hour are taken between 8.30 and 9.30 A.M. and at intervals thereafter for up to eight hours. The urine volume and osmolality are recorded as well as the osmolality of the plasma taken at the midpoint of each urine sample. At the end of the eight-hour period, 2 µg of desmopressin (DDAVP) is given intramuscularly and thereafter the patient may drink. Urine and blood samples are taken after this at two-hour intervals for four hours. If the test is carefully supervised, severe electrolyte and fluid depletion can be avoided.

Interpretation. In normal subjects after eight hours' dehydration, urine osmolality should be greater than 600 mOsm/kg. Plasma osmolality should remain below 300

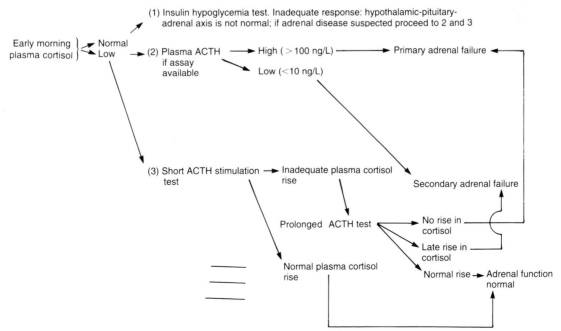

FIGURE 31–1. Biochemical diagnosis of adrenal insufficiency.

mOsm/kg. The urine flow rate should fall to below 0.5 ml/min. In patients with diabetes insipidus, the plasma becomes abnormally concentrated (>300 mOsm/kg) and the urine remains dilute (<270 mOsm/kg). Urine flow is not reduced to the expected degree. Urine flow/volume measurements alone, however, are inadequate, because they may fall in severe diabetes insipidus owing to excessive dehydration and a fall in GFR. The ratio of the osmolality of the urine to that of plasma does not rise above 1.9 in patients with moderate or severe diabetes insipidus. After DDAVP the maximal urine osmolality should become greater than 700 mOsm/kg in central diabetes insipidus. If there is no increase in urine osmolality after DDAVP, nephrogenic diabetes insipidus is present.

Compulsive water drinking (primary polydipsia) is rare. It can usually be differentiated from true diabetes insipidus with little difficulty, provided that the patient is denied access to water (it may be prudent to remove the tap handles in the room during the test). There may be a minor defect in urine concentration, but unlike patients with true diabetes insipidus, the plasma osmolality at the beginning of the test is normal (275 to 293 mOsm/kg) or low, and the clinical picture is one in which thirst rather than polyuria predominates. If during the water deprivation test 3 per cent or more of body weight is lost, a plasma osmolality estimation should be obtained. In the presence of a plasma osmolality greater than 305 mOsm/kg, a urine sample should be obtained and the test concluded early by giving DDAVP. Thereafter the urine osmolality is followed as in the full test. Cranial diabetes insipidus will have been established. A plasma osmolality of less than 280 mOsm/kg at this point usually indicates overdrinking before the test.

Prolonged Water Deprivation Test (Miller and Moses Test). In the prolonged water deprivation test, usually done in cases of mild diabetes insipidus when the results of a standard test are normal or equivocal, the patient has nothing to drink from the preceding night (6 P.M.). Basal urine and plasma are taken at 8 A.M., and hourly samples are taken for urine and plasma osmolality. The procedure is continued until a rise in urine osmolality of less than 30 mOsm/kg occurs over two succeeding samples. The patient is then given DDAVP as in the normal eight-hour water deprivation test, and the urine osmolality is followed for four hours.

In normal subjects a plateau of urine osmolality occurs and no further rise occurs after DDAVP. This means that as much urinary concentration occurs with maximal endogenous ADH secretion as can be achieved with exogenous hormone. This is not the case in patients with central diabetes insipidus, in which urine concentration after exogenous ADH rises markedly.

SYNDROMES OF PITUITARY HORMONE EXCESS

Acromegaly and Giantism (GH Excess)

BASAL TESTS. Measurement of basal serum GH on its own is not useful in acromegalic patients, as stress may cause elevation of GH in nonacromegalic patients,[30] and in acromegaly GH levels in blood may fluctuate markedly. The definitive diagnosis depends on the suppression of GH

values after oral glucose,[31] but as shown in Table 31–6, acromegaly is not the only condition associated with this abnormal GH response to oral glucose. IGF-I levels are a reliable indicator of excessive GH levels if raised, but a normal level of IGF-I does not exclude mild acromegaly.

DYNAMIC TESTS. *Oral Glucose Tolerance Test. Background.* Oral glucose in normal subjects results in elevation of blood glucose and suppression of GH release. It has been shown that hypothalamic neurons are electrically responsive to shifts in blood glucose, and these have been demonstrated in the ventromedial nucleus of the hypothalamus, one of the primary sites mediating GH secretion.[32] This fall is usually followed by a compensatory rebound of circulating GH. In acromegaly, elevated basal GH levels either do not suppress or even paradoxically increase after oral glucose.[33-35]

It is now accepted that GH levels should fall to less than 1 mU/L (0.5 ng/ml) at some time during the test to exclude active acromegaly. There are no contraindications to giving oral glucose apart from uncontrolled diabetes mellitus.

Procedure. After an overnight fast and 30 minutes after cannulation, 75 g of glucose are given (e.g., as cooled Lucozade to avoid nausea), and samples for blood glucose and GH are taken at 30-minute intervals for 150 minutes.

Interpretation. GH levels in serum should fall to less than 1 mU/L (0.5 ng/ml), but there are a number of causes of inadequate suppression besides acromegaly, including severe liver or renal disease, malnutrition, heroin addiction, and L-dopa ingestion (Table 31–6). In some patients confirmatory tests for acromegaly are required because there is a strong clinical suspicion of the disease in patients in whom the response during a glucose tolerance test is equivocal. In these cases TRH or dopamine may be used.

TRH Test. In 80 percent of patients with acromegaly, TRH causes GH release.[36] The reason for this is unclear, but in other circumstances in which basal GH is elevated (e.g., anorexia, liver disease), GH levels may also rise after intravenous TRH (Table 31–7). Again, therefore, the abnormal GH response to TRH is not diagnostic of acromegaly. In contrast, however, these patients usually have low circulating levels of IGF I, and it may be that lack of normal feedback initially is the underlying cause of these abnormal responses in nonacromegalic patients. It used to be thought that the GH rise after TRH seen in acromegalic patients was a result of abnormal receptors on the GH-producing pituitary tumor. This cannot be the case because such responses have been shown in patients with acromegaly caused by a GRF-secreting pancreatic tumor

TABLE 31–6. CONDITIONS ASSOCIATED WITH A FAILURE OF GH SUPPRESSION AFTER A GLUCOSE LOAD

Tall adolescents (>90 centile)
Acromegaly
Gigantism
Laron's syndrome
Diabetes mellitus (uncontrolled)
Hepatic cirrhosis and other liver diseases
Carcinoid syndrome
Renal failure
Malnutrition
Anorexia nervosa
Opiate addiction

TABLE 31–7. CONDITIONS ASSOCIATED WITH AN ABNORMAL GH RESPONSE TO TRH

Acromegaly
Gigantism
Malnutrition
Anorexia nervosa
Renal failure
Hepatic cirrhosis
Carcinoid syndrome
Endogenous depression
Diabetes mellitus

that causes pituitary hyperplasia[37] and in those with liver or renal disease.

Dopamine Infusion. Dopamine may also be used to diagnose acromegaly. As has been noted earlier, L-dopa causes a rise in GH levels in normal subjects.[38] In acromegaly, however, dopamine and dopamine-agonist compounds cause a paradoxical fall in circulating GH in at least 70 to 80 per cent of patients. Dopamine, when infused intravenously at a rate of 4 µg/kg/min for 90 minutes in patients with acromegaly, usually produces a fall in circulating GH levels throughout the period of the infusion, whereas in normal subjects a transient rise in circulating GH occurs.

Day Curve. In normal subjects, GH levels are undetectable for the majority of the day (in most routine assays <1mU/L[0.5 ng/ml]). In acromegalic patients there is always detectable GH in the circulation even though this may be low at times in mild cases. Samples for a "day curve" may be taken at 8.30 A.M., 1 P.M., 5 P.M., and 7 P.M. through an indwelling heparinized needle to assess GH secretion during the day in the ambulant patient.[39] The average level of GH determined in this way provides a more reliable measure of the general tissue exposure to GH than do the results of single blood samples.

The GRH Test. The GRH test is not diagnostically useful in acromegaly. Circulating GRH is elevated in a small proportion of acromegalics with nonpituitary tumors, usually of the pancreas or lung, causing hyperplasia of the pituitary.[40]

IGF-Binding Proteins (IGFBP). IGF I and IGF II circulate in the plasma attached to carrier or binding proteins. These function either as storage pools for IGF's or as a system to deliver IGF to the tissues. There are at least six IGFBP's. IGFBP-3, which exhibits constant levels in the serum throughout the day and corresponds to the acid stable subunit of the 140-kDa complex, does not cross the capillary barrier. IGFBP-3 is regulated by IGF I, and studies have shown IGFBP-3 is increased in acromegaly and conversely decreased in states of GH deficiency. It may thus prove to be a good clinical marker of GH status.

Prolactin Excess

Hyperprolactinemia

Physiological causes of hyperprolactinemia include pregnancy and lactation; drugs, particularly estrogens and dopamine antagonists like metoclopramide, domperidone, and haloperidol, may also have this effect. Patients with hypothyroidism may also have hyperprolactinemia, galactorrhea, and amenorrhea. Most frequent, however, are the

diseases of the hypothalamus and pituitary. Any hypothalamic lesion or pituitary tumor that may be ACTH- or GH-secreting or functionless but compresses the pituitary stalk may cause hyperprolactinemia up to about 2500 mU/L (125 ng/L) by interfering with the passage of dopamine down the pituitary stalk to the lactotropes. Levels above this usually indicate a primary prolactin-producing pituitary tumor, which is the most common cause of pathological hyperprolactinemia.[41]

Basal samples are adequate to diagnose hyperprolactinemia. Prolactin is a stress hormone; therefore, stress should be avoided during venipuncture. Several samples should be taken on three different occasions, because prolactin is secreted in a pulsatile fashion and basal levels may vary considerably in the same patient.

Dynamic tests of prolactin secretion do not aid diagnosis. Despite early suggestions to the contrary, the use of dopamine agonists and receptor antagonists such as nomifensine, L-dopa, chlorpromazine, and TRH do not differentiate reliably between hyperprolactinemia due to a pituitary tumor secreting prolactin and that due to other causes,[42] and the best indicator is an unstimulated serum prolactin level.

Adrenocorticotropin Excess

Details concerning all the tests utilized in Cushing's syndrome, its diagnosis and differential diagnosis with pituitary dependent disease, and causes of Cushing's syndrome are discussed in Chapter 100.

REFERENCES

1. Livesey JH, Hodgkinson SC, Roud HR, Donald RA: Effect of time, temperature and freezing on the stability of immunoreactive LH, FSH, TSH, growth hormone, prolactin and insulin in plasma. Clin Biochem 13:151–155, 1980.
2. Plotnick LP, Lee PA, Mijeon CJ, Kowarski A: Comparison of physiological tests of growth hormone function in children with short stature. J Clin Endocrinol Metab 48:811, 1979.
3. Clemmons DR, Van Wyk JJ: Factors controlling blood concentration of somatomedin-C. Clin Endocrinol Metab 13:113–143, 1984.
4. Furlanetto RW, Underwood LE, Van Wyk JJ, D'Ercole AJ: Estimation of somatomedin-C levels in normals and patients with pituitary disease by radioimmunoassay. J Clin Invest 60:648–657, 1977.
4a. Schonberg D: Diagnosis of growth hormone deficiency. Clin Endocrinol Metab 6:527–546, 1992.
5. Hindmarsh PC, Smith PJ, Taylor BJ, et al: Comparison between a physiological and pharmacological stimulus of growth hormone secretion: The response to stage IV sleep and insulin-induced hypoglycaemia. Lancet 2:1033–1035, 1985.
6. Roth J, Glick SM, Yalow RS, Berson SA: Hypoglycaemia: A potent stimulus to secretion of growth hormone. Science 140:987–988, 1963.
7. Landon J, Wynn V, James VHT: The adrenocortical response to insulin induced hypoglycaemia. J Endocrinol 27:183–192, 1963.
8. Greenwood FC, Landon J, Stamp TCP: The plasma sugar, free fatty acid, cortisol, and growth hormone response to insulin. 1. In control subjects. J Clin Invest 45:429–436, 1966.
9. Plumpton FS, Besser GM: The adrenocortical response to surgery and insulin-induced hypoglycaemia in corticosteroid-treatment and normal subjects. Br J Surg 56:216–219, 1969.
10. Fraser SD: A review of growth hormone stimulation tests in children. Paediatrics 53:929–937, 1974.
11. Raiti S, Davis WT, Blizzard RM: A comparison of the effects of insulin hypoglycaemia and arginine infusion on release of human growth hormone. Lancet 2:112, 1967.
12. Merimee TJ, Rabinowitz D, Fineberg SE: Arginine initiated release of human growth hormone: Factors modifying the response in normal men. N Engl J Med 280:1434–1438, 1969.

13. Jackson D, Grant DB, Clayton BE: A simple oral test of growth hormone secretion in children. Lancet 2:373–375, 1968.
14. Weldon VV, Gupta SK, Haymond MW, et al: The use of L-dopa in the diagnosis of hyposomatotropism in children. J Clin Endocrinol Metab 36:42, 1973.
15. Lazarus L: Growth hormone in endocrine disorders. *In* Donald RA (ed): A Guide to Diagnosis. New York, Marcel Dekker, 1984.
16. Lal S, Tobis G, Martin JB, et al: Effect of clonidine on growth hormone, prolactin, leutinising hormone, follicle stimulating hormone and thyroid stimulating hormone in the serum of normal men. J Clin Endocrinol Metab 41:827–832, 1975.
17. Gil'Ad I, Toffer E, Laron Z: Oral clonidine as a growth hormone stimulation test. Lancet 2:278–280, 1979.
18. Mitchell ML, Byrne MJ, Sanchez Y, Sawin CT: Detection of growth hormone deficiency: The glucagon stimulation test. N Engl J Med 282:539, 1970.
19. Fass B, Lippe BM, Kaplan SA: Relative usefulness of 3 growth hormone stimulation screening tests. Am J Dis Child 133:931–933, 1979.
20. Grossman A, Lytras N, Savage MO, et al: Growth hormone releasing factor: Comparison of two analogues and demonstration of hypothalamic defect in growth hormone release after radiotherapy. Br Med J 288:1785–1787, 1984.
21. Ross RJM, Grossman A, Davies PSW, et al: The effects of stilboestrol pre-treatment on the growth hormone response to insulin hypoglycaemia and GHRH; evidence from a hypothalamic site of action. J Endocrinol 108(Suppl):138, 1986.
22. Anderson DC, Marshall JC, Young JL, Russel Fraser T: Stimulation tests of pituitary-Leydig cell function in normal male subjects and hypogonadal men. Clin Endocrinol 1:127–140, 1972.
23. Ormston BJ, Garry R, Cryer RJ, et al: Thyrotropin-releasing hormone as a thyroid function test. Lancet 2:10–14, 1971.
24. Hall R, Ormston BJ, Besser GM, et al: Thyrotrophin releasing hormone test in diseases of the pituitary and hypothalamus. Lancet 1:759–763, 1972.
25. Drury PL, Belchetz PE, McDonald WI, et al: Transient amaurosis and headache after thyrotropin releasing hormone [letter]. Lancet 1:218–219, 1982.
26. Grossman A, Nieuwenhuyzen-Kruseman AC, et al: New hypothalamic hormone, corticotropin-releasing factor, specifically stimulates the release of adrenocorticotrophic hormone and cortisol in man. Lancet 1:921–922, 1982.
27. Liddle GW, Setep HL, Kendall JW, et al: Clinical application of a new test of pituitary reserve. J Clin Endocrinol Metab 19:875–894, 1959.
28. Dashe AM, Cramm RE, Crist CA, et al: A water deprivation test for the differential diagnosis of polyuria. JAMA 185: 699–703, 1963.
29. Miller M, Dalakos T, Moses AM, et al: Recognition of partial defects in anti-diuretic hormone secretion. Ann Intern Med 73:721–729, 1970.
30. Roth J, Glick SM, Yalow RJ, Bersen SA: Secretion of human growth hormone: Physiologic and experimental modification. Metabolism 21:577–579, 1963.
31. Earl JM, Sparks LL, Forsham PH: Glucose suppression of serum GH in the diagnosis of acromegaly. JAMA 201:134–136, 1967.
32. Oomura Y, Ono T, Ooyama H, Wamner MJ: Glucose and osmo-sensitive neurones of the rat hypothalamus. Nature 222:282–284, 1969.
33. Glick SM, Roth J, Yalow RJ, Bersen SA: The regulation of growth hormone secretion. Recent Prog Horm Res 21:241–283, 1965.
34. Hunter WM, Gillinham FJ, Harris PE, et al: Serial assays of plasma growth hormone in treated and untreated acromegaly. J Endocrinol 63:21–34, 1974.
35. Beck P, Parker ML, Daughaday WH: Paradoxical hypersecretion of growth hormone response to glucose. J Clin Endocrinol Metab 26:1463–1469, 1966.
36. Saito S, Abe K, Yoshida H, et al: Effects of synthetic thyrotrophin releasing hormone on plasma thyrotrophin, growth hormone and insulin levels in man. Endocrinol Jpn 17:101–108, 1971.
37. Thorner MO, Perryman RL, Krunen MJ, et al: Somatotroph hyperplasia: Successful treatment of acromegaly by removal of pancreatic islet tumour secreting a growth hormone releasing factor. J Clin Invest 70:965–977, 1982.
38. Boyd AE, Lebovitz HE, Pfeiffer JB: Stimulation of human growth hormone secretion by L-dopa. N Engl J Med 283:1425–1429, 1970.
39. Wass JAH, Thorner MO, Morris DV, et al: Long term treatment of acromegaly with bromocriptine. Br Med J 1:875–878, 1977.
40. Penny ES, Penman E, Price J, et al: Circulating growth hormone releasing factor concentrations in normal subjects and patients with acromegaly. Br Med J 25:453–455, 1984.
41. Ross RJM, Grossman A, Bouloux P, et al: The relationship between serum prolactin and immunocytochemical staining for prolactin in patients with pituitary macroadenomas. Clin Endocrinol 23:227–235, 1985.
42. Ho KY, Evans WS, Thorner MO: Disorders of prolactin and growth hormone secretion. Clin Endocrinol Metab 14:1–32, 1985.
43. Chang-DeMoranville BM, Jackson IMQ: Diagnosis and endocrine testing in acromegaly. Endocr Metab Clin North Am 21:649–668, 1992.
44. Abdulla AF, Holly JMP, Cotterill AC: Insulin-like growth factor binding proteins in acromegaly. Acta Endocrinol (Copenh) 124:87, 1991.

32

General Aspects of the Management of Pituitary Tumors by Surgery or Radiation Therapy

SHLOMO MELMED

TRANSSPHENOIDAL SURGERY

Although transcranial surgical removal of pituitary tumors had been advocated since the end of the nineteenth century, it was in 1909 that Harvey Cushing reported the cure of acromegaly by transsphenoidal resection of a pituitary adenoma.[1] Using the transsphenoidal approach, Oscar Hirsch, in 1910, successfully removed pituitary tumors using a transsinus approach.[2] However, the transcranial approach to surgically removing these tumors was subsequently favored for several decades until the development of the intraoperative microscope and its application by Hardy and co-workers.[3] The clear operative field and intense illumination provided by this technique facilitated the lucid visual distinction between adenomatous and normal pituitary tissue and allowed microdissection of very small tumors. The development of microinstrumentation as well as sophisticated head immobilization techniques further enhanced the utility of the transsphenoidal approach to tumor resection (Fig. 32–1).

The rapid improvement of MR imaging sensitivity and precision has likewise resulted in improved surgical efficacy for the pituitary mass. The role of accurate MR imaging in diagnosing the presence of a tumor, delineating its precise site and degree of invasiveness, and accurately assessing its size is pivotal in ensuring successful transsphenoidal surgery.

AIMS OF TRANSSPHENOIDAL SURGERY

Several important goals should be fulfilled to achieve successful resection of a pituitary mass. The primary pituitary lesion (that is, adenoma or other mass) should be carefully and selectively resected (Fig. 32–2). Neat and circumscribed resection may be difficult if the mass is poorly encapsulated, deeply embedded in the body of the adenohypophysis, or poorly discernible in the operative field. Clearly, manipulation or even excision of normal pituitary tissue should be performed only when these perturbations are essential for effective dissection of the lesion. Rarely, nonselective hemihypophysectomy or even total hypophysectomy may be required if no mass lesion is clearly discernible, if multifocal lesions are present, or if the remaining nontumorous pituitary tissue is clearly necrotic. Successful resection of a pituitary mass implies that endogenous pituitary trophic function not be compromised postoperatively. Retention or resumption of normal postoperative pituitary function is a major clinical goal for a surgical procedure. When preoperative compression including visual field defects or compromised trophic hormone secretion is present, surgery is expected to reverse these signs. When tumors are large and invasive, the skill of the experienced neurosurgeon will carefully determine the optimal balance between maximally effective tumor tissue removal and preservation of anterior pituitary function. In children and young adults this is especially important in preserving growth and reproductive function. Although pituitary hormone replacement is a well-proven and readily available option, it is usually a lifelong therapeutic commitment with careful and subtle control, especially of adrenal and reproductive function, being most difficult to achieve. Although residual tumor remnants in parasellar regions are not usually of major clinical importance in nonfunctional adenomas, these tissue remnants often remain hypersecretory, especially for prolactin-, growth hormone (GH)–, and the rare thyroid-stimulating hormone (TSH)–secreting adenomas, and may be difficult to access.

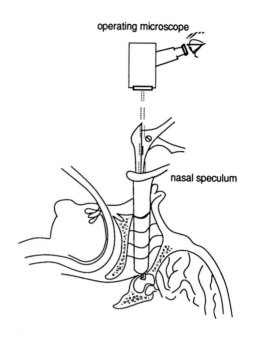

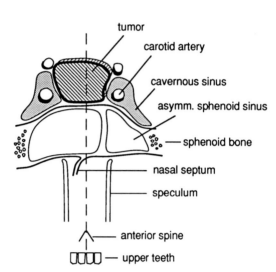

FIGURE 32–1. Schematic route for standard transsphenoidal midline approach. (From Fahlbusch R, Honegger J, Buchfelder M: Surgical management of acromegaly. Endocrinol Metab Clin North Am 21:669–692, 1992.)

INDICATIONS FOR TRANSSPHENOIDAL SURGERY

General

Naturally, the surgical benefits of not having to invade the cranium or directly manipulate brain tissue render the transsphenoidal approach to a pituitary lesion highly desirable if, in fact, therapeutic success can be achieved. This method is therefore highly favored and, with few exceptions, is the mainstay surgical approach for pituitary tumors.[4]

The general indications for pituitary surgery include the presence of a pituitary mass that may or may not be impinging on vital surrounding structures. The transsphenoidal approach to decompressing mass lesions of the pituitary is favored for several reasons. Most notably, the morbidity and mortality of the procedure are minimal. Most patients are ambulatory within six to nine hours after surgery, and length of hospital stay is generally less than five days. The low morbidity may be ascribed to the fact that the cranial fossa is not violated by the ventral sphenoid approach to the pituitary. Signs and symptoms of postoperative cerebral damage therefore do not occur, as direct

trauma to the brain is usually not encountered. Importantly, elderly and even critically ill patients are able to undergo the procedure with minimal added physical discomfort. The effective intraoperative use of the surgical microscope also allows clear microdissection of small tumors that may not be readily discernible on MR imaging.

Nevertheless, the procedure may not necessarily be optimal for resection of all pituitary mass lesions, especially those extending above the sella turcica, surrounding the frontal or middle fossa, or invading posteriorly behind the clivus. Occasionally, if the optic tracts are surrounded or impinged upon by large invasive tumors, visualization of these vital structures may be difficult from the ventral approach.

Symptoms and signs of an expanding pituitary mass, including persistent headache, progressive visual field defects or loss of acuity, cranial nerve palsies, internal hydrocephalus, and very rarely intrapituitary hemorrhage and apoplexy, all require surgical decompression and resection of the enlarging lesion. The closed bony pituitary fossa renders intrapituitary bleeding a major life-threatening hazard if not adequately decompressed. Pituitary hemorrhage, with resultant apoplexy and partial or complete infarction, is an indication for urgent surgical decompression. Persist-

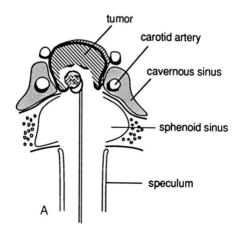

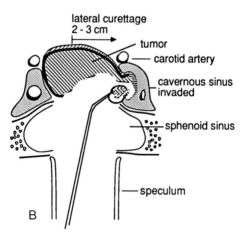

FIGURE 32–2. Midline (A) or lateral (B) tumor curettage. (From Fahlbusch R, Honegger J, Buchfelder M: Surgical management of acromegaly. Endocrinol Metab Clin North Am 21:669–692, 1992.)

ent CSF leakage after previous surgery may also require reoperation and transsphenoidal repair procedures. Finally, transsphenoidal surgery may rarely be indicated to perform a biopsy of pituitary tissue when a histological diagnosis is required.

Primary Indications

The specific lesions that require transsphenoidal resection are listed in Table 32–1.[4] The nonfunctioning pituitary adenoma is the most commonly encountered pituitary mass lesion. These tumors are often asymptomatic and may be diagnosed only after an incidental brain MR or other imaging procedures. As they grow inexorably and rarely undergo hemorrhage and infarction, they should be resected even if no obvious pituitary dysfunction is apparent. Adjuvant radiation therapy may be required.

Transsphenoidal resection is the primary treatment of choice for GH-secreting adenomas. Lower GH levels (less than 40 μg/L or 80 mU/L) and smaller tumors (less than 10 mm in diameter) are indication of the best surgical response rate.[5] It is unclear at present whether or not preoperative octreotide therapy will shrink these tumors, especially in patients harboring macroadenomas.[6] Furthermore, although it has been proposed that preoperative octreotide may in fact improve the surgical outcome, no prospective data are yet available to support this contention. The results of surgery for these tumors are difficult to deduce accurately from the literature, as the definition of biochemical remission is often inadequate. Currently, most endocrinologists insist upon a GH level less than 2 μg/L (4 mU/L) within two hours after an oral glucose load, as well as a normalized insulin-like growth factor (IGF)-I level.[7] Using a less stringent criterion of random GH of less than 5 μg/L (10 mU/L), about 60 per cent of patients worldwide appear to be in remission after transsphenoidal pituitary tumor resection.[5] After successful surgery, small microadenomas are in biochemical remission in more than 80 per cent of cases.[8] The long-term relapse rate of other patients is unclear at present. Although most of these patients appear to be in permanent clinical remission, GH levels fail to suppress after oral glucose in many patients who were apparently in remission.[9] Larger tumors and invasion of parasellar structures portend a poor surgical response.

Although transsphenoidal resection of ACTH adenomas

TABLE 32–1. INDICATIONS FOR TRANSSPHENOIDAL SURGERY

Primary
  Nonsecreting adenoma
  GH-secreting adenoma
  ACTH-secreting adenoma
  FSH/LH-secreting adenoma
  TSH-secreting adenoma
  Nonadenomatous pituitary mass
  Pituitary hemorrhage
  Tissue histology
Secondary
  Tumor recurrence after surgery
  PRL-secreting adenoma (bromocriptine "resistant")
  Nelson's syndrome
  Tumor recurrence after irradiation
  Persistent hormone hypersecretion

is the treatment of choice for Cushing's disease, these adenomas may be difficult to visualize by current MR imaging techniques. In fact, highly active ACTH-secreting tumors may be only approximately 2 mm in diameter. Often, hemihypophysectomy or complete hypophysectomy may be required if adequate tumor visualization is not achieved preoperatively or intraoperatively. Importantly, the success of surgery in these patients is highly dependent upon the expertise and skill of the neurosurgeon. More than 70 per cent of patients with Cushing's disease experience postoperative remission in experienced centers.[10] Intrasellar tumor localization and size of less than 5 mm portend a favorable surgical outcome. In fact, extrasellar extension results in the surgical cure rate dropping to less than 40 per cent. Clinical recurrences occur in about 5 per cent of patients in remission, with a mean recurrence time of less than four years.[10] Nelson's syndrome is now rarely encountered, as bilateral adrenalectomies are no longer routinely performed in the management of Cushing's disease. These tumors arise in up to one third of patients who have undergone bilateral adrenalectomy and may manifest many years later. They are often aggressively invasive, and consequently their surgical results are relatively unfavorable. Although surgery offers the best chance of cure, successful resection is apparent in only about a quarter of all patients. Most patients require postoperative irradiation as well as poorly successful adjuvant medical treatment.

Transsphenoidal surgery is also the primary treatment of choice for the very rare tumors secreting TSH, follicle-stimulating hormone, or luteinizing hormone.[11] These tumors are usually large, with resultant hypopituitarism and visual impairment. If α-subunit levels are elevated preoperatively, then postoperative recurrence may be detected biochemically by recurring increased α-subunit levels.

In considering the diagnosis of a pituitary mass, it may occasionally be necessary to perform transsphenoidal surgery either to resect a nonadenomatous intrasellar mass or to rely on the histology of the surgical specimen to confirm a diagnosis. For example, a secondary metastatic deposit to the pituitary may, at transsphenoidal resection, be diagnosed in a patient not previously suspected of harboring a primary extrapituitary carcinoma.

Secondary Indications

The role of transsphenoidal surgery in the management of prolactin-secreting adenomas has changed over the past decade. During a 20-year follow-up, most of these adenomas are stable and do not grow appreciably.[12] Because of the excellent biochemical and anatomical response of these tumors to dopamine agonists and because of their relatively benign natural history, it has become infrequent for transsphenoidal resection to be indicated in these patients. In fact, the tumor recurrence rate after apparently initially successful transsphenoidal resection is unacceptably high, with most tumors recurring within five years.[13] In patients in whom prolactin levels are greater than 100 ng/ml (2000 mU/L) or who are harboring macroadenomas, recurrences increase. Overall, up to 50 per cent of microadenomas and up to 80 per cent of macroadenomas either recur or fail to remit after surgery. Nevertheless, surgery offers a rapid resolution of the biochemical and clinical features of hyperprolactinemia, decompression of compromised parasellar vital structures, and, at least in the short term, avoidance of medication.[14]

Therefore, the indications for transsphenoidal surgery in patients harboring prolactinomas include those resistant to dopamine agonists or those intolerant of the medication's side effects. An expanding prolactinoma impinging upon vital structures should be resected if bromocriptine gives no immediate relief of pressure symptoms. Pregnancy is associated with swelling of the normal pituitary gland, and, in addition, prolactinoma growth may be directly stimulated by estrogen. A rapidly expanding prolactinoma during pregnancy may therefore require urgent decompression and resection via the transsphenoidal route. Importantly, some patients may prefer the surgical option to the long-term commitment to take regular medication. An informed choice with explanation of relative risks and benefits of available treatment modalities should be offered to these patients.

Role of Surgery for Recurrent Tumors

The most important causes of tumor recurrence after surgery include extrasellar tumor extension and cavernous sinus involvement. Significantly, prior surgery performed by a relatively less experienced neurosurgeon or a prior unsuccessful transfrontal approach accounts for over half of patients requiring reoperation in experienced centers.

SIDE EFFECTS

The side effects of transsphenoidal pituitary surgery are listed in Table 32–2.[4] CSF leakage, transient diabetes insipidus, and hypopituitarism may occur in up to 20 per cent of all patients, and permanent diabetes insipidus, cranial

TABLE 32–2. SIDE EFFECTS OF TRANSSPHENOIDAL SURGERY

Surgery-related mortality (1%)
  Hypothalamic injury
  Vascular damage
  Cardiac
  Meningitis
  Pneumocephalus
  Pulmonary embolism
  Anesthetic
Permanent complications (5%–10%)
  Visual loss
  Diabetes insipidus
  Hypopituitarism—total or partial
  Oculomotor palsy
  SIADH
  Hemiparesis
  Encephalopathy
Transient complications (6%–20%)
  Diabetes insipidus
  CSF rhinorrhea
  Inappropriate ADH secretion
  Meningitis
  Hematoma
  Vascular damage
  Pulmonary embolism
  Narcolepsy
  Epistaxis
  Gastrointestinal bleeding
  Abscess

nerve damage, or visual disturbances may be encountered in up to 10 per cent of patients. Although the nasal sinuses in fact provide a nonsterile operating field, infectious arachnoiditis or meningitis is rarely encountered after this procedure. The incidence of side effects clearly depends on the degree of tumor invasiveness and the technical difficulty of the procedure. In most large series reported, operative mortality has generally been about 1 per cent. Generally, permanent side effects are rarely encountered in patients after microadenoma resection.

Surgical Failure

Surgical failure may have several causes. Naturally, a non–pituitary-related event such as bleeding disorder, anesthetic-related accident, or systemic complication may result in unsuccessful surgery. The most important causes of surgical failure appear to be related to incomplete tumor tissue removal. False preoperative tumor identification and poor tumor localization by imaging also may account for an unsuccessful resection. Rarely, the presence of a second, previously undiagnosed pituitary tumor results in persistence of hormone hypersecretion postoperatively. The presence of an ectopic tumor hypersecreting pituitary trophic hormone, especially ACTH, may become evident only after "failed" pituitary surgery.

Approach to the Pituitary "Incidentaloma"

Incidental sellar masses are commonly encountered, and pituitary adenoma accounts for most of these lesions.[15] Autopsy reports, as well as careful imaging techniques, indicate that clinically silent pituitary microadenomas are incidentally present in up to 25 per cent of the population. Because of their very slow growth, benign natural history, and absence of hormone hypersecretion, these microadenomas can safely be observed by annual imaging, without resorting to surgery or irradiation. In fact, during a 22-month median follow-up, 14 such patients did not demonstrate visible tumor growth.[16] For larger masses (greater than 1 cm) it is important to recognize nonadenomatous mass lesions whose management is most likely to be surgical. For example, a meningioma is often associated with bony hyperostosis; craniophayngiomas may be calcified and are usually hypodense on T2-weighted MR images; and gliomas are hyperdense on T2 images. Incidentally discovered silent macroadenomas require surgical intervention after appropriate hormonal and visual field evaluation. These tumors may in fact become invasive and may be associated with local pressure effects. If hormone hypersecretion is diagnosed, specific therapies are directed against the adenoma, including surgical, medical, and radiation therapy.

RADIATION THERAPY OF PITUITARY TUMORS

Principles

Megavoltage radiation therapy has the capacity to deliver high-energy ionizing irradiation to deep tissues. The ideal balance of maximal localized irradiation with minimum irradiation of surrounding normal structures requires precise tumor localization. A focused homogeneous irradiation field is achieved by precise MR image localization, a high-voltage (6 to 15 MeV) linear accelerator, an effective simulation technique, and accurate isocentric rotational arcing. A major determinant of accurate focus of the irradiation is the ability to reproduce the position of the patient's head at exactly the same points. This need for pinpoint accuracy is especially critical when delivering high-energy particles at recurrent patient visits. Maintenance of absolute head immobility is also essential during the procedure. The preferred dosage schedule for irradiating pituitary tumors is less than a total of 5000 rads given as 180-rad daily fractions over about six weeks.[17]

Indications for Radiation Therapy

The indications for radiation therapy are listed in Table 32–3. Radiation may be used either as a primary therapy for pituitary or parasellar masses or as an adjunct to surgical or medical treatment. The indication for primary use of radiation therapy is a highly individualized choice that depends on the experience of the center, expertise of the radiation therapist, and willingness of the patient to choose the benefits of the procedure against its potential risks. For example, in some centers, radiation is the primary therapy of choice in the management of patients with GH-secreting adenomas, whereas in others this treatment is reserved for post-surgical management of these patients.[18–20] Prolactin-secreting adenomas, although managed medically in most centers, may be subjected to primary irradiation.[21] The main indication for radiation therapy, however, is as adjuvant therapy to surgery. After surgical resection of non-functioning macroadenomas, irradiation may be indicated for ablation of residual tumor mass which may be apparent. In these cases, radiation is indicated for preventing or reversing prolactinoma invasiveness rather than for managing the hyperprolactinemia per se. Similarly, surgical resection of craniopharyngioma or other parasellar masses may require follow-up irradiation to prevent regrowth of the mass or to shrink residual tumor tissue not resected by surgery. Relative benefits of the respective modes of therapy for each disorder are discussed fully in their respective chapters.

As a general principle, persistent pituitary hormone hypersecretion after surgical resection requires either irradiation or medical management to suppress undesirable high trophic hormone levels. Tumor bulk present after surgery may persist either within the sella or in adjacent structures. Irradiation offers the only effective means of ablation of residual tumor tissue, derived from nonfunctional tumors. Prolactin- and GH-secreting tumor tissues are, however, also amenable to shrinkage by dopaminergic agonists or somatostatin analogues. Whenever surgery is contraindicated, irradiation is clearly a primary therapeutic option.

SIDE EFFECTS OF IRRADIATION

Pituitary Hormone Disruption

The hormone-synthesizing cells of the anterior pituitary gland are sensitive to radiation. Failure of pituitary hormone synthesis occurs commonly in patients who have undergone pituitary irradiation.[22, 23] More than 50 per cent of patients irradiated for acromegaly do in fact develop failure of ACTH, TSH, and or gonadotrophin secretion within 10 years.[18] No difference in radiation sensitivity of pituitary function has been confirmed for acromegalic versus nonacromegalic patients. Patients who have undergone previous surgery have an increased risk of radiation-induced hypopituitarism, and women also have an increased risk of developing hypogonadism.[17] Patients who have undergone pituitary irradiation require lifelong endocrine follow-up, with regular testing of anterior pituitary hormone reserve and, if necessary, adequate replacement therapy.

Cranial Nerve Damage

Damage to the optic nerve with impaired or lost vision occurs in about 2 per cent of all patients undergoing pituitary irradiation.[24–26] The risk of cranial nerve damage has been considerably lowered by not exceeding a dose of 200 rads at any one treatment session, and achieving a maximum dose exposure of less than 5000 rads. Nevertheless, blindness was recently reported in two patients receiving 4500 rads in 180-rad fractions for pituitary adenoma.[26] The differing incidence of visual impairment reported from several centers emphasizes the need for scrupulous adherence to a highly rigid therapy protocol in order to minimize this distressing side effect. In his extensive review of the literature, Jones has stressed that, using carefully planned radiation therapy to the pituitary, with fraction doses of 180 rads per day or less, to a total dose of 4500 rads, the risks are negligible.[27]

Central Nervous System Damage

Radiation-induced brain necrosis occurs in less than 1 per cent of patients receiving pituitary irradiation and also appears to be dose-related. Recently, MR imaging was used to determine cerebral effects of pituitary irradiation, and 14 of 46 patients exhibited visible changes, including temporal lobe atrophy and cystic changes, as well as diffuse cerebral atrophy.[24] Although the functional implications of these observations are at present unclear, they may in fact substantiate the loss of intellectual function and memory often invoked as a side effect of radiation in children and adults.

TABLE 32–3. INDICATIONS FOR PITUITARY RADIATION THERAPY

GH adenoma
PRL adenoma
ACTH adenoma
Nonfunctional adenoma
Craniopharyngioma
Tumor recurrence
Hypersecretion recurrence
Parasellar mass
Nelson's syndrome

Neoplasia

Suspected malignancies arising following pituitary tumor irradiation were not documented in a review of more than 1000 cases.[17] Nevertheless, in a recent report, five of 334 patients developed a second brain tumor during a 3760 person-year follow-up.[28] The calculated cumulative risk of developing a brain tumor over the first 10 years after treatment was 1.3 per cent, and over 20 years 1.9 per cent. This implies a relative risk to patients of greater than 9 compared with the general population risk.[28] All these tumors arose within radiation field regions. When irradiation of craniopharyngioma was reviewed, 57 patients were found to have developed gliomas, sarcomas, or meningiomas within 7 to 14 years after surgery. Although the association of pituitary tumors with secondary brain tumors could potentially occur independently of irradiation, these compelling results warrant a controlled study of this very important question.

Effect on Subsequent Surgery

Radiation-induced fibrosis and scar formation may render subsequent pituitary surgery technically difficult. Postoperative CSF leaks, wound healing, and hemorrhage may also be more difficult to control in these patients.

PITUITARY REPLACEMENT THERAPY

The tests to determine the necessity for replacement therapy in pituitary disease are detailed in Chapter 31. Replacement of pituitary trophic hormone function may be required after pituitary surgery or irradiation. The determination of postoperative or postirradiation partial or complete pituitary dysfunction is usually followed by a lifelong commitment to adequately restore physiological pituitary function.

Adrenal Hormone Replacement

The diagnosis of ACTH deficiency is critical, as hypofunction of this axis may lead to adrenal crisis and death, especially during a stressful event. Replacement adrenal steroids are usually administered as a 30-mg daily dose of hydrocortisone (or 5 mg prednisone), usually given in a split dose of roughly 2:1 ratio in the morning and early evening. Because ACTH deficiency is rarely associated with mineralocorticoid deficiency, adequate hydrocortisone replacement should suffice for most patients. The dose of hydrocortisone should be increased two- to three-fold during stress, including dental procedures, anesthetics, and infections. Prominently displayed personal identification should indicate that patients are hypopituitary, and when traveling they should be encouraged to carry vials of injectable hydrocortisone.

Evaluation of efficient replacement is difficult and subjective. Patients' feelings of well-being, strength, and maintenance of body weight as well as important but subtle clinical features including serum sodium levels and blood pressure responses to postural changes should be followed.

Thyroid Hormone Replacement

Adequate physiological thyroid hormone replacement, traditionally administered as 0.1 to 0.2 mg synthetic T_4 daily, was traditionally monitored by measuring serum T_4 levels by RIA. Recently, several developments have challenged the accepted "mid" or "upper" level of derived T_4 as a determinant of replacement. The advent of ultrasensitive TSH assays has allowed replacement to be followed more precisely by the desired suppressed TSH levels. Clearly, most patients with post-surgical or irradiation pituitary damage have low or absent TSH levels; therefore, measuring serum T_4 or even T_3 by RIA provides a physiological reflection of the achieved blood levels. A further consideration is the recently emphasized notion of "over-replacement" of thyroid hormone, leading potentially to accelerated osteopenia in women.

Although compelling, these data require several years to be totally substantiated. Nevertheless, women receiving T_4 replacement should therefore not be "overtreated," and their desirable T_4 levels should be titrated to achieve appropriate ranges. This is usually accomplished by maintaining TSH in the range 0.4 to 1.0 μU/ml if TSH levels can be evaluated, or by maintaining serum T_4, or free thyroxine index, free T_4 levels in the high-normal or slightly elevated range. The use of desiccated or natural thyroid is not advocated for physiological replacement.

Gonadotropin Replacement

Gonadotropin requirements naturally differ in patients desirous of an active fertility span. The management of ovulation induction or testicular dysfunction to achieve fertility is fully considered in Chapter 119. In those women who do not wish to be fertile, conjugated estrogens should be replaced at a dose of 0.65 to 1.25 mg daily for the first 25 days of each month. Uterine shedding is facilitated by prescribing medroxyprogesterone (5 or 10 mg daily) from days 21 through 25 or 26. Recently, the availability of the estrogen skin patch has obviated the first hepatic pass of the hormones, with a potential for decreasing subsequent toxicity. This form of replacement may be preferred by some women, although long-term experience of efficacy and tolerability are still required.

Besides the well-described benefits of estrogen replacement, including maintenance of secondary sex characteristics, vaginal mucosal turgor, and breast tissue maintenance, the prevention of osteoporosis is of primary importance in these women. Patients on estrogen replacement should also be followed by a gynecologist every six months for pelvic evaluation and cervical cytology. The desired frequency of mammography requirements in premenopausal women on estrogen replacement therapy is currently under intense debate. A baseline mammogram is recommended, and the frequency of subsequent imaging depends on accepted community practice standards.

In males, testosterone replacement should be administered as an intramuscular injection of testosterone enanthate, 200 to 300 mg every two weeks. Frequency of shaving and potency are the two criteria used for assessing adequate replacement. Gynecomastia, acne, and accelerated baldness may be associated with excessive doses. Potency restoration may take several months, and patients and their partners should be counseled that their libido and lifestyles may in fact change dramatically; this is especially true in middle-aged men with long-standing hypogonadism.

Growth Hormone Replacement

Since the recent availability of adequate amounts of recombinant human growth hormone for study, it is apparent that at least some hypopituitary adult patients benefit from its administration. In fact, the central obesity, lethargy, muscle weakness, and lipid abnormalities associated with long-standing pituitary deficiency may be reversed by growth hormone administration (0.01 to 0.025 mg/kg/d subcutaneously). As the cost of this hormone is currently prohibitive, advocating its routine prescription is still premature.

Vasopressin Replacement

When posterior pituitary damage requires replacement of vasopressin, desmopressin (DDAVP) is administered as an intranasal spray (0.1-ml doses). The frequency of administration is usually determined by the patients' subjective need for regulating frequency of urination.

In summary, effective pituitary hormone replacement requires carefully balanced long-term clinical decisions. Subjective history, physical examination, and, where relevant, laboratory testing, provide an overall indication of the adequacy of therapy and requirements for its fine tuning.

REFERENCES

1. Cushing H: Intracranial Tumors. Notes upon a Series of Two-Thousand Verified Cases with Surgical-Mortality Percentages Pertaining Thereto. Springfield, IL, Charles C Thomas, 1932.
2. Hirsch O: Endonasal method of removal of hypophyseal tumours: With report of two cases. JAMA 55:772, 1910.
3. Hardy J: Transsphenoidal surgery of hypersecreting pituitary tumors. In Kohler PO, Ross GT (eds): Diagnosis and Treatment of Pituitary Tumors. International Congress Series, No. 303. New York, Elsevier, 1973, pp 179–194.
4. Wilson CB: Role of surgery in the management of pituitary tumors. Neurosurg Clin North Am 1:139–159, 1990.
5. Ross DA, Wilson CB: Results of transsphenoidal microsurgery for growth hormone–secreting pituitary adenoma in a series of 214 patients. J Neurosurg 68:854–867, 1988.
6. Ezzat S, Snyder PJ, Young WF, et al: Octreotide treatment of acromegaly: A randomized, multicenter study. Ann Intern Med 117:711–718, 1992.
7. Melmed S: Acromegaly. N Engl J Med 322:966–977, 1990.
8. Fahlbusch R, Honegger J, Buchfelder M: Surgical management of acromegaly. Endocrinol Metab Clin North Am 21:669–692, 1992.
9. Chang-DeMoranville B, Jackson IMD: Diagnosis and endocrine testing in acromegaly. Endocrinol Metab Clin North Am 21:649–668, 1992.
10. Mampalam TJ, Tyrrell JB, Wilson CB: Transsphenoidal microsurgery for Cushing disease: A report of 216 cases. Ann Intern Med 109:487–493, 1988.
11. Ebersold MY, Quast LM, Laws R: Long-term results in transsphenoidal removal of non-functioning pituitary adenomas. J Neurosurg 64:713–719, 1986.
12. Schlechte J, Dolank B, Sherman B, et al: The natural history of untreated hyperprolactinemia: A prospective analysis. J Clin Endocrinol Metab 68:412–418, 1989.
13. Serri O, Rasio E, Beuregard H, et al: Recurrence of hyperprolactinemia after selective transsphenoidal adenomectomy in women with prolactinoma. N Engl J Med 309:280–283, 1983.
14. Rodman EF, Molitch ME, Post KD, et al: Long-term follow-up of transsphenoidal selective adenomectomy for prolactinoma. JAMA 252:921–924, 1984.
15. Molitch ME, Russell EJ: The pituitary "incidentaloma." Ann Intern Med 112:925–931, 1990.
16. Reincke M, Allolio B, Saeger W, et al: The 'incidentaloma' of the pituitary gland: Is neurosurgery required? JAMA 263:2772–2776, 1990.
17. Eastman RC, Gorden P, Glatstein E, Roth J: Radiation therapy of acromegaly. Endocrinol Metab Clin North Am 21:693–712, 1992.
18. Eastman RC, Gorden P, Roth J: Conventional supervoltage irradiation is an effective treatment for acromegaly. J Clin Endocrinol Metab 48:931, 1979.
19. Macleod AF, Clarke DG, Pambakian H, et al: Treatment of acromegaly by external irradiation. Clin Endocrinol 30:303, 1989.
20. Wass JAH, Ciccarelli E, Corsello S, et al: External radiation therapy for acromegaly. In Lamberts SWJ (ed): Sandostatin® in the Treatment of Acromegaly. New York, Springer-Verlag, 1987, p 37.
21. Grossman A, Besser GM: Prolactinomas. BMJ 290:182–184, 1985.
22. Snyder PJ, Fowble BF, Schatz NJ, et al: Hypopituitarism following radiation therapy of pituitary adenomas. Am J Med 81:457, 1986.
23. Feek CM, McLelland J, Seth J, et al: Long term follow-up of external pituitary irradiation in the treatment of acromegaly. In Lamberts SWJ, Tilders FJH, van der Veen EA, et al (eds): Trends in Diagnosis and Treatment of Pituitary Adenomas. Amsterdam, Free University Press, 1984, p 235.
24. Al-Mefty O, Kersh JE, Routh A, et al: The long-term side effects of radiation therapy for benign brain tumors in adults. J Neurosurg 73:502, 1990.
25. Atkinson AB, Allen IV, Gordon DS, et al: Progressive visual failure in acromegaly following external pituitary irradiation. Clin Endocrinol 10:469, 1979.
26. Millar JL, Spry NA, Lamb DS, Delahunt J: Blindness in patients after external beam irradiation for pituitary adenomas: Two cases occurring after small fractional doses. Clin Oncol 3:291–294, 1991.
27. Jones A: Review: Radiation oncogenesis in relation to the treatment of pituitary tumors. Clin Endocrinol 35:379, 1991.
28. Brada M, Ford D, Ashley S, et al: Risk of second brain tumor after conservative surgery and radiotherapy for pituitary adenoma. BMJ 304:1343–1346, 1992.

PART III

THYROID GLAND

33

Anatomy and Development

RAGNAR EKHOLM

GROSS ANATOMY

In humans the thyroid gland weighs 15 to 20 g. The brownish red, highly vascular organ consists of right and left lobes connected by a narrow isthmus. The latter crosses the trachea in front of the second to fourth cartilage rings, and the conical or pear-shaped lobes extend upward to the middle of the thyroid cartilage and downward to the fifth and sixth tracheal rings. A pyramidal lobe exists in about 30 per cent of thyroid glands; it projects upward from the isthmus, usually near the left lobe. Accessory thyroid tissue may occur in the midline of the neck at any point between the tongue and the upper trachea.

The gland is enclosed by connective tissue that is continuous with the pretracheal fascia. This outer capsule is loosely connected to a deeper layer of connective tissue that forms an inner capsule. The space between the two capsules contains the vessels, the recurrent laryngeal nerves, and, in general, the parathyroid glands.

BLOOD SUPPLY

The ample blood supply of the thyroid is provided by the superior thyroid artery, generally arising from the external carotid artery, and the larger and more important inferior thyroid artery, a branch of the thyrocervical trunk. The close and variable relation of the inferior artery to the recurrent laryngeal nerve is of surgical importance. An inconstant artery, the thyroidea ima, is a branch of varying size from the brachiocephalic trunk or the aortic arch ascending on the front of the trachea. All the arteries have frequent anastomoses with one another and with the arteries of the trachea and the esophagus. The arteries ramify on the surface of the gland, forming a plexus from which branches enter the tissue, arborize, and eventually form a rich network of capillaries encapsulating the follicles.[1, 2] These capillaries are fenestrated and generally run close to the follicles without any intervening tissue.[1, 2] It has been estimated that about half of the surface of follicles is next to capillaries.[3] During thyroid hyperplasia the capillaries enlarge progressively, which eventually gives the gland a sponge-like texture.[3]

The veins form a plexus on the surface of the gland that is drained by the superior, middle, and inferior thyroid veins. The superior and middle veins end in the lateral jugular vein, and the inferior vein opens in the brachiocephalic vein.

LYMPHATICS

Lymph capillaries are found in close relation to the follicles, but they are rare compared with the blood capillaries. Most of the lymphatics in the thyroid occur in the interlobular connective tissue, where they are often seen surrounding the arteries. These deep lymphatics communicate with a network of lymph vessels in the capsule of the gland. The lymph vessels drain to nodes located on the thyroid, on the trachea and larynx, and in the groove between the trachea and the esophagus. They further drain to the deep cervical nodes along the internal jugular vein. Lymph drainage to the superior mediastinal nodes is also common.

INNERVATION

The thyroid has a rich supply of norepinephrine-storing and acetylcholinesterase-positive nerve fibers.[4, 5] The adre-

507

nergic nerve fibers originate in the stellate and superior cervical ganglia and reach the gland along with the arteries.[4, 6–8] The acetylcholinesterase-positive fibers in the thyroid are generally considered to represent cholinergic, postganglionic parasympathetic fibers.[9, 10] The parasympathetic fibers, together with sensory fibers, derive from the jugular-nodose ganglia and reach the gland via the superior laryngeal nerve and, to a small extent, via the recurrent nerve.[7, 11] Both the adrenergic and the cholinergic fibers are found around blood vessels as well as between and along follicles, and nerve terminals are seen by electron microscopy in close relation to follicle cells.[4]

With immunocytochemical methods a number of neuropeptides have been demonstrated in the thyroid of several species. The fibers containing these peptides are generally uniformly distributed throughout the gland, closely related to arteries and follicles, but the frequency of the various peptide-containing fibers varies considerably among species. (For a review of the thyroidal neuropeptides and their fibers, see ref. 12.)

Clear evidence exists that the autonomic nervous system is an integral part of the thyroid control apparatus. The picture of the neurogenic mechanism is, however, incomplete, at least partly because of a pronounced structural and functional interspecies variation in thyroid innervation.

THE THYROID FOLLICLE

In general, endocrine organs have a low level of fine structural organization showing cords of gland cells that are scattered in loose connective tissue and lack clear signs of polarity. The thyroid differs fundamentally from this pattern by displaying a highly organized structure, the characteristic element of which is the thyroid follicle. This unique structure corresponds to unique functional features.

The follicle is a spheroidal, hollow structure measuring between 20 and 500 μm in diameter (Fig. 33–1). The wall is formed of a single layer of epthelial cells (follicle cells)

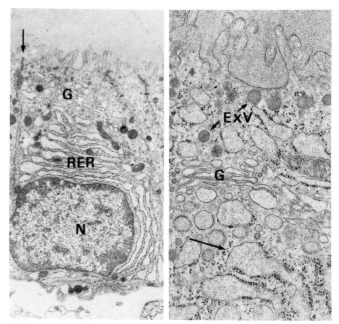

FIGURE 33–2. *Left,* **Electron micrograph of a follicle cell in a rat thyroid follicle.** The apical surface, facing the follicle lumen, is furnished with microvilli. The cell is separated from its neighbors by narrow intercellular spaces, bridged by cell junctions (*arrow*). The nucleus (N) has a basal location. The cytoplasm is dominated by the ribosome-carrying endoplasmic reticulum (RER). The apical region contains a Golgi complex (G) and small, dense vesicles (× 7000).

FIGURE 33–3. *Right,* **Electron micrograph showing the apical half of a rat follicle cell.** Golgi cisternae form a stack (G) that is surrounded by vesicles of various appearance. Note that the portions of the RER cisternae facing the Golgi complex lack ribosomes (*arrow*). Note also that small dense vesicles (exocytotic vesicles, ExV) occur only in the region between the Golgi complex and the apical cell surface. This picture corresponds to the notion that the light vesicles between the RER and the Golgi complex are formed by budding from the bare RER membrane and that the dense exocytotic vesicles emanate from the Golgi complex (× 26,000).

which encloses the follicle lumen; the lumen is filled with the colloid, a protein solution. Each follicle is surrounded by a thin basal lamina. The extrafollicular (interfollicular) space contains a rich network of blood vessels, some lymphatics, and numerous nerve fibers.

The follicle cells (Figs. 33–2 to 33–4) are distinctly polarized with an apical surface facing the follicle lumen and a basolateral surface facing the extrafollicular space and adjoining follicle cells. The cells vary in height among species and among follicles. In humans the cells are commonly squamous to cuboidal, whereas in rats they are usually cuboidal to low columnar. In general, the cell height is related to the functional condition, columnar cells being more active than low cells.

The cells are joined by three types of cell junctions (Fig. 33–5), common in all epithelia, which together form the junctional complex. The *tight junction (zonula occludens)* bridges the intercellular space close to the apical border of the cells. These junctions consist of anastomosing strands of junctional proteins which make contact across the intercellular space. The strands encircle the cells like a belt and make the epithelium a sealed monolayer that separates the follicle lumen from the extrafollicular space. The tight junctions restrict the lateral mobility of plasma membrane components and maintain a difference in qualities between the apical and basolateral plasma membrane.[13]

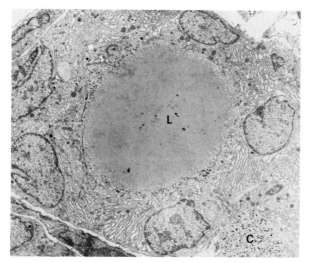

FIGURE 33–1. **Survey electron micrograph of a section through a rat thyroid follicle** showing the single layer of follicle cells enclosing the follicle lumen (L), filled with colloid. Part of a parafollicular cell (C cell) is seen in the lower right corner (C) (× 3000).

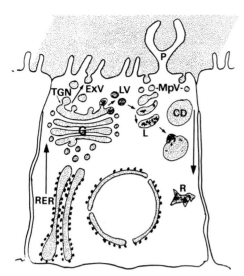

FIGURE 33-4. **Schematic representation of a follicle cell and adjacent follicle lumen** to show the structural basis of thyroid hormone synthesis (left half of the sketch) and secretion (right half). Left half: RER, rough endoplasmic reticulum; G, Golgi cisternae; TGN, *trans*-Golgi network; ExV, exocytotic vesicles carrying thyroglobulin; LV, vesicles containing lysosomal hydrolases. Right half: P, pseudopod; CD, colloid droplet; MpV, micropinocytotic vesicles; E, endosome; L, lysosome; R, residual of lysosome.

The *adherent junction* (*zonula adherens*) is located at a level just below the tight junction and also extends around the entire cell perimeter. This junction is composed of intracellular attachment proteins and the transmembrane linker glycoproteins, the latter connected with the linker glycoproteins of neighbor cells. The intracellular attachment proteins serve as anchorage to contractile actin filaments, most of which are arranged in a circumferential bundle running just inside the plasma membrane. In this way the actin bundles form a transcellular network of great importance for the maintenance of a complete epithelial layer.

The third type of junction is the *desmosome* or *macula adherens*. The desmosomes are spotlike structures that occur in varying number at all levels of the plasma membrane below the adherent junctions. The desmosome consists of a dense cytoplasmic plaque, to which bundles of intermediate filaments are anchored, and transmembrane linker glycoproteins, which interact with the linker proteins of an adjacent cell. The noncontractile intermediate filaments constitute, together with the microtubules, the structural framework for the cytoplasm. Via the desmosomes the intermediate filaments are connected with the filaments in adjacent cells and form a transcellular network throughout the epithelium.

The three types of junction are of crucial importance for the maintenance of the polarity of the follicle cells, which is a prerequisite for the normal function of the follicle. This polarity is expressed in the different properties of the apical and basolateral plasma membranes. Only the apical membrane bears microvilli and has the ability to form pseudopods, and some enzyme activities seem restricted to the apical domain of the membrane, e.g., peroxidase,[14] aminopeptidase,[15] and H_2O_2-generating capacity.[16] On the other hand, Na$^+$, K$^+$ ATPase has been demonstrated only in the basolateral plasma membrane,[17] and the same is true

of thyroid-stimulating hormone (TSH) receptors.[18] The polarity of the cells is also indicated by the defined pattern of organelle distribution.

The interrelation between the organization of the follicle and the structure of the follicle cell, on one hand, and the specific thyroid functions, on the other, may be outlined as follows (see Fig. 33-4): Thyroglobulin, the specific thyroid glycoprotein, is synthesized in the rough endoplasmic reticulum (RER) and transferred by small vesicles from the RER cisternae to the Golgi cisternae and carried from the latter to the apical cell surface by exocytotic vesicles; these vesicles discharge the thyroglobulin into the follicle lumen. During its intracellular transport, the thyroglobulin undergoes post-translational modifications but does not bind any iodine. Iodination of thyroglobulin and hormone formation take place outside the cell, in the follicle lumen, in close association with the apical plasma membrane. The hormones are formed by binding of iodine to tyrosyl residues in the thyroglobulin molecule and "coupling" of two iodotyrosyls so formed to iodothyronines. Secretion of hormones requires that the hormones be released from the thyroglobulin molecule, and this occurs inside the follicle cells. Thus, the first step in hormone secretion is reabsorption of hormone-containing thyroglobulin, which occurs by endocytosis. The endocytotic containers receive lysosomal enzymes, and these hydrolases degrade the thyroglobulin. The thyroid hormones thereby released move across the membrane of the endosome-lysosome and the basolateral plasma membrane and pass into the blood.

From this general outline of the structure-function interrelationship it should be clear that the organization in follicles—with follicle cells of normal polarity—is necessary for the normal synthesis, storage, and secretion of thyroid hormone; the follicle is, in fact, the smallest complete functional unit of the thyroid. The integration between thyroid structure and function is discussed in more detail later. Naturally, this discussion is based primarily on observations made on the thyroid. However, some aspects of structure-function integration have not been explored in the thyroid but are well studied in other cell systems. When applicable

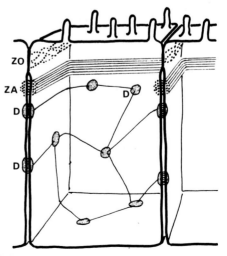

FIGURE 33-5. **Schematic representation of cell junctions and associated filaments in a follicle cell.** ZO, zonula occludens; ZA, zonula adherens with associated bundle of actin filaments; D, desmosomes interconnected by intermediate filaments.

to the thyroid, information from such studies has been used in the discussion.

PARAFOLLICULAR CELLS

Most of the parafollicular cells, or C cells, are assembled in groups in the interfollicular spaces, but they are also seen in the follicle wall where, however, they never reach the follicle lumen. The C cells are generally larger than the follicle cells and display a distinctly different electron microscopic structure.[19] Their most characteristic ultrastructural feature is an abundance of cytoplasmic granules, 100 to 200 nm in diameter and with a dense content, separated from the bounding membrane by a zone of low density. The granules are closely related to the large Golgi complex in which granules are seen at all stages of development. The parafollicular cells secrete the polypeptide hormone calcitonin, which is stored in the specific granules together with monoamines formed by the cells from precursor amino acids. The C cells also produce, at least in some species, a number of other peptides, like calcitonin gene-related peptide, somatostatin, gastrin-releasing peptide, and helodermin.[12] It cannot be excluded that C cells exert a paracrine function and act as modulators of follicle cell activity.

THE STRUCTURAL BASIS OF THYROID HORMONE BIOSYNTHESIS

Thyroglobulin Synthesis and Transport

Thyroglobulin, the principal iodoprotein of the thyroid, is a glycoprotein with a molecular weight of 660,000. The molecule contains about 10 per cent carbohydrates, which occur as two distinct types linked to asparagine residues in the polypeptide chain. One unit consists of N-acetylglucosamine and mannose; the other has the same core structure but, in addition, peripheral chains containing fucose, N-acetylglucosamine, galactose, and sialic acid.[20]

The dominant organelle in the follicle cells is the RER, which reflects a high capacity for protein synthesis. Most of this capacity is used in the production of thyroglobulin. Thyroglobulin is synthesized on ribosomes directed to the RER membrane at an early stage of synthesis by the signal sequence of the nascent chain; after attachment of the ribosome to the RER membrane, the peptide chain is translocated into the cisternae via a tunnel in the membrane.[21, 22] At this early stage of thyroglobulin synthesis the glycosylation is initiated: The first steps are assembly of an oligosaccharide on a lipid carrier and the transfer en bloc of this oligosaccharide to an asparagine in the nascent chain; this transfer is concomitant with the inward transit of the peptide across the RER membrane. The initial phases in the processing of the carbohydrate units (removal of some sugars) also take place in the RER cisternae (for a review, see ref. 20). In addition, the RER cisternae are the sites of incorporation of phosphate into thyroglobulin; at least some of these phosphates are present as mannose-6-phosphate, which is remarkable considering that this is the specific recognition marker of lysosomal hydrolases.[23, 24]

After their release from the ribosomes, the thyroglobulin monomers fold and assemble in the cisternae, where they mix with a number of other proteins targeted to the RER. The transfer of proteins from the RER cisternae to the Golgi cisternae probably requires that folding and assembly be completed.[25, 26] The exit of thyroglobulin from the RER cisternae seems also to be affected by the glycosylation of thyroglobulin. For example, observations indicate that inhibition of glycosylation by tunicamycin arrests thyroglobulin in the RER cisternae.[27, 28]

The glycosylation of thyroglobulin continues after its transfer to the Golgi complex: Studies on the thyroid have documented that the peripheral glycosylation occurs in this complex (for references, see ref. 29). More recent studies on cells other than thyrocytes have localized very precisely the Golgi sugar transferases catalyzing the attachment of individual monosaccharides in the peripheral chains of glycoproteins. These observations, combined with thorough electron microscopic analyses, are the basis of the current idea of the organization of the Golgi complex[30–33] (which very likely applies to the thyrocyte). According to this idea, the five or six flattened cisternae that form a Golgi stack in a typical mammalian cell can be divided into three groups—the cis, medial, and trans cisternae; the cis cisternae are those closest to the RER (see Figs. 33–3 and 33–4). On its basal and apical side the stack is flanked by tubular networks, the cis-Golgi network (CGN) and, respectively, the trans-Golgi network (TGN). The CGN is closely related to the RER and the TGN to the secretory vesicles. The sugar transferases in the membrane of the Golgi cisternae have a defined distribution: The enzymes catalyzing the binding of the most central components in the peripheral carbohydrate chains, that is, early events in peripheral glycosylation, are located toward the cis side of the Golgi stack, whereas enzymes involved in the incorporation of terminal sugars (late events) are located toward the trans side of the Golgi.[34–37] This distribution of the enzymes is in accord with a unidirectional transport of proteins across the Golgi complex—from the cis to the trans side—and a stepwise binding of the monosaccharides.

With respect to the mechanism of the one-way transport of thyroglobulin across the Golgi stack, evidence strongly suggests that the cisternae are stationary and that the protein is carried by vesicles budding from one cisterna and fusing with another cisterna closer to the trans side[38, 39] (see Figs. 33–3 and 33–4). Obviously, this transport is accompanied by an extensive membrane flow through the Golgi stack. Nevertheless, the specific protein composition of the membranes and the polarized distribution of enzymes remain. This may be achieved by exclusion of certain proteins from budding vesicles and/or selective retrieval of membrane (for a review, see ref. 40).

The transport of proteins across the Golgi stack appears to be a nonselective bulk transport, and the sorting of proteins is probably restricted to the TGN. It may be assumed that thyroglobulin is recognized by some sort of receptor concentrated in pits of the TGN membrane which pinch off and form exocytotic vesicles. The nature of the sorting signal of thyroglobulin (or other secretory proteins) recognized by a TGN receptor is not known. It has been suggested, however, that this signal is not a linear sequence, specific for each protein, but a "signal patch,"[26] that is, a surface region formed from separate regions of a polypeptide chain which have been brought together during protein folding.[26]

There have been speculations about the possible role of the carbohydrates in thyroglobulin as sorting signals, but no convincing evidence in favor of this idea has been presented. The role played in thyroglobulin sorting by the mannose-6-phosphate in the thyroglobulin molecule is obscure.[23]

The TGN is also the compartment where the lysosomal hydrolases are separated from other newly synthesized proteins.[41, 42] The sorting process begins with two phosphorylation reactions, by which the lysosomal acid hydrolases are furnished with mannose-6-phosphate residues. By these recognition markers the hydrolases are bound to mannose-6-phosphate receptors in the TGN membrane.[41–43] The receptors cluster in pits, which are pinched off to form vesicles carrying the hydrolases to prelysosomes (see Fig. 33–4).

The pits in the TGN forming vesicles that carry secretory proteins and those forming vesicles that carry lysosomal hydrolases are characterized by being clathrin-coated. Clathrin is a protein complex that assembles on the cytoplasmic face of TGN membrane and forms the outer layer of the coat. The inner layer is composed of protein molecules called adaptors. Clathrin and adaptors are present together in the TGN membrane, and specific adaptors are restricted to coated pits with specific receptors. When a specific protein has bound to the receptors in the pit, a vesicle is formed and pinched off. Once the coated vesicle is freed, the coat of clathrin and adaptors dissociate from the vesicle and the coat components return to the Golgi complex (for a review, see ref. 44).

The exocytotic vesicles formed in the TGN carry the newly synthesized thyroglobulin to the apical cell surface (see Figs. 33–3 and 33–4). The vesicle membrane fuses with the apical plasma membrane in the areas between the bases of the microvilli, an opening is formed in the membrane, and the vesicle content is emptied into the follicle lumen. The thyroglobulin in the vesicles is uniodinated and contains no hormones[45, 46] but seems to be complete in other respects, including glycosylation. The fusion of the membrane of the exocytotic vesicles with the apical plasma membrane implies that membrane-bound proteins manufactured in the RER are transferred to the apical plasma membrane.

Iodination of Thyroglobulin; Hormone Formation

Hormone formation takes place in the thyroglobulin molecule. It comprises two reactions—binding of iodine to tyrosyl residues and coupling of two iodotyrosyls to form iodothyronines. Both reactions are oxidative, catalyzed by thyroperoxidase in the presence of hydrogen peroxide that acts as an electron acceptor.

Thyroid hormone formation evidently requires four reactants; how these are distributed in the follicle is of interest for understanding the integration of structure and function in hormone synthesis. The bulk of the *thyroglobulin* is extracellular, in the follicle lumen, but thyroglobulin is also present intracellularly, at various stages of maturation, in all parts of the secretory pathway. *Iodine* is absorbed in the alimentary tract in the form of iodide, which is taken up by an active mechanism in the basolateral plasma membrane of the follicle cells and rapidly transported through the cells into the follicle lumen.[20] *Thyroid peroxidase* is present in the membranes of the RER, Golgi complex, and exocytotic vesicles and transferred from the latter to the apical plasma membrane in connection with exocytosis.[29] *Hydrogen peroxide* has been demonstrated cytochemically on the apical surface of follicle cells, and there is evidence that H_2O_2 is formed in the apical plasma membrane by an NADPH oxidase.[16, 47, 48] It is likely that this enzyme complex is synthesized in the RER and transported to the apical plasma membrane along the same route as the thyroperoxidase.

The wide distribution of the reactants in the iodination and coupling reactions indicates that these reactions could take place at several sites in the follicle cell. However, electron microscopic autoradiographs at very short intervals ($\cong$ 30 seconds) after intravenous administration of radioiodide (to rats) show a concentration of autoradiographic grains in a narrow ring over the follicle lumen close to the apical border of the follicle cells and practically no grains over the cytoplasm[49] (Fig. 33–6). These autoradiographs show the location of organified radioiodine as the unbound radioiodide is washed out by the fixation and embedding procedures. The very short interval between radioiodide administration and fixation guarantees that the bound radioiodine was immobilized at the site of iodine binding. Thus, this labeling pattern shows that iodination of thyroglobulin occurs in the follicle lumen and is related to the apical plasma membrane. The association of iodination with the apical plasma membrane is logical with respect to the presence of peroxidase as well as hydrogen peroxide–producing enzyme in this membrane.[49, 50] With increasing time after radioiodide administration, the ring of autoradiographic grains broadens and passes into a disk, which illustrates the diffusion of labeled thyroglobulin in the colloid.

A second site of in vivo iodination of thyroglobulin is the so-called intracellular lumina.[51] These lumina are closed cavities, limited by a membrane furnished with microvilli, and have a content similar to that of the follicle lumen. After radioiodide administration, the content of the intracellular lumina is labeled as fast as the colloid of the follicle lumen.[51] Although seen in several species, including humans, these lumina are very rare and the iodination occurring in them is unimportant from a practical point of view.

Theoretically, however, the iodination in the intracellular lumina is interesting as indicated by observations of iodination in vitro.[52] Brief incubations of well-preserved isolated follicles with ^{125}I results in an autoradiographic labeling pattern in full agreement with that in vivo. Similar incubations of follicle fragments, cell clusters, and dispersed cells yield autoradiographs characterized by a concentration of label in intracellular lumina which are much more frequent than in vivo (Fig. 33–7). Common to cells with an intracellular lumen is their lost polarity. The connection between development of lumina and polarity seems to be that loss of polarity disrupts the normal, directed movement of exocytotic vesicles from the Golgi complex to the apical cell surface (which no longer exists). As a consequence, exocytotic vesicles accumulate and then fuse and form intracellular lumina. Interestingly, the membrane of the fused vesicles develops microvilli, typical of

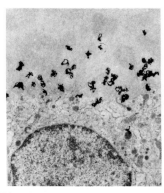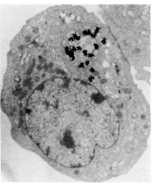

FIGURE 33–6. **Electron microscopic autoradiograph from a rat thyroid** about 30 seconds after intravenous injection of ^{125}I-iodide. The autoradiographic silver grains are concentrated over the peripheral zone of the follicle lumen; a single grain is seen over the cell (× 7000).

FIGURE 33–7. **Electron microscopic autoradiograph of follicle cell** almost detached from its neighbor and with lost polarity after incubation with ^{125}I-iodide for 30 seconds. The autoradiographic grains are concentrated over an intracellular lumen (× 5000).

the apical cell surface, and displays the ability to catalyze iodination, a functional quality characteristic of the apical plasma membrane. These observations indicate that the intracellular membranes have a potential capacity to catalyze iodination. A possible explanation of the fact that intracellular iodination is not a common phenomenon in vivo may be that the peroxidase and the H_2O_2-generating enzyme exist in inactivated forms intracellularly under normal conditions. If so, activation of the enzyme(s) can obviously occur when exocytic vesicles fuse to form intracellular lumina. The same activation mechanism should operate in the regular exocytosis at the apical cell surface.

STRUCTURAL BASIS OF THYROID HORMONE STORAGE AND RELEASE

The Follicle Lumen and the Colloid

The follicle lumen is completely filled with the colloid. Analyses of samples of colloid obtained by micropuncture of follicles in vivo have shown that practically all the protein is thyroglobulin.[53] The protein concentration of the colloid is very high (in the rat 10 to 20 per cent[53]) but varies with the functional state of the gland.

The water content and ion composition of the colloid are determined by the barrier functions of the thyroid epithelium. Observations on thyrocyte cultures forming a continuous, polarized monolayer on a semipermeable membrane show that the epithelium has a transepithelial resistance of about 3000 to 6000 ohms · cm^2,[54, 55] which indicates a very high tightness and low paracellular transport. The transepithelial potential difference, found to be 10 to 20 mV (apical side negative) in vitro[54, 55] as well as in vivo,[20] is the result of the pumping activity of the cells, which controls the ionic composition in the follicle lumen.

Endocytosis of Thyroglobulin

Hormone release requires degradation of the hormone-containing thyroglobulin molecule. This is accomplished by lysosomal enzymes, which necessitates that colloid re-enter the cells. The internalization occurs by endocytosis, which is of two types in the follicle cells—macropinocytosis and micropinocytosis (for reviews, see refs. 29 and 56).

MACROPINOCYTOSIS. Macropinocytosis[57-60] implies a bulk uptake of thyroglobulin and probably does not involve any receptor mechanism. The first step in macropinocytosis is the formation of pseudopods (Fig. 33–8) on the apical cell surface which is observed within five minutes after administration of TSH in vivo or in vitro[61, 62]: The pseudopods originate as broad, thin folds of the plasma membrane; when these flaps curl and their overlapping edges fuse, tube-like structures are formed.[62, 63] As the tubes grow, their apical aperture closes and they are transformed into cyst-like structures that enclose portions of the colloid. The pseudopods disappear from the cell surface by a retraction process whereby the cavities of the pseudopods are internalized and appear in the cell body as spherical inclusions (colloid droplets) limited by a single membrane and filled with colloid (Fig. 33–9). The colloid droplets show a great variation in size, the largest ones reaching a diameter of 2 μm or more. The pseudopods protrude up to 3 to 4 μm into the follicle lumen and, consequently, engulf colloid at some distance from the apical cell surface; this may prevent the immediate reuptake of hormone-poor thyroglobulin recently discharged onto the apical cell surface by exocytosis.[64]

The mechanisms of macropinocytosis are not well understood. An interesting phenomenon is that the pseudopod membrane differs in several respects, such as enzyme equipment, from the apical plasma membrane, which shows that the plasma membrane is not simply transferred into the pseudopod. The machinery responsible for the movement of membranes in macropinocytosis involves both microtubules and contractile filaments, but it is not clear how these structures interact in macropinocytosis in the follicle cells (for references, see ref. 29).

MICROPINOCYTOSIS. Micropinocytosis involves formation of small vesicles, 100 to 200 nm in diameter, by invagina-

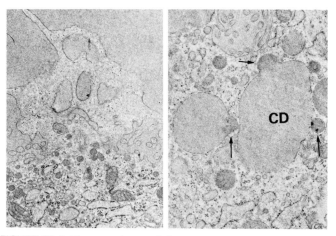

FIGURE 33–8. **Electron micrograph from a rat thyroid** 10 minutes after a TSH injection showing a pseudopod with several colloid inclusions (× 9000).

FIGURE 33–9. **Electron micrograph from a rat thyroid 20** minutes after a TSH injection. Two large colloid droplets (CD) and several lysosomes, three of which seem to have fused with the colloid droplets (*arrows*), are seen (× 18,000).

tions of the apical plasma membrane. In the follicle cells micropinocytosis was first demonstrated by microinjections of tracers (ferritin, Thorotrast, colloidal gold) into the follicle lumen of rat thyroids in vivo, followed by identification by electron microscopy of the tracers in pits and vesicles in the apical zone of the cells[58]; similar observations were later made with other tracers in in vitro experiments on open follicles.[65, 66] That thyroglobulin is also internalized by this route was supported by experiments in which endocytosis was studied with electron microscopic autoradiography after prelabeling of the colloid with ^{125}I-iodide.[60] These studies[60, 65, 66] also indicate that micropinocytotic vesicles may fuse and form droplets and, in addition, may communicate with vesicular and tubular structures belonging to the endosomes (see later). Further evidence that micropinocytosis is a mode of thyroglobulin internalization is the observation on thyroid slices that hormone secretion continues when macropinocytosis is inhibited.[67] In addition, coated microvesicles, apparently of endocytotic nature, have been isolated from reconstituted thyroid follicles and shown to contain iodinated thyroglobulin.[68]

INTRACELLULAR ROUTES OF INTERNALIZED THYROGLOBULIN. The intracellular route of internalized thyroglobulin depends on the mode of endocytosis. The route used by the colloid droplet thyroglobulin is well documented by electron microscopic observations. Soon after their appearance in the cell body, the colloid droplets become surrounded by small lysosomes; these are recognized by their electron-dense content separated from the limiting membrane by an electron-lucent rim. The lysosomes fuse with the droplets (Fig. 33–9) and empty their hydrolases into the droplet, a mechanism demonstrated by cytochemical technique to be a transfer of acid phosphatase activity from lysosomes to colloid droplets[57, 69–71] By this process the typical lysosomes are reduced in number, and the population of colloid droplets becomes heterogeneous with respect to size and morphology of the content. The fate of the lysosomes is uncertain; they may have a cyclic existence and regenerate from the colloid droplet–lysosome complex after completing hydrolysis.[72]

The intracellular route used by thyroglobulin internalized by micropinocytosis is less extensively studied. However, observations in the last few years on other cells have resulted in a notion of the micropinocytotic pathway that seems to have wide applicability.[73–75] According to this notion, the molecules taken up by micropinocytotic vesicles pass through a series of vesicotubular structures called *endosomes* (see Fig. 33–4) and are characterized by their acid pH. *Early endosomes* receive internalized material by fusion with micropinocytotic vesicles and are the site of uncoupling of ligand and receptor in receptor-mediated endocytosis. *Late endosomes* (or *prelysosomes*) contain, besides internalized material, some lysosomal enzymes transferred from the Golgi complex (TGN) and still bound to mannose-6-phosphate receptors. The *lysosomes*, respresenting the third compartment, develop from the late endosomes and are characterized by their content of lysosomal enzymes and absence of mannose-6-phosphate receptors.

In retrospect it is clear that structures corresponding to endosomal compartments were described in thyroid follicle cells several years ago as tubulovesicular structures containing various types of label exposed to the apical cell surface.[58, 65, 66] More recently, in studies on reconstituted thyroid follicles, it has been possible to identify endosomal compartments and demonstrate their involvement in the transport and degradation of internalized thyroglobulin.[76]

It has not been proven that the two routes of thyroglobulin endocytosis communicate, but some observations indicate that this is the case. For example, in isolated open follicles, cationized ferritin internalized by micropinocytosis has been observed in vacuoles corresponding to colloid droplets[65, 66] and autoradiographic observations after ^{125}I labeling in vivo indicate a gradual transfer of labeled material from microvesicles to colloid droplets.[60]

The relative importance of macro- and micropinocytosis of thyroglobulin is difficult to assess. In species with a high basal thyroid activity (e.g., the rat), macropinocytotic structures are common under normal conditions, whereas in species with a low basal activity (e.g., humans, guinea pigs) such structures are rare under the same conditions. But macropinocytosis can be induced by TSH in thyroids of low basal activity and increased in glands of high basal activity. On the other hand, micropinocytosis may also be stimulated by TSH,[68, 77] and observations indicate that a considerable acceleration of hormone secretion may occur without induction of macropinocytosis.[68]

The question of whether or not thyroglobulin endocytosis is a selective process has long been discussed. A number of observations considered to support the view that certain thyroglobulin molecules are preferentially internalized have been published but, as recently discussed in some detail,[29] no solid arguments in favor of this view have been produced. However, the recent demonstration[78] on reconstituted follicles that some internalized iodinated thyroglobulin is present in clathrin-coated vesicles is an interesting contribution to this question, as clathrin-coated vesicles are known to be generally involved in receptor-mediated transports.

DEGRADATION OF THYROGLOBULIN. The lysosomal hydrolases have an acidic pH optimum, which means that the degradation of thyroglobulin occurs exclusively in the endocytotic compartments where the pH is less than 6. The enzymes involved in the thyroglobulin hydrolysis (glycoside hydrolases and proteases) have been identified, and the degradation of thyroglobulin has been studied by following the hydrolysis of ^{125}I-labeled thyroglobulin inside lysosomal particles and by incubation of labeled thyroglobulin with purified thyroid hydrolases (for references, see ref. 20). On the basis of such studies, it has been suggested[79] that thyroglobulin normally in vivo is degraded to iodoamino acids and peptide fragments and not hydrolyzed completely to amino acids.

The fate of the products of thyroglobulin hydrolysis is only partially known. The iodotyrosines are almost completely deiodinated inside the follicle cells by a microsomal dehalogenase,[80] and the released iodide is reutilized in the follicle. The transport of the hormones from the lysosomes to the extracellular space has long been assumed to occur by passive diffusion. However, it has been demonstrated that monoiodotyrosine in FRTL-5 thyroid cells is transported across the lysosomal membrane by a carrier[81] and that the entrance of thyroid hormones into peripheral cells involves transport systems.[82] It seems possible, therefore, that the transport of thyroid hormones across the lysosomal membrane and across the plasma membrane is carrier-mediated.

Apical Plasma Membrane Turnover; Membrane Recycling

By exocytosis and endocytosis there is a continuous bidirectional transport of thyroglobulin across the apical surface of the follicle cells. The transports involve extensive movement of membrane, which is added to the apical plasma membrane during exocytosis and removed by endocytosis. Under normal conditions these membrane movements must balance each other. The size of the membrane areas involved in these redistributions has been estimated by two methods.[83–86] Both methods have shortcomings, but the figures obtained are of the same order of magnitude and indicate that the apical plasma membrane may be renewed one to several times per hour.

TSH has a rapid stimulatory effect on the turnover of the apical plasma membrane. The redistribution of membrane induced by a large TSH dose has been followed by quantitative electron microscopy on the rat thyroid in vivo.[77, 87] The earliest effect of TSH (during the first five minutes) was a transfer of membrane from exocytotic vesicles to the apical plasma membrane, whose surface area was transiently increased. During the next 15 minutes exocytotic vesicle membrane continued to be added to the apical plasma membrane, but plasma membrane was simultaneously and more rapidly transferred to endocytotic structures and the apical plasma membrane surface area returned to the prestimulatory level. The apical surface area was never reduced below the prestimulatory size, and pseudopods were not formed until the apical plasma membrane had received membrane by exocytosis. This indicates that the exocytotic vesicles—rather than the apical plasma membrane—represent the membrane store required for a large, acute endocytotic response to TSH. This interpretation is supported by observations on rats that the reduction of the pool of exocytotic vesicles before administration of TSH reduces the endocytotic response to TSH to a corresponding degree.[88–90]

The high turnover rate of the apical plasma membrane observed in the thyroid follicle cells is a phenomenon common to many cell types. It has long been agreed that these amounts of plasma membrane cannot be replaced by de novo synthesis, and reutilization of membrane by recycling of intact plasma membrane components to the cell surface has been suggested. Observations indicate that a certain recycling of membrane via the Golgi complex may occur in the thyroid, but the quantitative importance of this route is not clear.[65, 66]

ONTOGENESIS

The development of the thyroid conforms to the same general pattern in all mammals, but the stage of development at birth varies between species. The gland develops from an endodermal invagination in the floor of the primitive pharynx, in humans observable in the third week of gestation; the site of origin is indicated by the foramen cecum of the adult tongue. The invagination becomes a diverticulum that grows downward in front of the primitive pharynx but remains connected to its origin by the narrow thyroglossal duct. The distal end of the diverticulum gradually acquires a bilobed shape and, by cell proliferation, it soon becomes solid. The thyroglossal duct undergoes atrophy and disappears, but its most distal part may develop into a pyramidal lobe consisting of differentiated thyroid tissue still connected with the isthmus of the gland. The thyroglossal duct may also give rise to cysts, fistulae, and ectopic thyroid tissue located along the path of descent.

During the seventh week, the median thyroid anlage receives branchiogenic material, derived from the epithelium of the fourth branchial pouch, the ultimobranchial body.

The histogenesis of the thyroid begins by splitting of the solid primordium into plates and cords of epithelial cells by invading mesenchyme and blood vessels. The cell cords are divided by connective tissue septa into subunits that organize into follicles. The first step in the genesis of follicles seems to be the formation of junctional complexes. These devices keep neighboring cells together and seal the intercellular spaces at specific sites, thereby partitioning off the nascent follicle lumina. The calcitonin-producing parafollicular cells, or C cells, reach the thyroid from the ultimobranchial body. However, these cells have their origin in the neural crest (rhombencephalic level) and use the ultimobranchial body as an intermediate migration station. Small numbers of calcitonin-containing C cells may occur in other tissues derived from branchial epithelium, such as the thymus and parathyroid IV.

The development of the specific functions of the thyroid is closely related to the development of the thyroid structure. The ability to synthesize thyroglobulin is correlated with the development of the RER and is observed before the occurrence of a true follicle organization. Iodination of thyroglobulin and hormone synthesis are generally not manifest until follicles have been formed. In human embryos, iodinated thyroglobulin has been demonstrated in glands with early follicles in fetuses of about 75 days. The binding of iodine to thyroglobulin takes place in the follicle lumina. Thyroid hormones are present in the plasma of the fetus within hours after the first sign of thyroglobulin iodination, which indicates that the maturation of the hormone release mechanisms accompanies the development of the follicle. (For references, see review in ref. 92.)

REFERENCES

1. Fujita H: Functional morphology of the thyroid. Int Rev Cytol 113:145–181, 1988.
2. Ekholm R: The ultrastructure of the blood capillaries in the mouse thyroid gland. Z Zellforsch 46:139–146, 1957.
3. Wollman SH: Structure of the thyroid gland. In De Visscher M (ed): The Thyroid Gland, Comprehensive Endocrinology. New York, Raven Press, 1980, pp 1–19.
4. Melander A, Ericson LE, Sundler F, Westgren U: Intrathyroidal amines in the regulation of thyroid activity. Rev Physiol Biochem Pharmacol 73:39–71, 1975.
5. Melander A, Sundler F: Presence and influence of cholinergic nerves in the mouse thyroid. Endocrinology 105:7–9, 1979.
6. Grunditz T, Håkanson R, Rerup C, et al: Neuropeptide Y in the thyroid gland: Neuronal localization and enhancement of stimulated thyroid hormone secretion. Endocrinology 115:1537–1542, 1984.
7. Nonidez JF: Innervation of the thyroid gland. II. Origin and course of the thyroid nerves in the dog. Am J Anat 48:299–330, 1931.
8. Romeo HE, Gonzales-Solveyra C, Vacas MI, et al: Origins of the sympathetic projections to the rat thyroid and parathyroid glands. J Auton Nerv Syst 17:63–70, 1986.
9. Cauna N, Naik NT: The distribution of cholinesterases in the sensory

ganglia of man and some mammals. J Histochem Cytochem 11:129–138, 1963.

10. Erankö O, Härkönen M: Noradrenaline and acetylesterase in sympathetic ganglion cells in the rat. Acta Physiol Scand 61:299–300, 1964.

11. Nonidez JF: Innervation of the thyroid gland. III. Distribution and termination of the nerve fibers in the dog. Am J Anat 57:135–170, 1935.

12. Grunditz T, Sundler F, Håkansson R, Uddman R: Regulatory peptides in the thyroid gland. In Ekholm R, Kohn LD, Wollman SH (eds): Control of the Thyroid Gland. New York, Plenum Press, 1989, pp 121–149.

13. Gumbiner B: Structure, biochemistry and assembly of epithelial tight junctions. Am J Physiol 253:C749–C758, 1987.

14. Tice LW, Wollman SH: Ultrastructural localization of peroxidase on pseudopods and other structures of the typical thyroid epithelial cell. Endocrinology 94:1555–1567, 1974.

15. Hovsépian S, Foracci H, Maroux S, Fayet G: Kinetic studies of the localization of aminopeptidase N in monolayer and in follicle-associated cultures of porcine thyroid cells. Cell Tissue Res 224:601–611, 1982.

16. Björkman U, Ekholm R, Denef J-F: Cytochemical localization of hydrogen peroxide in isolated thyroid follicles. J Ultrastruct Res 74:105–115, 1981.

17. Gerard C, Gabrion J, Werrier B, et al: Localization of the Na^+/K^+-ATPase and of an amiloride sensitive Na^+ uptake on thyroid epithelial cells. Eur J Cell Biol 38:134–141, 1985.

18. Chambard MB, Verrier J, Gabrion J, Mauchamp J: Polarization of thyroid cells in culture: Evidence for the basolateral localization of the "iodide pump" and of the thyroid-stimulating hormone receptor-adenyl cyclase complex. J Cell Biol 96:1172–1177, 1983.

19. Ericson LE, Sundler F: Thyroid parafollicular cells: Ultrastructural and functional correlations. In Motta P (ed): Electron Microscopy in Biology and Medicine: Ultrastructure of Endocrine Cells and Tissue. Hague, The Netherlands, Martinus Nijhoff, 1983, pp 274–285.

20. Björkman U, Ekholm R: Biochemistry of thyroid hormone formation and secretion. In Green MA (ed): The Thyroid Gland, Comprehensive Endocrinology. New York, Raven Press, 1990, pp 83–125.

21. Gilmore R, Blobel G, Walter P: Protein translocation across the endoplasmic reticulum. I. Detection in the microsomal membrane of a receptor for the signal recognition particle. J Cell Biol 95:463–469, 1982.

22. Walter P, Blobel G: Translocation of proteins across the endoplasmic reticulum. II. Signal recognition protein (SRP) mediates the selective binding to microsomal membranes of in-vitro–assembled polysomes synthesizing secretory protein. J Cell Biol 91:551–556, 1981.

23. Herzog V, Neumüller W, Holzmann B: Thyroglobulin, the major and obligatory exportable protein of thyroid follicle cells, carries the lysosomal recognition marker mannose-6-phosphate. EMBO J 6:555–560, 1987.

24. Consiglio E, Acquaviva AM, Formisano S, et al: Characterization of phosphate residues on thyroglobulin. J Biol Chem 262:10304–10314, 1987.

25. Burgess TL, Kelly RB: Constitutive and regulated secretion of proteins. Annu Rev Cell Biol 3:243–293, 1987.

26. Pfeffer SR, Rothman JE: Biosynthetic protein transport and sorting by the endoplasmic reticulum and Golgi. Annu Rev Biochem 56:829–852, 1987.

27. Björkman U, Ekholm R: Effect of tunicamycin on thyroglobulin secretion. Eur J Biochem 125:585–591, 1982.

28. Kim PS, Arvan P: Folding and assembly of newly synthesized thyroglobulin occurs in a pre-Golgi compartment. J Biol Chem 266:12412–12418, 1991.

29. Ekholm R, Björkman U: Structural and functional integration of the thyroid gland. In Green MA (ed): The Thyroid Gland, Comprehensive Endocrinology. New York, Raven Press, 1990, pp 37–81.

30. Dunphy WG, Rothman JE: Compartmental organization of the Golgi stack. Cell 42:13–21, 1985.

31. Berger EG: How Golgi-associated glycosylation works. Cell Biol Int Rep 9:407–417, 1985.

32. Pavelka M: Functional morphology of the Golgi-apparatus. Adv Anat Embryol Cell Biol 106:1–94, 1987.

33. Rambourg A, Clermont Y: Three-dimensional electron microscopy: Structure of the Golgi apparatus. Eur J Cell Biol 51:189–200, 1990.

34. Dunphy WG, Brands R, Rothman JE: Attachment of terminal N-acetyl-glucosamine to asparagine-linked oligosaccharides occurs in central cisternae of the Golgi stack. Cell 40:463–472, 1985.

35. Roth J, Berger EG: Immunocytochemical localization of galactosyl-transferase in HeLa cells: Codistribution with thiamine pyrophosphatase in trans-Golgi cisternae. J Cell Biol 93:223–229, 1982.

36. Slot JW, Geuze HJ: Immunoelectron microscopic exploration of the Golgi complex. J Histochem Cytochem 31:1049–1056, 1983.

37. Roth J, Taatjes D, Lucocq J, et al: Demonstration of an extensive trans-tubular network continuous with the Golgi apparatus stack that may function in glycosylation. Cell 43:287–295, 1985.

38. Orci L, Glick BS, Rothman JE: A new type of coated vesicular carrier that appears not to contain clathrin: Its possible role in protein transport within the Golgi stack. Cell 46:171–184, 1986.

39. Rothman JE, Miller RL, Urbani LJ: Intercompartmental transport in the Golgi complex is a dissociative process: Facile transfer of membrane protein between two Golgi populations. J Cell Biol 99:260–271, 1984.

40. Duden R, Allan V, Kreis T: Involvement of β-COP in membrane traffic through the Golgi complex. Trends Cell Biol 1:14–19, 1991.

41. Kornfeld S: Trafficking of lysosomal enzymes in normal and disease states. J Clin Invest 77:1–6, 1986.

42. von Figura K, Hasilik A: Lysosomal enzymes and their receptors. Annu Rev Biochem 55:167–193, 1986.

43. Kaplan A, Ackord DT, Sly WS: Phosphohexosyl components of a lysosomal enzyme are recognized by pinocytosis receptors on human fibroblasts. Proc Natl Acad Sci USA 74:2026–2030, 1977.

44. Pearse MF, Robinson MS: Clathrin, adaptors, and sorting. Annu Rev Cell Biol 6:151–172, 1990.

45. Björkman U, Ekholm R, Ericson LE, Öfverholm T: Transport of thyroglobulin and peroxidase in the thyroid follicle cell. Mol Cell Endocrinol 5:3–17, 1976.

46. Ring P, Johanson V: Immunoelectron-microscopic demonstration of thyroglobulin and thyroid hormones in the rat thyroid gland. J Histochem Cytochem 35:1095–1104, 1987.

47. Björkman U, Ekholm R: Generation of H_2O_2 in isolated porcine thyroid follicles. Endocrinology 115:392–398, 1984.

48. Virion A, Michot JL, Deme D, et al: NADPH-dependent H_2O_2 generation and peroxidase activity in thyroid particular fraction. Mol Cell Endocrinol 36:95–105, 1984.

49. Ekholm R, Wollman SH: Site of iodination in the rat thyroid gland deduced from electron microscopic autoradiographs. Endocrinology 97:1432–1444, 1975.

50. Ekholm R: Iodination of thyroglobulin, an intracellular or extracellular process? Mol Cell Endocrinol 24:141–163, 1981.

51. Ericson LE: Intracellular lumens in thyroid follicle cells of thyroxine-treated rats. J Ultrastruct Res 69:297–305, 1979.

52. Ekholm R, Björkman U: Localization of iodine binding in the thyroid gland in vitro. Endocrinology 115:1558–1567, 1984.

53. Smeds S: A microgel electrophoretic analysis of the colloid proteins in single rat thyroid follicles. II. The protein concentration of the colloid in single rat thyroid follicles. Endocrinology 91:1300–1306, 1972.

54. Penel C, Gerard C, Mauchamp J, Verrier B: The thyroid cell monolayer in culture. A tight sodium absorbing epithelium. Pflügers Arch 414:509–515, 1989.

55. Nilsson M: Integrity of the occluding barrier in high resistant thyroid follicular epithelium in culture, I. Dependence of extracellular Ca^{2+} is polarized. Eur J Cell Biol 56:295–307, 1991.

56. Ericson LE: Exocytosis and endocytosis in the thyroid follicle cell. Mol Cell Endocrinol 22:1–24, 1981.

57. Wetzel BK, Spicer SS, Wollman SH: Changes in fine structure and acid phosphatase localization in rat thyroid cells following thyrotropin administration. J Cell Biol 25:593–618, 1965.

58. Seljelid R: Endocytosis in thyroid follicle cells. II. A microinjection study of the origin of colloid droplets. J Ultrastruct Res 17:401–420, 1967.

59. Seljelid R: Endocytosis in thyroid follicle cells. III. An electron microscopic study of the cell surface and related structures. J Ultrastruct Res 18:1–24, 1967.

60. Seljelid R, Reith A, Nakken KF: An early phase of endocytosis in rat thyroid follicle cells. Lab Invest 23:595–605, 1970.

61. Engström G, Ericson LE: Effect of graded doses of thyrotropin on exocytosis and early phase of endocytosis in the rat thyroid. Endocrinology 108:399–405, 1981.

62. Ketelbant-Balasse P, Rodesch F, Nève P, Pasteels JM: Scanning electron microscope observations of apical surfaces of dog thyroid cells. Exp Cell Res 79:111–119, 1973.

63. Wetzel B, Wollman SH: Scanning electron microscopy of pseudopod formation in rat thyroids. J Cell Biol 55:279a, 1972.

64. Ericson LE, Ring KM, Öfverholm T: Selective macropinocytosis of thyroglobulin in rat thyroid follicles. Endocrinology 113:1746–1753, 1983.

65. Herzog V, Miller F: Membrane retrieval in epithelial cells of isolated thyroid follicles. Eur J Cell Biol 19:203–215, 1979.

66. Denef J-F, Ekholm R: Membrane labelling with cationized ferritin in isolated thyroid follicles. J Ultrastruct Res 71:203–221, 1980.
67. Rocmans PA, Ketelbant-Balasse P, Dumont JE, Neve P: Hormonal secretion by hyperactive thyroid cells is not secondary to apical phagocytosis. Endocrinology 103:1834–1848, 1978.
68. Bernier-Valentin F, Kostrouch Z, Rabilloud R, Rousset B: Analysis of the thyroglobulin internalization process using in vitro reconstituted follicles: Evidence for a coated vesicle-dependent endocytic pathway. Endocrinology 129:2194–2201, 1991.
69. Wollman SH, Spicer SS, Burstone MS: Localization of esterase and phosphatase in granules and colloid droplets in rat thyroid epithelium. J Cell Biol 21:191–201, 1964.
70. Ekholm R, Smeds S: On dense bodies and droplets in the follicular cells of the guinea pig thyroid. J Ultrastruct Res 16:71–82, 1966.
71. Seljelid R: Endocytosis in thyroid follicle cells. I. Structure and significance of different types of single membrane-limited vacuoles and bodies. J Ultrastruct Res 17:195–219, 1967.
72. Wollman SH: Secretion of thyroid hormones. In Dingle JT, Fell HB (eds): Lysosomes in Biology and Pathology, vol 2. New York, American Elsevier Publishing Comp, 1969, pp 483–512.
73. Hubbard AL: Endocytosis. Curr Opinion Cell Biol 1: 675–683, 1989.
74. Van Deurs B, Petersen OW, Olsnes S, Sandvig K: The ways of endocytosis. Int Rev Cytol 117:131–177, 1989.
75. Bomsel M, Prydz K, Parton RG, et al: Endocytosis in filter-grown Madin-Darby canine kidney cell. J Cell Biol 109:3243–3258, 1989.
76. Kostrouch Z, Munari-Silem Y, Rajas F, et al: Thyroglobulin internalized by thyrocytes passes through early and late endosomes. Endocrinology 129:2202–2211, 1991.
77. Ericson LE, Engström G: Quantitative electron microscopic studies on exocytosis and endocytosis in the thyroid follicle cell. Endocrinology 103:883–892, 1978.
78. Bernier-Valentin F, Kostrouch Z, Rabilloud R, et al: Coated vesicles from thyroid cells carry iodinated thyroglobulin molecules. First indication for an internalization of the thyroid prohormone via a mechanism of receptor-mediated endocytosis. J Biol Chem 265:17373–17380, 1990.
79. Tokuyama T, Yoshinari M, Rawitch AB, Taurog A: Digestion of thyroglobulin with purified thyroid lysosomes: Preferential release of iodoamino acids. Endocrinology 121:714–721, 1987.
80. Rosenberg IN, Gorwanni A: Purification and characterization of a flavoprotein from bovine thyroid with iodotyrosine deiodinase activity J Biol Chem 254:12318–12325, 1979.
81. Tietze F, Kohn LD, Kohn AD, et al: Carrier mediated transport of monoiodotyrosine out of thyroid cell lysosomes. J Biol Chem 264:4762–4765, 1989.
82. Oppenheimer JH, Schwarz HL: Stereospecific transport of triiodothyronine from plasma to cytosol and from cytosol to nucleus in rat liver, kidney, brain, and heart. J Clin Invest 75:147–154, 1985.
83. Wollman SH, Loewenstein JE: Rates of colloid droplet and apical vesicle production and membrane turnover during thyroglobulin secretion and resorption. Endocrinology 93:248–252, 1973.
84. Öfverholm T, Ericson LE: Rate of protein transport in thyroid follicle cells of normal, thyroxine-treated and TSH-injected rats. Eur J Cell Biol 35:171–179, 1984.
85. Johanson V, Öfverholm T, Ericson LE: Turnover of apical plasma membrane in thyroid follicle cells of normal and thyroxine-treated rats. Eur J Cell Biol 35:165–170, 1984.
86. Wollman SH: Turnover of plasma membrane in thyroid epithelium and review of evidence for the role of micropinocytosis. Eur J Cell Biol 50:274–256, 1989.
87. Ekholm R: Thyroid hormone secretion. In Dumont JE, Nunez J (eds): Hormones and Cell Regulation. Amsterdam, Elsevier/North Holland, 1977, pp 91–110.
88. Ericson LE, Engström G, Ekholm R: Effects of long-term thyroxine treatment on thyrotropin-induced exocytosis and endocytosis in the rat thyroid. Endocrinology 104:704–710, 1979.
89. Ericson LE, Engström G, Ekholm R: Effect of cycloheximide on thyrotropin-stimulated endocytosis in the rat thyroid. Endocrinology 106:1119–1126, 1980.
90. Ericson LE, Johanson V: Effect of a second dose of thyrotropin on exocytosis and endocytosis in the rat thyroid gland. J Endocrinol Invest 7: 603–610, 1984.
91. Ericson LE, Fredriksson G: Phylogeny and ontogeny of the thyroid gland. In Greer MA (ed): The Thyroid Gland, Comprehensive Endocrinology. New York, Raven Press, 1990, pp 1–35.

Biosynthesis and Secretion of Thyroid Hormones

FABRIZIO GENTILE
ROBERTO DI LAURO
GAETANO SALVATORE

THYROID HORMONE BIOSYNTHESIS AND SECRETION: AN OVERVIEW

Most thyroid diseases are accompanied by alterations of the biosynthesis and/or secretion of thyroid hormones. Although iodine metabolism is still viewed as an essential part of thyroid hormone biosynthesis, emphasis has recently changed from iodine to the molecular site of hormonal synthesis, i.e., thyroglobulin (Tg). In this chapter thyroid hormone biosynthesis and secretion are viewed accordingly. Few areas of endocrinology have profited so much from advances in biochemistry and molecular biology as has clinical thyroidology. What follows is intended to be a critical appraisal of the subject from the viewpoint of the molecular endocrinologist.

Expression of Thyroid-Specific Functions

The thyroid gland is the site of synthesis, storage, and controlled secretion of thyroid hormones. Thyroid hormones are synthesized by the iodination and coupling of a small subset of tyrosyl residues within the peptide chains of Tg. This is a large glycoprotein synthesized and secreted by thyroid follicular cells into the lumen of the follicles that they surround and delimit. Iodination and coupling are catalyzed at the apical surface of follicular cells by thyroid peroxidase (TPO), a thyroid-specific, membrane-bound glycoprotein. For the newly formed hormones to reach the bloodstream, Tg must be reabsorbed and degraded by the follicular cells. Hypothalamic cells "sense" a decrease in the serum levels of thyroid hormones and secrete thyrotropin-releasing factor (TRH), a peptide that prompts specific cells in the anterior pituitary gland to secrete thyroid-stimulating hormone (TSH). The binding of TSH to its receptor on thyroid follicular cells triggers in these cells an increase of iodide uptake, Tg and TPO synthesis, and Tg reabsorption. Increased Tg degradation in lysosomes and hormone secretion lead to the restoration of normal serum hormone levels.

The unique capabilities of the thyroid follicular cells depend on the exclusive presence in these cells of Tg, TPO, and TSH receptor. The cell type–specific expression of the respective genes is coordinately induced during thyroid differentiation.[1] This suggests that common mechanisms are shared by a whole thyroid-specific "regulon." During embryonal development, these mechanisms are finely regulated in space and in time. Thyroid follicular cells derive from the downward proliferation of the endoderm paving the anterior pharyngeal cavity, in the area of the presumptive sublingual region called *thyroid anlage* (see Ch. 33). The differentiated functions of the follicular cells begin to be expressed only after the completion of migration. In rats, five days separate the commitment of the precursors of thyroid follicular cells, first detected at day 9.5 postcoitum (thyroid anlage stage), from the induction of the differentiated phenotype, beginning at day 14.5.[1]

Three factors are involved in the expression of the Tg and TPO genes: thyroid transcription factor 1 (TTF-1), thyroid transcription factor 2 (TTF-2),[2] and Pax-8.[3] These are DNA-binding proteins, capable of activating the transcription of both genes to different extents.[4, 5] The expression of TTF-1 and Pax-8 starts at the commitment step, before the onset of differentiation.[1] Thus TTF-1 and Pax-8 could play multiple roles during thyroid development. At an early stage, they could induce the commitment of the follicular cell precursors. Later, an unknown mechanism triggers their control on the thyroid-specific expression of the Tg and TPO genes. The roles of TTF-1, TTF-2, and Pax-8 in the expression of the TSH receptor gene are unknown.

Phylogenetic Aspects

Thyroid hormones T_4 and T_3 and the molecular site of their biosynthesis, Tg and Tg-like iodoproteins, as well as the follicle (the basic morphological unit of the thyroid gland), are present in all vertebrates from adult Cyclostomata to Mammalia. A typical thyroid gland is present in higher vertebrates, whereas only isolated thyroid follicles are found in lower vertebrates.[6] The *Ammocoetes,* which is the larval stage of the lamprey (a cyclostome), lacks both a thyroid gland and thyroid follicles. It has instead an elongated subpharyngeal glandular sac, sometimes improperly called the *endostyle,* originating from the floor of the pharynx. At metamorphosis, part of this sac separates from the primitive pharynx and becomes a nonencapsulated thyroid made of scattered follicles. Thus the subpharyngeal gland of the *Ammocoetes* is the anlage of the thyroid gland of the adult lamprey, as first suggested in 1886 by Dohrn.[7] The subpharyngeal gland concentrates iodide[8] and synthesizes iodoamino acids,[9] most likely within the polypeptide chain of a Tg-like iodoprotein.[10] By the end of metamorphosis,

Tg can be detected by immunocytochemistry in most follicles.[11]

The appearance of the molecular mechanism of hormone synthesis seems to have evolved earlier than that of the thyroid follicle.[12] Thyroid hormone biosynthesis occurs in the entire phylum of Chordata, to which Vertebrates belong, together with the more primitive subphyla of Tunicata and Cephalochordata, both referred to as "Protochordata." Sizeable amounts of thyroid hormones are present in Cephalochordata, e.g., *Amphioxus,* and in various Tunicata.[12] Protochordata, however, seem to lack the thyroid follicle and a typical Tg protein. There is only one report of a Tg-like molecule in *Styela clava.*[13] The midventral line of the pharynx of the Protochordata is marked by a hypobranchial groove, the "endostyle," whose dorsal part continues the epithelium of the branchial cavity and is considered by some authors[14, 15] the equivalent of a primitive thyroid region. Iodide binding was first detected in the endostyle of *Amphioxus*[14] and in *Ciona intestinalis,* a tunicate.[15] However, only a minute fraction of the radioiodine taken up by *C. intestinalis* was concentrated in the endostyle as free T_4, most of it being found in the tunic as protein-bound iodotyrosines and iodothyronines.[16] On the other hand, iodide binding and peroxidase activity were localized in restricted zones of the endostyle of Cephalochordata and Tunicata.[6] In summary, the molecular site of hormone biosynthesis in Protochordata has not been clearly established and the cellular site is also uncertain, despite the morphological analogy between the vertebrate thyroid and the protochordate endostyle.

Iodotyrosines (MIT and DIT), but not iodothyronines (T_3 and T_4), are present in several marine invertebrates.[12] However, neither iodotyrosine coupling nor the biosynthesis of Tg-like iodoproteins seems to occur below the phylum of Chordata.[12]

STRUCTURE OF THYROGLOBULIN

Physicochemical Properties

Tg is the most abundant protein of thyroid tissue. The molecular mass of bovine Tg, calculated from sedimentation measurements, is 669 kDa.[17] The isoelectric point of porcine Tg is 4.5.[18] The sedimentation coefficient, extrapolated to infinite dilution in water at 20°C ($S_{20,w}$), of bovine Tg is 19 S.[17] However, 19 S Tg is constituted by a microheterogeneous pool of molecules whose iodine content varies from 10 to 60 atoms per Tg molecule[19–21] and whose density and sedimentation coefficient increase linearly with the iodine content.[22] About 10 per cent of the Tg mass is made of carbohydrates.[23] 19 S Tg is a mixture of both noncovalent and covalent dimers of two subunits having a relative molecular mass (Mr) of 330 kDa and a sedimentation coefficient of 12 S.[24] The proportion of covalent dimers increases linearly with the average iodine content of Tg (see under Secondary, Tertiary, and Quaternary Structure). Thyroid follicles also contain in their lumina an iodoprotein sedimenting at 27 S whose proportion in the pool of thyroid iodoproteins increases with the iodine content.[25, 26] COOH-terminal analysis showed that this is a tetramer of the same 330-kDa oligomer that constitutes 19 S Tg dimers.[27] Iodinated albumin is a minor fraction of the thyroid iodoproteins in normal rats.[28] Albumin and albumin-like iodoproteins replace Tg in the congenital goiters of various animal species.[29, 30] Albumin in thyroid follicles originates from blood.[30a]

Molecular Structure

Primary Structure

Full-length sequences of the bovine[31] and human Tg mRNA's,[32] and a partial sequence for the rat,[33] have been determined from overlapping cDNA clones. The structure of the human mRNA consists of 8448 nucleotides, including an untranslated 5′-end, an open reading frame, and an untranslated 3′-end of 41, 8301, and 106 nucleotides, respectively. The corresponding segments of the bovine mRNA are 41, 8307, and 83 nucleotides long. The 3018 bases of the partial mRNA of rat Tg include a segment of 2901 bases, coding for 967 amino acids at the COOH-terminus of Tg, and an untranslated 3′-end of 117 bases.

The human Tg mRNA encodes a polypeptide of 2767 amino acids. The first 19 residues probably represent a hydrophobic signal sequence and are absent from the mature Tg polypeptide,[34] which is composed of 2748 residues and has an expected Mr of 302,773.[32] The bovine Tg mRNA encodes a polypeptide of 2769 amino acids, including 19 residues that are not present in the mature polypeptide,[35] and a mature chain of 2750 residues with an expected Mr of 302,253.[31] The similarity is 81 per cent between the human and bovine mRNA's, and 77 per cent between the deduced polypeptide sequences.

Two thirds of the Tg sequence at its amino-terminal side consist of tandemly repeated motifs (Fig. 34–1). The type 1 motif is 60 to 70 residues long, contains 6 cysteinyl residues, and is repeated 10 times. The type 2 motif consists of 14 to 17 amino acids, 2 of which are cysteines, and is repeated 3 times at the center of Tg. Five type 3 repeats,

subdivided into subtype 3a, with 8 cysteines each, and subtype 3b, with 6 cysteines each, follow in alternating order. There are also several glycyl and prolyl residues at invariant positions in the type 1 repeats. The type 1 motif of Tg is homologous with a cysteine-rich motif of the invariant chain associated with the class II major histocompatibility antigen,[36] and it shares partial sequence similarity with cysteine-rich motifs of entactin[37] and epithelial glycoprotein.[38]

The sequence of 570 amino acids at the COOH-terminus of Tg is very similar (up to 60 per cent in some regions) to those of the members of a superfamily of esterases, including the acetylcholinesterase of Torpedo californica,[39] human serum cholinesterase, and other esterases.[40] However, Tg and the esterases do not share any functional property. In fact, the hormonogenic tyrosyl residues of Tg are absent from the esterases, and the active site seryl and histidyl residues of the esterases are absent from Tg.[39, 40]

Some mRNA variants generated by alternative splicing are known.[41] Those with a possible functional significance are discussed later (see under Acceptor and Donor Sites for the Coupling Reaction).

Secondary, Tertiary, and Quaternary Structure

In secondary structure predictions for human and bovine Tg, β-turns and β-strands prevail in the cysteine-rich motifs, whereas α-helices, β-strands, and segments of irregular structure are interspersed in the regions interrupting or separating the cysteine-rich repeats and in the acetylcholinesterase-like domain.[42] These data agree with an earlier prediction and analysis with circular dichroism of the COOH-terminal third of rat Tg.[43] It was suggested that the repeated sequences of Tg probably have a rigid structure, due to the presence of several cysteinyl, glycyl, and prolyl residues at invariant positions.[44]

Most of the exon-intron junctions in the amino-terminal half of the Tg gene are located either at the borders of type 1 repeats or within or at the borders of the unrelated

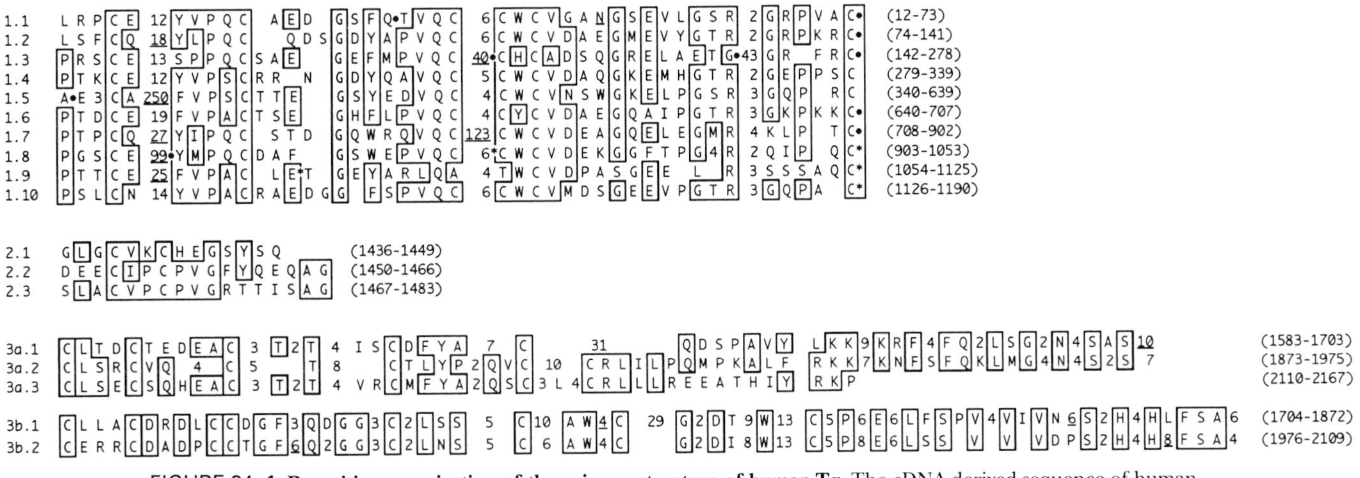

FIGURE 34–1. **Repetitive organization of the primary structure of human Tg.** The cDNA-derived sequence of human Tg[32] is reported in the one-letter amino acid code. Tandem repeats are aligned and the residues spanned by each repeat are indicated by the numbers in parentheses on the right. Insertions and deletions were introduced to optimize the homology. Conserved residues are boxed when present at least five times in type 1 and twice in type 2 and type 3 repeats. Numbers within the sequence indicate the length of segments showing no similarity between repeats. Underlined numbers or letters mark putative glycosylation sites. Exon-intron junctions are marked by dots if observed and asterisks if deduced from comparison to calf Tg.[45] Residues 1–11, the regions separating different kinds of repeat (residues 1191–1435 and 1484–1582) and the acetylcholinesterase-homologous domain (residues 2179–2748), are not shown.

inserts that interrupt some of the repeats.[45] Since exon-intron junctions often map at the surface of proteins[46] and coincide with regions of the sequence that display insertions and/or deletions and form loops at the surface of proteins,[47] it was suggested that some of the unrelated sequences that interrupt the cysteine-rich repeats of Tg may play a role in shaping the protein surface.[45] Limited proteolysis of Tg (see later) shows that several of these inserts correspond indeed to protease-labile regions of Tg.[42]

Some 19 S Tg dimers dissociate into 12 S monomers at alkaline pH[17] and in the presence of sodium dodecyl sulfate.[24, 48] Guinea pig is the only species in which Tg dissociates spontaneously into subunits at low temperature.[49] Other 19 S dimers are composed of monomers covalently linked by disulfide bonds and dissociate only upon reduction. Their proportion is linearly related to the iodine content of Tg.[50, 51] The 27 S tetramers of Tg dissociate into 19 S dimers upon mild treatment with alkali or heat, or at low ionic strength.[52]

Reducing electrophoresis of bovine 19 S Tg shows a doublet of two closely migrating bands that have a mobility similar to that of purified 12 S Tg.[53] Restriction mapping of the cDNA of bovine Tg reinforced the concept that there is only one elementary Tg chain.[54] It was suggested that the faster band of the electrophoretic doublet of reduced bovine Tg (F band) was of proteolytic origin[53, 55] and was produced after the secretion of Tg[56] by cleavage of the 330-kDa monomer at a protease-labile site.[57] Indeed, the F band of human and bovine Tg, which has an apparent mass of 270 kDa, derives from the cleavage of the slower band at residues 503 and 520, respectively.[58]

Antigenic Properties

Circulating anti-Tg antibodies are found in both healthy subjects and patients with autoimmune thyroid disorders.[59] Studies with monoclonal heterologous anti-Tg antibodies have shown that the antigenic determinants of Tg are clustered in antigenic regions, whose number varied from six in human Tg[60, 61] to seven in mouse Tg.[62] The autoantibodies of patients with autoimmune diseases recognized a single antigenic cluster of human Tg,[60] which was distinct from those recognized by the natural autoantibodies of healthy subjects.[63]

Heterologous epitopes of human Tg have been localized by studying the reaction of rabbit immune sera with Tg fragments obtained by inserting cDNA segments in expression vectors. Ten epitopes were identified using cDNA's primed from the 3'-tail of the Tg mRNA. Several of them were located near the COOH-terminus of Tg, and none was recognized by the sera of patients with autoimmune thyroid diseases.[64] Seven epitopes were found using the total human Tg cDNA. Five of them occurred in the center of Tg and one near each Tg extremity; several were recognized by the sera of patients with autoimmune diseases.[65] As cautioned by the authors, epitopes dependent on the tertiary and quaternary structure and on post-translational modifications may escape detection by this method.

Some heteroepitopes are destroyed by reduction[66] and denaturation.[67] The reactivity of proteolytic Tg fragments with serum antibodies of patients with autoimmune thyroid disorders was inversely related to the size of the Tg fragments[68, 69]; it was diminished by thermal denaturation and abolished by reduction.[69] The reactivity of the epitopes recognized by autoreactive T cells, on the other hand, was independent of fragment size, denaturation, or reduction. This suggests that the autoantibodies recognize conformational epitopes, whereas T cells recognize sequential epitopes.[69]

The antigenicity of Tg is influenced by its iodine content. The binding of some mouse monoclonal antibodies to human Tg increased with the iodine and hormone content of Tg.[67] Two of them were directed against the NH_2-terminal hormonogenic site, and one was directed against the COOH-terminal hormonogenic site of Tg[70] (see Acceptor and Donor Sites for the Coupling Reaction). Highly iodinated autologous Tg was more capable of inducing experimental autoimmune thyroiditis than noniodinated Tg both in the Cornell strain chickens, which are genetically susceptible to iodide-induced thyroiditis,[71] and in the mouse.[72] In the latter study, serum antibodies did not differentiate Tg molecules according to their iodine content, whereas autoreactive T cells were activated only by highly iodinated Tg.[72] Two iodination-dependent epitopes of mouse Tg recognized by autoreactive T cells were centered on the hormonogenic site corresponding to human Tg residue 2553[73] (see Acceptor and Donor Sites for the Coupling Reaction).

BIOSYNTHESIS OF THYROGLOBULIN

The Thyroglobulin Gene: Structure, Evolution, and Expression

The Tg gene is located on human chromosome 8 and rat chromosome 7.[74–76] An overall picture of the structure of this huge gene emerges from the data collected in humans,[45, 77] rat,[78] and calf.[79] The coding information is split into at least 42 exons and spans more than 200 kb pairs, making the Tg gene one of the largest known. About two thirds of Tg at its amino-terminal side consists of tandemly repeated cysteine-rich motifs of various kinds. The location of the exon-intron junctions determined so far in the amino-terminal half of the Tg gene correlates partially with the arrangement of these repetitive units. Out of 10 repeats found in the amino-terminal portion of the protein, four are encoded by a single exon, two are found together in one exon, and four are divided between two or three exons. These findings, together with the interspersion of unrelated sequences in the repeating units, suggested that this portion of the gene arose by duplication of an ancestral unit made of four exons. Subsequent unequal crossing-over events, and the partial "exonization" of some introns and the loss of several others, could have resulted in the present structure.[45] The carboxy-terminal third of Tg is very similar to acetylcholinesterase and appears to have originated from the duplication of an ancestral gene common to a superfamily of esterases.[39] Thus, Tg appears to be made of two moieties, an amino-terminal one and a carboxy-terminal one, that have different evolutionary histories.[78] It is noteworthy that both of them seem able to support the biosynthesis of thyroid hormones (see Acceptor and Donor Sites for the Coupling Reaction). The question is: Did one of these molecular sites of thyroid hormone synthesis precede the other in evolution or did they appear together in two different polypeptides?

The expression of the Tg gene is described in detail in Chapter 35. Suffice it to say here that such a large transcriptional unit is controlled by an amazingly small promoter, which is probably not larger than 2000 base pairs and could be as small as 200 base pairs. This small region, located before the transcription start site, contains the binding sites of the transcription factors described at the beginning of this chapter and is probably sufficient for both the hormonal[80, 81] and the developmental control of the Tg gene expression.[82–84]

Synthesis, Folding, and Assembly of the Elementary Polypeptide Chains of Thyroglobulin

The elementary chains of Tg are synthesized on polysomes bound on the rough endoplasmic reticulum.[85, 86] The folding and assembly of the Tg dimer, the major molecular species found in the follicle lumen, has recently been investigated in hog thyrocytes.[87, 87a] Newly synthesized Tg chains first form aggregates with and without interchain disulfide bonds. These are solubilized into unfolded monomers that are then folded and assembled into dimers. At this stage, none of the Tg dimers has a covalent nature because they all dissociate easily under nonreducing conditions. All these steps occur in a pre-Golgi compartment. Nascent Tg aggregates and unfolded free monomers are associated with the molecular chaperone BiP, which may be involved in driving the dissolution of the aggregates or presenting the polypeptides to other helper molecules that catalyze folding.[87, 87a]

Post-translational Modifications

Glycosylation

Carbohydrates contribute about 10 per cent of the Tg mass. Two kinds of oligosaccharide units (A and B) are attached by glycosylamine linkages to asparagine residues of Tg. High-mannose A units contain a variable number of mannose residues and two N-acetylglucosamine residues; 7 to 8 units of this type have been found per human Tg molecule and 5 to 6 per bovine Tg molecule. Complex B units contain three mannose residues and variable numbers of N-acetylglucosamine, galactose, fucose, and sialic acid residues; 22 of these units have been detected in human Tg and 13 to 14 in bovine Tg.[23] Carbohydrate units of porcine Tg also include five subtypes of A units, with 5 to 9 mannose residues,[88] and bi- and triantennary B units with sialic acid in the terminal position.[89] B units with terminal α-D-galactose occur in the Tg of some species.[90]

The synthesis of the carbohydrate units of Tg starts cotranslationally in the endoplasmic reticulum with the transfer of an oligosaccharide precursor containing N-acetylglucosamine, mannose, and glucose from a pyrophosphoryl lipid carrier to an asparagine residue of Tg.[91] Glucose residues must be present on this precursor for the transfer to occur, but they are removed soon after by a glucosidase.[92] Further processing probably follows the general scheme of the assembly of N-linked oligosaccharides.[93] The removal of one mannose residue in the endoplasmic reticulum and

of three mannose residues in the *cis*-Golgi cisternae yields the A units. The removal of mannose and the addition of N-acetylglucosamine in the mid-Golgi cisternae and of fucose, galactose, and sialic acid in the trans-Golgi cisternae produce the B units.

TSH promotes the capping with sialic acid of the oligosaccharide units of the Tg secreted by hog thyroid follicles in serum-free culture[94] and induces maturation of the B units of the Tg secreted by the rat thyroid cell line FRTL-5.[95] The maturing units are located in the NH$_2$-terminal part of Tg.[96]

Putative sites for N-linked glycosylation, characterized by the Asn-X-Ser/Thr sequence, in the cDNA-derived sequence of human[32] and bovine Tg[31] outnumber the oligosaccharide units found in Tg. The glycosidic units localized so far include one type A unit linked to an asparagine residue of bovine Tg, later identified as number 2562,[97] and two type B units linked to asparagines 57 and 91 of human Tg.[98]

Human Tg also contains C and D oligosaccharide units. C units are linked to serine and threonine by O-glycosidic bonds and contain galactosamine[23]; D units are chondroitin-6-sulfate–like oligosaccharides linked to serine and contain a repeating unit of glucuronic acid and galactosamine, plus xylose, galactose, and sulfate.[99–101]

Phosphorylation and Sulfation

Phosphate groups have been detected in the Tg of calf, rat, and humans.[102] About one half of them were phosphate groups phosphodiester- or phosphomonoester-linked to the mannose residues of N-linked A oligosaccharide units. Phosphate groups phosphomonoester-linked to mannose residues have been found also in A and B oligosaccharide units of hog Tg.[103] Phosphorylated mannose residues were not detected in earlier studies.[56, 104] The other phosphate groups reported were linked to residues of serine[56] or serine and tyrosine.[102]

Sulfate groups occur in three types of oligosaccharide units of human Tg: (1) biantennary B units, containing galactose-3-sulfate; (2) tri- and tetra-antennary B units, containing galactose-3-sulfate and N-acetylglucosamine-6-sulfate; and (3) chondroitin-6-sulfate–like C units.[100, 101] In bovine Tg, the presence of sulfate is restricted to a single type of multibranched B unit.[100] In some N-linked oligosaccharide units of human Tg, sulfate groups co-exist with sialic acid residues[100, 105] or with sialic acid residues and phosphodiester groups.[106]

The addition of sulfate to the B units of bovine Tg occurs in the Golgi compartment, late during Tg biosynthesis.[57] [^{35}S]sulfate is bound to the slower band of the electrophoretic doublet of bovine Tg and to a 60-kDa peptide released from it by mild tryptic treatment but is absent from the faster band of the doublet.[57] The finding that the faster band derives from the cleavage of bovine Tg at residue 520[58] (see Secondary, Tertiary, and Quaternary Structure) restricts the location of the sulfated oligosaccharides to the NH$_2$-terminus of Tg.

While two thirds of the [^{35}S]sulfate incorporated into the Tg from hog thyrocytes was linked to tyrosine,[107] 90 per cent of the sulfate incorporated into human Tg was in B and C oligosaccharide units.[101] Chemical analysis demonstrated the lack of sulfated tyrosines in the Tg of calf and man.[57]

Iodination

Iodoamino acids found in Tg include monoiodotyrosine (MIT), 3,5-diiodotyrosine (DIT), and the hormones T_3 and T_4. Tg contains also small amounts (about 1 per cent) of hormonally inactive 3,3',5'-triiodothyronine (reverse T_3) and 3',5'-diiodothyronine (3',5'-T_2) and traces of 3,3'-diiodothyronine (3,3'-T_2) and monoiodohistidine[108] (Fig. 34–2).

The iodoamino acid composition of Tg is related to the iodine content of Tg[19-21] (Fig. 34–3). Under normal conditions, the iodine level ranges from 0.2 to 1.2 per cent of the Tg weight (10 to 60 moles of iodine atoms per mole of Tg).[20] MIT, DIT, and T_4 appear sequentially during the course of iodination and appear to be in a precursor-product relationship in the same order (see Fig. 34–5). MIT and DIT are the most abundant iodoamino acids. In hog Tg, the molar ratio of DIT to MIT increases in proportion to the level of Tg iodination. The ratio of DIT to T_4 remains constant at 2 up to an iodine content of 0.7 per cent of the Tg weight, after which it rapidly increases in proportion to the iodine content of Tg.[20] For an iodine content of 0.5 per cent of the Tg weight (25 moles of iodine atoms per mole of Tg), 2.5 to 3 moles of T_4 and less than 1 mole of T_3 are formed per mole of human Tg[19] and porcine Tg.[20]

Tg molecules iodinated in vivo exhibit a wide range of iodine content. Several properties of Tg are affected by iodination. Iodination produces such increases in the density and thereby in the sedimentation rate of Tg, that subpopulations of 19 S molecules, differing by a few iodine atoms, can be separated by centrifugation in a rubidium chloride gradient.[22] Increasing Tg iodination is accompanied by increases both in the resistance of Tg to dissociation by conditions affecting noncovalent interactions, such as alkali, detergents, and other denaturants,[51] and in the

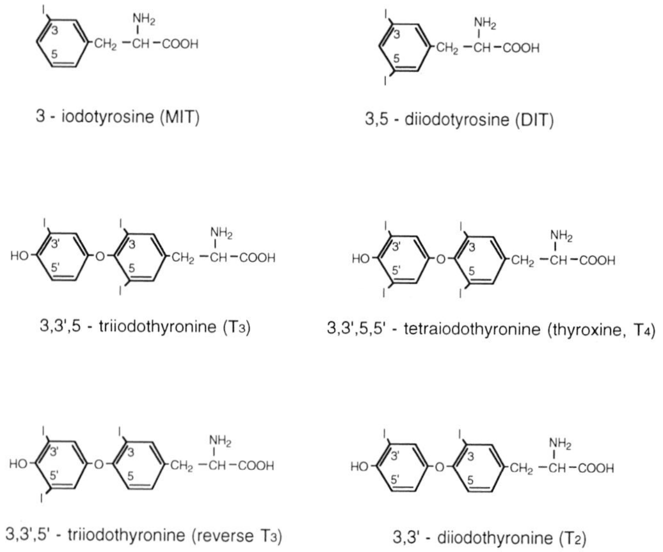

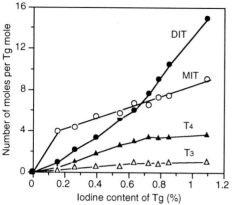

FIGURE 34–3. Iodoamino acid synthesis as a function of the iodine content of Tg. Various preparations of hog 19 S Tg with different iodine contents were hydrolyzed, and their iodoamino acid composition was determined after separation of the single iodoamino acids by anion-exchange chromatography.[20] The results are expressed as the number of iodoamino acid residues per Tg molecule. (Redrawn from Sorimachi K, Ui N: Comparison of the iodoamino acid distribution in various preparations of hog thyroglobulin with different iodine content and subunit structure. Biochim Biophys Acta 342:30–40, 1974).

fraction of 19 S Tg dimers whose subunits are covalently linked.[24, 50, 51] In the course of iodination, the noncovalent dimers appear to be converted into covalent dimers by the intermolecular oxidation of free sulfhydryl groups, whose number varies from 5 to 6 to 1 to 2 as the iodine content increases from 0.02 to 0.15 per cent of the Tg mass.[51, 109]

The iodination of the 27 S iodoprotein proceeds in vivo at a slower rate and to higher levels than that of 19 S Tg.[26] The formation of the tetramer is prevented by inhibitors of iodination, but not by inhibitors of de novo protein synthesis. This suggests that the 27 S iodoprotein is produced from a pre-existing pool of 19 S Tg via oxidative side reactions accompanying Tg iodination.[110]

Tg preparations of several animal species contain hormone-rich peptides that can be separated from the rest of Tg by reduction. In vitro iodination of human Tg to low and high iodination levels is accompanied by the formation of a 26-kDa and a 18-kDa peptide, respectively. These peptides contain a high fraction of the total T_4 content of Tg.[111] They both correspond to the NH_2-terminal end of Tg.[34, 112] Hormone-rich peptides of 20 and 15 kDa are formed during the iodination of rabbit and rat Tg.[113, 114] The amount of these peptides increases in proportion to their iodine and T_4 content. Therefore, it was proposed that their cleavage may be a consequence of iodination.[114] The human 26-kDa peptide is produced by the cleavage of Tg at the amino group of tyrosine 130.[115] Experiments in which iodination and coupling are partially dissociated suggest that the cleavage of the human 26-kDa peptide accompanies the coupling reaction. Apparently, tyrosine 130 donates an iodophenoxyl ring to tyrosine 5, and it has been suggested that such modification of tyrosine 130 is followed by the splitting of the peptide chain[116] (see Acceptor and Donor Sites for the Coupling Reaction).

Other T_4-enriched peptides corresponding to the NH_2-terminus of Tg include a 10-kDa peptide of calf Tg[35] ending at residue 80,[117] analogous 10-kDa peptides of sheep and hog Tg,[118] and a 30-kDa peptide of calf Tg ending at residue 234.[117]

3 - iodotyrosine (MIT)

3,5 - diiodotyrosine (DIT)

3,3',5 - triiodothyronine (T3)

3',3,5,5' - tetraiodothyronine (thyroxine, T4)

3,3',5' - triiodothyronine (reverse T3)

3,3' - diiodothyronine (T2)

FIGURE 34–2. Iodoamino acids found in Tg. Only 3,3',5-triiodothyronine (T_3) and 3,3',5,5'-tetraiodothyronine (T_4) possess hormonal activity. 3,3',5'-triiodothyronine (reverse T_3) and 3',5'-diiodothyronine (3',5'-T_2) are present in very low amounts.[108]

STRUCTURE-FUNCTION RELATIONSHIPS OF THYROGLOBULIN

Sequential Iodination of Tyrosyl Residues

Not all the tyrosyl residues of Tg are equally accessible to iodination, and their reactivity is largely determined by the secondary and tertiary structure of Tg.[119] At average levels of iodination, out of 134 tyrosyl residues per molecule of human Tg, only 25 to 30 are iodinated, and only 6 to 8 of these iodotyrosines form iodothyronines.[21, 108] When human goiter Tg iodinated in vitro with TPO and [^{125}I]-labeled iodine is mixed with noniodinated goiter Tg and the mixture is iodinated with [^{131}I]-labeled iodine, all the Tg molecules reach the same iodine content. This suggests that an order is followed in Tg iodination: the tyrosyl residues of noniodinated Tg, corresponding to those iodinated in prelabeled Tg, react with iodine before the other tyrosyl residues do.[120]

Preferential Synthesis of T$_4$ From Early Iodinated Tyrosyl Residues

The tyrosyl residues of Tg that are iodinated first are also those most readily converted to T$_4$.[121] In goiter Tg iodinated with TPO to low levels of iodine content with [^{131}I] and then to higher levels with [^{125}I], the tyrosyl residues labeled with [^{131}I] are preferentially used for T$_4$ synthesis. The preferential synthesis of T$_4$ from early iodinated tyrosyl residues is prevented by Tg denaturation in guanidine and is not observed with two proteins, casein and fibrinogen, which can form T$_4$ upon iodination with TPO.[121] Support for the idea that the tyrosyl residues most reactive toward iodination are also those most available for coupling comes from the finding that tyrosine 5, which is the main T$_4$-forming residue of Tg, is also the first tyrosyl residue to be iodinated in rat Tg.[122]

Acceptor and Donor Sites for the Coupling Reaction: The Hormonogenic Sites

T$_3$ and T$_4$ are formed in Tg via the iodination of some tyrosyl residues and the subsequent transfer of an iodophenoxyl group from a "donor" iodotyrosine, which provides the outer ring of the hormone, to an "acceptor" iodotyrosine, which provides the inner ring.[123] Hormonogenic acceptor tyrosines have been localized in the primary structure of Tg by sequencing various hormone-rich fragments of Tg and comparing their sequences to the cDNA-derived sequence of Tg (Fig. 34–4). The main T$_4$-forming site of Tg has been located at tyrosine 5 of the amino-terminal peptides of the Tg of humans,[34] calf,[35] sheep, hog,[118] rabbit,[124] and guinea pig.[125] These peptides contain up to 50 per cent of the T$_4$ of Tg. Tyrosine 5 is the most efficient T$_4$-forming residue at low levels of iodination during the in vitro iodination of human goiter Tg.[126] T$_4$ is also formed at two sites in hog Tg, corresponding to human tyrosines 2553 and 2567, with high and low efficiency, re-

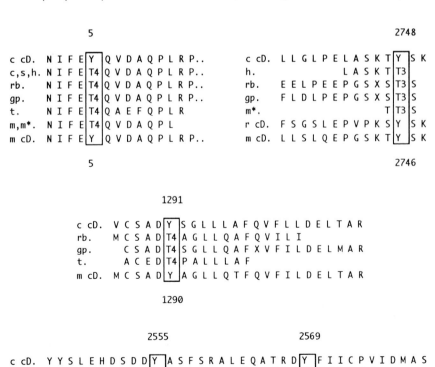

FIGURE 34–4. **Principal hormonogenic acceptor tyrosyl residues of Tg.** The amino acid sequences of the hormone-containing fragments of the Tg of various animal species are reported in the one-letter amino acid code. c cD, m cD, and r cD, cDNA-derived amino acid sequences of the Tg of calf,[31] humans,[32] and rat,[33] respectively. Hormone-forming tyrosyl residues are boxed and are numbered as in the Tg of calf (*top line*) and humans (*bottom line*). c, s, h, amino-terminal peptide sequences of three identical hormone-containing peptides of calf, sheep, and hog Tg.[35, 118] h, sequences of a peptide containing the preferential T$_3$-forming site (tyrosine 2746, numbered as in human Tg)[128] and of two other hormone-containing peptides at the COOH-terminus of hog Tg.[127] Variable proportions of MIT, DIT, T$_3$, and T$_4$ were found at residue number 2567 (numbered as in human Tg) in relation to the degree of Tg iodination.[127] The sequences are also shown of some hormone-bearing peptides of rb, rabbit,[124] gp, guinea pig,[125] and t, turtle Tg.[130] §, This peptide contained T$_4$ but was not sequenced far enough to detect it.[125] m, partial sequence of overlapping T$_4$-rich peptides of human Tg.[34, 112] m*, sequences of hormone-containing peptides of human Tg iodinated in vitro with lactoperoxidase.[129]

spectively.[127] In rabbit Tg, the tyrosine corresponding to human tyrosine 2553 is the second most efficient T_4-forming site.[124] The third T_4-forming site of rabbit Tg, in order of efficiency, corresponds to human residue 1290.[124] The corresponding tyrosine of guinea pig Tg is the most active site for new T_4 formation.[125] A site of preferential T_3 formation identified in fragments of hog,[128] rabbit,[124] and guinea pig Tg[125] corresponds to human tyrosine 2746. During in vitro low-level iodination of human Tg with lactoperoxidase (LPO), T_4 and T_3 are formed at residues 5, 2746, 2553, and 685, whereas only iodotyrosines are formed at tyrosines 1290 and 2567.[129] In rabbit and guinea pig Tg, TSH stimulates T_4 formation at tyrosine 1290 and T_3 formation at tyrosine 2746 and decreases T_4 synthesis at tyrosine 5.[125]

All the T_4-forming tyrosines occur in the Glu/Asp-Tyr sequence, whereas the Thr/Ser-Tyr-Ser sequence seems to favor the formation of T_3, with Ser in the first position being more favorable than Thr.[129] T_3 formation is scarce in turtle Tg, which lacks the Ser-Tyr-Ser sequence.[130] During in vitro iodination of human Tg with LPO, the Glu-Xaa-Tyr sequence is regularly associated with iodotyrosine formation.[129]

The transfer of an iodophenoxyl group in the coupling reaction results in the formation of dehydroalanine at the donor site.[131, 132] Dehydroalanine residues were identified at positions 2469 and/or 2522[133] and at positions 5, 926, 986 or 1008, and 1375 of bovine Tg.[134] T_4 formation in the isolated fragment 1-171 of human Tg appeared to involve tyrosine 5 as the acceptor site and tyrosine 130 as the donor site. Alanine was found in the place of tyrosine 130, and its formation was traced back to the formation of dehydroalanine during the coupling reaction[116] via a sequence of events that included the cleavage of the peptide chain of Tg at tyrosine 130.[115]

Various observations support the hypothesis that the amino- and carboxy-terminal ends of Tg are hormonogenic domains functionally independent of each other and of the rest of the Tg molecule.[43, 78] In a strain of Dutch goats with congenital goiter, a normal-sized Tg mRNA present at low concentrations in thyroid cells is translated into truncated Tg fragments of 40 and 32 kDa in vivo and of 35 kDa in vitro, all corresponding to the NH_2-terminal extremity of Tg.[135] These peptides synthesize T_4 and T_3 and, although present in low concentrations, they meet the thyroid hormone requirements of the goats, provided that the animals receive a high dietary intake of iodide.[136] The molecular defect consists in a point mutation in exon 8 creating a termination signal in the place of tyrosine 296.[136a] Two abnormal Tg-related polypeptides are found in a congenital goiter of Afrikander cattle.[137] The main one is a 75-kDa peptide that results from the abortive translation of a normal-sized Tg mRNA containing a nonsense mutation at codon 697 in exon 9. A minor translation product of 250 kDa derives from an alternatively spliced mRNA of 7.3 kilobases, lacking the region encoded by exon 9,[138] which is expressed at low levels in the normal population.[139] The euthyroid state of these animals may indicate that hormone synthesis occurs in the NH_2-terminal peptide of 75 kDa.[139] A 0.95-kb mRNA corresponding for most of its length to the first 5 exons of the Tg gene (rTg-2) abounds in rat thyrocytes in addition to the 9.0-kb mRNA (rTg-1).[140] It is not known whether rTg-2 is translated and whether its product is capable of synthesizing T_4. Finally, hormones

are efficiently formed upon in vitro iodination of a segment comprising the 224 COOH-terminal amino acids of rat Tg, fused to staphylococcal protein A.[141]

Figure 34–5 shows a diagram of the Tg monomer, with its sequence repeats, putative glycosylation sites, and hormonogenic tyrosyl residues.

Efficiency of Tg as a Thyroid Hormone–Forming Molecule

Thyroid hormones are formed in Tg with an efficiency unparalleled in other proteins. This appears already in DIT formation, a prerequisite for iodothyronine formation. Shortly after the incorporation of the first few atoms of iodine into Tg, the ratio between the rate constants for the formation of DIT and MIT exceeds the ratio calculated for the respective free iodinated derivatives of acetyltyrosine. The formation of DIT seems to be favored as iodination proceeds by changes in the interaction of some tyrosyl residues with the surface groups of Tg that limit the amount of water in the reaction phase. After Tg denaturation in urea, DIT formation is no longer favored.[142]

Thyroxine is formed with high efficiency during in vivo iodination of Tg. Even at iodination levels as low as 4 moles of iodine atoms per mole of Tg, T_4 is formed in the Tg from human goiters.[19] The proportion of iodine incorporated in vivo into iodothyronines in human Tg[143] and porcine Tg[20] is about 20 per cent for an iodine content of 1 to 5 moles of iodine atoms per mole of Tg and increases to 40 to 50 per cent when the iodine content reaches 25 moles of iodine atoms per mole of Tg. T_4 synthesis is abolished by Tg denaturation in guanidine.[143]

SECRETION OF THYROGLOBULIN

Polarized Secretion

All the steps of thyroid hormone synthesis and secretion display a vectorial character that depends on the polarity of thyroid follicles. These are monolayers of epithelial cells

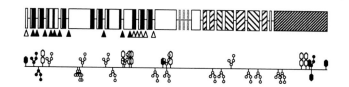

200 amino acids

FIGURE 34–5. **Diagrammatic representation of the Tg monomer.** The repeated motifs and the other parts of human Tg[32] are represented as follows: ■ type 1 repeats, ▨ type 2, ▨ type 3a, ◨ type 3b, ▨ acetylcholinesterase-similar domain, □ unrelated sequences interrupting a repeat or separating different kinds of repeats. Spaces have been introduced for clarity between contiguous motifs and bear no relationship to the gene introns. ▲, exon-intron junctions detected in the genomic sequence of the Tg of humans and △, calf[45]; ♀, putative and ♥, actual sites of glycosylation[97, 98] (symbols are upside down when the consensus asparagine has a negative hydrophilic score[32]); ♦, hormonogenic acceptor[34, 35, 112, 118, 124, 125, 127–130] and ♂, donor tyrosines,[115, 133, 134] as identified in the Tg of various animal species.

enclosing a central cavity. Tight junctions seal adjacent cells and separate their plasma membrane into an apical domain, facing the follicular lumen, and a basolateral domain, lying on a basement membrane.[144] TPO and the H_2O_2-generating system are at the apical cell pole (see Iodide Organification), whereas the iodide carrier and the TSH receptor are in the basolateral domain.[145]

Secretion of Tg into the follicular lumen conforms to the scheme of regulated apical secretion.[146] Newly synthesized Tg is concentrated in condensing vacuoles at the distal end of the Golgi apparatus to form apical vesicles, which are emptied into the follicular colloid.[147] Exocytic vesicles remain for days in the apical cytoplasm of rat follicle cells after the suppression of TSH secretion with T_4. TSH reinduces exocytosis within minutes[148] in a dose-related manner.[149]

Thyroid follicles form in primary suspension cultures of cell clusters isolated from rat thyroid.[150] In the presence of serum they acquire an inverted polarity,[151] with the apical cell poles facing the culture medium and the basal poles facing the internal lumen.[152] Embedding in collagen prevents or reverts the inversion.[153, 154] Normal follicles secrete Tg into their lumina, whereas inverted follicles secrete Tg into the culture medium.[155] In tight monolayers of polarized hog thyroid cells cultured on porous filters with separate apical and basal compartments, about 90 per cent of Tg is secreted into the apical medium and 10 per cent into the basal medium. Polarized secretion into the apical medium, but not into the basal medium, is stimulated by the addition of TSH to the basal compartment.[156, 157] Iodide concentrations from 0.5 μM in the basal medium inhibit the TSH-induced apical secretion of Tg.[157, 157a] Substantial secretion occurs in the absence of secretory stimuli. Eighty per cent of newly synthesized Tg is secreted into the apical medium, 7 per cent into the basal one, and 13 per cent is retained intracellularly, probably in regulated secretory vesicles, because further apical release can be stimulated by secretogogues.[158] It has been proposed that the regulated pathway of Tg secretion has a predetermined apical polarity and that also the Tg apically secreted in a "constitutive" manner is sorted to the same pathway but is rapidly diverted from immature secretory granules to the apical surface, instead of being stored in mature secretory vesicles.[158] The signals mediating the sorting of Tg to regulated and polarized secretion are unknown.

In primary cultures of open hog thyroid follicles, Tg secretion is stimulated by TSH and forskolin by means of a cAMP-dependent mechanism.[159] The secretion of Tg by sheep thyroid cells in primary culture is stimulated by TSH and forskolin, as well as by 12-O-tetradecanoyl phorbol-13-acetate (TPA), a protein kinase C activator, and by the Ca^{2+} ionophore A23187.[160] This effect of TPA contrasts with its ability to inhibit the synthesis of Tg and TPO in sheep[161] and dog thyroid cells.[162] In FRTL-5 cells Tg secretion is stimulated by forskolin, [8Br]-cAMP, and several protein kinase C activators.[163]

Tunicamycin, an inhibitor of the synthesis of the lipid-linked core oligosaccharide precursor of N-linked oligosaccharides, suppresses Tg secretion in hog[164] and sheep thyroid follicles.[165] Castanospermine, an inhibitor of the α-glucosidases of the endoplasmic reticulum that causes the accumulation of glucosylated high-mannose units, lowers the rate of Tg secretion.[166] Tg secretion is not modified by inhibitors of the synthesis of complex oligosaccharide

units, such as swainsonine, an inhibitor of mannosidase II,[167] and deoxymannojirimycin, an inhibitor of mannosidase I.[166]

The Tg present in low concentrations in the serum of humans[168] and rat[169] appears to be secreted from the basolateral pole of the follicular cells, without reaching the apical pole where iodination occurs, because serum Tg in humans[170] and rat[171] is almost entirely devoid of iodine. Tg secretion into the blood is stimulated by TSH in humans[172] and in rat.[169]

Site of Iodination

In normal rat thyroids[173] and in hypertrophic, chronically stimulated rat thyroids[174] labeled in vivo with radioiodine, the autoradiographic grains corresponding to protein-bound iodine form, a few seconds after administration of radioiodine, a ring at the apical border of the follicular cells along the surface of microvilli but the grains are absent from the distal part of pseudopods. Within minutes to hours, the protein-bound radioiodine diffuses over the follicular lumen, as Tg diffuses from the site of iodination into the colloid filling the lumen.[175]

In dispersed hog and rat thyroid follicles with closed, colloid-filled lumina, the protein-bound radioiodine concentrates over the lumina and none is seen over the cells. In open follicles that lack colloid, the label is associated with the microvilli at the apical surface of cells and over closed intracellular lumina in the apical cytoplasm. In isolated cells with lost polarity, intracellular lumina are common and are the major site of iodination.[176] The membrane of these structures is related to the apical plasma membrane because it has microvilli and the cytochemical reactivity of TPO.[177] Intracellular lumina increase in number after the disorganization of the follicles. They seem to be derived from the coalescence of secretory vesicles as a consequence of the loss of cell polarity and may be functionally equivalent, in isolated cells, to the apical plasma membrane of follicular cells in vivo.[176] Thus autoradiographic studies suggest that iodination occurs primarily at the apical surface of thyroid cells when follicles are preserved, whereas a minor fraction of Tg molecules is iodinated intracellularly in the absence of follicles.

The faster diffusion of [^{125}I], compared with [^{3}H]leucine label, toward the center of the follicular lumen suggests that some Tg molecules may also be iodinated intraluminally by a diffusible active iodine species, e.g., hypoiodous acid, produced by TPO at the apical cell surface[178] (see Molecular Mechanism of Iodination).

Studies with cultured cells suggest that follicular organization plays an important, albeit not obligate, role in iodide organification. Dog thyroid cells lose most of their differentiated functions, including iodide trapping and organification, when cultured as monolayers without TSH.[179, 180] The loss of iodide organification is accompanied by a decrease of TPO activity. The addition of TSH, cAMP analogues, forskolin, or cholera toxin partially restores TPO activity, without a comparable increase of iodinating ability.[181] The addition of TSH to preformed monolayers does not induce follicle formation and results in full restoration of iodide transport but only partial[179] or inefficient restoration of iodination,[180] whereas TSH addition to freshly isolated cells induces the formation of follicle-like structures that both trap and organify iodide.[179] Normal rat thyroid follicles in suspension culture secrete and iodinate Tg in their lumina, whereas inverted follicles secrete non-iodinated Tg into the medium. This suggests that the correct follicular polarity is required for iodination.[155] Polarized monolayers of hog thyrocytes on floating collagen gels concentrate iodide, but iodide organification is observed only when follicle formation is induced by embedding in collagen gels.[182] Instead, porcine monolayers on porous bottom chambers with separate basal and apical compartments iodinate Tg to levels not higher than 4 to 6 iodine atoms per Tg molecule, yet T_4 and T_3 are efficiently formed.[157, 157a] Intact[183] and reconstituted hog thyroid follicles[184] in primary culture organify iodide efficiently. However, intracellular T_4 formation, not requiring Tg secretion and endocytosis, was observed also in dispersed hog thyroid cells.[185] Sheep thyrocytes cultured in low serum and physiological TSH concentrations form follicles that secrete and iodinate Tg in their lumina,[165, 186] but culture conditions can be changed so that iodination persists in the absence of follicles.[187]

In intact hog thyroid follicles with normal polarity, cAMP induces the formation of thyroid hormones, while TPA disrupts thyroid follicles and inhibits cAMP-stimulated hormonogenesis.[183] In sheep thyroid cells, TSH stimulates iodide organification, while TPA and EGF cause a cAMP-independent inhibition of iodination.[161] In open hog thyroid follicles, iodination at the apical cell surface is independently stimulated by the Ca^{2+}-dependent increase of H_2O_2 production, and the cAMP-dependent increase of exocytosis, both of which are stimulated by TSH.[159]

Accumulation and Storage

Tg secreted by the follicular cells is stored in the follicular lumen as a concentrated colloidal solution of Tg and Tg-like iodoproteins whose abundance reflects the functional state of the thyroid. Persistent TSH stimulation and its suppression are accompanied, respectively, by a decrease and an increase in the size of the follicular lumina and in the amount and Tg concentration of the colloid.[188]

The colloid is a microheterogeneous pool composed mainly of 19 S Tg and of a minor fraction (10 per cent) of 27 S iodoprotein.[110] Tg molecules differ in their carbohydrate and iodine content. The proportion of covalent dimers and the density of Tg molecules vary in proportion with their iodination level.[22] This probably reflects the exposure of Tg to variable amounts of iodine during its synthesis and the continuing iodination of secreted Tg.

Tg in the colloid seems to be concentrated by the extrusion of water from the follicular lumen. A net transport of water from the apical to the basal side of follicular cells was observed in inverted rat thyroid follicles in suspension[189] and in polarized monolayers of hog thyroid cells.[156] Ca^{2+} ions are also concentrated in the lumen of follicles, to an extent (up to 5 mM) that is inversely related to the level of TSH stimulation of the gland, as in the case of Tg. It was suggested that Ca^{2+} ions are retained in the follicle lumen by their association with Tg, that high concentrations of Ca^{2+} ions and Tg cause the formation of Tg gels,[190] and that electrostatic interactions between Ca^{2+} ions and the

anionic phosphate and sulfate groups of Tg allow the compactation of Tg in the colloid.[107] Each 19 S Tg molecule binds from 18 to 50 Ca^{2+} ions at binding sites divided in two classes with different affinities.[191] Tg in calf thyroid follicles was reported to be stored in insoluble aggregates linked mostly by covalent, nondisulfide bonds. This contrasts with the ability of thyrocytes to endocytose rapidly huge amounts of colloid.[191a]

THE IODINATION PROCESS

Iodine Supply and Availability

An adequate dietary iodine intake is essential to maintain thyroid function. The desired intake is 150 µg per day.[192] Iodine is a rare element; although it is present in fairly constant amounts in sea water, it is unevenly distributed in the earth's crust. The best form of prophylaxis of iodine deficiency in some endemic areas is the use of iodized salt.[192]

The metabolic effects of chronic iodine deficiency in rats include decreases of thyroidal iodine, iodine in Tg and serum T_4, and increases of serum TSH, the MIT:DIT ratio in Tg, and the T_3:T_4 ratio in the thyroid.[193] The main adaptive change induced by iodine deficiency is a relative increase of the synthesis and secretion of T_3 versus T_4,[194] which reflects changes at several levels. One of these is the decrease of the T_4:T_3 ratio in Tg. TSH induces a decrease of the T_4:T_3 ratio and an increase in the synthesis of T_3 at the COOH-terminus of Tg.[125] TSH may also enhance the release of T_3 from Tg by way of the activation of cathepsin B[195] (see Degradation of Tg in Lysosomes). A prominent change is the increase of the intrathyroidal deiodination of T_4 to T_3. Under normal conditions, most of the T_3 comes from the deiodination of T_4 in peripheral tissues, whereas in severely iodine-deficient rats most of it is produced in the thyroid[194, 196] (see Intrathyroidal T_4-T_3 Conversion).

Iodide Transport: Mechanism and Regulation

So efficiently does the thyroid concentrate serum iodide that a 50- to 100-fold increase of the daily iodide intake is needed to restore thyroid function by passive diffusion in patients with congenital defects of iodide transport.[197] Thyroid iodide uptake can be measured in vivo and in vitro by determining the ratio between the iodide concentrations in thyroid tissue and serum (T/S[I^-]), in tissue and medium (T:M[I^-]), or in cells and medium (C/M[I^-]) after blocking iodine organification (see Inhibition of Iodination). The T:S ratio equals the ratio between the rate constants for the inward iodide flow from plasma to tissue (C/m, C being the thyroidal iodide clearance from plasma, in volume · min^{-1}, and m the tissue mass) and the outward flow from tissue to plasma (KTB, exit rate constant in min^{-1}).[198]

The ability to concentrate iodide has been demonstrated in isolated thyroid cells in culture.[199, 200] In polarized monolayers of hog thyroid cells, the iodide pump is located in the basolateral membrane of the cells.[145] Monolayers grown on collagen-coated filters translocate iodide from the basal medium to the apical medium.[201] The radioiodide taken up by the intact thyroid, in which iodine organification has been blocked, is found within both the follicular cells and the follicular lumen.[202] The apical plasma membrane constitutes an incomplete barrier to the diffusion of iodide into the follicular lumen, which can be overcome with time and TSH stimulation[202] (discussed in ref. 203).

The iodide pump has the properties of an active transport system[197, 204]: it concentrates iodide against a chemical and an electrical gradient; it uses metabolic energy from both oxidative and glycolytic sources and is inhibited by inhibitors of ATP production; it is temperature-dependent; it requires external Na^+ and K^+ and is inhibited by ouabain and other cardiac glycosides to an extent that parallels their inhibition of Na^+, K^+ ATPase; and it is saturable and exhibits a Michaelis-Menten type of kinetics that can be measured by its Km, i.e., the iodide concentration required for half-saturation of the carrier system. The Km was 30 $\mu mol/L$ in thyroid slices[204] and FRTL-5 cells,[200] whereas it was 5 $\mu mol/L$ in thyroid plasma membrane vesicles.[205, 206] The rate of iodide transport is proportional to the extracellular Na^+ concentration in isolated cells[199, 200] and in reconstituted thyroid membrane vesicles.[207] This suggests the existence of a Na^+-I^- cotransport system in which the iodide carrier must bind Na^+ ions on the external surface of the cells in order to transport I^- ions, while the Na^+, K^+ ATPase maintains the electric and chemical gradient that drives Na^+ reentry. The binding of more than one Na^+ ion to the carrier seems required for the transport of one I^- ion into thyroid membrane vesicles.[205, 206]

Several monovalent anions act as competitive inhibitors of iodide uptake. These are, in rank order of decreasing inhibitory potency, $TcO_4^- \geq ClO_4^- > ReO_4^- > BF_4^- > SCN^- > I^- > NO_3^- > Br^- > Cl^-$. This selection of anions by the thyroid transporter has the characteristics of an anion exchange process, in which the thyroid exchanger behaves like a large cationic group with weak field strength and strong basic character, and the hydration energies of the exchangeable anions determine the order by which they are selected.[197, 204] The charged group of the carrier may be the quaternary amino group of phosphatidyl-choline or the guanidinium group of arginine.[197, 204] The I^- carrier seems to be protein in nature.[207] ClO_4^- and SCN^- ions are used to induce radioiodine discharge from the thyroid of patients with defects of iodide organification. $^{99}TcO4^-$ ions are not organified and are used for thyroid scanning and for the study of thyroid anion transport.

All these anions are concentrated in salivary and mammary glands, gastric mucosa, choroid plexus, and ciliary body but are not metabolized and appear in such secretions as saliva and gastric juice. Extrathyroidal and thyroidal carriers are under the same genetic control.[197]

The iodide transport system of the thyroid is controlled by TSH. In dispersed bovine thyroid cells TSH elicits a biphasic response of iodide transport: an acute depression due to an increase of the iodide efflux, followed by a slow increase of the iodide influx above the initial value. The effect of TSH is mimicked by dibutyryl-cAMP, and its late phase is blocked by inhibitors of RNA and of protein synthesis.[208] Similar results were obtained with FRTL-5 cells.[200, 209] In these cells the initial stimulation of the iodide efflux is mediated by an increase of cytosolic Ca^{2+} ions[210] synergistically induced by TSH and norepinephrine.[211] TSH, norepinephrine, and the Ca^{2+} ionophore A23187

stimulate iodide efflux via arachidonic acid metabolites released from phospholipids upon the Ca^{2+}-dependent activation of phospholipase A_2.[212]

Thyroid iodide transport is regulated by iodide concentration. Excess iodide in the medium of dispersed thyroid cells suppresses iodide uptake and causes a concomitant increase in the Km of the iodide pump, i.e., a decrease in its affinity for I^- ions.[213] These effects are mediated by a mechanism that requires protein synthesis.[214]

Iodide Organification

Thyroid Peroxidase

MOLECULAR STRUCTURE. Thyroid peroxidase (TPO) is a heme-containing enzyme, but the nature of its prosthetic group is not clear. Spectral differences between TPO and other proteins containing ferriprotoporphyrine IX prompted the suggestions that the latter is not the prosthetic group of TPO[215] and that it is anomalously bound to the TPO apoprotein.[216] TPO is membrane-bound, and in fact early purification schemes included the use of detergents and trypsin.[215] TPO purified by immunoaffinity after solubilization from thyroid membrane fractions, in the absence of proteolytic enzymes, has an apparent mass of about 100 kDa in SDS-polyacrylamide gel electrophoresis.[217, 218] Ten per cent of the TPO mass consists of carbohydrates.[215] The TPO gene is located on the short arm of chromosome 2 in humans[219] and on chromosome 12 in mouse.[220] The human gene consists of 17 exons dispersed over 150-kb pairs.[221] The single or overlapping cDNA clones that have been sequenced represent the entire coding sequence of TPO of humans[219, 222, 223] and hog,[224] and most of that of rat.[220] The human and porcine TPO mRNA's encode proteins of 933 and 926 residues, respectively. An alternatively spliced human TPO mRNA encodes a polypeptide of 876 amino acids, lacking the 57 residues in the middle of the sequence encoded by exon 10.[219] The deduced amino acid sequence of TPO contains a putative signal peptide at the NH_2-terminus and 25 hydrophobic amino acids near the COOH-terminus (residues 847 to 871 in human TPO), which probably represent a trans-membrane domain anchoring TPO to the plasma membrane of the thyroid follicular cells. A mutated TPO lacking this domain is secreted by Chinese hamster ovary cells.[225] Four high-mannose oligosaccharide units have been localized and characterized in porcine TPO.[226]

The sequences of TPO and myeloperoxidase (MPO) have been compared.[227, 228] MPO is a soluble protein of the azurophylic granules of polymorphonuclear leukocytes, made of four chains, deriving from a single polypeptide of 745 amino acids. The average similarity between MPO and TPO is 44 per cent, and it reaches 74 per cent around the histidine residue (his 407 of TPO and his 416 of MPO) linking each apoenzyme to the iron center of its prosthetic group. The most striking difference is the presence of 197 additional amino acids at the COOH-terminus of TPO, which contain, besides the trans-membrane domain, two short regions of homology with the $C4b$-β_2 glycoprotein family and with the epidermal growth factor and the low-density lipoprotein receptor family. The similarity suggests that TPO and MPO may have evolved from a common ancestor, with TPO acquiring a COOH-terminal extension, which is responsible for its specific subcellular localization as a membrane-bound enzyme.[227, 228] Moreover, the region comprising residues 510 to 567 of human TPO is homologous to subunit I of cytochrome c oxidase, a polypeptide encoded by the mitochondrial genome. Thus, TPO appears to consist of a mosaic of nuclear and mitochondrial gene modules.[228] The TPO mRNA is present only in thyroid follicular cells,[1] which indicates that TPO has evolved as an enzyme specifically catalyzing the biosynthesis of thyroid hormones.

SUBCELLULAR LOCALIZATION. In rat thyroid cells, TPO is widely distributed in the membranes of the rough endoplasmic reticulum, the nuclear envelope, some cisternae of the Golgi apparatus, the exocytotic vesicles, and along the microvilli of the apical plasma membrane.[229, 230] TPO is absent from the membrane of the pseudopods protruding into the follicular lumen.[230] On the apical plasma membrane, TPO faces the follicular lumen, as shown by cytochemistry[230] and by immunofluorescence.[231] In membranous organelles TPO faces the internal lumen,[230] and in fact the release of TPO activity from microsomal fractions requires the use of detergents in addition to trypsin.[232] Thus, the localization of TPO parallels the localization of the TPO-dependent iodination of Tg at the apical cell surface of thyroid cells, and within the intracellular lumina deriving from the coalescence of exocytotic vesicles (see The Site of Iodination). TPO reacts with some autoimmune sera[217, 233] and with monoclonal antibodies directed against the microsomal antigen, an antigen triggering the autoaggression of the thyroid in Hashimoto's thyroiditis and Graves' disease.[234] The identity of TPO and the microsomal antigen has been established at the cDNA sequence level.[222] The cell surface localization of the microsomal antigen, determined with electron microscopy, closely parallels that of TPO.[235] Moreover, studies in patients having autoantibodies recognizing the gastric parietal cell antigen (PCA) suggest the existence of an epitope shared by TPO and the H^+, K^+ ATPase, a major component of PCA.[236]

CATALYTIC PROPERTIES AND SPECIFICITY OF TPO. Two reactions can be alternatively catalyzed by TPO with iodide as a substrate: the iodination of tyrosyl residues of Tg and the peroxidation of I^- ions to I_2. Although I_2 can iodinate Tg nonenzymatically,[123, 237] the catalytic role of TPO in the iodination of Tg is demonstrated by the finding that TPO-catalyzed iodination of Tg is inhibited at the iodide concentrations needed for enzymatic I_2 formation,[238, 239] and it has different pH requirements than do chemical iodination and enzymatic I_2 production.[240] The Km for iodide peroxidation, i.e., the iodide concentration required for I_2 formation with half-maximal velocity, is $6 \cdot 10^{-3}$ M, while the Km for iodide in Tg iodination is about $8 \cdot 10^{-5}$ M.[239]

TPO catalyzes also the coupling of iodotyrosines into iodothyronines. During TPO-catalyzed iodination of Tg in vitro, iodotyrosine formation is faster than iodothyronine formation, and a lag precedes the appearance of T_4.[241, 242] [^{125}I]-labeled hormones are formed when Tg preiodinated with [^{125}I]-labeled iodide, but devoid of hormones, is incubated with TPO and [^{131}I]-labeled iodide after removal of excess [^{125}I]-labeled iodide. Both iodide and an H_2O_2-generating system seem necessary for the coupling.[242] In another study, however, the hormone content of Tg increased markedly when chemically iodinated Tg was incubated with TPO and an H_2O_2-generating system in the absence of iodine.[243] Low concentrations of free DIT mark-

edly stimulate coupling, whereas high concentrations of DIT inhibit Tg iodination and iodide peroxidation.[244] The effects of free DIT do not involve its participation in coupling as a substrate[243, 244] but do require its oxidation.[237]

Both iodination and coupling can be catalyzed by such peroxidases as LPO,[245, 246] horseradish peroxidase (HPO),[246, 247] and myeloperoxidase (MPO).[248] TPO and LPO were reported to be equally effective in catalyzing iodotyrosine and T_4 formation at pH 7.0, although TPO was more effective at physiological iodide concentrations and had a pH optimum (6.6 to 7.0) that was closer to the physiological pH range than that of LPO (6.0 or less).[245] In another study, LPO and TPO were equally effective in catalyzing hormone formation at pH 7.4, whereas at pH 6.3 to 6.6 fewer iodothyronines were formed with LPO than with TPO.[246] Hormones are formed in human goiter Tg iodinated in vitro with LPO with only 7.8 moles of iodine atoms per Tg mole, and most of them are located at the same sites as in native Tg.[129] HPO has a pH optimum for iodination of 5.2 and two pH optima for coupling (pH 7.5 and 8.5) and is much less efficient than TPO in T_4 synthesis.[246, 247] MPO has a pH optimum for Tg iodination of 4.0 but is as efficient as TPO in iodination and coupling when iodination is performed at pH 7.0 with 0.1 N Cl^-.[248]

Nonenzymatic iodination and coupling can occur in the presence of iodine plus iodide, chloramine T plus iodide, and iodine monochloride.[123, 237] Much smaller amounts of hormones are formed in chemically versus enzymatically iodinated Tg at comparable levels of iodination.[108, 126, 241] In Tg iodinated with TPO, significant amounts of hormones are formed at iodination levels of less than 10 iodine atoms per Tg molecule, whereas in chemically iodinated Tg hormones are found only above 30 to 40 iodine atoms per Tg molecule. This suggests that most of the chemically iodinated tyrosyl residues are unable to undergo coupling.[246]

The H_2O_2 Generating System

H_2O_2 is an essential electron acceptor in the reactions catalyzed by TPO, and it has a limiting role in Tg iodination and hormone formation.[249, 250] The concentration of H_2O_2 controls the relative rates of iodination and coupling.[237, 251] The addition of a source of H_2O_2 to the medium of thyroid slices from a human goiter with an organification defect and normal TPO activity restores iodine organification.[252]

In open follicles from rat[253] and hog thyroid,[254] and in rat thyroid slices,[255] H_2O_2 is produced by an NADPH-dependent process on the external aspect of the apical plasma membrane of follicular cells. Although various enzyme systems, including cytochrome reductases, can support H_2O_2 production in the thyroid,[256] an NADPH-dependent, H_2O_2-generating system was detected in thyroid particulate fractions[257] that appears to be distinct from cytochrome c reductase.[258, 259] The activation of this NADPH oxidase requires Ca^{2+} ions.[260]

The mechanism of H_2O_2 formation is controversial (Fig. 34–6). There are data showing that the superoxide anion O_2^- is the primary product of the enzymatic conversion of O_2 and that H_2O_2 is secondarily generated via the dismutation of the O_2^- anion.[261] In intact follicular cells and in cell fragments, O_2^- anions seem to be produced on the inside of the apical membrane and released to the outside of the

A

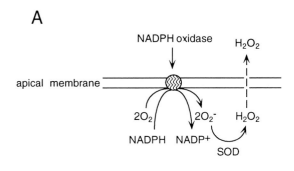

B

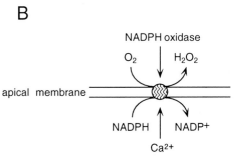

FIGURE 34–6. **Proposed mechanisms of H$_2$O$_2$ formation.** Two alternative mechanisms are shown. Panel A, the superoxide anion O$_2^-$ is first produced from O$_2$ by the superoxide dismutase and then converted to H$_2$O$_2$ by dismutation, on the inside of the apical membrane of thyroid follicular cells. H$_2$O$_2$ is then released to the outside.[261, 262] Panel B, H$_2$O$_2$ is produced from O$_2$ by the NADPH oxidase outside the cells.[258, 259]

cells only after conversion to H$_2$O$_2$.[262] Other data suggest that H$_2$O$_2$ is the primary product of NADPH oxidase and is produced outside the cells via the two-electron reduction of O$_2$.[258, 259]

In isolated hog thyroid follicles, the production of H$_2$O$_2$ at the apical cell surface is stimulated by the Ca^{2+} ionophore A23187 by means of increases of the intracellular Ca^{2+} concentration and by TSH through a cAMP-independent pathway.[254] H$_2$O$_2$ generation is stimulated by both the Ca^{2+}-phosphatidylinositol and the cAMP cascade in dog thyroid cells or slices[263, 264] and in FRTL-5 cells.[265] Cytosolic free calcium and protein kinase C synergistically stimulate H$_2$O$_2$ production in calf thyroid slices,[266] and in cultured hog[267] and dog thyroid cells.[263] Like the TSH-mediated stimulation of exocytosis, the stimulation of the H$_2$O$_2$ production in open hog thyroid follicles induces an increase of Tg iodination at the apical cell surface.[159]

The rate of H$_2$O$_2$ generation controls iodination and the activity of the pentose phosphate pathway. In fact, both the H$_2$O$_2$ production by NADPH oxidase and the H$_2$O$_2$ reduction in the cytosol by glutathione peroxidase use NADPH as a coenzyme and increase the NADP supply, which in turn drives the pentose phosphate pathway.[264]

Molecular Mechanism of Iodination

The primary catalytic intermediate formed upon addition of H$_2$O$_2$ to TPO and LPO is compound I; it catalyzes the iodination of the tyrosyl residues of Tg (Fig. 34–7). In the absence of iodide and in the presence of equimolar amounts of H$_2$O$_2$, compound I is spontaneously converted into a stable compound, compound II, which catalyzes the coupling of iodotyrosines into iodothyronines but not the

iodination reaction.[268, 269] Spectral studies suggest that both compound I and compound II of TPO and LPO possess two oxidizing equivalents above the native state. In compound I both are localized on the porphyrin ring, whereas in compound II one of them is localized over the apoprotein.[251, 269] In the presence of excess H$_2$O$_2$, compound II is converted to an inactive form, compound III. The formation of compound III is prevented by iodide.[268, 269]

One of the proposed mechanisms of the TPO-catalyzed iodination of Tg foresees the binding of iodide and of the tyrosyl residues of Tg at two distinct sites of TPO-compound I[239] and the one-electron oxidation of each of them to the respective free radicals I· and Tyr·.[270, 271] (Fig. 34–8). In this model the addition of these two radicals leads to the formation of MIT, while the addition of the MIT· radical produced by the one-electron oxidation of MIT to the I· radical generates DIT. At high iodide concentrations, two I$^-$ ions bind to one molecule of TPO; they are oxidized to I· radicals and are added together, forming I$_2$ (see Inhibition of Iodination). Alternative models imply the two-electron oxidation of iodide by TPO-compound I and the iodination of tyrosyl residues by electrophilic substitution (Fig. 34–9).[271] According to one hypothesis, a TPO-bound iodinium ion (I$^+$) is the active iodinating species.[268, 272] The transfer of this enzyme-bound I$^+$ ion is stimulated by iodotyrosines.[273] Another model postulates that the oxidation of I$^-$ by TPO-compound I produces the TPO-bound hypoiodite ion (IO$^-$). This would be the active intermediate in several reactions: iodination of tyrosyl residues with formation of OH$^-$ ions, evolution of O$_2$ from H$_2$O$_2$, oxidation of I$^-$ ions to I$_2$, and oxidation of thioureylene drugs (see Inhibition of Iodination). This model is supported by (1) the finding that catalytic degradation of H$_2$O$_2$ by TPO occurs in the presence of iodide and is inhibited by tyrosine, excess iodide, and thioureylene drugs,[274] and (2) stoichiometric and kinetic measurements.[275]

The two-electron model of iodide oxidation is not explicit as to whether the substitution reaction occurs while Tg is in contact with TPO or through a free form of the

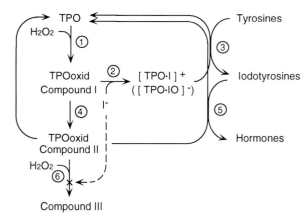

FIGURE 34–7. **Compounds of TPO and H$_2$O$_2$ and their reactions.** Compound I is formed upon addition of H$_2$O$_2$ to TPO (reaction 1) and oxidizes iodide (reaction 2) to an active iodinating form (represented here as either an iodinium ion or a hypoiodite ion bound to TPO), which catalyzes the iodination of the tyrosyl residues of Tg (reaction 3). In the absence of iodide, TPO compound I is converted to compound II (reaction 4), which catalyzes the coupling reaction (reaction 5). Excess H$_2$O$_2$ causes the conversion of TPO compound II to the inactive compound III (reaction 6). Inactivation is prevented by iodide.[268, 269]

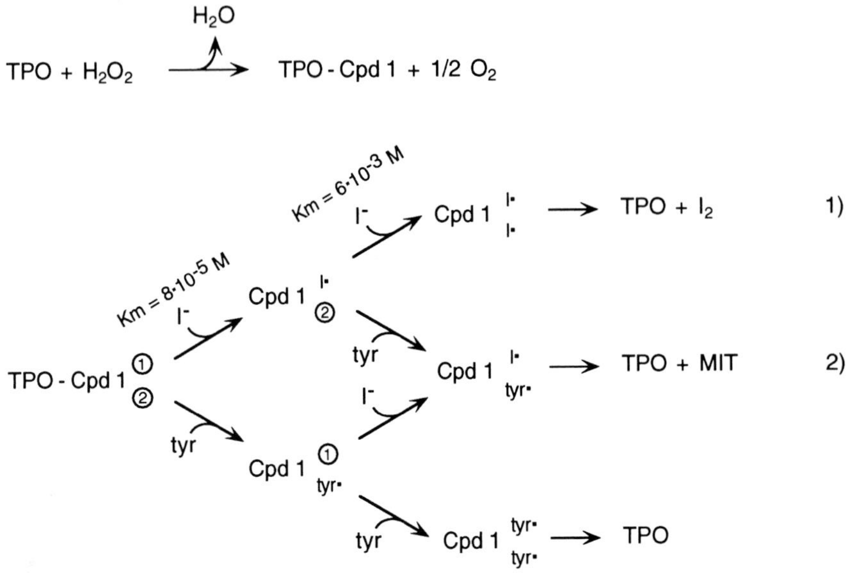

$$TPO + H_2O_2 \xrightarrow{\quad H_2O \quad} TPO\text{-}Cpd\ 1 + 1/2\ O_2$$

1)

2)

FIGURE 34–8. **Free radical model of the TPO-catalyzed iodination of Tg.** In this model, each molecule of TPO has two sites. Site 1 has a higher affinity for iodide ions, whereas site 2 has a higher affinity for tyrosine.[239] I_2 formation (reaction 1) is favored and the iodination of tyrosyl residues (reaction 2) is inhibited by high I^-:Tg concentration ratios (millimolar versus micromolar concentrations, respectively).[238, 239, 286] TPO-catalyzed iodination proceeds via a free-radical mechanism.[270, 271] The two oxidizing equivalents of TPO compound I serve to remove one electron from each ligand. I_2 is formed by the radical addition between two I· atoms (reaction 1), whereas MIT is formed by the radical addition between an I· atom and the free radical Tyr· (DIT is formed by the addition of I· and MIT·) (reaction 2). (Modified from Wolff J: Excess iodide inhibits the thyroid by multiple mechanisms. *In* Ekholm R, Kohn LD, Wollman SH (eds): Control of the Thyroid Gland. New York, Plenum Publishing Corporation, 1989, pp 211–244.

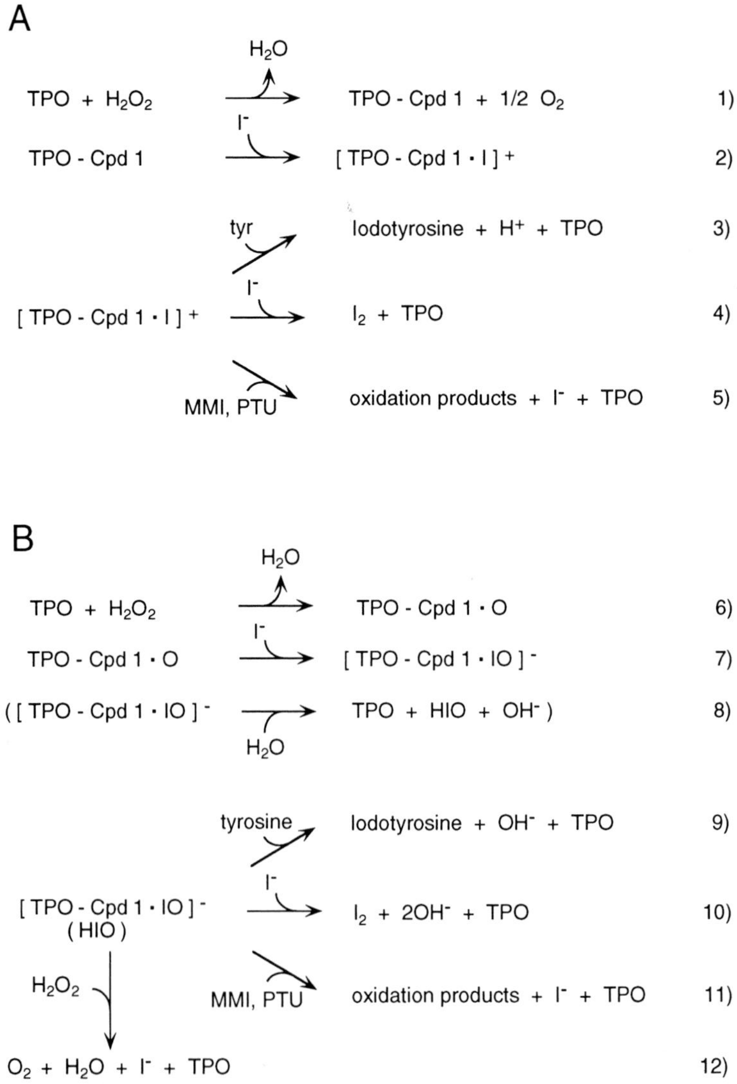

FIGURE 34–9. **Models of TPO-catalyzed iodination of Tg by the two-electron oxidation of iodide.** The models presented in panel A and panel B postulate that the TPO-catalyzed iodination of Tg proceeds via electrophylic substitution.[271] The two oxidizing equivalents of TPO compound I are used to remove two electrons from iodide, with the formation of an active oxidized species that substitutes the hydrogen atom in position 3 or 5 of a tyrosyl residue. Panel A, TPO compound I is formed (reaction 1) and oxidizes I^- to iodinium ion (I^+) (reaction 2),[268, 272] which is the active species in iodotyrosine formation (3), iodide peroxidation (4), and thioureylene drug oxidation (5). Panel B, an oxygen atom of H_2O_2 is retained in TPO compound I (6). Upon reaction with I^-, a TPO-bound hypoiodite ion (IO^-) is formed (7).[274] This hypoiodite ion, or the free hypoiodous acid (HIO) generated by its hydrolysis (8),[275] is the active intermediate in several reactions. These include the iodination of tyrosyl residues, with formation of OH^- ions (9), the peroxidation of I^- (10), the oxidation of thioureylene drugs (11), and the catalytic degradation of H_2O_2, with evolution of O_2 (12).[274, 275]

A

B

active iodinating species. Although there is evidence that the TPO-catalyzed iodination of Tg occurs at a specific site on the enzyme,[240, 246] studies with LPO suggest that iodination may occur through a diffusible intermediate, i.e., hypoiodous acid.[275]

The coupling reaction is a concerted succession of three steps: oxidation of two iodotyrosyl residues to an activated form, nonoxidative formation of a covalent bond linking them, and nonoxidative decomposition of the coupling product, leading to the formation of equimolar amounts of hormone and dehydroalanine residues within the polypeptide chain of Tg[123, 131, 132] (Fig. 34–10). Correct align-

FIGURE 34–10. **Proposed mechanisms of the coupling reaction.** Nonenzymatic coupling is probably ionic, and proceeds via the removal of two electrons from one of the two hormonogenic iodotyrosyl residues (reaction 1).[271] Whether the TPO-catalyzed coupling proceeds via an ionic or a free radical mechanism is unclear. In the latter case, one electron is removed from each iodotyrosyl residue (reaction 2).[271] In either case, the oxidation of the iodotyrosyl residues is followed by the formation of a charge transfer complex between the acceptor and the donor iodotyrosine. This is a zwitterion resonance hybrid (3) in ionic coupling, and a biradical resonance hybrid (4) in radical coupling.[123, 271] The reaction continues with the formation of a quinol ether intermediate (5).[123] Its splitting at the side chain of the donor iodotyrosyl residue causes the formation of dehydroalanine at the hormonogenic donor site,[123,131,132] and of T_4 or T_3 at the hormonogenic acceptor site, depending on whether the donor iodotyrosine was DIT or MIT.[239]

ment of two iodotyrosines is a prerequisite for coupling.[276] The coupling of two DIT residues may occur either through a free radical or an ionic mechanism. The latter probably prevails in nonenzymatic conditions, while it is not clear whether enzymatic coupling occurs by means of free radical formation.[271] The radical mechanism requires the formation of two DIT· radicals by the one-electron oxidation of two diiodotyrosines. The ionic mechanism requires the two-electron oxidation of one of the two iodotyrosyl residues. In either case, a charge transfer complex is formed, consisting of a zwitterion-biradical resonance hybrid. This is followed by the formation of a quinol ether intermediate and by its splitting at the side chain of one of the two former DIT residues, with the formation of a T_4 residue at the site of the acceptor iodotyrosine, and of a dehydroalanine residue at the site of the donor iodotyrosine.[123, 131, 132] The formation of T_3 occurs similarly, via the coupling between MIT, which contributes the outer ring, and DIT, which contributes the inner ring.[239]

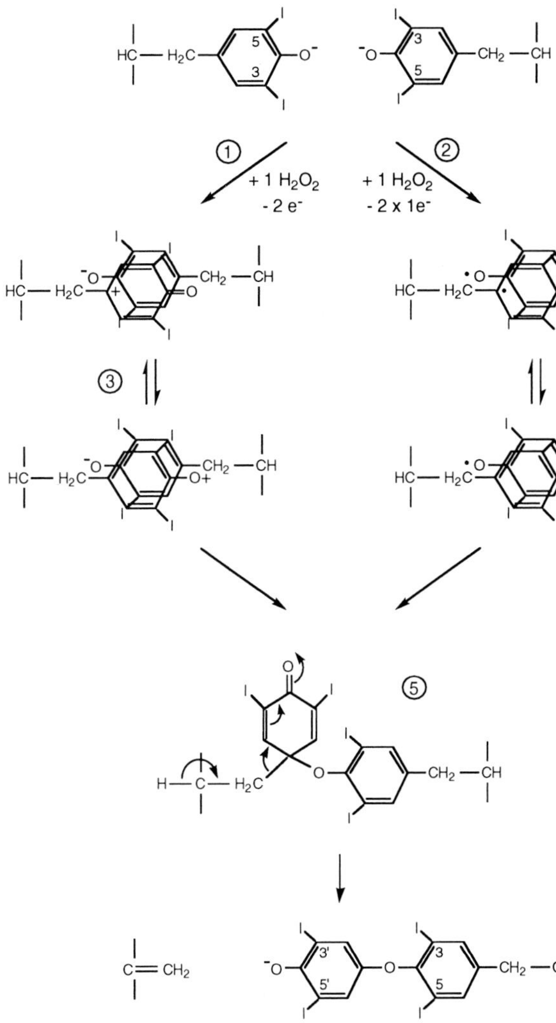

Inhibition of Iodination

Among the inhibitors of TPO-catalyzed iodination, the thioureylene drugs 6-propylthiouracil (PTU) and 1-methyl-2-mercaptoimidazole (MMI) are the ones whose effect has been best characterized.[277] Their effect in vitro depends on the iodide-to-drug concentration ratio, being transient and reversible at high ratios and apparently irreversible at low ratios.[278, 279] Preliminary incubation of TPO and H_2O_2 with oxidizable substrates such as iodide ions or guaiacol prevents the irreversible inactivation of TPO, suggesting that these drugs block iodination by trapping oxidized iodine.[280] The intrathyroidal metabolism of PTU and MMI is mediated by TPO and is iodide-dependent.[281] Thioureylene drugs seem favored over the tyrosyl residues of Tg for the oxidization by the active iodine species (TPO-bound I^+ or IO^- ion or free HIO) resulting from the oxidation of iodide by TPO compound I.[282, 283] High iodide-to-drug concentration ratios prevent irreversible TPO inhibition, because iodide is sufficient to oxidize MMI and PTU first to their disulfides and then to sulfate and sulfite, until they disappear and iodination can resume. In the presence of lower iodide concentrations, MMI and PTU are only oxidized to disulfides, from which the drugs are re-formed by disproportionation. In the absence of or after the consumption of iodide, irreversible TPO inactivation is caused by suicide reactions between the oxidized forms of the drugs and the heme group of TPO compound II.[282, 283]

MMI accelerates the conversion of TPO compound I to compound II, spontaneously occurring in the absence of iodide, and reacts with compound II to form an inactivated form of the enzyme.[216] However, it would seem that TPO inactivation by MMI and PTU in vivo involves only a reversible competition between the drug and the tyrosyl residues of Tg for oxidized iodine.[282, 284] PTU and MMI seem to inhibit iodination and coupling by different mechanisms. Indeed, selective inhibition of coupling, but not of iodination is observed in vitro with graded doses of the drugs.[278] Thioureylene and other drugs form charge transfer complexes with iodine, whose formation constants are related to the antithyroid activity of the respective drugs in vivo.[285]

Large doses of iodide transiently inhibit TPO-catalyzed iodination of Tg. This is known as the *Wolff-Chaikoff effect.*

Iodide probably competes with the tyrosyl residues of Tg for the active species of oxidized iodine and converts the latter to I_2.[238, 239, 286] In bovine thyroid slices, the inhibitory effect of excess iodine can be prevented by adding an H_2O_2 generator system. This suggests that the Wolff-Chaikoff effect may be due to decreased H_2O_2 availability.[287] The participation of iodide in the catalytic destruction of H_2O_2[274, 275] may not be the sole way by which excess iodide reduces the H_2O_2 level. In dog thyroid slices excess iodide inhibits the H_2O_2 generation in response to various stimulators. The inhibition is reversed by MMI and seems to involve the formation of oxidized derivatives of iodide, both at the level of the generation of the intracellular signals (Ca^{2+} and diacylglycerol, cAMP) and of their targets.[288] Iodide at concentrations above 0.5 μM in the medium bathing the basal poles of hog thyroid cell monolayers also inhibits iodination and hormone formation by a mechanism that does not seem to involve its competition with the tyrosyl residues of Tg for TPO.[157a]

REABSORPTION OF THYROGLOBULIN

Mechanisms and Selectivity of Endocytosis

For hormone secretion to occur, Tg must be reabsorbed from the follicular lumen and degraded. Two major mechanisms mediate the reabsorption of Tg.[177] Macropinocytosis consists of the nonselective reabsorption of large amounts of colloid by bulk fluid pinocytosis, and permits a rapid readjustment of the rate of Tg internalization and hormone secretion. Exocytotic vesicles fuse with the apical plasma membrane, thus producing a transient increase of its surface area. Large pseudopods are formed from the apical membrane, protrude into the follicular lumen, and enclose the colloid substance in large vacuoles or colloid droplets, up to 2.5 μm in diameter.[289] The number, size, and rate of formation of the pseudopods are related to the intensity of the TSH stimulus.[149] Morphological and functional studies[149, 177, 289] and theoretical estimates of the daily rate of Tg degradation[289a] indicate that macropinocytosis is the prevalent way of Tg internalization in the rat, whereas in other mammals it is observed only after acute stimulation with high concentrations of TSH.

Micropinocytosis is mediated by small heterogeneous vesicles formed by the invagination of the plasma membrane in the apical region. It is the main route of endocytosis in the thyroid gland of higher mammals (humans, dog, pig) chronically stimulated with physiological levels of TSH[289a, 290] and after moderate acute TSH stimulation. Moderate activation by TSH induces a rapid increase in the cellular uptake of Tg at both 20° and 37°C, which is not mediated by macropinocytosis, because pseudopod formation is not observed within the time required to obtain a full endocytic response at 37°C, nor at any time at 20°C.[184] Micropinocytosis of Tg seems mediated, at least in part, by a coated vesicle-dependent pathway. Tg is detected in coated vesicles isolated from reconstituted hog thyroid follicles.[291] The amount of Tg in purified coated vesicles increases upon stimulation with TSH at 20°C.[184] Whether the internalization via coated vesicles involves the binding of Tg to specific receptors is unclear. A role for mannose-6-phosphate residues in the reabsorption of Tg was pro-

posed,[292] because of the occurrence of mannose-6-phosphate groups in the high-mannose oligosaccharide units of the Tg of calf, rat,[102] and hog,[103] and of receptors for mannose-6-phosphate on the plasma membrane of hog thyroid cells[292]; such a role has been ruled out.[292a] Low-affinity binding sites for Tg on the plasma membrane of thyrocytes have been reported to be operating in the adsorptive endocytosis of Tg.[292a]

The selectivity of endocytosis was studied in rat by estimating the iodine distribution of the Tg molecules remaining in the colloid using isopicnic centrifugation in RbCl, and the relative proportions of 19 S Tg and 27 S iodoprotein using zonal centrifugation.[293] Tg molecules labeled to equilibrium in vivo with [^{125}I]-iodine are internalized randomly, at a rate that does not differ between 19 S Tg and 27 S iodoprotein or between 19 S molecules with different iodine contents. In contrast, newly iodinated Tg molecules pulse-labeled with [^{131}I]-iodine are reabsorbed faster than the pre-existing ones; among these, iodine-rich Tg molecules are reabsorbed faster than iodine-poor ones, and 27 S molecules are reabsorbed faster than 19 S molecules.[293] In rat thyroid hemilobes incubated with exogenous Tg, the uptake of homologous Tg is more active than the uptake of heterologous Tg, and is also selective. In fact, the rat Tg molecules having a higher density and a higher iodine content, within a pool of molecules equilibrium-labeled with radioiodine, are reabsorbed more actively than poorly iodinated ones.[294] A model mechanism, called *selective fluid pinocytosis*, postulated that only mature Tg molecules with a normal iodine content are internalized by fluid pinocytosis, whereas the newly synthesized, poorly iodinated molecules are retained at specific binding sites of the apical plasma membrane located near the site of iodination and far from the site of endocytosis.[294] Recent data suggest that, although Tg molecules are not selected at the step of endocytosis, they are sorted in early endosomes and partially recycled back to the follicular lumen. This may be at the base of the selective utilization of well-iodinated Tg in hormone production.[294a]

In inverted hog thyroid follicles, most of the labeled Tg added to the medium, in contact with the apical cell membranes, is transported to lysosomes, whereas a small fraction is transported unmodified to the basolateral membrane of the cells and accumulates in the lumen of the inverted follicles. Such vesicular transport from the apical to the basolateral plasma membranes of thyroid cells is called *transcytosis*. It is stimulated by TSH and inhibited by cooling to 15°C.[295]

Interaction of Thyroglobulin with the Thyroid Cell Membranes

Asialothyroglobulin binds to a specific receptor on isolated thyroid plasma membranes.[296] The efficiency of the binding is higher at pH 5.0 and 37°C than at pH 6.0 through 7.5 and 0°C and is inversely related, under the latter conditions, to the iodine content of Tg. It was suggested that the association between asialothyroglobulin and its membrane receptor may serve to direct the transport of asialothyroglobulin from the Golgi apparatus to the apical membrane of the follicular cells.[296] Studies with glycohydrolase-treated Tg showed that the best binding of Tg to thyroid plasma membranes, as well as to microsomal, lysosomal, and Golgi membranes, is obtained by stripping Tg of sialic acid and galactose. This suggested that the N-acetylglucosamine residues of type B carbohydrate units of Tg were involved in the interaction of Tg with thyroid membranes.[297] Noteworthy, the iodine content of Tg molecules separated by isopicnic centrifugation in RbCl was inversely related to the number of exposed N-acetylglucosamine residues and directly related to the number of sialic acid residues in their oligosaccharide units.[297] The discovery of an N-acetylglucosamine receptor that interacted with iodine-poor Tg molecules at acidic pH suggested that iodine-poor Tg molecules with exposed N-acetylglucosamine residues may remain bound to the receptor in the endosomes and be recycled back to the follicular lumen, while fully iodinated and sialylated molecules may progress to be graded in lysosomes.[297a] Such receptor recently has been further characterized.[297b] The participation of tyrosyl residues in the interaction of Tg with thyroid membranes is suggested by the decrease of Tg binding upon chemical modification of tyrosyl residues.[298] The 27 S iodoprotein also binds to thyroid membranes; its binding occurs at different sites than the binding of 19 S Tg.[299]

LYSOSOMAL DEGRADATION OF THYROGLOBULIN AND THYROID HORMONE RELEASE

Targeting of Thyroglobulin to Lysosomes

Once formed, thyroid hormones are released from Tg by proteolysis in secondary lysosomes.[177] Tg reaches this final destination after a complex cycle of secretion into the lumen of the follicles, storage in the colloid, and endocytotic recapture. Thus Tg has the properties of a protein destined for both export and lysosomes.

Secondary lysosomes, possibly resulting from the fusion of Tg-containing endocytotic vesicles with primary lysosomes, were isolated by subfractionating purified hog thyroid lysosomes.[300] More recently, three compartments involved in the transport of Tg to the site of degradation were resolved: early endosomes, located in the apical cytoplasm and representing a meeting compartment for micropinocytotic vesicles carrying internalized Tg; late endosomes or prelysosomes, enriched with the receptor of mannose-6-phosphate and lysosomal enzymes; and lysosomes. Tg appears to be first transported to early endosomes and then transferred to late endosomes, where Tg proteolysis possibly starts.[301] On the basis of these and other studies on the internalization of Tg[184, 289a, 291, 301] (see The Reabsorption of Thyroglobulin) the role of the colloid droplets and of the phagolysosomes formed by their fusion with lysosomes in Tg reabsorption and degradation, respectively, seems to be limited, in species other than rat, to rare cases of acute intense TSH stimulation.[301]

Mannose-6-phosphate functions as a marker for the targeting of acid hydrolases to lysosomes[302] and is present in the oligosaccharide units of the Tg of calf, rat,[102] and hog.[103] The presence of a secretory signal, dominating over mannose-6-phosphate, may explain why Tg is first exported and reaches the lysosomes only after endocytotic recapture.[103]

Thyroid Lysosomes and Lysosomal Proteases

Dense primary lysosomes have been isolated from preparations of hog thyroid lysosomes.[300] Several thyroid endopeptidases active in Tg degradation have been also isolated. The aspartic proteinase cathepsin D, a carboxyl endopeptidase with a preference for peptide bonds involving hydrophobic amino acids, was originally isolated from rabbit thyroids; it has a pH optimum of 3.5, is inhibited by pepstatin and hydrolizes Tg in vitro into a number of discrete peptide intermediates.[303] Two cysteine proteinases were purified from hog thyroid lysosomes: one of them, thiol-protease 1, is a cathepsin H–like enzyme that has both endo- and exopeptidase activities and induces the release of free T_4 from Tg and its peptides, while thiol-protease 2, a cathepsin B–like enzyme, has poor T_4-releasing ability.[304, 305] Cysteine proteinases isolated from human thyroid include cathepsin B, an endopeptidase inhibited by leupeptin and thiol-blocking agents, and an enzyme formerly designated cysteine proteinase 1[306] and later identified as cathepsin L.[307, 195] Cathepsins B and L have pH optima of 4.5 to 5.0 and 3.5 to 4.0, respectively, and preferentially cleave large, discrete hormone-containing fragments from both Tg extremities. Together, cathepsins B, D, and L represent most of the endopeptidase activity of the human thyroid.[195]

Degradation of Thyroglobulin in Lysosomes

Several observations suggest that the release of thyroid hormones in lysosomes in vivo depends on the synergistic activities of various endopeptidases and exopeptidases. The release of a limited number of hormone-containing fragments by endopeptidases cleaving Tg at specific sites seems to facilitate the release of the hormones by other endo- and exopeptidases.[195, 306, 307]

Analysis of the Tg degradation products in pig thyroid lysosomes by denaturing, nonreducing polyacrylamide gel electrophoresis reveals hormone-depleted Tg molecules that have the same mobility as intact Tg monomers and that resolve into several large fragments upon reduction. Apparently, limited endoproteolytic attack produces discrete fragments that remain bound by intrachain disulfide bonds, while the hormones at the Tg ends are removed by recurrent exopeptidase action or by the endoproteolytic cleavage of small peptides.[308]

In hog thyroid lysosomes, thiol protease 2 enhances the T_4-releasing ability of thiol protease 1 by reducing the size of the hormone-bearing protein substrate.[305] During the limited proteolysis of rabbit Tg, cathepsins B and L cleave hormone-containing peptides of 10 to 50 kDa from both the hormone-bearing Tg extremities, possibly making them more accessible to the action of other endo- and exopeptidases.[306, 307] Cathepsin B seems able to release a small T_3-containing peptide from the COOH-terminal end of Tg but has little endopeptidase activity against Tg when used by itself in purified form. Apparently, its action is facilitated by the earlier action of cathepsins D and L.[195] Cathepsin B is stimulated by TSH,[309] which may contribute to the enhanced thyroidal secretion of T_3 after TSH stimulation in vivo.[195] Rabbit Tg is cleaved at residues 532, 795, 2487 (hTg numbering) by cathepsin B, at residues 551, 1835, 2468 by cathepsin D, and at residues 2389, 2452, 2490 by cathepsin L. The peptides produced contain major hormonogenic sites at both Tg ends[195] (see Acceptor and Donor Sites for the Coupling Reaction). During extensive digestion of human and rat Tg with hog thyroid lysosomal proteases in reducing conditions, iodoamino acids are released at a higher rate than the other amino acids, and a substantial part of Tg remains undegraded in the form of small peptides.[310]

Limited Proteolysis of Thyroglobulin

When subjected to limited proteolysis with thermolysin, trypsin, and chymotrypsin, Tg of humans, calf, and rat presents well-localized and conserved regions highly sensitive to proteolysis.[42, 58] In all species, the most sensitive sites are concentrated in a restricted region after residue number 500 and are either identical or very close to the sites whose cleavage produces the faster band of the electrophoretic doublet of Tg (see Secondary, Tertiary, and Quaternary Structure). Cleavage consistently occurs also in the region surrounding residue 1800 and at residue 2513 (human Tg numbering).[42] Some of these cleavages produce hormone-bearing NH_2- and COOH-terminal fragments. In analogy with studies on the degradation of Tg by lysosomal proteases, the production of a limited number of hormonal peptides by selective endoproteolytic cleavages may facilitate the final release of the hormones. Many of the sites of cleavage by thermolysin and trypsin are not far from the sites of cleavage by human thyroid cathepsins.[195] Thus, the lysosomal degradation of Tg appears to be governed by the inherent proteolytic susceptibility of some regions of the primary structure of Tg. Most sites of cleavage by thermolysin and trypsin lie within the unrelated sequences that interrupt the cysteine-rich repeats of Tg, namely the inserts of repeats 1.3, 1.5, 1.8, 3a.1, and 3b.1.[42] Several circumstances, including the relationship of these regions with the splice junctions and with the pattern of sequence conservation among the cysteine-rich repeats, suggest that they may form loops at the surface of Tg.[45]

Release of Iodotyrosines and Iodothyronines from Lysosomes, Iodotyrosine Deiodination, and Iodide Recycling

Free iodoamino acids do not accumulate in lysosomes.[311] In FRTL-5 cells, the exit of MIT from lysosomes is carrier-mediated and competition experiments suggest that DIT, T_3, and T_4 might share the same transport system.[312] Countertransport experiments[313] indicate that this carrier coincides with system h, a TSH-responsive carrier that transfers tyrosine and other neutral amino acids into the cytosol.[314] Radioisotopic studies show very low amounts of iodotyrosines in the cells and in the medium of hog thyroid cells. This appears to be the result of the intracellular deiodination of iodotyrosines by iodotyrosine deiodinase. Indeed, [^{125}I]MIT and [^{125}I]DIT accumulate in the medium of thyroid cells labeled with [^{125}I]iodide in the presence of dini-

trotyrosine, an inhibitor of iodotyrosine deiodinase, which shows that iodotyrosines rapidly leak out of both lysosomes and cells.[311]

A flavoprotein purified after solubilization with steapsin from bovine thyroid mitochondria and microsomes catalyzed the deiodination of L-MIT and L-DIT. The purified enzyme was inactive in the presence of NADPH, its activator in microsomes. Inhibition of the particulate enzyme by iron chelators suggested that its activity required an iron-containing electron carrier.[315] An NADPH-dependent deiodinating activity was then reconstituted with ferredoxin and NADPH-ferredoxin reductase isolated from particulate fractions of bovine thyroid.[316]

Normally, the iodide released from MIT and DIT by thyroid deiodinase is recycled in situ through additional rounds of organification. The fraction that is not reused intracellularly "leaks out" of the cells to an extent that is directly related to the iodide intake from external sources. This mechanism probably contributes by regulating the amount of iodide that is available for hormonogenesis.[317] Unlike iodotyrosines, free iodothyronines are retained intracellularly after their exit from lysosomes[311] (see Secretory Products).

Intrathyroidal T_4-T_3 Conversion

T_4, the predominant product of hormone synthesis in Tg, has little biological activity compared to T_3. There is a growing agreement with the concept that T_3 is the active thyroid hormone being both synthesized in the thyroid and produced by deiodination of its precursor T_4 in the thyroid and in peripheral tissues (see Ch. 37). About 84 per cent of the T_4 secreted by the thyroid undergoes 5'- and 5-monodeiodination to T_3 and to the inactive rT_3, respectively, in peripheral tissues.[318] T_3 and rT_3 are secreted from perfused thyroid lobes of iodine-deficient rats in considerably higher amounts than could be expected from the relative amounts of T_4 and T_3 in the hydrolysate of a thyroid homogenate.[196] Such "preferential secretion of T_3 and rT_3" has suggested that T_4 underwent a partial deiodination in the thyroid by a process resembling its deiodination in peripheral tissues.[319] Iodothyronine deiodinase activities have been detected in the thyroid of rat,[320] humans,[321] dog,[322] and mouse.[323] In rat thyroid, these activities are similar to the type I T_4-deiodinases of liver, because they are inhibited by PTU and have a preference for rT_3 as a substrate. In fact, rT_3 is rapidly degraded to T_2 and competitively inhibits the 5'-deiodination of T_4 to T_3.[320] In dog thyroid microsomes, instead, PTU inhibits the conversion of T_4 to T_3 and to rT_3, but rT_3 does not inhibit significantly the deiodination of T_4.[322] Increases of the T_4:T_3 and T_4:rT_3 ratios are caused by the addition of PTU to the infusion medium of dog thyroid lobes.[324] The intrathyroidal production of T_3 is scarce under normal conditions but becomes important in severe iodine deficiency, in which the increase of the relative T_3 content of the thyroid secretion contributes to maintain an eumetabolic state.[194] The intrathyroidal T_4-T_3 conversion is regulated by TSH. Thyroid homogenates of rats hyperstimulated with TSH contain higher levels of T_4-deiodinating activity than those of hypophysectomized rats.[325] TSH stimulates thyroidal iodothyronine deiodinases of humans,[326] dog,[327] and mouse.[323]

THYROID HORMONE SECRETION

Secretory Products

Under normal conditions, T_4 is the main secretory product of the thyroid. About 80 to 90 μg (105 to 115 nmoles) of T_4 are secreted per day. Limited amounts of T_3 (3,5,3'-triiodothyronine) (8 μg) and of the inactive reverse T_3 (rT_3, 3,3',5'-triiodothyronine) (1 μg) are also secreted by the normal human thyroid. Indeed, in euthyroid subjects, most of the T_3 and rT_3 of serum are produced by 5'- and 5-monodeiodination of T_4 in peripheral tissues, respectively, and only 25 per cent of T_3 and 2.5 per cent of rT_3 are secreted as such by the thyroid.[318]

The factors influencing the ratio of T_4 to T_3 in the thyroidal secretion are discussed in detail elsewhere.[324] One of them is the $T_4:T_3$ ratio in Tg; this ratio decreases in rats subjected to restricted iodine intake[194] and in rabbits and guinea pigs given TSH.[125] Another factor of possible importance is the ratio between the rates of T_3 and T_4 release during the hydrolysis of Tg. Acute stimulation of secretion by perfused dog thyroid lobes causes increased T_4 and T_3 release accompanied by a transient decrease of the $T_4:T_3$ ratio that is independent of the intrathyroidal deiodination of T_4.[324] Enhanced T_3 release from Tg under hyperstimulation by TSH could result from increased proteolysis at the COOH-terminus of Tg by cathepsin B.[195] A prominent mechanism governing the ratio of T_4 to T_3 in thyroid secretion is the intrathyroidal conversion of T_4 to T_3, especially in severe iodine deficiency, in such cases of thyroid hyperfunction, as Graves' disease, and in primary hypothyroidism. Under these conditions, the fraction of total circulating T_3 of thyroidal origin increases markedly, through the action of a thyroid iodothyronine 5'-deiodinase, whose activity is controlled by TSH (see Intrathyroidal T_4-T_3 Conversion).

The thyroid releases small amounts of diiodothyronines[324] and variable amounts of iodide into the circulation.[317] Small amounts of Tg are secreted from the basolateral pole of follicular cells (see Polarized Secretion).

Mechanism and Regulation of Secretion

Thyroid cells contain an intracellular pool of free T_4, which functions as the intermediate compartment of a three-reactant system, whose precursor is the Tg-bound T_4 and whose product is the T_4 secreted in the medium. It has been hypothesized that this intracellular T_4 pool may function as a presecretory reservoir for the regulated release of the hormones.[311] The mechanism whereby thyroid hormones are released into the circulation is uncertain. In analogy with the entry of thyroid hormones into peripheral cells, it is probable that their secretion also involves facilitated or active transport (see Ch. 36). The need for a specific transport system has been sustained also in view of the fact that thyroid hormone secretion is probably a polarized process that occurs at the basolateral, but not at the apical pole of thyroid cells.[311]

Thyroid hormone secretion is controlled by TSH. The administration of TSH causes marked increases of thyroidal secretion in rat[169] and humans in vivo.[172] In sheep thyroid cells, the secretion of iodinated compounds is stim-

ulated not only by TSH and forskolin, via a cAMP-dependent mechanism but also by TPA, by means of the activation of protein kinase C and by the Ca^{2+} ionophore A23187.[160] As in the case of Tg secretion, the effects of TPA on thyroid hormone secretion contrast with its inhibitory action on various differentiated functions of thyroid cells in primary culture (see Secretion of Thyroglobulin). Two other activators of the adenylate cyclase–cAMP system that stimulate thyroid secretion are $beta_2$-adrenergic agonists[328] and vasointestinal peptide (VIP), a neuropeptide found in intrathyroidal nerves.[329]

In sheep thyroid cells, increasing iodide concentrations inhibit, in the order, iodide uptake, thyroid hormone secretion, and hormone formation, an effect that may serve to maintain an euthyroid state in times of moderate iodide excess by preventing the secretion of hormones while allowing their synthesis and storage.[330]

SUMMARY

A general scheme of thyroid hormone biosynthesis and secretion is illustrated in Figure 34–11. The iodide transporter located at the basolateral pole of the thyroid follicular cell co-transports I^- and Na^+ ions into the cell. Tg synthesized in the endoplasmic reticulum and glycosylated in the reticulum and in the Golgi apparatus is condensed

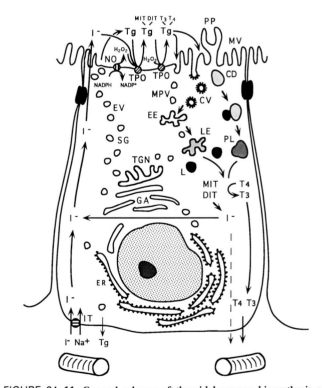

FIGURE 34–11. **General scheme of thyroid hormone biosynthesis and secretion.** See text (Summary) for explanation. Legend: IT, iodide transporter; ER, endoplasmic reticulum; GA, Golgi apparatus; TGN, trans-Golgi network; SG, secretory granules; EV, exocytotic vesicles; NO, NADPH oxidase; TPO, thyroid peroxidase; MV, microvilli (note that microvilli are present all over the apical surface but have been omitted for clarity over part of it); MPV, micropinocytotic vesicles; CV, coated vesicles; EE, early endosomes; LE, late endosomes; L, lysosomes; PP, pseudopods; CD, colloid droplets; PL, phagolysosomes. Iodotyrosine deiodination, iodide recycling and "leaking," T_4 to T_3 conversion and T_4 and T_3 secretion are also shown.

at the exit of the trans-Golgi network in secretory granules that undergo regulated secretion. The polarity of secretion is mostly apical and, for a minor part, basolateral. TPO catalyzes Tg iodination and T_4 and T_3 synthesis at the apical cell pole, using the I^- ions accumulated in the follicle lumen and the H_2O_2 formed by the NADPH oxidase. Hormone-bearing Tg is reabsorbed via micropinocytotic vesicles, some of which are coated and whose coalescence originates early endosomes, and via colloid droplets engulfed by pseudopods. Tg hydrolysis and iodoamino acid release seem to occur both in late endosomes, and in the phagolysosomes resulting from the fusion of colloid droplets and lysosomes. Free iodotyrosines are deiodinated, and the iodide is in part recycled and in part it "leaks" out of the cell. Part of T_4 is converted intracellularly to T_3. T_4 and T_3 are finally secreted.

REFERENCES

1. Lazzaro D, Price M, De Felice M, Di Lauro R: The transcription factor TTF-1 is expressed at the onset of thyroid and lung morphogenesis and in restricted regions of the foetal brain. Development 113:1093–1104, 1991.
2. Civitareale D, Lonigro R, Sinclair AJ, Di Lauro R: A thyroid specific nuclear protein essential for tissue-specific expression of the thyroglobulin promoter. EMBO J 8:2537–2542, 1989.
3. Plachov D, Chowdhury K, Walther C, et al: Pax8, a murine paired box gene expressed in the developing excretory system and the thyroid gland. Development 110:643–651, 1990.
4. Guazzi S, Price M, De Felice M, et al: Thyroid nuclear factor 1 (TTF-1) contains a homeodomain and displays a novel DNA binding specificity. EMBO J 9:3631–3639, 1990.
5. Zannini M, Francis-Lang H, Plachov D, Di Lauro R: Pax-8, a paired domain containing protein, binds to a sequence overlapping with the recognition site of an homeodomain and activates transcription from two thyroid specific promoters. Mol Cell Biol 12:4230–4241, 1992.
6. Ericson LE, Frederiksson G: Phylogeny and ontogeny of the thyroid gland. In Greer MA (ed): The Thyroid Gland. New York, Raven Press, 1990, pp 1–35.
7. Dohrn A: Thyroidea bei Petromyzon, Amphioxus, und den Tunicaten. Mitt Zool Sta Neapel 6:49–92, 1886.
8. Gorbman A, Creaser CW: Accumulation of radioactive iodine by the endostyle of larval lampreys and the problem of homology of the thyroid. J Exptl Zool 83:391–405, 1942.
9. Leloup J, Berg O: Sur la présence d'acides amines iodés (monoiodotyrosine diiodotyrosine et thyroxine) dans l'endostyle de l'Ammocoete. Compt Rend Acad Sci Ser D 238:1069–1071, 1954.
10. Aloj S, Salvatore G, Roche J: Isolation and properties of a native subunit of lamprey thyroglobulin. J Biol Chem 242:3810–3814, 1967.
11. Wright GM, Filosa MF, Youson JH: Immunocytochemical localization of thyroglobulin in the transforming endostyle of anadromous sea lampreys, Petromyzon marinus L, during metamorphosis. Gen Comp Endocrinol 42:187–194, 1980.
12. Salvatore G: Thyroid hormone biosynthesis in Agnatha and Protochordata. Gen Comp Endocrinol (Suppl 2):535–552, 1969.
13. Thorndyke MC: Evidence for a "mammalian" thyroglobulin in endostyle of the ascidian Styela clava. Nature 271:61–62, 1978.
14. Thomas IM: The accumulation of radioactive iodine by Amphioxus. J Marine Biol Assoc UK 35:203–210, 1956.
15. Barrington EJW, Franchi LL: Organic binding of iodine in the endostyle of Ciona intestinalis. Nature 177, 432, 1956.
16. Roche J, Salvatore G, Rametta G: Sur la présence et la biosynthèse d'hormones thyroïdiennes chez un Tunicier, Ciona intestinalis L. Biochim Biophys Acta 63:154–165, 1962.
17. Edelhoch H: The properties of thyroglobulin. I. The effects of alkali. J Biol Chem 235:1326–1334, 1960.
18. Ui N: Electrophoretic mobility and isoelectric point of hog thyroglobulin. Biochim Biophys Acta 257:350–364, 1972.
19. Rolland M, Montfort MF, Valenta L, Lissitzky S: Iodoaminoacid composition of the thyroglobulin of normal and diseased thyroid glands: Comparison with in vitro iodinated thyroglobulin. Clin Chim Acta 39:95–108, 1972.
20. Sorimachi K, Ui N: Comparison of the iodoamino acid distribution in various preparations of hog thyroglobulin with different iodine content and subunit structure. Biochim Biophys Acta 342:30–40, 1974.
21. Izumi M, Larsen PR: Triiodothyronine, thyroxine, and iodine in purified thyroglobulin from patients with Graves' disease. J Clin Invest 59:1105–1112, 1977.
22. Schneider AB, Edelhoch H: Equilibrium density centrifugation of thyroglobulin in RbCl. Effect of iodine. J Biol Chem 246:6592–6596, 1971.
23. Arima T, Spiro MJ, Spiro RG: Studies of the carbohydrate units of thyroglobulin. Evaluation of their microheterogeneity in the human and calf proteins. J Biol Chem 247:1825–1835, 1972.
24. Tarutani O, Ui N: Subunit structure of hog thyroglobulin. Dissociation by treatment with sodium dodecyl sulfate. Biochim Biophys Acta 181:116–135, 1969.
25. Salvatore G, Vecchio G, Salvatore M, et al: 27S iodoprotein. Isolation and properties. J Biol Chem 240:2935–2943, 1965.
26. Robbins J, Salvatore G, Vecchio G, Ui N: Thyroglobulin and 27-S iodoprotein. Iodination and ultracentrifugal heterogeneity. Biochim Biophys Acta 127:101–111, 1966.
27. Marriq C, Rolland M, Lissitzky S: Polypeptide chains of 19 S thyroglobulin from several mammalian species and of porcine 27S iodoprotein. Eur J Biochem 79:143–149, 1977.
28. Torresani J, Roques M, Peyrot A, Lissitzky S: Mise en evidence, purification et propriétés d'une iodoalbumine, constituant physiologique de la glande thyroide de rat. Acta Endocrinol 57:153–167, 1968.
29. Lissitzky S, Codaccioni JL, Bismuth J, Depieds R: Congenital goiter with hypothyroidism and iodo-serum albumin replacing thyroglobulin. J Clin Endocrinol Metab 27:185–196, 1967.
30. Dolling CE, Good BF: Congenital goiter in sheep: isolation of the iodoproteins which replace thyroglobulin. J Endocrinol 71:179–192, 1976.
30a. de Vijlder JJM, Veenboer GJM, van Dijk JE: Thyroid albumin originates from blood. Endocrinology 131:578–584, 1992.
31. Mercken L, Simons M-J, Swillens S, Massaer M, Vassart G: Primary structure of bovine thyroglobulin deduced from the sequence of its 8,431-base complementary DNA. Nature 316:647–651, 1985.
32. Malthièry Y, Lissitzky S: Primary structure of human thyroglobulin deduced from its 8448-base complementary DNA. Eur J Biochem 165:491–498, 1987.
33. Di Lauro R, Obici S, Condliffe D, et al: The sequence of 967 amino acids at the carboxyl-end of rat thyroglobulin. Location and surroundings of two thyroxine-forming sites. Eur J Biochem 148:7–11, 1985.
34. Lejeune P-J, Marriq C, Rolland M, Lissitzky S: Amino acid sequence around a hormonogenic tyrosine residue in the N-terminal region of human thyroglobulin after in vivo and in vitro iodination. Biochem Biophys Res Commun 114:73–80, 1983.
35. Rawitch AB, Chernoff SB, Litwer MR, Rouse JB, Hamilton JW: Thyroglobulin structure-function. The amino acid sequence surrounding thyroxine. J Biol Chem 258:2079–2082, 1983.
36. Koch N, Lauer W, Habicht J, Dobberstein B: Primary structure of the gene for the murine Ia antigen-associated invariant chains (Ii). An alternatively spliced exon encodes a cysteine-rich domain highly homologous to a repetitive sequence of thyroglobulin. EMBO J 6:1677–1683, 1987.
37. Durkin ME, Chakravarti S, Bartos BB, et al: Amino acid sequence and domain structure of entactin. Homology with epidermal growth factor precursor and low density lipoprotein receptor. J Cell Biol 107:2749–2756, 1988.
38. Simon B, Podolsky DK, Moldenhauer G, et al: Epithelial glycoprotein is a member of a family of epithelial cell surface antigens homologous to nidogen, a matrix adhesion protein. Proc Natl Acad Sci USA 87:2755–2759, 1990.
39. Schumacher M, Camp S, Maulet Y, et al: Primary structure of acetylcholinesterase: Implications for regulation and function. Fed Proc 45:2976–2981, 1986.
40. Takagi Y, Omura T, Go M: Evolutionary origin of thyroglobulin by duplication of esterase gene. FEBS Lett 282:17–22, 1991.
41. Mercken L, Simons M-J, Brocas H, Vassart G: Alternative splicing may be responsible for heterogeneity of thyroglobulin structure. Biochimie 71:223–226, 1989.
42. Gentile F, Salvatore S: Preferential sites of proteolytic cleavage of bovine, human and rat thyroglobulin. The use of limited proteolysis

to detect solvent-exposed regions of the primary structure. Eur J Biochem 218:603–621, 1993.

43. Formisano S, Moscatelli C, Zarrilli R, et al: Prediction of the secondary structure of the carboxy-terminal third of rat thyroglobulin. Biochem Biophys Res Commun 133:766–772, 1985.

44. Malthièry Y, Marriq C, Bergè-Lefranc J-L, et al: Thyroglobulin structure and function: Recent advances. Biochimie 71:195–210, 1989.

45. Parma J, Cristophe D, Pohl V, Vassart G: Structural organization of the 5′ region of the thyroglobulin gene. Evidence for intron loss and "exonization" during evolution. J Mol Biol 196:769–779, 1987.

46. Craik CS, Sprang S, Fletterick R, Rutter WJ: Intron-exon splice junctions map at protein surfaces. Nature 299:180–182, 1982.

47. Craik CS, Rutter WJ, Fletterick R: Splice junctions: Association with variation in protein structure. Science 220:1125–1129, 1983.

48. Edelhoch H, Lippoldt R: The properties of thyroglobulin. II. The effects of sodium dodecyl sulfate. J Biol Chem 235:1335–1340, 1960.

49. Schneider AB, Edelhoch H: The properties of thyroglobulin. XIX. The equilibrium between guinea pig thyroglobulin and its subunits. J Biol Chem 245:885–890, 1970.

50. Tarutani O, Ui N: Subunit structure of hog thyroglobulin. Dissociation of noniodinated and highly iodinated preparations. Biochim Biophys Acta 181:136–145, 1969.

51. Rossi G, Edelhoch H, Tenore A, et al: Characterization and properties of thyroid iodoproteins from severely iodine-deficient rats. Endocrinology 92:1241–1249, 1973.

52. Vecchio G, Edelhoch H, Robbins J, Weathers B: Studies on the structure of the 27 S thyroid iodoprotein. Biochemistry 5:2617–2620, 1966.

53. Van der Walt B, Kotzé B, Edelhoch H, Van Jaarsveld PP: Characterization of the major polypeptide chains of reduced bovine thyroglobulin. Biochim Biophys Acta 744:90–98, 1983.

54. Vassart G, Brocas H: Restriction mapping of synthetic thyroglobulin structural gene as a means of investigating thyroglobulin structure. Biochim Biophys Acta 610:189–194, 1980.

55. Van Jaarsveld PP, Van der Merwe MJ, Van der Walt B, Edelhoch H: Enzymatic conversion of the major polypeptide chains of thyroglobulin. Endocrinology 108:1285–1292, 1981.

56. Spiro MJ, Gorski KM: Studies on the posttranslational migration and processing of thyroglobulin: Use of inhibitors and evaluation of the role of phosphorylation. Endocrinology 119:1146–1158, 1986.

57. Spiro MJ, Spiro RG: Biosynthesis of sulfated asparagine–linked complex carbohydrate units of calf thyroglobulin. Endocrinology 122:56–65, 1988.

58. Gentile F, Palumbo G, Salvatore G: The origin of the electrophoretic doublet of thyroglobulin. Biochem Biophys Res Commun 186:1185–1191, 1992.

59. Ruf J, Carayon P, Lissitzky S: Various expressions of a unique anti-human thyroglobulin antibody repertoire in normal state and autoimmune disease. Eur J Immunol 15:268–272, 1985.

60. Ruf J, Carayon P, Sarles-Philip N, et al: Specificity of monoclonal antibodies against human thyroglobulin; comparison with autoimmune antibodies. EMBO J 2:1821–1826, 1983.

61. Piechaczyk M, Bouanani S, Salhi SL, et al: Antigenic domains on the human thyroglobulin recognized by autoantibodies in patient's sera and by natural autoantibodies isolated from the sera of healthy subjects. Clin Immunol Immunopathol 45:114–121, 1987.

62. Gleason SL, Gearhart P, Rose NR, Kuppers RC: Autoantibodies to thyroglobulin are encoded by diverse V-gene segments and recognize restricted epitopes. J Immunol 145:1768–1775, 1990.

63. Bouanani M, Piechaczyk M, Pau B, Bastide M: Significance of the recognition of certain antigenic regions on the human thyroglobulin molecule by natural autoantibodies from healthy subjects. J Immunol 143:1129–1132, 1989.

64. Dong Q, Ludgate M, Vassart G: Towards an antigenic map of human thyroglobulin: Identification of ten epitope-bearing sequences within the primary structure of thyroglobulin. J Endocrinol 122:169–176, 1989.

65. Henry M, Malthièry Y, Zanelli E, Charvet B: Epitope mapping of human thyroglobulin. Heterogeneous recognition by thyroid pathologic sera. J Immunol 145:3692–3698, 1990.

66. Kondo E, Kondo Y: Monoclonal antibodies to hog thyroglobulin recognizing disulfide-dependent conformational structures. Mol Immunol 21:581–588, 1984.

67. De Baets MH, Theunissen R, Kok K, et al: Monoclonal antibodies to human thyroglobulin as probes for thyroglobulin structure. Endocrinology 120:1104–1111, 1987.

68. Male DK, Champion BR, Pryce G, et al: Antigenic determinants of human thyroglobulin differentiated using antigen fragments. Immunology 54:419–427, 1985.

69. Shimojo N, Saito K, Kohno Y, et al: Antigenic determinants on thyroglobulin: Comparison of the reactivities of different thyroglobulin preparations with serum antibodies and T cells of patients with chronic thyroiditis. J Clin Endocrinol Metab 66:689–695, 1988.

70. Den Hartog MT, De Boer M, Veenboer GJM, de Vijlder JJM: Generation and characterization of monoclonal antibodies directed against noniodinated and iodinated thyroglobulin, among which are antibodies against hormonogenic sites. Endocrinology 127:3160–3165, 1990.

71. Sundick RS, Herdegen DM, Brown TR, Bagchi N: The incorporation of dietary iodine into thyroglobulin increases its immunogenicity. Endocrinology 120:2078–2084, 1987.

72. Champion BR, Rayner DC, Byfield PGH, et al: Critical role of iodination for T cell recognition of thyroglobulin in experimental murine thyroid autoimmunity. J Immunol 139:3665–3670, 1987.

73. Champion BR, Page KR, Parish N, et al: Identification of a thyroxine-containing self-epitope of thyroglobulin which triggers thyroid autoreactive T cells. J Exp Med 174:363–370, 1991.

74. Baas F, Bikker H, Geurts Van Kessel A, et al: The human thyroglobulin gene: A polymorphic marker localized distal to c-myc on chromosome 8 band q24. Hum Genet 69:138–143, 1985.

75. Brocas H, Szpirer J, Lebo RV, et al: The thyroglobulin gene resides on chromosome 8 in man and on chromosome 7 in the rat. Cytogenet Cell Genet 39:150–153, 1985.

76. Avvedimento VE, Di Lauro R, Monticelli A, et al: Mapping of human thyroglobulin gene on the long arm of chromosome 8 by in situ hybridization. Hum Genet 71:163–166, 1985.

77. Baas F, van Ommen G-JB, Bikker H, et al: The human thyroglobulin gene is over 300 kb long and contains introns of up to 64 kb. Nucl Acids Res 14:5171–5186, 1986.

78. Musti AM, Avvedimento EV, Polistina C. et al: The complete structure of the rat thyroglobulin gene. Proc Natl Acad Sci USA 83:323–327, 1986.

79. de Martynoff G, Pohl V, Mercken L, et al: Structural organization of the bovine thyroglobulin gene and of its 5′-flanking region. Eur J Biochem 164:591–599, 1987.

80. Lee NT, Kamikubo K, Chai K-J, et al: The deoxynucleic acid regions involved in the hormonal regulation of the thyroglobulin gene. Endocrinology 128:111–118, 1991.

81. Santisteban P, Polycarpou-Schwartz M, Acebron A, Di Lauro R: Insulin and insulin-Like growth factor I regulate a thyroid specific nuclear protein that binds to the thyroglobulin promoter. Mol Endocrinol 6:1310–1317, 1992.

82. Ledent C, Parmentier M, Vassart G: Tissue-specific expression and methylation of a thyroglobulin-chloramphenicol acetyltransferase fusion gene in transgenic mice. Proc Natl Acad Sci USA 87:6176–6180, 1990.

83. Sinclair AJ, Lonigro R, Civitareale D, et al: The tissue specific expression of the thyroglobulin gene requires interaction between thyroid specific and ubiquitous factors. Eur J Biochem 193:311–318, 1990.

84. Skinner CA, Kelly D, Kao L-R, et al: Thyroid-specific and hormone-dependent expression of rat Tg promoter fused with bacterial chloramphenicol acetyltransferase gene in transgenic mice. Mol Cell Endocrinol 90:33–38, 1992.

85. Vassart G, Dumont J: Identification of polysomes synthesizing thyroglobulin. Eur J Biochem 32:332–330, 1973.

86. Di Lauro R, Metafora S, Consiglio E, et al: In vitro synthesis of a thyroglobulin precursor by porcine membrane-bound ribosomes in a heterologous cell-free system. J Biol Chem 250:3267–3272, 1975.

87. Kim PS, Arvan P: Folding and assembly of newly synthesized thyroglobulin occurs in a pre-Golgi compartment. J Biol Chem 266:12412–12418, 1991.

87a. Kim PS, Bole D, Arvan P: Transient aggregation of nascent thyroglobulin in the endoplasmic reticulum: Relationship to the molecular chaperone, BiP. J Cell Biol 118:541–549, 1992.

88. Tsuji T, Yamamoto K, Irimura T, Osawa T: Structure of carbohydrate unit A of porcine thyroglobulin. Biochem J 195:691–699, 1981.

89. Yamamoto K, Tsuji T, Irimura T, Osawa T: The structure of carbohydrate unit B of porcine thyroglobulin. Biochem J 195:701–713, 1981.

90. Spiro RG, Bhoyroo VD: Occurrence of α-D-galactosyl residues in the thyroglobulins from several species. Localization in the saccharide chains of the complex carbohydrate units. J Biol Chem 259:9858–9866, 1984.

91. Godelaine D, Spiro MJ, Spiro RG: Processing of the carbohydrate units of thyroglobulin. J Biol Chem 256:10161–10168, 1981.

92. Spiro MJ, Spiro RG, Bhoyroo VD: Glycosylation of proteins by oligosaccharide-lipids. Studies on a thyroid enzyme involved in oligosac-

charide transfer and the role of glucose in this reaction. J Biol Chem 254:7668–7674, 1979.

93. Kornfeld R, Kornfeld S: Assembly of asparagine-linked oligosaccharides. Ann Rev Biochem 54:631–664, 1985.

94. Ronin C, Fenouillet E, Hovsepian S, et al: Regulation of thyroglobulin glycosylation. A comparative study of the thyroglobulins from porcine thyroid glands and follicles in serum-free culture. J Biol Chem 261:7287–7293, 1986.

95. Di Jeso B, Liguoro D, Ferranti P, et al: Modulation of the carbohydrate moiety of thyroglobulin by thyrotropin and calcium in Fisher rat thyroid line-5 cells. J Biol Chem 267:1983–1944, 1992.

96. Di Jeso B, Gentile F: TSH-Induced galactose incorporation at the NH₂-terminus of thyroglobulin secreted by FRTL-5 cells. Biochem Biophys Res Commun 189:1624–1630, 1992.

97. Rawitch AB, Liao TH, Pierce JG: The amino acid sequence of a tryptic glycopeptide from human thyroglobulin. Biochim Biophys Acta 160:360–367, 1968.

98. Franc J-L, Venot N, Marriq C: Characterization of the two oligosaccharides present in the preferential hormonogenic domain of human thyroglobulin. Biochem Biophys Res Commun 166:937–944, 1990.

99. Spiro MJ: Presence of a glucuronic acid–containing carbohydrate unit in human thyroglobulin. J Biol Chem 252:5424–5430, 1977.

100. Spiro RG, Bhoyroo VD: Occurrence of sulfate in the asparagine-linked complex carbohydrate units of thyroglobulin. Identification and localization of galactose 3-sulfate and N-acetylglucosamine 6-sulfate residues in the human and calf proteins. J Biol Chem 263:14351–14358, 1988.

101. Schneider AB, McCurdy A, Chang T, et al: Metabolic labeling of human thyroglobulin with [35S] sulfate: Incorporation into chondroitin 6-sulfate and endoglycosidase-F–susceptible carbohydrate units. Endocrinology 122:2428–2435, 1988.

102. Consiglio E, Acquaviva AM, Formisano S, et al: Characterization of phosphate residues on thyroglobulin. J Biol Chem 262:10304–10314, 1987.

103. Herzog V, Neumüller W, Holzmann B: Thyroglobulin, the major and obligatory exportable protein of thyroid follicle cells, carries the lysosomal recognition marker mannose-6-phosphate. EMBO J 6:555–560, 1987.

104. Yamamoto K, Tsuji T, Tarutani O, Osawa T: Phosphorylated high mannose-type and hybrid-type oligosaccharide chains of human thyroglobulin isolated from malignant thyroid tissue. Biochim Biophys Acta 838:84–91, 1985.

105. Sakurai S, Fogelfeld L, Ries A, Schneider A: Anionic complex–carbohydrate units of human thyroglobulin. Endocrinology 127:2056–2063, 1990.

106. Sakurai S, Fogelfeld L, Schneider A: Anionic carbohydrate groups of human thyroglobulin containing both phosphate and sulfate. Endocrinology 129:915–920, 1991.

107. Herzog V: Secretion of sulfated thyroglobulin. Eur J Cell Biol 39:399–409, 1985.

108. Ogawara H, Bilstad JM, Cahnmann HJ: Iodoamino acid distribution in thyroglobulin iodinated in vivo and in vitro. Biochim Biophys Acta 257:339–349, 1972.

109. Edelhoch H, Carlomagno MS, Salvatore G: Iodine and the structure of thyroglobulin. Arch Biochem Biophys 134:264–265, 1969.

110. Frati L, Bilstad J, Edelhoch H, et al: Biosynthesis of the 27 S thyroid iodoprotein. Arch Biochem Biophys 162:126–134, 1974.

111. Dunn JT, Kim PS, Dunn AD: Favored sites for thyroid hormone formation on the peptide chains of human thyroglobulin. J Biol Chem 257:88–94, 1982.

112. Marriq C, Lejeune P-J, Malthièry Y, et al: Precursor-product relationship between the 26-kDa and 18-kDa fragments formed by iodination of human thyroglobulin. FEBS Lett 175:140–146, 1984.

113. Dunn JT, Dunn AD, Heppner DG Jr, Kim PS: A discrete thyroxine-rich iodopeptide of 20,000 daltons from rabbit thyroglobulin. J Biol Chem 256:942–947, 1981.

114. Dunn JT, Kim PS, Dunn AD, et al: The role of iodination in the formation of hormone-rich peptides from thyroglobulin. J Biol Chem 258:9093–9099, 1983.

115. Marriq C, Lejeune P-J, Venot N, Vinet L: Hormone synthesis in human thyroglobulin: Possible cleavage of the polypeptide chain at the tyrosine donor site. FEBS Lett 242:414–418, 1989.

116. Marriq C, Lejeune P-J, Venot N, Vinet L: Hormone formation in the isolated fragment 1–171 of human thyroglobulin involves the couple tyrosine 5 and tyrosine 130. Mol Cell Endocrinol 81:155–164, 1991.

117. Gregg JD, Dziadik-Turner C, Rouse J, et al: A comparison of 30-kDa and 10-kDa hormone-containing fragments of bovine thyroglobulin. J Biol Chem 263:5190–5196, 1988.

118. Rawitch AB, Litwer MR, Gregg J, et al: The isolation of identical thyroxine containing amino acid sequences from bovine, ovine and porcine thyroglobulins. Biochem Biophys Res Commun 118:423–429, 1984.

119. Edelhoch H: The properties of thyroglobulin. VIII. The iodination of thyroglobulin. J Biol Chem 237:2778–2787, 1962.

120. Gavaret J-M, Déme D, Nunez J: Sequential reactivity of tyrosyl residues of thyroglobulin upon iodination catalyzed by thyroid peroxidase. J Biol Chem 252:3281–3285, 1977.

121. Lamas L, Taurog A, Salvatore G, Edelhoch H: Preferential synthesis of thyroxine from early iodinated tyrosyl residues in thyroglobulin. J Biol Chem 249:2732–2737, 1974.

122. Palumbo G, Gentile F, Condorelli GL, Salvatore G: The earliest site of iodination in thyroglobulin is residue number 5. J Biol Chem 265:8887–8892, 1990.

123. Gavaret J-M, Cahnmann HJ, Nunez J: Thyroid hormone synthesis in thyroglobulin. The mechanism of the coupling reaction. J Biol Chem 256:9167–9173, 1981.

124. Dunn JT, Anderson PC, Fox JW, et al: The sites of thyroid hormone formation in rabbit thyroglobulin. J Biol Chem 262:16948–16952, 1987.

125. Fassler CA, Dunn JT, Anderson PC, et al: Thyrotropin alters the utilization of thyroglobulin's hormonogenic sites. J Biol Chem 263:17366–17371, 1988.

126. Dziadik-Turner C, Hamilton JW, Taurog A, Rawitch AB: Hormone-containing peptides from normal and goiter human thyroglobulins. Arch Biochem Biophys 266:377–385, 1988.

127. Marriq C, Rolland M, Lissitzky S: Structure-function relationship in thyroglobulin: Amino acid sequence of two different thyroxine-containing peptides from porcine thyroglobulin. EMBO J 1:397–401, 1982.

128. Marriq C, Rolland M, Lissitzky S: Amino acid sequence of the unique 3,5,3′-triiodothyronine-containing sequence from porcine thyroglobulin. Biochem Biophys Res Commun 112:206–213, 1983.

129. Lamas L, Anderson PC, Fox JW, Dunn JT: Consensus sequences for early iodination and hormonogenesis in human thyroglobulin. J Biol Chem 264:13541–13545, 1989.

130. Roe MT, Anderson PC, Dunn AD, and Dunn JT: The hormonogenic sites of turtle thyroglobulin and their homology with those of mammals. Endocrinology 124:1327–1332, 1989.

131. Gavaret J-M, Cahnmann HJ, Nunez J: The fate of the "lost side chain" during thyroid hormonogenesis. J Biol Chem 254:11218–11222, 1979.

132. Gavaret J-M, Nunez J, Cahnmann HJ: Formation of dehydroalanine residues during thyroid hormone synthesis in thyroglobulin. J Biol Chem 255:5281–5285, 1980.

133. Palumbo G: Thyroid hormonogenesis. Identification of a sequence containing iodophenyl donor site(s) in calf thyroglobulin. J Biol Chem 262:17182–17188, 1987.

134. Ohmiya Y, Hayashi H, Kondo T, Kondo Y: Location of dehydroalanine residues in the amino acid sequence of bovine thyroglobulin. Identification of "donor" tyrosine sites for hormonogenesis in thyroglobulin. J Biol Chem 265:9066–9071, 1990.

135. Sterk A, van Dijk JE, Veenboer GJM, et al: Normal-sized thyroglobulin messenger ribonucleic acid in Dutch goats with a thyroglobulin synthesis defect is translated into a 35,000 molecular weight N-terminal fragment. Endocrinology 124:477–483, 1989.

136. Van Voorthuizen WF, de Vijlder JJM, van Dijk JE, Tegelaers WHH: Euthyroidism via iodide supplementation in hereditary congenital goiter with thyroglobulin deficiency. Endocrinology 103:2105–2111, 1978.

136a. Veenboer GJM, de Vijlder JJM: Molecular basis of the thyroglobulin synthesis defect in Dutch goats. Endocrinology 132:377–381, 1993.

137. Tassi VPN, Di Lauro R, Van Jaarsveld P, Alvino C: Two abnormal thyroglobulin-like polypeptides are produced from Afrikander cattle congenital goiter mRNA. J Biol Chem 259:10507–10510, 1984.

138. Ricketts MH, Pohl V, de Martynoff G, et al: Defective splicing of thyroglobulin gene transcripts in the congenital goitre of the Afrikander cattle. EMBO J 4:731–737, 1985.

139. Ricketts MH, Simons MJ, Parma J, Mercken L, Dong Q, Vassart G: A nonsense mutation causes hereditary goitre in the Afrikander cattle and unmasks alternative splicing of thyroglobulin transcripts. Proc Natl Acad Sci USA 84:3181–3184, 1987.

140. Graves PN, Davies TF: A second thyroglobulin messenger RNA species (rTg-2) in rat thyrocytes. Mol Endocrinol 4:155–161, 1990.

141. Asunciòn M, Ingrassia R, Escribano J, et al: Efficient thyroid hormone formation by in vitro iodination of a segment of rat thyroglobulin fused to staphylococcal protein A. FEBS Lett 297:266–270, 1992.

142. Van Zyl A, Edelhoch H: The properties of thyroglobulin. XV. The function of the protein in the control of diiodotyrosine synthesis. J Biol Chem 242:2423–2427, 1967.

143. Rolland M, Montfort M-F, Lissitzky S: Efficiency of thyroglobulin as a thyroid hormone-forming protein. Biochim Biophys Acta 303:338–347, 1973.

144. Tice LW, Wollman SH, Carter RC: Changes in tight junctions of thyroid epithelium with changes in thyroid activity. J Cell Biol 66:657–663, 1975.

145. Chambard M, Verrier B, Gabrion J, Mauchamp J: Polarization of thyroid cells in culture: Evidence for the basolateral localization of the iodide "pump" and of the thyroid-stimulating hormone receptor–adenyl cyclase complex. J Cell Biol 96:1172–1177, 1983.

146. Burgess TL, Kelly RB: Constitutive and regulated secretion of proteins. Ann Rev Cell Biol 3:243–293, 1987.

147. Paiement J, Leblond CP: Localization of thyroglobulin antigenicity in rat thyroid sections using antibodies labeled with peroxidase or ^{125}I-radioiodine. J Cell Biol 74:992–1015, 1977.

148. Ekholm R, Engström G, Ericson LE, Melander A: Exocytosis of protein into the thyroid follicle lumen: An early effect of TSH. Endocrinology 97:337–346, 1975.

149. Engström G, Ericson LE: Effect of graded doses of thyrotropin on exocytosis and early phase of endocytosis in the rat thyroid. Endocrinology 108:399–405, 1981.

150. Nitsch L, Wollman SH: Suspension culture of separated follicles consisting of differentiated thyroid epithelial cells. Proc Natl Acad Sci USA 77:472–476, 1980.

151. Nitsch L, Wollman SH: Ultrastructure of intermediate stages in polarity reversal of thyroid epithelium in follicles in suspension culture. J Cell Biol 86:875–880, 1980.

152. Garbi C, Wollman SH: Ultrastructure and some other properties of inverted thyroid follicles in suspension culture. Exp Cell Res 138:343–353, 1982.

153. Chambard M, Gabrion J, Mauchamp J: Influence of collagen gels on the orientation of epithelial cell polarity: Follicle formation from isolated thyroid cells and from preformed monolayers. J Cell Biol 91:157–166, 1981.

154. Garbi C, Nitsch L, Wollman SH: Embedding in a collagen gel stabilizes the polarity of epithelial cells in thyroid follicles in suspension culture. Exp Cell Res 151:458–465, 1984.

155. Tacchetti C, Zurzolo C, Monticelli A, Nitsch L: Functional properties of normal and inverted rat thyroid follicles in suspension culture. J Cell Physiol 126:93–98, 1986.

156. Chambard M, Mauchamp J, Chabaud O: Synthesis and apical and basolateral secretion of thyroglobulin by thyroid cell monolayers on permeable substrate: Modulation by thyrotropin. J Cell Physiol 133:37–45, 1987.

157. Gruffat D, Gonzalvez S, Chambard M, et al: Long-term iodination of thyroglobulin by porcine thyroid cells cultured in porous-bottomed culture chambers: Regulation by thyrotropin. J Endocrinol 128:51–61, 1991.

157a. Gruffat D, Venot N, Marriq C, Chabaud O: Thyroid hormone synthesis in thyroglobulin secreted by porcine thyroid cells cultured on porous bottom chambers. Effect of iodide. Endocrinology 131:2921–2927, 1992.

158. Arvan P, Lee J: Regulated and constitutive protein targeting can be distinguished by secretory polarity in thyroid epithelial cells. J Cell Biol 112:365–376, 1991.

159. Björkman U, Ekholm R: Accelerated exocytosis and H_2O_2-generation in isolated thyroid follicles enhance protein iodination. Endocrinology 122:488–494, 1988.

160. Eggo MC, Lippes H, Burrow GN: Control of thyroid secretion: Effects of stimulators of protein kinase C, thyrotropin, and calcium mobilization on secretion of iodinated compounds from sheep thyroid cells. Endocrinology 130:2274–2283, 1992.

161. Bachrach LK, Eggo MC, Mak WW, Burrow GN: Phorbol esters stimulate growth and inhibit differentiation in cultured thyroid cells. Endocrinology 116:1603–1609, 1985.

162. Roger PP, Reuse S, Servais P, et al: Stimulation of cell proliferation and inhibition of differentiation expression by tumor-promoting phorbol esters in dog thyroid cells in primary culture. Cancer Res 46:898–906, 1986.

163. Di Jeso B, Laviola L, Liguoro D, et al: P_2-purinergic agonists and 12-O-tetradecanoylphorbol-13-acetate, as well as protein kinase A activators, stimulate thyroglobulin secretion in FRTL-5 cells. Biochim Biophys Res Commun 191:385–391, 1993.

164. Björkman U, Ekholm R: Effect of tunicamycin on thyroglobulin secretion. Eur J Biochem 125:585–591, 1982.

165. Eggo MC, Burrow GN: Glycosylation of thyroglobulin—its role in secretion, iodination, and stability. Endocrinology 113:1655–1663, 1983.

166. Franc J-L, Giraud A, Lanet J: Effects of deoxymannojirimycin and castanospermine on the polarized secretion of thyroglobulin. Endocrinology 126:1464–1470, 1990.

167. Franc J-L, Hovsepian S, Fayet G, Bouchilloux S: Inhibition of N-linked oligosaccharide processing does not prevent the secretion of thyroglobulin. A study with swainsonine and deoxynojirimycin. Eur J Biochem 157:225–232, 1986.

168. Van Herle AJ, Uller RP, Matthews NL, Brown J: Radioimmunoassay for measurement of thyroglobulin in human serum. J Clin Invest 52:1320–1327, 1973.

169. Van Herle AJ, Klandorf H, Uller RP: A radioimmunoassay for serum rat thyroglobulin. Physiologic and pharmacological studies. J Clin Invest 56:1073–1081, 1975.

170. Schneider AB, Ikekubo K, Kuma K: Iodine content of serum thyroglobulin in normal individuals and patients with thyroid tumors. J Clin Endocrinol Metab 57:1251–1256, 1983.

171. Ikekubo K, Kishihara M, Sanders J, et al: Differences between circulating and tissue thyroglobulin in rats. Endocrinology 109:427–432, 1981.

172. Unger J, Van Heuerswyn B, Decoster C, et al: Thyroglobulin and thyroid hormone release after intravenous administration of bovine thyrotropin in man. J Clin Endocrinol Metab 51:590–594, 1980.

173. Ekholm R, Wollman SH: Site of iodination in the rat thyroid gland deduced from electron microscopic autoradiographs. Endocrinology 97:1432–1443, 1975.

174. Wollman SH, Ekholm R: Site of iodination in hyperplastic thyroid glands deduced from autoradiographs. Endocrinology 108:2082–2085, 1981.

175. Lowenstein JE, Wollman SH: Diffusion of thyroglobulin in the lumen of the rat thyroid follicle. Endocrinology 81:1086–1090, 1967.

176. Ekholm R, Björkman U: Localization of iodine binding in the thyroid gland in vitro. Endocrinology 115:1558–1567, 1984.

177. Ericson LE: Exocytosis and endocytosis in the thyroid follicle cell. Mol Cell Endocrinol 22:1–24, 1981.

178. Öfverholm T, Ericson LE: Intraluminal iodination of thyroglobulin. Endocrinology 114:827–835, 1984.

179. Wadeleux P, Etienne-Decerf J, Winand RJ, Kohn LD: Effects of thyrotropin on iodine metabolism of dog thyroid cells in tissue culture. Endocrinology 102:889–902, 1978.

180. Roger PP, Dumont JE: Thyrotropin and the differential expression of proliferation and differentiation in dog thyroid cells in primary culture. J Endocrinol 96:241–249, 1983.

181. Magnusson RP, Rapoport B: Modulation of differentiated function in cultured thyroid cells: Thyrotropin control of thyroid peroxidase activity. Endocrinology 116:1493–1500, 1985.

182. Chambard M, Verrier B, Gabrion J, Mauchamp J: Polarity reversal of inside-out thyroid follicles cultured within collagen gels: Reexpression of specific functions. Biol Cell 51:315–326, 1984.

183. Murakami S, Summer CN, Iida-Klein A, et al: Physiological de novo thyroid hormone formation in primary culture of porcine thyroid follicles: Adenosine 3',5'-monophosphate alone is sufficient for thyroid hormone formation. Endocrinology 126:1692–1698, 1990.

184. Bernier-Valentin F, Kostrouch Z, Rabilloud R, Rousset B: Analysis of the thyroglobulin internalization process using in vitro reconstituted thyroid follicles: Evidence for a coated vesicle-dependent endocytic pathway. Endocrinology 129:2194–2201, 1991.

185. Rousset B, Mornex R: Identification of an intracellular pathway of thyroxine synthesis by dispersed thyroid cells. Biochim Biophys Acta 675:8–18, 1981.

186. Mak WW, Errick JE, Chan RC, et al: Thyrotropin-induced formation of functional follicles in primary cultures of ovine thyroid cells. Exp Cell Res 164:311–322, 1986.

187. Eggo MC, Mak WW, Bachrach LK, et al: Cultured thyroids—is immortality the answer? In Eggo MC, Burrow GN (eds): Progress in Endocrine Research and Therapy, Vol 2. Thyroglobulin: The Prothyroid Hormone. New York, Raven Press, 1985, pp 201–210.

188. Tarutani O, Ui N: Accumulation of noniodinated thyroglobulin in the thyroid of goitrogen-treated hogs. Biochem Biophys Res Commun 33:733–738, 1968.

189. Nitsch L, Wollman SH: Cell polarity and water transport in thyroid epithelial cells in separated follicles in suspension culture. Scann Microsc 1:1279–1286, 1987.

190. Haeberli A, Millar FK, Wollman SH: Accumulation and localization of radiocalcium in the rat thyroid gland. Endocrinology 102:1511–1519, 1978.

191. Acquaviva R, Consiglio E, Di Jeso B, et al: Calcium interaction with bovine thyroglobulin: Stoichiometry and structural consequences of calcium binding. Mol Cell Endocrinol 82:175–181, 1991.

191a. Herzog V, Berndorfer U, Saber Y: Isolation of insoluble secretory product from bovine thyroid: Extracellular storage of thyroglobulin in covalently cross-linked form. J Cell Biol 118:1071–1083, 1992.

192. Dunn JT, Van der Haar F: A practical guide to the correction of iodine deficiency. International Council for Control of Iodine Deficiency Disorders, 1990.

193. Riesco G, Taurog A, Larsen PR, Krulich L: Acute and chronic responses to iodine deficiency in rats. Endocrinology 100:303–313, 1977.

194. Abrams GM, Larsen PR: Triiodothyronine and thyroxine in the serum and thyroid glands of iodine-deficient rats. J Clin Invest 52:2522–2531, 1973.

195. Dunn AD, Crutchfield HE, Dunn JT: Thyroglobulin processing by thyroidal proteases. Major sites of cleavage by cathepsins B, D, and L. J Biol Chem 266:20198–20204, 1991.

196. Inoue K, Grimm Y, Greer MA: Quantitative studies on the iodinated components secreted by the rat thyroid gland as determined by in situ perfusion. Endocrinology 81:946–964, 1967.

197. Wolff J: Congenital goiter with defective iodide transport. Endocr Rev 4:240–254, 1983.

198. Wolff J: Iodide concentrating mechanism. In Rall JE, Kopin IJ (eds): The Thyroid and Biogenic Amines. Amsterdam, North-Holland, 1972, pp 115–140.

199. Bagchi N, Fawcett DM: Role of sodium ion in active transport of iodide by cultured thyroid cells. Biochim Biophys Acta 318:235–251, 1973.

200. Weiss SJ, Philp NJ, Grollman EF: Iodide transport in a continuous line of cultured cells from rat thyroid. Endocrinology 114:1090–1098, 1984.

201. Nakamura Y, Kotani T, Ohtaki S: Transcellular iodide transport and iodination on the apical plasma membrane by monolayer porcine thyroid cells cultured on collagen-coated filters. J Endocrinol 126:275–281, 1989.

202. Andros GW, Wollman SH: Autoradiographic localization of radioiodide in the thyroid gland of the mouse. Am J Physiol 213:198–208, 1967.

203. Ekholm R: Biosynthesis of thyroid hormones. Int Rev Cytol 120:243–288, 1990.

204. Wolff J: Iodide transport. Anion selectivity and the iodide "trap." In Reinwein D, Klein E (eds): Diminished Thyroid Hormone Formation. Possible Causes and Clinical Aspects. Stuttgart, FK Schattauer Verlag, 1982, pp 3–15.

205. O'Neill B, Magnolato D, Semenza G: The electrogenic, Na⁺-dependent I⁻ transport system in plasma membrane vesicles from thyroid glands. Biochim Biophys Acta 896:263–274, 1987.

206. Nakamura Y, Ohtaki S, Yamazaki I: Molecular mechanism of iodide transport by thyroid plasmalemmal vesicles: Cooperative sodium activation and asymmetrical affinities for the ions on the outside and inside of the vesicles. J Biochem 104:544–549, 1988.

207. Saito K, Yamamoto K, Takai T, Yoshida S: Characteristics of the thyroid iodide translocator and of iodide-accumulating phospholipid vesicles. Endocrinology 114:868–872, 1984.

208. Tong W: Actions of thyroid-stimulating hormone. In Greer MA, Solomon DH (eds): Handbook of Physiology, Vol 3. Washington, DC, American Physiological Society, 1974, pp 255–283.

209. Weiss SJ, Philp NJ, Ambesi-Impiombato FS, Grollman EF: Thyrotropin-stimulated iodide transport mediated by adenosine 3′,5′-monophosphate and dependent on protein synthesis. Endocrinology 114:1099–1107, 1984.

210. Weiss SJ, Philp NJ, Grollman EF: Effect of thyrotropin on iodide efflux in FRTL-5 cells mediated by Ca²⁺. Endocrinology 114:1108–1113, 1984.

211. Corda D, Marcocci C, Kohn LD, et al: Association of the changes in cytosolic Ca²⁺ and iodide efflux induced by thyrotropin and by the stimulation of α₁-adrenergic receptors in cultured rat thyroid cells. J Biol Chem 260:9230–9236, 1985.

212. Marcocci C, Luini A, Santisteban P, Grollman EF: Norepinephrine and thyrotropin stimulation of iodide efflux in FRTL-5 thyroid cells involves metabolites of arachidonic acid and is associated with the iodination of thyroglobulin. Endocrinology 120:1127–1133, 1987.

213. Sherwin JR, Tong W: The actions of iodide and TSH on thyroid cells showing a dual control system for the iodide pump. Endocrinology 94:1465–1474, 1974.

214. Sherwin JR, Price DJ: Autoregulation of thyroid iodide transport: Evidence for the mediation of protein synthesis in iodide-induced suppression of iodide transport. Endocrinology 119:2553–2559, 1986.

215. Rawitch AB, Taurog A, Chernoff SB, Dorris ML: Hog thyroid peroxidase: Physical, chemical and catalytic properties of the highly purified enzyme. Arch Biochem Biophys 194:244–257, 1979.

216. Ohtaki S, Nakagawa H, Nakamura M, Yamazaki I: Reactions of hog thyroid peroxidase with H₂O₂, tyrosine, and methylmercaptoimidazole (goitrogen) in comparison with bovine lactoperoxidase. J Biol Chem 257:761–766, 1982.

217. Czarnocka B, Ruf J, Ferrand M, et al: Purification of the human thyroid peroxidase and its identification as the microsomal antigen involved in autoimmune thyroid diseases. FEBS Lett 190:147–152, 1985.

218. Ohtaki S, Kotani T, Nakamura Y: Characterization of human thyroid peroxidase purified by monoclonal antibody–assisted chromatography. J Clin Endocrinol Metab 63:570–576, 1986.

219. Kimura S, Kotani T, McBride OW, et al: Human thyroid peroxidase: Complete cDNA and protein sequence, chromosome mapping, and identification of two alternatively spliced mRNAs. Proc Natl Acad Sci USA 84:5555–5559, 1987.

220. Isozaki O, Kohn LD, Kozak CA, Kimura S: Thyroid peroxidase: Rat cDNA sequence, chromosomal localization in mouse, and regulation of gene expression by comparison to thyroglobulin in rat FRTL-5 cells. Mol Endocrinol 3:1681–1692, 1989.

221. Kimura S, Hong Y-S, Kotani T, Ohtaki S, Kikkawa F: Structure of the human thyroid peroxidase gene: Comparison and relationship to the human myeloperoxidase gene. Biochemistry 28:4481–4489, 1989.

222. Libert F, Ruel J, Ludgate M, et al: Complete nucleotide sequence of the human thyroperoxidase-microsomal antigen cDNA. Nucleic Acid Res 15:6735, 1987.

223. Magnusson RP, Chazenbalk GD, Gestautas J, et al: Molecular cloning of the complementary deoxyribonucleic acid for human thyroid peroxidase. Mol Endocrinol 1:856–861, 1987.

224. Magnusson RP, Gestautas J, Taurog A, Rapoport B: Molecular cloning of the structural gene for porcine thyroid peroxidase. J Biol Chem 262:13885–13888, 1987.

225. Foti D, Kaufman KD, Chazenbalk GD, Rapoport B: Generation of a biologically active, secreted form of human thyroid peroxidase by site-directed mutagenesis. Mol Endocrinol 4:786–791, 1990.

226. Rawitch AB, Pollock G, Yang SX, Taurog A: The location and nature of the N-linked oligosaccharide units in porcine thyroid peroxidase: studies on the tryptic glycopeptides. In Carayon P, Ruf J (eds): Thyroperoxidase and Thyroid Autoimmunity, Vol 207. London, Colloque INSERM, John Libbey Eurotext, 1990, pp 69–76.

227. Kimura S, Ikeda-Saito M: Human myeloperoxidase and thyroid peroxidase, two enzymes with separate and distinct physiological functions, are evolutionarily related members of the same gene family. Proteins Struct Funct Genet 3:113–120, 1988.

228. Libert F, Ruel J, Ludgate M, et al: Thyroperoxidase, an autoantigen with a mosaic structure made of nuclear and mitochondrial gene modules. EMBO J 6:4193–4196, 1987.

229. Tice LW, Wollman SH: Ultrastructural localization of peroxidase on pseudopods and other structures of the typical thyroid epithelium cell. Endocrinology 94:1555–1567, 1974.

230. Öfverholm T, Ericson LE: Diffusion artifacts and tissue fixation in thyroperoxidase cytochemistry. Histochemistry 81:1–8, 1984.

231. Kotani T, Ohtaki S: Characterization of thyroid follicular cell apical plasma membrane peroxidase using monoclonal antibody. Endocrinol Jpn 34:407–413, 1987.

232. Nakagawa H, Ohtaki S: Orientation of thyroid peroxidase in hog thyroid microsomes. J Biochem 94:155–162, 1983.

233. Portmann L, Hamada N, Heinrich G, DeGroot LJ: Antithyroid peroxidase antibody in patients with autoimmune thyroid disease: Possible identity with antimicrosomal antibody. J Clin Endocrinol Metab 61:1001–1003, 1985.

234. Portmann L, Fitch FW, Havran W, et al: Characterization of the thyroid microsomal antigen, and its relationship to thyroid peroxidase, using monoclonal antibodies. J Clin Invest 81:1217–1224, 1988.

235. Nilsson M, Mölne J, Karlsson FA, Ericson LE: Immunoelectron microscopic studies on the cell surface localization of the thyroid microsomal antigen. Mol Cell Endocrinol 53:177–186, 1987.

236. Elisei R, Mariotti S, Swillens S, et al: Studies with recombinant autoepitopes of thyroid peroxidase: Evidence suggesting an epitope shared between the thyroid and the gastric parietal cell. Autoimmunity 8:65–70, 1990.

237. Virion A, Dème D, Pommier J, Nunez J: The role of iodide and free diiodotyrosine in enzymatic and nonenzymatic thyroid hormone synthesis. Eur J Biochem 118:239–245, 1981.

238. Taurog A: Thyroid peroxidase–catalyzed iodination of thyroglobulin: Inhibition by excess iodide. Arch Biochem Biophys 139:212–220, 1970.

239. Pommier J, Dème D, Nunez J: Effect of iodide concentration on thyroxine synthesis catalyzed by thyroid peroxidase. Eur J Biochem 37:406–414, 1973.

240. Davidson B, Neary JT, Strout HV, et al: Evidence for a thyroid peroxidase–associated "active iodine" species. Biochim Biophys Acta 522:318–326, 1978.

241. Lamas L, Dorris ML, Taurog A: Evidence for a catalytic role of peroxidase in the conversion of diiodotyrosine to thyroxine. Endocrinology 90:1417–1426, 1972.

242. Dème D, Pommier J, Nunez J: Kinetics of thyroglobulin iodination and of hormone synthesis catalyzed by thyroid peroxidase. Role of iodide in the coupling reaction. Eur J Biochem 70:435–440, 1976.

243. Taurog A, Nakashima T: Dissociation between degree of iodination and iodoamino acid distribution in thyroglobulin. Endocrinology 103:632–640, 1978.

244. Dème D, Fimiani E, Pommier J, Nunez J: Free diiodotyrosine effects on protein iodination and thyroid hormone synthesis catalyzed by thyroid peroxidase. Eur J Biochem 51:329–336, 1975.

245. Taurog A, Dorris ML, Lamas L: Comparison of lactoperoxidase- and thyroid peroxidase–catalyzed iodination and coupling. Endocrinology 94:1286–1294, 1974.

246. Dème D, Pommier J, Nunez J: Specificity of thyroid hormone synthesis. The role of thyroid peroxidase. Biochim Biophys Acta 540:73–82, 1978.

247. Virion A, Pommier J, Nunez J: Dissociation of thyroglobulin iodination and hormone synthesis catalyzed by peroxidases. Eur J Biochem 102:549–554, 1979.

248. Taurog A, Dorris M: Myeloperoxidase catalyzed iodination and coupling. Arch Biochem Biophys 296:239–246, 1992.

249. Ahn CS, Rosenberg IN: Iodine metabolism in thyroid slices: Effects of TSH, dibutyrryl cyclic 3,5′-AMP, NaF and prostaglandin E1. Endocrinology 86:396–405, 1970.

250. Nagasaka A, DeGroot LJ, Hati R, Liu C: Studies on the biosynthesis of thyroid hormone: Reconstruction of a defined in vitro iodinating system. Endocrinology 88:486–490, 1971.

251. Virion A, Courtin F, Dème D, et al: Spectral characteristics and catalytic properties of thyroid peroxidase-H_2O_2 compounds in the iodination and coupling reactions. Arch Biochem Biophys 242:41–47, 1985.

252. Niepomniszcze H, Targovnik HM, Gluzman BE, Curutchet P: Abnormal H_2O_2 supply in the thyroid of a patient with goiter and iodine organification defect. J Clin Endocrinol Metab 65:344–348, 1987.

253. Björkman U, Ekholm R, and Denef J-F: Cytochemical localization of hydrogen peroxide in isolated thyroid follicles. J Ultrastruct Res 71:105–115, 1981.

254. Björkman U, Ekholm R: Generation of H_2O_2 in isolated porcine thyroid follicles. Endocrinology 115:392–398, 1984.

255. Mitzukami Y, Matsubara F, Matsukawa S: Cytochemical localization of peroxidase and hydrogen peroxide–producing NAD(P)H-oxidase in thyroid follicular cells of propylthiouracil-treated rats. Histochemistry 82:263–268, 1985.

256. DeGroot LJ, Niepomniszcze H: Biosynthesis of thyroid hormones: Basic and clinical aspects. Metabolism 26:665–718, 1977.

257. Virion A, Michot JL, Dème D, et al: NADPH-dependent H_2O_2 generation and peroxidase activity in thyroid particulate fraction. Mol Cell Endocrinol 36:95–105, 1984.

258. Dupuy C, Kaniewski J, Dème D, et al: NADPH-dependent H_2O_2 generation catalyzed by thyroid plasma membranes. Studies with electron scavengers. Eur J Biochem 185:597–603, 1989.

259. Dupuy C, Virion A, Ohayon R, et al: Mechanism of hydrogen peroxide formation catalyzed by NADPH oxidase in thyroid plasma membrane. J Biol Chem 266:3739–3743, 1991.

260. Dème D, Virion A, Hammou NA, Pommier J: NADPH-dependent generation of H_2O_2 in a thyroid particulate fraction requires Ca^{2+}. FEBS Lett 186:107–110, 1985.

261. Nakamura Y, Ohtaki S, Makino R, et al: Superoxide anion is the initial product in the hydrogen peroxide formation catalyzed by NADPH oxidase in porcine thyroid plasma membrane. J Biol Chem 264:4759–4761, 1989.

262. Nakamura Y, Makino R, Tanaka T, et al: Mechanism of H_2O_2 production in porcine thyroid cells: Evidence for intermediary formation of superoxide anion by NADPH-dependent H_2O_2-generating machinery. Biochemistry 30:4880–4886, 1991.

263. Raspé E, Laurent E, Corvilain B, et al: Control of the intracellular Ca^{2+}-concentration and the inositol phosphate accumulation in dog thyrocyte primary culture: evidence for different kinetics of Ca^{2+}-phosphatidylinositol cascade activation and for involvement in the regulation of H_2O_2 production. J Cell Physiol 146:242–250, 1991.

264. Corvilain B, Van Sande J, Laurent E, Dumont J: The H_2O_2-generating system modulates protein iodination and the activity of the pentose phosphate pathway in dog thyroid. Endocrinology 128:779–785, 1991.

265. Björkman U, Ekholm R: Hydrogen peroxide generation and its regulation in FRTL-5 and porcine thyroid cells. Endocrinology 130:393–399, 1992.

266. Lippes HA, Spaulding SW: Peroxide formation and glucose oxidation in calf thyroid slices: Regulation by protein kinase-C and cytosolic free calcium. Endocrinology 118:1306–1311, 1986.

267. Takasu N, Yamada T, Shimizu Y, et al: Generation of hydrogen peroxide in cultured porcine thyroid cells: Synergistic regulation by cytoplasmic free calcium and protein kinase C. J Endocrinol 120:503–508, 1989.

268. Ohtaki S, Nakagawa H, Kimura S, Yamazaki I: Analyses of catalytic intermediates of hog thyroid peroxidase during its iodinating reaction. J Biol Chem 256:805–810, 1981.

269. Courtin F, Dème D, Virion A, et al: The role of lactoperoxidase-H_2O_2 compounds in the catalysis of thyroglobulin iodination and thyroid hormone synthesis. Eur J Biochem 124:603–609, 1982.

270. Nunez J, Pommier J: Formation of thyroid hormones. Vitam Horm 39:175–229, 1982.

271. Nunez J: Thyroid hormones: Mechanism of phenoxyether formation. Methods Enzymol 107:476–488, 1984.

272. Nakamura M, Yamazaki I, Nakagawa H, Ohtaki S: Steady-state kinetics and regulation of thyroid peroxidase–catalyzed iodination. J Biol Chem 258:3837–3842, 1983.

273. Nakamura M, Yamazaki I, Nakagawa H, et al: Iodination and oxidation of thyroglobulin catalyzed by thyroid peroxidase. J Biol Chem 259:359–364, 1984.

274. Magnusson RP, Taurog A, Dorris M: Mechanism of iodide-dependent catalytic activity of thyroid peroxidase and lactoperoxidase. J Biol Chem 259:197–205, 1984.

275. Magnusson RP, Taurog A, Dorris ML: Mechanisms of thyroid peroxidase- and lactoperoxidase-catalyzed reactions involving iodide. J Biol Chem 259:13783–13790, 1984.

276. Cahnmann HJ, Pommier J, Nunez J: Spatial requirements for coupling of iodotyrosine residues to form thyroid hormones. Proc Natl Acad Sci USA 74:5333–5335, 1977.

277. Taurog A: Hormone synthesis: Thyroid iodine metabolism. In Braverman LE, and Utiger RD (eds): Werner and Ingbar's The Thyroid: A Fundamental and Clinical Text. Philadelphia, JB Lippincott Co, 1991, pp 51–97.

278. Engler H, Taurog A, Dorris ML: Preferential inhibition of thyroxine and 3,5,3′-triiodothyronine formation by propylthiouracil and methylmercaptoimidazole in thyroid peroxidase–catalyzed iodination of thyroglobulin. Endocrinology 110:190–197, 1982.

279. Engler H, Taurog A, Luthy C, Dorris ML: Reversible and irreversible inhibition of thyroid peroxidase–catalyzed iodination by thioureylene drugs. Endocrinology 112:86–95, 1983.

280. Davidson B, Soodak M, Neary JT, et al: The irreversible inactivation of thyroid peroxidase by methylmercaptoimidazole, thiouracil, and propylthiouracil in vitro and its relationship to in vivo findings. Endocrinology 103:871–882, 1978.

281. Nakashima T, Taurog A, Riesco G: Mechanism of action of thioureylene antithyroid drugs: Factors affecting intrathyroidal metabolism of propylthiouracil and methimazole in rats. Endocrinology 103:2187–2197, 1978.

282. Taurog A, Dorris M, Guziec, FS Jr: Metabolism of ^{35}S- and ^{14}C-labeled 1-methyl-2-mercaptoimidazole in vitro and in vivo. Endocrinology 124:30–39, 1989.

283. Taurog A, Dorris M, Guziec FS Jr, Uetrecht, JP: Metabolism of ^{35}S- and ^{14}C-labeled propylthiouracil in a model in vitro system containing thyroid peroxidase. Endocrinology 124:3030–3037, 1989.

284. Taurog A, Dorris M: A reexamination of the proposed inactivation of thyroid peroxidase in the rat thyroid by propylthiouracil. Endocrinology 124:3038–3042, 1989.

285. Raby C, Lagorce J-F, Jambut-Absil A-C, et al: The mechanism of action of synthetic antithyroid drugs: Iodine complexation during oxidation of iodide. Endocrinology:1683–1691, 1990.

286. Wolff J: Excess iodide inhibits the thyroid by multiple mechanisms. In Ekholm R, Kohn LD, Wollman SH (eds): Control of the Thyroid Gland. New York, Plenum, 1989, pp 211–244.

287. Chiraseveenuprapund P, Rosenberg IN: Effects of hydrogen peroxide–generating systems on the Wolff-Chaikoff effect. Endocrinology 109:2095–2101, 1981.

288. Corvilain B, Van Sande J, Dumont J: Inhibition by iodide of iodide binding to proteins: The "Wolff-Chaikoff" effect is caused by inhibition of H_2O_2 generation. Biochem Biophys Res Commun 154:1287–1292, 1988.

289. Ericson LE, Engström G: Quantitative electron microscopic studies on exocytosis and endocytosis in the thyroid follicle cell. Endocrinology 103:883–892, 1978.

289a. Rousset B: Endocytose et transport intracellulaire de la thyroglobuline. In Leclerc J, Orgiazzi J, Rousset B, et al: La Thyroïde: De la Physiologie Cellulaire aux Dysfonctions. Paris, Expansion Scientifique Française, 1992, pp 54–59.

290. Ketelbant-Balasse P, Rodesch F, Neve P, Pasteels JM: Scanning electron microscope observations of apical surfaces of dog thyroid cells. Exp Cell Res 79:111–119, 1973.

291. Bernier-Valentin F, Kostrouch Z, Rabilloud R, et al: Coated vesicles from thyroid cells carry iodinated thyroglobulin molecules. First indication for an internalization of the thyroid prohormone via a mechanism of receptor-mediated endocytosis. J Biol Chem 265:17373–17380, 1990.

292. Scheel G, Herzog V: Mannose-6-phosphate receptor in porcine thyroid follicle cells. Localization and possible implications for the intracellular transport of thyroglobulin. Eur J Cell Biol 49:140–148, 1989.

292a. Lemansky P, Herzog V: Endocytosis of thyroglobulin is not mediated by mannose-6-phosphate receptors in thyrocytes. Evidence for low-affinity-binding sites operating in the uptake of thyroglobulin. Eur J Biochem 209:111–119, 1992.

293. Cortese F, Schneider AB, Salvatore G: Isopycnic centrifugation of thyroid iodoproteins: Selectivity of endocytosis. Eur J Biochem 68:121–129, 1976.

294. Van den Hove MF, Couvreur M, DeVisscher M, Salvatore G: A new mechanism for the reabsorption of thyroid iodoproteins: Selective fluid pinocytosis. Eur J Biochem 122:415–422, 1982.

294a. Kostrouch Z, Bernier-Valentin F, Munari-Silem Y, et al: Thyroglobulin molecules internalized by thyrocytes are sorted in early endosomes and partially recycled back to the follicular lumen. Endocrinology 132:2645–2653, 1993.

295. Herzog V: Trancytosis in thyroid cells. J Cell Biol 97:607–617, 1983.

296. Consiglio E, Salvatore G, Rall JE, Kohn LD: Thyroglobulin interactions with thyroid plasma membranes. The existence of specific receptors and their potential role. J Biol Chem 254:5065–5076, 1979.

297. Consiglio E, Shifrin S, Yavin Z, et al: Thyroglobulin interactions with thyroid membranes. Relationship between receptor recognition of N-acetylglucosamine residues and the iodine content of thyroglobulin preparations. J Biol Chem 256:10592–10599, 1981.

297a. Miquelis R, Alquier C, Monsigny M: The N-acetylglucosamine receptor of the thyroid. Binding characteristics, partial characterization and potential role. J Biol Chem 262:15291–15298, 1987.

297b. Thibault V, Blanck O, Courageot J, et al: The N-acetylglucosamine-specific receptor of the thyroid: Purification, further characterization, and expression patterns on normal and pathological glands. Endocrinology 132:468–476, 1993.

298. Shifrin S, Kohn LD: Binding of thyroglobulin to bovine thyroid membranes. Role of specific amino acids in receptor recognition. J Biol Chem 256:10600–10605, 1981.

299. Shifrin S, Consiglio E, Laccetti P, et al: Bovine thyroglobulin. 27 S iodoprotein interactions with thyroid membranes and formation of a 27 S iodoprotein in vitro. J Biol Chem 257:9539–9547, 1982.

300. Selmi S, Rousset B: Identification of two subpopulations of thyroid lysosomes: Relation to the thyroglobulin proteolytic pathway. Biochem J 253:523–532, 1988.

301. Kostrouch Z, Munari-Silem Y, Rajas F, et al: Thyroglobulin internalized by thyrocytes passes through early and late endosomes. Endocrinology 129:2202–2211, 1991.

302. Von Figura K, Hasilik A: Lysosomal enzymes and their receptors. Ann Rev Biochem 55:167–193, 1986.

303. Dunn AD, Dunn JT: Thyroglobulin degradation by thyroidal proteases: Action of purified cathepsin D. Endocrinology 111:280–289, 1982.

304. Nakagawa H, Ohtaki S: Partial purification and characterization of two thiol proteases from hog thyroid lysosomes. Endocrinology 115:1433–1439, 1984.

305. Nakagawa H, Ohtaki S: Thyroxine (T_4) release from thyroglobulin and its T_4-containing peptide by thyroid thiol proteases. Endocrinology 116:33–40, 1985.

306. Dunn AD, Dunn JT: Cysteine proteinases from human thyroids and their actions on thyroglobulin. Endocrinology 123:1089–1097, 1988.

307. Dunn AD, Crutchfield HE, Dunn JT: Proteolytic processing of thyroglobulin by extracts of thyroid lysosomes. Endocrinology 128:3073–3080, 1991.

308. Rousset B, Selmi S, Bornet H, et al: Thyroid hormone residues are released from thyroglobulin with only limited alteration of the thyroglobulin structure. J Biol Chem 264:12620–12626, 1989.

309. Dunn AD: Stimulation of thyroidal thiol endopeptidases by thyrotropin. Endocrinology 114:375–382, 1984.

310. Tokuyama T, Yoshinari M, Rawitch AB, Taurog A: Digestion of thyroglobulin with purified thyroid lysosomes: Preferential release of iodoamino acids. Endocrinology 121:714–721, 1987.

311. Rousset B, Selmi S, Alquier C, et al: In vitro studies of the thyroglobulin degradation pathway: Endocytosis and delivery of thyroglobulin to lysosomes, release of thyroglobulin cleavage products—iodotyrosines and iodothyronines. Biochimie 71:247–262, 1989.

312. Tietze F, Kohn LD, Kohn AD, et al: Carrier-mediated transport of monoiodotyrosine out of thyroid cell lysosomes. J Biol Chem 264:4762–4765, 1989.

313. Andersson HC, Kohn LD, Bernardini I, et al: Characterization of lysosomal monoiodotyrosine transport in rat thyroid cells. Evidence for transport by system h. J Biol Chem 265:10950–10954, 1990.

314. Harper GS, Kohn LD, Bernardini I, et al: Thyrotropin stimulation of lysosomal tyrosine transport in rat FRTL-5 thyroid cells. J Biol Chem 263:9320–9325, 1988.

315. Goswami A, Rosenberg I: Characterization of a flavoprotein iodotyrosine deiodinase from bovine thyroid. Flavin nucleotide binding and oxidation-reduction properties. J Biol Chem 254:12326–12330, 1979.

316. Goswami A, Rosenberg I: Ferredoxin and ferredoxin reductase activities in bovine thyroid. Possible relationship to iodotyrosine deiodinase. J Biol Chem 256:893–899, 1981.

317. Fisher DA, Oddie TH, Thompson CS: Thyroidal thyronine and non-thyronine iodine secretion in euthyroid subjects. J Clin Endocrinol Metab 33:647–652, 1971.

318. Chopra IJ, Solomon DH, Chopra U, et al: Pathways of metabolism of thyroid hormones. In Greep RO (ed): Recent Progress in Hormone Research, Vol 34. New York, Academic Press, 1978, pp 521–567.

319. Greer MA, Haibach H: Thyroid secretion. In Greer MA, Solomon DH (eds): Handbook of Physiology, Vol 3. Washington, DC, American Physiological Society, 1974, pp 135–146.

320. Erickson VJ, Cavalieri RR, Rosenberg LL: Phenolic and nonphenolic ring iodothyronine deiodinases from rat thyroid gland. Endocrinology 108:1257–1264, 1981.

321. Ishii H, Inada M, Tanaka K, et al: Triiodothyronine generation from thyroxine in human thyroid: Enhanced conversion in Graves' thyroid tissue. J Clin Endocrinol Metab 52:1211–1217, 1981.

322. Laurberg P, Boye N: Outer and inner ring monodeiodination of thyroxine by dog thyroid and liver: A comparative study using a particulate cell fraction. Endocrinology 110:2124–2130, 1982.

323. Wu SY, Reggio R, Florsheim WH: Characterization of thyrotropin-induced increase in iodothyronine monodeiodinating activity in mice. Endocrinology 116:901–908, 1985.

324. Laurberg P: Mechanisms governing the relative proportions of thyroxine and 3,5,3'-triiodothyronine in thyroid secretion. Metabolism 33:379–392, 1984.

325. Erickson VJ, Cavalieri RR, Rosenberg LL: Thyroxine-5'-deiodinase of rat thyroid, but not that of liver, is dependent on thyrotropin. Endocrinology 111:434–440, 1982.

326. Ishii H, Inada M, Tanaka K, et al: Induction of outer and inner ring monodeiodinases in human thyroid gland by thyrotropin. J Clin Endocrinol Metab 57:500–505, 1983.

327. Wu SY: Thyrotropin-mediated induction of thyroidal iodothyronine monodeiodinases in the dog. Endocrinology 112:417–424, 1983.

328. Melander A, Ranklev E, Sundler F, Westgren U: Beta$_2$-adrenergic stimulation of thyroid hormone secretion. Endocrinology 97:332–336, 1975.

329. Ahrén B, Alumets J, Ericsson M, et al: VIP occurs in intrathyroidal nerves and stimulates thyroid hormone secretion. Nature 287:343–345, 1980.

330. Becks GP, Eggo MC, Burrow GN: Regulation of differentiated thyroid function by iodide: Preferential inhibitory effect of excess iodide on thyroid hormone secretion in sheep thyroid cell cultures. Endocrinology 120:2569–2575, 1987.

35

Thyroid Regulation

J. E. DUMONT
G. VASSART

Four major biological variables are regulated in the thyrocyte as in any other cell type: function, cell size, cell number, and differentiation. The first three variables are quantitative and the latter is qualitative. In this chapter we consider the factors involved in these controls in physiology and in pathology, the receptors and main regulatory cascades through which these factors exert their effects, and the regulated processes, which are function, proliferation and cell death, gene expression, and differentiation. Whenever possible, we describe what is known in humans.

THYROID REGULATORY FACTORS
(Table 35–1)

In Physiology

The two main factors that control the physiology of the thyroid are the requirement of thyroid hormones and the supply of its main and specialized substrate iodide. Thyroid hormone plasma levels and action are monitored by the hypothalamic supraoptic nuclei and mainly by the thyrotrophs of the anterior lobe of the pituitary, where they exert a negative feedback. The corresponding homeostatic control is expressed by the thyroid-stimulating hormone (TSH, thyrotropin). Iodide supply is monitored in part through its effects on the plasma level of thyroid hormone but mainly in the thyroid itself, where it depresses various aspects of thyroid function and the response of the thyrocyte to TSH. These two major physiological regulators control the function and the size of the thyroid—TSH positively, iodide negatively.[1-4] Although the thyroid contains receptors for thyroid hormones and a direct effect of these hormones on the thyrocytes would make sense,[5] there is as yet little evidence that such a control plays a role in physiology. Luteinizing hormone (LH) and human chorionic gonadotropin (hCG) at high levels directly stimulate the

thyroid, and this effect accounts for the elevated thyroid activity in pregnancy.[6-8]

The thyroid gland is also influenced by various other nonspecific hormones. Hydrocortisone exerts a differentiating action in vitro. Estrogens affect the thyroid by unknown mechanisms, directly or indirectly, as exemplified in the menstrual cycle and in pregnancy. Growth hormone induces thyroid growth, but its effects are thought to be

TABLE 35–1. THYROID REGULATORY FACTORS

	FUNCTION	DIFFERENTIATION	PROLIFERATION
		Specific	
Physiological			
TSH	↑	↑	↑
LH, hCG (high levels)	↑	↑	↑
I⁻	↓	?	↓ ?
T₃T₄	?	?	?
Pathological			
TSAb	↑	↑	↑
TBAb	↓	?	↓
(TGI?)	?	?	↑ ?
		Nonspecific	
Physiological			
Hydrocortisone	0	↑	0
IGF₁	?	↑	↑
EGF	↓ /0	↓	↑
FGF	?	↓ /0	↑
TGFβ	?	↓ /0	↓
Norepinephrine	↑	0	0
PGE	↑	0	0
ATP bradykinin TRH	↑ / ↓	?	?
Pathological			
IL₁	↓	↓	↓
TNF	↓	↓	↓
IFNγ	↓	↓	↓

TSAb, Thyroid stimulating immunoglobulins; TBAb, thyroid blocking immunoglobulins; TGI, thyroid growth immunoglobulins; PGE, prostaglandin E.
↑, Stimulation; ↓, inhibition; 0, no effect.

mediated by locally produced somatomedins. Effects of locally secreted neurotransmitters and growth factors on the thyrocytes have been demonstrated in vitro and sometimes in vivo, and the presence of some of these agents in the thyroid has been ascertained. However, there is no evidence that such controls have a physiological role. The set of neurotransmitters acting on the thyrocyte and their effects vary from species to species.[9, 10] In the human, well-defined direct but short-lived responses to norepinephrine, adenosine triphosphate (ATP), adenosine, bradykinin, and thyrotropin-releasing hormone (TRH) have been observed.[10–12] Similarly, effects of insulin-like growth factor I (IGF-I), epidermal growth factor (EGF), hepatocyte growth factor (HGF), tumor growth factor (TGF), and fibroblast growth factor (FGH) have been demonstrated on thyrocytes of human and other species in vitro.[2, 10, 13, 14] The facts that the thyroid is hypertrophied in acromegaly and does not develop into a goiter in endemic goiter areas in pygmies who have no receptors for IGF-I suggest that IGF-I might have a tonic physiological role on the growth of the human thyroid.[2]

In Pathology

Pathological extracellular signals play an important role in autoimmune thyroid disease. Thyroid-stimulating antibodies (TSAb's), which bind to the TSH receptor and activate it, reproduce the stimulatory effects of TSH on the function and growth of the tissue. Their abnormal generation is responsible for the hyperthyroidism and goiter of Graves' disease. Thyroid-blocking antibodies (TBAb's) also bind to the TSH receptor but do not activate it and hence behave as competitive inhibitors of the hormone. Such antibodies are responsible for some cases of hypothyroidism in thyroiditis. Both stimulating and inhibitory antibodies induce transient hyper- or hypothyroidism in newborns of mothers with positive sera.[1] The existence of thyroid growth immunoglobulins has been hypothesized to explain the existence of Graves' disease with weak hyperthyroidism and prominent goiter. The thyroid specificity of such immunoglobulins would imply that they recognize thyroid-specific targets. However, despite many reports on the subject, convincing evidence is still lacking.[15–17] Local cytokines have been shown to influence the function, growth, and differentiation of thyrocytes in vitro and thyroid function in vivo. As they are presumably secreted in loco in autoimmune thyroid diseases, these effects might play a role in the pathology of these diseases, but this has not yet been proved.[10, 18]

REGULATORY CASCADES

The great number of extracellular signals acting through specific receptors on cells in fact control a very limited number of regulatory cascades. We first outline these cascades, indicating for each the signals that control it, then describe in more detail the specific thyroid cell features: controls by iodide and the TSH receptor.

The Cyclic AMP Cascade

The cAMP cascade in thyroid corresponds, so far as it has been studied, to the canonical model of the B-adrenergic receptor cascade (Fig. 35–1).[1] It is activated in the human thyrocyte by the TSH and the β-adrenergic and prostaglandin E receptors. These receptors are classic seven-transmembrane receptors controlling transducing guanosine triphosphate (GTP)–binding proteins. The activated G proteins belong to the G_s class activating adenylate cyclase and are constituted of a distinct α_s subunit and nonspecific β and γ monomers. The activation of a G protein corresponds to its release of guanosine diphosphate (GDP) and binding of GTP and to its dissociation into α_{GTP} and β/γ dimers. α_{sGTP} directly binds to and activates adenylate cyclase. The inactivation of the G protein follows the spontaneous, more or less rapid hydrolysis of GTP to GDP by α_s GTPase activity and the reassociation of α_{GDP} with β/γ. The effect of the receptor stimulated by agonist binding is to increase the rate of GDP release and GTP binding, thus shifting the equilibrium of the cycle toward the α_{GTP} active form. One receptor can consecutively activate several G proteins (hit and run model). A similar system negatively controls through Gi (α_iβ γ), adenylate cyclase. It is stimulated in the human thyroid by norepinephrine through α^2 receptors and perhaps by adenosine through A1 receptors. The cAMP generated by adenylate cyclase binds to the regulatory subunit of protein kinase that is blocking the catalytic subunit and releases this now-active unit. The activated released catalytic unit of protein kinase phosphorylates serines in the set of proteins containing accessible specific peptides that it recognizes. These phosphorylations through more or less complicated cascades lead to the

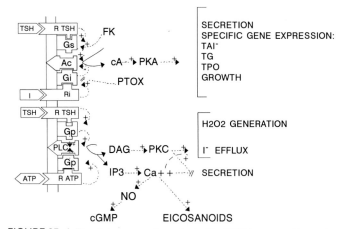

FIGURE 35–1. Regulatory cascades activated by TSH in human thyrocytes. In the human thyrocyte H_2O_2 generation is activated only by the PIP_2 cascade, i.e., by the Ca^{2+} and diacylglycerol (DAG) internal signals. In dog thyrocytes, it is activated also by the cAMP cascade. In dog thyrocytes and FRTL-5 cells TSH does not activate the PIP_2 cascade at concentrations 100 times higher than those required to elicit its other effects. Ac, adenylate cyclase; cA, 3'5'-cAMP; cGMP, 3'5'-cGMP; FK, forskolin; Gi, GTP-binding transducing protein–inhibiting adenylate cyclase; Gp, GTP-binding transducing protein–activating PIP_2 phospholipase C; Gs, GTP-binding transducing-protein activating adenylate cyclase; I, extracellular signal-inhibiting adenylate cyclase (e.g; adenosine through A1 receptors); IP_3, myoinositol 1,4,5-triphosphate; PKA, cAMP-dependent protein kinases; PKC, protein kinase C; PLC, phospholipase C; PTOX, pertussis toxin; R ATP, ATP purinergic P_2 receptor; R TSH, TSH receptor; Ri, receptor for I; TAI⁻, active transport of iodide; TG, thyroglobulin; TPO, thyroperoxidase.

observed effects of the cascade. There are two isoenzymes of cAMP-dependent kinases (I, II), the first of which is more sensitive to cAMP, but as yet no clear specificity of action of these kinases has been demonstrated.[1] In the case of the thyroid, this cascade is activated through specific receptors by TSH in all species and by norepinephrine (β receptors) and prostaglandins E in humans, with widely different kinetics: prolonged for TSH and short-lived (minutes) for norepinephrine and prostaglandins.[19-21] Other neurotransmitters have been reported to activate the cascade in thyroid tissue but not necessarily in the thyrocytes of the tissue.[12]

The Ca^{2+}-IP_3 Cascade

The Ca^{2+}-IP_3 cascade in the thyroid also corresponds, so far as it has been studied, to the canonical model of the muscarinic or α_1-adrenergic receptor–activated cascades. It is activated in the human thyrocyte by TSH, through the same receptors that stimulate adenylate cyclase and by ATP, bradykinin, and TRH—through specific receptors. In this cascade, as in the cAMP pathway, the activated receptor causes the release of GDP and the binding of GTP by the GTP-binding transducing protein (G_q) and its dissociation into α_q and $\beta\gamma$. GTP then stimulates phospholipase C. Phospholipase C hydrolyzes membrane phosphatidylinositol 4-5 biphosphate (PIP_2) into diacylglycerol and inositol 1-4-5 phosphate (IP_3). IP_3 enhances calcium release from its intracellular stores and later its influx from the extracellular medium. The rise in free ionized intracellular Ca^{2+} leads to the activation of several proteins, including calmodulin. The latter protein in turn binds to target proteins and thus stimulates them: cyclic nucleotide phosphodiesterase and most importantly calmodulin-dependent protein kinases. These kinases phosphorylate a whole set of proteins exhibiting specific peptides on their serines and threonines and thus modulate them and cause the observable effects of this arm of the cascade.[1] Calmodulin also activates constitutive nitric oxide (NO) synthase in thyrocytes. The generated NO itself enhances soluble guanylate cyclase activity in thyrocytes and perhaps in other thyroid cells and thus increases cGMP accumulation.[20] Nothing is yet known about the role of guanosine monophosphate (cGMP) in the thyroid cell.

Diacylglycerol released from PIP_2 also activates protein kinase C, or rather the family of protein kinases C, which by phosphorylating serines or threonines in specific accessible peptides in target proteins causes the effects of the second arm of the cascade.[22] It inhibits phospholipase C or its G_q thus creating a negative feedback loop. In the thyroid the PIP_2 cascade is stimulated through specific receptors by ATP, bradykinin, and TRH and in humans by TSH.[12, 23, 24] The effects of bradykinin and TRH are very short-lived. Acetylcholine, which is the main activator of this cascade in dog thyrocyte, is inactive on the human cell, although it activates nonfollicular (presumably endothelial) cells in this tissue.[12]

Other Phospholipid-Linked Cascades

In dog thyroid and in a functional rat thyroid cell line (FRTL5) cells, TSH activates PIP_2 hydrolysis weakly and at concentrations three orders of magnitude higher than those required to enhance cAMP accumulation. Of course, these effects have little biological significance. However, in dog cells at lower concentrations TSH increases the incorporation of labeled inositol and phosphate into phosphatidylinositol. Similar effects may exist in human cells, but they would be masked by the stimulation of the PIP_2 cascade. They may reflect increased turnover or increased synthesis. Increased turnover would be explained by the reported stimulation by TSH of the hydrolysis of phosphatidylinositol glycan with the release of inositol phosphate glycan as observed in pig cells.[25] No such release is observed in dog or human cells. This explanation therefore does not stand in these systems, and the possible role of inositol phosphate glycan in the mediation of TSH effects remains very doubtful. After elimination of other hypotheses, the only remaining mechanism for the increased incorporation is an increased synthesis perhaps coupled to and necessary for cell growth.[1]

Diacylglycerol can be generated by other cascades than the classic Ca^{2+} IP_3 pathway. Activation of phosphatidylcholine phospholipase D takes place in dog thyroid cells stimulated by carbamylcholine. As it is reproduced by phorbol esters, viz., stable analogues of diacylglycerol, it has been ascribed to phosphorylation of the enzyme by protein kinase C, which would represent a positive feedback loop. Although such mechanisms operate in many types of cells, their existence in human thyroid cells has not been demonstrated.[1]

The release of arachidonate from phosphatidylinositol by phospholipase A2 and the consequent generation by a substrate-driven process of prostaglandins is enhanced in various cell types directly through G protein–coupled receptors, by intracellular calcium, or by phosphorylation by protein kinase C. In dog thyroid all agents enhancing intracellular calcium concentration, including acetylcholine, also enhance the release of arachidonate and the generation of prostaglandins. In this species stimulation of the cAMP cascade by TSH inhibits this pathway. In pig thyrocytes TSH has been reported to enhance arachidonate release. In human thyroid, TSH, by stimulating the PIP_2 hydrolysis and intracellular calcium accumulation, might be expected to enhance arachidonate release and prostaglandin generation, but this has not yet been proved.[1, 19]

Regulatory Cascades Controlled by Receptor Tyrosine Kinases

Many growth factors and hormones act on their target cells by receptors that contain one transmembrane segment. They interact with the extracellular domain and activate the intracellular domain, which phosphorylates proteins on their tyrosines. Receptor activation involves in some cases a dimerization, in others a conformational change. The first step in the activation is interprotein tyrosine phosphorylation, followed by binding of various protein substrates on the peptides of the receptor, which include tyrosine phosphates. This binding through SRC homology domains (SH_2) leads to phosphorylation of these proteins on their tyrosines. In turn, this causes the sequential activation of *Ras* and *Raf* proto-oncogenes, mitogen-activated protein (MAP) kinase kinase, MAP kinase, and so on. The set of proteins phosphorylated by a receptor defines the pattern of action of this receptor. In thyroids of various species insulin, IGF-I, EGF, FGF, keratinocyte growth factor (KGF), HGF, but not platelet-derived growth factor (PDGF), activate such cascades, while TGFβ inhibits proliferation. In the human thyroid effects of insulin, IGF-I, EGF, FGF, HGF, and TGFβ have been demonstrated.[2, 26–28]

Cross-Signaling between the Cascades

Calcium, the intracellular signal generated by the PIP_2 cascade, activates calmodulin-dependent cyclic nucleotide phosphodiesterases and thus inhibits cAMP accumulation and cascade.[29] This represents a negative cross control between the PIP_2 and the cAMP cascades. Activation of protein kinase C enhances the cAMP response to TSH and inhibits the prostaglandin E response, which suggests opposite effects on the TSH and prostaglandin receptors.[30] There is no important effect of cAMP on the PIP_2 cascade. On the other hand, stimulation of protein kinase C by phorbol esters inhibits EGF action.

SPECIFIC CONTROL BY IODIDE

Iodide, the main substrate of the specific metabolism of the thyrocyte, is known to control the thyroid. Its main effects in vivo and in vitro are to decrease the response of the thyroid to TSH, to inhibit acutely its own oxidation (Wolff-Chaikoff effect), to reduce after a delay its trapping (adaptation to the Wolff-Chaikoff effect), and at high concentrations to inhibit thyroid hormone secretion (Fig. 35–2). The first effect is very sensitive, since small changes in iodine intake are sufficient to reset the thyroid system at different serum TSH levels without any other changes (e.g., thyroid hormone levels), suggesting that in physiological conditions the modulation by iodide of the thyroid response to TSH plays a major role in the negative feedback loop.[3] Iodide in vitro has also been reported to inhibit a number of metabolic steps in thyroid cells.[31, 32] These actions might be direct or indirect owing to an effect on an initial step of a regulatory cascade. Certainly iodide inhibits the cAMP cascade at the level of G_s or cyclase and the Ca^{2+}-PIP_2 cascade at the level of G_q or phospholipase C; such effects can account for the inhibition of many metabolic steps controlled by these cascades.[33–35] In one case in which this has been studied in detail, the control of H_2O_2, i.e., of iodide oxidation and thyroid hormone formation, iodide inhibited both the cAMP and the Ca^{2+}-PIP_2 cascades at their first step and the effects of the generated intracellular signaled cAMP, Ca^{2+}, and diacylglycerol on H_2O_2 generation.

The mechanism of action of iodide on all the metabolic steps besides secretion fits the "Xi" paradigm of Van Sande. These inhibitions are relieved by agents that block the trapping of iodide (e.g., perchlorate) and its oxidation (e.g., methimazole)—the Van Sande criteria. The effects are therefore ascribed to one or several postulated intracellular iodinated inhibitors Xi.[36] The identity of such signals is still unproved. At various times several candidates have been proposed for this role, e.g., thyroxine, iodinated ei-

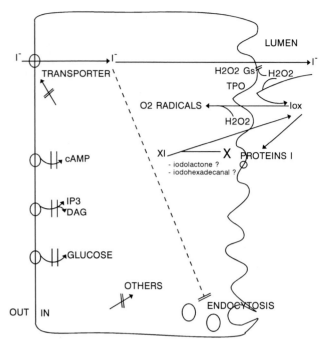

FIGURE 35–2. Effects of iodide on thyroid metabolism. All inhibitory effects of iodide, except in part the inhibition of secretion, are relieved by drugs that inhibit iodide trapping (e.g., perchlorate) or iodide oxidation (e.g., methimazole). Three possible mechanisms corresponding to this paradigm are outlined, the generation of O_2 radicals, the synthesis of an Xi compound, and the iodination of target proteins. Any of these mechanisms could account for the various steps inhibited by I^- (indicated by / /).

cosanoids (iodolactone),[37, 38] and iodohexadecanal,[39] but until now no clear proof has been reported of the role of one of these compounds in one of the inhibitions observed. It should be emphasized that iodination of the various enzymes, as well as a catalytic role of iodide in the generation of O_2 radicals (shown to be involved in the toxic effects of iodide), could account for the Van Sande criteria with no need of the Xi paradigm.[36, 40]

THE THYROID-STIMULATING HORMONE RECEPTOR

As the sensor for the main regulatory agent acting on the thyroid and the target of disease causing autoimmune reactions, the TSH receptor had been extensively studied before it was cloned. Studies from affinity-labeling experiments described the receptor quite accurately as an integral membrane protein inserted in the basolateral plasma membrane and consisting of a relatively large extracellular domain responsible for TSH binding linked to a membrane-spanning domain.[41] The number of receptors was estimated to be around 1000/cell. From its coupling to the generation of cAMP, it was classified as a member of the large family of G protein–coupled receptors interacting with G_s (see earlier). It was its belonging to this large receptor family, and the expectation that it would display significant sequence similarity with other members of the family (in particular with the FSH and LH receptors), that allowed the cloning of the TSH receptor cDNA.[42–46]

Structure of the Protein

The structure of the protein as it can be deduced from the sequence of the cDNA confirms that it belongs to the superfamily of G protein–coupled receptors (Fig. 35–3). Its 346-residue carboxyl-terminal half contains seven segments with the potential to constitute transmembrane helices, which is the hallmark of this protein family.[47] However, as predicted before cloning, it contains in addition a large amino-terminal extracellular domain, a characteristic that it shares with the other glycoprotein hormone receptors. The cDNA sequence revealed also that, contrary to most other G protein–coupled receptors, the TSH receptor (and the LH/chorionic gonadotropin and follicle-stimulating hormone [FSH] receptors as well) relies on a 20-residue signal peptide for its co-translational insertion in the membrane of the endoplasmic reticulum. The amino-terminal extracellular domain is about 398 residues in length. It is made of the loose repetition of 25 amino acid segments, referred to as *leucine repeats*. This kind of protein motif is found in a variety of intracellular as well as extracellular proteins, in which it is believed to serve in protein-protein or protein-membrane interactions.[48, 49] Six potential acceptor sites for N-glycosylation are distributed along the extracellular domain.

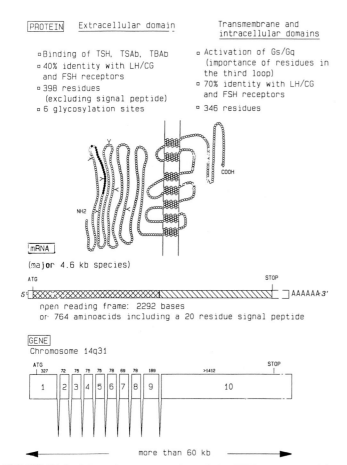

FIGURE 35–3. **Schematic representation of the TSH receptor and its chromosomal gene.** The potential N-glycosylation sites are represented by Y. The black portion of the extracellular domain represents one "leucine motif." The organization of the gene is not represented to scale except for the size of the exons, which are numbered and connected by introns schematized as V. Their sizes are indicated above individual boxes and are taken from Gross et al.[53]

The existence of structural variants of the receptor has been postulated from the cloning of several cDNA's with distinctive characteristics. In the dog, a cDNA lacking the potential to encode one leucine repeat is likely to arise from the differential splicing of exon Nr 3.[50] In humans, cDNA's coding for a truncated form of the receptor, lacking the transmembrane domains and carboxyl-terminal part, have been identified.[51, 52] From the comparison of these cDNA's with the structure of the chromosomal gene,[53] it is suggested that they originate from differential splicing and/or polyadenylation of the primary transcript (see later). Similar cDNA variants have been described for the LH/CG receptor.[54] It is presently unclear whether the corresponding truncated proteins do exist or if these cDNA's represent "noise" of the splicing/maturation pathway of gene expression.

It must be emphasized that the above description is that of a conceptual molecule derived from the mere translation of a reading frame (Fig. 35–3). Regarding the actual structure of the receptor, as it is inserted in the basolateral membrane of the thyrocyte, conflicting results have been reported. Some seem to validate the earlier suggestion that the receptor protein is made of two subunits held together by disulfide bonds. This implies maturation of the molecule by posttranslational cleavage.[55] Others support the view that the cleavage is artefactual in nature and occurs during the analysis procedure.[56] Sequence comparison of the primary structures of the glycoprotein hormone receptors reveals maximal conservation (about 70 per cent identity) within the carboxyl half of the molecules, containing the transmembrane segments. The amino-terminal extracellular domains display still highly significant similarities in the range of 40 per cent overall identity. A 50-residue insertion specific for the TSH receptor is found at the border between the extracellular domain and the first transmembrane segment. The pattern of these similarities within the glycoprotein hormone receptors immediately suggests that the extracellular domain would be responsible for the binding specificity. The carboxyl-terminal half of the molecules containing the transmembrane segments would play the role of a transducer leading to G_s protein activation. Structure function analyses of mutagenized receptors have since confirmed this hypothesis (see below).

Desensitization of some G protein–coupled receptors has been shown to involve phosphorylation of specific residues by beta-adrenergic receptor kinase (BARK)-like (homologous desensitization) or protein kinase A (heterologous desensitization) enzymes.[47] As compared with other G protein–coupled receptors, the TSH receptor contains few phosphorylatable serine or threonine residues in its intracellular loops and carboxyl-terminal tail, which probably accounts for the limited desensitization observed after stimulation by TSH.

Structure of the Gene

The gene coding for the human TSH receptor has been localized on the long arm of chromosome 14 (14q31)[57, 58] (see Fig. 35–3). It spreads over more than 60 kilobases and is organized into 10 exons displaying an interesting correlation with the protein structure.[53] The extracellular domain is encoded by a series of nine exons, each of which corresponds to one or an integer number of leucine repeats. The carboxyl-terminal half of the receptor containing the transmembrane segments is encoded by a single large exon. This is reminiscent of the fact that many G protein–coupled receptor genes are intronless. A likely evolutionary scenario derives from this gene organization[53]: The glycoprotein hormone receptor genes would have evolved from the condensation of an intronless classic G protein–coupled receptor with a mosaic gene encoding a protein with leucine repeats. Triplication of this ancestral gene and subsequent divergence led to the receptors for LH/CG, FSH, and TSH.

The gene promoter has been cloned and sequenced in humans and rats.[53, 59] It is too early to draw a precise picture of its structure and function relationships. However, the proximal promoter of the gene has characteristics of "housekeeping" genes, since it is guanine, cytosine (GC)-rich and devoid of TATA boxes; in rat it was shown to drive transcription from multiple start sites.[59]

Expression of the TSH receptor gene is largely thyroid-specific. Constructs made of a chloramphenicol acetyltransferase (CAT) reporter gene under the control of the 5′ flanking region of the rat gene show expression when transfected in FRTL5 cells and FRT cells but not in the nonthyroid HeLa or a rat liver cell line (BRL) cells.[59] If one excepts the clear demonstration of TSH receptor mRNA in fat tissue of the guinea pig,[60] reports showing its presence in lymphocytes and extraocular tissue by reverse polymerase chain reaction (PCR) are likely to correspond at best to illegitimate transcription,[61] since no functional activity has been clearly demonstrated in these cell types.

Functional Aspects

Activation by TSH

Binding to the receptor of TSH, its natural ligand, results mainly in the activation of Gs causing the stimulation of adenylyl cyclase. The EC_{50} for adenylyl cyclase activation by bovine TSH in human thyrocytes and in CHO cells transfected with the human cDNA is around 0.3 to 0.4 mU/ml.[23, 62] The dissociation constant for TSH binding (bovine TSH) expressed in biological units is close to the same value (1.5 to 1.8 mU/ml).[63] In the absence of a reliable knowledge of the bioactivity of pure intact human TSH,[64] it is difficult to translate this value in molar terms. The consensus is that it must be in the nanomolar range. The bioactivity of TSH is highly dependent on the glycosylation state of the hormone (see Ch. 12). In this respect it is interesting that artificially deglycosylated TSH behaves as a potent antagonist.[65]

In humans, but not in the dog, TSH is also able to activate phospholipase C, resulting in the accumulation of IP_3 and diacylglycerol (see earlier).[23, 24] The EC_{50} for the activation of this pathway is about one order of magnitude higher (about 5 mU/ml) than for the cAMP cascade. The ability to activate adenylyl cyclase and phospholipase C is an intrinsic property of the receptor, since the cloned molecule expressed in Chinese hamster ovary (CHO) cells displays both activities.[23] Interestingly, the cloned canine TSH receptor exhibits the same dual potential when expressed in CHO cells, even though it activates only cAMP accumulation in the dog thyrocyte. It is likely that it is the G

protein complement of cells that determines whether the receptor couples to one cascade or the other or both.

Activation by Chorionic Gonadotropin

The extensive sequence similarity between glycoprotein hormones and observations of hyperthyroidism in molar pregnancies led to the concept that LH/CG could stimulate the TSH receptor (for recent references, see ref. 8). Although the issue is still controversial, a detailed analysis of TSH and thyroid hormone levels during pregnancy suggests that physiological levels of CG can activate the thyroid.[6]

Activation by Autoantibodies

Autoantibodies found in Graves' disease and some idiopathic myxoedema can stimulate (TSAb) or block (TBAb) TSH receptor, respectively (see Ch. 43). On slices of human thyroid tissue, under the conditions tested, TSAb's have been found to stimulate only the cAMP cascade with no effect on phospholipase C activation.[66] However, experiments with the recombinant human TSH receptor expressed in CHO cells have shown that potent TSAb preparations are capable of activating both cascades, demonstrating that binding of TSH or TSAb's results in similar conformational changes within the TSH receptor.[67]

Structure-Function Relationships

It is tempting to exploit our knowledge of the primary structure of the TSH receptor and its belonging to the family of G protein–coupled receptors to try to answer the following questions: What are the domains involved in the recognition of the receptor by TSH or TSAbs? What are the mechanisms leading to the activation of the receptor and to subsequent activation of G_s? Before doing so, it is appropriate to summarize briefly what has been learned from the study of other G protein–coupled receptors and in particular from the adrenergic receptors.[47] The interaction between the ligand and the receptor takes place within the hydrophobic slit provided in the plasma membrane by the seven transmembrane alpha helices. Key hydrophilic residues of some of these helices are implicated in the actual binding: e.g., the Asp^{113} residue of the β-adrenergic receptor (or the homologue in the other receptors for charged amines) interacts with the amino group of norepinephrine. A still undefined change in conformation induced by the binding of agonists triggers activation of $G\alpha_s$. Residues of the amino and carboxyl portions of the third intracellular loop are known to play a crucial role in this interaction with G_s.

Considering their common evolutionary origin and extensive sequence similarities, the TSH receptor and the adrenergic receptor are likely to share basic mechanisms implicated in their activation. However, one faces the problem of the disproportion of the ligands. The huge dimeric TSH obviously cannot fit within the hydrophobic slit of the TSH receptor. Despite extensive site-directed mutagenesis studies,[68–80] the problem is still open. Domain-swapping experiments in which the extracellular domains of the LH/CG and TSH receptors were exchanged demonstrated clearly that the extracellular domain is responsible for the binding of the hormone.[78, 79] Since the chimeric receptors were competent for adenylyl cyclase stimulation, these experiments demonstrate also that whatever the mechanism of receptor activation, it is compatible with the exchange of the extracellular domain and hormone complex. Attempts to identify the hormone-binding domain on a few residues have been unsuccessful, the conclusion being that binding of TSH must involve large portions of tertiary structure. Nevertheless, TSH receptor–LH/CG receptor chimeric constructs led to the identification of short segments of the extracellular domain of the TSH receptor[78, 79] that take part in the interaction. The exact role of carbohydrate chains in the function of the receptor awaits further extension of site-directed mutagenesis experiments[77] to include mutation of each residues in the six potential acceptor sites for N-glycosylation.

The identification of the binding sites of TSAbs to the receptor (see Ch. 43) is an example of the difficulties of dealing with discontinuous epitopes.[81] A fair summary is that some epitopes implicated in Graves' disease can be separated from regions involved in the binding of TSH and that TSAbs seem to be heterogenous in their recognition sites.[76, 82]

Identification of the segments or residues of the receptor responsible for interaction with G_s or with its activation has been made difficult by the great sensitivity of the receptor to mutation of individual residues or segments of its intracellular loops. In agreement with results obtained with the adrenergic receptors, a detailed site-directed mutagenesis study indicated an important role for the carboxyl-terminal portion of the third intracellular loop.[72, 80] Recent data suggest that Ala[623] in this region would play a role in the coupling of the receptor to G_q, as its mutation to Glu or Lys in the rat receptor destroys its ability to stimulate the Ca^{2+}-IP_3 pathway, leaving intact stimulation of adenylyl cyclase.[83]

CONTROL OF THYROID FUNCTION

Thyroid Hormone Synthesis

Thyroid hormone synthesis requires the uptake of iodide by active transport, thyroglobulin biosynthesis, oxidation and binding of iodide to thyroglobulin, and, within the matrix of this protein, oxidative coupling of two iodotyrosines into iodothyronines. All these steps are regulated by the cascades just described.

Iodide Transport

Iodide is actively transported against the electrical gradient at the basal membrane of the thyrocyte and diffuses by a specialized channel from the cell to the lumen at the apical membrane. The opposite fluxes of iodide, from the lumen to the cell and from the cell to the outside, are generally considered to be passive and nonspecific. At least three types of control have been demonstrated[31, 32, 84]:

1. A rapid and transient stimulation of iodide efflux by TSH in vivo that might reflect a general increase in membrane permeability. The cascade involved is not known.

2. A rapid activation by TSH of iodide apical efflux from the cell to the lumen. This effect, which contributes to the concentration of iodide at the site of its oxidation, is mediated, depending on the species, by Ca^{2+} and/or cAMP.[85] In human cells it is mainly controlled by Ca^{2+} and therefore by the TSH effect on phospholipase C.

3. A delayed increase in the capacity (V_{max}) of the active iodide transport in response to TSH. This effect is inhibited by inhibitors of RNA and protein synthesis and is therefore ascribed to an activation of iodide transporter gene expression. However, as this transporter has not yet been cloned, this conclusion remains to be proved. This effect of TSH is reproduced by cAMP analogues in vitro and therefore is mediated by the cAMP cascade.[4] TSH enhancement of thyroid blood flow, more or less delayed depending on the species, also contributes to increase the uptake of iodide.[4] Iodine levels in the thyroid are also inversely related to blood flow.[86]

4. Iodide rapidly inhibits its own transport in vivo and in vitro. This inhibitory effect requires an intact transport and oxidation, i.e., it fulfills the criteria of an Xi effect. After several hours the capacity of the active transport mechanism is greatly impaired (adaptation to the Wolff-Chaikoff effect).[31] The mechanism of these effects is unknown but probably involves first a direct inhibition of the transport system itself (akin to the desensitization of a receptor) and later of its synthesis (akin to the down-regulation of a receptor).

Iodide Binding to Protein and Iodotyrosine Coupling

Iodide oxidation and binding to thyroglobulin and iodotyrosine coupling in iodothyronines are catalyzed by the same enzyme thyroperoxidase using H_2O_2 as a substrate.[87] The same regulations therefore apply to the two steps. H_2O_2 is generated by a still-undefined membrane system. The system is very efficient in the basal state, as little of the iodide trapped can be chased by perchlorate in vivo. Also, in vitro the amount of iodine bound to proteins mainly depends on iodide supply. Nevertheless in human thyroid in vitro stimulation of the iodination process takes place even at low concentrations of the anion, indicating that iodination is a secondary limiting step. Such stimulation is caused in all species by intracellular Ca^{2+} and therefore is a consequence of the activation of the Ca^{2+}-PIP_2 cascade. In many species phorbol esters and diacyglycerol, presumably through protein kinase C, also enhance iodination.[88] It is striking that in a species such as the human, in which TSH activates the PIP_2 cascade, cAMP does not stimulate iodination, whereas in a species (dog) in which TSH activates only the cAMP cascade, cAMP enhances iodination. Obviously in the latter species a supplementary cAMP control was necessary.[1, 88, 89]

Thyroperoxidase does not contain any obvious phosphorylation site in its intracellular tail. On the other hand, all the agents that activate iodination also activate H_2O_2 generation, and inhibition of H_2O_2 generation decreases iodination. This therefore suggests that iodination is a H_2O_2 substrate-driven process and that it is mainly controlled by H_2O_2 generation.[26, 88] Congruent with the relatively high Km of thyroperoxidase for H_2O_2, H_2O_2 is generated in disproportionate amounts with regard to the amount of iodide oxidized. Negative control of iodination by iodide (the Wolff-Chaikoff effect) is accompanied and mostly explained by the inhibition of H_2O_2 generation. This effect of I^- is relieved by perchlorate and methimazole and thus pertains to the Xi paradigm.[20, 36, 88]

Iodotyrosine coupling to iodotyrosines is catalyzed by the same system and therefore is subject to the same regulations as iodination. However, coupling requires that suitable tyrosyl groups in thyroglobulin are iodinated, i.e., that the level of iodination of the protein is sufficient. In the case of severe iodine deficiency or when thyroglubulin exceeds the iodine available, insufficient iodination of each thyroglobulin molecule will preclude iodothyronine formation whatever the activity of the H_2O_2 generating system and thyroperoxidase. On the other hand, when the iodotyrosines involved in the coupling are present, coupling is controlled by H_2O_2 concentration but independent of iodide.[87] In this case H_2O_2 control has a significance even at very low iodide concentrations.

H_2O_2 generation requires the reduced form of nicotinamide-adenine dinucleotide phosphate (NADPH) as a coenzyme and thus is accompanied by NADPH oxidation. As the activity of the pentose phosphate pathway is limited by $NADP^+$, this leads to a stimulation of this pathway. Also, excess H_2O_2 leaking back into the thyrocyte is reduced by glutathione (GSH) peroxidase and the GSSG produced is reduced by NADPH-linked GSH reductase. Thus both the generation of H_2O_2 and the disposal of excess H_2O_2 by pulling NADP reduction and the pentose pathway lead to activation of this pathway—historically one of the earliest and unexplained effects of TSH.[4, 88]

In long-term situations in vivo or in vitro the activity of the whole iodination system obviously also depends on the level of its constitutive enzymes. It is therefore not surprising that activation of the thyrocytes by the cAMP cascade increases the corresponding gene expressions while dedifferentiating treatments with EGF and phorbol esters inhibit these expressions and thus reduce the capacity and activity of the system. Apparent discrepancies in the literature about the effects of phorbol esters on iodination are mostly explained by the kinetics of these effects (acute stimulation of the system, delayed inhibition of the involved genes expression).

Thyroid Hormone Secretion

The secretion of thyroid hormone requires the endocytosis of human thyroglobulin, its hydrolysis, and the release of thyroid hormones from the cell. Thyroglobulin can be ingested by the thyrocyte by three mechanisms.[4, 90] In *macropinocytosis*, which is the first, pseudopods engulf clumps of thyroglobulin. In all species this process is triggered by the activation of the cAMP cascade and therefore by TSH. Stimulation of macropinocytosis is preceded and accompanied by an enhancement of thyroglobulin exocytosis and thus membrane surface.[4, 91–94] By *micropinocytosis*, the second process, small amounts of colloid fluid are ingested. This process does not appear to be greatly influenced by acute modulation of the regulatory cascades. It is enhanced in chronically stimulated thyroids. A third (hypothesized) process is *receptor-mediated endocytosis*; its existence is still controversial and its regulation unknown.[95, 96]

Contrary to the last named, the first two processes are not specific for the protein. They can be distinguished by the fact that macropinocytosis is inhibited by microfilament and microtubule poisons and by lowering of the temperature (below 23°C). Whatever its mechanism, endocytosis is followed by lysosomal digestion with complete hydrolysis of thyroglobulin. The main iodothyronine in thyroglobulin is thyroxine. However, during its secretion a small fraction is deiodinated by type I 5′ deiodinase to T_3, thus increasing the relative T_3 (the active hormone) secretion.[1, 4]

The free thyroid hormones are released by an unknown mechanism, which may be diffusion or transport. The iodotyrosines are deiodinated by specific desiodases and their iodide recirculated in the thyroid iodide compartments. Under acute stimulation a release (spillover) of amino acids and iodide from the thyroid is observed. A mechanism for uptake in lysosomes of poorly iodinated thryoglobulin on N-acetylglucosamine receptors and recirculation to the lumen has been proposed. Under normal physiological conditions endocytosis is the limiting step of secretion, but after acute stimulation, hydrolysis might become limiting with the accumulation of colloid droplets. Secretion by macropinocytosis is triggered by activation of the cAMP cascade and inhibited by Ca^{2+} at two levels: cAMP accumulation and cAMP action. It is also inhibited in some thyroids by protein kinase C downstream from cAMP. Thus the PIP_2 cascade negatively controls macropinocytosis.[1, 30]

The thyroid also releases thyroglobulin. As this thyroglobulin was first demonstrated by its iodine, at least part of this thyrogloblin is iodinated, thus it must originate from the colloid lumen. The release is inhibited in vitro by various metabolic inhibitors and therefore corresponds to active secretion.[5, 92] The most plausible mechanism is transcytosis from the lumen to the thyrocyte lateral membranes.[93] As for thyroid hormone, this secretion is enhanced by activation of the cAMP cascade and TSH and inhibited by Ca^{2+} and protein kinase C activation. As thyroglobulin secretion does not require its iodination, it reflects the activation state of the gland regardless of the efficiency of thyroid hormone synthesis. Thyroglobulin serum levels and their increase after TSH stimulation constitute a very useful index of the functional state of the gland when this synthesis is impaired, as in iodine deficiency, iodine metabolism congenital defects, treatment with antithyroid drugs, and the like. Regulated thyroglobulin secretion should not be confused with the release of this protein from thyroid tumors, which corresponds in large part to exocytosis of newly synthesized thyroglobulin in the extracellular space rather than in the nonexistent or disrupted follicular lumen. In inflammation or after even a mild trauma also, opening of the follicles can cause unregulated leakage of lumen thyroglobulin.

CONTROL OF THYROID-SPECIFIC GENE EXPRESSION

A positive effect of TSH on general protein synthesis has been well documented. This effect is mimicked by cAMP agonists and is part of the trophic effect of TSH on the thyrocyte. It involves stimulation of transcription and translation; however, the detailed mechanisms implicated are not known (see ref. 97 for references).

Thyroglobulin

The regulation of thyroglobulin gene expression has been studied in depth and reviewed in several publications.[97, 98] Clear evidence has been obtained for regulation by TSH via cAMP at the transcription level, with some evidence for the existence of translational control as well.[98-101] Continuous protein synthesis is required to sustain thyroglobulin gene transcription.[102] Together with the relatively long delay before stimulation by TSH or cAMP is observed (8 to 16 hours in primocultured cultured dog thyrocytes, depending on the conditions), this observation suggests that the TSH or cAMP transcriptional effects on thyroglobulin gene require synthesis of new proteins. However, provided that the thyroids have first been deprived of TSH, a rapid stimulatory effect on transcription is observed one hour after stimulation by TSH or cAMP in incubated tissue slices[102] and, following TSH administration in the rat, in vivo.[99]

It is likely that TSH or cAMP can exert effects at more than one level, depending on the differentiation state of the cell. In the fully differentiated thyrocyte, as present in vivo or in tissue slices, rapid stimulation may be achieved via a phosphorylation cascade involving pre-existing proteins. It is not clear whether de novo protein synthesis is required, since in the thyroid slices also, the protein synthesis inhibitor cycloheximide abolishes thyroglobulin gene transcription.[102] In the primocultured thyrocytes, TSH may need to bring the thyroglobulin gene and its complement of transcription factors to a state of differentiation (by mechanisms involving regulation at transcription and/or translation), on which it could exert its stimulatory action.[2] Another possibility is that one level of control is simply lost during adaptation of thyrocytes to primoculture. Coherent with this view is the observation that expression of the thyroglobulin gene is poorly controlled by TSH or cAMP in the FRTL5 cell line.[103] This immortalized rat thyroid cell line is expected to be one step further down in the scale of thyroid differentiation as compared with primocultured thyrocytes, which themselves would be less differentiated than thyroid slices or the tissue in vivo.

The 250 base pairs (bp) upstream from the transcription start contain DNA sequences implicated in both the stimulation by TSH or cAMP of thyroglobulin gene transcription[104] and elements responsible for its tissue-specific expression[104-113] (see Ch. 34). Contrary to the case in the majority of genes under rapid control by cAMP, thyroglobulin promoter does not contain target sequences for cAMP responsive element binding factor (CREB) (see Ch. 5). This fits with the relatively slow kinetics of cAMP action and with the dependence of the effect on protein synthesis. An important unanswered question is whether two transcription factors showing some specificity for expression in the thyroid (thyroid transcription factor 1 [TTF1], and Pax-8) and interacting with specific segments of the proximal gene promoter, play a role in the control of thyroglobulin gene transcription by cAMP[108, 109] (see Ch. 34). However, there is clear indication that regulation of

thyroglobulin gene transcription involves DNA segments situated further upstream. In the bovine species, an enhancer displaying thyroid-specific hypersensitivity to DNAase I has been identified between −1600 and −2000 from the CAP site.[112, 114] Gene constructs containing 2000 bp of 5′ flanking sequences of the thyroglobulin gene have been found very effective to target expression of a series of genes to the thyroid in transgenic mice.[115-117] In addition, a similarly positioned enhancer has recently been identified in humans. Whereas the bovine enhancer did not show any sensitivity to stimulation by cAMP, the human one does (V. Berg, D. Christophe et al., unpublished observation). This different behavior fits well with the observation that the human proximal promoter seems to be less efficiently controlled by cAMP than is its bovine counterpart, suggesting a different spatial organization of the regulatory segments in different species.[118]

It has recently been shown that under stimulation by TSH, a short 0.95 Kb thyroglobulin transcript accumulates in the rat thyroid. This results from differential splicing and polyadenylation of the primary transcript, yielding a protein limited to the first five exons.[119] The functional significance of this observation is not completely clear; it could mean that in conditions in which the balance of thyroid metabolism would favor hormone synthesis over iodine storage (e.g., shortage of iodine), the thyrocyte would manufacture a truncated thyroglobulin containing the major hormonogenic site at the aminoterminus (see Ch. 34) but devoid of the many nonhormonogenic tyrosines.

Thyroperoxidase

TSH has been shown to increase both thyroperoxidase enzymatic activity[120] and steady-state mRNA level in the thyrocyte of all species studied.[121-123] This effect is mimicked by cAMP analogues and by forskolin. There is still no consensus, however, whether thyroperoxidase mRNA accumulation observed after stimulation by TSH or forskolin is entirely due to transcriptional or posttranscriptional mechanisms. According to some data, no transcriptional regulation of thyroperoxidase gene expression is observed in the immortalized rat thyroid FRTL5 cell line.[122] On the contrary, in dog thyrocytes in primary culture, a clear transcriptional regulation of the gene has been demonstrated in run-on assays.[124, 125] As already stated, this difference may reflect the less differentiated phenotype of FRTL5 cells more than a true species difference. Contrary to the regulation of thyroglobulin gene, activation of thyroperoxidase gene transcription by cAMP is rapid and does not require ongoing protein synthesis.[102, 126] The thyroperoxidase gene thus behaves as most other genes under rapid control by cAMP. However, its proximal promoter region is conspicuous, as it does not contain any of the cAMP-responsive cis-acting sequences known to date (see Ch. 5). Nevertheless, it was shown that the 130 bp's 5′ flanking sequence of the gene contain targets for regulation by TSH-cAMP.[125] The TSH or cAMP-dependent interaction of transcription factors has been localized within this gene segment, which is able to confer regulation by cAMP agonists to reporter genes ligated downstream. Here also, the question remains whether thyroid transcription factor 1 (TTF-1) and/or Pax-

8, which also bind to thyroperoxidase gene promoter, have a role in the activation of the gene by cAMP or whether their role is limited to the establishment and maintenance of the differentiated phenotype of the cell[108, 127] (see Ch. 34). In keeping with this question, an enhancer with binding sites for TTF-1 has been identified 5.5 Kb upstream from the CAP site, but its role in cAMP-dependent regulation remains speculative.[128, 129]

Thyrotropin Receptor

It is generally accepted that low concentrations of TSH (<0.2 mU/ml) exert a positive control on TSH receptor number at the surface of thyrocytes, whereas high concentrations (>0.2 mU/ml) lead to partial desensitization.[130] The control of TSH receptor gene expression has been studied in the FRTL5,[131-134] the canine thyrocyte in primary culture,[135] cultured human thyrocytes,[136-138] and human thyroid cancer.[139, 140] The general conclusion emerging from these studies is the extreme robustness of TSH receptor gene expression as compared with the other markers of thyroid cell differentiation (thyroglobulin and thyroperoxidase). In the dog, levels of TSH receptor mRNA remain virtually unchanged in animals subjected for 28 days to hyperstimulation by TSH secondary to treatment with methimazole or to TSH withdrawal achieved by administration of thyroxine.[135] In the same study, the effect of TSH or forskolin has been studied on dog thyrocytes in primary culture. This experimental system has the advantage that the differentiation state of the cells can be manipulated at will: cAMP agonists maintain expression of the differentiated phenotype, whereas agents such as EGF, tetradecanoyl phorbol acetate (TPA), and serum lead to "dedifferentiation."[141] The results demonstrate that the dedifferentiating agents strongly reduce accumulation of the receptor mRNA. However, contrary to what is observed with thyroglobulin and thyroperoxidase mRNAs, the inhibition is never complete. TSH or forskolin is capable of promoting reaccumulation of the receptor message, a maximum being reached after 20 hours. As with thyroglobulin, but at variance with the thyroperoxidase gene, this stimulation requires ongoing protein synthesis.[135] Chronic stimulation of cultured dog thyrocytes by TSH for several days does not lead to an important down-regulation of the mRNA. Similar data have been obtained with human thyrocytes in primary culture.[135, 137, 138]

A negative regulation of the receptor mRNA accumulation has been observed in the immortal FRTL5 following treatment with TSH or TSAB.[131, 134] The significance of this difference with human and canine cells must probably be interpreted in the general framework of the other known differences in phenotype and regulatory behavior of this cell line as compared with primary cultured thyrocytes (see above). The effect of malignant transformation on the amounts of TSH receptor mRNA has been studied in spontaneous tumors in humans,[139, 140] in a murine transgenic model of thyroid tumor promoted by the expression of the SV40 large T oncogene,[116] and in the FRTL5 cells transformed with v-*ras*.[132] In the two last models, expression of the TSH receptor gene was suppressed: the tumor or cell growth became TSH-independent. In the transgenic animal model the loss of TSH receptor mRNA seemed to take

place gradually, with early tumors still displaying some TSH dependence for growth. In the human tumors a spectrum of phenotypes was observed. As expected, the anaplastic tumors had completely lost the receptor mRNA, as they had with those for the other markers of thyrocyte differentiation (thyroglobulin and thyroperoxidase). In papillary carcinoma variable amounts of TSH receptor mRNA were invariably found,[139] even in the tumors that had lost the capacity to express the thyroglobulin or thyroperoxidase genes.[139] These data agree well with the observations of thyrocytes in primary culture: expression of the TSH receptor gene is robust and it persists in the presence of agents (or after several steps in tumor progression) that promote extinction of the other markers of thyroid cell differentiation. This leads to the conclusion that the basic marker of the thyroid phenotype is probably the TSH receptor itself, which makes sense: the gene encoding the sensor of TSH—the major regulator of thyroid function, growth, and differentiated phenotype—is virtually constitutive in thyrocytes. From a pragmatic viewpoint, these data provide a rationale for the common therapeutic practice of suppressing TSH secretion in patients with a differentiated thyroid tumor.[142.]

CONTROL OF GROWTH AND DIFFERENTIATION

Thyroid Cell Turnover

The thyroid is constituted by thyrocytes (70 per cent), endothelial cells (20 per cent), and fibroblasts (10 per cent). In the normal adult the weight and composition of the tissue remain relatively constant. As a low but significant proliferation is demonstrated in all types of cells, it must be assumed that the generation of new cells is balanced by a corresponding rate of cell death.[2, 4, 143, 144] The resulting turnover is of the order of one per 5 to 10 years for human thyrocytes, i.e., 6 to 8 renewals in adult life, as in other species.[144] Cell population can therefore be modulated at the level of proliferation or cell death. In growth situations, i.e., either in normal development or after stimulation, the different cell types grow more or less in parallel, which implies a coordination between them.[22, 145] As TSH receptors and iodine metabolism and signaling exist only in the thyrocyte, this cell, sole receiver of the physiological information, must presumably control the other types of cells by paracrine factors such as FGF, IGF-I, NO, and the like.[2]

The Mitogenic Cascades

In the thyroid at least three distinct mitogenic pathways have been well-defined (Fig. 35–4): (1) the hormone receptor–adenylate cyclase–cAMP protein kinase system, (2) the hormone receptor–tyrosine protein kinase pathway, and (3) the hormone receptor–phospholipase C cascade.[2, 21, 146] The receptor–tyrosine kinase pathway may be subdivided into two branches; some growth factors, such as EGF, induce proliferation and repress differentiation expression; others, such as FGF or IGF-I and insulin, are either mitogenic or are necessary for the proliferation effect of

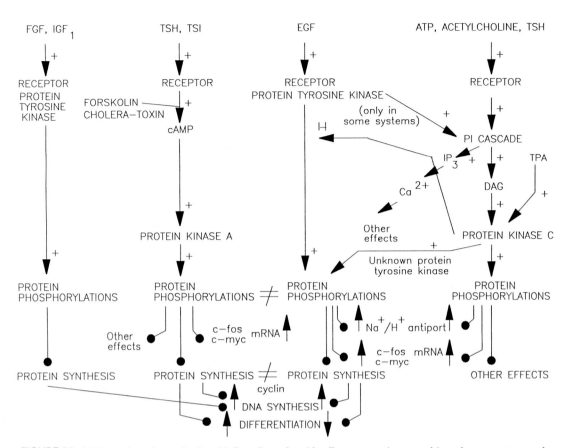

FIGURE 35–4. **Mitogenic pathways in thyroid.** Data from thyroid cell system are integrated into the present general scheme of cell proliferation cascades. In first line, known activators of various cascades in dog and human thyroid cells are shown. Various levels indicate a time sequence and postulated causal relations from initial interaction of extracellular signal with its receptor to end points: proliferation and differentiation expression. Cyclin is now called PCNA; proliferating cell nuclear antigen; DAG, diacylglycerol; IP_3, inositol (1,4,5) triphosphate; PI, phosphatidylinositol; TSI, thyroid-stimulating immunoglobulins; =, overlapping patterns; *arrow with plus*, stimulation; *arrow with bar*, inhibition; *line with dot*, time sequence; ≠, different patterns; ↑, stimulation; ↓, inhibition.

other factors without being mitogenic by themselves, but they do not inhibit differentiation expression.[147] In human[148] thyroid cells IGF-I or insulin is required for the mitogenic action of TSH or EGF but does not by itself stimulate proliferation. In FRTL5 and rat cells IGF-I is weakly stimulatory per se, whereas in pig thyroid cells it produces a strong mitogenic signal.[2, 13]

It should be noted that TSH directly stimulates proliferation while maintaining the expression of differentiation. Differentiation expression, as evaluated by iodide transport, or thyroperoxidase and thyroglobulin mRNA content or nuclear transcription, is induced by TSH, forskolin, cholera toxin, and cAMP analogues.[2] These effects are obtained in all the cells of a culture, as shown by in situ hybridization experiments.[147] They are reversible; they can be obtained either after the arrest of proliferation or during the cell division cycle.[147] Moreover, the expression of differentiation, as measured by iodide transport, is stimulated by concentrations of TSH lower than those required for proliferation.[2]

All the effects of TSH are mimicked by nonspecific modulators of the cAMP cascade, i.e., choleratoxin and forskolin (which stimulate adenylate cyclase), cAMP analogues (which activate the cAMP-dependent protein kinases), and even synergistic pairs of cAMP analogues acting on the different sites of these two kinases.[149] They are reproduced in vitro and in vivo by expression of the adenosine A2

receptor, which is constitutively activated by endogenous adenosine.[117] They are inhibited by antibodies blocking G_s.[150] There is therefore no doubt that the mitogenic and differentiating effects of TSH are mainly, and probably entirely, mediated by cAMP.[2, 148]

EGF also induces proliferation of thyroid cells from various species.[2, 148] However, the action of EGF is accompanied by a general and reversible loss of differentiation expression assessed as described above. The effects of EGF on differentiation can be dissociated from their proliferative action. Indeed, they are obtained in cells that do not proliferate in the absence of insulin and in human cells, in which the proliferative effects are weaker, or in pig cells at concentrations lower than the mitogenic concentrations.[2]

Finally, the tumor-promoting phorbol esters, the pharmacological probes of the protein kinase C system, and analogues of diacylglycerol also enhance the proliferation and inhibit the differentiation of thyroid cells (Table 35–1). These effects are transient owing to desensitization of the system by protein kinase C inactivation.[2, 148, 151] The activation of the PIP_2 cascade by physiological agents such as carbamylcholine and bradykinin in dog thyroid cells does not reproduce all the effects of phorbol esters. In particular, prolonged stimulation of the cascade inhibits rather than stimulates proliferation.[152] Thus, we cannot necessarily equate effects of phorbol esters and prolonged stimulation of the PIP_2 cascade. Similarly, prolonged enhancement of intracellular Ca^{2+} level might explain the mitogenic effects of IGF-I on FRTL5 cells but does not stimulate growth in dog thyroid cells. The dedifferentiating effects of phorbol esters do not require their mitogenic action, either. Thus the effects of TSH, EGF, and phorbol esters on differentiation expression are largely independent of their mitogenic action.[2]

In several thyroid cell models, very high insulin concentrations are necessary for growth even in the presence of EGF. We now know that this mainly reflects a requirement for IGF-I.[2, 13, 14, 153] It is interesting that in the FRTL5, as in cells from thyroid nodules, this requirement may disappear as the cells secrete their own somatomedins and thus become autonomous with regard to these hormones.[14, 154]

In the action of growth factors on receptor protein tyrosine kinase pathways the effects on differentiation expression vary depending on the species and on the factor involved: from a stimulation (e.g., insulin, and IGF II in dog and FRTL5 cells) to an absence of effect, to transitory inhibition of differentiation during growth (FGF and HGF in dog cells) and to full dedifferentiation effects (EGF in dog and human cells).[2, 148, 153, 154]

The kinetics of the induction of thymidine incorporation into nuclear DNA of dog thyroid cells is similar for TSH, forskolin, EGF, and TPA. Whatever the stimulant, there is a minimal delay of about 16 to 20 hours before the beginning of the labeling, i.e., of DNA synthesis. This is the minimal time required to prepare the necessary machinery. For the cAMP and EGF pathways the stimulatory agent has to be present during this whole prereplicative period: any interruption of the activation (e.g., by washing out the stimulatory forskolin) greatly delays the start of DNA synthesis. This explains why norepinephrine and prostaglandin E, which also activate the cAMP cascade, do not induce growth and differentiation: the rapid desensitization of their receptors does not allow a sustained rise in cAMP levels.

The three main types of mitogenic cascade, vis., growth factor protein tyrosine kinase, phorbol esters protein kinase C, TSH-cAMP cascade are fully distinct at the level of their primary intracellular signal and/or of the first signal-activated protein kinase.[2]

Iodide actually inhibits the cAMP and the Ca^{2+} phosphatidylinositol cascades and in a more delayed and chronic effect decreases the sensitivity of the thyroid to the TSH growth response. In FRTL5 cells it inhibits the TSH, IGF-I, and tumor promoters (TPA), i.e., phorbol myristate ester–induced cell proliferation; these effects are relieved, according to the general paradigm of Van Sande, by perchlorate and methimazole.[36, 155]

Steps in the Mitogenic Cascades

The phenomenology of EGF, TPA, and TSH proliferative action on dog quiescent cells has been partially elucidated.[2] Three biochemical aspects of the proliferative response occurring at different times of the prereplicative phase have been considered. The pattern of protein phosphorylation induced within minutes by TSH is reproduced by forskolin and cAMP analogues.[156] The serine-threonine phosphorylation of at least 11 proteins is increased or in-

duced. In EGF-stimulated cells, the phosphorylation of five proteins is stimulated, two of them phosphorylated on tyrosines (42k to 44k), the MAP kinases. Phorbol esters induce the phosphorylation of 19 proteins, including the tyrosine-phosphorylated MAP kinases already mentioned. There is no overlap in the patterns of protein phosphorylation induced by TSH and cAMP enhancers on the one hand and by EGF and phorbol esters on the other.[156] In particular the cAMP cascade does not involve the phosphorylation of MAP kinases.

As in other types of cells, EGF and TPA first enhance c-fos, then c-myc mRNA concentrations. On the other hand, TSH or forskolin enhances strongly but for a short period c-myc mRNA concentration and with the same kinetics as for EGF/TPA, c-fos mRNA concentration. In fact, cAMP first enhances and then decreases c-myc mRNA accumulation. This second phenomenon is akin to what has been observed in fibroblast, in which cAMP negatively regulates growth. As in fibroblasts, EGF and TPA enhance c-jun, junB and junD expression. However, as in fibroblasts, the activators of the cAMP cascade decrease c-jun expression. c-Jun is therefore not, as it has been claimed to be, a universal gene necessary for growth.[2, 157]

The pattern of proteins synthesized in response to the various proliferation stimuli has been studied.[21, 158, 159] Again two patterns emerge. TSH and forskolin induce the synthesis of at least eight proteins and decrease the synthesis of five proteins. EGF, phorbol ester, and serum induce the synthesis of at least two proteins and decrease the synthesis of two proteins. The only overlap between the two patterns concerns the decrease in the synthesis of a protein (18K), which is also reduced by EGF after proliferation has stopped. Only one protein has been shown to be synthesized in response to the three pathways: PCNA, the auxilliary protein of DNA polymerase δ. However, the kinetics of this synthesis are very different, with an early synthesis in the cAMP cascade (consistent with a role of signal) and a late S phase synthesis in the other cascades. Thus, obviously two different phenomenologies are involved in the proliferation response to TSH through cAMP on the one hand and EGF and phorbol ester, presumably through protein tyrosine phosphorylation, on the other. Although this conclusion needs to be further substantiated, it certainly suggests that the proliferation of dog thyroid cells is controlled by at least two largely independent pathways. The effects of TSH, EGF, and phorbol esters on protein synthesis can be obtained in the absence of insulin in the medium, except for the induction of PCNA synthesis; some are enhanced by insulin. Thus these effects also are not sufficient to induce mitogenesis.[2]

The studies of protein phosphorylation, proto-oncogene expression, and protein synthesis in the dog thyrocytes allow discrimination between two models of cAMP action on proliferation in this system: a direct effect on the thyrocyte or an indirect effect through the secretion and autocrine action of another growth factor. If the effect of TSH through cAMP involves such an autocrine loop, one would expect to find a faster kinetics of action of the growth factor and at least some common parts in the patterns of protein phosphorylation and protein synthesis induced by cAMP and the growth factor. The results do not support such a hypothesis, at least for the growth factors tested (Fig. 35–5).[2]

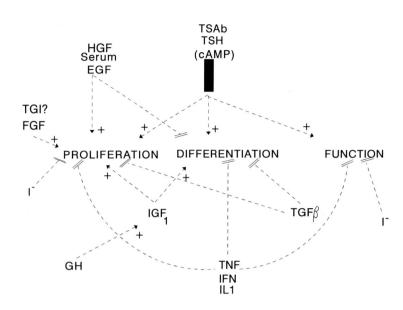

FIGURE 35–5. **Main controls of the main biological variables of the human thyrocyte.** EGF, Epidermal growth factor; FGF, fibroblast growth factor; GH, growth hormone; HGF, hepatocyte growth factor; I⁻, iodide; IGF-1, insulin-like growth factor 1; IFN, interferon; IL1, interleukin 1; TGI, thyroid growth immunoglobulins; TGFβ, tumor growth factor β; TNF, tumor necrosis factor; TSAb, thyroid-stimulating immunoglobulins. +, positive control (stimulation); −, negative control (inhibition).

Proliferation and Differentiation

The incompatibility at the cell level of a proliferation and differentiation program is commonly accepted in biology. In general, cells with a high proliferative capacity are poorly differentiated, and during development such cells lose this capacity as they progressively differentiate. Some cells even lose all potential to divide when reaching their full differentiation; this is called *terminal differentiation.* Conversely, in tumor cells there is an inverse relationship between proliferation and differentiation expression. It is therefore not surprising that in thyroid cells the general mitogenic agents and pathways, phorbol esters and the protein kinase C pathway, EGF, and in calf and porcine cells FGF, and the protein tyrosine kinase pathway induce both proliferation and the loss of differentiation expression. The effects of the cAMP cascade are in striking contrast to this general concept. Indeed TSH and cAMP induce proliferation of dog thyrocytes while maintaining differentiation expression; both proliferation and differentiation programs can be triggered by TSH in the same cells at the same time. This is by no means unique because neuroblasts in the cell cycle may simultaneously differentiate. It is tempting to relate this apparent paradox to the role and expression of proto-oncogenes in these cells. C-*fos* expression is enhanced in a great variety of cell stimulations leading to either proliferation or differentiation expression. On the other hand, if there is one generalization that could be made about proto-oncogenes, it is the dedifferentiating role of c-*myc* in all. A rapid and dramatic decrease in c-*myc* mRNA by antisense *myc* sequences induces differentiation of a variety of cell types. It is therefore striking that in the case of the thyrocyte in which the activation of the cAMP cascade leads to both proliferation and differentiation, the kinetics of c-*myc* gene appears tightly controlled. After a first phase of one hour of higher level of c-*myc* mRNA, c-*myc* expression is decreased below control levels. In this second phase, cAMP decreases c-*myc* mRNA levels, as it does in proliferation-inhibited fibroblasts. It even depresses EGF-induced expression. The first phase could be necessary for proliferation, whereas the second phase could reflect the stimulation of differentiation by TSH. This down-regulation is suppressed by cycloheximide,

which suggests the involvement of a neosynthesized or labile inhibitory protein at the transcriptional level or at the level of mRNA stabilization.[2]

REFERENCES

1. Vassart G, Dumont JE: The thyrotropin receptor and the regulation of thyrocyte function and growth. Endocr Rev 13:596–611, 1992.
2. Dumont JE, Lamy F, Roger P, Maenhaut C: Physiological and pathological regulation of thyroid cell proliferation and differentiation by thyrotropin and other factors. Physiol Rev 72:667–697, 1992.
3. Brabant G, Bergmann P, Kirsch CM, et al: Early adaptation of thyrotropin and thyroglobulin secretion to experimentally decreased iodine supply in man. Metabolism 41:1093–1096, 1992.
4. Dumont JE: The action of thyrotropin on thyroid metabolism. Vitam Horm 29:287–412, 1971.
5. Toyoda N, Nishikawa M, Horimoto M, et al: Synergistic effect of thyroid hormone and thyrotropin on iodothyronine 5'-adenosinase in FRTL-5 rat thyroid cells. Endocrinology 127:1199–1205, 1990.
6. Glinoer D, de Nayer P, Bourdoux P, et al: Regulation of maternal thyroid during pregnancy. J Clin Endocrinol Metab 71:276–287, 1990.
7. Hershman JM, Lee HY, Sugawara M, et al: Human chorionic gonadotropin stimulates iodide uptake, adenylate cyclase, and deoxyribonucleic acid synthesis in cultured rat thyroid cells. J Clin Endocrinol Metab 67:74–79, 1988.
8. Hershman JM: Role of human chorionic gonadotropin as a thyroid stimulator: editorial. J Clin Endocrinol Metab 74:258–259, 1992.
9. Ahren B: Regulatory peptides in the thyroid gland—a review on their localization and function. Acta Endocrinologica 124:225–232, 1991.
10. Dumont JE, Maenhaut C, Pirson I, et al: Growth factors controlling the thyroid gland. Baillière's Clinical Endocrinol Metab 5:727–754, 1991.
11. Van Sande J, Lamy F, Lecocq R, et al: Pathogenesis of autonomous thyroid nodules: in vitro study of iodine and adenosine 3', 5'-monophosphate metabolism. J Clin Endocrinol Metab 66:570–579, 1988.
12. Raspé E, Andry G, Dumont JE: Adenosine triphosphate, bradykinin, and thyrotropin-releasing hormone regulate the intracellular Ca²⁺ concentration and the 45Ca²⁺ efflux of human thyrocytes in primary culture. J Cell Physiol 140:608–614, 1989.
13. Tramontano D, Cushing G, Moses AC, Ingbar SH: Insulin-like growth factor–I stimulates the growth of rat thyroid cells in culture and synergizes the stimulation of DNA synthesis induced by TSH and Graves' IgG. Endocrinology 119:940–942, 1986.
14. Williams DW, Williams ED, Wyndford-Thomas D: Evidence for autocrine production of IGF-1 in human thyroid adenomas. Mol Cell Endocrinol 61:139–147, 1989.
15. Dumont JE, Roger PP, Ludgate M: Assays for the thyroid growth

immunoglobulins and their clinical implications: Methods, concepts and misconceptions. Endocr Rev 8:448–452, 1987.

16. Zakarija M, Jin S, McKenzie JM: Evidence supporting the identity in Graves's disease of thyroid-stimulating antibody and thyroid growth–promoting immunoglobulin G as assayed in FRTL5 cells. J Clin Invest 81:879–884, 1988.

17. Zakarija M, McKenzie JM: Do thyroid growth-promoting immunoglobulins exist? J Clin Endocrinol Metab 70:308–310, 1990.

18. Zakarija M, McKenzie JM: Influence of cytokines on growth and differentiated function of FRTL-5 cells. Endocrinology 125:1260–1265, 1989.

19. Van Sande J, Mockel J, Boeynaems JM, et al: Regulation of cyclic nucleotide and prostaglandin formation in normal human thyroid tissues and in autonomous nodules. J Clin Endocrinol Metab 50:776, 1980.

20. Esteves R, Van Sande J, Dumont JE: Nitric oxide as a signal in thyroid. Mol Cell Endocrinol 90:R1–R3, 1992.

21. Maenhaut C, Lefort A, Libert F, et al: Function, proliferation and differentiation of the dog and human thyrocyte. Horm Metab Res 23:51–61, 1990.

22. Munari-Silem Y, Audebet C, Rousset B: Protein kinase C in pig thyroid cells: Activation, translocation and endogenous substrate phosphorylating activity in response to phorbol esters. Mol Cell Endocrinol 54:81–90, 1987.

23. Van Sande J, Raspe E, Perret J, et al: Thyrotropin activates both the cyclic AMP and the PIP2 cascades in CHO cells expressing the human cDNA of TSH receptor. Mol Cell Endocrinol 74:R1–R6, 1990.

24. Laurent E, Mockel J, Van Sande J, et al: Dual activation by thyrotropin of the phospholipase C and cyclic AMP cascades in human thyroid. Mol Cell Endocrinol 52:273–278, 1987.

25. Jacquemin C: Glycosyl phosphatidylinositol in thyroid: Cell signalling or protein anchor? Biochimie 73:37–40, 1991.

26. Garbi C, Colletta G, Cirafici AM, et al: Transforming growth factor-β induces cytoskeleton and extracellular matrix modifications in FRTL-5 thyroid epithelial cells. Eur J Cell Biol 53:281–289, 1990.

27. Gärtner R, Bechtner G, Stübner D, Greil W: Growth regulation of porcine thyroid follicles in vitro by growth factors. Horm Metab Res 23:61–67, 1990.

28. Grübeck-Loebenstein B, Buchan G, Sadeghi R, et al: Transforming growth factor beta regulates thyroid growth. J Clin Invest 83:764–770, 1989.

29. Dumont JE, Miot F, Erneux C, et al: Negative regulation of cyclic AMP levels by activation of cyclic nucleotide phosphodiesterases: The example of the dog thyroid. Adv Cyclic Nucleotide Protein Phosphoryl Res 16:325, 1984.

30. Mockel J, Van Sande J, Decoster C, Dumont JE: Tumor promoters as probes of protein kinase C in dog thyroid cell: inhibition of the primary effects of carbamylcholine and reproduction of some distal effects. Metabolism 36:137–143, 1987.

31. Wolff J: Iodide goiter and the pharmacologic effect of excess iodide. Am J Med 47:101–124, 1991.

32. Wolff J: Congenital goiter with defective iodide transport. Endocrinol Rev 4:240, 1983.

33. Bray GA: Increased sensitivity of the thyroid in iodine-depleted rats to the goitrogenic effects of thyrotropin. J Clin Invest 47:1640–1647, 1968.

34. Cochaux P, Van Sande J, Swillens S, Dumont JE: Iodide-induced inhibition of adenylate cyclase activity in horse and dog thyroid. Eur J Biochem 170:435–442, 1987.

35. Laurent E, Mockel J, Takazawa K, et al: Stimulation of generation of inositol phosphates by carbamoylcholine and its inhibition by phorbol esters and iodide in dog thyroid cells. Biochem J 263:795–801, 1989.

36. Van Sande J, Grenier G, Willems C, Dumont JE: Inhibition by iodide of the activation of the thyroid cyclic 3′, 5′-AMP system. Endocrinology 96:781–786, 1975.

37. Boeynaems JM, Hubbard WC: Transformation of arachidonic acid into an iodolactone by the rat thyroid. J Biol Chem 255:9001–9004, 1980.

38. Dugrillon A, Bechtner G, Uedelhoven WM, et al: Evidence that an iodolactone mediates the inhibitory effect of iodide on thyroid cell proliferation but not on adenosine 3′, 5′-monophosphate formation. Endocrinology 127:337–343, 1990.

39. Pereira A, Braekman JC, Dumont JE, Boeynaems JM: Identification of a major iodolipid from the horse thyroid gland as 2-iodohexadecanal. J Biol Chem 265:17018–17025, 1990.

40. Many MC, Mestdagh C, Van Den Hove MF, Denef JF: In vitro study of acute toxic effects of high iodide doses in human thyroid follicles. Endocrinology 131:621–630, 1992.

41. Rees Smith B, McLachlan SM, Furmaniak J: Autoantibodies to the thyrotropin receptor. Endocr Rev 9:106–121, 1988.

42. Libert F, Lefort A, Gerard C, et al: Cloning, sequencing and expression of the human thyrotropin (TSH) receptor: Evidence for binding of autoantibodies. Biochem Biophys Res Commun 165:1250–1255, 1989.

43. Parmentier M, Libert F, Maenhaut C, et al: Molecular cloning of the thyrotropin receptor. Science 246:1620–1622, 1989.

44. Misrahi M, Loosfelt H, Atger M, et al: Cloning, sequencing and expression of human TSH receptor. Biochem Biophys Res Commun 166:394–403, 1990.

45. Nagayama Y, Kaufman KD, Seto P, Rapoport B: Molecular cloning, sequence and functional expression of the cDNA for the human thyrotropin receptor. Biochem Biophys Res Commun 165:1184–1190, 1989.

46. Frazier AL, Robbins LS, Stork PJ, et al: Isolation of TSH and LH/CG receptor cDNAs from human thyroid: Regulation by tissue specific splicing. Mol Endocrinol 4:1264–1276, 1990.

47. Raymond JR, Hnatowich M, Lefkowitz RJ, Caron MG: Adrenergic receptors. Models for regulation of signal transduction processes. Hypertension 15:119–131, 1990.

48. McFarland KC, Sprengel R, Phillips HS, et al: Lutropin-choriogonadotropin receptor: An unusual member of the G protein-coupled receptor family. Science 245:494–499, 1989.

49. Roth GJ: Developing relationships: Arterial platelet adhesion, glycoprotein Ib, and leucine-rich glycoproteins. Blood 77:5–19, 1991.

50. Libert F, Parmentier M, Maenhaut C, et al: Molecular cloning of a dog thyrotropin (TSH) receptor variant. Mol Cell Endocrinol 68:R15–R17, 1990.

51. Takeshita A, Nagayama Y, Fujiyama K, et al: Molecular cloning and sequencing of an alternatively spliced form of the human TSH receptor transcript. Biochem Biophys Res Commun 188:1214–1219, 1992.

52. Graves PN, Tomer Y, Davies TF: Cloning and sequencing of a 1.3 KB variant of human thyrotropin receptor mRNA lacking the transmembrane domain. Biochem Biophys Res Commun 187:1135–1143, 1992.

53. Gross B, Misrahi M, Sar S, Milgrom E: Composite structure of the human thyrotropin receptor gene. Biochem Biophys Res Commun 177:679–687, 1991.

54. Loosfelt H, Misrahi M, Atger M, et al: Cloning and sequencing of porcine LH-hCG receptor cDNA: Variants lacking transmembrane domain. Science 245:525–528, 1989.

55. Loosfelt H, Pichon C, Jolivet A, et al: Two-subunit structure of the human thyrotropin receptor. Proc Natl Acad Sci USA 89:3765–3769, 1992.

56. Russo D, Chazenbalk GD, Nagayama Y, et al: A new structural model for the thyrotropin (TSH) receptor, as determined by covalent cross-linking of TSH to the recombinant receptor in intact cells: Evidence for a single polypeptide chain. Mol Endocrinol 5:1607–1612, 1991.

57. Libert F, Passage E, Lefort A, et al: Localization of human thyrotropin receptor gene to chromosome region 14q3 by in situ hybridization. Cytogenet Cell Genet 54:82–83, 1990.

58. Rousseau-Merck MF, Misrahi M, Loosfelt H, et al: Assignment of the human TSH receptor gene to chromosome 14q31. Genomics 8:233–236, 1990.

59. Ikuyama S, Niller HH, Shimura H, et al: Characterization of the 5′-flanking region of the rat thyrotropin receptor gene. Mol Endocrinol 6:793–804, 1992.

60. Roselli Rehfuss L, Robbins LS, Cone RD: Thyrotropin receptor messenger ribonucleic acid is expressed in most brown and white adipose tissues in the guinea pig. Endocrinology 130:1857–1861, 1992.

61. Francis T, Burch HB, Cai WY, et al: Lymphocytes express thyrotropin receptor–specific mRNA as detected by the PCR technique. Thyroid 1:223–228, 1991.

62. Perret J, Ludgate M, Libert F, et al: Stable expression of the human TSH receptor in CHO cells and characterization of differentially expressing clones. Biochem Biophys Res Commun 171:1044–1050, 1990.

63. Costagliola S, Swillens S, Niccoli P, et al: Binding assay for thyrotropin receptor autoantibodies using the recombinant receptor protein. J Clin Endocrinol Metab 75:1540–1544, 1992.

64. Rapoport B, Seto P: Bovine thyrotropin has a specific bioactivity 5- to 10-fold that of previous estimates for highly purified hormone. Endocrinology 116:1379–1382, 1985.

65. Amr S, Menezez Ferreira M, Shimohigashi Y, et al: Activities of deglycosylated thyrotropin at the thyroid membrane receptor–adenylate cyclase system. J Endocrinol Invest 8:537–541, 1985.

66. Laurent E, Van Sande J, Ludgate M, et al: Unlike thyrotropin, thy-

roid-stimulating antibodies do not activate phospholipase C in human thyroid slices. J Clin Invest 87:1634–1642, 1991.

67. Van Sande J, Lejeune C, Ludgate M, et al: Thyroid stimulating immunoglobulins, as thyrotropin, activate both the cyclic AMP and PIP2 cascades in CHO cells expressing the TSH receptor. Mol Cell Endocrinol 88:R1–R5, 1992.

68. Nagayama Y, Rapoport B: Role of the carboxyl-terminal half of the extracellular domain of the human thyrotropin receptor in signal transduction. Endocrinology 131:548–552, 1992.

69. Wadsworth HL, Russo D, Nagayama Y, et al: Studies on the role of amino acids 38-45 in the expression of a functional thyrotropin receptor. Mol Endocrinol 6:394–398, 1992.

70. Kosugi S, Ban T, Akamizu T, Kohn LD: Identification of separate determinants on the thyrotropin receptor reactive with Graves' thyroid-stimulating antibodies and with thyroid-stimulating blocking antibodies in idiopathic myxedema: These determinants have no homologous sequence on gonadotropin receptors. Mol Endocrinol 6:168–180, 1992.

71. Nagayama Y, Rapoport B: The thyrotropin receptor 25 years after its discovery: New insight after its molecular cloning. Mol Endocrinol 6:145–156, 1992.

72. Chazenbalk GD, Nagayama Y, Wadsworth H, et al: Signal transduction by the human thyrotropin receptor: Studies on the role of individual amino acid residues in the carboxyl terminal region of the third cytoplasmic loop. Mol Endocrinol 5:1523–1526, 1991.

73. Kosugi S, Ban T, Akamizu T, Kohn LD: Further characterization of a high affinity thyrotropin binding site on the rat thyrotropin receptor which is an epitope for blocking antibodies from idiopathic myxedema patients but not thyroid stimulating antibodies from Graves' patients. Biochem Biophys Res Commun 180:1118–1124, 1991.

74. Kosugi S, Ban T, Akamizu T, Kohn LD: Site-directed mutagenesis of a portion of the extracellular domain of the rat thyrotropin receptor important in autoimmune thyroid disease and nonhomologous with gonadotropin receptors. Relationship of functional and immunogenic domains. J Biol Chem 266:19413–19418, 1991.

75. Nagayama Y, Russo D, Wadsworth HL, et al: Eleven amino acids (Lys-201 to Lys-211) and 9 amino acids (Gly-222 to Leu-230) in the human thyrotropin receptor are involved in ligand binding. J Biol Chem 266:14926–14930, 1991.

76. Nagayama Y, Wadsworth HL, Russo D, et al: Binding domains of stimulatory and inhibitory thyrotropin (TSH) receptor autoantibodies determined with chimeric TSH-lutropin/chorionic gonadotropin receptors. J Clin Invest 88:336–340, 1991.

77. Russo D, Chazenbalk GD, Nagayama Y, et al: Site-directed mutagenesis of the human thyrotropin receptor: Role of asparagine-linked oligosaccharides in the expression of a functional receptor. Mol Endocrinol 5:29–33, 1991.

78. Nagayama Y, Wadsworth HL, Chazenbalk GD, et al: Thyrotropin-luteinizing hormone/chorionic gonadotropin receptor extracellular domain chimeras as probes for thyrotropin receptor function. Proc Natl Acad Sci USA 88:902–905, 1991.

79. Nagayama Y, Russo D, Chazenbalk GD, et al: Extracellular domain chimeras of the TSH and LH/CG receptors reveal the mid-region (amino acids 171-260) to play a vital role in high affinity TSH binding. Biochem Biophys Res Commun 173:1150–1156, 1990.

80. Chazenbalk GD, Nagayama Y, Russo D, et al: Functional analysis of the cytoplasmic domains of the human thyrotropin receptor by site-directed mutagenesis. J Biol Chem 265:20970–20975, 1990.

81. Libert F, Ludgate M, Dinsart C, Vassart G: Thyroperoxidase, but not the thyrotropin receptor, contains sequential epitopes recognized by autoantibodies in recombinant peptides expressed in the pUEX vector. J Clin Endocrinol Metab 73:857–860, 1991.

82. Tahara K, Ban T, Minegishi T, Kohn LD: Immunoglobulins from Graves' disease patients interact with different sites on TSH receptor/LH-CG receptor chimeras than either TSH or immunoglobulins from idiopathic myxedema patients. Biochem Biophys Res Commun 179:70–77, 1991.

83. Kosugi S, Okajima F, Ban T, et al: Mutation of Alanine 623 in the third cytoplasmic loop of the rat TSH receptor results in a loss in the phosphoinositide but not cAMP signal induced by TSH and receptor autoantibodies. J Biol Chem 267:24153–24156, 1992.

84. Nilsson M, Björkman U, Ekholm R, Ericson LE: Polarized efflux of iodide in porcine thyrocytes occurs via a cAMP-regulated iodide channel in the apical plasma membrane. Acta Endocrinologica 126:67–74, 1992.

85. Nilsson M, Björkman U, Ekholm R, Ericson LE: Iodide transport in primary cultured thyroid follicle cells: Evidence of a TSH-regulated channel mediating iodide efflux selectively across the apical domain of the plasma membrane. Eur J Cell Biol 52:270–281, 1990.

86. Arntzenius AB, Smit LJ, Schipper J, et al: Inverse relation between iodine intake and thyroid blood flow: Color doppler flow imaging in euthyroid humans. J Clin Endocrinol Metab 73:1051–1055, 1991.

87. Nunez J, Pommier J: Formation of thyroid hormones. Vitam Horm 39:175–229, 1982.

88. Corvilain B, Van Sande J, Laurent E, Dumont JE: The H_2O_2-generating system modulates protein iodination and the activity of the pentose phosphate pathway in dog thyroid. Endocrinology 128:779–785, 1991.

89. Björkman U, Ekholm R: Hydrogen peroxide generation and its regulation in FRTL-5 and porcine thyroid cells. Endocrinology 130:393–399, 1992.

90. Bernier-Valentin F, Kostrouch Z, Rabilloud R, Rousset B: Analysis of the thyroglobulin internalization process using in vitro reconstituted thyroid follicles: Evidence for a coated vesicle-dependent endocytic pathway. Endocrinology 129:2194–2201, 1991.

91. Björkman U, Ekholm R: Accelerated exocytosis and H_2O_2 generation in isolated thyroid follicles enhance protein iodination. Endocrinology 122:488–494, 1988.

92. Chambard M, Depetris D, Gruffat D, et al: Thyrotropin regulation of apical and basal exocytosis of thyroglobulin by porcine thyroid monolayers. J Mol Endocrinol 4:193–199, 1990.

93. Herzog V: Pathways of endocytosis in thyroid follicle cells. Internat Rev Cytol 91:107–139, 1984.

94. Van Den Hove MF, Couvreur M, De Visscher M: A new mechanism for the reabsorption of thyroid iodoproteins: Selective fluid pinocytosis. Eur J Biochem 122:415–422, 1982.

95. Lemansky P, Herzog V: Endocytosis of thyroglobulin is not mediated by mannose-6-phosphate receptors in thyrocytes. Evidence for low-affinity binding sites operating in the uptake of thyroglobulin. Eur J Biochem 209:111–119, 1992.

96. Consiglio E, Shifrin S, Yavin Z, et al: Thyroglobulin interactions with thyroid membranes. Relationship between receptor recognition of N-acetylglucosamine residues and the iodine content of thyroglobulin preparations. J Biol Chem 256:10592–10599, 1981.

97. Dumont JE, Vassart G, Refetoff S: Thyroid disorders. In Scriver CR (ed): The Metabolic Basis of Inherited Diseases. New York, McGraw-Hill, 1989, pp 1843–1879.

98. Christophe D, Vassart G: The thyroglobulin gene: Evolutionary and regulatory issues. TEM 1:10–15, 1990.

99. Van Heuverswyn B, Streydio C, Brocas H, et al: Thyrotropin controls transcription of the thyroglobulin gene. Proc Natl Acad Sci USA 81:5941–5945, 1984.

100. Van Heuverswyn B, Leriche A, Van Sande J, et al: Transcriptional control of thyroglobulin gene expression by cyclic AMP. FEBS Lett 188:192–196, 1985.

101. Davies E, Dumont JE, Vassart G: Thyrotropin-stimulated recruitment of free monoribosomes on to membrane-bound thyroglobulin-synthesizing polyribosomes. Biochem J 172:227–231, 1978.

102. Gerard CM, Lefort A, Christophe D, et al: Control of thyroperoxidase and thyroglobulin transcription by cAMP: Evidence for distinct regulatory mechanisms. Mol Endocrinol 3:2110–2118, 1989.

103. Avvedimento VE, Tramontano D, Ursini MV, et al: The level of thyroglobulin mRNA is regulated by TSH both in vitro and in vivo. Biochem Biophys Res Commun 122:472–477, 1984.

104. Christophe D, Gerard C, Juvenal G, et al: Identification of a cAMP-responsive region in thyroglobulin gene promoter. Mol Cell Endocrinol 64:5–18, 1989.

105. Sinclair AJ, Lonigro R, Civitareale D, et al: The tissue-specific expression of the thyroglobulin gene requires interaction between thyroid-specific and ubiquitous factors. Eur J Biochem 193:311–318, 1990.

106. Donda A, Vassart G, Christophe D: Isolation and characterization of the canine thyroglobulin gene promoter region. Biochim Biophys Acta 1090:235–237, 1991.

107. Civitareale D, Lonigro R, Sinclair AJ, Di Lauro R: A thyroid-specific nuclear protein essential for tissue-specific expression of the thyroglobulin promoter. EMBO J 8:2537–2542, 1989.

108. Zannini M, Francis Lang H, Plachov D, Di Lauro R: Pax-8, a paired domain-containing protein, binds to a sequence overlapping the recognition site of a homeodomain and activates transcription from two thyroid-specific promoters. Mol Cell Biol 12:4230–4241, 1992.

109. Lazzaro D, Price M, de Felice M, Di Lauro R: The transcription factor TTF-1 is expressed at the onset of thyroid and lung morphogenesis and in restricted regions of the foetal brain. Development 113:1093–1104, 1991.

110. Javaux F, Bertaux F, Donda A, et al: Functional role of TTF-1 binding sites in bovine thyroglobulin promoter. FEBS Lett 300:222–226, 1992.

36

Thyroid Hormone Transport and Metabolism

SAMUEL REFETOFF
JOHN T. NICOLOFF

MECHANISM OF THYROID HORMONE
TRANSPORT
NATURE AND PROPERTIES OF THE
PRINCIPAL THYROID HORMONE–BINDING
PROTEINS
Thyroxine-Binding Globulin (TBG)
Asialo or Slow TBG (sTBG)
Transthyretin (TTR)

MECHANISM OF THYROID HORMONE TRANSPORT

In most vertebrates, the bulk of circulating thyroid hormone* is bound to serum proteins.[1, 2] In normal humans, approximately 0.03 per cent of the total serum T_4 and 0.3 per cent of the total serum T_3 are present in free or unbound form. The major serum thyroid hormone-binding proteins are thyroxine-binding globulin (TBG or thyropexin), thyroxine-binding prealbumin (TBPA or transthyretin TTR), and albumin (ALB).[3] The normal distribution of T_4 among these proteins is 75 to 80 per cent bound to TBG, 15 to 20 per cent bound to TTR, and 5 to 10 per cent bound to ALB. The proportion of the serum total T_3 bound to TBG is about the same as that of T_4 but TTR contributes little to the transport of T_3. Most of the information about the relative distribution of T_4 and T_3 among the three principal thyroid hormone-binding proteins has been derived from in vitro studies utilizing electrophoresis of serum enriched with isotope-labeled hormones. Despite the artificial conditions of such studies, it is believed that the data obtained are representative of the situation existing in vivo, and they have been confirmed by direct immunoadsorption techniques.[4] Several other serum proteins, in particular high density lipoproteins, bind T_4, T_3 as well as rT_3,[5, 6] but in both physiological and pathological situations their contribution to hormone transport is negligible. Thyroid hormone binding to γ-globulin may occur under pathological conditions.[7-10] Since serum proteins bind both

T_4 and T_3, as well as most of their metabolites, it would have been more accurate to designate them iodothyronine-binding proteins or thyroid hormone–binding proteins rather than T_4-binding proteins. Nevertheless, the latter term has been used over the years and is universally accepted.

The interaction of the hormone with the various binding proteins is noncovalent and reversible. It can be expressed in terms of multiple equilibria obeying the law of mass action.[11] The binding between T_4 and TBG can be written as

$$T_4 + uTBG \rightleftharpoons TBG\text{-}T_4 \qquad (1)$$

and the mass action relationship at equilibrium as

$$k_{T_4, TBG} = \frac{[TBG\text{-}T_4]}{[T_4][uTBG]} \qquad (2)$$

where [ ] represents the molar concentration; $k_{T_4.TBG}$ is the association constant representing the affinity of T_4 for TBG; TBG-T_4 is T_4-bound TBG; uTBG is unsaturated or unbound TBG, and T_4 is free or unbound T_4. Rearranging equation (2),

$$[T_4] = \frac{[TBG\text{-}T_4]}{k_{T_4, TBG}[uTBG]} \qquad (3)$$

Similar equations can be written for the interaction of T_4 with the other two major T_4-binding serum proteins, TTR and ALB. Hence,

$$[T_4] = \frac{[TBG\text{-}T_4]}{k_{T_4, TBG}[uTBG]} + \frac{[TTR\text{-}T_4]}{k_{T_4, TTR}[uTTR]} + \frac{[ALB\text{-}T_4]}{k_{T_4, ALB}[uALB]} \qquad (4)$$

or, in general, for n classes of binding sites

---

*The term *thyroid hormone* is used to designate the two naturally occurring, metabolically active hormones: L-3,5,3',5'-tetraiodothyronine or thyroxine (T_4) and L-3,5,3'-triiodothyronine or liothyronine (T_3).

Supported in part by United States National Institutes of Health Grants DK 15070 and DK 11727 and General Clinical Research Center Program Grants RR-55 and RR-43.

$$[T_4] = \frac{\sum\limits_{i}^{n} [Pi\text{-}T_4]}{\sum\limits_{i}^{n} k_{T_4, Pi} [uPi]} \qquad (5)$$

where Pi is any protein with a class of binding sites i.

Since the concentration of free T_4 is negligibly small, this relationship indicates that the molar concentration of free T_4 ($[T_4]$) is directly proportional to that of total serum T_4 ($[Pi\text{-}T_4]$), and inversely proportional to the sum of the products of each association constant (k_{T_4},Pi) and the molar concentration of the corresponding class of unsaturated T_4-binding protein [uPi]. Accordingly, an acute alteration in the concentration of a particular class of binding protein, and thus in the maximal T_4-binding capacity, will have an effect on the concentration of free T_4 proportional to the affinity of the protein for T_4. Alterations in the concentration of the weak T_4-binding proteins are initially buffered by the high-affinity T_4-binding proteins with minimal changes in the free T_4 concentration. In the presence of a normally functioning hypothalamic pituitary-thyroid axis, free T_4 concentration is gradually restored after appropriate but temporary changes in the rate of hormonal release and disposal (see below). Similar interactions and dynamic equilibria exist between T_3 and the various T_4-binding serum proteins. Equations expressing these interactions can be written by substituting the appropriate values of T_3 concentration and the association constants for the interaction of T_3 with the various classes of binding proteins (Pi). Because the molar concentration of total T_4 in serum is approximately 50-fold that of T_3, its occupancy of binding sites, particularly on TBG, must be taken into account in the calculation. Thus,

$$[uTBG] = [TBG] - [TBG\text{-}T_4] - [TBG\text{-}T_3] \qquad (6)$$

where [TBG] is the molar concentration of total TBG, both unsaturated and hormone bound. As [TBG-T_3] is usually negligibly small, it can be ignored in the estimation of [uTBG].

The three major T_4-binding proteins are synthesized in the liver.[12] Since wide fluctuations in their concentration or even their total absence does not appear to alter the hormonal economy or metabolic status of the subject,[13] their function is open to speculation. However, two effects may be of physiological consequence. First, they are responsible for the maintenance of a large extrathyroidal pool or reservoir of thyroid hormone of which only the minute fraction (less than 0.5 per cent) of free hormone is immediately available to tissues. It can be estimated that in the absence of binding proteins the small extrathyroidal T_4 pool would be significantly reduced, if not completely depleted, in a matter of hours following a sudden cessation of hormone secretion. In contrast, with normal concentrations of T_4-binding proteins in serum, a 24-hour arrest in hormonal secretion would bring about a diminution in the concentration of T_4 and T_3 in the order of only 10 and 40 per cent, respectively. Thus it seems logical to assume that one of the functions of T_4-binding proteins in serum is to safeguard the body from the effects of abrupt fluctuations in hormonal secretion. The second likely function of T_4-binding proteins in serum is to serve as an additional protection against iodine wastage by imparting macromolecu-

lar properties to the small iodothyronine molecules, thus limiting their direct urinary loss.[14] The lack of high-affinity T_4-binding proteins in fish,[2] for example, may be teleologically attributed to the greater iodine abundance in their natural habitat. Other mechanisms of iodine conservation include hormone storage in thyroglobulin and intrathyroidal iodide recirculation (see Ch. 34).

NATURE AND PROPERTIES OF THE PRINCIPAL THYROID HORMONE–BINDING PROTEINS

Thyroxine-Binding Globulin (TBG)

TBG is a 54-kDa acidic glycoprotein migrating in the inter-α-globulin zone on conventional paper electrophoresis at pH 8.6. Identified some 40 years ago by three independent groups of investigators,[15–17] TBG has been purified[18] and more recently its amino acid sequence has been deduced from the nucleotide sequence of the TBG gene.[19] Its properties are summarized in Table 36–1. The molecule, encoded by a single gene copy located in the long arm of the human X chromosome,[20] is composed of a single polypeptide chain of 359 amino acids and four heterosaccharide units with 5 to 9 terminal sialic acids.[21] The carbohydrate chains, of biantennary and triantennary structure, are not absolutely required for hormone binding.[22, 23] Rather, they appear to be important for the correct post-translational folding and secretion of the molecule[24, 25] and are responsible for the multiple TBG isoforms (microheterogeneity) present on isoelectric focusing.[26] Improper folding of the molecule due to faulty glycosylation or to changes in the polypeptide core alters not only the secretion of TBG but also its ability to bind the iodothyronine ligands and its immunoreactivity.[25, 27] In contrast, cleavage of the carbohydrate moieties from a properly folded and secreted TBG does not affect its hormone-binding and immunological properties.[23, 28]

The TBG molecule has a single iodothyronine binding site with a 10-fold higher affinity for T_4 than for T_3.[29] The

TABLE 36–1. SOME PROPERTIES AND METABOLIC PARAMETERS OF THE PRINCIPAL THYROID HORMONE-BINDING PROTEINS IN SERUM

	TBG	TTR	ALB
Molecular weight (k Da)	54*	55	66.5
Structure	Monomer	Tetramer	Monomer
Carbohydrate content (%)	20		
No. of binding sites for T_4, T_3	1	2	Several
Association constant, Ka (M^{-1})			
$\quad T_4$	1×10^{10}	2×10^{8}†	1.5×10^{6}†
$\quad T_3$	1×10^{9}	1×10^{7}	2×10^{5}
Concentration in serum (mean normal, mg/L [nM])	16[0.30]	250[4.5]	40,000[600]
Relative distribution of T_4 and T_3 in serum (%)			
$\quad T_4$	75	20	5
$\quad T_3$	75	5	20
In-vivo survival			
$\quad$ Half-life (days)	5‡	2	15
$\quad$ Degradation rate (mg/day)	15	650	17,000

*Apparent molecular weight on acrylamide gel electrophoresis 60 k Da.
†Value given is for the high-affinity binding site only.
‡Longer under the influence of estrogen.

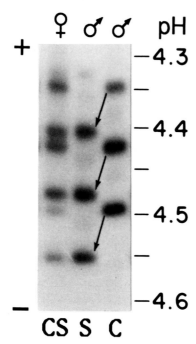

FIGURE 36–1. Microheterogeneity of TBG. Tracer amounts of ^{125}I-T4 were added to serum prior to submission to isoelectric focusing and radioautography. The common type TBG (TBG-C) exhibits 6 bands spanning from pH 4.18 to 4.58. Three of the six are major and shown here between pH 4.35 and 4.50. TBG-Slow (TBG-S) from a hemizygous male shows a cathodally shifted pattern relative to TBG-C (arrows). A mixed pattern occurs in heterogyzous females expressing both TBG-C and TBG-S. (From Waltz MR, Pullman TN, Takeda K, et al: Molecular basis for the properties of the thyroxine-binding globulin–slow variant in American Blacks. Endocrinol Invest 13:343, 1990.)

protein is very stable and can be preserved for many years at $-20°C$. It is stable even at room temperature and in dilute alkali but rapidly loses its binding activity by denaturation at temperatures above 55°C and pH below 4.[18, 28, 30] The half-life at 60°C is approximately 7 minutes but association with T_4 increases the stability of TBG and partially protects the molecule from denaturation.[22, 28, 30, 31] Denatured TBG does not bind iodothyronines but retains its molecular weight and can be detected with antibodies that recognize the primary structure of the molecule.[28] TBG is the least abundant iodothyronine-binding protein in serum, occurring in a molar ratio approximately 20- and 2000-fold lower than TTR and ALB, respectively, but it transports 70 to 75 per cent of the total serum T_4 and T_3. This is due to its high association constant for T_4, which is about 100-fold superior to TTR. Binding is stable over a wide range of pH from 6.4 to 10.4[18, 29] but declines markedly above and below this range. Under steady-state conditions, and for a tightly controlled constant level of free T_4, the concentration of total T_4 in serum depends on the concentration of TBG.

In euthyroid adults with normal TBG concentration, about one-third of the molecules carry thyroid hormone, mainly T_4. When fully saturated, it carries about 20 μg of T_4/dl of serum. The biological half-life is about 5 days, and the volume of distribution is similar to that of albumin.[32, 33] Its half-life is prolonged during pregnancy, which, at least in part, is responsible for higher TBG concentration in serum.[34] This effect of estrogen is mediated through an increase in the complexity of the oligosaccharide residues

of TBG resulting in an increase in the number of sialic acids.[35] Measurement of the amount of T_4 carried on TBG at saturation served for many years as the only method for the quantitation of serum TBG. This is being supplanted by immunological methods for direct quantitation (see Ch. 39). Nevertheless, results of the widely used in vitro hormone uptake tests usually provide the first clue for the existence of quantitative abnormalities in TBG. As discussed later, TBG concentration in serum may be altered by inherited defects, various drugs and hormones, and by a variety of diseases unrelated to thyroid gland pathology.

A number of compounds compete with iodothyronines for their binding site on TBG, presumably due to similarities in structure. Such binding competitors have been used to determine the conformational requirements for the interaction of T_4 with the protein. Based on studies with thyroid hormone analogues, optimal binding activity requires the presence of the L-alanine side chain, an unsubstituted 4'-hydroxyl group, a diphenyl ether bridge, and halogen (I or Br) constituents at the 3,5,3', and 5' positions.[36] A number of organic compounds, many of which are commonly used pharmaceutical agents, compete with thyroid hormone-binding to TBG. Although their affinity is usually inferior to that of T_4 by at least several orders of magnitude, when used in therapeutic doses, their concentration in serum is often high enough to occupy a significant portion of iodothyronine binding site on TBG. The drug most extensively studied in this regard is 5,5'-diphenylhydantoin (DPH).[37] DPH has additional but unrelated effects on thyroid hormone metabolism.[38] Other binding competitors include 1,8-anilinonaphthalenesulfonic acid (ANS) and salicylates.[39] The latter two compounds and DPH are used in vitro to release T_4 and T_3 from serum TBG for the immunometric quantitation of these hormones (see Ch. 39).

Asialo or Slow Thyroxine-Binding Globulin

A fourth protein capable of binding T_4 has been detected in some sera.[40, 41] Initially believed to represent an artifact arising from long periods of serum sample storage, it appears to be partially desialylated TBG, as earlier postulated by Premachandra et al.[41] The term slow TBG (sTBG) arose from its electrophoretic mobility cathodal to native TBG. sTBG can be generated from TBG by treatment with neuraminidase.[40, 41] Similar to intact TBG, sTBG has a single binding site for T_4 and also binds T_3, although with a slightly lower affinity. It is denatured by heat at the same rate as TBG and cross-reacts with antibodies produced in rabbits against intact human TBG.[22] The most striking difference from TBG is its very short biological half-life. While the $t_{1/2}$ of TBG in normal man is approximately 5 days, that of sTBG is 15 to 30 minutes. sTBG is rapidly trapped by the liver, in which it is partially degraded and excreted in the bile.[22] As it competes with other asialoglycoproteins for binding to liver plasma membranes,[42] sTBG, not surprisingly, has been found in serum of some patients with severe liver disease[40] and may be present in relatively higher proportion than TBG in serum of patients with a variety of nonthyroidal illnesses.[43] While it is known that TBG is synthesized and glycosylated by hepatocytes,[12] it is uncertain whether desialylation and formation of sTBG is a prerequisite in the normal pathway of TBG metabolism.

Transthyretin (TTR)

TTR, formerly named thyroxine-binding prealbumin for its electrophoretic mobility anodal to albumin, was first recognized to bind T_4 in 1958.[44] Subsequently, it was demonstrated that TTR also forms a complex with retinol-binding protein (RBP) and thus plays a role in the transport of vitamin A (retinol).[45, 46] Some of the properties of TTR are summarized in Table 36–1. TTR is a stable tetramer composed of four identical subunits as demonstrated by crystallographic[47, 48] and genetic[49, 50] studies. Each subunit contains 127 amino acids encoded by a single gene copy located on human chromosome 18.[51, 52] The complete molecule has a molecular weight of 55 kDa and is highly acidic but contains no carbohydrate. The four subunits form a symmetrical structure with a double-trumpeted channel that traverses the molecule forming the two iodothyronine binding sites.[47] Despite their apparent identity, TTR usually binds only one T_4 molecule because the binding affinity of the second site is greatly reduced through a negative cooperative effect.[53] RBP interaction with TTR does not influence binding of T_4, and vice versa.[54] On the other hand, formation of TTR-RBP complex stabilized the bond between vitamin A and RBP.

Although on a molar basis the relative abundance of TTR in serum is 20-fold that of TBG, it plays a lesser role in thyroid hormone transport. In fact, in the presence of normal levels of TBG, wide fluctuations in TTR concentration, or its removal from serum by specific antibodies has little influence on the concentration of free T_4.[4] While only 0.5 per cent of the circulating TTR is occupied by T_4, the molar ratio of RBP to TTR is 2.5:1. Thus, TTR seems to be more important for the transport of vitamin A than for thyroid hormone.

TTR can be measured by densitometry after its separation from the other serum proteins by electrophoresis, by hormone saturation, and by immunoassays (see Ch. 39). Normal average concentration is about 250 mg/liter of serum, corresponding to a maximal binding capacity of approximately 300 μg T_4/dl. The first T_4 molecule binds to TTR with a Ka of about 100-fold higher than that for ALB and about 100-fold less than that for TBG. Properties necessary for optimal binding activity include iodines at the 3′ and 5′ positions and a desamino acid side chain explaining the lower T_3 and higher tetraiodoacetic acid (TETRAC) affinities relative to that of T4.[36, 55] Among drugs that compete with T_4-binding to TTR are ethacrynic acid, salicylates, 2,4-dinitrophenol, and penicillin.[56, 57] Barbital also inhibits hormonal binding to TTR. Its former use as buffer for paper electrophoresis was in part responsible for the delay in the recognition of TTR as a T_4-binding protein.

TTR has a relatively rapid turnover ($t_{1/2}$ = 2 days) and a distribution space similar to that of ALB and TBG.[58, 59] Hence, acute diminution in the rate of synthesis, as typically occurs with undernutrition and systemic illness, is accompanied by a rapid decrease of its concentration in serum.

Albumin (ALB)

Albumin is a 66.5-kDa protein encoded by a single gene copy located on human chromosome 4.[60] It is composed of 585 amino acids with high content of cystine and charged amino acids but no carbohydrate.[61] The three structural domains of the molecule can be conceived as three tennis balls packaged in a cylindrical case. It has the property of associating with a wide variety of substances including fatty acids, hormones, and drugs possessing a hydrophobic region, and thus the association of thyroid hormone to ALB can be viewed as nonspecific. In spite of its weak affinity for T_4 and T_3, the large abundance in serum allows ALB to be a not totally negligible contributor to iodothyronines transport.[62] On the other hand, even extreme fluctuations in ALB concentration have little influence on the total concentration of thyroid hormone in serum. Of the several potential T_4 binding sites on the ALB molecule, only one possesses a high enough affinity to be significantly involved in the transport of T_4 and T_3. Fatty acids and chloride ions decrease their binding to ALB.[63] The biological $t_{1/2}$ of ALB is long compared with those of TBG and TTR.[64] Some of its properties are summarized in Table 36–1.

ALTERATIONS OF THYROID HORMONE TRANSPORT

Thyroid hormone effect depends on the quantity of the hormone that reaches peripheral tissues and the availability of unaltered thyroid hormone receptors in the cells nuclei (see Ch. 37). Since intracellular hormone is in equilibrium with the free thyroid hormone in serum, the latter rather than the concentration of total hormone is believed to determine the level of thyroid hormone–dependent processes. In the absence of abnormalities of thyroid secretion, changes in free hormone level are corrected by appropriate stimulation or suppression of hormone secretion and disposal. It is likely that the "sensor" controlling hormonal supply is not set to detect an optimal intracellular hormone concentration but actually responds to specific metabolic actions of the hormone. Such effect is, however, closely related to the intracellular hormone concentration, and hence, in practice, it is best quantitated by measuring the free hormone concentration in serum.

Hormone-binding proteins in serum are the principal intravascular factors influencing total hormone concentration (THC). Under normal conditions THC is kept at a level proportional to the concentration of carrier proteins and appropriate to maintain a constant free hormone level. Changes in THC can occur as a result of changes in the number or affinity of the available binding sites on the carrier proteins. Most carrier protein–dependent alterations in THC in serum are due to quantitative changes in the hormone-binding proteins. Less commonly, genetic defects producing carrier proteins with altered affinity for the hormone can be responsible for alterations in the concentration of hormone in serum.

Changes in Thyroxine-Binding Globulin

Various factors may bring about changes in the concentration of TBG. Irrespective of the specific factor or mechanism causing these changes, the consequences are the same. Figure 36–2 illustrates the sequence of events that follow an acute change in serum TBG concentration. If, for example, TBG concentration is increased, the resulting increase in unoccupied binding sites on this hormone-binding protein brings about a shift in the equilibrium between total and bound T_4, having as a net effect a diminution in the serum free T_4 concentration. The consequences are threefold. First, a re-equilibration of the exchangeable T_4 occurs with a shift from tissues to blood. Second, the resulting diminution in tissue supply of T_4 decreases its disposal. Third, activation of the hypothalamopituitary axis increases in thyroidal secretion of T_4. The latter two compensatory effects last until a new steady state is reached in which the increased TBG concentration is associated with a higher concentration of total and bound T_4 that is compatible with a normal concentration of free T_4, a normal tissue supply of hormone, and a return to the initial secretion and disposal rates that existed before the perturbation of the steady state. The total extrathyroidal T_4 pool is augmented due to an increase in the intravascular T_4 pool. The fractional turnover rate of T_4 is decreased, but because the intracellular T_4 pool is reduced relative to the blood T_4 pool, the total distribution space of T_4 is decreased. Under this new steady-state condition, the absolute amount of T_4 degraded and secreted each day remains normal.[11, 33, 65–67] The converse sequence of events occurs during an acute decrease in TBG concentration. With establishment of a new steady state, T_4 turnover kinetics show an increase in the fractional turnover rate and distribution space and a decrease in the extrathyroidal T_4 pool, but a normal daily disposal rate of the hormone[11, 33, 67] (Fig. 36–2). Similar alterations in T_3 concentration and

metabolism should be expected and indeed have been observed.[68] Accordingly, measurement of thyroid hormone transport parameters shows changes in serum total T_4 and T_3 concentrations that parallel the changes in total TBG concentration, and in the unsaturated binding sites of TBG, the latter manifested by reciprocal findings in the in-vitro hormone uptake test (see Ch. 39).

Conditions associated with changes in TBG concentration are either genetic or acquired. Acquired causes may be physiological or pathological, caused by diseases, hormones, or drugs. A list is provided in Table 36–2.

Acquired Thyroxine-Binding Globulin Abnormalities

TBG appears at about the 12th week of intrauterine life.[98] Serum TBG concentration in normal adults, expressed in terms of maximal T_4-binding capacity, ranges from approximately 14 to 26 μg T_4/dl (180 to 300 nM). Values from direct and indirect immunoassays vary at the extreme from 6 to 16 mg/liter to 15 to 35 mg/liter owing primarily to differences in purity of the reference standard. Furthermore, there are independent diurnal variations of TBG concentration that directly result from postural changes acting on the concentration of serum proteins.[99] Although estrogens increase TBG concentration, sex differences are small except during pregnancy.[71, 100] In the newborn infant, serum TBG is to about 1.5 times the normal adult concentration and remains at this level for the first two to three years of life.[28, 74, 76] It is lower in infants born prematurely and in infants small-for-gestational age born at term.[101] In addition, there are slight age-related

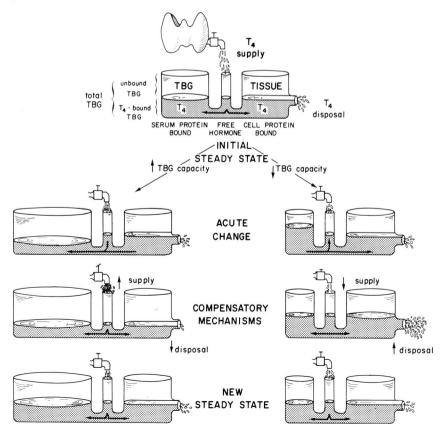

FIGURE 36–2. Graphic representation of the sequence of events following an acute change in serum TBG concentration in a subject with normally regulated thyroid hormone secretion and metabolism. The principle of communicating vessels is used for the purpose of illustration. The width of the two large vessels represents available T_4-binding sites in serum protein TBG (left vessel) and T_4-binding sites in intracellular (TISSUE) proteins (right vessel), which are partially saturated by T_4 (fluid level). The height of fluid in the small (central) vessel represents free T_4 concentration in equilibrium with bound T_4 in each of the large vessels. Free T_4 is proportional to the level of saturation of the T_4-binding sites in serum (TBG) and in cells (TISSUE). Thyroidal secretion of T_4 is represented by the input of fluid through the faucet (supply), and hormone metabolism by the overspill of the tissue reservoir (disposal). For further details see text.

changes in which TBG levels reach a nadir during mid-adulthood followed by a trend for a rise with further advance in age.[102] The latter changes may be related to the variable prevalence of intercurrent nonthyroidal illness.[103] The most striking physiological change in serum TBG concentration occurs during pregnancy. As indicated in the preceding section on the nature and properties of TBG, this increase is primarily due to an increase in the sialic acid content that prolongs its biological half-life in serum. An increase in TBG concentration may be observed as early as three weeks following implantation, usually reaching a maximum of 2.5-fold the normal value during the end of the second or the beginning of the third trimester.[74] Following delivery, levels decline to reach pregestational values within four to six weeks. Fetal distress and intrauterine death are often accompanied by a decrease in TBG concentration.

Hyperestrogenism, either endogenous (hydatidiform mole, estrogen-producing tumors) or exogenous (administration of estrogens) is the most common cause of an increase in TBG concentration other than pregnancy. The magnitude of the increase is, in part, dose-related and can even be caused by topical application of estrogen-containing compounds. It occurs both in women and in men. The concentration of other serum proteins, including several hormone-binding proteins such as cortisol-binding globulin, testosterone-binding globulin, ceruloplasmin, and transferrin, are also increased.[104] Androgens and anabolic steroids produce the opposite effect (Table 36–2).

Drugs competing with T_4 binding to TBG do not change the concentration of TBG but may affect the total T_4 concentration and tests measuring available binding sites in TBG (see Ch. 37). Some drugs can, however, alter the concentration of TBG in serum (Table 36–2).

Altered synthesis, degradation, or both are responsible for the majority of acquired TBG abnormalities.[33] Severe terminal illness is undoubtedly the most common cause for acquired decrease in TBG concentration.[86] It is probably caused, in part, by changes in hepatic function. Both the magnitude and frequency of disease-associated alterations in TBG concentration are variable.

TBG loss in urine occurs in some patients with nephrotic syndrome.[91, 92] Gastrointestinal loss of TBG may be the cause for reduced TBG in some patients with protein-losing enteropathy.[94] In vivo turnover studies of TBG in humans suggest that decreased turnover rate in hypothyroidism and an increased rate in hyperthyroidism may be the cause for the changes in TBG concentration in these two conditions.[32, 33]

Inherited Thyroxine-Binding Globulin Abnormalities

The occurrence of inherited TBG abnormality was first described in 1957 and consisted of familial TBG excess.[105] Five years later, TBG deficiency was reported in 6 of 13 family members.[106] Although the inheritance pattern in these two families was not incompatible with X-chromosome linkage, the authors proposed a mendelian dominant transmission. Evidence for X chromosome–linked inheritance of familial TBG abnormalities was independently presented in 1966 with the report of two additional families with TBG deficiency.[107, 108] Subsequent analysis of 24 pedigrees with altered TBG concentration strongly indicated that all inherited TBG abnormalities are X chromosome–linked.[67] Confirmation was secured only recently by the localization of the TBG gene to the long arm of the X chromosome followed by the demonstration of point mutation in its coding sequence.

Clinically, TBG defects are divided into three categories according to the level of TBG in serum of affected hemizygotes (XY males or XO females) who express only the mutant allele: complete TBG deficiency (TBG-CD), partial TBG deficiency, and TBG excess. Inherited TBG defects can be further characterized according to the level of denatured TBG (dn TBG) in serum and the physiocochemical properties of the molecule. The properties of variant TBG's can be determined easily without the need of purification from serum. These are: (1) immunological identity, (2) isoelectric focusing (IEF) pattern, (3) rate of inactivation when exposed to various temperatures or pH's,

TABLE 36–2. CONDITIONS ASSOCIATED WITH ALTERATIONS IN TBG CONCENTRATION

	INCREASED	DECREASED
Genetic	Inherited TBG excess (see Fig. 36–3)	Inherited, complete and partial TBG deficiency (see Fig. 36–3) Carbohydrate-deficient glycoprotein syndrome[69]
Acquired		
Hormonal	Estrogens (used as ovulatory suppressants), anticancer agents[35, 70, 71]	Androgens and anabolic steroids[72, 73]
	Hyperestrogenic states (pregnancy, newborn, molar pregnancy, estrogen-producing tumors[28, 34, 74, 75, 76])	Glucocorticoids (large doses)[77]
Drugs	Perphenazine (Trilafon)[78]	L-Asparaginase[79]
	Heroin and methadone addiction[80]	
	Clofibrate[81]	
	5-Fluorouracil[35, 82]	
	Nicotinic acid[83, 84]	
Diseases	Acute intermittent porphyria (especially in women)[85]	Major illness (nonspecific)[86]
	Acute viral and chronic active hepatitis,[35, 71, 87] primary biliary cirrhosis and hepatocellular carcinoma[88]	Protein-calorie malnutrition[89]
	Myeloma[71]	Galactosemia[90]
	Collagen diseases[71]	Nephrotic syndrome[91, 92]
	Hypogammaglobulinemia[93]	Protein-losing enteropathy[94]
	Hypothyroidism[28, 71, 95]	Liver cirrhosis[96]
		Active acromegaly[97]
		Hyperthyroidism[71, 95]

and (4) affinity for the ligands T_4 and T_3. More precise identification of TBG defects requires sequencing of the variant TBG gene.[13]

In families with completely TBG-deficient males, carrier females have on the average half the normal TBG concentration (Table 36–3). In families with partially TBG-deficient males, the mean TBG concentration in heterozygous females is usually above half-normal, suggesting that in addition to the half of the cell population expressing the normal TBG gene, the cells possessing the mutant gene contribute to the serum level of TBG as in the affected males. Similar conclusions can be drawn from data obtained in families with TBG excess because the mean concentration of TBG in heterozygous females suggests an approximately equal contribution of cells expressing the normal and mutant TBG genes.[67]

TBG deficiency or excess are uncovered most frequently by the incidental finding of abnormal serum T_4 or T_3 concentration and reciprocal changes of the in vitro hormone uptake test. The inherited nature of the defect, suspected by exclusion of factors known to cause acquired TBG abnormalities, can be easily confirmed by the finding of similar TBG abnormalities in members of the family. Inherited TBG abnormalities are not associated with changes in other serum proteins, including TTR, or in proteins involved in the transport of other hormones.[67] In fact, the absence of reciprocal or parallel changes of TTR in relation to TBG usually suggests that the TBG abnormality is inherited. Although a higher incidence of thyrotoxicosis has been reported in patients with inherited reduction of TBG,[109] in most patients euthyroidism is maintained by the integrity of the hypothalamopituitary axis.[110] Association with other disorders is believed to be fortuitous.[13] The association with thyroid dysfunction or goiter is not surprising considering that individuals with manifestations of thyroid hormone disorders are more likely to undergo thyroid testing leading to the detection of a TBG defect. On the other hand, associated X-linked defects are likely to cosegregate. For example, the occurrence of X-linked anhydrotic ectodermal dysplasia and TBG excess has been reported.[111]

The estimated prevalence of TBG deficiency of 1:5,000 is based on data from neonatal screening programs for congenital hypothyroidism.[112, 113] This is probably an underestimation due to limitation of total T_4 measurement to detect TBG deficiency in heterozygous females and even less likely to detect TBG excess, being out of limits for detecting high T_4 values.

Twelve TBG variants have been so far identified by gene sequencing. Their primary structure, some of their physical and chemical properties, and the resulting serum T_4 concentrations are summarized in Figures 36–3 and 36–4.

Three occur with high enough frequency in some populations to be considered as polymorphic. These are: (1) TBG-Poly, harboring a Phe-283 instead of Leu, has an allele frequency of 16 per cent in French Canadians[126] and 20 per cent in Japanese.[132] It has been also found to occur in association with other mutations in the TBG gene (Fig. 36–3). However, when occurring alone, it does not cause alterations in the physical or chemical properties of the molecule, and subjects expressing TBG-Poly have normal concentrations of TBG in serum. (2) TBG slow (TBG-S), first identified in 1981,[133] has an allele frequency of 5 to 16 per cent in black populations of African origin and 2 to 10 per cent in Pacific Islanders.[122] Not to be confused with the desialylated TBG (sTBG), it has an Asn instead of Asp in position 171 resulting in the loss of a negative charge; this loss is responsible for its slower mobility on polyacrylamide gel electrophoresis and cathodal shift on IEF (Fig. 36–1). It is associated with a very mild form of TBG deficiency.[121] (3) TBG-A, a variant having 51 per cent allele frequency in Australian Aborigines,[125] was first described in 1980.[134, 135] Affected individuals have reduced serum total T_4 and T_3 concentrations out of proportion to the level of TBG as measured by RIA or by binding capacity[123] (Fig. 36–4). Furthermore, because TBG-A has a 50 per cent reduction of the affinity for T_4 and 70 per cent reduction of the affinity to T_3, the concentration of free T_4 estimated from calculation of the free T_4 index using the in vitro hormone uptake tests gives a low value when sera containing TBG-C are used as a standard.[124] The TBG-A molecule has normal immunological properties but is more labile when exposed to high temperature and acid. The rate of serum TBG inactivation is useful in identifying TBG-A both in hemizygous and heterozygous individuals (Fig. 36–5). These characteristics of TBG-A are caused by a single amino acid substitution (Fig. 36–3).

Two additional polymorphic TBG variants have been identified but their molecular basis remains unknown. TBG-F has a slightly anodal (fast) mobility on IEF.[125a] It occurs in the Eskimo population with allele frequency of 3.2 per cent. A TBG variant (TBG-C1) with a small cathodal shift on IEF electrophoresis has been described in subjects inhabiting two Mali villages.[125b] Its allele frequency is 5.1 per cent. The ligand-binding and physical properties of TBG-F and TBG-C1 have not been reported.

COMPLETE TBG DEFICIENCY (TBG-CD). TBG-CD is defined as undetectable TBG in serum of affected hemizygous subjects. The current limit of detection is 5 μg/liter corresponding to 0.03 per cent of the average TBG concentration in serum of normal adults.[126] Heterozygous females have approximately half the normal concentration of TBG, and serum thyroid hormone levels are correspondingly intermediate between those of affected hemizygous subjects

TABLE 36–3. SERUM TBG CONCENTRATION IN SUBJECTS WITH INHERITED TBG ABNORMALITIES

CLINICAL TYPE	TBG MEAN ± SD PERCENTAGE OF AVERAGE NORMAL VALUE		
	Hemizygous Affected	Heterozygous Carriers	Unaffected Relatives
Complete deficiency (CD)	0	50 ± 15	107 ± 17
Partial deficiency (PD)	30 ± 11	62 ± 13	101 ± 10
Excess	326 ± 64	230 ± 56	102 ± 10

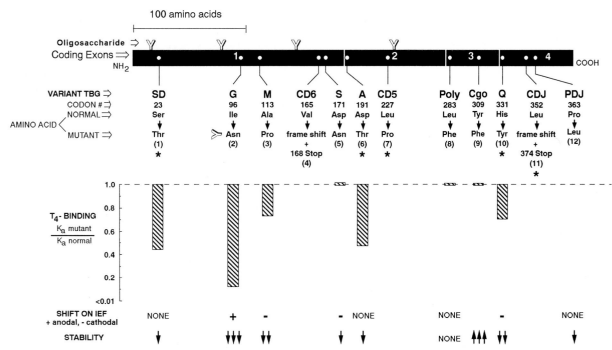

FIGURE 36–3. Known mutations in the TBG gene, their location, and effect on the properties of the molecule. The TBG variants are: −**SD**, San Diego; −**G**, Gary; −**M**, Montreal, −**CD6**, complete deficiency 6; −**S**, slow; −**A**, Aborigine; −**CD5**, complete deficiency 5; −**Cgo**, Chicago; −**Poly**, polymorphic; −**Q**, Quebec; −**CDJ**, complete deficiency Japan, and −**PDJ**, partial deficiency Japan. Asterisks indicate the coexistence of TBG-Poly. For detailed description, see refs. 25, 27, 114–131, and 135a.

and normal individuals (Table 36–3). The prevalence of TBG-CD is approximately 1:15,000 newborn males.[126]

Three distinct mutant TBG's have been identified in subjects with TBG-CD. Two, TBG-CD6 and TBG-CD Japan (TBG-CDJ), involve the deletion of a single, albeit a different, nucleotide in the coding sequence producing frameshifts and early termination codons (Fig. 36–3). The third variant TBG, TBG-CD5, has two nucleotide substitutions resulting in the replacements of the normal Leu-227 with Pro and the normal Leu-283 with Phe (Fig. 36–3). In vitro expression of this mutant TBG has shown that the Pro-227 alone is responsible for the failure of its secretion due to aberrant post-translational processing,[27] Phe-283 being a polymorphic variant that does not alter the properties of the molecule (see above). Similarly, the truncated TBG-CDJ molecule is retained within the endoplasmic reticulum, explaining the failure to be detected in serum by immunologic techniques.[131]

PARTIAL TBG DEFICIENCY. By definition, the variant TBG's comprised in this category are detected in serum of hemizygotes, albeit at a reduced level. When the TBG levels in affected males are above 15 per cent the mean normal value, those in heterozygous females often overlap the normal range, invalidating the assignment of genotype based solely on serum TBG concentration. Variants of this category constitute the most common types of TBG deficiency having a prevalence in white and mixed populations of 1:4000 newborns.[13] Two variant TBG's presenting as partial TBG deficiency, TBG-A and TBG-S, have been found with high frequency in some populations, as already described.

While, in general, the reduction in total T_4 and T_3 concentrations is proportional to that of TBG, this is not the case in TBG variants that, in addition, have reduced affinity for these hormone ligands. Most notable for such discrepancies are TBG-A and TBG-San Diego (TBG-SD) (Fig. 36–4). The decreased stability at 37°C and increased concen-

FIGURE 36–4. Serum T_4 bound to TBG, and TBG and denatured TBG (dn TBG) concentrations in hemizgyous subjects expressing the different TBG variants. Results, shown as mean ± SD, were normalized by expressing them as percentages of the TBG-C. For abbreviations used in the nomenclature of the TBG variants, see legend to Figure 36–3. (Adapted from Janssen OE, Bertenshaw R, Takeda K, et al: Molecular basis of inherited thyroxine-binding globulin defects. Trends Endocrinol Metab 3:49, 1992.)

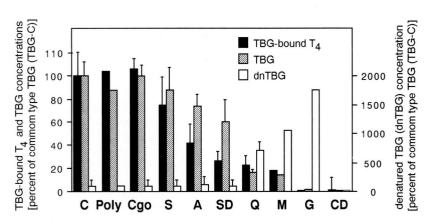

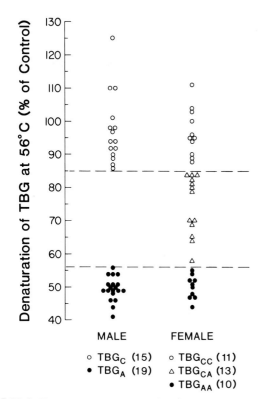

FIGURE 36–5. Phenotyping of the variant TBG-A in serum by the rate of its denaturation at 56°C. Results are expressed as percentages of the mean $t_{1/2}$ of denaturation of control sera expressing TBG-C, analyzed in the same assay. In parenthesis are the number of individuals having the indicated phenotype according to sex. (Reproduced from Takeda K, Mori Y, Sobieszczyk S, et al: Sequence of the variant thyroxine-binding globulin in serum of Australian Aborigines: Its physical, chemical and biological properties. J Clin Invest 83:1344, 1989, by copyright permission of the American Society for Clinical Investigation.)

tration of denatured TBG in serum of subjects expressing three TBG variants, TBG-Gary (TBG-G), TBG-Montreal (TBG-M), and TBG-Quebec (TBG-Q), suggested that an accelerated rate of degradation is likely responsible for their markedly reduced concentration in serum.[116, 118] In vitro expression of TBG-M has confirmed this hypothesis.[27] However, in the case of TBG-G, transfection experiments indicate that impaired secretion leading to excessive intracellular degradation is responsible for the low concentrations of TBG in subjects expressing this variant molecule.[25] This is caused by improper folding and thus faulty intracellular processing of the molecule due to the presence of an additional carbohydrate at a new site of N-linked glycosylation created by the replacement of the normal Ile-96 with an Asn.[117] TBG-G has a greatly reduced affinity for T_4, and the additional carbohydrate chain, which increases its overall content in sialic acid, produces a characteristic anodal shift on IEF. TBG-PDJ, manifesting as partial TBG deficiency in Japanese, has only mild reduction of heat stability, suggesting impaired secretion.[135a]

TBG EXCESS. Inherited TBG excess has a lower prevalence than TBG deficiency, being detected in 1:25,000 newborns.[13] Hemizygous subjects have serum TBG and total T_4 levels 2½ to 5 times the normal mean value and heterozygous females 1½ to 2½ times the normal mean value[13, 136] (Table 36–3). The TBG molecule has been found to have properties identical to those of TBG-C. No abnormalities in the coding sequence of the TBG gene have been identi-

fied; therefore, the defect is believed to reside at the promoter region of the gene.

TBG VARIANTS WITH UNALTERED BIOLOGICAL PROPERTIES AND CONCENTRATIONS. Three TBG variants have been identified that have normal or clinically insignificant alterations in their concentration in serum or hormone-binding properties. Two of the three variants, namely, TBG-Poly and TBG-S, occurring with high frequency in some population groups, have been described already. A third, TBG-Chicago (TBG-Cgo), is probably a rare variant that was detected fortuitously during the screening of serum samples for TBG's with reduced heat stability.[127] TBG-Cgo is relatively resistant to high temperatures. Its $t_{1/2}$ at 60°C is 90 minutes compared to that of 6.8 ± 1.1 min for TBG-C. Its concentration in serum is normal, as are the association constant for T_4 and IEF pattern (Fig. 36–3). A substitution of the normal Tyr-309 for Phe was recently found to be the cause of the increased resistance of TBG-Cgo to heat inactivation, presumably by stabilization of its tertiary structure through interaction of the mutant Phe-309 with one of the α-helixes of the molecule.[128]

Changes in Transthyretin

Acquired Abnormalities

Changes in TTR concentration exert relatively little effect on the serum concentrations of T_4 and T_3.[4, 137] Normal values for TTR in healthy individuals range from 150 to 400 mg/L or, expressed in terms of maximal T_4-binding capacity, from 240 to 380 μg T4/dl. There is a distinct reciprocal relationship between acquired changes in TBG and TTR concentration related to gender,[100] age,[102] glucocorticoids,[77] estrogen,[138] and androgens.[66] On the other hand, reductions in TTR parallel or surpass those of TBG when associated with major illness, nephrotic syndrome, liver disease, cystic fibrosis, hyperthyroidism, and protein-calorie malnutrition.[3, 96, 139, 140] Increased serum TTR concentration can occur in some patients with islet cell carcinoma.[141]

Studies on the metabolism of TTR in humans, utilizing radioiodinated purified human TTR, indicate that diminished TTR concentration associated with severe illness or stress is due to a decrease in the rate of synthesis or an increase in the rate of degradation or both.[58, 59] On the other hand, increase in TTR concentration induced by the administration of the anabolic steroid norethandrolone is caused by an enhanced rate of synthesis rather than a decreased rate of degradation of the protein.[142]

Inherited Abnormalities

VARIANTS WITH INCREASED AFFINITY FOR T_4. A family with elevated total T_4 that was predominantly bound to TTR was first described in 1982.[143] Affected family members were clinically euthyroid and had normal free T_4 levels measured by equilibrium dialysis. As in subjects with inherited albumin-like variant serum protein (see below), serum total reverse T_3 (rT_3) concentration was elevated and total T_3 levels were normal.[143, 144] However, in accordance with the thyroid hormone–binding properties of wild-type molecule, tetraiodothyroacetic acid bound to the variant TTR's with higher affinity than T_4. The inheritance pattern was

TABLE 36–4. TTR MUTATIONS ASSOCIATED WITH AMYLOIDOSES

AMINO ACID SUBSTITUTION (Normal → Mutant)	POSITION (Codon Number)	TYPE (Acronym)	CLINICAL PICTURE	GEOGRAPHIC ORIGIN
Cys → Arg	10		Heart, eye	US (PA)
Val → Met	30	FAP I	LLN, AN, Eye	Portugal/Japan/Sweden/US
Val → Ala	30		Heart, AN	US
Val → Leu	30			Japan
Phe → Ile	33	Jewish	LLN, Eye	Israel
Phe → Leu	33		LLN, Heart	US
Ala → Pro	36		Eye, CTS	US
Glu → Gly	42			Japan
Ala → Thr	45		Heart	US
Gly → Ala	47		Heart, AN	Italy
Gly → Arg	47		LLN, AN	Japan
Thr → Ala	49		Heart, CTS	France/Italy
Ser → Arg	50		AN, LLN	Japan
Ser → Ile	50			Japan
Leu → Pro	55		Heart, AN, Eye	US
Leu → His	58	FAP	CTS, Heart	US (MD)
Leu → Arg	58		CTS, AN, Eye	Japan
Thr → Ala	60	Appalachian	Heart, CTS	US
Phe → Leu	64		LLN, CTS, Heart	US
Ile → Leu	68		Heart	Germany
Tyr → His	69		Eye	US
Lys → Asp	70		Eye, CTS, LLN	US
Val → Ala	71		LLN, Eye, CTS	France
Ser → Tyr	77		Kidney	US (IL)
Ile → Ser	84	FAP II	Heart, CTS, Eye	US (IN)
Ile → Asp	84		Heart, Eye	US
Glu → Gln	89		LLN, Heart	Sicily
Asn → Asp	90		Heart, Eye, CTS	US
Leu → Met	111	Danish	Heart	Denmark
Tyr → Cys	114		Eye	Japan
Val → Ile	122	Senile cardiac	Heart	US

LLN, lower limb neuropathy; AN, autonomic neuropathy; CTS, carpal tunnel syndrome.
Adapted from Benson et al: Amyloidosis. *In* The Metabolic Basis of Inherited Diseases, 7th ed. New York, McGraw-Hill, 1993.

autosomal dominant. The defect appears to be caused by a single nucleotide substitution producing a replacement of the normal Ala-109 by Thr in the TTR.[145] A recent crystallographic analysis suggested that the increased affinity of this variant TTR for T_4 is due to the altered size of the T_4-binding pocket.[145a]

A more common mutation found in subjects with prealbumin-associated hyperthyroxinemia (PAH) is a point mutation in exon 4 of the TTR gene replacing the normal Thr-119 with a Met.[146] First described in a single individual with normal serum total and free T_4 levels,[146a] the majority of subsequently reported heterozygous individuals harboring Met-119 had an increase in the fraction of T_4 and rT_3 associated with TTR, only a few having T_4 levels above the upper limit of normal. Furthermore, the hyperthyroxinemia in subjects with Met-119 appears to be transient and associated with nonthyroidal illness. It remains unknown whether under such circumstances the variant TTR contributes to the hyperthyroxinemia, possibly through the formation of an increased proportion of mutant-normal heterotetramers of TTR. Furthermore, the normal Msp 1 restriction site in exon 2 of the TTR gene was not present in the individual with PAH.[147] This abnormality has not been further characterized. The variant TTR's associated with PAH are not amyloidogenic.

VARIANTS WITH REDUCED AFFINITY FOR T_4 ASSOCIATED WITH AMYLOIDOSIS. A growing number of variant TTR's have been shown to produce dominantly inherited familial amyloidotic polyneuropathy (FAP) (Table 36–4). Two of these variant TTR's, namely those associated with type I FAP (Val→30-Met) and type II FAP (Ile-84→Ser), have been shown to have a five- to six-fold reduced affinity for T_4.[148] In contrast, the TTR associated with the Appalachian type FAP (Thr-60±Ala) had normal affinity for T_4. As in the case of variant Met-119, the T_4-binding abnormality in variant TTR's with decreased affinity for T_4 does not produce significant changes in the concentration of serum total T_4 in serum. The increased incidence of hypothyroidism in patients with FAP is probably due to the destruction of the thyroid gland by amyloid deposits.[148]

VARIANTS WITHOUT KNOWN BIOLOGICAL EFFECTS. Several TTR variants have been found that do not alter the properties of the molecule and are thus of no clinical significance. Of interest is a TTR variant found in rhesus monkeys (*Macaca mulatta*) but not in humans.[49, 50] This variant has a slower electrophoretic mobility resulting in three phenotypes that exhibit: (1) a single rapidly migrating band similar to that found in human and other primates (PA^{FF}), (2) a single slowly migrating band cathodal to albumin (PA^{SS}), and (3) a five-banded form corresponding to the various tetrameric recombinants present in the heterozygous state possessing the two different subunits (PA^{FS}). This finding was important because the variant rhesus PA-S could be hybridized in vitro with human TTR yielding a five-banded pattern, hence demonstrating, for the first time, that human TTR is also a tetramer. All naturally occurring and hybrid polymorphic variants show no detectable alteration in the binding of either T_4 or retinol-binding protein.[149]

Changes in Albumin

Because of the low affinity and despite the high capacity of ALB for thyroid hormone, its contribution to hormone transport is relatively minor.[150] Thus, even the most marked fluctuations in serum concentration of this protein have no significant effects on thyroid hormone levels.

Inherited Albumin Abnormalities

FAMILIAL DYSALBUMINEMIC HYPERTHYROXINEMIA (FDH). First described in 1979,[151, 152] the abnormality appears to be quite common, accounting for 12 per cent of subjects with euthyroid hyperthyroxinemia.[153] Such individuals have clearly increased serum total T_4 levels, in the range of 12 to 25 μg/dl and normal or minimally elevated serum total T_3 values. Although they are clinically euthyroid, many have been inappropriately treated for presumed hyperthyroidism. The euthyroid status has been confirmed by normal TSH response to TRH, free T_4 concentration measured by equilibrium dialysis using appropriate buffer systems, and T_4 production rate.[152, 154–156]

The increased concentration of T_4 in serum is due to the presence of an inherited variant protein with immunological properties similar to ALB but approximately 10-fold higher affinity for T_4. As a consequence, the relative distribution of T_4 among the binding proteins in serum is altered, with a three- to four-fold increase in the proportion carried with the variant protein fraction relative to normal ALB. Because the binding affinity for T_3 is not proportionately increased, total T_3 concentration remains in the upper limit of normal and estimation of the free T_4 concentration by the T_3-uptake test gives spuriously high values. When free T_4 is measured by the single-step RIA methods employing T_4 analogues, values were also spuriously high.[157] Serum total rT_3 concentration is also commonly increased. T_4 binding to the variant serum protein is inhibited by chloride ions[158] and by the reducing agent, dithiothreitol.[159] The latter finding suggests that disulfide linkage in the variant protein is essential for T_4 binding.

The FDH phenotype is inherited as an autosomal dominant trait. The abnormality has not been yet localized to the ALB gene. While a mutant ALB is considered to be a strong candidate, it is surprising that in the presence of normal ALB concentration and a single copy of the ALB gene, the high T_4 affinity variant protein does not co-migrate on IEF with half of the total ALB as determined by staining.[160] A classification of FDH into subtypes I through VI, based on the relative concentration of total T_4, T_3, and rT_3 in serum, has been suggested.[161] However, it appears that the magnitude of increased concentration of these three iodothyronines in serum may be due to the quantity of the variant ALB-like protein in serum.[162]

BISALBUMINEMIA AND ANALBUMINEMIA. Of passing interest are the genetic variants of ALB, detected by electrophoresis and producing "bisalbuminemia" in the heterozygotes.[61] T_4 binding has been studied in subjects from unrelated families with a slow ALB variant. In two studies only the slow-moving ALB bound T_4[163, 164] and in another, both bound the hormone.[98] The differential binding of T_4 to one of the components of bisalbumin may be due to enhanced binding to the variant component with charged amino acid sequence. Bisalbuminemia does not seem to be associated with gross alterations in thyroid hormone concentration in serum.

Analbuminemia is extremely rare.[61] This homozygous condition has been studied only in two subjects with respect to T_4 transport.[150] The virtual absence of ALB had no clear effect on thyroid hormone concentration in serum, as judged by protein-bound iodine determination, despite increased binding capacity of TBG and TTR. The latter two normalized when serum ALB was restored to normal by multiple transfusions.

THYROID HORMONE METABOLISM

The human thyroid gland primarily secretes a rather weak hormone, T_4, and thereby must rely on its subsequent peripheral tissue conversion to T_3 to achieve full hormonal expression. This peripheral T_4 to T_3 conversion process, which increases hormonal activity on nuclear receptor proteins some 10-fold (see Ch. 37), appears to play the dominant role in prereceptor regulation of thyroid hormone action in man. Although similar peripheral tissue T_4 to T_3 conversion has been demonstrated in all vertebrate species thus far studied, alterations in TSH-mediated thyroid gland secretion generally assume a much greater role in determining circulating levels of serum T_4 and T_3 in nonhuman species.[165] This is particularly evident in smaller mammalian species, such as the rat, in which acute changes in TSH-mediated thyroid gland secretion occur in response to a variety of environmental stimuli.[166] In contrast, the T_4 secretion rate and free thyroxine concentrations remain remarkably stable in humans under similar conditions (see Ch. 40). This constancy is further enhanced by the presence of a large serum pool of extrathyroidal T_4 bound to TBG which serves to modulate or "buffer" any acute variations in T_4 secretion, as was discussed earlier. However, this large pool of extrathyroidal T_4 places a greater reliance on the peripheral tissue T_4 to T_3 conversion processes to adjust for moment-to-moment variations in hormonal requirements, as imposed by environmental influences such as altered nutrition and illness. Such a peripheral regulatory system also affords the theoretical opportunity for differential tissue and organ control of hormonal activation through regulation of local T_4 to T_3 conversion. Because peripheral thyroid hormone metabolism appears to play such an important role in determining thyroid status in humans, special emphasis is placed on this aspect of thyroid hormone metabolism in the subsequent discussion. The reader is encouraged to refer to other recent reviews concerning this subject.[167–172]

Hormone Production and Kinetics

Thyroxine, T_3, and rT_3 constitute the three major forms of the thyroid hormones found in the circulation. All three hormones are bound to a varying degree by TBG. The

TABLE 36–5. NORMAL THYROID HORMONE KINETICS IN HUMANS

	T_4	T_3	rT_3
Total serum concentration ($\mu g/dl$)	7.5	0.14	0.022
Distribution volume (L)	10	38	90
Metabolic clearance rates (L/d)	1.2	22	130
Production or disposal rate ($\mu g/d$)	90	31	19
Conversion factors:		T_4 / nmol = 0.78 μg	
		T_3 and rT_3 / nmol = 0.65 μg	

greater binding of T_4 by TBG accounts, in part, for the total serum T_4 concentration being substantially greater than that for T_3 and rT_3, as shown in Table 36–5. When the total serum hormone concentrations for T_4, T_3, and rT_3 are multiplied by their respective clearance rates, as determined independently by tracer kinetic studies, an estimate of the disposal rate can be obtained. This value also equals the hormone production rate because disposal and production rates are identical in steady-state conditions.

THYROXINE. Circulating T_4 originates solely from thyroid gland secretion because the thyroid is the only site where the synthesis of T_4 occurs. The average adult secretes and metabolizes approximately 90 μg or 116 nmols of T_4 daily.[173, 174] Two-thirds of this thyroidal T_4 secretion depends on circulating TSH levels, while the remaining one-third appears to reflect constitutive T_4 secretion.[175] The normal daily production and disposal of T_4 varies in direct relationship to body size and, more precisely, to body surface area.[173] As body surface area is proportional to liver size, and the liver appears to be the primary organ responsible for T_4 disposal, such a relationship is not surprising.[173] Thyroxine production remains relatively constant throughout adulthood with the exception of a modest increase with pregnancy and a slight decrease after the age of 60 years.[176, 177] In the former situation, the increased T_4 secretory demand reflects the added requirements of the conceptus,[176] while in the latter instance, there appears to be a decrease in the T_4 disposal rate associated with advancing age.[177] When these particular patient populations are receiving T_4 replacement therapy, appropriate adjustments in the T_4 dosage are recommended.

The kinetic turnover of the extrathyroidal T_4 pool is extremely slow, with the normal half-life in circulation averaging 7 to 8 days. This translates into a daily fractional turnover rate of about 10 per cent. The relatively slow turnover for the extrathyroidal T_4 pool is primarily the product of the intense extracellular binding of T_4 by TBG;

this allows only 0.03 per cent of circulating T_4 to exist in a free state. It is this free T_4 that is available for entry into peripheral tissues where it can initiate hormonal action or undergo enzymatic conversion to T_3, rT_3, and other metabolites, as shown in Figure 36–6.

TRIIODOTHYRONINE. The sources of circulating T_3 are more complex than those for T_4. Normally a total of 31 μg or 48 nmols of T_3 are produced daily in the average euthyroid adult.[174] About 80 per cent, or 38 nmols of T_3, originates from outer-ring monodeiodination of T_4 by deiodinase enzymes located in peripheral tissues. This approximates about one third of the total daily secretion of T_4. The remaining 20 per cent or 10 nmols of T_3 production is directly secreted by the thyroid gland. These estimates are largely based on analysis of the T_3 and T_4 residues present in normal human thyroglobulin.[178] It should be noted that normal total serum T_3 concentrations are 50-fold lower, the free hormone values 5-fold lower, the free fraction 10-fold higher (0.3 per cent), the serum half-life 7-fold shorter (1.0 day) and the fractional turnover rate 5-fold greater (50 per cent) than for T_4, as shown in Table 36–5. Also a much larger component of the total distribution volume of T_3 (38 L) resides intracellularly (85 per cent) compared to that for T_4 (10 L, 50 per cent, respectively). Thus, the extrathyroidal T_3 pool is primarily distributed intracellularly while T_4 is about equally divided between the intra- and extracellular compartments.

REVERSE TRIIODOTHYRONINE. The other major circulating thyroid hormone is reverse T_3. Circulating rT_3 originates almost entirely from inner-ring monodeiodination of T_4 by peripheral tissue deiodinases, as direct rT_3 secretion by the thyroid gland is negligible.[179] Since rT_3 possesses no inherent calorigenic activity and does not bind to the nuclear thyroid hormone receptors,[180] this peripheral production of rT_3 from T_4 may be considered as an inactivation step. The estimated daily rT_3 blood production rate approximates 19 μg or 29 nmols, which accounts for about 40 per cent of the total daily disposal of T_4. Although rT_3 and T_3 have similar binding affinities for TBG, the rT_3 clearance rate is three times greater than that of T_3. This difference in clearance rate presumably results from rT_3 being a superior substrate for hepatic deiodinase enzymes.[171]

ALTERNATE ROUTES OF METABOLISM. About 70 per cent of the total daily disposal of thyroxine can be accounted for by the combined blood production estimates of T_3 (38 nmols) and rT_3 (29 nmols). The remaining 30 per cent presumably occurs by alternate routes of metabolism, as

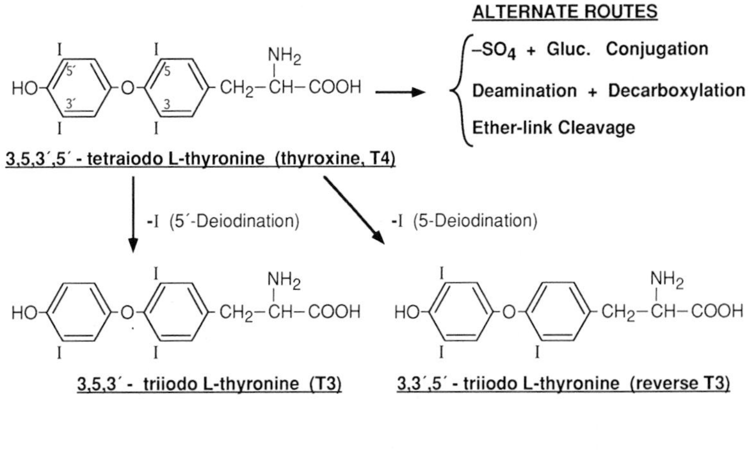

FIGURE 36–6. Graphic representation of the three major pathways for peripheral thyroxine metabolism which includes: (1) outer-ring monodeiodination by type I and II deiodinases, (2) inner-ring monodeiodination by type I and II deiodinases, and (3) alternate routes of hormone disposal by sulfo and glucuronyl conjugation; deamination combined with decarboxylation to form tetraiodothyroacetic acid and ether-link cleavage to form iodotyrosines.

shown in Figure 36–6. These alternate routes include (1) T_4 conjugation to form T_4 sulfate (T_4S)[181, 182] or T_4 glucuronide (T_4G),[183] (2) T_4 deamination and decarboxylation to form the acetic acid analogue tetrathyroacetic acid (tetrac),[184, 185] and (3) ether-link cleavage.[186–188] T_3 and rT_3 produced by peripheral tissue deiodinases that undergo further metabolism within the cell of origin and are not reflected in the circulating T_3 and rT_3 levels may also be considered an alternate disposal pathway. This occult source of T_3 and rT_3 formation has been termed a "hidden" pool.[190] Unfortunately, the amount of hormone produced within such hidden pools cannot be accurately quantified.

Another method of assessing the various routes of T_4 disposal is to evaluate the end products of its metabolism excreted in the urine. Following the initial monodeiodination of T_4 to form T_3 and rT_3, these metabolites undergo further sequential monodeiodination to form diiodothyronines (T_2), monoiodothyronines (T_1), and ultimately thyronine (T_0), the iodine-free form of the thyroxine molecule. Studies employing ^{14}C and ^{125}I T_4 tracers reveal that about 75 per cent of T_4 can be recovered in urine as either labeled T_0 or iodide.[191, 192] As this figure is 15 per cent higher than the 70 per cent obtained for the combined T_3 and rT_3 blood production rates, this indicates that other sources exist for these deiodinative end-products. It appears that sulfate or acetic acid derivatives of T_4 and T_3 are the most likely candidates because they serve as excellent substrates for deiodination and are major products of T_3 and T_4 metabolism. For example, it is projected that as much as one-half of T_3 disposal may occur through T_3S formation[168] and that two-thirds of urinary T_0 is excreted as the acetic acid derivative.[193] The role that these alternate routes may play in the regulation of thyroid hormone metabolism is further emphasized in the subsequent discussion.

Cellular Transport

Circulating T_3 and T_4 must pass through capillary, cellular, and nuclear membranes before undergoing further metabolism or exerting hormonal action. Because most of the circulating T_3 and virtually all of the rT_3 originate within peripheral tissues, this transport must be bidirectional. Presently, there are two general models explaining this transport: a passive model in which unbound hormone freely enters or exits the cell and an active model in which the hormone is bound to a specific cell membrane receptor involved with regulating transport.

Passive Transport Model

The passive model proposes that unbound thyronines, due to their inherent solubility in lipids, freely and rapidly cross cell membranes bidirectionally.[194–202] The magnitude of such transport appears to be limited by the exposure time of the blood passing through the capillary bed for any particular organ or tissue. In most tissues this exposure period is brief, approximating one second or less, which allows time only for complete exchange of free hormone but not hormone bound to serum carrier proteins. In contrast, in the hepatic portal circulation, where this exposure

interval is extended to about 10 seconds, there is sufficient time for occurrence of hormone debinding from serum carrier proteins, thereby allowing considerably greater hormone exchange between serum and tissues to take place. Additionally, there appears to be a "stripping" of hormone bound to serum proteins as blood slowly percolates through the hepatic sinusoidal system, which further increases the efficiency of this transfer process. These differences in circulatory characteristics are largely responsible for producing the so-called rapid and slow equilibrating tissue pools that have been described following the injection of labeled T_3 and T_4 tracers. It should be emphasized, however, that these differences in tissue and organ exchange do not appear to be rate limiting; they are several orders of magnitude greater than the rate at which hormonal disposal is believed to occur within those tissues. Another way of stating this proposition is that free hormone levels in the cytosol and nucleus would be essentially the same as in the serum. This supposition would also explain why there is such a close correlation between serum free hormone levels and hormone disposal rates.[203]

Active Transport Model

There are numerous reports describing the existence of specific binding sites for T_3 and T_4 situated on the outer surface of cell membranes. The cell types displaying such receptors are varied and include hepatocytes,[204] thymocytes,[205–207] glial and neuronal cells,[208, 209] fibroblasts,[210, 211] and erythrocytes.[212, 213] Most of these cellular binding sites demonstrate stereospecificity when tested. Some of these membrane receptors also seem to be involved with hormone transport, as monodansylcadaverine and other inhibitors known to interfere with endocytosis impair hormonal uptake. Several of these binding sites may also influence glucose uptake[214] and calcium pump activity and therefore may represent extranuclear sites of hormone action.[215] Although exceptions exist, the majority of studies purporting to demonstrate the existence of such plasma membrane receptors have been performed in vitro employing nonphysiological concentrations of T_3 and T_4. Therefore, caution should be exercised in interpreting the physiological relevance of these findings.

On the basis of current information it would appear that most cellular transport of T_3 and T_4 occurs by a passive transfer process. However, the abundance of evidence indicating the existence of membrane receptors raises the possibility that active transport may also occur. Perhaps active transport may play a role in regulating hormone concentrations at a subcellular level, while the bulk of hormone exchange remains passive in nature. Certainly higher local concentrations of T_3 resulting from intracellular deiodination of T_4 occur in pituitary, brain, and brown adipose tissue (BAT), indicating that a T_3 gradient can be maintained with the extracellular environment.[167, 216, 217] Further evidence for intracellular T_3 compartmentalization is provided by the reported differences observed between cytosol and nuclear distribution of D and L isomers of T_3.[218] In any case, the physiological role of these plasma membrane receptors and the processes involved with intracellular hormone compartmentalization remain subjects worthy of further investigation.

Intracellular Pathways for Iodothyronine Metabolism

With their entry into cells, T_3 and T_4 become bound to hydrophobic binding sites on cytoplasmic proteins in a manner similar to those observed in serum. The bulk of intracellular T_3 and T_4 remains situated in the cytoplasm while that contained in the nucleus generally accounts for less than 10 per cent of the total cell content. A clear exception to this rule is found in pituitary cells, in which approximately 50 per cent of intracellular T_3 resides in the nucleus.[167, 220] This large nuclear T_3 concentration in pituitary cells appears principally to be the consequence of higher levels of nuclear receptor proteins; however, a nuclear T_3 transport system has not been ruled out.[219] Although cytoplasmic binding proteins have not been as well characterized as their serum counterparts, they do seem to be qualitatively distinct from serum binding proteins.[215] A small fraction of this cytoplasmic T_3 and T_4 represents hormone bound to enzymes concerned with their metabolism. In the hepatocyte, these enzymes include members of the membrane-bound deiodinases and glucuronyl transferases, as well as cytosolic phenol sulfotransferases. The iodothyronine deiodinases may be considered to be the most important of the enzymatic systems because they are responsible for both hormonal activation through T_4 to T_3 conversion as well as thyronine deiodination, which is essential for recycling iodide into new hormone formation.

Iodothyronine Deiodinases

Iodothyronine deiodinases have been identified in a wide variety of tissues from experimental animals and, to a more limited degree, in humans. Based on a variety of functional criteria, their general catalytic properties, substrate preferences and co-factor requirements have been reasonably well defined. By convention, they have been classified into outer-ring or 5'-deiodinases (5'D), of which there are two major forms, type I and type II, and inner-ring or 5-deiodinases (5D), of which there is only a single class, type III.[167] A summary of the major properties of the three types of deiodinases are shown in Table 36–6.

TYPE I 5'DEIODINASE. The type I 5'D enzyme is widely distributed throughout most tissues but is most abundantly found in the liver, kidney, and the thyroid. In the liver it is limited to the hepatocyte, while in the kidney it appears to be localized to a portion of the proximal tubule.[222] The deiodinase found in the thyroid appears to be specialized in that it is activated by TSH.[221] The type I 5'D is also integrally associated with cellular membranes, either of the endoplasmic reticulum or plasma membrane, where it is oriented in such a manner as to have its catalytic unit freely accessible to the cytosolic iodothyronine pool. Substrate preference studies, as determined in homogenate systems with fixed thiol co-factor levels, reveal that rT_3 and sulfated or acetic acid derivatives of naturally occurring thyronines serve as optimal substrates for this enzyme.[182, 223, 224] Using the same kinetic criteria, T_3 and T_4 do not appear to serve as effective substrates for the type I 5'D at physiological concentrations. However, a certain degree of caution should also be exercised so as not to overinterpret the physiological relevance of such data obtained from in vitro studies. Optimal enzyme activation in vitro is achieved with the addition of dithiols with high redox potential, such as dithiothreitol (DTT), as co-factors.[225, 226] However, the exact character of the natural dithiol present in vivo is uncertain. Abundant data indicates that the deiodination process is a two-step mechanism commonly referred to as a "ping-pong" reaction.[226, 227] The first half-reaction produces the thyronine deiodination and an oxidized enzyme intermediate, while the second half-reaction leads to the reduction of the enzyme by a thiol co-factor. Thiourylenes such as PTU form a stable mixed disulfide with the oxidized enzyme, preventing the second half of this reaction from taking place.[226–228] Since uncompetitive PTU inhibition appears to be limited to the type I 5'D enzyme, it allows PTU administration to serve as a functional marker for this enzyme when in vivo and in vitro studies are performed. It is interesting to note that oral PTU given to euthyroid humans produces only a modest fall in circulating T_3 levels despite causing a substantial inhibition of the overall T_4 deiodination rate.[229, 230] This observation infers that serum T_3 originating from peripheral T_4 conversion is catalyzed by PTU-insensitive enzyme systems, possibly the type II 5'D. A similar situation is seen in the juvenile rat model.[231] In contrast, substantial reductions in serum T_3 levels can be produced with PTU therapy in hyperthyroxinemic states. In this respect, PTU therapy has proved to be beneficial adjunctive treatment for severe thyrotoxic states.[232] Thus the source of circulating T_3 originating from T_4 in humans is likely the product of more than one enzyme system depending on the serum T_4 level.

Major advances in the biochemical isolation and gene identification of the type I 5'D has been recently achieved, thereby allowing better definition of its physicochemical properties.[233–235] These studies indicate that the type I 5'D gene contains a crucial sequence coding for incorporation of seleno-methionine.[233, 235] This protein-bound selenium appears to be an integral part of the catalytic unit responsible for imparting deiodinase activity.[233, 235] This finding now explains the previous clinical observations that selenium therapy alone, when given to cretinous subjects with combined endemic selenium and iodine deficiency, results in decreased serum T_4 levels as well as worsening the hy-

TABLE 36–6. CLASSIFICATION OF IODOTHYRONINE DEIODINASES

	TYPE I 5'D	TYPE II 5'D	TYPE III 5'D
Dominant locations	Liver, kidney, thyroid	CNS, pituitary, placenta, Brown adipose tissue	Placenta, CNS
Substrate preference	$rT_3 > T_4 > T_3$	$T_4 > rT_3 > T_3$	$T_4 \geq rT_3$
PTU	Inhibits	No effect	No effect
Iopanoic acid	Inhibits	Inhibits	Inhibits
Selenium	Present	Absent	Absent
Km for T_4	High	Low	Low

pothyroid state.[236, 237] Presumably this is due to an acceleration of T_4 disposal produced by restoration of type I 5'D activity.[237] The marked reduction in both hepatic and renal type I 5'D activity observed in the selenium-deficient rat model supports this clinical observation.[238, 239] These advances in the molecular biological understanding of the type I 5'D also should provide further insights into its gene regulation, isoenzyme forms, and subcellular localization. They may also provide information relevant to the question of whether a specialized low Km (high-affinity) PTU-resistant 5'D subspecies exists in hepatocytes which may be primarily responsible for generating circulating T_3 from peripheral tissue T_4 to T_3 conversion, as has been proposed by several investigative groups.[240–242]

TYPE II 5'-DEIODINASE. The type II 5'D enzyme appears to be distinct from the type I 5'D in that it prefers T_4 over rT_3 as a substrate, possesses a much lower Km (higher affinity) for T_4, displays a sequential rather than a ping-pong deiodination mechanism, and is unaffected by dietary selenium deficiency.[167, 170, 171, 243] Most type II activity is found in the central nervous system, pituitary, and BAT, where it seems to be responsible for local autocrine and paracrine T_3 generation. In this regard, it is estimated that approximately 50 per cent of the T_3 in the pituitary and 75 per cent in the brain originates from local T_4 to T_3 conversion. Some type II 5'D activity can also be demonstrated in placenta, where its physiological role is uncertain.[244–246] Type II 5'D requires higher concentrations of reduced thiols than type I 5'D. This may explain its resistance to PTU effects because these high thiol levels interfere with the mixed-disulfide formation required for PTU inhibition.[171]

TYPE III 5'-DEIODINASE. It is reasonably certain that more than one enzyme is responsible for producing inner-ring deiodination of thyronines. In the liver and kidney, the type I enzyme serves this function of inner-ring deiodination for substrates such as 3,3' dioodothyronine and the sulfated or acetic acid analogues of all naturally occurring thyronine.[182, 223, 224] In other tissues, a distinct deiodinase, designated as type III 5D, appears responsible for inner ring deiodination. Its highest activity is found in brain and placenta, with T_3 and T_4 being are the preferred substrates.[245, 247, 248] The physiological role of type III 5D in iodothyronine metabolism is uncertain other than the possibility that it may reduce cellular T_3 content as seems to be the case in the placenta. The placental type III 5D may not only serve the function of isolating maternal from fetal thyroid systems but also appears to facilitate local iodide generation used in hormone formation by the fetal thyroid gland.[245] The type III 5D also seems to be responsible for generating most of the circulating rT_3 in humans from T_4 to rT_3 conversion.[229] It is noteworthy that the blood rT_3 production rates in humans are not influenced by PTU administration; this is consistent with in vitro observations that type III 5D is not inhibited by PTU. However, total serum rT_3 values do increase with PTU administration due to the slowing of rT_3 clearance resulting from inhibition of hepatic type I 5'D.[229] In contrast, glucocorticoids do increase rT_3 production by stimulating type III 5D enzyme activity.[229] This enzyme, as with other deiodinases, also requires reduced thiols as a co-factor to achieve full catalytic activity.[171]

Alternate Enzymatic Routes for Iodothyronine Metabolism

There are several enzymatic pathways other than deiodinases which are also responsible for T_4 disposal, as illustrated in Figure 36–1. As previously discussed, these alternate routes may account for as much as 30 per cent of total T_4 disposal and perhaps an even higher percentage for T_3. Recently increasing attention has been focused on the actions of phenol sulfotransferases to produce sulfate conjugates as a major enzymatic disposal pathway for both T_4 and T_3.[181, 182] Such sulfotransferases are abundant in liver and kidney but are also widely distributed in other tissues.[182, 249] As previously noted, both T_3S and T_4S serve as exceptionally good substrates for the hepatic type I 5'-deiodinase. With the recent development of an immunoassay for serum T_3S measurement[250] and the determination of T_3S kinetic turnover data,[251] it is now possible to estimate blood T_3S production rates. These data indicate that about 10 per cent of total T_3 disposal can be accounted for by T_3S formation. However, this may be a gross underestimate of total T_3S production because T_3S formed within the hepatocyte would not likely contribute to circulating T_3S due to its rapid deiodination by the hepatic type I 5'D. It also appears that increased T_4S formation takes place in association with high T_4 states, which shunt excess T_4 into disposal pathways rather than into T_3 formation.[182] This presumably explains the minimal increase in serum T_3 values observed following large doses of oral T_4.[252, 253] T_3S and T_4S formation is also probably increased with fasting and nonthyroidal illnesses, thereby maintaining normal T_4 and T_3 clearance rates despite evidence of hepatic type I 5'D inhibition. Sulfation of T_3 primarily represents a disposal mechanism—tracer T_3S kinetic studies in humans indicate that once T_3S enters the circulation, no detectable deconjugation and release of T_3 occur.[251] Glucuronidation of T_3 and T_4 by hepatic glucuronyl transferases represents an additional mechanism for hormonal inactivation and excretion both in animals and humans.[183, 185, 254] In contrast to sulfation, however, glucuronide conjugates are not effective substrates for deiodinases but typically pass directly into the bile and are excreted into the feces.[185] Although some deconjugation and enterohepatic recycling may occur in some animal species, such recycling appears to be minimal in humans.

Formation of acetic acid analogues of T_4 and T_3 by enzymatic actions of aminotransferases and oxidative decarboxylases found in liver, kidney, and other tissues provides an additional route for hormonal metabolism.[184, 185, 255–258] Although estimates of the blood production rates of tetrac and triiodothyroacetic acid (triac) are very modest,[257] more than half of the T_0 excreted in urine exists in the acetic acid form indicating that a much larger quantity of T_4 and T_3 may be converted into an acetic acid derivative than is reflected by their blood production rates. In addition, triac has been found to have an equal or greater biological activity to that of T_3 in activating nuclear thyroid hormone receptors.[259] However, triac is a much weaker systemic hormone than T_3, primarily due to its nearly 8-fold greater clearance from serum.[257] Thus the formation of triac, either as a hormonal disposal or activation mechanism, presently remains an enigma deserving further investigation. Ether bond cleavage of T_3 and T_4 to form mono- and diiodotyrosine is catalyzed by myeloperoxidases within activated leukocytes.[185, 186] However, the quantity of hormone normally undergoing this form of degradation is thought to be very low with the exception, perhaps, in severe bacterial infections.[188]

Regulation of Circulating and Tissue Iodothyronine Metabolism

It is not surprising that both circulating and tissue T_3 levels are precisely regulated because T_3 represents the most active form of thyroid hormone. Although many details still remain to be clarified, some general concepts have emerged as to how this control may be achieved. For example, in subjects receiving exogenous T_4 therapy, serum T_3 values are "defended" within a narrow range of values despite substantial differences in serum T_4 levels, as shown in Figure 36–7. This indicates that a peripheral regulatory process exists for controlling T_4 to T_3 conversion.[251, 252] On the other hand, tight regulation of serum T_3 levels is also seen in patients with severe iodine deficiency. High serum TSH values induced by the low serum T_4 levels act to increase T_3 secretion by the thyroid gland.[260] This suggests that a central mechanism may also be involved in maintaining serum T_3 values.[167] As the term *autoregulation* has been applied to both these central and peripheral autoregulatory mechanisms, it is helpful to subdivide them for discussion.

Peripheral Autoregulation

Several studies have demonstrated that serum T_3 levels do not parallel T_4 values in athyreotic subjects adminis-

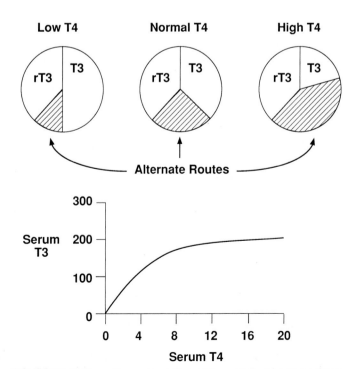

FIGURE 36–7. Shematic representation of the peripheral autoregulatory control of T_4 to T_3 conversion as it affects the major pathways of T_4 disposal *(upper panel)* and serum T_3 values. Normal serum T_3 values range between 80 and 220 ng/dl and serum T_4 between 4.5 and 11.5 µg/dl.

tered varying doses of exogenous T_4.[252, 253, 260] As can be seen from Figure 36–7, serum T_3 levels rapidly increase as T_4 values rise to the subnormal range and then increase more gradually as serum T_4 values undergo transition into the normal and supraphysiological ranges. The net effect of this response pattern is to maintain serum T_3 levels within the normal range except at the extremes of serum T_4 concentrations. This phenomenon likely explains why many patients appear tolerant to mild excesses or deficiencies in T_4 replacement therapy. The mechanism responsible for this peripheral autoregulation is revealed by tracer kinetic studies, which show that net T_4 to T_3 conversion efficiency progressively falls from a high of 50 per cent at serum low T_4 concentrations to less than 10 per cent at supraphysiological levels. It is interesting to note that the normal conversion efficiency of 32 per cent is about midway between these two extremes. In contrast, the T_4 to rT_3 conversion efficiency, which primarily reflects type III 5D activity, remains fixed regardless of the serum T_4 level. What also occurs, as is shown in the pie diagrams in the upper panel of Figure 36–7, is that the quantity of alternate metabolites formed from T_4 is reciprocally related to the T_4 to T_3 conversion efficiency. Thus the blood production of T_3 from T_4 appears to be further modulated by the quantity of T_4 or T_3 shunted into alternate metabolic pathways. As these alternate metabolites include sulfate, glucuronide, and acetic acid derivatives principally generated by the liver, it would indicate that the hepatocyte might be the primary site at which this peripheral autoregulatory process might occur. However, as it is uncertain which tissues or organs are responsible for generating circulating T_3 from T_4—either in humans or laboratory animal models—no firm conclusion can be reached.

Another form of peripheral T_4 to T_3 autoregulatory control also exists at the cellular level in those tissues that contain type II 5′D systems such as the cerebral cortex, pituitary, and BAT.[167, 171] In the cerebral cortex, type II 5′D system enzymes up-regulate their activity in response to low T_4 concentrations both in vivo and in vitro. The net effect of this is that intracellular T_3 concentrations are maintained constant over a broad range of extracellular free T_4 concentrations. As the brain derives the majority of its T_3 from local T_4 conversion, this intracellular T_3 autoregulation allows the brain to defend its T_3 content in the face of a T_4-deficient state. It is of some interest that rT_3, but not T_3, can also regulate the brain type II 5′D in a manner similar to that of T_4 and therefore may exert some additional regulatory control over T_4 to T_3 conversion at the cellular level.[171, 261] The BAT type II 5′D also displays a similar autoregulatory response to low T_4 states but additionally shows a stimulatory response to α-adrenergic agonists; apparently this accounts for the increased T_3 generation found in BAT with cold exposure.[167, 171, 262]

The overall effect of these circulatory and cellular autoregulatory mechanisms is to gain more precise control over tissue T_3 levels. It should once again be emphasized that this peripheral control of tissue T_3 levels appears to be a dominant mechanism for regulation of human thyroid hormone metabolism.

Central Autoregulation

The central autoregulatory system defends serum T_3 levels through the hypothalamic-pituitary-thyroid axis. The primary mechanism responsible for orchestrating this response appears to be focused at the level of the pituitary thyrotroph and its unique type II 5'D system. The thyrotroph type II 5'D enzyme, in contrast to those found in other tissues, appears *not* to be regulated by T_4 but rather generates T_3 proportionally to the extracellular free T_4 level.[167] By this mechanism, the thyrotroph becomes sensitized to even minor alterations in serum free T_4 values through its influence on intracellular T_3 generation. This ability of the thyrotroph to directly respond to changes in serum free T_4 is primarily responsible for the diagnostic utility of the serum TSH measurement in thyroid function testing (see Ch. 39). When serum TSH values rise secondary to a decline in serum free T_4 values, they act not only to stimulate overall thyroid gland secretion but additionally to activate the thyroidal type I 5'D system to generate T_3 through local T_4 to T_3 conversion. This increased TSH-mediated T_3 secretion complements that of the peripheral autoregulatory system in maintaining serum T_3 levels at normal. The effectiveness of these dual systems is probably best exemplified by the ability of inhabitants living in areas of severe endemic iodine deficiency to maintain normal serum T_3 values and an even metabolic status despite hypothyroid range serum T_4 and TSH values.[263] These autoregulatory systems can act in the opposite manner to maintain normal serum T_3 levels in high T_4 states as well.

Alterations in Serum T_3 Levels in Pathophysiological States

In view of the preceding discussion regarding the autoregulatory defense of circulating and tissue T_3 levels, it becomes even more significant that serum T_3 values are allowed to precipitously fall in a variety of conditions, including undernutrition, metabolic derangements, and a wide variety of systemic illnesses or injuries, without evoking either a peripheral or central autoregulatory response. These low T_3 states presumably represent an adaptive response designed to minimize tissue protein losses in the face of secondary to increased levels of gluconeogenesis which commonly accompany these conditions (see Ch. 40).

Although the mechanisms responsible for these changes are not well understood, a few interesting alterations in iodothyronine metabolism are worthy of note. The first relates to the maintenance of normal T_3 and T_4 clearance rates despite the presence of substantial inhibition of hepatic type I 5'D systems as reflected by elevated serum rT_3 values. In vitro studies confirm the reduced hepatic type I 5'D activity in response to fasting or metabolic derangements.[264] Presumably the maintenance of normal T_3 and T_4 clearances is accomplished by increased shunting of thyronine metabolites into the alternate pathways in a manner similar to that observed for high T_4 states (see Figs. 36–7 and 40–4). However, it is not understood how such a diversion is accomplished. The observation that serum TSH values either remain normal or fall in the face of declining serum T_3 levels in these states constitutes another notable paradox. This observation would indicate that a reset in thyrotroph negative feedback for T_3 has occurred.[265] The genesis of the reset is unknown, but it does not appear to be due to increases in local T_4 to T_3 generation by type II 5'D activity within the pituitary.[266, 267] It is noteworthy that

when pharmacological doses of glucocorticoids are administered to healthy subjects all the essential features seen with the low T_3 state are produced, including inhibition of the net conversion of T_4 to T_3, as well as transient reductions in serum TSH levels.[268] Although endogenous glucocorticoid secretion undoubtedly plays a significant role in the production of many low T_3 states associated with systemic nonthyroidal illness or injuries, it would not be sufficient to explain either the magnitude or the character of changes found in all such conditions (see Ch. 40).

Summary

This overview of human thyroid hormone metabolism indicates that the control of thyroid hormone availability to sites of action resides at the peripheral tissue level as well as through TSH-mediated thyroid gland secretion. This emphasis on peripheral rather than central control is enhanced by the existence of large extrathyroidal pools of T_3 and T_4 bound to TBG and other serum carrier proteins that modulate acute perturbations in thyroid gland secretion. As T_3 is the most active form of thyroid hormone, it is not surprising that the cellular T_3 levels are closely regulated by a combination of both local and systemic hormonal activation, transport, and disposal mechanisms. In certain specialized tissues, such as brain, pituitary, and BAT, intracellular T_3 content appears to be established by mechanisms that operate largely independently of circulating T_3 levels. By such independence, differential tissue hormonal expression is, in part, achieved. For other tissues that depend on circulating T_3, serum T_3 is controlled by varying the efficiency of systemic T_4 to T_3 conversion through an autoregulation mechanism which maintains near-normal T_3 levels in euthyroid healthy subjects despite changes in circulating T_4. This peripheral control of circulating T_3 is also complemented by a central system that alters thyroidal T_3 secretion via a TSH-dependent intrathyroidal type I 5'D. In contrast to this defense of serum T_3 seen in healthy individuals, a variety of catabolic conditions—including fasting, diabetes, systemic illness and glucocorticoid therapy—decrease serum T_3 by diminishing peripheral T_4 to T_3 conversion as well as preventing a compensatory increase in TSH secretion. As in healthy individuals, these lower levels also appear to be closely regulated.

These different patterns of pre-receptor regulation of thyroid hormone metabolism suggests the existence of two general classes of control over tissue T_3 levels: namely, those tissues that are capable of regulating their own level of T_3 and those that must depend on circulating T_3. It would seem that those tissues with specialized functions, such as brain, pituitary, and BAT, exert local control over their T_3 requirements, whereas those concerned with general somatic growth depend on circulating T_3 levels. In such a system, it makes sense that serum T_3 levels should fall in states of undernutrition and systemic illness when general growth and development would be retarded while still maintaining T_3 content in crucial organs such as the brain. Whether such a dualistic control of tissue T_3 levels exists in such low T_3 states is, at this point, only speculation. In any case, it would appear that the cellular control of thyroid hormone metabolism is a considerably more diversified and sophisticated process than has been generally appreciated.

REFERENCES

1. Farer LS, Robbins J, Blumberg BS, Rall JE: Thyroxine-serum protein complexes in various animals. Endocrinology 70:686–696, 1962.
2. Refetoff S, Robin NI, Fang VS: Parameters of thyroid function in serum of 16 selected vertebrate species: A study of PBI, serum T_4, free T_4, and the pattern of T_4 and T_3 binding to serum proteins. Endocrinology 86:793–805, 1970.
3. Oppenheimer JH: Role of plasma proteins in the binding, distribution, and metabolism of the thyroid hormones. N Engl J Med 278:1153–1162, 1968.
4. Woeber KA, Ingbar SH: The contribution of thyroxine-binding prealbumin to the binding of thyroxine in human serum, as assessed by immunoadsorption. J Clin Invest 47:1710–1721, 1968.
5. Freeman T, Pearson JD: The use of quantitative immunoelectrophoresis to investigate thyroxine-binding human serum proteins. Clin Chim Acta 26:365–368, 1969.
6. Benvenga S, Gregg RE, Robbins J: Binding of thyroid hormone to human plasma lipoproteins. J Clin Endocrinol Metab 67:6–16, 1988.
7. Robbins J, Rall JE, Rawson RW: An unusual instance of thyroxine-binding by human serum gamma globulin. J Clin Endocrinol Metab 16:573–579, 1956.
8. Premachandra BN, Blumenthal HT: Abnormal binding of thyroid hormone in sera from patients with Hashimoto's disease. J Clin Endocrinol Metab 27:931–936, 1967.
9. Beck-Peccoz P, Romelli PB, Cattaneo MG, et al: Evaluation of free thyroxine methods in the presence of iodothyronine-binding autoantibodies. J Clin Endocrinol Metab 58:736–739, 1984.
10. Benvenga S, Trimarchi F, Robbins J: Circulating thyroid hormone autoantibodies. J Endocrinol Invest 10:605–619, 1987.
11. Robbins J, Rall JE: Proteins associated with the thyroid hormones. Physiol Rev 40:415–489, 1960.
12. Bartalena L, Farsetti A, Flink IL, Robbins J: Effects of interleukin-6 on the expression of thyroid-hormone binding protein genes in cultured hepatoblastoma-derived (Hep G2) cells. Mol Endocrinol 6:935–942, 1992.
13. Refetoff S: Inherited thyroxine-binding globulin (TBG) abnormalities in man. Endocr Rev 10:275–293, 1989.
14. Chan V, Besser GM, Landon J: Effects of oestrogen on urinary thyroxine excretion. Br Med J 4:699–701, 1972.
15. Robbins J, Rall JE: Zone electrophoresis in filter paper of serum I^{131} after radioiodine administration. Proc Soc Exper Biol Med 81:530–536, 1952.
16. Gordon AH, Gross J, O'Connor D, Pitt-Rivers R: Nature of circulating thyroid hormone-plasma protein complex. Nature 169:19–20, 1952.
17. Larson F, Deiss WP, Albright EC: Localization of protein-bound radioactive iodine by filter paper electrophoresis. Science 115:626–627, 1952.
18. Marshall JS, Pensky J: Studies on thyroxine-binding globulin (TBG). III. Some physical characteristics of TBG and its interaction with thyroxine. Arch Biochem Biophys 146:76–83, 1971.
19. Flink IL, Bailey TJ, Gustefson TA, et al: Complete amino acid sequence of human thyroxine-binding globulin deduced from cloned DNA: Close homology to the serine antiproteases. Proc Natl Acad Sci (USA) 83:7708–7712, 1986.
20. Trent JM, Flink IL, Morkin E, et al: Localization of the human thyroxine-binding globulin gene to the long arm of the X chromosome (Xq21-22). Am J Hum Genet 41:428–435, 1987.
21. Zinn AB, Marshall JS, Carlson DM: Carbohydrate structures of thyroxine-binding globulin and their effects on hepatocyte membrane binding. J Biol Chem 253:6768–6773, 1978.
22. Refetoff S, Fang VS, Marshall JS: Studies on human thyroxine-binding globulin (TBG). IX. Some physical, chemical and biological properties of radioiodinated TBG and partially desialylated TBG (STBG). J Clin Invest 56:177–187, 1975.
23. Cheng SY, Morrone S, Robbins J: Effect of deglycosylation on the binding and immunoreactivity of human thyroxine-binding globulin. J Biol Chem 254:8830–8835, 1979.
24. Murata Y, Magner J, Refetoff S: The role of glycosylation in the molecular conformation and secretion of thyroxine-binding globulin. Endocrinology 118:1614–1621, 1986.
25. Kambe F, Seo H, Mori Y, et al: An additional carbohydrate chain in the variant thyroxine-binding globulin-Gary (TBG^{Asn-96}) impairs its secretion. Mol Endocrinol 6:443–449, 1992.
26. Gartner R, Henze R, Horn K, et al: Thyroxine-binding globulin: Investigation of microheterogeneity. J Clin Endocrinol Metab 52:657–664, 1981.
27. Janssen OE, Refetoff S: In-vitro expression of thyroxine-binding globulin (TBG) variants: Impaired secretion of the complete deficiency variant TBG$^{PRO-227}$ but not the partial deficiency variant TBG$^{PRO-113}$. J Biol Chem 267:13998–14004, 1992.
28. Refetoff S, Murata Y, Vassart G, et al: Radioimmunoassays specific for the tertiary and primary structures of thyroxine-binding globulin (TBG): Measurement of denatured TBG in serum. J Clin Endocrinol Metab 59:269–277, 1984.
29. Hocman G: Human thyroxine binding globulin. Rev Physiol Biochem Pharmacol 81:45–88, 1981.
30. Grimaldi S, Edelhoch H, Robbins J: Effects of thyroxine binding on the stability, conformation, and fluorescence properties of thyroxine-binding globulin. Biochemistry 21:145–150, 1982.
31. Takemura Y, Hocman G, Sterling K: Thermal stability of serum thyroxine-binding proteins. J Clin Endocrinol Metab 32:222–224, 1971.
32. Cavalieri RR, McMahon FA, Castle JN: Preparation of ^{125}I-labeled human thyroxine-binding alpha globulin and its turnover in normal and hypothyroid subjects. J Clin Invest 56:79–87, 1975.
33. Refetoff S, Fang VS, Marshall JS, Robin NI: Metabolism of thyroxine-binding globulin (TBG) in man: Abnormal rate of synthesis in inherited TBG deficiency and excess. J Clin Invest 57:485–495, 1976.
34. Ain KB, Mori Y, Refetoff S: Reduced clearance rate of thyroxine-binding globulin (TBG) with increased sialylation: A mechanism for estrogen induced elevation of serum TBG concentration. J Clin Endocrinol Metab 65:689–696, 1987.
35. Ain KB, Refetoff S: Relationship of oligosaccharide modification to the cause of serum thyroxine-binding globulin excess. J Clin Endocrinol Metab 66:1037–1043, 1988.
36. Cody V: Thyroid hormone interactions: Molecular conformation, protein binding and hormone action. Endocr Rev 1:140, 1980.
37. Oppenheimer JH, Tavernetti RR: Displacement of thyroxine from human thyroxine-binding globulin by analogues of hydantoin. Steric aspects of the thyroxine-binding site. J Clin Invest 41:2213–2220, 1962.
38. Smith PJ, Surks MI: Multiple effects of 5,5'-diphenylhydantoin on the thyroid hormone system. Endocr Rev 5:514–524, 1984.
39. Larsen PR: Salicylate-induced increases in free triiodothyronine in human serum: Evidence of inhibition of triiodothyronine binding to thyroxine-binding gloublin and thyroxine-binding prealbumin. J Clin Invest 51:1125–1134, 1972.
40. Marshall JS, Pensky J, Green AM: Studies on human thyroxine-binding globulin. IV. The nature of slow thyroxine-binding globulin. J Clin Invest 51:3173–3181, 1972.
41. Premachandra BN, Perlstein IB, Blumenthal HT: Studies on obesity. II. Slow-moving thyroxine-binding globulin in the sera of normal and obese subjects. J Clin Endocrinol Metab 30:752–762, 1970.
42. Marshall JS, Green AM, Pensky J, et al: Measurement of circulating desialylated glycoproteins and correlation with hepatocellular damage. J Clin Invest 54:555–562, 1974.
43. Reilly CP, Wellby ML: Slow thyroxine binding globulin in the pathogenesis of increased dialysable fraction of thyroxine in nonthyroidal illnesses. J Clin Endocrinol Metab 57:15–18, 1983.
44. Ingbar SH: A thyroxine-binding protein of human plasma. Endocrinology 63:256–259, 1958.
45. Kanai M, Raz A, Goodman D: Retinol-binding protein: The transport protein for vitamin A in human plasma. J Clin Invest 47:2025–2044, 1968.
46. Peterson PA: Characteristics of a vitamin A-transporting protein complex occurring in human serum. J Biol Chem 246:34–43, 1971.
47. Blake CCF, Oatley SJ: Protein-DNA and protein-hormone interactions in prealbumin: A model of the thyroid hormone nuclear receptor? Nature (London) 268:115–120, 1977.
48. Rerat C, Schwick HG: Données cristallographiques sur la préalbumine du plasma sanguin. Acta Cryst 22:441, 1967.
49. Alper CA, Robin NI, Refetoff S: Genetic polymorphism of rhesus thyroxine-binding prealbumin: Evidence for tetrameric structure in primates. Proc Natl Acad Sci (USA) 63:775–781, 1969.
50. Bernstein RS, Robbins J, Rall JE: Polymorphism of monkey thyroxine-binding prealbumin (TBPA): Mode of inheritance and hybridization. Endocrinology 86:383–390, 1970.
51. Tsuzuki T, Mita S, Maeda S, et al: Stucture of human prealbumin gene. J Biol Chem 260:12224–12227, 1985.

52. Wallace MR, Naylor SL, Kluve-Beckerman B, et al: Localization of the human prealbumin gene to chromosome 18. Biochem Biophys Res Comm 129:753–758, 1985.

53. Irace G, Edelhoch H: Thyroxine induced conformational changes in prealbumin. Biochemistry 17:5729–5733, 1978.

54. van Jaarsveld PP, Edelhoch H, Goodman DS, Robbins J: The interaction of human plasma retinol binding protein with prealbumin. J Biol Chem 248:4698–4705, 1973.

55. Pages RA, Robbins J, Edelhoch H: Binding of thyroxine and thyroxine analogs to human serum prealbumin. Biochemistry 12:2773–2779, 1973.

56. Wolff J, Standaert ME, Rall JE: Thyroxine displacement from serum proteins and depression of serum protein-bound iodine by certain drugs. J Clin Invest 40:1373–1379, 1961.

57. Munro SL, Lim CF, Hall JG, et al: Drug competition for thyroxine binding to transthyretin (Prealbumin): Comparison with effects on thyroxine-binding globulin. J Clin Endocrinol Metab 68:1141–1147, 1989.

58. Socolow EL, Woeber KA, Purdy RH, et al: Preparation of I^{131}-labeled human serum prealbumin and its metabolism in normal and sick patients. J Clin Invest 44:1600, 1965.

59. Oppenheimer JH, Surks MI, Bernstein G, Smith JC: Metabolism of iodine-131-labeled thyroxine-binding prealbumin in man. Science 149:748–751, 1965.

60. Hawkins JW, Dugaiczyk A: The human serum albumin gene: Structure of a unique locus. Gene 19:55–58, 1982.

61. Peters T Jr: Serum albumin. Adv Prot Chem 37:161–245, 1985.

62. Tabachnick M, Giorgio NA Jr: Thyroxine-protein interactions. II. The binding of thyroxine and its analogues to human serum albumin. Arch Biochem Biophys 105:563–569, 1964.

63. Tabachnick M: Thyroxine-protein interactions. III. Effect of fatty acids, 2,4-dinitrophenol and other anionic compounds on the binding of thyroxine by human serum albumin. Arch Biochem Biophys 106:415–421, 1964.

64. Beeken WL, Volwilier W, Goldsworthy PD, et al: Studies of I^{131}-albumin catabolism and distribution in normal young male adults. J Clin Invest 41:1312–1333, 1962.

65. Dowling JT, Freinkel N, Ingbar SH: The effect of estrogens upon the peripheral metabolism of thyroxine. J Clin Invest 39:1119–1130, 1960.

66. Braverman LE, Ingbar SH: Effects of norethandrolone on the transport in serum and peripheral turnover of thyroxine. J Clin Endocrinol Metab 27:389–396, 1967.

67. Refetoff S, Robin NI, Alper CA: Study of four new kindreds with inherited thyroxine-binding globulin abnormalities: Possible mutations of a single gene locus. J Clin Invest 51:848–867, 1972.

68. Sakurada T, Yamaguchi T, Yamamoto M, et al: Effect of estrogen on serum total and free thyroxine and triiodothyronine in a thyroxine-binding globulin deficient family. Tohoku J Exp Med 112:35–46, 1974.

69. Macchia PE, Harrison HH, Refetoff S, et al: Functional impairment of underglycosylated thyroxine-binding gloublin in patients with the carbohydrate-deficient glycoprotein syndrome. Thyroid 2(Suppl 1):S104, 1992.

70. Dowling JT, Freinkel N, Ingbar SH: Effect of diethylstilbestrol on binding of thyroxine in serum. J Clin Endocrinol Metab 16:1491–1506, 1956.

71. Refetoff S, Hagen S, Selenkow HA: Estimation of the T$_4$ binding capacity of serum TBG and TBPA by a single T$_4$ load ion exchange resin method. J Nucl Med 13:2–12, 1972.

72. Federman DD, Robbins J, Rall JE: Effects of methyl testosterone on thyroid function, thyroxine metabolism, and thyroxine-binding protein. J Clin Invest 37:1024–1030, 1958.

73. Barbosa J, Seal US, Doe RP: Effects of anabolic steroids on hormone-binding proteins, serum cortisol and serum nonprotein-bound cortisol. J Clin Endocrinol Metab 32:232–240, 1971.

74. Robbins J, Nelson JH: Thyroxine-binding by serum protein in pregnancy and in the newborn. J Clin Invest 37:153–159, 1958.

75. Galton VA, Ingbar SH, Jimenez-Fonseca J, Hershman JM: Alterations in thyroid hormone economy in patients with hydatidiform mole. J Clin Invest 50:1345–1354, 1971.

76. Stubbe P, Gatz J, Heidemann P, et al: Thyroxine-binding globulin, triiodothyronine, thyroxine and thyrotropin in newborn infants and children. Horm Metab Res 10:58–61, 1978.

77. Oppenheimer JH, Werner SC: Effect of prednisone on thyroxine-binding proteins. J Clin Endocrinol Metab 26:715–721, 1966.

78. Oltman JE, Friedman S: Protein-bound iodine in patients receiving perphenazine. JAMA 185:726–727, 1963.

79. Garnick MB, Larsen PR: Acute deficiency of thyroxine-binding globulin during L-asparaginase therapy. N Engl J Med 301:252–253, 1979.

80. Webster JB, Coupal JJ, Cushman P Jr: Increased serum thyroxine levels in euthyroid narcotic addicts. J Clin Endocrinol Metab 37:928–934, 1973.

81. McKerron CG, Scott RL, Asper SP, Levy RI: Effects of clofibrate (Atromid S) on the thyroxine-binding capacity of thyroxine-binding globulin and free thyroxine. J Clin Endocrinol Metab 29:957–961, 1969.

82. Beex L, Ross A, Smals P, Kloppenborg P: 5-Fluorouracil–induced increase of total thyroxine and triiodothyronine. Cancer Treat Rep 61:1291–1295, 1977.

83. Cashin-Hemphill L, Spencer CA, Nicoloff JT, et al: Alterations in serum thyroid hormonal indices with colestipol-niacin therapy. Ann Intern Med 107:324–329, 1987.

84. O'Brien T, Silverberg JD, Nguyen TT: Nicotinic acid–induced toxicity associated with cytopenia and decreased levels of thyroxine-binding globulin. Mayo Clin Proc 67:465–468, 1992.

85. Hollander CS, Scott RL, Tschudy DP, et al: Increased protein-bound iodine and thyroxine-binding globulin in acute intermittent porphyria. N Engl J Med 277:995–1000, 1967.

86. Bellabarba D, Inada M, Varsano-Aharon N, Sterling K: Thyroxine transport and turnover in major nonthyroidal illness. J Clin Endocrinol Metab 28:1023–1030, 1968.

87. Vannotti A, Beraud T: Functional relationships between the liver, the thyroxine-binding protein of serum, and the thyroid. J Clin Endocrinol Metab 19:466–477, 1959.

88. Kalk WJ, Kew MC, Danilewitz MD, et al: Thyroxine binding globulin and thyroid function tests in patients with hepatocellular carcinoma. Hepatology 2:72–76, 1982.

89. Ingenbleek Y, DeNayer P, DeVisscher M: Thyroxine-binding globulin in infant protein-calorie malnutrition. J Clin Endocrinol Metab 39:178–180, 1974.

90. Campbell S, Kulin HE: Transient thyroid binding globulin deficiency with classic galactosemia. J Pediatr 105:335–336, 1984.

91. Robbins J, Rall JE, Petermann ML: Thyroxine-binding by serum and urine proteins in nephrosis. Qualitative aspects. J Clin Invest 36:1333–1342, 1957.

92. Musa BU, Seal US, Doe RP: Excretion of corticosteroid-binding globulin, thyroxine-binding globulin and total protein in adult males with nephrosis: Effects of sex hormones. J Clin Endocrinol Metab 27:768–774, 1967.

93. Lever A, Bird D, Byfield PGH, et al: Increased serum concentration of T$_4$-binding globulin in patients with hypogammaglobulinaemia. Clin Endocrinol 18:195–199, 1983.

94. Hansen J: Increased fecal thyroxine losses: With protein-losing enteropathy. NY State J Med 74:1993–1995, 1974.

95. Inada M, Sterling K: Thyroxine transport in thyrotoxicosis and hypothyroidism. J Clin Invest 46:1442–1450, 1967.

96. Inada M, Sterling K: Thyroxine turnover and transport in Laennec's cirrhosis of the liver. J Clin Invest 1275–1282, 1967.

97. Inada M, Sterling K: Thyroxine turnover and transport in active acromegaly. J Clin Endocrinol Metab 27:1019–1027, 1967.

98. Andreoli M, Robbins J: Serum proteins and thyroxine-protein interaction in early human fetuses. J Clin Invest 41:1070–1077, 1962.

99. DeCostre P, Buhler U, DeGroot LJ, Refetoff S: Diurnal rhythm in total serum thyroxine levels. Metabolism 20:782–791, 1971.

100. Braverman LE, Foster AE, Ingbar SH: Sex-related differences in the binding in serum of thyroid hormone. J Clin Endocrinol Metab 27:227–232, 1967.

101. Brock Jacobsen B, Peitersen B, et al: Serum concentrations of thyroxine-binding globulin, prealbumin and albumin in healthy full-term, small-for-gestational age and preterm newborn infants. Acta Paediatr Scand 68:49–55, 1979.

102. Braverman LE, Dawber NA, Ingbar SH: Observations concerning the binding of thyroid hormones in sera of normal subjects of varying ages. J Clin Invest 45:1273–1279, 1966.

103. Kojima N, Sakata S, Nakamura S, et al: Age- and sex-related differences of serum thyroxine binding globulin (TBG) in healthy subjects. Acta Endocrinol 104:303–306, 1983.

104. Doe RP, Mellinger GT, Swaim WR, Seal JS: Estrogen dosage effects on serum proteins: A longitudinal study. J Clin Endocrinol Metab 27:1081–1086, 1967.

105. Beierwaltes WH, Robbins J: Familial increase in the thyroxine-binding sites in serum α globulin. J Clin Invest 38:1683–1688, 1959.

106. Nicoloff JT, Dowling JT, Patton DD: Inheritance of decreased thyroxine-binding by the thyroxine-binding globulin. J Clin Endocrinol Metab 24:294–298, 1964.

107. Marshall JS, Levy RP, Steinberg AG: Human thyroxine-binding globulin deficiency: A genetic study. N Engl J Med 274:1469–1473, 1966.
108. Nikolai TF, Seal US: X-chromosome linked familial decrease in thyroxine-binding globulin deficiency. J Clin Endocrinol Metab 25:835–841, 1966.
109. Horwitz DL, Refetoff S: Graves' disease associated with familial deficiency of thyroxine-binding globulin. J Clin Endocrinol Metab 44:242–247, 1977.
110. Hansen E, Kirkegaard C, Friis T, Siersbaek-Nielsen K: Normal response to thyrotrophin releasing hormone (TRH) in familial thyroxine-binding globulin deficiency. Acta Endocrinol 80:297–301, 1975.
111. Siersbaek-Nielsen K, Hansen JM, Hippe E: Familial elevation of serum thyroxine-binding globulin capacity. Acta Endocrinol 60:130–136, 1969.
112. Dussault JH: An update on screening for congenital hypothyroidism. Thyroid Today 8:1–5, 1985.
113. Pitt D, Connelly J, Francis I, et al: Genetic screening of newborns in Australia. Results for 1981. Med J Austr 1:333–335, 1983.
114. Sarne DH, Refetoff S, Nelson JC, Dussault J: A new inherited abnormality of thyroxine-binding globulin (TBG-San Diego) with decreased affinity for thyroxine and triiodothyronine. J Clin Endocrinol Metab 68:114–119, 1989.
115. Bertenshaw R, Sarne D, Tornari J, et al: Sequencing of the variant thyroxine-binding globulin (TBG)–San Diego reveals two nucleotide substitutions. Biochim Biophys Acta 1139:307–310, 1992.
116. Murata Y, Takamatsu J, Refetoff S: Inherited abnormality of thyroxine-binding globulin with no demonstrable thyroxine-binding activity and high serum levels of denatured thyroxine-binding globulin. N Engl J Med 314:694–699, 1986.
117. Mori Y, Seino S, Takeda K, et al: A mutation causing reduced biological activity and stability of thyroxine-binding globulin probably as a result of abnormal glycosylation of the molecule. Mol Endocrinol 3:575–579, 1989.
118. Takamatsu J, Refetoff S, Charbonneau M, Dussault JH: Two new inherited defects of the thyroxine-binding globulin (TBG) molecule presenting as partial TBG deficiency. J Clin Invest 79:833–840, 1987.
119. Li P, Janssen OE, Takeda K, et al: Complete thyroxine-binding globulin (TBG) deficiency caused by a single nucleotide deletion in the TBG gene. Metabolism 40:1231–1234, 1990.
120. Daiger SP, Wildin RS: Human thyroxine-binding globulin (TBG): Heterogeneity within individuals and among individuals demonstrated by isoelectric focusing. Biochem Genet 19:673–685, 1981.
121. Takamatsu J, Ando M, Weinberg M, Refetoff S: Isoelectric focusing variant thyroxine-binding globulin (TBG-S) in American Blacks: Increased heat lability and reduced concentration in serum. J Clin Endocrinol Metab 63:80–87, 1986.
122. Waltz MR, Pullman TN, Takeda K, et al: Molecular basis for the properties of the thyroxine-binding globulin–slow variant in American Blacks. J Endocrinol Invest 13:343–349, 1990.
123. Sarne DH, Refetoff S, Murata Y, et al: Variant thyroxine-binding globulin in serum of Australian Aborigines: A comparison with familial TBG deficiency in Caucasians and American Blacks. J Endocrinol Invest 8:217–224, 1985.
124. Murata Y, Refetoff S, Sarne DH, et al: Variant thyroxine-binding globulin in serum of Australian Aborigines: Its physical, chemical and biological properties. J Endocrinol Invest 8:225–232, 1985.
125. Takeda K, Mori Y, Sobieszczyk S, et al: Sequence of the variant thyroxine-binding globulin of Australian Aborigines: Only one of two amino acid replacements is responsible for its altered properties. J Clin Invest 83:1344–1348, 1989.
125a. Kamboh MI, Ferrell RE: A sensitive immunoblotting technique to identify thyroxine-binding globulin protein heterogeneity after isoelectric focusing. Biochem Genet 24:273–280, 1986.
125b. Constans J, Ribouchon MT, Govaillard C, et al: A new polymorphism of thyroxin binding globulin in three African groups (Mali) with endemic nodular goitre. Hum Genet 89:199–203, 1992.
126. Mori Y, Takeda K, Charbonneau M, Refetoff S: Replacement of Leu[227] by pro in thyroxine-binding globulin (TBG) is associated with complete TBG deficiency in three of eight families with this inherited defect. J Clin Endocrinol Metab 70:804–809, 1990.
127. Takamatsu J, Refetoff S: Inherited heat stable variant thyroxine-binding globulin (TBG-Chicago). J Clin Endocrinol Metab 63:1140–1144, 1986.
128. Janssen OE, Chen B, Büttner C, et al: Sequence analysis and in-vitro expression of the heat-resistant variant thyroxine-binding globulin–Chicago. Annual meeting of The Endocrine Society, Las Vegas, Nevada, 1993.
129. Bertenshaw R, Takeda K, Refetoff S: Sequencing of the variant thyroxine binding globulin (TBG)-Quebec reveals two nucleotide substitutions. Am J Hum Genet 48:741–744, 1991.
130. Yamamori I, Mori Y, Seo H, et al: Nucleotide deletion resulting in frameshift as a possible cause of complete thyroxine-binding globulin deficiency in six Japanese families. J Clin Endocrinol Metab 73:262–267, 1991.
131. Miura Y, Kambe F, Yamamori I, et al: Retention within the rough endoplasmic reticulum may be the cause of complete thyroxine-binding globulin deficiency in Japanese (TBG-CDJ): As evidenced by endoglycosidase H sensitivity. Thyroid 2 (Suppl 1):S–37, 1992.
132. Takeda K, Iyola I, Suehiro T, Hashimoto K: Gene screening in Japanese families with thyroxine-binding globulin complete deficiency (TBG-CD) demonstrates a race specific mutation. Thyroid 2 (Suppl 1):S–27, 1992.
133. Daiger SP, Rummel DP, Wang L, Cavalli-Sforza LL: Detection of genetic variation with radioactive ligands. IV. X-linked, polymorphic genetic variation of thyroxin-binding globulin (TBG). Am J Hum Genet 33:640–648, 1981.
134. Dick M, Watson F: Prevalent low serum thyroxine-binding globulin level in Western Australian Aborigines. Med J Aust 1:115–118, 1980.
135. Watson F, Dick M: Distribution and inheritance of low serum thyroxine-binding globulin levels in Australian Aborigines. Med J Aust 2:385–387, 1980.
135a. Miura Y, Mori Y, Yamamori I, et al: Sequence of a variant thyroxine-binding globulin (TBG) in a family with partial TBG deficiency in Japanese (TBG-PDJ). Endocrinol Jpn 40:127–132, 1993.
136. Burr WA, Ramsden DB, Hoffenberg R: Hereditary abnormalities of thyroxine-binding globulin concentration. Quart J Med 49:295–313, 1980.
136a. Hayashi Y, Mori Y, Janssen DE, et al: Human thyroxine-binding globulin gene: Complete sequence and transcription regulation. Mol Endocrinol 7:1049–1060, 1993.
137. Braverman LE, AvRuskin T, Cullen MJ, et al: Effects of norethandrolone on the transport and peripheral metabolism of thyroxine in patients lacking thyroxine-binding globulin. J Clin Invest 50:1644–1649, 1971.
138. Man EB, Reid WA, Hellegers AE, Jones WS: Thyroid function in human pregnancy. III. Serum thyroxine-binding prealbumin (TBPA) and thyroxine-binding globulin (TBG) of pregnant women aged 14 through 43 years. Am J Obstet Gynecol 103:338–347, 1969.
139. Ingenbleek Y, deVisscher M, deNayer P: Measurement of prealbumin as index of protein-calorie malnutrition. Lancet 2:106–108, 1972.
140. Smith FR, Underwood BA, Denning CR, et al: Depressed plasma retinol-binding protein levels in cystic fibrosis. J Lab Clin Med 80:423–433, 1972.
141. Rajatanavin R, Liberman C, Lawrence GD, et al: Euthyroid hyperthyroxinemia and thyroxine-binding prealbumin excess in islet cell carcinoma. J Clin Endocrinol Metab 61:17–21, 1985.
142. Braverman LE, Socolow EL, Woeber KA, Ingbar SH: Effect of norethandrolone on the metabolism of ^{125}I-labeled thyroxine-binding prealbumin. J Clin Endocrinol Metab 28:831–835, 1968.
143. Moses AC, Lawlor J, Haddow J, Jackson IMD: Familial euthyroid hyperthyroxinemia resulting from increased thyroxine binding to thyroxine-binding prealbumin. N Engl J Med 306:966–969, 1982.
144. Lalloz MRA, Byfield PGH, Himsworth RL: A prealbumin variant with an increased affinity for T4 and reverse T3. Clin Endocrinol 21:331–338, 1984.
145. Moses C, Rosen HN, Moller DE, et al: A point mutation in transthyretin increases affinity for thyroxine and produces euthyroid hyperthyroxinemia. J Clin Invest 86:2025–2033, 1990.
145a. Steinrauf LK, Hamilton JA, Braden BC, et al: X-ray crystal structure of the Ala-109 ± Thr variant of human transthyretin which produces euthyroid hyperthyroxinemia. J Biol Chem 268:2425–2430, 1993.
146. Scrimshaw BJ, Fellowes AP, Palmer BN, et al: A novel variant of transthyretin (prealbumin), Thr[119] to Met, associated with increased thyroxine binding. Thyroid 2:21–26, 1992.
146a. Harrison HH, Gordon ED, Nichols WC: Biochemical and clinical characterization of prealbumin[CHICAGO]: An apparently benign variant of serum prealbumin (transthyretin) discovered with high-resolution two-dimensional electrophoresis. Am J Med Genet 39:442–452, 1991.
147. Akbari MT, Fitch NJ, Farmer M, et al: Thyroxine-binding prealbumin gene: A population study. Clin Endocrinol 33:155–160, 1990.
148. Refetoff S, Dwulet FE, Benson MD: Reduced affinity for thyroxine in two of three structural thyroxine-binding prealbumin variants associated with familial amyloidotic polyneuropathy. J Clin Endocrinol Metab 63:1432–1437, 1986.
149. van Jaarsveld PP, Branch WT, Edelhoch H, Robbins J: Polymorphism of Rhesus monkey serum prealbumin. Molecular properties and

binding of thyroxine and retinol-binding protein. J Biol Chem 248:4706–4712, 1973.

150. Hollander CS, Bernstein G, Oppenheimer JH: Abnormalities of thyroxine binding in analbuminemia. J Clin Endocrinol Metab 28:1064–1066, 1968.

151. Lee WNP, Golden MP, Van Herle AJ, et al: Inherited abnormal thyroid hormone-binding protein causing selective increase of total serum thyroxine. J Clin Endocrinol Metab 49:292–299, 1979.

152. Henneman G, Krenning EP, Otten M, et al: Raised total thyroxine and free thyroxine index but normal free thyroxine. A serum abnormality due to inherited increased affinity of iodothyronines for serum binding protein. Lancet 1:639–642, 1979.

153. Croxson MS, Palmer BN, Holdaway IM, et al: Detection of familial dysalbuminaemic hyperthyroxinaemia. Br Med J 290:1099–1102, 1985.

154. DeNayer P, Malvaux P: Hyperthyroxinemia associated with high thyroxine binding to albumin in euthyroid subjects. J Endocrinol Invest 5:383–386, 1982.

155. Ruiz M, Rajatanavin R, Young RA, et al: Familial dysalbuminemic hyperthyroxinemia: A syndrome that can be confused with thyrotoxicosis. N Engl J Med 306:635–639, 1982.

156. Mendel CM, Cavalieri RR: Thyroxine distribution and metabolism in familial dysalbuminemic hyperthyroxinemia. J Clin Endocrinol Metab 59:499–504, 1984.

157. Stockigt JR, DeGaris M, Csicsmann J, et al: Limitations of a new free thyroxine assay (Amerlex Free T4). Clin Endocrinol 15:313–318, 1981.

158. Rajatanavin R, Young RA, Braverman LE: Effect of chloride on serum thyroxine binding in familial dysalbuminemic hyperthyroxinemia. J Clin Endocrinol Metab 58:388–391, 1984.

159. Barlow JW, Csicsmann JM, White EL, et al: Familial euthyroid thyroxine excess: Characterization of abnormal intermediate affinity thyroxine binding to albumin. J Clin Endocrinol Metab 55:244–250, 1982.

160. Yabu Y, Amir SM, Ruiz M, et al: Heterogeneity of thyroxine binding by serum albumins in normal subjects and patients with familial dysalbuminemic hyperthyroxinemia. J Clin Endocrinol Metab 60:451–459, 1985.

161. Lalloz MRA, Byfield PGH, Himsworth RL: A new and distinctive albumin variant with increased affinities for both triiodothyronines and causing hyperthyroxinaemia. Clin Endocrinol 22:521–529, 1985.

162. Takamatsu J, Meriden T, Ikegami Y, et al: Can the type of variant albumin in familial dysalbuminemic hyperthyroxinemia be determined by measuring iodothyronines in serum? Endocrinol Jpn 37:389–395, 1990.

163. Sarcione EJ, Aungst CW: Bisalbuminemia associated with albumin thyroxine-binding defect. Clin Chim Acta 7:297–298, 1962.

164. Tarnoky AL, Lestas AN: A new type of bisalbuminemia. Clin Chim Acta 9:551–558, 1964.

165. Chanoine JP, Braverman LE, Farwell AP, et al: The thyroid gland is a major source of circulating T3 in the rat. J Clin Invest 91:2709–2722, 1993.

166. Harris ARC, Fang S, Azizi F, et al: Effect of starvation on hypothalamic-pituitary-thyroid function of the rat. Metab Clin Exp 27:1074–1083, 1978.

167. Larsen PR, Silva JE, Kaplan MM: Relationships between circulating and intracellular thyroid hormones: Physiological and clinical implications. Endocr Rev 2:87–102, 1981.

168. Engler D, Burger AG: The deiodination of the iodothyronines and their derivatives in man. Endocr Rev 5:151–184, 1984.

169. Hennemann G (ed): Thyroid Hormone Metabolism. New York, Marcel Dekker, 1986.

170. Leonard JL: Identification and structure analysis of iodothyronine deiodinases. In Greer MA (ed): Comprehensive Endocrinology. The Thyroid Gland. New York, Raven Press, 1990, pp 285–305.

171. Kohrle J, Hesch D, Leonard JL: Intracellular pathways of iodothyronine metabolism. In Braver LE, Utiger RD (eds): The Thyroid. A Fundamental and Clinical Text. Philadelphia, JB Lippincott, 1991, pp 144–189.

172. Chopra IJ: Nature, Science and Relative Biologic Significance of Circulation Thyroid Hormones. In Braverman LE, Utiger RD (eds): The Thyroid. A Fundamental and Clinical Text. Philadelphia, JB Lippincott, 1991, pp 126–143.

173. Nicoloff JT, Dowling JT: Methods for the estimation of thyroxine distribution in man. J Clin Invest 47:26–37, 1968.

174. Nicoloff JT, Low JC, Dussault JH, Fisher DA: Simultaneous measurement of thyroxine and triiodothyronine peripheral turnover kinetics in man. J Clin Invest 51:473–483, 1972.

175. Duick DS, Stein RB, Warren DW, Nicoloff JT: The significance of partial suppressibility of serum thyroxine by triiodothyronine administration in euthyroid man. J Clin Endocrinol Metab 41:229–234, 1975.

176. Mandel SJ, Larsen LR, Seely EW, Brent GA: Increased need for thyroxine during pregnancy in women with primary hypothyroidism. N Engl J Med 323:91–96, 1990.

177. Gregerman RI, Goffney GW, Schck NW: Thyroxine turnover in euthyroid man with special reference to changes with age. J Clin Invest 41:2065–2074, 1962.

178. Chopra IJ, Fisher DA, Solomon DH, Beall GN: Thyroxine and triiodothyronine in the human thyroid. J Clin Endocrinol Metab 36:311, 1973.

179. LoPresti JS, Eigen A, Kaptein E, et al: Alterations in 3,3′,5′–triiodothyronine metabolism in response to propylthiouracil, dexamethasone, and thyroxine administration in man. J Clin Invest 84:1650–1656, 1989.

180. Pittman HA, Brown RW, Register HB Jr: Biological activity of 3,3′,5′-triiodo-DL-thyronine. Endocrinology 70:79, 1962.

181. DeHerder WW, Bonthuis F, Rutgers M, et al: Effects of inhibition of type I iodothyronine deiodinase and phenol sulfotransferase on the biliary clearance of triiodothyronine in rats. Endocrinology 122:153, 1988.

182. Visser TJ, van Buuren JCJ, Rutgers M, et al: The role of sulfation in thyroid hormone metabolism. Trends Endocrinol Metab 1:211, 1990.

183. Sato K, Robbins J: Thyroid hormone metabolism in primary cultured rat hepatocytes: Effects of glucose, glucagon, and insulin. J Clin Invest 68:475, 1981.

184. Pittman CS, Shimizu T, Burger A, Chambers JB Jr: The nondeiodinative pathways of thyroxine metabolism: 3,3′,5,5′-tetraiodothyroacetic acid turnover in normal and fasting subjects. J Clin Endocrinol Metab 50:712, 1980.

185. Rutgers M, Heusdens FA, Visser TJ. Metabolism of triiodothyroacetic acid (TA$_3$) in rat liver. I. Deiodination of TA$_3$ and TA$_3$ sulfate by microsomes. Endocrinology 125:424, 1989.

186. Balsam A, Sexton F, Borges M, Ingbar SH: Formation of diiodotyrosine from thyroxine: Ether-link cleavage, an alternate pathway of thyroxine metabolism. J Clin Invest 72:1234, 1983.

187. Burger AG, Engler D, Buergi U, et al: Ether link cleavage is the major pathway of iodothyronine metabolism in the phagocytosing human leukocyte and also occurs in vivo in the rat. J Clin Invest 71:935, 1983.

188. Meinhold H, Gramm H-J, Meissner W, et al: Elevated serum diiodotyrosine (DIT) in severe infections and sepsis: DIT, a possible new marker of leukocyte activity. J Clin Endocrinol Metab 72:945, 1991.

189. Van Doorn J, van der Heide D, Roelfsema F: Sources and quantity of 3,5,5′-triiodothyronine in several tissues of the rat. J Clin Invest 72:1778, 1983.

190. LoPresti JS, Anderson KP, Nicoloff JT: Does a hidden pool of reverse triiodothyronine (rT$_3$) production contribute to total thyroxine (T$_4$) disposal in high T$_4$ states in man. Clin Endocrinol Metab 70:1479, 1990.

191. Pittman CS, Buck MW, Chambers JB: Urinary metabolites of ^{14}C-labeled thyroxine in man. J Clin Invest 51:1759–1766, 1972.

192. Berson SA, Yalow RS: Quantitative aspects of iodine metabolism. The exchangeable organic iodine pool, and the rates of thyroidal secretion, peripheral degradation and fecal excretion of endogenously synthesized organically bound iodine. J Clin Invest 33:1533, 1954.

193. Chopra IJ, Boado RJ, Geffner DL, Solomon DH: A radioimmunoassay for measurement of thyronine and its acetic acid analog in urine. J Clin Endocrinol Metab 67:480, 1988.

194. Robbins J, Johnson ML: Theoretical considerations in the transport of the thyroid hormones in blood. In Ekins R, Faglia F, Pennisi F, Pinchera A (eds): Free Thyroid Hormones. Amsterdam, Excerpta Medica, 1979, pp 1–14.

195. Pardridge WM: Transport of protein-bound hormones into tissues in vivo. Endocr Rev 2:103–234, 1981.

196. Ekins R, Edwards P, Newman B: The role of binding-proteins in hormone delivery (appendix). In Albertini A, Ekins RP (eds): Free Hormones in Blood. Amsterdam, Elsevier Biomedical, 1982, pp 3–43.

197. Robbins J, Rall JE: The iodine containing hormones. In Gray CH, James VHT (eds): Hormone in Blood (ed 3). London Academic Press, 1983, pp 219–265.

198. Robbins J, Bartalena L: Plasma transport of thyroid hormones. In Hennemann G (ed): Thyroid Hormone Metabolism. New York, Marcel Dekker, 1986, pp 3.

199. Mendel CM, Cavalieri R: Transport of thyroid hormones in health

and disease: recent controversy surrounding the free hormone hypothesis. Thyroid Today 11:3, 1988.

200. Mendel CM, Cavalieri RR, Weisiger RA: Uptake of thyroxine by the perfused rat liver: Implications for the free hormone hypothesis. Endocrinology 123:1817, 1988.

201. Mendel CM, Cavalieri RA, Weisiger RA: On plasma-protein mediated transport of steroid and thyroid hormones. Am J Physiol 255:E221, 1988.

202. Mendel CM: The free hormone hypothesis: A physiologically based mathematical model. Endocr Rev 10:232, 1989.

203. Mendel CM, Cavalieri R: Transport of thyroid hormones in health and disease: recent controversy surrounding the free hormone hypothesis. Thyroid Today 11:3, 1988.

204. Blondeau JP, Osty J, Francon J: Characterization of the thyroid hormone transport system of isolated hepatocytes. J Biol Chem 263:2685, 1988.

205. Segal J: A rapid extranuclear effect of 3,5,3'-triiodothyronine on sugar uptake by several tissues in the rat in vivo: Evidence for a physiological role for the thyroid hormone action at the level of the plasma membrane. Endocrinology 122:2240, 1989.

206. Segal J: Calmodulin modulates thymocyte adenylate cyclase activity through the guanine nucleotide regulatory unit. Mol Cell Endocrinol 64:95, 1989.

207. Centanni M, Mancini G, Andreoli M: Carrier-mediated [^{125}I]T$_3$-uptake by mouse thymocytes. Endocrinology 124:243, 1989.

208. Goncalves E, Lakshmanan M, Pontecorvia A, Robbins J: Thyroid hormone transport in human glioma cell line. Mol Cell Endocrinol 69:157, 1990.

209. Lakshmanan M, Goncalves E, Lessly G, et al: The transport of thyroxine into mouse neuroblastoma cells. NB41A3: the effect of L-system amino acids. Endocrinology 126:3245, 1990.

210. Cheng S-Y: Characterization of binding and uptake of 3,3'-5-triiodo-L-thyronine in cultured mouse fibroblasts. Endocrinology 112:1754, 1983.

211. Docter R, Krenning EP, Bernard HF, Hennemann G: Active transport of iodothyronines into human cultured fibroblasts. J Clin Endocrinol Metab 65:624, 1987.

212. Holm A-C: Active transport of L-tri-iodothyronine through the red cell plasma membrane: True or false? Scand J Clin Lab Invest 47:185, 1987.

213. Osty J, Jego L, Francon J, Blondeau J-P: Characterization of triiodothyronine transport and accumulation in rat erythrocytes. Endocrinology 123:2303, 1988.

214. Krenning EP, Docter R, Bernard HF, et al: Decreased transport of thyroxine (T$_4$) 3,3',5-triiodothyronine (T$_3$) and 3,3',5'-triiodothyronine (rT$_3$) into rat hepatocytes in primary culture due to a decrease of cellular ATP content and various drugs. FEBS Lett 140:229–233, 1982.

215. Davis PJ: Cellular actions of thyroid hormones. In Braverman LE, Utiger RE (eds): The Thyroid. Philadelphia, JB Lippincott, 1991, pp 190–203.

216. Oppenheimer JH, Schwartz HL: Stereospecific transport of triiodothyronine from plasma to cytosol and from cytosol to nucleus in rat liver, kidney, brain and heart. J Soc Clin Invest 75:147–154, 1985.

217. Bianco AC, Silva JE: Nuclear 3,5,3'-triiodothyronine (T$_3$) in brown adipose tissue: Receptor occupancy and sources of T$_3$ as determined by in vivo techniques. Endocrinology 120:55–62, 1987.

218. Schwartz HL, Trence D, Oppenheimer JH, et al: Distribution and metabolism of L- and D-triiodothyronine (T$_3$) in the rat: Preferential accumulation of L-T$_3$ by hepatic and cardiac nuclei as a probable explanation of the differential biological potency of T$_3$ enantiomers. Endocrinology 113:1235–1243, 1983.

219. Mooradian AD, Schwartz HL, Mariash CN, Oppenheimer JH: Transcellular and transnuclear transport of 3,5,3'-triiodothyronine in isolated hepatocytes. Endocrinology 117:2449, 1985.

220. Oppenheimer JH, Schwartz HL, Surks MI: Tissue differences in the concentrations of triiodothyronine nuclear binding sites in the rat: Liver, kidney, pituitary, heart, brain, spleen, and testis. Endocrinology 95:897–903, 1974.

221. Erickson VJ, Cavalieri RR, Rosenberg LL: Thyroxine 5'-deiodinase of rat thyroid, but not that of liver, is dependent on thyrotropin. Endocrinology 111:434–440, 1982.

222. Leonard JL, Rosenberg IN: Subcellular distribution of thyroxine-5'-deiodinase in the rat kidney, a plasma membrane location. Endocrinology 103:274, 1978.

223. Otten MH, Mol JA, Visser TJ: Sulfation preceding deiodination of iodothyronines in rat hepatocytes. Science 221:81, 1983.

224. Mol JA, Visser TI: Thyroxine sulfate is rapidly inactivated by deiodination. Ann Endocrinol (Paris) 45:62, 1984.

225. Sato K, Robbins J: Glutathione deficiency induced by cysteine and/or methionine deprivation does not affect thyroid hormone deiodination in cultured rat hepatocytes and monkey carcinoma cells. Endocrinology 109:884, 1981.

226. Leonard JL, Visser TJ: Biochemistry of deiodination. In Henneman G (ed): Thyroid Hormone Metabolism. New York, Marcel Dekker, 1986, p 189.

227. Visser TJ: Mechanism of action of iodothyronine 5'-deiodinase. Biochim Biophys Acta 569:302, 1979.

228. Leonard JL, Rosenberg IN: Characterization of essential enzyme sulhydryl group of thyroxine-5'-deiodinase from rat kidney. Endocrinology 106:444, 1980.

229. LoPresti JS, Eigen A, Kaptein E, et al: Alterations in 3,3',5'-triiodothyronine metabolism in response to propylthiouracil, dexamethasone, and thyroxine administration in man. J Clin Invest 84:1650, 1989.

230. Nicoloff JT: A new method for the measurement of acute alterations in thyroxine deiodination rate in man. J Clin Invest 49:267–273, 1970.

231. Silva JE, Matthews PS: Thyroid hormone metabolism and source of plasma triiodothyronine in 2-week-old rat: Effect of thyroid status. Endocrinology 116:2394–2405, 1984.

232. Saberi M, Sterling FH, Utiger RD: Reduction in extrathyroidal triiodothyronine production by propylthiouracil in man. J Clin Invest 55:224–329, 1975.

233. Berry MJ, Banu L, Larsen PR: Type I iodothyronine deiodinase is a selenocysteine-containing enzyme. Nature 349:438–440, 1991.

234. Sharifi J, St Germain DL: The cDNA for the type I iodothyronine 5'-deiodinase encodes an enzyme manifesting both high Km and low Km activity. Evidence that rat liver and kidney contain a single enzyme which converts thyroxine to 3,5,3'-triiodothyronine. J Biol Chem 267:12539–12544, 1992.

235. Berry MJ, Larsen PR: The role of selenium in thyroid hormone action. Endocr Rev 13:207–219, 1992.

236. Goyens P, Golstein J, Nsombola B, et al: Selenium deficiency as a possible factor in the pathogenesis of myxedematous endemic cretinism. Acta Endocrinol (Copenh) 114:497–502, 1987.

237. Contempre B, Dumont JE, Ngo B, et al: Effect of selenium supplementation in hypothyroid subjects of an iodine and selenium deficient area: The possible danger of indiscriminate supplementation of iodine-deficient subjects with selenium. J Clin Endocrinol Metab 73:213–215, 1991.

238. Chanoine JP, Safran M, Farwell AP, et al: Effects of selenium deficiency on thyroid hormone economy in rats. Endocrinology 131:1787–1792, 1992.

239. Chanoine JP, Safran M, Farwell AP, et al: Selenium deficiency and type II 5'-deiodinase regulation in the euthyroid and hypothyroid rat: Evidence of a direct effect of thyroxine. Endocrinology 130:479–484, 1992.

240. Goswami A, Rosenberg IN: Purification and characterization of a cytosolic protein enhancing GSH-dependent microsomal iodothyronine 5'-monodeiodination. J Biol Chem 260:6012, 1985.

241. Bhat GB, Iwase K, Hummel BCW, Walfish PG: Kinetic characteristics of a thioredoxin-activated rat hepatic and renal low Km iodothyronien 5'-deiodinase. Biochem J 258:785, 1989.

242. Boado RJ, Chopra IJ: A study of hepatic low Km iodothyronine 5'-monodeiodinase. Endocrinology 124:2245, 1989.

243. Safran M, Farwell AP, Leonard JL: Evidence that type II 5'-deiodinase is not a selenoprotein. J Biol Chem 266:13477–13480, 1991.

244. Roti E, Fang SL, Green K, et al: Human placenta is an active site of thyroxine and 3,3',5'-triiodothyronine tyrosyl ring deiodination. J Clin Endocrinol Metab 53:498, 1981.

245. Roti E, Gnudi A, Braverman LE: The placental transport, synthesis and metabolism of hormones and drugs which affect thyroid function. Endocr Rev 4:131, 1983.

246. Kaplan MM, Shaw EA: Type II iodothyronine 5'-deiodination by human and rat placenta in vitro. J Clin Endocrinol Metab 59:253, 1984.

247. Kaplan MM, Yaskoski KA: Maturational patterns of iodothyronine phenolic and tryosyl ring deiodinase activities in rat cerebrum, cerebellum, and hypothalamus. J Clin Invest 67:1208, 1981.

248. Fay M, Roti E, Fang SH, et al: The effects of propylthiouracil iodothyronines, and other agents on thyroid hormone metabolism in human placenta. J Clin Endocrinol Metab 58:280, 1984.

249. Flock EV, David C, Stobie GH, Owen CA: 3,3'-5'-triiodothyronine and 3,3'-deiodothyronine: Partially deiodinated intermediates in the metabolism of the thyroid hormones. Endocrinology 73:442, 1963.

250. Chopra IJ, Wu SY, Teco GNC, Santini F: A radioimmunoassay for

measurement of 3,5,3'-triiodothyronine sulfate studies in thyroidal and nonthyroidal diseases, pregnancy, and neonatal life. J Clin Endocrinol Metab 75:189–194, 1992.

251. LoPresti JS, Mizuno L, Nimalsuryia A, et al: Characteristics of 3,5,3'-triiodothyronine sulfate metabolism in euthyroid man. J Clin Endocrinol Metab 73:703–709, 1991.

252. Nicoloff JT, Lum SMC, Spencer CA, Morris R: Peripheral autoregulation of thyroxine to triiodothyronine conversion in man. *In* Loos U, Wartofsky L (eds): Peripheral Metabolism of Thyroxine, Hormone, and Metabolic Research. Supplement No. 14. Stuttgart, Georg Thieme Verlag, 1984, pp 74–79.

253. Lum SMC, Nicoloff JT, Spencer CA, Kaptein EM: Peripheral tissue mechanism for maintenance of serum T_3 values in a T_4 deficient state in man. J Clin Invest 73:570–575, 1984.

254. Greer MA, Solomon DH (eds): Handbook of physiology. Sect 7 Vol 3. The Thyroid. Washington, DC, American Physiology Society, 1974, p. 215.

255. Souffer RL, Hechtman P, Savage M: L-triiodothyronine aminotransferase. J Biol Chem 248:1224–1230, 1973.

256. Fishman N, Huang YP, Tergis DC, Rivlin RS: Relation of triiodothyronine and reverse triiodothyronine administration in rats to hepatic-L-triiodothyronine aminotransferase activity. Endocrinology 100:105–109, 1977.

257. Gavin L, Castle J, McMahon F, et al: Extrathyroidal conversion of thyroxine to 3,3',5'-triiodothyronine (reverse T_3) and to 3,5,3'-triiodothyronine (T_3) in humans. J Clin Endocrinol Metab 44:733, 1977.

258. Siegrist-Kaiser CA, Bubloz C, Burger AG: Studies on L-amino acid oxidase, a renal enzyme converting 3,5,3'-triiodothyronine (T_3) to 3,5,3'-triiodothyroacetic acid (triac). 15th Annual Meeting of the Endocrine Society, Las Vegas, June 1993, 812.

259. Schueler PA, Schwartz HL, Strait KA, et al: Binding of 3,5,3'-triiodothyronine (T_3) and its analogues to the in vitro translational products of c-*erb* A protooncogenes: Differences in the affinity of the α and β forms for the acetic acid analogue and failure of the human testis and kidney α-2 products to bind T_3. Mol Endocrinol 4:227, 1990.

260. Braverman LE, Vagenakis A, Downes P, et al: Effect of replacement doses of sodium L-thyroxine on peripheral metabolism of thyroxine and triiodothyronine in man. J Clin Invest 52:1010–1017, 1973.

261. Visser TJ, Leonard JL, Kaplan MM, Larsen PR: Kinetic evidence suggesting two mechanisms for iodothyronine 5'-deiodinase in rat cerebral cortex. Proc Natl Acad Sci USA 79:5080, 1982.

262. Mills I, Raasmaja A, Moolten N, et al: Effect of thyroid status on catecholamine stimulation of thyroxine 5'-deiodinase in brown adipocytes. Am J Physiol 256:E74–E79, 1989.

263. Delange F, Camerz M, Ermans AM: Circulating thyroid hormones in endemic goiter. J Clin Endocrinol 34:891–895, 1972.

264. Kaplan MM: Subcellular alterations causing reduced hepatic thyroxine 5' monodeiodinase activity in fasted rats. Endocrinology 104:58–64, 1979.

265. Spencer CA, Lum SMC, Wilber JF, et al: Dynamics of serum TSH and thyroid hormone changes in fasting. J Clin Endocrinol Metab 56:883–888, 1983.

266. St. Germain DL, Carlton VA: Comparative study of pituitary-thyroid hormone economy in fasting and hypothyroid rats. J Clin Invest 75:679–688, 1985.

267. Kaplan MM: Thyroxine 5' monodeiodination in rat anterior pituitary homogenates. Endocrinology 106:567–576, 1980.

268. Nicoloff JT, Fisher DA, Appleman MD Jr: The role of glucocorticoids in the regulation of thyroid function in man. J Clin Invest 49:1922–1929, 1970.

Mechanisms of Thyroid Hormone Action

J. LARRY JAMESON
LESLIE J. DeGROOT

Thyroid hormone has myriad physiological effects, causing alterations in essentially all metabolic pathways and organs. Thyroid hormone modulates oxygen consumption and protein, carbohydrate, lipid, and vitamin metabolism. It also alters the synthesis and degradation rates of many other hormones and growth factors so that many of its effects occur through secondary influences on other endocrine pathways. The effects of thyroid hormone can be largely divided into two broad categories: (1) effects on cellular differentiation and development and (2) effects on metabolic pathways. Obviously, these two actions of thyroid hormone are interrelated in that alterations in growth and development require concomitant shifts in metabolism. Similarly, changes in cellular differentiation can alter patterns of gene expression, thereby influencing metabolic pathways. Thus, the effects of thyroid hormone represent a complex integration of pathways both at the cellular level and in terms of whole-animal physiology.

Some of the most prominent effects of thyroid hormone occur during fetal development and early childhood. In animal models, the developmental effects of thyroid hormone have been well documented. For example, in amphibians, the process of metamorphosis from tadpoles to frogs is strictly dependent upon thyroid hormone.[1, 2] In humans, the requirement for thyroid hormone during development is manifest dramatically in the syndrome of cretinism. Many of these developmental effects are not reversed by later treatment with hormone, suggesting that thyroid hormone acts during developmental windows in combination with other differentiation factors that may not be available later in life. Thyroid hormone continues to play a critical role during growth and development in childhood, as illustrated by the characteristic delayed growth curves that occur in hypothyroidism. In this case, many of the effects of thyroid hormone may be metabolic rather than developmental, as growth is restored rapidly with institution of treatment.

In adults, the primary effects of thyroid hormone are manifest by alterations in metabolism. The clinical features of hypothyroidism and hyperthyroidism serve as emphatic reminders that thyroid hormone causes pleiotropic effects that reflect its action on many different pathways and target organs. Alterations in oxygen consumption have long been recognized as one of the hallmarks of thyroid hormone action. Clinically, this aspect of thyroid hormone action forms the basis for measurements of basal metabolic rate, which is reduced in hypothyroidism and increased in hyperthyroidism. Measurements of oxygen consumption in individual tissues have provided an index of organs that are targets for thyroid hormone action. As shown in Figure 37–1, the metabolic effects of thyroid hormone are highly variable in different organs. Oxygen consumption is stimulated markedly by thyroid hormone in heart, skeletal muscle, liver, kidney, and gastrointestinal organs, whereas brain, spleen, and gonadal tissues are metabolically less responsive.[3–5] The pituitary gland exhibits a paradoxical response to thyroid hormone, with increased metabolic activity in hypothyroidism and decreased activity in hyperthyroidism. The reasons for the variable metabolic responses in different organs are not well understood. Each of these tissues depends upon aerobic metabolism and contains the enzymes necessary for increasing oxygen con-

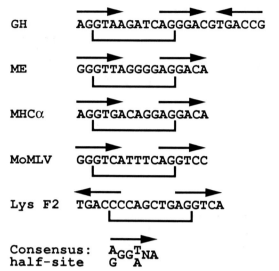

GH   AGGTAAGATCAGGGACGTGACCG

ME   GGGTTAGGGGAGGACA

MHCα AGGTGACAGGAGGACA

MoMLV GGGTCATTTCAGGTCC

Lys F2 TGACCCCAGCTGAGGTCA

Consensus: A GG T NA
half-site   G   A

FIGURE 37–5. Sequences of positive thyroid response elements (TRE's). Promoter regions involved in thyroid hormone stimulation are shown for several different genes, including rat growth hormone (GH),[161] rat malic enzyme (ME),[213] rat myosin heavy chain α,[108] Moloney murine leukemia virus (MoMLV),[214] and chicken lysozyme F2 silencer (Lys F2).[215] Although detailed mutagenesis has not been performed for each element, putative TRE half-sites are denoted by arrows, and a 10-bp interval between pairs of guanines is indicated by brackets. A "consensus" TRE half-site sequence is shown at the bottom of the figure. Of note, there is considerable diversity in the sequences of half-sites, orientation of half-sites, and bases that form the spacers between half-sites.

gene product is not required for thyroid hormone action.[66] Third, thyroid hormone receptor–binding sites have been identified in the promoter regions of the TSH α and β genes.[67–72] Lastly, mutant thyroid hormone receptors that cannot bind to DNA are unable to cause transcriptional repression.[67] Unlike positive TRE's, the proposed negative TRE's in these genes reside on either side of the transcriptional initiation site, leading to the hypothesis that negative regulation might involve receptor interference with basal transcription factors that interact with RNA polymerase.[73] Other mechanisms of transcriptional repression may also apply for these and other negatively regulated genes. Evidence suggests that a negative TRE from the TSHβ gene functions when inserted at an upstream promoter location rather than in its native site adjacent to the TATA box.[74, 75] In the case of the epidermal growth factor (EGF) receptor gene, a negative TRE is located in an upstream region of the promoter and appears to overlap a binding site for the positive transcription factor, Sp-1.[76–78] Thus, it is possible that the hormone-activated receptor interferes in some manner with the binding or action of Sp-1. In a related mechanism, the thyroid hormone receptor has been shown to inhibit the activity of AP-1, a heterodimeric transcription factor composed of jun and fos.[79] In this case, mutual inhibition occurs such that AP-1 also blocks thyroid hormone receptor activation of its target genes. Thus, the thyroid hormone receptor may interact with a variety of other classes of transcription factors, including NF-1, Oct-1, AP-1, Sp-1, and Pit-1, a pituitary specific factor involved in growth hormone (GH) and prolactin gene expression.[79–83] By binding to these or other positive transcription factors, the thyroid hormone receptor may be able to inhibit gene expression in a manner that does not explicitly require receptor binding to DNA. In the case of the alcohol dehy-

drogenase 3 gene, the thyroid hormone receptor causes inhibition, probably by blocking access of retinoic acid receptors to their DNA target sites.[84] The chicken ovalbumin upstream promoter (COUP) transcription factor, which is a member of the nuclear receptor superfamily, is also able to block thyroid hormone receptor action by binding to a subset of TRE's.[85, 86] Thus, competition for DNA-binding sites among related nuclear receptors may provide an important mechanism for altering gene expression in response to different hormonal signals.

Despite examples of genes that are regulated directly by thyroid hormone receptors, the majority of thyroid hormone–responsive genes may be regulated indirectly (see Fig. 37–4). This concept is supported by the fact that in some cases, the kinetics for changes in gene expression are relatively slow (requiring several hours). Moreover, experiments using cycloheximide to block the induction of intermediate gene products are consistent with an indirect mechanism for stimulation or repression of many thyroid hormone–responsive genes.[87]

Indirect mechanisms for thyroid hormone action provide a powerful means to alter patterns of gene expression. If thyroid hormone first causes induction of a transcription factor or kinase, this protein can in turn alter the expression of a number of different genes in a cascade type of mechanism. Analogously, thyroid hormone can ultimately change patterns of gene expression by participating in the process of cellular differentiation. Of course, indirect mechanisms do not preclude concomitant direct actions of thyroid hormone receptors for a given gene. Furthermore, it is possible that some effects of thyroid hormone are direct (e.g., transcription), whereas other effects may be mediated through an indirect pathway (e.g., mRNA stability).

Thyroid hormone also exerts indirect effects at the physiological level. For example, in the rat, thyroid hormone stimulates hepatic insulin-like growth factor (IGF)-I mRNA. Because thyroid hormone also causes marked stimulation of GH in this species, the effects of thyroid hormone on IGF-I are mediated largely by an indirect mechanism involving GH.[88, 89] In hypophysectomized animals, thyroid hormone has little or no effect on IGF-I mRNA, although it enhances GH stimulation of IGF-I, suggesting that it may also function in concert with GH at the hepatic level.[88] Similarly, thyroid hormone effects on cardiac proteins and enzymes may represent a combination of direct effects on target genes and secondary effects that are consequences of thyroid hormone–induced alterations in contractility and hemodynamics.[90]

The physiological setting in which the effects of thyroid hormone are analyzed can have a major impact on its action. For example, thyroid hormone and glucocorticoids stimulate rat GH gene expression in a synergistic manner.[91–93] Many of the effects of thyroid hormone on liver enzymes involve complex interactions with other hormones. Thyroid hormone enhances insulin or IGF-I stimulation of fatty acid synthetase.[94] Activation of protein kinase pathways can block thyroid hormone stimulation of several lipogenic enzymes, including malic enzyme, fatty acid synthetase, and acetyl CoA carboxylase.[94, 95] Nutritional states also have a profound effect on hepatic enzyme induction by T$_3$. For example, a high-carbohydrate diet amplifies T$_3$ effects on glucose 6-phosphate dehydrogenase production by 40-fold.[26, 96] Thus, for many if not most thyroid hormone–responsive genes, the level of transcriptional activity integrates many signaling pathways in addition to thyroid hormone. Indeed, thyroid hormone often plays the role of a modulator that amplifies the effects of other hormones. At a mechanistic level, these complex forms of regulation may reflect the large number of transcription factors that regulate a given gene. Many well-characterized genes have been shown to bind a daunting number of regulatory proteins in their promoter regions in addition to the basal transcription factors that are required by RNA polymerase to initiate transcription. An important area for future research is to better understand how thyroid hormone receptors interact with these other proteins to change levels of gene expression.

CLONING, STRUCTURE, AND EXPRESSION OF THYROID HORMONE RECEPTORS

Thyroid Hormone Receptors are Cellular Homologues of the v-*erb*A Oncogene

The thyroid hormone receptor cDNA's were cloned in 1986.[16, 17] Although two groups independently isolated receptor clones, neither group had set out explicitly to clone a thyroid hormone receptor. Rather, in the course of analyzing clones that were related to the v-*erb*A oncogene, thyroid receptor cDNA's were isolated based upon their high degree of sequence homology with the viral oncogene.

Sap et al[16] isolated a v-*erb*A–related cDNA from a chicken embryo library. The 46-kDa protein encoded by this cDNA was shown to bind thyroid hormones with high affinity and is referred to as the thyroid receptor α (TRα) isoform. As expected, the amino acid sequence of TRα was strikingly similar to that of the v-*erb*A oncogene, suggesting that the thyroid hormone receptor is the cellular homologue of the viral oncogene. There are, however, important differences between the v-*erb*A oncogene and the cellular TRα. Comparison of their sequences reveals that the v-*erb*A protein contains 17 amino acid substitutions, including two changes in the DNA-binding domain. In addition, deletion of nine amino acids at the carboxy-terminus of the v-*erb*A protein eliminates its ability to bind thyroid hormone.[16] These mutations in v-*erb*A likely account for its ability to

block cellular differentiation and to function together with the v-*erb*B oncogene to cause erythroleukemia.[97]

In parallel with the isolation of the TRα, Weinberger et al.[17] isolated a β form of the TR from a human placental library. Like TRα, TRβ binds thyroid hormones with high affinity and with a profile of binding to thyroid hormone analogues similar to that of thyroid hormone receptors in native tissues. The TRα and β isoforms are encoded by separate genes that are located on chromosomes 17 and 3, respectively.[98, 99]

Structure of the Thyroid Hormone Receptors

In addition to the thyroid hormone receptors, the v-*erb*A–related superfamily includes receptors for estrogen, progesterone, glucocorticoid, mineralocorticoid, androgen, vitamin D, and retinoic acid as well as a number of "orphan receptors" that may or may not bind specific ligand.[100, 101] (see also Ch. 6). The members of this receptor family are characterized by a central DNA-binding domain and a carboxy-terminal hormone or ligand-binding domain. Dimerization domains and nuclear localization signals are found in both the DNA and ligand-binding domains (Fig. 37–6). The amino-termini of the receptors are more variable between different classes of receptors (e.g., glucocorticoid versus thyroid) as well as within subgroups of receptors (e.g., TRα versus TRβ).

The DNA-binding domains of the nuclear receptors are composed of two distinct zinc fingers in which a single zinc atom is coordinated tetrahedrally with four cysteines. Each of the zinc fingers contains a loop of amino acids that forms the "finger" extending from the planar zinc coordinated complex. The fingers are separated by a 15- to 17-amino acid linker sequence. The crystal structure of the DNA-binding domain of the glucocorticoid receptor has been determined, allowing detailed understanding of the the structural features of this domain.[102] In addition, a number of elegant structure-function analyses of the DNA-binding domain have been performed. Exchanges of sequences between various receptors have been particularly informative to define the structural determinants for binding to specific DNA sequences.[103, 104] These experiments show that a small stretch of amino acids at the base of the

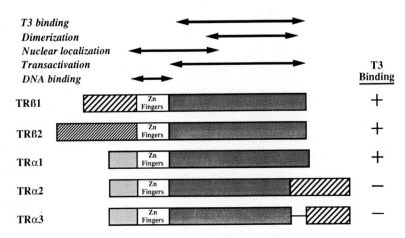

FIGURE 37–6. **Functional domains of thyroid hormone receptor isoforms.** The thyroid hormone receptor (TR) β and α isoforms are illustrated schematically. The zinc finger DNA-binding regions are indicated, and homologous regions of the α and β receptors are shown by stippled boxes. The TRβ isoform, which is expressed specifically in the pituitary and hypothalamus, contains a unique amino-terminus *(narrow stripes)*. The TRα2 and TRα3 isoforms *(broad stripes)* contain unique carboxy-terminal sequences that eliminate ligand binding. Some of the functional domains of the receptors are indicated by arrows at the top of the figure. These regions have not been mapped extensively, and other regions may be important in the three-dimensional context of the native receptor.

TABLE 37–5. SUBFAMILIES OF NUCLEAR RECEPTORS BASED UPON THEIR DNA-BINDING DOMAINS AND DNA RECOGNITION SEQUENCES

RECEPTOR	P-BOX	CONSENSUS HALF-SITE
Estrogen/thyroid subfamily		AGGTCA
Estrogen	EGCKA	
Thyroid α,β	EGCKG	
Rev-*erbA*	EGCKG	
Retinoic acid α,β,γ	EGCKG	
Retinoid X α,β,γ	EGCKG	
Vitamin D	EGCKG	
NGFI-B	EGCKG	
v-*erbA*	EGCKS	
COUP-TF	EGCKS	
ARP-1	EGCKS	
Glucocorticoid subfamily		AGAACA
Glucocorticoid	GSCKV	
Mineralocorticoid	GSCKV	
Progesterone	GSCKV	
Androgen	GSCKV	

The P-box refers to a 5-amino acid sequence (in single letter code) at the base of the first zinc finger in the DNA-binding domain of the nuclear receptors. The half-sites refer to a consensus nucleotide sequence recognized by the DNA-binding domains of the receptor subfamilies. ARP, Apolipoprotein A1 regulatory protein; COUP-TF, Chicken ovalbumin upstream promoter transcription factor; NGFI-B, Nerve growth factor induced gene-B. (Adapted from Umesono K, Evans RM: Determinants of target gene specificity for steroid/thyroid hormone receptors. Cell 57:1142, 1989. Copyright by Cell Press.)

first finger (referred to as the P-box) define the specificity for binding to DNA. As described below, the various nuclear receptors recognize specific hexameric nucleotide sequences that define the hormone response elements in target genes. Consistent with its role in defining DNA specificity, the P-box sequence is one of the most variable regions in the DNA-binding domain of the nuclear receptors. The P-box sequence is shared by certain receptor subfamilies that bind to similar or identical DNA recognition sites. This finding allows the nuclear receptors to be divided into subfamilies (Table 37–5). In the case of the thyroid hormone receptors, the P-box sequence (EGCKA) is also shared with the retinoic acid receptors, the retinoic acid X receptors, the Rev-*erbA* protein, the vitamin D receptor, and nerve growth factor–induced gene B (NGFI-B).

A second region of the DNA-binding domain (referred to as the D-box) is located between the first two cysteines of the second zinc finger.[104] The D-box is thought to be involved in spacing between receptor homodimers or, potentially, heterodimers. Because most DNA recognition sequences for receptors are either palindromic or direct repeats of the hexameric half-sites, the D-box likely represents one of the receptor determinants that defines recognition of the spacing between the half-sites. Thus, for receptor subfamilies that share a common P-box and hexameric half-site, distinct target DNA sequences may be defined by spacing between the half-sites rather than by the primary sequence of the receptor-binding sites. This hypothesis is supported by data that varying the number of nucleotide spacers alters the DNA sequence specificity for members of the thyroid hormone receptor subfamily, each of which binds to similar or identical half-sites (Fig. 37–7).[75, 105] The effects of sequence variation within the half-sites and in the spacer sequences have not been fully elucidated but may provide an important means for determining the affinity and specificity of receptor interactions with DNA.

Alternate Splicing Results in Multiple Thyroid Hormone Receptor Isoforms

The TRα gene is alternately spliced to result in a number of distinct protein products. In mammals, the splicing variants involve only the carboxy-terminal hormone-binding domain (see Fig. 37–6). One variant, referred to as α2, is identical to TRα1 through the first 370 amino acids, but then the sequences diverge completely, reflecting the splicing of alternative exons.[106–110] Another splicing variant, referred to as TRvII or α3, is similar to α2 except that it lacks the first 39 amino acids that are found in the unique region of α2.[107] The functional consequences of substituting the carboxy-terminal sequences of α1 with those of α2 are profound. First, α2 no longer binds thyroid hormone because of substitution of critical amino acids at the extreme carboxy-terminal end of the protein.[111] Consequently, α2 cannot modulate gene transcription in a manner analogous to its TRα1 and β receptor counterparts.[112–114] Second, the sequence substitutions in α2 alter a critical region in the receptor dimerization domain. Thus, even though the DNA-binding domain is not altered, the affinity of α2 interactions with DNA is reduced, presumably because dimerization is important for high-affinity binding to DNA.[115] The

FIGURE 37–7. Nuclear receptor specificity for DNA is defined by the sequences of DNA half-sites and by the spacing between half-sites. Receptor binding to DNA half-sites *(arrows)* is defined in part by the P-box region of the DNA-binding domain.[104] The orientation and spacing between the half-sites are also important determinants of receptor specificity. In the idealized example shown, the same half-site (AGGTCA) is arranged as direct repeats or inverted repeats spaced by a variable number of nucleotides.[75, 104] Binding by the retinoic acid X receptor (RXR), chicken ovalbumin upstream promoter (COUP), vitamin D receptor (VDR), thyroid hormone receptor (TR), retinoic acid receptor (RAR), and estrogen receptor (ER) is depicted by + + + (see text for details).

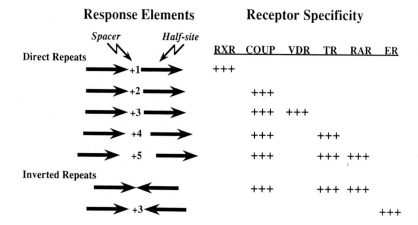

function of the α2 splicing variant is poorly understood. It is expressed in many tissues, and it is present at particularly high levels in brain, testis, kidney, and brown fat[46, 116–119] (Fig. 37–8). The α2 isoform has been proposed to be an endogenous inhibitor of thyroid hormone receptor function, in part because thyroid hormone action is thought to be blunted in some of the tissues in which α2 is highly expressed. Consistent with this view, α2 inhibits TRα and β receptor function in transient gene expression assays,[112, 113] but its inhibitory effects are not seen for all target genes.[114] It remains to be determined whether these effects of α2 have physiological significance.

In addition to splicing variants of the TRα gene, a number of isoforms appear to be generated by initiation of translation from internal AUG codons, at least in chickens.[120] Internal translation gives rise to a series of proteins that contain variable amounts of the amino-terminal and DNA-binding domains. These receptor fragments are of interest because of their potential to act as receptor antagonists by forming inactive dimers. When co-expressed with full-length receptors, the carboxy-terminal receptor fragments inhibit activation of receptor-dependent gene expression.[121, 122] Dimerization domains are required for the inhibitory activity of the carboxy-terminal fragments. Although carboxy-terminal fragments have not been demonstrated in mammals or for TRβ, it is important to consider such proteins because they can contribute to thyroid hormone–binding activity and potentially play a role in regulating the activity of the full-length receptor.

Surprisingly, a receptor-like molecule is also encoded on the opposite strand of the TRα genomic locus.[123, 124] This protein, Rev-*erb*A, is approximately 56 kDa and contains a DNA-binding domain that is homologous to thyroid hormone receptors (see Table 37–5). However, Rev-*erb*A does not bind thyroid hormone and exhibits little homology to other nuclear receptors in its putative ligand-binding domain. The function of Rev-*erb*A is unknown, and it is currently categorized as an "orphan receptor." One possibility is that it exerts direct transcriptional control of genes in a manner analogous to other nuclear receptors. Alternatively, because Rev-*erb*A shares a 269-bp exonic segment of the bidirectionally transcribed TRα gene, it might modulate expression or splicing of TRα1 and α2.[125, 126]

In contrast to the TRα gene, the splicing variants of the TRβ gene involve the amino-terminus of the receptor (see Fig. 37–6). One splicing variant, referred to as TRβ2, is expressed predominantly in the pituitary[127] and hypothalamus.[128] In TRβ2, the amino-terminal region of the receptor is distinct, probably reflecting use of a tissue-specific promoter as well as alternate splicing. The function of the amino-terminus of the thyroid hormone receptor is not known. The β1 and β2 isoforms function similarly in transient gene expression assays.[127] The significance of the TRβ2 isoform may be derived from its expression by a distinct promoter site rather than the presence of a unique amino-terminal protein sequence. As described below, expression of TRβ2 is down-regulated by thyroid hormone, whereas expression of TRβ1 is unaffected or increased by thyroid hormone.[127] Thus, expression from the TRβ2 promoter may provide a mechanism for an additional level of thyroid hormone regulation in tissues that control TSH production. It is notable that a large number of amino-terminal splicing variants of both TRα and TRβ have been found in *Xenopus*.[129] It is unclear why this degree of TR diversity exists in the frog and not in mammals. However, these findings raise the possibility of unrecognized functions for the amino-terminal domain of the receptors. Possibilities include modulation of translation efficiency, interactions with other cellular proteins, promoter-specific expression, and control of receptor turnover.

Regulation of Thyroid Hormone Receptor Expression during Development and by Thyroid Hormone

The distribution of thyroid hormone receptors in adult tissues has been assessed in several species.[46, 118, 130, 131] In general, the α and β receptor isoforms are distributed widely and exhibit overlapping patterns of expression (Fig. 37–8). Spleen and testis are notable for their relative lack of α1 and β1 receptors, a feature consistent with data indicating that these tissues have minimal metabolic responses to thyroid hormone. The α2 isoform is highly expressed in many tissues, particularly brain, kidney, and testis. Most studies of receptor isoform expression have involved mRNA analyses, and it is possible that expression of the proteins may be different from that predicted by studies of mRNA.[46]

Expression of thyroid hormone receptors during development is of great interest in view of the effects of T_3 on cellular differentiation and organogenesis. In particular,

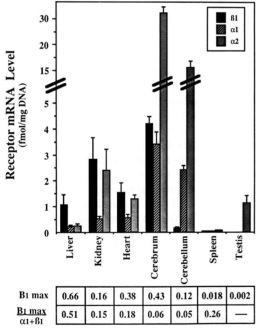

	Liver	Kidney	Heart	Cerebrum	Cerebellum	Spleen	Testis
B1 max	0.66	0.16	0.38	0.43	0.12	0.018	0.002
$\dfrac{\text{B1 max}}{\alpha1+\beta1}$	0.51	0.15	0.18	0.06	0.05	0.26	—

FIGURE 37–8. **Expression of thyroid hormone receptor mRNA's and thyroid hormone–binding activity in various rat tissues.** The mRNA levels for the thyroid hormone receptor β1 *(solid bars)*, α1 *(striped bars)*, and α2 *(stippled bars)* isoforms were quantitated in different tissues (note the broken scale for α2 expression in the cerebrum and cerebellum). T_3-binding capacity in isolated whole nuclei was used to determine B1 max. The relationship between T_3-binding capacity (ng T_3/mg DNA) and levels of thyroid hormone receptor mRNA's (α1 and β) that encode T_3-binding proteins are shown below the figure. (Adapted from Strait KA, Schwartz HL, Perez-Castillo A, Oppenheimer JH: Relationship of c-*erb*A mRNA content to tissue triiodothyronine nuclear binding capacity and function in developing and adult rats. J Biol Chem 265:10516, 1990.)

REFERENCES

1. Gudernatsch JF: Feeding experiments on tadpoles. 1. The influence of specific organs given as food on growth and differentiation. A contribution to the knowledge of organs with internal secretion. Arch Entw Mech Org 35:457, 1912.
2. Shellabarger CJ, Brown JR: The biosynthesis of thyroxine and 3,5,3′-triiodothyronine in larval and adult toads. J Endocrinol 18:98, 1959.
3. Barker SB, Klitgaard HM: Metabolism of tissues excised from thyroxine-injected rats. Am J Physiol 170:81–86, 1952.
4. Barker SB, Schwartz HS: Further studies on metabolism of tissues from thyroxine-injected rats. Proc Soc Exp Biol Med 83:500–502, 1953.
5. Barker SB: Physiological activity of thyroid hormone and analogues. In Pitt-Rivers R, Trotter WR (eds): The Thyroid Gland. London, Butterworths, 1964, pp 199–236.
6. Leonard JL, Kaplan MM, Visser TJ, et al: Cerebral cortex responds rapidly to thyroid hormones. Science 214:571–573, 1981.
7. Farsetti A, Mitsuhashi T, Desvergne B, et al: Molecular basis of thyroid hormone regulation of myelin basic protein gene expression in rodent brain. J Biol Chem 266:23226–23232, 1991.
8. Shanker G, Campagnoni AT, Pieringer RA: Investigations on myelinogenesis in vitro: Developmental expression of myelin basic protein mRNA and its regulation by thyroid hormone in primary cerebral cell cultures from embryonic mice. J Neurosci Res 17:220–224, 1987.
9. Munoz A, Rodriguez PA, Perez CA, et al: Effects of neonatal hypothyroidism on rat brain gene expression. Mol Endocrinol 5:273–280, 1991.
10. Magnus-Levey A: Ueber den respiratorischen gaswechsel unter dem einfluss der thyroidea sowie unter verschiedenen pathologische zustand. Berl Klin Wochenschr 32:650, 1895.
11. Davis FB, Cody V, Davis PJ, et al: Stimulation by thyroid hormone analogues of red blood cell Ca^{2+}-ATPase activity in vitro. Correlations between hormone structure and biological activity in a human cell system. J Biol Chem 258:12373–12377, 1983.
12. Nomura T, Borges M, Ingbar SH, Silva JE: Factors determining the differential tissue response of Na/K-ATPase to thyroid hormone in the neonatal rat. Metabolism 39:1049–1055, 1990.
13. Segal J, Hardiman J, Ingbar SH: Stimulation of calcium-ATPase activity by 3,5,3′-tri-iodothyronine in rat thymocyte plasma membranes. A possible role in the modulation of cellular calcium concentration. Biochem J 261:1073–1080, 1989.
14. Rohrer D, Dillmann WH: Thyroid hormone markedly increases the mRNA coding for sarcoplasmic reticulum Ca^{2+}-ATPase in the rat heart. J Biol Chem 263:6941–6944, 1988.
15. Chaudhury S, Ismail BF, Gick GG, et al: Effect of thyroid hormone on the abundance of Na,K-adenosine triphosphatase alpha-subunit messenger ribonucleic acid. Mol Endocrinol 1:83–89, 1987.
16. Sap J, Munoz A, Damm K, et al: The c-erb-A protein is a high-affinity receptor for thyroid hormone. Nature 324:635–640, 1986.
17. Weinberger C, Thompson CC, Ong ES, et al: The c-erb-A gene encodes a thyroid hormone receptor. Nature 324:641–646, 1986.
18. Brent GA, Moore DD, Larsen PR: Thyroid hormone regulation of gene expression. Annu Rev Physiol 53:17–35, 1991.
19. Larsen PR, Silva JE, Kaplan MM: Relationships between circulating and intracellular thyroid hormones: Physiological and clinical implications. Endocr Rev 2:87–102, 1981.
20. Selenkow HA, Asper SP: Biological activity of compounds structurally related to thyroxine. Physiol Rev 35:426, 1955.
21. Koerner D, Schwartz HL, Surks MI, Oppenheimer JH: Binding of selected iodothyronine analogues to receptor sites of isolated rat hepatic nuclei. High correlation between structural requirements for nuclear binding and biological activity. J Biol Chem 250:6417–6423, 1975.
22. Samuels HH, Stanley F, Casanova J: Relationship of receptor affinity to the modulation of thyroid hormone nuclear receptor levels and growth hormone synthesis by L-triiodothyronine and iodothyronine analogues in cultured GH1 cells. J Clin Invest 63:1229–1240, 1979.
23. Silva JE, Dick TE, Larsen PR: The contribution of local tissue thyroxine monodeiodination to the nuclear 3,5,3′-triiodothyronine in pituitary, liver, and kidney of euthyroid rats. Endocrinology 103:1196–1207, 1978.
24. Crantz FR, Larsen PR: Rapid thyroxine to 3,5,3′-triiodothyronine conversion and nuclear 3,5,3′-triiodothyronine binding in rat cerebral cortex and cerebellum. J Clin Invest 65:935–938, 1980.
25. Larsen PR, Frumess RD: Comparison of the biological effects of thyroxine and triiodothyronine in the rat. Endocrinology 100:980–988, 1977.
26. Oppenheimer JH, Schwartz HL, Mariash CN, et al: Advances in our understanding of thyroid hormone action at the cellular level. Endocr Rev 8:288–308, 1987.
27. Hennemann G, Krenning EP, Polhuys M, et al: Carrier-mediated transport of thyroid hormone into rat hepatocytes is rate-limiting in total cellular uptake and metabolism. Endocrinology 119:1870–1872, 1986.
28. Lakshmanan M, Goncalves E, Lessly G, et al: The transport of thyroxine into mouse neuroblastoma cells, NB41A3: The effect of L-system amino acids. Endocrinology 126:3245–3250, 1990.
29. Blondeau JP, Osty J, Francon J: Characterization of the thyroid hormone transport system of isolated hepatocytes. J Biol Chem 263:2685–2692, 1988.
30. Zhou Y, Samson M, Osty J, et al: Evidence for a close link between the thyroid hormone transport system and the aromatic amino acid transport system T in erythrocytes. J Biol Chem 265:17000–17004, 1990.
31. Osty J, Valensi P, Samson M, et al: Transport of thyroid hormones by human erythrocytes: Kinetic characterization in adults and newborns. J Clin Endocrinol Metab 71:1589–1595, 1990.
32. Segal J, Ingbar SH: Specific binding sites for the triiodothyronine in the plasma membrane of rat thymocytes. Correlation with biochemical responses. J Clin Invest 70:919–926, 1982.
33. Horiuchi R, Johnson ML, Willingham MC, et al: Affinity labeling of the plasma membrane 3,3′,5-triiodo-L-thyronine receptor in GH3 cells. Proc Natl Acad Sci USA 79:5527–5531, 1982.
34. Angel RC, Botta JA, Farias RN: High affinity L-triiodothyronine binding to right-side-out and inside-out vesicles from rat and human erythrocyte membrane. J Biol Chem 264:19143–19146, 1989.
35. Cheng SY, Gong QH, Parkison C, et al: The nucleotide sequence of a human cellular thyroid hormone binding protein present in endoplasmic reticulum. J Biol Chem 262:11221–11227, 1987.
36. Cheng S-Y, Hasumura S, Willingham MC, Pastan I: Purification and characterization of a membrane-associated 3,3′,5-triiodo-L-thyronine binding protein from a human carcinoma cell line. Proc Natl Acad Sci USA 83:947–951, 1986.
37. Kato H, Fukuda T, Parkison C, et al: Cytosolic thyroid hormone–binding protein is a monomer of pyruvate kinase. Proc Natl Acad Sci USA 86:7861–7865, 1989.
38. Ashizawa K, Fukuda T, Cheng SY: Transcriptional stimulation by thyroid hormone of a cytosolic thyroid hormone binding protein which is homologous to a subunit of pyruvate kinase M1. Biochemistry 31:2774–2778, 1992.
39. Oppenheimer JH, Schwartz HL: Stereospecific transport of triiodothyronine from plasma to cytosol and from cytosol to nucleus in rat liver, kidney, brain, and heart. J Clin Invest 75:147–154, 1985.
40. Freake HC, Mooradian AD, Schwartz HL, Oppenheimer JH: Stereospecific transport of triiodothyronine to cytoplasm and nucleus in GH1 cells. Mol Cell Endocrinol 44:25–35, 1986.
41. Tata JR, Widnell CC: Ribonucleic acid synthesis during the early action of thyroid hormone. Biochem J 98:604–620, 1966.
42. Shadlow AR, Surks MI, Schwartz HL, Oppenheimer JH: Specific triiodothyronine binding sites in the anterior pituitary of the rat. Science 176:1252–1254, 1972.
43. Samuels HH, Tsai JS, Casanova J, Stanley F: Thyroid hormone action: In vitro characterization of solubilized nuclear receptors from rat liver and cultured GH1 cells. J Clin Invest 54:853–865, 1974.
44. Schwartz HL, Trence D, Oppenheimer JH, et al: Distribution and metabolism of L- and D-triiodothyronine (T_3) in the rat: Preferential accumulation of L-T_3 by hepatic and cardiac nuclei as a probable explanation of the differential biologic potency of T_3 enantiomers. Endocrinology 113:1236–1243, 1983.
45. Oppenheimer JH, Schwartz HL, Surks MI: Tissue differences in the concentration of triiodothyronine nuclear binding sites in the rat: Liver, kidney, pituitary, heart, brain, spleen, testis. Endocrinology 95:897–903, 1974.
46. Strait KA, Schwartz HL, Perez-Castillo A, Oppenheimer JH: Relationship of c-erbA mRNA content to tissue triiodothyronine nuclear binding capacity and function in developing and adult rats. J Biol Chem 265:10514–10521, 1990.
47. Spindler SR, MacLeod KM, Ring J, Baxter JD: Thyroid hormone receptors: Binding characteristics and lack of hormonal dependency for nuclear localization. J Biol Chem 250:4113–4119, 1975.
48. Perlman AJ, Stanley F, Samuels HH: Thyroid hormone nuclear receptor: Evidence for multimeric organization in chromatin. J Biol Chem 257:930–938, 1982.

49. MacLeod KM, Baxter JD: Chromatin receptors for thyroid hormones: Interactions of the solubilized proteins with DNA. J Biol Chem 251:7380–7387, 1976.

50. Jump DB, Seelig S, Schwartz HL, Oppenheimer JH: Association of thyroid hormone receptor with rat liver chromatin. Biochemistry 20:6781–6789, 1981.

51. Casanova J, Horowitz ZD, Copp RP, et al: Photoaffinity labeling of thyroid hormone nuclear receptors. Influence of n-butyrate and analysis of the half-lives of the 57,000 and 47,000 molecular weight receptor forms. J Biol Chem 259:12084–12091, 1984.

52. Pascual A, Casanova J, Samuels HH: Photoaffinity labeling of thyroid hormone nuclear receptors in intact cells. J Biol Chem 257:9640–9647, 1982.

53. Latham KR, Ring JC, Baxter JD: Solubilized nuclear "receptors" for thyroid hormones: Physical characteristics and binding properties, evidence for multiple forms. J Biol Chem 251:7388–7397, 1976.

54. Ichikawa K, DeGroot LJ: Purification and characterization of rat liver nuclear thyroid hormone receptors. Proc Natl Acad Sci USA 84:3420–3424, 1987.

55. Samuels HH, Forman BM, Horowitz ZD, Ye ZS: Regulation of gene expression by thyroid hormone. J Clin Invest 81:957–967, 1988.

56. Simonet WS, Ness GC: Post-transcriptional regulation of 3-hydroxy-3-methylglutaryl-CoA reductase mRNA in rat liver. Glucocorticoids block the stabilization caused by thyroid hormones. J Biol Chem 264:569–573, 1989.

57. Simonet WS, Ness GC: Transcriptional and posttranscriptional regulation of rat hepatic 3-hydroxy-3-methylglutaryl-coenzyme A reductase by thyroid hormones. J Biol Chem 263:12448–12453, 1988.

58. Strobl W, Gorder NL, Lin LY, et al: Role of thyroid hormones in apolipoprotein A-I gene expression in rat liver. J Clin Invest 85:659–667, 1990.

59. Brent GA, Dunn MK, Harney JW, et al: Thyroid hormone aporeceptor represses T₃-inducible promoters and blocks activity of the retinoic acid receptor. New Biol 1:329–336, 1989.

60. Damm K, Thompson CC, Evans RM: Protein encoded by v-erbA functions as a thyroid-hormone receptor antagonist. Nature 339:593–597, 1989.

61. Graupner G, Wills KN, Tzukerman M, et al: Dual regulatory role for thyroid-hormone receptors allows control of retinoic-acid receptor activity. Nature 340:653–656, 1989.

62. Sap J, de Magistris L, Stunnenberg H, Vennstrom B: A major thyroid hormone response element in the third intron of the rat growth hormone gene. EMBO J 9:887–896, 1990.

63. Chin WW, Shupnik MA, Ross DS, et al: Regulation of the alpha and thyrotropin beta-subunit messenger ribonucleic acids by thyroid hormones. Endocrinology 116:873–878, 1985.

64. Shupnik MA, Ardisson LJ, Meskell MJ, et al: Triiodothyronine (T₃) regulation of thyrotropin subunit gene transcription is proportional to T₃ nuclear receptor occupancy. Endocrinology 118:367–371, 1986.

65. Shupnik MA, Chin WW, Habener JF, Ridgway EC: Transcriptional regulation of the thyrotropin subunit genes by thyroid hormone. J Biol Chem 260:2900–2903, 1985.

66. Shupnik MA, Ridgway EC: Thyroid hormone control of thyrotropin gene expression in rat anterior pituitary cells. Endocrinology 121:619–624, 1987.

67. Chatterjee VKK, Lee JK, Rentoumis A, Jameson JL: Negative regulation of the thyroid-stimulating hormone alpha gene by thyroid hormone: Receptor interaction adjacent to the TATA box. Proc Natl Acad Sci USA 86:9114–9118, 1989.

68. Burnside J, Darling DS, Carr FE, Chin WW: Thyroid hormone regulation of the rat glycoprotein hormone alpha-subunit gene promoter activity. J Biol Chem 264:6886–6891, 1989.

69. Carr FE, Burnside J, Chin WW: Thyroid hormones regulate rat thyrotropin beta gene promoter activity expressed in GH3 cells. Mol Endocrinol 3:709–716, 1989.

70. Wondisford FE, Farr EA, Radovick S, et al: Thyroid hormone inhibition of human thyrotropin beta-subunit gene expression is mediated by a cis-acting element located in the first exon. J Biol Chem 264:14601–14604, 1989.

71. Wood WM, Kao MY, Gordon DF, Ridgway EC: Thyroid hormone regulates the mouse thyrotropin beta-subunit gene promoter in transfected primary thyrotropes. J Biol Chem 264:14840–14847, 1989.

72. Bodenner DL, Mroczynski MA, Weintraub BD, et al: A detailed functional and structural analysis of a major thyroid hormone inhibitory element in the human thyrotropin beta-subunit gene. J Biol Chem 266:21666–21673, 1991.

73. Datta S, Magge SN, Madison LD, Jameson JL: Thyroid hormone receptor mediates transcriptional activation and repression of different promoters in vitro. Mol Endocrinol 6:815–825, 1992.

74. Carr FE, Kaseem LL, Wong NCW: Thyroid hormone inhibits thyrotropin gene expression via a position-independent negative L-triiodothyronine-responsive element. J Biol Chem 267:18689–18694, 1992.

75. Naar AM, Boutin JM, Lipkin SM, et al: The orientation and spacing of core DNA-binding motifs dictate selective transcriptional responses to three nuclear receptors. Cell 65:1267–1279, 1991.

76. Hudson LG, Santon JB, Glass CK, Gill GN: Ligand-activated thyroid hormone and retinoic acid receptors inhibit growth factor receptor promoter expression. Cell 62:1165–1175, 1990.

77. Hudson LG, Thompson KL, Xu J, Gill GN: Identification and characterization of a regulated promoter element in the epidermal growth factor receptor gene. Proc Natl Acad Sci USA 87:7536–7540, 1990.

78. Thompson KL, Santon JB, Shephard LB, et al: A nuclear protein is required for thyroid hormone receptor binding to an inhibitory half-site in the epidermal growth factor receptor promoter. Mol Endocrinol 6:627–635, 1992.

79. Zhang XK, Wills KN, Husmann M, et al: Novel pathway for thyroid hormone receptor action through interaction with jun and fos oncogene activities. Mol Cell Biol 11:6016–6025, 1991.

80. Voz ML, Peers B, Wiedig MJ, et al: Transcriptional regulation by triiodothyronine requires synergistic action of the thyroid receptor with another trans-acting factor. Mol Cell Biol 12:3991–3997, 1992.

81. Tansey WP, Catanzaro DF: Sp1 and thyroid hormone receptor differentially activate expression of human growth hormone and chorionic somatomammotropin genes. J Biol Chem 266:9805–9813, 1991.

82. Schaufele F, West BL, Reudelhuber TL: Overlapping Pit-1 and Sp1 binding sites are both essential to full rat growth hormone gene promoter activity despite mutually exclusive Pit-1 and Sp1 binding. J Biol Chem 265:17189–17196, 1990.

83. Schaufele F, West BL, Baxter JD: Synergistic activation of the rat growth hormone promoter by Pit-1 and the thyroid hormone receptor. Mol Endocrinol 6:656–665, 1992.

84. Harding PP, Duester G: Retinoic acid activation and thyroid hormone repression of the human alcohol dehydrogenase gene ADH3. J Biol Chem 267:14145–14150, 1992.

85. Tran P, Zhang X-K, Salbert G, et al: COUP orphan receptors are negative regulators of retinoic acid response pathways. Mol Cell Biol 12:4666–4676, 1992.

86. Cooney AJ, Tsai SY, O'Malley BW, Tsai M-J: Chicken ovalbumin upstream promoter transcription factor (COUP-TF) dimers bind to different GGTCA response elements, allowing COUP-TF to repress hormonal induction of the vitamin D₃, thyroid hormone, and retinoic acid receptors. Mol Cell Biol 12:4153–4163, 1992.

87. Kanamori A, Brown DD: The regulation of thyroid hormone receptor beta genes by thyroid hormone in Xenopus laevis. J Biol Chem 267:739–745, 1992.

88. Wolf M, Ingbar SH, Moses AC: Thyroid hormone and growth hormone interact to regulate insulin-like growth factor-I messenger ribonucleic acid and circulating levels in the rat. Endocrinology 125:2905–2914, 1989.

89. Harakawa S, Yamashita S, Tobinaga T, et al: In vivo regulation of hepatic insulin-like growth factor-1 messenger ribonucleic acids with thyroid hormone. Endocrinol Jpn 37:205–211, 1990.

90. Balkman C, Ojamaa K, Klein I: Time course of the in vivo effects of thyroid hormone on cardiac gene expression. Endocrinology 130:2001–2006, 1992.

91. Evans RM, Birnberg NC, Rosenfeld MG: Glucocorticoids and thyroid hormones transcriptionally regulate growth hormone gene expression. Proc Natl Acad Sci USA 79:7659–7663, 1982.

92. Martial JA, Baxter JD, Goodman HM, Seeberg PH: Regulation of growth hormone messenger RNA by thyroid and glucocorticoid hormones. Proc Natl Acad Sci USA 74:1816–1820, 1977.

93. Spindler SR, Mellon SH, Baxter JD: Growth hormone gene transcription is regulated by thyroid and glucocorticoid hormones in cultured rat pituitary tumor cells. J Biol Chem 257:11627–11632, 1982.

94. Stapleton SR, Mitchell DA, Salati LM, Goodridge AG: Triiodothyronine stimulates transcription of the fatty acid synthase gene in chick embryo hepatocytes in culture. Insulin and insulin-like growth factor amplify that effect. J Biol Chem 265:18442–18446, 1990.

95. Swierczynski J, Mitchell DA, Reinhold DS, et al: Triiodothyronine-induced accumulations of malic enzyme, fatty acid synthase, acetyl-coenzyme A carboxylase, and their mRNAs are blocked by protein kinase inhibitors. Transcription is the affected step. J Biol Chem 266:17459–17466, 1991.

96. Mariash CN, Seelig S, Schwartz HL, Oppenheimer JH: Rapid synergistic interaction between thyroid hormone and carbohydrate on mRNAS14 induction. J Biol Chem 261:9583–9586, 1986.

97. Zenke M, Munoz A, Sap J, et al: v-erbA oncogene activation entails the loss of hormone-dependent regulator activity of c-erbA. Cell 61:1035–1049, 1990.

98. Thompson CC, Weinberger C, Lebo R, Evans RM: Identification of a novel thyroid hormone receptor expressed in the mammalian central nervous system. Science 237:1610–1614, 1987.

99. Drabkin H, Kao FT, Hartz J, et al: Localization of human ERBA2 to the 3p22–3p24.1 region of chromosome 3 and variable deletion in small cell lung cancer. Proc Natl Acad Sci USA 85:9258–9262, 1988.

100. Evans RM: The steroid and thyroid hormone receptor superfamily. Science 240:889–895, 1988.

101. O'Malley BW, Conneally OM: Orphan receptors: In search of a unifying hypothesis for activation. Mol Endocrinol 6:1359–1361, 1992.

102. Luisi BF, Xu WX, Otwinowski Z, et al: Crystallographic analysis of the interaction of the glucocorticoid receptor with DNA. Nature 352:497–505, 1991.

103. Mader S, Kumar V, de VH, Chambon P: Three amino acids of the oestrogen receptor are essential to its ability to distinguish an oestrogen from a glucocorticoid-responsive element. Nature 338:271–274, 1989.

104. Umesono K, Evans RM: Determinants of target gene specificity for steroid/thyroid hormone receptors. Cell 57:1139–1146, 1989.

105. Umesono K, Murakami KK, Thompson CC, Evans RM: Direct repeats as selective response elements for the thyroid hormone, retinoic acid, and vitamin D receptors. Cell 65:1255–1266, 1991.

106. Lazar MA, Hodin RA, Darling DS, Chin WW: Identification of a rat c-erbAα-related protein which binds deoxyribonucleic acid but does not bind thyroid hormone. Mol Endocrinol 2:893–901, 1988.

107. Mitsuhashi T, Tennyson GE, Nikodem VM: Alternative splicing generates messages encoding rat c-erbA proteins that do not bind thyroid hormone. Proc Natl Acad Sci USA 85:5804–5808, 1988.

108. Izumo S, Mahdavi V: Thyroid hormone receptor alpha isoforms generated by alternative splicing differentially activate myosin HC gene transcription. Nature 334:539–542, 1988.

109. Nakai A, Seino S, Sakurai A, et al: Characterization of a thyroid hormone receptor expressed in human kidney and other tissues. Proc Natl Acad Sci USA 85:2781–2785, 1988.

110. Benbrook D, Pfahl M: A novel thyroid hormone receptor encoded by a cDNA clone from a human testis library. Science 238:788–791, 1987.

111. Schueler PA, Schwartz HL, Strait KA, et al: Binding of 3,5,3'-triiodothyronine (T₃) and its analogs to the in vitro translational products of c-erbA protooncogenes: Differences in the affinity of the α and β forms for the acetic acid analog and failure of the human testis and kidney products to bind T₃. Mol Endocrinol 4:227–234, 1990.

112. Lazar MA, Hodin RA, Chin WW: Human carboxy-terminal variant of α-type c-erbA inhibits trans-activation by thyroid hormone receptors without binding thyroid hormone. Proc Natl Acad Sci USA 86:7771–7774, 1989.

113. Koenig RJ, Lazar MA, Hodin RA, et al: Inhibition of thyroid hormone action by a non–hormone binding c-erbA protein generated by alternative mRNA splicing. Nature 337:659–661, 1989.

114. Rentoumis A, Chatterjee VK, Madison LD, et al: Negative and positive transcriptional regulation by thyroid hormone receptor isoforms. Mol Endocrinol 4:1522–1531, 1990.

115. Katz D, Berrodin TJ, Lazar MA: The unique C-termini of the thyroid hormone receptor variant, c-erbAα2, and thyroid hormone receptor α1 mediate different DNA-binding and heterodimerization properties. Mol Endocrinol 6:805–814, 1992.

116. Santos A, Freake HC, Rosenberg ME, et al: Triiodothyronine nuclear binding capacity in rat tissues correlates with a 6.0 kilobase (kb) and not a 2.6 kb messenger ribonucleic acid hybridization signal generated by a human c-erbA probe. Mol Endocrinol 2:992–998, 1988.

117. Mitsuhashi T, Nikodem VM: Regulation of expression of the alternative mRNAs of the rat alpha-thyroid hormone receptor gene. J Biol Chem 264:8900–8904, 1989.

118. Hodin RA, Lazar MA, Chin WW: Differential and tissue-specific regulation of the multiple rat c-erbA messenger RNA species by thyroid hormone. J Clin Invest 85:101–105, 1990.

119. Sakurai A, Nakai A, DeGroot LJ: Expression of three forms of thyroid hormone receptor in human tissues. Mol Endocrinol 3:392–399, 1989.

120. Bigler J, Eisenman RN: c-erbA encodes multiple proteins in chicken erythroid cells. Mol Cell Biol 8:4155–4161, 1988.

121. Bigler J, Hokanson W, Eisenman RN: Thyroid hormone receptor transcriptional activity is potentially autoregulated by truncated forms of the receptor. Mol Cell Biol 12:2406–2417, 1992.

122. Forman BM, Yang CR, Au M, et al: A domain containing leucine-zipper-like motifs mediate novel in vivo interactions between the thyroid hormone and retinoic acid receptors. Mol Endocrinol 3:1610–1626, 1989.

123. Miyajima N, Horiuchi R, Shibuya Y, et al: Two erbA homologs encoding proteins with different T₃ binding capacities are transcribed from opposite DNA strands of the same genetic locus. Cell 57:31–39, 1989.

124. Lazar MA, Hodin RA, Darling DS, Chin WW: A novel member of the thyroid/steroid hormone receptor family is encoded by the opposite strand of the rat c-erbA alpha transcriptional unit. Mol Cell Biol 9:1128–1136, 1989.

125. Munroe SH, Lazar MA: Inhibition of c-erbA mRNA splicing by a naturally occurring antisense RNA. J Biol Chem 266:22083–22086, 1991.

126. Lazar MA, Hodin RA, Cardona G, Chin WW: Gene expression from the c-erbA alpha/Rev-ErbA alpha genomic locus. Potential regulation of alternative splicing by opposite strand transcription. J Biol Chem 265:12859–12863, 1990.

127. Hodin RA, Lazar MA, Wintman BI, et al: Identification of a thyroid hormone receptor that is pituitary-specific. Science 244:76–79, 1989.

128. Cook CB, Kakucska I, Lechan RM, Koenig RJ: Expression of thyroid hormone receptor β2 in rat hypothalamus. Endocrinology 130:1077–1079, 1992.

129. Shi YB, Yaoita Y, Brown DD: Genomic organization and alternative promoter usage of the two thyroid hormone receptor beta genes in Xenopus laevis. J Biol Chem 267:733–738, 1992.

130. Nakai A, Sakurai A, Bell GI, DeGroot LJ: Characterization of a third human thyroid hormone receptor coexpressed with other thyroid hormone receptors in several tissues. Mol Endocrinol 2:1087–1092, 1988.

131. Forrest D, Sjoberg M, Vennstrom B: Contrasting developmental and tissue-specific expression of alpha and beta thyroid hormone receptor genes. EMBO J 9:1519–1528, 1990.

132. Mellstrom B, Naranjo JR, Santos A, et al: Independent expression of the α and β c-erbA genes in developing rat brain. Mol Endocrinol 5:1339–1350, 1991.

133. Bradley DJ, Towle HC, Young WS: Spatial and temporal expression of α- and β-thyroid hormone receptor mRNAs, including the β2-subtype, in the developing mammalian nervous system. J Neuroscience 12:2288–2302, 1992.

134. Forrest D, Hallbook F, Persson H, Vennstrom B: Distinct functions for thyroid hormone receptors alpha and beta in brain development indicated by differential expression of receptor genes. EMBO J 10:269–275, 1991.

135. Hodin RA, Lazar MA, Wintman BI, et al: Identification of a thyroid hormone receptor that is pituitary-specific. Science 244:76–79, 1989.

136. Nunez J: Effects of thyroid hormone during brain differentiation. Mol Cell Endocrinol 37:125–132, 1984.

137. Nicholson JL, Altman J: Synaptogenesis in the rat cerebellum: Effects of early hypo- and hyperthyroidism. Science 176:530–532, 1972.

138. Yaoita Y, Brown DD: A correlation of thyroid hormone receptor gene expression with amphibian metamorphosis. Genes Dev 4:1917–1924, 1990.

139. Samuels HH, Stanley F, Shapiro LE: Dose-dependent depletion of nuclear receptors by L-triiodothyronine: Evidence for a role in induction of growth hormone synthesis in cultured GH1 cells. Proc Natl Acad Sci USA 73:3877–3881, 1976.

140. Samuels HH, Stanley F, Shapiro LE: Modulation of thyroid hormone nuclear receptor levels by 3,5,3'-triiodo-L-thyronine in GH1 cells. J Biol Chem 252:6052–6060, 1977.

141. Beato M: Gene regulation by steroid hormones. Cell 56:335–344, 1989.

142. Klock G, Strahle U, Schutz G: Oestrogen and glucocorticoid responsive elements are closely related but distinct. Nature 329:734–736, 1987.

143. Kumar V, Chambon P: The estrogen receptor binds tightly to its responsive element as a ligand-induced homodimer. Cell 55:145–156, 1988.

144. Eriksson P, Wrange O: Protein-protein contacts in the glucocorticoid receptor homodimer influence its DNA binding properties. J Biol Chem 265:3535–3542, 1990.

145. Scwabe JWR, Neuhaus D, Rhodes D: Solution structure of the DNA binding domain of the oestrogen receptor. Nature 348:458–461, 1990.

146. Hard T, Kellenbach E, Boelens R, et al: Solution structure of the glucocorticoid receptor DNA binding domain. Science 249:157–160, 1990.

147. Hervas F, Morreale de Escobar G, Escobar Del Ray F: Rapid effects of single small doses of L-thyroxine and triiodo-L-thyronine on growth hormone as studied in the rat by radioimmunoassay. Endocrinology 97:91–101, 1975.

148. Samuels HH, Shapiro LE: Thyroid hormone stimulates *de novo* growth hormone synthesis in cultured GH1 cells: Evidence for the accumulation of a rate limiting RNA species in the induction process. Proc Natl Acad Sci USA 73:3369–3373, 1976.

149. Seo H, Vassart G, Brocas H, Refetoff S: Triiodothyronine stimulates specifically growth hormone mRNA in rat pituitary tumor cells. Proc Natl Acad Sci USA 74:2054–2058, 1977.

150. Yaffe BM, Samuels HH: Hormonal regulation of the growth hormone gene: Relationship of the rate of transcription to the level of nuclear thyroid hormone-receptor complexes. J Biol Chem 259:6284–6291, 1984.

151. Casanova J, Copp RP, Janocko L, Samuels HH: 5'-Flanking DNA of the rat growth hormone gene mediates regulated expression by thyroid hormone. J Biol Chem 260:11744–11748, 1985.

152. Nelson C, Crenshaw E, Franco R, et al: Discrete *cis*-active genomic sequences dictate the pituitary cell type-specific expression of rat prolactin and growth hormone genes. Nature 322:557–562, 1986.

153. Larsen PR, Harney JW, Moore DD: Sequences required for cell-type specific thyroid hormone regulation of rat growth hormone promoter activity. J Biol Chem 261:14373–14376, 1986.

154. Crew MD, Spindler SR: Thyroid hormone regulation of the transfected rat growth hormone promoter. J Biol Chem 261:5018–5022, 1986.

155. Wight PA, Crew MD, Spindler SR: Discrete positive and negative thyroid hormone–responsive transcription regulatory elements of the rat growth hormone gene. J Biol Chem 262:5659–5663, 1987.

156. Wight PA, Crew MD, Spindler SR: Sequences essential for activity of the thyroid hormone responsive transcription stimulatory element of the rat growth hormone gene. Mol Endocrinol 2:536–542, 1988.

157. Flug F, Copp RP, Casanova J, et al: *cis*-Acting elements of the rat growth hormone gene which mediate basal and regulated expression by thyroid hormone. J Biol Chem 262:6373–6382, 1987.

158. Ye ZS, Forman BM, Aranda A, et al: Rat growth hormone gene expression. Both cell-specific and thyroid hormone response elements are required for thyroid hormone regulation. J Biol Chem 263:7821–7829, 1988.

159. Koenig RJ, Brent GA, Warne RL, et al: Thyroid hormone receptor binds to a site in the rat growth hormone promoter required for induction by thyroid hormone. Proc Natl Acad Sci USA 84:5670–5674, 1987.

160. Glass CK, Franco R, Weinberger C, et al: A c-erb-A binding site in rat growth hormone gene mediates trans-activation by thyroid hormone. Nature 329:738–741, 1987.

161. Brent GA, Harney JW, Chen Y, et al: Mutations of the rat growth hormone promoter which increase and decrease response to thyroid hormone define a consensus thyroid hormone response element. Mol Endocrinol 3:1996–2004, 1989.

162. Brent GA, Larsen PR, Harney JW, et al: Functional characterization of the rat growth hormone promoter elements required for induction by thyroid hormone with and without a co-transfected beta type thyroid hormone receptor. J Biol Chem 264:178–182, 1989.

163. Williams GR, Harney JW, Forman BM, et al: Oligomeric binding of T3 receptor is required for maximal T3 response. J Biol Chem 266:19636–19644, 1991.

164. Danielson M, Hinck L, Ringold GM: Two amino acids within the knuckle of the first zinc finger specify response element activation by the glucocorticoid receptor. Cell 57:1131–1138, 1989.

165. Fawell SE, Lees JA, White R, Parker MG: Characterization and localization of steroid binding and dimerization activities in the mouse estrogen receptor. Cell 60:953–962, 1990.

166. Freedman LP: Anatomy of the steroid receptor zinc finger region. Endocr Rev 13:129–145, 1992.

167. Forman BM, Samuels HH: Interactions among a subfamily of nuclear hormone receptors: The regulatory zipper model. Mol Endocrinol 4:1293–1301, 1990.

168. Tsai SY, Carlstedt-Duke J, Weigel NL, et al: Molecular interactions of steroid hormone receptor with its enhancer element: Evidence for receptor dimer formation. Cell 55:361–369, 1988.

169. Tsai SY, Tsai M-J, O'Malley BW: Cooperative binding of steroid hormone receptors contributes to transcriptional synergism at target enhancer elements. Cell 57:443–448, 1989.

170. Klein-Hitpass L, Tsai SY, Weigel NL, et al: The progesterone receptor stimulates cell-free transcription by enhancing the formation of a stable preinitiation complex. Cell 60:247–257, 1990.

171. Habener JF: Cyclic AMP response element binding proteins: A cornucopia of transcription factors. Mol Endocrinol 4:1087–1094, 1990.

172. Landschulz WH, Johnson PF, McKnight SL: The leucine zipper: A hypothetical structure common to a new class of DNA binding proteins. Science 240:1759–1764, 1988.

173. Brent GA, Williams GR, Harney JW, et al: Capacity for cooperative binding of thyroid hormone (T3) receptor dimers defines wild type T3 response elements. Mol Endocrinol 6:502–514, 1992.

174. Forman BM, Casanova J, Raaka BM, et al: Half-site spacing and orientation determines whether thyroid hormone and retinoic acid receptors and related factors bind to DNA response elements as monomers, homodimers, or heterodimers. Mol Endocrinol 6:429–442, 1992.

175. Ribeiro RCJ, Kushner PJ, Apriletti JW, et al: Thyroid hormone alters in vitro DNA binding of monomers and dimers of thyroid hormone receptors. Mol Endocrinol 6:1142–1152, 1992.

176. Wahlstrom GM, Sjoberg M, Andersson M, et al: Binding characteristics of the thyroid hormone receptor homo- and heterodimers to consensus AGGTCA repeat motifs. Mol Endocrinol 6:1013–1022, 1992.

177. Yen PM, Darling DS, Carter RL, et al: Triiodothyronine (T3) decreases binding to DNA by T3-receptor homodimers but not receptor-auxiliary protein heterodimers. J Biol Chem 267:3565–3568, 1992.

178. Lazar MA, Berrodin TJ, Harding HP: Differential DNA binding by monomeric, homodimeric, and potentially heteromeric forms of the thyroid hormone receptor. Mol Cell Biol 11:5005–5015, 1991.

179. Murray MB, Towle HC: Identification of nuclear factors that enhance binding of the thyroid hormone receptor to a thyroid hormone response element. Mol Endocrinol 3:1434–1442, 1989.

180. Burnside J, Darling DS, Chin WW: A nuclear factor that enhances binding of thyroid hormone receptors to thyroid hormone response elements. J Biol Chem 265:2500–2504, 1990.

181. Beebe JS, Darlaing DS, Chin WW: 3,5,3'-Triiodothyronine receptor auxiliary protein (TRAP) enhances receptor binding by interactions within the thyroid hormone response element. Mol Endocrinol 5:85–93, 1991.

182. Darling DS, Beebe JS, Burnside J, et al: 3,5,3'-Triiodothyronine (T3) receptor-auxiliary protein (TRAP) binds DNA and forms heterodimers with the T3 receptor. Mol Endocrinol 5:73–84, 1991.

183. Glass CK, Lipkin SM, Devary OV, Rosenfeld MG: Positive and negative regulation of gene transcription by a retinoic acid–thyroid hormone receptor heterodimer. Cell 59:697–708, 1989.

184. Lazar MA, Berrodin TJ: Thyroid hormone receptors form distinct nuclear protein–dependent and independent complexes with a thyroid hormone response element. Mol Endocrinol 4:1627–1635, 1990.

185. O'Donnell AL, Rosen ED, Darling DS, Koenig RJ: Thyroid hormone receptor mutations that interfere with transcriptional activation also interfere with receptor interaction with a nuclear protein. Mol Endocrinol 5:94–99, 1991.

186. Glass CK, Devary OV, Rosenfeld MG: Multiple cell type–specific proteins differentially regulate target sequence recognition by the α retinoic acid receptor. Cell 63:729–738, 1990.

187. Sone T, Kerner S, Pike JW: Vitamin D receptor interaction with specific DNA. Association as a 1,25-dihyroxyvitamin D3–modulated heterodimer. J Biol Chem 266:23296–23305, 1991.

188. MacDonald PN, Haussler CA, Terpening CM, et al: Baculovirus-mediated expression of the human vitamin D receptor. Functional characterization, vitamin D response element interactions, and evidence for a receptor auxiliary factor. J Biol Chem 266:18808–18813, 1991.

189. Yu VC, Delsert C, Andersen B, et al: RXR beta: A coregulator that enhances binding of retinoic acid, thyroid hormone, and vitamin D receptors to their cognate response elements. Cell 67:1251–1266, 1991.

190. Leid M, Kastner P, Lyons R, et al: Purification, cloning, and RXR identity of the HeLa cell factor with which RAR or TR heterodimerizes to bind target sequences efficiently. Cell 68:377–395, 1992.

191. Zhang XK, Hoffmann B, Tran PB, et al: Retinoid X receptor is an auxiliary protein for thyroid hormone and retinoic acid receptors. Nature 355:441–446, 1992.

192. Kliewer SA, Umesono K, Mangelsdorf DJ, Evans RM: Retinoid X receptor interacts with nuclear receptors in retinoic acid, thyroid hormone and vitamin D3 signalling. Nature 355:446–449, 1992.

193. Bugge TH, Pohl J, Lonnoy O, Stunnenberg HG: RXRa, a promiscuous partner of retinoic acid and thyroid hormone receptors. EMBO J 11:1409–1418, 1992.

194. Marks MS, Hallenbeck PL, Nagata T, et al: H-2RIIBP (RXR beta) heterodimerization provides a mechanism for combinatorial diversity in the regulation of retinoic acid and thyroid hormone responsive genes. EMBO J 11:1419–1435, 1992.

195. Mangelsdorf DJ, Borgmeyer U, Heyman RA, et al: Characterization of three RXR genes that mediate the action of 9-cis retinoic acid. Genes Dev 6:329–344, 1992.

196. Wang LH, Tsai SY, Cook RG, et al: COUP transcription factor is a member of the steroid receptor superfamily. Nature 340:163–166, 1989.

197. Hermann T, Hoffmann B, Zhang X-K, et al: Heterodimeric receptor complexes determine 3,5,3′-triiodothyronine and retinoid signaling specificities. Mol Endocrinol 6:1153–1162, 1992.

198. Levin AA, Sturzenbecker LJ, Kazmer S, et al: 9-cis Retinoic acid stereoisomer binds and activates the nuclear receptor RXRα. Nature 355:359–361, 1992.

199. Heyman RA, Mangelsdorf DJ, Dyck JA, et al: 9-cis Retinoic acid is a high affinity ligand for the retinoid X receptor. Cell 68:397–406, 1992.

200. Zhang X-K, Lehmann J, Hoffmann B, et al: Homodimer formation of retinoid X receptor induced by 9-cis retinoic acid. Nature 358:587–591, 1992.

201. Refetoff S, DeWind LT, DeGroot LJ: Familial syndrome combining deaf-mutism, stippled epiphyses, goiter and abnormally high PBI: Possible target organ refractoriness to thyroid hormone. J Clin Endocrinol Metab 27:279–294, 1967.

202. Weiss RE, Refetoff S: Thyroid hormone resistance. Annu Rev Med 43:363–375, 1992.

203. Magner JA, Petrick P, Menezes-Ferreira M, et al: Familial generalized resistance to thyroid hormones: Report of three kindreds and correlation of patterns of affected tissues with the binding of [125I] triiodothyronine to fibroblast nuclei. J Endocrinol Invest 9:459–469, 1986.

203a. Hauser P, Zametkin AJ, Martinez P, et al: Attention deficit-hyperactivity disorder in people with generalized resistance to thyroid hormone. N Engl J Med 328:997–1001, 1993.

204. Sarne DH, Sobieszczyk S, Ain KB, Refetoff S: Serum thyrotropin and prolactin in the syndrome of generalized resistance to thyroid hormone: Responses to thyrotropin-releasing hormone and short term triiodothyronine suppression. J Clin Endocrinol Metab 70:1305–1311, 1990.

205. Usala SJ, Weintraub BD: Thyroid hormone resistance syndromes. Trends Endocrinol Metab 2:140–144, 1991.

206. Usala SJ, Tennyson GE, Bale AE, et al: A base mutation of the c-erbA beta thyroid hormone receptor in a kindred with generalized thyroid hormone resistance. Molecular heterogeneity in two other kindreds. J Clin Invest 85:93–100, 1990.

207. Sakurai A, Takeda K, Ain K, et al: Generalized resistance to thyroid hormone associated with a mutation in the ligand-binding domain of the human thyroid hormone receptor beta. Proc Natl Acad Sci USA 86:8977–8981, 1989.

208. Parilla R, Mixson J, McPherson JA, et al: Characterization of seven novel mutations of the c-erbAβ gene in unrelated kindreds with generalized thyroid hormone resistance. Evidence for two "hot spot" regions in the ligand binding domain. J Clin Invest 88:2123–2130, 1991.

209. Takeda K, Weiss RE, Refetoff S: Rapid localization of mutations in the thyroid hormone receptor β gene by denaturing gel electrophoresis in eighteen families with thyroid hormone resistance. J Clin Endocrinol Metab 74:712–719, 1992.

210. Chatterjee VK, Nagaya T, Madison LD, et al: Thyroid hormone resistance syndrome. Inhibition of normal receptor function by mutant thyroid hormone receptors. J Clin Invest 87:1977–1984, 1991.

211. Sakurai A, Miyamoto T, Refetoff S, DeGroot LJ: Dominant negative transcriptional regulation by a mutant thyroid hormone receptor-beta in a family with generalized resistance to thyroid hormone. Mol Endocrinol 4:1988–1994, 1990.

212. Nagaya T, Madison LM, Jameson JL: Thyroid hormone receptor mutations that cause resistance to thyroid hormone. Evidence for receptor competition for DNA sequences in target genes. J Biol Chem 267:13014–13019, 1992.

213. Petty KJ, Desvergne B, Mitsuhashi T, Nikodem VM: Identification of a thyroid hormone response element in the malic enzyme gene. J Biol Chem 265:7395–7400, 1990.

214. Sap J, Munoz A, Schmitt J, et al: Repression of transcription mediated at a thyroid hormone response element by the v-erb-A oncogene product. Nature 340:242–244, 1989.

215. Baniahmad A, Steiner C, Kohne AC, Renkawitz R: Modular structure of a chicken lysozyme silencer: Involvement of an unusual thyroid hormone receptor binding site. Cell 61:505–514, 1990.

216. Mooradian AD, Schwartz HL, Mariash CN, Oppenheimer JH: Transcellular and transnuclear transport of 3,5,3′-triiodothyronine in isolated hepatocytes. Endocrinology 117:2449–2456, 1985.

217. Davis PJ, Blas SD: In vitro stimulation of human red blood cell Ca^{2+}-ATPase by thyroid hormone. Biochem Biophys Res Commun 99:1073–1080, 1981.

218. Davis FB, Davis PJ, Blas SD: Role of calmodulin in thyroid hormone stimulation in vitro of human erythrocyte Ca^{2+}-ATPase activity. J Clin Invest 71:579–586, 1983.

219. Segal J, Buckley C, Ingbar SH: Stimulation of adenylate cyclase activity in rat thymocytes in vitro by 3,5,3′-triiodothyronine. Endocrinology 116:2036–2043, 1985.

220. Segal J, Ingbar SH: 3,5,3′-Triiodothyronine increases cellular adenosine 3′,5′-monophosphate concentration and sugar uptake in rat thymocytes by stimulating adenylate cyclase activity: Studies with the adenylate cyclase inhibitor MDL 12330A. Endocrinology 124:2166–2171, 1989.

221. Segal J, Gordon A: The effects of actinomycin D, puromycin, cycloheximide and hydroxyurea on 3′,5,3-triiodo-L-thyronine stimulated 2-deoxy-D-glucose uptake in chick embryo heart cells in vitro. Endocrinology 101:150–156, 1977.

222. Segal J, Ingbar SH: Studies of the mechanism by which 3,5,3′-triiodothyronine stimulates 2-deoxyglucose uptake in rat thymocytes in vitro. Role of calcium and adenosine 3′:5′-monophosphate. J Clin Invest 68:103–110, 1981.

223. Segal J, Ingbar SH: In vivo stimulation of sugar uptake in rat thymocytes. An extranuclear action of 3,5,3′-triiodothyronine. J Clin Invest 76:1575–1580, 1985.

224. Segal J, Ingbar SH: 3,5,3′-tri-iodothyronine enhances sugar transport in rat thymocytes by increasing the intrinsic activity of the plasma membrane sugar transporter. J Endocrinol 124:133–140, 1990.

225. Sterling K: Direct thyroid hormone activation of mitochondria: The role of adenine nucleotide translocase. Endocrinology 119:292–295, 1986.

226. Sterling K: Direct triiodothyronine (T$_3$) action by a primary mitochondrial pathway. Endocr Res 15:683–715, 1989.

227. Ashizawa K, Cheng S-Y: Regulation of thyroid hormone receptor–mediated transcription by a cytosol protein. Proc Natl Acad Sci USA 89:9277–9281, 1992.

228. Siegrist-Kaiser CA, Juge AC, Tranter MP, et al: Thyroxine-dependent modulation of actin polymerization in cultured astrocytes. A novel, extranuclear action of thyroid hormone. J Biol Chem 265:5296–5302, 1990.

229. Kumara-Siri MH, Surks MI: Regulation of growth hormone mRNA synthesis by 3,5,3′-triiodo-L-thyronine in cultured growth hormone-producing rat pituitary tumor cells (GC cells): Dissociation between nuclear iodothyronine receptor concentration and growth hormone mRNA synthesis during the deoxyribonucleic acid synthesis phase of the cell cycle. J Biol Chem 260:14529–14537, 1985.

230. Izumo S, Lompre AM, Matsuoka R, et al: Myosin heavy chain messenger RNA and protein isoform transitions during cardiac hypertrophy. Interaction between hemodynamic and thyroid hormone-induced signals. J Clin Invest 79:970–977, 1987.

231. Subramaniam A, Jones WK, Gulick J, et al: Tissue-specific regulation of the alpha-myosin heavy chain gene promoter in transgenic mice. J Biol Chem 266:24613–24620, 1991.

232. Tsika RW, Bahl JJ, Leinwand LA, Morkin E: Thyroid hormone regulates expression of a transfected human alpha-myosin heavy-chain fusion gene in fetal rat heart cells. Proc Natl Acad Sci USA 87:379–383, 1990.

233. Umeda PK, Darling DS, Kennedy JM, et al: Control of myosin heavy chain expression in cardiac hypertrophy. Am J Cardiol 59:49A–55A, 1987.

234. Song MK, Dozin B, Grieco D, et al: Transcriptional activation and stabilization of malic enzyme mRNA precursor by thyroid hormone. J Biol Chem 263:17970–17974, 1988.

235. Dozin B, Magnuson MA, Nikodem VM: Tissue-specific regulation of two functional malic enzyme mRNAs by triiodothyronine. Biochemistry 24:5581–5586, 1985.

236. Desvergne B, Petty KJ, Nikodem VM: Functional characterization and receptor binding studies of the malic enzyme thyroid hormone response element. J Biol Chem 266:1008–1013, 1991.

237. Morioka H, Tennyson GE, Nikodem VM: Structural and functional analysis of the rat malic enzyme gene promoter. Mol Cell Biol 8:3542–3545, 1988.

238. Magnuson MA, Nikodem VM: Molecular cloning of a cDNA se-

quence for rat malic enzyme. Direct evidence for induction in vivo of rat liver malic enzyme mRNA by thyroid hormone. J Biol Chem 258:12712–12717, 1983.

239. Towle HC, Mariash CN, Schwartz HL, Oppenheimer JH: Quantitation of rat liver messenger ribonucleic acid for malic enzyme during induction by thyroid hormone. Biochemistry 20:3486–3492, 1981.

240. Munoz A, Hoppner W, Sap J, et al: The chicken c-erbA alpha-product induces expression of thyroid hormone-responsive genes in 3,5,3'-triiodothyronine receptor- deficient rat hepatoma cells. Mol Endocrinol 4:312–320, 1990.

241. Salati LM, Ma XJ, McCormick CC, et al: Triiodothyronine stimulates and cyclic AMP inhibits transcription of the gene for malic enzyme in chick embryo hepatocytes in culture. J Biol Chem 266:4010–4016, 1991.

242. Jacoby DB, Engle JA, Towle HC: Induction of a rapidly responsive hepatic gene product by thyroid hormone requires ongoing protein synthesis. Mol Cell Biol 7:1352–1357, 1987.

243. Wong NC, Perez CA, Sanders MM, et al: Thyroid hormone and circadian regulation of the binding activity of a liver-specific protein associated with the 5'-flanking region of the S14 gene. J Biol Chem 264:4466–4470, 1989.

244. Zilz ND, Murray MB, Towle HC: Identification of multiple thyroid hormone response elements located far upstream from the rat S14 promoter. J Biol Chem 265:8136–8143, 1990.

245. Adan RA, Cox JJ, van Kats JP, Burbach JP: Thyroid hormone regulates the oxytocin gene. J Biol Chem 267:3771–3777, 1992.

246. Loose DS, Cameron DK, Short HP, Hanson RW: Thyroid hormone regulates transcription of the gene for cytosolic phosphoenolpyruvate carboxykinase (GTP) in rat liver. Biochemistry 24:4509–4512, 1985.

247. Hoppner W, Sussmuth W, Seitz HJ: Effect of thyroid state on cyclic AMP-mediated induction of hepatic phosphoenolpyruvate carboxykinase. Biochem J 226:67–73, 1985.

248. Giralt M, Park EA, Gurney AL, et al: Identification of a thyroid hormone response element in the phosphoenolpyruvate carboxykinase (GTP) gene. Evidence for synergistic interaction between thyroid hormone and cAMP cis-regulatory elements. J Biol Chem 266:21991–21996, 1991.

249. Hoppner W, Seitz HJ: Effect of thyroid hormones on glucokinase gene transcription in rat liver. J Biol Chem 264:20643–20647, 1989.

250. Minderop RH, Hoeppner W, Seitz HJ: Regulation of hepatic glucokinase gene expression. Role of carbohydrates, and glucocorticoid and thyroid hormones. Eur J Biochem 164:181–187, 1987.

251. Wall SR, van den Hove MF, Crepin KM, et al: Thyroid hormone stimulates expression of 6-phosphofructo-2-kinase in rat liver. FEBS Lett 257:211–214, 1989.

252. Miksicek RJ, Towle HC: Use of a cloned cDNA sequence to measure changes in 6-phosphogluconate dehydrogenase mRNA levels caused by thyroid hormone and dietary carbohydrate. J Biol Chem 258:9575–9579, 1983.

253. Izquierdo JM, Luis AM, Cuezva JM: Postnatal mitochondrial differentiation in rat liver. Regulation by thyroid hormones of the beta-subunit of the mitochondrial F1-ATPase complex. J Biol Chem 265:9090–9097, 1990.

254. Wiesner RJ, Kurowski TT, Zak R: Regulation by thyroid hormone of nuclear and mitochondrial genes encoding subunits of cytochrome-c oxidase in rat liver and skeletal muscle. Mol Endocrinol 6:1458–1467, 1992.

255. Orlowski J, Lingrel JB: Thyroid and glucocorticoid hormones regulate the expression of multiple Na,K-ATPase genes in cultured neonatal rat cardiac myocytes. J Biol Chem 265:3462–3470, 1990.

256. Bahouth SW: Thyroid hormones transcriptionally regulate the beta 1-adrenergic receptor gene in cultured ventricular myocytes. J Biol Chem 266:15863–15869, 1991.

257. Bianco AC, Sheng XY, Silva JE: Triiodothyronine amplifies norepinephrine stimulation of uncoupling protein gene transcription by a mechanism not requiring protein synthesis. J Biol Chem 263:18168–18175, 1988.

258. Weinstein SP, Watts J, Graves PN, Haber RS: Stimulation of glucose transport by thyroid hormone in ARL 15 cells: Increased abundance of glucose transporter protein and messenger ribonucleic acid. Endocrinology 126:1421–1429, 1990.

259. Fullerton MJ, Stuchbury S, Krozowski ZS, Funder JW: Altered thyroidal status and the in vivo synthesis of atrial natriuretic peptide in the rat heart. Mol Cell Endocrinol 69:227–233, 1990.

260. Hong BL, Deschepper CF: Effects of thyroid hormones on angiotensinogen gene expression in rat liver, brain, and cultured cells. Endocrinology 130:1231–1237, 1992.

261. Jonassen JA, Mullikin KD, McAdam A, Leeman SE: Thyroid hormone status regulates preprotachykinin-A gene expression in male rat anterior pituitary. Endocrinology 121:1555–1561, 1987.

262. Murata Y, Seo H, Sekiguchi K, et al: Specific induction of fibronectin gene in rat liver by thyroid hormone. Mol Endocrinol 4:693–699, 1990.

263. Leidig F, Shepard AR, Zhang WG, et al: Thyroid hormone responsiveness in human growth hormone–related genes. Possible correlation with receptor-induced DNA conformational changes. J Biol Chem 267:913–921, 1992.

264. Black MA, Pope L, Lefebvre FA, et al: Thyroid hormones precociously increase nerve growth factor gene expression in the submandibular gland of neonatal mice. Endocrinology 130:2083–2090, 1992.

265. Kasayama S, Yoshimura M, Oka T: The regulation by thyroid hormones and androgen of epidermal growth factor synthesis in the submandibular gland and its plasma concentrations in mice. J Endocrinol 121:269–275, 1989.

266. Strait KA, Schwartz HL, Seybold VS, et al: Immunofluorescence localization of thyroid hormone receptor protein beta 1 and variant alpha 2 in selected tissues: Cerebellar Purkinje cells as a model for beta 1 receptor–mediated developmental effects of thyroid hormone in brain. Proc Natl Acad Sci USA 88:3887–3891, 1991.

267. Ross DS, Ellis MF, Ridgway EC: Acute thyroid hormone withdrawal rapidly increases the thyrotropin beta and alpha-subunit messenger ribonucleic acids in mouse thyrotropic tumors. Endocrinology 118:1006–1010, 1986.

268. Shupnik MA, Ridgway EC: Triiodothyronine rapidly decreases transcription of the thyrotropin subunit genes in thyrotropic tumor explants. Endocrinology 117:1940–1946, 1985.

269. Sarapura VD, Wood WM, Gordon DF, et al: Thyrotrope expression and thyroid hormone inhibition map to different regions of the mouse glycoprotein hormone alpha-subunit gene promoter. Endocrinology 127:1352–1361, 1990.

270. Franklyn JA, Lynam T, Docherty K, et al: Effect of hypothyroidism on pituitary cytoplasmic concentrations of messenger RNA encoding thyrotrophin beta and alpha subunits, prolactin and growth hormone. J Endocrinol 108:43–47, 1986.

271. Kesavan P, Mukhopadhayay S, Murphy S, et al: Thyroid hormone decreases the expression of epidermal growth factor receptor. J Biol Chem 266:10282–10286, 1991.

272. Zhang W, Brooks RL, Silversides DW, et al: Negative thyroid hormone control of human growth hormone gene expression is mediated by 3'-untranslated / 3'-flanking DNA. J Biol Chem 267:15056–10563, 1992.

273. Koller KJ, Wolff RS, Warden MK, Zoeller RT: Thyroid hormones regulate levels of thyrotropin-releasing–hormone mRNA in the paraventricular nucleus. Proc Natl Acad Sci USA 84:7329–7333, 1987.

274. Segerson TP, Kauer J, Wolfe HC, et al: Thyroid hormone regulates TRH biosynthesis in the paraventricular nucleus of the rat hypothalamus. Science 238:78–80, 1987.

275. Taylor T, Wondisford FE, Blaine T, Weintraub BD: The paraventricular nucleus of the hypothalamus has a major role in thyroid hormone feedback regulation of thyrotropin synthesis and secretion. Endocrinology 126:317–324, 1990.

276. Rapiejko PJ, Watkins DC, Ros M, Malbon CC: Thyroid hormones regulate G-protein beta-subunit mRNA expression in vivo. J Biol Chem 264:16183–16189, 1989.

277. Thompson J, Moore SE, Walsh FS: Thyroid hormones regulate expression of the neural cell adhesion molecule in adult skeletal muscle. FEBS Lett 219:135–138, 1987.

278. Ouafik L, May V, Saffen DW, Eipper BA: Thyroid hormone regulation of peptidylglycine alpha-amidating monooxygenase expression in anterior pituitary gland. Mol Endocrinol 4:1497–1505, 1990.

38

Control of Thyroid Function: The Hypothalamic-Pituitary-Thyroid Axis

JOHN F. WILBER

The constancy of circulating concentrations of thyroxine (T_4) and triiodothyronine (T_3) is achieved by a dynamic regulatory system involving the hypothalamus, the pituitary, and the thyroid gland. The prepotent regulator of the production and secretion of pituitary thyroid-stimulating hormone (TSH) is hypothalamic thyrotropin-releasing hormone (TRH).[1] The secretion and pituitary actions of TRH are, in turn, inhibited by thyroid hormones. Additional peptide and neurotransmitter influences act upon the hypothalamus, the pituitary thyrotrope, and the thyroid gland itself, exemplified by the unique autoregulatory actions of iodine ion. Thyroid hormone formation and secretion are regulated during life from infancy to old age and are affected by a number of illnesses, environmental substances, and pharmacological agents.

HYPOTHALAMIC REGULATION BY THYROTROPIN-RELEASING HORMONE

TRH is the primary regulator of both the synthesis and secretion of pituitary TSH in humans.[1] TRH was the first hypothalamic-releasing hormone to be characterized, and since 1969 its actions both upon pituitary TSH regulation and in other extrahypothalamic loci have been extensively studied.[2]

TRH stimulates TSH in a dose-responsive manner over a wide range of TRH concentrations, and in humans, administered doses from 15 to 500 µg cause progressively higher increments in circulating TSH, with peak plasma TSH concentrations at 20 to 30 minutes following TRH administration.[3] TRH is found in the hypophyseal portal circulation in animals at concentrations in the nanomolar range, and

TRH antibody neutralization dramatically reduces TSH secretion. Of importance is that TRH not only activates TSH biosynthesis and TSH secretion, but also modulates the post-translational glycosylation of the TSH molecule, such that TRH participates in stimulating full glycosylation of the TSH molecule required for optimal biological activity.[4] In clinical situations in which TRH secretion is deficient (tertiary hypothyroidism), insufficient TSH glycosylation results in a lower than normal biological/immunological ratio of circulating TSH forms, leading to paradoxical elevations of serum TSH immunological activity in the face of decreased TSH thyroid-stimulatory activity.[5]

Initially it was postulated that TRH, pGluHisProamide, was synthesized enzymatically, analogous to glutathione.[1] However, with the advent of molecular biological tools, it has become clear that TRH is processed proteolytically from a much larger precursor protein with multiple copies of TRH. Recently, the human gene encoding prepro (pp) TRH has been cloned, sequenced, and characterized. The cardinal features of this gene, located on chromosome 3, are summarized briefly because they hold implications for regulation by T_4, T_3, and other modulators in humans.[6-9]

The gene encoding human ppTRH possesses a transcriptional unit of 3.3 kb, made up of three exons, interrupted by two introns of 1050 and 650 bp, respectively (Fig. 38–1).[9] Exon 1 encodes the 5' untranslated region of the mRNA; exon 2, the signal sequence and the initial portion of the ppTRH peptide; and exon 3, the remainder of this peptide (242 amino acids). The protein encoded by the human gene contains six identical copies of TRH, in contrast to five copies in the homologous rat ppTRH gene. There are 73.3 and 59.5 per cent homologies between the human and rat TRH genes at the nucleic acid and amino

c DNA

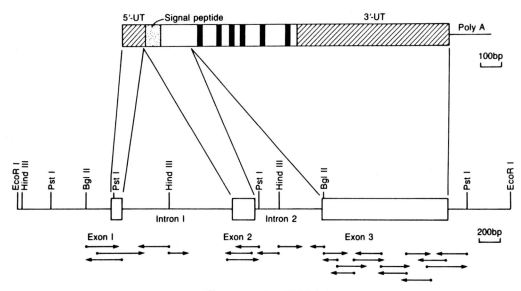

Genomic DNA

FIGURE 38–1. **Structure of human preproTRH cDNA and gene and the sequencing strategy.** The top line shows a schematic diagram of the human preproTRH cDNA, the 5′-untranslated region (5′-UT), the signal peptide–encoding region, the preproTRH encoding region, the 3′-untranslated region (3′-UT), and the poly(A) tail *(solid line)*. Solid boxes represent the TRH coding sequences. The bottom line shows a representation of the human preproTRH gene. Exons are represented by open boxes. Vertical connecting lines indicate relationships between structural regions of the cDNA and genomic DNA. The horizontal arrows beneath the genomic DNA indicate the direction and extent of sequence determinations. (From Yamada M, Radovick S, Wondisford FE, et al: Cloning and structure of human genomic DNA and hypothalamic cDNA encoding human prepro thyrotropin-releasing hormone. Mol Endocr 4:552, 1990. © The Endocrine Society.)

acid levels, respectively. The 5′ flanking region of the human TRH gene contains several features of interest with regard to regulation of gene transcription. First, in regard to inhibitory control by thyroid hormones, the 5′ flanking region contains several potential thyroid hormone regulatory element (TRE) elements that could interact with T_3.[9] The first, at base pairs (bp) −191 to −184, is identical to that in the rat TSH β chain gene sequence at +12 to +19 bp, which is a negative TRE. A second TRH gene sequence, at −158 to −166 bp (GGTCCCCAC), is homologous to a second human TSH β TRE sequence between +2 and +11 bp. The conservation of these particular sequences suggests their potential importance for thyroid hormone regulation of gene transcription.

A second feature of the 5′ flanking sequence in the human TRH gene is the enhancer sequence for the cAMP-response DNA-binding (CREB) protein, at −53 to −60 bp (TGACGTCA), suggesting regulatory influences by cAMP. Possible homology between the TRH and other peptide genes has revealed that the human ppTRH gene shares 52 per cent homology at the nucleic acid level with the human chromagranin A gene over the 700-bp reading frame of the TRH gene.[9] This is intriguing because chromagranin A is a protein found in most endocrine tissues, including the adrenal medulla, parathyroid gland, pituitary, hypothalamus, and pancreas. Further investigation is needed to explore the possible physiological significance of this homology in relation to thyroid regulation.

Finally, because genomic Southern analyses have established that human TRH gene is a single-copy gene located on human chromosome 3,[10] studies of potential abnormalities in TRH gene structure and/or regulation in patients with hereditary TRH deficiency can now be undertaken using white blood cell genomic DNA from such patients as a source for mutational analysis.

Abundant evidence indicates that TRH secretion is activated by hypothalamic α_2 adrenergic stimulation of the paraventricular nucleus (PVN). In studies with neuropharmacological agents that modify either neurotransmitter biosynthesis or actions, TRH secretory physiology has been examined in vivo both under basal conditions and in response to a physiological stimulus of TSH secretion, cold exposure.[6, 11] TRH was administered also to animals bearing indwelling atrial cannulae to assess the impact of these various pharmacological manipulations upon pituitary thyrotrope reserve. Cold exposure caused significant increments in TSH concentrations. Administration of the catecholaminergic-depleting drug, reserpine, completely inhibited this cold activation of serum TSH. Administration of α-methyl-P-tyrosine, an inhibitor of the rate-limiting step in norepinephrine biosynthesis, *tyrosine hydroxylase,* also blocked such cold activation partially[11] (Fig. 38–2). Moreover, blocking the conversion of dopamine to norepinephrine with diethyldithiocarbamate (DDC), an inhibitor of *dopamine β hydroxylase,* resulted in diminished TSH response to cold (Fig. 38–2). Finally, pimozide, a dopaminergic receptor site antagonist, failed to reverse the TSH inhibition caused by DDC, indicating that deficiency of norepinephrine, rather than an accumulation of its precursor, dopamine, was responsible for pimozide's effect. Experiments with α- and β-adrenergic blocking agents have revealed that cold responses in rats can be inhibited by the

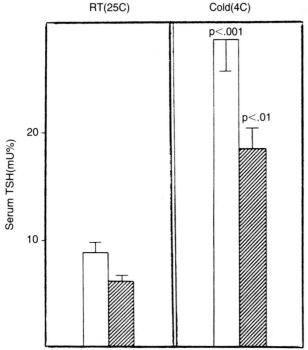

FIGURE 38–2. **Effect of a α-methyl-p-tyrosine (250 mg/kg) upon basal and cold-activated TSH secretion.** Drug-treated animals are denoted by the cross-hatched bars and control animals by the open bars. Vertical lines above the bars represent 1 SEM. (From Montoya E, Wilber JF, Lorincz M: Catecholaminergic control of thyrotropin secretion. J Lab Clin Med 93:889, 1979.)

α-adrenergic blocking agent phentolamine. Conversely, stimulation with the α-adrenergic agonist clonidine results in a enormous augmentation of cold-evoked TSH release. Thus, from these pharmacological studies, it is clear that cold-mediated TSH secretion is regulated primarily by α-adrenergic stimulation.

The primary inhibitory regulators of TSH secretion are thyroid hormones, which have been well established in animals and humans to block the pituitary (thyrotroph) actions of TRH.[1] Careful examination of quantitative relationships between TSH and intrapituitary thyroid hormone concentrations have documented that intrapituitary T_3, 50 per cent of which is generated from peripheral T_4, is the

major regulator of pituitary TSH secretion.[2] In addition, there is now strong experimental evidence that thyroid hormones can inhibit hypothalamic TRH gene transcription and TRH secretion both in vitro and in vivo.[12] Minute quantities of T_3, for example, can suppress TSH secretion when administered intracerebroventricularly, whereas identical amounts of T_3 given peripherally do not.[1] Moreover, TRH secretion from hypothyroid rat hypothalami is augmented in vitro, whereas L-T_3 can prevent completely such ouabain-activated TRH secretion.[1] Finally, it has been established by dot-blot hybridization that experimental hypothyroidism and hyperthyroidism reciprocally alter ppTRH RNA density in the rat PVN, but not in whole hypothalami.[13] On the basis of these observations, potential T_3 inhibitory influences on the human TRH gene have been examined, using chimeric plasmid constructs containing the 5′ flanking region of TRH and the reporter gene *luciferase*. In a transient transfection system with pituitary GH_3 cells, T_3 concentrations between 10^{-11} and 10^{-9} M inhibited TRH activation significantly[12] (Fig. 38–3). Such inhibition was absent when the plasmid constructs were devoid of the TRH gene 5′ flanking region (−900 to +54 bp). Future studies will be required to establish exactly what nucleotide sequences (TRE's) participate in this inhibition of the TRH gene by T_3 and what potential trans-acting factors may be operative in the hypothalamic PVN which permit T_3 inhibition selectively in this nucleus but not in other hypothalamic nuclei, or in other structures throughout the CNS and in extra-CNS structures, such as in the rat testis.[14, 15]

Minor TRH inhibition is exerted also in the PVN by such neurotransmitters as somatostatin and dopamine. Dopamine acts at both the hypothalamic level and at thyrotrope cells through pituitary D_2 receptors.[16]

Other neurotransmitters and peptides have been implicated in TRH regulation in animal studies, but their role in humans at present remains unclear. Opioids can stimulate TRH secretion experimentally,[17] and galanin in pharmacological quantities can inhibit TRH release.[18] Serotonin appears to possess both stimulatory and inhibitory effects, depending on dosages and schedules used in experimental models.[3] Other factors demonstrated experimentally to modulate TRH-dependent TSH secretion include neurotensin, vasopressin, oxytocin, substance P,

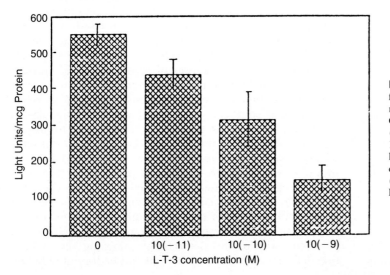

FIGURE 38–3. The effect of L-T_3 in vitro upon the activity of transfected chimeric construct, "pSVO-TRH-LUC" (containing the human ppTRH 5′ flanking sequence −900 to +54 bp) in cultured GH_3 cells. Significant inhibition was seen at all L-T_3 concentrations (10^{-11}M, −24 per cent, $P < 0.02$; 10^{-10}M, −45 per cent, $P < 0.01$; 10^{-9}M, −71 per cent, $P < 0.001$). (From Yamada M, Wilber J: The human preproTRH (ppTRH) gene: Inhibition of expression in GH_3 cells of plasmid chimeric luciferase constructs by L-triiodothyronine (L-T_3). *In* Gordon A, Gross J (eds): Progress in Thyroid Research. Rotterdam, Balkema, 1991, p 92.)

cholecystokinin, tumor necrosis factor α, and interleukin-1. Their functions in human thyroid regulation, however, have not been established.

Indirect evidence from recent studies of TRH measurements in spinal fluid in selected patients suggests that TRH may inhibit its own secretion. Adinoff et al.[19] stimulated TSH secretion with exogenous TRH in 13 abstinent alcoholic subjects and identified an inverse relationship between the pituitary TSH responses to TRH and CSF TRH concentrations, supporting the hypothesis that increasing CSF TRH concentrations may lower pituitary TRH responses, possibly via reductions in TRH pituitary receptor number.

An important feature of TSH secretion in man is its diurnal and circhoral rhythms. The role of TRH in the central generation of pulsatile thyrotropin secretion has been supported recently by studies of Brabant et al.,[20] who have investigated the influences of dopamine and somatostatin on the pulsatile release of TSH in healthy human volunteers. TSH pulses were found to persist during TSH inhibition by dopamine and somatostatin treatment. Moreover, in patients with surgically caused hypothalamic destruction after craniopharyngioma resection, in whom TSH pulsatility was abolished, repetitive TRH intravenous challenge led to restoration of a pulsatile TSH release pattern, simulating closely normal circhoral variations of TSH in intact subjects. In contrast, the reciprocal physiological pattern of glucocorticoid rhythmicity does not appear to be the modulator of such TSH rhythmicity, even though pharmacological quantities of glucocorticoids can inhibit TSH secretion.[21]

Recently TRH mRNA has been identified, using reverse transcriptase polymerase chain reaction (PCR), in both the normal and adenomatous human pituitary.[22] Previous studies have demonstrated that TRH is present in long-term primary cultures of anterior pituitary tissue.[23] The potential role of such pituitary TRH in local regulatory events concerning TSH metabolism is not currently known. However, there is good evidence now, as discussed below, that TRH can directly activate TSH β chain gene transcription.

MECHANISM OF ACTIONS OF TRH

Stimulation of TSH secretion and synthesis by TRH is initiated by TRH binding to a specific, high-affinity plasma membrane receptor on the thyrotroph cell. This receptor protein is a 393-amino acid protein that exhibits a seven-transmembrane spanning region, the major feature of other guanine-nucleotide–binding protein–coupled receptors.[24] After TRH binding, TRH activates its biochemical actions by stimulating the rapid hydrolysis of phosphatidylinositol via phospholipase C, which leads to the formation of inositol 1,4,5 triphosphate, an elevation of cytosolic free calcium, and 1,2-diacylglycerol, a protein kinase C agonist.[25] TRH signal transduction involves not only protein kinase C stimulation, but also activation of protein kinase A via cAMP formation.[26] Murine TRH-R gene transcription can be down-regulated by TRH; by phorbol myristate acetate, a stimulator of protein kinase C; and also by epidermal growth factor (EGF), which causes a 60 per cent reduction in the amount of binding of ^{3}H-CH$_3$-TRH to specific TRH receptors.[27] Subsequent events in TRH-catalyzed stimulus-secretion coupling likely involve the phosphorylation of critical protein kinase systems necessary for the TSH exocytotic process.

PITUITARY THYROTROPIN (TSH)

Pituitary TSH is a glycoprotein hormone with a molecular weight of approximately 28,000 kDa formed from two noncovalently linked subunit chains, α and β. The α chain is common to the other three glycoprotein hormones—luteinizing hormone (LH), follicle-stimulating hormone (FSH), and chorionic gonadotropin (CG). The β subunit in each hormone confers the unique biological activity and binding properties of each glycoprotein hormone molecule. TSH is 200 times larger than T_4 and T_3, whose secretion and synthesis TSH regulates. The human α and β apoprotein chains have 92 and 112 amino acids, respectively. During post-translational processing, TSH acquires three complex oligosaccharide chains, two on the α chain and one on the β chain, which are N-linked via asparagine. The oligosaccharide antennae of these units contain mannose, galactose, fucose, N-acetylglucosamine, and N-acetylgalactosamine moieties. Each carbohydrate chain is capped terminally with either a sulfate or sialic acid moiety. These complex carbohydrate additions have important implications for the formation, metabolic clearance rate, and biological activity of TSH (see under Post-translational Glycosylation of the TSH Apoprotein Chains).

TSH BIOSYNTHESIS

Genes located on separate chromosomes encode the TSH subunit chains. The TSH α chain gene is located on chromosome 6 and the TSH β chain gene is on chromosome 1.[28] The human α chain gene of 9.4 kb has four exons, three introns, and a single transcription start site.[29] The TSH β chain gene has three exons separated by two introns. The first exon encodes 37 untranslated bases, the second exon encodes the leader peptide and the initial 34 amino acids of the N-terminal end of the TSH β chain, and the third exon codes for the remaining amino acids and the 3′ untranslated sequence. The human TSH β subunit gene contains only one transcriptional start site, in contrast to two such sites in rats and mice. A puzzling feature of the human β-subunit gene is that it encodes a 118-amino acid chain, whereas human TSH, after chemical extraction and purification of cadaveric pituitary gland extracts, contains only 112 amino acids. The chemically prepared TSH forms may have been cleaved by proteolytic enzymes during purification and may not represent physiological circulating TSH. TSH preparations containing either 112 or 118 residues generated by recombinant techniques, however, show comparable biological activity in vitro.[30] The potential significance of this discrepancy between the predicted β-subunit protein size and the smaller purified subunit remains unclear.

REGULATION OF TSH BIOSYNTHESIS

Thyroid hormone (predominantly as intrapituitary T_3) has been established to be the major inhibitory regulator of TSH. As indicated earlier, however, there is abundant evidence now that thyroid hormones antagonize also the hypothalamic synthesis and secretion of TRH.[12] Thyroid hormones can suppress the transcription of both the β and α subunits. The TSH β subunit mRNA, however, is suppressed faster and more completely than the α subunit mRNA.[28] Such inhibition has been shown by nuclear run-on assays by Shupnick and colleagues to be due to T_3 actions at the level of gene transcription.[31] Two sequences of particular interest in the TSH β chain are thought to be involved as TRE's, to which thyroid hormone–receptor proteins (c-erbAα₁, c-erbAβ₁, c-erbAβ₂) can attach. These two TRE's in the human TSH β gene have been localized to +3 to +37 bp in the first exon.[32] The more upstream TRE is located between +2 and +15 bp of exon 1, and the second half-site between +30 and +37 bp. Of interest is that within these sequences bp +3 to +7 and +31 to +36 share homology with the TRE consensus sequence proposed by Brent et al.: AGGTC/AA.[33] Because these half-sites are distal to the initiation site of gene transcription, transcriptional inhibition by thyroid hormones may involve interference with initiation complex formation. Although the predominant effect of thyroid hormones upon TSH is inhibitory, it has been demonstrated in vivo that TSH concentrations in human peripheral blood may increase during early T_3 treatment, reflecting positive stimulation of pituitary protein synthesis prior to development of specific inhibitory effects on TSH synthesis.[34]

The major stimulator of TSH biosynthesis is TRH, which exerts direct transcription effects upon 5' flanking elements between −128 to +8 bp in the TSH β chain gene. Elegant deletion analysis studies have defined two discreet TRH-responsive regions at −128 to −92 bp and −28 to +8 bp.[35] Each sequence can mediate a twofold enhancement of transcription by TRH. The upstream site contains a DNA sequence with high homology to the DNA-binding site for the pituitary-specific transcriptional factor, Pit-1/GHF-1. Moreover, DNAase 1 footprinting analyses, using mouse thyrotropin tumor extracts or an expression vector for N-terminally deleted Pit-1/GHF-1 cDNA, indicate that either Pit-1 or a related protein mediates TRH responsiveness of the TSH β chain gene. Moreover, the more downstream cis sequence overlaps the thyroid hormone inhibitory elements, suggesting that the TRH stimulatory element and the TRE may interact in TSH β chain regulation.

In addition to thyroid hormones, three classes of steroid hormones can exert minor effects upon TSH gene transcription post-transcriptional events: glucocorticoids, estrogens (E_2), and testosterone.[35] Although the effects of glucocorticoids have been studied by several groups, uncertainty remains concerning the direction of glucocorticoid regulatory influences. Moreover, dexamethasone actions on TSH formation may be mediated at the translational stage of TSH biosynthesis because dexamethasone reduces TSH synthesis without significantly reducing TSH-subunit mRNA concentrations in experimental animals.[36] With regard to estrogens, E_2 can amplify inhibitory effects of T_3, implying their inhibitory role upon TSH β gene transcription.[28] Similarly, because testosterone can blunt the rise in TSH β and α subunit mRNA's in hypothyroidism, an inhibitory role in transcriptional regulation has been assigned to testosterone.[37] In other studies, however, testosterone has been shown to increase TSH β mRNA in pituitaries of both castrated male animals and hypothyroid

murine hosts bearing pituitary TSH-secreting tumors (TtT97).[38]

Other modulators of TSH gene transcription include cAMP and dopamine. TSH β gene stimulation of transcription by cAMP depends upon cis sequences situated between −128 to −28 bp of the 5' flanking region.[39] These sequences, surprisingly, do not share homology with elements recognizing the CREB protein. Dopamine also is known to inhibit basal concentrations of TSH and to inhibit TRH-mediated TSH secretion in humans,[40] and dopamine antagonists increase TSH concentrations in primary hypothyroidism.[41] Dopamine is thought to lower TSH β chain gene transcription by decreasing intracellular cAMP concentrations, which pre-empt cAMP activation of TSH subunit transcription. Somatostatin plays only a minor inhibitory role in TSH β chain transcription.

POST-TRANSLATIONAL GLYCOSYLATION OF THE TSH APOPROTEIN CHAINS

An important characteristic of TSH is its high carbohydrate content, and the TSH α and β chains have 21 and 12 per cent carbohydrate by weight, respectively. The first event in the post-translational addition of carbohydrate to the two TSH apoprotein chains is the addition of high-mannose oligosaccharides, which contain three glucose, nine mannose, and two N-acetylglucosamine residues (Glc_3 Man_9 $GlcNAc_2$). These carbohydrates are preassembled in the endoplasmic reticulum and are linked by phosphates to a compound with 20 polypyrene units.[28] Two high-mannose chains are added to the TSH α-subunit and one is joined to the β-subunit, where these oligosaccharides are covalently bound to asparagine residues in the sequence asparagine-x-serine or asparagine-x-threonine (where x is any amino acid). The function of these initial high-mannose forms is thought to be facilitation of appropriate disulfide bond formation and shaping of the tertiary structure of TSH because inhibition of mannose incorporation by tunacamycin results in proteolysis of unglycosylated α and β chains and an absence of normal TSH heterodimer formation.[42, 43] The pathway for the biogenesis of such sulfated and sialylated Asn-linked oligosaccharides is schematized in Figure 38–4. These initial oligosaccharide forms are modified rapidly. Two glucose residues are removed, followed by slower cleavage of the third glucose residue and progressive deletion of the mannose residues, leaving a core oligosaccharide of three mannose residues. This structure is then extended by two Glc NAc, and either galactose itself or Gal NAc, to create the final complex oligosaccharide chains, fucosylated on the most inner Glc NAc moiety which is capped with either sialic acid or sulfate. The composition of the final complex oligosaccharides in human TSH indicates a unique pattern: 18 per cent contain two sulfate residues, 25 per cent have one sulfate, 21 per cent have both one sulfate and one sialic acid residue, 12 per cent have two sialic acids, and 5 per cent have one sialic acid.[44, 45] These varied glycosylated TSH forms are probably responsible for the observed heterogeneity of TSH molecules during isoelectric focusing.

The potential function(s) of these complex and TSH-specific oligosaccharides involve both the bioactivity and metabolic clearance of TSH. That oligosaccharide units

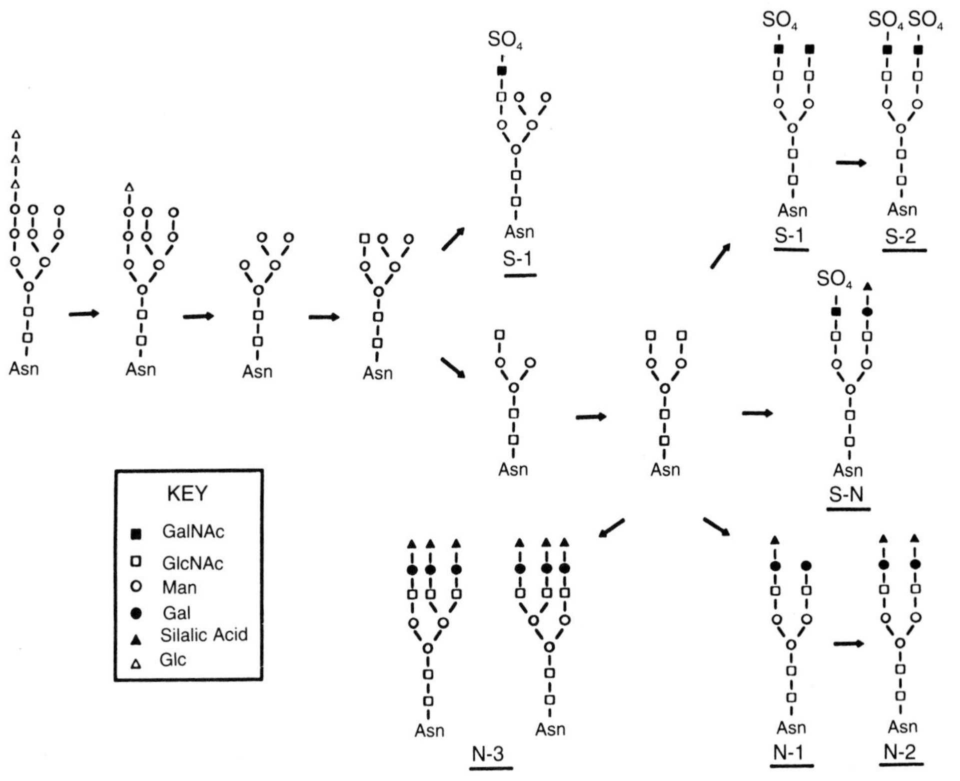

FIGURE 38-4. **Pathway for biosynthesis of sulfated and sialylated Asn-linked oligosaccharides.** Asn residues are glycosylated with high mannose units that contain three glucose residues. Two glucose residues are then rapidly trimmed, followed by removal of the final glucose and then several mannose residues; *N*-acetylglucosamine residues are then added to the three core mannoses. A key branch point is the addition of Gal versus GalNAc residues; Gal residues may then have sialic acid attached, whereas GalNAc residues may become sulfated. S-1, S-2, and S-3 refer to the number of sulfates, and N-1, N-2, and N-3 refer to the number of sialic acid residues present. S-N refers to an oligosaccharide in which one antenna is capped with sulfate and the other with sialic acid. (From Wondisford FE, Magner JA, Weintraub BD: Chemistry and biosynthesis of thyrotropin. *In* Braverman LE, Utiger RD (eds): The Thyroid. New York, Elsevier, 1991, p 268.)

KEY

- ■ GalNAc
- □ GlcNAc
- ○ Man
- ● Gal
- ▲ Silalic Acid
- △ Glc

contribute to the intrinsic biological activity of the TSH molecule has been shown by enzymatic cleavage studies. After incubation with the enzyme endoglycosidase F, bovine TSH exhibits markedly reduced bioactivity of the order of five- to ten-fold after deglycosylation.[46] The role of TRH in modulating TSH bioactivity via glycosylation in man is illustrated by the observations of Faglia et al.,[47] and Beck-Peccoz et al.,[48] which demonstrate that patients with tertiary (TRH-deficiency type) hypothyroidism have circulating TSH forms with a decreased biological or receptor-binding activity/immunological activity ratio. These differences, moreover, can be largely restored with either acute or chronic TRH administration. The reciprocal phenomenon of increased biological/immunological activity ratios has been reported in thyrotoxic individuals with TSH-producing tumors, and normal TSH bioactivity is restored following pituitary adenomectomy.[49]

The second and perhaps more important role of TSH oligosaccharides is their contribution to the metabolic clearance of human TSH.[50] Human TSH is cleared predominantly by the kidney experimentally, with less hepatic and virtually no thyroidal clearance.[51] The clearance of TSH is greatly accelerated by deglycosylation of TSH.[52]

The concept that the oligosaccharides of glycoprotein hormones from the pituitary or other sources have a role in determining clearance has been postulated previously. New data now indicate that glycoprotein hormones, like LH and TSH, with the terminal $SO_4GalNAc$ signal, can be rapidly cleared by a specific receptor on nonparenchymal liver cells described recently by Fiete et al.[53] This type of receptor recognizes the oligosaccharide structure $SO_4$4GalNAc4GlcNAc2Man α and is distinct from that which mediates the biological activity of TSH. This new type of receptor could provide a mechanism for generating a short burst of circulating hormone, as opposed to a sus-

tained unregulated secretory process. Moreover, no hormone processing would be required initially to expose these clearance signals, because TSH is synthesized with its signals fully exposed.

The process of TSH glycosylation is regulated during neonatal development.[54] It has been observed in developing rodents that the sialylated forms are increased relative to sulfated oligosaccharides, with an increment in oligosaccharide forms that have three or more negatively charged terminal moieties. These developmental events, thought to be mediated by TRH, have implications for TSH physiology during the neonatal period. Studies in vitro have demonstrated that TRH can augment the quantity of biantennary compared with triantennary TSH oligosaccharides.[55] The importance of these TRH-regulated changes in oligosaccharide structure has been underscored in the studies of Taylor et al.[56-59] Animals with selective lesions of the hypothalamic PVN to produce experimental TRH deficiency were investigated, and such TRH-deficient animals were found to have TSH forms characterized by diminished biantennary structures compared with normals. In contrast, when animals are rendered experimentally hypothyroid by thyroidectomy, circulating TSH has more biantennary structures, and TRH administration to animals with hypothalamic hypothyroidism also causes an increase in multiantennary structures. This enhancement of complex antennary structures results in a slower clearance rate of plasma TSH in human primary hypothyroidism, where the TSH $T_{1/2}$ of disappearance is approximately 80 min, compared with 60 min in euthyroid subjects. The glycosylation process may be modified also by factors other than TRH, as illustrated by one aggressive, autonomous pituitary adenoma that had more multiantennary oligosaccharide chains than those from a less active pituitary adenoma.[60]

AUTOREGULATION OF THYROID FUNCTION

The thyroid gland has the unique capacity also to alter its synthesis and secretion of thyroid hormones independently of TSH through autoregulatory processes, and the most important autoregulatory system involves iodide.[61] In the presence of iodine deficiency, the thyroid gland can increase its iodide uptake and also the ratio of monoiodotyrosine (MIT) to diiodotyrosine (DIT) in thyroglobulin. This ratio favors the preferential synthesis of T_3 vis-à-vis T_4, optimizing metabolic effects in the context of a limited iodide supply. In addition, iodine deficiency can activate glucose oxidation or thyrocytes independently of TSH.[62] When iodine deficiency is sufficiently severe that circulating thyroid hormone concentrations remain below normal despite autoregulatory compensation, serum TSH then rises in response to reduced free T_4 concentrations to stimulate further thyroidal iodine uptake, thyroid hormonogenesis with preferential T_3 secretion, and thyroid cell growth. The characteristic preferential production of T_3 in iodide deficiency tends to maintain euthyroidism at the expense of thyromegaly.

Excess iodide, conversely, has the capacity to inhibit thyroid organification, a process termed the Wolff-Chaikoff effect[63] (Fig. 38–5). Although the mechanism of this effect has not been completely elucidated, it depends on the generation of a sufficiently high concentration of intrathyroidal iodide such that the reactive form of iodide generated by oxidizing processes can react with additional iodide to produce an iodide species relatively inefficient in iodinating thyroglobulin tyrosine residues. The degree of inhibition of iodide organification is not a simple linear function of progressive quantities of iodide ion. When iodide is administered acutely, small to moderate amounts of iodide do not result in any alteration in thyroid uptake. However, when progressively larger doses of iodide are given acutely, there is initially a progressive increase in organification followed by decreasing organification as the result of the Wolff-Chaikoff effect. Qualitative changes, as well as quantitative ones, occur in thyroid hormonogenesis. A smaller amount of organified iodide is incorporated into T_4 and T_3, and a subnormal proportion appears in the form of

DIT, such that MIT becomes the major iodotyrosine. Thus, the Wolff-Chaikoff effect prevents the thyroid gland quantitatively and qualitatively from undergoing the very large increase in thyroid hormonogenesis that would have resulted from excess iodide if autoregulation did not supervene. Susceptibility to the Wolff-Chaikoff effect is increased by stimulation of the thyroid gland by either the thyroid-stimulating immunoglobulin (TSI) of Graves' disease or by TSH itself. Enhanced susceptibility to the Wolff-Chaikoff effect also occurs during treatment with propylthiouracil and in individuals with chronic lymphocytic thyroiditis (Hashimoto's thyroiditis). When iodide is given in excess chronically, partial escape from the inhibition of iodide organification occurs owing to reduced iodide transport. Thus, the resultant intrathyroidal iodide is too low to maintain the Wolff-Chaikoff effect. It has recently been reported that iodolipids may be the mediators of the effects of excess iodide. Krawiec and co-workers have demonstrated that 14-iodo-15-hydroxy-5,8,11, eicosatrienoic acid (I-HO-A) and its omega lactone (IL-W) can mimic the inhibitory actions of excess iodide upon several parameters of thyroid metabolism.[64] The inhibitory effects of I-HO-A and IL-W were quantitatively similar to those of KI upon TSH stimulation of the thyroidal Na^+, K^+-ATPase system. The effects were tissue specific as well because no inhibition was observed in liver or kidney.[64]

In addition to inhibiting thyroid hormone formation, acute pharmacological doses of iodide can inhibit hormone *release*. This has been demonstrated by prelabeling the thyroid with ^{131}I, in conjunction with large quantities of antithyroid drugs to preclude recycling of radioiodine released from the thyroid gland. Under these conditions, iodide administration causes an acute slowing of the rate of ^{131}I disappearance from the thyroid gland. This effect is easily seen in hyperfunctioning thyroid gland but can occur also in the normal thyroid gland when stimulated by TSH. Secretory inhibition of T_4 and T_3 by [127]I is used in the emergency treatment of thyroid storm. The biochemical mechanism(s) responsible for iodide inhibition of thyroid hormone secretion is not known. It is mediated at the level of the thyroid, however, and does not depend on pituitary TSH itself because it can occur in Graves' disease and in autonomously hyperfunctioning thyroid nodules.[65]

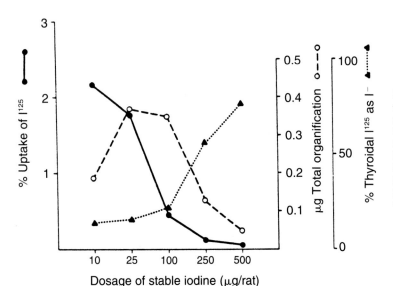

FIGURE 38–5. Wolff-Chaikoff block of thyroid iodine synthesis. Rats were given increasing doses of stable iodide, from 10 to 500 μg, with tracer radioactive [125]I. Per cent iodide uptake is shown in the solid lines, per cent of thyroidal iodine present as free iodide is shown in the dotted line, and total organified iodine is shown in the dashed line. As the dosage of stable iodide increases, there is an augmentation of protein-bound (organified) iodide, but above the level of 100 μg iodide per rat there is a marked inhibition of binding and a progressive decrease in total organic iodine formed. This phenomenon is referred to as the Wolff-Chaikoff block.

A third aspect of thyroid autoregulation by iodide is the capacity of iodide to reverse thyroidal hyperplasia and hypervascularity.[66] This effect is not an invariable consequence of iodide excess. The effect of iodine probably involves thyroid intermediary metabolism, because intrathyroidal iodine can lower glucose oxidation and ^{32}P incorporation into phospholipids stimulated by a variety of agents. These effects of iodide involve ionic transport processes, because preloading of dog thyroid slices with ^{32}P or ^{14}C-glucose prevents such iodide inhibition.[67] Other metabolic sequelae include lowered incorporation of precursors into nucleic acids and diminished amino acid incorporation into protein. Thus, decreased energy metabolism by iodides may restrain those anabolic events required for thyroid cell hyperplasia.

A new aspect of thyroid autoregulation involves the capacity of those hormones (TSH, insulin, insulin-like growth factor [IGF] I) required for thyrocyte growth and function to autoregulate the abundance of TSH receptor (R) mRNA levels in FRTL-5 thyroid cells.[68] In the studies of Saji et al., TSH down-regulated the level its own of receptor mRNA levels via cAMP. These changes are preceded by TSH-dependent reductions in TSH-R pre-mRNA levels (nuclear run-on assays) to the same quantitative degree evidenced by decreased TSH-R mRNA densities in Northern analyses, indicating autoregulation at a transcriptional level.[68]

THE ROLE OF THE AUTONOMIC NERVOUS SYSTEM IN THYROID REGULATION

Adrenergic nerve fibers terminate in the human thyroid on arterioles and thyroid follicles.[69–71] Similar anatomic arrangements are seen in mice, in which stimulation of the cervical sympathetic trunks, after prelabeling with radioiodine, induces the formation of colloid droplets and an increase in radiolabeled thyroid hormone blood levels. Similarly, direct effects of catecholamines on intermediatory metabolism of the mouse thyroid gland have been demonstrated. Such catecholamine effects are mediated through protein kinase A systems with a rise in thyrocyte cAMP.[71] However, in contrast to the effects of TSH, catecholamine stimulation of adenylyl cyclase is inhibited by adrenergic antagonists.

Comparable effects of catecholamines upon thyroid economy in humans are not nearly as well characterized. Thus, no significant changes in thyroid function are seen in individuals given pharmacological doses of adrenergic blocking drugs, although propranolol, in contrast to other adrenergic antagonists, may impair peripheral conversion of T_4 to T_3. Depending on the magnitude and temporal sequence of catecholamine dosage, administration of epinephrine can either increase or decrease radioactive iodine uptake,[71] but thyroid function is usually normal in most patients with pheochromocytomas. Therefore, the autonomic system does not seem to play a major role in human thyroid regulation.

GLUCOCORTICOIDS AND GONADAL STEROIDS

Glucocorticoids have the capacity to inhibit thyroid function at multiple regulatory levels, including inhibition of

TRH synthesis, reduction of TSH secretion, and pituitary responsiveness to TRH.[72] This decreased response to TRH may be important in Cushing's syndrome, and glucocorticoid excess may play a role in the genesis of inappropriately low serum TSH concentrations during acute illness in other stress states. The preferential reduction in serum T_3 by pharmacological quantities of glucocorticoids in normal and thyrotoxic individuals is probably due to inhibition of the hepatic 5' monodeiodinase system because this occurs in hypothyroid patients receiving exogenous thyroxine. The decrease in serum T_3 is accompanied by a reciprocal rise in serum rT_3 concentrations, suggesting inhibition of outer-ring T_4 deiodination. Pharmacological quantities of glucocorticoids may also decrease the concentrations of thyroxine-binding globulin (TBG) and thyroxine-binding prealbumin (TBPA), but these effects do not influence concentrations of free T_4.[73]

The possibility that the thyroid gland is regulated by gonadal steroids as well has been raised by the well-established observation that thyroid disorders of all types are more frequent in women than in men, and by the increased prevalence of goiter in the setting of puberty, pregnancy, and the menopause.[71] Many studies have, therefore, been conducted to assess the possible role of sex steroids in thyroid function. It has been shown, however, that the production, secretion, and peripheral metabolism of thyroid hormones is virtually identical in normal men and women. Moreover, no variation has been found in radioactive iodine uptake during the menstrual cycle. A greater secretory response of TSH to TRH in women than in men, especially in individuals over the age of 40, has been noted.[74] Estrogens, moreover, can augment the TSH response to TRH, probably by increasing the number of TRH receptors in the thyrotroph cell. This enhancement by estrogen and possible reduction of pituitary TSH responsiveness to TRH by androgens probably permit the larger TSH responses to TRH seen in women than in men.

THE EFFECTS OF GROWTH HORMONE UPON THE THYROID FUNCTION IN THYROID GROWTH

The diminished response of TSH secretion to TRH in acromegalic subjects is well known,[75] and the development of secondary (TSH-deficient) hypothyroidism following growth hormone (GH) administration to GH-deficient individuals has been well documented.[76] This has been attributed to augmented secretion of somatostatin, although direct pituitary influences of somatomedins have not been ruled out. Thyroid enlargement, both diffuse and nodular, is observed in about one quarter of acromegalic subjects.[77] These changes are postulated to reflect increased IGF-1 levels.

THYROID FUNCTION AND AGE

The human thyroid gland begins to synthesize and secrete thyroid hormones at about the 12th week of intrauterine life.[73] Prior to that time, fetal tissues derive their thyroid hormone exclusively from the maternal circulation.[77] Maternal thyroid hormone access to the fetal circulation is limited after the first trimester, however, because of the high activity of placental deiodinases. It is clear that T_4 and T_3 can cross the placenta to some extent, however, because athyeotic infants have concentrations of circulating thyroid hormones nearly half the maternal level. Fetal TSH concentrations are below normal at the 12th week of gestation and increase rapidly between weeks 18 to 20, suggesting enhanced pituitary TRH stimulation at that time.[79] The fetal thyroid is regulated in utero, as reflected by elevated TSH concentrations in amniotic fluid of congenitally hypothyroid fetuses. Moreover, maternal T_4 administration 24 hours prior to delivery reduces cord TSH levels and inhibits the normal acute postnatal elevation of TSH.[80, 81] Between 18 weeks and term, TBG concentrations rise gradually to values slightly higher than in the adult at term.[82] Circulating T_4 concentrations rise disproportionately to these increments in TBG concentration without parallel rises in TSH, implying increased fetal thyroid sensitivity to prevailing TSH. Moreover, fetal thyroid function is preserved in anencephalic infants, suggesting that the fetal thyroid is not completely dependent upon hypothalamic-pituitary regulation prior to delivery.[83] Serum T_3 concentrations become detectable later than T_4, at about 30 weeks, and increase to concentrations at term slightly lower than those seen in the adult.[84] At delivery, both fetal TSH and T_4 are slightly higher than the corresponding maternal values, whereas T_3 is below normal with a reciprocally elevated rT_3, indicating low Type I deiodinase activity in the newborn. During the first 24 hours of life, serum TSH concentrations rise rapidly to peak at about 30 minutes after birth, returning toward normal at 48 hours. This acute activation of TSH secretion at birth is thought to be due in part to the ambient cooling that follows exposure to the extrauterine milieu.[84] TSH stimulates the secretion of both T_4 and T_3, which rise into the hyperthyroid range by 24 hours of life, to return toward adult levels gradually after day 10. The rapid rises in T_3 are due primarily to extrathyroidal conversion of T_4 to T_3.[85, 86] Thyroid hormone production rates are higher in children than in adults, and higher dosages of thyroid hormone are required, therefore, in the therapy for congenital hypothyroidism.[87] When expressed per unit body weight, the T_4 requirement is approximately 10 μg/kg in the newborn, compared with 1.6 μg/kg in adults. In adulthood, thyroid hormone dosage requirements remain constant, except for the increased thyroxine needed during pregnancy and a reduction in requirement for T_4 replacement by 10 to 20 per cent in the seventh and eighth decades in men.[71]

The function of fetally derived thyroid hormones during ontogeny is not entirely clear. In the total absence of fetal thyroid function, there are minimal alterations in in utero fetal growth, and the athyreotic fetus is typically without hypothyroid signs and is detected only by thyroid function testing.[86] This, of course, may be due to the protective effect of maternally derived hormones. On the other hand, neonates with severe hypothyroidism secondary to maternal iodide deficiency are larger at birth, with signs of fetal immaturity, jaundice, and retarded bone age. It has been speculated that fetal CNS maturation may be abnormal, but this has not been rigorously established except for impaired otic development in experimental animals.[88] In contrast to endemic cretinism, the athyreotic infant born to a euthyroid mother does not exhibit neurological abnormalities characteristic of cretinism, so that T_4 contributions

from the normal maternal plasma seem to protect the fetus to a considerable extent from profound hypothyroidism. It is also probable that the brain is partially protected by highly active iodothyronine deiodinase so that the low amount of T_4 available is fully converted to T_3.

After year one of life the neonatal elevated T_4 values approach the normal adult range, whereas serum T_3 concentrations remain higher through early adolescence.

Two features of alterations in thyroid function with later age are the reductions in T_4 turnover rate in individuals over 65 and the reduced or absent TSH response to TRH in elderly individuals, primarily men.[89] Serum concentrations of T_3 and its turnover are also reduced in some elderly men, but these changes may be related to underlying illnesses with the euthyroid sick syndrome. In elderly subjects, both free T_4 and free T_3 concentrations tend to be at the lower end of normal or below normal values for younger individuals. The radioactive iodine uptake also decreases slightly with age owing to both lower T_4 clearance and decreased renal iodide clearance.[89]

NONTHYROIDAL ILLNESS

A variety of alterations in thyroid function occur in nonthyroidal illnesses (NTI), and these changes can make the interpretation of thyroid status quite difficult.[90, 91] The most common abnormalities include a decrease in the circulating concentrations of T_3, accompanied by a reciprocal rise in rT_3, the so-called low-T_3 syndrome. These changes are identical to those seen during experimental caloric restriction and are presumed to be due to a coordinate reduction in the $5'$ monodeiodination of T_4 and reverse T_3. This low-T_3 state can occur in a variety of illnesses, including infectious diseases, uremia, starvation, acute myocardial infarction, acute febrile illnesses, and uncontrolled diabetes, including diabetic ketoacidosis. Similar changes also occur following surgery. There is a quantitative relationship between the degree of severity of the illness and the magnitude of the T_3 reductions. The low T_3 syndrome is easily distinguished from true primary hypothyroidism because TSH concentrations are not elevated and serum T_4 concentrations are not reduced.

In the context of more severe illness, thyroid function can be characterized by a reduction of T_4 as well as a reduction in T_3 concentrations. Whereas a small reduction in total T_4 is commonly noted as well in the low T_3 syndrome, due to reductions in TBG or TBPA-binding capacity, more severely ill patients have an authentic fall in T_4 out of proportion to the reductions in serum T_4-binding capacity. Interpretation of these findings is complicated because such individuals are often receiving glucocorticoids and dopamine, which can affect thyroxine production. Reductions in T_4 to 30 to 50 nM (2 to 4 μg/dl) can occur. Such patients have a poor prognosis for recovery from the acute illness process. In these patients the lack of appropriate elevations in TSH in response to reduced free T_3 and free T_4 levels are due to unidentified inhibitory factors, although to some extent this may represent TSH depression by dopamine or glucocorticoids. NTI is difficult to distinguish from hypothalamic or pituitary hypothyroidism that may occur in such settings as bone marrow transplantation.[92] In two excellent but limited studies in which either T_4 or T_3 was administered therapeutically, there was no amelioration or worsening of the underlying condition.[93, 94] Free T_4 concentrations decline approximately 10 to 40 per cent, as quantified by ultrafiltration. Analogue methods, by contrast, give reductions of less than 30 per cent. The normal to slightly below normal concentrations of TSH seen in hospitalized patients without primary hypothyroidism become elevated above the normal range during recovery from the NTI syndrome.[71] Thus, an unidentified suppressor of hypothalamic-pituitary function disappears during recovery, allowing the system to respond in an appropriate, adaptive manner. These postrecovery, elevated TSH concentrations often persist until circulating free T_4 and free T_3 concentrations are normalized.

The pathophysiology of the low free T_4 concentrations in those individuals with systemic illness with suppression of the pituitary thyroid axis is not entirely clear. Some reductions in T_4 may be due to circulating fatty acid inhibitors of T_4 and T_3 binding to thyroid hormone–binding proteins.[71] Several additional mechanisms have been proposed to account for the altered thyroid function tests as seen in the euthyroid sick syndrome. First, it has been demonstrated in a dog model that glucagon infusion can induce a decline in T_3 and a reciprocal rise in rT_3.[95] Because the elevation in levels of stress hormones that occur during anesthesia do not occur during a conscious resting state, it is postulated that hyperglucagonemia may be a contributor of thyroid hormone alterations observed in several euthyroid sick states associated with stress.[95] Chopra and co-workers[96] have studied the serum concentrations of immunoassayable tumor necrosis factor-α (TNF-α) and iodothyronines (T_4, T_3, and rT_3) in normal subjects and patients with NTI's (n = 13). The slight elevation of TNF-α in NTI patients of 84 ± 38 fmol/ml, compared with normals of 45, 54 in hyperthyroidism, and 50 in hypothyroidism, did not reach statistical significance. However, free T_4 concentrations correlated positively with NTI TNF-α concentrations, a feature of a rarer variant of this syndrome (see below).[97] In a related study, Van Der Poll et al. examined the potential role of TNF-α by administration of human recombinant TNF (50 µg/m²) to five healthy males.[98] During the 10.5-hour study, TNF-α produced changes in circulating thyroid hormones characteristic of the euthyroid sick syndrome. Compared with saline-receiving controls, TNF-α was capable of inducing significant decreases in T_3 (−36 ± 2 per cent) and TSH levels (−68 ± 3 per cent) and a significant increase in rT_3 values (+48 ± 11 per cent versus saline of −12 ± 7 per cent; $P < 0.05$). Free T_4 did not become elevated statistically in this study. Recently another feature has been described involving impaired nocturnal elevations in TSH in NTI patients. This feature has been explored in 26 NTI patients, and a nocturnal surge was present in only 11, compared with 100 per cent of the control subjects. The absence of the TSH nocturnal surge is not related to ambient T_4, T_3, or TSH concentrations, or pituitary TSH responsiveness to TRH, suggesting that a dysregulation in hypothalamic TRH secretion may be operative in this setting.[99]

A rarer variant of NTI includes patients in whom serum T_3 is subnormal but serum T_4 concentration is increased transiently during illness.[71] These patients are characterized by an elevation free T_4 and free T_4 index and a reduction in free T_3 index. This thyroid function pattern has been identified in hyperemesis gravidarum and in some patients with acute psychoses, in whom the serum T_3 levels may also be elevated. These subjects are difficult to differentiate from those with authentic thyrotoxicosis with elevations in T_4 only, or with Graves' disease complicated by serious illness in which there may occur a selective T_4 elevation. Patients, however, who are not truly hyperthyroid exhibit T_3 concentrations of the order of 50 to 80 ng/dl, in contrast to the preferentially elevated values of T_3 in most thyrotoxic states.[71]

REGULATION OF THE MATERNAL THYROID GLAND DURING PREGNANCY

Changes in the maternal hormonal milieu during pregnancy result in important alterations in thyroid function.[98] First, an elevation in T_4-binding globulin (TBG) concentration is induced by the increased gestational production of estrogen. Secondly, a reduction in circulating iodide occurs, resulting from a smaller iodine pool and an increase in the renal clearance of iodine. Because radioactive iodine uptake depends on the size of the ^{125}I pool in addition to TSH activity, thyroid radioactive uptake is elevated in pregnancy, although it is not measured because of isotope contraindications during pregnancy.

An interesting recent observation is that human chorionic gonadotropin (hCG) plays a physiological role in pregnancy as an ancillary thyroid-stimulating hormone, as shown in a prospective study of 606 healthy mildly iodine deficient women by Glinoer and colleagues.[99] This study addressed changes in maternal thyroid economy, and four major observations emerged. First, when thyroid hormone concentrations are adjusted for the marked increase in TBG-binding capacity, free T_4 and T_3 levels are actually lower than during the prepartum period, although in most cases free hormone levels remain within the normal range. In approximately one third of the women, however, there was relative hypothyroxinemia with higher T_3/T_4 ratios, indicative of preferential T_3 secretion. A second feature was that high levels of hCG were associated with thyroid stimulation, both functionally, in association with lower serum TSH concentrations, and anatomically, by an increase in thyroid size (Fig. 38–6). There was also a significant elevation in thyroglobulin concentrations throughout gestation, most marked in the third trimester. Finally, there was an increase in goiter formation, identified in 9 per cent of women at parturition.

These new data indicate that pregnancy in an area of mild iodine deficiency is accompanied by an overall TBG desaturation with lower free T_4 and free T_3 levels, 30 per cent of which are below the lower limit of normal. Moreover, thyrotropic regulation of the maternal thyroid is complex because both elevated hCG primarily in the first half of gestation and increasing TSH in the second half of gestation participate in thyroid stimulation. These findings of Glinoer become particularly relevant in environments of marginally low iodine intake, because pregnancy constitutes a goitrogenic stimulus. The implications of these findings made in Belgium, for an American cohort, remain uncertain at the present time. Studies are needed, moreover, to confirm the reversibility of these features during the postpartum period, because if they were to be repeated during subsequent pregnancies, these data would provide

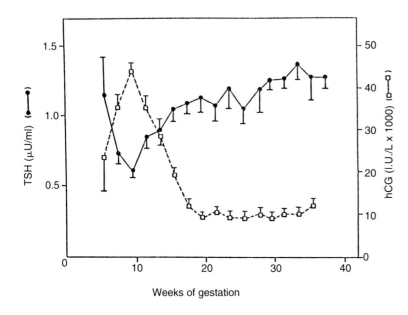

FIGURE 38–6. **Serum TSH and hCG as a function of gestational age.** Serum hCG was determined at initial evaluation, and TSH at initial evaluation and during late gestation. The symbols give the mean value ($\pm$ SE) for samples pooled for two weeks of gestation. Each point corresponds to the average of 33 determinations for hCG and 49 for TSH. (From Glinoer D, DeNayer P, Bourdoux P, et al: Regulation of maternal thyroid during pregnancy. J Clin Endocrinol Metab 71:282, 1990. © The Endocrine Society.)

insight into the higher prevalence of thyroid disorders in women than in men.

EFFECTS OF PHYSICAL FACTORS UPON THYROID REGULATION

Stress

Acute stress has been reported previously to raise thyroid hormone levels in experimental animals. Transient elevations of thyroid hormones have been noted in patients with acute psychiatric illnesses (see above under Nonthyroidal Illness). More recently, it has become clear that thyroid hormone concentrations may decline during intense physical exercise. The effects of a one-week, extremely intense, strength-training period on maximal muscle strength and pituitary-thyroid regulation were investigated in eight male weight lifters.[100] These investigators found that decreased concentrations of TSH, T_4, and T_3 occurred during the training period. However, there were no statistically significant changes that occurred in free T_4, reverse T_3, or TBG concentrations. The authors concluded that intense physical training may lead to a conditioned reduction in TRH secretion with secondary reductions in the pituitary TSH secretion. Similar changes of pituitary and thyroid function have also been described after cardiopulmonary bypass surgery, in which serum concentrations of free T_3, free T_4, and TSH decrease after open-heart surgery, with recovery of TSH and free T_4 on the second to third postoperative day.[101] These changes are characteristic of the severe NTI syndrome. The response of the pituitary to TRH testing was progressively impaired in relation to the duration of the bypass procedure.[102] Recently, it has been found that in severely injured patients there is an inverse relationship between concentrations of circulating norepinephrine and depressed T_3 levels.[102] Moreover, this relationship disappears in the absence of intact CNS systems as a result of head injury or barbiturate intoxication.

Cold Exposure

Acute and chronic cold exposure in experimental animals leads to pituitary-thyroid activation and thyroid hyperplasia secondary to increased TSH stimulation. This response depends, in turn, on an α-adrenergic stimulation of TRH release.[103] Until recently augmented thyroid activity by environmental cold has been seen only during infancy or in young children subjected to hypothermic cardiovascular surgery.[104] The effects of cold exposure on serum free T_4, free T_3, TSH, and TBG have now been investigated in 82 euthyroid factory workers by Solter et al.[105] Twenty-five workers were exposed intermittently for 3.5 hours daily to extreme cold ($-20°$ to $-40°C$) (Group I) and 47 were exposed to moderate cold ($8°$ to $-10°C$) for the entire eight-hour period (Group II). After cold exposure, serum total T_4, but not free T_4, decreased only in Group I, exposed to the lower temperatures. Serum total T_3 and reverse T_3 decreased significantly in both groups, but free T_3 did not decline in either group. Thus, cold exposure may have opposite effects upon total thyroid hormones and free fractions, consistent with cold-induced alterations of serum thyroid hormone–binding capacities. These results raise the possibility that decreased thyroid hormone–binding capacity is an adaptive response to cold exposure, effecting a new higher equilibrium between extracellular and intracellular free T_4 and T_3.

Hypoxia

Thyroid hormone regulation is known to be affected by high altitude, which causes an elevation of plasma T_4 and T_3, accelerated T_4 turnover, and elevations in serum TSH and its response to TRH.[71]

Recently Drucker et al. have investigated circulating levels of thyroid hormones and TSH, as well as TSH response to TRH, in healthy euthyroid residents at sea level, compared with those exposed either acutely (3 weeks) or chronically (3 months to 10 years) to a high altitude of 3500 meters.[106] High altitude natives and euthyroid men were also examined during intermittent exposure to a simulated 3500-meter altitude in a hypobaric oxygen chamber. It was found that hypoxic stress, either natural or simulated, caused a marked elevation in plasma T_4 and T_3 within four hours that was maintained through the entire exposure period. There was no change in TBG or TPBA-binding capacities. Serum T_4 and T_3 returned to sea level values when the transient or chronically adapted high altitude individuals were returned to sea level environmental conditions.

It has been observed that in premature hypothyroid infants, the degree of severity of hypothyroidism is adversely influenced by hypoxia as well as gestational age.[107]

ANTITHYROID DRUGS AND FOODSTUFFS

A number of pharmacological agents, including most importantly those used for the treatment of hyperthyroidism, can lead to inhibition of thyroid hormone transport, hormonogenesis, or release, resulting in a rise in circulating TSH and the induction of goiter[108] (Fig. 38–7). Hence, these drugs and other chemical compounds considered in this section are called goitrogens. Goitrogens fall into two main categories: (1) those that inhibit organification and/or coupling of iodine in thyroglobulin and (2) monovalent cations that inhibit the transport of iodide from blood into the thyroid follicle. Two members of this group, thiocyanate and perchlorate, have been used in the treatment of hyperthyroidism but are no longer used routinely because of toxicity.[71] An additional drawback is that they depend on plasma iodide concentrations, and therefore in the presence of iodine abundance their efficacy is preempted.

The inhibitors of organification fall into three classes. The thionamides, exemplified by propylthiouracil and methimazole, are the mainstay of therapy for hyperthyroidism, particularly Graves' disease.[106] In contrast to the ion transport inhibitors, these compounds are affected minimally by iodide abundance. The aminoheterocyclic goitrogenic compounds include tolbutamide, carbutamide, and the sulfonamides. Sulfonamides have not been shown to cause goiter in humans, and their potency, in contrast to that of the hypoglycemic agents, is enhanced by increased thyroidal iodide.

The third group are the substituted phenols, exemplified by resorcinol, a skin antiseptic. Closely related compounds are analogues of salicylic acid. Resorcinol has been known to cause goitrous hypothyroidism in humans. A number of other chemical structures possess antithyroid activity, such as phenylbutazone, which both decreases thyroid iodide uptake and causes goitrous hypothyroidism in humans. Antithyroid activity has also been ascribed to ethionamide and 6-mercaptopurine, which both contain thionamide groupings.[106] Goiter, which may be accompanied by hypothyroidism, is sometimes encountered in manic-depressive patients treated with the monovalent cation lithium. Like iodide, lithium inhibits thyroid hormone release. In extremely high concentrations intracellularly lithium can inhibit organification of iodine also. It is not entirely clear what distinguishes individuals who develop goiter during lithium therapy, but it is possible that those

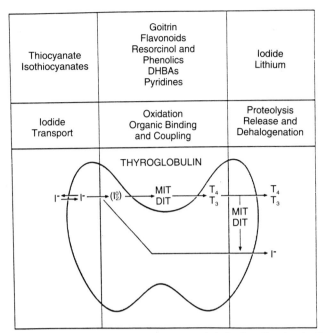

FIGURE 38–7. **Environmental goitrogens and their site of action in the thyroid gland.** Abbreviations: goitrin, L,5-vinyl-2-thiooxazolidone; DHBA's, dihydroxibenzoic acids; I, iodide; MIT, monoiodotyrosine; DIT, diiodotyrosine; T_4, thyroxine; T_3, triiodothyronine. (From Gaitan E: Goitrogens in food and water. Ann Rev Nutr 10:23, 1990. Reproduced, with permission, from the Annual Review of Nutrition, Vol. 10, © 1990 by Annual Reviews Inc.)

more susceptible to lithium's effects have underlying impairment of thyroid reserve due to chronic lymphocytic thyroiditis.[107]

A number of antithyroid chemical agents occur naturally in foodstuffs.[108] The most celebrated of those are in the cruciferous plant family, including cabbages, turnips, rutabaga, kale, and a number of plants used for animal nutrition. One chemical responsible for the goitrogenic effect of these foods is thiocyanate, especially in cabbage leaves. In addition, there are a variety of other progoitrins, in the form of thioglycosides, which become goitrogenic when catalyzed by thioglycosidase or by intestinal bacteria glycosidases.[108] The active goitrogen in turnips is 5-vinyl-2-thiooxazolidone. Thiocyanates have been isolated from other foodstuffs, including cassava meal, a common dietary supplement in many parts of the world. Cassava contains linamarin, which is metabolized to thiocyanate. Cassava consumption is thought to be an important factor in goiter formation in regions of endemic iodine deficiency. Plant goitrogens, except for thiocyanate, act by blocking iodide organification, identically to the action of thionamide goitrogens.

The pathogenic role of dietary goitrogens in human goiter formation is not established, but their effect(s) probably depends in large part on the concomitant intake of environmental iodide. Goitrogenic food consumption is rarely sufficient to cause goiter. Gaitan's group has shown recently that water-borne sulfur-containing goitrogens of mineral origin contribute importantly to the development of endemic goiter in certain parts of the world such as Colombia, South America.[108]

REFERENCES

1. Wilber JF, Yamada M: Thyrotropin-releasing hormone: Current concepts. *In* Greer MA (ed): The Thyroid Gland. New York, Raven Press, 1990, pp 127–145.
2. Wu P: Identification and characterization of JRH-precursor peptides. *In* Jackson IMD, Metcalf J (eds): Thyrotropin Releasing Hormone: Biomedical Significance. New York, Elsevier, 1989, pp 60–70.
3. Scanlon MF, Hall R: Thyroid-stimulating hormone: Synthesis, control of release, and secretion. *In* DeGroot LJ (ed): Endocrinology. Philadelphia, WB Saunders, 1989, pp 337–383.
4. Faglia G, Bitensky L, Pinchera A, et al: Thyrotropin secretion in patients with central hypothyroidism: Evidence for reduced biological activity of immunoreactive thyrotropin. J Clin Endocrinol Metab 48:989–998, 1979.
5. Faglia G, Beck-Peccoz P, Ballabio M, Nava C: Excess of β-subunit of thyrotropin (TSH) in patients with idiopathic central hypothyroidism due to the secretion of TSH with reduced biological activity. J Clin Endocrinol Metab 56:908–914, 1983.
6. Richter K, Kawashima E, Egger R, Kriel G: Biosynthesis of thyrotropin releasing hormone in the skin of *Xenopus laevis:* Partial sequence of the precursor deduced from cloned cDNA. EMBO J 3:617–621, 1984.
7. Lechan RM, Wu P, Jackson IMD, et al: Thyrotropin-releasing hormone precursor: Characterization in rat brain. Science 231:159–161, 1986.
8. Lee SL, Stewart K, Goodman RH: Structure of the gene encoding rat thyrotropin releasing hormone. J Biol Chem 263:16604–16609, 1988.
9. Yamada M, Radovick S, Wondisford FE, et al: Cloning and structure of human genomic DNA and hypothalamic cDNA encoding human prepro thyrotropin-releasing hormone. Mol Endocr 4:551–556, 1990.
10. Yamada M, Wondisford FE, Radovick S, et al: Assignment of human prepro thyrotropin-releasing hormone (TRH) gene to chromosome 3. Somat Cell Mol Genet 17:97–100, 1991.
11. Montoya E, Wilber JF, Lorincz M: Catecholaminergic control of thyrotropin secretion. J Lab Clin Med 93:887–894, 1979.
12. Yamada M, Wilber JF: The human preproTRH (ppTRH) gene: Inhibition of expression in GH$_3$ cells of plasmid chimeric luciferase constructs by L-triiodothyronine (L-T$_3$). *In* Gordon A, Gross J (eds): Progress in Thyroid Research. Rotterdam, A. A. Balkema, 1991, pp 89–94.
13. Yamada M, Wilber JF: Reciprocal regulation of prepro thyrotropin-releasing hormone (TRH) mRNA in the rat anterior hypothalamus by thyroid hormone: Dissociation from TRH concentrations during hypothyroidism. Neuropeptides 15:49–53, 1990.
14. Feng P, Gu J, Kim UJ, et al: Identification, localization, and developmental studies of rat prepro thyrotropin-releasing hormone mRNA and TRH in rat testis. Neuropeptides 24:63–69, 1993.
15. Feng P, Kim U, Yamada M, et al: Rat preproTRH gene expression: Selective alterations by thyroid status in the paraventricular nucleus (PVN) but not in testis—a new extra-CNS locus for ppTRH gene expression. *In* Gordon A, Gross J (eds): Progress in Thyroid Research. Rotterdam, A. A. Balkema, 1991, pp 83–87.
16. Foord SM, Peters JR, Dieguez C, et al: Hypothyroid pituitary cells in cultures: An analysis of TSH and PRL responses to dopamine and dopamine receptor binding. Endocrinology 115:407–415, 1984.
17. Grossman A, Stubbs WA, Gaillard RC, et al: Studies of the opiate control of prolactin, GH and TSH. Clin Endocrinol 14:381–386, 1981.
18. Hooi SC, Maiter DM, Martin JB, Koenig JI: Galaninergic mechanisms are involved in the regulation of corticotropin and thyrotropin secretion in the rat. Endocrinology 127:2281–2289, 1990.
19. Adinoff B, Nemeroff CB, Bissette G, et al: Inverse relationship between CSF TRH concentrations and the TSH response to TRH in abstinent alcohol-dependent patients. Am J Psychiatry 148:1586–1588, 1991.
20. Brabant G, Ocran K, Ranft U, et al: Physiological regulation of thyrotropin. Biochimie 71:293–301, 1989.
21. Wilber JF, Utiger RD: The effect of glucocorticoids on thyrotropin secretion. J Clin Invest 48:2096–2103, 1969.
22. Pagesy P, Croissandeau G, LeDafniet M, et al: Detection of thyrotropin-releasing hormone (TRH) mRNA in the reverse transcription-polymerase chain reaction in the human normal and tumoral anterior pituitary. Biochem Biophys Res Commun 182:182–187, 1992.
23. May V, Wilber JF, U'Prichard DC, Childs GV: Persistence of immunoreactive TRH and GnRH in long-term primary anterior pituitary cultures. Peptides 8:543–558, 1987.
24. Straub RE, Frech GC, Joho RH, Gershengorn MC: Expression cloning of a cDNA encoding the mouse pituitary thyrotropin-releasing hormone receptor. Proc Natl Acad Sci USA 87:9514–9518, 1990.
25. Kolesnick RN: Thyrotropin-releasing hormone and phorbol esters induce phosphatidylcholine synthesis in GH3 pituitary cells. Evidence for stimulation via protein kinase C. J Biol Chem 262:14525–14530, 1987.
26. Paulssen RH, Paulssen EJ, Gautvik KM, Gordeladze JO: The thyroliberin receptor interacts directly with a stimulatory guanine-nucleotide-binding protein in the activation of adenylyl cyclase in GH3 rat pituitary tumor cells. Evidence obtained by the use of antisense RNA inhibition and immunoblocking of the stimulatory guanine-nucleotide-binding protein. Eur J Biochem 204:413–418, 1992.
27. Hinkle PM, Shanshala ED II, Yan ZF: Epidermal growth factor decreases the concentration of thyrotropin-releasing hormone (TRH) receptors and TRH responses in pituitary GH4C1 cells. Endocrinology 129:1283–1288, 1991.
28. Dracopoli NC, Retting WJ, Whitfield GK, et al: Assignment of the gene for the β subunit of thyroid-stimulating hormone to the short arm of human chromosome 1. Proc Natl Acad Sci USA 83:1822–1826, 1986.
29. Wondisford FE, Magner JA, Weintraub BD: Chemistry and biosynthesis of thyrotropin. *In* Braverman LE, Utiger RD (eds): The Thyroid. Philadelphia, JB Lippincott, 1991, pp 257–276.
30. Takata K-I, Watanabe S, Hirono M, et al: The role of the carboxyterminal 6 amino acid extension of human TSH β-subunit. Biochem Biophys Res Commun 165:1035–1042, 1989.
31. Shupnik MA, Greenspan SL, Ridgway EC: Transcriptional regulation of thyrotropin subunit genes by thyrotropin-releasing hormone and dopamine in pituitary cell culture. J Biol Chem 261:12675–12679, 1986.
32. Wondisford FE, Farr EA, Radovick S, et al: Thyroid hormone inhibition of human thyrotropin subunit gene expression is mediated by a *cis*-acting element located in the first exon. J Biol Chem 264:14601–14604, 1989.
33. Brent GA, Harney JW, Chen Y, et al: Mutations of the rat growth hormone promoter which increase and decrease response to thyroid hormone define a consensus thyroid hormone response element. Mol Endocrinol 3:1996–2004, 1989.
34. Ridgway EC, Kourides IA, Chin WW, et al: Augmentation of pituitary thyrotropin response to thyrotropin releasing hormone during subphysiological triiodothyronine therapy in hypothyroidism. Clin Endocrinol 10:343–353, 1979.
35. Sarne DH, DeGroot LJ: Hypothalamic and neuroendocrine regulation of thyroid hormone. *In* DeGroot LJ (ed): Endocrinology. Philadelphia, WB Saunders, 1989, pp 574–589.
36. Ross DS, Ellis MF, Milbury P, Ridgway EC: A comparison of changes in plasma thyrotropin and subunits, and mouse thyrotropic tumor thyrotropin and subunit mRNA concentrations after in vivo dexamethasone of T$_3$ administration. Metabolism 36:799–803, 1987.
37. Franklyn JA, Ahlquist N, Balfour N, et al: Testosterone and effects of thyroid status on pituitary and hepatic messenger (m)RNAs. Program of the 62nd Annual Meeting of the American Thyroid Association, Washington, DC, 1987 (abstract T69).
38. Ross DS: Testosterone increases TSHβ mRNA and modulates α-subunit mRNA differentially in the thyrotrope and the gonadotrope. Program of the 67th Annual Meeting to the Endocrine Society, New Orleans, LA 1988, p 177 (abstract 705).
39. Weintraub BD, Wondisford FE, Farr EA, et al: Pretranslational and post-translational regulation of TSH synthesis in normal and neoplastic thyrotrophs. Horm Res 32:22–24, 1989.
40. Cooper DS, Klibanski A, Ridgway EC: Dopaminergic modulation of TSH and its subunits: In vivo and in vitro studies. Clin Endocrinol (Oxf) 18:265–275, 1983.
41. Scanlon MF, Weightman DR, Shale DJ, et al: Dopamine is a physiological regulator of thyrotropin secretion in man. Clin Endocrinol (Oxf) 10:7–15, 1979.
42. Strickland TW, Pierce JG: The α-subunit of pituitary glycoprotein hormones: Formation of three-dimensional structure during cell-free biosynthesis. J Biol Chem 258:5927–5932, 1983.
43. Weintraub BD, Stannard BS, Meyers L: Glycosylation of thyroid-stimulating hormone in pituitary tumor cells: Influence of high-mannose oligosaccharide units on subunit aggregation, combination and intracellular degradation. Endocrinology 112:1331–1345, 1983.
44. Green ED, Baenziger JU: Asparagine-linked oligosaccharides on lu-

tropin, follitropin, and thyrotropin. I. Structural elucidation of the sulfated and sialylated oligosaccharides on bovine, ovine, and human pituitary glycoprotein hormones. J Biol Chem 263:25–35, 1988.

45. Green ED, Baenzigr JU: Asparagine-linked oligosaccharides on lutropin, follitropin, and thyrotropin. II. Distributions of sulfated and sialylated oligosaccharides on bovine, ovine, and human pituitary glycoprotein hormones. J Biol Chem 263:36–44, 1988.

46. Thotakura NR, LiCalzi L, Weintraub BD: The role of carbohydrate in thyrotropin action assessed by a novel method of enzymatic deglycosylation. J Biol Chem 265:11527–11534, 1990.

47. Faglia G, Bittensky L, Pinchera A, et al: Thyrotropin secretion in patients with central hypothyroidism: Evidence for reduced biological activity of immunoreactive thyrotropin. J Clin Endocrinol Metab 48:989–998, 1979.

48. Beck-Peccoz P, Amr S, Menezes-Ferreira MM, et al: Decreased receptor binding of biologically inactive thyrotropin in central hypothyroidism: Effect of treatment with thyrotropin-releasing hormone. N Engl J Med 312:1085–1090, 1985.

49. Nissim M, Lee KO, Petrick PA, et al: A sensitive thyrotropin (TSH) bioassay based on iodide uptake in rat FRTL-5 thyroid cells: Comparison with the adenosine 3',5''-monophosphate response to human serum TSH and enzymatically deglycosylated bovine and human TSH. Endocrinology 121:1278–1287, 1987.

50. Drickamer K: Clearing up glycoprotein hormones. Cell 67:1029–1032, 1991.

51. Ridgway EC, Singer FR, Weintraub BD, et al: Metabolism of human thyrotropin in the dog. Endocrinology 95:1181–1185, 1974.

52. Constant RB, Weintraub BD: Differences in the metabolic clearance of pituitary and serum thyrotropin (TSH) derived from euthyroid and hypothyroid rats: Effects of chemical deglycosylation of pituitary TSH. Endocrinology 119:2720–2727, 1986.

53. Fiete D, Srivastava V, Hindsgaul O, Baenziger JU: A hepatic reticuloendothelial cell receptor specific for SO₄-4GalNAcβ1, 4GlcNAcβ1, 2Manα that mediates rapid clearance of lutropin. Cell 67:1103–1110, 1991.

54. Ronin C, Stannard BS, Weintraub BD: Differential processing and regulation of thyroid-stimulating hormone subunit carbohydrate chains in thyrotropic tumors and in normal and hypothyroid pituitaries. Biochemistry 24:5626–5631, 1985.

55. Gesundheit N, Fink DL, Silverman LA, Weintraub BD: Effect of thyrotropin-releasing hormone on the carbohydrate structure of secreted mouse thyrotropin: Analysis by lectin affinity chromatography. J Biol Chem 262:5197–5203, 1987.

56. Taylor T, Gesundheit N, Gyves PW, et al: Hypothalamic hypothyroidism caused by lesions in rat paraventricular nuclei alters the carbohydrate structure of secreted thyrotropin. Endocrinology 122:283–290, 1988.

57. Taylor T, Gesundheit N, Weintraub BD: Effects in in vivo bolus versus continuous TRH administration on TSH secretion, biosynthesis, and glycosylation in normal and hypothyroid rats. Mol Cell Endocr 46:253–261, 1986.

58. Taylor T, Weintraub BD: Altered thyrotropin (TSH) carbohydrate structures in hypothalamic hypothyroidism created by paraventricular nuclear lesions are corrected by in vivo TSH-releasing hormone. Endocrinology 125:2198–2203, 1989.

59. Taylor T, Wondisford FE, Blaine T, Weintraub BD: The paraventricular nucleus of the hypothalamus has a major role in thyroid feedback regulation of thyrotropin synthesis and secretion. Endocrinology 126:317–324, 1990.

60. Gesundheit N, Petrick PA, Taylor T, et al: Comparison of a pituitary TSH-secreting micro- versus macroadenoma. In Medeiros-Neto G, Gaitan E (eds): Frontiers in Thyroidology. New York, Plenum Press, 1986, pp 259–265.

61. Silva JF: Effects of iodine and iodine-containing compounds on thyroid function. Med Clin North Am 69:881–898, 1985.

62. Green WL, Ingbar SH: Effects of inorganic iodide on the intermediary carbohydrate metabolism of surviving sheep thyroid slices. J Clin Invest 42:1802–1815, 1963.

63. Hershman JM: Inhibition of organic binding of iodine with graded doses of iodide in euthyroid men. J Clin Endocrinol Metab 27:1607–1615, 1967.

64. Krawiec L, Chester HA, Bocanera LV, et al: Thyroid autoregulation: Evidence for an action of iodoarachidonates and iodide at the cell membrane level. Horm Metab Res 23:321–325, 1991.

65. Uchimura H, Chiu SC, Kuzaya N, et al: Effects of iodine enrichment in vitro on the adenylate-cyclase adenosine, 3'',5'-monophosphate system in thyroid glands from normal subjects and patients with Graves' disease. J Clin Endocrinol Metab 50:1066–1070, 1980.

66. Michalkiewicz M, Huffman LJ, Connors JM: Alterations in thyroid blood flow induced by varying levels of iodine intake in the rat. Endocrinology 125:54–60, 1989.

67. Tseng FY, Rani CS, Field JB: Effect of iodide on glucose oxidation and ³²P incorporation into phospholipids stimulated by different agents in dog thyroid slices. Endocrinology 124:1450–1455, 1989.

68. Saji M, Akamizu T, Sanchez M, et al: Regulation of thyrotropin receptor gene expression in rat FRTL-5 thyroid cells. Endocrinology 130:520–533, 1922.

69. Melander A, Sundler F: Presence and influence of cholinergic nerves in the mouse thyroid. Endocrinology 105:7–9, 1979.

70. Melander A, Ericson LE, Ljunggren J-G, et al: Sympathetic innervation of the normal human thyroid. J Clin Endocrinol Metab 39:713–718, 1974.

71. Larsen PR, Ingbar SH: The thyroid gland. In Wilson JD, Foster DW (eds): Textbook of Endocrinology. Philadelphia, WB Saunders, 1992, pp 357–487.

72. Morley JE: Neuroendocrine control of thyrotropin secretion. Endocr Rev 2:396–436, 1981.

73. Gamstedt A, Jarnerot G, Kagedal B: Dose related effects of betamethasone on iodothyronines and thyroid hormone-binding proteins in serum. Acta Endocrinol 96:484–490, 1981.

74. Sawin CT, Hershman JM, Boyd AE III, et al: The relationship of changes in serum estradiol and progesterone during the menstrual cycle to the thyrotropin and prolactin responses to thyrotropin-releasing hormone. J Clin Endocrinol Metab 47:1296–1302, 1978.

75. Cobb WE, Reichlin S, Jackson IMD: Growth hormone secretory status is a determinant of the thyrotropin response to thyrotropin-releasing hormone in euthyroid patients with hypothalamic-pituitary disease. J Clin Endocrinol Metab 52:324–329, 1981.

76. Porter BA, Refetoff S, Rosenfield RL, et al: Abnormal thyroxine metabolism in hyposomatotrophic dwarfism and inhibition of responsiveness to TRH during GN therapy. Pediatrics 51:668–674, 1973.

77. Corrigan DF, Wartofsky L, Dimond RC, et al: Parameters of thyroid function in patients with active acromegaly. Metabolism 27:209–216, 1978.

78. Shepard TH: Onset of function in the human fetal thyroid: Biochemical and radioautographic studies from organ culture. J Clin Endocrinol 27:945–958, 1967.

79. Fisher DA, Hobel CJ, Garza R, Pierce CA: Thyroid function in the preterm fetus. Pediatrics 46:208–216, 1970.

80. Kourides IA, Berkowitz RL, Pang S, et al: Antepartum diagnosis of goitrous hypothyroidism by fetal ultrasonography and amniotic fluid thyrotropin concentration. J Clin Endocrinol Metab 59:1016–1018, 1984.

81. Klein AH, Hobel CJ, Sack J, Fisher DA: Effect of intraamniotic fluid thyroxine injection on fetal serum and amniotic fluid iodothyronine concentrations. J Clin Endocrinol Metab 47:1034–1037, 1978.

82. Greenberg AH, Czernichow P, Reba RC, et al: Observations on the maturation of thyroid function in early fetal life. J Clin Invest 49:1790–1803, 1970.

83. Allen JP, Greer MA, McGilvra R, et al: Endocrine function in an anencephalic infant. J Clin Endocrinol Metab 38:94–98, 1974.

84. Fisher DA, Hobel CJ, Garza R, Pierce CA: Thyroid function in the preterm fetus. Pediatrics 46:208–216, 1970.

85. Abuid J, Stinson DA, Larsen PR: Serum triiodothyronine and thyroxine in the neonate and the acute increases in these hormones following delivery. J Clin Invest 52:1195–1199, 1973.

86. Fisher DA, Klein AH: Thyroid development and disorders of thyroid function in the newborn. N Engl J Med 304:702–712, 1981.

87. Cavalieri RR, Castle JN, McMahon FA: Effects of dexamethasone on kinetics and distribution of triiodothyronine in the rat. Endocrinology 114:215–221, 1984.

88. Bargman GJ, Gardner LI: Experimental production of otic lesions with antithyroid drugs. In Stanburg JB, Kroc RL (eds): Human Development and the Thyroid Gland: Relation to Endemic Cretinism. New York, Plenum Press, 1972, pp 305–323.

89. Ingbar SH: The influence of aging on human thyroid hormone economy. In Greenblatt R (ed): Geriatric Endocrinology. New York, Raven, 1978, pp 13–32.

90. Kaplan MM, Larsen PR, Crantz FR, et al: Prevalence of abnormal thyroid function test results in patients with acute medical illnesses. Am J Med 72:9–16, 1982.

91. Brent GA, Hershman JM: Effects of nonthyroidal illness on thyroid function tests. In Van Middlesworth L (ed): The Thyroid Gland: A Practical Treatise. Chicago, Year Book Medical Publishers, 1986, pp 83–110.

92. Wehmann RE, Gregerman RI, Burns WH, et al: Suppression of thyrotropin in the low-thyroxine state of severe nonthyroidal illness. N Engl J Med 312:546–552, 1985.

93. Brent GA, Hershman JM: Thyroxine therapy in patients with severe nonthyroidal illnesses and low serum thyroxine concentration. J Clin Endocrinol Metab 63:1–8, 1986.

94. Becker RA, Vaughan GM, Ziegler MG, et al: Hypermetabolic low triiodothyronine syndrome of burn injury. Crit Care Med 10:870–875, 1982.

95. Kabadi UM, Dragstedt LR II: Glucagon-induced changes in plasma thyroid hormone concentrations in healthy dogs resemble euthyroid sick syndrome. J Endocrinol Invest 14:269–275, 1991.

96. Chopra IJ, Sakane S, Teco GN: A study of the serum concentration of tumor necrosis factor-alpha in thyroidal and nonthyroidal illnesses. J Clin Endocrinol Metab 72:1113–1116, 1991.

97. Romijn JA, Wiersinga WM: Decreased nocturnal surge of thyrotropin in nonthyroidal illness. J Clin Endocrinol Metab 70:35–42, 1990.

98. Van Der Poll T, Romijn JA, Wiersinga WM, et al: Tumor necrosis factor: A putative mediator of the sick euthyroid syndrome in man. J Clin Endocrinol Metab 71:1567–1572, 1990.

99. Glinoer D, de Nayer P, Bourdoux P, et al: Regulation of maternal thyroid during pregnancy. J Clin Endocrinol Metab 71:276–287, 1990.

100. Pakarinen A, Hakkinen K, Alen M: Serum thyroid hormones, thyrotropin and thyroxine binding globulin in elite athletes during very intense strength training of one week. J Sports Med Phys Fitness 31:142–146, 1991.

101. Kodama H: Changes of hypothalami-pituitary-thyroid function after open heart surgery—especially evaluated by TRH test. Nippon Kyobu Geka Gakkai Zasshi 39:1139–1146, 1991.

102. Ziegler MG, Morrissey EC, Marshall LF: Catecholamine and thyroid hormones in traumatic injury. Crit Care Med 18:253–258, 1990.

103. Montoya E, Wilber JF, Lorincz M: Catecholaminergic control of thyrotropin secretion. J Lab Clin Med 93:887–894, 1979.

104. Wilber JF, Baum D: Elevation of plasma TSH during surgical hypothermia. J Clin Endocrinol Metabol 31:372–375, 1970.

105. Solter M, Brkic K, Petek M, et al: Thyroid hormone economy in response to extreme cold exposure in healthy factory workers. J Clin Endocrinol Metab 68:168–172, 1989.

106. Drucker D, Eggo MC, Salit IE, et al: Ethionamide-induced goitrous hypothyroidism. Ann Intern Med 100:837–839, 1984.

107. Kniazev I, Tabolin V, Tikhonov V, et al: Effects of hypoxia on the functional state of the thyroid gland in premature infants of different gestational age. Pediatria 10:24–28, 1989.

108. Gaitan E: Goitrogens in food and water. Annu Rev Nutr 10:21–39, 1990.

109. Transbol I, Christiansen C, Baastrup PC, et al: Endocrine effects of lithium. Hypothyroidism, its prevalence in long-term patients. Acta Endocrinol 87:759–767, 1978.

Thyroid Function Tests

DAVID H. SARNE
SAMUEL REFETOFF

Over the past three decades, clinical thyroidology has witnessed the introduction of a profusion of diagnostic procedures. These laboratory procedures provide greater choice, sensitivity, and specificity that have enhanced the possibility of early detection of occult thyroid diseases that present with only marginal clinical findings or are obscured by coincidental nonthyroid diseases as well as the exclusion of thyroid dysfunction in the presence of symptoms that closely mimic a thyroid ailment. On the other hand, the wide choice of complementary and overlapping tests indicates that each procedure has its limitations and that no single test is always reliable. Finally, the trend in clinical medicine to place a greater reliance on laboratory aids has depreciated the value of the conventional history and physical findings, which are still crucial in the overall management and in the physician-patient relationship. Thus it should be remembered that the tests discussed in this chapter serve as tools to validate a clinical impression and that one should be cautious in using tests alone

Supported in part by U.S. National Institutes of Health Grant DK 15,070 and Public Health Service Grant RR 00,055.

to make a diagnosis or choose a particular mode of therapy.

In the evaluation of thyroid diseases, two fundamental questions should be considered. The first involves the metabolic status of the patient. Is the patient hormonally deficient (hypothyroid) or hormonally sufficient (euthyroid), or is there hormonal excess (thyrotoxicosis)? Second, what is the etiology of the disease process responsible for the hormonal imbalance or thyroid gland abnormality in the absence of hormonal perturbation?

Thyroid tests can be classified into categories according to the information they provide at the functional, etiological and anatomical levels. Tests such as thyroidal radioiodide uptake and perchlorate discharge are performed in vivo to directly assess the level of the gland activity and integrity of hormone biosynthesis. Tests that measure hormone concentration and its transport in blood are carried out in vitro and are basic for the indirect assessment of the level of metabolic activity. Another category of tests attempts to measure more directly the impact of thyroid hormone on peripheral tissues. Tests available to assess this important parameter are nonspecific because they often are altered by various nonthyroidal processes. In contrast to the foregoing, the presence of several substances, such as thyroid autoantibodies, usually absent in healthy people, is useful in establishing the cause of some thyroid illness. Occasionally, definite establishment of a diagnosis requires invasive procedures, such as biopsy, for histological examination or enzymatic studies. Gross abnormalities of the thyroid gland, detected by palpation, can be assessed by scintiscanning and by ultrasonography. The integrity of the hypothalamo-pituitary-thyroid axis can be evaluated by (1) the response of the pituitary to thyroid hormone excess of deficiency; (2) the capacity of the thyroid gland to respond to thyrotropin (TSH); and (3) the pituitary responsiveness to thyrotropin-releasing hormone (TRH). These tests are intended to identify the primary organ affected by the disease process that manifests as thyroid dysfunction—in other words, primary (thyroid), secondary (pituitary), or tertiary (hypothalamic) malfunction. Finally, a number of special tests are briefly described. Some are invaluable in the elucidation of the rare inborn errors of hormone biosynthesis and others are mainly research tools.

Each test has inherent limitations, and no single procedure is diagnostically adequate for the entire spectrum of possible thyroid abnormalities. The choice, execution, application, and interpretation of each test require an understanding of thyroid physiology and biochemistry dealt with in the preceding chapters. Thyroid tests serve not only in the diagnosis and management of thyroid illnesses but also to better understand the pathophysiology underlying a specific disease.

IN VIVO TESTS OF THYROID GLAND ACTIVITY AND INTEGRITY OF HORMONE SYNTHESIS AND SECRETION

Common to these tests is the administration of radioisotopes that cannot be distinguished by the body from the naturally occurring stable iodine (^{127}I) isotope. In contrast to all other tests, these procedures provide a means to directly evaluate thyroid gland function. Formerly of common use in the diagnosis of hypothyroidism and thyrotoxicosis, this particular application has been supplanted by measurement of TSH and thyroid hormone concentrations in blood. Furthermore, alterations in thyroid gland activity and in handling of iodine are not necessarily coupled to the amount of hormone produced and secreted. The tests are time-consuming and relatively expensive, and they expose the patient to irradiation that may not always be inconsequential. Nevertheless, they still have an important application in the field of investigative medicine and in the diagnosis of inborn errors of thyroid hormonogenesis. Measurement of the thyroidal radioiodide uptake is useful in establishing the etiology of thyrotoxicosis and is the only means for estimating the dose of radioiodide to be delivered in the treatment of thyrotoxicosis and thyroid carcinoma.

To understand the physiological basis of this category of tests, one should remember the following facts. Iodine constitutes an integral part of the thyroid hormone molecule. Although several other tissues, including the salivary glands, mammary glands, lacrimal glands, choroid plexus, and parietal cells of the stomach, can extract iodide from blood and generate a positive tissue to serum iodide gradient, only the thyroid gland stores iodine for an appreciable period of time.[1] Because the kidneys continually filter blood iodide, the final fate of most iodine atoms is either to be trapped by the thyroid gland or to be excreted in the urine. When a tracer of iodide is administered to the patient, it rapidly becomes mixed with the stable extrathyroidal iodide pool and is thereafter handled identically as the stable isotope. Thus the thyroidal content of radioiodide gradually increases and that in the extrathyroidal body pool gradually declines, until virtually none is left. This end point normally occurs between 24 and 72 hours.

From data of the radioiodide uptake by the thyroid and/or urinary excretion and/or stable iodide concentration in plasma and urine, the following pertinent parameters can be derived: (1) rate of thyroidal iodine uptake (thyroid iodide clearance), (2) fractional thyroid radioactive iodide uptake (RAIU), (3) absolute iodide uptake, and (4) urinary excretion of radioiodide, or iodide clearance. After the complete removal of the administered radioiodide from the circulation, depletion of the radioisotope from the thyroid gland can be monitored by direct counting over the gland. Reappearance of the radioiodine in the circulation bound to proteins can be measured to estimate the intrathyroidal turnover of iodine and the secretory activity of the thyroid gland.

The foregoing tests can be combined with the administration of agents known either to normally stimulate or to inhibit thyroid gland activity, thus providing information on the control of thyroid gland activity. Administration of radioiodide followed by scanning provides a means to examine the anatomy of the thyroid gland in terms of topical function. The latter two applications of in vivo tests utilizing radioiodide are discussed under their respective headings.

The potential irradiation hazard from administered radioisotopes should always be kept in mind. Children are particularly vulnerable, and doses of x-rays as small as 20 rad to the thyroid are associated with an increased risk of developing thyroid cancers,[2] but there is no proven danger from isotopes used for the diagnosis of thyroid diseases. In vivo administration of radioisotopes is contraindicated dur-

TABLE 39–1. COMMONLY USED ISOTOPES FOR IN VIVO STUDIES AND RADIATION DOSE DELIVERED

| NUCLIDE | PRINCIPAL PHOTON ENERGY (KeV) | PHYSICAL DECAY | | ESTIMATED RADIATION DOSE (m rads/μCi) ADMINISTERED | | AVERAGE DOSE GIVEN FOR SCANNING PURPOSES (μCi) |
		Mode	Half-Life (days)	Thyroid*	Total Body	
[131]I–	364	β (0.606 Mev)	8.1	1340	0.08	50
[125]I–	28	Electron capture	60	825	0.06	50
[123]I–	159	Electron capture	0.55	13	0.03	200
[132]I–	670	β (2.12 MeV)	0.10	15	0.1	50†
[99m]TcO$_4$–	141	Isometric transition	0.25	0.2	0.01	2,500

*Calculations take into account the rate of maximal uptake and residence time of the isotope as well as gland size. For the iodine isotopes, average data for adult euthyroid people used were t½ of uptake 5 hours, biological t½ 50 days, maximal uptake 20%, and gland size 15 g (see also refs. 4–6).

†Dose used for early thyroidal uptake studies.

ing pregnancy and in breastfeeding mothers.[3] Studies should be deferred if pregnancy is likely.

A number of radioisotopes are now available. Furthermore, provision of more sophisticated and sensitive detection devices has substantially decreased the dose required for the completion of the studies. Table 39–1 lists the isotopes most commonly used for in vivo studies of the thyroid. Isotopes with slower physical decay, such as ^{125}I and ^{131}I, are particularly suitable for long-term studies. Isotopes with faster decay, such as ^{123}I and [132]I, usually deliver a lower irradiation dose and are advantageous in short-term and repeated studies. The peak photon energy gamma emission differs among isotopes, allowing the execution of simultaneous studies with two isotopes.

Thyroidal Radioiodide Uptake

The RAIU is the most commonly used thyroid test that requires the administration of a radioisotope. The radioisotope usually is given orally in a capsule or in liquid form, and the quantity accumulated by the thyroid gland at various intervals of time is measured by epithyroid counting, using a gamma scintillation counter. Correction for the amount of isotope circulating in the blood of the neck region, done by subtracting counts obtained over the thigh, is particularly important early after its administration. A dose of the same radioisotope placed in a neck "phantom" is also counted as a "standard." The percentage of RAIU is calculated from the counts cumulated per constant time unit.

The percentage of RAIU 24 hours after the administration of radioiodide is most useful because in most instances, the thyroid gland has reached the plateau of isotope accumulation and because it has been shown that at this time the best separation between high, normal, and low uptake is obtained. Normal values for 24-hour RAIU in most parts of North America range from 5 to 30 per cent. In many other parts of the world, normal values range from 15 to 50 per cent. Lower normal values are caused by the increase in dietary iodine intake after the enrichment of foods, particularly mass-produced bread (150 μg of iodine per slice), with this element.[7] The inverse relation between the daily dietary intake of iodine and the RAIU test is clearly shown in Figure 39–1. The intake of large amounts of iodide (>5 mg/day)—mainly from the use of iodine-containing radiologic contrast media, antiseptics, vitamins,

and drugs—completely suppresses the RAIU values to a level hardly detectable, using the usual equipment and doses of the isotope. Depending on the type of iodine preparation and the period of exposure, depression of RAIU can last for weeks, months, and even years. Most notorious is Lipiodol, formerly used in myelography. Even external application of iodide may suppress thyroidal radioiodide uptake. The need to inquire about individual dietary habits and sources of excess iodide intake is obvious.

The test does not measure hormone production and release but merely the avidity of the thyroid gland for io-

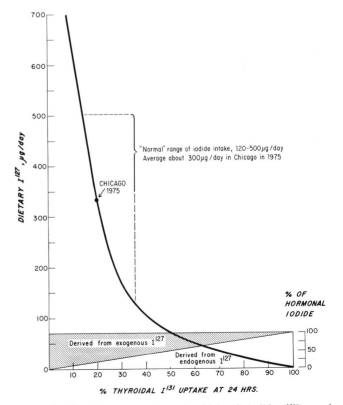

FIGURE 39–1. Relation of 24-hour thyroidal radioiodide (^{131}I) uptake (RAIU) to dietary content of stable iodine (^{125}I). The uptake increases with decreasing dietary iodine. With iodine intake below the amount provided from thyroid hormone degradation, the latter contributes a larger proportion of the total iodine taken up by the thyroid. Under dietary habits in the United States, the average 24-hour thyroidal RAIU is below 20 per cent. (From DeGroot et al: The Thyroid and Its Diseases. New York, John Wiley, 1984, with permission.)

dide and its rate of clearance relative to the kidney. Disease states resulting in excessive production and release of thyroid hormone are most often associated with increased thyroidal RAIU and those causing hormone underproduction with decreased thyroidal RAIU (Fig. 39–2). Important exceptions include high uptake values in some hypothyroid patients and low values in some hyperthyroid patients. Increased thyroidal RAIU occurs with hormonal insufficiency in the presence of severe iodide deficiency and in most inborn errors of hormonogenesis. In the former a lack of substrate and in the latter a specific enzymatic block of hormone synthesis cause hypothyroidism poorly compensated by TSH-induced thyroid gland overactivity. Decreased thyroidal RAIU with hormonal excess typically is encountered in the syndrome of transient thyrotoxicosis (both de Quervain's disease and painless thyroiditis),[8] ingestion of exogenous hormone (thyrotoxicosis factitia), and iodide-induced thyrotoxicosis (jodbasedow),[9] as well as in patients with thyrotoxicosis on moderately high intake of iodide. High or low thyroid as a result of low or high dietary iodine intake, respectively, may not be associated with significant changes in thyroid hormone secretion.

Factors that affect the value of the 24-hour thyroidal RAIU are listed in Table 39–2. Minor changes related to sex and age may be disregarded. Surreptitious spitting and vomiting within hours after administration of the radioisotope could significantly reduce the RAIU.

Several variations of the test have been devised that have particular value under special circumstances but are rarely used. For the sake of completeness, some are briefly described.

Early Thyroid RAIU and ⁹⁹ᵐPertechnetate Uptake Measurements

In some patients with severe thyrotoxicosis and low intrathyroidal iodine concentration, the turnover rate of iodine

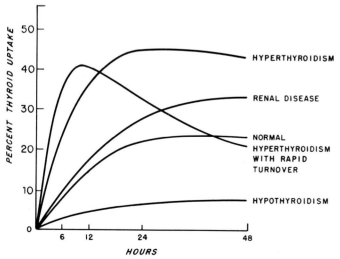

FIGURE 39–2. Examples of thyroidal RAIU curves under various pathological conditions. Note the prolonged uptake in renal disease caused by decreased urinary excretion of the isotope and the early decline in thyroidal radioiodide content in some patients with thyrotoxicosis associated with a small but rapidly turning over intrathyroidal iodine pool. (From DeGroot et al: The Thyroid and Its Diseases. New York, John Wiley, 1984, with permission.)

TABLE 39–2. DISEASES AND OTHER FACTORS THAT AFFECT THE 24-HOUR THYROIDAL RAIU

INCREASED RAIU
Hyperthyroidism (Graves' disease, Plummer's disease, toxic adenoma, trophoblastic disease, predominantly pituitary resistance to thyroid hormone, TSH-producing pituitary adenoma)
Nontoxic goiter (endemic, inherited biosynthetic defects, generalized resistance to thyroid hormone, Hashimoto's thyroiditis)
Excessive hormonal loss (nephrosis, chronic diarrhea, hypolipidemic resins, diet high in soybean)
Decreased renal clearance of iodine (renal insufficiency, severe heart failure)
Recovery of the suppressed thyroid (withdrawal of thyroid hormone and antithyroid drug administration, subacute thyroiditis, iodine-induced myxedema)
Iodine deficiency (endemic or sporadic dietary deficiency, excessive iodine loss as in pregnancy or in the dehalogenase defect)
TSH administration

DECREASED RAIU
Hypothyroidism (primary or secondary)
Defect in iodide concentration (inherited trapping defect, early phase of subacute thyroiditis, transient hyperthyroidism)
Suppressed thyroid gland caused by thyroid hormone (hormone replacement, thyrotoxicosis factitia, struma ovarii)
Iodine excess (dietary, drugs, and other iodine contaminants)
Miscellaneous drugs and chemicals (see Tables 39–10 and 39–12)

may be accelerated, causing a rapid initial uptake of the radioiodide that reaches a plateau before six hours, followed by a decline through release of the isotope in hormonal or other forms (see Fig. 39–2). Although this phenomenon is rare, some laboratories choose to routinely measure early RAIU. Early measurements require the accurate determination of background activity contributed by the circulating isotope. Radioisotopes with a shorter half-life, such as ¹²³I and ¹³²I, are more suitable.

Because thyroidal uptake in the early period after administration of radioiodide mainly reflects trapping activity, ⁹⁹ᵐTc as the pertechnetate ion (⁹⁹ᵐTcO₄⁻) may be used. In euthyroid patients, thyroid trapping is maximal at about 20 minutes and is about 1 per cent of the administered dose.[10] This test, when coupled with the administration of T₃, can be used to evaluate thyroid gland suppressibility in thyrotoxic patients treated with antithyroid drugs (see below).

Other In Vivo Tests of Thyroid Gland Activity

A number of parameters of thyroid gland activity can be derived from the RAIU combined with measurement in blood and urine after the administration of radioiodide. They are (1) thyroidal iodide clearance, (2) absolute iodide uptake by the thyroid gland, (3) urinary radioiodide excretion, (4) thyroidal radioiodine release, and (5) serum protein-bound radioiodide or radioiodide conversion ratio. Formerly routinely used in clinical practice, these tests have been replaced by in vitro measurements carried out on serum samples. They remain important tools for clinical investigation.

Perchlorate Discharge Test

This test, which is used to detect defects in intrathyroidal iodide organification, is based on the following physiological principle. Iodide is trapped by the thyroid gland through an energy-requiring active transport mechanism. Once in the gland, it is rapidly bound to thyroglobulin and retention no longer requires active transport. Several ions, such as thiocyanate (SCN^-) and perchlorate (ClO_4^-), inhibit active iodide transport and cause the release of the intrathyroidal iodide not bound to thyroid protein. Thus measurement of intrathyroidal radioiodine loss after the administration of an inhibitor of iodide trapping would indicate the presence of an iodine-binding defect.

In the standard test, epithyroid counts are obtained at frequent intervals (every 10 or 15 minutes) after the administration of radioiodide. Two hours later 1 g of $KClO_4^-$ is administered orally, and epithyroid counts continue to be obtained for an additional two hours. In normal individuals radioiodide accumulation in the thyroid gland ceases after the administration of the iodide transport inhibitor, but there is little loss of the thyroidal radioactivity accumulated before induction of the trapping block. A loss of 5 per cent or more indicates an organification defect.[11] The severity of the defect is proportional to the extent of radioiodide discharged from the gland and is complete when virtually all the activity accumulated by the gland is lost. The test is positive in the inborn defect of iodide organification, which can be associated with deafness (Pendred's syndrome); during the administration of iodide organification blocking agents; in some cases of Hashimoto's thyroiditis[12]; or after treatment with radioactive iodide.[13]

Several modifications of this test have been devised to increase its sensitivity, thus allowing the detection of minor defects of iodide organification. For example, in the 20-minute perchlorate discharge test, $NaClO_4^-$ is given intravenously 10 minutes after an intravenous dose of radioiodide.[14] In the iodide-perchlorate discharge test, 0.5 mg of stable iodide is given along with the tracer isotope.[15]

Saliva-Plasma Radioiodide Ratio

The saliva-plasma (S:P) ratio of radioiodide evaluates the iodide trapping function, and its principal application is in the diagnosis of congenital defects of this step of iodine metabolism. Like the thyroid gland, some organs, including the salivary glands, concentrate iodide to several times the plasma level.[1] In patients unable to concentrate iodide in the thyroid gland, this defect is shared with other tissues that normally possess this transport process. The test involves the administration of radioiodide followed one hour later by the simultaneous collection of saliva and blood. The S:P of isotope in an equal volume of these fluids normally is greater than 10; it is 1 or less in patients with congenital trapping defect.[16]

MEASUREMENT OF HORMONE CONCENTRATION AND OTHER IODINATED COMPOUNDS AND THEIR TRANSPORT IN BLOOD

Measurements of T_4 and T_3 in serum and the estimation of their free concentration have become the most commonly used tests for the evaluation of the thyroid hor-

mone–dependent metabolic status. This approach has been espoused as a result of the development of simple, sensitive, and specific methods for measuring these iodothyronines and because of the lack of specific tests for the direct measurement of the metabolic effect of these hormones. Other advantages are the requirement of only a small blood sample and the large number of determinations that can be completed by a laboratory during a regular workday.

The thyroid gland is the principal source of all hormonal iodine–containing compounds or their precursors. Their chemical structures and normal concentrations in serum are given in Figure 39–3. Importantly, the concentration of each substance depends on not only the amount synthesized and secreted but also its affinity for carrier proteins, its distribution in tissues, its rate of degradation, and finally its clearance.

The main secretory product of the thyroid gland is T_4, T_3 being next in relative abundance. Both compounds are metabolically active when administered in vivo. They are synthesized and stored in the thyroid gland as part of a larger molecule, thyroglobulin (Tg), which must be degraded to release the two thyronines in a ratio favoring T_4 by 10- to 20-fold.[17] Under normal circumstances only minute amounts of Tg escape into the circulation; on a molar basis it is the least abundant iodine-containing compound in blood. With the exception of T_4, Tg, and small amounts of diiodotyrosine (DIT) and monoiodotyrosine (MIT), all other iodine-containing compounds found in the serum of normal humans are produced mainly in extrathyroidal tissues by a stepwise process of deiodination of T_4.[18] An alternative pathway of T_4 metabolism that involves deamination and decarboxylation but retention of the iodine residues gives rise to tetraiodothyroacetic acid (TETRAC or T_4 A) and 3,5,3'-triiodothyroacetic acid (TRIAC or T_3 A).[19, 20] Circulating iodoalbumin is generated by intrathyroidal iodination of serum albumin.[21] Small amounts of iodoproteins may be formed in peripheral tissues[22] or serum[23, 24] by covalent linkage of T_4 and T_3 to soluble proteins. Although the physiological function of circulating iodine compounds other than T_4 and T_3 remains unknown, measurement of changes in their concentration occasionally are of diagnostic value.

Measurement of Total Thyroid Hormone Concentration in Serum

Iodometry

Iodine constitutes an integral part of the thyroid hormone molecule. It is thus not surprising that determination of iodine content in serum was the first method suggested almost five decades ago for the identification and quantitation of thyroid hormone.[25]

Measurement of the protein-bound iodine (PBI) was the earliest method used routinely for the estimation of thyroid hormone concentration in serum. The test measures the total quantity of iodine precipitable with the serum proteins,[26] 90 per cent of which is T_4. Efforts to measure serum thyroid hormone levels with greater specificity and with lesser interference from nonhormonal iodinated compounds led to the development of the butanol extractable iodine (BEI) and T_4I by column techniques. In the BEI

NAME	Abbre-viation	Mole-cular Weight	FORMULA	NORMAL CONCENTRATION[a] (range)	
				ng / dl	pmol / L
3,5,3',5'-tetraiodothyronine (Thyroxine)	T_4	777	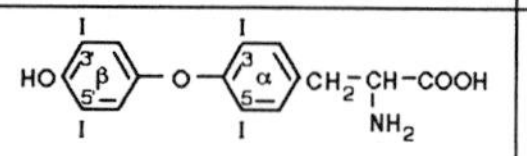	5,000 - 12,000	64,000 - 154,000
3,5,3'-triiodothyronine (Liothyronine)	T_3	651	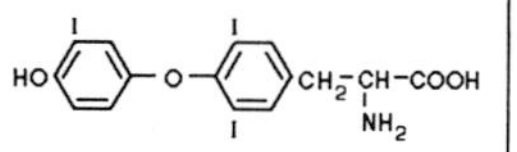	80 - 190[b]	1,200 - 2,900
3,3',5'-triiodothyronine (ReverseT$_3$)	rT_3	651	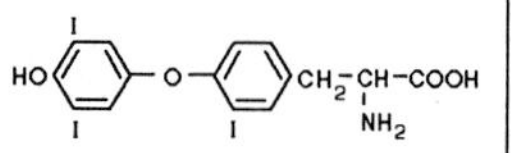	14 - 30	220 - 480
3,5-diiodothyronine	$3,5$-T_2	525	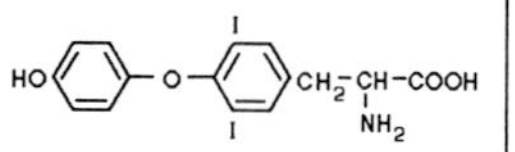	0.20- 0.75[b]	3.8 - 14
3,3'-diiodothyronine	$3,3'$-T_2	525	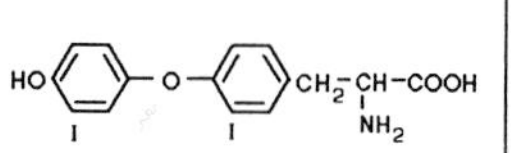	1 - 8[b]	19 - 150
3'5'-diiodothyronine	$3'5'$-T_2	525	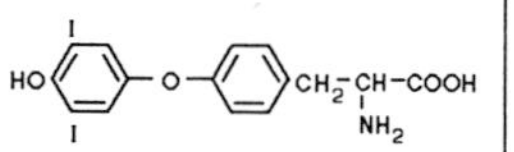	1.5 - 9.0[b]	30 - 170
3'-monoiodothyronine	$3'$-T_1	399	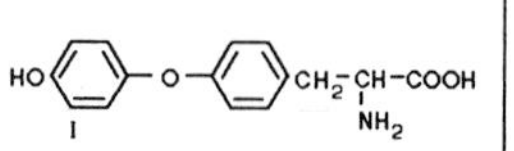	0.6 - 4	15 - 100
3-monoiodothyronine	3-T_1	399	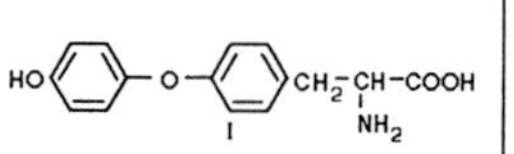	< 0.5 - 7.5	< 13 - 190
3,5,3',5'-tetraiodothyroacetic acid (TETRAC)	T_4A	748	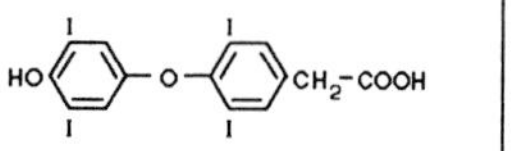	< 8 - 60	< 105 - 800
3,5,3'-triiodothyroacetic acid (TRIAC)	T_3A	622	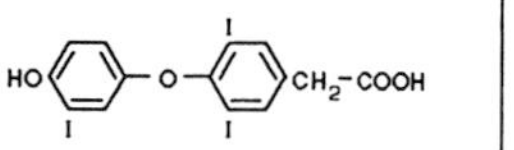	1.6 - 3	26 - 48
3,5-diiodotyrosine	DIT	433	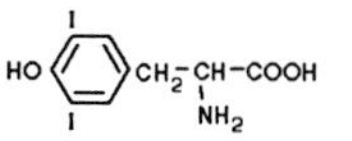	1 - 23	23 - 530
3-monoiodotyrosine	MIT	307	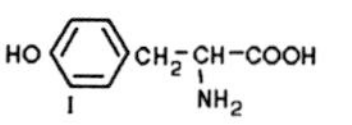	90 - 390[c]	2,900 - 12,700
thyroglobulin	Tg	660,000	glycoprotein maid of two identical subunits	< 100 - 2,500	1.5 - 38

FIGURE 39–3. Iodine-containing compounds in serum of healthy adults.

[a]Iodothyronine concentrations in the euthyroid population are not normally distributed. Thus calculation of the normal range on the basis of 95 per cent confidence limits for a Gaussian distribution is accurate.

[b]Significant decline with old age.

[c]Probably an overestimation because of cross-reactivity by related substances.

method sequential extractions with acidified butanol and washes with alkali result in the isolation of iodothyronines. The T_4I by column measures the iodine content in iodothyronines after their isolation from serum by columns of anion exchange resin. All chemical methods for the measurement of thyroid hormone in serum have been replaced by the ligand assays, which are devoid of interference by even large quantities of nonhormonal iodine–containing substances.

Iodometry is used experimentally to measure the iodine content in thyroglobulin (Tg) and in special clinical conditions such as inborn defects of hormonogenesis, when the production and secretion of nonhormonal iodine-containing compounds are suspected.

Radioligand Assays

Naturally occurring iodide-containing compounds in serum are measured by radioimmunoassay (RIA). The principle of these assays is the competition of a substance (S) being measured with the same isotopically labeled compound (S*) for binding to a specific class of IgG molecules present in the antiserum (antibody [Ab]). S is the ligand and the Ab is either a polyclonal antiserum to S or a mono-

clonal IgG. The reaction obeys the law of mass action. Thus, at equilibrium, the amount of S* bound to Ab to form the complex Ab-S* is inversely proportional to the concentration of S, forming the complex Ab-S, provided that the amounts of Ab and S* are kept constant.

$$Ab\text{-}S^* + [S] \rightleftharpoons Ab\text{-}S + S^*$$

The radioisotope content in Ab-S* or in the unbound (free) S* is determined after their separation by precipitation of the antibody-ligand complex or adsorption of the free ligand. Some RIA's are carried out with the Ab fixed to a solid support, reacting with S and S* in solution. Increments of known amounts of S are added to a series of reactions to construct a standard curve that describes the curvilinear stoichiometric relation between Ab-S* and S. It can be converted to a straight line by a number of mathematical transformations, such as the logit-log plot. Blank reactions contain S* but not specific Ab or a large excess of S in a full reaction.[27] The sensitivity of the assay depends on the affinity of the Ab and specific activity of S*. Under optimal conditions as little as 1 pg of S can be measured.

Production of antisera requires that iodoamino acids be rendered antigenic by conjugation to albumin or to some other large molecule or particle.[28] In the assay the iodoamino acids need to be liberated from their association to serum binding proteins, mainly thyroxine-binding globulin (TBG), because of affinity constants often equal to those of the antisera. Methods include extraction, competitive displacement of the iodoamino acid being measured, and inactivation of TBG.[29-32] Ideally, binding competitors should displace the iodoamino acid from TBG but interfere little or not at all with the specific immune reaction. This technique allows measurements in samples of whole unprocessed serum. Although there is no interference by nonhormonal iodine–containing compounds, some cross-reactivity among related naturally occurring iodoamino acids does exist.[33] Thus antibodies that possess little or no cross-reactivity should be selected for each assay. This is of particular importance when the concentration of the measured substance is lower than that of the cross-reacting congeners. Antisera seldom are able to differentiate the L- from the D-isomers,[34, 35] but this is less crucial in clinical assays. Rarely, some patients develop circulating antibodies against thyronines that interfere with the RIA carried out on unextracted serum samples. Depending on the method used for the separation of bound from free ligand, values obtained may be either spuriously low or high in the presence of such antibodies.[36, 37]

A wide choice of commercial kits is available for most RIA procedures, making these assays accessible to all medical centers. RIA's have been adapted for the measurement of T_4 in small samples of dried blood spots on filter paper and are used in screening for neonatal hypothyroidism.[38]

The first method developed to measure an iodoamino acid using the principle just described did not make use of antiserum.[39] The native serum protein, TBG, was used instead of an antibody to measure T_4 in extracted serum. The method, competitve protein-binding assay, was gradually supplanted by the RIA.

Other Methods

Another group of assays has been developed that are based on the principle of the radioligand assay but that do not use radioactive material. These assays, which use ligand conjugated to an enzyme, are likely to replace RIA's. The enzyme-linked ligand competes with the ligand being measured for the same binding sites on the antibody. Quantitation is carried out by spectrophotometry of the color reaction developed after the addition of the enzyme substrate.[40] Both homogeneous (enzyme-multiplied immunoassay technique [EMIT]) and heterogeneous (enzyme-linked immunosorbent assay [ELISA]) assays for T_4 have been developed.[41-43] In the homogeneous assays no separation step is required, thus providing easy automation.[41] In one such assay T_4 is linked to malate dehydrogenase, inhibiting the enzyme activity. The enzyme is activated when the T_4-enzyme conjugate is bound to T_4-specific antibody. Active T_4 conjugates to other enzymes, such as peroxidase[42] and alkaline phosphatase,[43] have also been developed. The assay has been adapted for the measurement of T_4 in dried blood samples used in mass screening programs for neonatal hypothyroidism.[43] Other nonradioisotope immunoassays use fluorescence excitation for detection of the labeled ligand and radial diffusion for the separation of antibody bound from free ligand on a solid matrix.

Several techniques distinct from iodometry, radioligand assays, and enzyme-linked immunologic assays have been devised for measurement of T_4 and T_3 in serum and other biological materials. They include gas-liquid chromatography,[44] neutron activation,[45] and double isotope derivative[46] assays. These methods are likely to remain strictly research tools. A modified version of liquid chromatography can distinguish between D- and L-isomers.[47]

Serum Total Thyroxine

The usual concentration of total thyroxine (TT_4) in adults ranges from 5 to 12 µg/dl (64–154 nmol/L). When concentrations are below or above this range in the absence of thyroid dysfunction, they usually are the result of an abnormal level of serum TBG (see Ch. 36). The hyperestrogenic state of pregnancy and the administration of estrogen-containing compounds are the most common causes of a significant elevation of serum TT_4 levels in euthyroid people. Serum TT_4 is virtually undetectable in the fetus until midgestation. Thereafter it rapidly increases, reaching high normal adult levels during the last trimester. A further acute but transient rise occurs within hours after delivery.[48] Values remain above the adult range until six years of age,[49] but subsequent age-related changes are minimal and not a uniform finding.[50-52] In clinical practice the same normal range of TT_4 applies to both sexes and all ages above six years.

Small seasonal variations and changes related to high altitude, cold, and heat have been described. Rhythmic variations in serum TT_4 concentration are of two types: variations related to postural changes in serum protein concentration[53] and true circadian variation.[29] Postural changes in protein concentration do not alter the free T_4 (FT_4) concentration.

Although levels of serum TT_4 below the normal range usually are associated with hypothyroidism and above this range with thyrotoxicosis, it must be remembered that the TT_4 level may not always correspond to the FT_4 concentration, which represents the metabolically active fraction (see below). The TT_4 concentration in serum may be altered by independent mechanisms: (1) an increase or decrease in the supply of T_4, as seen in most cases of thyrotoxicosis and hypothyroidism, respectively; (2) changes caused solely by alterations in T_4 binding to serum proteins; and (3) compensatory changes in serum TT_4 concentration caused by high or low serum levels of T_3. Conditions associated with changes in serum TT_4 and their relation to the metabolic status of the patient are listed in Table 39–3.

Serum TT_4 levels are low in conditions associated with decreased TBG concentration (see Ch. 36) or the presence of abnormal TBG's with reduced binding affinity or when the available T_4-binding sites on TBG are partially saturated by competing drugs present in blood in high concentrations (Table 39–4). Conversely, TT_4 levels are high when the serum TBG concentration is high (see Ch. 36). The person remains euthyroid, provided that the feedback regulation of the thyroid gland is intact.

Although changes in transthyretin (TTR) concentration seldom give rise to significant alterations in TT_4 concentration (see Ch. 36), the presence in serum of a variant protein with high affinity for T_4 and albumin-like properties[80] or antibodies against T_4[36, 37] produce elevations in the TT_4 concentration, whereas the FT_4 level and metabolic status remain normal. The variant albumin-like protein is inherited as an autosomal dominant trait termed familial dysalbuminemic hyperthyroxinemia (FDH; see Ch. 36).

Another possible cause of discrepancy between the ob-

TABLE 39–3. CONDITIONS ASSOCIATED WITH CHANGES IN SERUM TT$_4$ CONCENTRATION AND RELATION TO THE METABOLIC STATUS

METABOLIC STATUS	SERUM TT$_4$ CONCENTRATION		
	High	Low	Normal
Thyrotoxic	Hyperthyroidism (all causes, including Graves' disease, Plummer's disease, toxic thyroid adenoma, early phase of subacute thyroiditis) Thyroid hormone leak (early stage of subacute thyroiditis, transient thyrotoxicosis) Excess of exogenous or ectopic T$_4$ (thyrotoxicosis factitia, struma ovarii) Predominantly pituitary resistance to thyroid hormone	Intake of excessive amounts of T$_3$ (thyrotoxicosis factitia)	Low TBG (congenital or acquired) T$_3$ thyrotoxicosis (untreated or recurrent post therapy); more common in iodine-deficient areas Drugs competing with T$_4$ binding to serum proteins (see also entry under euthyroid with low TT$_4$) Hypermetabolism of nonthyroidal origin (Luft's syndrome)

Euthyroid	High TBG (congenital or acquired)
	 T$_4$ binding albumin-like variant
	 Endogenous T$_4$ antibodies
	 Replacement therapy with T$_4$ only
	 Treatment with D-T$_4$
	 Generalized resistance to thyroid hormone
		Low TBG (congenital or acquired)
		 Endogenous T$_4$ antibodies
		 Mildly elevated or normal T$_3$
		    T$_3$ replacement therapy
		    Iodine deficiency
		    Treated thyrotoxicosis
		    Chronic thyroiditis
		    Congenital goiter
		 Drugs competing with T$_4$ binding to serum proteins (see Table 39–4)
			Normal state

Hypothyroid	Severe generalized resistance to thyroid hormone	Thyroid gland failure
		    Primary (all causes, including gland destruction, severe iodine deficiency, inborn error of hormonogenesis)
		    Secondary (pituitary failure)
		    Tertiary (hypothalamic failure)
			High TBG (congenital or acquired)
			 ? Isolated peripheral tissue resistance to thyroid hormone

TABLE 39–4. COMPOUNDS THAT AFFECT THYROID HORMONE SERUM TRANSPORT PROTEINS

SUBSTANCE	COMMON USE
Increase TBG Concentration	
Estrogens[54, 55]	Ovulation suppressants and anticancer
Heroin and methadone[56]	Opiates (in addicts)
Clofibrate[57]	Hypolipidemic
5-Fluorouracil[58]	Anticancer
Perphenazine[59]	Tranquilizer
Decrease TBG Concentration	
Androgens and anabolic steroids[60, 61]	Virilizing, anticancer, and anabolic
Glucocorticoids[62]	Anti-inflammatory and immunosuppressive; decrease intracranial pressure
L-Asparaginase[63]	Antileukemic
Nicotinic acid[64]	Hypolipidemic
Interfere With Thyroid Hormone Binding to TBG and/or TTR	
Salicylates and salsalate[65–67]	Anti-inflammatory, analgesic, and antipyrexic
Diphenylhydantoin and analogues[66, 68]	Anticonvulsive and anti-arrhythmic
Diazepam[69]	Anti-anxiety
Furosemide[70]	Diuretic
Sulfonylureas[71]	Hypoglycemic
Dinitrophenol[65]	Uncouples oxidative phosphorylation
Free fatty acids[72]	
o,p′-DDD[73]	Anti-adrenal
Phenylbutazone[74]	Anti-inflammatory
Halofenate[75]	Hypolipidemic
Fenclofenac[76]	Antirheumatic
Orphenadrine[77]	Spasmolytic
Monovalent anions (SCN$^-$, ClO$_4^-$)[78]	Antithyroid
Thyroid hormone analogues, including dextroisomers[79]	Cholesterol reducing

served serum TT$_4$ concentration and the metabolic status of the patient is divergent changes in the serum TT$_3$ and TT$_4$ concentrations with alterations in the serum T$_3$:T$_4$ ratio. The most common situation is that of elevated TT$_3$ concentration. The source of T$_3$ may be endogenous, as in T$_3$ thyrotoxicosis, or exogenous, as during ingestion of T$_3$. In the former situation, contrary to the common variety of thyrotoxicosis, elevation in the serum TT$_3$ concentration is not accompanied by an increase in the TT$_4$ level. In fact, the serum TT$_4$ level is normal and occasionally low.[81] This finding indicates that in T$_3$ thyrotoxicosis, the hormone is predominantly secreted as such rather than arising from the peripheral conversion of T$_4$ to T$_3$. Ingestion of pharmacological doses of T$_3$ results in thyrotoxicosis associated with severe depression of the serum TT$_4$ concentration. A moderate hypersecretion of T$_3$ can be associated with euthyroidism and a low serum TT$_4$ concentration. This circumstance, occasionally referred to as T$_3$ euthyroidism, may be more prevalent than T$_3$ thyrotoxicosis. It is believed to constitute a state of compensatory T$_3$ secretion as a physiological adaptation of the failing thyroid gland, such as after treatment for thyrotoxicosis, in some cases of chronic thyroiditis, or during iodine deprivation.[82, 83] Serum TT$_4$ concentration is also low in normal people receiving replacement doses of T$_3$. Conversely, serum TT$_4$ levels are above the upper limit of normal in 15 to 50 per cent of patients rendered eumetabolic by administration of T$_4$ alone.[84] Because of the relatively slow rate of metabolism and large extrathyroidal T$_4$ pool, the serum concentration of the hormone varies little with the time of sampling in relation to ingestion of the daily dose.[85]

Two conditions also characteristically occur with a discrepancy between the clinical status and the serum concen-

TABLE 39–5. CONDITIONS THAT MAY BE ASSOCIATED WITH DISCREPANCIES BETWEEN THE CONCENTRATION OF SERUM TT_3 AND TT_4

SERUM			METABOLIC STATUS		
TT_3:TT_4 Ratio	TT_3	TT_4	*Thyrotoxic*	*Euthyroid*	*Hypothyroid*
↑	↑	N	T_3-thyrotoxicosis (endogenous)	Endemic iodine deficiency (T_3 autoantibodies)†	—
↑	N	↓	—	Treated thyrotoxicosis (T_4 autoantibodies)†	Endemic cretins (severe iodine deficiency)
↑	↑	↓	Pharmacological doses of T_3 (exogenous T_3-toxicosis) Partially treated thyrotoxicosis	T_3 replacement (especially 1 to 3 h after ingestion) Endemic iodine deficiency	(T_3 autoantibodies)†
↓	↓	N	—	Most conditions associated with reduced conversion of T_4 to T_3 Chronic or severe acute illness* Trauma (surgical, burns) Fasting and malnutrition Drugs‡ (T_3 autoantibodies)†	—
↓	N	↑	Severe nonthyroidal illness associated wtih thyrotoxicosis	Neonates (first three weeks of life) T_4 replacement Familial hyperthyroxinemia resulting from T_4 binding albumin-like variant (T_4 autoantibodies)†	—
↓	↓	↑	—	At birth Acute nonthyroidal illness with transient hyperthyroxinemia	(T_4 autoantibodies)†

*Hepatic and renal failure, diabetic ketoacidosis, myocardial infarction, infectious and febrile illness, cancers.
†Artefactual values dependent on the method of hormone determination in serum.
‡Glucocorticoids, iodinated contrast agents, amiodarone, propranolol, propylthiouracil.

tration of TT_4: (1) the syndrome of generalized resistance to thyroid hormone associated with elevated TT_4 as well as FT_4 and TT_3 levels and usually clinical euthyroidism[86] and (2) the syndrome of hypermetabolism in the absence of thyroid dysfunction described by Luft et al.[87] The latter is a rare mitochondrial defect that produces thyroid hormone–independent hypermetabolism.

Serum Total Triiodothyronine

Normal serum total triiodothyronine (TT_3) concentrations in the adult are 80 to 190 ng/dl (1.2–2.9 nmol/L). Although sex differences are small, those with age are more dramatic. In contrast to serum TT_4, TT_3 concentration at birth is low, about one half the normal adult level. It rises within 24 hours to about double the normal adult value followed by a rapid decrease over the subsequent 24 hours to a level in the upper adult range, which persists for the first year of life.[48] A steady decline in the mean TT_3 level has been observed covering the entire life span from early childhood to old age.[50-52] It is possible that the change is related to the prevalence of nonthyroidal illness rather than to age alone.[88] The interpretation of borderline values should take into account the patient's age. Although a positive correlation between serum TT_3 level and body weight has been observed, it may be related to overeating.[89] Rapid and profound reductions in serum TT_3 level can be produced within 24 to 48 hours of total calorie or only carbohydrate deprivation.[90-92]

Most conditions that cause serum TT_4 levels to increase are associated with high TT_3 concentrations. Thus serum TT_3 levels usually are elevated in thyrotoxicosis and reduced in hypothyroidism. In both conditions the TT_3:TT_4 ratio is elevated relative to normal euthyroid people. This elevation is caused by the disproportionate increase in serum TT_3 concentration in thyrotoxicosis and a lesser diminution in hypothyroidism relative to the TT_4 concentration.[28, 34, 93] Accordingly, measurement of the serum TT_3 level is a more sensitive test for the diagnosis of hyperthyroidism and that of TT_4 is more useful in the diagnosis of hypothyroidism.

Under some circumstances discrepancies between the serum TT_3 and TT_4 concentrations are either disproportionate or in opposite direction (Table 39–5). In such conditions the measurement of T_3 has been most useful. It has helped to explain the syndrome of thyrotoxicosis with normal TT_4 and FT_4 levels (T_3 thyrotoxicosis), and in some cases only the free T_3 may be elevated.[81, 94] In some patients with Graves' disease the treatment of thyrotoxicosis with antithyroid drugs may normalize the serum TT_4 but not TT_3 level, producing a high TT_3:TT_4 ratio. Such patients with T_3-predominant Graves' disease and TT_3:TT_4 >20 ng/μg are believed to be less prone to remission.[95] In areas of limited iodine supply[83] and in patients with limited thyroidal ability to process iodide,[82] euthyroidism can be maintained at low serum TT_4 and FT_4 levels by increased direct thyroidal secretion of T_3. Although these changes have a rational physiological explanation, the significance of discordant serum TT_4 and TT_3 levels under other circumstances is less well understood.

The most common cause of discordant serum concentrations of TT_3 and TT_4 is a selective decrease of serum TT_3 caused by decreased conversion of T_4 to T_3 in peripheral tissues. This reduction is an integral part of the pathophysiology of a number of nonthyroidal acute and chronic illnesses and calorie deprivation (see Ch. 40). In these conditions the serum TT_3 level often is lower than that commonly found in patients with frank primary hypothyroidism. Yet these people do not present clear clinical evidence of hypometabolism. In some people decreased T_4-to-T_3 conversion in the pituitary gland[96] or peripheral tissues[97] is an inherited condition.

Various drugs may also produce changes in the serum TT_3 concentration without apparent metabolic consequences (see below). Drugs that compete with hormone binding to serum proteins decrease serum TT_3 levels, presumably without affecting the FT_3 concentration (see Table 39–4). Some drugs, such as glucocorticoids,[98] depress the serum TT_3 concentration by interfering with the peripheral conversion of T_4 to T_3. Others, such as phenobarbital,[99] depress the serum TT_3 concentration by stimulating the rate of intracellular hormone degradation. Most have multiple effects that are combinations of those just described, and they also inhibit the hypothalamic-pituitary axis and thyroidal hormonogenesis.[100]

Changes in serum TBG concentration have an effect on the serum TT_3 concentration similar to that on TT_4 (see Ch. 36). The presence of endogenous antibodies to T_3 may result in an elevation of the serum TT_3, but as in the case of high TBG, the concentration of FT_3 is normal and does not cause hypermetabolism.[36]

Administration of commonly used replacement doses of T_3, usually in the order of 75 μg/day or 1 μg/kg body weight per day,[101] results in serum TT_3 levels in the thyrotoxic range. Furthermore, because of the rapid gastrointestinal absorption and relatively fast degradation rate, the serum level varies considerably according to the time of sampling in relation to hormone ingestion.[85]

Estimation of Free Thyroid Hormone Concentration

A minute amount of thyroid hormone circulates in the blood in a free form, not bound to serum proteins. It is in reversible equilibrium with the bound hormone and represents the diffusible fraction of the hormone capable of traversing cellular membranes to exert its effects on body tissues.[102] Although changes in serum hormone-binding proteins affect both the total hormone concentration and the corresponding fraction circulating free, in the euthyroid person the absolute concentration of free hormone remains constant. This finding is in agreement with the theoretical concept of hormone transfer from blood to tissue. It is thus not surprising that the concentration of free hormone in serum correlates better with the tissue hormone level and the metabolic status of the person.[103] Information concerning this value is probably the most important parameter in the evaluation of thyroid function because it relates to the metabolic status of the patient.

With few exceptions, the free hormone concentration is high in thyrotoxicosis, low in hypothyroidism, and normal in euthyroidism even in the presence of changes in TBG concentration,[104, 105] provided that the patient is in a steady state (see Fig. 36–4). Notably, FT_4 concentration may be normal or even low in patients with T_3 thyrotoxicosis and in those ingesting pharmacological doses of T_3. On occasion, the concentration of FT_4 may be outside the normal range in the absence of an apparent abnormality in the thyroid hormone–dependent metabolic status. This frequently is observed in severe nonthyroidal illness during which both high[104-106] and low[107, 108] values have been reported. As expected, when a euthyroid state is maintained by the administration of T_3 or by predominant thyroidal secretion of T_3, the FT_4 level is also depressed. More consistently, patients with a variety of nonthyroidal illnesses have

low FT_3 levels.[109] This decrease is characteristic of all conditions associated with depressed serum TT_3 concentrations caused by a diminished conversion of T_4 to T_3 in peripheral tissues (see Ch. 40). Both FT_4 and FT_3 values may be out of line in patients receiving a variety of drugs (see below). Marked elevations in both FT_4 and FT_3 concentrations in the absence of hypermetabolism are typical of patients with generalized resistance to thyroid hormone.[86] The FT_3 concentration usually is normal or even high in hypothyroid people living in areas of severe endemic iodine deficiency. Their FT_4 levels, however, are normal or low.[83]

Direct Measurement of FT_4 and FT_3

The precise measurements of the absolute FT_4 and FT_3 concentrations are technically difficult and until recently have been limited to research assays. To minimize perturbations of the relation between the free and bound hormone, these must be separated by ultrafiltration or by dialysis involving minimal dilution and little alteration of the pH or electrolyte composition. The separated free hormone is then measured directly in an RIA.[105] These assays are probably the most accurate available, but small, weakly bound dialyzable substances or drugs may be removed from the binding proteins, and the free hormone concentration measured in their presence may not fully reflect the free concentration in vivo. The broad normal range varies among laboratories and is between 0.8 and 2.7 ng/dl (10–35 pmol/L).

Isotopic Equilibrium Dialysis

Isotopic equilibrium dialysis has been the gold standard for the estimation of the FT_4 or FT_3 concentration for more than 30 years. It is based on the determination of the proportion of T_4 or T_3 that is unbound, or free, and is thus able to diffuse through a dialysis membrane (i.e., the dialyzable fraction [DF]). To carry out the test, a sample of serum is incubated with a tracer amount of labeled T_4 or T_3. The labeled tracer rapidly equilibrates with the respective bound and free endogenous hormones. The sample is then dialyzed against buffer at a constant temperature until the concentrations of free hormone on either side of the dialysis membrane have reached equilibrium. The DF is calculated from the proportion of labeled hormone in the dialysate. The contribution from radioiodide present as contaminant in the labeled tracer hormone should be eliminated by careful purification[106] and by various techniques of precipitation of the dialyzed hormone.[104, 110] FT_4 and FT_3 levels can be measured simultaneously by addition to the sample of T_4 and T_3 labeled with two different radioiodine isotopes.[54] Ultrafiltration is a modification of the dialysis technique.[106] Results are expressed as the fraction (DFT_4 or DFT_3) or percentage (%FT_4 or %FT_3) of the respective hormones that dialyzed, and the absolute concentrations of FT_4 and FT_3 are calculated from the product of the total concentration of the hormone in serum and its respective DF. Typical normal values for FT_4 in the adult range from 1 to 3 ng/dl (13–39 pmol/L) and for FT_3, from 0.25 to 0.65 ng/dl (3.8–10 nmol/L).

Results by these techniques are comparable to those determined with the direct methods but are more likely to differ with extremely low or extremely high TBG concentrations or in the presence of circulating inhibitors of protein binding.[111] The measured DF may be altered by the temperature at which the assay is run, the degree of dilution, the time allowed for equilibrium to be reached, and the composition of the diluting fluid.[112] The calculated value depends on an accurate measurement of total T_4 or T_3 and may be incorrect in patients with T_4 or T_3 autoantibodies.

Index Methods

Because the determination by isotopic equilibrium dialysis is cumbersome and technically demanding, most clinical laboratories have used a method by which an FT_4 index (FT_4I) or FT_3 index (FT_3I) is derived from the product of the TT_4 or TT_3 (determined by immunoassay) and a measurement of in vitro uptake (see below). Although not always in agreement with the values obtained by dialysis, these techniques are rapid and inexpensive. They are more likely to fail at extremely low or extremely high TBG concentrations, in the presence of abnormal binding proteins, in patients with nonthyroidal illness, or in the presence of circulating inhibitors of protein binding.

The theoretical contention that the FT_4I is an accurate estimate of the absolute FT_4 concentration can be confirmed by the linear correlation between these two parameters. This is true, provided that results of the in vitro uptake test (T_3U or T_4U) are expressed as the thyroid hormone–binding ratio, determined by dividing the tracer counts bound to the solid matrix by counts bound to serum proteins.[113] Values are corrected for assay variations using appropriate serum standards and are expressed as the ratio of a normal reference pool.[113, 114] The normal range is slightly narrower than the corresponding TT_4 in healthy euthyroid patients with a normal TBG concentration; it is 6.0 to 10.5 when calculated from TT_4 values measured by RIA and expressed in micrograms per deciliter. In thyrotoxicosis FT_4I is high and in hypothyroidism it is low irrespective of the TBG concentration. Euthyroid patients with TT_4 values outside the normal range as a result of TBG abnormalities have a normal FT_4I.[115] Lack of correlation between the FT_4I and the metabolic status of the patient has been observed under the same circumstances as those described for similar discrepancies when the FT_4 concentration was measured by dialysis.

Methods for the estimation of the FT_3I are also available[54, 116] but seldom are used in routine clinical evaluation of thyroid function. Like the FT_4I, it correlates well with the absolute FT_3 concentration. The test corrects for changes in TT_3 concentration secondary to variations in TBG concentration.

Estimation of FT_4 and FT_3 Based on TBG Measurements

Because most T_4 and T_3 are bound to TBG, FT_4I can be calculated from the affinity constant of T_4-binding to TBG and the molar concentrations of T_4 and TBG.[117] Similarly, FT_3I can be calculated from the affinity constant T_3-binding to TBG and the molar concentrations of T_3 and TBG.[118] A simpler calculation of the T_4:TBG and T_3:TBG ratios yields values that are similar to but less accurate than the FT_4I and FT_3I, respectively.[113]

Two-Step Immunoassays

In these assays the free hormone is first immunoextracted by a specific bound antibody (first step); the antibody frequently is fixed to the tube (coated tube).[119, 120] After washing, labeled tracer is added and binds to the unoccupied sites. The free hormone concentration will be inversely related to the antibody-bound tracer, and values are determined by comparison with a standard curve. Values obtained with this technique are comparable to those determined with the direct methods. They are more likely to differ in the presence of circulating inhibitors of protein binding and in sera from patients with nonthyroidal illness.

Analogue (One-Step) Immunoassays

In these assays a labeled analogue of T_4 or T_3 directly competes with the endogenous free hormone for binding by antibodies.[121] In theory, these analogues are not bound by the thyroid hormone–binding proteins in serum. Various studies, however, have found significant protein binding to the variant albumin-like protein,[103] to transthyretin, and to iodothyronine autoantibodies.[122] This results in discrepant values to other assays in a number of conditions, including nonthyroidal illness and pregnancy, and in people with FDH.[103] Commercial kits have been modified to minimize these problems, but their accuracy remains controversial.

In another method the antibody to which the labeled T_4 is attached is contained in nylon microcapsules through which FT_4 from the sample can penetrate (i.e., a form of dialysis). The displacement of the labeled T_4 from the antibody is proportional to the FT_4 concentration in the test sample of serum.[123]

Considerations in Selection of Methods for the Estimation of Free Thyroid Hormone Concentration

None of the available methods for the estimation of the free hormone concentration in serum are infallible in the evaluation of the thyroid hormone–dependent metabolic status. Each test possesses inherent advantages and disadvantages, depending on specific physiological and pathological circumstances. For example, methods based on the measurement of the total thyroid hormone and TBG concentrations cannot be used in patients with absent TBG caused by inherited TBG deficiency. Under such circumstances the concentration of free thyroid hormone depends on the interaction of the hormone with serum proteins that normally play a negligible role (TTR and albumin). When alterations of thyroid hormone binding do not equally affect T_4 and T_3, discrepant results of FT_4I are obtained when using labeled T_4 or T_3 in the in vitro uptake test. For example, euthyroid patients with the inherited albumin-like variant serum protein or having endogenous antibodies with greater affinity for T_4 will have high TT_4 but a normal T_3U test, which will result in an overestimation of the calculated FT_4I. In such instances calculation of the FT_4I from a T_4U test may provide more accurate results. Conversely, reduced overall binding affinity for T_4, which affects T_3 to a lesser extent, underestimates the FT_4I derived from a T_3U test. Similarly, use of the T_4U and T_3U for estimation of the free hormone concentration is satisfactory in the presence of alterations in TBG concentration but not alterations of the affinity of TBG for the hormone.[124, 125] A different range of normal values for free hormone indices must be established for each TBG variant with altered affinity for thyroid hormone to serve as means to correct for variations in TBG concentration. Methods based on dialyzable fractions of the hormones are most appropriate in the estimation of the free thyroid hormone level in patients with all varieties of abnormal binding to serum proteins, provided that the true concentration of total hormone has been accurately determined. Notwithstanding the in vivo experiments of Pardridge et al.,[126] all methods for the estimation of the FT_4 concentration may give either high or low values in patients with severe nonthyroidal illness who are believed to be euthyroid.[104–108, 127, 128] This has been attributed, at least in part, to the presence of inhibitors of thyroid hormone binding to serum proteins as well as to the various adsorbents used in the test procedures.[129, 130] Some of these inhibitors allegedly leak from the tissues of the diseased patient.[131, 132] Such discrepancies are even more pronounced during transient states of hyperthyroxinemia or hypothyroxinemia associated with acute illness, after withdrawal of treatment with thyroid hormone, and in acute changes in TBG concentration (see Chs. 36 and 40).

The contribution of various drugs that interfere with binding of thyroid hormone to serum proteins or with the in vitro tests should also be taken into account in the choice and interpretation of tests (see Table 39–4 and below). Although the free thyroid hormone concentration in serum seems to determine the amount of hormone available to body tissues, less well understood factors that govern its intracellular binding and metabolism may alter its action. For these reasons and because of technical problems, serum measurements of free hormone in serum occasionally need to be supplemented by tests that measure the effect of thyroid hormone and its pathway of intracellular metabolism. Bioassays that measure the amount of thyroid hormone entering the cell (bioavailable T_4)[133] may find clinical application in the future.

Measurement of Total and Unsaturated Thyroid Hormone–Binding Capacity in Serum

Because the concentration of thyroid hormone in serum depends on its supply as well as on the abundance of hormone-binding sites on serum proteins, the estimation of the latter is useful in the correct interpretation of values obtained from the measurement of the total hormone concentration. These results may be used to estimate the free hormone concentration, which is important in differentiating changes in serum total hormone concentration caused by alterations of binding proteins in euthyroid patients from those caused by abnormalities in thyroid gland activity giving rise to hypermetabolism or hypometabolism.

In Vitro Uptake Tests

In vitro uptake tests measure the unoccupied thyroid hormone–binding sites on TBG. They use labeled T_3 or T_4 and some form of synthetic absorbent to measure the pro-

portion of radiolabeled hormone that is not tightly bound to serum proteins. Because ion exchange resins often are used as absorbents, the test became known as the resin T_3 or T_4 uptake test (T_3U or T_4U), describing the technique rather than the entity measured. Sometimes this name has led to confusion with the in vivo iodine uptake test. Sometimes the T_3U test is referred to as the T_3 test. This name is inappropriate and should be reserved to indicate measurement of T_3 concentration.

The test usually is carried out by incubation of a sample of the patient's serum with a trace amount of RAI-labeled T_3 or T_4. The labeled hormone, not bound to available binding sites on TBG present in the serum sample, is absorbed onto an anion exchange resin and measured as resin-bound radioactivity. Values correlate inversely with the concentration of unsaturated TBG. Various methods use different absorbing materials to remove the hormone not tightly bound to TBG. The original test used red blood cells,[134] which were soon replaced by anion exchange resin in the form of beads or sponges.[135] Labeled T_3 usually is used because of its less firm yet preferential binding to TBG. Similar results can be obtained with T_4 after appropriate serum dilution and addition of T_4. The addition of barbital buffer allows selective binding of T_4 to TBG.[115] Irrespective of the materials used, the various assay requirements must be standardized and kept constant. Although the test is not affected by the presence of most nonhormonal iodine-containing compounds, it has been reported that Oragrafin[136] and, to a limited extent, heparin[137] increase the uptake of tracer by particular absorbents. Depending on the method, typical normal results for T_3U are 25 to 35 per cent or 45 to 55 per cent. Thus it is more valuable to express results of the uptake tests as a ratio of the result obtained in a normal control serum run in the same assay as the test samples. Normal values then range on either side of 1, usually 0.85 to 1.15.

The uptake of the tracer by the absorbent is inversely proportional to the amount of unsaturated binding sites (unoccupied by endogenous thyroid hormone) in serum TBG. Thus the uptake is increased when the amount of unsaturated TBG is reduced as a result of excess endogenous thyroid hormone or a decrease in the concentration of TBG. In contrast, the uptake is decreased when the amount of unsaturated TBG is increased as a result of a low serum thyroid hormone concentration or an increase in the concentration of TBG. As a rule, parallel increases or decreases in both serum TT_4 concentration and the T_3U test indicate hyperthyroidism or hypothyroidism, respectively, whereas discrepant changes in serum TT_4 and T_3U suggest abnormalities in TBG binding. Abnormalities in hormone and TBG concentrations may coexist in the same patient. For example, a hypothyroid patient with a low TBG level typically shows a low TT_4 level and normal T_3U result (Fig. 39–4). Several nonhormonal compounds caused by structural similarities compete with thyroid hormone for its binding site on TBG. Some are used as pharmacological agents and may thus alter the in vitro uptake test as well as the total thyroid hormone concentration in serum. A list is provided in Table 39–4.

TBG and TTR Measurements

The concentrations of TBG and TTR in serum can be either estimated by measurement of their total T_4-binding

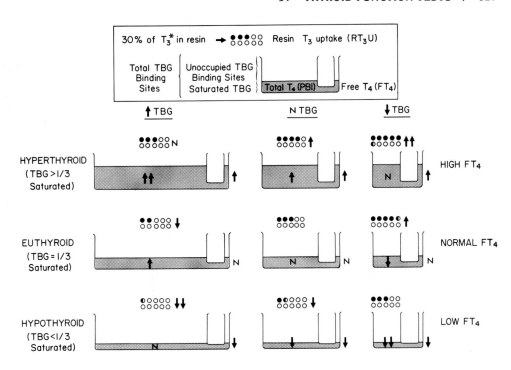

FIGURE 39–4. Graphic representation of the relation between the serum total T_4 concentration, the RT3U test, and the free T_4 (FT_4) concentration in various metabolic states and in association with changes in TBG. The principle of communicating vessels is used as an illustration. The height of fluid in the small vessel represents the level of FT_4; the total amount of fluid in the large vessel, the total T_4 concentration; and the total volume of the large vessel, the TBG capacity. Dots represent resin beads and black dots, those carrying the radioactive T_3 tracer (T_3*). The RT3U test result (black dots) is inversely proportional to the unoccupied TBG binding sites represented by the unfilled capacity of the large vessel.

capacity at saturation[138] or measured directly by immunological techniques.[139, 140] Although the saturation methods provide accurate information on the total binding capacity of individual carrier proteins, they are tedious. They are based on the partition of labeled T_4 among the carrier proteins in serum (TBG, TTR, and albumin) separated by electrophoresis and determined at several increments of added T_4. Values may vary according to the conditions of electrophoresis, in particular the type of buffer and pH. Generally accepted normal values in the adult are 14 to 27 µg T_4/dl serum (180–350 nmol/L) for TBG capacity and 220 to 360 µg T_4/dl serum (2.8–4.6 µmol/L) for TTR capacity. A simple saturation method, using anion exchange resin rather than electrophoresis, is available for routine use in clinical laboratories.[115]

Immunological methods for the direct measurement of the proteins are also available. TBG concentration in serum can be determined by RIA,[140] and both TBG and TTR can be measured by Laurell's rocket immunoelectrophoresis,[141, 142] by radial immunodiffusion,[143] or by enzyme immunoassay.[139] Another method combines hormone binding to TBG and immunological techniques.[144] Commercial kits are available for the quantitation of serum TBG that use, with various modifications, the technical principles described above. Some use a competitive partition of the radioiodinated hormone between endogenous TBG and added antiserum against the hormone; others use a specific TBG antiserum and T_4 or radioiodinated TBG as label. Absolute concentrations in the serum of normal adults vary according to the purity of the standard preparation. The true mean value for TBG is 1.6 mg/dl (260 nmol/L), with a range of 1.1 to 2.2 mg/dl (180–350 nmol/L) serum. In adults the normal range for TTR is 16 to 30 mg/dl (2.7–5.0 µmol/L).

The concentrations of TBG and TTR in serum vary with age, sex, pregnancy, and posture (see Ch. 36). Determination of the concentration of these proteins in serum is particularly helpful in the evaluation of extreme deviations from normal, as in congenital abnormalities of TBG. In most instances the in vitro uptake test, in conjunction with the serum TT_4 level, gives an estimation of the TBG concentration. A numerical value can be derived from the ratio of the T_3U test expressed as a percentage of the normal control and the serum TT_4, known as the TBG index.[145]

Measurements of Iodine-Containing Hormone Precursors and Products of Degradation

RIA's have been developed for the measurement of a number of naturally occurring iodine-containing substances that possess little, if any, thyromimetic activity. Some of these substances are products of T_4 and T_3 degradation in peripheral tissues. Others are predominantly, if not exclusively, of thyroidal origin. Because they are devoid of significant metabolic activity, measurement of their concentration is of value only in detecting abnormalities in the metabolism of thyroid hormone in peripheral tissues as well as defects of hormone synthesis and secretion. Such knowledge often is helpful in defining the cause of some thyroid illnesses or hormonal imbalance. They may be collectively viewed as diagnostic markers.

3,3',5'-Triiodothyronine or Reverse T_3

Reverse T_3 (rT_3) is principally a product of T_4 degradation in peripheral tissues (see Ch. 36). It is also secreted by the thyroid gland, but the amounts are practically insignificant.[146] Thus measurement of its concentration in serum reflects both tissue supply and metabolism of T_4 and identifies conditions that favor this particular pathway of T_4 degradation.

When total rT_3 (TrT_3) is measured in unextracted serum, a competitor of rT_3 binding to serum proteins must be added.[147] Several chemically related compounds may cross-react with the antibodies. The strongest cross-reactivity is observed with 3,3'-diiodothyronine (3,3'-T$_2$) but because of its relatively low levels in human serum, it does not present a serious methodological problem. Although of lesser cross-reactivity, T$_3$ and T$_4$ are more often the cause of rT$_3$ overestimation because of their relative abundance, particularly in thyrotoxicosis.[148] Free fatty acids interfere with the measurement of rT$_3$ by RIA.[149]

The normal range in adult serum for TrT$_3$ is 14 to 30 ng/dl (0.22–0.46 nmol/L), although values ranging from 25 to 65 ng/dl have been reported.[109, 146, 147, 150, 151] It is elevated in subjects with high TBG and in some people with FDH.[152] Serum TrT$_3$ levels are normal in hypothyroid patients treated with T$_4$, indicating that peripheral T$_4$ metabolism is an important source of circulating rT$_3$.[146, 153] Values are high in thyrotoxicosis and low in untreated hypothyroidism. High values are normally found in cord blood and in neonates.[153, 154]

It has been clearly demonstrated that with only a few exceptions, notably uremia, serum TrT$_3$ concentrations are elevated in all circumstances that cause low serum T$_3$ levels in the absence of obvious clinical signs of hypothyroidism. These conditions include, in addition to the neonatal period, various acute and chronic nonthyroidal illnesses,[151] calorie deprivation, and the influence of a growing list of clinical agents and drugs (Table 39–6). Clinical application of TrT$_3$ measurement in serum is in the differential diagnosis of conditions associated with alterations in serum T$_3$ and T$_4$ concentrations when thyroid gland and metabolic abnormalities are not readily apparent.

The dialyzable fraction of rT$_3$ in normal adult serum is 0.2 to 0.32 per cent, or about the same as that of T$_3$. The corresponding serum FrT$_3$ concentration is 50 to 100 pg/dl (0.77–1.5 pmol/L). In the absence of gross TBG abnormalities, variations in serum FrT$_3$ concentration closely follow those of TrT$_3$.[109]

3,5-Diiodothyronine

The normal adult range for total 3,5-diiodothyronine (3,5-T$_2$) in serum measured by direct RIA's is 0.20 to 0.75

TABLE 39–6. AGENTS THAT ALTER THE EXTRATHYROIDAL METABOLISM OF THYROID HORMONE

SUBSTANCE	COMMON USE
Inhibit Conversion of T$_4$ to T$_3$	
PTU[155-157]	Antithyroid
Glucocorticoids (hydrocortisone, prednisone, dexamethasone)[98, 158]	Anti-inflammatory and immunosuppressive; decrease intracranial pressure
Propranolol[159, 160]	Adrenergic blocker (anti-arrhythmic, antihypertensive)
Iodinated contrast agents: ipodate (Oragrafin), iopanoic acid (Telepaque)[161, 162]	Radiological contrast media
Amiodarone[163, 164]	Anti-anginal and antiarrhythmic
Clomipramine[165]	Tricyclic antidepressant
Stimulators of Hormone Degradation or Fecal Excretion	
Diphenylhydantoin[166-168]	Anticonvulsive and anti-arrhythmic
Carbamazepine[168]	Anticonvulsant
Phenobarbital[99, 168]	Hypnotic, tranquilizing and anticonvulsive
Cholestyramine[169] and colestipol[170]	Hypolipidemic resins
Soybeans[171, 172]	Diet
Rifampin[173]	Antituberculosis drug

ng/dl (3.8–14 pmol/L).[174] That 3,5-T$_2$ is derived from T$_3$ is supported by the observations that conditions associated with high and low serum T$_3$ levels have elevated and reduced serum concentrations of 3,5-T$_2$, respectively.[175] Thus high serum 3,5-T$_2$ levels have been reported in hyperthyroidism and low levels, in the serum of hypothyroid patients and neonates, during fasting, and in patients with liver cirrhosis.

3,3'-Diiodothyronine

Normal concentrations of 3,3' diiodothyronine (3,3'-T$_2$) in adults probably range from 1 to 8 ng/dl (19–150 pmol/L).[51, 176] Levels are clearly elevated in hyperthyroidism and in the neonate.[151] Values have been found to be either normal or depressed in nonthyroidal illnesses,[151, 176] in agreement with the demonstration of reduced monodeiodination of rT$_3$ to 3,3'-T$_2$.[177] In vivo turnover kinetic studies and measurement of 3,3'-T$_2$ in serum after the administration of T$_3$ and rT$_3$ have clearly shown that 3,3'-T$_2$ is the principal metabolic product of these two triiodothyronines.

3',5'-Diiodothyronine

Reported concentrations of 3',5'-diiodothyronine (3',5'-T$_2$) in serum of normal adults have a mean overall range of 1.5 to 9.0 ng/dl (30 to 170 pmol/L).[51, 151, 176, 178, 179] Values are high in hyperthyroidism and in the neonate.[178, 179] Administration of dexamethasone also produces an increase in the serum 3',5'-T$_2$ level.[178] Being the derivative of rT$_3$ monodeiodination,[178] 3',5'-T$_2$ levels are elevated in serum during fasting[179, 180] and in nonthyroidal illnesses[153] in which the level of the rT$_3$ precursor is also high.

3'-Monoiodothyronine

The concentration of 3'-monoiodothyronine (3'-T$_1$) in serum of normal adults, measured by RIA, has been reported to range from 0.6 to 2.3 ng/dl (15 to 58 pmol/L)[153] and from <0.9 to 6.8 ng/dl (<20 to 170 pmol/L).[151] The cross-reactants in the RIA are its two immediate precursors, 3,3'-T$_2$ and 3',5'-T$_2$. Serum levels are very high in hyperthyroidism and low in hypothyroidism. The concentration of 3'-T$_1$ in serum is elevated in all conditions associated with high rT$_3$ levels, including nonthyroidal illness and fasting, as well as in neonates.[151, 154] This finding is not surprising because the immediate precursor at 3'-T$_1$ is 3',5'-T$_2$,[181] a product of rT$_3$ deiodination, which is also present in serum in high concentration under the same circumstances. The elevated serum levels of 3'-T$_1$ in renal failure are attributed to decreased clearance because the concentrations of its precursors are not increased.[151]

3-Monoiodothyronine

Experience with the measurement of 3-monoiodothyronine (3-T$_1$) in serum is limited. Normal values in serum of adult humans using ^{3}H-labeled 3-T$_1$ in a specific RIA ranged from <0.5 to 7.5 ng/dl (<13 to 190 pmol/L).[182] The mean concentration of 3-T$_1$ in serum of thyrotoxic patients and in cord blood was significantly higher. 3-T$_1$ appears to be a product of in vivo deiodination of 3,3'-T$_2$.

Tetraiodothyroacetic Acid and Triiodothyroacetic Acid

The iodoamino acids T_4A and T_3A, products of deamination and oxidative decarboxylation of T_4 and T_3, respectively, have been detected in serum by direct RIA measurements.[20, 97, 183] Reported mean concentrations in the serum of healthy adults have been 8.7 ng/dl[183] and 2.6 ng/dl (range, 1.6 to 3.0 ng/dl or 26 to 48 pmol/L)[20] for T_3A and 28 ng/dl (range <8 to 60 mg/dl or <105 to 800 pmol/L)[97] for T_4A. Serum T_4A levels are reduced during fasting and in patients with severe illness,[184] although the percentage of conversion of T_4 to T_4A is increased.[19, 185] The concentration of serum T_3A remains unchanged during the administration of replacement doses of T_4 and T_3.[20] It has been suggested that intracellular rerouting of T_3 to T_3A during fasting is responsible for the maintenance of normal serum TSH levels in the presence of low T_3 concentrations.[186]

Diiodotyrosine and Monoiodotyrosine

Although RIA's for the measurement of DIT and MIT in serum have been developed, because of limited experience their value in clinical practice remains unknown. Early reports gave a normal mean value for DIT in serum of normal adults of 156 ng/dl (3.6 nmol/L),[187] with progressive decline resulting from refinement of techniques to values as low as 7 ng/dl with a range of 1 to 23 ng/dl (0.02 to 0.5 nmol/L).[188] Thus the normal range for MIT of 90 to 390 ng/dl (2.9 to 12.7 nmol/L)[189] is undoubtedly an overestimation. Iodotyrosine that has escaped enzymatic deiodination in the thyroid gland appears to be the principal source of DIT in serum. Iodothyronine degradation in peripheral tissues is probably a minor source of iodotyrosines because administration of large doses of T_4 to normal subjects produces a decline rather than an increase in the serum DIT level.[188] DIT is metabolized to MIT in peripheral tissues. Serum levels of DIT are low during pregnancy and high in cord blood.

Thyroglobulin

RIA methods are now used routinely for measurement of Tg in serum.[190, 191] They are specific and, depending on the sensitivity of the assay, capable of detecting Tg in the serum of about 90 per cent of the euthyroid healthy adults. When antisera are used in high dilutions, there is virtually no cross-reactivity with iodothyronines or iodotyrosines. Results obtained from the analysis of sera containing Tg autoantibodies are inaccurate, limiting the applicability of the assay.[191] Thus interpretation of the test requires prior screening for the presence of such autoantibodies. The presence of thyroid peroxidase antibodies does not interfere with the Tg RIA.

Tg concentration in serum of normal adults ranges from <1 to 25 ng/ml (<1.5 to 38 pmol/L), with mean levels of 5 to 10 ng/ml.[190, 192–194] On a molar basis these concentrations of Tg are minute relative to the circulating iodothyronines, 5000-fold lower than the corresponding concentration of T_4 in serum. Values tend to be slightly higher in women than in men.[190] In the neonatal period and during the third trimester of pregnancy, mean values are about fourfold and twofold higher.[193, 195] They gradually decline throughout infancy, childhood, and adolescence.[196] The

positive correlation between the levels of serum Tg and TSH indicates that pituitary TSH regulates the secretion of Tg.

Elevated serum Tg levels reflect increased secretory activity by stimulation of the thyroid gland or damage to thyroid tissue, whereas values below or at the level of detectability indicate a paucity of thyroid tissue or suppressed activity. Tg levels in a variety of conditions that affect the thyroid gland have been reviewed[197] and are listed in Table 39–7.

Interpretation of a serum Tg value should take into account the fact that Tg concentrations may be high under normal physiological conditions or altered by drugs. Administration of iodine and antithyroid drugs increase the serum Tg level, as do states associated with hyperstimulation of the thyroid gland by TSH or other substances with thyroid-stimulating activity. This is caused by increased thyroidal release of Tg rather than by changes in its clearance.[198] Administration of TRH and TSH also transiently increases the serum level of Tg.[199] Trauma to the thyroid gland, such as that occurring during diagnostic and therapeutic procedures, including percutaneous needle biopsy, surgery, and ^{131}I therapy, can produce a striking, although short-lived, elevation in the Tg level in serum.[193, 200, 201] Pathological processes with destructive effect on the thyroid gland also produce transient, although more prolonged, increases.[202] Tg is undetectable in serum after total ablation of the thyroid gland as well as in normal people who receive suppressive doses of thyroid hormone.[197] It is thus a useful test in the differential diagnosis of thyrotoxicosis factitia,[203] especially when transient thyrotoxicosis with a low RAIU or suppression of thyroidal RAIU by iodine are alternative possibilities.

TABLE 39–7. CONDITIONS ASSOCIATED WITH CHANGES IN SERUM Tg CONCENTRATION LISTED ACCORDING TO THE PRESUMED MECHANISM

INCREASED

TSH-Mediated
Acute and transient (TSH and TRH administration, neonatal period)
Chronic stimulation
   Iodine deficiency, endemic goiter, goitrogens
   Reduce thyroidal reserve (lingual thyroid)
   TSH-producing pituitary adenoma
   Resistance to thyroid hormone
   TBG deficiency

Non–TSH-Mediated
Thyroid stimulators
   IgG (Graves' disease)
   hCG (trophoblastic disease)
Trauma to the thyroid (needle aspiration and surgery of the thyroid gland, ^{131}I therapy)
Destructive thyroid pathology
   Subacute thyroiditis
   Painless thyroiditis
   Postpartum thyroiditis
Abnormal release
   Thyroid nodules (toxic, nontoxic, multinodular goiter)
   Differentiated nonmedullary thyroid carcinoma
Abnormal clearance (renal failure)

DECREASED

TSH Suppression
Administration of thyroid hormone

Decreased Synthesis
Athyreosis (postoperative, congenital)
Tg synthesis defect

The most striking elevations in serum Tg concentrations have been observed in patients with metastatic differentiated nonmedullary thyroid carcinoma even after total surgical and radioiodide ablation of all normal thyroid tissue.[193, 204] It usually persists despite full thyroid hormone suppressive therapy, suggesting excessive autonomous release of Tg by the neoplastic cells. The determination is thus of particular value in the follow-up and management of metastatic thyroid carcinomas, particularly when they fail to concentrate radioiodide.[192, 204] Follow-up of such patients with sequential serum Tg determinations helps the early detection of tumor recurrence or growth and the assessment of treatment effect. Measurement of serum Tg is also useful in patients with metastases, particularly to bone, in whom there is no evidence of a primary site and thyroid cancer is being considered in the differential diagnosis.[193, 204] On the other hand, serum Tg levels are of no value in the differential diagnosis of primary thyroid cancer because levels may be within the normal range in the presence of differentiated thyroid cancer and high in a variety of benign thyroid nodules.[192, 194, 204] Whether early detection of recurrent thyroid cancer after initial ablative therapy could be achieved by serum Tg measurement without cessation of hormone replacement therapy is still debatable.[205–207] The problem stems from the fact that Tg secretion by the tumor is modulated by TSH and could be suppressed by the administration of thyroid hormone.[205, 207]

Tg levels are high in the early phase of subacute thyroiditis.[202] Declining serum Tg levels during the course of antithyroid drug treatment of patients with Graves' disease may indicate the onset of a remission.[201, 208] Tg may be undetectable in the serum of neonates with dyshormonogenetic goiters caused by defects in Tg synthesis,[209] but levels are very high in some hypothyroid infants with thyromegaly or ectopic gland.[210] Measurement of serum Tg in hypothyroid neonates is useful in the differentiation of infants with complete thyroid agenesis from those with hypothyroidism resulting from other causes and, thus, in most cases obviates the need for the diagnostic administration of radioiodide.[210, 211]

MEASUREMENT OF THYROID HORMONE AND ITS METABOLITES IN OTHER BODY FLUIDS AND IN TISSUES

Clinical experience with measurement of thyroid hormone and its metabolites in body fluids other than serum and in tissues is limited for several reasons. Analyses carried out in urine and saliva do not appear to give additional information to that obtained from measurements carried out in serum. Amniotic fluid (AF), cerebrospinal fluid (CSF), and tissues are less readily accessible for sampling. Their likely application in the future will depend on information they could provide beyond that obtained from similar analyses in serum.

Urine

Because thyroid hormone is filtered in the urine predominantly in free form, measurement of the total amount excreted over 24 hours offers an indirect method for the estimation of the free hormone concentration in serum. The 24-hour excretion of T_4 in normal adults ranges from 4 to 13 μg and from 1.8 to 3.7 μg, depending on whether total or only conjugated T_4 is measured. Corresponding normal ranges for T_3 are 2 to 4 μg and 0.4 to 1.9 μg.[212–214] Striking seasonal variations have been shown for the urinary excretion of both hormones, with a nadir during the hot summer months, in the absence of significant changes in serum TT_4 and TT_3. As expected, values are normal in pregnancy and nonthyroidal illnesses, high in thyrotoxicosis, and low in hypothyroidism.[35, 213, 214] The test may not be valid in the presence of gross proteinuria and impairment of renal function.[215]

Amniotic Fluid

All iodothyronines measured in blood have also been detected in AF. With the exception of T_3, $3,3'-T_2$, and $3'-T_2$, the concentration at term is lower than that in cord serum.[178, 179, 181, 216–218] This fact cannot be fully explained by the low TBG concentration in AF. Although the source of iodothyronines in AF is unknown, the general pattern more closely resembles that found in the fetal than in the maternal circulation.

The TT_4 concentration in AF averages 0.5 μg/dl (65 nmol/L) with a range of 0.15 to 1.0 μg/dl and is thus very low when compared with values in maternal and cord serum.[216–218] The FT_4 concentration is, however, twice as high in AF relative to serum. The TT_3 concentration also is low relative to maternal serum, being on the average 30 ng/dl (0.46 nmol/L) in both AF and cord serum.[218] rT_3, on the other hand, is very high in AF—on average 330 ng/dl (5.1 nmol/L) during the first half of gestation—declining precipitously at about the 30th week of gestation to an average of 85 ng/dl (1.3 nmol/L), which is also found at term.[217, 218]

Cerebrospinal Fluid

T_4, T_3, and rT_3 concentrations have been measured in human CSF.[219–221] The concentrations of both TT_4 and TT_3 are about 50-fold lower than those found in serum. However, the free concentrations are similar to those in serum. In contrast, the level of TrT_3 in CSF is only 2.5-fold lower than that in serum, whereas that of FrT_3 is 25-fold higher. All the thyroid hormone–binding proteins present in serum are also found in CSF, although in lower concentrations.[220] The concentrations of TT_4 and FT_4 are increased in thyrotoxicosis and depressed in hypothyroidism. Severe nonthyroidal illness gives rise to increased TrT_3 and FrT_3 levels.[221]

Milk

TT_4 concentration in human milk is of the order of 0.03 to 0.5 μg/dl.[222] Analytical artefacts were responsible for the much higher values formerly reported.[222, 223] TT_3 concentrations range from 10 to 200 ng/dl (0.15 to 3.1 nmol/L).[223, 224] The concentration of TrT_3 ranges from 1 to 30 ng/dl (15 to 460 pmol/L).[223] Thus it is unlikely that milk would provide a sufficient quantity of thyroid hormone to alleviate hypothyroidism in the infant.

Saliva

It has been suggested that only the free fraction of small nonpeptide hormones that circulate predominantly bound to serum proteins would be transferred to saliva and that their measurement in this easily accessible body fluid would provide a simple and direct means to determine their free concentration in blood. This hypothesis was confirmed for steroid hormones[225] not tightly bound to serum proteins. Levels of T_4 in saliva range from 4.2 to 35 ng/dl (54 to 450 pmol/L) and do not correlate with the concentration of free T_4 in serum.[226] This finding is in part a result of the transfer of T_4 bound to the small but variable amounts of serum proteins that reach the saliva.

Effusions

TT_4 measured in fluid obtained from serous cavities bears a direct relation to the protein content and the serum concentration of T_4. Limited experience with Tg measurement in pleural effusions from patients with thyroid cancer metastatic to lungs suggests that it may be of diagnostic value.[204]

Tissues

Because the response to thyroid hormone is expressed at the cell level, it is logical to assume that hormone concentration in tissues should correlate best with its action. Methods for extraction, recovery, and measurement of iodothyronines from tissues have been developed, but for obvious reasons data from thyroid hormone measurements in human tissues are limited. Preliminary work has shown that under several circumstances, hormonal levels in tissues such as liver, kidneys, and muscle usually correlate with those found in serum.[227]

Measurements of T_3 in cells most accessible for sampling in humans—red blood cells—gave values of 20 to 45 ng/dl (0.31 to 0.69 nmol/L), or one fourth those found in serum.[228] They are higher in thyrotoxicosis and lower in hypothyroidism.

The concentrations of all iodothyronines have been measured in thyroid gland hydrolysates.[17, 153, 178] In normal glands the molar ratios relative to the concentration of T_4 are, on average, as follows: $T_4{:}T_3 = 10$; $T_4{:}rT_3 = 80$; $T_4{:}3{,}5'{-}T_2 = 1400$; $T_4{:}3{,}3'{-}T_2 = 350$; $T_4{:}3'{,}5'{-}T_2 = 1100$; and $T_4{:}3'{-}T_1 = 4400$. Information concerning the content of iodothyronines in hydrolysates of abnormal thyroid tissue is limited, and the diagnostic value of such measurements has not been established.

TESTS THAT ASSESS THE EFFECTS OF THYROID HORMONE ON BODY TISSUES

Thyroid hormone exerts its effect through the regulation of various biochemical reactions in virtually all tissues.

Thus, ideally, the adequacy of hormonal supply should be assessed by the tissue responses rather than by parameters of thyroid gland activity or serum hormone concentration, which are several steps removed from the site of thyroid hormone action. The tissue responses (metabolic indices) that are easily measured are nonspecific because of their alteration by various physiological and pathological mechanisms unrelated to thyroid hormone deprivation or excess. For this reason these tests have been replaced by direct measurements of thyroid gland activity and hormone concentration in serum that provide greater sensitivity, specificity, and diagnostic accuracy. Yet none of the specific tests are true substitutes for tests that measure metabolic and biochemical responses of tissues to thyroid hormone. Although mild degrees of thyroid dysfunction may be measured by alterations in the serum concentration of TSH or the TSH response to TRH, it is uncertain whether the pituitary threshold of response to the hormonal supply reflects the status of other tissues. Furthermore, in certain conditions, serum TSH levels may be elevated to maintain a normal hormone supply to peripheral tissue. Similar reasoning, backed by concrete examples, could be used to depreciate the reliance on tests measuring thyroid hormone concentration in serum. In practice such arguments do not improve the reliability of available tests of hormone action. As a consequence they are primarily used as confirmatory tests in patients with unusual or uncertain diagnoses.

The following review of biochemical and physiological changes mediated by thyroid hormone has a dual purpose: to review some of the changes that may be used as clinical tests in the evaluation of the metabolic status and to point out the changes in various determinations commonly used in the diagnosis of a variety of nonthyroidal illnesses, which may be affected by the concomitant presence of thyroid hormone deficiency or excess.

Basal Metabolic Rate

The basal metabolic rate (BMR) has a long history in the evaluation of thyroid function. It measures the oxygen consumption under basal conditions of overnight fast and rest from mental and physical exertion. Because standard equipment for the measurement of BMR may not be readily available, it can be estimated from the oxygen consumed over a timed interval by analysis of samples of expired air.[229] The test indirectly measures metabolic energy expenditure or heat production.

Results are expressed as the percentage of deviation from normal after appropriate corrections have been made for age, sex, and body surface area. Low values are suggestive of hypothyroidism, and high values reflect thyrotoxicosis. The various nonthyroidal illnesses and other factors that affect the BMR, including sources of errors, have been reviewed.[230] Although this test is no longer part of the routine diagnostic armamentarium, it is still useful in research and in the evaluation of patients suspected of having resistance to thyroid hormone.[86]

Deep Tendon Reflex Relaxation Time (Photomotography)

A delay in the relaxation time of the deep tendon reflexes, visible to the experienced eye, occurs in hypothyroidism. Several instruments have been devised to quantitate various phases of the Achilles tendon reflex. Although normal values vary according to the phase of the tendon reflex measured, the apparatus used, and individual laboratory standards, the approximate adult normal range for the half-relaxation time is 230 to 390 msec. Diurnal variation, differences with sex, and changes with age, cold exposure, fever, exercise, obesity, and pregnancy have been reported. The main reason for the failure of this test as a diagnostic measure of thyroid dysfunction is the large overlap with values obtained in euthyroid patients and alterations caused by nonthyroidal illnesses.[231] These illnesses include myotonic disorders, pernicious anemia, diabetes mellitus, uremia, neurosyphilis, Parkinson's disease, sarcoidosis, local edema, and psychiatric disorders. Also, hypoglycemia and the administration of glucose, epinephrine, reserpine, β-adrenergic blockers, potassium, and large doses of salicylates, amphetamines, glucocorticoids, and estrogens cause alterations in the relaxation time.[231] The test is of little value in the diagnosis of thyrotoxicosis and is less reliable in the diagnosis of hypothyroidism in children than in adults. It has no value in cases of mild hypothyroidism.

Tests Related to Cardiovascular Function

Thyroid hormone–induced changes in the cardiovascular system can be measured by noninvasive techniques. One such test measures the time interval between the onset of the electrocardiographic QRS complex (Q) and the arrival of the pulse wave at the brachial artery, detected by the Korotkoff sound (K) at the antecubital fossa. This QK interval can be measured at various cuff pressures from systolic (QKs) to diastolic (QKd), the latter being more commonly used.[232] Normal adult values for QKd range from 185 to 235 msec. It is shorter in thyrotoxicosis and prolonged in hypothyroidism, but changes also occur with age and after exercise. Related tests that determine the systolic time interval (STI) measure the pre-ejection period (PEP), obtained by subtraction of the left ventricular ejection time (LVET) from the total electromechanical systole (Q-A₂).[233] The left ventricular shortening fraction (LVET), which is also affected by the thyroid status, can be measured by M-mode echocardiography.[234] As with other tests of thyroid hormone action, the principal deficiency of these measurements is their alteration in various nonthyroidal illnesses. These conditions include high-output states such as acute febrile illnesses or anemia, pheochromocytoma, aortic valvular stenosis, and ventricular conduction defects. Drugs such as epinephrine and β-adrenergic blocking agents also affect the test results.

Miscellaneous Biochemical and Physiological Changes Related to the Action of Thyroid Hormone on Peripheral Tissues

Thyroid hormone affects the function of various peripheral tissues. Thus hormone deficiency or excess may alter a number of determinations used in the diagnosis of illnesses unrelated to thyroid hormone dysfunction. Knowledge of the determinations that may be affected by thyroid hormone is important in the interpretation of laboratory data (Table 39–8).

MEASUREMENT OF SUBSTANCES ABSENT IN NORMAL SERUM

Tests that measure substances present in the circulation only under pathological circumstances do not provide information on the level of thyroid gland function. They are of value in establishing the cause of the hormonal dysfunction or thyroid gland pathology.

Thyroid Autoantibodies

Humoral antithyroid antibodies most commonly measured in clinical practice are directed against Tg or thyroid cell microsomal (MC) proteins. The latter is principally represented by the thyroid peroxidase (TPO).[333–335] Assays have recently been developed that use purified and recombinant TPO.[336] Other circulating immunoglobulins, which are less frequently used as diagnostic markers, are those directed against a colloid antigen, T₄ and T₃. Antibodies against nuclear components are not tissue-specific. Immunoglobulins that possess the property of stimulating the thyroid gland are discussed in the next section.

Various techniques are available for the measurement of Tg and MC antibodies. These procedures include a precipitation reaction, the Ouchterlony diffusion technique, immunoelectro-osmophoresis, cytotoxic assay, competitive binding radioassay, complement fixation reaction,[337] tanned red cell agglutination assay,[338] the Coon's immunofluorescent technique,[339] and ELISA.[336, 340] Although the competitive binding radioassay[341, 342] appears to be the most sensitive of these tests, the new-generation agglutination methods best combine sensitivity and simplicity and have found the widest clinical application. Current commercial kits use synthetic beads rather than red cells.

In the assay of Tg and MC antibodies by hemagglutination (TgHA and MCHA), particulate material is coated with either human Tg or solubilized thyroid MC proteins (TPO) and exposed to serial dilutions of the patient's serum. Agglutination of the coated particulates occurs in the presence of antibodies specific to the antigen attached to their cell surface. Results are expressed in terms of the highest serum dilution, or titer, showing persistent agglutination. The presence of immune complexes, particularly in patients with high serum Tg levels, may mask the presence of Tg antibodies. Assays for the measurement of such Tg–anti-Tg immune complexes have been developed.[343]

The test response normally is negative, but results may be positive in up to 10 per cent of the adult population. The frequency of positive test results is higher in women and with advancing age. The presence of thyroid autoantibodies in the apparently healthy population is thought to represent subclinical autoimmune thyroid disease rather than false-positive reactions. TPO antibodies are detectable in about 95 per cent of patients with Hashimoto's thyroiditis and 85 per cent of those with Graves' disease, irrespective of the functional state of the thyroid gland. Similarly, Tg antibodies are positive in about 60 and 30 per cent of

TABLE 39–8. BIOCHEMICAL AND PHYSIOLOGICAL CHANGES RELATED TO THYROID HORMONE DEFICIENCY AND EXCESS

ENTITY MEASURED	DURING HYPOTHYROIDISM	DURING THYROTOXICOSIS
Metabolism of various substances and drugs		
Fractional turnover rate (antipyrine,[235] dipyrone,[236] PTU, and methimazole,[235] albumin,[237] low-density lipoproteins,[238] cortisol,[239, 240] and Fe[241, 242])	↓	↑
Serum		
Amino acids		
Tyrosine (fasting level and afterload)[243, 244]	↓	↑
Glutamic acid[243]	N	↑
Proteins		
Albumin[245]	↓	↓
Sex hormone–binding globulin[13, 246, 247]	↓	↑↑
Ferritin[248, 249]	↓	↑
Low-density lipoproteins[238]	↓	↑
Fibronectin[250]		↑
Factor VIII–related antigen[250]		↑
Tissue plasminogen activator[250]		↑
TBG[115]	↑	
TBPA[55]	N	↓
Hormones		
Insulin		
Response to glucose[251]	↓	↓
Response to glucagon[252]	↑	↓
Estradiol-17β,[253] testosterone,[13, 246, 253] and gastrin[254]	↓ or N	↑
Parathyroid hormone concentration[255, 256]	↑	↓
Response to PTH administration[256]	↓	↑
Calcitonin[257]	↓	↑
Calcitonin response to Ca²⁺ infusion[258]	↓	
Renin activity and aldosterone[259, 260]	↓	↑
Catecholamines[261] and noradrenaline[262]	↑	↓
Atrial naturetic peptide[263, 264]	↓	↑
Erythropoietin[242]	N or ↓	↑
LH[253]		N or ↑
Response to GnRH[265]	↑	N
Prolactin and response to stimulation with TRH, arginine, and chlorpromazine[266, 267]	↑ or N	↓
Growth hormone		
Response to insulin[268, 269]	↓	N or ↓
Response to TRH[270]		No change
Epidermal growth factor[271]	N	↑
Enzymes		
Creatine phosphokinase,[272, 273] lactic dehydrogenase,[273] and glutamic oxaloacetic transaminase[273]	↑	↓
Adenylate kinase[274]	N	
Dopamine β-hydroxylase[275]	↑	↓
Alkaline phosphatase[256, 276]	↓ *	↑
Malic dehydrogenase[277]	↑↑	↑
Angiotensin-converting enzyme,[250, 278] alanine aminotransferase,[279] and glutathione S-transferase[279, 280]	N	↑
Coenzyme Q₁₀[281]		↓
Others		
1,25,OH-vitamin D₃[282]	↑	N or ↓
Carotene, vitamin A[283]	↑	↓
cAMP,[284] cGMP,[285] and Fe[241, 286]	N or ↓	N or ↑
K[287]		↓
Na[288]	↓	
Mg[289]	↑	↓
Ca[256, 290]	↓	↑
P[255, 256]		↑
Glucose		
Concentration[252, 268]	↓	↑
Fractional turnover during IV tolerance test[251]	↓	
Insulin hypoglycemia[268]	prolonged	
Bilirubin[291, 292]	↑†	↑
Creatinine[293]	N or ↑	↓
Creatine[293]	N or ↑	↑
Cholesterol,[283, 294] carotene,[283, 294] phospholipids and lethicin,[283, 294] and triglycerides[294, 295]	↑	↓

ENTITY MEASURED	DURING HYPOTHYROIDISM	DURING THYROTOXICOSIS
Lipoprotein*[296]	↑	↓
Apolipoprotein B[296]	↑	↓
Type IV collagen[297]	↓	↓
Type III Pro-collagen[297]	↓	↑
Free fatty acids[298]		↑
Carcinoembryonic antigen[299]	↑	
Osteocalcin[257]	↓	↑
Urine		
cAMP[300]	↓	↑
after epinephrine infusion[301]	No change	↑
cGMP[285]	N or ↓	↑
Mg[289]	↓	↑
Creatinine[293]	N	↓
Creatine[293]	N	↑↑
Tyrosine[244]	N or ↓	↑↑
MIT (after) administration of ¹³¹IMIT[302]		
Glutamic acid[244]	N	↑↑
Taurine[303]	↓	
Carnitine[304]	↓	
Tyramine, tryptamine, and histamine[305]		↑
17-hydroxycorticoids and ketogenic steroids[306]	↓	↑
Pyridinoline (PYD), deoxypyridinoline (DPD)[307]		↑
Hydroxyproline[308] and hydroxylysyl glycoside[309]		↑
Red blood cells		
Fe[241, 286]	↓	↑
Na[310]	N	↑
Zn[311]	N	↓
Hemoglobin[241, 286]	↓	↓
Glucose-6-phosphate dehydrogenase activity[312]	N or ↓	↑
Reduced glutathione[313] and carbonic anhydrase[314]	↑	↓
Ca-ATPase activity[315]	↓	↑
White blood cells		
Alkaline phosphatase[316]	? ↑	↓
ATP production in mitochondria[317]	N	↓
Adipose tissue		
cAMP[284]		
Lipoprotein lipase[295]	↓	
Skeletal muscle		
cAMP[284]		↑
Sweat glands		
Sweat electrolytes[318]	↑	N
Sebium excretion rate[319]	↓	N
Intestinal system and absorption		
Basic electrical rhythm of the duodenum[320]	↓	↑
Riboflavin absorption[321]	↑ *	↓ *
Ca absorption[322]		
Intestinal transit and fecal fat[323, 324]		↑
Pulmonary function and gas exchange		
Dead space,[325] hypoxic ventilatory drive,[326] and arterial pO₂[325]	↓	
Neurological system and CSF		
Relaxation time of deep tendon reflexes (photomotography)[327]	↑	↓
CSF proteins[328]	↑	
Cardiovascular and circulatory system		
Timing of the arterial sounds (QKd)[232]	↑	↓
Pre-ejection period (PEP), left ventricular ejection time (LVET) ratio[233]	↑	↓
ECG[329, 330]	↓	↑
Heart rate and QRS voltage	↓	↑
Q-Tc interval		↓
PR interval		
T wave	Flat or inverted	Transient abnormalities
Common arrhythmias	Atrioventricular block	Atrial fibrillation
Bones		
Osseous maturation (bone age by x-ray film)[331, 332]	Delayed (epiphysial dysgenesis)	Advanced

N, normal; ↑, increased; ↓, decreased.
*In children.
†In neonates.

adult patients with Hashimoto's thyroiditis and Graves' disease, respectively.[342, 344–346] Tg antibodies are less frequently detected in children with autoimmune thyroid disease.[347] Although higher titers are more common with Hashimoto's thyroiditis, quantitation of the antibody titer carries little diagnostic implication. The tests are of particular value in the evaluation of patients with atypical or selected manifestations of autoimmune thyroid disease (ophthalmopathy and dermopathy). Positive antibody titers are predicative of postpartum thyroiditis.[348] Low antibody titers occur transiently in some patients after an episode of subacute thyroiditis.[349] There is no increased incidence of thyroid autoantibodies in patients with multinodular goiter, thyroid adenomas, or secondary hypothyroidism. In some patients with Hashimoto's thyroiditis and undetectable thyroid autoantibodies in their serum, intrathyroidal lymphocytes have been demonstrated to produce TPO antibodies.

Other antibodies directed against thyroid components or other tissues have been described in the serum of some patients with autoimmune thyroid disease. They are less frequently measured, and their diagnostic value in thyroid disease has not been fully evaluated. A small proportion of patients with Hashimoto's thyroiditis and undetectable Tg antibodies may have circulating antibodies against a distinct antigen present in the thyroid colloid.[350] Circulating antibodies capable of binding T_4 and T_3 have also been demonstrated in patients with autoimmune thyroid diseases, which may interfere with the measurement of T_4 and T_3 by RIA techniques.[36, 37, 351]

Antibodies that react with nuclear components, which are not tissue-specific, and with cellular components of parietal cells and adrenal, ovarian, and testicular tissues are more commonly encountered in patients with autoimmune thyroid disease.[352] Their presence reflects the frequency of coexistence of several autoimmune disease processes in the same patient (see Ch. 43). Increased incidence of circulating antibodies against *Yersinia enterocolitica* has been observed in patients with various pathological conditions of the thyroid gland.[353]

Thyroid-Stimulating Immunoglobulins

A large number of names have been given to tests that measure abnormal γ-globulins present in the serum of some patients with autoimmune thyroid disease, in particular Graves' disease.[354] The interaction of these immunoglobulins with thyroid follicular cells usually results in a global stimulation of thyroid gland activity and only seldom causes inhibition. It has been recommended that these assays all be called TSH receptor antibodies (TRAb) with a phrase "measured by _____ assay to identify the type of method used for their determination.[113] The tests are described under three general categories: those measuring the thyroid-stimulating activity using in vivo or in vitro bioassays; tests based on the competition of the abnormal immunoglobulin with binding of TSH to its receptor; and measurement of thyroid growth-promoting activity of immunoglobulins. Tests use both human and animal tissue material.

Thyroid-Stimulation Assays

The earliest assays used various modifications of the McKenzie mouse bioassay.[355, 356] The abnormal γ-globulin with TSH-like biological properties has relatively longer in vivo activity, hence its name long-acting thyroid stimulator (LATS). The assay measures the LATS-induced release of thyroid hormone from the mouse thyroid gland prelabeled with radioiodide. The presence of LATS in serum is pathognomonic of Graves' disease. However, depending on the assay sensitivity, a variable percentage of untreated patients show a positive LATS response. LATS may be found in the serum of patients with Graves' disease even in the absence of thyrotoxicosis. Although it is more commonly present in patients with ophthalmopathy, especially when accompanied by pretibial myxedema,[357] LATS does not appear to cause or correlate with the severity or course of these complications. LATS crosses the placenta and may be found transiently in neonates from mothers possessing the abnormal γ-globulin.[358]

Attempts to improve the ability to detect thyroid-stimulating antibodies (TSAb) in autoimmune thyroid disease led to the development of several in vitro assays using animal as well as human thyroid tissue. In a cytological assay the ability of human serum to stimulate endocytosis in fresh human thyroid tissue is measured by direct count of intracellular colloid droplets formed. Using such a technique human thyroid stimulator activity has been demonstrated in serum samples from patients with Graves' disease that were devoid of LATS activity measured by the standard mouse bioassay.[359] TSAb can be detected by measuring the accumulation of cAMP or stimulation of adenylate cyclase activity in human thyroid cell cultures and thyroid plasma membranes, respectively.[360] Accumulation of cAMP in the cultured rat thyroid cell line FRTL5 has also been used as an assay for TSAb.[361] Stimulation of release of T_3 from human[362] and porcine[363] thyroid slices is another form of in vitro assay for TSAb. An in vitro bioassay using a cytochemical technique depends on the ability of thyroid-stimulating material to increase lysosomal membrane permeability to a chromogenic substrate, leucyl-β-naphthylamide, which then reacts with the enzyme naphthylamidase. Quantitation is by scanning and integrated microdensitometry.[364]

The recent cloning of the TSH receptor[365, 366] led to the development of an in vitro assay of TSAb using cell lines that express the recombinant TSH receptor.[367, 368] This assay, based on the generation of cAMP, is specific for the measurement of human TSH receptor antibodies that have thyroid-stimulating activity and thus contrasts with assays based on binding to the TSH receptor (see below) that cannot distinguish between antibodies with thyroid-stimulating and TSH-blocking activity. Accordingly, the recombinant human TSH receptor assay measures antibodies relevant to the pathogenesis of autoimmune thyroid disease and is more sensitive than formerly used TSAb assays. For example, 94 per cent of serum samples were positive for TSAb compared with 74 per cent when the same samples were assayed using FRTL5 cells.[369]

Thyrotropin-Binding Inhibition Assays

The principal of binding inhibition assays dates to the discovery of another class of abnormal immunoglobulins in patients with Graves' disease—those that prevent human thyroid gland extract from neutralizing the bioactivity of LATS tested in the mouse.[370] This material, known as LATS protector, is species-specific, having no biological effect on the mouse thyroid gland but capable of stimulating the human thyroid.[371] The original assay was cumbersome, limiting its clinical application.

Techniques used currently, which may be collectively termed radioreceptor assays, are based on the competition of the abnormal immunoglobulins and TSH for a common receptor binding site on thyroid cells. The test is akin in principle to the radioligand assays, in which a natural membrane receptor takes the place of the binding proteins or antibodies. Various sources of TSH receptors are used, including human thyroid cells,[372] their particulate or solubilized membrane,[373, 374] and cell membranes from porcine thyroids[375] or from guinea pig fat cells.[376] Because the assays do not directly measure thyroid-stimulating activity, the abnormal immunoglobulins determined have been given various names, such as thyroid-binding inhibitory immunoglobulins or antibodies and thyrotropin-displacing immunoglobulins.

Thyroid Growth-Promoting Assays

New assays have been developed that measure the growth-promoting activity of abnormal immunoglobulins. One such assay is based on the staining by the Feulgen reaction of nuclei from guinea pig thyroid cells in S-phase.[377] Another assay measures the incorporation of ³H-thymidine into DNA in FRTL cells.[378] Whether the thyroid growth-stimulating immunoglobulins measured by these assays represent a population of immunoglobulins distinct from that with stimulatory functional activity remains a subject of active debate.

Clinical Applications

Measurement of abnormal immunoglobulins that interact with thyroid tissue by any of the methods just described is not indicated as a routine diagnostic test for Graves' disease. It is useful, however, in a few selected clinical conditions: (1) in the differential diagnosis of exophthalmos, particularly unilateral exophthalmos, when the origin of this condition is otherwise not apparent; the presence of thyroid-stimulating immunoglobulins would obviate the necessity to undertake more complex diagnostic procedures described elsewhere[379]; (2) in the differential diagnosis of pretibial myxedema or other forms of dermopathy when the cause is unclear and it is imperative that the cause of the skin lesion be ascertained; (3) in the differentiation of Graves' disease from toxic nodular goiter when both are being considered as the possible cause of thyrotoxicosis, when other tests such as thyroid scanning and thyroid autoantibody tests have been inconclusive, and particularly when such a distinction would play a role in determining the course of therapy; (4) in Graves' disease during pregnancy when high maternal levels of TSAb are a warning for the possible occurrence of neonatal thyrotoxicosis; (5) in neonatal thyrotoxicosis when serial TSAb determinations may be helpful to distinguish between intrinsic Graves' disease in the infant and transient thyrotoxicosis resulting from passive transfer of maternal TSAb.[358, 380] Some investigators have found the persistence of TSAb's to be predicative of the relapse of Graves' thyrotoxicosis after a course of antithyroid drug therapy.[381]

Other Substances With Thyroid-Stimulating Activity

Some patients with trophoblastic disease develop hyperthyroidism as a result of the production and release of a thyroid stimulator known as molar or trophoblastic thyrotropin or big placental TSH.[382] This material can be detected in the standard mouse bioassay and is distinguished from LATS and TSH by its intermediate length of biological action. Furthermore, in contrast to LATS, it can be detected in the chick bioassay, which is based on the incorporation of radioactive phosphorus in the thyroid of day-old chicks.[383] It is likely that the thyroid-stimulating activity in patients with trophoblastic disease results from the presence of high levels of human chorionic gonadotropin (hCG).[384] Thus the RIA of hCG can be useful in the differential diagnosis of thyroid dysfunction.

Exophthalmos-Producing Substance

Various tests have been developed for measuring exophthalmogenic activity in serum.[385–388] Although a great uncertainty still exists regarding the pathogenesis of thyroid-associated eye disease, the role of the immune system appears to be central. Exophthalmogenic activity has also been detected in IgG fractions of some patients with Graves' ophthalmopathy. The role of assays to detect specific antibodies is discussed further in Chapter 42.

Tests of Cell-Mediated Immunity

Delayed-hypersensitivity reactions to thyroid antigens are present in autoimmune thyroid diseases (see Chs. 41 through 43). Cell-mediated immunity can be measured in several ways: (1) the migration inhibition test, which measures the inhibition of migration of sensitized leukocytes when exposed to the sensitizing antigen; (2) the lymphotoxic assay, which measures the ability of sensitized lymphocytes to kill target cells when exposed to the antigen; (3) the blastogenesis assay, which scores the formation of blast cells after exposure of lymphocytes to a thyroid antigen; and (4) thymus-dependent lymphocyte subset quantitation, using monoclonal antibodies. The tests require fresh leukocytes from the patient, are variable in their response, and are difficult to perform.

ANATOMICAL AND TISSUE DIAGNOSES

The purpose of the procedures described in this section is to evaluate the anatomical features of the thyroid gland, localize and determine the nature of abnormal areas, and eventually provide a pathological or tissue diagnosis. All these tests are performed in vivo. They cause inconvenience and, at times, discomfort and thus require the patient's understanding and cooperation.

Thyroid Scintiscanning

Normal and abnormal thyroid tissue can be externally imaged by three scintiscanning methods: (1) with radionuclides that are concentrated by normal thyroid tissues, such as iodide isotopes, and ^{99m}Tc given as the pertechnetate ion; (2) by administration of radiopharmaceutical agents that are preferentially concentrated by abnormal thyroid tissues; and (3) by fluorescent scanning, which uses an external source of ^{241}Am and does not require administration of radioactive material. Each has specific indications, advantages, and disadvantages.

The physical properties, dosages, and radiation delivered by the most commonly used radioisotopes are listed in Table 39–1. The choice of scanning agents depends on the purpose of the scan, the age of the patient, and the equipment available. Radioiodide scans cannot be performed in patients who have recently ingested iodine-containing compounds. ^{123}I and ^{99m}TcO$_4^-$ are the radionuclides of choice because of the low radiation exposure.[389–391] Iodine 131 is still used for the detection of functioning metastatic thyroid carcinoma by total body scanning.

A wide variety of imaging instruments are available. Rectilinear scanners have been largely replaced by stationary pinhole collimated Anger-type scanner γ-cameras that view the entire field being scanned. The image is displayed on an oscilloscope, and a Polaroid photograph is obtained for a permanent record. The data can also be stored on magnetic tape. The camera provides better resolution, but greater attention should be given to positioning because magnification and distortion may cause significant problems.[391] Regardless of the display format, the scan should reproduce as accurately as possible the anatomical configuration of the tissue and the relative concentration of the radioactivity. Oblique and lateral views are helpful for demonstration of cold nodules that may be obscured by overlying functioning tissue. If retrosternal goiter is suspected, the proper isotope should be chosen to allow penetration through bony structures.

One of the most critical aspects in the correct interpretation of scans is the provision of anatomical landmarks that allow orientation of position and provide a scale for estimation of size. Palpable abnormalities must also be marked in the scanning position. With the γ-camera, landmarks are recorded by obtaining a scan record with small ^{57}Co marker sources placed over the areas of interest.

Radioiodide and ^{99m}Pertechnetate Scans

^{99m}TcO$_4^-$ is concentrated and all iodide isotopes are concentrated and bound by thyroid tissue. Depending on the isotope used, scans are carried out at different times after administration: 20 minutes for ^{99m}TcO$_4^-$; 4 or 24 hours for ^{123}I$^-$; 24 hours for ^{125}I$^-$ and ^{131}I$^-$; and 48, 72, and 96 hours when ^{131}I$^-$ is used in the search for metastatic thyroid carcinoma. The appearance of the normal thyroid gland on scan may be best described as a narrow-winged butterfly. Each wing represents a thyroid lobe, which in the adult measures 5 ± 1 cm in length and 2.3 ± 0.5 cm in width.[392] Common variants include the absence of a connecting isthmus, a large isthmus, asymmetry between the two lobes, and trailing activity extending to the cricoid cartilage (pyramidal lobe). The latter is more commonly found in conditions associated with diffuse thyroid hyperplasia. Collection of saliva in the esophagus during ^{99m}TcO$_4^-$ scanning may simulate a pyramidal lobe, but this artefact can be eliminated by drinking water.

TABLE 39–9. INDICATIONS FOR RADIONUCLIDE SCANNING

Detection of anatomical variants and search for ectopic thyroid tissue (thyroid hemiagenesis, lingual thyroid, struma ovarii)
Diagnosis of congenital athyreosis
Determination of the nature of abnormal neck or chest (mediastinal) masses
Evaluation of solitary thyroid nodules (functioning or nonfunctioning)
Evaluation of thyroid remnants after surgery
Detection of functioning thyroid metastases
Evaluation of focal functional thyroid abnormalities (suppressed or nonsuppressible tissue)

The indications for scanning are listed in Table 39–9. In clinical practice scans are most often requested for evaluation of the functional activity of solitary nodules. The isotope is homogeneously distributed throughout both lobes of the thyroid gland. This distribution occurs in the enlarged gland of Graves' disease and may be seen in Hashimoto's thyroiditis. A mottled appearance may be noted in Hashimoto's thyroiditis and occasionally can be seen in Graves' disease, especially after therapy with radioactive iodine. Irregular areas of relatively diminished and occasionally increased uptake are characteristic of large multinodular goiters. The traditional nuclear medicine jargon classifies nodules as hot, warm, and cold, according to their isotope-concentrating ability relative to the surrounding normal parenchyma. Hot, or hyperfunctioning, nodules typically are benign, although the presence of cancer has been reported.[393, 394] Cold, or hypofunctioning, nodules may be solid or cystic. Some may prove to be malignant, but the great majority are benign. This differentiation cannot be made by scanning.[98, 395] A nodule that is functional on a ^{99m}TcO$_4^-$ scan occasionally is found to be cold on an iodine scan; this pattern is found with both benign and malignant nodules. The scan is of particular value in identifying autonomous thyroid nodules because the remainder of the gland is suppressed. The search for functioning thyroid metastases is best accomplished by using 2 to 10 mCi of ^{131}I after ablation of the normal thyroid tissue and cessation of hormone therapy to allow TSH to increase above the upper limit of normal. Administration of bovine TSH is not recommended; however, recombinant human TSH may prove to be useful in allowing scanning without requiring cessation of hormone therapy.[396] Uptake is also found outside the thyroid gland in patients with lingual thyroids and in the rare ovarian dermoid tumor that contains functioning thyroid tissue.

The scan can be used as an adjunct during TSH stimulation and T_3 suppression tests to localize suppressed normal thyroid tissue or autonomously functioning areas, respectively (see below). Applications other than those listed in Table 39–9 are of doubtful benefit and seldom are justified considering the radiation exposure, expense, and inconvenience. ^{123}I single-photon emission computed tomography may also be useful in the evaluation of thyroid abnormalities.[397]

Other Isotope Scans

Because most test procedures, short of direct microscopic examination of thyroid tissue, fail to detect thyroid cancer with any degree of certainty, efforts have been made to find other radioactive materials that may be of diagnostic use. Several such agents that are concentrated by a metabolically active tissue irrespective of whether it has iodide-concentrating ability have been tried. Despite claims to the contrary, they have had only limited value or their diagnostic usefulness has not been fully evaluated. These agents include ^{75}Se methionine, [125]Ce, ^{67}Ga, citrate, ^{32}P, pyrophosphate ^{99m}Tc, and [201]Tl.[398]

Scanning with ^{131}I-labeled anti-Tg for the detection of occult metastatic thyroid cancer that fails to concentrate ^{131}I showed early promising results,[399] but the procedure has not proved clinically useful.

Fluorescent Scans

Fluorescent scans allow thyroid scanning without the administration of radioisotopes. Scanning involves the focal irradiation of the thyroid gland with a 60-KeV γ-ray derived from a [241]Am source. Its interaction with stable iodine ([127]I) within the gland produces the emission of a characteristic 28.5-KeV K-alpha (fluorescent) x-ray that is picked up by a lithium-drifted silicon detector.[400] The resulting scan shows the distribution of stable iodine within the gland, the content of which can be quantified by the use of appropriate iodide standards. Because the procedure is independent of the iodide-concentrating mechanism of the thyroid gland, fluorescent scanning is not hampered by excess iodide ingestion or treatment with thyroid hormone, situations under which a radionuclide scan cannot be obtained. Furthermore, because administration of radioisotopes is not required, the scan is safe for children and for women during pregnancy and lactation.

The information derived relates to iodine storage and distribution within the gland, thus differing from that obtained from scans using radionuclides. Nevertheless, nodules that appear to be cold by isotope scanning usually also show decreased [127]I content by fluorescent scan. The procedure is of particular value in the demonstration of suppressed thyroid tissue, with potential functioning capability, in patients who have been taking replacement thyroid hormone treatment for a prolonged period.[401] Despite its apparent usefulness, this technique is not available in most centers.

Ultrasonography

Ultrasonography, or echography, is used to outline the thyroid gland and to characterize lesions differing in density from the surrounding tissue. The technique differentiates interphases of different acoustic densities, using sound frequencies in the megahertz range that are above audible sound. A transducer fitted with a piezoelectric crystal produces and transmits the signal and receives echo reflections. Interfaces of different acoustic densities reflect dense echoes, liquid transmits sound without reflections, and air-filled spaces do not transmit the ultrasound.[402]

In one-dimensional, or A-mode, ultrasonography the transducer is held in one position for each image. The echoes, a series of spikes recorded on an oscilloscope, are of height proportional to the intensity of the echo and of distance corresponding to the actual space of echo interphases. Two-dimensional, or B-mode, ultrasonography is performed using a scanner that moves the transducer in a horizontal plane across the neck. A composite image of echoes represented by lines and dots in a scale of shades from black to white (gray-scale scan) proportional to the intensity of generated echoes is assembled electronically. Because air is a poor conductor of ultrasound, contact with the skin is secured using special gels, oil, or water. This contact as well as maintenance of the transducer in a perpendicular position to the skin are essential to avoid artefacts.

One of the most useful applications of the ultrasonogram is the differentiation of solid from cystic lesions.[402, 403] Purely cystic lesions are entirely sonolucent, whereas solid lesions produce multiple echoes because of multiple sonic interphases. Many lesions are mixed (solid and cystic), called complex lesions. Some tumors may have the same acoustic characteristics as the surrounding normal tissue, thus escaping echographic detection. Although high-resolution ultrasonography can detect thyroid nodules of the order of a few millimeters,[404] lesions need to be larger than 1 cm to allow differentiation between solid and cystic structures. A sonolucent pattern frequently is noted in glands with Hashimoto's thyroiditis, but this has also been described in multinodular glands and in patients with Graves' disease.[402, 405, 406]

Because sonography localizes the position as well as the depth of lesions, the procedure has been used to guide the needle during aspiration biopsy.[407] In complex lesions the sonographic guiding ensures sampling from the solid portion of the nodule. With experience and proper calibration, sonography can be used for the estimation of thyroid gland size.[408, 409] Several reports have described treatment of toxic nodules by the injection of alcohol under sonographic guidance.[410] Although ultrasonography has found virtually the same applications as scintiscanning, claims that the former may differentiate benign from malignant lesions are unfounded. Also, the test cannot be used for the assessment of substernal goiters because of interference from overlying bone.

The procedure is simple and painless and at the frequencies of sound used do not produce tissue damage. Because it does not require the administration of isotopes, it can be safely used in children and during pregnancy. Also, because the procedure is independent of iodine-concentrating mechanisms, it is valuable in the study of suppressed glands.

X-Ray Procedures

A simple x-ray film of the neck and upper mediastinum may provide valuable information regarding the location, size, and effect of the goiter on surrounding structures. Roentgenograms may show an asymmetric goiter, an intrathoracic extension of the gland, and displacement or narrowing of the trachea. If there is any suggestion of posterior extension of the mass, it is useful to take films while the patient swallows x-ray contrast material. The soft tissue x-ray technique may disclose calcium deposits. Large deposits in flakes or rings are typical of an old multinodular goiter, whereas foci of finely stippled flecks of calcium are pathognomonic of papillary adenocarcinoma.

Information not related to anatomical abnormalities of the thyroid gland may be obtained from x-ray studies. In children with a history of hypothyroidism, an x-ray film of the hand to determine the bone age could aid in estimating the onset and duration of thyroid dysfunction.[331, 332] Hypothyroidism leads to retardation in bone age and in infants produces a dense calcification of epiphyseal plates most easily seen at the distal end of the radius. Long-standing myxedema produces pituitary hypertrophy, which, especially in children but also in adults, causes enlargement of the sella turcica demonstrable on skull x-ray films.[411]

Computed Tomography and Magnetic Resonance Imaging

Computed tomography (CT) provides useful information on the location and architecture of the thyroid gland as well as its relation to surrounding tissues.[412] The test is too costly relative to other procedures that provide similar information. An important application of CT is the assessment and delineation of obscure mediastinal masses and large substernal goiters.[413] In such instances the substernal location limits the use of ultrasonography and the lack of function, especially during suppressive therapy, of radionuclide scanning. The necessity to infuse iodine-containing contrast agents limits the application of CT in patients being considered for radioiodide therapy.

CT and magnetic resonance imaging (MRI) have found firm application in another area of thyroid diseases—the evaluation of ophthalmopathy.[379] As is the case with CT, MRI is also useful in delineating mediastinal masses.[413]

Other Procedures

Several unrelated methods for the anatomical delineation and characterization of thyroid pathological conditions have been used. Their usefulness and level of sophistication are variable and have limited clinical application. These procedures include (1) angiography with selective injection of radiological contrast material for the delineation of tumor masses[414]; (2) lymphography by injection of contrast material[415] or radionuclide-tagged colloid material[416] directly into the thyroid tissue that is rapidly transported to local lymph nodes by hyperplastic glands; and (3) thermography,[417] to differentiate between malignant and benign thyroid lesions, based on the assumption that malignant lesions are more active metabolically and would thus increase in infrared energy emission from the overlying dermis. A barium swallow may be useful in evaluating impingement of a goiter on the esophagus, and a flow-volume loop may be useful in documenting functional impingement on the upper airway.

Biopsy of the Thyroid Gland

Histological examination of thyroid tissue for diagnostic purposes requires some form of an invasive procedure. The biopsy procedure depends on the intended type of microscopic examination. Core biopsy for histological examination of tissue with preservation of architecture is obtained by closed needle or open surgical procedure; aspiration biopsy is performed to obtain material for cytological examination.

Core Biopsy

Closed core biopsy is an office procedure carried out under local anesthesia. A large (about 15-gauge) cutting needle of the Vim-Silverman type is most commonly used.[418] The needle is introduced under local anesthesia through a small skin nick, and firm pressure is applied over the puncture site for 5 to 10 minutes after withdrawal of the needle. In experienced hands complications are rare but may include transient damage to the laryngeal nerve, puncture of the trachea, laryngospasm, jugular vein phlebitis, and bleeding.[419] Because of the fear of disseminating malignant cells, biopsy was restricted for many years to the differential diagnosis of diffuse benign diseases. With the improvement of cytology and biopsy techniques, open biopsy carried out under local or general anesthesia has been virtually abandoned.[419]

Percutaneous Fine-Needle Aspiration

The development of more sophisticated staining techniques for cytological examination and the realization that fear of tumor dissemination along the needle tract was not well founded[420, 421] are responsible for the revival and increasing popularity of percutaneous fine-needle aspiration.[419, 422]

The procedure is exceedingly simple and safe. The patient lays supine with the neck hyperextended by placing a small pillow under the shoulders. Local anesthesia usually is not required. The skin is prepared with an antiseptic solution. The lesion, fixed between two gloved fingers, is penetrated with a fine (22- to 27-gauge) needle attached to a syringe. Suction is then applied while the needle is moved within the nodule. A nonsuction technique using capillary action has also been developed. The small amount of aspirated material, usually contained within the needle or its hub, is applied to glass slides and spread. Some slides are air-dried and others are fixed before staining. Because biopsy of small nodules may be technically more difficult, the use of ultrasound to guide the needle has been suggested.[407, 410] It is important that the slides be properly prepared, stained, and read by a cytologist experienced in the interpretation of material from thyroid gland aspirates.

The yield of false-positive and false-negative results is variable from one center to another, but both are acceptably low. Various centers have reported that the accuracy of this technique in distinguishing benign from malignant lesions may be as high as 95 per cent.[419, 422] In one clinic in which the procedure is used routinely, the number of patients operated on decreased by one third, whereas the percentage of thyroid carcinomas among the patients who underwent surgery doubled.[423] When results are suggestive of a follicular neoplasia, surgery is required because follicular adenoma cannot be differentiated from follicular cancer by cytology alone. Because the sample obtained may not always be representative of the lesion, surgical treatment is indicated for lesions highly suspicious of being malignant on clinical grounds. In such instances some physicians recommend repeated aspiration biopsies. Other uses of aspiration biopsy include presumed lymphoma or invasive anaplastic carcinoma when biopsy may spare the patient an unnecessary neck exploration. Another application of needle aspiration is in the confirmation and treatment of thyroid cysts.

EVALUATION OF THE HYPOTHALAMIC-PITUITARY-THYROID AXIS

The development of an RIA for the routine measurement of TSH in serum and the availability of synthetic TRH[424, 425] have placed increased reliance on tests that assess the hypothalamic-pituitary control of thyroid function. These tests allow the diagnosis of mild and subclinical forms of thyroid dysfunction and provide a means to differentiate between thyroprivic (primary) and trophoprivic, either pituitary (secondary) or hypothalamic (tertiary), thyroid gland failure. Furthermore, as a result of these methodological advances, classic theories of the feedback mechanisms regulating thyroid gland function have been confirmed.[424–427]

Thyrotropin

Efforts to improve existing assays for the measurement of TSH have produced more than 100 bioassay systems.[428, 429] Despite general agreement of results among assays,[429] none were sensitive enough for the routine measurement of pituitary TSH in serum. The more sensitive bioassays developed[359, 360, 362–364, 369–378, 430] are still technically demanding and unsuitable for routine use. The clinical use of these assays is restricted to the measurement of thyroid-stimulating substances of other than pituitary origin (see previous section) and in the characterization of TSH with reduced or increased bioactivity.[431, 432]

The routine measurement of TSH in clinical practice initially used RIA techniques. These first-generation assays had a sensitivity level of 1 mU/L, which did not allow the separation of normal and reduced values. A major problem with early TSH RIA's was cross-reactivity with gonadotropins (LH, FSH, and hCG) sharing with TSH a common α-subunit.[433] Despite potential errors from immunological cross-reactivity and the possibility of detecting immunological material with altered biological activity,[431, 432, 434] under the usual circumstances even older RIA methods for measurement of pituitary TSH correlated well with values obtained using bioassay techniques.[435] Another uncommon source of error is the presence in the serum sample of heterophilic antibodies induced by vaccination with materials contaminated with animal serum,[436] or endogenous TSH antibodies.[437] RIA techniques for measurement of TSH in dry blood spots on filter paper are used for the screening of neonatal hypothyroidism.[31]

Newer techniques have been developed using multiple antibodies to produce a sandwich-type assay in which one antibody (usually directed against the α-subunit) serves to anchor the TSH molecule and others (usually monoclonal antibodies directed against the β-subunit) either are radioiodinated (immunoradiometric assay) or are conjugated with an enzyme (immunoenzymometric assay) or a chemiluminescent compound (chemiluminescent assay).[120, 438] In these assays the signal should be directly related to the amount of the ligand present rather than being inversely related as in an RIA.[439] This results in decreased background noise and a greater sensitivity, decreased interference from related compounds, and an expanded useful range.[120, 438, 440] Initial improvements of the TSH assay resulted in assays with sensitivity limit of 0.1 mU/L, a normal range of about 0.5 to 4.5 mU/L, and the ability to distinguish between low and normal TSH values.[120, 438, 440] Commercial assays have been developed with even higher sensitivity limit of 0.005 to 0.01 mU/L and a similar normal range but an expanded range between the lower limit of normal and the lower limit of sensitivity.[441, 442]

The nomenclature for differentiating these various assays has not been standardized with manufacturers applying various combinations of high(ly), ultra, and sensitive. It has been recommended that the sensitivity limit be used in defining the assays with the early RIA's detecting values ≥ 1 mU/L designated first-generation assays, those with a lower sensitivity limit of 0.1 mU/L designated as second-generation assays, and those with a lower sensitivity limit of ≤ 0.01 mU/L designated as third-generation assays.[120] The determination of the appropriate sensitivity level has also been controversial. Some define it based on the level with a coefficient of variation less than 20 per cent, and others, as the lowest level that can be reliably differentiated from the zero TSH standard.[120, 440] At a minimum, for a TSH assay to be considered sensitive, the overlap of TSH values in sera from groups of clinically hyperthyroid with those of euthyroid individuals should be less than 5 per cent and preferably less than 1 per cent.[120]

In a number of third-generation assays, TSH detected in clinically toxic patients and elevated values found in euthyroid subjects were not confirmed when the samples were measured in other assays. In some cases this has been attributed to the presence of antibodies directed against the animal immunoglobulins used in the assay.[443–445] These act to bind the anchoring and detecting antibodies and lead to an overestimation of TSH. In some cases this effect may be blocked by the addition of an excess of nonspecific immunoglobulin of the same species.[445]

TSH appears abruptly in the pituitary and serum of the fetus at midgestation and can also be detected in amniotic fluid.[48, 446, 447] Mean TSH is higher in cord than in maternal blood. A substantial increase to levels severalfold above the upper range in adults is observed during the first 30 minutes of life.[447] Levels decline to the normal adult range by the third day of life. Minimal changes reported to occur during adult life and in early adolescence[448] have no significant effect on the overall range of normal. In the absence of pregnancy no significant sex differences have been observed. Although early studies failed to show diurnal TSH variation,[449] significantly higher values have been recorded during the late evening and early night, which are partially inhibited by sleep.[450] The diurnal rhythm of TSH is superimposed on continuous high-frequency, low-amplitude variations. The nocturnal TSH surge persists in patients with mild primary hypothyroidism,[451, 452] and is abolished in hypothalamic hypothyroidism[451, 453] and in some patients during fasting[454] and with nonthyroidal illness.[455, 456] It is enhanced by oral contraceptives[457] and abolished by high levels of glucocorticoids.[458] The presence of seasonal variation has not been a uniform finding, but it is unlikely to affect the clinical interpretation of serum values.[459] Various types of stressful stimuli have no significant effect on the basal serum TSH level, except for a rise during surgical hypothermia in infants but not in adults.[460] Various stimuli, such as administration of insulin, vasopressin, glucagon, bacterial pyrogens, arginine, prostaglandins, and chlorpromazine, which elicit in normal humans a secretory response of some pituitary hormones, have no effect on serum TSH. However, administration of any of a growing list of drugs has been found to alter the basal concentration of serum TSH and/or its response to exogenous TRH (Table 39–10).

In the presence of a normally functioning hypothalamic-

TABLE 39–10. AGENTS THAT MAY AFFECT TSH SECRETION

SUBSTANCE	COMMON USE
Increase Serum TSH Concentration and/or Its Response to TRH	
Iodine (iodide and iodine-containing compounds)[161, 461, 462]	Radiologic contrast media, antiseptic, expectorants, anti-arrhythmic and anti-anginal
Lithium[463]	Treatment of bipolar psychoses
Dopamine antagonists	
Dopamine receptor blockers (metcropramide,[464, 465] domperidone[465])	Antiemetic
Dopamine-blocking agent (sulpiride[466])	Tranquilizer
Decarboxylase inhibitor (benserazide[467])	—
Dopamine-depleting agent (monoiodotyrosine[465])	—
L-Dopa inhibitors (chloropromazine,[468] biperiden,[469] haloperidol[469])	Neuroleptic
Cimetidine (histamine receptor blocker)[470]	Treatment of peptic ulcers
Clomiphene (antiestrogen)[471]	Induction of ovulation
Spironolactone[472]	Antihypertensive
Amphetamines[473]	Anticongestants and antiappetite
Increase Serum TSH Concentration and/or Its Response to TRH	
Thyroid hormones (T4 and T3)	Replacement therapy, antigoitrogenic and anticancer
Thyroid hormone analogues (DT4,[474] 3,3′,5-TRIAC,[475] etiroxate-HCl,[476] dimethyl-3 isopropyl-L-thyronine)[477]	Cholesterol-lowering and weight-reducing
Dopaminergic agents (agonists)	
Dopamine[464, 478]	Antihypotensive
L-Dopa[266] (dopamine precursor)	Diagnostic agent and antiparkinsonian
Bromocriptine[479]	Antilactation and pituitary tumor suppression
Fusaric acid (inhibitor of dopamine hydroxylase)[480]	—
Pyridoxine (coenzyme of dopamine synthesis)[481]	Vitamin and antineuropathic
Other dopaminergic agents (pirbidil,[482] apomorphine,[482] lisuride[483])	Treatment of cerebrovascular diseases and migraine
Dopamine antagonist (pimozide)[484]	Neuroleptic
α-Noradrenergic blockers (phentolamine,[485] thioridazine[486])	Neuroleptic
Serotonin antagonists (metergoline,[487] cyproheptadine,[488] methysergide[489])	Antimigraine and appetite stimulators
Serotonin agonist (5-hydroxytryptophan)[490]	—
Glucocorticoids[491, 492]	Anti-inflammatory, immunosuppressive, and anticancer; reduction of intracranial pressure
Acetylsalicylic acid[493]	Anti-inflammatory, antipyrexic and analgesic
Growth hormone[494]*	Growth-promoting
Somatostatin[495]	—
Opiates (morphine,[496] leucine-eukephaline,[497] heroin[498])	Analgesic
Clofibrate[499]	Hypolipidemic
Fenclofenac[76]	Nonsteroidal anti-inflammatory drug

*In hyposomatotrophic dwarfs.

pituitary system, there is an inverse correlation between the serum concentration of FT4 and TSH. Changes in the serum concentration of TT4 as a result of TBG abnormalities or drugs competing with T4 binding to TBG have no effect on the level of serum TSH. The pituitary is exquisitely sensitive to both minimal decreases and increases in thyroid hormone concentration, with a logarithmic change in TSH levels in response to changes in T4[438, 442, 461, 500] (Fig. 39–5). Thus serum TSH levels should be elevated in patients with primary hypothyroidism and low or undetectable in thyrotoxicosis. Indeed, in the absence of hypothalamic pituitary disease, illness, or drugs, TSH is an accurate indicator of thyroid hormone status and the adequacy of thyroid hormone replacement.[438, 501]

In patients with primary hypothyroidism of whatever cause, levels may reach 1000 μU/ml or higher. The magnitude of serum TSH elevation grossly correlates with the severity and in part with the duration of thyroid hormone deficiency.[502, 503] TSH concentrations above the upper limit of normal have been observed in the absence of clinical symptoms and signs of hypothyroidism and in the presence of serum T4 and T3 levels well within the normal range.[502, 504] Discrepancies between TSH and T4 and T3 levels are listed in Table 39–11. This condition most commonly is encountered in patients who develop hypothyroidism as a result of Hashimoto's thyroiditis or in those with limited ability to synthesize thyroid hormone because of prior thyroid surgery, radioiodide treatment, or severe iodine deficiency.[502, 505] There is disagreement on whether such patients have subclinical hypothyroidism or represent compensated states in which euthyroidism is maintained by chronic stimulation of a reduced amount of functioning thyroid tissue through hypersecretion of TSH. Transient hypothyroidism may occur in some infants during the early neonatal period.[506] There are two circumstances in which the usual reverse relation between the serum level of TSH and T4 is not maintained in patients with proven primary hypothyroidism. Treatment with replacement doses of T4 may normalize or even produce serum levels of thyroid hormone above the normal range before the high TSH

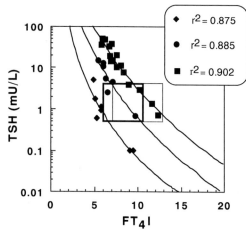

FIGURE 39–5. Correlation of the serum TSH concentration and the free thyroxine index (FT4I) in three persons given increasing doses of L-T4. Note the logarithmic correlation between TSH and FT4I and the variable individual requirement of T4 to normalize the TSH level. Normal ranges are included in the heavy lined box and those for subjects on L-T4 replacement in the light lined box.

TABLE 39–11. DISCREPANCIES BETWEEN TSH AND FREE THYROID HORMONE LEVELS

Elevated Serum TSH Value Without Low FT₄ or FT₃ Values
Subclinical hypothyroidism (inadequate replacement therapy, mild thyroid gland failure)
Recent increase in thyroid hormone dosage
Drugs
Inappropriate TSH secretion syndromes
Laboratory artefact

Subnormal Serum TSH Value Without Elevated FT₄ or FT₃ Values
Subclinical hyperthyroidism (excessive replacement therapy, mild thyroid gland hyperfunction, autonomous nodule)
Recent decrease in suppressive thyroid hormone dosage
Recent treatment of thyrotoxicosis (Graves' disease, toxic multinodular goiter, toxic nodule)
Resolution thyrotoxic phase of thyroiditis
Nonthyroidal illness
Drugs
Central hypothyroidism

levels have reached the normal range.[438, 503, 507] This is particularly true in patients with severe or long-standing primary hypothyroidism, who may require three to six months of hormone replacement before TSH levels are fully suppressed. Conversely, serum TSH concentration may remain low or normal for up to five weeks after withdrawal of thyroid hormone replacement when serum levels of T_4 and T_3 have already declined to values well below the lower range of normal.[438, 508] It is uncertain what TSH level is appropriate for suppressive thyroid hormone therapy. The frequency with which patients have subnormal but detectable TSH values depends on both the population studied and the sensitivity of the assay (Fig. 39–6). Using an assay with a sensitivity limit of 0.1 mU/L, 3 to 4 per cent of hospitalized patients have been noted to have a subnormal TSH.[504, 509] When patients with an undetectable TSH level in such an assay were re-evaluated in an assay with a sensitivity limit of 0.005 mU/L, 3 of 77 (4 per cent) with thyrotoxicosis and 32 of 37 (86 per cent) with nonthyroidal illness or on drugs were found to have a subnormal but detectable TSH level.[441] Thus the more sensitive the assay, the more likely that patients with clinical thyrotoxicosis will have undetectable serum TSH levels, whereas those with illness will have subnormal but detectable levels. With progressively more sensitive assays, the likelihood of a clinically toxic patient having a detectable TSH level increases, and if patients on suppressive therapy are treated until the TSH is undetectable, the more likely they will have symptoms of thyrotoxicosis.

A persistent absence of a reverse correlation between serum thyroid hormone and TSH concentration has a different connotation. A low serum level of thyroid hormone without clear elevation of the serum TSH concentration is suggestive of trophoprivic hypothyroidism, especially when associated with obvious clinical stigmata of hypothyroidism.[505] In some cases a mild elevation of the serum TSH level measured by RIA is probably caused by the presence of immunoreactive TSH with reduced biological activity.[431] Distinction between pituitary and hypothalamic hypothyroidism can be made on the basis of the TSH response to the administration of TRH (see below).

In another group of pathological conditions, serum TSH levels may not be suppressed despite a clear elevation of serum free thyroid hormone levels. Because such a finding is incompatible with a normal thyroregulatory control mechanism of the pituitary, which is preserved in the more common forms of thyrotoxicosis, it has been termed inappropriate secretion of TSH.[510] It implicitly suggests that thyroidal hypersecretion is driven by TSH. When associated with clinical and metabolic changes compatible with thyrotoxicosis, it is usually caused by one of two entities: TSH-secreting pituitary adenoma or pituitary resistance to the feedback regulation by thyroid hormone.[510] The existence of hypothalamic hyperthyroidism can be questioned.[511] Precise diagnosis requires further studies, including radiological examination of the pituitary gland and a TRH test. In addition, the presence of high circulating levels of the α-subunit of pituitary glycoprotein hormones (α-SU), giving rise to a disproportionately high α-SU:TSH molar ratio in serum, is characteristic, if not pathognomonic, of TSH-secreting pituitary tumors.[510, 512] Normal and occasionally high serum TSH levels associated with a clear elevation in serum FT₄ and FT₃ but no clear clinical evidence of hypothyroidism are typical of generalized resistance to thyroid hormone (GRTH).[86, 513]

Although TSH has been implicated in the pathogenesis of simple, nontoxic goiter, unless hypothyroidism supervenes or iodide deficiency is severe, TSH levels are characteristically normal. Elevated TSH levels may occur in the presence of normal thyroid hormone levels and apparent euthyroidism in nonthyroidal diseases[509, 514] and with primary adrenal failure.[515] A more common occurrence in severe acute and chronic illnesses is a normal or low serum TSH concentration despite low levels of T_3 and even low T_4 levels.[441, 501, 516] TSH values may be transiently elevated during the recovery phase.[517] Various hypotheses to explain these anomalous findings have been proposed, but a perfectly satisfactory explanation is not at hand.

A specific RIA for the β-subunits of human TSH is also available but has not found clinical application.[518]

Thyrotropin-Releasing Hormone

TRH (protirelin) plays a central role in the regulation of pituitary TSH secretion.[425, 426, 453] It is thus not surprising that attempts have been made to measure its concentration

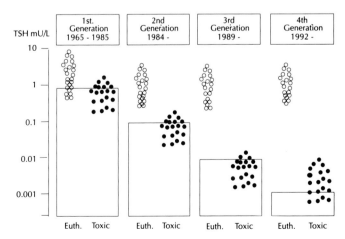

FIGURE 39–6. The effect of serum TSH assay sensitivity on the discrimination of euthyroid subject (Euth) from those with thyrotoxicosis (Toxic). (From Spencer C: Clinical Diagnostics. Rochester, NY, Eastman Kodak Co., 1992.)

in various body fluids, with the purpose of deriving information relevant to the function of the thyroid gland in health and in disease. Several methods have been used for quantitation of TRH, but for many reasons measurement in humans has failed to provide information of diagnostic value. These include high dilution by the time it reaches the systemic circulation, rapid enzymatic degradation, and ubiquitous tissue distribution.[426]

TRH Test

The TRH test measures the increase of pituitary TSH in serum in response to the administration of synthetic TRH. The magnitude of the TSH response to TRH is modulated by the thyrotroph response to active thyroid hormone and is thus almost always proportional to the concentration of free thyroid hormone in serum. The response is exquisitely sensitive to minor changes in the level of circulating thyroid hormones, which may not be detected by direct measurement.[461, 500] A direct correlation between basal serum TSH values and the maximal response to TRH has been observed even in the absence of thyroid hormone abnormalities, suggesting that there may be a fine modulation of pituitary sensitivity to TRH in the euthyroid state.[519]

TRH normally stimulates pituitary prolactin secretion and, under certain pathological conditions, the release of growth hormone and ACTH.[425, 426] Accordingly, the test has been used for the assessment of various endocrine functions, some unrelated to the thyroid. In clinical thyroidology the TRH test is used mainly to assess the functional integrity of the pituitary thyrotrophs, and thus to aid in differentiating hypothyroidism resulting from intrinsic pituitary disease from hypothalamic dysfunction, and in the diagnosis of mild hypothyroidism and mild thyrotoxicosis when results of other tests are equivocal.

TRH is effective when given intravenously as a bolus or by infusion,[448, 520] intramuscularly,[521] or orally[522] in single or repeated doses. Doses as small as 6 μg can elicit a significant TSH response, and there is a linear correlation between the incremental changes in serum TSH concentrations and the logarithm of the TRH doses.[448] The standard test uses a single TRH dose of 400 μg/1.73 m² body surface area, given by rapid intravenous injection. Serum is collected before and at 15 minutes and then at 30-minute intervals over 120 to 180 minutes, although many clinicians chose to obtain a single postinjection sample at 15, 20, or 30 minutes. In normal people there is a prompt increase in serum TSH with a peak level at 15 to 40 minutes, which is, on average, 16 μU/ml, or fivefold the basal level. The decline is more gradual with a return of serum TSH to the pre-injection level by three to four hours.[448, 520] Results can be expressed in terms of the peak level of TSH achieved, the maximal increment above the basal level (TSH), the peak TSH value expressed as a percentage of the basal value, or the integrated area of the TSH response curve. Determination of TSH before and 30 minutes after the injection of TRH provides information concerning the presence or absence of TSH responsiveness but cannot detect delayed or prolonged responses.

The stimulatory effect of TRH is specific for pituitary TSH, its free α- and β-subunits,[518] and prolactin. Under normal circumstances no significant changes are observed in the serum levels of other pituitary hormones[523] or potential thyroid stimulators.[524] Responsiveness is present at birth,[525] is greater in women than in men, particularly in the follicular phase of the menstrual cycle,[526] and may be blunted in older men,[448, 521, 522] but this is not a consistent finding.[527] On average, the magnitude of the response is greater at 11 P.M. than at 11 A.M.,[519] in accordance with the diurnal pattern of the basal TSH level, which correlates to its response to TRH. Repetitive administration of TRH to the same subject at daily intervals causes a gradual obtundation of the TSH response,[520] presumably because of the increase in thyroid hormone concentration[528] and, in part, TSH exhaustion.[529] More than one hour must elapse between the increase in thyroid hormone concentration and TRH administration for inhibition of the TSH response to occur. A number of drugs (see Table 39–10) and nonendocrine diseases (see Ch. 40) may affect to various extents the magnitude of the response.

TRH-induced secretion of TSH is followed by a release of thyroid hormone that can be detected by direct measurement of serum TT_4 and TT_3 concentrations.[199] Peak levels are normally reached about four hours after the administration of TRH and are accompanied by an increase in serum Tg concentration. The incremental rise in serum TT_3 is relatively greater, and the peak is, on average, 50 per cent above the basal level. Measurement of changes in serum thyroid hormone concentration after the administration of TRH has been proposed as an adjunctive test and is useful in the evaluation of the integrity of the thyroid gland or bioactivity of endogenous TSH.[530] Increase in RAIU is minimal and occurs only with high doses of TRH given orally.[522]

Adverse effects from the intravenous administration of TRH, in decreasing order of frequency, include nausea, flushing or a sensation of warmth, desire to micturate, peculiar taste, light-headedness or headache, dry mouth, urge to defecate, and chest tightness. They usually are mild, begin within one minute after the injection of TRH, and last for a few seconds to several minutes. A transient rise in blood pressure has been observed on occasion, but there are no other changes in vital signs, urine analysis, blood count, or routine blood chemistry tests.[523, 531] The occurrence of circulatory collapse is exceedingly rare.[532]

The test provides a means to distinguish between secondary (pituitary) and tertiary (hypothalamic) hypothyroidism (Fig. 39–7). Although the diagnosis of primary hypothyroidism can be easily confirmed by the presence of elevated basal serum TSH levels, secondary and tertiary hypothyroidism typically are associated with TSH levels that are low or normal. The serum TSH concentration may be slightly elevated because of the secretion of biologically less potent molecules,[431] but it remains inappropriately low for the degree of thyroid hormone deficiency. Differentiation between secondary and tertiary hypothyroidism cannot be made with certainty without the TRH test. A TSH response is suggestive of a hypothalamic disorder, and a failure to respond is compatible with intrinsic pituitary dysfunction.[533] Furthermore, the typical TSH response curve in hypothalamic hypothyroidism shows a delayed peak with a prolonged elevation of serum TSH before return to the basal value (see Fig. 39–7). The lack of a TSH response in association with normal prolactin stimulation may be a result of isolated pituitary TSH deficiency.[534] Caution should be exercised in the interpretation of the test result after

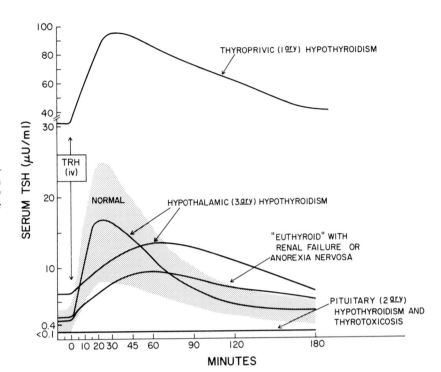

FIGURE 39–7. Typical serum TSH responses to the administration of a single intravenous bolus of TRH at time 0 in various conditions. The normal response is represented by the shaded area. Data used for this figure are the average of several studies.

withdrawal of suppressive doses of thyroid hormone or after treatment of thyrotoxicosis when, despite a low serum thyroid hormone concentration, TSH may remain low and not respond to TRH for several weeks.[438, 505, 508, 535]

In the most common forms of thyrotoxicosis, the mechanism of feedback regulation of TSH secretion is intact but is appropriately suppressed by the excessive amounts of thyroid hormone. Thus both the basal TSH level and its response to TRH are suppressed unless thyrotoxicosis is TSH-induced.[438, 441, 451] With the development of more sensitive TSH assays, the TRH test is not needed in the evaluation of a thyrotoxic patient with undetectable TSH.[441] Differential diagnosis of conditions leading to inappropriate secretion of TSH may be aided by the TRH test result. Elevated basal TSH values that do not respond by a further increase to TRH are typical of TSH-secreting pituitary adenomas.[510, 512] Patients with inappropriate secretion of TSH resulting from resistance to thyroid hormone have a normal or exaggerated TSH response to TRH that, in most instances, is suppressed with supraphysiological doses of thyroid hormone.[513]

Because of the high sensitivity of the pituitary gland to the feedback regulation by thyroid hormone, small changes in the latter profoundly affect the response of TSH to TRH. Thus patients with non–TSH-induced thyrotoxicosis of the mildest degree have a reduced TSH response to TRH, whereas those with primary hypothyroidism exhibit an accentuated response that is prolonged (see Fig. 39–7). These changes may occur in the absence of clinical or other laboratory evidence of thyroid dysfunction.

The TSH response to TRH is subnormal or absent in one third of apparently euthyroid patients with autoimmune thyroid disease, and even members of their family may not respond to TRH.[536, 537] Most patients with reduced TSH response to TRH also show thyroid activity that is nonsuppressible by thyroid hormone. A common dissocia-

tion between these two tests is typified by a normal TRH response in a nonsuppressible patient. This finding is not surprising because patients with nonsuppressible thyroid glands often have limited capacity to synthesize and secrete thyroid hormone because of prior therapy or partial destruction of their glands by the disease process. Clinically, euthyroid patients who do not respond to TRH admittedly have a slight excess of thyroid hormone. It is less easy to reconcile the rare occurrence of TRH unresponsiveness in a patient who is suppressible by exogenous thyroid hormone. It should be remembered, however, that a suppressed pituitary may take a variable amount of time to recover, a phenomenon that may be the basis of such discrepancies.[438, 508, 535] Despite discrepancies between the results of the TRH and T_3 suppression tests,[536, 537] the use of the former is much preferred, particularly in elderly patients in whom administration of T_3 can produce untoward effects.

Other Tests of TSH Reserve

It has been reasoned that by virtue of different mechanisms of action, testing the TSH response by means other than TRH may provide information of diagnostic value not obtainable from the stimulation and suppression of the pituitary by TRH and thyroid hormone, respectively.[427] Many trials using various drugs such as metoclopramide, L-dopa, and dexamethasone have been carried out but so far have provided only limited additional information and, thus, have not found a place in clinical practice. These tests have a limited application in the study of patients with inappropriate secretion of TSH, in whom the distinction of autonomous secretion of TSH as compared with a selective unresponsiveness to thyroid hormone inhibition is of diagnostic value.[86]

Other tests indirectly measure pituitary TSH reserve during the rebound period after suppression of thyroid hormone synthesis or pituitary TSH secretion. Assessment of thyroid gland activity after withdrawal of antithyroid drugs or T$_3$ replacement has been proposed.[538, 539]

Thyroid Stimulation Test

The thyroid stimulation test, also known as the TSH stimulation test, measures the ability of thyroid tissue to respond to exogenous TSH by an increase in iodide accumulation and/or hormone release. Formerly used to differentiate hypothyroidism caused by thyroid gland failure from that caused by TSH deficiency, the test is now almost exclusively done in conjunction with a scintiscan to localize areas of suppressed thyroid tissue. It requires the intramuscular administration of one or three 5- to 10-U doses of bovine TSH. The response is assessed from the change in the 24-hour RAIU or the incremental change in serum TT$_4$ or TT$_3$ measured before and after the course of TSH treatment.[540, 541] The presence of normal but nonfunctioning thyroid tissue suppressed by excess hormone from a functioning thyroid nodule, ectopic thyroid tissue, or hormone administration is best demonstrated by scanning after a three-day course of TSH.

The test may cause discomfort, and some of the reactions to the heterologous TSH may be serious.[541] Repeated administration of bovine TSH can also lead to the production of antibodies that may neutralize its action.[542] This is the main reason for not recommending the routine use of exogenous TSH in the search for functioning metastases in patients with thyroid cancer. Whether similar problems will occur with recombinant human TSH remains to be determined.

Thyroid Suppression Test

The maintenance of thyroid gland activity that is independent of TSH can be demonstrated by the thyroid suppression test. Under normal conditions administration of thyroid hormone in quantities sufficient to satisfy the body requirement suppresses endogenous TSH, resulting in reduction of thyroid hormone synthesis and secretion. Because thyrotoxicosis resulting from excessive secretion of hormone by the thyroid gland implies that the feedback control mechanism is not operative or has been perturbed, it is easy to understand why under such circumstances the supply of exogenous hormone would also be ineffective in suppressing thyroid gland activity. The test is of particular value in patients who are euthyroid or only mildly thyrotoxic but suspected of having abnormal thyroid gland stimulation or autonomy.

The test usually is carried out with 100 μg of L-T$_3$ (liothyronine) given daily in two divided doses over 7 to 10 days. Twenty-four-hour RAIU is obtained before and during the last two days of T$_3$ administration.[543] Normal people show a suppression of the RAIU by at least 50 per cent compared with the pre–L-T$_3$ treatment value. No change or lesser reduction is not only typical of Graves' disease but also other forms of endogenous thyrotoxicosis, including toxic adenoma, functioning carcinoma, and thyrotoxicosis resulting from trophoblastic diseases. The presence of nonsuppressibility indicates thyroid gland activity independent of TSH but not necessarily thyrotoxicosis. Euthyroid patients with autonomous thyroid function have a normal TSH response to TRH before the administration of L-T$_3$. However, inhibition of TSH secretion by the exogenous T$_3$ does not suppress the autonomous activity of the thyroid gland. This is the most commonly encountered discrepancy between the results of the two related tests. When the T$_3$ suppression test is used in conjunction with the scintiscan, localized areas of autonomous function can be identified. The test can be carried out without the administration of radioisotopes by measuring serum T$_4$ before and two weeks after the ingestion of L-T$_3$. Although total suppression of T$_4$ secretion never occurs, even after prolonged treatment with L-T$_3$, a reduction by at least 50 per cent is normal.[544]

A return to thyroid gland suppressibility in patients with autoimmune thyroid disease under treatment with antithyroid drugs can be demonstrated by the suppression of the 20-minute thyroidal uptake of $^{99m}TcO_4^-$ or $^{123}I^-$ during the administration of L-T$_3$.[545] The test has limited prognostic value in relation to long-term remission or outcome of therapy.[536, 546]

Variants of the test have been proposed to reduce the potential risks of L-T$_3$ administration in elderly patients and in those with angina pectoris or congestive heart failure. With the availability of sensitive TSH determinations and the TRH test, which are less dangerous, thyroid suppression tests are used infrequently.

SPECIALIZED THYROID TESTS

A number of specialized tests are available for the evaluation of specific aspects of thyroid hormone biosynthesis, secretion, turnover, distribution, and absorption. Their primary application is of investigative nature. Some are rather simple, others are complex. They are mentioned only briefly here for the sake of completeness. Most of these tests require in vivo administration of radioisotopes.

Iodotyrosine Deiodinase Activity

The test involves the intravenous administration of tracer MIT or DIT labeled with radioiodide. Urine collected over a period of four hours is analyzed by chromatography. Only 4 to 8 per cent of the radioactivity normally is excreted as such; the remainder appears in the urine in the form of iodide.[547] Excretion of larger amounts of the parent compound indicates inability to deiodinate iodothyrosine. The test is useful in the diagnosis of a dehalogenase defect (see Ch. 52).

Test for Defective Hormonogenesis

After administration of RAI the isotopically labeled compounds synthesized in the thyroid gland and those secreted into the circulation can be analyzed by immunological, chromatographic, electrophoretic, and density gradient centrifugation techniques.[548] Such tests serve to evaluate the synthesis and release of thyroid hormone as well as to delineate the formation of abnormal iodoproteins.

Iodine Kinetic Studies

The iodine kinetic procedure is used to evaluate overall iodide metabolism and to elucidate the pathophysiology of thyroid diseases. The analysis involves follow-up of the fate of administered radioiodide tracer by measurement of thyroidal accumulation, secretion into blood, and excretion in the urine and feces.[549]

Absorption of Thyroid Hormone

Failure to achieve normal serum thyroid hormone concentration after administration of replacement doses of thyroid hormone usually is the result of poor compliance occasionally to the use of inactive preparations and seldom to malabsorption. The last can be evaluated by the simultaneous oral and intravenous administration of the hormone labeled with two iodine isotope tracers. The ratio of the two isotopes in blood is proportional to the net absorbed fraction of the orally administered hormone.[550, 551] Under normal circumstances about 80 per cent of T_4 and 95 per cent of T_3 administered orally are absorbed. Hypothyroidism and various other, unrelated conditions have little effect on the intestinal absorption of thyroid hormones. Absorption may be diminished in patients with steatorrhea, in some cases of hepatic failure, during treatment with cholestyramine, and with diets rich in soybeans. The absorption of thyroid hormone can also be evaluated by the administration of a single oral dose of 100 μg T_3 or 1 mg T_4, followed by their measurement in blood sampled at various intervals.[552, 553]

Turnover Kinetics of T_4 and T_3

Turnover kinetic studies require the intravenous administration of isotope-labeled tracer T_4 or T_3.[554–558] The half-time (t½) of disappearance of the hormone is calculated from the rate of decrease in serum trichloroacetic acid precipitable, ethanol extractable, or antibody precipitable isotope counts. Compartmental analysis can be used for the calculation of the turnover parameters.[555, 556] The calculated daily degradation or production rate (PR) is the product of the fractional turnover rate (K), the extrathyroidal distribution space (DS), and the average concentration of the hormone in serum. Noncompartmental analysis may be used for the calculation of kinetic parameters.[555] The metabolic clearance rate (MCR) is defined as the dose of the injected labeled tracer divided by the area under its curve of disappearance. The PR is then calculated from the product of the MCR and the average concentration of the respective nonradioactive iodothyronine measured in serum over the period of the study. Simultaneous studies of the T_4 and T_3 turnover kinetics can be carried out by injection of both hormones labeled with different iodine isotopes.[555, 557, 558]

Average normal values in adults for T_4 and T_3, respectively, are t½ = 7.0 and 0.8 days; K = 10 per cent and 90 per cent per day; DS = 11 and 30 L of serum equivalent; MCR = 1.1 and 25 L/day; and PR = 90 and 25 μg/day.

The hormonal PR is accelerated in thyrotoxicosis and diminished in hypothyroidism.[554] In euthyroid patients with TBG abnormalities, the PR remains normal because changes in the serum hormone concentration are accompanied by compensatory changes in the fractional turnover rate and the extrathyroidal hormonal pool.[559] Various nonthyroidal illnesses may alter hormone kinetics[558, 560] (see Ch. 40).

Metabolic Kinetics of Thyroid Hormones and Their Metabolites

The kinetics of production of various metabolites of T_4 and T_3 in peripheral tissues and their further metabolism can be studied. Most methods use radiolabeled iodothyronine tracers injected intravenously.[18, 174, 176, 556–558] Their disappearance is followed in serum samples obtained at various intervals of time after injection of the tracers by means of chromatographic and immunological techniques of separation.[19, 176] Kinetic parameters can be calculated by noncompartmental analysis[555, 557] or by two- or multiple-compartment analysis.[554, 556] Estimates have been made by the differential measurement in urine of the isotopes derived from the precursor and its metabolite. They are in agreement with measurements carried out in serum.[561] Conversion rates (CR) of iodothyronines, principally generated in peripheral tissues, can be calculated from the ratio of their PR and that of their respective precursors. Some iodothyronines, such as T_3, are secreted by the thyroid gland as well as generated in peripheral tissues. Studies to calculate the CR require administration of thyroid hormone to block thyroidal secretion.[560]

On average, 35 and 45 per cent of T_4 are converted to T_3 and rT_3, respectively, in peripheral tissues. The conversion of T_4 to T_3 is greatly diminished in a variety of illnesses (see Ch. 40) of nonthyroidal origin and in response to many drugs (see Table 39–6). Degradation and monodeiodination of iodothyronines can be estimated without the administration of isotopes. They are, however, less accurate. The conversion of T_4 to T_3 can be estimated semiquantitatively by the measurement of serum TT_3 concentration after treatment with replacement doses of T_4.[560] Data can be also derived by measurement of the iodothyronine in serum after the administration of its precursor to athyreotic patients.[175, 181] Measurements of an iodothyronine in samples of serum obtained at intervals after its administration as a single, large intravenous or oral dose have also been used to estimate the MCR.[189]

Measurement of the PR and Metabolic Kinetics of Other Compounds

The metabolism and PR's of various compounds related to thyroid physiology can be studied using their radiolabeled congeners and application of the general principles of turnover kinetics. Studies of TSH have demonstrated changes related not only to thyroid dysfunction but also associated with age and kidney and liver disease.[562, 563] Studies of the turnover kinetics of TBG have shown that the slight increases and decreases of serum TBG concentration associated with hypothyroidism and thyrotoxicosis, respectively, are caused by changes in the degradation rate of TBG rather than by synthesis.[559]

Transfer of Thyroid Hormone From Blood to Tissues

Transfer of hormone from blood to tissues can be estimated in vivo by two techniques. A direct method follows the accumulation of the administered labeled hormone tracer by surface counting over the organ of interest.[564] An indirect method follows the early disappearance from plasma of the simultaneously administered hormone and albumin labeled with different radioisotope tracers.[565] The difference between the rates of disappearance of the hormone and albumin represents the fraction of hormone that has left the vascular (albumin) space and, presumably, has entered the tissues.

Applications of Molecular Biology in the Diagnosis of Thyroid Diseases

Recombinant technology has already produced new, highly purified reagents for the detection of anti-TSH receptor[367, 368] and peroxidase antibodies.[336] Human TSH has also been made by recombinant techniques and is being tested as a diagnostic agent.[396] Restriction fragment length polymorphisms have proved useful in the identification of inherited defects linked to chromosome 3 in kindreds with GRTH[566] and linked to chromosome 10 in patients having increased risk for the inheritance of medullary cancer as part of the multiple endocrine neoplasia 2A syndrome.[567] Detection of specific gene abnormalities by various techniques has been used to identify people with qualitative TBG abnormalities[568] and patients with GRTH as the result of an abnormal thyroid receptor.[86] With the characterization of specific gene abnormalities, it will be possible to identify people who are likely to develop the inherited form of medullary carcinoma and to enhance the diagnostic value of fine-needle aspirates of thyroid lesions.

EFFECTS OF DRUGS ON THYROID FUNCTION

A large number of compounds may affect thyroid function and economy.[100, 569] The list has rapidly grown with the introduction of new diagnostic agents, drugs, and food additives. This section is not intended to provide an all-encompassing review. Rather, the more commonly encountered compounds are listed, and those enjoying wider use or helpful in understanding the mechanism of drug interaction are described in greater detail.

Mechanisms of Action

Drugs affect the thyroid system at all levels of the hypothalamic-pituitary-thyroid axis. In addition to modulating thyroid hormone synthesis, drugs may alter the transport, metabolism, and excretion of T_4 and its derivatives. Some drugs and hormones, such as estrogens and androgens, affect thyroid hormone transport in blood by altering the concentration of the binding proteins in serum (see Ch. 36). Thyroid hormone transport may also be affected by substances that compete with the binding of thyroid hormone to its carrier proteins (see Table 39–4). The most extensively studied compounds that interfere competitively with thyroid hormone binding to the carrier proteins in serum are salicylates and diphenylhydantoin.[65, 66, 68] In general, the effect is a diminution in the serum concentration of total (bound) T_4 and, less often, T_3 with lesser effect on the absolute concentration of their metabolically active free fractions. In the steady state the quantity of thyroid hormone reaching peripheral tissues and the pathways and amount of hormone degradation remain unaltered. Before this steady state is reached, an acute perturbation in the equilibrium between free and bound hormone brings about transient changes in thyroid hormone secretion and degradation. The hypothalamic-pituitary-thyroid axis participates in the re-establishment of the new steady state (see Ch. 36).

Some of the agents that may alter the extrathyroidal metabolism of thyroid hormone are listed in Table 39–6. Several drugs widely used in clinical practice inhibit the conversion of T_4 to T_3 in peripheral tissues. Glucocorticoids, amiodarone, and propranolol are examples. As expected, their most profound effect on thyroid function is a decrease in the serum concentration of T_3, usually with a concomitant increase in the rT_3 level.[98, 159, 163, 164] An increase in the serum T_4 concentration has also been observed on occasion.[160, 163, 164] When intrapituitary T_4-to-T_3 conversion is inhibited, the serum TSH concentration may also rise.[163] In the absence of inherent abnormalities in thyroid hormone secretion or in its regulation, TSH levels should return to normal and hypothyroidism should not ensue from the chronic administration of compounds that only partially interfere with T_4 monodeiodination.

Other mechanisms by which some compounds affect the extrathyroidal metabolism of thyroid hormone are acceleration of the overall rates of the deiodinative and non-deiodinative routes of hormone disposal. An example of a drug acting principally through the former mechanism is phenobarbital[99] and by way of the latter, diphenylhydantoin.[167] Increase in thyroid hormone secretion is required to compensate for the enhanced hormonal loss through degradation or fecal excretion. Thyroid hormone concentration in blood should remain unaltered. Furthermore, it has been anticipated as well as observed that hypothyroid patients receiving such drugs require higher doses of exogenous hormone to maintain a eumetabolic state. Some drugs have multiple effects.

There has been a prodigious growth in the list of substances that act on the hypothalamic-pituitary axis (see Table 39–10). Although many of these compounds occupy an important place in the modern pharmaceutical armamentarium, only a few have significant effect on thyroid function by way of this central mechanism. Furthermore, people under drug treatment who have no thyroid disease seldom show important changes in basal serum TSH concentration. The response of TSH to the administration of TRH may be altered or the high levels of serum TSH in primary hypothyroidism may undergo a further increase or a significant diminution.

Although the aim of the next three paragraphs is to provide general information on the mechanism of action of these compounds, because of some inconsistencies in available information, it is premature to draw definite conclusions. A major problem in interpretation is the variability of experimental designs. These variables include doses, routes of administration, duration and time of treatment, drug combinations, age and sex of subjects, hormonal status at the time of testing, and time of blood sampling. Furthermore, observed responses are biased not only by the technical constraints of serum TSH measurements but also by the method of data analysis. For example, results of TSH responses to TRH have been expressed in terms of changes in the absolute value, increments or decrements from the basal level, and the percentage of the basal value at either the peak and nadir of the response or the integrated area over the duration of the response.

The most potent suppressors of pituitary TSH secretion are thyroid hormone and its analogues. They act on the pituitary by blocking TSH secretion through mechanisms discussed in Chapter 38. Some of the TSH-inhibiting agents listed in Table 39–10—fenclofenac and salicylates—may act by increasing the free thyroid hormone level by interference with its binding to serum proteins. Other agents appear to have a direct inhibitory effect on the pituitary and, possibly, the hypothalamus. The most notable is dopamine and its agonists. They have been shown to suppress the basal TSH levels in the euthyroid person[266, 478] and in patients with primary hypothyroidism.[266, 478–481] They also suppress the TSH response to TRH.[266] It is thus not surprising that a great number of dopamine antagonists amplify TSH secretion.[464–469, 570] Increases in the basal TSH and in its response to TRH have been observed in euthyroid people[464, 466] who have been given these drugs. A notable exception to this rule, which casts some doubt on the assumed mechanism of action of dopamine antagonists, is pimozide. This neuroleptic dopamine blocker has been shown to reduce the elevated serum TSH level in patients with primary hypothyroidism.[484]

Iodide and some iodine-containing organic compounds cause a rapid increase in the basal and TRH-stimulated levels of serum TSH. This effect is undoubtedly caused by a decrease in the serum thyroid hormone concentration either by inhibition of hormone synthesis and secretion by the thyroid gland[461] or by a selective decrease in the intrapituitary concentration of T_3 as with iopanoic acid and amiodarone.[462] Indeed, a predominant block on the intrapituitary conversion of T_4 to T_3 has been demonstrated.[499] It should be noted that iodide and iodine-containing compounds do not stimulate TSH secretion in patients in whom they induce excessive secretion of thyroid hormone.[571, 572] A decrease in the free thyroid hormone concentration in serum, albeit minimal in magnitude, may also be responsible for the increase in TSH levels observed during treatment with clomiphene.[471] An increase in serum TSH concentration during lithium therapy is also believed to be caused by reduced thyroid hormone levels rather than by a direct effect of this ion on the pituitary.[463]

It has been postulated that some agents may act by modifying the effect of TSH on its target tissue. For example, theophylline may potentiate the action of TSH through its inhibitory effect on phosphodiesterase, which may lead to an increase in the intracellular concentration of cAMP.[573] In fact, the presence of the pituitary is required to demonstrate that methylxanthines augment the goitrogenic effect of a low-iodine diet in the rat.[574]

A handful of drugs seem to act by blocking some of the peripheral tissue effects of thyroid hormone. Others appear to mimic one or several manifestations of the thyroid hormone effect on tissues. Guanethidine, which releases catecholamines from tissues, has a beneficial effect in thyrotoxicosis, decreasing the BMR, pulse rate, and tremulousness.[575, 576] This agent probably has no direct effect on the thyroid gland but may depress those manifestations of thyrotoxicosis that are mediated by sympathetic pathways. The sympatholytic agents phentolamine and Dibenzyline have been reported to both depress and stimulate thyroid function in animals. Their action is not clear, and clinically, it is not impressive. Among a number of α-adrenergic blocking agents tested, only phentolamine showed an inhibitory effect on the TSH response to TRH.[485]

Among the multiple effects of the β-adrenergic blocker propranolol on thyroid hormone economy is a reduction of peripheral tissue responses to thyroid hormone. In contrast, dinitrophenol enhances oxygen consumption by a direct effect on tissues and thus mimics one of the actions of thyroid hormone.[577]

Specific Agents

Estrogens

Hyperestrogenism caused by pregnancy, hydatidiform moles, tumors, or treatment with estrogens is the most common cause of TBG elevation.[55, 117] The magnitude of the increase is dose-related and occurs in women as well as in men. Estrogens increase the complexity of oligosaccharide side chains and, as a consequence, the number of sialic acids in the TBG molecule, which in turn prolongs its survival in serum.[578] The concentrations of other serum proteins, ceruloplasmin, transferrin, and several that bind hormones (cortisol-binding globulin and testosterone-binding globulin) are also increased.[579]

The consequences of increased TBG concentration in serum are higher serum levels of T_4 and T_3 and, to a lesser extent, other metabolites of T_4 deiodination. The fractional turnover rate of T_4 is depressed principally because of an increase in the intravascular T_4 pool. On the other hand, the FT_4 and FT_3 concentrations and the absolute amount of hormone degraded each day remain normal.[559, 580]

The effect of estrogen, if any, on the control of TSH secretion is controversial. Although women show a greater TSH responsiveness to TRH than men,[457, 520] administration of pharmacological doses of estrogens does not appear to have a significantly enhancing effect.[581] In addition to the consequences of high serum TBG levels, pregnancy also independently increases the thyroidal and renal iodide clearance and BMR.

Androgens

Androgens decrease the concentration of TBG in serum and thereby reduce the level of T_4 and T_3.[60, 61] The TTR concentration is increased.[60] As with estrogens, the concentration of free hormone remains unaffected, and the degradation rate of T_4 is normal at the expense of an accelerated turnover rate.[60] TSH levels are normal.[582] Anabolic steroids with weaker androgenic action have the same effect, although similar changes observed during danazol therapy have been attributed to its androgen-like properties.[583]

Salicylates

Salicylate and its noncalorigenic congeners compete for thyroid hormone–binding sites on TTR and TBG in serum, causing a decline of T_4 and T_3 concentrations and an increase of their free fractions.[65, 66] The turnover rate of T_4 is accelerated but degradation rates remain normal.[584, 585] Furthermore, they suppress the thyroidal RAIU but do not retard iodine release from the thyroid gland.[586] Thus the impaired response of TSH to TRH and the hypermetabolic effect of this drug were attributed to the increase in the FT_4 and FT_3 fractions.[493] If this proposed explanation were correct, hormonal release from the serum-binding proteins should produce only a temporary suppression of the thyroidal RAIU and transient hypermetabolism. In fact, both effects have been observed during chronic administration of salicylates.[584, 585] In addition, this mechanism of action does not explain the lack of calorigenic effect of some salicylate congeners despite their ability also to displace thyroid hormone from its serum-binding proteins.

In vitro studies have demonstrated an inhibitory effect of salicylate on the outer-ring monodeiodination of both T_4 and rT_3,[587] but lack of typical changes in the relative levels of serum iodothyronine suggests that this action is less important in vivo.

Acetylsalicylic acid mimics in several ways the action of thyroid hormone. For example, it lowers the serum cholesterol level,[588] but it does not provide a therapeutic effect in myxedema or lower TSH levels.[589] Administration of 8 g aspirin daily raises the BMR and accelerates the circulation, suggesting that the changes of blood flow in thyrotoxicosis and myxedema are secondary to heat production rather than primary effects of the hormone on the circulation.

Because of some analogies between the effects of salicylates and nitrophenol, uncoupling of oxidative phosphorylation has been suggested as a possible mechanism of action. If this were the case, direct chemical action does not appear to be involved because analogues of salicylate that do not uncouple oxidative phosphorylation in vitro are active in vivo.[590]

p-Aminosalicylic acid and p-aminobenzoic acid are closely related chemically to salicylate. They inhibit iodide binding in the thyroid gland and are goitrogenic.[591, 592]

Glucocorticoids

Physiological amounts of glucocorticoids as well as pharmacological doses influence thyroid function. The effects are variable and multiple, depending on the dose and on the endocrine status of the person. The type of glucocorticoid and the route of administration may also influence the magnitude of the effect.[593] Known effects include decrease in the serum concentration of TBG and increase in that of TTR[63]; inhibition of the outer-ring deiodination of T_4 and probably rT_3[98, 158]; suppression of TSH secretion[491]; a possible decrease in hepatic binding of T_4; and increase in renal clearance of iodide.[594]

The decrease in the serum concentration of TBG caused by the administration of pharmacological doses of glucocorticoids results in a decrease in the serum TT_4 concentration and an increase in its free fraction and the in vitro uptake test result. The absolute concentration of FT_4 and the FT_4I remain normal.

The more profound decrease in the concentration of serum T_3 compared with T_4 associated with pharmacological doses of glucocorticoids cannot be ascribed to the reduced serum TBG level. It is caused by decreased conversion of T_4 to T_3 in peripheral tissues. Thus the reduced $T_3{:}T_4$ ratio also occurs in hypothyroid patients receiving replacement doses of T_4. It is accompanied by an increase in the serum level of rT_3.[98] This effect of the steroid is rapid and may be seen within 24 hours.[98, 158]

Earlier observations of cortisone-induced depression of uptake and clearance of iodide by the thyroid gland[594] can now be attributed to the effect of this steroid on TSH secretion. Pharmacological doses of glucocorticoids suppress the basal TSH level in euthyroid subjects and in patients with primary hypothyroidism and decrease their TSH response to TRH.[491, 492] Normal adrenocortical secretion appears to have a suppressive influence on pituitary TSH secretion because patients with primary adrenal insufficiency have a significant elevation of TSH.[515]

No single change in thyroid function can be ascribed to a specific mode of action of glucocorticoids. For example, a diminished thyroidal RAIU may be caused by the combined effects of TSH suppression and increased renal clearance of iodide. Similarly, a low serum TT_4 level is the result of suppressed thyroidal secretion caused by diminished TSH stimulation as well as the decreased serum level of TBG. One of the common problems in clinical practice is to separate the effect of glucocorticoid action on pituitary function from that of other agents and those caused by acute and chronic illness. This situation arises often because steroids are commonly used in various autoimmune and allergic disorders as well as in the treatment of septic shock. The diagnosis of coexisting true hypothyroidism is difficult. Because of the suppressive effects of glucocorticoids on the hypothalamic-pituitary axis, the low levels of serum T_4 and T_3 may not be accompanied by an increase in the serum TSH level, which would otherwise be diagnostic of primary hypothyroidism. In such circumstances a depressed rather than an elevated serum rT_3 level may be helpful in the detection of coexistent primary thyroid failure.

Pharmacological doses of glucocorticoids induce a prompt decline in serum T_4 and T_3 concentrations in thyrotoxic patients with autoimmune thyroid disease.[98] Amelioration of the symptoms and signs in such patients may also be accompanied by a decrease in the elevated thyroidal RAIU and a diminution of the TSH receptor antibody titer.[595] This effect of glucocorticoids may be caused in part by its immunosuppressive action because it has been shown that administration of dexamethasone to hypothyroid patients with Hashimoto's thyroiditis causes an increase in the serum concentration of both T_4 and T_3.[596]

Diphenylhydantoin

Diphenylhydantoin (DPH) competes with thyroid hormone binding to TBG.[66, 69] This effect of DPH and diazepam, a related compound, has been exploited to study the conformational requirements for the interaction of thyroid hormone with its serum carrier protein.[68, 69] Although the affinity of DPH for TBG is far below that of T_4, when used in therapeutic doses the serum concentration achieved is high enough to cause a significant occupancy of the hormone binding sites on TBG. This effect of DPH is only partly responsible for the decrease in the total concentration of T_4 and T_3 in serum.

DPH reduces the intestinal absorption of T_4 and increases its nondeiodinative metabolism.[167] At the usual therapeutic concentrations this effect of the drug is probably more important than competition with T_4 for binding to TBG and is, by and large, responsible for the reduced concentration of T_4 in serum. Yet basal and TRH-stimulated TSH levels are within the range of normal[597] or only slightly elevated.[167, 168] This is partly the result of the increased generation of T_3 from T_4.[166, 167]

Both DPH and diazepam are commonly used in clinical practice, the former as an anticonvulsant and anti-arrhythmic agent and the latter as an anxiolytic. Reduced serum levels of thyroid hormone in patients having therapeutic blood levels of DPH should not be viewed as indicative of thyroid dysfunction unless the TSH level is elevated. DPH may slightly increase the required dose for thyroid hormone replacement in athyreotic subjects.[598]

Phenobarbital

Chronic administration of phenobarbital to animals induces increased binding of thyroid hormone to liver microsomes and enhanced deiodinating activity.[599] Phenobarbital administration reduces the biological effectiveness of the hormone by diverting it to microsomal degradative pathways. In humans phenobarbital augments fecal T_4 clearance by nearly 100 per cent,[99] but serum T_4 and FT_4I levels remain near normal because of compensatory increases in T_4 secretion. It is not apparent that barbiturates have an important effect on thyroid-mediated metabolic action in normal humans. The augmented hepatic removal of T_4 induced by phenobarbital increases T_4 clearance and lowers T_4 and FT_4I in patients with Graves' disease but has no effect on clinical response.[99]

Propranolol

Propranolol, a β-adrenergic blocker, often is used as an adjunct in the treatment of thyrotoxicosis. It is also used, in its own right, in the treatment of cardiac arrhythmias and hypertension.

Propranolol does not affect the secretion or overall turnover rate of T_4 or TSH release or its regulatory mechanisms.[99] A small to moderate lowering effect on serum T_3 has been reported in euthyroid subjects as well as in patients with hyperthyroidism or in those with myxedema under L-T_4 replacement therapy.[159, 160] Such data, combined with the findings of reciprocal increases in rT_3 and minimal increases in serum T_4 levels, suggest a mild blocking effect of this drug on the 5′-deiodination of iodothyronines in peripheral tissue.[160] This effect does not appear to be related to the β-adrenergic blocking action of propranolol because other β-blocking agents do not share the deiodinase-blocking property.[600, 601]

Clearly, the amelioration of the clinical manifestations of thyrotoxicosis are related to the β-adrenergic blocking action of propranolol rather than to its effect on thyronine metabolism. The reduction of tachycardia, anxiety, and tremor is useful in the management of patients.[602] Whether it in fact alters the hypermetabolism of thyrotoxicosis is debatable.

Nitrophenols

2,4-Dinitrophenol elevates the BMR, lowers the serum T_4 concentration, accelerates the peripheral metabolism of T_4, and depresses the thyroidal RAIU and secretion.[577, 603] The action is probably complex. Like T_4, the drug stimulates metabolism by uncoupling oxidative phosphorylation in the mitochondria.[604] Part of the effect of dinitrophenol may be to mimic the action of thyroid hormone on hypothalamic or pituitary receptor control centers; this effect would account for the diminished thyroid activity. Dinitrophenol also displaces thyroid hormone from T_4-binding serum proteins[65]; this action could lower the total hormone concentration in serum but should have no persistent effect on thyroid function. Dinitrophenol increases biliary and fecal excretion of T_4, and this action largely accounts for the rapid removal of hormone from the circulation.[605] Deiodination of T_4 is also increased. 2,4-Dinitrophenol does not share some of the most important properties of T_4. It cannot initiate metamorphosis of tadpoles[606] or provide substitution therapy in myxedema.

Dopaminergic Agents

It is now reasonably well established that endogenous brain dopamine plays a physiological role in the regulation of TSH secretion through its effect on the hypothalamic-pituitary axis.[464, 607] Dopamine exerts a suppressive effect on TSH secretion and can be regarded as antagonistic to the stimulatory action of TRH at the pituitary level.[478, 607] Much of the information regarding the role of dopamine in the control of TSH secretion in humans has been derived from observations made during the administration of agents with dopamine-agonistic and -antagonistic activity (see Table 39–10).

Dopamine infusion commonly is used in acutely ill hypotensive patients. It lowers the basal serum TSH level in both euthyroid and hypothyroid patients and blunts its response to the administration of TRH.[464, 478, 608] L-Dopa, the precursor of dopamine, used in the treatment of Parkinson's disease and as a test agent in the diagnosis of pituitary diseases, also suppresses the basal and TRH-stimulated serum TSH level in euthyroid subjects as well as in patients with primary hypothyroidism.[266] A similar effect has been observed during the administration of bromocriptine, a dopamine agonist used in the treatment of some pituitary tumors and to suppress lactation during the puerperal period. Although the agent has been shown to definitely diminish the high serum TSH levels in patients with primary hypothyroidism,[479] chronic administration does not produce a significant inhibitory effect on TRH-induced TSH secretion.[609]

Although some authors have cautioned that prolonged infusion of dopamine may induce secondary hypothyroidism and thus worsen the prognosis of severely ill patients,[610] there is no evidence that chronic treatment with dopaminergic drugs induces hypothyroidism in less critically ill patients. These drugs have been used in the treatment of pituitary-induced thyrotoxicosis.[510] When measurements of the basal or stimulated serum TSH levels are used in the differential diagnosis of primary and secondary hypothyroidism, the concomitant use of drugs with dopamine-agonistic or -antagonistic activity should be taken into account in the interpretation of results.

Iodide and Iodine-Containing Compounds

Iodine is an integral part of thyroid hormone, and its presence is thus critical for the maintenance of normal thyroid function. Administration of milligram quantities of iodide usually causes transient reduction in thyroid hormone secretion associated with an increase in serum TSH.[461] Under special circumstances it can cause a more permanent state of hypothyroidism, thyrotoxicosis or goiter. These and the effects of other minerals are discussed elsewhere in this book.

IODINATED CONTRAST AGENTS. The principal effect of some iodine-containing radiological contrast media is inhibition of T_4-to-T_3 conversion. In fact, they may be the most potent of all agents known to interfere with this step of iodothyronine metabolism. A triiodo- and a monoamino-benzene ring with a proprionic acid chain appear to be required because iodinated contrast agents without this chemical structure have little or no effect.[161] Several of these agents—ipodate (Oragrafin) and iopanoic acid (Telepaque)—are used for cholecystography.

A decrease in the rate of deiodination of the outer ring of thyronines causes a profound decrease in the serum T_3 concentration and an increase in the rT_3 and T_4 levels.[161, 162] The serum T_4 concentration may reach values well within the thyrotoxic range.[161] These changes are accompanied by an increase in serum TSH secretion.[462] The latter is particularly notable, if not characteristic, of these agents probably because of their potent inhibitory effect on T_3 generation in pituitary tissue.[611] The changes induced by these compounds usually persist for at least two weeks after their administration.[161]

Iodocontrast agents also decrease the hepatic uptake of T_4[612] and inhibit T_3 binding to its nuclear receptors.[613] The antithyroidal effect of the iodine present in these agents is believed to be responsible for the falling T_4 level and the amelioration of the symptoms and signs of thyrotoxicosis when they are administered to patients with Graves' thyrotoxicosis.[162]

AMIODARONE. Changes in thyroid function observed during the administration of this drug are similar to those seen with iodine-containing contrast agents. They include a marked decrease in serum T_3, an increase in rT_3, and a more modest elevation in the T_4 concentration.[163, 164] Basal and TRH-stimulated TSH levels are increased. The principal mechanism of action is believed to be inhibition of T_3 generation from T_4.

Amiodarone also contains iodine (37 per cent), a characteristic shared with the iodine-containing contrast media, but the principal effect on thyroid function appears to be caused by its structural resemblance to thyroid hormone rather than by its iodine content. In contrast, the rarer occurrence of amiodarone-induced thyrotoxicosis is caused by the excess iodine release from the drug and is observed more frequently in areas of mild iodine deficiency.[572] Drug-induced thyroiditis may also cause thyrotoxicosis, which often is followed by transient hypothyroidism.[614]

The use of this drug as an anti-anginal and anti-arrhythmic agent has increased. Amiodarone metabolites compete with thyroid hormone for its receptor, but it is uncertain to what extent this action is of physiological relevance at the concentrations achieved at the level of tissues. The bradycardia that almost invariably occurs when the drug is used in high doses may suggest the presence of

hypothyroidism.[164] Measurement of serum TSH, the most useful test in the differential diagnosis of this condition, may also give misleading results. If hypothyroidism is suspected, it is appropriate to obtain a measurement of the serum rT_3 concentration. A failure to show high serum levels of this iodothyronine in a patient receiving amiodarone can be considered indicative of hypothyroidism and a low serum TSH value with a normal serum T_3 concentration, as possibly thyrotoxicosis.

Antithyroid Drugs

Agents that act principally by inhibiting thyroid hormone synthesis are called collectively goitrogens or antithyroid drugs. A number of these compounds occur naturally in foodstuffs. Others are used in the treatment of thyrotoxicosis. A list of substances that inhibit thyroid hormone synthesis and secretion is provided in (Table 39–12). The reader is referred to Chapter 38 for details on their use and mechanism of action.

TABLE 39–12. AGENTS THAT INHIBIT THYROID HORMONE SYNTHESIS AND SECRETION

SUBSTANCE	COMMON USE
Block Iodide Transport Into the Thyroid Gland	
Monovalent anions (SCN^-, ClO_4^-, NO_3^-)	Not in current use; ClO_4 test agent
Complex anions (monofluorosulfonate, difluorophosphate, fluoroborate)	—
Minerals	In diet
Lithium	Treatment of manic-depressive psychosis
Ethionamide	Antituberculosis drug
Impair TG Iodination and Iodotyrosine Coupling	
Thionamides and thiourylenes (PTU, methimazole, carbimazole)	Antithyroid drugs
Sulfonamides (acetazolamide, sulfadiazine, sulfisoxazole)	Diuretic, bacteriostatic
Sulfonylureas (carbutamide, tolbutamide, metahexamide, ? chlorpropamide)	Hypoglycemic agents
Salicylamides (aminosalicylic acid)	Antituberculosis drugs
Ethionamide (P-aminobenzoic acid)	
Resorcinol	Cutaneous antiseptic
Amphenone and aminoglutethimide	Anti-adrenal and anticonvulsive agents
Thiocyanate	No current use; in diet
Antipyrine (phenazone)	Anti-asthmatic
Aminotriazole	Cranberry poison
Amphenidone	Tranquilizer
2,3-Dimercaptopropanol (BAL)	Chelating agent
Ketoconazole	Antifungal agent
Inhibitors of Thyroid Hormone Secretion	
Iodide (in large doses)	Antiseptic, expectorant, and others
Lithium	
Mechanism Unknown	
p-Bromdylamine maleate	Antihistaminic
Phenylbutazone	Anti-inflammatory agent
Minerals (calcium, rubidium, cobalt)	—
Interleukin II	Chemotherapeutic agent
γ-Interferon	Antiviral and chemotherapeutic agent

REFERENCES

1. Brown-Grant K: Extrathyroidal iodide concentrating mechanisms. Physiol Rev 4I:189–211, 1961.
2. Modan B, Mart H, Baidatz D: Radiation-induced head and neck tumors. Lancet 1:277–299, 1974.
3. Bland EP, Crawford JS, Docker MF, Farr RF: Radioactive iodine uptake by thyroid of breast-fed infants after maternal blood-volume measurements. Lancet 2:1039–1041, 1969.
4. Quimby EH, Feitelberg S, Gross W: Radioactive nuclides in medicine and biology (ed 3). Philadelphia, Lea & Febiger, 1970.
5. MIRD: Dose Estimate Report No. 5: Summary of current radiation dose estimates to humans from ^{123}I, ^{124}I, ^{126}I, ^{130}I, ^{131}I, and ^{132}I as sodium iodide. J Nucl Med 16:857–860, 1975.
6. MIRD: Dose Estimate Report No. 8: Summary of current radiation dose estimates to normal humans from ^{99m}Tc as sodium pertechnetate. J Nucl Med 17:74–77, 1976.
7. Pittman JA Jr, Dailey GE III, Beschi RJ: Changing normal values for thyroidal radioiodine uptake. N Engl J Med 280:1431–1434, 1969.
8. Gluck FB, Nusynowitz ML, Plymate S: Chronic lymphocytic thyroiditis, thyrotoxicosis, and low radioactive iodine uptake: Report of four cases. N Engl J Med 293:624–628, 1975.
9. Savoie JC, Massin JP, Thomopoulos P, Leger F: Iodine-induced thyrotoxicosis in apparently normal thyroid glands. J Clin Endocrinol Metab 41:685–691, 1975.
10. Higgins HP, Ball D, Estham S: 20-min ^{99m}Tc thyroid uptake: A simplified method using the gamma camera. J Nucl Med 14:907–911, 1973.
11. Baschieri L, Benedetti G, deLuca F, Negri M: Evaluation and limitations of the perchlorate test in the study of thyroid function. J Clin Endocrinol Metab 23:786–791, 1963.
12. Morgans ME, Trotter WR: Defective organic binding of iodine by the thyroid in Hashimoto's thyroiditis. Lancet 1:553–554, 1957.
13. Ford HC, Cooke RR, Keightley EA, Feek CM: Serum levels of free and bound testosterone in hyperthyroidism. Clin Endocrinol 36:187–192, 1992.
14. Gray HW, Hooper LA, Greig WR, McDougall IR: A 20-minute perchlorate discharge test. J Clin Endocrinol Metab 34:594–597, 1972.
15. Suzuki H, Mashimo K: Significance of the iodide-perchlorate discharge test in patients with ^{131}I-treated and untreated hyperthyroidism. J Clin Endocrinol Metab 34: 332–338, 1972.
16. Stanbury JB, Chapman EM: Congenital hypothyroidism with goiter. Absence of an iodide-concentrating mechanism. Lancet 1:1162–1165, 1960.
17. Chopra IJ, Fisher DA, Solomon DH, Beall GN: Thyroxine and triiodothyronine in the human thyroid. J Clin Endocrinol Metab 36:311–316, 1973.
18. Engler D, Burger AG: The deiodination of iodothyronines and of their derivatives in man. Endocr Rev 5:151–184, 1984.
19. Pittman CS, Shimizu T, Burger A, Chambers JB Jr: The nondeiodinative pathways of thyroxine metabolism: 3,5,3′,5′-tetraiodothyroacetic acid turnover in normal and fasting human subjects. J Clin Endocrinol Metab 50:712–716, 1980.
20. Gavin LA, Livermore BM, Cavalieri RR, et al: Serum concentration, metabolic clearance, and production rates of 3,5,3′-triiodothyroacetic acid in normal and athyreotic man. J Clin Endocrinol Metab 51:529–534, 1980.
21. deVijlder JJM, Veenboer GJM: Thyroid albumin originates from blood. Endocrinology 131:578–584, 1992.
22. Surks MI, Oppenheimer JH: Formation of iodoprotein during the peripheral metabolism of 3,5,3′-triiodo-L-thyronine-^{125}I in the euthyroid man and rat. J Clin Invest 48:685–695, 1969.
23. Refetoff S, Matalon R, Bigazzi M: Metabolism of L-thyroxine (T_4) and L-triiodothyronine (T_3) by human fibroblasts in tissue culture: Evidence for cellular binding proteins and conversion of T_4 to T_3. Endocrinology 91:934–947, 1972.
24. Koerner D, Surks MI, Oppenheimer JH: In vitro formation of apparent covalent complexes between L-triiodothyronine and plasma protein. J Clin Endocrinol Metab 36:239–245, 1973.
25. Trevorrow V: Studies on the nature of the iodine in blood. J Biol Chem 127:737–750, 1939.
26. Barker SB: Determination of protein-bound iodine. J Biol Chem 173:715–724, 1948.
27. Refetoff S: Principles of competitive binding assay and radioimmunoassay. In Gottschalk A, Potchen EJ (eds): Diagnostic Nuclear Medicine (Golden's Diagnostic Radiology). Baltimore, Williams & Wilkins, 1976, pp 215–236.
28. Mitsuma T, Colucci J, Shenkman L, Hollander CS: Rapid simultaneous radioimmunoassay for triiodothyronine and thyroxine in unextracted serum. Biochem Biophys Res Commun 46:2107–2113, 1972.
29. O'Connor JF, Wu GY, Gallagher TF, Hellman L: The 24-hour plasma thyroxine profile in normal man. J Clin Endocrinol Metab 39:765–771, 1974.
30. Fang VS, Refetoff S: Radioimmunoassay for serum triiodothyronine: Evaluation of simple techniques to control interference from binding proteins. Clin Chem 20:1150–1154, 1974.
31. Larsen PR, Dockalova J, Sipula D, Wu FM: Immunoassay of thyroxine in unextracted human serum. J Clin Endocrinol Metab 37:117–182, 1973.
32. Sterling K, Milch PO: Thermal inactivation of thyroxine-binding globulin for direct radioimmunoassay of triiodothyronine in serum. J Clin Endocrinol Metab 38:866–875, 1974.
33. Mitsuma T, Nihei N, Gershengorn MC, Hollander CS: Serum triiodothyronine: Measurements in human serum by radioimmunoassay with corroboration by gas-liquid chromatography. J Clin Invest 50:2679–2688, 1971.
34. Lieblich J, Utiger RD: Triiodothyronine radioimmunoassay. J Clin Invest 51:157–166, 1972.
35. Gaitan JE, Wahner HW, Gorman CA, Jiang NS: Measurement of triiodothyronine in unextracted urine. J Lab Clin Med 86:538–546, 1975.
36. Ikekubo K, Konishi J, Endo K, et al: Anti-thyroxine and anti-triiodothyronine antibodies in three cases of Hashimoto's thyroiditis. Acta Endocrinol 89:557–566, 1978.
37. Sakata S, Nakamura S, Miura K: Autoantibodies against thyroid hormones or iodothyronine. Implications in diagnosis, thyroid function, treatment, and pathogenesis. Ann Intern Med 103:579–589, 1985.
38. Canadian Task Force on the Periodic Health Examination: Periodic health examination, 1990 Update. I. Early detection of hyperthyroidism and hypothyroidism in adults and screening of newborns for congenital hypothyroidism. J Can Med Assoc 142:955–961, 1990.
39. Murphy BEP, Pattee CJ: Determination of thyroxine utilizing the property of protein-binding. J Clin Endocrinol Metab 24:187–196, 1964.
40. Schuurs AWM, Van Weemen BK: Enzyme-immunoassay. Clin Chim Acta 81:1–40, 1977.
41. Galen RS, Forman D: Enzyme immunoassay of serum thyroxine with AutoChemist multichannel analyzer. Clin Chem 23:119–121, 1977.
42. Schall RF, Fraser AS, Hausen HW, et al: A sensitive manual enzyme immunoassay for thyroxine. Clin Chem 24:1801–1804, 1978.
43. Miyai K, Ishibashi K, Kawashima M: Enzyme immunoassay of thyroxine in serum and dried blood samples on filter paper. Endocrinol Jpn 27:375–380, 1980.
44. Nihei NN, Gershengorn MC, Mitsuma T, et al: Measurements of triiodothyronine and thyroxine in human serum by gas-liquid chromatography. Anal Biochem 43:433–445, 1971.
45. Hoch FL, Kuras RA, Jones JD: Iodine analysis of biological samples by neutron activation of ^{127}I, with scintillation counting of Cerenkov radiation. Anal Biochem 40:86–94, 1971.
46. Hagen GA, Diuguid LI, Kliman B, Stanbury JB: Double-isotope derivative assay of serum iodothyronines. III. Triiodothyronine. Biochem Med 7:191–202, 1973.
47. Hay ID, Annesley TM, Jiang NS, Gorman CA: Simultaneous determination of D- and L-thyroxine in human serum by liquid chromatography with electrochemical detection. J Chromatogr 226:383–390, 1981.
48. Abuid J, Klein AH, Foley TP Jr, Larsen PR: Total and free triiodothyronine and thyroxine in early infancy. J Clin Endocrinol Metab 39:263–268, 1974.
49. Roger M, Soldat MC, Laffi E, et al: La thyroxine plasmatique chez l'enfant: Variations du taux avec l'âge et applications au diagnostic des dysthyroïdies. Ann Pediatr 22:27–33, 1975.
50. Westgren U, Burger A, Ingemanssons S, et al: Blood levels of 3,5,3′-triiodothyronine and thyroxine: Differences between children, adults, and elderly subjects. Acta Med Scand 200: 493–495, 1976.
51. Nishikawa M, Inada M, Naito K, et al: Age-related changes in serum 3,3′-diiodothyronine, 3′,5′-diiodothyronine, and 3,5-diiodothyronine concentrations in man. J Clin Endocrinol Metab 52:517–522, 1981.
52. Herrmann J, Rusche HJ, Kröll HJ, et al: Free triiodothyronine (T_3) and thyroxine (T_4) serum levels in old age. Horm Metab Res 6:239–240, 1974.
53. DeCostre P, Buhler U, DeGroot LJ, Refetoff S: Diurnal rhythm in total serum thyroxine levels. Metabolism 20:782–791, 1971.
54. Snyder SM, Cavalieri RR, Ingbar SH: Simultaneous measurement of percentage free thyroxine and triiodothyronine: Comparison of

equilibrium dialysis and Sephadex chromatography. J Nucl Med 17:660–664, 1976.

55. Oppenheimer JH: Role of plasma proteins in the binding, distribution, and metabolism of the thyroid hormones. N Engl J Med 278:1153–1162, 1968.

56. Azizi F, Vagenakis AG, Portnay GI, et al: Thyroxine transport and metabolism in methadone and heroin addicts. Ann Intern Med 80:194–199, 1974.

57. McKerron CG, Scott RL, Asper SP, Levy RI: Effects of clofibrate (Atromid S) on the thyroxine-binding capacity of thyroxine-binding globulin and free thyroxine. J Clin Endocrinol Metab 29:957–961, 1969.

58. Beex L, Ross A, Smals P, Kloppenborg P: 5-Fluorouracil-induced increase of total thyroxine and triiodothyronine. Cancer Treat Rep 61:1291–1295, 1977.

59. Oltman JE, Friedman S: Protein-bound iodine in patients receiving perphenazine. JAMA 185:726–727, 1963.

60. Braverman LE, Ingbar SH: Effects of norethandrolone on the transport in serum and peripheral turnover of thyroxine. J Clin Endocrinol Metab 27:389–396, 1967.

61. Barbosa J, Seal US, Doe RP: Effects of anabolic steroids on hormone-binding proteins, serum cortisol and serum nonprotein-bound cortisol. J Clin Endocrinol Metab 32:232–240, 1971.

62. Oppenheimer JH, Werner SC: Effect of prednisone on thyroxine-binding proteins. J Clin Endocrinol Metab 26:715–721, 1966.

63. Garnick MB, Larsen PR: Acute deficiency of thyroxine-binding globulin during L-asparaginase therapy. N Engl J Med 301:252–253, 1979.

64. O'Brien T, Silverberg JD, Nguyen TT: Nicotinic acid-induced toxicity associated with cytopenia and decreased levels of thyroxine-binding globulin. Mayo Clin Proc 67:465–468, 1992.

65. Christensen LK: Thyroxine-releasing effect of salicylate and of 2,4-dinitrophenol. Nature 183:1189–1190, 1959.

66. Larsen PR: Salicylate-induced increases in free triiodothyronine in human serum: Evidence of inhibition of triiodothyronine binding to thyroxine-binding globulin and thyroxine-binding prealbumin. J Clin Invest 51:1125–1134, 1972.

67. McConnell RJ: Abnormal thyroid function in patients taking salsalate. JAMA 267:1242–1243, 1992.

68. Oppenheimer JH, Tavernetti RR: Displacement of thyroxine from human thyroxine-binding globulin by analogues of hydantoin. Steric aspects of the thyroxine-binding site. J Clin Invest 41:2213–2220, 1962.

69. Schussler GC: Diazepam competes for thyroxine binding. J Pharmacol Exp Ther 178:204–209, 1971.

70. Stockigt JR, Lim CF, Barlow JW, et al: Interaction of furosemide with serum thyroxine-binding sites: In vivo and in vitro studies and comparison with other inhibitors. J Clin Endocrinol Metab 60:1025–1031, 1985.

71. Hershman JM, Craane TJ, Colwell JA: Effect of sulfonylurea drugs on the binding of triiodothyronine and thyroxine to thyroxine-binding globulin. J Clin Endocrinol Metab 28:1605–1610, 1968.

72. Tabachnick M, Hao YL, Korcek L: Effect of oleate, diphenylhydantoin, and heparin on the binding of ¹²⁵I-thyroxine to purified thyroxine-binding globulin. J Clin Endocrinol Metab 36:392–394, 1973.

73. Marshall JS, Tompkins LS: Effect of o,p'-DDD and similar compounds on thyroxine-binding globulin. J Clin Endocrinol Metab 28:386–392, 1968.

74. Abiodun MO, Bird R, Havard CW, Sood NK: The effects of phenylbutazone on thyroid function. Acta Endocrinol 72:257–264, 1973.

75. Davis PJ, Hsu TH, Bianchine JR, Morgan JP: Effects of a new hypolipidemic agent, MK-185, on serum thyroxine-binding globulin (TBG) and dialyzable fraction thyroxine. J Clin Endocrinol Metab 34:200–208, 1972.

76. Taylor R, Clark F, Griffiths ID, Weeke J: Prospective study of effect of fenclofenac on thyroid function tests. BJM 281:911–912, 1980.

77. Wiersinga WM, Fabius AJ, Touber JL: Orphenadrine, serum thyroxine and thyroid function. Acta Endocrinol 86:522–532, 1977.

78. Michajlovskij N, Langer P: Increase of serum free thyroxine following the administration of thiocyanate and other anions in vivo and in vitro. Acta Endocrinol 75:707–716, 1974.

79. Pages RA, Robbins J, Edelhoch H: Binding of thyroxine and thyroxine analogs to human serum prealbumin. Biochemistry 12:2773–2779, 1973.

80. Stockigt JR, Topliss DJ, Barlow JW, et al: Familial euthyroid thyroxine excess: An appropriate response to abnormal thyroid binding associated with albumin. J Clin Endocrinol Metab 53:353–359, 1981.

81. Sterling K, Refetoff S, Selenkow HA: T₃ toxicosis: Thyrotoxicosis due to elevated serum triiodothyronine levels. JAMA 213:571–575, 1970.

82. Sterling K, Brenner MA, Newman ES, et al: The significance of triiodothyronine (T₃) in maintenance of euthyroid status after treatment of hyperthyroidism. J Clin Endocrinol Metab 33:729–731, 1971.

83. Delange F, Camus M, Ermans AM: Circulating thyroid hormones in endemic goiter. J Clin Endocrinol Metab 34:891–895, 1972.

84. Fish LH, Schwartz HL, Cavanaugh MD, et al: Replacement dose, metabolism, and bioavailability of levothyroxine in the treatment of hypothyroidism. N Engl J Med 316:764–770, 1987.

85. Saberi M, Utiger RD: Serum thyroid hormone and thyrotropin concentrations during thyroxine and triiodothyronine therapy. J Clin Endocrinol Metab 39:923–927, 1974.

86. Refetoff S, Weiss RE, Usala SJ: The syndromes of resistance to thyroid hormone. Endocr Rev 14:348–399, 1993.

87. Luft R, Ikkos D, Palmieri G, et al: A case of severe hypermetabolism of nonthyroid origin with a defect in the maintenance of mitochondrial respiratory control: A correlated clinical, biochemical, and morphological study. J Clin Invest 41:1776–1803, 1962.

88. Olsen T, Laurberg P, Weeke J: Low serum triiodothyronine and high serum reverse triiodothyronine in old age: An effect of disease not age. J Clin Endocrinol Metab 47:1111–1115, 1978.

89. Welle S, O'Connell M, Danforth D Jr, Campbell R: Decreased free fraction of serum thyroid hormones during carbohydrate over-feeding. Metabolism 33:837–839, 1984.

90. Portnay GI, O'Brian JT, Bush J, et al: The effect of starvation on the concentration and binding of thyroxine and triiodothyronine in serum and on the response to TRH. J Clin Endocrinol Metab 39:191–194, 1974.

91. Azizi F: Effect of dietary composition on fasting-induced changes in serum thyroid hormones and thyrotropin. Metabolism 27:935–942, 1978.

92. Scriba PC, Bauer M, Emmert D, et al: Effects of obesity, total fasting and re-alimentation of L-thyroxine (T₄), 3,5,3'-L-triiodothyronine (T₃), 3,3',5'-L-triiodothyronine (rT₃), thyroxine-binding globulin (TBG), cortisol, thyrotrophin, cortisol binding gloublin (CBG), transferrin, α₂-haptoglobin and complement C′3 in serum. Acta Endocrinol 91:629–643, 1979.

93. Larsen PR: Triiodothyronine: Review of recent studies of its physiology and pathophysiology in man. Metabolism 21:1073–1092, 1972.

94. Hollander CS, Stevenson C, Mitsuma T, et al: T₃ toxicosis in an iodide-deficient area. Lancet 2:1276–1278, 1972.

95. Takamatsu J, Kuma K, Mozai T: Serum triiodothyronine/thyroxine ratio: A newly recognized predictor of the outcome of hyperthyroidism due to Graves' disease. J Clin Endocrinol Metab 62:980–983, 1986.

96. Rösler A, Litvin Y, Hage C, et al: Familial hyperthyroidism due to inappropriate thyrotropin secretion successfully treated with triiodothyronine. J Clin Endocrinol Metab 54:76–82, 1982.

97. Maxon HR, Burman KD, Premachandra BN, et al: Familial elevation of total and free thyroxine in healthy, euthyroid subjects without detectable binding protein abnormalities. Acta Endocrinol 100:224–230, 1982.

98. Chopra IJ, Williams DE, Orgiazzi J, Solomon DH: Opposite effects of dexamethasone on serum concentrations of 3,3',5'-triiodothyronine (reverse T₃) and 3,3',5-triiodothyronine (T₃). J Clin Endocrinol Metab 41:911–920, 1975.

99. Cavalieri RR, Sung LC, Becker CE: Effects of phenobarbital on thyroxine and triiodothyronine kinetics in Graves' disease. J Clin Endocrinol Metab 37:308–316, 1973.

100. Wenzel KW: Pharmacological interference with in vitro tests of thyroid function. Metabolism 30:717–732, 1981.

101. Busnardo B, Vangelista R, Girelli ME, et al: TSH levels and TSH response to TRH as a guide to the replacement treatment of patients with thyroid carcinoma. J Clin Endocrinol Metab 42:901–906, 1976.

102. Ekins R: Measurement of free hormones in blood. Endocr Rev 11:5–6, 1990.

103. Ekins R: The free hormone hypothesis and measurement of free hormones. Clin Chem 38:1289–1293, 1992.

104. Sterling K, Brenner MA: Free thyroxine in human serum: Simplified measurement with aid of magnesium precipitation. J Clin Invest 45:153–163, 1966.

105. Nelson JC, Tomel RT: Direct determination of free thyroxine in undiluted serum by equilibrium dialysis/radioimmunoassay. Clin Chem 34:1737–1744, 1988.

106. Surks MI, Hupart KH, Pan C, Shapiro LE: Normal free thyroxine in critical nonthyroidal illnesses measured by ultrafiltration of undiluted serum and equilibrium dialysis. J Clin Endocrinol Metab 67:1031–1039, 1988.

107. Melmed S, Geola FL, Reed AW, et al: A comparison of methods for

assessing thyroid function in non-thyroidal illness. J Clin Endocrinol Metab 54:300–306, 1982.

108. Wong TK, Pekary E, Hoo GS, et al: Comparison of methods for measuring free thyroxine in nonthyroidal illness. Clin Chem 38:720–724, 1992.

109. Chopra IJ, Chopra U, Smith SR, et al: Reciprocal changes in serum concentration of 3,3′,5′-triiodothyronine (reverse T₃) and 3,3′,5-triiodothyronine (T₃) in systemic illnesses. J Clin Endocrinol Metab 41:1043–1049, 1975.

110. Oppenheimer JH, Squef R, Surks MI, Hauer H: Binding of thyroxine by serum proteins evaluated by equilibrium dialysis and electrophoretic techniques. Alterations in nonthyroidal illness. J Clin Invest 42:1769–1782, 1963.

111. Nelson JC, Bruce WR, Pandian MR: Dependence of free thyroxine estimates obtained with equilibrium tracer dialysis on the concentration of thyroxine-binding globulin. Clin Chem 38:1294–1300, 1992.

112. Van der Sluijs Veer G, Vermes I, Bonte HA, Hoorn RKJ: Temperature effects on free-thyroxine measurements: Analytical and clinical consequences. Clin Chem 38:1327–1331, 1992.

113. Larsen PR, Alexander NM, Chopra IJ, et al: Revised nomenclature for test of thyroid hormones and thyroid-related proteins in serum. Clin Chem 33:2114–2116, 1987.

114. Felicetta JV, Green WL, Mass LB, et al: Thyroid function and lipids in patients with chronic liver disease treated by hemodialysis with comments on the free thyroxine index. Metabolism 28:756–763, 1979.

115. Refetoff S, Hagen S, Selenkow HA: Estimation of the T₄ binding capacity of serum TBG and TBPA by a single T₄ load ion exchange resin method. J Nucl Med 13:2–12, 1972.

116. Konno N: Evaluation of free triiodothyronine index as a measure of thyroid function. Folia Endocrinol Jpn 50:711–718, 1974.

117. Glinoer D, Fernandez-Deville M, Ermans AM: Use of direct thyroxine-binding globulin measurement in the evaluation of thyroid function. J Endocrinol Invest 1:329–335, 1978.

118. Attwood EC: The T₃/TBG ratio and the biochemical investigation of thyrotoxicosis. Clin Biochem 12:88–92, 1979.

119. Nuutila P, Koskinen P, Irjala K, et al: Two new two-step immunoassays for free thyroxine evaluated: Solid-phase radioimmunoassay and time-resolved fluoroimmunoassay. Clin Chem 36:1355–1360, 1990.

120. Hay ID, Bayer MF, Kaplan MM, et al: American Thyroid Association assessment of current free thyroid hormone and thyrotropin measurements and guidelines for future clinical assays. Clin Chem 37:2002–2008, 1991.

121. Wilkins TA, Midgley JEM, Barron N: Comprehensive study of a thyroxine-analog–based assay for free thyroxine (Amerlex FT₄). Clin Chem 31:1644–1653, 1985.

122. John R: Autoantibodies to thyroxin and interference with free-thyroxine assay. Clin Chem 29:581–582, 1983.

123. Ashkar FS, Buehler RJ, Chan T, Hourani M: Radioimmunoassay of free thyroxine with prebound anti-T₄ microcapsules. J Nucl Med 20:956–960, 1979.

124. Sarne DH, Refetoff S, Murata Y, et al: Variant thyroxine-binding globulin in serum of Australian aborigines. A comparison with familial TBG deficiency in Caucasians and American blacks. J Endocrinol Invest 8:217–224, 1985.

125. Murata Y, Refetoff S, Sarne DH, et al: Variant thyroxine-binding globulin in serum of Australian aborigines: Its physical, chemical and biological properties. J Endocrinol Invest 8:225–232, 1985.

126. Pardridge WM, Slag MF, Morley JE, et al: Hepatic bioavailability of serum thyroid hormones in nonthyroidal illness. J Clin Endocrinol Metab 53:913–916, 1981.

127. Keptein EM, Macintyre SS, Weiner JM, et al: Free thyroxine estimates in nonthyroidal illness: Comparison of eight methods. J Clin Endocrinol Metab 52:1073–1077, 1981.

128. Lehotay DC, Weight CW, Seltman JH, et al: Free thyroxine: A comparison of direct and indirect methods and their diagnostic usefulness in nonthyroidal illness. Clin Chem 28:1826–1829, 1982.

129. Oppenheimer JH, Schwartz HL, Mariash CN, Kaiser FE: Evidence for a factor in the sera of patients with nonthyroidal illness which inhibits iodothyronine binding by solid matrices, serum proteins, and rat hepatocytes. J Clin Endocrinol Metab 54:757–766, 1982.

130. Woeber KA, Maddux BA: Thyroid hormone binding in nonthyroidal illness. Metabolism 30:412–416, 1981.

131. Chopra IJ, Solomon DH, Teco GNC, Eisenberg JB: An inhibitor of the binding of thyroid hormones to serum proteins is present in extrathyroidal tissues. Science 215:407–409, 1982.

132. Chopra IJ, Chua Teco GN, Mead JF, et al: Relationship between serum free fatty acids and thyroid hormone binding inhibitor in nonthyroidal illnesses. J Clin Endocrinol Metab 60:980–984, 1985.

133. Sarne DH, Refetoff S: Measurement of thyroxine uptake from serum by cultured human hepatocytes as an index of thyroid status: Reduced thyroxine uptake from serum of patients with non-thyroidal illness. J Clin Endocrinol Metab 61:1046–1052, 1985.

134. Hamolsky MW, Stein M, Freedberg AS: The thyroid hormone-plasma protein complex in man. II. A new in vitro method for study of "uptake" of labeled hormonal components by human erythrocytes. J Clin Endocrinol Metab 17:33–44, 1957.

135. Sterling K, Tabachnick M: Resin uptake of ¹³¹I triiodothyronine as a test of thyroid function. J Clin Endocrinol Metab 21:456–464, 1961.

136. Braverman LE, Foster AE, Arky RA: Oragrafin and the triiodothyronine uptake test of thyroid function. J Nucl Med 8:209–212, 1967.

137. Schatz DL, Sheppard RH, Steiner G, et al: Influence of heparin on serum free thyroxine. J Clin Endocrinol Metab 29:1015–1022, 1969.

138. Elzinga KE, Carr EA Jr, Beierwaltes WH: Adaptation of standard Durrum-type cell for reverse-flow electrophoresis. Am J Clin Pathol 36:125–131, 1961.

139. Miyai K, Ito M, Hata N: Enzyme immunoassay of thyroxine-binding globulin. Clin Chem 28:2408–2411, 1982.

140. Refetoff S, Murata Y, Vassart G, et al: Radioimmunoassays specific for the tertiary and primary structures of thyroxine-binding globulin (TBG): Measurement of denatured TBG in serum. J Clin Endocrinol Metab 59:269–277, 1984.

141. Freeman T, Pearson JD: The use of quantitative immunoelectrophoresis to investigate thyroxine-binding human serum proteins. Clin Chim Acta 26:365–368, 1969.

142. Nielsen HG, Buus O, Weeke B: A rapid determination of thyroxine-binding globulin in human serum by means of the Laurell Rocket immunoelectrophoresis. Clin Chim Acta 36:133–138, 1972.

143. Mancini G, Carbonara AO, Heremans JF: Immunochemical quantitation of antigens by single radial immunodiffusion. Immunochemistry 2:235–254, 1965.

144. Chopra IJ, Solomon DH, Ho RS: Competitive ligand-binding assay for measurement of thyroxine-binding globulin (TBG). J Clin Endocrinol Metab 35:565–573, 1972.

145. Marshall JS, Levy RP, Steinberg AG: Human thyroxine-binding globulin deficiency: A genetic study. N Engl J Med 274:1469–1473, 1966.

146. Chopra IJ: An assessment of daily production and significance of thyroidal secretion of 3,3′,5′-triiodothyronine (reverse T₃) in man. J Clin Invest 58:32–40, 1976.

147. Nicod P, Burger A, Staeheli V, Vallotton MB: A radioimmunoassay for 3,3′,5′-triiodo-L-thyronine in unextracted serum: Method and clinical results. J Clin Endocrinol Metab 42:823–829, 1976.

148. Chopra IJ: A radioimmunoassay for measurement of 3,3′,5′-triiodothyronine (reverse T₃). J Clin Invest 54:583–592, 1974.

149. O'Connell M, Robbins DC, Bogardus C, et al: The interaction of free fatty acids in radioimmunoassays for reverse triiodothyronine. J Clin Endocrinol Metab 55:577–582, 1982.

150. Burman KD, Dimond RC, Wright FD, et al: A radioimmunoassay for 3,3′,5′-L-triiodothyronine (reverse T₃): Assessment of thyroid gland content and serum measurements in conditions of normal and altered thyroidal economy and following administration of thyrotropin releasing hormone (TRH) and thyrotropin (TSH). J Clin Endocrinol Metab 44:660–672, 1977.

151. Kirkegaard C, Faber J, Cohn D, et al: Serum 3′-monoiodothyronine levels in normal subjects and in patients with thyroid and non-thyroid disease. Acta Endocrinol 97:454–460, 1981.

152. Lalloz MRA, Byfield PGH, Himsworth RL: Hyperthyroxinaemia: Abnormal binding of T₄ by an inherited albumin variant. Clin Endocrinol 18:11–24, 1983.

153. Chopra IJ: A radioimmunoassay for measurement of 3′-monoiodothyronine. J Clin Endocrinol Metab 51:117–123, 1980.

154. Chopra IJ, Sack J, Fisher DA: Circulating 3,3′,5′-triiodothyronine (reverse T₃) in the human newborn. J Clin Invest 55:1137–1141, 1975.

155. Escobar del Rey F, Morreale de Escobar G: The effect of propylthiouracil, methylthiouracil and thiouracil on the peripheral metabolism of L-thyroxine in thyroidectomized L-thyroxine maintained rats. Endocrinology 69:456–465, 1961.

156. Furth ED, Rives K, Becker DV: Nonthyroidal action of propylthiouracil in euthyroid, hypothyroid, and hyperthyroid man. J Clin Endocrinol Metab 26:239–246, 1966.

157. Oppenheimer JH, Schwartz HL, Surks MI: Propylthiouracil inhibits the conversion of L-thyroxine to L-triiodothyronine. An explanation of the antithyroxine effect of propylthiouracil and evidence supporting the concept that triiodothyronine is the active hormone. J Clin Invest 51:2493–2497, 1972.

158. Duick DS, Warren DW, Nicoloff JT, et al: Effect of a single dose of

159. dexamethasone on the concentration of serum triiodothyronine in man. J Clin Endocrinol Metab 39:1151–1154, 1974.

159. Faber J, Friis T, Kirkegaard C, et al: Serum T_4, T_3 and reverse T_3 during treatment with propranolol in hyperthyroidism, L-T_4 treated myxedema and normal man. Horm Metab Res 11:34–36, 1979.

160. Wiersinga WM, Touber JL: The influence of β-adrenoreceptor blocking agents on plasma thyroxine and triiodothyronine. J Clin Endocrinol Metab 45:293–298, 1977.

161. Bürgi H, Wimpfheimer C, Burger A, et al: Changes of circulating thyroxine, triiodothyronine and reverse triiodothyronine after radiographic contrast agents. J Clin Endocrinol Metab 43:1203–1210, 1976.

162. Wu SY, Chopra IJ, Solomon DH, Bennett LR: Changes in circulating iodothyronines in euthyroid and hyperthyroid subjects given Ipodate (Oragrafin), an agent for oral cholecystography. J Clin Endocrinol Metab 46:691–697, 1978.

163. Burger A, Dinichert D, Nicod P, et al: Effects of amiodarone on serum triiodothyronine, reverse triiodothyronine, thyroxine and thyrotropin. J Clin Invest 58:255–259, 1976.

164. Nademanee K, Piwonka RW, Singh BN, Hershman JM: Amiodarone and thyroid function. Prog Cardiovascul Dis 31:427–437, 1989.

165. Schlienger JL, Kapfer MT, Singer L, Stephan F: The action of clomipramine on thyroid function. Horm Metab Res 12:481–482, 1980.

166. Larsen PR, Atkinson AJ, Wellman HN, Goldsmith RE: The effect of diphenylhydantoin on thyroxine metabolism in man. J Clin Invest 49:1266–1279, 1970.

167. Faber J, Lumholtz IB, Kirkegaard C, et al: The effects of phenytoin (diphenylhydantoin) on the extrathyroidal turnover of thyroxine, 3,5,3'-triiodothyronine, 3,3',5'-triiodothyronine and 3',5'-diiodothyronine in man. J Clin Endocrinol Metab 61:1093–1099, 1985.

168. Rootwelt K, Ganes T, Johannessen SI: Effect of carbamazepine, phenytoin and phenobarbitone on serum levels of thyroid hormones and thyrotropin in humans. Scand J Clin Lab Invest 38:731–736, 1978.

169. Northcutt RC, Stiel MN, Nollifield JW, Stant EG Jr: The influence of cholestyramine on thyroxine absorption. JAMA 208:1857–1861, 1969.

170. Witztum JL, Jacobs LS, Schonfeld G: Thyroid hormone and thyrotropin levels in patients placed on colestipol hydrochloride. J Clin Endocrinol Metab 46:838–840, 1978.

171. Van Wyk JJ, Arnold MB, Wynn J, Pepper F: The effects of a soybean product on thyroid functions in humans. Pediatrics 24:752–760, 1959.

172. Pinchera A, MacGillivray MH, Crawford JD, Freeman AG: Thyroid refractoriness in an athyrotic cretin fed soybean formula. N Engl J Med 273:83–86, 1965.

173. Isley WL: Effect of rifampin therapy on thyroid function tests in a hypothyroid patient on replacement L-thyroxine. Ann Intern Med 107:517–518, 1987.

174. Engler D, Markelbach U, Steiger G, Burger AG: The monodeiodination of triiodothyronine and reverse triiodothyronine in man: A quantitative evaluation of the pathway by the use of turnover rate techniques. J Clin Endocrinol Metab 58:49–61, 1984.

175. Pangaro L, Burman KD, Wartofsky L, et al: Radioimmunoassay for 3,5-diiodothyronine and evidence for dependence on conversion from 3,5,3'-triiodothyronine. J Clin Endocrinol Metab 50:1075–1081, 1980.

176. Faber J, Kirkegaard C, Lumholtz IB, et al: Measurements of serum 3',5'-diiodothyronine and 3,3'-diiodothyronine concentrations in normal subjects and in patients with thyroid and nonthyroid disease: Studies of 3',5'-diiodothyronine metabolism. J Clin Endocrinol Metab 48:611–617, 1979.

177. Geola F, Chopra IJ, Geffner DL: Patterns of 3,3',5'-triiodothyronine monodeiodination in hypothyroidism and nonthyroidal illnesses. J Clin Endocrinol Metab 50:336–340, 1980.

178. Chopra IJ, Geola F, Solomon DH, Maciel RMB: 3',5'-diiodothyronine in health and disease: Studies by a radioimmunoassay. J Clin Endocrinol Metab 47:1198–1207, 1978.

179. Burman KD, Wright FD, Smallridge RC, et al: A radioimmunoassay for 3',5'-diiodothyronine. J Clin Endocrinol Metab 47:1059–1064, 1978.

180. Jaedig S, Faber J: The effect of starvation and refeeding with oral versus intravenous glucose on serum 3,5-3,3'- and 3',5'-diiodothyronine and 3'-monoiodothyronine. Acta Endocrinol 100:388–392, 1982.

181. Smallridge RC, Wartofsky L, Green BJ, et al: 3'-L-monoiodothyronine: Development of a radioimmunoassay and demonstration of in vivo conversion from 3',5'-diiodothyronine. J Clin Endocrinol Metab 48:32–36, 1979.

182. Corcoran JM, Eastman CJ: Radioimmunoassay of 3-L-monoiodotyronine: Application in normal human physiology and thyroid disease. J Clin Endocrinol Metab 57:66–70, 1983.

183. Nakamura Y, Chopra IJ, Solomon DH: An assessment of the concentration of acetic acid and proprionic acid derivatives of 3,5,3'-triiodothyronine in human serum. J Clin Endocrinol Metab 46:91–97, 1978.

184. Burger A, Suter P, Nicod P, et al: Reduced active thyroid hormone levels in acute illness. Lancet 1:163–655, 1976.

185. Pittman CS, Suda AK, Chambers JB Jr, et al: Abnormalities of thyroid hormone turnover in patients with diabetes mellitus before and after insulin therapy. J Clin Endocrinol Metab 48:854–860, 1979.

186. Dlott RS, LoPresti JS, Nicoloff JT: Evidence that triiodoacetate (TRIAC) is the autocrine thyroid hormone in man. Thyroid 2(Suppl):S–94, 1992.

187. Nelson JC, Weiss RM, Lewis JE, et al: A multiple ligand-binding radioimmunoassay of diiodotyrosine. J Clin Invest 53:416–422, 1974.

188. Nelson JC, Lewis JE: Radioimmunoassay of iodotyrosines. In Abraham GE (ed): Handbook of Radioimmunoassay. New York, Marcel Dekker, 1979, p 705.

189. Meinhold H, Beckert A, Wenzel W: Circulating diiodotyrosine: Studies of its serum concentration, source, and turnover using radioimmunoassay after immunoextraction. J Clin Endocrinol Metab 53:1171–1178, 1981.

190. Van Herle AJ, Uller RP, Matthews NL, Brown J: Radioimmunoassay for measurement of thyroglobulin in human serum. J Clin Invest 52:1320–1327, 1973.

191. Schneider AB, Pervos R: Radioimmunoassay of human thyroglobulin: Effect of antithyroglobulin antibodies. J Clin Endocrinol Metab 47:126–137, 1978.

192. Schneider AB, Favus MJ, Stachura ME, et al: Plasma thyroglobulin in detecting thyroid carcinoma after childhood head and neck irradiation. Ann Intern Med 86:29–34, 1977.

193. Pacini F, Pinchera A, Giani C, et al: Serum thyroglobulin in thyroid carcinoma and other thyroid disorders. J Endocrinol Invest 3:283–292, 1980.

194. Black EG, Cassoni A, Gimlette TMD, et al: Serum thyroglobulin in thyroid cancer. BMJ 3:443–445, 1981.

195. Pezzino V, Filetti S, Belfiore A, et al: Serum thyroglobulin levels in the newborn. J Clin Endocrinol Metab 52:364–366, 1981.

196. Penny R, Spencer CA, Frasier D, Nicoloff JT: Thyroid-stimulating hormone and thyroglobulin levels decrease with chronological age in children and adolescents. J Clin Endocrinol Metab 56:177–180, 1983.

197. Refetoff S, Lever EG: The value of serum thyroglobulin measurement in clinical practice. JAMA 250:2352–2357, 1983.

198. Izumi M, Kubo I, Taura M, et al: Kinetic study of immunoreactive human thyroglobulin. J Clin Endocrinol Metab 62:400–412, 1986.

199. Uller RP, Van Herle AJ, Chopra IJ: Comparison of alterations in circulating thyroglobulin, triiodothyronine and thyroxine in response to exogenous (bovine) and endogenous (human) thyrotropin. J Clin Endocrinol Metab 37:741–745, 1973.

200. Lever EG, Refetoff S, Scherberg NH, Carr K: The influence of percutaneous fine needle aspiration on serum thyroglobulin. J Clin Endocrinol Metab 56:26–29, 1983.

201. Uller RP, Van Herle AJ: Effect of therapy on serum thyroglobulin levels in patients with Graves' disease. J Clin Endocrinol Metab 46:747–755, 1978.

202. Smallridge RC, DeKeyser FM, Van Herle AJ, et al: Thyroid iodine content and serum thyroglobulin: Clues to the national history of destruction-induced thyroiditis. J Clin Endocrinol Metab 62:1213–1219, 1986.

203. Mariotti S, Martino E, Cupini C, et al: Low serum thyroglobulin as a clue to the diagnosis of thyrotoxicosis factitia. N Engl J Med 307:410–412, 1982.

204. Van Herle AJ, Uller RP: Elevated serum thyroglobulin: A marker of metastases in differentiated thyroid carcinoma. J Clin Invest 56:272–277, 1975.

205. Schneider AB, Line BR, Goldman JM, Robbins J: Sequential serum thyroglobulin determinations, ^{131}I scans, and ^{131}I uptakes after triiodothyronine withdrawal in patients with thyroid cancer. J Clin Endocrinol Metab 53:1199–1206, 1981.

206. Colacchio TA, LoGerfo P, Colacchio DA, Feind C: Radioiodine total body scan versus serum thyroglobulin levels in follow-up of patients with thyroid cancer. Surgery 91:42–45, 1982.

207. Barsano CP, Skosey C, DeGroot LJ, Refetoff S: Serum thyroglobulin in the management of patients with thyroid cancer. Arch Intern Med 142:763–767, 1982.

208. Kawamura S, Kishino B, Tajima K, et al: Serum thyroglobulin changes in patients with Graves' disease treated with long term antithyroid drug therapy. J Clin Endocrinol Metab 56:507–512, 1983.

209. Black EG, Bodden SJ, Hulse JA, Hoffenberg R: Serum thyroglobulin in normal and hypothyroid neonates. Clin Endocrinol 16:267–274, 1982.

210. Heinze HJ, Shulman DI, Diamond FB Jr, Bercu BB: Spectrum of serum thyroglobulin elevation in congenital thyroid disorders. Thyroid 3:37–40, 1993.

211. Czernichow P, Schlumberger M, Pomarede R, Fragu P: Plasma thyroglobulin measurements help determine the type of thyroid defect in congenital hypothyroidism. J Clin Endocrinol Metab 56:242, 1983.

212. Burke CW, Shakespear RA, Fraser TR: Measurement of thyroxine and triiodothyronine in human urine. Lancet 2:1177–1179, 1972.

213. Chan V, Landon J: Urinary thyroxine excretion as index of thyroid function. Lancet 1:4–6, 1972.

214. Chan V, Besser GM, Landon J, Ekins RP: Urinary triiodothyronine excretion as index of thyroid function. Lancet 2:253–256, 1972.

215. Burke CW, Shakespear RA: Triiodothyronine and thyroxine in urine. II. Renal handling and effect of urinary protein. J Clin Endocrinol Metab 42:504–513, 1976.

216. Sack J, Fisher DA, Hobel CJ, Lam R: Thyroxine in human amniotic fluid. J Pediatr 87:364–368, 1975.

217. Chopra IJ, Crandall BF: Thyroid hormones and thyrotropin in amniotic fluid. N Engl J Med 293:740–743, 1975.

218. Burman KD, Read J, Dimond RC, et al: Measurement of 3,3',5'-triiodothyronine (reverse T₃), 3,3'-L-diiodothyronine, T₃, and T₄ in human amniotic fluid and in cord and maternal serum. J Clin Endocrinol Metab 43:1351–1359, 1976.

219. Siersbaek-Nielsen K, Hansen JM: Tyrosine and free thyroxine in cerebrospinal fluid in thyroid disease. Acta Endocrinol 64:126–132, 1970.

220. Hagen GA, Elliott WJ: Transport of thyroid hormones in serum and cerebrospinal fluid. J Clin Endocrinol Metab 37:415–422, 1973.

221. Nishikawa M, Inada M, Naito K, et al: 3,3',5'-Triiodothyronine (reverse T₃) in human cerebrospinal fluid. J Clin Endocrinol Metab 53:1030–1035, 1981.

222. Mallol J, Obregón MJ, Morreale de Escobar G: Analytical artifacts in radioimmunoassay of L-thyroxine in human milk. Clin Chem 28:1277–1282, 1982.

223. Varma SK, Collins M, Row A, et al: Thyroxine, triiodothyronine, and reverse triiodothyronine concentrations in human milk. J Pediatr 93:803–806, 1978.

224. Jansson L, Ivarsson S, Larsson I, Ekman R: Triiodothyronine and thyroxine in human milk. Acta Paediatr Scand 72:703–705, 1983.

225. Riad-Fahmy D, Read GF, Walker RF, Griffiths K: Steroids in saliva for assessing endocrine function. Endocr Rev 3:367–395, 1982.

226. Elson MK, Morley JE, Shafer RB: Salivary thyroxine as an estimate of free thyroxine: Concise communication. J Nucl Med 24:700–702, 1983.

227. Reichlin S, Bollinger J, Nejad I, Sullivan P: Tissue thyroid hormone concentration of rat and man determined by radioimmunoassay: Biologic significance. Mt Sinai J Med 40:502–510, 1973.

228. Ochi Y, Hachiya T, Yoshimura M, et al: Determination of triiodothyronine in red blood cells by radioimmunoassay. Endocrinol Jpn 23:207–213, 1976.

229. Lim VS, Zavata DC, Flanigan MJ, Freeman RM: Basal oxygen uptake: A new technique for an old test. J Clin Endocrinol Metab 62:863–868, 1986.

230. Becker DV: Metabolic indices. In Werner SC, Ingbar SH (eds): The Thyroid: A Fundamental and Clinical Text. New York, Harper & Row, 1971, pp 524–533.

231. Waal-Manning HJ: Effect of propranolol on the duration of the Achiles tendon reflex. Clin Pharmacol Ther 10:199–206, 1969.

232. Rodbard D, Fujita T, Rodbard S: Estimation of thyroid function by timing the arterial sounds. JAMA 201:884–887, 1967.

233. Nuutila P, Irjala K, Saraste M, et al: Cardiac systolic time intervals and thyroid hormone levels during treatment of hypothyroidism. Scand J Clin Lab Invest 52:467–477, 1992.

234. Lewis BS, Ehrenfeld EN, Lewis N, Gotsman MS: Echocardiographic LV function in thyrotoxicosis. Am Heart J 97:460–468, 1979.

235. Vesell ES, Shapiro JR, Passananti GT, et al: Altered plasma half-lives of antipyrine, propylthiouracil, and methimazole in thyroid dysfunction. Clin Pharmacol Ther 17:48–56, 1975.

236. Brunk SF, Combs SP, Miller JD, et al: Effects of hypothyroidism and hyperthyroidism on dipyrone metabolism in man. J Clin Pharmacol 14:271–279, 1974.

237. Kekki M: Serum protein turnover in experimental hypo- and hyperthyroidism. Acta Endocrinol (Suppl) 91:1–139, 1964.

238. Walton KW, Scott PJ, Dykes PW, Davies JWL: The significance of alterations in serum lipids in thyroid dysfunction. II. Alterations of the metabolism and turnover of ¹³¹I-low-density lipoproteins in hypothyroidism and thyrotoxicosis. Clin Sci 29:217–238, 1965.

239. Hellman L, Bradlow HL, Zumoff B, Gallagher TF: The influence of thyroid hormone on hydrocortisone production and metabolism. J Clin Endocrinol Metab 21:1231–1247, 1961.

240. Gallagher TF, Hellman L, Finkelstein J, et al: Hyperthyroidism and cortisol secretion in man. J Clin Endocrinol Metab 34:919–927, 1972.

241. Kiely JM, Purnell DC, Owen CA Jr: Erythrokinetics in myxedema. Ann Intern Med 67:533–538, 1967.

242. Das KC, Mukherjee M, Sarkar TK, et al: Erythropoiesis and erythropoietin in hypo- and hyperthyroidism. J Clin Endocrinol Metab 40:211–220, 1975.

243. Rivlin RS, Melmon KL, Sjoerdsma A: An oral tyrosine tolerance test in thyrotoxicosis and myxedema. N Engl J Med 272:1143–1148, 1965.

244. Bélanger R, Chandramohan N, Misbin R, Rivlin RS: Tyrosine and glutamic acid in plasma and urine of patients with altered thyroid function. Metabolism 21:855–865, 1972.

245. Lamberg BA, Gräsbeck R: The serum protein pattern in disorders of thyroid function. Acta Endocrinol 19:91–100, 1955.

246. Anderson DC: Sex-hormone-binding globulin. Clin Endocrinol 3:69–96, 1974.

247. DeNayer P, Lambot MP, Desmons MC, et al: Sex hormone–binding protein in hypothyroxinemic patients: A discriminator for thyroid status in thyroid hormone resistance and familial dysalbuminemic hyperthyroxinemia. J Clin Endocrinol Metab 62:1309–1312, 1986.

248. Macaron CI, Macaron ZG: Increased serum ferritin levels in hyperthyroidism. Ann Intern Med 96:617–618, 1982.

249. Takamatsu J, Majima M, Miki K, et al: Serum ferritin as a marker of thyroid hormone action on peripheral tissues. J Clin Endocrinol Metab 61:672–676, 1985.

250. Graninger W, Pirich KR, Speiser W, et al: Effect of thyroid hormones on plasma protein concentration in man. J Clin Endocrinol Metab 63:407–411, 1986.

251. Shah JH, Cechio GM: Hypoinsulinemia of hypothyroidism. Arch Intern Med 132:657–661, 1973.

252. Levy LJ, Adesman JJ, Spergel G: Studies on the carbohydrate and lipid metabolism in thyroid disease: Effects of glucagon. J Clin Endocrinol Metab 30:372–379, 1970.

253. Chopra IJ, Tulchinsky D: Status of estrogen-androgen balance in hyperthyroid men with Graves' disease. J Clin Endocrinol Metab 38:269–277, 1974.

254. Seino Y, Matsukura S, Miyamoto Y, et al: Hypergastrinemia in hyperthyroidism. J Clin Endocrinol Metab 43:852–855, 1976.

255. Bouillon R, DeMoor P: Parathyroid function in patients with hyper- or hypothyroidism. J Clin Endocrinol Metab 38:999–1004, 1974.

256. Castro JH, Genuth SM, Klein L: Comparative response to parathyroid hormone in hyperthyroidism and hypothyroidism. Metabolism 24:839–848, 1975.

257. Kojima N, Sakata S, Nakamura S, et al: Serum concentrations of osteocalcin in patients with hyperthyroidism, hypothyroidism and subacute thyroiditis. J Endocrinol Invest 15:491–496, 1992.

258. Body JJ, Demeester-Mirkine N, Borkowski A, et al: Calcitonin deficiency in primary hypothyroidism. J Clin Endocrinol Metab 62:700–703, 1986.

259. Hauger-Klevene JH, Brown H, Zavaleta J: Plasma renin activity in hyper- and hypothyroidism: Effect of adrenergic blocking agents. J Clin Endocrinol Metab 34:625–629, 1972.

260. Ogihara T, Yamamoto T, Miyai K, Kumahara Y: Plasma renin activity and aldosterone concentration of patients with hyperthyroidism and hypothyroidism. Endocrinol Jpn 20:433–438, 1973.

261. Stoffer SS, Jiang NS, Gorman CA, Pikler GM: Plasma catecholamines in hypothyroidism and hyperthyroidism. J Clin Endocrinol Metab 36:587–589, 1973.

262. Christensen NJ: Plasma noradrenaline and adrenaline in patients with thyrotoxicosis and myxoedema. Clin Sci Mol Med 45:163–171, 1973.

263. Zimmerman RS, Gharib H, Zimmerman D, et al: Atrial naturetic peptide in hypothyroidism. J Clin Endocrinol Metab 64:353–355, 1987.

264. Rolandi E, Santaniello B, Bagnasco M, et al: Thyroid hormones and atrial natriuretic hormone secretion: Study in hyper- and hypothyroid patients. Acta Endocrinol 127:23–26, 1992.

265. Distiller LA, Sagel J, Morley JE: Assessment of pituitary gonadotropin reserve using luteinizing hormone–releasing hormone (LRH) in states of altered thyroid function. J Clin Endocrinol Metab 40:512–515, 1975.

266. Refetoff S, Fang VS, Rapoport B, Friesen HG: Interrelationships in the regulation of TSH and prolactin secretion in man: Effects of L-DOPA, TRH and thyroid hormone in various combinations. J Clin Endocrinol Metab 38:450–457, 1974.

267. Honbo KS, Van Herle AJ, Kellett KA: Serum prolactin levels in untreated primary hypothyroidism. Am J Med 64:782–787, 1978.

268. Brauman H, Corvilain J: Growth hormone response to hypoglycemia in myxedema. J Clin Endocrinol Metab 28:301–304, 1968.

269. Rosenfield PS, Wool MS, Danforth E Jr: Growth hormone response to insulin-induced hypoglycemia in thyrotoxicosis. J Clin Endocrinol Metab 29:777–780, 1969.

270. Hamada N, Uoi K, Nishizawa Y, et al: Increase of serum GH concentration following TRH injection in patients with primary hypothyroidism. Endocrinol Jpn 23:5–10, 1976.

271. Kung AEC, Hui WM, Ng ESK: Serum and plasma epidermal growth factor in thyroid disorders. Acta Endocrinol 127:52–57, 1992.

272. Graig FA, Smith JC: Serum creatine phosphokinase activity in altered thyroid states. J Clin Endocrinol Metab 25:723–731, 1965.

273. Fleisher GA, McConahey WM, Pankow M: Serum creatine kinase, lactic dehydrogenase, and glutamic-oxalacetic transaminase in thyroid diseases and pregnancy. Mayo Clin Proc 40:300–311, 1965.

274. Doran GR, Wilkinson JH: Serum creatine kinase and adenylate kinase in thyroid disease. Clin Chim Acta 35:115–119, 1971.

275. Stolk JM, Hurst JH, Nisula BC: The inverse relationship between serum dopamine-β-hydroxylase activity and thyroid function. J Clin Endocrinol Metab 51:259–264, 1980.

276. Talbot NB, Hoeffel G, Schwachman H, Tuohy EL: Serum phosphatase as an aid in the diagnosis of cretinism and juvenile hypothyroidism. Am J Dis Child 62:273–278, 1941.

277. Lieberthal AS, Benson SG, Klitgaard HM: Serum malic dehydrogenase in thyroid disease. J Clin Endocrinol Metab 23:211–214, 1963.

278. Yotsumuto H, Imai Y, Kuzuya N, et al: Increased levels of serum angiotensin-converting enzyme activity in hyperthyroidism. Ann Intern Med 96:326–328, 1982.

279. Gow SMG, Caldwell G, Toft AD, et al: Relationship between pituitary and other target organ responsiveness in thyroid patients receiving thyroxine replacement. J Clin Endocrinol Metab 64:364–370, 1987.

280. Beckett GJ, Kellett HA, Gow SM, et al: Elevated plasma glutathione S-transferase concentrations in hyperthyroidism and in hypothyroid patients receiving thyroxine replacement: Evidence for hepatic damage. BMJ 2:427–429, 1985.

281. Ogura F, Morii H, Ohmo M, et al: Serum coenzyme Q_{10} levels in thyroid disorders. Horm Metab Res 12:537–540, 1980.

282. Bouillon R, Muls E, DeMoor P: Influence of thyroid function on the serum concentration of 1,25-dihydroxy vitamin D_3. J Clin Endocrinol Metab 51:793–796, 1980.

283. Walton KW, Campbell DA, Tonks EL: The significance of alterations in serum lipids in thyroid function. I. The relation between serum lipoproteins, carotenoids, and vitamin A in hypothyroidism and thyrotoxicosis. Clin Sci 29:199–215, 1965.

284. Karlberg BE, Henriksson KG, Andersson RGG: Cyclic adenosine 3′,5′-monophosphate concentration in plasma, adipose tissue and skeletal muscle in normal subjects and in patients with hyper- and hypothyroidism. J Clin Endocrinol Metab 39:96–101, 1974.

285. Peracchi M, Bamonti-Catena F, Lombardi L, et al: Plasma and urine cyclic nucleotide levels in patients with hyperthyroidism and hypothyroidism. J Endocrinol Invest 6:173–177, 1983.

286. Rivlin RS, Wagner HN Jr: Anemia in hyperthyroidism. Ann Intern Med 70:507–516, 1969.

287. Feldman DL, Goldberg WM: Hyperthyroidism with periodic paralysis. Can Med Assoc J 101:667–671, 1969.

288. Pettinger WA, Talner L, Ferris TF: Inappropriate secretion of antidiuretic hormone due to myxedema. N Engl J Med 272:362–364, 1965.

289. Jones JE, Deser PC, Shane SR, Flink EB: Magnesium metabolism in hyperthyroidism and hypothyroidism. J Clin Invest 45:891–900, 1966.

290. Baxter JD, Bondy PK: Hypercalcemia of thyrotoxicosis. Ann Intern Med 65:429–442, 1966.

291. Weldon AP, Danks DM: Congenital hypothyroidism and neonatal jaundice. Arch Dis Child 47:469–471, 1972.

292. Greenberger NJ, Milligan FD, DeGroot LJ, Isselbacher KJ: Jaundice and thyrotoxicosis in the absence of congestive heart failure: A study of four cases. Am J Med 36:840–846, 1964.

293. Kuhlbäch B: Creatine and creatinine metabolism in thyrotoxicosis and hypothyroidism. Acta Med Scand (Suppl) 331:1–70, 1957.

294. Adlkofer F, Armbrecht U, Schleusener H: Plasma lecithin: Cholesterol acyltransferase activity in hypo- and hyperthyroidism. Horm Metab Res 6:142–146, 1974.

295. Pykälistö O, Goldberg AP, Brunzell JD: Reversal of decreased human adipose tissue lipoprotein lipase and hypertriglyceridemia after treatment of hypothyroidism. J Clin Endocrinol Metab 43:591–600, 1976.

296. De Bruin TWA, Van Barlingen H, Van Linde-Sibenius Trip M, et al: Lipoprotein (a) and apolipoprotein B plasma concentrations in hypothyroid, euthyroid, and hyperthyroid subjects. J Clin Endocrinol Metab 76:121–126, 1993.

297. Inui T, Ochi Y, Chen W, et al: Increased serum concentration of type IV collagen peptide and type III collagen peptide in hyperthyroidism. Clin Chim Acta 205:181–186, 1992.

298. Rich C, Bierman EL, Schwartz IL: Plasma nonesterified fatty acids in hyperthyroid states. J Clin Invest 38:275–278, 1959.

299. Amino N, Kuro R, Yabu Y, et al: Elevated levels of circulating carcinoembryonic antigen in hypothyroidism. J Clin Endocrinol Metab 52:457–462, 1981.

300. Tucci JR, Kopp L: Urinary cyclic nucleotide levels in patients with hyper- and hypothyroidism. J Clin Endocrinol Metab 43:1323–1329, 1976.

301. Guttler RB, Shaw JW, Otis CL, Nicoloff JT: Epinephrine-induced alterations in urinary cyclic AMP in hyper- and hypothyroidism. J Clin Endocrinol Metab 41:707–711, 1975.

302. MacFarlane S, Papadopoulos S, Harden RM, Alexander WD: [131]I and MIT-^{131}I in human urine, saliva and gastric juice: A comparison between euthyroid and thyrotoxic patients. J Nucl Med 9:181–186, 1968.

303. Hellström K, Schuberth J: The effect of thyroid hormones on the urinary excretion of taurine in man. Acta Med Scand 187:61–65, 1970.

304. Maebashi M, Kawamura N, Sato M, et al: Urinary excretion of carnitine in patients with hyperthyroidism and hypothyroidism: Augmentation by thyroid hormone. Metabolism 26:351–356, 1977.

305. Levine RJ, Oates JA, Vendsalu A, Sjoerdsma A: Studies on the metabolism of aromatic amines in relation to altered thyroid function in man. J Clin Endocrinol Metab 22:1242–1250, 1962.

306. Copinschi G, Leclercq R, Bruno OD, Cornil A: Effects of altered thyroid function upon cortisol secretion in man. Horm Metab Res 3:437–442, 1971.

307. Harvey RD, McHardy KC, Reid IW, et al: Measurement of bone collagen degradation in hyperthyroidism and during thyroxine replacement therapy using pyridinium cross-links as specific urinary markers. J Clin Endocrinol Metab 72:1189–1194, 1991.

308. Kivirikko KI, Laitinen O, Lamberg BA: Value of urine and serum hydroxyproline in the diagnosis of thyroid disease. J Clin Endocrinol Metab 25:1347–1352, 1965.

309. Askenasi R, Demeester-Mirkine N: Urinary excretion of hydroxylysyl glycosides and thyroid function. J Clin Endocrinol Metab 40:342–344, 1975.

310. Golden AWG, Bateman D, Torr S: Red cell sodium in hyperthyroidism. Br Med J 2:552–554, 1971.

311. Weinstein M, Sartorio G, Stalldecker GB, et al: Red cell zinc in thyroid dysfunction. Acta Endocrinol 20:147–152, 1972.

312. Pearson HA, Druyan R: Erythrocyte glucose-6-phosphate dehydrogenase activity related to thyroid activity. J Lab Clin Med 57:343–349, 1961.

313. Vuopio P, Viherkoski M, Nikkilä E, Lamberg BA: The content of reduced glutathione (GSH) in the red blood cells in hypo- and hyperthyroidism. Ann Clin Res 2:184–186, 1970.

314. Kiso Y, Yoshida K, Kaise K, et al: Erythrocyte carbonic anhydrase-I concentrations in patients with Graves' disease and subacute thyroiditis reflect integrated thyroid hormone levels over the previous few months. J Clin Endocrinol Metab 72:515–518, 1991.

315. Dube MP, Davis FB, Davis PJ, et al: Effects of hyperthyroidism and hypothyroidism on human red blood cells Ca^{2+}-ATPase activity. J Clin Endocrinol Metab 62:253–257, 1986.

316. Gwinup G, Ogundip O: Decreased leukocyte alkaline phosphatase in hyperthyroidism. Metabolism 62:253–257, 1974.

317. Jemelin M, Frei J, Scazziga B: Production of ATP in leukocyte mitochondria from hyperthyroid patients before and after treatment with a β-adrenergic blocker and antithyroid drugs. Acta Endocrinol 66:606–610, 1971.

318. Strickland AL: Sweat electrolytes in thyroid disorders. J Pediatr 82:284–286, 1973.

319. Goolamali SK, Evered D, Shuster S: Thyroid disease and sebaceous function. BMJ 1:432–433, 1976.

320. Christensen J, Schedl HP, Clifton JA: The basic electrical rhythm of the duodenum in normal human subjects and in patients with thyroid disease. J Clin Invest 43:1659–1667, 1964.

321. Levy G, MacGillivray MH, Procknal JA: Riboflavin absorption in children with thyroid disorders. Pediatrics 50:896–900, 1972.

322. Singhelakis P, Alevizaki CC, Ikkos DG: Intestinal calcium absorption in hyperthyroidism. Metabolism 23:311–321, 1974.

323. Thomas FB, Caldwell JH, Greenberger NJ: Steatorrhea in thyrotoxicosis: Relation to hypermotility and excessive dietary fat. Ann Intern Med 78:669–675, 1973.

324. Wegener M, Wedmann B, Langhoff T, et al: Effect of hyperthyroidism on the transport of a solid-liquid meal through the stomach, intestine, and the colon in man. J Clin Endocrinol Metab 75:745–749, 1992.

325. Scherrer M, König MP: Pulmonary gas exchange in hypothyroidism. Pneumonologie 151:105–113, 1974.

326. Zwillich CW, Pierson DJ, Hofeldt FD, et al: Ventilatory control in myxedema and hypothyroidism. N Engl J Med 292:662–665, 1975.

327. Lawson JD: The free Achilles reflex in hypothyroidism and hyperthyroidism. N Engl J Med 259:761–764, 1958.

328. Hall R, Owen SG: Thyroid antibodies in cerebrospinal fluid. BMJ 2:710–711, 1960.

329. Hoffman I, Lowrey RD: The electrocardiogram in thyrotoxicosis. Am J Cardiol 6:893–904, 1960.

330. Lee JK, Lewis JA: Myxoedema with complete A-V block and Adams-Stokes disease abolished with thyroid medication. Br Heart J 24:253–265, 1962.

331. Wilkins L: Epiphysial dysgenesis associated with hypothyroidism. Am J Dis Child 61:13–34, 1941.

332. Bonakdarpour A, Kirkpatrick JA, Renzi A, Kendall N: Skeletal changes in neonatal thyrotoxicosis. Radiology 102:149–150, 1972.

333. Mariotti S, Anelli S, Ruf J, et al: Comparison of serum thyroid microsomal and thyroid peroxidase autoantibodies in thyroid diseases. J Clin Endocrinol Metab 65:987–993, 1987.

334. Portmann L, Hamada N, Neinrich G, DeGroot LJ: Antithyroid peroxidase antibody in patients with autoimmune thyroid disease: Possible identity with antimicrosomal antibody. J Clin Endocrinol Metab 61:1001–1003, 1985.

335. Rinke R, Seto P, Rapoport B: Evidence for the highly conformational nature of the epitope(s) on human thyroid peroxidase that are recognized by sera from patients with Hashimoto's thyroiditis. J Clin Endocrinol Metab 71:53, 1990.

336. Kaufman KD, Filetti S, Seto P, Rapoport B: Recombinant human thyroid peroxidase generated in eukaryotic cells: A source of specific antigen for the immunological assay of antimicrosomal antibodies in the sera of patients with autoimmune thyroid disease. J Clin Endocrinol Metab 70:724–728, 1990.

337. Trotter WR, Belyavin G, Waddams A: Precipitating and complement fixing antibodies in Hashimoto's disease. Proc R Soc Med 50:961–962, 1957.

338. Boyden SV: The adsorption of proteins on erythrocytes treated with tannic acid and subsequent hemagglutination by antiprotein sera. J Exp Med 93:107–120, 1951.

339. Holborrow EJ, Brown PC, Roitt IM, Doniach D: Cytoplasmic localization of complement-fixing auto-antigen in human thyroid epithelium. Br J Exp Pathol 40:583–588, 1959.

340. Hamada N, Jaeduck N, Portmann L, et al: Antibodies against denatured and reduced thyroid microsomal antigen in autoimmune thyroid disease. J Clin Endocrinol Metab 64:230–238, 1987.

341. Mori T, Kriss JP: Measurements by competitive binding radioassay of serum antimicrosomal and antithyroglobulin antibodies in Graves' disease and other thyroid disorders. J Clin Endocrinol Metab 33:688–698, 1971.

342. Mariotti S, Pinchera A, Vitti P, et al: Comparison of radioassay and haemagglutination methods for anti-thyroid microsomal antibodies. Clin Exp Immunol 34:118–125, 1978.

343. Ohtaki S, Endo Y, Horinouchi K, et al: Circulating thyroglobulin-antithyroglobulin immune complex in thyroid diseases using enzyme-linked immunoassays. J Clin Endocrinol Metab 52:239–246, 1981.

344. Amino N, Hagen SR, Yamada N, Refetoff S: Measurement of circulating thyroid microsomal antibodies by the tanned red cell haemagglutination technique: Its usefulness in the diagnosis of autoimmune thyroid disease. Clin Endocrinol 5:115, 1976.

345. Roitt IM, Doniach D: Thyroid auto-immunity. Br Med Bull 16:152–158, 1960.

346. Anderson JW, McConahey WM, Alcarón-Segovia D, et al: Diagnostic value of thyroid antibodies. J Clin Endocrinol Metab 27:937–944, 1967.

347. Loeb PB, Drash AL, Kenny FM: Prevalence of low-titer and "negative" antithyroglobulin antibodies in biopsy-proved juvenile Hashimoto's thyroiditis. J Pediatr 82:17–21, 1973.

348. Tamaki H, Katsumaru H, Amino N, et al: Usefulness of thyroglobulin antibody detected by ultrasensitive enzyme immunoassay: A good parameter for immune surveillance in healthy subjects and for prediction of postpartum thyroid dysfunction. Clin Endocrinol (Oxf) 37:266–273, 1992.

349. Volpé R, Row VV, Ezrin C: Circulating viral and thyroid antibodies in subacute thyroiditis. J Clin Endocrinol Metab 27:1275–1284, 1967.

350. Balfour BM, Doniach D, Roitt IM, Couchman KG: Fluorescent antibody studies in human thyroiditis: Auto-antibodies to an antigen of the thyroid distinct from thyroglobulin. Br J Exp Pathol 42:307–316, 1961.

351. Staeheli V, Vallotton MB, Burger A: Detection of human anti-thyroxine and anti-triiodothyronine antibodies in different thyroid conditions. J Clin Endocrinol Metab 41:669–675, 1975.

352. Bastenie PA, Bonnyns M, Vanhaelst L, Nève P: Diseases associated with autoimmune thyroiditis. In Bastenie PA, Ermans A (eds): Thyroiditis and Thyroid Function. Oxford, Pergamon Press, 1972.

353. Bech K, Nerup J, Larsen JH: Yersinia enterocolitica infection and thyroid diseases. Acta Endocrinol 84:87–92, 1977.

354. Gupta MK: Thyrotropin receptor antibodies: Advances and importance of detection techniques in thyroid disease. Clin Biochem 25:193–199, 1992.

355. McKenzie JM: The bioassay of thyrotropin in serum. Endocrinology 63:372–381, 1958.

356. Furth ED, Rathbun M, Posillico J: A modified bioassay for the long-acting thyroid stimulator (LATS). Endocrinology 85:592–593, 1969.

357. Kriss JP, Pleshakov V, Rosenblum AL, et al: Studies on the pathogenesis of the ophthalmopathy of Graves' disease. J Clin Endocrinol Metab 27:582–593, 1967.

358. Sunshine P, Kusumoto H, Kriss JP: Survival time of circulating long-acting thyroid stimulator in neonatal thyrotoxicosis: Implications for diagnosis and therapy of the disorder. Pediatrics 57:869–876, 1965.

359. Onaya T, Kotani M, Yamada T, Ochi Y: New in vitro tests to detect the thyroid stimulator in sera from hyperthyroid patients by measuring colloid droplet formation and cyclic AMP in human thyroid slices. J Clin Endocrinol Metab 36:859–866, 1973.

360. Hinds WE, Takai N, Rapoport B, et al: Thyroid-stimulating activity and clinical state in antithyroid treatment of juvenile Graves' disease. Acta Endocrinol 94:46–52, 1981.

361. Leedman PJ, Frauman AG, Colman PG, Michelangeli VP: Measurement of thyroid-stimulating immunoglobulins by incorporation of tritiated-adenine into intact FRTL-5 cells: A viable alternative to radioimmunoassay for the measurement of cAMP. Clin Endocrinol (Oxf) 37:493–499, 1992.

362. Takata I, Suzuki Y, Saida K, Sato T: Human thyroid-stimulating activity and clinical state in antithyroid treatment of juvenile Graves' disease. Acta Endocrinol 94:46–52, 1980.

363. Kendall-Taylor P, Atkinson S: A biological method for the assay of TSAb in serum. In Stockigt JR, Nagataki S (eds): Thyroid Research VIII. Canberra, Australian Academy of Science, 1980, p 763.

364. Petersen V, Rees Smith B, Hall R: A study of thyroid-stimulating activity in human serum with the highly sensitive cytochemical bioassay. J Clin Endocrinol Metab 41:199–202, 1975.

365. Libert F, Lefort A, Gerard C, et al: Cloning, sequencing and expression of the human thyrotropin (TSH) receptors: Evidence for binding of autoantibodies. Biochem Biophys Res Commun 165:1250–1255, 1989.

366. Nagayama Y, Kaufman KD, Seto P, Rapoport B: Molecular cloning, sequence and functional expression of the cDNA for the human thyrotropin receptor. Biochem Biophys Res Commun 165:1184–1190, 1989.

367. Ludgate M, Perret J, Parmentier M, et al: Use of the recombinant human thyrotropin receptor (TRHr) expressed in mammalian cell lines to assay TSHr autoantibodies. Mol Cell Endocrinol 73:R13–R18, 1990.

368. Filetti S, Foti D, Costante G, Rapoport B: Recombinant human thyrotropin (TSH) receptor in a radioreceptor assay for the measurement of TSH receptor antibodies. J Clin Endocrinol Metab 72:1096–1101, 1991.

369. Vitti P, Elisei R, Tonacchera M, et al: Detection of thyroid-stimulating antibody using Chinese hamster ovary cells transfected with cloned human thyrotropin receptor. J Clin Endocrinol Metab 76:499–503, 1993.

370. Adams DD, Kennedy TH: Occurrence in thyrotoxicosis of a gamma globulin which protects LATS from neutralization by an extract of thyroid gland. J Clin Endocrinol Metab 27:173–177, 1967.

371. Shishiba Y, Shimizu T, Yoshimura S, Shizume K: Direct evidence for human thyroidal stimulation by LATS-protector. J Clin Endocrinol Metab 36:517–521, 1973.

372. Rapoport B, Greenspan FS, Filetti S, Pepitone M: Clinical experience with a human thyroid cell bioassay for thyroid-stimulating immunoglobulins. J Clin Endocrinol Metab 58:332–338, 1984.

373. Smith BR, Hall R: Thyroid-stimulating immunoglobulins in Graves' disease. Lancet 2:427–431, 1974.

374. Zakarija M, McKenzie JM, Munro DS: Evidence of an IgG inhibitor of thyroid-stimulating antibody (TSAb) as a cause of delay in the onset of neonatal Graves' disease. J Clin Invest 72:1352–1356, 1983.

375. Shewring G, Smith BR: An improved radioreceptor assay for TSH receptor antibodies. Clin Endocrinol 17:409–417, 1982.

376. Endo K, Amir SM, Ingbar SH: Development and evaluation of a method for the partial purification of immunoglobulin specific for Graves' disease. J Clin Endocrinol Metab 52:1113–1123, 981.

377. Drexhage HA, Bottazzo GF, Doniach D: Thyroid growth stimulating and blocking immunoglobulins. In Chayen J, Bitensky L (eds): Cytochemical Bioassays. New York, Marcel Dekker, 1983, p 153.

378. Valente WA, Vitti P, Rotella CM, et al: Autoantibodies that promote thyroid growth: A distinct population of thyroid stimulating antibodies. N Engl J Med 309:1028–1034, 1983.

379. Grove AS Jr: Evaluation of exophthalmos. N Engl J Med 292:1005–1013, 1975.

380. McKenzie JM, Zakarija M: Fetal and neonatal hyper- and hypothyroidism due to maternal TSH receptor antibodies. Thyroid 2:155–159, 1992.

381. Cho Y, Shong MH, Yi KH, et al: Evaluation of serum basal thyrotrophin levels and thyrotrophin receptor antibody activities as prognostic markers for discontinuation of antithyroid drug treatment in patients with Graves' disease. Clin Endocrinol (Oxf) 36:585–590, 1992.

382. Hershman JM: Hyperthyroidism induced by trophoblastic thyrotropin. Mayo Clin Proc 47:913–918, 1972.

383. Greenspan FS, Kriss JP, Moses LE, Lew W: An improved bioassay method for thyrotropin hormone using thyroid uptake of radiophosphorus. Endocrinology 58:767–776, 1956.

384. Nisula BC, Ketelslegers JM: Thyroid-stimulating activity and chorionic gonadotropin. J Clin Invest 54:494–499, 1974.

385. Sobonya RE, Dobyns BM: Comparison of the responses of native Ohio fish and two species of salt-water Fundulus to the exophthalmos-producing substance (EPS) of the pituitary gland. Endocrinology 80:1090–1096, 1967.

386. Singh SP, McKenzie JM: ^{35}S-sulfate uptake by mouse harderian gland: Effect of serum from patients with Graves' disease. Metabolism 20:422–427, 1971.

387. Winand RJ, Kohn LD: Stimulation of adenylate cyclase activity in retro-orbital tissue membranes by thyrotropin and an exophthalmogenic factor derived from thyrotropin. J Biol Chem 250:6522–6526, 1975.

388. Kodama K, Sikorka H, Bandy-Dafoe P, et al: Demonstration of a circulating antibody against a soluble eye-muscle antigen in Graves' ophthalmopathy. Lancet 2:1353–1356, 1982.

389. Ryo UY, Arnold J, Colman M, et al: Thyroid scintigram: Sensitivity with sodium pertechnetate Tc 99m and gamma camera with pinhole collimator. JAMA 235:1235–1238, 1976.

390. Atkins HL, Klopper JF, Lambrecht RM, Wolf AP: A comparison of technetium 99m and iodine 123 for thyroid imaging. Am J Roentgenol Radium Ther Nucl Med 117:195–201, 1973.

391. Nishiyama H, Sodd VJ, Berke RA, Saenger EL: Evaluation of clinical value of ^{123}I and ^{131}I in thyroid disease. J Nucl Med 15:261–265, 1974.

392. Tong ECK, Rubenfeld S: Scan measurements of normal and enlarged thyroid glands. Am J Roentgenol Radium Ther Nucl Med 115:706–708, 1972.

393. Miller JM, Hamburger JI: The thyroid scintigram. I. The hot nodule. Radiol 84:66–74, 1965.

394. Becker FO, Economou PG, Schwartz TB: The occurrence of carcinoma in ''hot'' thyroid nodules: Report of two cases. Ann Intern Med 58:877–882, 1963.

395. Miller JM, Hamburger JI, Mellinger RC: The thyroid scintigram. II. The cold nodule. Radiology 85:702–710, 1965.

396. Meier CA, Braverman LE, Ebner SA, et al: Diagnostic use of recombinant human thyrotropin in patients with thyroid carcinoma (Phase I/II study). J Clin Endocrinol Metab 78:188–196, 1994.

397. Chen JJS, LaFrance ND, Allo MD, et al: Single photon emission computed tomography of the thyroid. J Clin Endocrinol Metab 66:1240, 1988.

398. Corstens F, Huysmans D, Kloppenborg P: Thallium-210 scintigraphy of the suppressed thyroid: An alternative for iodine-123 scanning after TSH stimulation. J Nucl Med 29:1360–1363, 1988.

399. Fairweather DS, Bradwell AR, Watson-James SF, et al: Deletion of thyroid tumours using radiolabeled thyroglobulin. Clin Endocrinol 18:563–570, 1983.

400. Hoffer HP: Fluorescent thyroid scanning. Am J Roentgenol 105:721–727, 1969.

401. Hoffer PB, Gottschalk A, Refetoff S: Thyroid scanning technics: The old and the new. Curr Probl Radiol 2:1–26, 1972.

402. Barki Y: Ultrasonographic evaluation of neck masses—sonographic pattern in differential diagnosis. Isr J Med Sci 28:212–216, 1992.

403. Watters DAK, Ahuja AT, Evans RM, et al: Role of ultrasound in the management of thyroid nodules. Am J Surg 164:654–657, 1992.

404. Scheible W, Leopold GR, Woo VL, Gosink BB: High resolution real-time ultrasonography of thyroid nodules. Radiology 133:413–417, 1979.

405. Sostre S, Reyes MM: Sonographic diagnosis and grading of Hashimoto's thyroiditis. J Endocrinol Invest 14:115–121, 1991.

406. Brander A, Viikinkoski P, Nickels J, Kivisaari L: Thyroid gland: US screening in a random adult population. Radiology 181:683–687, 1991.

407. Jensen F, Rasmussen SN: The treatment of thyroid cysts by ultrasonically guided fine needle aspiration. Acta Chir Scand 142:209–211, 1976.

408. Szebeni A, Beleznay EJ: New simple method for thyroid volume determination by ultrasonography. Clin Ultrasound 20:329–337, 1992.

409. Jarlov AE, Hegedus L, Gjorup T, Hansen JEM: Accuracy of the clinical assessment of thyroid size. Dan Med Bull 38:87–89, 1991.

410. Paracchi A, Ferrari C, Livraghi T, et al: Percutaneous intranodular ethanol injection: A new treatment for autonomous thyroid adenoma. J Endocrinol Invest 15:353–362, 1992.

411. Yamada T, Tsukui T, Ikerjiri K, et al: Volume of sella turcica in normal subjects and in patients with primary hypothyroidism and hyperthyroidism. J Clin Endocrinol Metab 42:817–822, 1976.

412. Blum M, Reede DL, Seltzer TF, Burroughs VJ: Computerized axial tomography in the diagnosis of thyroid and parathyroid disorders. Am J Med Sci 287:34–39, 1984.

413. Brown LR, Aughenbaugh GL: Masses of the anterior mediastinum: CT and MR imaging. Am J Radiol 157:1171–1180, 1991.

414. Damascelli B, Cascinelli N, Terno G, et al: Second thoughts on the value of selective thyroid angiography. Am J Roentgenol Radium Ther Nucl Med 114:822–829, 1972.

415. Matoba N, Kikuchi T: Thyroidolymphography: A new technic for visualization of the thyroid and cervical lymph nodes. Radiology 92:339–342, 1969.

416. Chamla-Soumenkoff J, Frühling J, Mahaux JE: Mise en évidence des ganglions de drainage lymphatique de la thyroïde par la caméra à scintillation après injection intrathyroïdienne d'un microcolloïde de 198 Au. Communication préliminaire. Ann Endocrinol 32:203–209, 1971.

417. Clark H, Greenspan FS, Coggs GC, Goldman L: Evaluation of solitary cold thyroid nodules by echography and thermography. Am J Surg 130:206–211, 1976.

418. Wang C, Vickery AL Jr, Maloof F: Needle biopsy of the thyroid. Surg Gynecol Obstet 143:365–368, 1976.

419. Ashcraft MW, Van Herle AJ: Management of thyroid suppressive therapy, and fine needle aspiration. Head Neck Surg 3:297–322, 1981.

420. Crill C Jr: The danger of surgical dissemination of papillary carcinoma of the thyroid. Surg Gynecol Obstet 102:161–165, 1956.

421. Crill G Jr, Esselstyn CB, Hawk WA: Needle biopsy in the diagnosis of thyroid nodules appearing after radiation. N Engl J Med 301:997–998, 1979.

422. Matos-Godilho L, Kocjan G, Kurtz A: Contribution of fine needle aspiration cytology to diagnosis and management of thyroid disease. J Clin Pathol 45:391–395, 1992.

423. Hamberger B, Gharib H, Melton LJ III, et al: Fine-needle aspiration biopsy of thyroid nodules: Impact on thyroid practice and cost of care. Am J Med 73:381–384, 1982.

424. Odell WD, Wilber FJ, Utiger RD: Studies on thyrotropin physiology by means of radioimmunoassay. Recent Prog Horm Res 23:47–85, 1967.

425. Jackson IMD: Thyrotropin-releasing hormone. N Engl J Med 306:145–155, 1982.

426. Wilber JF: Thyrotropin releasing hormone: Secretion and actions. Ann Rev Med 24:353–364, 1973.

427. Scanlon MF, Rees Smith B, Hall R: Thyroid-stimulating hormone: Neuroregulation and clinical applications. Clin Sci Mol Med 55:1–10, 129–138, 1978.

428. Brown JR: The measurement of thyroid stimulating hormone (TSH) in body fluids: A critical review. Acta Endocrinol 32:289–309, 1959.

429. Bakke JL: Assay of human thyroid-stimulating hormone by 18 different assay laboratories using 12 different methods. J Clin Endocrinol Metab 25:545–550, 1965.

430. Ambesi-Impiombato FS, Parks LAM, Coons HG: Culture of hormone dependent epithelial cells from rat thyroids. Proc Natl Acad Sci USA 77:3444–3459, 1980.

431. Beck-Peccoz P, Amr S, Menezes-Ferreira M, et al: Decreased receptor binding of biologically inactive thyrotropin in central hypothyroidism. Effect of treatment with thyrotropin-releasing hormone. J Clin Endocrinol Metab 312:1085–1090, 1985.

432. Beck-Peccoz P, Piscitelli G, Amr S, et al: Endocrine, biomedical, and morphological studies of a pituitary adenoma secreting growth hormone thyrotropin (TSH), and α-subunit: Evidence for secretion of TSH with increased bioactivity. J Clin Endocrinol Metab 62:704–711, 1986.

433. Pierce JG: The subunits of pituitary thyrotropin: Their relation to other glycoprotein hormones. Endocrinology 89:1331–1344, 1971.

434. Spitz IM, LeRoith D, Hirsch H, et al: Increased high-molecular-weight thyrotropin with impaired biologic activity in a euthyroid man. N Engl J Med 304:278–282, 1981.

435. Miyai K, Fukuchi M, Kumahara Y: Correlation between biological and immunological potencies of human serum and pituitary thyrotropin. J Clin Endocrinol Metab 29:1438–1442, 1969.

436. Gendrel D, Feinstein MC, Grenier J, et al: Falsely elevated serum thyrotropin (TSH) in newborn infants: Transfer from mothers to infants of a factor interfering in the TSH radioimmunoassay. J Clin Endocrinol Metab 52:62–65, 1981.

437. Chaussain JL, Binet E, Job JC: Antibodies to human thyrotrophin in the serum of certain hypopituitary dwarfs. Rev Eur Etud Clin Biol 17:95–99, 1972.

438. Nicoloff JT, Spencer CA: The use and misuse of the sensitive thyrotropin assays. J Clin Endocrinol Metab 71:553–558, 1990.

439. Kricka LJ: Chemiluminescent and bioluminescent techniques. Clin Chem 37:1472–1481, 1991.

440. Klee GG, Hay ID: Assessment of sensitive thyrotropin assays for an expanded role in thyroid function testing: Proposed criteria for analytic performance and clinical utility. J Clin Endocrinol Metab 64:461–471, 1987.

441. Spencer CA, LoPresti JS, Patel A: Applications of a new chemiluminometric thyrotropin assay to subnormal measurement. J Clin Endocrinol Metab 70:453–460, 1990.

442. Ross DS, Ardisson LJ, Meskell MJ: Measurement of thyrotropin in clinical and subclinical hyperthyroidism using a new chemiluminescent assay. J Clin Endocrinol Metab 69:684–688, 1989.

443. Brennan MD, Klee GG, Preissner CM, Hay ID: Heterophilic serum antibodies: A cause for falsely elevated serum thyrotropin levels. Mayo Clin Proc 62:894–898, 1987.

444. Wood JM, Gordon DL, Rudinger AN, Brooks MM: Artifactual elevation of thyroid-stimulating hormone. Am J Med 90:261–262, 1991.

445. Zweig MH, Csako G, Reynolds JC, Carrasquillo JA: Interference by iatrogenically induced anti-mouse IgG antibodies in a two-site immunometric assay for thyrotropin. Arch Pathol Rad Metab 1165:164–168, 1991.

446. Kourides IA, Heath CV, Ginsberg-Fellner F: Measurement of thyroid-stimulating hormone in human amniotic fluid. J Clin Endocrinol Metab 54:635–637, 1982.

447. Fisher DA, Klein AH: Thyroid development and disorders of thyroid function in the newborn. N Engl J Med 304:702–712, 1981.

448. Snyder PJ, Utiger RD: Response to thyrotropin releasing hormone (TRH) in normal man. J Clin Endocrinol Metab 34:380–385, 1972.

449. Hershman JM, Pittman JA Jr: Utility of the radioimmunoassay of serum thyrotropin in man. Ann Intern Med 74:481–490, 1971.

450. Brabant G, Prank K, Ranft U, et al: Physiological regulation of circadian and pulsatile thyrotropin secretion in normal man and woman. J Clin Endocrinol Metab 70:403–409, 1990.

451. Bartalena L, Martino E, Falcone M, et al: Evaluation of the nocturnal serum thyrotropin (TSH) surge, as assessed by TSH ultrasensitive assay, in patients receiving long term L-thyroxine suppression therapy and in patients with various thyroid disorders. J Clin Endocrinol Metab 65:1265–1271, 1987.

452. Ria AG, Brabant K, Prank E, et al: Circadian changes in pulsatile TSH release in primary hypothyroidism. Clin Endocrinol 37:504–510, 1992.

453. Brabant G, Prank C, Hoang-Vu C, et al: Hypothalamic regulation of pulsatile thyrotropin secretion. J Clin Endocrinol Metab 72:145–150, 1991.

454. Romijn JA, Adriaanse G, Brabant K, et al: Pulsatile secretion of thyrotropin during fasting: A decrease of thyrotropin pulse amplitude. J Clin Endocrinol Metab 70:1631–1636, 1990.

455. Bartalena L, Pacchiarotti A, Palla R, et al: Lack of nocturnal serum thyrotropin (TSH) surge in patients with chronic renal failure undergoing regular maintenance hemofiltration: A case of central hypothyroidism. Clin Nephrol 34:30–34, 1990.

456. Romijn JA, Wiersinga WM: Decreased nocturnal surge of thyrotropin in nonthyroidal illness. J Clin Endocrinol Metab 70:35–42, 1990.

457. Van Cauter E, Golstein J, Vanhaelst L, Leclercq R: Effects of oral contraceptive therapy on the circadian patterns of cortisol and thyrotropin (TSH). Eur J Clin Invest 5:115–121, 1975.

458. Brabant G, Brabant A, Ranft U, et al: Circadian and pulsatile thyrotropin secretion in euthyroid man under the influence of thyroid hormone and glucocorticoid administration. J Clin Endocrinol Metab 65:83–88, 1987.

459. Simoni M, Velardo A, Montanini V, et al: Circannual rhythm of plasma thyrotropin in middle-aged and old euthyroid subjects. Horm Res 33:184–189, 1990.

460. Wilber JF, Baum D: Elevation of plasma TSH during surgical hypothermia. J Clin Endocrinol Metab 31:372–375, 1970.

461. Vagenakis AG, Rapoport B, Azizi F, et al: Hyper-response to thyrotropin-releasing hormone accompanying small decreases in serum thyroid hormone concentration. J Clin Invest 54:913–918, 1974.

462. Kleinman RE, Vagenakis AG, Braverman LE: The effect of iopanoic acid on the regulation of thyrotropin secretion in euthyroid subjects. J Clin Endocrinol Metab 51:399–403, 1980.

463. Lazarus JH, Joh R, Bennie EH, et al: Lithium therapy and thyroid function: A long term study. Psychiatr Med 11:85–92, 1981.

464. Scanlon MF, Weightman DR, Shale DJ, et al: Dopamine is a physiological regulator of thyrotropin (TSH) secretion in normal man. Clin Endocrinol 10:7–15, 1979.

465. Scanlon MF, Rodriguez-Arnao MD, Pourmand M, et al: Catecholaminergic interactions in the regulation of thyrotropin (TSH) secretion in man. J Endocrinol Invest 3:125–129, 1980.

466. Massara F, Camanni F, Belforte L, et al: Increased thyrotropin secretion induced by sulpiride in man. Clin Endocrinol 9:419–428, 1978.

467. Delitala G, Devilla L, Lotti G: TSH and prolactin stimulation by the decarboxylase inhibitor benserazide in primary hypothyroidism. Clin Endocrinol 12:313–316, 1980.

468. Kirkegaard C, Bjoerum CN, Cohn D, et al: Studies of the influence of biogenic amines and psychoactive drugs on the prognostic value of the TRH stimulation test in endogeneous depression. Psychoneuroendocrinology 2:131–136, 1977.

469. Kirkegaard C, Bjoerum N, Cohn D, Lauridsen UB: TRH stimulation test in manic-depressive illness. Arch Gen Psychiatry 35:1017–1021, 1978.

470. Nelis GF, Van DeMeene JG: The effect of oral cimetidine on the basal and stimulated values of prolactin, thyroid stimulating hormone, follicle stimulating hormone and luteinizing hormone. Postgrad Med J 56:26–29, 1980.

471. Feldt-Rasmussen U, Lange AP, Date J, Kern-Hansen M: Effect of clomifen on thyroid function in normal men. Acta Endocrinol 90:43–51, 1979.

472. Smals AG, Kloppenborg PW, Hoefnagesl WH, Drayer JM: Pituitary-thyroid function in spironolactone treated hypertensive women. Acta Endocrinol 90:577–584, 1979.

473. Morely JE, Shafer RB, Elson MK, et al: Amphetamine-induced hyperthyroxinemia. Ann Intern Med 93:707–709, 1980.

474. Gloebel B, Weinheimer B: TRH-test during D-T₄ application. NucCompact 8:44, 1977.

475. Medeiros-Neto G, Kallas WG, Knobel M, et al: TRIAC (3,5,3′-triiodothyroacetic acid) partially inhibits the thyrotropin response to thyrotropin-releasing hormone in normal and thyroidectomized hypothyroid patients. J Clin Endocrinol Metab 50:223–225, 1980.

476. Emrich D: Untersuchungen zum einfluss von Etiroxat-HCL auf den Jodstoffwechsel beim menschen. Arzneim Forsch 27:422–426, 1977.

477. Tamagna EI, Hershman JM, Jorgensen EC: Thyrotropin secretion by 3,5-dimethyl-3′-isopropyl-L-thyronine in man. J Clin Endocrinol Metab 48:196–200, 1979.

478. Delitala G: Dopamine and TSH secretion in man. Lancet 2:760–761, 1977.

479. Miyai K, Onishi T, Hosokawa M, et al: Inhibition of thyrotropin and prolactin secretions in primary hypothyroidism by 2-Br-α-ergocryptine. J Clin Endocrinol Metab 39:391–394, 1974.

480. Yoshimura M, Hachiya T, Ochi Y, et al: Suppression of elevated serum TSH levels in hypothyroidism by fusaric acid. J Clin Endocrinol Metab 45:95–98, 1977.

481. Delitala G, Rovasio P, Lotti G: Suppression of thyrotropin (TSH) and prolactin (PRL) release by pyridoxine in chronic primary hypothyroidism. J Clin Endocrinol Metab 45:1019–1022, 1977.

482. Masala A, Delitala G, Devilla L, et al: Effect of apomorphine and piribedil on the secretion of thyrotropin and prolactin in patients with primary hypothyroidism. Metabolism 27:1608–1612, 1978.
483. Delitala G, Wass JAH, Stubbs WA, et al: The effect of lisurgide hydrogen maleate, an ergot derivative on anterior pituitary hormone secretion in man. Clin Endocrinol 11:1–9, 1979.
484. Collu R, Jéquier JC, Leboeuf G, et al: Endocrine effects of pimozide, a specific dopaminergic blocker. J Clin Endocrinol Metab 41:981–984, 1975.
485. Nilsson KO, Thorell JI, Hökfelt B: The effect of thyrotrophin releasing hormone on the release of thyrotrophin and other pituitary hormones in man under basal conditions and following adrenergic blocking agents. Acta Endocrinol 76:24–34, 1974.
486. Lamberg BA, Linnoila M, Fogelholm R, et al: The effect of psychotropic drugs on the SH-response to thyroliberin (TRH). Neuroendocrinology 24:90–97, 1977.
487. Delitala G, Rovasio PP, Masala A, et al: Metergoline inhibition of thyrotropin and prolactin secretion in primary hypothyroidism. Clin Endocrinol 8:69–73, 1978.
488. Ferrari C, Paracchi A, Rondena M, et al: Effect of two serotonin antagonists on prolactin and thyrotropin secretion in man. Clin Endocrinol 5:575–578, 1976.
489. Collu R: The effect of TRH on the release of TSH, PRL and GH in man under basal conditions and following methysergide. J Endocrinol Invest 2:121–124, 1978.
490. Yoshimura M, Ochi Y, Miyazaki T, et al: Effect of intravenous and oral administration of L-DOPA on HGH and TSH release. Endocrinol Jpn 19:543–548, 1972.
491. Re RN, Kourides IA, Ridgway EC, et al: The effect of glucocorticoid administration on human pituitary secretion of thyrotropin and prolactin. J Clin Endocrinol Metab 43:338–346, 1976.
492. Dussault JH: The effect of dexamethasone on TSH and prolactin secretion after TRH stimulation. Can Med Assoc J 111:1195–1197, 1974.
493. Dussault JH, Turcotte R, Guyda H: The effect of acetylsalicylic acid on TSH and PRL secretion after TRH stimulation in the human. J Clin Endocrinol Metab 43:232–235, 1976.
494. Porter BA, Refetoff S, Rosenfield RL, et al: Abnormal thyroxine metabolism in hyposomatotrophic dwarfism and inhibition of responsiveness to TRH during GH therapy. Pediatrics 51:668–674, 1973.
495. Weeke J, Hansen AP, Lundbaek K: Inhibition by somatostatin of basal levels of serum thyrotropin (TSH) in normal men. J Clin Endocrinol Metab 41:168–171, 1975.
496. Thomas JA, Shahid-Salles KS, Donovan MP: Effects of narcotics on the reproduction system. Adv Sex Horm Res 3:169–195, 1977.
497. May P, Mittler J, Manougian A, Erte N: TSH release-inhibiting activity of leucine-enkephalin. Horm Metab Res 11:30–33, 1979.
498. Chan V, Wang C, Yeung RT: Effects of heroin addiction on thyrotropin, thyroid hormones and prolactin secretion in men. Clin Endocrinol 10:557–565, 1979.
499. Kobayashi I, Shimomura Y, Maruta S, et al: Clofibrate and a related compound suppress TSH secretion in primary hypothyroidism. Acta Endocrinol 94:53–57, 1980.
500. Snyder PJ, Utiger RD: Inhibition of thyrotropin response to thyrotropin releasing hormone by small quantities of thyroid hormones. J Clin Invest 51:2077–2084, 1972.
501. Ehrmann DA, Weinberg M, Sarne DH: Limitations to the use of a sensitive assay for serum thyrotropin in the assessment of thyroid status. Arch Intern Med 149:369–372, 1989.
502. Ridgway EC, Cooper DS, Walker H, et al: Peripheral responses of thyroid hormone before and after L-thyroxine therapy in patients with subclinical hypothyroidism. J Clin Endocrinol Metab 53:1238–1242, 1981.
503. Aizawa T, Koizumi Y, Yamada T, et al: Difference in pituitary-thyroid feedback regulation in hypothyroid patients, depending on the severity of hypothyroidism. J Clin Endocrinol Metab 47:560–565, 1978.
504. Spencer CA: Clinical utility and cost-effectiveness of sensitive thyrotropin assays in ambulatory and hospitalized patients. Mayo Clin Proc 63:1214–1222, 1988.
505. Surks MI, Chopra IJ, Mariash CN, et al: American Thyroid Association guidelines for use of laboratory tests in thyroid disorders. JAMA 263:1529–1532, 1990.
506. Delange F, Dodion J, Wolter R, et al: Transient hypothyroidism in the newborn infant. J Pediatr 92:974–976, 1978.
507. Brown ME, Refetoff S: Transient elevation of serum thyroid hormone concentration after initiation of replacement therapy in myxedema. Ann Intern Med 92:491–495, 1980.
508. Sanchez-Franco F, Cacicedo GL, Martin-Zurro A, et al: Transient lack of thyrotropin (TSH) response to thyrotropin-releasing hormone (TRH) in treated hyperthyroid patients with normal or low serum thyroxine (T₄) and triiodothyronine (T₃). J Clin Endocrinol Metab 38:1098–1102, 1974.
509. Spencer CA, Elgen A, Shen D, et al: Specificity of sensitive assays of thyrotropin (TSH) used to screen for thyroid disease in hospitalized patients. Clin Chem 33:1301–1396, 1987.
510. Weintraub BD, Gershengorn MC, Kourides IA, Fein H: Inappropriate secretion of thyroid stimulating hormone. Ann Intern Med 95:339–351, 1981.
511. Mihailovic V, Feller MS, Kourides IA, Utiger RD: Hyperthyroidism due to excess thyrotropin secretion: Follow-up studies. J Clin Endocrinol Metab 50:1135–1138, 1980.
512. Kourides IA, Ridgway EC, Weintraub BD, et al: Thyrotropin-induced hyperthyroidism: Use of alpha and beta subunit levels to identify patients with pituitary tumors. J Clin Endocrinol Metab 45:534–543, 1977.
513. Sarne DH, Sobieszczyk S, Ain KB, Refetoff S: Serum thyrotropin and prolactin in the syndrome of generalized resistance to thyroid hormone: Responses to thyrotropin-releasing hormone stimulation and short term triiodothyronine suppression. J Clin Endocrinol Metab 70:1305–1311, 1990.
514. Brent GA, Hershman JM, Braunstein GD: Patients with severe nonthyroidal illness and serum thyrotropin concentrations in the hypothyroid range. Am J Med 81:463–466, 1986.
515. Topliss DJ, White EL, Stockigt JR: Significance of thyrotropin excess in untreated primary adrenal insufficiency. J Clin Endocrinol Metab 50:52–56, 1980.
516. Wehmann RE, Gregerman RI, Burns WH, et al: Suppression of thyrotropin in the low-thyroxine state of severe nonthyroidal illness. N Engl J Med 312:546–552, 1985.
517. Bacci V, Schussler GC, Kaplan TB: The relationship between serum triiodothyronine and thyrotropin during systemic illness. J Clin Endocrinol Metab 54:1229–1235, 1982.
518. Kourides IA, Weintraub BD, Ridgway EC, Maloof F: Pituitary secretion of free alpha and beta subunit of human thyrotropin in patients with thyroid disorders. J Clin Endocrinol Metab 40:872–885, 1975.
519. Weeke J: The influence of the circadian thyrotropin rhythm on the thyrotropin response to thyrotropin-releasing hormone in normal subjects. Scand J Clin Lab Invest 33:17–20, 1974.
520. Haigler ED Jr, Hershman JM, Pittman JA Jr, Blaugh CM: Direct evaluation of pituitary thyrotropin reserve utilizing thyrotropin releasing hormone. J Clin Endocrinol Metab 33:573–581, 1971.
521. Azizi F, Vagenakis AG, Portnay GE, et al: Pituitary-thyroid responsiveness to intramuscular thyrotropin-releasing hormone based on analyses of serum thyroxine, tri-iodothyronine and thyrotropin concentration. N Engl J Med 292:273–277, 1975.
522. Haigler ED Jr, Hershman JM, Pittman JA Jr: Response to orally administered synthetic thyrotropin-releasing hormone in man. J Clin Endocrinol Metab 35:631–635, 1972.
523. Ormston BJ, Kilborn JR, Garry R, et al: Further observations on the effect of synthetic thyrotropin-releasing hormone in man. BMJ 2:199–202, 1971.
524. Hershman JM, Kojima A, Friesen HG: Effect of thyrotropin-releasing hormone on human pituitary thyrotropin, prolactin, placental lactogen, and chorionic thyrotropin. J Clin Endocrinol Metab 36:497–501, 1973.
525. Jacobsen BB, Andersen H, Dige-Petersen H, Hummer L: Thyrotropin response to thyrotropin-releasing hormone in fullterm, euthyroid and hypothyroid newborns. Acta Paediatr Scand 65:433–438, 1976.
526. Sanchez-Franco F, Garcia MD, Cacicedo L, et al: Influence of sex phase of the menstrual cycle on thyrotropin (TSH) response to thyrotropin-releasing hormone (TRH). J Clin Endocrinol Metab 37:736–740, 1973.
527. Harman SM, Wehmann RE, Blackman MR: Pituitary-thyroid hormone economy in healthy aging men: Basal indices of thyroid function and thyroid responses to constant infusions of thyrotropin releasing hormone. J Clin Endocrinol Metab 58:320–326, 1984.
528. Wilber J, Jaffer A, Jacobs L, et al: Inhibition of thyrotropin releasing hormone (TRH) stimulated thyrotropin (TSH) secretion in man by a single oral dose of thyroid hormone. Horm Metab Res 4:508, 1972.
529. Wartofsky L, Dimond RC, Noel GL, et al: Effect of acute increases in serum triiodothyronine on TSH and prolactin responses to TRH, and estimates of pituitary stores of TSH and prolactin in normal subjects and in patients with primary hypothyroidism. J Clin Endocrinol Metab 42:443–458, 1976.

530. Shenkman L, Mitsuma T, Suphavai A, Hollander CS: Triiodothyronine and thyroid-stimulating hormone response to thyrotropin-releasing hormone: A new test of thyroidal and pituitary reserve. Lancet 1:111–113, 1972.

531. Anderson MS, Bowers CY, Kastin AJ, et al: Synthetic thyrotropin-releasing hormone: A potent stimulator of thyrotropin secretion in man. N Engl J Med 285:1279–1283, 1971.

532. McFarland KF, Strickland AL, Metzger WT, Smith JS: Thyrotropin-releasing hormone test: An adverse reaction. Arch Intern Med 142:132–133, 1982.

533. Fleischer N, Lorente M, Kirkland J, et al: Synthetic thyrotropin releasing factor as a test of pituitary thyrotropin reserve. J Clin Endocrinol Metab 34:617–624, 1972.

534. Sachson R, Rosen SW, Cuatrecasas P, et al: Prolactin stimulation by thyrotropin-releasing hormone in a patient with isolated thyrotropin deficiency. N Engl J Med 287:972–973, 1972.

535. Vagenakis AG, Braverman LE, Azizi F, et al: Recovery of pituitary thyrotropic function after withdrawal of prolonged thyroid-suppression therapy. N Engl J Med 293:681–684, 1975.

536. Tamai H, Nakagawa T, Ohsako N, et al: Changes in thyroid function in patients with euthyroid Graves' disease. J Clin Endocrinol Metab 50:108–112, 1980.

537. Tamai H, Suematsu H, Ikemi Y, et al: Responses to TRH and T_3 suppression tests in euthyroid subjects with a family history of Graves' disease. J Clin Endocrinol Metab 47:475–479, 1978.

538. Stein RB, Nicoloff JT: Triiodothyronine withdrawal test—a test of thyroid-pituitary adequacy. J Clin Endocrinol Metab 32:127–129, 1971.

539. Mornex R, Berthezene F: Comments on a proposed new way of measuring thyrotropin (TSH) reserve. J Clin Endocrinol Metab 31:587–590, 1970.

540. Taunton OD, McDaniel HG, Pittman JA Jr: Standardization of TSH testing. J Clin Endocrinol Metab 25:266–277, 1965.

541. Burke G: The thyrotropin stimulation test. Ann Intern Med 69:1127–1139, 1968.

542. Hays MT, Solomon DH, Beall GN: Suppression of human thyroid function by antibodies to bovine thyrotropin. J Clin Endocrinol Metab 27:1540–1549, 1967.

543. Werner SC, Spooner M: A new and simple test for hyperthyroidism employing L-triiodothyronine and the twenty-four hour I-131 uptake method. Bull NY Acad Med 31:137–145, 1955.

544. Duick DS, Stein RB, Warren DW, Nicoloff JT: The significance of partial suppressibility of serum thyroxine by triiodothyronine administration in euthyroid man. J Clin Endocrinol Metab 41:229–234, 1975.

545. Alexander WD, Harden RM, McLarty D, Shimmins J: Thyroidal suppressibility after stopping long-term treatment of thyrotoxicosis with anti-thyroid drugs. Metabolism 18:58–62, 1969.

546. Lowry RC, Lowe D, Hadden DR, et al: Thyroid suppressibility: Follow-up for two years after antithyroid treatment. BMJ 2:19–22, 1971.

547. Stanbury JB, Kassenaar AAH, Meijer JWA: The metabolism of iodotyrosines. I. The fate of mono- and di-iodotyrosine in normal subjects and in patients with various diseases. J Clin Endocrinol Metab 16:735–746, 1956.

548. Lissitzky S, Codaccioni JL, Bismuth J, Depieds R: Congenital goiter with hypothyroidism and iodo-serum albumin replacing thyroglobulin. J Clin Endocrinol Metab 27:185–196, 1967.

549. DeGroot LJ: Kinetic analysis of iodine metabolism. J Clin Endocrinol Metab 26:149–173, 1966.

550. Hays MT: Absorption of oral thyroxine in man. J Clin Endocrinol Metab 28:749–756, 1968.

551. Hays MT: Absorption of triiodothyronine in man. J Clin Endocrinol Metab 30:675–677, 1970.

552. Valente WA, Goldiner WH, Hamilton BP, et al: Thyroid hormone levels after acute L-thyroxine loading in hypothyroidism. J Clin Endocrinol Metab 53:527–529, 1981.

553. Ain KB, Refetoff S, Fein HG, Weintraub BD: Pseudomalabsorption of levothyroxine. JAMA 266:2118–2120, 1991.

554. Sterling K, Chodos RB: Radiothyroxine turnover studies in myxedema thyrotoxicosis and hypermetabolism without endocrine disease. J Clin Invest 35:806–813, 1956.

555. Oppenheimer JH, Schwartz HL, Surks MI: Determination of common parameters of iodothyronine metabolism and distribution in man by noncompartmental analysis. J Clin Endocrinol Metab 41:319–324, 1172–1173, 1975.

556. Curti GI, Fresco GF: A theoretical five-pool model to evaluate triiodothyronine distribution and metabolism in healthy subjects. Metabolism 41:3–10, 1992.

557. Bianchi R, Mariani G, Molea N, et al: Peripheral metabolism of thyroid hormones in man. I. Direct measurement of the conversion rate of thyroxine to 3,5,3'-triiodothyronine (T_3) and determination of the peripheral and thyroidal production of T_3. J Clin Endocrinol Metab 56:1152–1163, 1983.

558. Faber J, Heaf J, Kirkegaard C, et al: Simultaneous turnover studies of thyroxine, 3,5,3'- and 3,3',5-triiodothyronine, and 3'-monoiodothyronine in chronic renal failure. J Clin Endocrinol Metab 56:211–217, 1983.

559. Refetoff S, Fang VS, Marshall JS, Robin NI: Metabolism of thyroxine-binding globulin (TBG) in man: Abnormal rate of synthesis in inherited TBG deficiency and excess. J Clin Invest 57:485–495, 1976.

560. Lim VS, Fang VS, Katz AI, Refetoff S: Thyroid dysfunction in chronic renal failure: A study of the pituitary-thyroid axis and peripheral turnover kinetics of thyroxine and triiodothyronine. J Clin Invest 60:522–534, 1977.

561. LoPresti JS, Warren DW, Kaptein EM, et al: Urinary immunoprecipitation method for estimation of thyroxine and triiodothyronine conversion in altered thyroid states. J Clin Endocrinol Metab 55:666–670, 1982.

562. Ridgway EC, Weintraub BD, Maloof F: Metabolic clearance and production rates of human thyrotropin. J Clin Invest 895–903, 1974.

563. Cuttelod S, Lemarchand-Beraud T, Magnenat P, et al: Effect of age and role of kidneys and liver on thyrotropin turnover in man. Metabolism 23:101–113, 1974.

564. Cavalieri RR, Searle GL: The kinetics of distribution between plasma and liver of ^{131}I-labeled L-thyroxine in man: Observations of subjects with normal and decreased serum thyroxine-binding globulin. J Clin Invest 45:939–949, 1966.

565. Oppenheimer JH, Bernstein G, Hasen J: Estimation of rapidly exchangeable cellular thyroxine from the plasma disappearance curves of simultaneously administered thyroxine-^{131}I and albumin-^{125}I. J Clin Invest 46:762–777, 1967.

566. Usala SJ, Tennyson GE, Bale AE, et al: A base mutation of the c-erbAβ thyroid hormone receptor in a kindred with generalized thyroid hormone resistance. Molecular heterogeneity in two other kindreds. J Clin Invest 85:93–100, 1990.

567. Lairmore TC, Howe JR, Korte JA, et al: Familial medullary thyroid carcinoma and multiple endocrine neoplasia type 2B map to the same region of chromosome 10 as multiple endocrine neoplasia type 2A. Genomics 9:181–192, 1991.

568. Janssen OE, Bertenshaw R, Takeda K, et al: Molecular basis of inherited thyroxine-binding globulin defects. Trends Endocrinol Metab 3:49–53, 1991.

569. Cavalieri RR: The effects of nonthyroid disease and drugs on thyroid function tests. Med Clinics North Am 75:27, 1991.

570. Delitala G, Devilla L, Lotti G: Domperidone, an extracerebral inhibitor of dopamine receptors, stimulates thyrotropin and prolactin release in man. J Clin Endocrinol Metab 50:1127–1130, 1980.

571. Vagenakis AG, Wang CA, Burger A, et al: Iodide-induced thyrotoxicosis in Boston. N Engl J Med 287:523–527, 1972.

572. Martino E, Safran M, Aghini-Lombardi F, et al: Environmental iodine intake and thyroid dysfunction during chronic amiodarone therapy. Ann Intern Med 101:28–34, 1984.

573. Faglia G, Ambrosi B, Beck-Peccoz P, et al: The effect of theophylline on plasma thyrotropin response (HTSH) to thyrotropin releasing factor (TRF) in man. J Clin Endocrinol Metab 34:906–909, 1972.

574. Wolff J, Varrone S: The methyll xanthines—a new class of goitrogens. Endocrinology 85:410–414, 1969.

575. Gaffney TE, Braunwald E, Kahler RL: Effects of guanethidine on triiodothyronine induced hyperthyroidism in man. N Engl J Med 265:16–20, 1961.

576. Lee WY, Bronsky D, Waldstein SS: Studies of thyroid and sympathetic nervous system interrelationships. II. Effect of guanethidine on manifestations of hyperthyroidism. J Clin Endocrinol Metab 22:879–885, 1962.

577. Cutting WC, Rytand DA, Tainter ML: Relationship between blood cholesterol and increased metabolism from dinitrophenol and thyroid. J Clin Invest 13:547–552, 1934.

578. Ain KB, Mori Y, Reetoff S: Reduced clearance of thyroxine-binding globulin (TBG) with increased sialylation: A mechanism for estrogen induced elevation of serum TBG concentration. J Clin Endocrinol Metab 65:689–696, 1987.

579. Doe RP, Mellinger GT, Swaim WR, Seal JS: Estrogen dosage effects on serum proteins: A longitudinal study. J Clin Endocrinol Metab 27:1081–1086, 1967.

580. Dowling JT, Frienkel N, Ingbar SH: The effect of estrogens upon the peripheral metabolism of thyroxine. J Clin Invest 39:1119–1130, 1974.

581. Rutlin E, Haug E, Torjesen PA: Serum thyrotrophin, prolactin and growth hormone, response to TRH during oestrogen treatment. Acta Endocrinol 84:23–35, 1977.
582. Gross HA, Appelman MD, Nicoloff JT: Effect of biologically active steroids on thyroid function in man. J Clin Endocrinol Metab 33:242–248, 1971.
583. Graham RL, Gambrell RD: Changes in thyroid function tests during danazol therapy. Obstet Gynecol 55:395–397, 1980.
584. Austen FK, Rubini ME, Meroney WH, Wolff J: Salicylates and thyroid function. I. Depression of thyroid function. J Clin Invest 37:1131–1143, 1958.
585. Wolff J, Austen FK: Salicylates and thyroid function. II. The effect on the thyroid-pituitary interrelation. J Clin Invest 37:1144–1165, 1958.
586. Woeber KA, Barakat RM, Ingbar SH: Effects of salicylate and its noncalorigenic congeners on the thyroidal release of ^{131}I in patients with thyrotoxicosis. J Clin Endocrinol Metab 224:1163–1168, 1964.
587. Chopra IJ, Solomon DH, Chua Teco GN, Nguyen AH: Inhibition of hepatic outer ring monodeiodination of thyroxine and 3,3′,5′-triiodothyronine by sodium salicylate. Endocrinology 106:1728–1734, 1980.
588. Alexander WD, Johnson KWM: A comparison of the effects of acetylsalicylic acid and DL-triiodothyronine in patients with myxoedema. Clin Sci 15:593–600, 1956.
589. Yamamoto T, Woeber KA, Ingbar SH: The influence of salicylate on serum TSH concentration in patients with primary hypothyroidism. J Clin Endocrinol Metab 34:423–426, 1972.
590. Woeber KA, Ingbar SH: The effects of noncalorigenic congeners of salicylate on the peripheral metabolism of thyroxine. J Clin Invest 43:931–942, 1964.
591. Christensen K: The metabolic effect of p-aminosalicylic acid. Acta Endocrinol 31:608–610, 1959.
592. MacGregor AG, Somner AR: The antithyroid action of para-amino salicylic acid. Lancet 2:931–936, 1954.
593. Gemstedt A, Jarnerot A, Kagedal B, Soderholm B: Corticosteroids and thyroid function. Acta Med Scand 205:379–383, 1979.
594. Ingbar SH: The effect of cortisone on the thyroidal and renal metabolism of iodine. Endocrinology 53:171–181, 1953.
595. Benoit FL, Greenspan FS: Corticoid therapy for pretibial myxedema. Observations on the long-acting thyroid stimulator. Ann Intern Med 66:711–720, 1967.
596. Yamada T, Ikejiri K, Kotani M, Kusakabe T: An increase of plasma triiodothyronine and thyroxine after administration of dexamethasone to hypothyroid patients with Hashimoto's thyroiditis. J Clin Endocrinol Metab 46:784–790, 1978.
597. Cavalieri RR, Gavin LA, Wallace A, et al: Serum thyroxine, free T_4, triiodothyronine, and reverse-T_3 in diphenylhydantoin treated patients. Metabolism 28:1161–1165, 1979.
598. Blackshear JL, Schultz AL, Napier JS, Stuart DD: Thyroxine replacement requirements in hypothyroid patients receiving phenytoin. Ann Intern Med 99:341–359, 1983.
599. Schwartz HL, Kozyreff V, Surks MI, Oppenheimer JH: Increased deiodination of L-thyroxine and L-triiodothyronine by liver microsomes from rats treated with phenobarbital. Nature 221:1262–1263, 1969.
600. Murchison LE, How J, Bewsher PD: Comparison of propranolol and metoprolol in the management of hyperthyroidism. Br J Clin Pharmacol 8:581, 1979.
601. How ASM, Khir AN, Bewsher PD: The effect of atenolol on serum thyroid hormones in hyperthyroid patients. Clin Endocrinol 13:299–302, 1980.
602. Zwillich CW, Matthay M, Potts DE, et al: Thyrotoxicosis: Comparison of effects of thyroid ablation and beta-adrenergic blockage on metabolic rate and ventilatory control. J Clin Endocrinol Metab 46:491–500, 1978.
603. Goldberg RC, Wolff J, Greep RO: The mechanism of depression of plasma protein-bound iodine by 2,4-dinitrophenol. Endocrinology 56:560–566, 1955.
604. Lardy HA, Wellman H: Oxidative phosphorylations: Role of inorganic phosphate and acceptor systems in control of metabolic rates. J Biol Chem 195:215–224, 1952.
605. Escobar del Rey F, Morreale de Escobar G: Studies on the peripheral disappearance of thyroid hormone. IV. The effect of 2,4-dinitrophenol on the ^{131}I distribution in thyroidectomized, L-thyroxine maintained rats, 24 hours after the injection of ^{131}I-labeled L-thyroxine. Acta Endocrinol 29:161–175, 1958.
606. Cutting CC, Tainter ML: Comparative effects of dinitrophenol and thyroxine on tadpole metamorphosis. Proc Soc Exp Biol Med 31:97–100, 1933.
607. Morley JE: Neuroendocrine control of thyrotropin secretion. Endocr Rev 2:396–436, 1981.
608. Kaptein EM, Spencer CA, Kamiel MB, Nicoloff JT: Prolonged dopamine administration and thyroid hormone economy in normal and critically ill subjects. J Clin Endocrinol Metab 51:387–393, 1980.
609. Kobberling J, Darrach A, Del Pozo E: Chronic dopamine receptor stimulation using bromocryptine: Failure to modify thyroid function. Clin Endocrinol 11:367–370, 1979.
610. Heinen E, Herrmann J, Konigshausen T, Kruskemper HL: Secondary hypothyroidism in severe non-thyroidal illness? Horm Metab Res 13:284–288, 1981.
611. Larsen PR, Silva JE, Kaplan MM: Relationships between circulating and intracellular thyroid hormones: Physiological and clinical implications. Endocr Rev 2:87–102, 1981.
612. Felicetta JV, Green WL, Nelp WB: Inhibition of hepatic binding of thyroxine by cholecystographic agents. J Clin Invest 65:1032–1040, 1980.
613. DeGroot LJ, Rue PA: Roentgenographic contrast agents inhibit triiodothyronine binding to nuclear receptors in vitro. J Clin Endocrinol Metab 49:538–542, 1979.
614. Roti E, Minelli R, Gardini E, et al: Thyrotoxicosis followed by hypothyroidism in patients treated with amiodarone. Arch Intern Med 153:886–892, 1993.

40

Nonthyroidal Illnesses

JOHN T. NICOLOFF
JONATHAN S. LoPRESTI

Alterations in serum thyroid hormone indices commonly occur in patients suffering from a wide variety of nonthyroidal illnesses (NTI) in whom no pre-existing intrinsic thyroid glandular disease appears to exist. This phenomenon has been collectively termed the "low T$_3$ state" of NTI, primarily because both total and apparently free serum T$_3$ values are consistently depressed. Alternatively, this condition has also been referred to as the "euthyroid sick syndrome" because it appears that there is little clinical or biochemical evidence that these patients are truly hypothyroid in a conventional sense. Although this phenomenon has been extensively investigated and documented in the medical literature over the past four decades,[1–4] the basic mechanisms responsible for its genesis and its metabolic-endocrine consequences remain uncertain.

The diseases giving rise to these changes are quite diverse, including a variety of acute and chronic systemic illnesses[5–9] and injuries such as major burns, trauma, and surgery.[10–12] The changes in thyroid indices resulting from these illnesses and injuries are probably triggered by cytokines released from macrophages and monocytes, as a part of a systemic immune response, as shown in Figure 40–1. Indeed, the administration of cytokines to human volun-

teers (interleukin-2 [IL-2] and tumor necrosis factor [TNF]) is capable of inducing the characteristic changes observed in the low T$_3$ state.[13, 14] In addition to illness and injury, a similar low T$_3$ state can be observed in a variety of catabolic conditions including fasting,[15] diabetes,[16] ketogenic diets,[17] liver and kidney disease,[8, 18] and pharmacological glucocorticoid administration.[19] Interestingly, it can also be seen in otherwise apparently healthy aged populations.[20] In view of the character of these aforementioned conditions, it is somewhat surprising that a similar low T$_3$ pattern is also seen in the normal healthy growing fetus.[21] Taken together, these low T$_3$ states in all their various forms account for the most common alteration from the normal pattern of thyroid function observed in adult humans.

The cardinal feature defining the low T$_3$ state of NTI, as the name implies, is depressed serum T$_3$ values. When studied, this reduction in serum T$_3$ likely originates from a decrease in the conversion of T$_4$ to T$_3$ by peripheral tissue 5'-deiodinase (5'D) enzyme systems.[22] In addition, serum reverse T$_3$ (rT$_3$) levels are usually reciprocally increased.[23] This rise in the serum rT$_3$ is not, however, the result of augmented rT$_3$ production but rather caused by a reduction in hormonal clearance resulting from inhibition of hepatic 5'D enzyme systems.[24] As rT$_3$ is a hormonally inactive isomer of T$_3$,[25] these serum rT$_3$ elevations are not believed to have any metabolic impact. In contrast to these

Supported in part by United States National Institutes of Health Grants DK 11727 and General Clinical Research Center Program Grant MO1-RR-43.

FIGURE 40–1. A schematic diagram of the cascade of events describing the development of the low T$_3$ and low T$_3$-T$_4$ states of nonthyroidal illness, fasting, and diabetes.

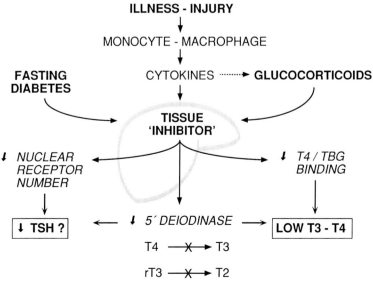

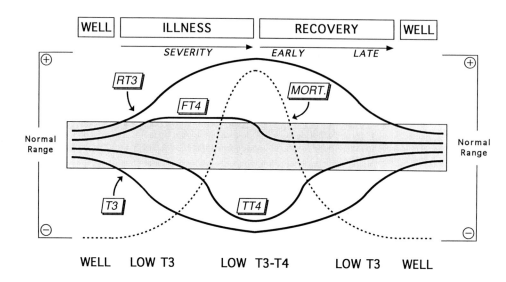

FIGURE 40–2. A description of the pattern of alterations in serum thyroid hormone indices and TSH occurring during the development and recovery from a typical nonthyroidal illness (NTI). The interrupted line portrays the predicted mortality rate (MORT) associated with the development of the low T_3-T_4 state of NTI.

dramatic changes in serum T_3 and rT_3, total and free T_4 values generally remain within the normal limits, although there is a tendency, as determined by some newer in vitro methods,[26] to observe mild to moderate free T_4 elevations.[27, 28] Despite such elevations in free T_4, however, serum T_4 production rates generally remain within normal limits.[29]

Serum TSH values in NTI are usually in the normal range, which is consistent with the finding of a normal thyroidal T_4 secretion rate. Such normal serum TSH values may be considered somewhat paradoxical, however, because the reduced serum T_3 values should, by reduction in negative feedback on the pituitary thyrotrophs, result in elevated serum TSH levels. In fact, producing a low T_3 state by inhibiting peripheral T_4 to T_3 conversion with the competitive deiodinase inhibitor iopanoic acid produces the expected elevation in serum TSH levels that further underscores this point.[30] In fact, newer and more sensitive TSH assays have shown that serum TSH values are usually transiently suppressed into the hyperthyroid range during the early phases of NTI's.[31] The mechanism responsible for the resetting of pituitary TSH secretion is not understood, but it seems likely to be coordinated with the alterations in peripheral T_4 to T_3 conversion so that normal TSH and T_4 production rate values are maintained.[29]

As the severity of an illness, injury, or metabolic derangement becomes more extreme, serum total T_4 values often decline into the hypothyroid range.[29] This syndrome is appropriately termed the "low T_3-T_4 state" and appears to result from the acquisition of a defect in T_4 binding to its serum carrier protein, thyroxine-binding globulin (TBG), as a secondary consequence of severe systemic NTI.[32] Despite dramatic falls in total T_4, however, free T_4 values usually remain normal or are even modestly elevated.[26, 27] The cause of the TBG binding defect is not well understood, but it is believed to result from the presence of either a circulating binding inhibitor[32] or an acquired intrinsic structural alteration in the T_4-binding site on TBG,[33] or from a combination of the two. The development of this low T_3-T_4 state is usually associated with severe life-threatening illnesses. In fact, a close inverse correlation exists between the magnitude of the T_4 fall and the mortality rate.[34, 35] Thus, there seems to be a continuum of responses by which a patient may pass from a low T_3 to a low T_3-T_4

state as a systemic illness or injury becomes more severe. The reverse of this sequence is seen during recovery from NTI, with the TBG-binding defect first being rectified, thereby normalizing serum total T_4 values, followed by a progressive fall in the elevated serum rT_3 levels, and last by a gradual normalization of serum T_3 levels. This pattern of entry and recovery from NTI is diagrammatically shown in Figure 40–2. Our descriptive understanding of the complexity and temporal dynamics of the development and recovery from the low T_3 and T_3-T_4 states of NTI has progressed substantially from its original descriptions four decades ago.[1-3] This has been largely accomplished by the development of improved assay methods for the measurement of T_4, FT_4, T_3, FT_3, rT_3, TBG, and TSH.[15, 27, 28, 31] In contrast, our understanding of the basic mechanisms responsible for this complex sequence of events has been marginal. As discussed later in the text, several theories exist regarding the genesis of these changes, but none of them has provided a satisfactory explanation of the observed phenomena. It is also important to emphasize that the low T_3 state of NTI undoubtedly takes place as a component of a more complex systemic endocrine-nutritional response. This endocrine signaling interplay is probably present whether the low T_3 state is caused by an NTI, a catabolic-metabolic state, or an in utero environment. Therefore, to focus on the thyroid system in isolation undoubtedly provides an incomplete and potentially misleading picture of the entire process.

Although it is clear that the low T_3 state represents circumstances in which distinct alterations from the normal pattern of thyroid metabolism have occurred, it is uncertain what effect it exerts on the general metabolic state of the affected individual. Probably the most widely held view is that the reduction in serum T_3 plays an important role in minimizing body protein losses during fasting or caloric restriction.[36] This conclusion is based on the observation that nitrogen losses promptly increase in fasted subjects when serum T_3 levels are normalized by the concurrent administration of exogenous oral T_3.[36, 37] How these observations relate to the low T_3 state of NTI or in utero is less evident.

The foregoing remarks have provided a brief overview of the subject. The remaining portion of this chapter is directed to a more detailed description of this process, its

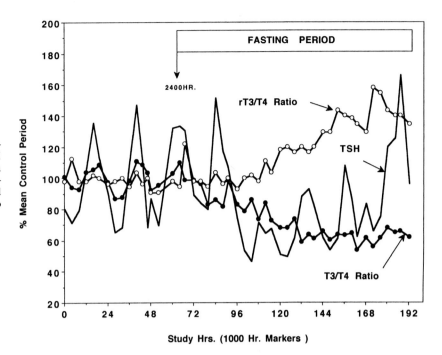

FIGURE 40-3. The temporal sequence of the relative alterations in serum thyroid hormone indices and TSH which occur in healthy nonobese subjects undergoing a voluntary fast. (Adapted from Spencer CA, Lum SMC, Wilber JF, et al: Dynamics of serum thyrotropin and thyroid hormone changes in fasting. J Clin Endocrinol Metab 56:883–888, © 1983 by the Endocrine Society.)

possible genesis, common variants, and potential adaptive significance, if any.

THE LOW T₃ STATE OF FASTING AND OTHER CATABOLIC CONDITIONS

Caloric restriction and fasting provide perhaps the most predictable and useful model for studying the development of the low T_3 state. However, it must be kept in mind that the low T_3 state produced by caloric restriction probably cannot be considered to be fully analogous with the low T_3 state of NTI. Despite this limitation, it is useful to describe the temporal sequence and character of the changes observed in thyroid indices as they occur with a voluntary fast or caloric restriction in otherwise healthy individuals in order to gain a more precise understanding of the process.

When normal healthy nonobese human subjects are fasted, the first detectable alterations are observed at about 12 to 16 hours into the fast, when an abrupt rise in serum free T_4 levels and a gradual decline in serum T_3 values occur, as shown in Figure 40–3.[15] Subsequently, the modest free T_4 elevation is sustained, whereas the serum T_3 level

NORMAL   NTI / FASTING

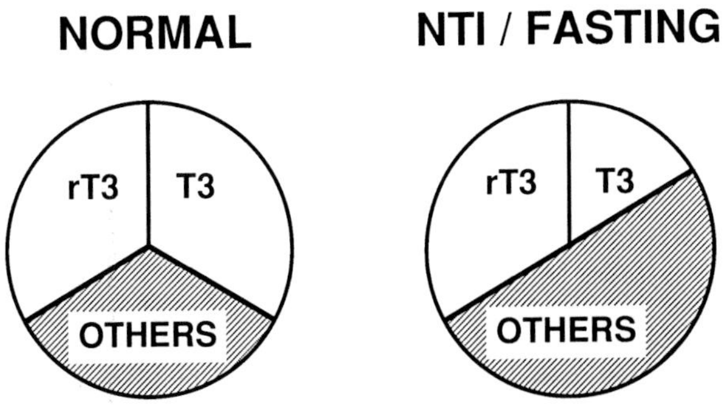

FIGURE 40–4. The overall partition of thyroxine deiodinated metabolites T_3 and rT_3, which occurs in fasting and nonthyroidal illness.

gradually falls over the next four days, achieving a new stable value at about one-half the concentration observed in the fed state. Despite an apparent 20 per cent increase in free T_4 levels, as measured in vitro, T_4 production rates, T_4 deiodination rates, and clearance values remain unaltered.[38, 39] Despite this apparent normality of T_4 secretion and metabolism, a progressive decrease in serum T_3 levels secondary to a diminished blood T_3 production rate implies that a major diversion of T_4 metabolism away from T_3 formation has taken place, as shown in Figure 40–4. In fact, the 50 per cent reduction in T_3 production produced by fasting probably occurs just as abruptly as the increase in FT_4 but requires three to four days to become fully expressed owing to the one day half-life of T_3 in the circulation. As serum total and free T_3 levels fall, sulfate conjugates of T_3 (T_3S) and the acetic acid analogue of T_3, triiodothyroacetic acid (triac) also appear as alternate products of T_3 metabolism.[40] This increased production of T_3S and triac as metabolites of T_3 is currently being proposed as the cause of the reduced T_3 blood production rate by acting as a shunting mechanism for redirecting T_3 production away from the circulation.[41]

The second major event in this sequence occurs at about 24 hours into the fast, when an abrupt fall in serum TSH takes place. This drop in serum TSH can be considered inappropriate in view of the concurrent decline in serum T_3 values, as noted previously. Subsequently, serum TSH values gradually return to the normal range as the serum T_3 levels stabilize at their lower fasting levels, indicating the achievement of a new homeostatic state.[15] This sequence of events is consistent with the concept that pituitary thyrotrophs have gained increased negative feedback sensitivity to circulating T_3 in fasting. Indeed, several reported studies appear to support this hypothesis.[36] The third and final event is marked by a rise in serum rT_3, which becomes apparent at about 48 hours into the fast. Note also that the rise in serum rT_3 does not temporally coincide with the fall in T_3, indicating that the genesis of these changes is not linked to the inhibition of the same deiodinase system.

Subsequently, rT_3 values progressively increase to about two to three times basal levels over the next two weeks.[42] If the fast is continued beyond two weeks, however, serum rT_3 values have a tendency to gradually decline and may even achieve normal concentrations after several weeks.[42] With the cessation of the fast, serum rT_3 values precipitously fall, achieving normal or even subnormal levels in a few days. Kinetic studies reveal that rT_3 production is unaffected during the first two weeks of a fast but is promptly reduced during the early refeeding period.[43, 44] In fact, the rapid fall in serum rT_3 with refeeding appears to result principally from a decline in rT_3 production rather than an increase in rT_3 clearance.[44] Whether the trend for rT_3 levels to normalize during a prolonged fast results from changes in rT_3 clearance and/or production is unknown.

The source of circulating rT_3 is believed to originate from deiodination of T_4 by a specific inner-ring 5-D, type III, enzyme system located in a variety of extrahepatic tissues.[45] The activity of this inner-ring deiodinase seems to be relatively constant except for the aforementioned decrease observed during the early refeeding period and an increase produced by the administration of pharmacological doses of glucocorticoids.[45] Although the hepatic 5'-deiodinase is capable of converting T_4 to rT_3 in vitro,[47] it does not appear to contribute to the overall blood rT_3 production rate in vivo.[47] Rather, the hepatic 5'-deiodinase is believed to be principally responsible for rT_3 disposal.[45] In this context, alterations in serum rT_3 levels indirectly reflect a reciprocal change in hepatic 5'-deiodinase activity in vivo.[44] For example, the two- to three-fold rise in serum rT_3 seen in fasting primarily reflects a proportionate decline in hepatic 5'-deiodinase activity.

Patients with uncontrolled diabetes mellitus display the same general pattern of thyroid hormone indices as observed in fasted or calorically deprived subjects.[16] This low T_3 state may be, in part, the product of a form of "metabolic starvation" caused by an absolute or relative lack of insulin action in which fatty acids and ketones serve as the primary body fuel. In this context, it is relevant to note that the use of a high-fat "ketogenic" diet also produces a low T_3 state in healthy subjects regardless of caloric intake.[17] Control of serum glucose levels with insulin therapy alone may not be sufficient to entirely reverse this low T_3 state.[16] This is particularly evident if conventional "weight maintenance" diets are employed, as is traditional in treatment of obese, non–insulin-dependent diabetic patients.[16] Rather, it appears that supplemental carbohydrate and/or protein intake is required to reverse the catabolic state of prolonged uncontrolled diabetes as well as to normalize thyroid indices. Thus, the integration of nutrition, insulin, and thyroid hormones may be required to achieve an optimal anabolic state. A similar integrative response has been described for T_3, insulin, and glucose acting at the postreceptor level on carbohydrate-sensitive enzyme systems of the hepatocyte.[48] Thus, the reversal of the low T_3 state may serve as an indicator of anabolism. Unfortunately, the use of thyroid function testing for this purpose in the clinical nutrition field has been very limited to date.

Severely obese subjects also display a low T_3 state when fasted or calorically restricted, but the pattern differs from that of the nonobese in that the decline of serum T_3 takes place at a much slower pace and no abrupt reset of serum TSH levels occurs, as is seen for nonobese individuals shown in Figure 40–3.[44]

Baseline serum T_3 values in obese patients are generally in the normal range, although some severely obese patients may display marginally low values.[42] In either case, these T_3 values may be considered to be inappropriately low because hyperalimentation of lean healthy subjects predictably increases both serum T_3 and T_3/T_4 ratio values.[49] By this standard, obese patients appear to have their thyroid status altered toward a low T_3 state even before undergoing weight reduction. This view is further supported by the finding that obese patients who display lower basal serum T_3 and T_3/T_4 ratio values sustain lower initial nitrogen losses during caloric restriction than do those with more normal T_3 values.[50] This observation is again consistent with the concept that the low T_3 state may play a role in minimizing lean body protein losses during caloric restriction or fasting. However, why some obese subjects assume such an apparent conservation mode in their thyroid hormone metabolism prior to caloric restriction is unknown. Upon breaking a fast or calorically restricted diet, obese subjects often display persistently depressed serum T_3 values for weeks and sometimes months. These altered response patterns in severely obese subjects before, during, and after weight reduction should be studied further, as they may provide important insights into the mechanisms underlying the genesis and adaptation to obesity.

Glucocorticoid excess represents another but probably distinct metabolic condition, which predictably produces a low T_3 state. As with fasting, the reduction in serum T_3 levels produced by pharmacological glucocorticoid administration results from diminished T_3 production from T_4. However, the glucocorticoid-induced low T_3 state differs in that the reduction in TSH, as well as the rise in serum rT_3, occurs abruptly within a few hours of administering glucocorticoids rather than being delayed as is seen with fasting. Further, the reduction in serum TSH appears to be produced by a reduction in endogenous TRH action on the pituitary rather than by a direct inhibition of pituitary TSH release, as appears to be the case with fasting.[51] The mechanism by which T_4 to T_3 conversion is reduced by glucocorticoids also displays some subtle differences from that seen with fasting. This relates primarily to the array of the urinary metabolites of T_3 that are produced.[52] With cessation of glucocorticoid therapy, serum rT_3 and T_3 values rapidly normalize, and a prompt rebound in serum TSH occurs which may transiently achieve elevated values.[52] This reversal pattern again occurs more rapidly than is usually observed with refeeding of the fasted subject. Therefore, both central and peripheral mechanisms of the glucocorticoid-induced low T_3 state appear to differ qualitatively from that produced by fasting.

LOW T_3 AND LOW T_3-T_4 STATES OF NTI AND INJURY

The overall pattern of the development and recovery from the low T_3 state of NTI is grossly similar to that observed for fasting. However, it is inherently more variable, reflecting, in part, the diversity of underlying illnesses and injuries responsible for its genesis. As with fasting, an initial phase occurs in which both serum T_3 and TSH levels fall in association with variable increases in rT_3 and decreases in total T_4 values while free T_4 values usually remain within the normal range.[16] However, instead of proceeding in a deliberate and predictable time sequence, as with fasting and caloric restriction, these changes can occur abruptly similar to the pattern seen with pharmacological glucocorticoid administration. As might be expected, this sudden response is most evident in those instances associated with major acute illnesses and injuries in which endogenous ACTH-induced adrenal cortical stimulation might be expected to have taken place.[53] Also, the magnitude of changes observed in serum TSH, T_3 and rT_3 are frequently greater than those seen with fasting and metabolic disorders.[10, 54] As previously proposed, this response may represent the combined effects of cytokine-induced catabolism and endogenous glucocorticoid action, as shown in Figure 40–1. Whether such a dual mechanism is sufficient to produce the magnitude of changes observed in some cases of severe illness is unknown. As patients recover from NTI's, the sequence reverses, with serum TSH levels often transiently rebounding into the supranormal range as depressed serum T_3 values gradually normalize.[55]

With more severe systemic illnesses and injuries, the low T_3 state may progress into what has been termed the "low T_3-T_4 state" in which total serum T_4 values become profoundly depressed, as shown in Figure 40–2. This low T_3-T_4 pattern may develop over a few days or within a few hours following catastrophic events such as major burns, cardiac arrest, or septic shock.[10, 11, 56] Despite reductions in serum T_4 concentrations into the hypothyroid range, however, free T_4 levels usually remain normal or are even elevated, depending on the assay method employed.[26–28] Concurrent T_4 kinetic measurements performed in such severely ill patients reveal that T_4 production rates remain normal or are slightly depressed.[22, 29] This tendency for lower T_4 production rates in some cases may reflect concurrent reductions in serum TSH levels and/or a diminished thyroid glandular responsiveness to TSH secondary to a direct inhibitory effect of TNF.[57] In any case, the tissue availability of T_4 as judged by free T_4 levels appears to be adequate; therefore, such patients probably should not be considered to be in a T_4-deficient state.

It is not unusual for considerable diagnostic confusion to result when subnormal free T_4 values are reported in patients with the low T_3-T_4 state when a variety of free thyroxine index or analogue techniques are used to estimate free thyroxine levels.[26] As these sera may provide normal or even elevated free T_4 values when using more physiological methods such as dialysis or ultrafiltration, this clearly represents a technical limitation of these more widely employed clinical methods.[26–28] Fortunately, many of these methods have undergone modifications in an attempt to overcome this deficiency, but this problem still persists to some degree, particularly when patients exhibit very low total T_4 values. In a few instances, total T_4 production and free T_4 values may actually be depressed. The most commonly encountered situation occurs when patients are receiving dopamine infusions for the treatment of hypotension. Pharmacological levels of dopamine directly inhibit TSH release and thereby reduce both thyroidal T_4 secretion and free T_4 levels.[58]

Both total T_3 and T_3 blood production rates are characteristically reduced in all forms of the low T_3 state. However, this reduction in T_3 production alone is not sufficient to produce a low circulating T_3 level unless T_3 clearance is maintained. In this context, it is important to note that

serum T_3 clearance remains essentially unaltered in NTI, which contrasts with the marked reduction characteristically seen for rT_3 clearance.[22, 24] This is best explained by the fact that T_3 clearance, unlike rT_3, is relatively independent of hepatic 5'-deiodinase activity. Indeed, T_3 kinetic tracer studies have revealed that fully one half of T_3 disposal normally occurs by nondeiodinative pathways primarily involving T_3S and triac formation.[59] Further, these alternate pathways are likely stimulated in low T_3 states, thereby maintaining normal T_3 clearance rates despite the inhibition of hepatic 5'-deiodinase observed in NTI.[22, 24, 40, 41] Therefore, the increased formation of T_3S and triac from T_3 may not only account for the apparent lowering of T_4 to T_3 conversion but also appear to play a crucial role in maintaining T_3 clearance in NTI and other low T_3 states.

In general, sick patients display normal serum TSH values. However, some subsets of patients may present with abnormal serum TSH levels, as shown in Figure 40–5. About 10 per cent of all patients have depressed TSH values, whereas 5 per cent display elevated levels.[31] However, most of these changes are marginal, as only 3 per cent of values are less than 0.1 mU/L and 1 per cent above 15 mU/L. Thus, only about 4 per cent of hospitalized patients display serum TSH alterations that suggest a major alteration in thyroid status. Further, NTI-induced TSH alterations are transient, usually normalizing within a few days.[31] Therefore, repeating the serum TSH value is often helpful in resolving a diagnostic question regarding the meaning of altered TSH values in NTI. For patients presenting with TSH values below 0.1 mU/L, it may be useful to employ a third-generation serum TSH assay that is capable of measuring TSH values down to the level of 0.01 mU/L, in which case, nearly all sick patients display detectable values. In contrast, truly thyrotoxic patients display values consistently below this level.[31] Alternatively, TRH stimulation testing can be performed, in which case a detectable TSH response would support the diagnosis of NTI rather than hyperthyroidism.[31] Finally, as most spontaneously occurring thyroid disorders result from an underlying autoimmune disease, measurement of serum anti-thyroperoxidase antibody levels (anti-TPO antibodies) may provide additional diagnostic information in difficult cases. When elevated values are encountered in sick patients, repetition of the serum TSH usually shows a progressive fall. However, full normalization may require several days to weeks to occur in certain instances.[31] Additionally, the finding of a normal serum free T_4 and negative anti-TPO antibody value indicates that NTI is the most likely cause.

Fully one half of the hospitalized patients presenting with abnormal TSH values also provide a history of recent glucocorticoid therapy.[31] As pharmacological levels of glucocorticoids inhibit endogenous TSH secretion through a TRH-mediated mechanism,[51] glucocorticoid use readily explains such depressed serum TSH levels. On the other hand, the finding of an elevated serum TSH value may well represent a rebound response following the recent cessation of glucocorticoids.[51, 52] It is also conceivable that many of the abnormal TSH values observed in patients without a history of glucocorticoid therapy may represent the influence of endogenous cortisol secretion induced by the stress of illness.[53]

It should again be emphasized, however, that the bulk of patients present with normal serum TSH values. This may be true even when the characteristic hormonal pattern of

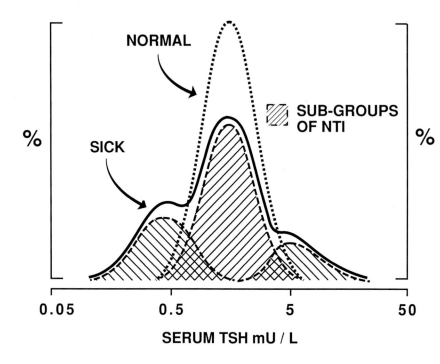

FIGURE 40–5. Comparison of the frequency of alterations in serum TSH values which occur in patients hospitalized with nonthyroidal illnesses (NTI's). Note that distinct subgroups of NTI patients present with transiently depressed or elevated serum TSH values but that the majority of the NTI population have normal serum TSH values on presentation. (Adapted from Spencer CA, Eigen A, Shen D, et al: Sensitive TSH tests—specificity limitations for screening for thyroid disease in hospitalized patients. Clin Chem 33:1391–1396, 1987.)

low T_3 or low T_3-T_4 states is observed. Presumably, such patients have passed through the initial phase of the NTI when TSH values are unstable and have achieved a new state.

PATHOGENESIS

At present, no generally agreed-upon theory explains the origin of the low T_3 state of NTI. For that matter, the same may be said for low T_3 levels associated with fasting, caloric deficiency, and various metabolic derangements, as well as the in utero environment. As illustrated in Figure 40–1, a diversity of pathways appears to exist by which the low T_3 state may be initiated. There seems to be, however, a strong likelihood that some features are common to its production regardless of the inciting cause. Further, it seems probable that some circulating humoral factor is required to initiate the diversity of alterations in both central and peripheral thyroid hormone metabolism. In the case of injuries and NTI's, cytokines, such as TNF and interleukins, are the likely candidates. Although cytokine-mediated ACTH and cortisol release would explain some aspects of the low T_3 state, the mechanisms responsible for the impairment in serum T_4 binding, inhibition of hepatic deiodinases, and activation of alternate pathways of T_3 metabolism are less apparent.

A considerable body of evidence exists regarding the possible presence of a serum T_4-binding inhibitor that may be responsible for many of the characteristic features of NTI.[32] In even the mildest forms of the low T_3 state of NTI, some degree of serum T_4 binding inhibition appears to be exhibited, which is reflected by variable increases in serum free T_4 levels, as assessed by dialysis or ultrafiltration methods.[27, 28] Further, T_4 binding to intracellular cytosolic proteins also appears to be impaired. This is particularly apparent for the "rapidly equilibrating" tissues such as liver and kidney, as demonstrated by compartmental tracer T_4 kinetic distribution analysis.[22] In fact, the intracellular

T_4-binding defect is probably more severely affected than that observed in serum. Thus, T_4-binding inhibition appears to be a combined intracellular and extracellular event. How and why this T_4-binding defect occurs is, however, less clear.

A lipid-like material can be extracted from sera of NTI patients that is capable of inhibiting T_4 binding to TBG when added back to normal sera in vitro.[32] As might be expected, the quantity of this serum inhibitor generally increases in critically ill patients displaying the low T_3-T_4 state.[32] Further, the finding of normal TBG concentrations, as determined by direct immunoassay, in patients presenting with the low T_3-T_4 of NTI is fully consistent with this binding inhibitor theory.[29] A similar binding inhibitor may also be extracted from normal liver, as well as other tissues.[32] The exact chemical nature of this binding inhibitor has, however, proved to be elusive. This inhibitor appears to possess many of the properties of a fatty acid, such as oleic acid.[60] However, it is doubtful that oleic acid itself can be responsible for such inhibition in vivo, as serum albumin appears to be its preferred serum-binding protein. However, in some severely stressed patients who may have hypoalbuminemia, unbound serum oleic acid levels may rise to a sufficient degree to theoretically produce such T_4-binding inhibition.[60]

An important and perhaps more provocative extension of this theory is that this putative inhibitor may also be responsible for inhibiting hepatic 5'-deiodinase activity, as well as interfering with phagocytic activity of leukocytes.[61, 62] The former would be responsible for the characteristic elevations in serum rT_3, whereas the latter could explain the high mortality rates observed in patients displaying the low T_3-T_4 state. Obviously, the identification of such an inhibitor and the development of methods for its removal from the circulation would be of potential therapeutic importance.

An alternate explanation for the serum T_4-binding inhibition phenomenon of NTI is provided by data indicating that TBG may become structurally altered; this, in turn, impairs its T_4-binding properties.[33] Such a structurally altered TBG, which has been termed "slow TBG" because of its retarded migration on protein electrophoresis, appears to have approximately one tenth the binding affinity of normal TBG for T_4 and thereby might provide a satisfactory alternative or additional explanation for the T_4-binding inhibition in illness. Unfortunately, this observation has been reported from only one laboratory and therefore needs further confirmation. Another recent study indicates that serum free T_3 levels may be normal in NTI even though serum T_3 values and production rates are depressed.[28] Employing what might be considered a more physiological ultrafiltration method to assess free T_3 and free T_4, entirely normal free T_3 values were measured in patients displaying the low T_3-T_4 response secondary to severe liver failure, respiratory insufficiency, cancer, and stroke.[28] Obviously, such data would readily explain why serum TSH values remain normal in NTI. However, it would not provide a mechanistic explanation for the binding inhibition or how free T_3 levels are maintained while T_3 production rates are depressed. These data require further verification.

Additional insights into the cause of the low T_3 state may be gained by studying the alterations in peripheral thyroid hormone metabolism that occur in NTI. Clearly, the low T_3 state produces major changes in the peripheral metabolism of T_4, as shown in Figures 40–2 and 40–4. It also appears to stimulate the formation of the T_3S at the apparent expense of circulating T_3 by activating sulfotransferase enzyme systems, primarily located in the liver and kidney.[63] As T_3S lacks any inherent thyromimetric activity[64, 65] and is not deconjugated in vivo when it is administered either systemically or orally to humans,[65] T_3S formation appears to represent primarily an inactivation pathway. Interestingly, as T_3S serves as a substantially better substrate for deiodination by hepatic deiodinase enzyme systems than does its precursor T_3,[46] iodide recovery from the deiodination of T_3 is efficiently recycled for new hormone formation despite the impaired hepatic deiodinase activity accompanying NTI. In addition, conversion of T_3 to triac also appears to be increased in low T_3 states of fasting and presumably NTI.[40, 41] This triac formation results from the deamination of T_3 by specific aminotransferase enzyme systems primarily found in liver and kidney but present in other tissues as well.[66] Although in vivo formation of triac from T_3 has been known to occur since the mid 1950's, it was not considered to play a significant role in thyroid hormone economy, as it exhibited approximately one-twentieth the systemic hormonal potency of T_3 when given systemically.[67, 68] This reduced potency of triac compared with T_3 was thought to be due primarily to the rapid clearance of triac from blood.[69–71] Recently, however, triac has been shown to display an equal or even greater potency in activating the nuclear thyroid hormone receptors responsible for mediating thyroid hormone action.[72, 73] This is particularly true of the β form of the nuclear thyroid hormone receptor, which is the dominant form found in liver, kidney, and pituitary.[73] It has been recently proposed that triac produced locally from T_3 could serve as a potent hormone in these tissues rich in β receptors and thereby might play an autocrine role in countering the effects of the lower circulating T_3 levels found in NTI and other low T_3 states.[40, 41] Such a putative autocrine action of triac in

liver and kidney might also be important in fostering gluconeogenesis in calorically deprived states.

NTI VARIANTS

Nonthyroidal illnesses usually produce very consistent and predictable responses in serum thyroid hormone indices, as shown in Figure 40–2. However, several situations result in very distinct patterns of thyroid function of which the clinician should be aware. These situations include kidney and liver disease, infection with the human immunodeficiency virus (HIV), pregnancy, psychiatric disorders, and aged populations.

Compensated liver disease, both acute and chronic, produces variable elevations in serum total T_4 values. This increase in T_4 appears to be entirely secondary to the elevation of serum TBG levels as free T_4 and T_4 production rates remain normal.[74] The cause of the increased TBG production by the liver is presumably a manifestation of the chronic inflammatory process acting on the hepatocyte to increase TBG synthesis.[74] The serum T_3 levels, in contrast, generally remain within the normal range, whereas rT_3 concentrations show a tendency to be depressed.[75] Such alterations occur in a variety of liver diseases, including acute and chronic viral hepatitis, compensated alcoholic cirrhosis, and acute intermittent porphyria.[76] These distortions in serum thyroid indices are most evident when a flare in the underlying inflammatory disease occurs.[75] However, when frank liver failure intervenes, manifested as jaundice and ascites, serum T_3 values fall and the classic picture of the low T_3 state is produced. In particular, a fall in T_3 values has been recognized as a particularly sensitive indicator of a poor prognosis in patients with alcoholic cirrhosis.[77] In addition, serum TSH levels may be mildly elevated in chronic liver disease, with values below 20 mU/L being seen most frequently.[78] The cause and consequences of these TSH elevations are not well understood and need to be confirmed with more sensitive and specific second- and third-generation TSH assays.

Chronic renal disease frequently produces a variant pattern in serum T_3 values that fail to increase despite low serum T_3 levels.[18] Kinetic studies reveal that rT_3 clearance rates remain normal rather than being reduced, as is characteristic in other low T_3 states. Although the mechanism for maintenance of rT_3 clearance has not been fully elucidated, it is believed that some factor unique to renal disease, possibly elevated parathyroid hormone levels, may be responsible.[79] As these alterations in rT_3 metabolism also occur in the nephrotic syndrome, in which glomerular filtration rates are relatively normal, such alterations do not simply represent a consequence of diminished renal filtration.[80] As with liver disease, serum TSH values may, on occasion, become modestly elevated.[81] Again, these observations need to be confirmed with more sensitive and specific TSH assays.

Patients chronically infected with HIV usually present with an aberrant pattern of thyroid indices, mimicking those of chronic liver disease in that they display elevated serum T_4 and TBG levels and low rT_3 values while maintaining a normal serum T_3.[82] These changes appear to become more pronounced as the HIV infection progresses. However, with the onset of life-threatening intercurrent illnesses, the typical pattern of the low T_3 state is usually seen. Because the low T_3 state serves as a harbinger of serious intercurrent illnesses, a low serum T_3 value has been proposed as a prognostic indicator in HIV-infected patients.[83] It is extremely uncommon, however, for a low T_3-T_4 state to develop even in the most severely ill HIV-infected patient. Unlike in liver disease, serum TSH values are unaffected.

Serum thyroid hormone indices in pregnant women are remarkably unresponsive to intervening illness. For example, women with hyperemesis gravidarum fail to display the characteristic low T_3 state despite substantial weight loss and ketonuria.[84] Further, the administration of pharmacological glucocorticoids will not lower T_3 serum despite altering the thyroid indices in the fetus via transplacental passage.[85] Additionally, minimal alterations in thyroid indices accompany intercurrent systemic illnesses. Therefore, one must conclude that pregnant women have a blunted response to NTI or to other stimuli that normally produce the low T_3 state. As both pregnant and HIV-infected patients have suppressed immune systems, these changes may be secondary to an aberrant cytokine response to illness.

Acute psychosis is a common, but not well understood, cause of a variant pattern of thyroid indices. Psychotic patients often display significant elevations in both total T_4 and free T_4 values in association with normal T_3 levels when admitted to a psychiatric facility.[86, 87] In most cases, serum TSH levels are mildly depressed but are detectable when more sensitive second- and third-generation TSH assays are employed, thereby ruling out thyrotoxicosis.[87] The cause of the increased circulating levels of T_4 and free T_4 is unknown, but the syndrome rapidly resolves in most cases within a few days after hospitalization and appropriate therapy. Because these alterations in thyroid indices in acute psychosis are transient, it appears advisable to defer a complete thyroid evaluation for several days after hospitalization and with appropriate therapeutic intervention.

Aging may be the most prevalent cause for the low T_3 state. Surveys of large populations of apparently healthy aged individuals reveal an increasing incidence of the low T_3 state with advancing age.[20] Currently, there is a debate as to whether such a low T_3 state represents an intrinsic element of the aging process or is a subtle manifestation of an unrecognized illness.[88] However, it also should be noted that in highly selected physically active healthy elderly populations, serum T_3 values are identical to those seen in normal healthy young adults.[88] A small subset of apparently euthyroid patients over the age of 65 have been reported to display persistently depressed serum TSH levels in the face of both normal total and free T_4 values.[92] By all other criteria, however, these individuals appear to be euthyroid, suggesting that a "reset" in pituitary feedback may have occurred. Alternatively, this may represent an unrecognized state of subclinical hyperthyroidism. Because the clinical manifestations of hyperthyroidism are very subtle in the elderly, this may be a troublesome diagnostic dilemma.

OVERVIEW AND CONCLUSIONS

The low T_3 state of NTI clearly represents an altered or different state of thyroid hormone metabolism distinct from that seen in a well-fed, healthy adult population. As shown in Figure 40–1, activation of the cytokine system appears to play an important role in initiating the complex series of alterations that occur in both the peripheral and central regulation of thyroid hormone metabolism. Although T_3 production rates and total serum T_3 values are suppressed in this condition, no compelling evidence indicates that these states represent a condition of true thyroid hormone deficiency. This conclusion is based on the findings that serum TSH levels are usually normal, there is an absence of clinical features suggestive of hypothyroidism, and, perhaps most importantly, serum free T_3 as well as free T_4 values appear to be normal when applying more advanced testing methods.[27, 28] Therefore, the term "euthyroid sick state" may be a more appropriate assignation for this condition than the "low T_3 state." Whether the low T_3 state observed in association with fasting and undernutrition or that seen with glucocorticoid excess represents a similar process, or even serves as an element in producing the NTI response, has yet to be defined.

The low T_3 state may, however, play a more well-defined role in defending protein body stores and regulating gluconeogenesis in subjects who are fasting or calorically deprived. In this context, the low T_3 state appears to foster protein conservation. Undoubtedly, such conservation is the result of the interaction of multiple hormonal systems, including cortisol and circulating growth factors such as growth hormone, IGF-1, and insulin.[90] It is also probable that these other hormonal influences acting in concert with the low T_3 state are responsible for orchestrating the anabolic processes taking place in the fetus in utero.

The liver, as depicted in Figure 40–1, conceivably plays a central role in orchestrating many of the alterations observed in the low T_3 state, whether caused by NTI, fasting, or other conditions, because it has been implicated in such phenomena as T_4 to T_3 conversion, rT_3 clearance, T_4 binding inhibitor generation, the synthesis of a putative "slow TBG," and further metabolism of T_3 to form T_3S or triac. Additionally, the hepatocyte has clearly been identified as having the capacity to produce integrated responses to nutritional factors, thyroid hormone, insulin, growth hormone and cytokines.[48] Although it appears evident that the liver, and perhaps the kidney as well, is deeply involved in this process, it is uncertain how they mechanistically carry out these functions.

We presently have a limited understanding of how the changes in serum thyroid hormone indices associated with NTI affect the action and expression of T_3-mediated events. Indeed, changes in the serum T_3 indices undoubtedly represent only indirect reflections of more complex events occurring at the receptor and postreceptor levels of T_3 expression. Further, it is apparent that, on closer inspection, the low T_3 states in fasting and glucocorticoid therapy are distinctly different processes that produce essentially the same alterations in thyroid indices. Undoubtedly, the situation with illness is even more complex and varied.

With this obvious lack of knowledge, it would seem prudent not to be too dogmatic regarding conclusions relevant to the role of thyroid hormones in these conditions. However, a few generalizations regarding the use of thyroid hormone therapy in these disorders would appear to be appropriate. Firstly, it would not seem advisable to administer triiodothyronine to "correct" a low T_3 state in patients undergoing weight reduction for treatment of obesity because it would likely accelerate the loss of lean body protein stores.[36, 37] Even when such therapy is combined with high protein intake, there is no evidence that such T_3 treatment would not be deleterious. Secondly, it is not apparent that the exogenous use of either T_4 or T_3 has a role in the treatment of severely ill patients presenting with low T_3 or T_3-T_4 states. This recommendation is based both on theoretical considerations that demonstrate that both free T_3 and T_4 are likely to be normal[27, 28] and on the negative clinical impact when thyroid hormone therapy has been empirically administered to such patients.[36, 37] Thirdly, it would appear, on the whole, that the alterations in serum thyroid hormone indices observed in sickness and with caloric deprivation are likely to be adaptive in nature or should be considered to be so until proved otherwise. In this latter context, it is important to keep in mind that certain pathological states could be associated with maladaptive responses. For example, the failure to develop the low T_3 state in an HIV-infected patient may contribute to the wasting present in these individuals. Therefore, one should keep an open mind and consider the role of these changes in thyroid indices on a case-by-case basis.

Despite the general confusion over what the various low T_3 states represent, there are a few recent observations that may allow a better understanding of the basic cellular events that may occur in these conditions. These relate to the finding that all low T_3 states appear to be associated with the increased generation of both active and inactive metabolites of T_3, namely triac and T_3S, respectively. As triac appears to dominantly act as an autocrine hormone and to be more potent than T_3 in activating the beta form of the nuclear receptor, it is tempting to speculate that these multiple low T_3 states may represent an altered prereceptor state in which thyroid hormone action has been switched from an endocrine to an autocrine mode. Such an autocrine hypothesis might then explain the varied pictures in which the low T_3 state occurs and, in particular, why it might be important in producing the selective thyroid hormone effects observed in fetal development.[21, 40, 41] We can hope that the future pursuit of such insights will provide a more concrete picture of why and how these altered states of thyroid function occur.

REFERENCES

1. Ingbar SH, Freinkl N: Regulation of the peripheral metabolism of thyroid hormones. Recent Prog Horm Res 16:353–403, 1960.
2. Oppenheimer JH, Squef R, Surks MI, Hauer H: Binding of thyroxine by serum proteins evaluated by equilibrium dialysis and electrophoretic techniques: Alterations in nonthyroidal disease. J Clin Invest 42:1769–1782, 1963.
3. Wartofsky L, Burman KD: Alterations in thyroid function in patients with systemic illnesses: The "euthyroid sick syndrome." Endocr Rev 3:164–217, 1982.
4. Tibaldi JM, Surks MI: Effect of nonthyroidal illness on thyroid function. Med Clin North Am 69:899–911, 1985.
5. Smith SJ, Bas G, Gerbrandy J, et al: Lowering of serum 3,3',5-triiodothyronine thyroxine ratio in patients with myocardial infarction: Relationship with extent of tissue injury. Eur J Clin Invest 8:99–102, 1978.
6. Lutz JH, Gregerman RF, Spaulding SW, et al: Thyroxine binding proteins, free thyroxine and thyroxine turnover interrelationships during acute infectious illness in man. J Clin Endocrinol Metab 35:230–249, 1972.
7. Talwar KK, Sawhney RC, Rastogi RK: Serum levels of thyrotropin, thyroid hormones and their response to thyrotropin-releasing hormone in infective febrile illness. J Clin Endocrinol Metab 44:398–403, 1977.
8. Chopra IJ, Solomon DH, Chopra U, et al: Alterations in circulating thyroid hormones and thyrotropin in hepatic cirrhosis: Evidence for euthyroidism despite subnormal serum triiodothyronine. J Clin Endocrinol Metab 39:501–511, 1974.
9. Chopra IJ, Smith SR: Circulating thyroid hormones and thyrotropin in adult patients with protein-calorie malnutrition. J Clin Endocrinol Metab 40:221–227, 1975.
10. Becker RA, Wilmore DW, Goodwin CW, et al: Free T_4, free T_3 and reverse T_3 in critically ill, thermally injured patients. J Trauma 20:713–721, 1980.
11. Vitek V, Shatney CH: Thyroid hormone alterations in patients with shock and injury. Injury 18:336–341, 1987.
12. Brandt MR, Skovsted L, Kehlet H, Hansen JM: Rapid decrease in plasma triiodothyronine during surgery and epidural anesthesia independent of afferent neurogenic stimuli and cortisol. Lancet 2:1333–1335, 1976.
13. Atkins MB, Mier JW, Parkinson DR, et al: Hypothyroidism after treatment with interleukin-2 and lymphokine-activated killer cells. N Engl J Med 318:1557–1563, 1988.
14. vanderPall T, Romijn JA, Wiersinga WM, Sauerwein HP: Tumor necrosis factor: A putative mediator of the sick euthyroid syndrome in man. J Clin Endocrinol Metab 71:1567–1572, 1990.
15. Spencer CA, Lum SMC, Wilber JF, et al: Dynamics of serum thyrotropin and thyroid hormone changes in fasting. J Clin Endocrinol Metab 56:883–888, 1983.
16. Alexander CM, Kaptein EM, Lum SMC, et al: Pattern of recovery of thyroid hormone indices associated with treatment of diabetes mellitus. J Clin Endocrinol Metab 54:362–366, 1982.
17. Otten MH, Hennemann G, Docter R, Visser TJ: The role of dietary fat in peripheral thyroid hormone metabolism. Metabolism 29:930–935, 1980.
18. Kaptein EM, Feinstein EI, Nicoloff JT, Massry SG: Serum reverse triiodothyronine and thyroxine kinetics in patients with chronic renal failure. J Clin Endocrinol Metab 57:181–189, 1983.
19. Chopra IJ, Williams DE, Orgiazzi J, Solomon DH: Opposite effects of dexamethasone on serum concentrations of 3,3',5'-triiodothyronine (reverse T_3) and 3,3',5-triiodothyronine (T_3). J Clin Endocrinol Metab 41:911–920, 1975.
20. Lipson A, Nickoloff EL, Hsu TH, et al: A study of age-dependent changes in thyroid function tests in adults. J Nucl Med 20:1124–1130, 1979.
21. Fisher DA, Klein AH: Thyroid development and disorders of thyroid function in newborn. N Engl J Med 304:702–712, 1981.
22. Kaptein EM, Robinson WJ, Grieb DA, Nicoloff JT: Peripheral serum thyroxine, triiodothyronine, and reverse triiodothyronine kinetics in the low thyroxine state of acute nonthyroidal illness. J Clin Invest 69:526–535, 1982.
23. Chopra IJ, Chopra U, Smith SR, et al: Reciprocal changes in serum concentration of 3,3',5'-triiodothyronine (reverse T_3) and 3,3',5-triiodothyronine (T_3) in systemic illnesses. J Clin Endocrinol Metab 41:1043–1049, 1975.
24. Faber J, Francis-Thomsen H, Lumholtz IB, et al: Kinetic studies of thyroxine, 3,5,3'-triiodothyronine, 3,3',5'-triiodothyronine, 3',5'-diiodothyronine, 3,3'-diiodothyronine and 3'-monoiodothyronine in patients with liver cirrhosis. J Clin Endocrinol Metab 53:978–984, 1981.
25. Shulkin BL, Utiger RD: Reverse triiodothyronine does not alter pituitary-thyroid function in normal subjects. J Clin Endocrinol Metab 58:1184–1187, 1984.
26. Kaptein EM, Macintyre SS, Weiner JM, et al: Free thyroxine estimations in nonthyroidal illness: Comparison of eight methods. J Clin Endocrinol Metab 52:1073–1077, 1981.
27. Nelson JC, Weiss RM: The effect of serum dilution on free thyroxine (T_4) concentration in the low T_4 syndrome of nonthyroidal illness. J Clin Endocrinol Metab 61:239–246, 1985.
28. Faber J, Kirkegaard C, Rasmussen B, et al: Pituitary-thyroid axis in critical illness. J Clin Endocrinol Metab 65:315–320, 1987.
29. Kaptein EM, Grieb DA, Spencer CA, et al: Thyroxine metabolism in the low thyroxine state of critical nonthyroidal illness. J Clin Endocrinol Metab 53:764–771, 1981.
30. Kleinmann RE, Vagenakis AG, Braverman LE: The effect of iopanoic acid on the regulation of thyrotropin secretion in euthyroid subjects. J Clin Endocrinol Metab 51:399–403, 1980.
31. Spencer CA, Eigen A, Shen D, et al: Sensitive TSH tests—specificity limitations for screening for thyroid disease in hospitalized patients. Clin Chem 33:1391–1396, 1987.
32. Chopra IJ, Huang TS, Hurd RE, et al: A competitive ligand binding

assay for measurement of thyroid hormone-binding inhibitor in serum and tissues. J Clin Endocrinol Metab 58:619–628, 1984.

33. Reilly CP, Welley ML: Slow thyroxine binding globulin in the pathogenesis of increased dialyzable fraction of thyroxine in nonthyroidal illness. J Clin Endocrinol Metab 57:15–18, 1983.

34. Slag MF, Morley JE, Elson MK, et al: Hypothyroxinemia in critically ill patients as a predictor of high mortality. JAMA 245:43–45, 1981.

35. Kaptein EM, Weiner JM, Robinson WJ, et al: Relationship of altered thyroid hormone indices to survival in nonthyroidal illness. Clin Endocrinol 16:565–579, 1982.

36. Gardner DR, Kaplan MM, Stanley CA, Utiger RD: Effect of triiodothyronine replacement on the metabolic and pituitary responses to starvation. N Engl J Med 300:579–584, 1979.

37. Burman KD, Wartofsky L, Dinterman RE, et al: The effect of T_3 and reverse T_3 administration on muscle protein catabolism during fasting as measured by 3-methylhistidine excretion. Metabolism 28:805–813, 1979.

38. Vagenakis AG, Portnoy GI, O'Brian JT, et al: Effect of starvation on the production and metabolism of thyroxine and triiodothyronine in euthyroid obese subjects. J Clin Endocrinol Metab 45:1305–1309, 1977.

39. LoPresti J, Spencer CA, Nicoloff JT: Search for a missing deiodinative metabolite of T_4 in fasting man. Annual Meeting of the Endocrine Society 745, Atlanta, GA, June 20–23, 1990.

40. LoPresti JS, Dlott RS: Augmented conversion of T_3 to triac (T_3AC) is the major regulator of the low T_3 state in fasting man. Am Thyroid Assoc, Rochester, MN, Sept. 23–26, 1992.

41. LoPresti JS, Dlott R, VanderVelden D, Nicoloff JT: Triac's role in the production of the low T_3 state of fasting in man. AFCR 239A, 1993.

42. Sciba PC, Bauer M, Emmert D, et al: Effect of obesity, total fasting and re-alimentation on L-thyroxine (T_4), 3,5,3'-triiodothyronine (T_3), 3,3',5'-triiodothyronine (rT_3), thyroxine binding globulin (TBG), cortisol, thyrotropin, cortisol binding globulin (CBG), transferrin, α^2-haptoglobin and complement C3 in serum. Acta Endocrinol (Copenh) 91:629–643, 1979.

43. Eisenstein Z, Haag S, Vagenakis AG, et al: Effect of starvation on the production and peripheral metabolism of 3,3',5'-triiodothyronine in euthyroid obese subjects. J Clin Endocrinol Metab 47:889–893, 1978.

44. LoPresti JS, Gray D, Nicoloff JT: Influence of fasting and refeeding on 3,3',5'-triiodothyronine metabolism in man. J Clin Endocrinol Metab 72:130–136, 1991.

45. LoPresti JS, Eigen A, Kaptein E, et al: Alterations in 3,3',5'-triiodothyronine metabolism in response to propylthiouracil, dexamethasone, and thyroxine administration in man. J Clin Invest 84:1650–1656, 1989.

46. Visser TJ, Kaptein E, Terpstra OT, Krenning EP: Deiodination of thyroid hormone by human liver. J Clin Endocrinol Metab 67:17–24, 1988.

47. Faber J, Faber OK, Lund B, et al: Hepatic extraction and renal production of 3,3'-diiodothyronine in man. J Clin Invest 66:941–945, 1980.

48. Oppenheimer JH, Schwartz HL, Mariash CN, et al: Advances in our understanding of thyroid hormone action at the cellular level. Endocr Rev 8:288–308, 1987.

49. Danforth E Jr, Horton ES, O'Connell M, et al: Dietary-induced alterations in thyroid hormone metabolism during overnutrition. J Clin Invest 64:1336–1347, 1979.

50. Fisler JS, Kaptein EM, Drinick EJ, et al: Metabolic and hormonal factors as predictors of nitrogen retention in obese men consuming very low calorie diets. Metabolism 34:101–105, 1985.

51. Brabant G, Brabant A, Ranft U, et al: Circadian and pulsatile thyrotropin secretion in euthyroid man under the influence of thyroid hormone and glucocorticoid administration. J Clin Endocrinol Metab 65:83–88, 1987.

52. LoPresti JS, Dlott RS, Nicoloff JT: Dexamethasone (DEX): an important in vivo regulator of triac (TA_3) production in man. Am Thyroid Assoc 76, Boston, MA, Sept 12–15, 1991.

53. Zipser RD, Davenport MW, Martin KL, et al: Hyperreninemic hypoaldosteronism in the critically ill: A new entity. J Clin Endocrinol Metab 53:867–873, 1981.

54. Phillips RH, Valente WA, Caplan ES, et al: Circulating thyroid hormone changes in acute trauma: Prognostic implications for clinical outcome. J Trauma 24:116–119, 1984.

55. Hamblin PS, Dyer SA, Mohr VS, et al: Relationship between thyrotropin and thyroxine changes during recovery from severe hypothyroxinemia of critical illness. J Clin Endocrinol Metab 62:717–722, 1986.

56. Worstman J, Premachandra BN, Chopra IJ, Murphy JE: Hypothyroxinemia in cardiac arrest. Arch Intern Med 147:245–248, 1987.

57. Pang X-P, Hershman JM, Mirell CJ, Pekary EA: Impairment of hypothalamic-pituitary-thyroid function in rats treated with human recombinant tumor necrosis factor-α (cachectin). Endocrinology 125:76–84, 1989.

58. Kaptein EM, Spencer CA, Kamiel MB, Nicoloff JT: Prolonged dopamine administration and thyroid hormone economy in normal and critically ill patients. J Clin Endocrinol Metab 51:387–393, 1980.

59. LoPresti JS, Nicoloff JT: 3,5,3'-triiodothyronine sulfate: A major metabolite in 3,5,3'-triiodothyronine metabolism in man. J Clin Endocrinol Metab 1993 (submitted).

60. Chopra IJ, Teco GN, Mead JF, et al: Relationship between serum free fatty acids and thyroid hormone binding inhibitor in nonthyroid illnesses. J Clin Endocrinol Metab 60:980–984, 1985.

61. Chopra IJ, Huang TS, Beredo A, et al: Evidence for an inhibitor of extrathyroidal conversion of thyroxine to 3,5,3'-triiodothyronine in serum of patients with nonthyroidal illnesses. J Clin Endocrinol Metab 60:666–672, 1985.

62. Huang TS, Hurd RE, Chopra IJ, et al: Inhibition of phagocytosis and chemiluminescence in human leukocytes by a lipid soluble factor in normal tissues. Infect Immun 46:544–550, 1984.

63. Young WF, Gorman CA, Weinshilboum RM: Triiodothyronine: A substrate for thermostabile and thermolabile forms of human phenol sulfotransferase. Endocrinology 122:1816–1824, 1988.

64. Spaulding SW, Smith TJ, Hinkle PM, et al: Studies on the biological activity of triiodothyronine sulfate. J Clin Endocrinol Metab 74:1062–1067, 1992.

65. LoPresti JS, Mizuno L, Nimalysuria A, et al: Characteristics of 3,5,3'-triiodothyronine sulfate metabolism in euthyroid man. J Clin Endocrinol Metab 73:703–709, 1991.

66. Fishman N, Huang YP, Tergis DC, Rivlin RS: Relation of triiodothyronine and reverse triiodothyronine administration in rats on hepatic L-triiodothyronine aminotransferase activity. Endocrinology 100:1055–1059, 1977.

67. Lerman J: Dissociation of response of triiodothyroacetic acid in myxedema: comparison with response to thyroid substance. J Clin Endocrinol Metab 21:1044–1051, 1961.

68. Medeiras-Neto G, Kallas WG, Knabel M, et al: Triac (3,5,3'-triiodothyroacetic acid) partially inhibits the thyrotropin response to synthetic thyrotropin-releasing hormone in normal and thyroidectomized hypothyroid patients. J Clin Endocrinol Metab 50:223–225, 1980.

69. Gavin LA, Livermore BA, Cavalieri RR, et al: Serum concentration, metabolic clearance, and production rates of 3,5,3'-triiodothyroacetic acid in normal and athyreotic man. J Clin Endocrinol Metab 51:529–534, 1980.

70. Menegay C, Juge C, Burger AG: Pharmacokinetics of 3,5,3'-triiodothyroacetic acid and its effects on serum TSH levels. Acta Endocrinologica 121:651–658, 1989.

71. Dlott RS, Nicoloff JT, LoPresti JS: Does triiodothyroacetic acid (T_3AC) formation mediate the low T_3 state (LT_3S) in man? Annual Meeting of the Endocrine Society 338, San Antonio, TX, June 24–27, 1992.

72. Samuels HH, Stanley F, Cassanova J: Relationship of receptor affinity to the modulation of thyroid hormone nuclear receptor levels and growth hormone synthesis by L-triodothyronine and iodothyronine analogues in cultured growth hormone 1 cells. J Clin Invest 63:1229–1240, 1979.

73. Lazar MA, Chin WW: Nuclear thyroid hormone receptors. J Clin Invest 86:1777–1782, 1990.

74. Schussler GC, Schaffner F, Karn F: Increased serum thyroid hormone binding and decreased free hormone in chronic active liver disease. N Engl J Med 299:510–515, 1978.

75. Yamanaka T, Ido K, Kumura K, Saito T: Serum levels of thyroid hormones in liver disease. Clin Chim Acta 101:45–55, 1980.

76. Herrick AL, McColl KEL, Michael Wallace A, et al: Elevation of hormone binding globulins in acute intermittent porphyria. Clin Chim Acta 187:141–148, 1990.

77. Walfish PG, Orrego H, Israel Y, et al: Serum triiodothyronine and other clinical and laboratory indices of alcoholic liver disease. Ann Intern Med 91:13–16, 1979.

78. Chopra IJ, Solomon DH, Chopra U, et al: Alterations in circulating thyroid hormones and thyrotropin in hepatic cirrhosis: evidence for euthyroidism despite subnormal serum triiodothyronine. J Clin Endocrinol Metab 39:501–511, 1974.

79. Kaptein EM, Massry SG, Quion-Verde H, et al: Serum thyroid hormone indexes in patients with primary hyperparathyroidism. Arch Int Med 1448:313–315, 1984.

80. Feinstein EI, Kaptein EM, Nicoloff JT, Massry SG: Thyroid function in patients with nephrotic syndrome and normal renal function. Am J Nephrol 2:70–76, 1982.

81. Soffer E, Pelet D, Segal S, Bar-Khayim Y: Thyroid function in hemodialysis. Israel J Med Sci 15:836–839, 1979.

82. LoPresti JS, Fried JC, Spencer CA, Nicoloff JT: Unique alterations of thyroid hormone indices in the acquired immunodeficiency syndrome (AIDS). Ann Intern Med 110:970–975, 1989.

83. Fried JC, LoPresti JS, Micon M, et al: Serum triiodothyronine values. Prognostic indicators of acute mortality due to pneumocystis carinii pneumonia associated with acquired immunodeficiency syndrome. Arch Intern Med 150:406–409, 1990.

84. Goodwin TM, Montoro M, Mestman JH, et al: The role of chorionic gonadotropin in transient hyperthyroidism of hyperemesis gravidarum. J Clin Endocrinol Metab 75:1333–1337, 1992.

85. Osathanondh R, Chopra IJ, Tulchinsky D: Effects of dexamethasone on fetal and maternal thyroxine, triiodothyronine, and reverse triiodothyronine and thyrotropin levels. J Clin Endocrinol Metab 47:1236–1239, 1978.

86. Spratt DI, Pont A, Miller MB, et al: Hyperthyroxinemia in patients with acute psychiatric disorders. Am J Med 73:41–48, 1982.

87. Hein MD, Jackson IM: Review: Thyroid function in psychiatric illness. General Hospital Psychiatry 12:232–244, 1990.

88. Kabadi UM, Rosman PM: Thyroid hormone indices in adult healthy subjects: no influence of aging. J Am Geriat Soc 36:312–316, 1988.

89. Lewis GF, Alessi CA, Imperial JG, Refetoff S: Low serum free thyroxine index in ambulating elderly is due to a resetting of the threshold of thyrotropin feedback suppression. J Clin Endocrinol Metab 73:843–849, 1991.

90. Grunfeld C, Sherman BM, Cavalieri RR: The acute effects of growth hormone administration on thyroid function in normal man. J Clin Endocrinol Metab 67:1111–1114, 1988.

41

Hyperthyroidism

J. MAXWELL McKENZIE
MARGITA ZAKARIJA

DEFINITIONS

There are various types of hyperthyroidism, although only two are common. Before dealing at length with those, i.e., Graves' disease and toxic adenoma, we shall outline the rarer syndromes, most of which have been reviewed recently as "unusual types of thyrotoxicosis."[1]

THYROTOXICOSIS FACTITIA. In this syndrome the patient may chronically ingest an excess of thyroid hormone (knowingly or because of its presence in a weight-reduction preparation) in a deliberate attempt to control obesity or a physician may wish to suppress thyrotropin unequivocally in instances of thyroid carcinoma. Neurotic impulses may underlie self-administration of excess hormone, the resulting illness serving to command needed attention of physicians, family, or associates. Occasionally a patient is inadvertently rendered hyperthyroid by a physician whose prescription is wrongly followed or who errs in an attempt to "treat" a laboratory test result. An example of this mistake occurs when T_3 is given in increasing dosage to "correct" a low or low-normal serum T_4 concentration. As thyroid function is progressively suppressed, the serum T_4 value falls lower, leading to more T_3 being prescribed; eventually thyrotoxicosis factitia ensues.

In 1985 the number of prescriptions for thyroid hormone preparations filled in the United States was estimated to be over 18 million.[2] The potential for accidental ingestion of excess thyroid hormone—especially by children—must be considerable. Indeed, in an earlier report,[3] ingestion of a thyroid hormone preparation was found to be the third most common cause of acute accidental poisoning in children, surpassed only by aspirin and laxatives. As reviewed by Cohen et al.,[4] the clinical course in children may be surprisingly benign.

As a result of exemplary clinical investigative effort—truly classified as fine medical detective work—an epidemic of hyperthyroidism in several communities in the midwestern United States was shown to be a form of thyrotoxicosis factitia.[5, 6]

It was established by painstaking epidemiological review that the "epidemic" was directly related to the practice in a few meat-processing plants of including bovine neck muscles in the meat destined to be hamburger patties; this was heavily contaminated with thyroid tissue. One calculation was that an average quarter-pound hamburger could provide as much as 1300 μg T_4 and 76 μg T_3. The appropriate regulations having been established, there ought to be no further outbreak of this variety of thyrotoxicosis factitia, at least in the United States.

FUNCTIONING METASTATIC THYROID CARCINOMA. This rare disease, first reported in 1946,[7] probably produces hyperthyroidism when the mass of tissue, of low inherent hormone-producing capacity, is sufficiently great to provide an excess of thyroid hormones. There have been only about 30 reported cases of this syndrome.[8–10] A unique circumstance—hyperthyroidism associated with anaplastic thyroid carcinoma—was reported in 1983[11]; this was seen as reflecting tissue necrosis, akin to hyperthyroidism in subacute thyroiditis, since the carcinomatous lesion was nonfunctioning with regard to thyroid hormone synthesis. No similar clinical report has appeared in the intervening 10 years.

HYPERTHYROIDISM DUE TO MOLAR THYROTROPIN. Synthesis and release of thyrotropin by nonendocrine malignant tumors, such as bronchial carcinoma, has not yet been unequivocally reported as a cause of hyperthyroidism, although extraction of thyrotropic activity from adenocarcinoma of the bronchus has been described.[12] However, placental extracts were found to contain two thyrotropic activities, human placental thyrotropin and molar thyrotropin[13]; the latter is the substance also found in high concentration in hydatidiform mole and choriocarcinoma. While the biological significance of placental thyrotropin is uncertain, and its existence was subsequently related by the original investigators to probable assay artifacts,[14] it is clear that some instances of hyperthyroidism have occurred as a result of secretion of molar thyrotropin from hydatidiform mole,[15] choriocarcinoma,[16] and even testicular embryonal

676

carcinoma.[17] Cure of the hyperthyroidism has been effected by removal of the trophoblastic tumor. Molar thyrotropin is probably identical to human chorionic gonadotropin (hCG),[16] although doubt was raised in view of the findings that more-purified hCG was less thyrotropic than a cruder preparation.[18] Additional data,[19] acquired in studies with serum from normal pregnant women, provided mixed support for hCG as a thyroid stimulator; in early pregnancy there was a good correlation between concentrations of hCG and in vitro thyroid stimulation by the patients' sera but there was evidence for the continued presence of a thyroid stimulator in the third term of the pregnancy when hCG was in much lower titer. Arguments in favor of hCG being a thyroid stimulator were recently reviewed,[20] and the expectation was expressed that the recent cloning of both the TSH and LH receptors will settle the uncertainty. In fact, in a publication a few weeks later,[21] evidence was presented for direct binding of purified hCG to recombinant human TSH receptor in transfected Chinese hamster ovary cells; increased cAMP release in a concentration-related manner was documented. The concept that hCG is a (weak) thyroid stimulator would seem to be validated. It has been suggested that hCG may also produce the elevated T_4 and T_3 levels and suppressed TSH seen in many patients with hyperemesis gravidarum.

INAPPROPRIATE SECRETION OF THYROTROPIN. Two major categories of the disorder that shows as inappropriate secretion of TSH have been recognized: the first involves resistance to thyroid hormone (either generalized or restricted to the pituitary) and the second involves a pituitary adenoma that is autonomously secreting TSH. In a massive review in 1993[22] Refetoff and colleagues analyzed data on 347 subjects with resistance. They also summarized 156 reported instances of TSH-secreting pituitary adenoma. Some clinical aspects of these two categories of abnormalities follow (see Ch. 37).

(1) TSH-producing tumor of the anterior hypophysis: these patients have been identified as secreting abnormally only TSH or TSH in conjunction with growth hormone (leading to associated acromegaly), prolactin (usually with galactorrhea), or LH and/or FSH.[22]

(2) Non-neoplastic pituitary resistance to the feedback effect of thyroid hormone; this may be part of generalized (including pituitary) resistance to thyroid hormone, but in these patients a euthyroid or hypothyroid state exists. If only the pituitary shows resistance to thyroid hormone, TSH is secreted in supranormal concentrations and thus hyperthyroidism ensues.

There is increasing evidence that separate categorization of pituitary and generalized resistance may be somewhat artificial, and they may represent ends of a spectrum of thyroid hormone resistance that reflects variable organ distribution of the disorder. The thyroid hormone receptors (TR) have been cloned and shown to exist in four forms, viz., TRα-1, TRα-2, TRβ-1, and TRβ-2 (see Chapter 37 for details). These show differential tissue expression and regulation, and resistance occurs as a mutation that may involve only one nucleotide in the relevant gene, usually in the T_3-binding domain of the receptor. There is no single mutation common to all subjects who inherit this syndrome. This area of knowledge is rapidly expanding and application to treatment will inevitably follow.

Characteristically, in instances of tumor, there is both resistance of TSH secretion to the administration of thy-

roid hormone, even in excess, and little or no response of TSH to the injection of thyrotropin-releasing hormone. In the non-neoplastic syndromes, on the other hand, most reports have shown TSH hypersecretion to be at least partially responsive to normal stimulatory and inhibitory factors. A major diagnostic distinction between tumorous and nontumorous syndromes is the fact that in the former category, there has been, in most (88 per cent) patients, disproportionately increased secretion of α-subunit with an α-to-TSH molar ratio higher than 1; in the latter (non-neoplastic) state, TSH and the free α-subunit are increased proportionately, with a ratio of less than 1.

Therapeutically there are also major differences. For a TSH-secreting tumor, removal of the lesion by the transsphenoidal route has been successfully accomplished[23]; pituitary irradiation has also been attempted with limited success.[23] On the other hand, pharmacological manipulation appears to be the major hope for therapy of the pituitary-resistant states (TSH secretion may be suppressed by administration of excessive amounts of thyroid hormone in some of these patients,[24] but this is obviously not appropriate as treatment of hyperthyroidism.) Glucocorticoid has been shown to suppress the abnormal secretion,[24, 25] but this is also unacceptable as long-term therapy. TRIAC (3,5,3'-triiodothyroacetic acid), in a dosage of 3 mg per day, has been reported to result in TSH, T_4, and T_3 all reverting to a normal level without evidence of hypermetabolism occurring from the drug itself.[26] A similar outcome was reported with dextrothyroxine (DT_4).[25] These interesting findings must be confirmed by others. Meanwhile the most frequently reported successful agents are the dopamine agonist bromocriptine[24] and the long-acting somatostatin analogue octreotide.[27] A direct comparison, in a patient with pituitary resistance to thyroid hormone, of the efficacy of TRIAC with that of bromocriptine was recently reported.[28] In that assessment the results favored bromocriptine as the superior therapeutic agent. Obviously, however, the optimal regimen for these and the other potential medications and the long-term benefits or hazards still have to be defined.[29] The two medications have also been shown to have suppressive effects on TSH-producing tumors in instances of regrowth after resection or when surgery as initial therapy was declined[27]; clearly their role in the therapy of pituitary adenomas will be an evaluation of interest to many.

STRUMA OVARII. This rare syndrome has been well reviewed.[30] It comprises differentiated thyroid tissue in an ovarian teratoma. Hyperthyroidism does not always ensue, since this would require a critical minimal mass of tissue to produce enough hormone to result in a hyperthyroid state. Of 25 instances of the syndrome reported from the Mayo Clinic (culled from 40 years of patient records), only eight subjects were hyperthyroid.[30] Radioisotope imaging showed uptake in the pelvis and limited, if any, evidence for active thyroid tissue in the neck.

IODIDE-INDUCED HYPERTHYROIDISM AND SILENT THYROIDITIS. Two varieties of hyperthyroidism that have achieved increasing prominence since the first edition of this text are iodide-induced hyperthyroidism and silent thyroiditis. The former subject was well reviewed in 1983 by Fradkin and Wolff.[31] As they pointed out, three circumstances have recently highlighted the problem. In the last few years numerous case reports have appeared, especially from Germany, describing hyperthyroidism apparently precipitated by the administration of radiocontrast dyes for diagnostic purposes. The advent of amiodarone, 37.2 per cent of which by weight is iodine, as a widely used cardiac medication has also been associated with episodes of hyperthyroidism. There have been proposals to use potassium iodide (KI) prophylactically in the event of nuclear reactor accidents.

Despite the renewed interest in *iodide-induced hyperthyroidism,* this condition is probably quite rare and the underlying mechanism is unclear. In some instances there is adequate reason to accept that the administered iodide merely acts as substrate for formation of excess hormone by an adenoma or Graves' disease gland that was, for whatever reason, ''starved'' of the essential element. However, as eloquently argued by Fradkin and Wolff,[31] there are many reports in which this does not appear to be the case, and a defective autoregulation of hormone biosynthesis may be involved. Nevertheless, considering available data, it appears that iodide-induced hyperthyroidism occurs predominantly in populations with modest to low intake of iodine (therefore excluding most of the United States), and it is usually a self-limited syndrome, even with continued exposure to the increased iodine load.

From 1970 to 1980 many names were given to a syndrome now generally accepted as *silent thyroiditis.*[32] Clinical features include hyperthyroidism, commonly a nontender small goiter, no other components such as ophthalmopathy or pretibial myxedema or relevant family history to suggest Graves' disease, a low or even zero thyroid uptake of radioactive iodine, and spontaneous remission within 3 to 6 months; most of the reported instances of this syndrome have occurred in postpartum women.[32a] Although these features, apart from the lack of tenderness of the thyroid, are identical to those of subacute (De Quervain's) thyroiditis (reviewed in Ch. 44) and there has been a tendency to link the conditions pathogenetically, available evidence points to the syndrome having an autoimmune basis. As reviewed by Woolf,[32] thyroid biopsy material (from 23 patients in 6 reports) showed prominent lymphocytic infiltration, both focal and diffuse, occasionally seen as lymphoid follicles. Secondly, circulating antibodies to the thyroid microsomal antigen are not uncommon. A subsequent report[33] confirmed an undue incidence of serum antibodies, there being 70 per cent of 50 patients with antibody to the microsomal antigen in titers >1:400. This study also showed a statistically significant increased frequency of HLA-DR3 in these patients, i.e., 24 of 50 versus 19 of 80 in a control population. Similar data were reported more recently.[33a] HLA-B8 and DR3, with or without A1, were more frequently found in patients. DR3 is the gene product commonly found in patients with autoimmune disorders.

The incidence of silent thyroiditis varied in four reports from 3.6 to 23 per cent of all causes of hyperthyroidism (reviewed in reference 32).

The practical conclusion from this burgeoning recognition of a syndrome that was apparently unknown 25 years ago is that all patients with hyperthyroidism who have a small or nonsignificant goiter and no other features of Graves' disease should have measurement of the thyroid uptake of radioiodine so as to confirm or exclude a diagnosis of silent thyroiditis. The subject is more extensively reviewed in Chapter 43.

Histological features of thyroiditis, termed *multifocal*

granulomatous folliculitis, have been described as a consequence of manual palpation of the thyroid gland.[34] Perhaps akin to that phenomenon are two recent reports of transient mild hyperthyroidism, with suppressed TSH and low radioiodine uptake by the thyroid, following aspiration of a thyroid cyst in six patients[35] and after parathyroidectomy in three subjects.[36] In both sets of observations, the hyperthyroidism was mild, developed within a few days of the putative insult, and remitted spontaneously within two[35] to eight[36] weeks. It seems reasonable that the physical trauma, in ways undefined, precipitated evanescent inflammatory reactions in the thyroid in these subjects, making this syndrome an unintended model of subacute thyroiditis.

In some texts the syndrome of hyperthyroidism associated with Hashimoto's disease is given the status of a distinct entity: ''Hashitoxicosis.'' As indicated below, in our opinion this is simply a variant of Graves' disease and need not be separately identified.

To turn from the rarities (although silent thyroiditis apparently is not rare in some centers), one must still clearly distinguish two varieties of hyperthyroidism—that caused by single or multiple hyperfunctioning adenoma of the thyroid and that resulting from Graves' disease. The former may be viewed as benign neoplasia associated with excess secretion of thyroid hormone; the disease is thus a strictly localized entity, although with whole-body consequences resulting from the excess thyroid hormone.

On the other hand, Graves' disease is a syndrome that has a variable expression. The full-blown presentation includes goiter with hyperthyroidism, exophthalmos with or without inflammation of periorbital and bulbar tissues, pretibial myxedema (which may be better termed dermopathy,[37] since it is often not pretibial), and, least common, acropachy (see Fig. 41–5). Any or even all of these features may be absent in an individual situation, since Graves' disease is truly a ''constitutional disorder,''[38] reflecting disturbances of autoimmune mechanisms not yet clearly identified. However, on a practical level, the presence of any of these features may merit the diagnosis, and by far the most common is *hyperthyroidism.* This is usually associated with goiter, although one study, based upon ultrasonic measurement of the thyroid gland, found 21 out of 90 consecutive Graves' disease patients had a normal volume of tissue.[39] Notwithstanding, the characteristic of the thyroid is that, microscopically, it shows diffuse hyperplasia, and on scanning with radioiodine, there is generalized hyperfunction. Neither of these features excludes the possible presence of nodules, functioning or not, in the midst of otherwise more uniform tissue, and such incidental nodules become common in the over-40 age group.

Some would subscribe to a third major category within the common varieties of hyperthyroidism, i.e., toxic multinodular goiter, especially as seen in the elderly. There appears, however, to be no justification for this if one salient fact is recognized: either an adenomatous process or Graves' disease, both resulting in hyperthyroidism, may develop in patients with preceding nodularity of the thyroid gland. Considering the increasing frequency with age of incidental nodularity of the thyroid, it would be surprising if this were not the case. As shown in studies of an endemic goiter population,[40] the multinodular gland of a hyperthyroid patient may have function in paranodular tissue (and variably in the nodules). The patient may adequately fulfill criteria for a diagnosis of Graves' disease or have the function largely confined to one or more identifiable nodules and thus be classified as having toxic adenoma or adenomata. Similar conclusions have been reached in other extensive series. Consequently, although various texts classify toxic multinodular goiter as a separate clinical entity, we fail to see the rationale, either from clinical presentation or considerations of pathogenesis, and prefer to offer only two major categories of hyperthyroidism, i.e., those associated with adenomatous processes and Graves' disease.

INCIDENCE

Exploiting an epidemiological program of unusual extent, investigators at the Mayo Clinic established the incidence of Graves' disease in Rochester, Minnesota, and its neighboring county for the years 1935 to 1967.[41] They found that 36.8 females and 8.3 males per 100,000 of the female and male population developed Graves' disease annually during that period; this is equivalent to about 23 per 100,000 overall population, and it established a sex ratio of 4 to 5:1 (females/males).

Subsequent studies from Britain and Scandinavia regarding hyperthyroidism (not specifically Graves' disease) have provided comparable figures. Tunbridge et al. in England found a prevalence of 1.9 per cent for females and 0.16 per cent for males with an annual incidence rate for females of 2 to 3 per 1000[42]; these figures are approximately 10 times higher than those from the United States.[41] The difference presumably is partly related to the fact that the English study assessed a total population (i.e., 2779 people or 82.4 per cent of the population available) and the United States one was hospital-based. However, another population-based British study established a prevalence, for the year 1982, of 35.5 per 100,000 women and 9.2 per 100,000 men,[43] figures remarkably similar to those from the United States.[41] From 1972 to 1974 annual incidence rates per 100,000 persons in a region of Denmark were 46.5 for women and 8.7 for men[44]; an interesting extrapolation from this study was that the lifetime risk of developing hyperthyroidism was 5 per cent for women and 1 per cent for men and that the prevalence of existing and previously diagnosed hyperthyroidism at the time of the analysis was 1.4 and 0.3 per cent, respectively. Screening a Swedish female population age 26 to 72 years, there was an incidence of hyperthyroidism of 1 to 3 cases/year per 1000 women,[44a] similar to the British[42] and Danish experiences.[44]

Although one may find significant differences among these, and other, sets of epidemiological data, it is clear that hyperthyroidism is a not uncommon disease. Some of the studies addressed the question of the age-specific incidence of the disease. For hyperthyroidism, i.e., not specifically Graves' disease, both the British[43] and Danish[44] observations indicated that the greatest incidence was in the geriatric population, with the former report[43] also showing a striking earlier, slightly lower, peak in the 50 to 64 age group. The data from the Mayo Clinic,[41] dealing solely with Graves' disease, indicated that in women the rate was 59 per 100,000 at age 20 to 30 years and only 38 per 100,000 in the 60 and older population.

The relative incidence of adenomatous hyperthyroidism and Graves' disease varies geographically, although precise assessment of this is complicated by differing diagnostic criteria. In Britain 5 per cent of the hyperthyroid patients may have toxic adenoma,[45] whereas in Austria 46 per cent of patients were given this diagnosis.[46] A careful study encompassing experience in both Hamburg and Zurich gave figures of 30 per cent for the proportion of adenomatous goiters producing hyperthyroidism, and 75 per cent of these patients had a single toxic adenoma.[47] For the United States, figures have varied from 31 per cent[48] to 86 per cent[49] for the incidence of "toxic nodular goiter" but, again, the criteria for diagnosis seem to vary. A problem with figures coming out of the studies in North America is always the proportion of immigrants included in a given population, especially that proportion attending a hospital clinic, and the geographic areas from which they have come, quite apart from the viewpoint of the clinicians regarding the concept of Graves' disease occurring in a gland that harbors nodules. It is therefore of particular interest that in a retrospective study of patients with hyperthyroidism seen in two clinics, one in Cardiff, Wales, and the other in Toronto, Canada, the incidence of Graves' disease was approximately the same, viz., 70 per cent; "toxic multinodular goiter" and toxic adenoma occurred more frequently in Cardiff (25 versus 8 per cent), whereas thyroiditis predominated in Toronto (17 versus 1 per cent).[50]

TOXIC ADENOMA

Pathogenesis

Understanding of toxic adenoma is the understanding of benign neoplasia, so it is obvious that in discussing pathogenesis, little definitive data may be offered, although studies of the possible involvement of oncogenes are increasingly reported.[51] Recently, it has been recognized that mutations in G proteins (Gs and Gi) can render them oncogenic, and activating somatic point mutations have been found in certain endocrine tumors, including mutations in Gs in toxic adenomas (reviewed in ref. 51a). The importance of cAMP generation for thyroid growth and function has been shown in an elegant study with transgenic mice.[52] The thyroid expression of a canine A_2 adenosine receptor, which activates adenylyl cyclase through the G_s protein, led to uncontrolled growth of the gland and severe hyperthyroidism. Surprisingly, the latest report by Selzer et al.[52a] identified constitutive TSH-independent expression of the adenylyl cyclase inhibitory $Gi\alpha$-1 in toxic adenomas. The authors speculated that this may lead to autonomous growth of thyroid cells "by a yet unidentified signaling pathway."[52a] Associated with these developments is recognition that many of the human functioning neoplasms are monoclonal.[53] Obviously, pathogenesis of this disorder remains uncertain, but it is slowly being clarified.

A gradual transition from inordinate (in comparison with neighboring thyroid tissue) sensitivity to thyrotropin to autonomous function has been hypothesized but remains a largely descriptive concept. It has been suggested that an adenoma has to be of a minimum size before it will produce enough hormone for hyperthyroidism to develop, which is a hypothesis that seems reasonable but has still to be proved.

Natural History

Not infrequently, a functioning adenoma of the thyroid that does not produce hyperthyroidism may be recognized. This has been referred to as a "warm" (distinct from "hot") nodule or a "compensated" (distinct from "decompensated") adenoma. The requirements for these designations are a more-or-less uniform radioiodine scan, including the nodule under consideration, and nonsuppression of function of the nodule by administration of thyroid hormone that suppresses thyroid-stimulating hormone (TSH) and thus the paranodular tissue. The interpretation of such findings is that the autonomous hormone output of the adenoma is not enough to suppress thyrotropin nor, as would be therefore expected, to produce hyperthyroidism. It is a simple concept that a warm nodule is the forerunner of a toxic adenoma, and this is probably true. There are, however, few reports of prolonged observations on patients with a warm nodule confirming the progression to true toxic adenoma; a study by Silverstein et al.[54] in fact failed to produce such evidence, but the concept appears so rational that more evidence would be required to refute it fully. Indeed, from a longitudinal study of 58 patients with compensated adenoma, it was concluded that the rate of decompensation, i.e., development of clinical thyrotoxicosis, was 4.1 per cent/year; there was an associated average increase in adenoma size of about 50 per cent.[55]

There is a possibility that a toxic adenoma may "self-ablate" by infarction or cyst formation as has been shown in at least one report.[56] To wait for such an uncertain event clearly cannot be recommended as a therapeutic modality.

Clinical Features

If the clinical features of hyperthyroidism due to toxic adenoma are compared with those due to Graves' disease, many points of difference are discernible. These include, in adenomatous disease, the typically slower rate of recognition of symptoms, the older age group affected (especially in multinodular disease), and the more common predominance of cardiac symptoms. However, the only clinical aspect that clearly differentiates one from the other is the presence of ophthalmopathy, pretibial myxedema, or acropachy in patients with Graves' disease. Otherwise, the Graves' disease subject who is less-than-average hyperkinetic may be indistinguishable from the patient with toxic adenoma, and the correct diagnosis rests upon the character of the goiter, both on physical examination and on imaging. When there is a single toxic adenoma, paranodular tissue and the contralateral lobe are functionally suppressed and usually are minimally, if at all, palpable. If the adenoma has developed in a multinodular goiter or if there are multiple adenomata, the clinical character of the goiter may be no different from that of the diffuse hyperplasia of Graves' disease being superimposed on preceding irregular enlargement. The diagnosis then rests upon a thyroid scan with ancillary tests, as described below.

If there is a family history of Hashimoto's or Graves' disease, extrathyroid features typical of Graves' disease, or thyroid antibodies in the blood, toxic adenoma becomes very unlikely and, if present, represents a most unusual coincidence of anomalies. Two such patients have been seen by us; in one, typical unilateral exophthalmos of Graves' disease, settling with time and conservative management, was associated with a toxic adenoma of the thyroid, proved by successful surgical excision of the adenoma. In the other patient, hyperthyroidism due to a toxic adenoma was treated adequately with radioiodine, and then ophthalmopathy, indistinguishable from that of Graves' disease, developed bilaterally and required treatment with corticosteroids. To re-emphasize the fact, however, the coincidence of these two diseases is rare.

Diagnosis

The diagnosis is suggested by thyroid scanning after administration of radioiodine or pertechnetate, giving the characteristic appearance as shown in Figure 41–1A. A similar appearance may be given by a gland in which the contralateral lobe does not take up radioiodine due to disease, congenital absence, or surgical ablation. In a patient who is clinically hyperthyroid, there is little need for a suppression test (Fig. 41–1A), but when the diagnosis is in doubt, this can be a useful procedure (i.e., repeating the uptake and scan measurements after 10 days of administration of triiodothyronine, 25 μg four times per day), since the scan of a nontoxic nodular goiter may appear very similar (Fig. 41–2); all functioning tissue should be suppressed in the case of the latter diagnosis (Fig. 41–2). More important usually, and commonly sufficient to confirm the diagnosis, is a repeat uptake and scan after administration of thyrotropin. Although one injection (5 to 10 U) may be sufficient, unequivocal evidence of the presence of stimulable (i.e., normal but suppressed) para-adenoma tissue ought to be obtained with injections of 5 to 10 U thyrotropin IM every day for three days. Radioiodine may be given 18 hours after the last injection and the uptake and scan obtained 24 hours later. A typical result with this procedure is shown in Figure 41–1A. Figure 41–3 illustrates that a similar sequence of investigation can confirm the diagnosis of multiple toxic adenomata. This test is also rarely needed.

It is not uncommon to find a patient with a confirmed hot nodule apparently asymptomatic and with normal results for a 24-hour radioiodine uptake and serum T_4 concentration. The fact that the adenoma secretes sufficient thyroid hormone to suppress release of thyrotropin is tantamount to there being a supraphysiological rate of secretion of thyroid hormone, i.e., there is hyperthyroidism. This conclusion may be supported by measurement of the serum T_3 concentration, which is usually mildly increased in these instances of "subclinical" hyperthyroidism. In our experience, ablation of the adenoma and subsequent return of the thyroid to normal function may lead to identification of previous symptoms recognized only on their disappearance.

Treatment

Although the hyperthyroidism of toxic adenoma may be controlled by antithyroid drugs, it would be irrational to consider this as definitive therapy. There is no evidence

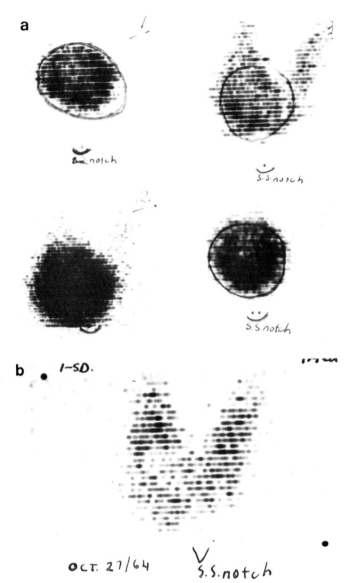

in a Graves' disease gland, may be given to effect a "one-dose cure"; because of possible relative radioresistance this means at least 1000 rads and repeated treatments with ¹³¹I may be required if these considerations are not acknowledged by the therapist in calculating the initial dose.

It has generally been accepted that development of hypothyroidism after ¹³¹I ablation of a toxic adenoma is unlikely. One report puts this conclusion in doubt.[57] Of 23 patients with autonomous adenoma (i.e., all with "hot" nodules but only 7 considered clinically to be hyperthyroid) who were evaluated 4 to 16.5 years after treatment with ¹³¹I, 8 (36 per cent) had become hypothyroid. Of the 7 hyperthyroid subjects, 2 (29 per cent) became hypothyroid. The length of time (mean 8.5 years) elapsing between treatment and evaluation is greater than described by others, and this no doubt should be kept in mind by those treating patients in this way. On the other hand, another group[58] used a standard dose of 20 mCi of ¹³¹I in 52 patients with toxic adenoma and found, with a follow-up period of 4 to 17.5 years, that hyperthyroidism recurred in 1 patient and hypothyroidism developed in only 3.

Individuals with coincident heart disease and toxic adenomata may have an exacerbation of the cardiac problem if radioactive ¹³¹I therapy causes temporary elevation of circulating thyroid hormones. To prevent this, such patients may be treated by multiple small doses of radioactive ¹³¹I given at 3- to 6-month intervals or by a conventional dose given after the hormone content of the adenoma has been depleted by antithyroid drug administration.

Because of the age of the patient or for individual preference, a decision may be made for surgical treatment. For a single adenoma, the mortality and morbidity to be expected from excision of the lesion by an experienced surgeon are negligible. The eventual postoperative development of hypothyroidism is a consideration certainly no more likely with surgery than with radioiodine therapy and may be even less in view of the aforementioned data.[57] When there are multiple adenomata, a subtotal thyroidectomy may be indicated; the operative problems will be greater, but the outcome is likely to be satisfactory. Naturally, hypothyroidism may be expected if too little normal tissue is left, but many recommend permanent postoperative treatment with thyroxine on the thought that this will prevent compensatory growth of remaining tissue.

FIGURE 41–1. *A,* **Radioiodine (¹³¹I) scans of the thyroid of patient with toxic adenoma.** Top left, activity is localized to the area of the palpable nodule. Bottom left, repeat scan after one injection of 10 U thyrotropin, and top right, after injections of 10 U thyrotropin daily for each of three days, showing evidence of responsive para-adenoma tissue in both right and left lobes; bottom right, repeat scan after administration of triiodothyronine, 100 μg per day for 10 days, establishing nonsuppression of the adenoma function. *B,* **Radioiodine scan of thyroid of the same patient 18 months after treatment with 25 mCi ¹³¹I;** the area of the former toxic adenoma now shows as "cold" nodule and the remaining thyroid tissue is functioning normally; the patient was euthyroid. (From McKenzie JM: Hyperthyroidism caused by thyroid adenomata. J Clin Endocrinol Metab 26:779, 1966; © by the Endocrine Society.

that drugs such as propylthiouracil exert a direct permanent effect on thyroid function so that in toxic adenoma cessation of therapy inevitably is followed by relapse. Ablation of the neoplasm or neoplasms is the only course to be offered these patients.

When para-adenoma tissue is not completely suppressed or when ablation of a warm nodule is intended, therapy with ¹³¹I may be preceded by a week of administration of triiodothyronine (e.g., 75 to 100 μg/day) to ensure that minimal isotope will be taken up by normal cells. With complete suppression of normal tissue, a dose of ¹³¹I, larger than would be calculated for an equivalent mass of tissue

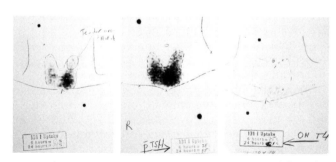

FIGURE 41–2. **Thyroid scans of a patient with nontoxic nodular goiter.** *Left,* Initial scan showing uptake predominantly in a clinically palpable solitary nodule. *Center,* repeat scan after injections of thyrotropin, 10 U daily for each of three days, outlining more functioning thyroid tissue. *Right,* Repeat scan after administration of triiodothyronine, 100 μg/day for 10 days, establishing complete suppression of gland function and confirming the diagnosis of nontoxic nodular goiter.

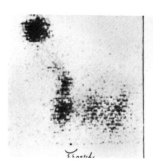
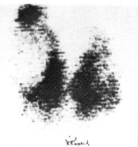
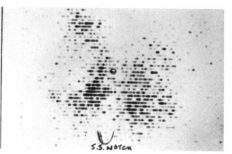

FIGURE 41–3. **Thyroid scans of a patient with multiple toxic adenomata.** Clinically the patient was hyperthyroid and had a large multinodular goiter. The scan shows, from left to right, the initial pattern, the appearance after three injections of thyrotropin, and the final scan after successful treatment with 40 mCi [131]I. (From McKenzie JM: Hyperthyroidism caused by thyroid adenomata. J Clin Endocrinol Metab 26:779, 1966; © by the Endocrine Society.)

Prognosis

Whichever form of ablation is chosen, the expectation is that the para-adenoma tissue, if the patient is not further treated with thyroxine (see above), will become active and maintain the patient in a euthyroid state, at least for several years.[57] The thyroid scan with radioiodine can be used to confirm this, as shown in Figure 41–1*B*. The "cold" area seen in the postradioiodine scan clearly reflects residual scar tissue of the ablated adenoma, but this might lead to subsequent surgery for fear of carcinoma if full details of the earlier procedure are not known to a future diagnostician. An obvious precaution is that patients should be made fully cognizant of their medical management.

The time between ablation of an adenoma and return of the normal tissue to full physiological function is variable. Recent studies have shown that a year or more may elapse before the pituitary thyrotrope is normally responsive to injected thyrotropin-releasing hormone (TRH), and the patient may be symptomatic of hypothyroidism for all or part of that period. However, an early recovery of the thyroid-pituitary axis and little, if any, intervening hypothyroidism is probably the rule.

GRAVES' DISEASE

Etiology

Genetic Factors

A hereditary component of the etiology of Graves' disease has been recognized for many years, with one of the first analyses of the familial incidence of the syndrome being that of Bartels.[59] Currently one may consider four lines of evidence, namely family studies of clinical thyroid disease, the incidence of more subtle abnormalities such as thyroid autoantibodies in blood, the occurrence in family members of other autoimmune but nonthyroid disease, and the frequency in Graves' disease of specific HLA antigens and other genetic markers—all are indicators of the significance of heredity in Graves' disease.

FAMILIAL INCIDENCE OF GRAVES' DISEASE. Isolated examples of families notably affected by what may be accepted as Graves' disease have been on record for almost 100 years. However, Bartels[59] was the first to provide substantial data backing the view that Graves' disease has a significant familial component; subsequent reports resulted in similar

conclusions. For instance, Heimann,[60] studying families in western Sweden (an area that he emphasized was without endemic goiter), found that of 109 patients with "toxic struma" 48 per cent had familial features and 9 per cent had more than 3 goitrous family members. The incidence of goiter in the families of these presumably Graves' disease patients is remarkably close to that found by Bartels, who studied 69 patients' families and noted a history of goiter in 42 per cent. Impressively, in a study that was important by itself and was further distinguished by a "genetical note" added by the doyen of statisticians, R.A. Fisher, the incidence of familial goiter was 40 per cent.[61]

A problem that is obvious in review of these studies—that all took place before the general acceptance of Graves' disease as an autoimmune thyroid disorder—is the matter of definition of Graves' disease and in particular the categorization of thyrotoxic patients with a nodular goiter. Although there are limited diagnostic criteria given in all of these papers, it is probably safe to accept a positive diagnosis of "Graves' disease"[59] and "exophthalmic goiter"[61] under today's definition. It is the meaning in the minds of various authors of "toxic adenoma,"[59] "toxic goiter,"[61] and "toxic struma"[60] that may lead to misinterpretation. Nonetheless the remarkable closeness of the familial incidence data is reassuring and leads to acceptance of a consensus that goiter runs in the families of Graves' disease patients.

The controls for these epidemiological studies were nonhyperthyroid patients with thyroid disorders other than Graves' disease. It is an acknowledged deficiency that the incidence of goiter in families of nongoitrous propositi is not known for the populations under study, and we may presume that this would be less than 40 per cent in a geographic area not recognized for endemic goiter. Regarding the reported "control" data, however, it is impressive that Martin and Fisher[61] found that 47 per cent of their patients with nodular goiter (both toxic and nontoxic) had goiter in the family and Heimann's[60] figure was 41 per cent.

This feature was further analyzed by Martin and Fisher, who showed that, first, patients with exophthalmic goiter tend to have relatives with that disease whereas relatives of patients with (presumably non-Graves') nodular goiter more often were "affected by simple or nondescript goiters."[61] Second, they found that of patients with exophthalmic goiter, the relatives with that disease were predominantly siblings (10 per cent of 160 were affected) rather than parents (0.6 per cent of 180), without the undoubted female preponderance of affected subjects influencing the conclusions. Contrariwise, 8 per cent of mothers and 8 per cent of sisters of nodular goiter patients suffered from a similar disorder. These findings led Fisher to conclude that "there is evidence strongly suggestive of a single recessive factor favorable to the disease (i.e., exophthalmic goiter) and perhaps necessary for its occurrence. . . ."[61]

FAMILIAL INCIDENCE OF THYROID ANTIBODIES IN GRAVES' DISEASE. Since recognition of the importance of autoimmunity in Graves' disease, family studies have concentrated more on measurement of serum antibodies than on clinical expression of the disease. One early careful study[62] showed that both thyroid and gastric parietal cell antibodies occurred with undue frequency in families of thyrotoxic subjects. Specifically they identified, with appropriate age- and sex-matched controls, that both sisters and mothers of the propositi had significantly greater frequencies of antibodies to thyroglubulin and to the microsomal antigen, whereas mothers alone had an undue incidence of antibody to the gastric parietal cell. There are more reports dealing with these aspects of Hashimoto's disease than there are for Graves' disease, but in the latter condition the fact of a familial incidence of antithyroid antibodies, perhaps greater than the frequency of clinical thyroid disease, appears to be entirely acceptable. The precise genetic nature of the inheritance has been subject to some debate. Early, there was a concept that the familial incidence of antibody production might reflect an intrauterine passage of maternal antibody that would in some way sequester antigen at an important time for the immune system to recognize "self." However, this conjecturing was answered by examples of paternal transmission of the antibody-forming tendency.

CO-INCIDENCE OF OTHER AUTOIMMUNE DISEASES. The incidence of other autoimmune endocrine disorders, such as Type I diabetes mellitus and Addison's disease, in patients with Graves' disease and especially in their families also is greater than in the general population. Similarly, nonendocrine disease of autoimmune pathogenesis occurs with undue frequency in Graves' disease patients and in their families; these disorders include pernicious anemia, myasthenia gravis, rheumatoid arthritis, Sjögren's syndrome, vitiligo, idiopathic thrombocytopenic purpura, and chronic active hepatitis. It is now accepted that a common genetic link underlying these associations is the occurrence of HLA antigens, specifically of the D series, in the individuals concerned, although that relationship is far from absolute (see below).

HLA ANTIGEN ASSOCIATIONS WITH GRAVES' DISEASE. In 1974 Grumet and colleagues reported that the HLA antigen B_8 occurred in Graves' disease with approximately twice the incidence that was observed in a control population.[63] This was one of the earliest recognized links between an autoimmune disease and the HLA system. Since then the relationship has been better defined, but without full explanation of etiological implications. Early data indicated that in white populations DR3 was the antigen most closely related to Graves' disease. There were claims that it is an even more specific marker for those who relapse after a course of antithyroid drugs,[64] but this was not confirmed.[65] In the most recent analysis[65a] the association was with DQA1*0501.

Data from nonwhite populations also show specific associations, but with different antigens. For example, in Japanese increased frequencies of HLA-A2 and DPB1*0501

have been reported recently, with an odds ratio for the risk to develop Graves' disease of 10.5 in individuals positive for both alleles.[66] A similar survey in Singapore Chinese revealed an association with B46 and DR9, with a twist that this was observed primarily in males.[67]

It is important to note that there is no recognition of an antigen of the HLA series that approaches 100 per cent incidence in Graves' disease or any other autoimmune disease. There is increasing evidence for the importance of other gene products that are significant genetic factors in autoimmune thyroid disease, but their roles have not yet been identified.

Current interpretation of the function of the class II antigens is developed below in relation to the production of antibodies to the TSH receptor.

These considerations regarding the genetic background of Graves' disease deserve to be placed in the perspective of work on the genetic defects underlying related experimental animal models, viz., of immune thyroiditis. As reviewed by Rose et al.[68] from their studies and those of others in experimentally produced thyroiditis in mice and rats and spontaneous autoimmune thyroiditis in rats and chickens, at least three genetically determined components may participate in triggering the immune response. First there is the immune-response gene, involvement of which is implied from inbreeding studies in rats and actual histocompatibility complex data in both mice and chickens. Interpretation is that the disease susceptibility gene predisposes to vigorous antibody response to the antigenic challenge, the experimental immunogen in these studies being thyroglobulin.

Particularly compelling data for this conclusion were presented from studies in mice. It was shown with generally genetically pure, in-bred mice that good responders (making high antibody titer to thyroglobulin) and poor responders (low titer animals) were dependent on the thymus for these characteristics. The animals were thymectomized and given a lethal dose of irradiation but restored, in terms of lymphocytes, by injections of bone marrow (B) and thymus (T) cells. The important determinant, effective regardless of the strain of mouse or the source of B cells, was the origin of the injected T cells; if these were from good responder mice, the reconstituted animal produced high titers of antibody to thyroglobulin.

A second crucial role of the thymus is seen in the result of neonatal thymectomy in either obese-strain chickens[69] or BUF rats[70]; the spontaneous thyroiditis characteristics of both colonies is significantly increased in severity by the operation. It is of interest that titers of antibody to thyroglobulin are not decreased by thymectomy, implying that sufficient helper T cells have left the thymus before birth. The implication of these findings was that suppressor T cells delay the onset of the spontaneous disease and the significant variable might be the ratio of suppressor to helper cells.

Finally, there is evidence for a genetic defect in the thyroid gland itself that was most clearly shown in the obese-strain chicks. For instance, Wick and his colleagues[71] showed that the thyroid of this strain, on the day of hatching, had a higher rate of uptake of injected radioiodine than had the glands of control nonobese chicks. Even more telling was the fact that when the test and control glands were co-cultured for six days, the thyroids from the obese-strain chickens still showed a greater rate of uptake of radioiodine.[72] This topic was reviewed recently with additional supportive data.[72a] So far there is no compelling evidence of a primary defect in the thyroid in Graves' disease. It is unfortunate that animal models for this condition do not exist.

Emotion

Parry's first description of a patient with the condition we now call Graves' or Basedow's disease included a "psychic trigger" to the illness; immediately before the onset of symptoms "she was thrown out of a wheelchair in coming fast downhill."[73] In the almost 170 years since that report, myriad similar descriptions of emotional trauma preceding the onset of Graves' disease have appeared, but little that has led to understanding of a role for emotion. In part, uncertainty of the significance of these reports is due to the existence of a similar frequency of comparable stressful episodes in control subjects[74]; this objection is readily answered by the recognition that, to lead to Graves' disease, a stress effect presumably must be imposed on a genetically prone individual. Over the years, various interpretations and descriptions of "stress triggers" have been expressed.

1. There is no characteristic premorbid personality and psychosomatic aberrations in Graves' disease reflect the influence of the hyperthyroidism rather than the underlying personality.

2. Although a few reports indicate an increase in the incidence of Graves' disease in wartime, others fail to confirm this; such epidemiological data do not support an etiological role for stress.

3. Thyroid stimulation in humans[75] and other large animals[76] as a result of acute stress was reported. (Acute stress in small animals seems to cause inhibition of thyroid function.[77]) Evidence of concomitant increased adrenal medullary secretion in humans was also obtained. Since catecholamines are known to enhance the rate of synthesis and secretion of thyroid hormones,[78] it may be that the thyroid stimulation seen with acute stress is mediated by adrenal medulla secretions.

4. Although TSH is now known not to be involved in active hyperthyroidism of Graves' disease, the possibility perhaps should be borne in mind that it conceivably may be a factor in initiation of the disorder. This concept may be seen to gain support from a recent report of an increase in the remission rate associated with antithyroid drug therapy if thyroxine is given to maintain suppression of TSH.[79] Thus, an emotion-induced activation of the suprahypothalamo-hypophyseal axis might have etiological importance.

Most persuasive to us is the possibility that emotion might have an important role in Graves' disease through influences on the immune system. There is evidence that emotional stress can be related to increased susceptibility to infection and cancer, depression of homograft rejection, reduction of antibody production, enhanced development of autoimmune disease, decreased sensitivity to anaphylaxis, reduction in serum concentrations of interferon, and atrophy of thymus and spleen. We reported that rats showed alterations (both increase and decrease, depending on the sex of the animals) of lymphocyte function related to the stresses of overcrowding and isolation.[80] We also observed in stressed rats that thyroidectomy or hypophysectomy may, in turn, affect the function of peripheral lymphocytes.[81] Whether such influences of stress on lymphocyte function are mediated by the central or autonomic nervous systems, to what degree they may be modulated by the endocrine systems, and what role, if any, they play in Graves' disease all remain to be determined. Nonetheless, the theory just expounded seems a promising approach for linking the time-honored anecdotal literature on emotional stress in Graves' disease and the current evidence for the central importance of autoimmunity in its pathogenesis.

Other Factors

In addition to the general etiological factors already discussed, certain specific agents may have been identified in several circumstances. The best documented of these is the exhibition of iodide in excess of that formerly available to the individual or population concerned. The condition applicable to this concept has long been known as *Jod-Basedow's disease*, although priority of description might advocate *Coindet's syndrome*.[82] In more recent times, relevant observations have been reported from Boston, Massachusetts,[83] in the United States, and from Tasmania.[84] In the former study, of eight subjects with nontoxic goiter four became hypothyroid after taking iodide.[83] Tasmanians experienced an unprecedented epidemic of hyperthyroidism coincident with iodination of bread.[84]

Possible explanations for the syndrome have been reviewed. Support for the concept that simple availability of sufficient iodide is important may be seen in the experience reported from Glasgow, Scotland,[85] where patients who were relatively iodine deficient as measured by plasma inorganic iodide, having been treated for hyperthyroidism by a course of antithyroid drug, were given an iodide supplement of 200 μg potassium iodide per day and compared with a similar group maintained on their normal diet. The iodide-supplemented group (16 patients) had a relapse rate of hyperthyroidism of 56 per cent compared with 27 per cent for the 41 control patients. However, this cannot be a universal explanation, as shown by a patient reported from Helsinki.[86] In this instance, excess iodide intake on top of iodine sufficiency apparently led to an episode of "diffuse toxic goiter" that regressed on cessation of the iodide excess. Similarly, the aforementioned Boston patients[83] were not considered to suffer from prior iodine deficiency, and one can only conclude that those patients who became thyrotoxic while taking excess iodide had glands lacking normal (unknown) homeostatic control mechanisms for reasons not apparent.

In another group of patients with an apparently identifiable trigger for their episodes of hyperthyroidism, thyroid hormone was prescribed shortly before endogenous hyperthyroidism developed.[87] The dosage of thyroid hormone was usually not enough to produce thyrotoxicosis factitia, and many were being treated for obesity. Perhaps a variant of the group is those patients whose anamnesis includes a preceding episode of weight reduction accomplished by dieting. There are no studies of thyroid function in these various patients either before or after their hyperthyroidism to facilitate formation of hypotheses to explain these

"triggers," which have occurred with sufficient frequency for one to accept that more than coincidence is involved.

More recently the existence of the TSH receptor in infectious agents has been reported. *Yersinia enterocolitica* has been shown to have a surface molecule that binds TSH,[88] and thyroid-stimulating antibody (TSAb) can compete with the hormone.[89] From these findings the hypothesis has been developed that infection with *Yersinia* (which is a common event) may induce the production of cross-reacting antibodies and thus initiate the syndrome. So far no proof of this concept has been published.

Another tantalizing finding was the description of retroviral sequences in human thyroid tissue[90]; that was not confirmed.[91, 92] However, some homology between the TSH receptor and the HIV-1 *nef* protein was found.[92a] In short, a valid hypothesis exists, viz., that autoimmunity could be initiated by bacterial or viral infections.[92b] This remains a research area of major interest.

In summary, it is probable that there are many components to the etiology of Graves' disease. Environmental factors such as iodine supply, emotions, and infections may interact with the genetic features that control metabolic and immunological systems, and this might lead to the clinical presentation of Graves' disease.

Pathogenesis

Hyperthyroidism

THYROID-STIMULATING ANTIBODY. From the 1930's to the 1950's the pituitary was thought to be the causative organ for both the hyperthyroidism and ophthalmopathy of Graves' disease. That is, thyrotropin was accepted as the offending agent, even if increasing knowledge of endocrine physiology made understanding of involved mechanisms progressively more difficult. Now, owing to application of highly sensitive immunoassays, it is clear that thyrotropin is not increased in hyperthyroidism, and the pituitary thyrotrope is, in a normal physiological manner, functionally suppressed by the high circulating concentration of thyroid hormone. In 1956 Adams and Purves made the initial observation that led, over the next eight years, to the recognition that in many instances of Graves' disease there was a circulating thyroid-stimulating IgG that could be measured by an in vivo mouse bioassay; this was the substance known as the *long-acting thyroid stimulator* (LATS), which was shown to be an immunoglobulin, IgG.

In the intervening years since 1964, advances in understanding of the role of the humoral immune system include the following:

1. Numerous assays were developed to detect and quantitate the thyroid-stimulating antibody, resulting in a confusing proliferation of methods, with varying sensitivity and specificity, and ambiguous terminology; the essence of the main characteristics of currently applied assays is shown in Table 41–1. As shown, there are two basic procedures, involving either direct stimulation of a thyroid preparation or inhibition of the binding of ^{125}I-TSH to its receptor. For data acquired by the former technique we shall use the term *thyroid-stimulating antibody* (TSAb) and for the latter, *TSH-binding inhibition* (TBI). A major difference in the two types of assay is that the TSAb procedure is specific for

TABLE 41–1. BASES OF CURRENT ASSAYS OF TSAb

Thyroid Stimulation
A. Cyclic AMP in
  1. Human thyroid cells*
  2. Rat thyroid cells (FRTL5)*
  3. Porcine thyroid cells
  4. CHO cells stably transfected with recombinant human TSH receptor
B. Iodide uptake in
  1. Rat thyroid cells (FRTL5)
  2. Porcine thyroid cells
C. Cytochemical bioassay in guinea pig thyroid fragments

Inhibition of Receptor Binding of ^{125}I-TSH
  Receptor preparation
  1. Solubilized porcine thyroid membranes*
  2. Particulate or solubilized human thyroid membranes

*Commercially available
Critical discussion of most of these methods is presented in reference 100.

what the term indicates, i.e., thyroid stimulation. The TBI procedure is nonspecific in that many instances are now recognized in which an IgG that inhibits TSH binding does not stimulate the thyroid gland.[92c] TBIAb probably also inhibits the binding of TSAb, since it inhibits the action of both TSH and TSAb.[92c] TSAb and TBIAb may co-exist in patients with autoimmune thyroid disease,[92c, 92d] with a clinical presentation reflecting the action of the predominant antibody. Two additional stimulating antibodies, distinct from TSAb, have been described,[92c, 92d] but their prevalence is unknown.

2. As far as LATS is concerned, the old data may be viewed as reflecting TSAb's action on a nonhuman thyroid. The assay was insensitive; therefore, positive data reflected a high titer or affinity of TSAb in the patient's serum.[93] The TSH receptor from the mouse has not yet been cloned, but the nucleotide sequences for the human, canine, and rat TSH receptor have been described in detail.[94–97] There is a high homology across the species for these receptors. Although the structure-function relationship of the TSH receptor is not fully understood, it appears that TSH, TSAb, and TBIAb all bind to multiple discontinuous epitopes on the receptor.[98, 98a] Some of the epitopes, but not all, may be shared and this presumably underlies the mechanism of interactions of these ligands.[98, 98a] Furthermore, as shown by the use of chimeric TSH receptors,[98b] TSAb derived from different patients may not bind to identical epitopes. These findings provide corroborative data for the recognition of multiple stimulating antibodies.[92c, 92d]

3. Although not all laboratories report identical results, no doubt related to individual assay sensitivities, it appears that in active Graves' disease TSAb can be measured in over 90 per cent of patients.[99] This applies to patients with the thyroid disorder; there is no significant correlation of the presence or titer of TSAb with ophthalmopathy *per se*. TBI assays are also usually positive in hyperthyroidism, but, as noted above, there is a significant incidence of false-positive and false-negative results. However, the clinical usefulness of TSAb or TBI values is limited.[100] They should not be required for the diagnosis of Graves' disease in most patients. Even in the more subtle presentations, such as euthyroid ophthalmopathy, measurement of the antibody to the microsomal antigen (thyroid peroxidase) is probably

just as relevant.[99] There may be a role, which is still to be thoroughly evaluated, for assay of TSAb in determining prognosis at the end of a course of antithyroid drugs; a positive result after 6 to 12 months of therapy appears to presage relapse, and absence of TSAb indicates that remission is highly likely.[99] Less well documented, but of greater use if confirmed, is the suggestion that a high value on initial diagnosis of hyperthyroidism indicates that remission on antithyroid drug therapy will not occur and that ablative treatment is indicated.[99] As detailed subsequently, there is good evidence that a high titer of TSAb in a woman in the third trimester of pregnancy forecasts neonatal hyperthyroidism.[93, 101, 102]

4. What has remained poorly understood is the underlying disorder that permits the emergence of TSAb to cause hyperthyroidism or, contrariwise, that explains the disappearance of TSAb eventually in the majority of patients. As reviewed above, class II antigens of the HLA series are thought to be implicated. They are functionally related to autoimmune responses. Helper T lymphocytes recognize the antigen bound to class II product on the surface of the antigen-presenting cell; this class II-restricted recognition of antigen results in activation of T helper cells with a subsequent cascade of events leading to, among others, antibody production. As well summarized by Martin and Davies,[103] many cytokines, which can affect thyroid function and antigen expression by thyroid cells, are produced by thyroid-infiltrating lymphocytes (e.g., interferon-γ, tumor necrosis factor α, interleukins). Thyroid cells themselves secrete IL-1, IL-6, IL-8,[104] and transforming growth factor β (TGFβ) and can be induced to express adhesion molecules such as ICAM-1. Autocrine and paracrine effects of these cytokines, as well as possible increased adhesion of T cells to thyroid epithelium, must play a role in the autoimmune process, but a coherent sequence of events has yet to be elaborated.

Formerly, class II antigens were thought to be expressed only on cells that have legitimate business interacting with helper T cells, viz., macrophages, dendritic cells, and B cells. There is now recognition that class II molecules can be ectopically expressed,[105] including on thyroid follicular cells.[106] These cell-surface molecules occur in autoimmune thyroid disease and may be induced in normal thyroid cells in vitro by the action, for instance, of γ-interferon.[106] To relate these developments in understanding of the autoimmune process to the production of TSAb and hyperthyroidism, it was hypothesized that expression of the class II gene product on the surface of the thyroid follicular cell permits presentation to lymphocytes of the TSH receptor as antigen leading to the induction of TSAb synthesis.[105, 106] However, most investigators now view the presence of class II antigen on thyroid cells in Graves' disease as a consequence of initial (poorly understood) pathogenic events and believe that, at best, it may be a component of a process that leads to perpetuation of the disorder.

TSAb-IgG, if not monoclonal, at least shows a major degree of restricted heterogeneity, particularly in patients with high titers of the autoantibody.[107–109] The evidence, based on study of patient serum, includes identification of a constant isoelectric point for TSAb, and the findings that its biological activity is associated with only one type of light chain (overwhelmingly λ) and, similarly, the activity is restricted to IgG subclass I. Furthermore, there is restriction

of the T cell receptor usage by thyroid-infiltrating lymphocytes,[103] pointing to the contribution of both immunoglobulin and T cell receptor genes to the pathogenesis of hyperthyroidism in Graves' disease.

Somehow these observations will have to be accommodated by any theory that explains the autoimmune events leading to production of TSAb. An antigen-specific deficiency of T-suppressor cells has been postulated, and the evidence was reviewed by Volpe.[110] He finds support for a concept invoking a defect in thyroid antigen–specific suppressor T cells, perhaps through defective HLA-related gene function that leads to failure of proper antigen presentation to the antigen-specific suppressor T-lymphocytes. Although there are arguments against such a putative defect,[103] this is a hypothesis that merits full evaluation.

To summarize, a mass of data has accumulated in recent years regarding mechanisms of autoimmunity and much is obviously relevant to autoimmune thyroid disease. However, a clear-cut scheme has not yet appeared that integrates these findings into a model to accommodate what is currently known about the pathogenesis of hyperthyroidism in Graves' disease.

Ophthalmopathy, Pretibial Myxedema, Acropachy

The pathogenesis of ophthalmopathy in Graves' disease is even less understood than that of hyperthyroidism; the subject is reviewed in Chapter 42. Regarding other features of Graves' disease, little of pathogenesis can profitably be presented. Trauma seems indeed to be a "trigger" to the location of pretibial myxedema (see Fig. 41–7). On the other hand, tissue specificity was invoked by studies of fibroblast-stimulating factor.[111] Fibroblasts from the pretibial area of normal individuals, as well as from patients with pretibial myxedema, responded to serum from pretibial myxedema patients by increasing the rate of synthesis of glycosaminoglycans; in contrast, fibroblasts from the skin of the back or prepuce did not. These findings still have to be confirmed, but other investigators emphasize the importance of the fibroblast as studied at the ultrastructural level.[112] Otherwise, perhaps the only comment to make is that in the histologically similar condition of lichen myxedematosus, a circulating IgM (M protein of myeloma) has been identified in a few instances; such observations are more tantalizing than informative. For acropachy, even less may be said. The condition is so rare that probably no clinic has sufficient experience to aid understanding of pathogenetic mechanisms.

Clinical Features

Hyperthyroidism

As intimated earlier, there is a characteristic constitution often recognized in Graves' disease patients that can influence clinical features. This opinion is supported by the generally accepted difference in symptoms between patients thyrotoxic from toxic adenoma or from Graves' disease. The major additional symptom component in hyperthyroidism of Graves' disease may be seen as an autonomic lability that leads, through synergism with excess thyroid hormone, to a greater degree of nervousness, heat intolerance and sweating, tachycardia, and "intestinal hurry" than is commonly found in the other forms of thyrotoxicosis. One consequence of the autonomic lability is that patients may retain symptoms such as flushing and excess perspiration at a time when they are, by all other criteria, euthyroid.

The majority of patients with hyperthyroidism are readily diagnosed clinically. The complaints of nervousness, heat intolerance, weight loss (often despite increased appetite), sweating, palpitations, and diarrhea make a characteristic anamnesis. Emotional lability is common, and mental change may be so extreme as to be termed a psychosis; in these instances the thyrotoxic state probably uncovers an underlying psychiatric trait. Even without ophthalmopathy, the supporting clinical signs of stare, lid lag, tachycardia, tremor of fingers and tongue, hot moist skin, and diffuse goiter create an unmistakable constellation. However, not every patient presents the total picture, and even goiter may not be a significant feature.[39] Excluding the syndrome of euthyroid ophthalmopathy, there are still many oligosymptomatic hyperthyroid patients. Particularly in the elderly, because of the likelihood of coincident myocardial inadequacy, cardiac symptoms may predominate. Occasionally the muscle weakness and wasting may be so extreme as to obscure, or render comparatively insignificant, other features of the disease. *Apathetic hyperthyroidism* is a term often applied in these situations, but it should be reserved for a distinct clinical picture that is quite rare. Generally, in oligosymptomatic patients, if the diagnosis of hyperthyroidism is given adequate consideration, multiple diagnostic criteria will be confirmed. On the other hand, in the syndrome of apathetic hyperthyroidism, weight loss and apathy may be solitary stigmata.

The nervousness and associated excitability, ill-temper, and lack of ability to concentrate may be reflected in the patient being fidgety or restless during interrogation and speaking with uncharacteristic rapidity; he or she is, in a common lay term, "hyper." Tremor of the fingers may be documented as a change in the smoothness of handwriting, as a newly recognized difficulty in using a typewriter or word processor or lighting a cigarette, or by the embarrassment of rattling a cup in the saucer; there is also a telltale clumsiness in manipulating buttons on clothing. There is no specific physiopathological explanation for these features. Since they are especially characteristic of the patient with Graves' disease rather than toxic adenoma, may be mimicked to a large extent by the existence of a pheochromocytoma, and are commonly much improved by administration of propranolol or similar agent that blocks the β-adrenergic nervous system, they are, at least in part, due to the synergistic effect of thyroid hormones on sympathetic tone. In the normal individual, ingestion of excess quantities of triiodothyronine is known to shorten the average evoked potential produced by a standard stimulus (light in this experiment), indicating a reduction in selective attention,[113] so that a direct effect of thyroid hormones on nervous tissue is probably also involved. However, since the biochemical bases for either normal or abnormal behavior are so poorly known, it is inevitable that the mediation of superimposed effects of hyperthyroidism is inadequately understood.

A highly characteristic feature is one often recognized on initial handshake with a patient, i.e., the warm, moist skin, so distinct from the cold, clammy feel of the anxious, neurotic person who may otherwise have many features difficult to distinguish from those shown by the hyperthyroid subject. The warmth of the skin may literally radiate, causing comment from the patient's bed companion. Related to this, when there is an appropriate sleeping arrangement, a useful yardstick exists of the development of hyperthyroidism: i.e., contrary to previous habit, the patient may prefer fewer covers and a lower bedroom temperature than does the roommate. These signs and symptoms are due to dilation of skin blood vessels, but once again, the degree to which this reflects thyroid hormone–catecholamine synergism or thyroid hormone effect itself is uncertain. Changes in skin color, as in vitiligo or hyperpigmentation, are other integumentary features, usually minimal but occasionally striking. Vitiligo is the more common and may be seen as a variably accompanying autoimmune disease, occurring also with Hashimoto's thyroiditis and in Addison's disease. Hyperpigmentation, which may be generalized similar to that in adrenocortical failure, is said to be secondary to an ACTH response to an enhanced rate of cortisol turnover. However, there are no published data in support of the thesis, and, in our experience, excess pigmentation may occur in euthyroid ophthalmopathy, i.e., in the absence of hypermetabolism.

Hair and nail changes are common. Characteristically the hair is fine and silky in texture and, especially in males, may show premature graying; hair "coming out in handfuls" is a frequent complaint and may persist, or occur for the first time, after treatment has restored a euthyroid state or even has induced hypothyroidism, a circumstance that may strain physician-patient rapport to a greater extent than many other consequences of the disease of greater import to physical well-being. Apart from acropachy, discussed later, a nail change typical of severe hyperthyroidism is onycholysis (Fig. 41–4), wherein a separation of the distal nail from its bed (also seen when there is malnutrition) may be visually accentuated by the presence in the space of dirt that is difficult to remove.

The hyperdynamic cardiovascular state was the earliest clinical component to attract attention[73] and is frequently both the basis of the presenting symptom (palpitations) and the most striking finding on physical examination. The pulse is typically full, bounding, and rapid, even in sleep; because of the dilated skin vessels, individual fingers may be felt to pulsate. The precordial impulse is so forceful as commonly to be visible, even with a moderately thick chest wall, and to be spontaneously recognized by the patient;

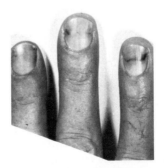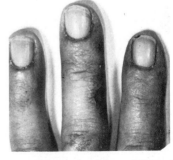

FIGURE 41–4. Onycholysis in a patient with hyperthyroidism of Graves' disease before (left) and after restoration to a euthyroid state. Note subungual dirt on the left. (Courtesy of Dr. M. M. Hoffman.)

often there is a complaint of insomnia due to an awareness of heart action that may be in the chest, ears, or more rarely, in the head. It has been said that it is a characteristic of the hyperthyroid patient who is breast-feeding a child that the right breast is preferred owing to the child's reaction to the (left-sided) hyperdynamic cardiac action. Palpitations are made prominent by the development of arrhythmia, that, as a sporadic premature ventricular contraction, may be even more evident to the patient than the clinically more significant atrial fibrillation; the latter occurs in about 10 per cent of patients and is more common in the older patient. On physical examination, all these features may be recognized, and the forceful, diffuse apex beat may suggest a heart size greater than actually exists. There is a widened pulse pressure as a result of the diastolic component being low and the systolic high, but hypertension persisting after restitution of euthyroidism is not to be expected. A common auscultatory finding during the hyperdynamic phase of the disease is a short, high-pitched systolic murmur to the left of the sternal border, especially in the "pulmonary valve area." Functional mitral valve insufficiency, reversible with therapy of thyrotoxicosis, is also known to occur, as is mitral valve prolapse. The cardiac output is almost always greater than normal, and high-output cardiac failure may occur directly related to hyperthyroidism, but, in most instances of myocardial decompensation, there is associated heart disease, e.g., coronary vascular inadequacy. Dependent edema is a frequent occurrence in severe hyperthyroidism of Graves' disease and ought not to be taken as a sign of heart failure, since it appears to be related to increased capillary permeability, perhaps aggravated by the decreased concentration of plasma albumin that is commonly associated.

Several studies have shown that the normal heart subjected to the state of hyperthyroidism responds with enhanced performance. For instance, echocardiographic and Doppler assessments of diastolic function showed shorter isovolumic relaxation times that were unaffected by propranolol but reverted to normal when the subjects were euthyroid.[114] These investigators suggested, similar to our interpretation of reasons for dyspnea on exertion,[115] that such symptoms may be more related to generalized (but specifically respiratory) muscle weakness rather than to myocardial inadequacy.

As noted earlier, increased appetite despite weight loss is a hallmark of hyperthyroidism, but anorexia may occur, especially in severe instances of the disease. Bowel function is disturbed, usually showing as an increased frequency of defecation and the passage of soft stools; frank diarrhea is not common and when it occurs is an indication of particularly severe disease. On physical examination of the abdomen, tissue wasting is often obvious, and hepatomegaly may be found but usually only with prolonged and extreme examples of the syndrome in which there may also be associated jaundice. Testing of hepatic function not uncommonly reveals abnormalities, including increased serum transaminases and alkaline phosphatase levels (which may be related to effects of excess thyroid hormone on bone; see below). Histologically, there are probably only modest changes to be found in the majority of instances, with some degree of fatty infiltration of the central areas of lobules occurring in severe disease; at the level of electron microscopy, characteristic—though minor—effects of hyperthyroidism on the liver have been described.[116] Hepatic

disorders are reversible with control of the hyperthyroidism, except for the most severe disease, usually meriting the term *crisis*, when the hepatic damage may, at least in part, be secondary to failure of other organs, e.g., in cardiac decompensation.

Abdominal examination may also disclose splenomegaly that is probably generally present in Graves' disease, particularly as judged radiologically. This is part of a generalized lymphoid hyperplasia in Graves' disease recognized over 60 years ago[38] and is associated with thymus hyperplasia and lymph node enlargement, especially cervical. The explanation for these changes is still debated in that some investigators would have them reflecting mild adrenal insufficiency or a direct effect of excess thyroid hormone; since similar changes do not occur in toxic adenoma, it seems to us that they have more pathogenic significance. Frequently the histological pattern is of germinal center formation, indicating B-cell hyperplasia, which would be in keeping with the pathogenic mechanisms discussed earlier. Peripheral lymphocytosis is said to be common in Graves' disease, but we have not found it to be so. Nonetheless, leukemia, especially acute disease, occurs with a greater than normal incidence,[117] and at least one episode of severe neutropenia has been described, responding (somewhat ironically) to control of hyperthyroidism with a potentially leukopenogenic drug, propylthiouracil. Regarding red cell metabolism, true pernicious anemia appears to occur with Graves' disease in 2 to 3 per cent of patients. (Gastric achlorhydria exists more commonly, but in most instances there is return to a normal secretion of acid when the hyperthyroidism is controlled.) This is an example of the coincidence of two autoimmune diseases. Serum antibodies to gastric parietal cells and to intrinsic factor occur with a greater frequency than does pernicious anemia itself. Rarely a normochromic, normocytic anemia (previously termed *achrestic*) occurs in the hyperthyroid state, and this may respond to administration of pyridoxine.

At least two aspects of red cell function are altered in hyperthyroidism, and both may be directly related to thyroid hormone action. The erythrocyte sodium content and concentration are enhanced, associated with a reduction in the rate constant for active sodium flux. This, in turn, appears to be due to a decrease in the activity of the enzyme responsible for sodium transport, viz., the ouabain-sensitive Na^+-K^+–activated component of the adenosine triphosphate (ATP)–hydrolyzing system of the erythrocyte membrane.[118] In one patient studied longitudinally, the abnormality regressed in parallel with control of the hyperthyroidism.[118] Second, the concentration of 2,3-diphosphoglyceric acid in the erythrocyte is supranormal, and the rate of synthesis of this compound is extremely sensitive in vitro to the action of thyroid hormones.[119] The biological significance of these facts, especially as related to the patient with hyperthyroidism, is not clear. It has been hypothesized that thyroid calorigenesis is mediated by stimulation of active Na^+ transport, and compatible experimental data[120] have shown, however, an activation of Na^+ extrusion from liver and diaphragm related to injection of thyroid hormone, rather than the reduction noted above in studies of patients' erythrocytes. There is so far no ready explanation for these apparently incompatible data. The observations regarding synthesis of 2,3-diphosphoglyceric acid can, however, be related to other physiological events. There is a decrease in the affinity of hemoglobin for oxygen in the erythrocytes of hyperthyroid subjects, i.e., there is "a shift to the right" in the oxygen dissociation curve, presumably enhancing rates of oxygenation of perfused tissues. This change of the affinity of hemoglobin for oxygen can be reproduced in solution by addition of 2,3-diphosphoglyceric acid, so that the clinical observation may well be explained by the actions of thyroid hormones, described above, on its synthesis.

Another component of peripheral blood, the thrombocyte, is rarely, but perhaps still too frequently, abnormal in Graves' disease. Idiopathic thrombocytopenic purpura occurring together with hyperthyroidism may again be viewed as the coincidence of two autoimmune diseases. The surprising finding in a few patients has been the apparent alleviation of the thrombocytopenia by control of the hyperthyroidism, an occurrence for which there is no obvious explanation, unless it is that there is a general improvement in the immune disorder that underlies both ailments.

Respiratory distress is often a complaint of the hyperthyroid patient and may result from any of several mechanisms, such as in association with cardiac decompensation. A typical symptom is extreme shortness of breath on climbing stairs (which should be distinguished from fatigue, particularly of quadriceps muscles, that may also exist). This may be a reflection of weakness of respiratory muscles. In detailed ventilatory studies of subjects who were either hyperthyroid spontaneously or as a result of ingestion of 300 μg T_3 daily, it was shown that the respiratory demand per increment of work load was normal, except that hyperthyroid subjects, of course, started from an abnormally high rate of oxygen consumption.[115] There was a reduction in vital capacity and increase in residual lung volume that was due to a lowered expiratory reserve volume, since the functional residual capacity approximated the predicted value. Thus, those functions that depend on a sustained and forceful muscular effort were reduced, and therefore if muscle weakness limited tidal volume, the patient with hyperthyroidism would be able to maintain alveolar ventilation only by increasing respiratory frequency. These data and interpretations may explain the rapid, shallow breathing typically observed both at rest and on exercise. Therefore, the complaint of dyspnea on exertion is probably partly due to the patient's awareness that a greater frequency of respiration is required in comparison with the pattern in a former euthyroid state.

Thyrotoxic periodic paralysis is a rare syndrome, seen only with Graves' disease and with greater frequency in Orientals, perhaps particularly Japanese. It has the same clinical associations as hypokalemic periodic paralysis, which occurs apart from Graves' disease. There is a tendency for an attack of paralysis that may be generalized or localized to be brought on by exercise or by meals containing much carbohydrate or sodium; in the former instance, it may be only the exercised muscles that are affected. The attack may last minutes, hours, or even days and occurs with a lowering, not always to an abnormal level, of the serum concentration of potassium; there is associated renal retention, rather than loss, of potassium. The episodes are usually aborted by administration of potassium and may be reduced in incidence by avoidance of recognized precipitants such as particular foods or exercises. The unique characteristic of periodic paralysis associated with Graves' disease is that it does not recur once the hyperthyroidism is controlled. The topic was conveniently reviewed by Engel, who summarized much of his contribution to our knowledge of the condition,[121] and more recently by Ober,[122] who concentrated on patients reported in the United States.

Even rarer than periodic paralysis are other neuromuscular disorders including peripheral nerve involvement (with or without entrapment in areas of pretibial myxedema),[123] and pyramidal tract dysfunction. An interesting report emphasized one patient's deficits mimicking amyotrophic lateral sclerosis.[124]

The generalized myopathy of the typical Graves' disease patient was quantitated recently and the response to propranolol evaluated.[125] Before thionamide the patients were treated with the β-blocker for two weeks. This was associated with highly significant improvement in muscle strength that increased further when a euthyroid state was achieved. No such change occurred with a control group given propranolol. The rational conclusion was that "thyroid hormone and catecholamines in concert mediate the muscle dysfunction of hyperthyroidism" in Graves' disease.

Abnormalities of nonthyroid endocrine function are common in hyperthyroidism. In patients with uncomplicated disease, polydipsia or polyuria are not marked, so that a complaint of increased thirst should lead to consideration of concurrent diabetes mellitus. If this is the diagnosis, it is probably an example of latent diabetes becoming overt, and restoration of euthyroidism commonly ameliorates the diabetes. On the other hand, modest polyuria occurs with a much greater frequency and may reflect rapid intestinal absorption of carbohydrate, although the peak of glycemia, when an oral glucose tolerance test is conducted, is often delayed. The degree to which insulin antagonism by thyroid hormones is important (blood insulin levels are commonly high) is uncertain, and there is a paucity of studies of the secretion of other carbohydrate-influencing hormones of the gastrointestinal tract in this disease. Similarly, precise knowledge of the effects of hyperthyroidism on growth hormone secretion is lacking. While in hyperthyroidism both hyperglycemia and insulin-induced hypoglycemia are said to result in inadequate responses of growth hormone (i.e., suppression in the former state and increased secretion in the latter), there are insufficient data available properly to interpret the significance of these observations. For instance, study of the diurnal pattern of blood growth hormone concentrations and the responses to stimuli known to enhance or suppress its secretion (somatostatin, bromocriptine, and thyrotropin-releasing hormone) is required to facilitate proper assessment of possible abnormalities of secretion of this pituitary hormone. Nevertheless, diabetes mellitus may be made overt or established glucose intolerance worsened by the onset of hyperthyroidism, and this will probably necessitate the initiation or modification of antidiabetes therapy. Part of the problem may be related to increased food intake, so that with control of the hyperthyroidism this exogenous variable in diabetes management should revert to normal.

On physical examination of the hyperthyroid male gynecomastia may be found that apparently, as assessed by histology of biopsy material, is present in most.[126] The explanation for this is no doubt related to excess estrogen or at least to a supranormal ratio of available estrogen to available androgen, but the precise endocrine events are not clear. An increase in the plasma sex steroid binding globulin occurs, and as a result, total testosterone concentration is enhanced but metabolic clearance is reduced, resulting in a normal production rate. There is less unanimity regarding the metabolism of the main estrogen, 17-β-estradiol, which is said by some to be in normal concentration and normal production rate and by others to be increased in both total (protein-bound) and free concentration. To complicate the situation further, the metabolism of both androgens and estrogens is affected by excess thyroid hormones; with the former there is accentuation of the pathway involving reduction of the 5α position (rather than 5β) and with the latter the appearance in the urine of predominantly 2-methoxy compounds instead of estriol. Most investigators have found serum luteinizing hormone to be in increased concentration in hyperthyroidism, although whether this is due to or despite alterations in gonadal steroid secretion and metabolism is not clear.

Much more common than clinically significant gynecomastia and doubtlessly related to these poorly understood disturbances in metabolism of gonadal steroids and gonadotropins is upset of menstrual function and, in both men and women, changes in the pattern of sexual activity. Commonly, menstruation becomes relatively scanty and sometimes less frequent. In either sex, libido may be enhanced but is, in our experience, more commonly decreased, at times severely. Furthermore, since the oligomenorrhea may be associated with failure to ovulate, the reduced fertility rate of hyperthyroid women is not unexpected. Spontaneous abortion is common in those who do achieve conception, although the precise reason for this is unclear.

The skeletal system is another site frequently affected by hyperthyroidism. Hypercalciuria is common and may contribute to the polyuria; hypercalcemia is less common but can occasionally be sufficiently prominent to cause primary investigation of that abnormality. The cause of the disturbance is probably a direct effect of thyroid hormone on bone that results in an increased rate of bone resorption. In addition, there may well be synergistic effects of parathyroid hormone, not necessarily directly but through an influence on the metabolism of vitamin D. Alternatively, hypomagnesemia is a feature of hyperthyroidism (even though the cause is unknown), and this can be a stimulant for the release of parathyroid hormone from the parathyroid glands. However, the few data available indicate that the blood level of parathyroid hormone is probably low or normal in hyperthyroidism. Further confusion in consideration of the mechanism of hypercalcemia comes from reports that the disorder responds favorably and acutely to the administration of propranolol.

Ophthalmopathy

The criteria and classification endorsed by the five Thyroid Associations for the eye features of Graves' disease[127] may merit criticism, but they incidentally serve a useful function of implying a continuum of changes in the eyes from mere stare and lid lag to complete visual loss from corneal or optic nerve involvement; examples of various degrees of ophthalmopathy are shown in Figures 41–5 to 41–8. Diagnostic difficulty arises when the ophthalmopathic process occurs in a patient who is euthyroid or has minimal or unrecognized symptoms and signs of hyperthyroidism, especially if the eye involvement is unilateral; then the diagnosis becomes one of exclusion of all other potential causes, particularly retrobulbar space-occupying lesions. The clinical picture of euthyroid ophthalmopathy includes the full gamut of that which is associated with hyperthyroidism and may progress from unilateral to bilateral (usually unequal in severity) with or without the development of thyroid hyperfunction. That unilateral lid retraction, or *lagophthalmos,* may occur in an unequivocally euthyroid (or even hypothyroid) subject serves to emphasize that this feature is not simply a reflection of hyperthyroidism, as older classifications would have it, but is indeed part of a wide spectrum of ophthalmological change within the syndrome. The degree of proptosis or exophthalmos that occurs varies greatly and is a measurement that can readily be made with the use of a Hertel or equivalent exophthalmometer. Although the upper limit of normal protrusion varies with race, 20 mm is commonly accepted in North America. (Orientals have lower limits and black races higher than do white Occidentals.) Exophthalmometry entails a minimal pressure on the lateral margin of the orbital cavity, and in a patient with major proptosis, especially if there is also significant lid retraction, care must be taken to avoid the eyelids slipping behind the equator of the globe. Such an event can also happen spontaneously or with minor, normal exertion by the patient (such as jumping out of bed in the morning as occurred with one of our patients). Obviously, with such an eye, the normal position of the lids must be restored as soon as possible to minimize the risk of damage to the exposed globe.

Inflammatory components of ophthalmopathy range from a complaint of "sand in the eye," with comparatively mild involvement of the palpebral conjunctiva or chemosis, to the sight-threatening panophthalmitis illustrated in Figure 41–8. The danger to sight lies in either corneal infection with subsequent scarring or in retro-orbital pressure from inflammatory edema and other space-occupying accumulations of fluid and swollen tissue causing damage to the optic nerve; rarely, retinal vein thrombosis may develop affecting sight on that account. With or without obvious inflammatory changes, external ocular muscle paresis can occur with dramatic suddenness, causing distressing diplopia; at the extreme, there may be virtual fixation of the eye. Although several millimeters of proptosis per se can disturb extraocular movements, the major abnormality causing paresis is an inflammatory swelling of the muscles, which can acquire three to four times their normal girth. These abnormalities may be well documented by CT scan, ultrasonography, or magnetic resonance imaging. Histologically, there is fragmentation and swelling of muscle fibers, "lymphorrhages," and a variable degree of fibrosis. It is when the fibrosis is established that little improvement can be expected from medical therapy. An uncommon feature, most distressing to the patient, which we have seen in one case, is blepharospasm, which was probably a response to diplopia, the sensation of grittiness that is otherwise a common symptom, and anxiety.

Pretibial Myxedema

This condition is rarer than ophthalmopathy, occurring possibly in 4 per cent of the Graves' disease population, but is akin to it in being usually, though not always, associ-

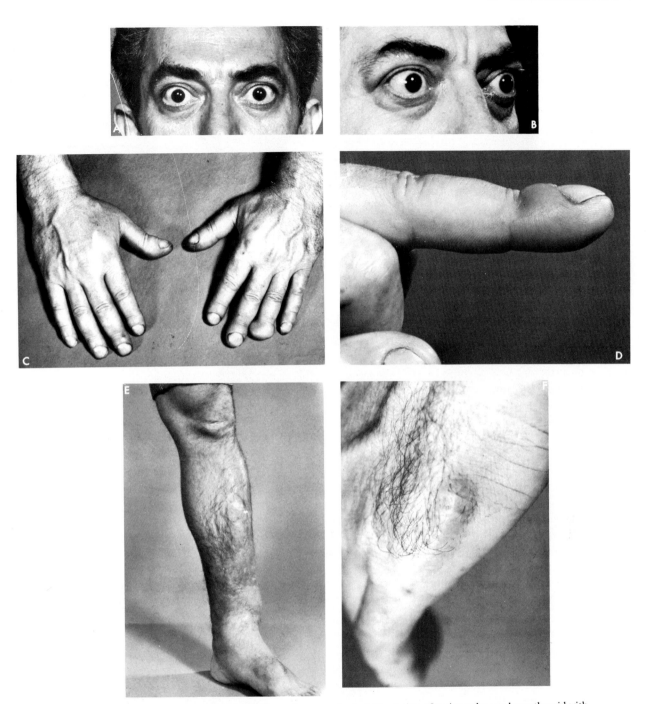

FIGURE 41-5. **Multiple aspects of Graves' disease in one patient.** *A*, Front view of patient who was hyperthyroid with goiter and lid retraction. *B*, Oblique view, illustrating bilateral exophthalmos. *C*, Hands showing acropachy. The "drumstick" appearance of the left fourth finger resulted from the acropachic process being superimposed on an old traumatic amputation of the terminal phalanx. *D*, Side view of one digit with swelling of the nail bed and terminal phalanx. *E*, Pretibial myxedema. *F*, "Pretibial myxedema" of the site of incision for biopsy of the fifth left metacarpal. Radiographs of the hands and photomicrographs of the bone biopsy are shown in Figures 43–10 and 43–11. (From McKenzie JM, Zakarija M, Bonnyns M: Graves' disease. Med Clin North Am 59:1177, 1975.)

ated with hyperthyroidism. As illustrated in Figure 41–5, it is not restricted to the pretibial region, and trauma seems to determine the site in many instances. A cigarette burn on the arm was another site of "pretibial" myxedema in one patient (Fig. 41–5). As advocated by Lipman et al,[37] "dermopathy" might be a more useful, noncommittal term, but it seems likely that the traditional phrase will linger. Whichever the area involved, the appearance of the skin is unmistakable. There is thickening, accentuation of hair follicles, erythema and itching, and sometimes pain, and a clear-cut edge to the lesion. Nodule formation is not unusual. The histological change in the dermis and epidermis is shown in Figure 41–9. An unusual complication[123] was entrapment of peroneal nerves in pads of pretibial myxedema, producing a bilateral foot drop, with recovery on satisfactory treatment of the myxedema.

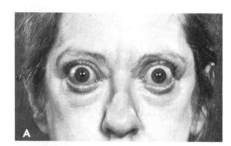
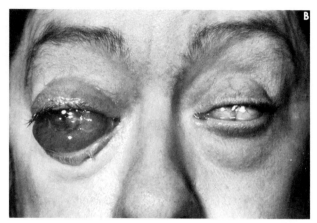
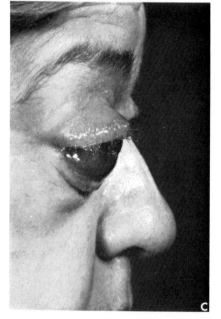
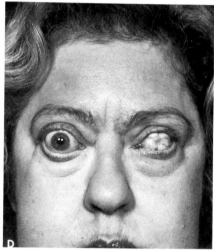
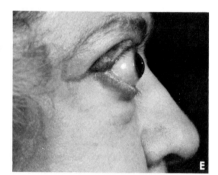

FIGURE 41–6. **Severe ophthalmopathy of Graves' disease.** *A,* Appearance when hyperthyroid with bilateral proptosis and moderate inflammatory changes; the patient was rendered euthyroid by treatment with [131]I. *B,* Appearance of eyes four years later. Two years previously the left eye became acutely inflamed, more proptotic, and was destroyed before medical attention was sought. The right eye acutely developed similar features in the 48 hours before the photograph was taken. Vision was reduced to distinguishing light and dark. *C,* Side view of right orbit. *D* and *E,* Views of the eyes after high-dosage corticosteroid therapy (initially 100 mg hydrocortisone IV every six hours, and subsequently prednisone, 100 mg daily orally, progressively withdrawn over three months). At this time, the patient has been without corticosteroid administration for over seven years and has normal vision and movement of the right eye. (From McKenzie JM, Zakarija M, Bonnyns M: Graves' disease. Med Clin North Am 59:1177, 1975.)

Acropachy

As shown in Figure 41–10, acropachy includes soft tissue swelling and underlying bone changes that may be seen on x-ray and may not be as rare as is usually considered.[128] When the bone is involved, there is subperiosteal new bone formation that may be identified both radiologically and histologically (Fig. 41–11).

Diagnostic Tests

Hyperthyroidism

Currently, the simplest, most cost-effective way of excluding hyperthyroidism of Graves' disease is by measurement of serum TSH (see Ch. 39); a normal value is incompatible with that diagnosis. On the other hand, while a suppressed value is to be expected in hyperthyroidism, there is a variable time period before TSH returns to normal after a euthyroid state has been achieved. Further confirmation of the diagnosis is usually readily achieved by measurement of circulating thyroid hormone concentrations, i.e., serum T_4 and T_3, together with a T_3 uptake test to estimate thyroxine-binding globulin (TBG). Elevated serum T_4 may reflect an increase in TBG that is familial, or due to estrogen as in pregnancy, or the use of an oral contraceptive preparation.

Many diagnosticians now rely on assessment of free hormones—fT_3 and/or fT_4—although there is still a problem of specificity of some of the methods used for their meas-

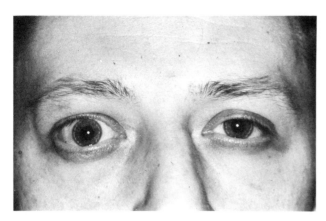

FIGURE 41–7. **Minimal degree of ophthalmopathy of Graves' disease.** Patient was a 23-year-old male with hyperthyroidism. There was lid retraction of the right eye with no other abnormality seen. Successful remission of hyperthyroidism followed treatment with propylthiouracil, and the lid retraction regressed spontaneously.

urement. If a reliable procedure is available, a supranormal value for fT_4 and/or fT_3, together with a suppressed value for TSH, unequivocally establishes the diagnosis of hyperthyroidism.

In hyperthyroidism the serum concentration of T_3 is almost always enhanced; the frequency of hyperthyroidism due to excess T_3 with a normal concentration of T_4 is uncertain but is clearly great enough (especially in patients who have been treated previously for the disease) to warrant measurement of T_3 in all those in whom clinical suspicion remains despite a normal value of serum T_4. On the other hand, the clinical picture of "T_3 toxicosis" is no different from that of the usual variety of hyperthyroidism, in which a supranormal concentration of T_4 in serum is found.

There is now no role for the measurement of the thyroid uptake of radioiodine in the routine confirmation of hyperthyroidism of Graves' disease; measurement of serum TSH, T_3, and T_4 is more cost-effective and convenient and less affected by extraneous influences such as iodide intake. However, it is an appropriate test when silent thyroiditis has to be confirmed or excluded, since the uptake in that syndrome should be approximately zero.

A thyroid suppression test, whether of uptake or release of radioiodine, is now rarely indicated. When more elaborate testing is required to establish or refute a diagnosis of hyperthyroidism of Graves' disease, a TRH test is convenient and, within limitations, effective. An increase in serum TSH within 15 to 30 min of the IV injection of 100 to 500 µg TRH indicates that the pituitary thyrotrope is not encountering an excess of thyroid hormone, i.e., there is no hyperthyroidism *at that time* (Fig. 41–12). Documenting a response has no relevance to prior status and is of restricted prognostic value. Furthermore, while it is typical of the hyperthyroid patient to show no response, the euthyroid subject similarly shows no increase in TSH for a variable time after hyperthyroidism has been treated. Thus the TRH test has to be used and results interpreted with due cognizance of the total clinical situation and pertinent laboratory data.

A hyperthyroid pregnant woman should have a suppressed serum TSH, as does the nonpregnant hyperthyroid subject. If further testing is indicated, a TRH test may be considered, but to reemphasize, current highly sensitive TSH assays have made this test virtually obsolete.

There are many other tests that have been applied to the diagnosis of hyperthyroidism. The basal metabolic rate (BMR) was among the most prestigious and still could serve a useful function, were not tests of greater accessibility and higher specificity readily available. BMR measure-

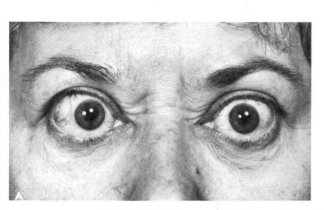
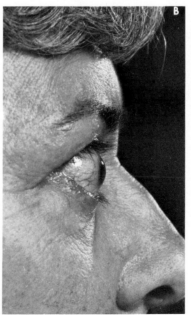
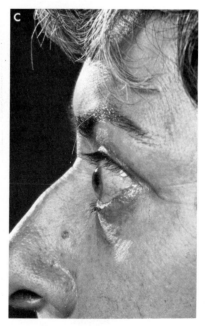

FIGURE 41–8. **Severe exophthalmos of Graves' disease.** There were minimal inflammatory changes but unequal proptosis, i.e., left eye 23 mm, right eye 28 mm. Treatment with oral prednisone, 60 mg daily, did not lead to improvement but to marked cushingoid features. Vision in the right eye was reduced to distinguishing finger movements. Return to normal vision, with little change in proptosis, was associated with four monthly injections of 40 mg methyl prednisolone into the right retro-orbital space.

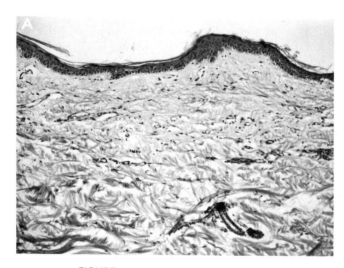
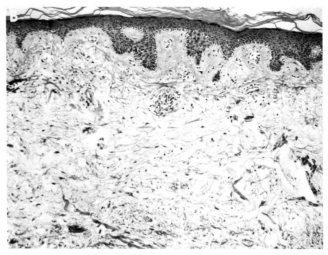

FIGURE 41–9. **Photomicrographs of skin** (hematoxylin and eosin, × 100). *A*, Normal skin. *B*, Skin from area of pretibial myxedema. Threads and granules of mucin are discernible, and there is separation of collagen bundles and individual fibers by mucin; the empty spaces are caused by shrinkage of the mucin during fixation and dehydration. (Courtesy of Dr. P. Schlopflocher.)

ment for diagnosis of hyperthyroidism, introduced over 60 years ago, was the standard diagnostic laboratory test in many centers for at least 30 years. The term is a misnomer in that the conditions under which the test is carried out are more "defined" than truly "basal," and it is oxygen consumption, not directly the rate of whole body metabolism, that is measured. Thus, while a common functional

definition of "basal" may be that the patient has fasted overnight and has rested, warm, quiet, and supine for at least 30 minutes, this does not prevent patient anxiety that can falsely elevate the measurement. It was common experience that values obtained on successive days, or at even longer intervals, in a euthyroid subject progressively fell for the first few readings. A "sedated" or "somnolent" meta-

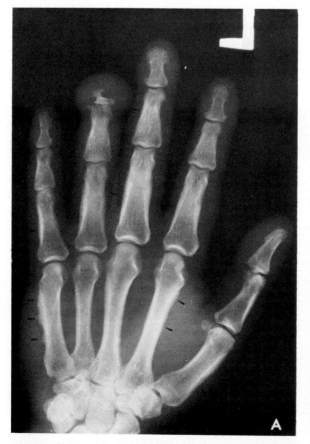
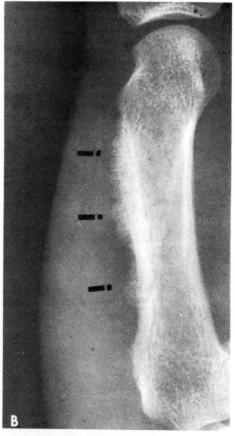

FIGURE 41–10. Radiographs of the left hand *(A)* and left fifth metacarpal *(B)* of the patient shown in Figure 41–5. Swelling of the terminal soft tissues and subperiosteal new bone formation are illustrated. (From McKenzie JM, Zakarija M, Bonnyns M: Graves' disease. Med Clin North Am 59:1177, 1975.)

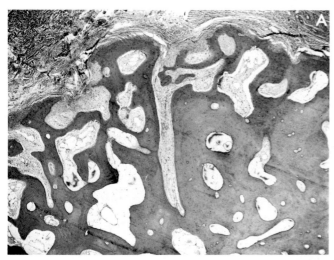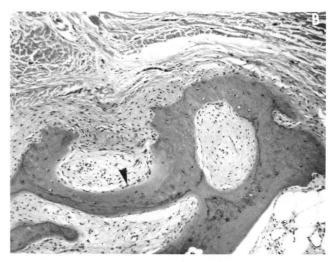

FIGURE 41–11. *A,* Photomicrograph of metacarpal cortex of the patient with acropachy shown in Figure 41–5. The outer surface of the cortex is irregular and presents spurlike processes (hematoxylin and eosin, × 25). *B,* Higher power (× 100) view. Formation of bone from the cambium layer is seen (arrowhead). (Courtesy of Dr. G. Tremblay.)

bolic rate, i.e., a measurement with the patient having ingested a sedative, was popular at one time. In any case, because of problems of reproducibility, diagnostic efficiency, and "through-put" time, costs, and patient convenience, the venerable BMR has been replaced by measurements of TSH, T_4, and T_3.

Of other tests that assess the peripheral effects of circulating thyroid hormones, the first is (mentioned only to be discarded) the determination of serum cholesterol, a time-honored test not otherwise meriting consideration in this context. Certainly any patient can have a lower concentration of blood cholesterol when hyperthyroid, but the other nonthyroid factors affecting this measurement are so numerous, and other tests are so much more specific, as now to render it worthless. Not much more useful is the record-

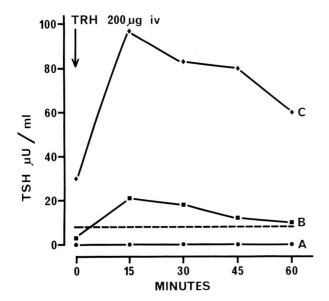

FIGURE 41–12. **Examples of thyrotropin (TSH) responses to thyrotropin-releasing hormone (TRH).** The interrupted line indicates the upper limit of the normal concentration of thyrotropin. Line A is typical of the absence of response seen in hyperthyroidism; line B is a normal response; and line C is the hyper-response found in primary thyroid insufficiency. TRH was given as a bolus injection IV.

ing of the ankle, or Achilles tendon, reflex time. Instruments are available to measure accurately, commonly in the form of a contraction-relaxation tracing, the rates of the various components of the reflex time. Usually the interval from the tapping of the tendon to the point of the curve denoting half-relaxation is measured. Normally, this phase takes from 270 to 330 msec. Although the procedure may have a place in confirming hypothyroidism, wherein the phase is prolonged, it is not clear that the discrimination is significantly greater than simple visual or tactile observation of the slowing of relaxation of the ankle or biceps jerk. The measure has minimal merit in confirming hyperthyroidism, even though the ankle jerk relaxation time is usually reduced.

More diagnostically efficacious are two indices of the effects of thyroid hormones on the cardiovascular system. The first to be described was the timing of Korotkoff arterial sounds with reference to the QRS complex of a simultaneously recorded electrocardiogram (EKG).[129] The QKd is the interval between the onset of the Q wave of the EKG and the beginning of the Korotkoff (K) sounds for that heartbeat; the latter is recorded by the microphone of a phonoarteriogram placed immediately distal to a sphygmomanometer cuff wrapped around the upper arm and inflated to the equivalent of the diastolic pressure. QKd thus reflects cardiac and vascular factors, i.e., myocardial contractility and the time for transmission of the pulse wave to the brachial artery, and therefore is an assessment of the effect of thyroid hormones on myocardium, peripheral arterial vessels, and blood viscosity. In normal subjects the range is from 186 to 235 msec. Similar data were published in Japan,[130] and QKd in hyperthyroidism was shown to correlate inversely with total or free T_4 or T_3 to a minimal value of about 165 msec.

A somewhat comparable noninvasive technique concentrates on measurements of myocardial contractility.[131] By simultaneous recordings of the carotid pulse, EKG and phonocardiogram, systolic time intervals corrected for heart rate can be readily assessed (Fig. 41–13). It was shown that the period between electrical depolarization of the left ventricle, i.e., beginning of the Q wave on the EKG, and the first heart sound was affected by hyperthyroidism

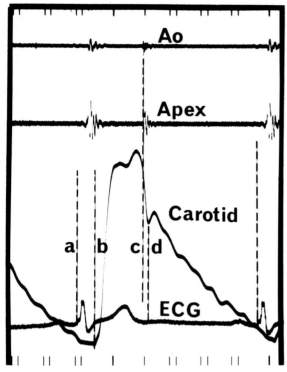

FIGURE 41–13. **Measurement of systolic time intervals.** From top to bottom, the tracings are as follows: Phonocardiograms with the microphone placed over the aortic valve (Ao) or apical (Apex) areas of the heart; carotid artery pulse tracing; lead 2 of the electrocardiogram (ECG). The vertical lines along the top and bottom edges indicate time in intervals of 0.04 sec. The interrupted vertical lines were drawn to intercept specific events on the tracing to facilitate measurements; a, q wave of ECG; b, opening of aortic valve; c, beginning of second aortic sound; d, closure of aortic valve, i.e., dicrotic notch. Left ventricular ejection time (LVET) = b to d; this may be corrected for heart rate by adding 0.0016 × heart rate. Pre-ejection period = (a to c) less LVET. (Data courtesy of Dr. L. Dragatakis.)

in Graves' disease,[136] there is the added convenience of simultaneously examining the heart for this lesion, the presence of which may in itself be associated with palpitations, tachycardia, and other cardiac arrhythmias that potentially complicate the clinical evaluation.

These measures of cardiovascular responses (QKd, systolic time intervals, and the velocity of circumferential fiber shortening) appear to be meaningful assessments of end-organ effects of thyroid hormones. However, their roles in diagnostic evaluation of the borderline hyperthyroid patient have not been established. In the reported observations,[129–135] apparently unequivocally hyperthyroid subjects were studied. There has been no description of use of these tests in the patient in whom the diagnosis is uncertain and no attempt to compare diagnostic efficiency of the procedures in marginal clinical states with more commonly used measurements such as serum TSH and T_4, although a linear correlation was shown between the velocity of circumferential fiber shortening and serum T_3 and T_4 concentrations. Furthermore, the techniques are not seen as specific for the consequences of hyperthyroidism; a short pre-ejection period is recognized in aortic valvular disease and as a consequence of the action of epinephrine.[131] Similarly, QKd is apparently affected by catecholamines and is known to be altered in aortic valvular and some other cardiovascular diseases.[129] However, if more information regarding the significance of these tests accrues, one area of therapy of hyperthyroidism in which either might be particularly useful could be in the pregnant hyperthyroid patient. As discussed below, minimal antithyroid drug therapy is the aim, and this can be difficult to achieve in view of the metabolic consequences of pregnancy. As of this writing no such studies have been

to only a minor degree, but the isovolumic contraction time (interval from the beginning of the first heart sound to the opening of the aortic valve) was impressively shortened. These measures reflect myocardial contractility known to be specifically enhanced by thyroid hormones. Thus, calculation of the isovolumic contraction time or of the total pre-ejection period (beginning of the Q wave to the opening of the aortic valve) was applied to the assessment of thyroid status. The pre-ejection period was shown[131] to vary directly with the concentration of serum T_4 in a group of patients studied when hyperthyroid and then when euthyroid and also longitudinally in individual subjects assessed as they responded to therapy.

Echocardiography has similarly been applied to assess left ventricular systolic and diastolic function in thyroid disease[132–135] with comparable measurements (Fig. 41–14) and conclusions. Although one group did not find statistically significant shortening of the pre-ejection period in hyperthyroidism by this technique,[133] unlike observations by others,[132, 134, 135] there is overall agreement that systolic time intervals and other measurements, such as the velocity of circumferential fiber shortening, well reflect the thyroid status. Because echocardiography, carried out by trained technical personnel, is so readily available, it is probably the procedure of choice for these assessments. Moreover, since prolapsed mitral valve occurs with undue frequency

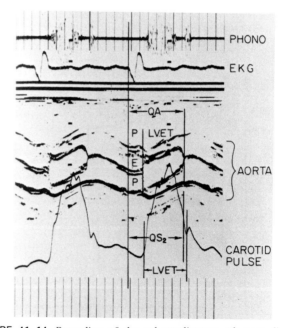

FIGURE 41–14. Recording of the echocardiogram, phonocardiogram (phono), electrocardiogram (EKG), and carotid pulse illustrates the **STI derived from echo and carotid pulse tracing** at a paper speed of 125 mm sec. QA, Electromechanical systole by echo; QS_2, electromechanical systole by carotid pulse tracing; LVET, left ventricular ejection times; PEP, pre-ejection period. (From Hirschfeld S, Meyer R, Schwartz DC, et al: Measurement of right and left ventricular systolic time intervals by echocardiography. Circulation 51:304, 1975. Reprinted by permission of the American Heart Association, Inc.)

reported, but it seems likely that these assessments could have a worthwhile role in the management of such patients, if normal values for the euthyroid pregnant subject are established.

A laboratory procedure that is of minimal diagnostic benefit but that is commonly used to evaluate hyperthyroid patients is the measurement of antithyroid antibodies. Although several antibodies, both organ-specific (to thyroglobulin, to the second colloid antigen, and to the thyroid microsomal antigen [thyroid peroxidase]) and non–organ-specific (to nuclei and mitochondria), have been described, assays of only two, i.e., antibodies to thyroglobulin and to thyroid peroxidase (TPO), are widely used. There is widespread use of kits that provide an effective procedure for antibodies to both of these antigens. Experience has shown that most patients with hyperthyroidism of Graves' disease test positive for antibody to TPO, and the incidence of antibody to thyroglobulin as so measured is appreciably lower in both Graves' and Hashimoto's diseases. Indeed, the occurrence of antibody to thyroglobulin and not to TPO is so infrequent that it probably is appropriate in routine clinical practice to test solely for anti-TPO.

The interpretation of antibody titers in the blood of a patient with hyperthyroidism is, as already stated, of limited clinical use. If there is uncertainty as to whether the diagnosis is toxic adenoma or Graves' disease, the presence of antibodies strongly substantiates the latter. Circumstantial support for a diagnosis of Graves' disease in instances of euthyroid ophthalmopathy also is useful, as elaborated below. However, the identification of antithyroid antibodies per se in no way reflects the degree of thyroid function, be that enhanced or reduced, and the only manner in which knowledge of the titer of circulating antibodies affects clinical management is that a high titer of either system identifies the coexistence of significant Hashimoto's thyroiditis. If Hashimoto's disease is present, this may indicate that hypothyroidism will follow ablative therapy for hyperthyroidism even more rapidly than usual. It does not appear, however, that the existence of Hashimoto's disease influences the outcome of a course of antithyroid therapy of conventional duration (see below). Consequently, since a decision for or against ablative therapy of hyperthyroidism is probably made from more cogent considerations than the possible hastening of inevitable hypothyroidism, the measurement of antithyroid antibodies has little but a curiosity role in routine management of the hyperthyroid patient with Graves' disease.

Ophthalmopathy (reviewed in detail in Ch. 42)

As implied earlier, exophthalmos occurs as a diagnostic problem essentially only when there is no hyperthyroidism. In such cases, the existence of alternative pathology must be excluded; at the same time, accrual of evidence supporting the presence of Graves' disease is comforting for the physician. Thus, sometimes a TRH test or measure of TSAb or other thyroid antibodies may be indicated. A positive test (i.e., no response to TRH, or the presence in serum of TSAb or of antibodies to TPO) is circumstantial support for the diagnosis. In our experience measurement of the antibody to TPO is the most cost-effective and correlates well with the other data. One group[137] has explored

the feasibility of measuring circulating antibody to eye muscle antigen to confirm autoimmune ophthalmopathy or even to predict its appearance. This is an interesting area that no doubt will be thoroughly evaluated in the next few years.

Orbital sonography, CT, and magnetic resonance imaging are now routine effective procedures in identifying enlargement of extraocular muscles (Figs. 41–15 and 41–16). The techniques can establish abnormalities in advance of overt symptoms or signs of ophthalmopathy. They are, thus, extremely useful in confirming that proptosis and extraocular muscle paresis are due to changes typical of Graves' disease or are related to other orbital or intracranial pathology.

Although little experience has yet been reported, it is most likely that magnetic resonance imaging will contribute information regarding metabolic activity in the underlying inflammatory processes, i.e., enable a decision as to whether ophthalmopathy is in a still-progressive or "burnt-out" phase. This is an important conclusion in that corrective eye muscle surgery is likely to be most successful when it is carried out on tissue that is fibrotic rather than the site of ongoing inflammation.

A mistaken associated diagnosis, not uncommonly made in the patient with ophthalmopathic disease, particularly when inferior oblique muscles are fibrosed and shortened, is increased intraocular pressure or glaucoma. This misdiagnosis results from the pressure measurement being taken with the patient having to try to rotate the globe superiorly against the inextensible muscle, and indeed the pressure is supranormal. However, if care is taken to measure intraocular pressure with the globe in the neutral position, a true reading may be obtained.

Pretibial Myxedema and Acropachy

Figures 41–5, 41–10, and 41–17 illustrate examples of these conditions. Unusual enough in themselves, these conditions very rarely occur in the absence of other features of Graves' disease. The histological appearance of either state is said to be characteristic (Figs. 41–9 and 41–11), but probably too little experience of atypical examples has been gathered for a dogmatic opinion to be given with total assurance.

In the absence of hyperthyroidism and ophthalmopathy, the differential diagnosis of pretibial myxedema includes a variety of papular mucinoses, including lichen myxedematosus. As noted earlier, this condition is often associated with the presence in serum of an abnormal immunoglobulin. On the other hand, pretibial myxedema usually occurs with TSAb in the blood, although there are no reports of attempts to measure TSAb in a series of patients with the skin condition occurring in the absence of other features of Graves' disease.

For acropachy, the differential diagnosis includes acromegaly, pulmonary hypertrophic osteoarthropathy, and the similar states associated with malignancy. The other features of these diseases and the close association of acropachy with hyperthyroidism, ophthalmopathy, and pretibial myxedema ought to render the diagnosis clear, at least after appropriate investigations are undertaken. One diagnostic procedure that apparently provides fairly specific indications of acropachy is scintigraphic scanning of the

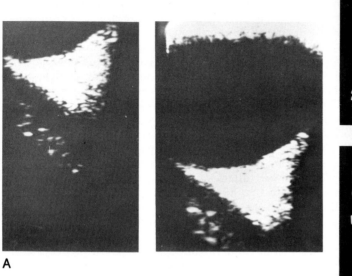

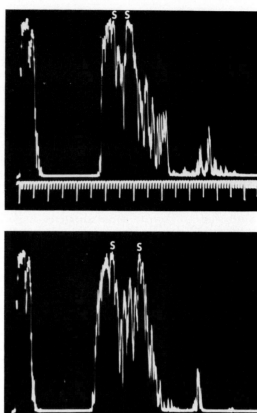

FIGURE 41–15. *A,* **Retro-orbital sonograms (B mode) in two patients with ophthalmopathy of Graves' disease.** The large triangular white patches reflect the retro-orbital fat pads and the oblique sequences of white spots the orbital wall. Normally there is no appreciable space between these structures and in these examples the space signifies swollen extraocular muscles. *B,* Retro-orbital sonogram (A mode) showing normal diameter of medial rectus *(top)* and enlarged medial rectus *(bottom)* in patient with ophthalmopathy. S, Muscle sheath. (*B* courtesy of Dr. Joel Glaser.)

appropriate regions after the intravenous injection of (99m) Tc-pyrophosphate.[138] The findings that distinguish it from other possibly similar abnormalities of the extremities include localization of the radioactive tracer to the diaphyseal regions of the bones, not the articular zones, and the rarity of involvement of the long bones. This skeletal scintigraphy was shown to be more sensitive than conventional radiography in that uptake of tracer occurred in phalangeal regions that were normal by x-ray. Of additional interest was the fact that areas of pretibial myxedema were found to concentrate (99m) Tc-pyrophosphate.[138]

Treatment

Hyperthyroidism

For treatment of hyperthyroidism five possibilities may be entertained: antithyroid drugs, radioiodine, surgical partial resection of the thyroid, iodide, and a combination of β-blockade and sedation. The last is probably indicated only in the mildest instances of hyperthyroidism, as is the use of iodide alone. Since long-term iodide administration can lead to exacerbation of hyperthyroidism, the use of an agent such as propranolol that blocks β-adrenergic receptors is probably safer for the symptomatic management of

the mild case. An attempt has been made to use propranolol as definitive therapy in an unselected group of patients,[139] but the outcome of that experience was not encouraging; only 4 of 21 adequately treated patients entered remission. As will be referred to again, propranolol, in addition to reducing heart rate by an effect in the myocardium, also decreases the rate of peripheral deiodination of T_4; this is an action duplicated by other β-blockers such as alprenolol, atenolol, and metoprolol, but not sotalol.[140] This peripheral effect is of therapeutic advantage only in the initial stages of treatment of the more severely thyrotoxic patient.

Iodide continues to have a place in the immediate preoperative care of patients about to undergo subtotal thyroidectomy for Graves' disease. Another indication for its use has been identified in the control of hyperthyroidism in patients to whom a therapeutic dose of ^{131}I has been given; the response to the radioisotope therapy may be delayed several weeks, and during this phase the thyroid appears to be particularly sensitive to the quieting effect of iodide and does not readily escape from that influence.[141] Sensitivity is such that the patient may become hypothyroid while taking the iodide. The dose commonly prescribed may more often be dictated by tradition than by objective evidence of that required for a desired effect. One milliliter of Lugol's solution or about 10 drops of saturated solution of potassium iodide per day is commonly prescribed.

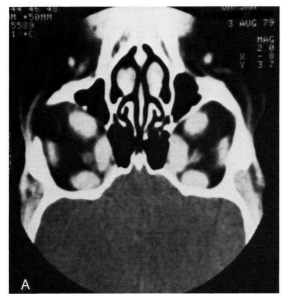

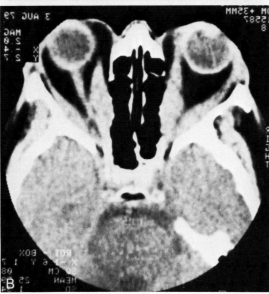

FIGURE 41–16. CT scans of orbital muscles of patient with ophthalmopathy. *A,* Coronal view, showing bilateral enlarged medial, inferior, and superior oblique and lateral recti. *B,* Axial view, showing bilateral enlarged medial and lateral recti. (Courtesy of Dr. Joel Glaser.)

The optimal quantity required to suppress thyroid function in hyperthyroidism was shown 40 years ago to be about 6 mg/day.[142] Since Lugol's solution contains 100 mg KI/ml and 50 mgI_2/ml and saturated solution of potassium iodide contains 750 mg/ml, the usual daily prescriptions result in approximately 150 mg and 375 mg, respectively. Even 1 drop twice daily of saturated solution of potassium iodide (i.e., about 75 mg iodide) will provide a major excess over that required for a satisfactory therapeutic response but will cause less comment than the prescribing of a smaller dose.

An interesting approach to treatment with iodide has been the use of a radiopaque dye, ipodate (Oragrafin), that was shown to influence thyroid function apparently directly but also to reduce the rate of peripheral production of T_3 from T_4.[143] The latter action presumably is due to the organic molecule itself and the former, i.e., the slowing of the release of hormone from the thyroid gland, reflects iodide availability from the metabolism of the ipodate. Although ipodate, or the related compound opanoate, has indeed been shown to control thyroid function in Graves' disease, this has been in only a minority of the patients studied[144, 145]; a beneficial long-term effect, particularly the induction of permanent remission, seems unlikely.

Lithium carbonate has been used for decades in the treatment of manic-depressive disease. Within the last 20 years an antithyroid effect of the cation has been recognized, and there has been study of its possible use in hyperthyroidism.[146] In a dosage of 900 to 1500 mg/day, resulting in 0.6 to 1.2 mEq lithium per liter of serum, effects comparable to those expected from the administration of iodide were observed; that is, the release of thyroid hormone was abruptly slowed with consequent decrease in the serum concentrations of T_4 and T_3. There was also an effect not seen with iodide, namely a slowing of the rate of metabolism of circulating hormones. It seems clear that the lithium ion can be used effectively, preferably in combination with a thionamide, to bring hyperthyroidism rapidly under control. However, the required serum concentration is about 1 mEq/L, at which level toxic effects such as nausea and vomiting, changes in the EKG, and other reactions are common; more serious toxicity, including coma and grand mal seizures, has been reported with little more than twice this concentration.[146] Consequently, it seems that lithium salts ought to be retained as therapy of hyperthyroidism only for the exceptional patient requiring rapid return to a euthyroid state and in whom iodide hypersensitivity rules out the use of that agent. Since the use of lithium specifically in thyroid storm has not been assessed, one would be most loath to administer the cation in that situation, in which undue sensitivity to the toxic effects might exist.

For the three major forms of treatment—antithyroid drugs, radioiodine, and surgery—the choice is influenced greatly by individual experience. This was recently emphasized by comparison of the reported preferences in the United States, Japan, and Europe.[147] For instance, administration of ^{131}I was chosen as primary therapy by 69 per cent of surveyed Americans, 22 per cent of European physicians, and only 11 per cent of those in Japan. Antithyroid drug was the preferred treatment by 30, 77, and 90 per cent of these groups, respectively. The one point of unanimity was in the lack of enthusiasm for subtotal thyroidectomy in all three geographic areas. These variations, which certainly do not reflect significantly different qualities of care, emphasize the fact that there is no absolute "right" in therapeutic decisions.

Even internationally these three major forms of treatment have need for an experienced therapist, but this is most evident with surgical partial resection of the thyroid. Apart from the outcome with regard to the hyperthyroidism, the morbidity, including hypoparathyroidism and recurrent laryngeal nerve damage, resulting from operation by other than the truly competent thyroid surgeon is unacceptable.[148] When an experienced surgeon is available, results judged as "euthyroid after 10 years" are probably as good as for therapy with ^{131}I,[149] that is, by either treatment, approximately 60 per cent of patients will be euthyroid, the remainder suffering relapse or becoming hypothyroid. Therefore, if ablative therapy is called for, the decision for either surgery or ^{131}I will usually be reached on largely nonclinical grounds, including the local surgical

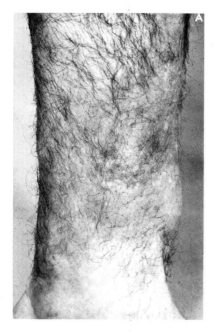
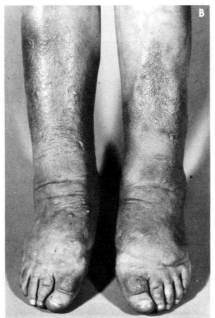
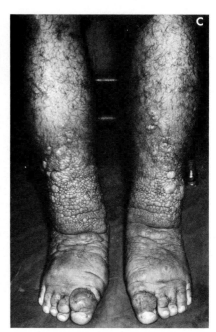
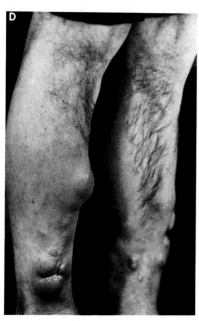

FIGURE 41–17. **Legs of patients with pretibial myxedema.** All are characteristic in being bilateral and fairly symmetrical. Extension to the dorsa of the feet *(B and C)* is unusual. *A,* Typical appearance showing prominent hair follicles in the plaque of involved skin and sharp demarcation with normal skin. *B,* The shiny appearance of the indurated skin is characteristic. *C,* Unusual micronodular form. Exaggeration of the joint creases (also seen in *B*) is common. *D,* The tuberous or macronodular form is also unusual. (From McKenzie JM, Zakarija M, Bonnyns M: Graves' disease. Med Clin North Am 59:1177, 1975.)

prowess, the patient's often already established fear of either surgery or radioiodine, and economic and family factors. Of the clinical contributions to the choice, the size of the goiter is, at times, decisive in that reduction of a large, especially multinodular, gland is not to be expected with radioiodine therapy. One other consideration might be the recognition of a "cold" nodule within a Graves' disease goiter. This has been reported[150] to have an incidence of malignancy almost twice that found in non-Graves' subjects with similar lesions, so that subtotal thyroidectomy may be the preferred therapy in this situation.

Preoperative preparation of the hyperthyroid patient generally includes a combination of thionamide and iodide, and although it may be considered a routine prescription, it must be individualized. The thionamide (the choice of which drug and the dosage are discussed later) ought to be given until the patient is euthyroid; since this varies from at least 3 to 6 weeks and may take longer, it is

clear that the intended date for the operation ought to be calculated only provisionally at the initiation of therapy. Treatment with thionamides has the reputation of increasing thyroid vascularity, but it may be that this view is based on examples of overtreatment. Certainly the stimulus of endogenous thyrotropin, when thionamide action is excessive and induces hypothyroidism, complementing effects of TSAb, results in increased vascularity, but whether this occurs with more controlled therapy is not clear. However, we may accept that the very vascular Graves' disease gland does not have reduced blood supply as a result of administration of thionamides, so that additional therapy to diminish vascularity is desirable. Iodide has been the empirical therapy for this purpose for generations, but objective quantitative assessment of its efficiency is comparatively recent. By use of the thyroid uptake of thallium-201, thyroid vascular perfusion was estimated to fall an average of 33 per cent with iodide administration in patients with

Graves' disease.[151] In practice, iodide (e.g., 1 drop saturated solution of KI twice daily) is usually given as well as thionamide for 7 to 10 days immediately preoperatively. To re-emphasize the point, it is only with the decision to initiate iodide therapy that operation should be scheduled.

Propranolol has been used both as adjuvant and as sole preoperative therapy. In a dose of 10 to 30 mg every 8 hours, it will slow the heart rate if this has not already been achieved by thionamide and iodide, but it probably has no effect on thyroid vascularity. Thus, its role in this context is in the rare patient who is so hypersensitive to thionamides or iodide or both that the conventional preparation for surgery is not feasible or when for adjunctive circumstance operation is needed before thionamide and iodide can produce their effects. If propranolol is to be used preoperatively, it is important that the anesthesiologist be so informed in order to accommodate the cardiovascular consequences of anesthesia.

It is now recognized that the majority of patients treated by either radioiodine or subtotal thyroidectomy can expect to become hypothyroid if they live long enough,[149] and this constitutes the major argument for the use of antithyroid drugs initially in those with good life expectancy—patients less than 40 years old. Unfortunately, probably no more than 25 per cent of those treated with antithyroid drugs for 6 months or more will enter long-term remission, and the major drawback is the apparent impossibility of identifying the "remitters" or "relapsers" in advance. A thyroid suppression test was used to try to identify those who will remain in remission after a course of antithyroid drugs. Experience from this laboratory is probably representative.[152] As shown in Figure 41–18, we found that at the end of a course of antithyroid drugs, 50 per cent of patients with suppressible thyroid function had relapse, usually within a few months; of those with nonsuppressible function, 78 per cent had relapse, so that such a result offers a fairly reliable index of prognosis, i.e., relapse, but the overall return from the test is such that it cannot be recommended as a routine procedure. As a possible alternative to a suppression test for prognosis, attempts have been made to use the TRH test at the end of a course of propylthiouracil therapy.

In this instance the TRH test is carried out at least 1 week after cessation of antithyroid drug therapy; a normal thyrotropin response is taken as indicating a physiological situation, and a subnormal or absent response indicates persistence of abnormality. Unfortunately, experience has failed to confirm initial indications of this test's value in prognostication and it probably has no more reliability than a suppression test. Moreover, current assays for TSH have a sensitivity that makes it possible to separate values into three important categories.[153, 154] These comprise a range of normal concentrations, subnormal values that indicate TSH suppression (as may be intended in treatment of goiter), and unmeasurable TSH. The last category is expected in hyperthyroidism; it is also the aim in thyroxine therapy of thyroid cancer, and, in either situation, there is no TSH response to injected TRH.[153]

As described earlier, measurements of TSAb at the end of a course of antithyroid drugs is a significantly better procedure for forecasting outcome, at least with the thyroid-stimulation type of assay.[99] With increasing commercial availability of TSAb measurements, no doubt its use in management of patients in this way will become more common. However, for the majority, there is probably little to be gained over the conventional practice of completing a course of antithyroid drug and then maintaining clinical evaluation to assess relapse, which most commonly occurs within two to three months, or long-term remission.

Initially the choice of a particular antithyroid drug of the thionamide type was of little consequence; familiarity with dosage and adverse reactions (fairly common to all of them) was of more importance. Now, however, there is a significant difference in action to be considered, exemplified by comparison of propylthiouracil with methimazole. It has been known for over 30 years that in addition to actions on the thyroid gland that interfere with synthesis of thyroid hormones, propylthiouracil reduces the rate of peripheral deiodination of thyroxine. In the last 20 years this pharmacological effect has come into renewed focus with the recognition of the major significance of such deiodination in the extrathyroid production of triiodothyronine, an action that is enhanced in hyperthyroidism.[155] The implications of these facts have been proved and quantitated, showing that propylthiouracil administration reduces the peripheral concentration of triiodothyronine in hyperthyroidism faster than does methimazole.[155] While this effect may be of little clinical significance in long-term management of the hyperthyroid subject, the advisability of taking advantage of the antideiodinating property of propylthiouracil in severe hyperthyroidism (especially thyroid storm) seems obvious.

The optimal dosage of antithyroid drug, on average, was early established, and for the drugs commonly used in North America, 300 mg propylthiouracil or 30 mg methimazole per day is generally effective in controlling the clinical state within four to eight weeks. For hyperthyroidism that is especially severe, a larger dosage, up to, for instance, 800 mg propylthiouracil per day, may be instituted. Practices differ in the timing in which the initial dosage is reduced or in which thyroid hormone is added. Certainly, any patient may be rendered hypothyroid by a large enough dosage of antithyroid drug for a sufficient length of time, but how rapidly this occurs appears to vary widely. Our routine has been to start patients on 100 mg propylthiouracil every 8 hours, 150 or 200 mg being reserved for the more severely ill patients. (A six-hourly dosage does not seem to be advisable in view of the therapeu-

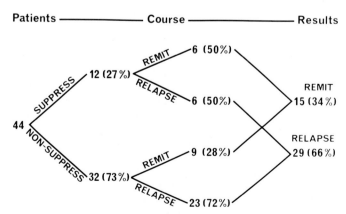

FIGURE 41–18. **Diagrammatic synopsis of experience with thyroid suppression tests** in the management of patients with hyperthyroidism of Graves' disease. All patients were treated with propylthiouracil for 6 to 12 months.

tic benefit of "a good night's sleep" that might have to be interrupted for the medication). Whether it is the initial dosage or one that is reached early in the course of therapy after an earlier higher dosage, up to 300 mg propylthiouracil is appropriate for many patients for a full course that is currently defined by us as lasting twelve months. Perhaps the earliest sign of overdosage is increase in the size of goiter, which no doubt reflects pituitary secretion of thyrotropin in response to a crucial reduction in the concentration of circulating thyroid hormones; at this point the prescription of thyroid hormone, e.g., 0.1 mg L-T_4 per day, is added to the regimen for the rest of the course. (Reduction in the dose of propylthiouracil is as logical but often more difficult to quantitate.)

One group has claimed a significantly higher rate of remission of hyperthyroidism by continued use for up to two years of three to four times the conventional dosage of thionamide and preventing hypothyroidism by the concomitant administration of T_4.[156] This approach is largely based on the indications that antithyroid drugs may influence Graves' disease by being concentrated in the thyroid gland and there having an immunosuppressive effect on the production of TSAb[157] through an action on accessory cells.[158] This implies that the thyroid is an important, if not the major, site of synthesis of TSAb (a debatable point) and the high-dose routine[156] is compatible with the concept that a larger intrathyroid concentration of thionamide is more effective as an immunosuppressant. However, until the theory is better substantiated and the clinical data are confirmed by others, the use of high-dose thionamide cannot be recommended as routine clinical practice. Indeed an alternate theory of a favorable thionamide effect on the immune system, postulating the development of anti-idiotype to TSAb associated with an increase in peripheral T-helper cells, was formulated from data obtained with use of a conventional dose of thionamide.[159] Another group reported that thyroxine administration, starting six months after the initiation of thionamide therapy and continuing for three years after cessation of that drug, led to a major increase in the remission rate, associated with a decrease in circulating TSAb.[79] The hypothesis was offered that suppression of TSH by the thyroxine, so "reducing the expression of thyroid antigens"—including the TSH receptor, resulted in the better rate of remission. This is an intriguing approach that no doubt will be tested by others in the near future.

Other theories have been promulgated in an attempt to understand a thionamide-induced remission of Graves' hyperthyroidism. For instance, in one study[159a] activated, i.e., DR expressing, T cells in the peripheral blood of patients with Graves' disease were monitored during therapy. A reduction in helper cells and an increase in suppressor cells were noted as the patients' hyperthyroidism came under control. While such observations could be attributed to the effect of methimazole on the immune system, other investigators[110] have emphasized that such changes may be due to the restoration of a euthyroid state, rather than a direct effect of the thionamide. Distributing the dosage of propylthiouracil over equal intervals of time throughout the day was warranted by early evidence that the average duration of action of the drug as measured by inhibition of radioiodine uptake was only a few hours. However, Greer and colleagues reported several years ago[160] that 300 mg propylthiouracil once a day was appropriate for effective therapy of most hyperthyroid patients; they have continued to have success with this routine (or 30 mg methimazole once daily), as have a few other clinics. A possible explanation for this experience might be that in thyroid hormonogenesis the point most sensitive to the action of propylthiouracil is the coupling of iodotyrosines; a continuing action of the drug (that is actively concentrated by the thyroid gland) at this step over most of 24 hours would effectively reduce thyroid hormone formation but would not be reflected for the same length of time in changes in the uptake of radioiodine. Certainly the routine of a once-a-day dosage has much to recommend it in the management of probably a majority of patients.

The possibility of identifying in advance those patients who can have their hyperthyroidism controlled by a single daily dose of antithyroid drug has been examined.[161] Persistence of a block of organification of iodide was confirmed by performing a perchlorate test 12 or 20 hours after a dose of propylthiouracil or methimazole. The studies showed that if 69 per cent of thyroid radioiodine was discharged by perchlorate at the 12-hour point, or 25 per cent at the 20-hour point, a single daily dose of thionamide was appropriate; in the series of 62 patients, the condition in 42 (68 per cent) was found to be adequately controlled by the once-a-day routine.

A course of antithyroid medication has never been defined on the basis of objective data that show the merit of a particular duration of administration of the drugs. Somehow it has become accepted that one to two years of control of hyperthyroidism is probably required to have a reasonable expectation of the patient remaining in remission when the medication is finally stopped. A few investigators have questioned the wisdom of the course of treatment routinely being of such duration. Alexander and colleagues[162] showed that the incidence of development of suppressible thyroid function in patients treated with carbimazole and triiodothyronine was as great after only six months of therapy as with longer treatment. Greer and his colleagues have described long-term remission of hyperthyroidism after antithyroid drugs were taken only for the few weeks required to produce and confirm a euthyroid state.[163] Thus, it seems very likely that most patients who are treated for one to two years gain little from a more prolonged course of therapy.

At present, when antithyroid drugs are used, it is common practice to accept that relapse after one course of therapy means that the likelihood of permanent remission after a second or subsequent course has sufficiently low expectation that alternate treatment, i.e., radioiodine therapy or subtotal thyroidectomy, is indicated. For those following this design of patient management, it is obvious that a decision regarding the probable success of the initial course of therapy ought to be reached as soon as possible. If the implication of the aforementioned reports[162, 163] that six months or less of drug therapy is as efficacious as longer courses is confirmed, there would be little justification for the regimens of 1 to 2 years currently in vogue.

If a laboratory index were available to identify, before stopping therapy, those patients who were truly cured, i.e., who would remain in remission without drugs, there would be a rational basis for choosing the duration of antithyroid drugs. As indicated earlier, a thyroid suppression or TRH test seems to have limited applicability in this regard. There is major expectation, however, that one of the methods for measuring TSAb will develop into the desired index of prognostication, in which case the following plan of management might be established: Antithyroid drugs will be prescribed to achieve a euthyroid state and then maintained for up to a year with, at the end, measurement of TSAb or some other, if more sensitive, marker of a continuing autoimmune state. Disappearance of the antibody from the patient's serum will be taken as a sign that remission (in fact, an immunological remission) has occurred, whereas persistence of the antibody will indicate the advisability of seriously considering a change to radioiodine therapy or subtotal thyroidectomy. However, until research developments provide the methods for both validating and making readily available such management, we recommend the following regimen in the routine care of patients with hyperthyroidism of Graves' disease.

1. Administer propylthiouracil (or similar thionamide) in appropriate dosage as discussed above, i.e., usually 100 mg every 8 hours or 300 mg once daily, for 12 months with care to identify the development of hypothyroidism, which seldom occurs within the first three months.

2. Stop therapy and maintain observation, with decreasing frequency of patient visit, for the relapse of hyperthyroidism. In our experience, of those destined to suffer relapse, 75 per cent have done so within three months and 90 per cent within two years. Thereafter, it might be more appropriate to refer to a recurrence, rather than a relapse, of the disease if hyperthyroidism appears.

The incidence of relapse (or recurrence) after antithyroid drug therapy is frequently a topic of debate, and it may be that it truly varies according to many factors apart from the natural course of the disease. The selection of the type of patient to be so treated is one; if only those with milder symptoms, with a small goiter, and having hyperthyroidism for the first time are offered antithyroid drug therapy, the incidence of prolonged remission will be greater than if there is no selection. Patients with more severe disease (including the complications of troublesome ophthalmopathy and pretibial myxedema), with a larger goiter, or with a previous episode of hyperthyroidism are more likely to have relapse after antithyroid drug treatment. Second, the iodine intake of the patient population studied appears to be an important influence, as was shown in a controlled investigation by Alexander and colleagues[85]; the incidence of relapse in 16 patients given an iodide supplement on stopping thionamide was 56 per cent, whereas only 27 per cent of 41 non–iodide-supplemented patients, otherwise identically treated, had relapse. In a similar vein, increasing intake of iodine by the North American population over the preceding 10 years was an explanation offered by Wartofsky[164] for the steady drop in the rate of remission reported over that length of time (Fig. 41–19). A more recent report from the same group[165] indicated that this trend may have been reversed; average iodine intake in the United States has decreased and the proportion of patients who are treated with a thinonamide and who enter remission may have increased. Thus, there may be a geographic influence on iodine intake that affects success, that is, the rate of long-term remission, in the use of antithyroid drugs.

As alluded to earlier, the incidence of adverse reactions to the thionamide drugs commonly used today—i.e., pro-

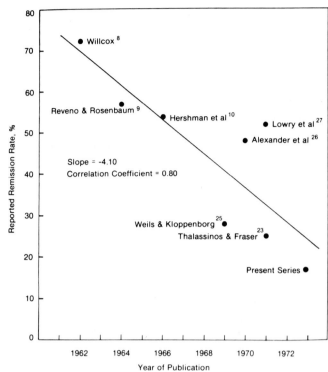

FIGURE 41–19. Falling incidence of remission rate as reported in publications from 1962 through 1973. (From Wartofsky L: Low remission after therapy for Graves' disease. Possible relation of dietary iodine with antithyroid therapy results. JAMA 226:1083, 1973. Copyright 1973, American Medical Association, with permission. The small superscripts in the figure identify the publications as quoted in that paper.)

pylthiouracil, methylthiouracil, methimazole, and carbimazole—is of a closely similar low frequency, especially if only the more serious complications are considered. Pruritus, with or without a skin eruption, may be alleviated by administration of antihistamines and change to an alternate thionamide. As may be judged from Figure 41–20, there is more likelihood of success if the change is from a uracil compound (methylthiouracil or propylthiouracil) to an imidazole (methimazole or carbimazole), or vice versa, rather than within the two subgroups of thionamides. The major side effect of these drugs is granulocytopenia, which may advance to agranulocytosis and which usually seems to occur early in a patient's exposure to the drug. No precise cause of this complication, occurring in about 0.02 per cent of patients, is known in that no evidence has been found for direct cytotoxicity on either circulating granulo-

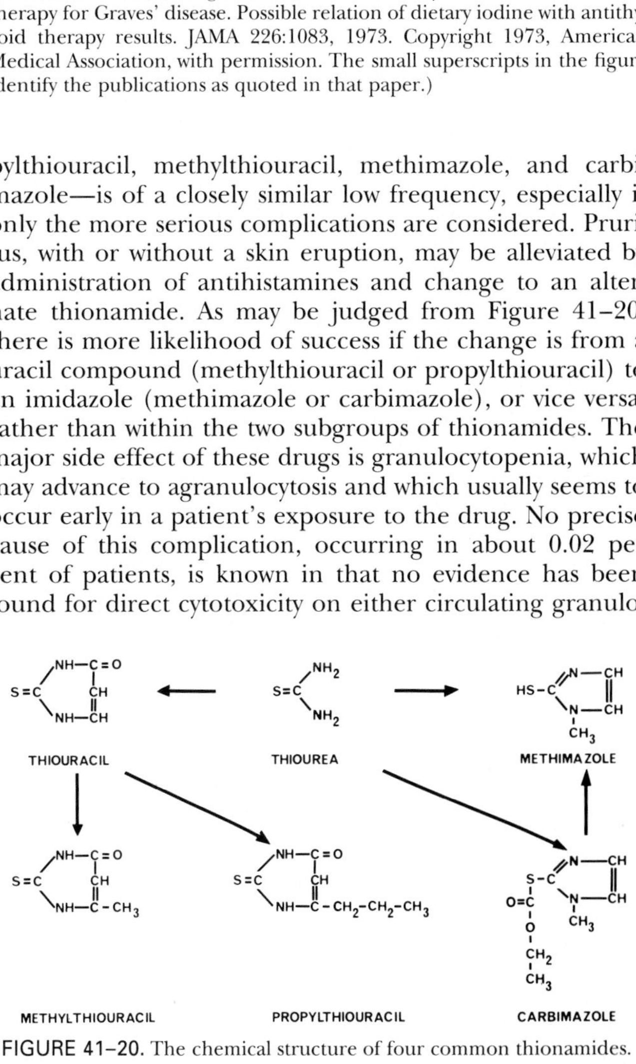

FIGURE 41–20. The chemical structure of four common thionamides.

cytes or bone marrow. If the offending drug is stopped when the granulocytopenia or even the agranulocytosis is recognized, full recovery is to be expected. In a patient recently observed by us (in an experience of over 35 years, the first true agranulocytosis attributable to an antithyroid drug, in this case propylthiouracil) there was virtually complete absence of stem cells from the bone marrow; recognizable recovery occurred within four days and complete restoration of a normal concentration of circulating granulocytes occurred within 10 days without any pharmacological attempt at marrow stimulation.

There is an extensive list of rare adverse effects to thionamides: cholestatic hepatitis, arthralgia, neuritis, lymph node enlargement, loss of hair, and dependent edema have all been described. We have had a patient with severe migraine-like headache temporarily associated with propylthiouracil therapy that cleared immediately on change to an equivalent dosage of methimazole. The cause of these problems is unknown. The few reports of a syndrome of periarteritis in patients taking propylthiouracil have prompted the suggestion that such patients may have circulating immune complexes related to the drug ingestion. A survey of patients with Graves' disease, half of whom were taking propylthiouracil, failed to show any correlation between the presence or titer of immune complexes in blood and the administration of the drug.[166] Whatever the basis of the complications, their occurrence dictates the need for at least a change to another thionamide and, if symptoms persist, to another form of therapy.

[131]I Therapy. If radioiodine is the therapy of preference, ^{131}I is the isotope of choice. Because of the aforementioned high incidence of hypothyroidism occurring after therapy, attempts were made to treat with ^{125}I to make use of its more limited range of tissue-destructive radiation. [131]I exerts its therapeutic effect primarily through its β-particle emissions, with an average tissue penetration of 2.2 mm; ^{125}I acts through k capture and a radiation effect of only 0.5 μm. Consequently, in theory, radiation from the latter isotope sequestered in the follicular lumen might effectively damage important hormone-synthesizing organelles but spare the nucleus, which is all-important for cell regeneration, and so reduce the incidence of hypothyroidism. In practice, this did not turn out to be the case.[167, 168]

A common therapeutic dose of ^{131}I has been estimated to irradiate the thyroid with 6000 to 7000 rads. On recognition of the high rate of post-^{131}I hypothyroidism, several groups, exemplified by Smith et al.,[169] evaluated the effect of a lower dosage. The incidence of hypothyroidism following an estimated 3500 rads, compared with 7000 rads, was impressively less, as shown in Figure 41–21, although the interval before control of hyperthyroidism occurred was appreciably longer. The combined experience of 26 centers, organized by the U.S. Public Health Service, seemed to confirm the findings[149] (Fig. 41–22). Although individual groups have reported less satisfactory results, it seems to us that an estimated 3000 to 4000 rads to the gland can be recommended for most patients. As adjuvant to this radiotherapy, a course of antithyroid drugs of two to three months' duration is often appropriate, or symptoms may be controlled initially with a β-blocking sympatholytic agent such as propranolol. For the more severe episode of hyperthyroidism, for the patient with additional complications such as cardiac disease (which make avoidance of relapse of hyperthyroidism especially crucial), or for the

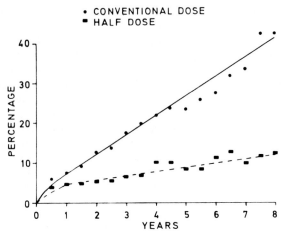

FIGURE 41–21. **Incidence of development of hypothyroidism in patients treated with [131]I.** The "conventional dose" was an estimated 7000 rads and was given to 326 patients; 312 patients had an estimated 3500 rads (half dose). (From Smith RN, Munro DS, Wilson GM: Two clinical trials of different doses of radio-iodine (^{131}I) in the treatment of thyrotoxicosis. *In* Fellinger K, Hofer R (eds): Further Advances in Thyroid Research. Vienna, Verlag der Weiner Medizinischen Akademie, 1971, p 611.)

patient over 60 years of age (in whom the development of post-^{131}I hypothyroidism within a normal life expectancy is of sufficiently low probability), the larger dose of 6000 to 7000 rads is advisable.

If the patient treated with radioiodine is still not euthyroid without adjuvant drug therapy six months later, a second dose of radioisotope is indicated in that although a continuing radiation effect from the initial dose may be presumed, a euthyroid state probably will not be reached without an unacceptable delay. In our experience, if a high blood level of TSAb is present on assay of the serum IgG, a second dose of ^{131}I is more likely to be required; if this impression is borne out by more data, it may become routine to give such patients a larger initial dose. Until then, when a second dose of ^{131}I is required, it is probably best to prescribe at least as many calculated rads as given previously.

Thyroid storm is now an infrequent medical emergency. It may be defined as a threat to life occasioned by an episode of hyperthyroidism and thus may encompass severe hyperthyroidism leading to critical failure of a number of organ systems, including cardiac, gastrointestinal, hepatic, renal, and cerebral. Usually there is underlying disease of the system or systems primarily affected, and cerebral coma, for instance, may develop without there being recognizable abnormality if and when recovery ensues. Therapy is partly specific and partly generally supportive. Administration of an antithyroid drug, e.g., 200 mg propylthiouracil every 4 hours by mouth or gavage; iodide (intravenously if necessary) in a dose of 10 to 20 mg/day; and propranolol, 20 to 40 mg every 4 hours, which may be given intravenously in 1- to 2-mg doses if necessary, constitutes specific therapy. If a β-blocker with greater specificity for cardiac receptors is required, e.g., in a patient with a history or signs of asthma, the effect on peripheral production of T_3 may still be obtained by use of either atenolol or metoprolol. Maintenance of fluid, electrolyte, and caloric balance and sedation are important supportive measures. Adrenal corticosteroids are commonly given but probably are seldom

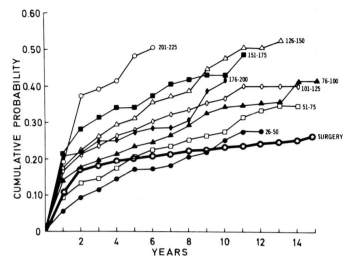

FIGURE 41–22. Experience of the Cooperative Thyrotoxicosis Therapy Follow-up Study initiated by the Bureau of Radiological Health of the U.S. Public Health Service. The 6000 patients included in this study had had no previous treatment for hyperthyroidism and received a single dose of ^{131}I; the number of patients in each dose category averaged 750. The cumulative probability of becoming hypothyroid is plotted on the ordinate and on the abscissa is the interval in years from the time of administration of ^{131}I. Radioiodine dosage is indicated on the chart from the lowest of 26 to 50 μCi per estimated gram of thyroid to the highest dose of 201 to 225 μCi/g; these assessments refer to μCi of ^{131}I delivered to the thyroid and not to the oral dose. The heavy line shows the appearance of hypothyroidism following surgical treatment in 5200 patients. After the third year the probability of becoming hypothyroid if less than 125 μCi per estimated gram of gland had been given was 2.3 per cent per year; from the second year after surgery the average probability of becoming hypothyroid was 0.7 per cent (From Becker DV, McConahey WM, Dobyns BM, et al: The results of radioiodine treatment of hyperthyroidism. A preliminary report of the Thyrotoxicosis Therapy Follow-up Study. In Fellinger K, Hofer R (eds): Further Advances in Thyroid Research. Vienna, Verlag der Wiener Medizinishchen Akademie, 1971, p 603.)

indicated and are more of a comfort to the physician than a need of the patient.

Radioiodine-induced thyroid storm is a complication often discussed but seldom seen. In a review published in 1983 an incidence, culled from reports critically analyzed, of 10 instances in 2975 treated patients (0.3 per cent), was deduced.[170] The most obvious approach to prevention of this rare complication is adequate therapy of any complicating illness that, by chance, is accompanying the hyperthyroidism.

Treatment of Ophthalmopathy. There has been considerable effort to relate thyroid pathogenesis in Graves' disease to the cause of the frequently clinically associated ophthalmopathy. In general, ophthalmopathy occurs most frequently in close proximity to the onset of hyperthyroidism. However, it is not unusual for ophthalmopathy to become a problem months or years after the presentation of hyperthyroidism, or to occur in advance of the thyroid disturbance, making co-pathogenesis a hypothesis difficult to support. The patient illustrated in Figure 41–6 exemplifies dramatically the possible discordance of thyroid and ophthalmic presentations in Graves' disease. This patient, sequentially over a decade, showed hyperthyroidism (with mild bilateral exophthalmos) successfully treated with ^{131}I, followed years later by malignant ophthalmopathic change in the left eye and two years after that a similar development in the right eye. Even a single clinical presentation

of this nature—and there are many similar anecdotes to be quoted—makes close pathogenetic mechanisms difficult to follow. Clearly this type of temporal dissociation of the thyroid and eye disease has to be accommodated by any of the pathogenetic theories currently being developed. The major link obviously is that both aspects of the syndrome reflect disturbances of autoimmunity. In time, any individual and shared autoimmune mechanisms will be disclosed. For now, an important clinical question has to be addressed: Does the therapy of the hyperthyroidism have any bearing on the course of the ophthalmopathy? Case reports abound, but there is limited information or experience to support the common clinical view that ^{131}I therapy of hyperthyroidism might exacerbate the accompanying ophthalmopathy.

In a retrospective study of 537 patients treated for hyperthyroidism there was no significant difference in the occurrence or progression of ocular signs whether treatment was by surgery, with thionamides, or by ^{131}I.[171] This publication also contained a careful review of previous reports and emphasized the lack of agreement on this subject. More recently a prospective study of the problem involved 168 patients. ^{131}I treatment was considered more likely than the other therapies to have caused or exacerbated the ophthalmopathy.[172] That conclusion was supported by valid statistical analyses; the relative risk for adverse change in the ophthalmological status was, on average, 0.8 to 1.5 in the groups not treated with ^{131}I and 3.2 in the 39 patients who were. However, the 95 per cent confidence limits for these means ranged from 0.2 to 5.0 in the non-^{131}I groups and from 1.1 to 8.8 in the patients treated with ^{131}I. Since no patient's ophthalmopathy worsened to the extent that orbital decompression or eye muscle surgery was needed, and there was major overlap of the relative risk data, the danger in use of ^{131}I cannot be seen as overwhelming.

HYPERTHYROIDISM DURING PREGNANCY. Radioiodine is contraindicated, and propranolol must be used with caution. If subtotal thyroidectomy is chosen, the second trimester is the period when the risk is lowest. Our preference is to treat with antithyroid drugs, usually propylthiouracil, for the following reasons. First, in some patients, hyperthyroidism seems to be associated with the event of pregnancy itself, and remission on antithyroid drug therapy may occur postpartum. (On the other hand, in patients who were hyperthyroid before conception, the pregnancy may ameliorate the condition, and a severe exacerbation may occur in the puerperium.) Second, the main argument against their use has been the danger of producing fetal goiter and hypothyroidism; this seems to be an avoidable risk with proper supervision as discussed below.

The aim of antithyroid drug therapy should be to maintain the mother euthyroid with the minimal required dose of thionamide. For this purpose a monthly evaluation is recommended. In most patients, control can be achieved initially with 300 mg propylthiouracil per day or the equivalent of another thionamide. As soon as euthyroidism ensues, attempts should be made to reduce the dosage, e.g., to 50 mg every 8 hours. It is generally accepted that the clinical diagnosis of hyperthyroidism can be especially difficult in pregnancy owing to the goiter, tachycardia, and hypermetabolism that occur in the euthyroid pregnant woman.[172a] Therefore, ancillary aids provided by the thyroid diagnostic laboratory become especially pertinent in this situation. A combination of serum thyroxine assay and assessment of the saturation of TBG permits the calculation of a free T_4 index. Alternatively, the concentration of free thyroxine (fT_4) may be measured directly. The aim should be to maintain these indices at the upper limit of normal, which is best to avoid the risk of hypothyroidism, and thus treat the mother with the minimal dose of antithyroid drug. Measurement of serum thyrotropin is advocated as a reliable monitor for hypothyroidism in this situation; while this is good advice, it is not necessarily the optimal approach for identifying the desired minimal dose of antithyroid drug, distinct from avoiding overdosage. A low or even subnormal level of serum thyrotropin should be the aim of treatment. Together with knowledge of the TSH concentration, a combination of clinical appraisal and the laboratory aid of free thyroxine assessment should lead to the recognition of the dosage of antithyroid drug that is appropriate for the pregnant thyrotoxic woman.

When the child of a patient being treated for hyperthyroidism is born, two different questions enter into clinical decisions: What is the thyroid status of the neonate? and, Should the mother's therapy be modified postpartum? The neonate in question may be hypothyroid as a result of maternal antepartum therapy. This may be on the basis of iodide given to the mother (a therapy that we specifically do not recommend) or due to maternal antithyroid drug. In our experience, management of the thyrotoxic mother, as just outlined, has not resulted in a hypothyroid infant in patients seen by us over 35 years. On the other hand, the child may be hyperthyroid, either at birth or within the first weeks of life. Over 100 cases have been reported[93, 101, 173] since the first description in 1910. The incidence is thus quite low but may in fact be higher if the possibility is kept in mind and milder clinical examples of the syndrome are identified by appropriate blood tests of the neonate. Although there is an alternate view,[174] we believe that the condition is due to the transplacental transfer of thyroid stimulating antibody from the mother; this theory is supported by several observations:

1. In only one report[175] did the mother have not even a history of Graves' disease, if not active hyperthyroidism, at the time of pregnancy; in the single exception to that relationship, the mother had LATS in the blood. There are insufficient data available to do more than theorize explanations for the absence of hyperthyroidism in this woman.

2. The clinical course of the majority of reported patients is compatible with the known rate of disappearance of maternal IgG from the neonatal circulation; in most instances this means that there is no need for antithyroid therapy beyond two to three months. The development of hyperthyroidism later in childhood[176] presumably represents the spontaneous emergence of Graves' disease in a genetically prone individual.

3. The likelihood of neonatal hyperthyroidism is directly related to the level of TSAb in the maternal blood during the third trimester of pregnancy.[101, 173] Accumulating experience indicates that although perhaps the majority of neonatal hyperthyroidism develops within the first few days of life and lasts only two to three months, exceptions to this pattern may exist. An extreme example is when development of the hyperthyroidism was delayed for about six weeks and the condition then persisted for up to six months.[177, 178] This pattern was explicable in terms of a mixture of maternal antibodies crossing the placenta and

their interaction at the receptor level in the child's thyroid.[92d] The frequency of such clinical situations occurring is unclear, and the proper interpretation of the available data[92d, 178] will have to await more sophisticated and discriminating assays. Current TSAb and TBI assays are sensitive enough to monitor in the third trimester a pregnant woman who has, or who has a history of, autoimmune thyroid disease.[101, 173] In this regard it should be emphasized that TSAb may be of sufficient titer in the mother's blood to induce neonatal Graves' disease even in women whose hyperthyroidism was treated by thyroid ablation years before or who have never had overt clinical Graves' disease but presented initially with Hashimoto's thyroiditis and hypothyroidism.[173]

Neonatal hyperthyroidism is short-lived, and treatment when indicated is similar to that given to the adult but with a reduced dosage. Thus, thionamide and iodide may be given to control thyroid function and propranolol to reduce the tachycardia and perhaps alleviate the diarrhea that may be particularly severe and dangerous in the newborn. The duration of the syndrome is probably directly related to the concentration of TSAb in the blood at the time of parturition and the rate of metabolism of this IgG. The half-time of clearance of maternal IgG is usually about 20 days, but this may be shortened by the influence of hyperthyroidism in the neonate.

Another aspect of the subject of Graves' disease in pregnancy that should be kept in mind is the possibility of fetal hyperthyroidism, with sometimes dire consequences. If the mother is under adequate (as defined above) treatment for hyperthyroidism, the transplacental passage of a thionamide should result in control of the fetal thyroid function. The problem arises when the mother is euthyroid, often on thyroxine, having had Graves' disease treated in the past,[101] or who has a primary diagnosis of Hashimoto's thyroiditis.[101, 178] In these instances, if the fetus is thought to be hyperthyroid,[173] treatment by giving the mother thionamide is a possibility (reviewed in ref. 178).

Management of the mother in the postpartum phase also requires specific consideration. It is important that maternal thyroid function continues to be controlled, in that exacerbation of hyperthyroidism often occurs in the puerperium; in our experience, one patient whose thionamide therapy was stopped antepartum suffered a severe relapse associated with puerperal depression and eventual suicide. At nine to twelve months postpartum, preferably when the child is sleeping all night and thus the mother is also able to get adequate rest, antithyroid drugs may be discontinued and routine clinical observation initiated.

Childhood hyperthyroidism is relatively uncommon. Rapid gain in height, not necessarily associated with the pubertal growth spurt, is a feature unique to this age group; otherwise signs and symptoms may be entirely as seen in adults except for the rare development of premature craniosynostosis. This has been reported both in childhood Graves' disease and in the treatment of hypothyroidism with presumably excessive dosages of thyroid hormone.[179] There is no consensus regarding therapy of hyperthyroidism in this age group, but probably most would advocate prolonged administration of thionamide in the first place. It may be that what has been said earlier about there being little to gain from a course of therapy longer than six months does not apply to prepubertal patients. Too little is known of the influence on the immune system of growth and the endocrinological changes of childhood and puberty for one to be dogmatic on the therapy of an autoimmune syndrome such as Graves' disease. It is said that at least 76 per cent of children treated medically will achieve a permanent remission,[180] which is a rate considerably greater than is expected for the adult population, and reported surgical experience has not been as satisfactory as in the older age groups.[181] We advocate a prolonged trial, one to two years, of thionamide therapy in the first instance. Many clinics are not prepared to use radioiodine therapy in the growing child because of the uncertainty of both potential genetic and carcinogenic hazards. Careful calculation of the gonadal irradiation to be expected from a conventional therapeutic dose of ^{131}I has shown that it is of the order seen with several routine radiological techniques, including barium enema and excretory pyelography.[182] Perhaps the correct interpretation of this information, however, is that all these procedures, including radioiodine therapy, should be used in the younger age groups (and that includes up to age 40) only when specifically indicated. The genesis of thyroid carcinoma after ^{131}I therapy is also a theoretical concern but one given considerable support by the recognition of thyroid neoplasia developing in adults subjected in childhood to external irradiation of the thyroid area.[183] However, a basic difference between external radiotherapy and the ablative use of ^{131}I may be important in this context. The former does not kill thyroid cells, and a mutagenic effect may persist in the putatively damaged but surviving thyrocytes. Use of ^{131}I, on the other hand, clearly kills the cells that therefore will not become malignant. Consequently, the recognition of a carcinogenic effect of external radiotherapy on the thyroid probably has little or no relevance to the use of [131]I. Nonetheless, until the issue is totally clarified, we do not advocate radioiodine for the treatment of childhood hyperthyroidism.

The coexistence of thyroid cancer and Graves' disease was recently reviewed. Of 132 patients subjected to subtotal thyroidectomy for Graves' disease, Belfiore et al.[184] found 13 (9.8 per cent) with thyroid cancer. Compared with cancer in patients with toxic adenoma (9 of 227 or 4 per cent) these tumors were, on average, larger and more aggressive. The possibility was raised that TSAb present in the Graves' disease patients was instrumental in these findings.[184, 184a] In an accompanying editorial Mazzaferri[185] supported the view that cancer in a Graves' disease thyroid is not rare. One review combined reports dealing with a total of 28,863 surgically treated Graves' disease patients. The incidence of cancer in the various publications was 0.06 to 8.7 per cent.[186] At present it is difficult to assess the importance of these data because of variables such as prior exposure to external radiation in these subjects. One conclusion that might be drawn is that when a cold nodule is found in a Graves' disease thyroid, it should be carefully evaluated as a possible malignant lesion.

Ophthalmopathy (reviewed in detail in Ch. 42)

The majority of patients with ophthalmopathy require no heroic measures for a condition that is self-limiting and one that will variably regress.

Total surgical thyroidectomy and absolute ablation by massive doses of ^{131}I are techniques that have been recommended[187]; others have failed to confirm the claim of satisfactory regression of ophthalmopathy following thyroid ablation.[188] Because spontaneous remission may occur and has followed, for example, retrobulbar decompression of the contralateral eye,[189] occasional improvement following thyroid ablation is to be expected. In any case, the original postulate—that the thyroid gland is involved in production of LATS or a similar agent, which in turn gives rise to ophthalmopathy[187]—becomes even more specious with current indications that specific antigens are associated with the autoimmune phenomena seen in ophthalmopathy.[137] Therefore, on the basis of current theories of pathogenesis, and since there has been no confirmatory report by others, total ablation of the thyroid as treatment of ophthalmopathy cannot be recommended.

Pretibial Myxedema

At times this condition may not be severe enough to merit much attention, but when treatment is required, good results often follow use of a corticosteroid cream such as 0.1 per cent triamcinolone. This may be applied in a water-soluble base without bandages or, for more severe lesions, under a cover of plastic film such as Saran Wrap. Eventual resolution of the lesions is the usual outcome. Resection of the exuberant tissue with autologous transplantation from another site has been attempted, with resultant pretibial myxedema of both operated areas.

Severe skin lesions were reported to clear rapidly in a patient who was subjected to plasmapheresis as therapy for ophthalmopathy,[190] but this cannot be seen as realistic therapy for pretibial myxedema per se.

Prognosis

The prognosis of hyperthyroidism and the other aspects of Graves' disease is discussed above under treatment. For patients not treated by modern methods, there is little information. McLarty and colleagues[139] studied 21 hyperthyroid patients treated solely with propranolol and found only four entering a phase of prolonged remission, perhaps an indication that spontaneous cure is unlikely. From a massive review of the literature published until 1907, Sattler[191] estimated that Basedow's disease had a mortality of about 11 per cent, and death occurred most often in patients who had an acute onset of severe symptoms; chronic ill health was to be expected in the majority of survivors. A different assessment might be made from experience reported by Bram in 1920[192]; he treated his patients by secluding them for up to a year in a sanatorium and administering therapy that would otherwise now be considered as nonspecific. The rate of remission was over 90 per cent. Perhaps, however, it is not correct to view isolation from the strains and stresses of everyday life as nonspecific therapy; as discussed earlier, emotional influences on the immune system may be all-important etiological factors in Graves' disease.

REFERENCES

1. Cavalieri RR, Gerard SK: Unusual types of thyrotoxicosis. Adv Intern Med 36:271–286, 1991.

2. Kulig K, Golightly LK, Rumack BH: Levothyroxine overdose associated with seizures in a young child. JAMA 254:2109–2110, 1985.

3. Stanage WF, Henski JA: Accidental ingestion of poisons. J Pediat 47:470–474, 1955.

4. Cohen JH, III, Ingbar SH, Braverman LE: Thyrotoxicosis due to ingestion of excess thyroid hormone. Endocr Rev 10:113–124, 1989.

5. Hedberg CW, Fishbein DB, Janssen RS, et al: An outbreak of thyrotoxicosis caused by the consumption of bovine thyroid gland in ground beef. N Engl J Med 316:993–998, 1987.

6. McMillin JM: Hamburger thyrotoxicosis: The endocrinologist as sleuth. Thyroid Today, April-June, XI:1–9, 1988.

7. Leiter L, Seidlin SM, Marinelli LD, Baumann EJ: Adenocarcinoma of the thyroid with hyperthyroidism and functional metastases. I. Studies with thiouracil and radioiodine. J Clin Endocrinol Metab 6:247–261, 1946.

8. Federman DD: Hyperthyroidism due to functioning metastatic carcinoma of the thyroid. Medicine 43:267–274, 1964.

9. Sung LC, Cavalieri RR: T$_3$ thyrotoxicosis due to metastatic thyroid carcinoma. J Clin Endocrinol Metab 36:215–217, 1973.

10. Bowden WD, Jones RE: Thyrotoxicosis associated with distant metastatic follicular carcinoma of the thyroid. South Med J 79:483–486, 1986.

11. Oppenheim A, Miller M, Anderson GHA Jr, et al: Anaplastic thyroid carcinoma presenting with hyperthyroidism. Am J Med 75:702–704, 1983.

12. Hennen G: Thyrotropin-like factor in a non endocrine cancer tissue. Arch Int Physiol Biochim 74:701–704, 1966.

13. Hershman JM, Higgins HP: Hydatidiform mole—A cause of clinical hyperthyroidism. N Engl J Med 284:573–577, 1971.

14. Harada A, Hershman JM: Extraction of human chorionic thyrotropin (hCT) from term placentas: Failure to recover thyrotropic activity. J Clin Endocrinol Metab 47:681–685, 1978.

15. Kenimer JG, Hershman JM, Higgins HP: The thyrotropin in hydatidiform moles is human chorionic gonadotropin. J Clin Endocrinol Metab 40:482–491, 1975.

16. Odell WD, Bates RW, Rivlin RS, et al: Increased thyroid function without clinical hyperthyroidism in patients with choriocarcinoma. J Clin Endocrinol Metab 23:658–664, 1963.

17. Steigbigel NH, Oppenheim JJ, Fishman LM, Carbone PL: Metastatic embryonal carcinoma of the testis associated with elevated plasma TSH-like activity and hyperthyroidism. N Engl J Med 271:345–349, 1964.

18. Amir SM, Uchimura H, Ingbar SH: Interactions of bovine thyrotropin and preparations of human chorionic gonadotropin with bovine thyroid membranes. J Clin Endocrinol Metab 45:280–292, 1977.

19. Kennedy RL, Darone J, Cohn M, et al: Human chorionic gonadotropin may not be responsible for thyroid-stimulating activity in normal pregnancy serum. J Clin Endocrinol Metab 74:260–265, 1992.

20. Hershman JM: Editorial: Role of human chorionic gonadotropin as a thyroid stimulator. J Clin Endocrinol Metab 74:258–259, 1992.

21. Tomer Y, Huber GK, Davies TF: Human chorionic gonadotropin (hCG) interacts directly with recombinant human TSH receptors. J Clin Endocrinol Metab 74:1477–1479, 1992.

22. Refetoff S, Weiss RE, Usala SJ: The syndrome of resistance to thyroid hormone. Endocr Rev 14:348–399, 1993.

23. Smallridge RC, Smith CE: Hyperthyroidism due to thyrotropin secreting pituitary tumors. Diagnostic and therapeutic considerations. Arch Intern Med 143:503–507, 1983.

24. Kourides IA: A patient with thyroid-stimulating hormone hypersecretion. Medical Grand Rounds 2:222–226, 1983.

25. Krawczynska H, Wojcik-Musialek K, Illig R: 10 years of successful treatment with dextrothyroxine in a girl with TSH-induced hyperthyroidism. Horm Res 35:213–216, 1991.

26. Beck-Peccoz P, Piscitelli G, Cattanea M, Faglia G: Successful treatment of hyperthyroidism due to nonneoplastic pituitary TSH hypersecretion with 3,5,3′-triiodothyroacetic acid (TRIAC). J Endocrinol Invest 6:217–223, 1983.

27. Beckers A, Abs R, Mahler C, et al: Thyrotropin-secreting pituitary adenomas: Report of seven cases. J Clin Endocrinol Metab 72:477–483, 1991.

28. Dulgeroff AJ, Geffner ME, Royal SN, et al: Bromocriptine and Triac therapy for hyperthyroidism due to pituitary resistance to thyroid hormone. J Clin Endocrinol Metab, 75:1071–1075, 1992.

29. Wynne AG, Gharib H, Scheithauer BW, et al: Hyperthyroidism due to inappropriate secretion of thyrotropin in 10 patients. Am J Med 92:15–24, 1992.

30. Kempers RD, Dockerty MB, Hoffman DL, Bartholomew LG: Struma ovarii-ascitic, hyperthyroid, and asymptomatic syndromes. Ann Intern Med 72:883–893, 1970.

31. Fradkin JE, Wolff J: Iodide-induced thyrotoxicosis. Medicine 62:1–20, 1983.

32. Woolf PD: Transient painless thyroiditis with hyperthyroidism: a variant of lymphocytic thyroiditis? Endocr Rev 1:411–420, 1980.

32a. Amino N, Mori H, Iwatani Y, et al: High prevalence of transient postpartum thyrotoxicosis and hypothyroidism. N Engl J Med 306:849–852, 1982.

33. Farid NR, Hawe BS, Walfish PG: Increased frequency of HLA-DR3 and 5 in the syndromes of painless thyroiditis with transient thyrotoxicosis: Evidence for an autoimmune etiology. Clin Endocrinol 19:699–704, 1983.

33a. Kologlu M, Fung H, Darke C, et al: Postpartum thyroid dysfunction and HLA status. Eur J Clin Invest 20:56–60, 1990.

34. Carney AG, Moore SB, Northcutt RC, et al: Palpation thyroiditis (multifocal granulomatous folliculitis). Am J Clin Pathol 64:639–648, 1973.

35. Kobayashi A, Kuma K, Matsuzuka F, et al: Thyrotoxicosis after needle aspiration of thyroid cyst. J Clin Endocrinol Metab 75:21–24, 1992.

36. Walfish PG, Caplan D, Rosen IB: Post parathyroidectomy transient thyrotoxicosis. J Clin Endocrinol Metab 75:224–227, 1992.

37. Lipman LM, Green DE, Snyder NJ, et al: Relationship of long-acting thyroid stimulator to the clinical features and course of Graves' disease. Am J Med 43:486–498, 1967.

38. Warthin AS: Constitutional entity of exophthalmic goiter and so-called toxic adenoma. Ann Intern Med 2:553–570, 1928.

39. Hegedüs L, Mølholm Hansen J, Karstrup S: High incidence of normal thyroid gland volume in patients with Graves' disease. Clin Endocrinol 19:603–607, 1983.

40. Lamberg BA, Gordin A, Viherkoski M, Kvist G: Long-acting thyroid stimulator (LATS) in toxic nodular goiter, toxic adenoma and Graves' disease. Acta Endocrinol 62:199–209, 1969.

41. Furszyfer J, Kurland LT, McConahey WM, et al: Epidemiologic aspects of Hashimoto's thyroiditis and Graves' disease in Rochester, Minnesota (1935-1967), with special reference to temporal trends. Metabolism 21:197–204, 1972.

42. Tunbridge WMG, Evered DC, Hall R, et al: The spectrum of thyroid disease in a community: The Whickham Survey. Clin Endocrinol 7:481–493, 1977.

43. Barker DJP, Phillips DIW: Current incidence of thyrotoxicosis and past prevalence of goitre in 12 British towns. Lancet 2:567–570, 1984.

44. Mogensen EF, Green A: The epidemiology of thyrotoxicosis in Denmark. Incidence and geographical variation in the Funem Region 1972-1974. Acta Med Scand 208:183–186, 1980.

44a. Nyström E, Bengtsson C, Lindquist O, et al: Serum triiodothyronine and hyperthyroidism in a population sample of women. Clin Endocrinol 20:31–42, 1984.

45. Hall R: Hyperthyroidism, pathogenesis, and diagnosis. Br Med J 1:743–745, 1970.

46. Pohl G, Galvan G, Steiner H, Salis-Samader R: Das autonome adenom der schilddrüse im struma-endemiegebiet. Deutsche Med Wchnsch 98:189–193, 1973.

47. Horst W, Rosler H, Schneider C, et al: 306 cases of toxic adenoma: Clinical aspects, findings in radioiodine diagnostics, radiochromatography and histology. Results of ^{131}I and surgical treatment. J Nucl Med 8:515–528, 1967.

48. Frantz VK, Quimby EH, Evans TC: Radioactive iodine studies of functional thyroid carcinoma. Radiology 51:532–552, 1948.

49. Reveno WS: Thyroidectomy at Harper Hospital: A 20 year survey. Harper Hosp Bull 5:131–134, 1947.

50. Williams I, Ankrett VO, Lazarus JH, Volpe R: Aetiology of hyperthyroidism in Canada and Wales. J Epidem Commun Health 37:245–248, 1983.

51. Suarez HG, du Villard JA, Severino M, et al: Presence of mutations in all three ras genes in human thyroid tumors. Oncogene 5:565–570, 1990.

51a. Spada A, Vallar L, Faglia G: G-protein oncogenes in endocrine disorders. Prog Neuro Endocrin Immunol 5:80–94, 1992.

52. Ledent C, Dumont JE, Vassart G, Parmentier M: Thyroid expression of an A$_2$ adenosine receptor transgene induces thyroid hyperplasia and hyperthyroidism. EMBO J 11:537–542, 1992.

52a. Selzer E, Wilfing A, Schiferer A, et al: Stimulation of human thyroid growth via the inhibitory guanine nucleotide binding (G) protein Gi: Constitutive expression of the G-protein α subunit Giα-1 in autonomous adenoma. Proc Natl Acad Sci USA 90:1609–1613, 1993.

53. Namba H, Matsuo K, Fagin JA: Clonal composition of benign and malignant human thyroid tumors. J Clin Invest 86:120–125, 1990.

54. Silverstein GE, Burke G, Cogan R: The natural history of the autonomous hyperfunctioning thyroid nodule. Ann Intern Med 67:539–548, 1967.

55. Schaller U, Holzel D, Kirsch C, et al: Natural history of compensated autonomous adenomata of the thyroid. Klin Wochenschr 69:786–792, 1991.
56. Blum M, Nocero MA Jr.: Spontaneous resolution of a euthyroid autonomous nodule of the thyroid. Am J Med Sci 264:49–54, 1972.
57. Goldstein R, Hart IR: Follow-up of solitary autonomous thyroid nodules treated with ¹³¹I. N Engl J Med 309:1473–1476, 1983.
58. Huysmans DA, Corstens FH, Kloppenborg PW: Long-term follow-up in toxic solitary autonomous thyroid nodules treated with radioactive iodine. J Nucl Med 32:27–30, 1991.
59. Bartels ED: Heredity in Graves' Disease. Copenhagen, Enjar Monksgaard Forlag, 1941.
60. Heimann P: Familial incidence of thyroid disease and anamnestic incidence of pubertal struma in 449 consecutive struma patients. Acta Med Scand 179:113–119, 1966.
61. Martin L, Fisher RA: Heredity and familial aspects of exophthalmic goitre and nodular goitre. Quart J Med 14:207–219, 1945.
62. Howell-Evans AW, Woodrow JC, McDougall CD, et al: Antibodies in the families of thyrotoxic patients. Lancet 1:637–641, 1967.
63. Grumet FC, Payne RO, Konishi J, Kriss JP: HL-A antigens as markers for disease susceptibility and autoimmunity in Graves' disease. J Clin Endocrinol Metab 39:1115–1119, 1974.
64. McGregor AM, Rees-Smith B, Hall R, et al: Prediction of relapse in hyperthyroid Graves' disease. Lancet 1:1101–1103, 1980.
65. Schernthaner G, Schleusener H, Kotulla P, et al: Prediction of relapse or long-term remission in hyperthyroid Graves' disease. Lancet 2:373–374, 1981.
65a. Yanagawa T, Mangklabruks A, Chang Y-B, et al: Human histocompatibility leukocyte antigen–DQA1*0501 allele associated with genetic susceptibility to Graves' disease in a Caucasian population. J Clin Endocrinol Metab 76:1569–1574, 1993.
66. Dong R-P, Kimura A, Okubo R, et al: HLA-A and DPB1 loci confer susceptibility to Graves' disease. Hum Immunol 35:165–172, 1992.
67. Yeo PPB, Chan SH, Thai AC, et al: HLA Bw46 and DR9 associations in Graves' disease of Chinese patients are age- and sex-related. Tissue Antigens 34:179–184, 1989.
68. Rose NR, Bacon LD, Sundick RS: Genetic determinants of thyroiditis in the OS chicken. Transplant Rev 31:264–285, 1976.
69. Wick G, Kite JH Jr, Witebsky E: Spontaneous thyroiditis in the obese strain of chickens. J Immunol 104:54–62, 1970.
70. Welch P, Rose NR, Kite JH Jr.: Neonatal thymectomy increases spontaneous autoimmune thyroiditis. J Immunol 110:575–577, 1973.
71. Wick G, Sundick RS, Albini B: A review. The obese strain (OS) of chickens: An animal model with spontaneous autoimmune thyroiditis. Clin Immunol Immunopathol 3:272–300, 1974.
72. Sundick RS, Wick G: Increased ¹³¹I-uptake by the thyroid glands of obese strain (OS) chickens derived from non-protamone-supplemented hens. Clin Exp Immunol 18:127–139, 1974.
72a. Sundick RS: The role of iodine in thyroid autoimmunity: from chickens to humans: A review. Autoimmunity 13:61–68, 1992.
73. Parry CH: Collections from the unpublished medical papers of the late Caleb Hillier Parry, M.D., F.R.S. Vol. 2, p 111. London, Underwoods, 1825.
74. Hermann HT, Quarton GC: Psychological changes and psychogenesis in thyroid hormone disorders. J Clin Endocrinol Metab 25:327–338, 1965.
75. Levi L: Stress and distress in response to psychosocial stimuli. Acta Med Scand 191 (suppl) 528:1–166, 1972.
76. Mason JW: A review of psychoendocrine research on the pituitary-thyroid system. Psychosom Med 30:666–681, 1968.
77. Gerwing J, Long DA, Pitt-Rivers R: The influence of bacterial exotoxins on the activity of the thyroid gland in different species. J Physiol 144:229–242, 1958.
78. Melander A, Ericson LE, Ljunggren JG, et al: Sympathetic innervation of the normal human thyroid. J Clin Endocrinol Metab 39:713–718, 1974.
79. Hashizume K, Ichikawa K, Sakurai A, et al: Administration of thyroxine in treated Graves' disease. N Engl J Med 324:947–953, 1991.
80. Joasoo A, McKenzie JM: Stress and the immune response in rats. Int Arch Allerg Appl Immunol 50:659–663, 1976.
81. Bonnyns M, McKenzie JM: Interactions of stress and of endocrine status on rat peripheral blood lymphocyte responsiveness to phytomitogens. Psychoneuroendocrinology 4:67–73, 1979.
82. Coindet JR: Nouvelles recherches sur les effects de l'iode. Ann Chim Phys 16:2525, 1821.
83. Vagenakis AG, Wang C, Burger A, et al: Iodide-induced thyrotoxicosis in Boston. N Engl J Med 287:523–527, 1972.
84. Stewart JC, Vidor GI, Buttfield IH, Hetzel BS: Epidemic thyrotoxicosis in northern Tasmania: Studies of clinical features and iodine nutrition. Aust NZ J Med 1:203–211, 1971.
85. Alexander WD, Harden R McG, Koutras DA, et al: Influence of iodine intake after treatment with antithyroid drugs. Lancet 2:866–868, 1965.
86. Liewendahl K, Gordin A: Iodine-induced toxic diffuse goitre. Acta Med Scand 196:237–239, 1974.
87. Bartels EC, Higgins GK: Graves' disease following thyroid administration. Lahey Clin Bull 9:81–87, 1955.
88. Weiss M, Ingbar SH, Winblad S, Kasper DL: Demonstration of a saturable binding site for thyrotropin in Yersinia enterocolitica. Science 219:1331–1333, 1983.
89. Heyma P, Harrison LC, Robins-Browne R: Thyrotropin (TSH) binding sites on Yersinia enterocolitica recognized by immunoglobulins from humans with Graves' disease. Clin Exp Immunol 64:249–254, 1986.
90. Ciampolillo A, Marini V, Mirakian R, et al: Retrovirus-like sequences in Graves' disease: Implications for human autoimmunity. Lancet 1:1096–1100, 1989.
91. Humphrey M, Mosca J, Baker JR, et al: Absence of retroviral sequences in Graves' disease. Lancet 337:17–18, 1991.
92. Tominaga T, Katamine S, Namba H, et al: Lack of evidence for the presence of human immunodeficiency virus type 1-related sequences in patients with Graves' disease. Thyroid 1:307–314, 1991.
92a. Burch HB, Nagy EV, Lukes YG, et al: Nucleotide and amino acid homology between the human thyrotropin receptor and the HIV-1 nef protein: Identification and functional analysis. Biochem Biophys Res Commun 181:498–505, 1991.
92b. Tomer Y, Davies TF: Infection, thyroid disease, and autoimmunity. Endocr Rev 14:107–120, 1993.
92c. Zakarija M, McKenzie JM, Edison MS: Transient neonatal hypothyroidism: Characterization of maternal antibodies to the thyrotropin receptor. J Clin Endocrinol Metab 70:1239–1246, 1990.
92d. Zakarija M, Garcia A, McKenzie JM: Studies on multiple thyroid cell membrane directed antibodies in Graves' disease. J Clin Invest 76:1855–1891, 1985.
93. McKenzie JM, Zakarija M: Pathogenesis of neonatal Graves' disease. J Endocrinol Invest 2:183–189, 1978.
94. Parmentier M, Libert F, Maenhaut C, et al: Molecular cloning of the thyrotropin receptor. Science 246:1620–1622, 1989.
95. Nagayama Y, Kaufman KD, Seto P, Rapoport B: Molecular cloning, sequence and functional expression of cDNA for the human thyrotropin receptor. Biochem Biophys Res Commun 165:1184–1190, 1989.
96. Misrahi M, Loosfelt H, Atger M, et al: Cloning, sequencing, and expression of human TSH receptor. Biochem Biophys Res Commun 166:394–403, 1990.
97. Akamizu T, Ikuyama S, Saji M, et al: Cloning, chromosomal assignment, and regulation of the rat thyrotropin receptor: Expression of the gene is regulated by thyrotropin, agents that increase cAMP levels, and thyroid autoantibodies. Proc Natl Acad Sci USA 87:5677–5681, 1990.
98. Nagayama Y, Wadsworth HL, Russo D, et al: Binding domains of stimulatory and inhibitory thyrotropin (TSH) receptor antibodies determined with chimeric TSH-lutropin/chorionic gonadotropin receptors. J Clin Invest 88:336–340, 1991.
98a. Kosugi S, Ban T, Kohn LD: Identification of thyroid-stimulating antibody-specific interaction sites in the N-terminal region of the thyrotropin receptor. Mol Endocrinol 7:114–130, 1993.
98b. Nagayama Y, Rapoport B: Thyroid stimulatory autoantibodies in different patients with autoimmune thyroid disease do not all recognize the same components of the human thyrotropin receptor: Selective role of receptor amino acids Ser₂₅-Glu₃₀. J Clin Endocrinol Metab 75:1425–1430, 1992.
99. Zakarija M, McKenzie JM, Banovac K: Clinical significance of assay of thyroid-stimulating antibody in Graves' disease. Ann Intern Med 93:28–32, 1980.
100. McKenzie JM, Zakarija M: Clinical review 3. The clinical use of thyrotropin receptor antibody measurements. J Clin Endocrinol Metab 69:1093–1096, 1989.
101. Zakarija M, McKenzie JM: Pregnancy-associated changes in the thyroid-stimulating antibody of Graves' disease and the relationship to neonatal hyperthyroidism. J Clin Endocrinol Metab 57:1036–1040, 1983.
102. Dirmikis SM, Munro DS: Placental transmission of thyroid-stimulating immunoglobulin. Br Med J 2:665–666, 1975.
103. Martin A, Davies TE: T cells and human autoimmune thyroid disease: Emerging data show lack of need to invoke suppressor T cells problems. Thyroid 2:247–261, 1992.

104. Weetman AP, Bennett GL, Wong WLT: Thyroid follicular cells produce interleukin-8. J Clin Endocrinol Metab 75:328–330, 1992.

105. McDevitt HO: The HLA system and its relation to disease. Hosp Pract 20:57–72, 1985.

106. Bottazzo GF, Pujol-Borrell R, Hanafusa T, Feldmann M: Role of aberrant HLA-DR expression and antigen presentation in induction of endocrine autoimmunity. Lancet 2:115–119, 1983.

107. Zakarija M: Immunochemical characterization of thyroid-stimulating antibody (TSAb) of Graves' disease: Evidence for restricted heterogeneity. J Clin Lab Immunol 10:77–85, 1983.

108. Knight J, Ling P, Knight A, et al: Thyroid-stimulating autoantibodies usually contain only lambda-light chains: Evidence for the "forbidden clone" theory. J Clin Endocrinol Metab 62:342–347, 1986.

109. Williams RC Jr., Marshall NJ, Kilpatrick K, et al: Kappa/lambda immunoglobulin distribution in Graves' thyroid-stimulating antibodies. J Clin Invest 82:1306–1312, 1988.

110. Volpe R: Immunology of human thyroid disease. In Volpe R (ed): Autoimmune Diseases of the Endocrine System. Boca Raton, CRC Press, 1990, pp 73–239.

111. Cheung HS, Nicoloff JT, Kamiel MB, et al: Stimulation of fibroblast biosynthetic activity by serum of patients with pretibial myxedema. J Invest Dermatol 71:12–17, 1978.

112. Konrad K, Brenner W, Pehamberger H: Ultrastructural and immunological findings in Graves' disease with pretibial myxedema. J Cutan Pathol 7:99–108, 1980.

113. Kopell BS, Wittner WK, Lunde D, et al: Influence of triiodothyronine on selective attention in man as measured by the visual averaged evoked potential. Psychosom Med 32:495–502, 1970.

114. Mintz G, Pizzarello R, Klein I: Enhanced left ventricular diastolic function in hyperthyroidism: Noninvasive assessment and response to treatment. J Clin Endocrinol Metab 73:146–150, 1991.

115. Massey DG, Becklake MR, McKenzie JM, Bates DV: Circulatory and ventilatory response to exercise in thyrotoxicosis. N Engl J Med 276:1104–1112, 1967.

116. Klion FM, Segal R, Schaffner F: The effect of altered thyroid function on the ultrastructure of the human liver. Am J Med 50:317–324, 1971.

117. Saenger EL, Thoma GE, Tompkins EA: Incidence of leukemia following treatment of hyperthyroidism. JAMA 205:855–862, 1968.

118. Cole CH, Waddell RW: Alteration in intracellular sodium concentration and ouabain-sensitive ATPase in erythrocytes from hyperthyroid patients. J Clin Endocrinol Metab 42:1056–1063, 1976.

119. Snyder LM, Reddy WJ: Thyroid hormone control of erythrocyte 2,3-diphosphoglyceric acid concentrations. Science 169:879–880, 1970.

120. Edelman IS: Thyroid thermogenesis. N Engl J Med 290:1303–1308, 1974.

121. Engel AG: Neuromuscular manifestations of Graves' disease. Mayo Clin Proc 47:919–925, 1972.

122. Ober KP: Thyrotoxic periodic paralysis in the United States—Report of 7 cases and review of the literature. Medicine 71:109–120, 1992.

123. Siegler M, Refetoff S: Pretibial myxedema—A reversible cause of foot drop due to entrapment of the peroneal nerve. N Engl J Med 294:1383–1384, 1976.

124. Fisher M, Mateer JE, Ullrich I, Gutrecht JA: Pyramidal tract deficits and polyneuropathy in hyperthyroidism. Combination clinically mimicking amyotrophic lateral sclerosis. Am J Med 78:1041–1044, 1985.

125. Olson BR, Klein I, Benner R, et al: Hyperthyroid myopathy and the response to treatment. Thyroid 1:137–144, 1991.

126. Becker KL, Matthews MJ, Higgins GA, Mohamadi M: Histologic evidence of gynecomastia in hyperthyroidism. Arch Pathol 98:257–260, 1974.

127. Classification of eye changes of Graves' disease. Thyroid 2:235–236, 1992.

128. Nixon DW, Samols E: Acral changes associated with thyroid diseases. JAMA 212:1175–1181, 1970.

129. Rodbard D, Fujita T, Rodbard S: Estimation of thyroid function by timing the arterial sounds. JAMA 201:884–887, 1967.

130. Konno N: The relationship between the timing of the Korotkoff sound (QKd) and the serum thyroid hormone concentrations. Fol Endocrinol Jpn 52:158–168, 1976.

131. Parisi AF, Hamilton BP, Thomas CN, Mazzaferri EL: The short cardiac pre-ejection period. An index to thyrotoxicosis. Circulation 49:900–904, 1974.

132. Hirschfeld S, Meyer R, Schwartz DC, et al: Measurement of the right and left ventricular systolic time intervals by echocardiography. Circulation 51:304–309, 1975.

133. Lewis BS, Ehrenfeld EN, Lewis N, Gotsman MS: Echocardiographic LV function in thyrotoxicosis. Am Heart J 97:460–468, 1979.

134. Cohen MV, Schulman IC, Spenillo A, Surks MI: Effects of thyroid hormone on left ventricular function in patients treated for thyrotoxicosis. Am J Cardiol 48:33–38, 1981.

135. Friedman MJ, Okada RD, Ewy GA, Hellman DJ: Left ventricular systolic and diastolic function in hyperthyroidism. Am Heart J 104:1303–1308, 1982.

136. Channick BJ, Adlin EV, Marks AD, et al: Hyperthyroidism and mitral-valve prolapse. N Engl J Med 305:497–500, 1981.

137. Miller A, Arthurs B, Boucher A, et al: Significance of antibodies reactive with a 64 kDa eye muscle membrane antigen in patients with thyroid autoimmunity. Thyroid 2:197–202, 1992.

138. Seigel RS, Thrall JH, Sisson JC: 99mTc-pyrophosphate scan and radiographic correlation in thyroid acropachy: Case report. J Nucl Med 17:791–793, 1976.

139. McLarty DG, Brownlie BEW, Alexander WD, Papapetrou PD: Remission of thyrotoxicosis during treatment with propranolol. Br Med J 2:332–334, 1973.

140. Perrild H, Mølholm Hansen J, Skovsted L, Christensen LK: Different effects of propranolol, alprenolol, sotalol, atenolol and metoprolol on serum T₃ and serum rT₃ in hyperthyroidism. Clin Endocrinol 18:139–142, 1983.

141. Braverman LE, Woeber KA, Ingbar SH: Induction of myxedema by iodide in patients euthyroid after radioiodine or surgical treatment of diffuse toxic goiter. N Engl J Med 281:816–821, 1969.

142. Riggs DS: Quantitative aspects of iodine metabolism in man. Pharmacol Rev 4:284–370, 1952.

143. Shen D-C, Wu S-Y, Chopra IJ, et al: Long term treatment of Graves' hyperthyroidism with sodium ipodate. J Clin Endocrinol Metab 61:723–727, 1985.

144. Wang Y-S, Tsou C-T, Lin W-H, Hershman JM: Long term treatment of Graves' disease with iopanoic acid (Telepaque). J Clin Endocrinol Metab 65:679–682, 1987.

145. Shen D-C, Wu S-Y, Chopra IJ, et al: Further studies on the long-term treatment of Graves' hyperthyroidism with ipodate: Assessment of a minimal effective dose. Thyroid 1:143–146, 1991.

146. Temple R, Berman M, Carlson HE, et al: The use of lithium in Graves' disease. Mayo Clin Proc 47:872–878, 1972.

147. Wartofsky L, Glinoer D, Solomon B, et al. Differences and similarities in the diagnosis and treatment of Graves' disease in Europe, Japan, and the United States. Thyroid 1:129–135, 1991.

148. Parfitt AM: The incidence of hypoparathyroidism tetany after thyroid operations: Relationship to age, extent of resection and surgical experience. Med J Aust 1:1103–1107, 1971.

149. Becker DV, McConahey WM, Dobyns BM, et al: The results of radioiodine treatment of hyperthyroidism. A preliminary report of the thyrotoxicosis therapy follow-up study. In Fellinger K, Höfer R (eds): Further Advances in Thyroid Research. Vienna, Verlag der Wiener Medizinischen Akademie, 1971, pp 603–609.

150. Livadas D, Psarras A, Koutras A: Malignant cold thyroid nodules in hyperthyroidism. Br J Surg 33:726–728, 1976.

151. Marigold JH, Morgan AK, Earle DJ, et al: Lugol's iodine: Its effect on thyroid blood flow in patients with thyrotoxicosis. Br J Surg 72:45–47, 1985.

152. McKenzie JM: Does LATS cause hyperthyroidism in Graves' disease? (A review biased toward the affirmative). Metabolism 21:883–894, 1972.

153. Spencer CA, Schwarzbein D, Guttler RB, et al: Thyrotropin (TSH)-releasing hormone stimulation test responses employing third and fourth generation TSH assays. J Clin Endocrinol Metab 76:494–498, 1993.

154. Klee GG, Hay ID: Assessment of sensitive thyrotropin assays for an expanded role in thyroid function testing: Proposed criteria for analytic performance and clinical utility. J Clin Endocrinol Metab 64:461–471, 1987.

155. Abuid J, Larsen PR: Triiodothyronine and thyroxine in hyperthyroidism. Comparison of the acute changes during therapy with antithyroid agents. J Clin Invest 54:201–208, 1974.

156. Romaldini JH, Bromberg N, Werner RS, et al: Comparison of effects of high and low dosage regimens of antithyroid drugs in the management of Graves' hyperthyroidism. J Clin Endocrinol Metab 57:563–570, 1983.

157. McGregor AM, Petersen MM, McLachlan SM, et al: Carbimazole and the autoimmune response in Graves' disease. N Engl J Med 303:302–307, 1980.

158. Weetman AP, McGregor AM, Hall R: Methimazole inhibits thyroid autoantibody production by an action on accessory cells. Clin Immunol Immunopathol 28:39–45, 1983.

159. Charreire J, Karsenty G, Bouchard P, Schaison G: Effect of carbima-

zole treatment on specific and nonspecific immunological parameters in patients with Graves' disease. Clin Exp Immunol 57:633–638, 1984.

159a. Tötterman TH, Karlsson FA, Bengtsson M, Mandel-Hartvig I: Induction of circulating activated suppressor-like T cells by methimazole therapy for Graves' disease. N Engl J Med 316:15–22, 1987.

160. Greer MA, Meihoff WC, Studer H: Treatment of hyperthyroidism with a single daily dose of propylthiouracil. N Engl J Med 272:888–891, 1965.

161. Barnes HV, Bledsoe T: A simple test for selecting the thionamide schedule in thyrotoxicosis. J Clin Endocrinol Metab 35:250–255, 1972.

162. Alexander WD, McLarty DG, Robertson J, et al: Prediction of the long-term results of antithyroid drug therapy for thyrotoxicosis. J Clin Endocrinol Metab 30:540–543, 1970.

163. Greer MA, Kammer H, Bouma DJ: Short-term antithyroid drug therapy for the thyrotoxicosis of Graves' disease. N Engl J Med 297:173–176, 1977.

164. Wartofsky L: Low remission after therapy for Graves' disease. Possible relation of dietary iodine with antithyroid therapy results. JAMA 226:1083–1088, 1973.

165. Solomon BL, Evaul JE, Burman KD, Wartofsky L: Remission rates with anti-thyroid drug therapy: Continuing influence of iodine intake? Ann Intern Med 107:510–512, 1987.

166. Cano PO, Chertman MM, Jerry LM, McKenzie JM: Circulating immune complexes in Graves' disease. Endocr Res Commun 3:307–317, 1976.

167. Weidinger P, Johnson PM, Werner SC: Five years' experience with iodine 125 therapy of Graves' disease. Lancet 2:74–77, 1974.

168. Bremner WF, McDougall IR, Greig WR: Results of treating 297 thyrotoxic patients with 125I. Lancet 2:281–282, 1973.

169. Smith RB, Munro DS, Wilson GM: Two clinical trials of different doses of radio-iodine (131I) in the treatment of thyrotoxicosis. In Fellinger K, Höfer R (eds): Further Advances in Thyroid Research. Vienna, Verlag der Wiener Medizinischen Akademie, 1971, pp 611–618.

170. McDermott MT, Kidd GS, Dodson LE Jr, Hofeldt FD: Radioiodine-induced thyroid storm. Case report and literature review. Am J Med 75:353–359, 1983.

171. Sridama V, DeGroot LJ: Treatment of Graves' disease and the course of ophthalmopathy. Am J Med 87:70–73, 1989.

172. Tallstedt L, Lundell G, Torring O, et al: Occurrence of ophthalmopathy after treatment for Graves' hyperthyroidism. N Engl J Med 326:1733–1738, 1992.

172a. Burrow GN: Thyroid function and hyperfunction during gestation. Endocr Rev 14:194–202, 1993.

173. McKenzie JM, Zakarija M: Fetal and neonatal hyperthyroidism and hypothyroidism due to maternal TSH receptor antibodies. Thyroid 2:155–159, 1992.

174. Hollingsworth DR, Mabry CC: Congenital Graves' disease. Four familial cases with long-term follow-up and perspective. Am J Dis Child 130:148–155, 1976.

175. Brookfield DSK, McCandless AE, Smith CS: Thyrotoxicosis in a neonate of a mother with no history of thyroid disease. Arch Dis Child 51:314–316, 1976.

176. Hollingsworth DR, Mabry CC, Eckerd J: Hereditary aspects of Graves' disease in infancy and childhood. J Pediatr 81:446–459, 1972.

177. Zakarija M, McKenzie JM, Munro DS: Immunoglobulin G inhibitor of thyroid-stimulating antibody is a cause of delay in the onset of neonatal Graves' disease. J Clin Invest 72:1352–1356, 1983.

178. Zakarija M, McKenzie JM, Hoffman WH: Prediction and therapy of intrauterine and late-onset neonatal hyperthyroidism. J Clin Endocrinol Metab 62:368–371, 1986.

179. Menking M, Wiebel J, Schmid WU, et al: Premature craniostenosis associated with hyperthyroidism in 4 children with reference to 5 further cases in the literature. Wschr Kinderheilk 120:106–110, 1972.

180. Hung W, Wilkins L, Blizzard R: Medical therapy of thyrotoxicosis in children. Pediatrics 30:17–26, 1962.

181. Hayles AB, Kennedy RLJ, Beahrs OH, Woolner LB: Exophthalmic goiter in children. J Clin Endocrinol Metab 19:138–151, 1959.

182. Robertson JS, Gorman CA: Gonadal radiation dose and its genetic significance in radioiodine therapy of hyperthyroidism. J Nucl Med 17:826–835, 1976.

183. DeGroot LJ, Paloyan E: Thyroid carcinoma and radiation. A Chicago endemic. JAMA 225:487–491, 1973.

184. Belfiore A, Garofalo MR, Giuffrida D, et al: Increased aggressiveness of thyroid cancer in patients with Graves' disease. J Clin Endocrinol Metab 70:830–835, 1990.

184a. Filetti S, Belfiore A, Amir SM, et al: The role of thyroid-stimulating antibodies of Graves' disease in differentiated thyroid cancer. N Engl J Med 318:753–759, 1988.

185. Mazzaferri EL: Editorial: Thyroid cancer and Graves' disease. J Clin Endocrinol Metab 70:826–829, 1990.

186. Behar R, Arganini M, Wu TC, et al: Graves' disease and thyroid cancer. Surgery 100:1121–1127, 1986.

187. Bauer RK, Catz B: Radioactive iodine therapy for progressive malignant exophthalmos. Acta Endocrinol (Copenhagen) 51:15–22, 1966.

188. Volpe R, Desbarats-Schonbaum ML, Schonbaum E, et al: The effect of radioablation of the thyroid gland in Graves' disease with high levels of long-acting thyroid stimulator (LATS). Am J Med 46:217–226, 1969.

189. Brain R: Pathogenesis and treatment of endocrine exophthalmos. Lancet 1:109–111, 1959.

190. Dandona P, Marshall NJ, Bidey SP, et al: Successful treatment of exophthalmos and pretibial myxedema with plasmapheresis. Br Med J 1:374–376, 1979.

191. Sattler H: Basedow's Disease. New York, Grune and Stratton, 1952.

192. Bram I: Exophthalmic Goiter and Its Nonsurgical Treatment. St. Louis, CV Mosby, 1920.

42

Ophthalmopathy

COLUM A. GORMAN
ARMIN E. HEUFELDER
GEORGE B. BARTLEY

The peripheral manifestations of Graves' disease include ophthalmopathy, dermopathy, and acropachy. Of these, Graves' ophthalmopathy is the most common. It is subtly present in at least 70 per cent of patients with Graves' hyperthyroidism,[1] although it may be overtly manifest in only about 3 per cent of Graves' patients when thyrotoxicosis is diagnosed.[2] Onset of ophthalmopathy may precede or follow the diagnosis of hyperthyroidism. Most commonly, however, the conditions commence concurrently (Fig. 42–1).

In the absence of Graves' hyperthyroidism, patients with thyroid-associated ophthalmopathy usually have some demonstrable immunological feature of underlying autoimmune thyroid disease (e.g., stimulating or blocking antibodies directed against the thyroid-stimulating hormone [TSH] receptor,[3] or antibodies directed against thyroglobulin,[4] thyroid peroxidase,[5] or thyroid membranes),[6] or they have histological evidence for thyroiditis.[7] Depending on the prevailing functional activity of these antibodies and the degree of immune-mediated damage to the thyroid gland, thyroid function in these patients tends to vary over time and may include periods of hyperthyroidism, hypothyroidism, and euthyroidism.[8, 9]

Models developed to explain the pathogenetic mechanisms leading to thyroid-associated ophthalmopathy must address the unique clinical links between ophthalmopathy, pretibial dermopathy, and autoimmune thyroid disease, including their frequent temporal synchronism,[8, 9] the striking—although not absolute—predilection for certain extraocular muscles,[10] asymmetrical ophthalmopathy,[1] and the reasons why severe ophthalmopathy develops in only a small minority of patients with Graves' hyperthyroidism.[2]

Although the pathogenesis of Graves' ophthalmopathy remains incompletely understood, we do understand the proximate mechanisms underlying the clinical symptoms. At the heart of the matter is a discrepancy between the volume of swollen retrobulbar soft tissues and the space in the bony orbit.[1] In this chapter, we review the essential elements of the eye examination, describe the clinical features of Graves' ophthalmopathy, discuss pressure-volume relationships in the orbit, explore what is known of pathogenesis, and recommend approaches to the diagnosis and treatment of this disorder.

INCIDENCE AND PREVALENCE

Tunbridge performed a cross-sectional study of the community of Whickham in England.[11] In this mixed urban and rural area, a 1 in 6 sample of the adult population was taken, which is considered to be representative of the British general population. The prevalence of previously undiagnosed hyperthyroidism was 4.7 per 1000 women. Previously diagnosed hyperthyroidism was found in 20 women per 1000 population. The incidence was about three cases per 1000 women annually. The condition was 10 times more common in women than in men, and mean age at diagnosis was 48 years. In a study from the United States in which serum free thyroxine index was used as the method of diagnosis, a similar incidence of hyperthyroidism was detected in a health screening program.[12]

The number of patients within a population who have ophthalmopathy is a matter of definition. Clinically apparent ophthalmopathy is present in about 3 per cent of the patients with Graves' disease.[2] When more subtle imaging techniques, such as ultrasonography,[13] MR imaging,[14] or CT scanning,[1] are used to identify early ophthalmopathy, a majority of Graves' patients, ranging from 60 to 90 per cent in different studies, show changes diagnostic of Graves' ophthalmopathy.

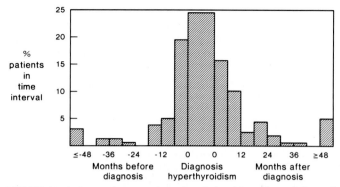

FIGURE 42–1. **Onset of eye symptoms in relationship to time of diagnosis of hyperthyroidism** (0 on horizontal axis). Number of patients who first experienced eye symptoms within a given six-month period is expressed as a percentage of the entire group. (From Gorman CA: Temporal relationship between onset of Graves' ophthalmopathy and diagnosis of thyrotoxicosis. Mayo Clin Proc 58:517, 1983.)

PATHOGENESIS

Mechanical Factors

In mechanical terms, the central problem in Graves' ophthalmopathy is a discrepancy between increased volume of retrobulbar soft tissues and the inexpansible space of the bony orbit (Fig. 42–2). The orbit is cone-shaped and open only to the front. An increase in volume of extraocular muscle and connective tissue can be accommodated without a pressure increase by forward displacement of the globe. As proptosis develops, however, the anterior movement of the globe is limited by the orbital septum and eyelids and by the tethering effect of the extraocular muscles. The stage is therefore set, by increased soft tissue volume posteriorly and restricted globe motion anteriorly, for a pressure rise in the orbital cavity.[15] It is important to note that not all of the pain, swelling, and conjunctival erythema seen in Graves' ophthalmopathy are due to inflammation. The rapidity of resolution following orbital decompression suggests that at least some of these findings are due to congestion.[16]

Abundant indirect and rather limited direct evidence[17] suggests that retrobulbar extradural pressure is increased in Graves' ophthalmopathy. The correlation between proptosis and direct intraconal pressure measurements in cadavers within 24 hours of death has been studied by Stanley et al.[16] An intraconal extradural balloon was expanded, and

simultaneous pressure and proptosis measurements revealed that proptosis increased with as little as 1 ml increase in balloon volume. Pressure increased rapidly when a critical increment in orbital balloon volume was reached. Stanley and co-workers[16] then subjected the orbits to a variety of decompression techniques and established that intraorbital pressure reduction correlated with the amount of bony orbital wall removed. In patients with Graves' ophthalmopathy, volume expansion of retrobulbar tissues appears to be due mainly to deposition of glycosaminoglycans (GAG's), which are potent water-binding molecules, in the retrobulbar space.[18]

Predisposing Factors

Several immunogenetic factors may predispose an individual with Graves' disease to develop severe ophthalmopathy.[19] These include susceptibility genes encoding certain HLA-DR genotypes, immunoglobulin allotypes, and T-cell receptor polymorphisms.[20, 21] Although some geographical and racial variations in HLA-DR genotypes have been reported,[22] no consistent major differences in genetic susceptibility among patients with Graves' disease with and without severe ophthalmopathy have been confirmed. The ratio of females to males in patients with Graves' hyperthyroidism is approximately 10:1.[11] Among patients with severe ophthalmopathy the female:male ratio is 2.3:1.[23] Cigarette smoking is a potential environmental risk factor for ophthalmopathy.[24–26] Because more men smoke cigarettes, this factor may contribute to the relatively higher incidence of ophthalmopathy in men. Asian smokers appear to have a lower incidence of ophthalmopathy than do Europeans.[24]

Although it has been suggested that the manner in which hyperthyroidism is treated may define the later development of ophthalmopathy,[27–32] the evidence to date is not entirely convincing. Marcocci et al.[198] found similar rates of progression of ophthalmopathy in patients treated with radioiodine and those who had thyroidectomy. Corticosteroids ameliorated the eye changes. Tallstedt et al.[199] observed that ophthalmopathy developed or worsened more frequently in patients who received radioiodine than in those who received antithyroid drugs or surgery. Sridama and DeGroot found approximately equal incidence of clinically significant ophthalmopathy among patients treated with ^{131}I, surgery, and antithyroid drugs.[31] Because the time courses of treated hyperthyroidism and ophthal-

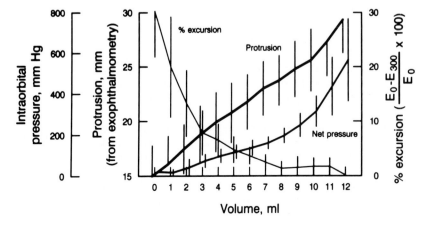

FIGURE 42–2. Mean (± SD) orbital protrusion, intraorbital pressure, and percentage of excursion as functions of added intraorbital volume. (From Stanley RJ, et al: Space-occupying orbital lesions: Can critical increases in intraorbital pressure be predicted clinically? Laryngoscope 99:22, 1989.)

mopathy are different, in some patients ophthalmopathy inevitably worsens following treatment directed to the thyroid. In the view of the authors, to ascribe such worsening to the treatment seems unwise.

Humoral Autoimmunity

The pathogenesis of the hyperthyroidism of Graves' disease is well explained by the presence of circulating immunoglobulins directed against the TSH receptor, causing unregulated production of excessive amounts of thyroid hormone.[33–35, 90] In contrast, it has been difficult to define a similar role for TSH receptor–stimulating immunoglobulins in the pathogenesis of Graves' ophthalmopathy. Serum concentrations of thyroid-stimulating immunoglobulin (TSI) measured by the cAMP generation assay in FRTL-5 cells show a general correlation with severity of ophthalmopathy.[33, 36] In the authors' experience (unpublished), a diagnosis of Graves' ophthalmopathy should be seriously questioned if TSI activity is absent from the serum when measured by this method.

Stimulation of collagen synthesis in fibroblasts by monoclonal TSH receptor antibodies has been reported[37]; however, excessive production of collagen does not seem to play a major role in this ophthalmopathy, and purified IgG's from sera with high TSI activity have failed to consistently stimulate GAG synthesis in cultured Graves' retro-ocular or pretibial fibroblasts.[38, 39] Patients with pretibial dermopathy reportedly have a subset of TSH receptor antibodies capable of potently stimulating thyroid follicular cell and fibroblast growth and protein synthesis.[38] Additionally, TSH-stimulated thyroid cells secrete an undefined factor that can potentiate the mitogenic activity of insulin-like growth factor (IGF) I for fibroblasts.[40] Graves' IgG's of potential relevance to Graves' ophthalmopathy have recently been shown to be capable of stimulating a 72-kDa heat shock protein (HSP) in thyroid cells and in Graves' retro-ocular fibroblasts[41, 42] and also of stimulating intercellular adhesion molecule-1 (ICAM-1) in Graves' retro-ocular fibroblasts.[43] Further research is necessary to define the nature of these stimulating antibodies and their pathogenic role.

Little evidence exists to suggest a pathogenic role in Graves' ophthalmopathy for circulating antibodies against other thyroidal antigens such as thyroglobulin or thyroid peroxidase.[88, 90] Many investigators have sought to identify an antigen unique to orbital tissues or shared between the thyroid gland and the orbit using techniques such as immunoblotting and enzyme-linked immunosorbent assay (ELISA).[3, 34, 44, 89] The presence of tissue-specific autoantibodies against a 64-kDa porcine eye muscle membrane protein was initially reported in two thirds of sera from patients with clinically overt thyroid-associated eye disease, and not in controls.[45] Subsequent studies by several groups have failed to confirm the specificity and sensitivity of this report[46–48, 89] and, in fact, have suggested that the 64-kDa eye muscle protein lacks pathogenic relevance.[49, 50] Recently, screening of a human thyroid cDNA expression library with sera from patients with Hashimoto's thyroiditis has revealed another potentially relevant cross-reactive epitope localized on a novel 64-kDa autoantigen.[51] Among the tissues studied, restriction of mRNA for this protein to human thyroid and eye muscle tissue has been reported, but its cellular localization within retro-ocular muscle and its functional relevance in Graves' ophthalmopathy remain to be established. Antibodies to a 23-kDa orbital fibroblast antigen have been found to lack specificity for Graves' ophthalmopathy.[46] Finally, the constitutive expression of a 72-kDa HSP (HSP 72) in cultured human retro-ocular and pretibial fibroblasts from patients with severe Graves' ophthalmopathy and pretibial dermopathy and its stress-enhanced expression on the cell surface of Graves' retro-ocular fibroblasts have been described.[52, 53] No expression of HSP 72 was found in abdominal fibroblasts of these same patients or in any fibroblast site of normal individuals. Strong expression of HSP 72 has also been reported in thyroid tissues from patients with Graves' disease and Hashimoto's thyroiditis but not in normal or goitrous thyroid glands.[54] The importance of these findings is not known, but it may be relevant, with respect to the proposed immunoregulatory functions of the 70-kDa HSP family,[55] that HSP 72 can be induced by purified Graves' IgG's both in rat thyroid follicular cells (FRTL-5) (Heufelder et al., unpublished observation) and in retro-ocular fibroblasts from patients with Graves' ophthalmopathy.[41, 42]

In view of its intriguing sequence homology with acetylcholinesterase, thyroglobulin has been implicated as a candidate antigen for epitope sharing and antibody cross-reactivity between homologous orbital and thyroidal epitopes.[56] However, serum thyroglobulin levels are not consistently elevated in Graves' ophthalmopathy, and conditions such as subacute thyroiditis, in which thyroglobulin levels are increased, are not associated with ophthalmopathy.

Cellular Autoimmunity

Studies exploring T-cell responses to orbital antigens have traditionally suffered from their confinement to peripherally circulating or thyroid-derived T cells, which may not reflect the autoimmune response within the retro-ocular space in Graves' ophthalmopathy. Assays of T-cell proliferation[50] and production of migration inhibition factor[57] have been used, with some problems concerning reproducibility. As with humoral studies, the observed T-cell responses have lacked specificity and were not confined to patients with thyroid-associated ophthalmopathy. Specific cytotoxic T-cell reactivity that is directed against a defined retro-ocular tissue and is unique to patients with Graves' ophthalmopathy has not been described. One study has suggested that antibody-dependent, natural killer cell–mediated cytotoxicity against extraocular muscle cells can be uniquely demonstrated in approximately 50 per cent of patients with thyroid-associated ophthalmopathy.[58] However, this observation has remained unconfirmed, and no cell damage to extraocular muscle is obvious in situ even when electron microscopic techniques are employed[59] or when well-preserved formalin-fixed or snap-frozen tissue sections through Graves' extraocular muscle bodies are studied.[60]

Histology

Imaging studies indicate that the extraocular muscle bodies, as well as the retro-ocular connective tissue spaces, are enlarged in Graves' ophthalmopathy.[1, 10, 14] CT images reveal that extraocular muscle tendons are relatively spared, in contrast to orbital myositis.[1, 10] Although the extraocular muscle tissue is grossly enlarged in Graves' ophthalmopathy, the muscle fibers themselves are morphologically and functionally normal.[60–63] The histological analysis of retro-ocular tissues in such patients has revealed two major abnormalities: (1) the presence of a mixed mononuclear cell population (including lymphocytes, monocytes, macrophages, and mast cells) that infiltrates predominantly the interstitial connective tissue within and around extraocular muscles but can also be detected in the retro-ocular connective and adipose tissue at a distance from extraocular muscle and in the lacrimal gland[59, 64–67] (Fig. 42–3), and (2) the expansion of the connective tissue compartment and the presence of large quantities of hydrophilic extracellular matrix components (GAG's, mainly hyaluronic acid) in retro-ocular tissues, including extraocular muscles.[18, 59, 66, 69]

Recent studies have characterized the mononuclear cell infiltrate as consisting mainly of CD8+ T cells (suppressor/cytotoxic) and CD4+ (helper/inducer) T cells (CD4/CD8 ratio approximately 1:1.5) (Fig. 42–4), a significant proportion of which carry the CD45RO + phenotype characteristic of memory T cells.[61, 65, 67, 70] Macrophages, mast cells, and a few B lymphocytes are also present. This infiltration is accompanied by strong co-expression of various adhesion molecules and HLA-DR molecules in endothelial cells, connective tissue cells, and perimysial fibroblasts, reflecting both the activated state of these cells and their capacity to perform functions relevant to antigen processing, presentation, and interaction with lymphocytes (Fig. 42–5).[67] Surprisingly, extraocular muscle cells do not express these adhesion and HLA-DR molecules in situ. Further, deposition of IgE and IgA has been detected in the perimysial connective tissue of Graves' extraocular muscles.[71, 72] Recently, immunoreactivity for C3Bi has been detected in the connective tissue interstitium and perimysium of extraocular muscles in patients with Graves' ophthalmopathy, whereas extraocular muscle fibers themselves were spared.[73]

Despite efforts by many investigators, a true eye muscle–

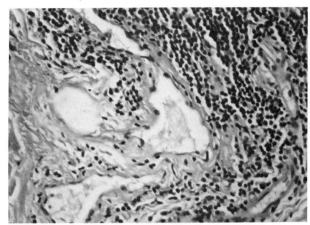

FIGURE 42–4. **Immunoperoxidase staining of a formalin-fixed retro-ocular connective tissue specimen** (obtained from a patient with severe Graves' ophthalmopathy during orbital decompression surgery). A monoclonal antibody directed against the CD8+ subset of T lymphocytes was used. Positive immunoreactivity is detected in the majority of mononuclear cells infiltrating the perivascular space. (Original magnification, × 160.)

specific protein that is recognized exclusively by sera from patients with thyroid-related ophthalmopathy, and not by normal or autoimmune control sera, has not been identified. It is possible and even probable that antibodies against orbital proteins detected to date arise as a result of the local autoimmune process within the inflamed retro-ocular tissues and do not possess primary pathogenic significance. These observations suggest that connective tissue cells such as fibroblasts, and not extraocular muscle, may be important targets for lymphocytes and thus actively contribute to the retro-ocular autoimmune processes in Graves' ophthalmopathy.

The Role of Cytokines

Cytokines and inflammatory mediators, released by infiltrating immunocompetent cells and residential connective

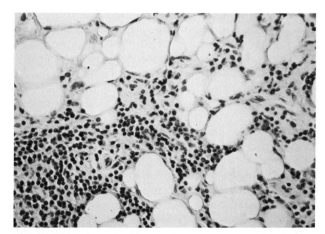

FIGURE 42–3. **Hematoxylin and eosin stain of formalin-fixed retro-ocular connective tissue** (obtained from a patient with severe Graves' ophthalmopathy during orbital decompression surgery). Mononuclear cell infiltration is present throughout the retro-ocular connective tissue. (Original magnification, × 160.)

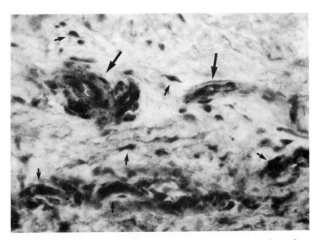

FIGURE 42–5. **Immunoperoxidase staining of a cryostat section of retro-ocular connective tissue** (obtained from a patient with severe Graves' ophthalmopathy during orbital decompression). A monoclonal antibody directed against the HLA-DR antigen was used. Strong HLA-DR immunoreactivity is present throughout the retro-ocular connective tissue and is detected in blood vessels and perivascular areas (*large arrows*) as well as in connective tissue cells (*small arrows*) and their surrounding extracellular matrix. (Original magnification, × 320.)

tissue cells, may influence a variety of processes that are pertinent to the pathogenesis.[52, 64, 67, 68, 74, 75] Various cytokines and growth factors are capable of stimulating proliferation and replication of retro-ocular fibroblasts.[93] Co-culture with mitogen-activated lymphocytes, incubation with lymphocyte-conditioned medium, and exposure to various cytokines such as interferon-γ (IFN-γ), interleukin-1α (IL-1α), and transforming growth factor-β (TGF-β) stimulate GAG synthesis in retro-ocular fibroblasts.[76–79, 85] Thus, lymphocyte-derived cytokines or autocrine mechanisms likely contribute to the local accumulation of GAG's in Graves' ophthalmopathy and pretibial dermopathy. Interferon-γ and tumor necrosis factor-α (TNF-α) are particularly effective in stimulating the expression of HLA-DR molecules in cultured retro-ocular and pretibial fibroblasts from patients with Graves' ophthalmopathy and pretibial dermopathy.[74] A similar spectrum of cytokines is capable of up-regulating the expression of a functional ICAM-1 in retro-ocular fibroblasts, thus facilitating their ICAM-1–mediated binding to and interaction with lymphocytes via their ICAM-1 counter-receptor, lymphocyte-associated adhesion molecule-1.[43, 80] In situ immunoreactivity for each of these cytokines has been demonstrated in mononuclear cell infiltrates, connective tissue, and vascular endothelium in retro-ocular tissues from patients with severe Graves' ophthalmopathy (Fig. 42–6).[67] Thus, the cytokine-mediated coordinate expression of certain adhesion receptors and MHC class II molecules by vascular endothelium, connective tissue, and perimysial fibroblasts may not only control the access of inflammatory cells to the retro-ocular space but also facilitate their migration, targeting, and effector functions, such as antigen processing and presentation,[80, 81] within the retro-ocular space. Development of site-specific extrathyroidal manifestations that are strongly associated with Graves' disease requires a certain cell type, a particular antigen, or a pathogenic mechanism that is common to all anatomical areas involved. Antigen specific to extraocular muscle does not fulfill these requirements. Both in situ and in vitro studies support the evolving concept of Graves' ophthal-mopathy as a locally controlled disease process, in which a network of paracrine and autocrine factors mediates and sustains the autoimmune process within the inflammatory retro-ocular microenvironment.[18, 64, 68, 80, 83–85]

Extraocular Muscles as Targets

Extraocular muscles reveal more muscle spindles, more interstitial connective tissue, richer nerve supply, and greater blood flow than skeletal muscle,[35, 86] and some of these factors may vary between and within individuals. Any such variable or several in combination may play a role in the unique involvement of extraocular muscle tissue in Graves' ophthalmopathy. Although some histological and sonographic results suggest a more uniform involvement of all seven extraocular muscles, the predilection of the disease process for the inferior and medial recti muscles is difficult to explain. Based on their immediate anatomical proximity to the ethmoid and maxillary sinuses and the relatively thin bony walls that may easily be transgressed, it is tempting to speculate that an infectious or toxic agent (viruses, tobacco-derived compounds) might reach the orbits via the paranasal sinuses.

Fibroblasts as Target Cells

Although fibroblasts may qualify as common pathogenic mediators, there are site-specific differences between fibroblasts from involved and uninvolved anatomical areas.[77] Apart from morphological differences in cell culture,[79] Graves' retro-ocular and pretibial fibroblasts are particularly sensitive to IFN-γ and TNF-α in terms of expressing HLA-DR molecules[18, 74] and in terms of glucocorticoid modulation of cytokine-induced HLA-DR expression[91, 92] and cell proliferation.[93] Similarly, fibroblasts from these particular locations constitutively express a 72-kDa HSP and appear to be uniquely sensitive to HSP 72–enhancing mechanisms.[52, 53, 75] IFN-γ stimulates GAG production by retro-ocular connective tissue fibroblasts and does not affect GAG production by fibroblasts derived from pretibial and abdominal skin.[77] Compared with dermal fibroblasts, retro-ocular fibroblasts are more susceptible to the inhibitory effects of triiodothyronine and dexamethasone in terms of GAG production.[87] Thus, certain morphological and functional differences appear to exist between fibroblasts from different anatomical sites that may render fibroblasts in certain sites particularly susceptible to the immunopathological process associated with Graves' disease.

In summary, to our perception, histological and immunological data support a role for retro-ocular fibroblasts both as targets and as metabolically and immunologically active cells in Graves' ophthalmopathy. Cytokine-activated adhesion molecules in the vascular endothelium may allow certain circulating immunocompetent cells to gain access to the extravascular space within the orbit. Expression of adhesion molecules by retro-ocular connective tissue cells or recognition of cross-reacting antigens may then further direct T-cell migration and targeting. Based on their unique and differential expression of certain surface molecules, fibroblasts residing in extraocular muscle interstitium and retro-ocular connective tissue, upon contact with

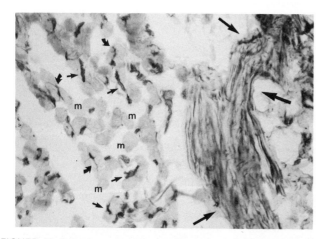

FIGURE 42–6. **Immunoperoxidase staining of a cryosat section through the belly of the inferior rectus muscle,** derived at autopsy from a patient with severe Graves' ophthalmopathy. A monoclonal antibody directed against intercellular adhesion molecule-1 (ICAM-1) was used. ICAM-1 immunoreactivity is detected in cells residing in the retro-ocular connective tissue (*large arrows*), in the extraocular muscle interstitium (*straight small arrows*), and in perimysial connective tissue (*curved small arrows*) surrounding extraocular muscle fibers(m). No ICAM-1 immunoreactivity is detected in extraocular muscle tissue itself. (Original magnification, × 160.)

infiltrating lymphocytes and macrophages, may become activated to process and present antigen and to produce GAG's in response to the evolving network of inflammatory mediators within the orbit (Fig. 42–7). Chronicity of the ongoing inflammatory activities within the orbit may eventually lead to progressive fibrosis of extraocular muscle interstitia, intraorbital septae, and retro-ocular connective tissue. Further study is indicated of interactions between lymphocytes and target/effector cells in the orbit.

Effect of Abnormal Thyroid Function on Severity of Graves' Ophthalmopathy

A close temporal relationship exists between the onset of eye changes and hyperthyroidism. Among 163 patients, 81 per cent first noted their eye changes within 18 months of the diagnosis of hyperthyroidism[9] (see Fig. 42–2). Wiersinga et al.[94] found that in 23 per cent of their patients, eye disease developed before the hyperthyroidism, and in 77 per cent, it developed concomitantly with or after the onset of Graves' thyroid disease. In 2.4 per cent of Graves' ophthalmopathy patients, autoimmune thyroid disease was first manifest as hypothyroidism.[94]

When sensitive tests of thyroid function and regulation are performed, very few patients are found to have true "euthyroid Graves' disease." Salvi et al.[5] and Marcocci et al.[95] found evidence for abnormal thyroid function or regulation in all of their presumably euthyroid Graves' ophthalmopathy patients.

History and Examination

In order to diagnose the clinical features of Graves' ophthalmopathy, it is helpful for the physician to be familiar with a problem-focused ophthalmic history and examination.[96, 97]

The History of Present Illness

The most important element of an ophthalmic history is to determine if the patient has noted a decrease in visual acuity. If so, is the disturbance of vision monocular or binocular and is it acute or chronic? Is the patient aware of any blind spots (scotomata) in the visual field? Double vision is a frequent symptom of dysthyroid ophthalmopathy. If the patient is having diplopia, one should ascertain whether the two images are separated horizontally, vertically, or a combination of the two. Is the double vision constant or intermittent, and is the patient able to fuse the disparate images with effort? Although it is unusual, double vision may occur in only one eye because of ocular media abnormalities, so one should question the patient as to whether the diplopia is relieved if one eye is occluded. The examiner should inquire about ocular comfort; patients with Graves' eyes often complain of light sensitivity (photophobia) or tearing (epiphora) because of exposure, or a vague feeling of "fullness" or "pressure" behind the globes because of the increase in retrobulbar tissue volume.

The Past Ophthalmic History

Patients should be questioned about previous ophthalmic surgical procedures or treatments to help determine if recent eye complaints are related to previous disorders. Specifically, has the patient undergone cataract extraction, strabismus operations, retinal detachment repair, or laser surgery? Some patients with a history of strabismus may not recall that they had crossed eyes during childhood or had extraocular muscle surgery; this historical detail may imply the presence of amblyopia (lazy eye), which many patients surprisingly are not aware of until unrelated ophthalmic problems develop in adulthood. A history of ocular trauma or treatment for glaucoma is of obvious importance, and the past or present use of topical ophthalmic medications, several of which have systemic side effects, should be recorded.

An Ophthalmic Examination for the Nonophthalmologist

Much useful information may be gleaned from a simplified 10-part eye examination, without using the specialized equipment needed for a formal ophthalmic evaluation.

VISUAL ACUITY. Quantitation of visual acuity is usually measured as a Snellen fraction (e.g., 20/30) for distance vision. During bedside or office examinations, however, one may use a near vision acuity card, several of which are commercially available. In the absence of a standardized card, the patient may be asked to read any available printed material, for example, the smallest type possible in a newspaper; the size of the print can be recorded, or the material itself can be taped in the patient's record. Of course, the patient should wear his glasses when visual acuity is being checked, and each eye should be evaluated separately.

COLOR VISION. Because loss of color perception may be

Connective tissue autoimmunity in GO

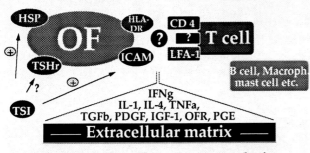

Glycosaminoglycan accumulation

proptosis, diplopia, periorbital edema, inflammation

FIGURE 42–7. The authors' current concept of pathogenesis of Graves' ophthalmopathy (GO). The progress of events is from top to bottom. Activated immunocompetent cells infiltrate the orbit and interact with each other and with orbital fibroblasts (OF), which are known to express HLA-DR, intercellular adhesion molecule-1 (ICAM-1), and heat shock protein (HSP). The presence of thyroid-stimulating hormone (TSH) receptor on orbital fibroblasts is presumed but not proven. Thyroid-stimulating immunoglobulins enhance HSP and ICAM-1 expression on the orbital fibroblasts and presumably interact with the putative TSH receptor. A variety of cytokines are produced (designated in the open triangle) as a result of these cellular interactions. The cytokines increase glycosaminoglycan production in the confined orbital space, and the resultant soft tissue swelling evokes the clinical symptoms and findings.

an early sign of optic neuropathy, color vision evaluation is an important diagnostic test.[98–100] A Farnsworth-Munsell panel is preferred for the detection of subtle acquired defects because most pseudoisochromatic color plate systems are designed to evince congenital color vision abnormalities.[101] One should remember that approximately 7 per cent of the male population has some degree of congenital red-green color "blindness." If color vision screening tests are not available, one simple method of detecting possible early optic neuropathy is to check whether the patient perceives a difference between the two eyes in the color intensity of a red object; the top of a bottle of mydriatic eyedrops is commonly used for this purpose.

PUPILS. The direct and consensual pupillary responses should be checked. An afferent pupillary defect (Marcus Gunn pupil) may indicate optic neuropathy.

EYELIDS. Upper eyelid retraction is the single most useful finding in establishing the diagnosis of Graves' ophthalmopathy.[102] Lid retraction may be unilateral or bilateral and may be subtle in some instances. The upper lid usually rests approximately 1 to 2 mm below the junction of the cornea and sclera; therefore, if the white of the eye is seen above the corneoscleral limbus, eyelid retraction of at least 1.5 mm is present. The level of the lower eyelid is typically at the inferior corneoscleral limbus. Lower eyelid retraction is a less constant and specific finding and usually is not seen in Graves' ophthalmopathy without concomitant retraction of the upper lids. Early in the course of thyroid disease the eyelid malpositions may result from increased sympathetic activity; with chronicity, however, the eyelid retractors (levator palpebrae superioris and Müller's muscle) become hypertrophic, eventually fibrotic, and adherent to orbital tissues.[103] Lid lag (Figs. 42–8 and 42–9), which is diagnosed by asking the patient to look down and observing delayed or restricted excursion of the upper eyelids as they follow the globes, and lagophthalmos (Fig. 42–10), which is the inability to close the eyelids completely, are suggestive of Graves' ophthalmopathy. Eyelid retraction, lid lag, and lagophthalmos frequently interfere with the maintenance of an adequate tear film on the eye. The result is ocular irritation and dryness, reflex tearing, and corneal scarring or even ulceration in severe cases.

CONJUCTIVA AND CORNEA. The conjunctiva is the clear, thin tissue that covers the sclera. It normally is transparent, except for the small blood vessels that course within it. In Graves' ophthalmopathy, the conjunctiva may become hyperemic (usually termed injection) or edematous (chemo-

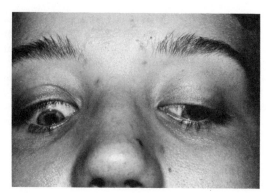

FIGURE 42–9. Lid lag of the right upper eyelid, a common sign of Graves' ophthalmopathy.

sis) from exposure or from decreased venous drainage due to orbital suffusion. A characteristic conjunctival finding in patients with Graves' eyes is focal injection over the insertions of the lateral or medial rectus muscles (Fig. 42–11). The engorged blood vessels do not extend to the corneoscleral limbus. This is in contrast to the prominent corkscrew vessels that may be seen secondary to a dural–cavernous sinus fistula, an entity that may be confused with Graves' ophthalmopathy.

The cornea normally should appear transparent and lustrous. Dryness resulting from exposure is difficult to detect without slit-lamp biomicroscopy. Corneal ulceration, which is an ophthalmic emergency, usually can be seen grossly with a penlight and typically is accompanied by severe pain.[104]

EXOPHTHALMOMETRY. Proptosis may be quantitated with an exophthalmometer, an instrument that measures the position of the globes in relation to a stable reference point (usually the lateral orbital rim). The device is easy to use and is helpful in documenting the results of treatment. Exophthalmometry in most adult eyes measures 22 mm or less, and the difference between the patient's two eyes usually does not exceed 2 mm.[105] Most Caucasians have Hertel exophthalmometry measurements of less than 18 mm.

OCULAR MOTILITY. The range of movement should be evaluated for each eye separately and then with the eyes together, during which time the patient should be asked to state whether double vision is noted. Diplopia is most likely to occur in upgaze or in extremes of lateral gaze because of restriction of the inferior recti or medial recti. Any or

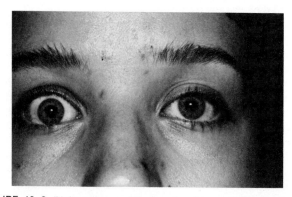

FIGURE 42–8. Right upper eyelid retraction in a patient with Graves' ophthalmopathy.

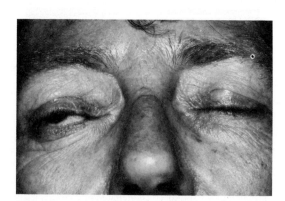

FIGURE 42–10. Lagophthalmos (an inability to close the eyelids completely) often causes exposure keratopathy (dryness of the cornea and conjunctiva).

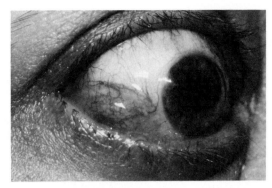

FIGURE 42–11. Chemosis (conjunctival edema) and focal injection (conjunctival blood vessel dilation) over the lateral rectus muscle insertion in a patient with Graves' ophthalmopathy.

all of the extraocular muscles may be involved in Graves' ophthalmopathy, however, and unusual patterns of incomitant strabismus may occur (Fig. 42–12).

VISUAL FIELDS. As noted above, scotomata may appear in the visual field from optic neuropathy. Formal perimetry is the most sensitive method of detecting early defects, which often involve the inferior visual field or the paracentral region or cause generalized constriction.[99] An Amsler grid, a hand-held card with a pattern of perpendicular crossed lines, may be used in the office or at the bedside as a simple screening tool. Gross visual field defects may be detected with careful confrontation testing.

INTRAOCULAR PRESSURE. Although most internists do not routinely measure intraocular pressure, the technique is simple to learn and practitioners with an interest in thyroid disease may wish to consider obtaining a hand-held tonometer for this purpose. Elevation of the intraocular pressure in upgaze, in comparison with the measurement in primary (straight ahead) gaze, occurs in normal persons[106] but is augmented in patients with Graves' ophthalmopathy because of external pressure on the globe from the enlarged, tight extraocular muscles. Although the finding has been considered by some authors[107, 108] to be an adjunctive feature of the diagnostic portrait, other investigators have questioned its usefulness.[109, 110]

OPHTHALMOSCOPY. Examination of the posterior pole of the retina may show a swollen optic disc from compressive optic neuropathy or choroidal folds (a slat-like, corrugated pattern) that occasionally accompany mechanical orbital

processes. Visually significant disorders such as opacities of the ocular media (corneal irregularities or cataracts) or macular degeneration also may be noted easily with the direct ophthalmoscope.

Differential Diagnosis

The diagnosis of Graves' ophthalmopathy is straightforward in a hyperthyroid patient with proptosis, eyelid retraction, restriction of ocular motility, and evidence of enlarged extraocular muscles on CT. In many patients the entire constellation of clinical and laboratory features is not present, making diagnosis more difficult.[111] Conditions that mimic Graves' ophthalmopathy usually may be categorized into one of three groups: inflammatory/infectious, vascular, or neoplastic.

Inflammatory disorders of the orbit include several entities referred to as "pseudotumor" (more specifically, myositis, dacryoadenitis, or scleritis), Wegener's granulomatosis, and sarcoidosis.[112] Inflammations may cause one or both eyes to protrude and often are associated with extraocular muscle enlargement on CT.[113, 114] Many authors have written that two important differential diagnostic CT features in favor of orbital inflammatory processes and against Graves' orbitopathy are bilaterality and involvement of the extraocular muscle tendons. A recent report, however, found that in orbital inflammations the process was bilateral in 40 per cent of patients and the tendons were involved in only 47 per cent of cases.[115] Orbital infections such as cellulitis, sinus mucoceles, or mucormycosis do not often cause diagnostic confusion.[116]

Vascular anomalies of the orbit that may simulate the clinical features of Graves' ophthalmopathy include dural–cavernous sinus fistulae (low-flow shunts), carotid–cavernous sinus fistulae (high-flow shunts),[117] and orbital varices. Historical features and appropriate radiographic studies usually facilitate proper diagnosis.

Neoplasms of the orbit, whether primary, secondary, or metastatic, often cause proptosis but infrequently are bilateral.[118] Lymphoma, however, may occur in both orbits, but the absence of extraocular muscle enlargement or eyelid retraction should help to differentiate it from Graves' ophthalmopathy.

Myasthenia gravis should always be considered in the evaluation of a patient with presumed dysthyroid ophthalmopathy.[119] Both disorders involve a disturbance of autoimmunity, and both may cause unusual patterns of strabismus and eyelid position.

Therapy

Treatment early in Graves' ophthalmopathy is directed toward protection of the cornea, relief of discomfort, and shrinkage of orbital soft tissues by immunosuppressive drugs or radiation therapy. Later in the course, surgical expansion of the bony orbital space is frequently necessary. Correction of extraocular muscle dysfunction and restoration of normal eyelid position complete the patient's rehabilitation. Frequently the condition is mild and spontaneously improves. Often one manifestation is prominent, for example, extraocular muscle dysfunction or eyelid re-

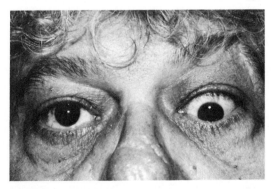

FIGURE 42–12. Hypotropia of the left eye secondary to contraction of the left inferior rectus muscle in Graves' ophthalmopathy. Unusual patterns of strabismus are characteristic of both Graves' ophthalmopathy and myasthenia gravis, diseases that may occur concomitantly.

traction, and treatment may be directed at the single problem. Patients with severe disease usually need all three modalities—correction of the soft tissue volume-space discrepancy in the orbit, strabismus surgery, and eyelid repair. These treatments usually are performed in the order listed, that is, orbital decompression precedes extraocular muscle surgery, which should, in turn, precede eyelid surgery. In all patients it is important to restore thyroid hormone levels to normal before any type of orbital surgery is done. The single exception to this rule is when very severe ophthalmopathy threatens vision and requires urgent orbital decompression.

Clinical Decisions

In deciding upon a course of therapy for these patients, clinicians should consider first whether the diagnosis is firmly established. As outlined in the section on differential diagnosis, many other conditions can mimic Graves' ophthalmopathy. In doubtful cases, orbital CT can be very helpful. Is the patient hyperthyroid, hypothyroid, or euthyroid? If thyroid dysfunction is present, it should be corrected before specific eye therapy is advised (local measures to relieve discomfort and protect the cornea are always appropriate). Is the ophthalmopathy still worsening, which is characteristically true in the first six months or so from the point of onset? Are the findings and symptoms stable and, if so, for how long and what is the patient's tolerance of the current symptoms? Is there evidence for spontaneous improvement in recent months? Which eye symptom or finding is of greatest concern to the patient, and which is viewed as most significant by the physician? Physician and patient need to establish common goals. At times, appearance and minor degrees of diplopia are high on the list of patient concerns, whereas physician concerns may be directed toward the presence of mild optic neuropathy. At this point, also, the overall treatment plan leading to the patient's complete rehabilitation should be established and coordinated with other consultants participating in the patient's care. The sequence of treatments should be agreed upon by patient and physicians. Again, we emphasize that decompressions should precede extraocular muscle surgery, which, in turn, should be completed before eyelid surgery is undertaken.[120]

Medical Treatment

All patients with Graves' ophthalmopathy should be instructed in simple measures to protect the cornea. These include the use of eye protection in windy, dusty, or industrial workplace environments and the use of dark glasses to relieve photophobia. Artificial tears may be employed liberally by patients who complain of dry eye symptoms. Taping the eyelids shut at night may prevent unpleasant exposure symptoms. Elevation of the head of the bed and diuretics are seldom of much help.

Corticosteroids and Immunosuppressives

Corticosteroids may be injected into the retrobulbar space, applied as topical eye drops, or taken orally. Retrobulbar injections originally held promise of achieving high local concentrations of corticosteroids in affected areas while minimizing systemic side effects.[121, 122] They are usually given twice weekly using a depocorticosteroid preparation. In practice, patients quickly tire of the repetitive injections and, in time, alternative treatment must be offered. In the short term, retrobulbar corticosteroids, especially for optic neuropathy, achieve comparable degrees of symptomatic relief, as do systemic steroids.[123]

Oral corticosteroids are particularly effective when the eyes are visibly reddened, swollen, congested, and painful.[101, 124] The major limitation to their use in high doses for long periods is their inevitable and sometimes severe side effects. Effective therapy frequently involves administration of 60 to 80 mg of prednisone daily for weeks at a time.[125] Such therapy commonly results in weight gain, redistribution of fat, gastric irritation, hyperglycemia, and osteoporosis. The combination of corticosteroids and radiation therapy is more effective than is treatment with corticosteroids alone.[126]

So-called burst therapy with corticosteroids has been advocated for patients with very severe ophthalmopathy, particularly when complicated by optic neuropathy.[127] Usually 1 g methylprednisolone sodium succinate is infused intravenously for 60 minutes daily on three successive days, and this course may be repeated several times at intervals of one week. Modest improvements in periorbital soft tissue swelling, size and function of extraocular muscles, and proptosis have been reported.[127]

In a comparative trial of cyclosporine and prednisone in treatment of severe Graves' ophthalmopathy, Prummel et al.[124] used 7.5 mg of cyclosporine per kilogram of body weight per day in comparison with prednisone, 60 mg/day initially, subsequently tapered to 20 mg/day. During a 12-week treatment period, 11 prednisone-treated and 4 cyclosporine-treated patients responded to therapy. The response was manifested by decreases in eye muscle enlargement and proptosis and improved visual acuity. The authors concluded that single-drug therapy with prednisone was more effective than cyclosporine and that the combination could be effective in patients who did not respond to either drug alone. The subject of immunosuppressant therapy for thyroid eye disease has been extensively reviewed by Kahaly and Beyer.[128]

Orbital Radiation Therapy

Pinchera et al.[129] have reviewed the many uncontrolled studies of orbital radiation therapy that have been published since the early 1930's. During this era, radiation therapy techniques have varied widely, and many of the studies were retrospective. The interval between treatment and observation of results varied widely, and the raw data were sometimes obscured by inclusion in aggregated therapeutic indices.[130] Patients were frequently treated concurrently with corticosteroids, and patients with abnormal and varying thyroid function were often included.

From these early studies some general statements can be made. Radiation therapy seldom corrects either proptosis or extraocular muscle dysfunction.[131] Periorbital soft tissue changes respond best.[132] Radiation dose should not exceed 2000 cGy in 200-cGy fractions.[133] At this dose level radiation retinopathy appears to be a rare complication.[134, 135] Recently, Prummel et al.[136] performed a randomized clinical trial using sham irradiation and included untreated patients with moderately severe ophthalmopathy who were euthyroid for two months before entry and who remained so during the study. Radiation therapy was compared with oral prednisone therapy. At 24 weeks, a similar response rate to prednisone and radiation therapy was observed (50 per cent versus 46 per cent). Neither prednisone nor radiation therapy improved eye muscle enlargement on CT scan, but prednisone had a slightly greater effect on soft tissue swelling, whereas radiation therapy appeared to be somewhat more effective in improving eye muscle motility. Neither treatment had a significant effect on proptosis. Orbital radiation therapy, usually in conjunction with simultaneously administered corticosteroids, has been effective in controlling Graves' optic neuropathy. A direct comparison of orbital radiation therapy with no therapy has not yet been performed.

The Surgical Treatment of Graves' Ophthalmopathy

A tripartite approach is most commonly used in the surgical therapy of Graves' ophthalmopathy: orbital decompression to relieve optic neuropathy or proptosis, extraocular muscle surgery to reduce diplopia, and eyelid procedures to treat retraction and cosmetic disfigurement. Although only a small fraction of patients with Graves' disease require operative intervention, some patients with severe ophthalmopathy need multiple procedures to achieve satisfactory functional and esthetic results.

ORBITAL DECOMPRESSION. The orbit is decompressed by removing one or more of its bony walls, which expands the eye socket and increases the potential space for the orbital contents. Indications for the procedure include optic neuropathy, severe proptosis (which in some patients may cause subluxation of the globe anterior to the lids), vision-threatening ocular exposure, debilitating retrobulbar and periorbital pain, or intolerable corticosteroid side effects.[137] Additionally, because some extraocular muscle procedures used in Graves' ophthalmopathy patients may worsen exophthalmos, preliminary orbital decompression may be useful in patients with severe proptosis. Finally, orbital expansion may be considered in some of these patients who do not have functional ocular disease but desire enhanced cosmesis.

Optic neuropathy is the most common indication for orbital decompression. In most instances, the optic nerve is compressed by the enlarged or noncompliant extraocular muscles at the crowded orbital apex (Fig. 42–13)[138–142]; in some patients, however, the muscles are of essentially normal size.[143] By removing one or more walls of the bony orbit, pressure on the nerve is reduced. Numerous approaches to orbital decompression have been described; variations include the number of walls removed (one, two, three, or four)[144, 145] and the avenue for surgical access—lateral,[146–148] medial,[149–151] transpalpebral,[98, 152–157] transantral,[159–163] transcranial,[164–166] through a bicoronal incision,[167] endoscopically,[168] or with a combination of procedures.[169, 170] Transantral orbital decompression with removal of a portion of the medial wall and the orbital floor has been the preferred method at our institution over the past 25 years.[171–174] Potential complications of orbital decompression include worsened diplopia, hypoglobus, numbness in the distribution of the infraorbital nerve, eye-

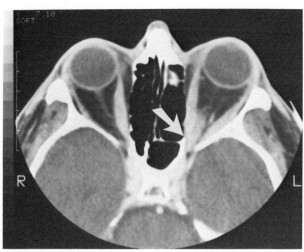

FIGURE 42–13. CT is useful to demonstrate the fusiform enlargement of the extraocular muscles in Graves' ophthalmopathy. In the left orbital apex, the optic nerve is compressed by the hypertrophied muscles (*arrow*).

lid malpositions, nasolacrimal duct obstruction, CSF leakage, meningitis, and even death in rare instances.[175–182]

It is important to recognize that patients with optic neuropathy often have less exophthalmos than patients without optic nerve compromise, as proptosis may function as the body's way of "autodecompressing" the orbit.[183] Needle aspiration of the orbital contents, previously recommended as a preliminary adjunct to orbital decompression,[184] should be avoided.

EXTRAOCULAR MUSCLE SURGERY. Diplopia resulting from extraocular muscle involvement in Graves' ophthalmopathy often is difficult to treat. When the disease is active, ocular alignment may vary from hour to hour, precluding prism spectacle correction or surgical repair. If the inflammation has stabilized and double vision cannot be corrected with glasses, then strabismus surgery is indicated.[185, 186] Because the underlying problem usually is a restrictive myopathy (not paralysis, as suggested in older reports) from tight, hypertrophied, and eventually fibrotic muscles, strabismus procedures for Graves' ophthalmopathy most frequently involve weakening the muscles by recessing their insertions onto the globe. The goal of surgery is to allow single vision in primary (straight ahead) gaze as well as in the reading position; postoperative diplopia in

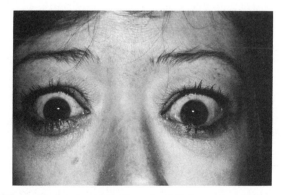

FIGURE 42–14. A patient with Graves' ophthalmopathy who has undergone bilateral transantral orbital decompression and strabismus surgery; treatment for upper eyelid retraction is indicated both to reduce ocular exposure and to enhance cosmesis.

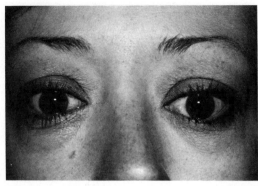

FIGURE 42–15. Same as in patient in Figure 42–14 after recession of Müller's muscle and the levator palpebrae superioris muscle in each upper eyelid.

extremes of lateral gaze or in upgaze is common and does not signify an unsuccessful procedure.

EYELID SURGERY. Eyelid surgery for Graves' ophthalmopathy is typically performed after orbital decompression and strabismus procedures, if either or both are needed (Figs. 42–14 and 42–15).[187] The retractors of the upper eyelid, the levator palpebrae superioris and Müller's muscle, undergo pathological changes similar to those seen in the extraocular muscles.[188, 189] Upper lid retraction is relieved by weakening (recessing) the muscles; lower lid retraction is treated with analogous procedures, although spacers of hard palate mucosa,[190, 191] tarsus,[192] donor sclera,[193–196] or cartilage[197] often are grafted into the lids to counteract the tendency of gravity to pull the lids inferiorly during the postoperative period. Blepharoplasty (removal of excess eyelid and orbital tissue that prolapses anteriorly from the increase in orbital volume) may be helpful in selected patients to reduce the unappealing esthetic sequelae of Graves' ophthalmopathy.

SUMMARY

Patients with severe Graves' ophthalmopathy can, in most instances, be given comfortable functional eyes and a very satisfactory appearance through energetic application of a coordinated, properly sequenced medical and surgical treatment plan. Best results are achieved when medical and surgical specialists collaborate to achieve goals defined in advance as attainable by patient and physicians.

REFERENCES

1. Forbes G, Groman CA, Bernnan MD, et al: Ophthalmopathy of Graves' disease: Computerized volume measurements of orbital fat and muscle. AJNR 7:651–656, 1986.
2. Hamilton RD, Mayberry WE, McConahey WM, Hanson KC: Ophthalmopathy of Graves' disease: A comparison between patients treated surgically and patients treated with radioiodine. Mayo Clin Proc 42:812–818, 1967.
3. Weetman AP: Thyroid associated eye disease: Pathophysiology. Lancet 338:24–28, 1991.
4. Ludgate M, Swillens S, Mercken L, Vassart G: Homology between thyroglobulin and acetylcholinesterase: An explanation for pathogenesis of Graves' ophthalmopathy. Lancet 2:219–220, 1986.
5. Salvi M, Zhang ZG, Haegert D, et al: Patients with endocrine ophthalmopathy not associated with overt thyroid disease have multiple

6. thyroid immunological abnormalities. J Clin Endocrinol Metab 70:89–94, 1990.
6. Kendall-Taylor P, Perros P, Weightman D, Taylor P: The nature and role of eye muscle autoantibodies. In Wall JR, How J (eds): Graves' Ophthalmopathy. Boston, Blackwell Scientific Publications, 1990, pp 17–28.
7. Christy JH, Morse RS: Hypothyroid Graves' disease. Ann Intern Med 62:291–296, 1977.
8. Wiersinga WM, Smit T, van der Gaag R, Koornneef L: Temporal relationship between onset of Graves' ophthalmopathy and onset of thyroidal Graves' disease. J Endocrinol Invest 11:615–619, 1988.
9. Gorman CA: Temporal relationship between onset of Graves' ophthalmopathy and diagnosis of thyrotoxicosis. Mayo Clin Proc 58:515–519, 1983.
10. Feldon SE, Lee CP, Muramatsu K, Weiner JM: Quantitative computed tomography of Graves' ophthalmopathy. Arch Ophthal 103:213–215, 1985.
11. Tunbridge WMG: The epidemiology of thyroid diseases. In Ingbar SH, Braverman LE (eds): The Thyroid. Philadelphia, JB Lippincott, 1986, pp 625–633.
12. dos Remedios LV, Weber PM, Feldman R, et al: Detecting unsuspected thyroid dysfunction by the free thyroxine index. Arch Intern Med 140:1045–1049, 1980.
13. Werner SC, Coleman DJ, Franzen LA: Ultrasonographic evidence for a consistent eye involvement in Graves' disease. N Engl J Med 290:1447–1450, 1974.
14. Just M, Kahaly G, Higer HP, et al: Graves' ophthalmopathy: Role of MR imaging in radiation therapy. Radiology 179:187–190, 1991.
15. Garrity JA, McCaffrey TV, Gorman CA: Compression and decompression of orbital contents in Graves' ophthalmopathy. Acta Endocrinol (Copenh) 12(Suppl 2):160–168, 1989.
16. Stanley RJ, McCaffrey TV, Offord KP, DeSanto LW: Superior and transantral orbital decompression procedures: Effects on increased orbital pressure and orbital dynamics. Arch Otolaryngol Head Neck Surg 115:369–373, 1989.
17. Otto AJ: Effects of volume, force and pressure alterations in the orbit. Academisch Proefschrift, University of Amsterdam Press, 1991.
18. Smith T, Bahn RS, Gorman CA: Connective tissue, glycosaminoglycans and diseases of the thyroid. Endocr Rev 10:366–391, 1989.
19. Kendall-Taylor P, Stephenson A, Stratton A, et al: Differentiation of autoimmune ophthalmopathy from Graves' hyperthyroidism by analysis of genetic markers. Clin Endocrinol 28:601–610, 1988.
20. Weetman AP, So Ak, Warner CA, et al: Immunogenetic markers in Graves' ophthalmopathy. Clin Endocrinol 28:619–628, 1988.
21. Frecker M, Stenszky V, Balazs C, et al: Genetic factors in Graves' ophthalmopathy. Clin Endocrinol 25:479–485, 1986.
22. Sridama V, Hars Y, Fauchet R, DeGroot LJ: HLA immunogenetic heterogeneity in black American patients with Graves' disease. Arch Intern Med 147:229–231, 1987.
23. Fatourechi V, Bartley G, DeSanto L, et al: Efficacy of transantral orbital decompression for treatment of Graves' optic neuropathy. Thyroid 1:S27, 1991.
24. Tellez M, Cooper J, Edmonds C: Graves' ophthalmopathy in relation to cigarette smoking and ethnic origin. Clin Endocrinol 36:291–294, 1992.
25. Shine B, Fells P, Edwards OM, Weetman AP: Association between Graves' ophthalmopathy and smoking. Lancet 335:1261–1264, 1990.
26. Bartalena L, Martino E, Marcocci C, et al: More on smoking habits and Graves' ophthalmopathy. J Endocrin Invest 12:733–737, 1989.
27. Bartalena L, Marcocci C, Bogazzi F, et al: Use of corticosteroids to prevent progression of Graves' ophthalmopathy after radioiodine treatment for hyperthyroidism. N Engl J Med 321:1349–1351, 1989.
28. Aranow H, Day RM: Management of thyrotoxicosis in patients with ophthalmopathy: Antithyroid regimen determined primarily by ocular manifestations. J Clin Endocrinol Metab 25:1–10, 1965.
29. Prummel MF, Wiersinga WM, Mourits MP, et al: Effect of abnormal thyroid function on severity of Graves' ophthalmopathy. Arch Intern Med 150:1098–1101, 1990.
30. Solem JH, Segaard E, Ytteborg J: The course of endocrine ophthalmopathy during antithyroid therapy in a prospective study. Acta Med Scand 205:111–114, 1979.
31. Sridama V, DeGroot LJ: Treatment of Graves' disease and the cause of ophthalmopathy. Am J Med 87:70–73, 1989.
32. Calissendorf BM, Soderstrom M, Alveryd A: Ophthalmopathy and hyperthyroidism: A comparison of patients receiving different antithyroid treatment. Acta Ophthalmol 64:698–703, 1986.
33. Pinchera A, Fenzi GF, Macchia E, et al: Thyroid stimulating immunoglobulins. Horm Res 16:317–328, 1982.

34. McGregor AM: Immunoendocrine interactions and autoimmunity. N Engl J Med 322:1739–1741, 1990.
35. Jacobson DH, Gorman CA: Endocrine ophthalmopathy: Current ideas concerning etiology, pathogenesis and treatment. Endocr Rev 5:200–220, 1984.
36. Morris JC, Hay ID, Nelson RE, Jiang NS: Clinical utility of thyrotropin receptor antibody assays: Comparison of radioreceptor and bioassay methods. Mayo Clin Proc 63:707, 1988.
37. Rotella CM, Zonefrati R, Toccafondi R, et al: Ability of monoclonal antibodies to the thyrotropin receptor to increase collagen synthesis in human fibroblasts: An assay which appears to measure exophthalmogenic immunoglobulins in Graves' sera. J Clin Endocrinol Metab 62:357–367, 1986.
38. Tao T-W, Leu S-L, Kriss JP: Biological activity of autoantibodies associated with Graves' dermopathy. J Clin Endocrinol Metab 69:90–99, 1989.
39. Westermark K, Lilja K, Karlsson FA: Effects of sera and immunoglobulin preparations from patients with endocrine ophthalmopathy on the production of hyaluronate and the incorporation of tritiated thymidine in fibroblasts. Acta Endocrinol (Copenh) 121 (Suppl 2):85–89, 1989.
40. Takahashi SI, Conti M, Van Wyk JJ: Thyrotropin potentiation of insulin-like growth factor-I dependent deoxyribonucleic acid synthesis in FRTL-5 cells: Mediation by an autocrine amplification factor(s). Endocrinology 126:736–745, 1990.
41. Heufelder AE, Wenzel BE, Bahn RS: Graves' immunoglobulins induce and bind to stress-induced proteins in retroocular fibroblasts from patients with Graves' ophthalmopathy. Thyroid 1 (Suppl 1):S21, 1991.
42. Heufelder AE, Bahn RS: Evidence for the presence of a functional TSH-receptor in retroocular fibroblasts from patients with Graves' ophthalmopathy. Exp Clin Endocr 100:62–67, 1992.
43. Heufelder AE, Bahn RS: Modulation of intercellular adhesion molecule-1 (ICAM-1) by cytokines and Graves' IgGs in cultured Graves' retroocular fibroblasts. Eur J Clin Invest 22:529–537, 1992.
44. Perros P, Kendall-Taylor P: Pathogenic mechanisms in thyroid-associated ophthalmopathy. J Intern Med 231:205–211, 1992.
45. Hiromatsu Y, Fukazawa H, Guinard F, et al: A thyroid cytotoxic antibody that cross-reacts with an eye muscle cell surface antigen may be the cause of thyroid-associated ophthalmopathy. J Clin Endocrinol Metab 67:565–570, 1988.
46. Bahn RS, Gorman CA, Johnson CM, Smith TJ: Presence of antibodies in the sera of patients with Graves' disease recognizing a 23 kilodalton fibroblast antigen. J Clin Endocrinol Metab 69:622–628, 1989.
47. Schifferdecker E, Ketzler-Sasse U, Boehm BO, et al: Reevaluation of eye muscle autoantibody determination in Graves' ophthalmopathy: Failure to detect a specific antigen by use of enzyme-linked immunosorbent assay, indirect immunofluorescence, and immunoblotting techniques. Acta Endocrinol 121:643–650, 1989.
48. Ahmann A, Baker JR, Weetman AP, et al: Antibodies to porcine eye muscle in patients with Graves' ophthalmopathy; identification of serum immunoglobulins directed against unique determinants by immunoblotting and enzyme-linked immunosorbent assay. J Clin Endocrinol Metab 64:454–460, 1987.
49. Kendler DL, Rootman J, Huber GK, Davies TF: A 64 kDa membrane antigen is a recurrent epitope for natural autoantibodies in patients with Graves' thyroid and ophthalmic diseases. Clin Endocrinol 35:539–547, 1991.
50. Weetman AP, Fells P, Shine B: T and B cell reactivity to extraocular and skeletal muscle in Graves' ophthalmopathy. Br J Ophthalmol 73:323–327, 1989.
51. Dong Q, Ludgate M, Vassart G: Cloning and sequencing of a novel 64 kDa autoantigen recognized by patients with autoimmune thyroid disease. J Clin Endocrinol Metab 72:1375–1381, 1991.
52. Heufelder AE, Wenzel BE, Gorman CA, Bahn RS: Detection, cellular localization and modulation of heat shock proteins in cultured fibroblasts from patients with extrathyroidal manifestations with Graves' disease. J Clin Endocrinol Metab 73:739–745, 1991.
53. Heufelder AE, Wenzel BE, Bahn RS: Cell surface localization of a 72 kDa heat shock protein in retroocular fibroblasts from patients with Graves' ophthalmopathy. J Clin Endocrinol Metab 74:732–736, 1992.
54. Heufelder AE, Goellner JR, Wenzel BE, Bahn RS: Immunohistochemical detection and localization of a 72 kDa heat shock protein in autoimmune thyroid disease. J Clin Endocrinol Metab 74:724–731, 1992.
55. Vanbuskirk A, Crump BL, Margoliash E, Pierce SK: A peptide binding protein having a role in antigen presentation is a member of the 70 kDa heat shock protein family. J Exp Med 170:1799–1809, 1989.
56. Ludgate M, Dong Q, Dreyfus PA, et al: Definition at the molecular level of a thyroglobulin-acetylcholinesterase shared epitope: Study of its pathophysiological significance in patients with Graves' ophthalmopathy. Autoimmunity 3:167–176, 1989.
57. Munro DE, Lamki L, Row VV, Volpe R: Cell mediated immunity in the exophthalmos of Graves' disease as demonstrated by the MIF test. J Clin Endocrinol Metab 37:286–292, 1973.
58. Zhang ZG, Medeiros-Neto G, Iacona A, et al: Studies of cytotoxic activities against eye muscle antigens in patients with thyroid-associated ophthalmopathy. Acta Endocrinol (Copenh) 121 (Suppl 2):23–30, 1989.
59. Hufnagel TJ, Hockey WF, Cobbs WH, et al: Immunohistochemical and ultrastructural studies on the exenterated orbital tissues of a patient with Graves' disease. Ophthalmology 91:1411–1419, 1989.
60. Heufelder AE, Bahn RS: Elevated expression in situ of selection and immunoglobulin superfamily type adhesion molecules in retroocular connective tissues from patients with Graves' ophthalmopathy. Thyroid 1(Suppl 2):S32, 1992.
61. Campbell RJ: Immunology of Graves' ophthalmopathy: Retrobulbar histology and histochemistry. Acta Endocrinol (Copenh) 121 (Suppl 2):9–16, 1989.
62. Kroll AJ, Kuwabara T: Dysthyroid ocular myopathy: Anatomy, histology and electron microscopy. Arch Ophthalmol 76:244–256, 1966.
63. Tallstedt L, Norberg R: Immunohistochemical staining of normal and Graves' extraocular muscle. Invest Ophthalmol Vis Sci 29:175–184, 1988.
64. Weetman AP: Thyroid-associated eye disease: Pathophysiology. Lancet 388:25–28, 1991.
65. Weetman AP, Cohen S, Gatter KC, et al: Immunohistochemical analysis of the retrobulbar tissues in Graves' ophthalmopathy. Clin Exp Immunol 75:222–227, 1989.
66. Riley FC: Orbital pathology in Graves' disease. Mayo Clin Proc 47:975–979, 1972.
67. Heufelder AE, Bahn RS: Role of connective tissue autoimmunity in Graves' ophthalmopathy. Autoimmunity 13:75–79, 1992.
68. Bahn RS, Heufelder AE: Retrocular fibroblasts—important effector cells in Graves' ophthalmopathy. Thyroid 2:89–94, 1992.
69. Wegelius O, Asboe-Hansen G, Lamberg BA: Retrobulbar connective tissue changes in malignant exophthalmos. Acta Endocrinol (Copenh) 25:452–456, 1957.
70. Van der Gaag R, Vernimmen R, Fiebelkorn N, et al: Graves' ophthalmopathy: What is the evidence for extraocular muscle specific antibodies? Int Ophthalmol 14:25–30, 1990.
71. Raikow RB, Dalbow MH, Kennerdell JS, et al: Immunohistochemical evidence for IgE involvement in Graves' orbitopathy. Ophthalmology 97:629–635, 1990.
72. Rosen CE, Raikow RB, Burde RM, et al: Immunohistochemical evidence for IgA1 involvement in Graves' ophthalmopathy. Ophthalmology 99:146–152, 1992.
73. Rosen CE, Parisi F, Raikow R, et al: Immunohistochemical evidence for C3Bi involvement in Graves' ophthalmopathy. Ophthalmology 99(Suppl 8):132–133, 1992.
74. Heufelder AE, Smith TJ, Gorman CA, Bahn RS: Increased induction of HLA-DR by interferon-gamma in cultured retroocular fibroblasts derived from patients with Graves' ophthalmopathy and pretibial dermopathy. J Clin Endocrinol Metab 73:307–313, 1991.
75. Heufelder AE, Wenzel BE, Bahn RS: Enhanced induction of a 72 kDa heat shock protein in cultured retroocular fibroblasts. J Invest Ophthalmol Vis Sci 33:466–470, 1992.
76. Bahn RS, Gorman CA, Woloschak GE, et al: Human retroocular fibroblasts in vitro: A model for the study of Graves' ophthalmopathy. J Clin Endocrinol Metab 65:665–670, 1987.
77. Smith TJ, Bahn RS, Gorman CA, Cheavens M: Stimulation of glycosaminoglycan accumulation by interferon-gamma in cultured human retroocular fibroblasts. J Clin Endocrinol Metab 72:1169–1171, 1991.
78. Korducki JM, Loftus SJ, Bahn RS: Stimulation of glycosaminoglycan production in cultured human retrocular fibroblasts. Invest Ophthalmol Vis Sci 33:209–214, 1992.
79. Bahn RS, Smith TJ, Gorman CA: The central role of the fibroblast in the pathogenesis of extrathyroidal manifestations of Graves' disease. Acta Endocrinol (Copenh) 121:75–81, 1989.
80. Altmann DM, Hogg N, Trowsdale J, Wilkinson D: Cotransfection of ICAM-1 and HLA-DR reconstitutes human antigen-presenting function in mouse L cells. Nature 338:512–514, 1989.
81. Makgoba MW, Sanders ME, Guther-Luce GE, et al: Functional evidence that intercellular adhesion molecule-1 (ICAM-1) is a ligand for LFA-1-dependent adhesion in T-cell-mediated cytotoxicity. Eur J Immunol 18:637–640, 1988.

82. Heufelder AE, Bahn RS: Detection and localization of cytokine immunoreactivity in retroocular connective tissue in Graves' ophthalmopathy. Eur J Clin Invest 23:10–17, 1993.

83. Hannson HA: Aspects on growth factors in exophthalmos. Acta Endocrinol 121(Suppl 2):107–111, 1989.

84. Heufelder AE, Wenzel BE, Bahn RS: Methimazole and propylthiouracil inhibit the oxygen free radical–induced retroocular fibroblasts. J Clin Endocrinol Metab 74:737–742, 1992.

85. Sisson JC: Stimulation of glucose utilization and glycosaminoglycan production by fibroblasts derived from retrobulbar tissue. Exp Eye Res 12:285–292, 1971.

86. Sevel D: Extraocular muscles: Their development and peculiarities. In Gorman CA, Waller RR, Dyer JA (eds): The Eye and Orbit in Thyroid Disease. New York, Raven Press, 1984, pp 33–42.

87. Smith TJ, Bahn RS, Gorman CA: Hormonal regulation of hyaluronate synthesis in cultured human fibroblasts: Evidence for differences between retrobulbar and dermal fibroblasts. J Clin Endocrinol Metab 69:1019–1023, 1989.

88. Bech K: Thyroid antibodies in endocrine ophthalmopathy. A review. Acta Endocrinol (Copenh) 121 (Suppl 2):117–122, 1989.

89. Weightman D, Kendall-Taylor P: Cross-reaction of eye muscle antibodies with thyroid tissue in thyroid-associated ophthalmopathy. Acta Endocrinol (Copenh) 122:201–206, 1989.

90. Weetman AP: Autoimmune thyroiditis: Predisposition and pathogenesis. Clin Endocrinol 36:307–323, 1992.

91. Heufelder AE, Bahn RS, Smith TJ: Glucocorticoid regulation of interferon-gamma-induced HLA-DR expression in human retroocular fibroblasts. Clin Endocrinol 37:59–63, 1992.

92. Heufelder AE, Gorman CA, Bahn RS: Modulation of HLA-DR expression on retroocular fibroblasts from patients with thyroid-related ophthalmopathy: In vitro effects of agents used in the management of hyperthyroidism and ophthalmopathy. J Clin Exp Endocrinol 97:206–211, 1991.

93. Heufelder AE, Bahn RS: Stimulation of human retroorbital fibroblast proliferation by paracrine/autocrine factors in its antagonism by glucocorticoid receptor agonists. Proceeding of the Endocrine Society, 74th Annual Meeting, San Antonio, TX, 1992, p 6.

94. Wiersinga WM, Smith T, van der Gaag R, Koornneef L: Temporal relationship between onset of Graves' ophthalmopathy and onset of thyroidal Graves' disease. J Endocrinol Invest 11:615–619, 1988.

95. Marcocci C, Bartalena L, Bogazzi F, et al: Studies on the occurrence of ophthalmopathy in Graves' disease. Acta Endocrinol (Copenh) 120:473–478, 1989.

96. Erie JC: Ophthalmic history and examination. In Bartley BG, Liesegang TJ (eds): Essentials of Ophthalmology. Philadelphia, JB Lippincott, 1992, pp 3–25.

97. Bartley GB, Waller RR: Graves' ophthalmopathy. In van Heerden JA (ed): Common Problems in Endocrine Surgery. Chicago, Year Book Medical Publishers, 1989, pp 25–29.

98. Fells P: Management of dysthyroid eye disease. Br J Ophthalmol 75:245–246, 1991.

99. Carter KD, Frueh BR, Hessburg TP, Musch DC: Long-term efficacy of orbital decompression for compressive optic neuropathy of Graves' eye disease. Ophthalmology 98:1435–1442, 1991.

100. Neigel JM, Rootman J, Belkin RI, et al: Dysthyroid optic neuropathy. The crowded orbital apex syndrome. Ophthalmology 95:1515–1521, 1988.

101. Mourits MPh, Koornneef L, Wiersinga WM, et al: Clinical criteria for the assessment of disease activity in Graves' ophthalmopathy: A novel approach. Br J Ophthalmol 73:639–644, 1989.

102. Bahn RS, Garrity JA, Bartley GB, Gorman CA: Diagnostic evaluation of Graves' ophthalmopathy. Endocrinol Metab Clin North Am 17:527–545, 1988.

103. Feldon SE, Levin L: Graves' ophthalmopathy: V. Aetiology of upper eyelid retraction in Graves' ophthalmopathy. Br J Ophthalmol 74:484–485, 1991.

104. Bahn RS, Bartley GB, Gorman CA: Emergency treatment of Graves' ophthalmopathy. Ballieres Clin Endocrinol Metab 6:95–105, 1992.

105. Bogren HG, Franti CE, Wilmarth SS: Normal variations of the position of the eye in the orbit. Ophthalmology 93:1072–1077, 1986.

106. Reader AL III: Normal variations of intraocular pressure on vertical gaze. Ophthalmology 89:1084–1087, 1982.

107. Sergott RC, Glaser JS: Graves' ophthalmopathy. A clinical and immunologic review. Ophthalmology 26:1–21, 1981.

108. Gamblin GT, Harper DG, Galentine P, et al: Prevalence of increased intraocular pressure in Graves' disease: Evidence of frequent subclinical ophthalmopathy. N Engl J Med 308:420–424, 1983.

109. Spierer A, Eisenstein Z: The role of increased intraocular pressure on upgaze in the assessment of Graves' ophthalmopathy. Ophthalmology 98:1491–1494, 1991.

110. Hudson HL, Levin L, Feldon SE: Graves' exophthalmos unrelated to extraocular muscle enlargement. Superior rectus muscle inflammation may induce venous obstruction. Ophthalmology 98:1495–1499, 1991.

111. Spector RH, Carlisle JA: Minimal thyroid ophthalmopathy. Neurology 37:1803–1808, 1987.

112. Barzel US, Kolbert GS, Edberg SC, et al: Ocular sarcoidosis and Graves' ophthalmopathy. Ann Ophthalmol 18:186–187, 1986.

113. Trokel SL, Hilal SK: Recognition and differential diagnosis of enlarged extraocular muscles in computed tomography. Am J Ophthalmol 87:503–512, 1979.

114. Rothfus WE, Curtin HD: Extraocular muscle enlargement: A CT review. Radiology 151:677–681, 1984.

115. Patrinely JR, Osborn AG, Anderson RL, Whiting AS: Computed tomographic features of nonthyroid extraocular muscle enlargement. Ophthalmology 96:1038–1047, 1989.

116. Sander MP, Brown P: Acute presentation of thyroid ophthalmopathy. Trans Ophthalmol Soc UK 105:720–722, 1986.

117. Merlis AL, Schaiberger CL, Adler R: External carotid-cavernous sinus fistula simulating unilateral Graves' ophthalmopathy. J Comput Assist Tomogr 6:1006–1009, 1982.

118. Mann AS: Bilateral exophthalmos in seminoma. J Clin Endocrinol Metab 27:1500–1502, 1967.

119. Cohen JS: Optic neuropathy of Graves' disease, hyperthyroidism, and ocular myasthenia gravis. Arch Ophthalmol 90:131–132, 1973.

120. Bahn RS, Garrity JA, Gorman CA: Diagnosis and management of Graves' ophthalmopathy. J Clin Endocrinol Metab 71:559–563, 1990.

121. Stubbs SS, Morrell RM: Intravenous methylprednisolone sodium succinate: Adverse reactions reported in association with immunosuppressive therapy. Transplant Proc 5:1145–1146, 1973.

122. Garrett R, Paulus H: Complications of intravenous methylprednisolone pulse therapy. Arthritis Rheum 23:677, 1980.

123. Guy JR, Fagien S, Donovan JP, Rubin ML: Methylprednisolone pulse therapy in severe dysthyroid optic neuropathy. Ophthalmology 96:1048–1053, 1989.

124. Prummel MF, Mourits MPh, Berghout A, et al: Prednisone and cyclosporine in the treatment of severe Graves' ophthalmopathy. N Engl J Med 321:1353–1359, 1989.

125. Apers RCL, Oosterhuis JA, Goslings BM, Bierlaagh JJM: Prednisone treatment in endocrine ophthalmopathy. Mod Prob Ophthalmol 14:414, 1975.

126. Pinchera A, Marcocci C, Bartalena L, et al: Orbital cobalt radiotherapy and systemic or retrobulbar corticosteroids for Graves' ophthalmopathy. Hormone Res 26:177–183, 1987.

127. Nagayama Y, Izumi M, Kiriyama T, et al: Treatment of Graves' ophthalmopathy with high dose intravenous methylprednisolone pulse therapy. Acta Endocrinol (Copenh) 116:513–518, 1987.

128. Kahaly G, Beyer J: Immunosuppressant therapy of thyroid eye disease. Klin Wochenschr 66:1049–1059, 1988.

129. Pinchera A, Bartalena L, Chiovato L, Marcocci C: Radiotherapy of Graves' ophthalmopathy. In Gorman CA, Waller RR, Dyer JA (eds): The Eye and Orbit in Thyroid Disease. New York, Raven Press, 1984, pp 301–316.

130. Gorman CA: Clever is not enough: NOSPECS is form in search of function. Thyroid 1(Suppl 84):353–355, 1991.

131. Teng CS, Crombie AL, Hall R, Ross WM: An evaluation of supervoltage orbital irradiation for Graves' ophthalmopathy. Clin Endocrinol 13:545–551, 1980.

132. Petersen IA, Kriss JP, McDougall IR, Donaldson S: Prognostic factors in radiotherapy of Graves' ophthalmopathy. Int J Rad Oncol Bio Physics 19:259–264, 1990.

133. Nikoskelainen E, Joensuu H: Retinopathy after irradiation for Graves' ophthalmopathy [letter]. Lancet 2:690–691, 1989.

134. Brown GC, Shields JA, Sanborn G, et al: Radiation retinopathy. Ophthalmology 89:1494–1501, 1982.

135. Miller ML, Goldberg SH, Bullock JD: Radiation retinopathy after standard therapy for thyroid related ophthalmopathy. Am J Ophthal 112:600–601, 1991.

136. Prummel MF, Mourits MPh, Blank L, et al: A prospective double blind comparison of prednisone and retrobulbar radiotherapy in the treatment of moderately severe Graves' ophthalmopathy. PhD Thesis, University of Amsterdam, 1992.

137. Kazim M, Trokel S, Moore S: Treatment of acute Graves' orbitopathy. Ophthalmology 98:1443–1448, 1991.

138. Kennerdell JS, Rosenbaum AE, El-Hoshy MH: Apical optic nerve compression of dysthyroid optic neuropathy on computed tomography. Arch Ophthalmol 99:807–809, 1981.

139. Trobe JD: Optic nerve involvement in dysthyroidism. Ophthalmology 88:488–492, 1981.

140. Feldon SE, Muramatsu S, Weiner JM: Clinical classification of Graves' ophthalmopathy. Identification of risk factors for optic neuropathy. Arch Ophthalmol 102:1469–1472, 1984.

141. Hallin ES, Feldon SE: Graves' ophthalmopathy: I. Simple CT estimates of extraocular muscle volume. Br J Ophthalmol 72:674–677, 1988.

142. Hallin ES, Feldon SE: Graves' ophthalmopathy: II. Correlation of clinical signs with measures derived from computed tomography. Br J Ophthalmol 72:678–682, 1988.

143. Anderson RL, Tweeten JP, Patrinely JR, et al: Dysthyroid optic neuropathy without extraocular muscle involvement. Ophthalmic Surg 20:568–574, 1989.

144. McCord CD Jr: Current trends in orbital decompression. Ophthalmology 92:21–33, 1985.

145. Kennerdell JS, Maroon JC, Buerger GF: Comprehensive surgical management of proptosis in dysthyroid orbitopathy. Orbit 6:153–179, 1987.

146. Dollinger J: Die Druckentlastung der Augenhöhle durch Entfernung der aüsseren Orbitalwand bei hochgradigem Exophthalmus (Morbus Basedowii) und konsekutiver Hornhauterkrankung. Dtsch Med Wochenschr 37:1888–1890, 1911.

147. Long JC, Ellis GD: Temporal decompression of the orbit for thyroid exophthalmos. Am J Ophthalmol 62:1089–1098, 1966.

148. Hurwitz JJ, Birt D: An individualized approach to orbital decompression in Graves' orbitopathy. Arch Ophthalmol 103:660–665, 1985.

149. Sewall EC: Operative control of progressive exophthalmos. Arch Otolaryngol 24:621–624, 1936.

150. Leone CR Jr, Piest KL, Newman RJ: Medial and lateral wall decompression for thyroid ophthalmopathy. Am J Ophthalmol 108:160–166, 1989.

151. Fells P: Orbital decompression for severe dysthyroid eye disease. Br J Ophthalmol 71:107–111, 1987.

152. Leone CR Jr, Bajandas FJ: Inferior orbital decompression for thyroid ophthalmopathy. Arch Ophthalmol 98:890–892, 1980.

153. Linberg JV, Anderson RL: Transorbital decompression. Indications and results. Arch Ophthalmol 99:113–119, 1981.

154. Anderson RL, Linberg JV: Transorbital approach to decompression in Graves' disease. Arch Ophthalmol 99:120–124, 1981.

155. McCord CD Jr: Orbital decompression for Graves' disease. Exposure through lateral canthal and inferior fornix incision. Ophthalmology 88:533–541, 1981.

156. Wilson WB, Manke WF: Orbital decompression in Graves' disease. The predictability of reduction of proptosis. Arch Ophthalmol 109:343–345, 1991.

157. Olivari N: Transpalpebral decompression of endocrine ophthalmopathy (Graves' disease) removal of intraorbital fat: Experience with 147 operations over 5 years. Plast Reconstr Surg 87:627–641, 1991.

158. Garrity JA, Bartley GB: Transpalpebral decompression of Graves' ophthalmopathy. Plast Reconstr Surg 89:574–575, 1992.

159. Walsh TE, Ogura JH: Transantral orbital decompression for malignant exophthalmos. Laryngoscope 67:544–568, 1957.

160. Ogura JH: Surgical results of orbital decompression for malignant exophthalmos. J Laryngol Otol 92:181–196, 1978.

161. Baylis HI, Call BN, Shibata CS: The transantral orbital decompression (Ogura technique) as performed by the ophthalmologist. A series of 24 patients. Ophthalmology 87:1005–1012, 1980.

162. Warren JD, Spector JG, Burde R: Long-term follow-up and recent observations on 305 cases of orbital decompression for dysthyroid orbitopathy. Laryngoscope 99:35–40, 1989.

163. Hallin ES, Feldon SE, Luttrell J: Graves' ophthalmopathy: III. Effect of transantral orbital decompression on optic neuropathy. Br J Ophthalmol 72:683–687, 1988.

164. Naffziger HC: Progressive exophthalmos following thyroidectomy: Its pathology and treatment. Ann Surg 94:582–586, 1931.

165. Kennerdell JS, Maroon JC: An orbital decompression for severe dysthyroid exophthalmos. Ophthalmology 89:467–472, 1982.

166. Strang M, West M: A four-wall orbital decompression for dysthyroid orbitopathy. J Neurosurg 68:671–677, 1988.

167. Mourits MPh, Koornneef L, Wiersinga WM, et al: Orbital decompression for Graves' ophthalmopathy by inferomedial, by inferomedial plus lateral, and by coronal approach. Ophthalmology 97:636–641, 1990.

168. Kennedy DW, Goodstein ML, Miller NR, Zinreich SJ: Endoscopic transnasal orbital decompression. Arch Otolaryngol Head Neck Surg 116:275–282, 1990.

169. Small RG, Meiring NL: A combined orbital and antral approach to surgical decompression of the orbit. Ophthalmology 88:542–547, 1981.

170. Wulc AE, Popp JC, Bartlett SP: Lateral wall advancement in orbital decompression. Ophthalmology 97:1358–1369, 1990.

171. DeSanto LW, Gorman CA: Selection of patients and choice of operation for orbital decompression in Graves' ophthalmopathy. Laryngoscope 83:945–959, 1973.

172. DeSanto LW: The total rehabilitation of Graves' ophthalmopathy. Laryngoscope 90:1652–1678, 1980.

173. Gorman CA, DeSanto LW, MacCarty CS, Riley FC: Optic neuropathy of Graves's disease. Treatment by transantral or transfrontal orbital decompression. N Engl J Med 290:70–75, 1974.

174. Garrity JA, Bartley GB, DeSanto LW, et al: Orbital decompression: Long-term results. In Wall JR, How J (eds): Graves' Ophthalmopathy. Cambridge, MA, Blackwell Scientific Publications, 1990, pp 171–182.

175. Trokel SL, Cooper WC: Orbital decompression: Effect on motility and globe position. Ophthalmology 86:2064–2070, 1979.

176. Shorr N, Neuhaus RW, Baylis HI: Ocular motility problems after orbital decompression for dysthyroid ophthalmopathy. Ophthalmology 89:323–328, 1982.

177. Goldberg RA, Shorr N, Cohen MS: The medial orbital strut in the prevention of postdecompression dystopia in dysthyroid ophthalmopathy. Ophthalmic Plast Reconstr Surg 8:32–34, 1992.

178. Goldberg SH, Bullock JD, Guyton DL: Esotropia following bilateral lateral orbital decompressions for Graves' disease. Ophthalmic Plast Reconstr Surg 6:190–192, 1990.

179. Long JA, Baylis HI: Hypoglobus following orbital decompression for dysthyroid ophthalmopathy. Ophthalmic Plast Reconstr Surg 6:185–189, 1990.

180. Goldberg RA, Christenbury JD, Shorr N: Medial entropion following orbital decompression for dysthyroid ophthalmopathy. Ophthalmic Plast Reconstr Surg 4:81–85, 1988.

181. Colvard DM, Waller RR, Neault RW, DeSanto LW: Nasolacrimal duct obstruction following transantral-ethmoidal orbital decompression. Ophthalmic Surg 10:25–28, 1979.

182. Seiff SR, Shorr N: Nasolacrimal drainage system obstruction after orbital decompression. Am J Ophthalmol 106:204–209, 1988.

183. Frueh BR, Musch DC, Garber FW: Exophthalmometer readings in patients with Graves' eye disease. Ophthalmic Surg 17:37–40, 1986.

184. Hamburger JI, Sugar HS: What the internist should know about the ophthalmopathy of Graves' disease. Arch Intern Med 129:131–139, 1972.

185. Dyer JA: Ocular muscle surgery in Graves' disease. Trans Am Ophthalmol Soc 76:126–139, 1978.

186. Dyer JA: The oculorotary muscles in Graves' disease. Trans Am Ophthalmol Soc 74:425–456, 1976.

187. Waller RR: Eyelid malpositions in Graves' ophthalmopathy. Trans Am Ophthalmol Soc 80:855–930, 1982.

188. Small RG: Upper eyelid retraction in Graves' ophthalmopathy: A new surgical technique and a study of the abnormal levator muscle. Trans Am Ophthalmol Soc 86:725–793, 1988.

189. Small RG: Enlargement of levator palpebrae superioris muscle fibers in Graves' ophthalmopathy. Ophthalmology 96:424–430, 1989.

190. Bartley GB, Kay PP: Posterior lamellar eyelid reconstruction with a hard palate mucosal graft. Am J Ophthalmol 107:609–612, 1989.

191. Kersten RC, Kulwin DR, Levartovsky S, et al: Management of lower-lid retraction with hard-palate mucosa grafting. Arch Ophthalmol 108:1339–1343, 1990.

192. Gardner TA, Kennerdell JS, Buerger GF: Treatment of dysthyroid lower lid retraction with autogenous tarsus transplants. Ophthalmic Plast Reconstr Surg 8:26–31, 1992.

193. Moutis MP, Koornneef L: Lid lengthening by sclera interposition for eyelid retraction in Graves' ophthalmopathy. Br J Ophthalmol 75:344–347, 1991.

194. Flanagan JC: Eye bank sclera in oculoplastic surgery. Ophthalmic Surg 5:45–53, 1974.

195. Dryden RM, Soll DB: The use of scleral transplantation in cicatricial entropion and eyelid retraction. Ophthalmology 83:669–678, 1977.

196. Flanagan JC: Retraction of the eyelids secondary to thyroid ophthalmopathy—its surgical correction with sclera and the fate of the graft. Trans Am Ophthalmol Soc 78:657–685, 1980.

197. Marks MW, Argenta LC, Friedman RJ, Hall JD: Conchal cartilage and composite grafts for correction of lower lid retraction. Plast Reconstr Surg 83:629–635, 1989.

198. Marcocci C, Bartalena L, Bogazzi F, et al: Relationship between Graves' ophthalmopathy and type of treatment of Graves' hyperthyroidism. Thyroid 2:171–178, 1992.

199. Tallstedt L, Lundell G, Torring O, et al: Occurrence of ophthalmopathy after treatment for Graves' hyperthyroidism. N Engl J Med 326:1733–1738, 1992.

43

Autoimmune Thyroid Disease/Thyroiditis

NOBUYUKI AMINO
HISATO TADA

Thyroid autoimmunity leads to two major disorders, Hashimoto's disease and Graves' disease. Hashimoto's disease is a lifelong autoimmune disease of the thyroid gland, also called *autoimmune thyroiditis* or *chronic thyroiditis*. In some patients, an enlarged thyroid gland gradually atrophies in association with development of hypothyroidism. Patients with Hashimoto's disease may show transient thyrotoxicosis during the clinical course. This is caused by thyroid destruction induced by autoimmune thyroid inflammation and differs from Graves' thyrotoxicosis.

AUTOIMMUNE THYROIDITIS: CURRENT CONCEPTS

The first variety of autoimmune thyroiditis, struma lymphomatosa, was described by Hakaru Hashimoto in 1912[1] and has since been called *Hashimoto's disease.* Hashimoto described four patients with diffuse goiter and clarified the four histological characteristics: diffuse lymphocytic infiltration, formation of lymphoid follicles, destruction of epithelial cells, and proliferation of fibrous tissue. Some of his patients developed hypothyroidism after partial thyroidectomy. Thus the association of Hashimoto's disease with hypothyroidism was described in the original article. The term *Hashimoto's disease* or *thyroiditis* is used to refer only to goitrous thyroiditis in some countries but is used synonymously with *autoimmune thyroiditis,* including the atrophic nongoitrous type, in the other countries, just as Graves' disease is often used to cover nonexophthalmic and nongoitrous hyperthyroidism.

Autoimmune thyroiditis or Hashimoto's disease can be classified into four subgroups according to the stage of disease progress (Table 43–1). In the early stage, patients only show a positive reaction for antithyroid antibodies.

Postmortem histological examination has revealed that positive tests for serum antithyroid antibodies, especially antithyroid microsomal antibodies, in subjects without overt thyroid disease indicate the presence of lymphocytic infiltration into the thyroid gland, presumably reflecting subclinical autoimmune thyroiditis.[2] When the disease progresses, patients show a firm, diffuse goiter of small to moderate size and are generally said to have chronic autoimmune thyroiditis. Their thyroid function is variable, from euthyroidism to thyrotoxicosis. Patients develop a large, firm goiter when the disease is more advanced, and this is the classical or goitrous Hashimoto's disease. When a cytotoxic autoimmune reaction is predominant, patients finally get atrophic thyroiditis associated with hypothyroidism. This is the final stage of Hashimoto's disease.

In the general population, antithyroid microsomal antibodies are found in 10.0 per cent of adult women and in 5.3 per cent of adult men.[3] Interestingly, 32 per cent of these women with antithyroid antibodies are found to have slight enlargement of the thyroid gland when the neck is palpated carefully by a specialist, but only 4.8 per cent of men with antibodies are found to have a small goiter. Subclinical autoimmune thyroiditis in these subjects is further evidenced by the fact that thyroid dysfunction develops after delivery in about half of these women, although functional abnormalities are usually transient.[4] Therefore, 1 of 10 to 30 adult females in the general population has autoimmune thyroiditis.

PATHOLOGY

Hashimoto's Thyroiditis

In the classical form of Hashimoto's thyroiditis (struma lymphomatosa) with a firm, enlarged thyroid, there is ex-

TABLE 43–1. CLASSIFICATION OF AUTOIMMUNE THYROIDITIS (HASHIMOTO'S DISEASE)

	SUBCLINICAL AUTOIMMUNE THYROIDITIS	CHRONIC AUTOIMMUNE THYROIDITIS	CLASSICAL HASHIMOTO'S DISEASE	ATROPHIC THYROIDITIS
Stage	Early	Mild	Advanced	Final
Antithyroid antibodies (agglutination methods)	Positive	Positive	Positive	Positive
Goiter	None or very small, soft to firm	Small or moderate, firm	Large, firm	None
Thyroid function	Euthyroid	Euthyroid Hypothyroid Destructive thyrotoxicosis	Euthyroid Hypothyroid Destructive thyrotoxicosis	Hypothyroid

tensive replacement of the normal follicular structure by lymphocytic and plasma cell infiltration with formation of lymphoid germinal centers[1] (Fig. 43–1). Thyroid follicles remain isolated or in small clusters, are small or atrophic, and are empty or contain sparse colloid. Some persistent follicular epithelial cells are transformed into Askanazy cells, which have an eosinophilic granular cytoplasm. These cells are found in many other thyroid diseases, probably representing a damaged state of the epithelial cells. Fibrosis of various extents and lymphocytic infiltration are found in the interstitial tissue.

Focal Thyroiditis

Focal thyroiditis was first recognized by Woolner et al.[5] as a mild form of Hashimoto's disease. In focal thyroiditis, the destruction of the normal thyroid structure is mild, and lymphocytes infiltrate focally into the disrupted follicles and interstitial tissues. Many follicles are preserved intact and viable. Fibrosis may exist to some extent. Focal thyroiditis is common and is found in association with various thyroid diseases. In subclinical autoimmune thyroiditis, found in about 10 per cent of females in the general population with positive microsomal antibodies,[3] this type of thyroiditis is seen (Fig. 43–2).

Silent Thyroiditis

The histological characteristics of silent thyroiditis are similar to those of chronic thyroiditis. Although lymphocytic infiltration and fibrosis may be less in silent thyroiditis, one cannot distinguish it from chronic thyroiditis histologically.[6] This is one of the reasons to consider this type of thyroiditis to be autoimmune in nature. Histological examination of the needle biopsy specimens reveals focal or diffuse infiltration of lymphocytes and collapsed thyroid follicles (Fig. 43–3). Fibrosis may be minimal. In contrast to subacute thyroiditis, a granulomatous reaction is not noted. After recovery from the acute inflammation, the histological findings spontaneously improve, leaving well-preserved thyroid follicles and slight focal lymphocytic infiltration.[7]

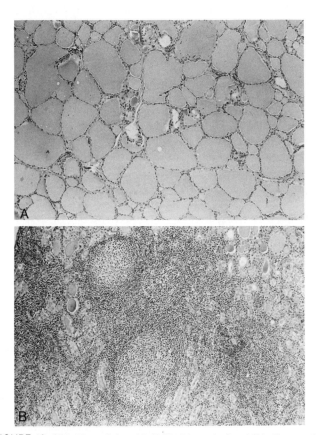

FIGURE 43–1. *A*, Normal thyroid. *B*, Hashimoto's thyroiditis. Destruction of normal follicular architecture by lymphocytic and plasma cell infiltration with formation of lymphoid germinal centers. A few atrophic thyroid follicles are seen (Hematoxylin and eosin stain; × 100).

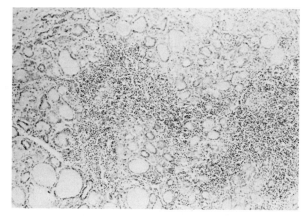

FIGURE 43–2. Focal thyroiditis. Lymphocytic infiltration is less extensive and is observed focally in the area of disrupted follicles and interstitial tissues. Many follicles are preserved (Hematoxylin and eosin stain; × 100).

728 / PART III—THYROID GLAND

AUTOIMMUNE ABNORMALITIES

Initiation of Thyroid Autoimmunity

Autoimmune thyroiditis may arise from a defect in self tolerance to thyroid antigens.[8] Immunological self tolerance is thought to be induced during the perinatal period when immature lymphocytes are exposed to self antigens.[9] At this critical point, clonal deletion or induced anergy of autoreactive T cells in the thymus provides self tolerance to autoantigens. If there is an abnormality during this period, self tolerance may not be induced,[9] and autoimmune thyroiditis may develop. An abnormality of thyroid-specific suppressor T lymphocytes is proposed to cause a partial defect of immunoregulation.[10] This genetically induced organ-specific suppressor T-lymphocyte defect may deregulate a thyroid-specific helper T-cell population. There also may be additional effects of environmental factors.[10] Further breakdown of self tolerance may be induced by altered self antigen, exposure to environmental antigens which mimic a self antigen, polyclonal immune activation, or idiotype cross-reaction of self antigens. These factors may augment low levels of autoimmune thyroiditis. For example, infection, drugs, or other factors may activate the autoreactive helper T lymphocytes, which activate thyroid-specific B lymphocytes, thyroid-specific cytotoxic T lymphocytes, nonspecific Tγδ cells, and killer (K) lymphocytes (Fig. 43–4). These cells and antithyroid antibodies attack the target thyroid epithelial cells. Locally produced interferon-γ may induce MHC class II antigen expression on thyroid cell surfaces. Class II MHC antigen expression may suppress the autoimmune reaction, possibly through activation of suppressor T lymphocytes or by inhibiting helper T-cell function within the thyroid gland,[8] although the first reports on aberrant expression of class II MHC antigen suggested that it induced autoimmunity.[11] Patients with autoimmune thyroiditis may have a defect in this local immunosuppressive circuit.[8]

Antibodies to Thyroid Antigens

Thyroglobulin

A classical experimental autoimmune thyroiditis with histological findings similar to Hashimoto's thyroiditis can be induced in animals by immunization with human thyroglobulin in an adjuvant. It was proposed that thyroglobulin is isolated from the immune system in the thyroid follicles and that exposure of thyroglobulin to the immune system by the destruction of the follicles could give rise to autoimmune thyroiditis. This is not the case, however, for thyroglobulin was found, in fact, not to be isolated but to be normally present in the circulation of humans.[12] Thyroglobulin-binding lymphocytes also can be detected in the fetus.[13]

Thyroglobulin is a glycoprotein with molecular weight 670,000 Da. Its cDNA shows that thyroglobulin contains a domain analogous to acetylcholinesterase. At least seven epitopes on human thyroglobulin are recognized by antithyroglobulin antibodies. Most are located on the middle part (in the region of 1097 to 1560 amino acids) of thyroglobulin. Interestingly, antithyroglobulin antibodies found in sera from the patient with autoimmune thyroiditis rec-

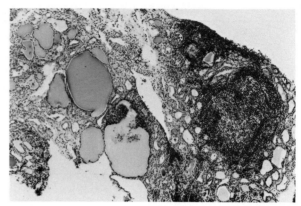

FIGURE 43–3. Silent thyroiditis. Lymphocytic infiltration with formation of a lymphoid follicle surrounded by atrophic or disrupted thyroid follicles is seen. A few thyroid follicles are persistent with slight damage (Hematoxylin and eosin stain; × 25). (Courtesy of Dr. F. Matsuzuka, Kuma Hospital, Kobe, Japan.)

ognize most frequently a particular epitope in the region of 1149 to 1250, whereas the antibodies from healthy subjects recognize more frequently another region.[14–16] The epitopes recognized by the T-cell receptor (TCR) are also reported.[17] Antithyroglobulin antibodies rarely have complement-fixing cytotoxicity.

Serum concentrations of antithyroglobulin antibodies are usually measured by the hemagglutination (TGHA) or particle agglutination (TGPA) technique.[18] Figure 43–5 shows TGHA titers in various thyroid diseases. The frequency of positive TGHA in Hashimoto's thyroiditis is 56 per cent, and that in Graves' disease is 29 per cent (Table 43–2). These frequencies are lower than those of positive antithyroid microsomal antibodies. However, using a more sensitive radioimmunoassay, 70 per cent of TGHA-negative patients with Hashimoto's disease showed positive antithyroglobulin antibody titers[19] (Fig. 43–6). The detection of thyroglobulin antibody (TGAb) by RIA is proving effective in diagnosing the existence of autoimmune thyroid abnormalities in both TGHA- and MCHA-negative Hashimoto's disease and in predicting postpartum thyroid dysfunction.

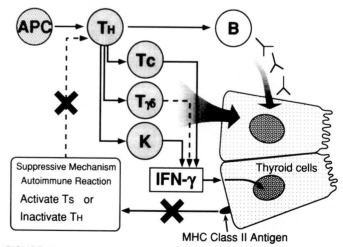

FIGURE 43–4. Possible mechanism of initiation of thyroid autoimmunity (APC, antigen-presenting cells; TH, helper T cells; B, B lymphocytes; TC, cytotoxic T cells; Tγδ, T gamma delta cells; K, killer cells; TS, suppressor T cells; INF-γ, interferon-gamma).

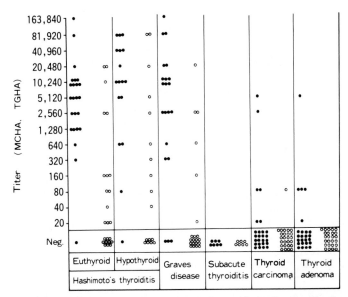

FIGURE 43–5. Titers of microsomal hemagglutination antibodies (MCHA) and thyroglobulin hemagglutination antibodies (TGHA) in patients with various thyroid diseases. (From Amino N, Hagan SR, Yamada N, Refetoff S: Measurement of circulating thyroid microsomal antibodies by the tanned red cell haemagglutination technique: Its usefulness in the diagnosis of autoimmune thyroid diseases. Clin Endocrinol 5:115–125, 1976.)

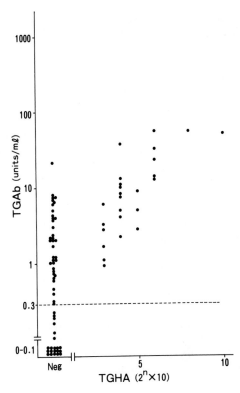

FIGURE 43–6. Titers of antithyroglobulin antibodies in patients with Hashimoto's disease measured by both hemagglutination technique (TGHA) and radioimmunoassay (TGAb). Antithyroglobulin antibodies were detectable by RIA in 63 per cent of TGHA-negative sera.

Thyroid Peroxidase

Thyroid peroxidase (TPO) is the major antigen of thyroid microsomes recognized by antithyroid microsomal antibodies.[20] Thyroid microsomal antigen is the antigen contained in the microsomal fraction separated by ultracentrifugation from thyroid cell homogenates. It consists of the proteins in exocytotic vesicle membrane including newly synthesized thyroglobulin. Thus antithyroid microsomal antibodies also may include antibodies to thyroglobulin and other proteins in the membrane. However, because these antibodies are a small population, we can consider that anti-TPO antibodies are effectively identical to antithyroid microsomal antibodies.

TPO is a glycoprotein anchored to the plasma membrane, with molecular weight 107,000 Dal. Molecular cloning of the protein showed it consists of 993 amino acids. B-cell epitopes of TPO,[21–23] most of which are in the extra-

cellular portion of the molecule, seem to be highly comformational and are formed by several discontinuous regions. Some of these B-cell epitopes are reported to be cross-reactive with epitopes of thyroglobulin and are recognized by both autoantibodies from patients with autoimmune thyroiditis.[24] Several T-cell epitopes that seem responsible for antigen-specific T-cell activation have been reported.[25] Anti-TPO antibodies are reported to be able to induce complement-dependent cytotoxicity.[26] Anti-idiotypic antibodies against antimicrosomal antibodies are occasionally found in sera of patients with autoimmune thyroid disease and might be involved in regulation of autoimmunity.[27]

The titers of anti-TPO antibodies are reported to corre-

TABLE 43–2. INCIDENCE OF THYROID AUTOANTIBODIES IN DIFFERENT THYROID DISORDERS

| DISORDER | ANTITHYROGLOBULIN | | ANTI-CA2 | ANTIMICROSOMAL | | ANTI-TSH RECEPTOR ANTIBODY (TBII) | ANTIBODIES TO THYROID HORMONES | |
	TGHA	RIA		MCHA	RIA		T₄	T₃
Graves' disease	29	89	41	86	98	95	5.9	20.5
Hashimoto's disease	56	100	74	95	100	7*		34.9
Primary hypothyroidism	59	94	16	94	100	14	14	34.9
Subacute thyroiditis	0	33†	33†	0		0		
Thyroid adenoma	0			20		0		
Thyroid carcinoma	3.8			23		0		
Normal population								
Male	1.8	4.2	3	6.0	8.4	0	0	0
Female	5.3			10.0			0	0

Values are percentages and are cited from reports described in the text. TBII = TSH-binding inhibitor immunoglobulin.
*Incidence in hypothyroid Hashimoto's disease with goiter.
†One of three patients.
Modified from Amino N: Antithyroid antibodies. *In* Ingbar SH, Braverman LE (eds): The Thyroid (ed. 5). Philadelphia, JB Lippincott, 1986, pp 546–559.

late with the severity of Hashimoto's thyroiditis,[28] and these antibodies may play an important role in pathogenesis. However, the significance of anti-TPO antibody in vivo is not definite. Microsomal antibodies transferred passively from mothers with Hashimoto's thyroiditis do not seem to affect thyroid function of the fetus or neonate.[29] Presently the clinical importance of anti-TPO antibodies lies in the diagnosis of the presence of thyroid autoimmunity. It is reported that positive serum anti-TPO antibodies always accompany the lymphocyte infiltration to the thyroid and thus the existence of autoimmune thyroid disease.[2]

Serum concentrations of antithyroid microsomal antibodies are usually measured by hemagglutination (MCHA) or particle agglutination (MCPA) in clinical practice.[18] Figure 43–5 shows MCHA titers in various thyroid diseases. MCHA is positive in more than 90 per cent of patients with Hashimoto's thyroiditis regardless of hypothyroidism or euthyroidism (see Table 43–2). The incidence of positive MCHA in patients with Graves' disease is 86 per cent. Thus MCHA can be positive in any type of autoimmunity in the thyroid. Ten per cent of adult females in the general population have positive MCHA titers and are thought to have subclinical autoimmune thyroiditis (Fig. 43–7). A more sensitive radioimmunoassay for the measurement of anti-TPO antibodies using human TPO as an antigen is presently available.[19]

TSH Receptor

The primary amino acid structure of the human thyroid-stimulating hormone (TSH) receptor (TSH-R) was revealed after its molecular cloning.[30–32] TSH receptor belongs to a subgroup of the superfamily of guanine nucleotide regulatory (G) protein–coupled receptors, which

have seven transmembrane regions. The human TSH-R cDNA codes for a protein of 764 amino acids, including a 20-amino acid signal peptide.[33] The calculated molecular weight of TSH-R is approximately 84,500 Da. The amino-terminal half of the mature TSH-R (398 amino acids) is generally hydrophilic and encodes a large extracellular region. The structure of the carboxyl-terminal half of the TSH-R (346 amino acids) is quite different from the amino terminus and contains the characteristic seven hydrophobic membrane-spanning segments.[33]

Thyroid-stimulating antibodies (TSAb's) to TSH-R are responsible for hyperthyroidism in Graves' disease, and TSH stimulation–blocking antibodies (TSBAb's) to TSH-R cause atrophic hypothyroidism in autoimmune thyroiditis.[34] TSH and TSH-R antibodies may bind to the same regions but with different affinities. TSH-R antibodies do not recognize linear epitopes, and the specific domain of epitopes for TSAb or TSBAb is still uncertain. Amino acids 38 to 45 in the TSH-R may be important in stimulating TSH-R antibody action.[33] In vitro conversion from TSBAb to TSAb after addition of antihuman IgG antibody suggests that the TSAb and TSBAb bind to the same epitope(s) of TSH-R, and the same TSH-R antibody may act as a stimulator or blocker by the influence of other factors.[35] As a routine test, TSH-R antibodies are measured by radioreceptor assay. The prevalence of TSH-binding inhibitory immunoglobulins (TBII) in various thyroid conditions is shown in Figure 43–8.

Thyroid Hormones

Antibodies to thyroxine (T_4) and triiodothyronine (T_3) are sometimes found in patients with autoimmune or other thyroid diseases.[36] They are seen in 14 and 35 per cent of patients with primary hypothyroidism, in most of whom TGHA's are found in high titers[3, 37] (see Table 43–2). The pathogenetic significance of these antibodies is not known, and probably they are of little importance as long as the thyroid can produce enough thyroid hormone to keep adequate levels of serum-free hormones. These antibodies are important in clinical practice because they interfere with the measurements of serum T_4 and T_3, especially in the assays of free T_4 and free T_3 concentrations.[38] This influence is dependent on the particular method of assay, and falsely high or low levels of free hormones compared with TSH are obtained.

Other Antigens

Anti-(bovine)-TSH autoantibodies, occasionally found in Graves' disease, are also reported in Hashimoto's thyroiditis.[39] Their pathogenetic significance is unclear. They are speculated to be anti-idiotypic antibodies to anti-TSH receptor antibodies (TRAb's) in Graves' disease. They may interfere with the measurement of TRAb's and give unusual high or negative titers.

Autoantibodies against several other thyroid components are reported. Antibodies to second colloid antigen (CA2) are detected by a diffuse immunofluorescence of colloid. This antigen is distinct from thyroglobulin. Antibodies to cell surface antigen are detected by the patchy immunofluorescent staining of the cell surface or by mixed hemabsorption. The antigen is distinct from thyroid per-

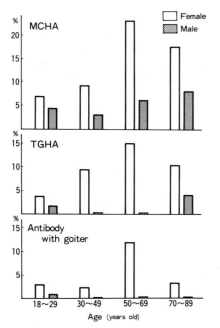

FIGURE 43–7. Incidence of antithyroid microsomal hemagglutination (MCHA) and antithyroglobulin hemagglutination (TGHA) antibodies in 1015 subjects from the general population shown in relation to age, sex, and thyroid enlargement. (From Amino N: Antithyroid antibodies. In Ingbar SH, Braverman LE (eds): The Thyroid (ed 5). Philadelphia, JB Lippincott, 1986, pp 546–559.)

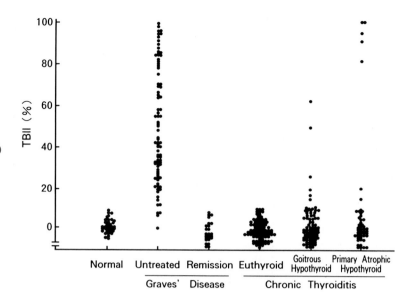

FIGURE 43–8. TSH-binding inhibitory immunoglobulins (TBII) in various types of autoimmune thyroid disease.

oxidase. Growth-stimulating immunoglobulins and growth-blocking immunoglobulins are reported. The former antibody is found in sera from the patients with goitrous Hashimoto's thyroiditis and may cause goiter formation. Growth-blocking antibodies, found in primary myxedema, may cause thyroid atrophy. They do not bind to TSH receptors nor activate adenylate cyclase. However, evidence for the presence of such antibodies is not widely accepted because of the lack of reproducibility of the detection methods.[40]

Autoantibodies against other cellular components (not always thyroid cell–specific) are also reported. Antinuclear and anti-DNA antibodies are sometimes found in autoimmune thyroiditis. Anti-DNA antibodies in patients with Hashimoto's thyroiditis increase during postpartum exacerbation.[41] Antibodies to cytoplasmic components such as tubulin and calmodulin are also seen.[42] Antibodies to the ganglioside asialo-G_{M1}, present in the plasma membrane of human thyroid cells, were detected by complement fixation in autoimmune thyroid disease.[43] Anti-α-galactosyl antibodies, which react with the carbohydrate structure Galα1→ 3Galβ1→ 4GlcNAcR, which is not expressed on the surface of normal human thyroid cells, may bind if aberrant expression of this epitope occurs, as in cancer.[44] Antibodies to other organs (e.g., islet cells, adrenal cortex, gastric mucosa, parathyroid) are found in autoimmune thyroiditis in higher incidence than expected in the general population.[42]

Cytotoxic Immune Reaction

It is important to understand the mechanism for development of hypothyroidism in patients with Hashimoto's disease. Several in vitro cytotoxic mechanisms have been demonstrated, as shown in Figure 43–9.[45] Complement-dependent cytotoxic antibodies are found in almost all sera from patients with Hashimoto's disease[46] and are thought to be identical to microsomal antibody. However, these antibodies do not act on intact thyroid cells in vitro.[47] Microsomal antibodies passively transferred from mothers with Hashimoto's disease have no effect on neonatal thyroid function.[29] Therefore, this antibody may have little

cytotoxic effect in vivo. K lymphocytes have a potential for killing antibody-coated target cells in vitro by the mechanism described as antibody-dependent cell-mediated cytotoxicity (ADCC).[48] ADCC activity was found in the sera from patients with Hashimoto's disease,[49] and the cytotoxic effect was correlated with microsomal antibody titers.[50] On the other hand, reports on the activity or number of peripheral K lymphocytes in Hashimoto's disease are conflicting. Using a plaque-forming cell assay, increased K lymphocyte counts were found at the time of thyroid destruction in Hashimoto's disease.[51] Furthermore, the percentage and absolute count of K lymphocytes were inversely correlated with serum thyroid hormone levels in autoimmune thyroid disease. Thus the higher number of K cells and increased ADCC activity may lead to reduced thyroid function in autoimmune thyroid disease.

Natural killer (NK) cells, which show cytotoxicity against target cells without prior sensitization, are nonadherent and nonphagocytic and bear Fc receptors for IgG. NK cell populations are rather heterogeneous, and it now seems established that the same cells, NK/K cells, are able to mediate both NK cell activity and ADCC. NK cell activity

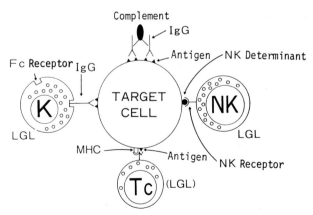

FIGURE 43–9. Cytotoxic immune reactions in Hashimoto's disease (LGL, large granular lymphocyte; Tc, cytotoxic T lymphocytes; K, killer cell; NK, natural killer cell; MHC, major histocompatibility complex). (From Amino N: Autoimmunity and hypothyroidism. In Lazarus JH, Hall R (eds): Baillière's Clinical Endocrinology and Metabolism, Vol 2, No 3. London, Baillière Tindall, 1988, pp 591–617.)

is measured by ^{51}Cr release, and cells are detected by monoclonal antibodies such as anti-Leu 7 (HNK-1) and anti-CD16 (NK-15, Leu 11) and are recognized as large granular lymphocytes (LGLs) with typical morphological characteristics.[52] The percentages of circulating HNK-positive cells and LGLs were reported to be normal in Hashimoto's disease.[53, 54] Conflicting results are reported on the activity of NK cells in peripheral blood. Schleusener and Bogner[55] reported increased activity, but Sack et al.[55a] observed normal activity. More recently, increased activity of peripheral NK cells was reported both in Hashimoto's and Graves' diseases.[56] Moreover, NK activity was found to increase during postpartum aggravation of autoimmune thyroiditis.[56] These data indicate that an increase in NK activity is associated with exacerbations of autoimmune thyroid disease, both in Hashimoto's thyroiditis and in Graves' disease, and suggest that NK cells may have an important role in control of disease activity in autoimmune thyroid disease.

Significant amounts of lymphotoxin, a soluble mediator of NK cytotoxicity, now termed *tumor necrosis factor* (TNF-β), is released from thyroid antigen–stimulated lymphocytes from patients with Hashimoto's disease.[57] The strongest activity of lymphotoxin was obtained from patients with associated hypothyroidism, suggesting that NK/K cell cytotoxicity, through lymphotoxin, plays an important role in the progress of Hashimoto's disease to hypothyroidism. Antigen-specific cytotoxic T lymphocytes recognize antigen in combination with the expression of MHC class I antigens. Cells in this category also have morphological features of LGL's. There is little information, however, on the thyroid antigen–specific MHC-restricted cytotoxic T lymphocytes, and thus the pathological role of these cells is ill defined in Hashimoto's disease. Using a clonal expansion technique, it was found recently that the majority of T-cell clones established from thyroid infiltrates in Hashimoto's thyroiditis were the precursors of CD8+ T lymphocytes with NK cell activity,[58] which may induce tissue damage in the thyroid gland. In vivo all these cytotoxic reactions might work together to induce thyroid cell atrophy.

Cellular Abnormalities

Several abnormalities in cellular populations and functions are observed in autoimmune thyroiditis. Some may be the direct representation of specific thyroid autoimmunities, and others may be reflections of thyroid dysfunction or of the general condition of autoimmunity.[25, 59]

Aberrant expression of HLA-DR molecules has been recognized on thyrocytes in autoimmune thyroid disease. This phenomenon, together with the expression of adhesion molecule ICAM-1,[60] might lead to T-cell activation by antigen presentation and the initiation of thyroid autoimmunity. However, another interpretation is that HLA-DR expression might have a protective role under normal conditions.[8] Thyroid cells in autoimmune thyroid disease are also reported to produce several cytokines (e.g., interleukin 1, interleukin 6, TNF-β) that might influence lymphocytic responses.

In studies of intrathyroid infiltrating lymphocytic populations, T lymphocytes are predominant over B cells, and CD8+ T lymphocytes are increased[25] in Hashimoto's thy-

roiditis. An analysis of the gene for the variable region of the α chain of the TCR (Vα gene) suggests that the infiltrating T cells are of a highly restricted population,[61] although this has been disputed. In these cells, activated (HLA-DR+) cells are increased when compared with the peripheral blood, especially DR+CD8+ and NK/K cells [CD57+ (= Leu7+)].[62] Some reports suggest an antigen-specific defect in suppressor T-lymphocyte[63] function in these cells, although this is not always accepted.[25] Functionally, there are increased frequencies of T lymphocytes that secrete interferon-γ and interleukin 2 (IL-2) and that proliferate when stimulated by thyroid antigens (e.g., TPO). MHC-restricted cytolytic activities and NK activities of intrathyroidal lymphocytes are also reported.

For the lymphocytic populations in the peripheral circulation, activated T cells (HLA-DR+CD3+) are increased,[64] and ordinary αβTCR+ T cells (Tαβ) are decreased in Hashimoto's thyroiditis. The more prominent changes are observed at the time of exacerbation of Hashimoto's thyroiditis. CD8+ cells decrease, and unusual subsets, such as γδTCR+ T cells (Tγδ), are decreased and CD4+CD8+ cells are increased during this thyrotoxic period.[65] The decrease in CD8+ and Tγδ cells may reflect their accumulation in the thyroid to cause cell lysis. An increase in CD5+ B cells,[66] which produce autoantibodies and have immunoregulatory functions, has been reported, but a more obvious increase is observed in Graves' disease.[67] NK/K cells (CD57+) are also increased at the time of exacerbation in Hashimoto's disease. NK cells are found to change in the course of normal pregnancy in number and activity,[68] and this may influence the clinical course during pregnancy and the postpartum period. The aforementioned changes in peripheral lymphocytes are summarized in Table 43–3. Because there are circulating lymphocytes reactive to thyroid antigen in peripheral blood, T-cell clones derived from these peripheral lymphocytes are utilized for the functional analysis of cellular autoimmunity in thyroid disease.

Cytokines

Cytokines are known to have a wide variety of inflammatory and immunomodulatory effects, and so it might be thought that many steps in thyroid autoimmunity are mediated and/or modulated by cytokines.[69] Indeed, administration of IL-2 or IFN-γ to animals can induce thyroid

TABLE 43–3. LYMPHOCYTE SUBSETS IN PERIPHERAL BLOOD IN AUTOIMMUNE THYROID DISEASE

| | | HASHIMOTO'S DISEASE | | GRAVES' DISEASE |
		Stable	Active	
T	Tαβ	↓	↓↓	→
	Tγδ	→	↓↓↓	→
	TH/I (CD4)	→	→	→
	Ts/c (CD8)	—	↓↓	→
B	CD5–B	—	—	→
	CD5+	↑	—	↑↑↑
NK		—	—	→
K	ADCC	—	↑↑	↓↓

→, no change; ↑, increase; ↓, decrease.

autoimmunity, and autoimmunity occurs in humans who received IL-2 for the treatment of cancer.[70]

IFN-γ, which is produced by T lymphocytes and NK cells infiltrated into the thyroid, is reported to have several effects on thyrocytes and lymphocytes. Acting directly on thyrocytes, it stimulates both HLA class I and class II expression on their surface. In cultured thyroid cells, IFN-γ reduces the content of TPO[71] and thyroglobulin mRNA and the secretion of thyroglobulin[72] and thyroid hormones in response to TSH. IFN-γ also causes morphological changes in thyrocytes, which is thought to represent dedifferentiation.[72] Acting on lymphocytes, IFN-γ induces B-cell proliferation and NK cell activation.

Tumor necrosis factor α (TNF-α), which is mainly produced by monocytes, has cytotoxic and cytostatic effects on many kinds of cultured cells, including thyrocytes. It can induce HLA class I antigen expression on thyrocytes. It cannot activate HLA class II expression alone, but acting synergically with IFN-γ, TNF-α enhances HLA class II expression.

Interleukins 1 (IL-1) and 6 (IL-6) are produced by thyrocytes as well as by lymphocytes. Thus interleukins produced by thyrocytes would stimulate the intrathyroidal lymphocytes. IL-1 stimulates T cells to release lymphokines and has many other inflammatory effects. IL-6 is known as a B-cell stimulatory factor. Antithyroid drugs are reported to reduce the production of these interleukins by thyrocytes attacked by complement and may have immunomodulatory effects.[73] IL-1 is also reported to have direct stimulatory effects on thyrocyte proliferation. Table 43–4 summarizes the effect of these cytokines on thyroid cells.[69]

GENETIC FACTORS

It is widely known that autoimmune thyroid diseases (both Hashimoto's thyroiditis and Graves' disease) occur in families. This fact could reveal the existence of genetic predisposition as well as environmental influences. Studies of the genetic predisposition revealed that autoimmune thyroid diseases are often associated with particular genetic markers. These markers include histocompatibility lymphocytic antigens (HLA's), allotypes of immunoglobulin heavy chains, variations in TCR and thyroid peroxidase, and so on. The associations have been examined serologically and recently by analysis of restriction fragment length polymorphisms (RFLP's), which allow more direct DNA-defined typing of genetic markers. The reports are not always consistent with each other, probably because of the subjects chosen and the small sizes of some studies.

The association of HLA genes, especially class II HLA (DR, DQ, DX, and the like) genes, has been examined extensively. In Caucasians,[42] goitrous Hashimoto's thyroiditis is associated with HLA-DR3 and -DR5 and atrophic autoimmune thyroiditis with HLA-DR3 and HLA-B8. By RFLP analysis, association with HLA-DQw2 was detected, probably because of its linkage disequilibrium with HLA-DR3.[74] HLA-DR3 is also associated with Graves' disease, which might reflect genetic effects in common with Hashimoto's thyroiditis. Postpartum thyroid dysfunction is reported to be associated with HLA-DR5.[75] In Japanese, Hashimoto's thyroiditis is reported to be associated with HLA-DRw53[76] and -B-51,[77] and in Shanghai Chinese, with HLA-DR9 and -Bw46,[78] indicating racial differences. In Japanese, patients with postpartum hypothyroidism are likely to develop permanent hypothyroidism when they show HLA-DRw9 and/or -B51 genotypes, and thus HLA typing is helpful during observation of patients.[79]

Linkage of specific TCR genes to inheritance of Hashimoto's thyroiditis is also reported. A specific TCRβ RFLP was increased in Hashimoto's thyroiditis as well as in Graves' disease,[77] and a TaqI RFLP for Vα gene of TCR also was increased.[80] These findings were not reproduced in another report.[74] The inheritance of specific allotypes of immunoglobulin G heavy chain (Gm) is also reported to relate to autoimmune thyroiditis,[81] as in Graves' disease.[82] These associations may not prove that the examined genes are causative, since another gene near the examined locus actually may be causative. To settle this, further studies are necessary.

CLINICAL FEATURES

Thyroid Dysfunction

Autoimmune thyroiditis progresses slowly and is not self-limited. Therefore, there is an age dependency in the development of thyroid dysfunction. With time, some patients progress from the metabolically normal stage to hypothyroidism, often associated with disappearance of the goiter. The prevalence of hypothyroidism is therefore higher in the elderly[45] (Fig. 43–10). Approximately 10 per cent of Hashimoto's patients who visited the clinic show overt hypothyroidism[45] (Table 43–5). An important recent finding is that about 5 per cent of patients have an associated

TABLE 43–4. EFFECT OF CYTOKINES ON THE FUNCTION AND GROWTH OF THYROID CELLS

	SECRETION		GENE EXPRESSION		DNA SYNTHESIS	MHC CLASS II ANTIGEN EXPRESSION
	T_3	Tg	TPO	Tg		
IFN-α	→	→	→	→	→	→
IFN-β	→	→	→	→	→	↑
IFN-γ	↓	↓	↓	↓	→	→
IL-1 α/β	↓	↓	↓	↓	↑	→
IL-2	→	→	→	→	→	→
IL-6	→	?	↓	?	→	→
TNF-α	↓	↓	↓	↓	→	→

T_3, triiodothyronine; Tg, thyroglobulin; TPO, thyroid peroxidase; →, no change; ↑, increase; ↓, decrease.
Data from Nagataki S, Eguchi K: Cytokines and immune regulation in thyroid autoimmunity. Autoimmunity 13:27–34, 1992.

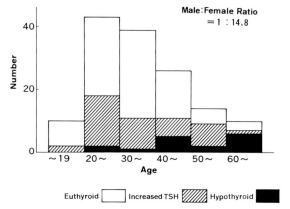

FIGURE 43–10. Age distribution and thyroid functional state in patients with Hashimoto's disease. (From Amino N: Autoimmunity and hypothyroidism. *In* Lazarus JH, Hall R (eds): Baillière's Clinical Endocrinology and Metabolism, Vol 2, No 3. London, Baillière Tindall, 1988, pp 591–617.)

destructive thyrotoxicosis. This condition is otherwise called *silent* or *painless thyroiditis* (see below).

Hawkins et al.[28] reported that thyroid microsomal antibodies provide a useful diagnostic test given the high predictive value for a raised serum TSH in a randomly selected population. They found a raised TSH in 36 to 44 per cent of subjects who were positive for thyroid microsomal antibodies. Using a hemagglutination method, we found positive thyroid microsomal antibodies (MCHA) in 64 (10.2 per cent) of 629 adult females and in 24 (6.0 per cent) of 395 adult males in the general population in Japan, but a raised serum TSH (>6 μIU/ml) was found in only 9.1 per cent of subjects with positive MCHA.[84] In subjects with MCHA who were less than 50 years old, the prevalence of increased TSH was only 2.2 per cent, and the mean serum TSH was not significantly different from that of age- and sex-matched controls without MCHA. A high TSH, however, was found in 16.2 per cent of older subjects with positive MCHA. Thus an age effect should be considered when assessing the predictive value of MCHA for a raised serum TSH. As shown in Figure 43–5, about 90 per cent of patients with Hashimoto's disease have positive MCHA, but there is no difference in titers and prevalence of antibodies between euthyroid and hypothyroid patients.

When the patients have an acute aggravation of thyroid autoimmunity, destruction-induced thyrotoxicosis occurs. These episodes are usually followed by transient hypothyroidism (see next section). High iodine ingestion may aggravate autoimmune thyroiditis and thus induce hypothyroidism. Therefore, whenever we examine patients, it is important to consider a recent excess of iodine ingestion. In children, Hashimoto's disease is less common, and titers of antithyroid antibodies are usually lower than those in adult patients. They usually present with a small symptomless goiter, and hypothyroidism is uncommon.

Silent and Postpartum Thyroiditis

Silent thyroiditis is a syndrome that has a clinical course of thyroid dysfunction similar to subacute thyroiditis but with no anterior neck pain and no tenderness of the thyroid.[85] Initially, patients have a thyrotoxic phase, later passing through euthyroidism to hypothyroidism and, finally, return to euthyroidism. Postpartum thyroiditis occurs within 6 months after delivery and runs an identical clinical course.[4] Postpartum thyroiditis is now considered to be identical to silent thyroiditis, and this term is used for patients who developed silent thyroiditis in the postpartum period.[4] After delivery, other forms of autoimmune thyroid dysfunction also occur, including Graves' disease, transient hypothyroidism without preceding destructive thyrotoxicosis, and persistent hypothyroidism. To include all these conditions, the term *postpartum autoimmune thyroid syndrome,* or simply *postpartum syndrome,* is often used.[86]

In recent years, the term *painless thyroiditis* also has been used frequently, and the same disorder has been described using different names, such as thyrotoxicosis with painless thyroiditis,[87] occult subacute thyroiditis,[88] hyperthyroiditis,[89] lymphocytic thyroiditis with spontaneously resolving hyperthyroidism,[90] and transient hyperthyroidism with lymphocytic thyroiditis.[91] The thyrotoxicosis in this disorder is different from that in Graves' disease and is induced by leakage of intrathyroidal hormones into the circulation caused by damage to thyroid epithelial cells from inflammation. Thus the thyroid radioactive iodine uptake (RAIU) is low. Therefore, the early phase of thyrotoxicosis in silent thyroiditis, postpartum thyroiditis, and subacute thyroiditis can be grouped together as destruction-induced thyrotoxicosis or simply as destructive thyrotoxicosis.[92]

Much evidence, including histopathological and immunological studies, indicates that this disorder is an autoimmune thyroid disease. During the clinical course of subclinical[2] or very mild autoimmune thyroiditis, aggravating factors cause exacerbation of the destructive process. Table 43–6[92a] summarizes clinical data on patients with destruction-induced thyrotoxicosis. We find that all women with subclinical autoimmune thyroiditis and antithyroid microsomal antibodies of more than 1:5120 before pregnancy develop postpartum thyroiditis.[4] A significant percentage of patients with silent thyroiditis have personal or family histories of autoimmune thyroid disease. Most patients have a complete remission, but some develop persistent hypothyroidism.[93, 94] Recurrence of disease is common in silent thyroiditis but very rare in subacute thyroiditis. Considering all these data, we assume that silent thyroiditis is caused by the exacerbation of autoimmune thyroiditis induced by aggravating factors.

An immune rebound mechanism (Fig. 43–11) has been established for the induction of postpartum thyroiditis.[4] Postpartum thyroid destruction is associated with an increase in NK cell counts and activity.[56] Cessation of steroid therapy has initiated silent thyroiditis in a patient with

TABLE 43–5. THYROID FUNCTION STATE IN HASHIMOTO'S DISEASE

T₄	T₃	TSH	CASES	PER CENT
→	→	→	77	54.2
→	→	↑	22	15.5
↓	→	↑	20	14.1
↓	↓	↑	16	11.3
↑	↑	↓	7	4.9
			142	100

→, normal; ↑, high; ↓, low.

From Amino N: Autoimmunity and hypothyroidism. *In* Lazarus JH, Hall R (eds): Hypothyroidism and Goiter. Baillière's Clinical Endocrinology and Metabolism, Vol 2, No 3. London, Baillière Tindall, 1988, pp 591–617.

TABLE 43–6. CLINICAL DATA ON PATIENTS WITH DESTRUCTION-INDUCED THYROTOXICOSIS

	SILENT THYROIDITIS		SUBACUTE THYROIDITIS
	Postpartum	Spontaneous	
No. examined	29	27	57
Female patients	29 (100)	25 (93)	52 (91)
Age less than 30 years	24 (83)†	7 (26)*	2 (4)
Antibodies			
Positive TGHA‡	11 (38)*	11 (41)†	0 (0)
Positive MCHA‡	24 (83)†	23 (85)†	0 (0)
Goiter			
Palpable at thyrotoxic state	26 (90)	27 (100)	57 (100)
Persistence	26 (90)†	26 (96)†	0 (0)

Values in parentheses indicate the percentage.
*Significantly different from subacute thyroiditis ($p < 0.01$, chi-square test).
†Significantly different from subacute thyroiditis ($p < 0.001$, chi-square test).
‡TGHA antithyroglobulin hemagglutination antibody; MCHA antithyroid microsomal hemagglutination antibody.
From Amino N: Postpartum and silent thyroiditis. In Monaco F, Satta MA, Shapiro B, Troncone L (eds): Thyroid Diseases. Clinical Fundamentals and Therapy. Boca Raton, FL, CRC Press, 1993, pp 239–249.

autoimmune thyroiditis and rheumatoid arthritis,[95] presumably because this also allows immune rebound. In patients with Cushing's syndrome who have associated subclinical autoimmune thyroiditis, silent thyroiditis has occurred after unilateral adrenalectomy.[96] Silent thyroiditis frequently recurs, and seasonal allergic rhinitis is reported to be an initiation factor.[97] Physically vigorous massage on the neck also was reported to be a contributing factor for silent thyroiditis.[98] Table 43–7 shows the incidence of various types of thyrotoxicosis in the outpatient clinic in Osaka University Hospital. The prevalence of silent thyroiditis, including postpartum disease, is 4.9 per cent of all types of thyrotoxicosis. Spontaneous silent thyroiditis is three times more frequent than postpartum thyroiditis.

The incidence of postpartum thyroiditis has been defined by prospective screening studies[99] (Fig. 43–12 and Table 43–8). Typically, painless thyroiditis or destructive thyrotoxicosis occurs at 1 to 3 months postpartum. Painless transient thyrotoxicosis was found in 20 (2.9 per cent) of 680 consecutive postpartum women. When patients with transient hypothyroidism are included, the incidence increases to 4.1 per cent. The range of incidence of postpartum thyroiditis was reported to be from 1.2 to 16.7 per cent. The reason for the variability is not clear but may be attributed to differences in the analytical methods, ethnic groups, or environmental or genetic risk factors. Most probably, the prevalence of postpartum thyroiditis ranges from 3 to 6 per cent.

The autoimmune inflammation only involves the thyroid gland, symptoms are usually mild, and the usual clinical features are attributed to thyroid dysfunction. The clinical course of a representative case with postpartum thyroiditis is shown in Figure 43–13. At 2 months postpartum this patient developed silent destructive thyrotoxicosis, passing through a euthyroid state to hypothyroidism. In the early thyrotoxic phase, goiter size increased slightly due to intrathyroidal autoimmune inflammation. During the hypothyroid phase, thyroid size enlarged further due to stimulation by increased serum TSH in association with an increase in titers of antithyroid microsomal antibody (MCAb). At 8 months postpartum, thyroid function finally returned to the normal range.

It is important to recognize that 5 to 10 per cent of thyrotoxic patients with diffuse goiter have silent thyroiditis. The principal diagnostic features are mild to moderate thyrotoxicosis, painless thyroid enlargement, and a low thyroid RAIU. However, RAIU is not always readily available. It is not practical for every patient with thyrotoxicosis to have a RAIU to exclude silent thyroiditis. As shown in Table 43–7, nearly 90 per cent of thyrotoxic patients have Graves' disease. Therefore, it is essential to differentiate this disorder from Graves' thyrotoxicosis. As shown in Table 43–9, Graves' thyrotoxicosis lasts for more than 3 months, but increased thyroid hormone levels in silent thyroiditis usually disappear within 3 months. Patients with Graves' disease have anti-TSH receptor antibody, and TSH-binding inhibitory immunoglobulin (TBII), measured by radioreceptor assay, is positive in about 90 per cent of

FIGURE 43–11. Immune rebound hypothesis regarding the onset of postpartum thyroiditis. Possible immunosuppression in pregnancy may disappear at delivery, and "transient enhancement" of the immune reactions may occur after delivery. (From Amino N, Miyai K: Postpartum autoimmune endocrine syndromes. In Davies TF (ed): Autoimmune Endocrine Disease. New York, John Wiley & Sons, 1983, pp 247–272.)

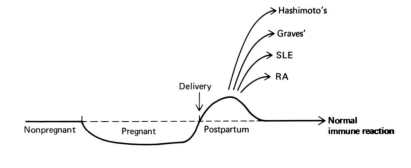

TABLE 43–7. PREVALENCE OF SILENT THYROIDITIS AMONG VARIOUS TYPES OF THYROTOXICOSES

	NO. OF PATIENTS	PER CENT
Graves' disease	372	88.4
Destructive thyrotoxicosis		
Subacute thyroiditis	27	6.4
Silent thyroiditis		
Postpartum	5	1.2
Spontaneous	15	3.7
Hyperfunctioning thyroid nodule	2	0.5
TOTAL	421	100

Reproduced with permission from Amino N: Postpartum and silent thyroiditis. *In* Monaco F, Satta MA, Shapiro B, Troncone L (eds): Thyroid Diseases. Clinical Fundamentals and Therapy. Boca Raton, FL., CRC Press, 1993, pp 239–249.

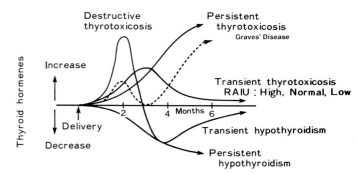

FIGURE 43–12. Various types of postpartum thyroid dysfunction. (From Amino N, Miyai K: Postpartum autoimmune endocrine syndromes. *In* Davies TF (ed): Autoimmune Endocrine Disease. New York, John Wiley & Sons, 1983, pp 247–272.)

patients. These antibodies are usually negative in silent thyroiditis, although there are some exceptions.[100] The serum T_3/T_4 ratio (ng/μg) is a simple indicator for differentiation between the two types of thyrotoxicosis. Eighty per cent of Graves' thyrotoxicosis shows a ratio of more than 20, but it is less than 20 in destructive thyrotoxicosis, including silent thyroiditis. After complete remission of Graves' disease, the same patients sometimes develop silent thyroiditis. Therefore, the previous history is not useful for differentiation.

Since the thyrotoxicosis is usually mild and self-limited, special treatment may not be required. An important point is to explain the nature of disease to the patient in order to allay anxiety. When thyrotoxic symptoms are severe enough to require treatment, patients may be given beta-adrenergic antagonists, sedatives, or tranquilizer therapy. A beta blocker such as propranolol, 10 mg three times a day, is often useful to reduce thyrotoxic symptoms. Steroid therapy reduces the inflammatory process,[85] but the optimal starting dose or duration of therapy has not been established. Since symptoms are controlled easily by beta blockers, use of steroids is not generally recommended.[101] About 10 to 20 per cent of patients have recurrent episodes of thyroiditis, but thyroid suppression therapy is not effective for prevention. In rare patients who have frequent recurrences, surgical removal of the gland or ^{131}I therapy has been recommended.[85, 91]

Relation to Graves' Disease

After treatment, patients with thyrotoxic Graves' disease often progress to hypothyroidism,[102] possibly due to the autoimmune destructive mechanisms described above. Development of hypothyroidism in Graves' disease may be induced in two ways,[103] autoimmune thyroid destruction or the appearance of predominant TSBAb. Macchia et al.[104] found that 15 of 135 thyrotoxic patients with Graves' disease (11.1 per cent) had blocking activity to TSH-induced adenylate cyclase stimulation but no TSAb activity. These data strongly suggest that many patients with Graves' disease have both stimulating and blocking antibodies. When the patients have predominantly stimulating antibodies, they develop hyperthyroidism. If they have predominantly blocking antibodies, they progress to hypothyroidism. The dominance between stimulation and blocking may change in some patients.[105] Simultaneous determination of TSAb

and TSBAb may be helpful in patients with Graves' disease who show spontaneous fluctuations in thyroid function.

The clinical features of patients depend on the balance between stimulating, blocking, and destructive aspects of humoral and cellular immunity[45] (Fig. 43–14). When stimulating factors are predominant, patients develop Graves' thyrotoxicosis. Predominance of destructive factors, such as ADCC, T-lymphocyte cytotoxicity, lymphotoxin (TNF), and cytotoxic antibody, may produce Hashimoto's disease or myxedema. Blocking factors such as TSBAb also cause a reduction in thyroid function. Once thyroid cells are destroyed completely, stimulating factors are ineffective.[106] From the clinical point of view, it is important to clarify the nature of the destructive factors in autoimmune thyroid disease.

Relation to Other Autoimmune Diseases

Patients with some other autoimmune diseases are often found to have positive MCHA and/or TGHA and thus to be associated with autoimmune thyroid diseases.[10] The incidence is higher than expected in the general population (Table 43–10). On the other hand, the frequency with

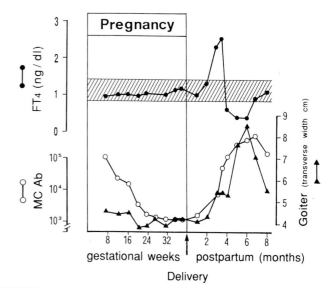

FIGURE 43–13. A case of postpartum thyroiditis (MCAb, antithyroid microsomal antibody; FT₄, free thyroxine).

TABLE 43–8. PREVALENCE OF POSTPARTUM THYROID DYSFUNCTION AMONG 680 CONSECUTIVE POSTPARTUM WOMEN

TYPE OF THYROID ABNORMALITY	NO. OF PATIENTS (%)	NUMBER OF CASES		
		Goiter	TGHA*	MCHA*
Transient thyrotoxicosis	13 (1.91)	6	5	11
Transient thyrotoxicosis followed by transient hypothyroidism	7 (1.03)	4	3	6
Persistent thyrotoxicosis	1 (0.15)	1	0	0
Transient hypothyroidism	8 (1.18)	8	3	7
Persistent hypothyroidism	1 (0.15)	1	1	1
TOTAL	30 (4.41)	19	12	25

*TGHA, antithyroglobulin hemagglutination antibody; MCHA, antithyroid microsomal hemagglutination antibody.
Reproduced with permission from Amino A, Mori H, Iwatani Y, et al: High prevalence of transient postpartum thyrotoxicosis and hypothyroidism. N Engl J Med 306:849–852, 1982.

which the patients with autoimmune thyroid disease suffer from an association with another autoimmune disease is low, except for autoimmune gastritis.[107] Anti-parietal cell antibodies and/or anti-intrinsic factor antibodies are found in about a third of patients with autoimmune thyroid disease. Conversely, in 80 per cent of patients with autoimmune gastritis, thyroid antibodies are found. Association of autoimmune thyroid disease is found both with organ-specific autoimmune diseases (e.g., vitiligo, myasthenia gravis, thrombocytopenic purpura, alopecia, Sjögren's syndrome[108]) and with systemic autoimmune diseases (e.g., rheumatoid arthritis, systemic lupus erythematosus, and progressive systemic sclerosis).

An association with other endocrine autoimmune diseases (such as insulin-dependent diabetes mellitus, autoimmune adrenalitis, autoimmune hypoparathyroidism, autoimmune hypophysitis) is also found in autoimmune thyroiditis. Such autoimmunity may occur simultaneously in multiple organs (polyendocrine autoimmune disease).

DIAGNOSIS

The diagnosis of autoimmune thyroiditis is usually simple by clinical observation and serological tests, especially in overt hypothyroidism. A diffuse goiter and positive anti-thyroid antibodies (antithyroglobulin antibodies and/or anti-TPO antibodies) without any evidence of other thyroid disease leads to the diagnosis of goitrous Hashimoto's thyroiditis. Tests for thyroid function (FT_4, FT_3, and TSH) may not be helpful, because thyroiditis is subclinical in about 90 per cent of patients. In patients who seem to have primary hypothyroidism with an atrophic thyroid, the existence of blocking-type anti-TSH receptor antibodies (TSBAb's) should be assessed, although their prevalence is low.[109]

Histological examination is confirmative but not necessary for the diagnosis and management of the thyroiditis, since lymphocytic infiltration into the thyroid is observed in all seropositive patients.[2] Conversely, either TGHA or MCHA is detectable in more than 95 per cent of histologically confirmed cases of Hashimoto's disease. Indeed, detection of the antibodies is sufficient for diagnosis of the existence of autoimmune thyroid disease. Antibodies are also found in about 10 per cent of individuals in the general population without any clinical manifestation, and these individuals should be considered to have subclinical autoimmune thyroiditis. For the small number of seronegative patients who have overt or latent hypothyroidism, the diagnosis of Hashimoto's thyroiditis is likely, but histological examination is the only way to prove its existence. Thyroid biopsy will be truly necessary if the goiter is rapidly increasing, is very hard or fixed—that is, when thyroid tumors are suspected.

TABLE 43–9. DIFFERENTIAL DIAGNOSIS OF THYROTOXICOSIS BETWEEN SILENT THYROIDITIS AND GRAVES' DISEASE

	SILENT THYROIDITIS	GRAVES' DISEASE
Duration of symptoms	<3 months	>3 months
Eye signs	No	30% yes
Radioactive iodine uptake	Low	High
Anti-TSH receptor antibody	Negative	Positive
T_3/T_4 ratio (ng/μg)	<20	80% >20
Thyrotoxicosis	Transient	Persistent

Reproduced with permission from Amino N: Postpartum and silent thyroiditis. In Monaco F, Satta MA, Shapiro B, Toncone L (eds): Thyroid Diseases. Clinical Fundamentals and Therapy. Boca Raton, FL, CRC Press, 1993, pp 239–249.

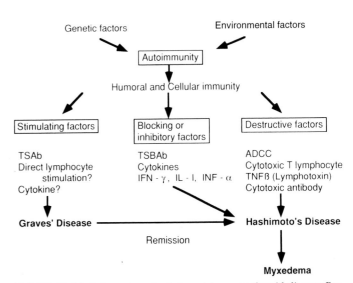

FIGURE 43–14. Balance hypothesis in autoimmune thyroid disease. Predominant stimulating factors produce Graves' thyrotoxicosis, and predominant destructive factors produce Hashimoto's disease and myxedema. Blocking factors induce the reduction of thyroid function. (From Amino N: Autoimmunity and hypothyroidism. In Lazarus JH, Hall R (eds): Baillière's Clinical Endocrinology and Metabolism, Vol 2, No 3. London, Baillière Tindall, 1988, pp 591–617.)

TABLE 43–10. INCIDENCE OF ANTITHYROGLOBULIN (TGHA) AND ANTITHYROID MICROSOMAL HEMAGGLUTINATION (MCHA) ANTIBODIES IN OTHER AUTOIMMUNE DISEASES

	NUMBER EXAMINED	TGHA TITER		MCHA TITER	
		20 and Over	More Than 10⁴	20 and Over	More Than 10⁴
Systemic lupus erythematosus	104	19* (41)†	4 (4)	43 (41)	5 (5)
Rheumatoid arthritis	38	8 (21)	2 (5)	15 (39)	5 (13)
Progressive systemic sclerosis	37	4 (11)	0 (0)	13 (35)	3 (8)
Sjögren's syndrome	19	4 (21)	0 (0)	10 (53)	4 (21)
Myasthenia gravis	183	18 (10)	2 (1)	52 (28)	5 (3)
Idiopathic thrombocytopenic purpura	64	9 (14)	5 (8)	26 (41)	11 (17)

*Indicates number of patients.
†Indicates percentage of patients.
From Amino N: Antithyroid antibodies. In Ingbar SH, Braverman LE (eds): The Thyroid (ed 5). Philadelphia, JB Lippincott, 1986, pp 546–559.

During the thyrotoxic phase of acute exacerbations of Hashimoto's thyroiditis and in silent thyroiditis, it is necessary to rule out Graves' disease, subacute thyroiditis, and toxic nodular goiter. In differentiation from Graves' disease, it is essential to verify decreased RAIU. Observation of a decreased T₃/T₄ ratio (< 20 ng/μg) is helpful when the RAIU is not available.[92] The history (period of thyrotoxicosis < 3 months), physical examination (no eye signs, no neck tenderness), and autoantibodies (TGHA, MCHA, TBII, TSAb) are also informative. Subacute thyroiditis, which is accompanied by a tender goiter, fever, and inflammatory reactions, is usually not associated with thyroid autoantibodies. The goiter disappears after recovery from subacute thyroiditis, whereas the goiter in autoimmune thyroiditis remains.

TREATMENT

There is no practical way to manipulate the autoimmune abnormality itself. The major approach is to treat the associated hypothyroidism or to attempt to shrink the goiter to release pressure symptoms or simply for cosmetic reasons. T₄ replacement therapy is usually not necessary in euthyroid patients with small or moderate goiters. These patients should be examined once a year to recognize later development of hypothyroidism. When patients develop hypothyroidism, they should be treated with T₄. The daily replacement dose is 100 to 200 μg/day (2 to 2.5 μg/kg/day). In patients with long-standing hypothyroidism, replacement therapy should be initiated with a small dose of thyroxine and built up gradually until a satisfactory maintenance dose is achieved. Hypothyroidism in patients with large goiters and high iodine uptake is often transient,[110] especially in patients younger than age 30. Restriction of high iodine ingestion may be effective in these patients. Hypothyroidism in patients with postpartum thyroiditis is usually transient. In these patients, lifelong T₄ therapy is not necessary. T₃ therapy, rather than T₄, is useful for a short period to quickly relieve the hypothyroid symptoms. In patients with silent and postpartum thyroiditis, the thyrotoxicosis is usually mild and self-limited, and special treatment may not be required. To relieve thyrotoxic symptoms, beta-adrenergic antagonists are sometimes effective. A painful subacute exacerbation of goitrous Hashimoto's disease is rare, and corticosteroid therapy is useful in these cases. Surgical resection of goiter is rarely necessary but may be required in patients with "active" Hashimoto's goiter who do not respond to steroid therapy or who have severe pressure symptoms.

NATURAL HISTORY

Most patients with Hashimoto's thyroiditis are either euthyroid or have latent hypothyroidism with goiter in their youth. As time passes, some progress to overt hypothyroidism. The goiter becomes smaller and occasionally atrophies. Histologically, fibrosis spreads, and few thyroid follicles remain in this stage of thyroiditis. Thus elderly patients with Hashimoto's thyroiditis are more likely to be found hypothyroid. It is appropriate for patients with subclinical autoimmune thyroiditis to be observed periodically (once or twice a year), although the incidence of developing hypothyroidism is not high.

Patients may experience periods of transient hypothyroidism under certain conditions. In some cases of Hashimoto's thyroiditis, hypothyroidism seems to be reversible.[110] This transient hypothyroidism may occur in the course of Hashimoto's thyroiditis when there is slow destruction of the thyroid. The hypothyroidism is often transient when goiter is present and serum thyroglobulin is high.[111] The thyroid response to TSH in response to TRH administration can be used to evaluate potential recovery from hypothyroidism in patients under thyroxine therapy.[112] Of patients with postpartum hypothyroidism, about 70 per cent recover in several months, whereas 30 per cent develop permanent hypothyroidism.[79]

About 5 per cent of patients experience destructive thyrotoxicosis.[92] Acute inflammatory symptoms (such as high fever and spontaneous pain in the thyroid) may be present. After the thyrotoxic phase, a period of transient hypothyroidism follows, and then such patients usually recover to euthyroidism.

In a region where iodine-containing foods (such as seaweeds) are common, as in Japan, excessive dietary iodine intake (1000 μg/day or more) may cause transient hypothyroidism in patients with subclinical autoimmune thyroiditis. This condition is easily reversible with reduction in iodine intake.[113]

A rare but important complication of Hashimoto's thyroiditis is malignant lymphoma. The frequency of malignant lymphoma of the thyroid origin is increased in patients with Hashimoto's thyroiditis.[114]

REFERENCES

1. Hashimoto H: Zur Kenntniss der lymphomatösen Veränderung der Schilddrüse (Struma lymphomatosa). Arch Klin Chir 97:219–248, 1912.
2. Yoshida H, Amino N, Yagawa K, et al: Association of serum antithyroid antibodies with lymphocytic infiltration of the thyroid gland: Study of 70 autopsied cases. J Clin Endocrinol Metab 46:859–862, 1978.
3. Amino N: Antithyroid antibodies. In Ingber SH, Braverman LE (eds): The Thyroid (ed 5). Philadelphia, JB Lippincott, 1986, pp 546–559.
4. Amino N, Miyai K: Postpartum autoimmune endocrine syndromes. In Davies TF (ed): Autoimmune Endocrine Disease. New York, John Wiley & Sons, 1983, pp 247–272.
5. Woolner LB, McConahey WM, Beahrs OH: Struma lymphomatosa (Hashimoto's thyroiditis and related thyroidal disorders). J Clin Endocrinol 19:53, 1959.
6. Gluck FB, Nusygnowitz ML, Plymate S: Chronic lymphocytic thyroiditis, thyrotoxicosis and low radioactive iodine uptake: Report of four cases. N Engl J Med 293:624–628, 1975.
7. Inada M, Nishikawa M, Oishi M, et al: Transient thyrotoxicosis associated with painless thyroiditis and low radioactive iodine uptake. Arch Intern Med 139:597–599, 1979.
8. Iwatani Y, Amino N, Miyai K: Peripheral self-tolerance and autoimmunity: The protective role of expression of class II major histocompatibility antigens on nonlymphoid cells. Biomed Pharmacother 43:593–605, 1989.
9. Nossal GJV, Pike BL: Evidence for the clonal abortion theory of B-lymphocyte tolerance. J Exp Med 141:904–917, 1975.
10. Volpé R: Immunology of human thyroid disease. In Volpé R (ed): Autoimmunity in Endocrine Diseases. Boca Raton, FL, CRC Press, 1990, pp 73–220.
11. Bottazzo GF, Pujol-Borrell R, Hanafusa T, Feldmann M: Role of aberrant HLA-DR expression and antigen presentation in induction of endocrine autoimmunity. Lancet 2:115, 1983.
12. Roitt IM, Torrigiani G: Identification and estimation of undegraded thyroglobulin in human serum. Endocrinology 81:421–429, 1967.
13. Roberts IM, Whittingham S, MacKay IR: Tolerance to an autoantigen-thyroglobulin: Antigen-binding lymphocytes in thymus and blood in health and autoimmune disease. Lancet 2:936–940, 1973.
14. Piechaczyk M, Bouanani M, Salhi SL, et al: Antigenic domains on the human thyroglobulin molecule recognized by autoantibodies in patients' sera and by natural autoantibodies isolated from the sera of healthy subjects. Clin Immunol Immunopathol 45:114–121, 1987.
15. Bouanani M, Piechaczyk M, Pau B, Bastide M: Significance of the recognition of certain antigenic regions on the human thyroglobulin molecules by natural auto antibodies from healthy subjects. J Immunol 143:1129–1132, 1989.
16. Henry M, Zanelli E, Piechaczyk M, et al: A major human thyroglobulin epitope defined with monoclonal antibodies is mainly recognized by human autoantibodies. Eur J Immunol 22:315–319, 1992.
17. Champion BR, Page KR, Parish N, et al: Identification of a thyroxine-containing self-epitope of human thyroglobulin which triggers thyroid autoreactive T cells. J Exp Med 174:363–370, 1991.
18. Amino N, Hagan SR, Yamada N, Refetoff S: Measurement of circulating thyroid microsomal antibodies by the tanned red cell hemagglutination technique: Its usefulness in the diagnosis of autoimmune thyroid diseases. Clin Endocrinol 5:115–125, 1976.
19. Tamaki H, Amino N, Iwatani Y, et al: Detection of thyroid microsomal and thyroglobulin antibodies by new sensitive radioimmunoassay in Hashimoto's disease: Comparison with conventional hemagglutination assay. Endocrinol Jpn 38:97–101, 1991.
20. Portmann L, Hamada N, Heinrich G, DeGroot LJ: Anti-thyroid peroxidase antibody in patients with autoimmune thyroid disease: Possible identity with anti-microsomal antibody. J Clin Endocrinol Metab 61:1001–1003, 1985.
21. Finke R, Seto P, Ruf J, et al: Determination at the molecular level of a B-cell epitope on thyroid peroxidase likely to be associated with autoimmune thyroid disease. J Clin Endocrinol Metab 73:919–921, 1991.
22. Frorath B, Abney CC, Scanarini M, et al: Mapping of a linear autoantigenic epitope within the human thyroid peroxidase using recombinant DNA techniques. J Biochem Tokyo 111:633–637, 1992.
23. Ewins DL, Barnett PS, Tomlinson RW, et al: Mapping epitope specificities of monoclonal antibodies to thyroid peroxidase using recombinant antigen preparations. Autoimmunity 11:141–149, 1992.

24. Kohno Y, Naito N, Hiyama N: Thyroglobulin and thyroid peroxidase share common epitopes recognized by autoantibodies in patients with chronic autoimmune thyroiditis. J Clin Endocrinol Metab 67:899–907, 1988.
25. Martin A, Davies TF: T cell and human autoimmune thyroid disease: Emerging data show lack of need to invoke suppressor T cell problems. Thyroid 2:247–261, 1992.
26. Khouney EL, Hammond L, Bottazzo GF, Donach D: Presence of the organ-specific "microsomal" autoantigen on the surface of human thyroid cells in culture: Its involvement in complement-mediated cytotoxicity. Clin Exp Immunol 45:316–328, 1981.
27. Tandon N, Jayne DRW, McGregor AM, Weetman AP: Analysis of anti-idiotypic antibodies against anti-microsomal antibodies in patients with thyroid autoimmunity. J Autoimmun 5:557–570, 1992.
28. Hawkins BR, Creah PS, Burger HG, et al: Diagnostic significance of thyroid microsomal antibodies in randomly selected population. Lancet 2:1057–1059, 1980.
29. Tamaki H, Amino N, Aozasa M, et al: Effective method for prediction of transient hypothyroidism in neonates born to mothers with chronic thyroiditis. Am J Perinatol 6:296–303, 1989.
30. Nagayama Y, Kaufman KD, Seto P, Rapoport B: Molecular cloning, sequence and functional expression of the cDNA for human thyrotropin receptor. Biochem Biophys Res Commun 165:1184–1190, 1989.
31. Libert F, Lefort A, Gerard C, et al: Cloning sequencing and expression of the human thyrotropin (TSH) receptor: Evidence for binding of auto-antibodies. Biochem Biophys Res Commun 165:1250–1255, 1989.
32. Misrahi M, Loosfelt H, Atger M, et al: Cloning, sequencing and expression of human TSH receptor. Biochem Biophys Res Commun 166:394–403, 1990.
33. Nagayama Y, Rapoport B: The thyrotropin receptor 25 years after its discovery: New insight after its molecular cloning. Mol Endocrinol 6:145–156, 1992.
34. Konishi J, Iida Y, Kasagi E, et al: Primary myxedema with thyrotropin-binding inhibitor immunoglobulins. Ann Intern Med 103:26–31, 1985.
35. Amino N, Watanabe Y, Tamaki H, et al: In vitro conversion of blocking type anti-TSH receptor antibody to the stimulating type by anti-human IgG antibodies. Clin Endocrinol 27:615–624, 1987.
36. Sakata S, Nakamura S, Miura K, et al: Autoantibodies against thyroid hormones or iodothyrosine. Ann Intern Med 103:579–589, 1985.
37. Staeheli V, Vallotton MB, Burger A: Detection of human anti-thyroxine and anti-triiodothyronine antibodies in different thyroid conditions. J Clin Endocrinol Metab 41:669–675, 1975.
38. Konishi J, Iida Y, Kousaka T, et al: Effect of anti-thyroxine autoantibodies on radioimmunoassay of free thyroxin in serum. Clin Chem 28:1389–1391, 1982.
39. Sakata S, Takuno H, Nagai K, et al: Anti-bovine thyrotropin autoantibodies in patients with Hashimoto's thyroiditis, subacute thyroiditis, and systemic lupus erythematosus. J Endocrinol Invest 14:123–130, 1991.
40. Zakaria M, MacKenzie J: Do thyroid growth-promoting immunoglobulins exist? J Clin Endocrinol Metab 70:308–310, 1990.
41. Tachi J, Amino N, Iwatani Y, et al: Increase in antideoxyribonucleotic acid antibody titer in postpartum aggravation of autoimmune thyroid disease. J Clin Endocrinol Metab 67:1049–1053, 1988.
42. DeGroot LJ, Quintans J: The causes of autoimmune thyroid disease. Endocr Rev 10:537–562, 1989.
43. Sawada K, Sakurami T, Imura H, et al: Antiasialo-G_{M1} antibody in sera from patients with Graves' disease and Hashimoto's thyroiditis. Lancet 2:198, 1980.
44. Thall A, Etienne-Decerf J, Winand RJ, Galli U: The α-galactosyl epitope on mammalian thyroid cells. Acta Endocrinol (Copenh) 124:692–698, 1991.
45. Amino N: Autoimmunity and hypothyroidism. In Lazarus JH, Hall R (eds): Hypothyroidism and Goiter. Ballière's Clin Endocrinol Metab, Vol 2, No. 3, 1988.
46. Iwatani Y, Amino N, Mori H, et al: A microcytotoxicity assay for thyroid-specific cytotoxic antibody, antibody-dependent cell-mediated cytotoxicity and direct lymphocyte cytotoxicity using human thyroid cells. J Immunol Methods 48:241–250, 1982.
47. Pulvertaft RJV, Doniach D, Roitt IM: The cytotoxic factor in Hashimoto's disease and its incidence in other thyroid diseases. Br J Exp Pathol 42:496–503, 1961.
48. Perlmann P, Perlmann H, Larsson A, Wahlin B: Antibody-dependent cytotoxic effector lymphocytes (K cells) in human blood. J Reticuloendothel Soc 17:241, 1975.

49. Calder EA, McLeman D, Irvine WJ: Lymphocyte cytotoxicity induced by preincubation with serum from patients with Hashimoto's thyroiditis. Clin Exp Immunol 15:467–470, 1973.

50. Bogner U, Schleusener H, Wall JR: Antibody-dependent cell-mediated cytotoxicity against human thyroid cells in Hashimoto's thyroiditis but not Graves' disease. J Clin Endocrinol Metab 59:734–738, 1984.

51. Amino N, Mori H, Iwatani Y, et al: Peripheral K lymphocytes in autoimmune thyroid disease: Decrease in Graves' disease and increase in Hashimoto's disease. J Clin Endocrinol Metab 54:587–591, 1982.

52. Iwatani Y, Amino N, Kabutomori O, et al: Effect of different sample preparations on enumeration of large granular lymphocytes (LGLs), and demonstration of a sex difference of LGLs. Am J Clin Pathol 90:674–678, 1988.

53. Wall JR, Baur R, Schleusener H, Bandy-Dafoe P: Peripheral blood and intrathyroidal mononuclear cell populations in patients with autoimmune thyroid disorders enumerated using monoclonal antibodies. J Clin Endocrinol Metab 56:164–169, 1983.

54. Iwatani Y, Amino N, Kabutomori O, et al: Decrease in peripheral large granular lymphocytes in Graves' disease. Clin Exp Immunol 55:239–244, 1984.

55. Schleusener H, Bogner U: Cytotoxic mechanisms in autoimmune thyroiditis. In Walfish PG, Wall JR, Volpé R (eds): Autoimmunity and the Thyroid. Orlando, FL, Academic Press, 1985, pp 95–107.

55a. Sack J, Baker JR, Weetman AP, et al: Killer cell activity and antibody-dependent cell-mediated cytotoxicity are normal in Hashimoto's disease. J Clin Endocrinol Metab 62:1059–1064, 1986.

56. Hidaka Y, Amino N, Iwatani Y, et al: Increase in peripheral natural killer cell activity in patients with autoimmune thyroid disease. Autoimmunity 11:239–246, 1992.

57. Amino N, DeGroot LJ: Insoluble particulate antigen(s) in cell-mediated immunity of autoimmune thyroid disease. Metabolism 24:45–56, 1975.

58. Del Prete GF, Maggi E, Mariotti S, et al: Cytolytic T lymphocytes with natural killer activity in thyroid infiltrate of patients with Hashimoto's thyroiditis: Analysis at clonal level. J Clin Endocrinol Metab 62:52–57, 1986.

59. Volpé R: Autoimmune thyroid disease. In Volpé R (ed): Autoimmunity and Endocrine Disease. New York, Marcel Dekker, 1985, pp 109–285.

60. Weetman AP, Freeman M, Borysiewicz LK, Macgoba MW: Functional analysis of intercellular adhesion molecule 1–expressing human thyroid cells. Eur J Immunol 20:271–275, 1990.

61. Davies TF, Martin A, Conception ES, et al: Evidence of limited variability of antigen receptors on intrathyroidal T cells in autoimmune thyroid disease. N Engl J Med 325:238–244, 1991.

62. Aozasa M, Amino N, Iwatani Y, et al: Intrathyroidal HLA-DR–positive lymphocytes in Hashimoto's disease: Increase in CD8 and Leu7 cells. Clin Immunol Immunopathol 52:516–522, 1989.

63. Volpé R, Iitaka M: Evidence for an antigen-specific T-lymphocyte in autoimmune thyroid disease. Exp Clin Endocrinol 97:133–138, 1991.

64. Ohashi H, Okugawa T, Itoh M: Circulating activated T cell subsets in autoimmune thyroid diseases: Differences between untreated and treated patients. Acta Endocrinol (Copenh) 125:502–509, 1991.

65. Iwatani Y, Amino N, Hidaka Y, et al: Decreases in αβ T cell receptor–negative T cells and CD8 cells, and an increase in CD4 + CD8 + cells in active Hashimoto's disease and subacute thyroiditis. Clin Exp Immunol 87:444–449, 1992.

66. Suranyi P, Szegedi G, Damjanovich S, et al: B lymphocyte subsets in Hashimoto's thyroiditis. Immunol Lett 22:147–150, 1989.

67. Iwatani Y, Amino N, Kaneda T, et al: Marked increase of CD5 + B cells in hyperthyroid Graves' disease. Clin Exp Immunol 78:196–200, 1989.

68. Hidaka Y, Amino N, Iwatani Y, et al: Changes in natural killer cell activity in normal pregnant and postpartum women: Increases in the first trimester and postpartum period and decrease in late pregnancy. J Reprod Immunol 20:73–83, 1991.

69. Nagataki S, Eguchi K: Cytokines and immune regulation in thyroid autoimmunity. Autoimmunity 13:27–34, 1992.

70. Kaplan MM: Hypothyroidism after treatment with interleukin-2 and lymphokine-activated killer cells. N Engl J Med 318:1157–1563, 1988.

71. Asakawa H, Hanafusa T, Kobayashi T, et al: Interferon-γ reduces the thyroid peroxidase content of cultured human thyrocytes and inhibits its increase induced by thyrotropin. J Clin Endocrinol Metab 74:1331–1335, 1992.

72. Kung AWC, Lau LMA, Lau KS: The role of interferon-gamma in lymphocytic thyroiditis: Its functional and pathological effect on human thyrocytes in culture. Clin Exp Immunol 87:261–265, 1992.

73. Weetman AP, Tandon N, Morgan BP: Antithyroid drugs and release of inflammatory mediators by complement-attacked thyroid cells. Lancet 340:633–636, 1992.

74. Mangklabruks A, Cox N, DeGroot LJ: Genetic factors in autoimmune thyroid disease analyzed by restriction fragment length polymorphisms of candidate genes. J Clin Endocrinol Metab 73:236–244, 1991.

75. Vargas MT, Briones-Urbina R, Gladman D, et al: Antithyroid microsomal autoantibodies and HLA-DR5 are associated with postpartum thyroid dysfunction: Evidence supporting an autoimmune pathogenesis. J Clin Endocrinol Metab 67:327–333, 1988.

76. Honda K, Tamai H, Morita T, et al: Hashimoto's thyroiditis and HLA in Japanese. J Clin Endocrinol Metab 69:1268–1273, 1989.

77. Ito M, Tanimoto M, Kamura H, et al: Association of HLA antigen and restriction fragment length polymorphism of T cell receptor β-chain gene with Graves' disease and Hashimoto's thyroiditis. J Clin Endocrinol Metab 69:100–104, 1989.

78. Wang FW, Yu ZQ, Xy JJ, et al: HLA and hypertrophic Hashimoto's thyroiditis in Shanghai Chinese. Tissue Antigens 33:235–236, 1988.

79. Tachi J, Amino N, Tamaki H, et al: Long term follow-up and HLA association in patients with postpartum hypothyroidism. J Clin Endocrinol Metab 66:480–484, 1988.

80. Weetman AP, So AK, Roe C, et al: T-cell receptor alpha V region polymorphism linked to primary autoimmune hypothyroidism but not Graves' disease. Hum Immunol 20:167–173, 1987.

81. Tamai H, Uno H, Hirota Y, et al: Immunogenetics of Hashimoto's and Graves' disease. J Clin Endocrinol Metab 60:62–66, 1985.

82. Uno H, Sasazuki T, Tamai H, Matsumoto H: Two major genes, linked to HLA and Gm, control susceptibility to Graves' disease. Nature 292:768–770, 1981.

83. Nikolai TF: Silent thyroiditis and subacute thyroiditis. In Braverman LE, Utiger RD (eds): The Thyroid. Philadelphia, JB Lippincott, 1991, pp 710–727.

84. Amino N, Mori H, Iwatani Y, et al: Significance of thyroid microsomal antibodies. Lancet 2:1369, 1980.

85. Nikolai TF, Coombs GJ, McKenzie AK, et al: Treatment of lymphocytic thyroiditis with spontaneously resolving hyperthyroidism (silent thyroiditis). Arch Intern Med 142:2281–2283, 1982.

86. Amino N, Iwatani Y, Tamaki H, et al: Postpartum autoimmune thyroid syndromes. In Walfish PG, Wall JR, Volpé R (eds): Autoimmunity and Thyroid. New York, Academic Press, 1985, pp 289–314.

87. Woolf PD, Daly R: Thyrotoxicosis with painless thyroiditis. Am J Med 60:73–79, 1976.

88. Hamburger JI: Occult subacute thyroiditis: Diagnostic challenge. Mich Med 70:1125, 1976.

89. Woolf PD: Transient painless thyroiditis with hyperthyroidism: A variant of lymphocytic thyroiditis? Endocr Rev 4:411–420, 1980.

90. Nikolai TF, Brosseau J, Kettrick MA, et al: Lymphocytic thyroiditis with spontaneously resolving hyperthyroidism (silent thyroiditis). Arch Intern Med 140:478–482, 1980.

91. Gorman CA, Duick DS, Woolner LB, et al: Transient hyperthyroidism in patients with lymphocytic thyroiditis. Mayo Clin Proc 53:359–365, 1978.

92. Amino N, Yabu Y, Miyai K, et al: Differentiation of thyrotoxicosis induced by thyroid destruction from Graves' disease. Lancet 2:344–346, 1978.

92a. Amino N: Postpartum and silent thyroiditis. In Monaco F, Satta MA, Shapiro B, Troncone L (eds): Thyroid Diseases. Clinical Fundamentals and Therapy. Boca Raton, FL, CRC Press, 1993, pp 239–249.

93. Amino N, Mori H, Iwatani Y, et al: High prevalence of transient postpartum thyrotoxicosis and hypothyroidism. N Engl J Med 306:849–852, 1982.

94. Nikolai TF, Coombs GJ, McKenzie AK: Lymphocytic thyroiditis with spontaneously resolving hyperthyroidism (silent thyroiditis) and subacute thyroiditis: Long term follow-up. Arch Intern Med 141:1455, 1981.

95. Maruyama H, Kato M, Mizuno O, et al: Transient thyrotoxicosis occurred after cessation of steroid therapy in a patient with autoimmune thyroiditis and rheumatoid arthritis. Endocrinol Jpn 29:583–588, 1982.

96. Takasu N, Komiya I, Nagasawa Y, et al: Exacerbation of autoimmune thyroid dysfunction after unilateral adrenalectomy in patients with Cushing's syndrome due to an adrenocortical adenoma. N Engl J Med 322:1708, 1990.

97. Yamamoto M, Shibuya N, Che LC, Ogata E: Seasonal recurrence of transient hypothyroidism in a patient with autoimmune thyroiditis. Endocrinol Jpn 35:135–142, 1988.

98. Tachi J, Amino N, Miyai K: Massage therapy on neck: A contributing factor for destructive thyrotoxicosis? Thyroidology 2:25–27, 1990.

99. Amino N: Postpartum thyroid disease. *In* Bercu BB, Shulam DI (eds): Advances in Perinatal Thyroidology. New York, Plenum Press, 1991, pp 167–180.

100. Morita T, Tamai H, Oshima A, et al: The occurrence of thyrotropin binding-inhibiting immunoglobulins and thyroid-stimulating antibodies in patients with silent thyroiditis. J Clin Endocrinol Metab 71:1051–1055, 1990.

101. Dorfman S, Sachson R, Feld S: The rationale for treatment of lymphocytic thyroiditis with spontaneously resolving hyperthyroidism: Prednisone therapy v chicken soup. Arch Intern Med 142:2261–2262, 1982.

102. Wood LC, Ingbar SH: Hypothyroidism as a late sequela in patients with Graves' treated with antithyroid agents. J Clin Invest 64:1429–1436, 1979.

103. Tamai H, Hirota Y, Kasagi K, et al: The mechanism of spontaneous hypothyroidism in patients with Graves' disease after antithyroid drug treatment. J Clin Endocrinol Metab 64:718–722, 1987.

104. Macchia E, Concetti R, Carone G, et al: Demonstration of blocking immunoglobulins G, having a heterogeneous behaviour in sera of patients with Graves' disease: Possible coexistence of different autoantibodies directed to the TSH receptor. Clin Endocrinol 28:147–156, 1988.

105. Miyauchi A, Amino N, Tamaki H, Kuma K: Coexistence of thyroid stimulating and blocking antibodies in a patient with Graves' disease who had transient hypothyroidism. Am J Med 85:418–420, 1988.

106. Tamaki H, Amino N, Iwatani Y, Miyai K: Improvement of infiltrative ophthalmopathy in parallel with decrease of thyroid-stimulating antibody (TSAb) activity in two patients with hypothyroid Graves' disease. J Endocrinol Invest 12:47–54, 1989.

107. Irvine WJ: Immunogenic aspects of pernicious anemia. N Engl J Med 273:432, 1965.

108. Karsh J, Pavlidis N, Weintraub BD, Moutsopoulus HM: Thyroid disease in Sjögren syndrome. Arthritis Rheum 23:1326–1329, 1980.

109. Tamaki H, Amino N, Kimura M, et al: Low prevalence of thyrotropin receptor antibody in primary hypothyroidism in Japan. J Clin Endocrinol Metab 71:1382–1386, 1990.

110. Yoshinari M, Okamura K, Tokuyama T, et al: Clinical importance of reversibility in primary goitrous hypothyroidism. Br Med J 287:720–722, 1983.

111. Sato K, Okamura K, Ikenoue H, et al: TSH-dependent elevation of serum thyroglobulin in reversible primary hypothyroidism. Clin Endocrinol 29:231–237, 1988.

112. Takasu N, Komaya I, Asawa T, et al: Test for recovery from hypothyroidism during thyroxine therapy in Hashimoto's thyroiditis. Lancet 2:1084–1086, 1990.

113. Tajiri J, Higashi K, Morita M, et al: Studies of hypothyroidism in patients with high iodine intake. J Clin Endocrinol Metab 63:412–417, 1986.

114. Hamburger JI, Miller JM, Kiri SR: Lymphoma of the thyroid. Ann Intern Med 99:685–693, 1983.

44

Subacute and Sclerosing Thyroiditis

ROBERT VOLPÉ

SUBACUTE THYROIDITIS

Subacute thyroiditis is a term that has come to describe a well-defined clinical entity, characterized by a generally painful self-limiting inflammatory process of the thyroid gland (probably of viral origin).[1-3] For the purposes of the following discussion, it is separated from a disorder having certain similarities but associated with no pain or tenderness and a different pathological picture, namely, painless or silent thyroiditis (see Ch. 43). It is clear that the term *subacute thyroiditis* connotes a temporal quality that might apply to any inflammatory process of intermediate severity and duration. However, as the term is generally employed, it specifically includes only those patients showing a pseudogranulomatous pathological picture (which is virtually specific for the disease) and a clinical syndrome in which the painful tender goiter is also associated with considerable malaise, fever, and evidence of thyroid dysfunction to be described more fully below.[1-3] This condition can sometimes be observed in men but is overwhelmingly seen in women.[1-3]

The name of DeQuervain has traditionally been associated with this condition because he described the pathology of this condition in 1904 and again in 1936.[4, 5] However, the credit for the first description ought to go to Mygind, who described 18 cases of "thyroiditis akuta simplex" in 1895.[6] This disorder has a multiplicity of synonyms, largely relating to early misconceptions and later conceptions about its nature. These synonyms include acute simple thyroiditis, noninfectious thyroiditis, DeQuervain's thyroiditis, acute or subacute diffuse thyroiditis, granulomatous thyroiditis, struma granulomatosa, pseudogranulomatous thyroiditis, giant cell thyroiditis, pseudo–giant cell thyroiditis, migratory "creeping" thyroiditis, pseudotuberculous thyroiditis, and viral thyroiditis. As noted below, the "giant cells" or "granulomata" actually only simulate such structures.[1]

Incidence

Subacute thyroiditis is relatively uncommon, occurring at the rate of about one case per five cases of Graves' disease and one case per 15 or 20 cases of chronic lymphocytic thyroiditis.[7] It seems to be most prevalent in the temperate zone, having been observed frequently in North America, Europe, and Japan, although rarely reported from many other parts of the world. It is not clear whether this apparent concentration in the aforementioned areas reflects its true prevalence or merely its ascertainment. It occurs most commonly between the second and fifth decades, is rare in children, seems to occur seasonally, and the female:male ratio is 3 to 6:1.[7]

Etiology

Considerable indirect evidence suggests that subacute thyroiditis represents a viral infection of the thyroid gland. Fraser and Harrison[8] were the first to propose this theory in 1952. Indeed, the malady is often preceded by an upper respiratory tract infection, and if such an infection cannot be recognized, there at least is frequently a prodromal phase characterized by musculoskeletal aches and pains, malaise, and fatigue.[1-3] Moreover, the illness may occur at the time of the outbreak of a specific viral infection, and its highest seasonal occurrence coincides with peaks of summer enterovirus infections.[7] After some weeks or months, complete recovery is the rule. A moderate leukocytosis may be encountered.

During the course of a mumps epidemic in Israel, 11 patients suffering subacute thyroiditis were reported who had circulating antibodies to the mumps virus without clinical evidence of mumps.[9] Subacute thyroiditis has also been reported in association with mumps in other reports.[10-13] Still other reports associate subacute thyroiditis with measles,[13-17] influenza,[17] the common cold,[18] adenovirus,[19] infectious mononucleosis,[18, 20, 21] Coxsackievirus,[22] myocarditis,[23] cat scratch fever,[24] and St. Louis encephalitis.[25] A virological study in 28 patients with this disease carried out in 1975 resulted in the isolation in five patients of a cytopathic virus that might have been of pathogenic significance.[26-28] However, viral inclusion bodies have not been observed within sections of thyroid tissue in this disorder.[2]

A study of viral antibodies in the acute and convalescent phase of this disease has implicated a variety of viruses, including Coxsackievirus, adenovirus, influenza, and mumps.[29] However, in a study of 10 patients in Singapore, such antibodies were not observed.[30] In any event, it is possible that the presence of such antibodies may not reflect pathogenic significance but may instead result from an anamnestic response to the inflammatory thyroid lesion.[29]

Certain nonviral infections such as Q fever and malaria have also been associated with subacute thyroiditis.[1] Moreover, epidemics of subacute thyroiditis have been described.[18]

Although subacute thyroiditis is not a primary autoimmune disease, secondary immunological phenomena are seen in the condition which are transitory in nature.[31] Significant levels of thyroid autoantibodies are found in a variable number of patients in the early phase, but the antibodies generally disappear several months after the onset of the process.[3, 29, 32–34] In one study, the transient phase of hypothyroidism correlated with the presence of microsomal antibodies, although this was not true for the rare development of permanent hypothyroidism.[33]

Antibodies to the thyroid-stimulating hormone (TSH) receptor have been observed during the course of subacute thyroiditis by several workers.[35–38] The method employed in most of those studies is the radioreceptor assay, in which the antibody (thyrotropin-binding inhibitory immunoglobulin [TBII, TBIAb]) prevents the binding of TSH to thyroid cell membranes. This assay does not measure the ability of the antibody to stimulate thyroid cells (thyroid-stimulating antibody, TSAb). In one study there was a good correlation between the presence of TBII and the hyperthyroid phase of the disorder, suggesting that the antibody might be pathogenetically related to the hyperthyroidism that occurs in thyroiditis.[38] However, in other studies no correlation was found between the presence or absence of this antibody and thyroid status.[35–37] The test result was positive in some patients in the hypothyroid phase and negative in others; when positive, it ultimately became negative without respect to the status of thyroid function. When TSAb was studied specifically, once again, a good correlation with thyroid function status did not exist.[37] However, when thyroid-blocking antibody was measured, at least some correlation with the development of hypothyroidism was noted.[37]

There is also evidence of T-lymphocyte sensitization to thyroid antigens.[1, 3, 31, 39] Moreover, the thyroid tissue in this disorder has been shown to contain large numbers of antigen-reactive T lymphocytes.[41] The overall percentage of T lymphocytes in the peripheral blood is low in subacute thyroiditis.[43] Finally, the thyrocytes have been shown to manifest HLA-DR on their cell surfaces during the active inflammatory stage,[44] and unpublished observations from our own laboratory have shown that this clears as the inflammatory process recedes.

Ultimately, following recovery, all elements of the immune response disappear, in contrast to the continuing presence of these abnormalities in patients with autoimmune thyroid disease (AITD).[1, 31] These observations are of considerable importance, however, in understanding AITD. In subacute thyroiditis, the immunological observations appear to be secondary to the release of antigenic material from the thyroid and do not appear to be related to the pathogenesis of this condition. The finding of thyrotropin-receptor antibodies, including thyroid-stimulating antibody, would also fit into this concept. The corollary is consistent with the view that antigen-driven events can produce a transient immunological disturbance, but this does not culminate in chronic AITD. This is thus evidence against a purely antigen-driven causation for AITD and fits with the concept that AITD is primarily a disorder of the immune system. This concept has relevance in relation to the proposal that bacterial antigens, such as *Yersinia*, which have homology for thyroid antigens, might somehow be causative factors in AITD. In the light of the above observations, this seems very unlikely. Moreover, the fact that many patients with subacute thyroiditis do display thyrotropin-receptor antibodies makes it clear that many normal people have the appropriate genes to be able to produce such antibodies, which they are then capable of doing under the circumstances of this condition, but are otherwise prevented from doing so by normal immunoregulation.[45]

An association between subacute thyroiditis and HLA-Dw35 has been found in all ethnic groupings.[46–49] The nature of this genetic relationship to the disorder has not yet been clarified but may indicate a particular susceptibility to viral infections of the thyroid in those populations. The incidence is approximately 72 per cent.

There is no direct association with AITD, and it is rare for this condition to progress to either Hashimoto's or Graves' disease,[1, 31] although this has happened in a few cases. Werner[50] reported a case of painful thyroiditis that progressed to Graves' disease and reviewed the literature in 1979. He argued that such inflammatory lesions of the thyroid gland could produce an antigenic alteration and initiate Graves' disease. Wartofsky and Schaaf[51] have recently published a similar case with similar arguments. However, because this development occurs so rarely and Graves' disease usually occurs de novo, this possibility seems very remote. It is possible that subacute thyroiditis could occasionally act as a nonspecific stress in precipitating hyperthyroidism.

Pathology[1–3, 52] (Fig. 44–1)

The thyroid gland is enlarged and somewhat edematous and may be slightly adherent to adjacent structures, although it can be freed from these without difficulty. Micro-

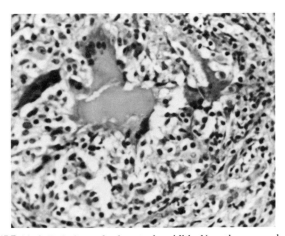

FIGURE 44–1. **Pathology of subacute thyroiditis.** Note the severe destruction of the thyroid follicle, with the remaining colloid being surrounded by large numbers of histiocytes giving a picture of a giant cell (pseudo giant cell). Marked interstitial edema is also present with a cellular infiltration and considerable destruction of the thyroid parenchyma.

scopically, the process may be diffuse or irregular in its involvement, with various stages of the disease sometimes present within the same specimen. The follicular cells sometimes virtually disappear, leaving a fragile and fine follicular lining. The initial phase is characterized by the appearance of neutrophils, followed by large mononuclear cells and lymphocytes. The follicles appear much larger than normal with disruption of the epithelial lining and hyperplasia of the surviving follicular cells. Histiocytes congregate around masses of colloid both within the follicles and in the interstitial tissue, producing "giant cells." These "cells" actually consist of masses of colloid surrounded by large numbers of individual histiocytes, thus earning the name *pseudo giant cells*. These are also seen in the interstitial tissue. There is considerable edema with histiocytes and lymphocytes in the interstitial tissue as well.

The process is often irregularly distributed in either lobe or throughout the thyroid gland. With recovery the inflammatory reaction begins to recede and a variable amount of fibrosis may then occur. Areas of follicular regeneration may appear, but there is no caseation, hemorrhage, or calcification. Aside from some residual fibrosis, the degree of recovery is almost always complete. Only in rare instances is there complete destruction of the thyroid parenchyma leading to permanent hypothyroidism. Viral inclusion bodies have not been demonstrated in the few electron microscopic studies that have been reported.[3] There is marked thickening of the basement membrane and some evidence to suggest increased cellular activity, although no apical pseudopods with colloid droplets are seen after TSH stimulation.[3]

Fine-needle aspiration biopsies often show large numbers of histiocytes, which can be misinterpreted. As mentioned earlier, the thyrocytes are found to express HLA-DR on their cell surfaces during the active phase of the inflammatory process.[44]

Clinical Features

The mode of onset and severity of the disorder vary widely.[1-3, 53-56] A prodromal phase often occurs, characterized by malaise and feverishness or by an upper respiratory tract infection. Pain in the region of the thyroid gland may be moderate or severe but in a few cases is entirely lacking. Similarly, tenderness may be moderate or severe (or even exquisite) or, conversely, may also be lacking. Either one of the lobes may be initially involved, or the condition may commence in one lobe and ultimately spread to the opposite lobe ("creeping thyroiditis") or may involve both lobes from the onset. The systemic reaction may be minimal or marked, and fever may reach as high as 40°C. Although patients without pain may often be categorized as having "silent thyroiditis," surgical thyroidectomy or biopsy has demonstrated the typical pseudogranulomatous picture in some of the specimens.

Patients can generally localize the pain to the region of the thyroid gland over one or both lobes. They may refer to their symptoms as a "sore throat," but with appropriate questioning, it should become apparent that the pain is not within the pharynx.[56] Typically the pain radiates from the region of the thyroid up to the angle of the jaw to the ear on the affected side or sides. The pain may also radiate

to the anterior chest or may be centered only over the thyroid. Moving the head, swallowing, or coughing may aggravate the pain. Many patients also become aware of the presence of swelling in the same region.

Although some patients have no systemic symptoms, most complain of such symptoms; these include malaise, fatigue, myalgia, and mild feverishness. The malaise may sometimes be extreme; some patients may also manifest arthritic complaints. In addition, many patients suffer mild or moderate nervousness, tremulousness, some weight loss, intolerance to heat, and rapid heart beat.

On examination most patients appear uncomfortable and flushed, with a variable fever, varying from just above normal values to as high as 40°C. Characteristically the thyroid gland is only slightly to moderately enlarged, with one lobe larger than the other. Indeed, if the thyroid gland is much larger than this, a diagnosis of subacute thyroiditis should be considered unlikely. The consistency of the involved area is usually quite firm to almost hard, with tenderness in the involved area of moderate to severe magnitude. Even after the tenderness subsides, the gland may maintain its size and consistency for several weeks. Cervical lymphadenopathy is rare. Physical signs of mild to moderate hyperthyroidism are often demonstrable. About 8 to 16 per cent of patients with this malady are noted to have a pre-existent goiter.[1-3, 53, 55]

Course of the Disease

The duration of subacute thyroiditis is quite variable; it may last two to five months without treatment.[1-3, 53-55] In about one fifth of patients following initial recovery, recurrences tend to prolong the course.

More than half of the patients have a phase of hyperthyroidism.[1-3, 53-57] This may not be apparent clinically in some instances, is usually mild when it is clinically evident, and can be detected by biochemical means. This is due to a disruptive process within the thyroid gland with continuous leakage of the colloid into the interstitial tissue, where it is broken down into its component parts, liberating thyroid hormones, thyroglobulin, and other iodoaminoacids into the circulation.[52] Because the thyroid cells during this phase are virtually incapable of producing new thyroid hormone, the colloid that has been stored within the follicles is depleted within two to three months, resulting in a phase of transient hypothyroidism in those patients in whom the process has persisted over the interval. Because disruption of the thyroid parenchyma can persist for some months, the hypothyroidism may persist for several weeks or months.[1-3, 33, 53-55] With recovery, the thyroid gland is finally reconstituted and repleted with colloid, and thyroid function is subsequently restored. Transient hypothyroidism of this nature may be subclinical or overt and occurs in about two thirds of patients.[33]

Only rarely does subacute thyroiditis progress to permanent hypothyroidism.[1-3, 33, 54, 58] In these cases, the progression may be due to total destruction of the thyroid gland with consequent fibrosis; in even more rare instances, the disorder may seem to culminate in autoimmune thyroiditis with hypothyroidism. Indeed, a few patients have developed Graves' disease following recovery from subacute thyroiditis, as mentioned earlier.[50, 51]

Because this occurs in far less than 1 per cent, it is very unlikely that thyrocyte HLA-DR expression (which does occur in the active phase of subacute thyroiditis)[44] plays a significant role in bringing about AITD under these circumstances. The thyroid inflammation may have acted as a nonspecific stress in susceptible individuals in inducing the subsequent AITD.

Thyroid Function Studies

Studies of thyroid function (Fig. 44–2) show dynamic changes consequent to the pathological process.[1-3, 57, 59-64] The initial inflammatory destruction of the thyroid gland results in leakage of the colloid from the damaged follicles into the interstitial tissue and thence into the circulation and includes a variety of iodinated material—protein, proteases, peptides, and amino acids.[57, 59-64] This results in an increase in the serum thyroxine (T_4) and triiodothyronine (T_3) resulting from cleavage of the thyroid hormones from the discharged colloid. The increase in serum T_4 and T_3

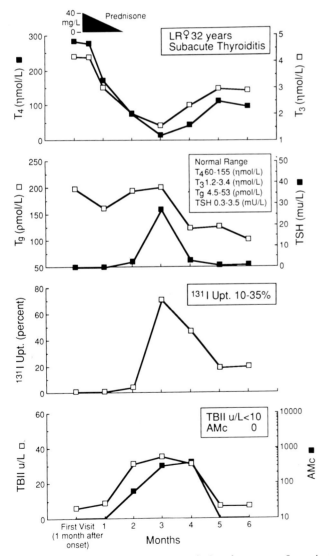

FIGURE 44–2. Salient laboratory features during the course of a patient with subacute thyroiditis. TBII, thyrotropin-binding inhibitory immunoglobulin; AMc, antimicrosomal antibody; Tg, thyroglobulin; T_4, thyroxine; T_3, triiodothyronine.

consequent to the thyroid inflammation accounts for the manifestations of hyperthyroidism.[57, 59-64] The increased amounts of T_3 that appear in the circulation are only proportional to the amount of T_4 released into the circulation, and thus *not* disproportionately elevated, as is seen in Graves' disease.[61, 62] This may well account for the mildness of the clinical manifestations of hyperthyroidism in subacute thyroiditis, because the severity of the clinical manifestations of Graves' disease relates closely to the levels of circulating T_3.

In addition, iodoproteins such as thyroglobulin and iodoalbumin are discharged from the gland into the circulation.[59-62] Indeed, plasma thyroglobulin may remain elevated long after all evidence of the inflammatory process has subsided.[61]

The fall in plasma T_4 is exponential during the first week.[64] As mentioned earlier, this phase of hyperthyroidism can continue only until the gland is depleted of its preformed colloid. At the same time, the damaged thyroid follicular cells cannot function adequately and cannot trap iodide; the 24-hour radioactive iodine uptake is characteristically suppressed to 0 to 1 per cent.[1-3, 55, 57, 62]

Even if only part of the gland is actually involved, the uptake may be similarly depressed as a result of suppression of pituitary TSH owing to the elevated levels of thyroid hormone.[65] Thus, subacute thyroiditis is one of the hyperthyroid conditions associated with high levels of serum thyroid hormones but a very low radioactive iodine uptake, and such observations are characteristic in the early phase of this disorder. Under these circumstances, only very minimal thyroid hormone biosynthesis is sustained, and what is produced leaks out.[59]

Isotope scans of the thyroid gland in the early stages of the malady reveal a patchy and irregular pattern of distribution of the tracer or no uptake whatsoever.[65, 66] The TSH is usually undetectable because of high concentrations of circulating thyroid hormones,[62, 64] and TSH response to TRH is concomitantly diminished at this time.[57-70] Perchlorate or thiocyanate administration generally does not cause release of excessive amounts of iodine from the gland.[59, 60, 71] Large doses of TSH generally do not cause a rise in the radioactive iodine uptake, except when some parts of the gland are uninvolved.[65]

This lack of response to exogenous TSH administration persists during the first weeks of the disease, reflecting continuing thyroid cell impairment and failure of the iodide-concentrating mechanism.[60] Indeed, the radioactive iodine uptake may remain suppressed for several weeks after the onset of the disorder.[57, 59, 60] There is complete suppression of the various stages of intrathyroidal iodide metabolism during the interval.[1-3] As mentioned earlier, when recovery of cellular function is delayed, a consequent phase of transient hypothyroidism may last for months.[1, 3, 57, 59, 60] This phase is, of course, associated with an elevated TSH.[62, 64] Ultimate recovery is the general rule; conversely, permanent hypothyroidism is unusual.[1-3] In my own experience, such permanent hypothyroidism occurs in about 1 per cent of patients, although other reports put it as high as 5 per cent.[33] There is often a lag between the re-establishment of the iodide-concentrating process within the thyroid gland and the resumption of hormone synthesis, secretion, and repletion within the gland.[72]

Erythrocyte sedimentation rate (ESR) is characteristically markedly elevated in the painful form of thyroiditis, often to values of 80 to 100 mm/h.[1-3] Indeed, if the ESR is normal, the diagnosis should be suspect. The leukocyte count is usually normal but has been reported as high as 18×10^9/L in this illness.[1-3] There may be a mild normochromic anemia. An increase in α-2-globulin is a nonspecific inflammatory response.[73] The alkaline phosphatase and other hepatic enzyme levels may be elevated in the early phase.[68] It has been suggested that subacute thyroiditis actually represents a multisystem disease also affecting the thyroid gland.[74] The serum ferritin has recently been demonstrated to be elevated in this condition.[75]

Tests of thyroid autoantibodies are positive in a minority of cases; these develop several weeks after the onset and tend to decline and disappear thereafter.[29, 32, 33] However, an antibody directed against an unpurified thyroid antigen has been shown to persist for up to two years following the disappearance of the clinical disorder.[34] Antibodies directed against the TSH receptor are often found during the course of the disease as another transitory thyroid autoantibody, and some of these are of the blocking, or conversely, thyroid-stimulatory category.[37] However, they do not correspond well to the thyroid functional state.[37] Ultrasonography of the thyroid often reveals hypoechogenicity of the involved areas.[76, 77]

Diagnosis

The diagnosis of subacute thyroiditis should present no difficulties in patients with fairly typical manifestations. Because "sore throat" is a frequent complaint, however, many patients are initially misdiagnosed with pharyngitis.[56] It is thus important that the thyroid gland be carefully palpated in patients presenting with upper respiratory infections or complaints of sore neck or throat or ear ache.

Occasionally patients with Hashimoto's thyroiditis have painful, tender thyroid enlargement that is virtually indistinguishable initially from subacute thyroiditis.[78] The radioactive iodine uptake is rarely completely suppressed in Hashimoto's thyroiditis as it is with subacute thyroiditis, and the titers of thyroid autoantibodies are usually high enough to suggest lymphocytic thyroiditis. Rarely thyroid lymphoma (which often emanates from Hashimoto's thyroiditis) may present with similar symptoms and signs.

Acute suppurative thyroiditis may be initially difficult to distinguish from subacute thyroiditis.[1] However, when clinical signs of suppuration appear, the diagnosis should become evident. In globus hystericus, patients complain of a sense of pressure or a feeling of a "ball" in the throat, and this may be associated with mild diffuse tenderness. There is no specific thyroid enlargement or tenderness.[1]

Severe pain and tenderness may occur in a rapidly growing anaplastic carcinoma of the thyroid, but this disorder is usually obvious by virtue of its large size, adherence to adjacent structures, lymphadenopathy, and characteristic progressive course.[79] Hemorrhage into the thyroid nodule may also cause thyroid pain and tenderness, but its very localized nature and nodule usually suffice to mark it as separate. An enlarging painful thyroid lymphoma can be confused with subacute thyroiditis.

As mentioned above, the most important laboratory tests consistent with subacute thyroiditis include an increased ESR, increased serum T_4 and T_3 levels, and a low radioactive iodine uptake.[1-3] The plasma thyroglobulin is also elevated.[61] Fine-needle aspiration biopsies may be useful[7] but may show large numbers of histiocytes and may thus be misleading. Occasionally a large-needle biopsy may be required for a definitive diagnosis.

Other possible erroneous diagnoses include hyperthyroidism and hypothyroidism, respectively,[1-3, 56] but a proper history should suffice to place the thyroid function into its proper context.

Therapy

Although the cause and pathogenesis of painful subacute thyroiditis are still not fully understood, treatment (while empirical) is highly effective.[1-3, 23] The use of corticosteroids has proven to be valuable in the management of the vast majority of patients.[1-3, 23, 54, 55] Relief of symptoms occurs often within 24 hours. The basic disease process may not be altered, but the inflammatory response is clearly suppressed, thus allowing the pathological process to run its now subclinical course.

Generally, prednisone or a similar analogue of cortisol is prescribed. The treatment is initiated with pharmacological dosages (e.g., 10 mg four times daily). The dosage levels are gradually diminished over four to six weeks and can then be discontinued altogether in most instances. In about 20 per cent of patients, however, as the dosage is reduced, recurrences necessitate the restoration of a higher dose once again. It is sometimes necessary to provide repeated courses of treatment before recovery ultimately occurs. In most instances, exacerbations do not occur and patients go on to full recovery.

There have been reports that triiodothyronine can bring about rapid relief of symptoms in the acute phase.[63, 80] In my own experience, it has not been of benefit when patients are chemically hyperthyroid at the time of therapy. However, after repeated exacerbations, the addition of thyroxine or triiodothyronine may often result in amelioration of the condition and appear to prevent further recurrences.[1-3, 54, 55] Endogenous TSH may play some role in maintaining the disorder under these circumstances; indeed, exogenous TSH may aggravate or precipitate thyroiditis.[55]

In the past generation, radiation therapy was employed effectively for subacute thyroiditis.[1-3, 56] Dosages varied between 200 and 2000 rads of external radiation. There was a failure rate of about 25 per cent, and the response was considerably slower than with corticosteroids and thus less predictable. Perhaps because of the major concern about the effects of low-dose radiation in inducing late thyroid carcinoma, such therapy is no longer used.[81]

In milder cases of this malady, salicylates and other nonsteroidal anti-inflammatory drugs have been administered with some success.[1-3, 60] For more severe cases of this illness, however, corticosteroids are far more rapid in their effect and are dramatically more effective.

Thiouracil and TSH have been reported to be beneficial, but such drugs have not found general favor.[55] Antibiotics are of no value. The high incidence of postoperative hypothyroidism has discouraged thyroidectomy as treatment for subacute thyroiditis, and because recovery is almost certain, thyroidectomy almost never needs to be recommended. Only in the unusual situation of a very prolonged course, with malaise and local distress continuing almost indefinitely, should thyroidectomy be considered.[3, 55]

After complete recovery, late recurrences are rare in the painful form of the disease. As mentioned earlier, permanent hypothyroidism is a rare complication.

SCLEROSING THYROIDITIS

Background and Definition

Sclerosing thyroiditis (invasive fibrous thyroiditis, Riedel's struma) is a rare disorder of unknown cause, characterized pathologically by dense fibrous tissue, which replaces the normal thyroid parenchyma and extends into adjacent tissues, such as muscles, blood vessels, and nerves.[82–85] The first description was by Riedel[86–88] in 1896 who described cases of chronic sclerosing thyroiditis primarily affecting women, which frequently caused pressure symptoms in the neck and tended to progress ultimately to complete destruction of the thyroid gland. Riedel's interesting description was that of a "specific inflammation of mysterious nature producing an iron-hard tumefaction of the thyroid."[86–88] Synonyms for the term *chronic invasive fibrous thyroiditis* include Riedel's struma, struma fibrosa, ligneous (Eisenharte) struma, chronic fibrous thyroiditis, and chronic productive thyroiditis.[82–84]

Incidence

This condition is quite rare. In thyroidectomies performed for all disorders, an incidence between 0.03 and 0.98 per cent for Riedel's struma has been reported from a small number of centers.[89, 90] At the Mayo Clinic, the operative incidence over 64 years was 0.06 per cent, and the overall incidence in outpatients was 1.06 per 100,000.[91–94] Because the manifestations associated with this disorder are likely to lead to surgery, the incidence of Riedel's thyroiditis among patients with thyroidectomies is much higher than the incidence in patients with goiters in general.

Etiology

The cause of this disorder remains unknown. A generation ago, chronic lymphocytic thyroiditis was considered to be an earlier stage of invasive fibrous thyroiditis.[95–99] Although this view was not sustained thereafter for several years, several cases of Riedel's struma have actually clearly progressed from Hashimoto's thyroiditis.[95–103] Thus, once again, the possibility must be seriously entertained that the two disorders can be associated. Of course, patients with lymphocytic thyroiditis, when followed for many years, almost never show progression to Riedel's struma. However, lymphocytic thyroiditis is quite common, whereas Riedel's struma is quite rare; thus, a link between these disorders is difficult to verify. In the past, thyroid autoantibodies were reported to be unusual in cases of Riedel's thyroiditis, but one recent report[92] stated that appreciable titers of thyroid autoantibodies may be found in 45 per cent of patients,

again suggesting a possible relationship between the two disorders. Moreover, three patients with Graves' disease ultimately developing Riedel's thyroiditis have been described.[104, 105] Very recently, Neufelder and Hays[106] demonstrated expression of HLA-DR and HSP (72 kDa) in the fibrosclerotic tissue of Riedel's struma and suggested a role for an active cell-mediated immune response early in the evolution of this condition.

Subacute nonsuppurative thyroiditis has also been suggested as a possible precursor of Riedel's struma.[107–109] However, these two disorders appear with rare exceptions to be quite separate. Preservation of the thyroid capsule in subacute thyroiditis is in marked contrast to capsular invasion in chronic fibrous thyroiditis. Patients with Riedel's struma almost never have histories of the type of pain in the thyroid region that is observed in subacute thyroiditis. The histological appearances of the two disorders are quite different. Perhaps, however, subacute thyroiditis may serve as a rare inducer of Riedel's struma, as the few such cases reported might suggest.

At present there is no adequate explanation for the type of fibroblastic proliferation seen in this disorder. Moreover, Riedel's struma is well known to occur in association with extracervical fibrosclerosis, first noted as early as 1885.[110] These associations include salivary gland fibrosis, fibrous mediastinitis, retroperitoneal fibrosis, sclerosing cholangitis, pseudotumors of the orbits, and lacrimal gland fibrosis. Long-term follow-up of patients with Riedel's struma (follow-up time 10 years) has shown that about one third develop fibrosing disorders of the retroperitoneal space (often leading to ureteral obstruction),[103, 104] chest, or orbits.[82–84, 103, 104, 111–121] DeLange et al.[104] have cited all of the available literature on this point. On the other hand, two thirds of patients with Riedel's struma do *not* develop extracervical fibrosis within the ensuing 10 years, and it is rare for one patient to have extracervical fibrosis in more than one site.[104] Conversely, less than 1 per cent of patients with retroperitoneal fibrosis have Riedel's thyroiditis.[103] It is quite possible that these apparently disparate fibrotic lesions may be different manifestations of the same generalized fibrosing disease, or, on the other hand, the extracervical fibrosis may result from some secondary factor emanating from Riedel's struma.

The established association of certain drugs with retroperitoneal fibrosis has not been observed with Riedel's struma.[103] The suggestion, as mentioned above, that autoimmune factors are involved in the cause would certainly be consistent with those cases that have a clear link with AITD,[103–106] but such evidence is lacking in many cases. Aside from one example of two brothers, children of consanguineous parents who developed fibrosclerosis in multiple sites (including Riedel's thyroiditis in one of the brothers),[112] there does not seem to be a genetic predisposition to this condition. The association of Riedel's struma with extracervical fibrotic lesions has recently been reviewed.[85]

Clinical Features

The age of onset has varied between 23 and 78 years, although most cases are diagnosed in the fourth to sixth decades. The female:male ratio has been reported to be between 2:1 and 4:1[82–84, 92, 93, 99] (Table 44–1).

A gradually or rapidly increasing goiter is a constant feature of this condition, precipitating the local symptoms within the neck. These include a marked sense of pressure or severe dyspnea, with symptoms often out of proportion to the size of the goiter.[82–84] Sensations of suffocation, cough, and dysphagia and a sense of heaviness in the neck are common. Recurrent laryngeal nerve palsy with hoarseness is described. Pain is unusual, although the sense of pressure may be inappropriately described as pain by the patient. The presence or degree of obstruction varies with the extent to which the surrounding structures have been invaded. Some patients have only mild and infrequent symptoms with minimal dysphagia and dyspnea. Others may have stridor, severe dyspnea, or attacks of suffocation.[82–84] In some patients, the entire gland is involved with the fibrotic process, and hypothyroidism develops with a recorded prevalence rate of 25 to 29 per cent.[93, 94, 103, 104] Even without hypothyroidism, however, there may be general malaise and fatigue. Rarely, tetany due to hypoparathyroidism may be observed.[103]

On examination, the thyroid gland is variable in size, from small to very large.[82–84] The lesion may be limited to one lobe, may be present in both, or (as mentioned above) may involve the entire gland. The goiter is stony hard and is densely adherent to adjacent cervical structures (such as muscles, blood vessels, and nerves) and may thus move poorly on swallowing. It has a harder consistency than carcinoma and is only rarely tender. Although adjacent lymph nodes are occasionally enlarged, when they are present and associated with a hard thyroid mass, a diagnosis of carcinoma is often suspected.[82–84]

As previously mentioned, hypothyroidism may occur if the whole gland is involved.[93, 94, 103, 104] Indeed, for similar reasons, the parathyroid glands can be involved with the fibrotic process, and five examples of hypoparathyroidism associated with Riedel's struma have been reported.[103, 104, 109] Because of the frequency of fibrotic lesions elsewhere in the body, the examination must include careful search for such associated disorders, with retroperitoneal fibrosis causing ureteral obstruction a not unusual feature.

Laboratory Findings

Usually the patient is clinically euthyroid, and thyroid function tests generally provide correspondingly normal values. However, as mentioned above, some patients develop hypothyroidism due to complete fibrosis of the entire thyroid gland.[93, 94, 103, 104, 109] Thyroid autoantibodies may be detected; Hay reported that 45 per cent of patients have significant titers of thyroid autoantibodies.[92] Indeed, as previously mentioned, in a small number of patients, AITD seems to have preceded the development of Riedel's struma.[95–103] Additionally, in a few cases, as previously mentioned, the serum calcium levels were found to be low and serum phosphate levels high, indicating hypoparathyroidism, and in such instances in which it has been measured, the serum parathyroid hormone levels have been low.[103, 104, 109] Although this is unusual, the serum calcium and phosphorus should certainly be measured in all patients. Thyroid scintiscans may show "cold" areas, corresponding to the extent of the lesions.[82–84] Axial CT and ultrasound examinations would likewise show the extent of the goiter.[103] The white blood cell count may be normal or elevated, and the ESR is usually elevated, although not to the high rates seen in subacute thyroiditis.[82–84] In one report, antinuclear factor was demonstrable.[103]

Pathology

Pathology consists of an exuberant fibrosing process involving part or all of the thyroid gland.[82–88, 93, 94] It may be unilateral or bilateral and has been described as woody or very hard. The term *Eisenharte* applied to this lesion signifies its "iron hard" quality. Extension of the fibrosis beyond the capsule of the thyroid into adjacent structures such as nerves, muscles, and blood vessels is a characteristic feature and also undoubtedly accounts for the small number of instances in which the parathyroid glands have been obliterated by this fibrosing process. There are no tissue planes, making surgical extirpation virtually impossible. An adenoma may occur in the midst of the fibrous mass.[82–84] Isolated thyroid amyloidosis has been described in one case of Riedel's struma.

Woolner et al.[93, 94] described microscopic criteria for this disorder. These include complete destruction of involved thyroid tissue with absence of normal lobulation; lack of granulomatous reaction; and extension of the fibrosis beyond the thyroid into adjacent structures such as nerves, blood vessels, fat, and skeletal muscle. Lymphocytes and Hürthle cells are sparse, in contrast to the findings in Hashimoto's thyroiditis, although occasionally a few foci of lymphocytes may be observed. An associated arteritis and phlebitis with intimal proliferation, medial destruction, adventitial inflammation, and frequent thrombosis may also occur.[82–84, 93, 94] An immunohistochemical comparison between Riedel's struma and Hashimoto's thyroiditis has been made by Schwaegerle et al.[85] and is reproduced herein in Table 44–2. Similar features are also observed in the extracervical fibrosclerotic lesions in the retroperitoneal or mediastinal regions, in the orbit or lacrimal glands, or in cholangitis.[82–85, 93, 94]

TABLE 44–1. CLINICAL FEATURES OF THYROIDITIS

	RIEDEL'S THYROIDITIS	HASHIMOTO'S THYROIDITIS
Age incidence	23–70 years (mostly over 50 years)	Any age (mostly over 20 years, gradually increasing with age)
Sex incidence (F:M)	2–4:1	4–10:1
Symptoms	Pressure, goiter	± Goiter
Thyroid involvement	May be unilateral or diffuse Goiter may be very large	Generally diffuse, occasionally goiter quite large
Thyroid status	Only rarely hypothyroid	Hypothyroid most commonly, may be euthyroid or hyperthyroid
Thyroid autoantibodies	Possibly 45%	Almost invariably
Follow-up	Hypoparathyroidism occasionally may recur following treatment, stabilize, or regress	Usually proceeds to hypothyroidism

TABLE 44–2. IMMUNOHISTOCHEMISTRY OF RIEDEL'S AND HASHIMOTO'S THYROIDITIS

ANTIBODY	ANTIBODY SPECIFICITY	RIEDEL'S THYROIDITIS	HASHIMOTO'S THYROIDITIS
CD3 (Leu-4)	Pan-T	Positive	Positive
CD4 (T4)	T-helper, inducer	Positive	Positive
CD8 (T8)	T-suppressor, cytotoxic	Positive	Positive
CD22 (Leu-14)	Pan-B	Scattered positivity	Germinal centers
CD20 (B1)	B-cells of mantle, germinal centers, medullary cords	Germinal centers	Germinal centers
PCA	Plasma cells	Negative	Scattered positivity
CD15 (Leu-M1)	Granulocytes, monocytes	Scattered positivity	Scattered positivity
CD11C (Leu-M5)	Monocytes, granulocytes	Negative	Scattered positivity

From Schwaegerle SM, Bauer TW, Esselstyn CB: Reidel's thyroiditis. Am J Clin Pathol 90:715–722, 1988.

Diagnosis and Treatment

Invasive fibrous thyroiditis may appear as a painless, fixed, hard goiter, with either slow or rapid growth. Whether it is associated with local lymphadenopathy or not, it may be impossible to differentiate this lesion from carcinoma or lymphoma of the thyroid on the basis of clinical findings alone.[82-84] The disorder can normally be distinguished from classic Hashimoto's thyroiditis or subacute thyroiditis, as indicated in Tables 44–1 and 44–2. Hashimoto's thyroiditis is not associated with any extension of the lesion beyond the capsule; the goiters are usually larger and lobulated, although Riedel's struma may sometimes be quite large. The antibody titers are generally markedly elevated in Hashimoto's thyroiditis and are usually not as elevated or may be negative in Riedel's thyroiditis.[82-84] Subacute thyroiditis is associated with severe pain and tenderness, frequent fever, and a rapidly evolving course. There is no extension of the lesion beyond the capsule. Closed biopsy findings in Riedel's struma may be difficult to interpret, although open biopsy findings are quite useful.

Anecdotal reports of improvement during glucocorticoid therapy and relapses reversed by the reinstitution of steroids suggest that glucocorticoids may be warranted in selected cases.[102, 108, 113, 114] However, in other instances in which glucocorticoids have been prescribed, there has been no significant amelioration.[103, 104] Thyroid hormone suppressive therapy has also been recommended. Although adequate assessment has not been carried out, this therapy does not seem to add much to the management of this rare disease in the absence of hypothyroidism.[82, 103] Of course, thyroxine therapy is necessary in those cases in which hypothyroidism has resulted from the disorder.[103] In addition, calcium and vitamin D therapy is indicated in those few cases with associated hypoparathyroidism.[103]

When surgical intervention is under consideration for pressure symptoms or for the diagnosis or treatment of a hard goiter, the possibility of chronic fibrous thyroiditis must be kept in mind so as to limit the extent of the surgery if no malignancy is found. Surgical intervention is indicated on two grounds: (1) to exclude malignancy and (2) to relieve tracheal compression.[82-84] Operation is limited to excising a wedge of thyroid isthmus when the process is diffuse.[82-84] Extensive resection is not indicated, particularly because the course of Riedel's struma often tends to be benign and self-limiting. Moreover, an extensive procedure may add considerable risk of injury to adjacent involved vital structures within the neck such as the carotid artery and the recurrent laryngeal nerve. Indeed, without actual impingement by the surgeon on the recurrent laryngeal nerves, the edema occurring with the surgery, acting upon an already partially compromised structure, can result in transient palsies, and occult hypoparathyroidism may be converted into overt hypoparathyroidism by this means. Subtotal lobectomy may be performed, however, if the process is localized to one lobe of the thyroid gland.

Prognosis

The course of the lesion may be slowly progressive, may stabilize, or may remit. Following surgery, the disease sometimes subsides or takes a benign, self-limiting course.[82-84] Spontaneous remissions without surgery may occur, and secondary surgery is only rarely required. The mortality rate has been reported to range from 6 to 10 per cent, with deaths usually attributed to asphyxia secondary to tracheal compression or laryngospasm.[82-84] However, the mortality rates mentioned are derived from older literature and may not reflect the (presumably lower) current rates. Hypothyroidism is relatively uncommon, and hypoparathyroidism is unusual. In many instances the condition is self-limiting, and improvement often persists after an isthmic wedge resection. As mentioned above, the disorder may be further complicated by fibrotic lesions elsewhere in the body, and these require appropriate treatment, including the possibility of surgical management.

REFERENCES

1. Volpé R: Subacute thyroiditis. *In* Burrow GN, Oppenheimer JH, Volpé R (eds): Thyroid Function and Disease. Philadelphia, WB Saunders, 1989, pp 179–190.
2. Bastenie PA, Ermans AM: Thyroiditis and thyroid function. Clinical, morphological and physiological studies. International Series of Monographs in Pure and Applied Biology. Modern Trends in Physiological Sciences, Vol. 36. New York, Pergamon Press, 1972.
3. LiVolsi JA, LoGerfo R: Thyroiditis. Boca Raton, FL, CRC Press, 1981.
4. DeQuervain F: Die akute nicht Eiterige Thyreoiditis und die Beteiligung der Schilddruse und akuten intoxikationen und infectionen Uberhaupt. Mitteilungen aus der Grenzgeheiten der Medizin und Chirurgie 2 (Suppl Bd):1–165, 6 pt., 1904.
5. DeQuervain F, Giordandengo G: Die akute und subakute nicht Eiteige Thyreoiditis. Mittielungen aus der Grenzgeheiten der Medizin und Chirurgie 44:538–590, 1936.
6. Mygind H: Thyroiditis akuta simplex. J Laryngol 91:181–193, 1895.
7. Nikolai TF: Silent thyroiditis and subacute thyroiditis. *In* Braverman

LE, Utiger R (eds): Werner and Ingbar's The Thyroid, A Fundamental and Clinical Text (ed 6). Philadelphia, JB Lippincott, 1991, pp 720–727.

8. Fraser R, Harrison RJ: Subacute thyroiditis. Lancet 1:382–386, 1952.

9. Eylan E, Zmucky R, Sheba C: Mumps virus and subacute thyroiditis. Evidence of a causal association. Lancet 1:1062–1063, 1957.

10. Felix-Davis D: Autoimmunization in subacute thyroiditis. Lancet 1:880–883, 1958.

11. Hung W: Mumps thyroiditis and hypothyroidism. J Pediatr 74:611–613, 1969.

12. McArthur AM: Subacute giant cell thyroiditis associated with mumps. Med J Australia 1:116–117, 1964.

13. Sheba C, Bank H: Prevention of mumps thyroiditis. N Engl J Med 279:108–109, 1968.

14. Candel S: Acute non-suppurative thyroiditis following measles. US Navy Med Bull 46:1109–1113, 1946.

15. McQuillan AS: Thyroiditis. Transactions of the 3rd International Goiter Conference and American Association for the Study of Goiter, 1938, pp 212–219.

16. Robertson WS: Acute inflammation of the thyroid gland. Lancet 1:930–931, 1911.

17. Saito S: Clinical studies of subacute thyroiditis. Gunma J Med Sci 8(Suppl 17):1–2, 1959.

18. Hintze G, Fortelius P, Railo J: Epidemic thyroiditis. Acta Endocrinol 45:381–401, 1964.

19. McWhinney IR: Incidence of DeQuervain's thyroiditis: Ten cases from one general practice. Br Med J 1:1225–1226, 1964.

20. Fennell JS, Tomkin GH: Subacute thyroiditis and hepatitis in a case of infectious mononucleosis. Postgrad Med J 54:351–352, 1978.

21. Volpé R: Subacute thyroiditis. In Soto RL, DeNichola A, Blaquier J (eds): Physiopathology of Endocrine Diseases and Mechanisms of Hormone Action. New York, Alan R. Liss, 1981, pp 115–134.

22. Liberman U, Djaldetti M, DeVries A: A case of herpangina, pleurodynia and subacute thyroiditis. Harefuah 67:342–345, 1964.

23. Schultz AL: Subacute diffuse thyroiditis: Clinical and laboratory findings in 24 patients and the effect of treating with adrenal corticoids. Postgrad Med 29:76–85, 1961.

24. Schumway M, Davis PL: Catscratch thyroiditis treated with thyrotropin hormone. J Clin Endocrinol Metab 14:742–743, 1964.

25. Goldman J, Bockna AJ, Becker FO: St. Louis encephalitis and subacute thyroiditis. Ann Intern Med 87:250, 1977.

26. Stancek D, Gressnerova M: A viral agent isolated from a patient with subacute DeQuervain type thyroiditis. Acta Virol (Praha) 18:365, 1974.

27. Stancek D, Stancekova M, Gressnerova M, et al: Isolation and some serological and epidemilogical data on the viruses recovered from patients with subacute thyroiditis DeQuervain. Med Microbiol Immunol 161:133–144, 1975.

28. Stancek D, Ciampor E, Mucha V, et al: Morphological, cytological and biological observations on viruses isolated from patients with subacute thyroiditis of DeQuervain. Acta Virol (Praha) 20:183, 1976.

29. Volpé R, Row VV, Ezrin C: Circulating viral and thyroid antibodies in subacute thyroiditis. J Clin Endocrinol Metab 27:1275–1284, 1967.

30. Yeo PPB, Rauff A, Chan SW, et al: Subacute (DeQuervain's) thyroiditis in the tropics. In Stockigt JR, Nagataki S (eds): Thyroid Research VIII. Canberra, Australian Academy of Science, 1980, pp 570–574.

31. Volpé R: Immunology of the thyroid. In Autoimmune Diseases of the Endocrine System. Boca Raton, FL, CRC Press, 1990, pp 73–240.

32. Bech K, Feldt-Rasmussen U, Bliddal H, et al: Persistence of autoimmune reactions during recovery of subacute thyroiditis. In Pinchera A, Ingbar SH, McKenzie JM, Fenzi GF (eds): Thyroid Autoimmunity. New York, Plenum Press, 1987, pp 623–625.

33. Lio S, Pontecorvi A, Caruso M, et al: Transitory subclinical and permanent hypothyroidism in the course of subacute thyroiditis (DeQuervain). Acta Endocrinol 106:67–70, 1984.

34. Weetman AP, Smallbridge RC, Nutman TB, Burman KD: Persistent thyroid autoimmunity after subacute thyroiditis. J Clin Lab Immunol 23:1–6, 1987.

35. Strakosch CR, Joyner D, Wall JR: Thyroid stimulating antibodies in subacute thyroiditis. J Clin Endocrinol Metab 46:345–348, 1978.

36. Wall JR, Strakosch CR, Bandy P, Bayly R: Nature of thyrotropin displacement activity in subacute thyroiditis. J Clin Endocrinol Metab 54:349–353, 1982.

37. Tamai H, Nozaki T, Mukuta T, et al: The incidence of thyroid stimulating blocking antibodies during the hypothyroid phase in patients with subacute thyroiditis. J Clin Endocrinol Metab 73:245–250, 1991.

38. Hashizume K, Roudebush CP, Fenzi G, DeGroot LJ: Effect of antithyroid therapy and thyroid stimulating immunoglobulin phase in

Graves' disease. Proceedings of the 53rd Meeting, American Thyroid Association, Cleveland, Ohio, Sept. 7–10, 1977.

39. Wall JR, Fang SL, Ingbar SH, Braverman LE: Lymphocyte transformation in response to human thyroid extract in patients with subacute thyroiditis. J Clin Endocrinol Metab 43:587–590, 1976.

40. Galluzo A, Giordano C, Andronica F, et al: Leucocyte migration test in subacute thyroiditis; hypothetical role of cell-mediated immunity. J Clin Endocrinol Metab 59:1038–1041, 1980.

41. Totterman TH: Distribution of T,B and thyroglobulin binding lymphocytes infiltrating the thyroid gland in Graves' disease, Hashimoto's thyroiditis and DeQuervain's thyroiditis. Clin Immunol Immunopathol 10:270–277, 1978.

42. Wall JR, Gray B, Greenwood DM: Total and "activated" peripheral blood T lymphocytes in patients with thyroid disorders. Acta Endocrinol 85:753–759, 1977.

43. Chartier B, Brandy P, Wall JR: Fc receptor bearing blood mononuclear cells in thyroid disorders: Increased levels in patients with subacute thyroiditis. J Clin Endocrinol Metab 51:1014–1018, 1980.

44. Leclere J, Faure C, Bene MC, et al: In situ immunological disorders in DeQuervain's thyroiditis. In Medeiros-Neto G, Gaitan E (eds): Frontiers of Thyroidology, Vol 2, New York, Plenum Press, 1986, pp 1365–1368.

45. Volpé R: Autoimmunity causing thyroid dysfunction. Endocr Metab Clin North Am 20:565–578, 1991.

46. Bech K, Nerup J, Thomsen M, et al: Subacute thyroiditis deQuervain: A disease associated with HLA-B antigen. Acta Endocrinol 86:504–509, 1977.

47. Nyulassy S, Hnilica P, Buc M, et al: Subacute (deQuervain's) thyroiditis: Association with HLA-Bw35 antigen and abnormalities of the complement system, immunoglobulins and other serum proteins. J Clin Endocrinol Metab 45:270–274, 1977.

48. Tamai H, Goto H, Uno H, et al: HLA in Japanese patients with subacute (DeQuervain's) thyroiditis. Tissue Antigens 24:58–59, 1984.

49. Yeo PPB, Chan SH, Aw TC, et al: HLA and Chinese patients with subacute (DeQuervain's) thyroiditis. Tissue Antigens 17:249–250, 1981.

50. Werner SC: Graves' disease following subacute thyroiditis. Arch Intern Med 139:1313–1315, 1979.

51. Wartofsky L, Schaaf M: Graves' disease with thyrotoxicosis following subacute thyroiditis. Am J Med 83:761–764, 1987.

52. Hazard JB: Thyroiditis: A review. Am J Clin Pathol 25:289–298, 399–426, 1955.

53. Harland WA, Frantz VK: Clinicopathologic study of 261 surgical cases of so-called thyroiditis. J Clin Endocrinol Metab 16:1433–1437, 1956.

54. Steinberg FU: Subacute granulomatous thyroiditis. A review. Ann Intern Med 52:1014–1025, 1960.

55. Greene JN: Subacute thyroiditis. Am J Med 51:97–108, 1971.

56. Volpé R, Johnston MW: Subacute thyroiditis: A disease commonly mistaken for pharyngitis. Can Med Assoc J 77:297–307, 1957.

57. Volpé R, Johnston MW, Haber N: Thyroid function in subacute thyroiditis. J Clin Endocrinol Metab 18:65–78, 1958.

58. Jay HK: Permanent myxedema: An unusual complication of granulomatous thyroiditis. J Clin Endocrinol Metab 21:1384–1387, 1961.

59. Ingbar SH, Freinkel N: Thyroid function and metabolism of iodine in patients with subacute thyroiditis. Arch Intern Med 101:339–346, 1958.

60. Dorta T, Beraud T: New investigations on subacute thyroiditis. Helv Med Acta 28:19–41, 1961.

61. Izumi M, Larsen PR: Correlation of sequential change in serum thyroglobulin, triiodothyronine, and thyroxine in patients with Graves' disease and subacute thyroiditis. Metabolism 27:449–460, 1978.

62. Larsen PR: Serum triiodothyronine and thyrotropin during hyperthyroid, and recovery phases of subacute non-suppurative thyroiditis. Metabolism 23:467–471, 1974.

63. Weihl AC, Daniels GH, Ridgeway ED, Maloof F: Thyroid function during the early days of subacute thyroiditis. J Clin Endocrinol Metab 44:1107–1114, 1977.

64. Glinoer D, Puttemans N, Van Herle AJ, et al: Sequential study of the impairment of thyroid function in the early stage of subacute thyroiditis. Acta Endocrinol 77:26–39, 1974.

65. Lewitus W, Rechnic J, Lubin E: Sequential scanning of the thyroid as an aid to the diagnosis of subacute thyroiditis. Israel J Med Sci 3:847–854, 1967.

66. Hamburger JL, Kadian G, Rossin HW: Subacute thyroiditis—evaluations depicted by serial ^{131}I scintigrams. J Nucl Med 6:560–565, 1965.

67. Berthezine F, Kressmann J, Olivier J, Fournier M: Le fonctionnement de l'axe hypophyso-thyroidien au cours de thyroidites subaiques. Ann Endocrinol 36:169–170, 1975.

68. Demeester-Mirkine N, Brauman H, Corvilain J: Delayed adjustment of the pituitary response in circulating thyroid hormones in a case of subacute thyroiditis. Clin Endocrinol 5:9–14, 1976.
69. Lebacq EG, Therasse G, Schmitz A, et al: Subacute thyroiditis. Acta Endocrinol 82:705–715, 1976.
70. Staub JJ: The TRH test in subacute thyroiditis. Lancet 1:868–870, 1975.
71. Leboeuf G, Ducharme JR: Thyroiditis in children. Diagnosis and management. Pediatr Clin North Am 13:19–42, 1966.
72. Kamio N, Kobayashi I, Mori M, et al: Permissive role of thyrotrophin in thyroid radioiodine uptake during the recovery phase of subacute thyroiditis. Metabolism 26:295–299, 1977.
73. Skillern PG, Lewis LA: Fractional plasma protein values in subacute thyroiditis. J Clin Invest 36:780–783, 1957.
74. Hamada S, Yagura T, Ishii H, et al: Subacute thyroiditis as a systemic multisystem disease. In Nagatai S, Torizuka K (eds): The Thyroid 1988, Excerpta Medica International Congress Series 796, Amsterdam, Elsevier, 1988, pp 521–525.
75. Sakata S, Nagai K, Maekawa H, et al: Serum ferritin concentration in subacute thyroiditis. Metabolism 40:683–688, 1991.
76. Benker G, Olbricht TH, Windeck R, et al: The sonographical and functional sequelae of deQuervain's subacute thyroiditis. Acta Endocrinol 117:435–441, 1988.
77. Tokuda Y, Kasagi K, Iida Y, et al: Sonography of subacute thyroiditis: Changes in the findings during the course of the disease. J Clin Ultrasound 18:21–26, 1990.
78. Volpé R: Autoimmune thyroiditis. In Braverman LE, Utiger R (eds): Werner and Ingbar's The Thyroid, A Fundamental and Clinical Text (ed 6). Philadelphia, JB Lippincott, 1991, pp 921–933.
79. Rosen F, Row VV, Volpé R, Ezrin C: Anaplastic carcinoma of thyroid with abnormal circulating iodoprotein. A case simulating subacute thyroiditis. Can Med Assoc J 95:1039–1041, 1966.
80. Higgins HP, Bayley TA, Diosy A: Suppression of endogenous TSH; a treatment of subacute thyroiditis. J Clin Endocrinol Metab 23:235–242, 1963.
81. Walfish PG, Volpé R: Irradiation related thyroid cancer. Ann Intern Med 88:261–262, 1978.
82. Volpé R: Invasive fibrous (Riedel's) thyroiditis. In Burrow GN, Oppenheimer JH, Volpé R (eds): Thyroid Function and Disease. Philadelphia, WB Saunders, 1989, pp 208–213.
83. Bastenie PA: Invasive fibrous thyroiditis (Riedel). In Bastenie PA, Ermans AM: Thyroiditis and thyroid function. International Series of Monographs in Pure and Applied Biology. Modern Trends in Physiological Sciences, Vol 36. Oxford, Pergamon Press, 1972, pp 99–108.
84. Livolsi VA: Riedel's struma. In Livolsi VA, LoGerfo PA: Thyroiditis. Boca Raton, FL, CRC Press, 1981, pp 133–146.
85. Schwaegerle SM, Bauer TW, Esselstyn CB: Riedel's thyroiditis. Am J Clin Pathol 90:715–722, 1988.
86. Riedel BM: Ueber Verlauf und Ausgang der Chronischer Chronica. Munch Med Wocherschr 57:1946–1947, 1910.
87. Riedel BM: Vorstellung eines Kranken mit Chronischer Strumitis. Verh Ges Chir 26:127–129, 1897.
88. Riedel BM: Die Chronische Zur Bildung eisenharter Tumoren fuhrende Entzundung der Schilddruse. Verh Ges Chir 25:101–105, 1896.
89. DeCourcy JL: A new theory concerning the etiology of Riedel's struma. Surgery 12:754–762, 1942.
90. Goodman HI: Riedel's thyroiditis: Review and report of two cases. Am J Surg 54:472–478, 1941.
91. Hay ID, McConahey WM, Carney JA, Woolner LB: Invasive fibrous thyroiditis (Riedel's struma) and associated extracervical fibrosclerosis: Bowlby's disease revisited. Ann Endocrinol 43:29A, 1982.
92. Hay ID: Thyroiditis: A clinical update. Mayo Clin Proc 60:836–843, 1985.
93. Woolner LB, McConahey WM, Beahrs O: Invasive fibrous thyroiditis (Riedel's struma). J Clin Endocrinol Metab 17:201–220, 1957.
94. Woolner LB: Thyroiditis: Classification and clinicopathologic correlations. In Hazard JB, Smith DE (eds): The Thyroid. Baltimore, Williams & Wilkins, 1964, pp 123–142.
95. Ewing J: Neoplastic Diseases: A Treatise on Tumors. Philadelphia, WB Saunders, 1922, pp 908–909.
96. Goetsch E, Kammer M: Chronic thyroiditis and Riedel's struma: Etiology and pathogenesis. J Clin Endocrinol 15:1010–1034, 1955.
97. Reist A: Uber Chronische Thyroiditis. Frankf Z Pathol 28:141–200, 1922.
98. Williamson GS, Pearse IH: Lymphadenoid goitre and its clinical significance. Br Med J 1:4–8, 1929.
99. Beierwaltes W: Thyroiditis. Ann NY Acad Sci 124:586–604, 1965.
100. Merrington WR: Chronic thyroiditis: A case showing features of both Riedel's and Hashimoto's thyroiditis. Br J Surg 35:423–426, 1948.
101. Baker TJ: Riedel's struma and struma lymphomatosa (Hashimoto). South Med J 46:1168–1171, 1953.
102. Thomson JA, Jackson IMD, Duguid WP: The effect of steroid therapy on Riedel's thyroiditis. Scot Med J 13:13–16, 1968.
103. Best TB, Munro RE, Burwell S, Volpé R: Riedel's thyroiditis associated with Hashimoto's thyroiditis, hypoparathyroidism, and retroperitoneal fibrosis. J Endocrinol Invest 14:767–772, 1991.
104. DeLange WE, Freling NJM, Molenaar WM, Doarenbos H: Invasive fibrous thyroiditis (Riedel's struma): A manifestation of multifocal fibrosclerosis: A case report with review of the literature. Q J Med 268:709–717, 1989.
105. Neufelder AE, Hay ID, Carney JA, Gorman CA: Coexistence of Graves' disease (GD) and Riedel's (invasive fibrous) thyroiditis: Further evidence for a link between Riedel's thyroiditis and organ-specific autoimmunity. Clin Res 39:377A, 1991.
106. Neufelder AE, Hays ID: Expression of HLA-DR and heat shock protein 72 in Riedel's invasive fibrous thyroiditis. Clin Res 40:49A, 1992.
107. Rose E, Rayster HP: Invasive fibrous thyroiditis (Riedel's struma). JAMA 176:224–226, 1961.
108. Katsikas D, Shorthouse AJ, Taylor S: Riedel's thyroiditis. Br J Surg 63:929–931, 1976.
109. Chopra D, Wool MS, Crosson A, Sawin CT: Riedel's struma associated with subacute thyroiditis, hypothyroidism, and hypoparathyroidism. J Clin Endocrinol Metab 46:869–871, 1978.
110. Bowlby AA: Diseases of the ductless glands. I. Infiltrating fibroma (?sarcoma) of the thyroid gland. Trans Pathol Soc (London) 36:420–423, 1885.
111. Turner-Warwick R, Nabarro JDN, Doniach D: Riedel's thyroiditis and retroperitoneal fibrosis. Proc R Soc Med 59:596–598, 1966.
112. Comings DE, Skubi KB, VanEyes J, Motulsky AG: Familial multifocal fibrosclerosis. Ann Intern Med 66:884–892, 1967.
113. Hines RC, Scheuermann HA, Royster HP, Rose E: Invasive fibrous (Riedel's) thyroiditis with bilateral fibrous parotitis. JAMA 213:869–871, 1970.
114. Amorosa LF, Shear MK, Spiera H: Multifocal fibrosis involving the thyroid, face and orbits. Arch Intern Med 136:221–223, 1976.
115. Meijer S, Hausman R: Occlusive phlebitis, a diagnostic feature in Riedel's thyroid. Virchows Arch 337:349–354, 1978.
116. Hellstrom HR, Perez-Stable EC: Retroperitoneal fibrosis with disseminated vasculitis and intrahepatic sclerosing cholangitis. Am J Med 40:184–188, 1966.
117. Schneider RJ: Orbital involvement in Riedel's struma. Can J Ophthalmol 11:87–90, 1976.
118. Anderson SR, Seedorff H, Halberg P: Thyroiditis with myxoedema and orbital pseudotumor. Acta Ophthalmol 41:120–125, 1963.
119. Arnott EJ, Greaves OP: Orbital involvement in Riedel's thyroiditis. Br J Ophalmol 49:1–4, 1965.
120. Bartholomew LG, Cain JC, Woolner LB, et al: Sclerosing cholangitis: Its possible association with Riedel's struma and fibrous retroperitonitis: Report of two cases. N Engl J Med 269:8–12, 1963.
121. Sclare G, Luxton W: Fibrosis of the thyroid and lacrimal glands. Br J Ophthalmol 51:173–177, 1967.

45

Hypothyroidism

ROBERT D. UTIGER

Hypothyroidism is the clinical and biochemical syndrome that results when thyroidal production of T_4 and T_3 is decreased and serum T_4 and T_3 concentrations are low and that is ameliorated by administration of thyroid hormone. The decreases in serum T_4 and T_3 concentrations that occur in patients with nonthyroidal illness are the result of transient decreases in extrathyroidal T_3 and less often thyroidal T_4 and T_3 production and are not accompanied by clinical manifestations of hypothyroidism, so that thyroid hormone treatment is not indicated (see Ch. 40). This chapter is devoted to a discussion of the causes, clinical manifestations, diagnosis, and treatment of hypothyroidism, as traditionally defined.

The severity of hypothyroidism varies greatly. Some patients have no symptoms or signs of hypothyroidism and normal serum T_4 and T_3 concentrations, but slightly to moderately elevated serum thyrotropin (TSH) concentrations; this is known as subclinical hypothyroidism. In other patients, hypothyroidism is overt, causing symptoms and signs indicating abnormal function of one or more organ systems; the serum TSH concentrations in these patients are usually elevated more than fivefold. Rarely, hypothyroidism is a medical emergency (myxedema coma).

The frequency of hypothyroidism also varies widely, depending on the definition used and the population studied. The prevalence rates of overt hypothyroidism in community surveys vary from 1 to 2 per 1000 persons but are as high as 18 per 1000 in elderly persons.[1, 2] In patients seeking medical care, 5 to 20 per 1000 have overt hypothyroidism. Subclinical hypothyroidism is found in 20 to 120 per 1000 persons in the community.[1, 2] The higher rates are in older women, most of whom have antithyroid antibodies. The ratio of women to men with either overt or subclinical hypothyroidism ranges from 2 to 8:1, and increases with age.

PATHOPHYSIOLOGY OF HYPOTHYROIDISM

Hypothyroidism is most often a result of thyroid disease, but occasionally it results from thyroid atrophy secondary to TSH or thyrotropin-releasing hormone (TRH) deficiency. Figure 45–1 shows a comparison of thyroidal and extrathyroidal hormone production and serum hormone concentrations in a normal subject and a patient with hypothyroidism. The daily rate of T_4 production in patients with overt hypothyroidism is about 25 per cent of normal. That of T_3 is decreased to a lesser extent, and the proportion of T_3 originating in the thyroid is increased and that originating in extrathyroidal tissues is decreased.[3, 4]

Several mechanisms limit or even prevent the development of hypothyroidism in patients with thyroid disease. Among them, the most important is increased secretion of

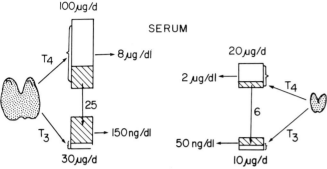

FIGURE 45–1. Comparison of thyroidal and peripheral production and serum concentrations of thyroxine (T₄) and triiodothyronine (T₃) in normal subjects and patients with hypothyroidism. Conversion factors for Systeme International units: T₄, μg/day × 1.28 = nmol/day; serum T₄, μg/dl × 12.8 = nmol/L; T₃, μg/day × 1.5 = nmol/day; serum T₃, ng/dl × 0.015 = nmol/L.

TSH. TSH secretion increases in response to very small decreases in thyroid secretion, and the increase not only limits the decrease in thyroid secretion but may even restore it to normal by stimulating thyroid hyperplasia and hypertrophy. Even if TSH hypersecretion does not restore thyroid secretion to normal, several of its actions serve to maintain the secretion of T_3 in preference to that of T_4. TSH stimulates the synthesis of T_3 more than that of T_4, and it also stimulates thyroidal T_4-5'-deiodinase activity.[5,6] As a result, thyroidal secretion of T_3 is decreased less than is that of T_4, and the thyroidal contribution to overall T_3 production is increased. Other mechanisms that serve to defend against the development of hypothyroidism are an increase in the overall fractional rate of extrathyroidal conversion of T_4 to T_3 and an increase in production of T_3 in some tissues, notably the brain and pituitary (but likely excluding the thyrotrophs, as an increase in those cells would limit the TSH response to hypothyroidism).[7] These changes serve to maintain the production of T_3, the more efficiently produced and biologically active of the two hormones, and therefore minimize the severity of hypothyroidism.

Patients with nonthyroidal illness, in contrast, have greater reductions in the production rate and serum concentration of T_3 than of T_4. The most common abnormality in these patients is decreased extrathyroidal T_3 production.[8] They also may have decreased TSH secretion, decreased thyroidal T_4 and T_3 secretion, and decreased serum T_4 concentrations, especially those who are severely ill (see also Ch. 40).

CAUSES OF HYPOTHYROIDISM

The causes of hypothyroidism are listed in Table 45–1. Among them, primary hypothyroidism is by far the most common, accounting for more than 98 per cent of cases. Worldwide, the most common cause is iodine deficiency. In iodine-sufficient regions, the most common causes of hypothyroidism are chronic autoimmune thyroiditis and previous ^{131}I therapy for thyrotoxicosis. An attempt should always be made to determine the cause of hypothyroidism, especially because hypothyroidism may be the predominant or only manifestation of hypothalamic-pituitary disease. History and physical examination alone are usually sufficient for this purpose, particular attention being devoted to obtaining information about previous thyroid disease, treatment for it, and current drug use and to palpation of the thyroid gland.

Hypothyroidism Caused by Loss of Functional Thyroid Tissue

Chronic Autoimmune Thyroiditis

Chronic autoimmune thyroiditis most commonly occurs in middle-aged or older women but can occur in men and in children. Both an atrophic (nongoitrous) form and a goitrous form of the disease occur. The former also has been called idiopathic hypothyroidism and primary myxedema, and the latter Hashimoto's disease. The two forms differ clinically only in the absence or presence of goiter. Pathologically, atrophic autoimmune thyroiditis is characterized by atrophy of thyroid follicles, lymphocytic infiltration and fibrosis, and goitrous autoimmune thyroiditis by thyroid follicular hyperplasia, lymphocytic and plasma cell infiltration, lymphoid germinal centers, and fibrosis.

Patients with either atrophic or goitrous autoimmune thyroiditis may be euthyroid or have subclinical or overt hypothyroidism. The extent of thyroid enlargement, when present, varies greatly, and rarely the goiter is tender. The spectrum of chronic autoimmune thyroiditis probably extends even further, to include painless thyroiditis and postpartum thyroiditis, both of which cause thyrotoxicosis followed by hypothyroidism (see also Ch. 43).

The thyroid dysfunction and destruction that characterize chronic autoimmune thyroiditis are probably both antibody- and cell-mediated (Fig. 45–2).[9,10] The types of autoantibodies found in these patients are listed in Table 45–2. Most of the information about the biological activity of these antibodies is based on the results of in vitro studies,[11–12] but in some patients their presence or absence correlates with the presence or absence of hypothyroidism.

TABLE 45–1. CAUSES OF HYPOTHYROIDISM

Primary (thyroidal) hypothyroidism
  Loss of functional thyroid tissue
    Chronic autoimmune thyroiditis
    Transient autoimmune thyroiditis
    [131]I and external radiation therapy
    Postoperative hypothyroidism
    Transient hypothyroidism
    Infiltrative and other diseases of the thyroid
    Thyroid dysgenesis (sporadic nongoitrous cretinism)
  Biosynthetic defects in thyroid hormonogenesis
    Congenital defects
    Iodine deficiency
    Iodine excess
    Antithyroid agents
Central (secondary) hypothyroidism
  Pituitary hypothyroidism
  Hypothalamic hypothyroidism
Generalized resistance to thyroid hormone
Drugs: dopamine, amiodarone, lithium

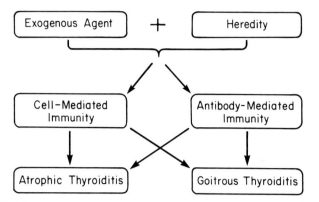

FIGURE 45–2. **Schematic outline of pathogenesis of chronic autoimmune thyroiditis.** In this scheme, exogenous agent(s) and hereditary factors interact to initiate cell- and antibody-mediated immunity to thyroid tissue, which in turn causes thyroid injury and hypothyroidism. Whether the result is atrophic or goitrous thyroiditis depends on the nature and extent of thyroid cell injury and on the types of antibodies produced.

For example, some hypothyroid patients who have antibodies that block the binding and action of TSH become euthyroid after the antibodies disappear.[13] Variations in the type(s) and amounts of these antibodies, therefore, can be important determinants of the extent of thyroid dysfunction and enlargement and also of the natural history of the disorder. The proportion of hypothyroid patients with either atrophic or goitrous autoimmune thyroiditis who have antibodies with biological activity varies from about 10 to 40 per cent.[12–14] The production of these antibodies by B lymphocytes is presumably stimulated by cytokines produced by T helper-inducer (CD4) cells that have been activated by binding complexes of thyroid antigens and HLA Class II molecules on antigen-presenting cells, which can include thyroid cells.

The permanent thyroid injury that occurs in most patients with autoimmune thyroiditis is probably the result of activation of cellular immunity.[9, 10] The postulated steps in this process are formation of complexes between thyroid antigens and HLA Class I molecules on antigen-presenting cells, including thyroid cells, binding of the complexes to T suppressor-cytotoxic (CD8) cells, thereby activating these cells, and then T-cell secretion of cytokines that have cytotoxic actions or T-cell differentiation into natural killer cells.

The factor(s) that initiates either antibody- or cell-mediated thyroid autoimmunity is not known. It could be an infectious agent or toxin that has properties similar to those of some component of thyroid cells (molecular mim-

TABLE 45–2. Types of Antithyroid Autoantibodies Found in Patients with Chronic Autoimmune Thyroiditis

Antibody	Biological Activity
Thyroid peroxidase*	Sometimes inhibits thyroid peroxidase activity
TSH-binding inhibitory	Inhibits TSH binding to its receptor
TSH-blocking†	Inhibits biological actions of TSH
Growth-stimulating‡	Stimulates growth of thyroid cells
Cytotoxic	Cytotoxic to thyroid cells
Thyroglobulin	No known biological activity

*Formerly known as thyroid microsomal antibody.
†Inhibition of TSH stimulation of cAMP generation, iodide transport, and thyroid growth; probably the same antibody as TSH-binding inhibitory antibody.
‡May be a property of thyroid-stimulating antibodies.

ickry) or that damages thyroid cells, rendering them immunogenic.[15] The result would depend on the antigen, its manner of presentation, and therefore the type of T cell activated. Another variable is the ability to regain tolerance, which would determine the natural history of the disorder, at least in those patients in whom the thyroid was not destroyed.

The risk factors for autoimmune thyroiditis include female sex, age, and heredity.[9, 10] Women outnumber men 6 to 8:1. Older women outnumber younger women about 4:1. Up to 50 per cent of siblings or offspring of patients with chronic autoimmune thyroiditis have antithyroid antibodies, and the frequency of Graves' disease in siblings and other relatives also may be increased. The frequency of certain isotypes of T-cell antigen receptors is increased in these patients, as is that of some HLA haplotypes, notably HLA-DR3 and -DR5, in affected patients in some ethnic groups.

Among patients who have atrophic autoimmune thyroiditis and subclinical hypothyroidism, from 5 to 20 per cent develop overt hypothyroidism each year.[16, 17] Similarly, most patients with goitrous autoimmune thyroiditis who are initially euthyroid eventually become hypothyroid. Treatment with T_4 decreases goiter size in about half of patients, but repeated biopsies show little change with time.[18] Both forms of chronic autoimmune thyroiditis, therefore, usually cause progressive and persistent thyroid failure, although remissions do occur, and in a few patients remissions followed by the development of Graves' hyperthyroidism, with the appearance of thyroid-stimulating antibodies, have been reported.[12, 18–20] Conversely, chronic autoimmune thyroiditis may follow Graves' disease.[21] Chronic autoimmune thyroiditis is an important risk factor for thyroid lymphoma.[22]

Transient Autoimmune Thyroiditis

Painless thyroiditis with thyrotoxicosis and postpartum thyroiditis are probably variant forms of chronic autoimmune thyroiditis. They differ from it in that the thyroid injury is transient and more intense, but thyroid follicular cells are not destroyed; immune activation seemingly develops more rapidly, but likewise tolerance is regained more quickly (see also Ch. 43).

Painless thyroiditis is characterized by transient thyrotoxicosis, followed in about half of the patients by transient hypothyroidism.[23] The latter lasts from two to eight weeks and is usually asymptomatic. Postpartum thyroiditis occurs in approximately 5 per cent of women after pregnancy, as determined by serial biochemical testing.[24, 25] About 75 per cent have hypothyroidism, preceded in about half by thyrotoxicosis. Whether preceded by thyrotoxicosis or not, the hypothyroidism usually occurs three to eight months after delivery and lasts from two to eight weeks. The proportion of affected women who have symptoms is about 50 per cent.

Painless thyroiditis and postpartum thyroiditis differ from each other in that patients with the latter more often have thyroid antibodies before, during, and after their thyroid illness and are more likely to have recurrences and to develop chronic autoimmune thyroiditis later.[23, 26] Thyroid biopsies in both disorders show lymphocytic thyroiditis, but less cellular infiltration than in chronic autoimmune thyroiditis and no germinal centers or fibrosis.

Hypothyroidism after Radioiodine Therapy for Thyrotoxicosis and after External Radiation Therapy

Among patients with thyrotoxicosis caused by Graves' disease, hypothyroidism occurs in a substantial proportion (from 40 to 90 per cent) within the first year after therapy with [131]I (see Ch. 41).[27–30] This high rate reflects the current use of large doses of ^{131}I, so as to minimize the risk of recurrent thyrotoxicosis. Thereafter, from 0.5 to 2 per cent of patients become hypothyroid each year, nearly always after having had subclinical hypothyroidism for several years.[31, 32] The occurrence of hypothyroidism within the first year after treatment depends on the dose of [131]I. Late hypothyroidism is caused by failure of surviving thyroid cells to replicate or by chronic autoimmune thyroiditis and is less ^{131}I dose dependent. Hypothyroidism is unusual after ^{131}I therapy for toxic uninodular or multinodular goiter, because these patients have some atrophic thyroid tissue that does not concentrate the radionuclide and therefore is not destroyed and can resume function later.

External neck irradiation, in doses of 2500 rads or more (25 Gy), as used for the treatment of patients with lymphoma or carcinoma of the larynx or nasopharynx also causes hypothyroidism.[33, 34] Its effect is dose dependent; about 50 per cent of patients who receive 4000 rads (40 Gy) ultimately develop hypothyroidism. The thyroid is also exposed in patients with tumors of the posterior fossa who are treated with radiation therapy and in those who receive total body irradiation before bone marrow transplantation.[35] External irradiation–induced overt hypothyroidism is usually preceded by a long period of subclinical hypothyroidism.

Postoperative Hypothyroidism

Serum TSH concentrations increase within one week, and overt hypothyroidism occurs within one month after total thyroidectomy.[36] The frequency of hypothyroidism after subtotal thyroidectomy for hyperthyroid Graves' disease varies, ranging from as low as 2 per cent to as high as 75 per cent in the first several years after surgery.[28–30, 37] The high rates are the result of aggressive surgery, undertaken to minimize the likelihood of postoperative recurrence of thyrotoxicosis. Hypothyroidism occurring soon after surgery is not invariably permanent; the remaining thyroid tissue may be sufficient to maintain normal thyroid secretion after a period of TSH stimulation.[38] Hypothyroidism occurs at a rate of about 0.5 to 1 per cent per year in patients who remain euthyroid for one to two years after surgery, probably as a result of autoimmune destruction of the thyroid remnant.

Patients with thyroid nodular disease treated by surgery should not develop permanent hypothyroidism, unless most of the thyroid is removed or the remaining thyroid is abnormal. Transient subclinical hypothyroidism, however, may occur after removal of as little as one lobe of the thyroid.

Transient Hypothyroidism

Transient hypothyroidism may occur within several weeks or months after subtotal thyroidectomy and occasionally ^{131}I therapy. It is part of the usual course of subacute thyroiditis, painless thyroiditis, and postpartum thyroiditis and can occur after discontinuation of thyroid therapy in patients who are euthyroid.[23, 25, 39, 40] In these situations, serum T_4 and T_3 concentrations decline and may remain low for several weeks or months. Initially, serum TSH concentrations may be low because of preceding thyrotoxicosis. TSH secretion usually recovers in several weeks, but several months may be required in patients who were thyrotoxic for prolonged periods. If the thyroid is injured or the remaining thyroid mass is small, serum TSH concentrations may rise to supranormal levels until thyroid recovery occurs. Transient hypothyroidism, therefore, may be associated with either low or high serum TSH concentrations.

Infiltrative and Other Diseases of the Thyroid

Hypothyroidism may result from destruction of the thyroid by cellular infiltration or fibrosis or intrathyroidal deposition of various substances. Among the disorders reported to involve the thyroid in these ways are amyloidosis, sarcoidosis, scleroderma, leukemia, fibrous invasive thyroiditis (Reidel's thyroiditis), cystinosis, and iron deposition diseases.[41] Infections of the thyroid, including *Pneumocystis carinii* infections, can occasionally damage the gland sufficiently to cause hypothyroidism.[42]

Thyroid Dysgenesis (Sporadic Nongoitrous Cretinism)

Developmental defects of the thyroid gland are the most common cause of hypothyroidism in newborn infants (see Ch. 47). Some patients have virtually complete thyroid agenesis, but about half have some thyroid tissue detectable by radionuclide scan. The cause is not known.

Biosynthetic Defects in Thyroid Hormonogenesis

Normal thyroid hormone production depends on the availability of iodine and the ability of thyroid tissue to carry out the multiple reactions needed to synthesize and secrete T_4 and T_3. Not surprisingly, therefore, decreased thyroid hormone production has multiple genetic, nutritional, and pharmacological causes.

Congenital Defects

The multiple rare genetic defects in thyroid hormone biosynthesis have provided much insight into the normal mechanisms of thyroid hormone production (see Ch. 52). Most of these defects are inherited as autosomal recessive traits. Affected homozygotes have severe hypothyroidism that is apparent at birth or in early infancy. The compensatory increase in TSH secretion leads to thyroid enlargement, which may be minimal initially but becomes obvious in childhood or later. In heterozygotes, the abnormality is usually mild, resulting only in subclinical hypothyroidism and variable degrees of thyroid enlargement.

IODIDE TRANSPORT DEFECT. This very rare abnormality is characterized by partial or complete lack of ability of thyroid tissue to transport iodide. Thyroid radioiodine uptake is therefore very low despite the presence of goiter.

IODIDE ORGANIFICATION DEFECTS. Several defects in iodine oxidation and organification have been described, including quantitative deficiency of thyroid peroxidase, qualitative abnormalities such as defective binding of heme prosthetic groups to the enzyme and abnormal intracellular localization of the enzyme, and deficient generation of hydrogen peroxide. Thyroid iodide transport is increased, but little further intrathyroidal metabolism of iodide occurs, so that inorganic iodide accumulates in the thyroid. This accumulation can be detected by a perchlorate discharge test; when transport of iodide into thyroid cells is inhibited by perchlorate, the outward diffusion of iodide that has accumulated can be detected.

In some families, goiter, usually with minimal hypothyroidism, occurs along with congenital sensorineural deafness (Pendred's syndrome). Perchlorate discharge tests are positive in these patients, but the defect seems to be more one of iodotyrosine coupling than of iodide organification.

DEFECTS IN THYROGLOBULIN BIOSYNTHESIS. Thyroglobulin production may be inadequate but its structure normal. It may be produced in adequate quantities but be structurally abnormal, so that organification of iodine or coupling of iodotyrosyl residues within it is poor or it cannot be secreted into the thyroid follicular lumen. The latter abnormalities may result from synthesis of thyroglobulin that is abnormal in either amino acid or carbohydrate composition.

IODOTYROSINE DEIODINASE DEFICIENCY. Thyroid iodotyrosine deiodinase plays an important role in the recirculation and therefore conservation of iodide. Iodotyrosine deiodinase deficiency results in release of large quantities of mono- and diiodotyrosine from the thyroid gland; these iodotyrosines then are excreted in the urine. Thus, iodide that normally becomes available for reuse within the thyroid is lost.

THYROID INSENSITIVITY TO TSH. The unique clinical feature of this disorder is the absence of goiter. Thyroid tissue is present but is unresponsive to either endogenous or exogenous TSH. Thyroid tissue from these patients binds TSH in vitro, but the cAMP response to TSH is poor, suggesting a postreceptor defect.

These disorders can be differentiated in a general way by the presence or absence of goiter, measurements of serum thyroglobulin and of thyroid radioiodine uptake, and perchlorate discharge testing. Identification of specific defects requires detailed in vitro studies of thyroid iodine metabolism, thyroglobulin structure, or DNA analysis.

Iodine Deficiency

Dietary iodide deficiency results in inadequate thyroid hormone production despite the presence of normal thyroid tissue. The presence of hypothyroidism (cretinism) in inhabitants of regions where iodine deficiency is endemic has long been recognized (see Ch. 49). Many more inhabitants of these regions are euthyroid but have goiter, abnormalities in thyroid iodide metabolism and in T_4 and T_3 secretion, and increased serum TSH concentrations. Although the degree of iodine deficiency is the major determinant of these abnormalities, other factors may modify the frequency or severity of endemic goiter, including genetic factors, dietary and water-borne goitrogens, and other nutritional deficiencies, in particular that of selenium.[43]

Iodine Excess

Iodine excess, in addition to iodine deficiency, can cause subclinical or overt hypothyroidism. The antithyroid action of iodide results from its ability, if present in sufficient quantities within the thyroid, to inhibit iodide organification. In normal subjects, inorganic iodide, in doses of 500 μg daily or more, has a weak antithyroid effect that is transient.[44] The effect is transient because the high intrathyroidal iodide concentrations needed to inhibit organification are not maintained, so that there is "escape" from the antithyroid action of iodide. Escape does not occur, and therefore the antithyroid action of iodide is sustained, in patients whose thyroid glands are abnormal, whether because of chronic autoimmune thyroiditis, previous painless or postpartum thyroiditis, or previous ^{131}I or surgical therapy for Graves' thyrotoxicosis.[45]

The iodine may be used as either inorganic iodide or an organic iodine compound that can be deiodinated in vivo, as most are. It may be in the diet or in medication that is ingested, applied to the skin or mucous membranes, or administered as a radiographic contrast agent.[45] Overt hypothyroidism induced by iodide is rare, because exposure usually is brief, except in regions where dietary iodine intake is very high, such as Japan.[46] A few iodine-containing drugs, notably amiodarone, accumulate in adipose tissue and are deiodinated very slowly, and so may cause persistent hypothyroidism.[45, 47]

Antithyroid Agents

A number of inorganic and organic compounds, both naturally occurring and synthetic, have antithyroid actions. These compounds inhibit thyroidal T_4 and T_3 synthesis and secretion, usually by inhibiting iodide transport or iodide organification and coupling, and therefore can cause hypothyroidism and goiter. The most potent antithyroid agents are propylthiouracil and methimazole; they are used only to treat hyperthyroidism, and their usage should be evident. The most commonly used drug that may cause hypothyroidism and goiter is lithium carbonate. Among patients treated with lithium, up to 20 per cent have increased serum TSH concentrations, and 1 per cent develop overt hypothyroidism.[48] Autoimmune thyroid disease may be a risk factor for lithium-induced thyroid disease.

Many other drugs, chemicals, and constituents of naturally occurring foodstuffs have antithyroid actions and occasionally have been implicated as the cause of hypothyroidism or goiter in individual patients.[41] None of these substances is an important cause of hypothyroidism, because they are very weak antithyroid agents and are not widely used.

The cytokines interferon (IFN)-α and interleukin-2, now being used to treat patients with a variety of tumors and viral diseases, can induce a syndrome much like painless thyroiditis, either thyrotoxicosis followed by transient hypothyroidism or transient hypothyroidism alone or by permanent hypothyroidism.[49, 50] Thyroid antibodies appear or, if present initially, their titers increase, especially in patients who develop thyroid dysfunction, indicating that pre-existing chronic autoimmune thyroiditis is a risk factor for cytokine-induced thyroid disease. These agents probably stimulate autoreactive cytotoxic T cells, B cells capable of producing thyroid antibodies, or both; they may also have direct cytotoxic actions on thyroid cells. In contrast, IFN-γ has no thyroidal effects.[51]

A few drugs inhibit TSH secretion (see Ch. 12). Among them are dopamine, the long-acting somatostatin analogue octreotide, and glucocorticoids. Prolonged infusions of dopamine can lower serum TSH and T_4 concentrations,[52] but are used only in critically ill patients who already have major abnormalities in thyroid function and in whom T_4 therapy is not beneficial.[8, 53] Octreotide is a much less potent inhibitor of TSH than of growth hormone secretion. Glucocorticoids inhibit TSH secretion, probably by inhibiting TRH secretion. Neither of these agents causes hypothyroidism, perhaps because any decline in TSH secretion is counterbalanced by the powerful stimulatory effect of decreased thyroid secretion on it.

Central (Secondary) Hypothyroidism

Pituitary Hypothyroidism

TSH is required for normal thyroid secretion, and TSH deficiency causes decreased thyroid secretion and thyroid atrophy. It is much less common than primary (thyroidal) hypothyroidism. Among patients with pituitary macroadenomas, 10 to 25 per cent have hypothyroidism, whereas nearly all patients with pituitary microadenomas are euthyroid. After pituitary adenomectomy, some initially euthyroid patients become TSH-deficient, and some initially hypothyroid patients become euthyroid.[54] Other causes of TSH deficiency include postpartum pituitary necrosis, trauma, hemochromatosis, lymphocytic hypophysitis, and metastatic cancer (see Ch. 29). In any of these situations, TSH deficiency may occur alone or in combination with other tropic hormone deficiencies. In infants and children, TSH deficiency may be caused by the same diseases and also by inherited structural defects in the gene for the β subunit of TSH.[55]

Hypothyroidism accompanied by pituitary enlargement does not always indicate the presence of a primary pituitary tumor and pituitary hypothyroidism. The compensatory increase in TSH secretion that occurs in all patients with primary hypothyroidism is accompanied by hyperplasia and hypertrophy of the thyrotrophs, which in a few patients is sufficient to cause radiologically and occasionally clinically evident pituitary enlargement, including impaired vision.[56] It is very important to recognize that primary hypothyroidism can cause pituitary enlargement, so that unnecessary pituitary surgery is avoided. These patients have very high serum TSH concentrations, which decline when T_4 therapy is given, and the pituitary gland diminishes in size.

Hypothalamic Hypothyroidism

TRH deficiency also causes hypothyroidism. It may be isolated or coexist with other hypothalamic hormone deficiencies. It is even less common than pituitary hypothyroidism. Its causes include cranial irradiation therapy, traumatic, infiltrative, and neoplastic diseases of the hypothalamus, or pituitary lesions that interrupt the hypothalamic-pituitary portal circulation (see Ch. 29).

Most hypothyroid patients with pituitary or hypothalamic disease have low or normal serum TSH concentrations (Fig. 45–3). Even when daytime serum TSH concentrations are normal, nocturnal TSH secretion is usually decreased.[57] Characteristically, serum TSH concentrations increase little after administration of TRH in patients with pituitary hypothyroidism, whereas the increase is normal or delayed in those with hypothalamic hypothyroidism, but the responses are too variable for the test to be useful in an individual patient. Rare patients with central hypothyroidism have increased serum TSH concentrations; their TSH is immunoreactive but biologically inactive, and its biological activity increases when they are given TRH.[58]

Generalized Resistance to Thyroid Hormone

Generalized resistance to thyroid hormones is a rare hereditary disorder characterized by few or no symptoms and signs of thyroid dysfunction, thyroid enlargement, increased serum total and free T_4 and T_3 concentrations, and normal or slightly increased serum TSH concentrations (see Ch. 52). Some patients have had abnormalities, such as deafness, stippled epiphyses and short stature, indicative of hypothyroidism in infancy. Others have had tachycardia

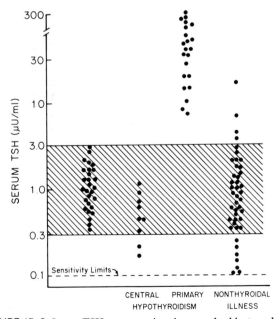

FIGURE 45–3. **Serum TSH concentrations in normal subjects and patients with central (secondary) hypothyroidism, primary hypothyroidism, and nonthyroidal illness.** The high values in the latter group were obtained during the recovery period. The stripped area indicates the range of serum TSH concentrations in normal subjects. (Modified from Felig P, Baxter JD, Frohman LA (eds): Endocrinology and Metabolism (ed 3). New York, McGraw-Hill, 1993.)

or hyperactivity that suggested the presence of excessive thyroid hormone action.

Most reported patients have been adolescents or adults, but the disorder can be recognized soon after birth by the finding of increased serum T_4, T_3, and TSH concentrations; the latter falls as thyroid secretion increases in the first months of life. The disorder is inherited as an autosomal recessive trait in most families. Patients with generalized resistance to thyroid hormone are euthyroid because they produce large amounts of T_4 and T_3; the pituitary is resistant to the same extent as other tissues, and the resistance is not complete in any tissue. Additional thyroid hormone evokes little additional response unless very large doses are given.[59] Most of these patients have point mutations of the gene for the β form of the T_3 nuclear receptor (see Ch. 37).[60] The mutant receptors have reduced affinity for T_3 and also inhibit the binding of the normal receptors to the T_3 response elements of DNA.[61]

CLINICAL MANIFESTATIONS OF HYPOTHYROIDISM

The clinical manifestations of hypothyroidism vary, depending on its cause, duration, and severity. The spectrum extends from subclinical hypothyroidism to overt hypothyroidism to myxedema coma. The characteristic change in organ system function is slowing; thus, there is slowing of physical and mental activity, and of cardiovascular, gastrointestinal, and neuromuscular function.

The more common symptoms and signs of hypothyroidism are listed in Table 45–3.[62-64] Among them, few are specific; the most discriminating are slow movements, decreased sweating, hoarseness, paresthesia, cold intolerance, periorbital edema, and delayed reflexes. A history of a cause of hypothyroidism, for example previous ^{131}I therapy or treatment with lithium carbonate, may be an important clue to its presence.

Spontaneously occurring hypothyroidism usually develops slowly because the thyroid injury is gradual and the decline in thyroid secretion is limited by the resulting rise in TSH secretion. When hypothyroidism develops more rapidly, for example soon after ^{131}I therapy or subtotal thyroidectomy, patients recognize the changes more readily, and symptoms such as muscle cramps, muscle tenderness, stiffness, and paresthesiae are more prominent. Patients with central hypothyroidism tend to have few symptoms and signs, because their hypothyroidism usually is not se-

vere or because they have other hormonal deficiencies that ameliorate or mask the manifestations of hypothyroidism.

The characteristic pathological finding in patients with hypothyroidism is the accumulation of hyaluronic acid and other glycosaminoglycans in interstitial tissue.[65] These substances accumulate because their synthesis is increased, and their hydrophilic properties lead to the mucinous edema (myxedema) characteristic of the disorder. Mucinous edema of the dermis produces some of the most obvious clinical manifestations of hypothyroidism, and in fatal cases, has been found in the interstitial tissue of most organs.[66]

General Appearance

Patients with hypothyroidism often appear normal but may have obvious myxedema of the face and extremities or may be comatose. The major manifestations often are subjective. The patient complains of being tired and weak or of decreasing physical energy or mental activity, changes often attributed to aging by the patient or the patient's relatives. Cold intolerance may be marked, the patient using extra clothing even in summer.

Skin and Appendages

The classic (but now rare) appearance of a patient with primary hypothyroidism (Fig. 45–4) is caused by nonpitting periorbital and peripheral mucinous edema. The facial features become coarse, the upper eyelids extend downward (blepharoptosis), and the skin becomes rough, scaly, and thickened.

Usually the patient's appearance is less altered. The skin may be dry but is not thickened or rough, and periorbital and peripheral edema is mild or absent. The edema may be pitting, particularly in the legs; such a finding need not

TABLE 45–3. COMMON SYMPTOMS AND SIGNS OF HYPOTHYROIDISM

Symptom	Signs
Weakness and fatigue	Slow movements
Dry skin	Coarse skin and hair
Cold intolerance	Cold skin
Hoarseness	Periorbital puffiness
Weight gain	Slow reflex relaxation
Constipation	Bradycardia
Decreased sweating	
Paresthesia	
Decreased hearing	

Data from References 62 to 64.

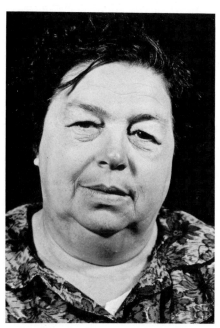

FIGURE 45–4. Appearance of a patient with primary hypothyroidism. Note the periorbital edema, blepharoptosis, and coarsened facial features.

indicate the presence of cardiac or other disease. The skin is often pale owing to thickening of the dermis and epidermis, decreased skin blood flow, and sometimes anemia; it may be yellowish owing to carotenemia; and it feels cold because it is thick and blood flow is decreased.

Decreased sebaceous and sweat gland function adds to the dryness of the skin. The hair may be coarse, dry, and brittle, and hair growth may slow or cease. Hair may be lost on the scalp, the extremities, or the eyebrows. The nails also grow slowly and may be thickened yet brittle.

Thyroid Gland

Palpation of the thyroid may not only suggest the cause of hypothyroidism but also its presence, because thyroid enlargement may be its first manifestation. Goitrous autoimmune thyroiditis is characterized by diffuse thyroid enlargement, although the surface may feel irregular or even nodular, and the consistency of the thyroid gland is often described as firm or rubbery. The thyroid gland initially is diffusely enlarged in patients with hypothyroidism caused by iodine deficiency, congenital defects in thyroid hormone biosynthesis, or any antithyroid agent, but it eventually becomes irregular or overtly nodular. It is not palpable in atrophic autoimmune thyroiditis or central hypothyroidism.

Nervous System

Symptoms of mental dysfunction are common in hypothyroid patients. Cerebral vascular resistance is increased and cerebral blood flow is reduced in proportion to the decrease in cardiac output. CNS glucose and oxygen consumption are normal.[67] The reduced delivery of oxygen to tissue utilizing it at a normal rate results in some degree of cerebral hypoxia.

The psychological and behavioral symptoms of hypothyroidism include slowing of movement and thought, decreased alertness and attention span, loss of ambition, and impaired memory. There may be some cognitive impairment,[68] and overt dementia may occur. The patient may sleep longer at night or sleep fitfully at night and frequently during the day because of sleep apnea. Some patients accept substantial limitations of activity with equanimity, whereas others become anxious and depressed; rarely there is severe anxiety and agitation ("myxedema madness").[69] Speech is slow and hesitant as well as hoarse, and physical movements may be clumsy. Headache or hearing loss may be prominent complaints.

Hypothyroid patients often complain of paresthesias but usually have no objective neurological findings other than slow deep tendon reflexes. Both the contraction and relaxation phases of the reflexes are prolonged, the latter more than the former. Several neurological syndromes that are reversible may occur. The most common is the carpal tunnel syndrome; others are a symmetrical sensorimotor polyneuropathy and cerebellar dysfunction, with ataxia, intention tremor, and nystagmus.[69,70]

Musculoskeletal System

Many hypothyroid patients have myalgia, muscle cramps, and muscle stiffness.[71] Their movements may be slow and clumsy, and complaints of muscle weakness and fatigability are common, but objective muscle weakness is uncommon. Rarely, chronic hypothyroid myopathy results in increased muscle mass (pseudohypertrophy), muscle spasm, and pseudomyotonia. Serum creatine kinase (MM fraction) concentrations are often elevated, even in the absence of muscle symptoms, owing to increased sarcolemmal permeability and also slowed clearance. Serum lactate dehydrogenase and aminotransferase concentrations may be increased as well. Muscle biopsies show interstitial edema and muscle fiber enlargement, loss of striations, and sarcoplasmic degeneration.

Hypothyroid patients may complain of arthralgia and joint stiffness. Other joint abnormalities include synovial thickening and synovial effusions, usually of the knees.

Cardiovascular-Pulmonary System

Hypothyroidism results in decreases in the rate and force of cardiac contractility and also in peripheral oxygen requirements.[72] Peripheral resistance increases, and cerebral, cutaneous, and renal blood flow and blood volume are reduced. The consequences are decreased cardiac output, but ventricular end-diastolic pressure and peripheral arteriovenous oxygen differences are normal. During exercise, cardiac output increases and peripheral resistance decreases appropriately, indicating normal cardiac reserve. In fatal cases, the myocardial fibers are edematous and vacuolated.[66]

The clinical manifestations of cardiovascular dysfunction in hypothyroid patients include bradycardia, evidence of poor peripheral circulation such as pallor and cold skin, dyspnea, decreased exercise tolerance, fatigability, distant heart sounds, and cardiac enlargement. The lethargy, puffiness, edema, and diminished cardiac activity may suggest the presence of cardiac failure, but it is rare; when it occurs, it is most likely due to the hemodynamic changes of hypothyroidism combined with pre-existing cardiac disease, although T_4-reversible cardiomyopathy has been described.[72] There is occasionally clinical and radiographic evidence of cardiac muscle enlargement or pericardial effusion; the effusions, which are both cholesterol- and protein-rich, rarely have any hemodynamic effects. The electrocardiogram shows bradycardia and low-amplitude P waves and QRS complexes and sometimes nonspecific QRS and T-wave abnormalities and conduction disturbances. Echocardiography may reveal pericardial effusion, varying degrees of ventricular septal and wall thickening, or diminished myocardial relaxation.[73]

About 20 per cent of hypothyroid patients are hypertensive.[74] Although undoubtedly coincidental in most patients, hypertension is aggravated by the increase in peripheral resistance that occurs in hypothyroidism. Some patients, however, become hypertensive as they become hypothyroid, and the hypertension disappears with T_4 treatment.

The coexistence of ischemic heart disease and hypothyroidism in some patients warrants mention. Serum creatine kinase measurements must be interpreted cautiously in hypothyroid patients with chest pain, because the values may be high as a result of hypothyroidism alone. Although hypothyroidism causes hypercholesterolemia,[75, 76] there is little evidence for accelerated atherogenesis in hypothyroid patients. Hypothyroidism may ameliorate angina pectoris, whether because cardiac work and thus myocardial oxygen requirements are reduced or simply because the patient becomes less active.[77] The management of patients with ischemic heart disease and hypothyroidism is discussed under "Treatment of Hypothyroidism."

Respiratory system complaints include nasal congestion, hoarseness, shortness of breath, and sleep apnea. The first two are caused by mucinous edema of the nasal mucosa and larynx, respectively. Shortness of breath may be caused by cardiac disease, pleural effusion, or generalized impairment of pulmonary function. Some patients have symptomatic sleep apnea, and it can be demonstrated by polysomnography in many others. It is caused by enlargement of the tongue and oropharyngeal muscles, respiratory muscle weakness, and central respiratory depression.[78]

Lung volumes, vital capacity, and arterial blood oxygen and carbon dioxide content are normal in hypothyroid patients. Maximum breathing capacity, compliance, and ventilatory drive may be reduced, owing to respiratory muscle weakness or depression of the respiratory center.[79] Pleural effusion(s) may be present with no other evidence of lung disease.[80]

Fluid and Electrolyte Metabolism and Renal Function

Hypothyroid patients often appear puffy, even edematous, and total body water and sodium content are increased as a result of extravascular accumulation of hydrophilic glycosaminoglycans, increased vascular permeability, and decreased lymph flow.[81] Plasma volume is decreased, and plasma renin activity and serum atrial natriuretic hormone and aldosterone concentrations are normal or slightly decreased.[82, 83]

Renal blood flow is reduced in proportion to the decrease in cardiac output, and the glomerular filtration rate is usually slightly reduced. Serum urea and creatinine concentrations are normal.

Free water clearance is decreased, as is excretion of a water load, resulting in hyponatremia in some patients. Vasopressin secretion, both basally and in response to saline infusion, is normal in most patients but may be increased.[83, 84]

Gastrointestinal System

The tongue may be enlarged. Gastric emptying may be impaired, causing nausea and vomiting, and intestinal motility slowed, causing constipation and abdominal distention. Intestinal motility may be so slow that the patient develops paralytic ileus or megacolon, with clinical manifestations of intestinal obstruction.[85] Liver size and function are usually normal, but the elevated serum enzyme concentrations mentioned previously may be caused in part by reduced hepatic clearance of the enzymes. A few patients have ascites, probably caused by abnormal capillary perme-

ability and reduced hepatic lymph flow. The gallbladder may be dilated and empty poorly.

Intestinal absorption is usually normal. Some patients have gastric atrophy and achlorhydria, which can be associated with vitamin B_{12} malabsorption. About 25 per cent of patients with chronic autoimmune thyroiditis have antiparietal cell antibodies; defects in gastric acid secretion and vitamin B_{12} malabsorption are more frequent in patients with this type of hypothyroidism.

Hematopoietic System

About 25 per cent of hypothyroid patients are slightly anemic. Reduction in red cell mass is more frequent but is masked by decreased plasma volume.[86] The anemia is usually normocytic, and the hemoglobin concentration is rarely less than 10 g/dl (100 g/L). Serum erythropoietin concentrations are low; those of iron, iron-binding capacity, vitamin B_{12}, and folate are usually normal. The bone marrow is hypocellular, and iron clearance and incorporation in erythroid cells are decreased. Occasional patients, however, have iron, folic acid, or vitamin B_{12} deficiency, with the appropriate peripheral blood and bone marrow findings. Iron deficiency may be caused by excessive menstrual bleeding or poor iron absorption secondary to decreased gastric acid secretion. Megaloblastic anemia may be caused by folic acid or vitamin B_{12} malabsorption due to the hypothyroidism itself or to pernicious anemia in patients with chronic autoimmune thyroiditis.

Granulocyte, lymphocyte, and platelet counts are usually normal in hypothyroidism. Platelet function may be abnormal, bleeding time prolonged, and the concentrations of some clotting factors slightly decreased.[85, 87] A few patients bruise easily, but the correlation between bruising and abnormalities in platelet function and clotting factors is poor.

Energy, Nutrient, and Drug Metabolism

The decreases in energy expenditure and oxygen consumption in hypothyroid patients are accompanied by decreased utilization of a variety of substrates. The result is decreased heat production, probably the major cause of the cold intolerance that is so characteristic of hypothyroidism. Decreased resting metabolic activity and substrate utilization, together with physical inactivity and mental depression, cause decreased appetite and food intake. Body weight may increase slightly,[88] but marked increases are unusual. Weight gain, when it does occur, is due to retention of salt and water in interstitial tissue as well as to fat deposition.

Patients with hypothyroidism have normal carbohydrate tolerance, although glucose absorption may be delayed.[89] Insulin secretory responses after oral glucose ingestion are appropriate for the rise in glucose that occurs. Hepatic stores of glycogen are normal, as is hepatic gluconeogenesis; blood glucose concentrations, therefore, are maintained normally during fasting. Overall glucose utilization is normal. In patients with insulin-dependent diabetes, exogenous insulin is degraded more slowly than normal; thus, sensitivity to exogenous insulin may increase.

The synthesis of proteins of all types—structural proteins, secreted proteins, and enzymes—is impaired in many tissues in hypothyroid patients. This impairment is perhaps most evident in hypothyroid children, in whom growth is very poor (see Ch. 47). Protein catabolism also is impaired. For several proteins, such as albumin and lipoproteins, catabolism is impaired more than synthesis. Serum albumin concentrations, however, are normal, because the excess albumin is largely in the interstitial space.[81]

The serum concentrations of total and low-density lipoprotein (LDL) cholesterol and, less often, triglycerides are elevated.[75, 76] Triglyceride synthesis is decreased, as is triglyceride clearance, because the activity of adipose tissue and hepatic lipase is decreased. The increase in serum LDL cholesterol concentrations and those of its apoprotein B constituent are due to decreases in receptor-mediated uptake of cholesterol and clearance and conversion of cholesterol to bile acids. Serum high-density lipoprotein (HDL) cholesterol concentrations may be normal, increased, or decreased and do not change consistently in response to T_4 treatment, whereas serum LDL cholesterol concentrations decrease.

The metabolism or renal clearance of many drugs, including digoxin, phenytoin, and morphine, is slowed by hypothyroidism, so that their actions may be prolonged or exaggerated. The effect of warfarin may be decreased because the catabolism of vitamin K–dependent clotting factors is slowed.

Endocrine System

Hypothyroidism alters the dynamics of secretion of other endocrine organs and in some patients causes clinically evident abnormalities in endocrine function. Characteristically, the rates of hormone clearance are decreased and there is compensatory reduction in the rates of hormone secretion, so that serum hormone concentrations are normal.

Pituitary Function

Nocturnal growth hormone (GH) secretion and serum GH responses to provocative stimuli such as GH–releasing hormone, hypoglycemia, and arginine infusion may be reduced.[90, 91] Serum insulin-like growth factor I (IGF I) concentrations tend to be low but increase normally in response to exogenous GH. The decrease in nocturnal GH secretion is probably sufficient to account for the decrease in production of IGF I.

Prolactin secretion is usually normal but may be increased; a few women have had serum prolactin concentrations as high as 200 ng/ml (200 μg/L).[76, 92, 93] Hyperprolactinemia is most likely to occur in women with long-standing hypothyroidism and may result in amenorrhea and galactorrhea, as it does in women with other disorders that cause hyperprolactinemia.

These abnormalities of pituitary hormone secretion are reversed by treatment of hypothyroidism. Pituitary hormone deficiencies also may occur as a result of any of the hypothalamic or pituitary diseases that cause hypothyroidism.

Adrenocortical and Sympathoadrenal Function

Twenty-four hour mean serum cortisol concentrations are normal or slightly increased.[94] Although cortisol clearance is slowed, cortisol production is nearly normal, suggesting that the sensitivity of ACTH secretion to cortisol is decreased. Urinary cortisol excretion is normal, whereas that of steroid metabolites tends to be low, corresponding with the decrease in cortisol clearance. Pituitary-adrenal responses to metyrapone, hypoglycemia, corticotropin-releasing hormone (CRH), and ACTH are normal or, in the case of CRH, increased.[95] Serum cortisol concentrations increase normally in hypothyroid patients who have other illnesses.

Some patients with hypothyroidism caused by chronic autoimmune thyroiditis have adrenal insufficiency caused by autoimmune adrenalitis (autoimmune polyglandular syndromes), and hypothyroidism can occur in patients with other forms of adrenal insufficiency.[96] Glucocorticoid replacement alone may result in restoration of normal thyroid function, indicating the sensitivity of autoimmune disease mechanisms to glucocorticoids.

The serum concentrations and production rates of norepinephrine are increased, whereas those of epinephrine are normal.[97] Responses to adrenergic stimulation are impaired.[98]

Parathyroid–Vitamin D–Bone System

Hypothyroid patients have normal serum calcium and phosphate concentrations, whereas those of parathyroid hormone and 1,25-dihydroxyvitamin D may be increased.[99] Calcium absorption is decreased, as are bone formation and resorption, suggesting resistance to the actions of parathyroid hormone and 1,25-dihydroxyvitamin D. Calcitonin secretion is decreased, not only in patients who have had a thyroidectomy but also in those with chronic autoimmune thyroiditis or after ^{131}I therapy; the decrease has no known clinical consequences.[100] Bone turnover is decreased; radial, femoral, and lumbar spine bone mineral density is normal.

Gonadal Function

In women with hypothyroidism, serum estradiol concentrations may be decreased, because sex hormone–binding globulin production is decreased; serum free estradiol concentrations usually are normal. Follicle-stimulating hormone (FSH) and luteinizing hormone (LH) secretions are usually in the normal range for the follicular phase of the menstrual cycle, but there is no ovulatory surge. The women, therefore, tend to have irregular, anovulatory cycles and excessive menstrual bleeding.[101] Postmenopausal women with hypothyroidism have serum FSH and LH concentrations somewhat lower than expected.

In men, serum testosterone concentrations may be low, because of decreased sex hormone–binding globulin production, but serum free testosterone is usually normal. Serum FSH and LH concentrations also are usually normal, but may be slightly increased or decreased. Little is known about reproductive capacity. Impotence is common, but may not respond to T_4 therapy.[102]

Pregnancy in Hypothyroidism

Although women with hypothyroidism tend to be infertile, they can conceive. The outcome of pregnancy may be normal, but the likelihood of abortion, stillbirth, or premature delivery is increased.[103] Even if the pregnancy is successful, the growth of the fetus may be retarded. The frequency of hypothyroidism (mostly subclinical) and antibodies to thyroid peroxidase among pregnant women in the first trimester is about 2 per cent, similar to that of nonpregnant women of the same age.[104] The presence of these antibodies alone early in pregnancy may be a risk factor for spontaneous abortion.[105]

Nonthyroidal Illness and Surgery in Hypothyroid Patients

Whether hypothyroidism alters the course or outcome of nonthyroidal illness is not known. Serum T_3 concentrations decline in hypothyroid patients who have nonthyroidal illness, as they do in normal subjects.[106] The patients' high serum TSH concentrations do not change during mild nonthyroidal illness, but fall during severe illness or when glucocorticoids or dopamine is given.[52, 107]

The overall morbidity or mortality of surgery is not increased in hypothyroid patients, although some postoperative complications, such as hypotension, cardiac failure, and gastrointestinal dysfunction, may be more common.[108–110] Hypothyroid patients should be given anesthetic, analgesic, and sedative drugs very cautiously, because drug clearance is likely to be impaired.

LABORATORY DIAGNOSIS OF HYPOTHYROIDISM

Serum TSH and Thyroid Hormone Concentrations

The best test for recognition of primary hypothyroidism and differentiation of primary from central hypothyroidism is measurement of the serum TSH concentration (see Fig. 45–3). Serum TSH concentrations are increased not only in all patients with overt primary hypothyroidism but also, by definition, in those with subclinical hypothyroidism, indicative of the sensitivity of TSH secretion to even minor decreases in thyroid secretion. In patients with primary hypothyroidism, a rough inverse correlation exists between serum TSH and T_4 concentrations. Although the vast majority of patients with high serum TSH concentrations have primary hypothyroidism, high concentrations also occur in patients with TSH-induced thyrotoxicosis (see Ch. 41), rare patients with central hypothyroidism, and transiently during recovery from nonthyroidal illness.[111] Spurious elevations have been identified in persons who had serum antibodies that reacted with mouse immunoglobulins (used in most TSH assays); most of these persons had been exposed extensively to rodents or had autoimmune disease.[112]

Serum TSH concentrations are normal or low in nearly all patients with hypothyroidism due to pituitary or hypothalamic disease (see "Central Hypothyroidism"). Measurement of serum TSH, therefore, is not only an extremely sensitive test for the recognition of primary hypothyroidism but also may provide the first evidence that hypothyroidism in an individual patient is due to pituitary or hypothalamic disease, thus indicating the need for neuroradiological studies and testing of pituitary function. Furthermore, even in patients with evidence of hypothalamic-pituitary disease, such as hyperprolactinemia, enlargement of the sella turcica, or even visual impairment, serum TSH must be measured because any of those findings may be caused by primary hypothyroidism and improve with T_4 therapy. Serum TSH concentrations also are normal or low in most patients with nonthyroidal illness,[8, 113] so TSH measurements cannot be used to differentiate between it and central hypothyroidism (see Fig. 45–3). The slight increases, rarely to more than 20 μU/ml (20 mU/L), that occur in some patients during recovery from nonthyroidal illness probably result from lessening of the illness-related suppression of the thyrotropes by nonthyroid factors.

Most patients who have symptomatic hypothyroidism have decreased serum total and free T_4 concentrations, but low serum T_4 concentrations do not necessarily indicate the presence of hypothyroidism. Low serum total T_4 concentrations may be caused by decreased production of thyroxine-binding globulin (TBG) or drugs such as salicylate that competitively inhibit T_4 binding to TBG or other binding proteins. In patients with low TBG, the thyroid hormone–binding ratio (determined by T_3-resin uptake tests) indicates decreased numbers of unoccupied T_4 binding sites, and serum free T_4 concentrations and free T_4 index values are normal. Serum total T_4, and sometimes free T_4, concentrations also are decreased in some patients who are seriously ill as a result of nonthyroidal illness (see Chs. 39 and 40).

Serum T_3 concentrations are usually low in patients with hypothyroidism. About 20 to 30 per cent, however, have normal serum T_3 concentrations as a result of both TSH-induced stimulation of thyroidal T_3 secretion and an increase in the fractional extrathyroidal conversion of T_4 to T_3.[5–7] Nearly all patients with nonthyroidal illness have low serum T_3 concentrations.

A scheme for the evaluation of patients with suspected hypothyroidism is shown in Figure 45–5. The first step should be measurement of the serum TSH concentration and free T_4 index. If the serum TSH concentration is high and the serum free T_4 index value is low, the diagnosis of primary hypothyroidism is confirmed. If the serum TSH concentration is normal or low and the serum free T_4 index value is low, the diagnosis is central hypothyroidism or severe nonthyroidal illness. Distinguishing between these two disorders in a severely ill patient at any one time may be very difficult but may be possible based on the presence or absence of clinical or biochemical evidence of hypothyroidism and of other pituitary hormone deficiencies, the fact that central hypothyroidism is rare, and the results of measurements in serum of thyroid hormone–binding ratios (which are low in hypothyroidism and normal or high in nonthyroidal illness) and of free T_4 (which are low in hypothyroidism and low, normal, or high in nonthyroidal illness).

In contrast to evaluation of patients suspected to have hypothyroidism, screening for hypothyroidism is best done simply by measurement of serum TSH concentrations. A normal serum TSH concentration provides very strong evidence against the presence of any thyroid dysfunction in

LABORATORY DIAGNOSIS OF HYPOTHYROIDISM

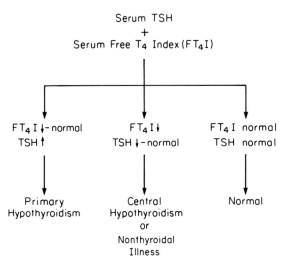

FIGURE 45–5. Scheme for the evaluation of patients suspected to have hypothyroidism. (From Felig P, Baxter JD, Frohman LA (eds): Endocrinology and Metabolism (ed 3). New York, McGraw-Hill, 1993.)

an asymptomatic person. Patients who should be screened for hypothyroidism include not only those whose risk is clearly increased, for example, patients who have received ^{131}I therapy and those taking lithium carbonate, but perhaps also the elderly and patients admitted to psychiatric units.[1] Screening for hypothyroidism in the general population is not warranted, except in newborn infants.

Other Laboratory Procedures

Determination of the serum TSH response to TRH is not useful for distinguishing between pituitary and hypothalamic hypothyroidism, because the responses are too variable. The distinction must be based on the results of neuroradiological imaging tests, the presence or absence of hyperprolactinemia, and the results of other hormonal tests. Similarly, central hypothyroidism and nonthyroidal illness cannot be distinguished by TRH testing; most patients with either disorder have poor serum TSH responses to TRH.*

Serum thyroglobulin concentrations are low in most hypothyroid patients but may be increased in those who have goitrous hypothyroidism. The presence of antithyroid peroxidase or other antithyroid antibodies indicates the presence of autoimmune thyroiditis but provides no information about thyroid secretion. The thyroidal uptake of radioiodine is low in most patients with hypothyroidism, but can be normal or high in patients with chronic autoimmune thyroiditis, iodine deficiency, and congenital defects of thyroid hormone biosynthesis.

TREATMENT OF HYPOTHYROIDISM

The treatment of hypothyroidism is T_4 replacement therapy, with rare exceptions. Occasionally, discontinuation of

iodide, lithium carbonate, or some other medication is all that is required, or the hypothyroidism is expected to be transient. Most patients, however, require lifelong T_4 treatment. The goal is simple—to restore and maintain the euthyroid state. In addition to prescription of an adequate dose of T_4, patients must be educated concerning the need for lifelong therapy and for periodic follow-up to evaluate the response to therapy and confirm compliance.

The initial T_4 dosage in young or middle-aged adults should be 0.075 to 0.1 mg/day orally. For elderly patients, the initial dosage should be smaller, 0.05 mg/day, because of the small risk of precipitation of angina pectoris, cardiac arrhythmia, or cardiac failure, and it should be even smaller (0.025 mg/day) if the patient is known to have cardiac disease. Hypothyroid patients should not be denied treatment because they might develop symptoms of ischemic heart disease, and indeed they may benefit. In a group of 55 hypothyroid patients with pre-existing angina, the angina improved or disappeared during thyroid hormone therapy in 21 patients, did not change in 25, and worsened in only 9.[114] Among about 1400 other patients, angina appeared in 6 during the first month of thyroid therapy, later in the first year in 6, and after that in 23. Antianginal therapy can be added if necessary, and coronary revascularization, if otherwise indicated, can be done safely in untreated hypothyroid patients.[77, 115] In a group of patients monitored for 24 hours before and during T_4 therapy, no patient developed any sustained arrhythmia, and the frequency of ventricular premature beats did not change, although the frequency of atrial premature beats increased slightly.[116]

Patients can be informed that they should notice increases in well-being and improvement in some symptoms within one to two weeks after initiation of moderate doses of T_4, and they should be re-examined after four to six weeks of treatment. The dosage should not be increased sooner, because this amount of time is needed for the full effects of an individual oral dose; even this period may not be sufficient to obtain the full effect on TSH secretion if the baseline serum TSH concentration was very high. Most symptoms and signs disappear within one to two months, although some neuropsychological and biochemical abnormalities may persist for four to six months.

About 80 per cent of an oral dose of T_4 is absorbed,[117] but because absorption is slow and the volume of distribution is large a usual dose does not result in appreciable between-dose fluctuations in serum T_4, T_3, or TSH concentrations.[118] The potency or bioavailability of different T_4 preparations may vary slightly, but the variations are rarely clinically important. Very rare patients have cutaneous allergy to T_4 or to the dye used to color the tablets.

The goal of treatment is to maintain well-being and normal serum TSH concentrations. An adequate replacement dose of T_4 in most patients is 0.075 to 0.125 mg (1.0 to 1.8 μg/kg) orally each day, and it is roughly proportional to the degree of initial serum TSH elevation.[119] The dose needed for adequate replacement may be altered, although usually by no more than 0.025 to 0.05 mg daily, by a number of factors (Table 45–4).[120–131] Women with hypothyroidism receiving T_4 therapy who become pregnant may need an increase in dosage during either the first or the second trimester.[125, 126] The most important factor seemingly necessitating changes in dosage is noncompliance.

After the initial follow-up visit and one or two additional

*Editor's note: Responsiveness to TRH in hypothalamic disease and failure to respond in pituitary destruction may differentiate these conditions.

TABLE 45–4. FACTORS ALTERING THE DOSAGE OF REPLACEMENT THYROXINE (T₄) FOR HYPOTHYROIDISM

Increased dosage requirement
  Decreased gastrointestinal absorption of T_4
    Malabsorption and short-bowel syndromes
    Therapy with agents that bind T_4
      Bile acid–sequestering agents, sucralfate, ferrous sulfate, aluminum hydroxide
  Increased production of T_4
    Pregnancy
    Obesity
  Increased clearance of T_4
    Therapy with phenytoin, carbamazepine, rifampin
    Younger age
  Decreased extrathyroidal T_4 conversion to T_3.*
    Amiodarone
  Apparent increased dosage requirement (pseudomalabsorption)
    Noncompliance
Decreased dosage requirement
  Residual nonsuppressible thyroid secretion
    Previous ablative treatment for Graves' hyperthyroiism
    Previous ablative treatment for toxic multinodular goiter
  Decreased clearance of T_4
    Older age

*Inhibition of Type II T_4-5'-deiodinase.
Data from references 119–131.

visits at approximately two-month intervals, the patient should be examined at six-month or yearly intervals. The adequacy of therapy should be based on the clinical response and the serum TSH concentration. No other test is such a sensitive indicator of either overtreatment or undertreatment. Most T_4-treated patients who have normal serum TSH concentrations also have normal serum T_4 and T_3 concentrations, but the former may be slightly elevated.* Very minor increases or decreases in serum TSH concentrations do not necessitate a change in T_4 dosage; the serum TSH concentration may be normal when retested soon thereafter.[117] If the serum TSH concentration is more abnormal, for example, 0.1 μU/ml (0.1 mU/L) or less, or 10 μU/ml (10 mU/L) or more (normal range 0.3 to 3.0 μU/ml [0.3 to 3.0 mU/L]), the serum T_4 concentration should be measured, and a change in dosage may be needed.† An increased serum TSH concentration indicates that the dose of T_4 is too small or compliance is poor. In the former situation, the serum T_4 concentration should be low. In the latter, it may be low or high, depending on whether the patient had taken little or no T_4 or a large dose, for example 0.6 to 0.8 mg, before the test.[132] A low serum TSH concentration indicates that treatment is excessive. One must rely on serum T_4 measurements in patients with central hypothyroidism.

The diverse consequences of slightly inadequate or excessive T_4 therapy have led to debate about which is potentially more harmful, and therefore whether it is better to err on the opposite side in choosing the dosage of T_4. Inadequate therapy may be associated with minimal hypercholesterolemia,[133] and excessive therapy with decreased bone density.[134, 135] There is, however, no evidence of in-creased risk of ischemic symptomatic heart disease in slightly undertreated patients or of fracture in those slightly overtreated.[136] Because these risks are hypothetical and frequent changes in T_4 dosage are inconvenient and tend to lead to overzealous testing, as noted in the preceding paragraph the dosage should not be changed merely because the serum TSH concentration is slightly abnormal at the time of a follow-up visit. The long-term mortality and morbidity of patients treated with T_4 are normal.[137]

A patient who cannot take T_4 orally, because of illness or an operation, need not be given T_4 for five to seven days. If oral treatment cannot then be resumed, 50 to 75 per cent of the usual T_4 dose should be given intravenously each day.

Other thyroid hormone preparations available for the treatment of hypothyroidism are T_3, combinations of T_4 and T_3, desiccated thyroid, and thyroglobulin. Serum T_3 concentrations fluctuate widely in patients treated with T_3,[118] but serum T_4 concentrations remain low; similar although less marked changes occur in patients receiving the other preparations. Treatment with such preparations can be monitored with serum TSH measurements; serum T_4 measurements greatly underestimate the dosage and often lead to administration of larger doses than needed. These preparations have disadvantages, and no advantages, compared with T_4.

SPECIAL CLINICAL SITUATIONS

For a discussion of hypothyroidism in infants and children, see Chapter 47.

Subclinical Hypothyroidism

Patients with subclinical hypothyroidism by definition have normal serum T_4 concentrations but increased serum TSH concentrations, the latter reflecting the effects of small decreases in thyroid secretion. The decreases may be caused by any of the disorders listed in Table 45–1; among them the most common are chronic autoimmune thyroiditis, previous ¹³¹I therapy for thyrotoxicosis, and iodine deficiency.

Some of these patients have thyroid enlargement. With regard to manifestations of hypothyroidism, they may have a few nonspecific symptoms such as fatigue, loss of energy, or constipation. They also may have slightly increased serum total and LDL cholesterol concentrations, diminished cardiac contractility, and hearing loss.[76, 138]

Whether or not patients with subclinical hypothyroidism should be treated is controversial. Treatment is not necessary merely to forestall the development of overt hypothyroidism, because it is not inevitable and progression to it is slow (5 to 20 per cent per year).[17, 31, 32] Treatment may reduce thyroid enlargement, if present, or the vague symptoms described earlier. In controlled trials of T_4 therapy in patients with subclinical hypothyroidism, these symptoms improved somewhat more during T_4 than during placebo therapy, as did cardiac contractility in one study, but serum cholesterol concentrations changed little.[139, 140] These results suggest that T_4 therapy is indicated for patients with subclinical hypothyroidism who have thyroid enlargement

Editor's note: In about one fourth of patients on T_4 replacement, T_4 and free T_4 values are just above the usual normal range when patients' TSH levels are in the normal range and their dosage is apparently appropriate.

†*Editor's note:* The editor believes that patients on replacement therapy are benefited by increased T_4 dosage if the TSH is consistently over 4 μU/ml.

or nonspecific symptoms, but not merely because their serum TSH concentrations are increased.

Discontinuation of Thyroid Hormone Therapy

Patients taking thyroid hormone therapy, or their physicians, may sometimes question the need for the therapy because of suspicion that the hypothyroidism has remitted or that the patient was not hypothyroid to begin with. The finding of an increased serum TSH concentration confirms the need for treatment, but if it is normal or low the need for continued treatment can be determined only by discontinuation of it. Normal subjects recover pituitary and thyroid function within one month after thyroid withdrawal, although they may have symptoms of hypothyroidism and subnormal serum T_4 concentrations transiently during the intervening weeks (Fig. 45–6).[39, 40] In contrast, virtually all patients who have hypothyroidism develop symptoms and unequivocal biochemical evidence of it within one month after treatment is discontinued.

Myxedema Coma

The development of coma in a patient with primary or central hypothyroidism is a life-threatening emergency. Myxedema coma occurs most often in the winter in elderly patients. In some patients it develops spontaneously, as the end-stage of prolonged severe hypothyroidism, due to respiratory center depression and decreased cardiac output and cerebral blood flow. In others it is precipitated by cold exposure, infection, cardiovascular or respiratory disease, and inappropriate administration of narcotic and analgesic drugs.[141, 142]

Patients with myxedema coma usually have overt hypothyroidism. Nearly all have progressive stupor, coma, and hypothermia; other important findings are hypoventilation with hypercapnia and respiratory acidosis, hyponatremia, hypotension, seizures, and hypoglycemia (Table 45–5). The hypothermia is due to severe hypometabolism and may precede the development of coma; any situation that hastens heat loss hastens the development not only of hypothermia but also of coma in these patients. Hypothermia may be overlooked or underestimated if the thermometer used does not register more than 1 to 2 degrees below normal. Hypoventilation may be caused by respiratory muscle weakness, upper airway obstruction from the large tongue, or impairment of the function of the respiratory center. Hyponatremia and water intoxication are caused by excess vasopressin secretion or a direct renal effect of thyroid hormone deficiency. Hypoglycemia usually indicates the presence of cortisol deficiency but may result from severe hypothyroidism alone.

Patients suspected to have myxedema coma must be treated aggressively because the mortality rate is high. After blood samples for serum T_4, TSH, and cortisol determinations are obtained, a large dose of T_4 should be administered. The initial dose should be 0.3 to 0.4 mg, followed by 0.1 mg daily, given intravenously because of the possibility of gastric retention or malabsorption. Such a large initial dose should rapidly restore the serum free T_4 concentra-

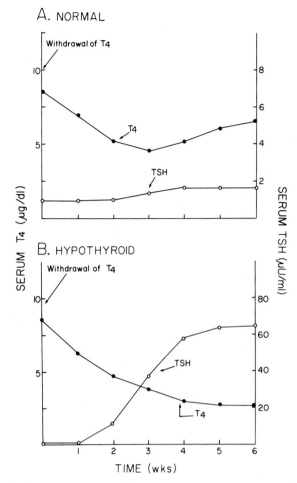

FIGURE 45–6. Serum T_4 and TSH concentrations after discontinuation of T_4 therapy in a normal subject *(A)* and a patient with primary hypothyroidism *(B)*. The serum concentrations of both hormones were within the normal range four weeks after discontinuation in the normal subject, whereas the serum T_4 concentration was low and the serum TSH concentration was high at that time in the patient with hypothyroidism. Conversion factors for Systeme International units: T_4, µg/dl × 12.8 = nmol/L; TSH, µU/ml = mU/L.

tion to normal, so that a substantial quantity of unbound T_4 is available to the tissues.[143] With the use of large doses of T_4, pulse rate, cardiac index, blood pressure, and temperature increase and mental status improves within 24 hours.[144, 145] Use of T_3, alone or in combination with T_4, has been advocated.[141] T_3 acts more rapidly and extrathyroidal conversion of T_4 to T_3 is decreased in these seriously ill patients, and T_3 for parenteral use is now available. However, some evidence suggests that rapid increases in serum T_3 concentrations are more likely to be accompanied by a fatal outcome.[142] Hydrocortisone or a synthetic glucocorticoid should be given intravenously along with T_4, because the patient may have concomitant adrenal insufficiency.

Supportive therapy is as important as hormonal therapy. Ventilatory assistance may be needed. Infection should be

TABLE 45–5. CLINICAL FEATURES OF MYXEDEMA COMA

Hypothermia	Hypotension
Hypoventilation and respiratory acidosis	Seizures
Hyponatremia	Hypoglycemia

sought and treated appropriately. Fluid replacement should be given cautiously, because insensible loss is decreased and water loads are excreted poorly. Water intoxication and hyponatremia should be treated by fluid restriction. Further heat loss should be prevented by adequate covering, but active rewarming is not indicated because it can cause vasodilatation and vascular collapse. These measures result in recovery of more than 50 per cent of patients with myxedema coma.

REFERENCES

1. Helfand M, Crapo LM: Screening for thyroid disease. Ann Intern Med 112:840–849, 1990.
2. Tunbridge WMG, Caldwell G: The epidemiology of thyroid diseases. *In* Braverman LE, Utiger RD (eds): The Thyroid: A Fundamental and Clinical Text (ed 6). Philadelphia, JB Lippincott, 1991, pp 578–587.
3. Nicoloff JT, Low JC, Dussault JH, Fisher DA: Simultaneous measurement of thyroxine and triiodothyronine peripheral turnover kinetics in man. J Clin Invest 51:473–483, 1972.
4. Bianchi R, Pilo A, Mariani G, et al: Comparison of plasma and urinary methods for the direct measurement of the thyroxine to 3,5,3'-triiodothyronine conversion rate in man. J Clin Endocrinol Metab 58:993–1002, 1984.
5. Laurberg P: Mechanisms governing the relative proportions of thyroxine and 3,5,3'-triiodothyronine in thyroid secretion. Metabolism 33:379–392, 1984.
6. Ishii H, Inada M, Tanaka K, et al: Induction of outer and inner ring monodeiodinases in human thyroid gland by thyrotropin. J Clin Endocrinol Metab 57:500–505, 1983.
7. Lum SM, Nicoloff JT, Spencer CA, Kaptein EM: Peripheral tissue mechanism for maintenance of serum triiodothyronine values in a thyroxine-deficient state in man. J Clin Invest 73:570–575, 1984.
8. Griffin JE: The dilemma of abnormal thyroid function tests—Is thyroid disease present or not? Am J Med Sci 289:76–99, 1985.
9. De Groot LJ, Quintans J: The causes of autoimmune thyroid disease. Endocr Rev 10:537–562, 1989.
10. Weetman AP: Autoimmune thyroiditis: predisposition and pathogenesis. Clin Endocrinol 36:307–323, 1992.
11. Okamoto Y, Hamada N, Saito H, et al: Thyroid peroxidase activity–inhibiting immunoglobulins in patients with autoimmune thyroid disease. J Clin Endocrinol Metab 68:730–734, 1989.
12. Takasu N, Yamada T, Takasu M, et al: Disappearance of thyrotropin-blocking antibodies and spontaneous recovery from hypothyroidism in autoimmune thyroiditis. N Engl J Med 326:513–518, 1992.
13. Chiovato L, Vitti P, Santini F, et al: Incidence of antibodies blocking thyrotropin effect *in vitro* in patients with euthyroid or hypothyroid autoimmune thyroiditis. J Clin Endocrinol Metab 71:40–45, 1990.
14. Sato K, Okamura K, Yoshinari M, et al: Goitrous hypothyroidism with blocking or stimulating thyrotropin binding inhibitor immunoglobulins. J Clin Endocrinol Metab 71:855–860, 1990.
15. Tomer Y, Davies TF: Infection, thyroid disease, and autoimmunity. Endocr Rev 14:107–120, 1993.
16. Parle JV, Franklyn JA, Cross KW, et al: Prevalence and follow-up of abnormal thyrotrophin (TSH) concentrations in the elderly in the United Kingdom. Clin Endocrinol 34:77–83, 1991.
17. Tunbridge WMG, Brewis M, French JM, et al: Natural history of autoimmune thyroiditis. Br Med J 282:258–262, 1981.
18. Hayashi Y, Tamai H, Fukata S, et al: A long term clinical, immunological, and histological follow-up study of patients with goitrous chronic lymphocytic thyroiditis. J Clin Endocrinol Metab 61:1172–1178, 1985.
19. Nikolai TF: Recovery of thyroid function in primary hypothyroidism. Am J Med Sci 297:18–21, 1989.
20. Takasu N, Yamada T, Sato A, et al: Graves' disease following hypothyroidism due to Hashimoto's disease: Studies of eight cases. Clin Endocrinol 33:687–698, 1990.
21. Tamai H, Kasagi K, Takaichi Y, et al: Development of spontaneous hypothyroidism in patients with Graves' disease treated with antithyroidal drugs: Clinical, immunological, and histological findings in 26 patients. J Clin Endocrinol Metab 69:49–53, 1989.
22. Holm L-E, Blomgren H, Lowhagen T: Cancer risks in patients with chronic lymphocytic thyroiditis. N Engl J Med 312:601–604, 1985.
23. Nikolai TF: Silent thyroiditis and subacute thyroiditis. *In* Braverman LE, Utiger RD (eds): The Thyroid: A Fundamental and Clinical Text (ed 6). Philadelphia, JB Lippincott, 1991, pp 710–727.
24. Gerstein HC: How common is postpartum thyroiditis? A methodologic overview of the literature. Arch Intern Med 150:1397–1400, 1990.
25. Learoyd DL, Fung HYM, McGregor AM: Postpartum thyroid dysfunction. Thyroid 2:73–80, 1992.
26. Othman S, Phillips DIW, Parkes AB, et al: A long-term follow-up of postpartum thyroiditis. Clin Endocrinol 32:559–564, 1990.
27. Cunnien AJ, Hay ID, Gorman CA, et al: Radioiodine-induced hypothyroidism in Graves' disease: Factors associated with the increasing incidence. J Nucl Med 23:978–983, 1982.
28. Sridama V, McCormick M, Kaplan EL, et al: Long-term follow-up study of compensated low-dose ^{131}I therapy for Graves' disease. N Engl J Med 311:426–432, 1984.
29. Orgiazzi J: Management of Graves' hyperthyroidism. Endocrinol Metab Clin North Am 16:365–389, 1987.
30. Franklyn JA, Daykin J, Droic Z, et al: Long-term follow-up of treatment of thyrotoxicosis by three different methods. Clin Endocrinol 34:71–76, 1991.
31. Toft AD, Irvine WJ, Seth J, et al: Thyroid function in the long-term follow-up of patients treated with iodine-131 for thyrotoxicosis. Lancet 2:576–578, 1975.
32. Davies PH, Franklyn JA, Daykin J, Sheppard MC: The significance of TSH values measured in a sensitive assay in the follow-up of hyperthyroid patients treated with radioiodine. J Clin Endocrinol Metab 74:1189–1194, 1992.
33. Schimpff SC, Diggs CH, Wiswell JG, et al: Radiation-related thyroid dysfunction. Implications for the treatment of Hodgkin's disease. Ann Intern Med 92:91–98, 1980.
34. Hancock SL, Cox RS, McDougall IR: Thyroid diseases after treatment of Hodgkin's disease. N Engl J Med 325:599–605, 1991.
35. Littley MD, Shalet SM, Morgenstern GR, Deakin DP: Endocrine and reproductive dysfunction following fractionated total body irradiation in adults. Q J Med 78:265–274, 1991.
36. Tamai H, Suemastu H, Kurokawa N, et al: Alterations in circulating thyroid hormones and thyrotropin after complete thyroidectomy. J Clin Endocrinol Metab 48:54–58, 1979.
37. Maier WP, Derrick BM, Marks AD, et al: Long-term follow-up of patients with Grave's disease treated by subtotal thyroidectomy. Am J Surg 147:266–268, 1984.
38. Toft AD, Irvine WJ, Sinclair I, et al: Thyroid function after surgical treatment of thyrotoxicosis. A report of 100 cases treated with propranolol before operation. N Engl J Med 298:643–647, 1978.
39. Vagenakis AG, Braverman LE, Azizi F, et al: Recovery of pituitary thyrotropic function after withdrawal of prolonged thyroid-suppression therapy. N Engl J Med 293:681–684, 1975.
40. Krugman LG, Hershman JM, Chopra IJ, et al: Patterns of recovery of the hypothalamic-pituitary axis in patients taken off chronic thyroid therapy. J Clin Endocrinol Metab 41:70–80, 1975.
41. Barsano CP: Other forms of primary hypothyroidism. *In* Braverman LE, Utiger RD (eds): The Thyroid: A Fundamental and Clinical Text (ed 6). Philadelphia, JB Lippincott, 1991, pp 956–967.
42. Ragni MV, Dekker A, DeRubertis FR, et al: *Pneumocystis carinii* infection presenting as necrotizing thyroiditis and hypothyroidism. Am J Clin Pathol 95:489–493, 1991.
43. Contempre B, Duale NL, Dumont JE, et al: Effect of selenium supplementation on thyroid hormone metabolism in an iodine and selenium deficient population. Clin Endocrinol 36:579–583, 1992.
44. Chow CC, Phillips DIW, Lazarus JH, Parkes AB: Effect of low dose iodide supplementation on thyroid function in potentially susceptible subjects: Are dietary iodide levels in Britain acceptable? Clin Endocrinol 34:413–416, 1991.
45. Roti E, Vagenakis AG: Effect of excess iodide: Clinical aspects. *In* Braverman LE, Utiger RD (eds): The Thyroid: A Fundamental and Clinical Text (ed 6). Philadelphia, JB Lippincott, 1991, pp 390–402.
46. Tajiri J, Higashi K, Morita M, et al: Studies of hypothyroidism in patients with high iodine intake. J Clin Endocrinol Metab 63:412–417, 1986.
47. Figge HL, Figge J: The effects of amiodarone on thyroid hormone function: A review of the physiology and clinical manifestations. J Clin Pharmacol 30:588–595, 1990.
48. Perrild H, Hegedus L, Baastrup PC, et al: Thyroid function and ultrasonically determined thyroid size in patients receiving long-term lithium treatment. Am J Psychiatry 147:1518–1521, 1990.
49. Ronnblom LE, Alm GV, Oberg KE: Autoimmunity after alpha-interferon therapy for malignant carcinoid tumors. Ann Intern Med 115:178–183, 1991.

50. Schwartzentruber DJ, White DE, Zweig MH, et al: Thyroid dysfunction associated with immunotherapy for patients with cancer. Cancer 68:2384–2390, 1991.

51. Kung AWC, Jones BM, Lai CL: Effects of interferon-γ therapy on thyroid function, T-lymphocyte subpopulations and induction of autoantibodies. J Clin Endocrinol Metab 71:1230–1234, 1990.

52. Kaptein EM, Spencer CA, Kamiel MB, Nicoloff JT: Prolonged dopamine administration and thyroid hormone economy in normal and critically ill subjects. J Clin Endocrinol Metab 51:387–393, 1980.

53. Brent GA, Hershman JM: Thyroxine therapy in patients with severe nonthyroidal illnesses and low serum thyroxine concentration. J Clin Endocrinol Metab 63:1–8, 1986.

54. Comtois R, Beauregard H, Somma M, et al: The clinical and endocrine outcome to transsphenoidal microsurgery of nonsecreting pituitary adenomas. Cancer 68:860–866, 1991.

55. Hayashizaki Y, Hiraoka Y, Tatsumi K, et al: Deoxyribonucleic acid analyses of five families with familial inherited thyroid stimulating hormone deficiency. J Clin Endocrinol Metab 71:792–796, 1990.

56. Lecky BRF, Williams TDM, Lightman SL, et al: Myxoedema presenting with chiasmal compression: Resolution after thyroxine replacement. Lancet 1:1347–1350, 1987.

57. Adriaanse R, Romijn JA, Endert E, Wiersinga WM: The nocturnal thyroid-stimulating hormone surge is absent in overt, present in mild primary and equivocal in central hypothyroidism. Acta Endocrinol 126:206–212, 1992

58. Beck-Peccoz P, Amr S, Menezes-Ferreira MM, et al:: Decreased receptor binding of biologically inactive thyrotropin in central hypothyroidism. Effect of treatment with thyrotropin-releasing hormone. N Engl J Med 312:1085–1090, 1985.

59. Sarne DH, Refetoff S, Rosenfield RL, Farriaux JP: Sex hormone-binding globulin in the diagnosis of peripheral tissue resistance to thyroid hormone: The value of changes after short term triiodothyronine administration. J Clin Endocrinol Metab 66:740–746, 1988.

60. Takeda K, Balzano S, Sakurai A, et al: Screening of nineteen unrelated families with generalized resistance to thyroid hormone for known point mutations in the thyroid hormone receptor B gene and the detection of a new mutation. J Clin Invest 87:496–502, 1991.

61. Chatterjee VKK, Nagaya T, Madison LD, et al: Thyroid hormone resistance syndrome: Inhibition of normal receptor function by mutant thyroid hormone receptors. J Clin Invest 87:1977–1984, 1991.

62. Wayne EJ: Clinical and metabolic studies in thyroid disease. Br Med J 1:1–11 and 78–90, 1960.

63. Watanakunakorn C, Hodges RH, Evans TC: Myxedema: A study of 400 cases. Arch Intern Med 116:183–190, 1965.

64. Billewicz WZ, Chapman RS, Crooks J, et al: Statistical methods applied to the diagnosis of hypothyroidism. Q J Med 38:255–266, 1969.

65. Smith TJ, Bahn RS, Gorman CA: Connective tissue, glycosaminoglycans, and diseases of the thyroid. Endocr Rev 10:366–391, 1989.

66. Douglas RC, Jacobson SD: Pathologic changes in adult myxedema: Survey of 10 necropsies. J Clin Endocrinol 17:1354–1363, 1957.

67. Sensenbach W, Madison L, Eisenberg S, Ochs L: The cerebral circulation and metabolism in hyperthyroidism and myxedema. J Clin Invest 33:1434–1440, 1954.

68. Osterweil D, Syndulko K, Cohen SN, et al: Cognitive function in nondemented older adults with hypothyroidism. J Am Geriatr Soc 40:325–335, 1992.

69. Swanson JW, Kelly JJ Jr, McConahey WM: Neurologic aspects of thyroid dysfunction. Mayo Clin Proc 56:504–512, 1981.

70. Beghi E, Delodovici ML, Bogliun G, et al: Hypothyroidism and polyneuropathy. J Neurol Neurosurg Psychiatry 52:1420–1423, 1989.

71. Khaleeli AA, Griffith DG, Edwards RHT: The clinical presentation of hypothyroid myopathy and its relationship to abnormalities in structure and function of skeletal muscle. Clin Endocrinol 19:365–376, 1983.

72. Ladenson PW, Sherman SI, Baughman KL, et al: Reversible alterations in myocardial gene expression in a young man with dilated cardiomyopathy and hypothyroidism. Proc Natl Acad Sci USA 89:5251–5255, 1992.

73. Shenoy MM, Goldman JM: Hypothyroid cardiomyopathy: Echocardiographic documentation of reversibility. Am J Med Sci 294:1–9, 1987.

74. Klein I: Thyroid hormone and the cardiovascular system. Am J Med 88:631–637, 1990.

75. Kuusi T, Taskinen M-R, Nikkila EA: Lipoproteins, lipolytic enzymes, and hormonal status in hypothyroid women at different levels of substitution. J Clin Endocrinol Metab 66:51–56, 1988.

76. Staub J-J, Althaus BU, Engler H, et al: Spectrum of subclinical and overt hypothyroidism: Effect on thyrotropin, prolactin, and thyroid reserve, and metabolic impact on peripheral target tissues. Am J Med 92:631–649, 1992.

77. Becker C: Hypothyroidism and atherosclerotic heart disease: Pathogenesis, medical management, and the role of coronary artery bypass surgery. Endocr Rev 6:432–440, 1985.

78. Grunstein RR, Sullivan CE: Sleep apnea and hypothyroidism: Mechanisms and management. Am J Med 85:775–779, 1988.

79. Siafakas NM, Salesiotou V, Filadativaki V, et al: Respiratory muscle strength in hypothyroidism. Chest 102:189–194, 1992.

80. Gottehrer A, Roa J, Stanford GG, et al: Hypothyroidism and pleural effusions. Chest 98:1130–1132, 1990.

81. Parving H-H, Hansen JM, Nielsen SL, et al: Mechanism of edema formation in myxedema—Increased protein extravasation and relatively slow lymphatic drainage. N Engl J Med 301:460–465, 1979.

82. Zimmerman RS, Gharib H, Zimmerman D, et al: Atrial natriuretic peptide in hypothyroidism. J Clin Endocrinol Metab 64:353–355, 1987.

83. Iwasaki Y, Oiso Y, Yamauchi K, et al: Osmoregulation of plasma vasopressin in myxedema. J Clin Endocrinol Metab 70:534–539, 1990.

84. Skowsky WR, Kikuchi TA: The role of vasopressin in the impaired water excretion of myxedema. Am J Med 64:613–621, 1978.

85. Tachman MC, Guthrie GP Jr: Hypothyroidism: Diversity of presentation. Endocr Rev 5:456–465, 1984.

86. Das KC, Mukherjee M, Sarkar TK, et al: Erythropoiesis and erythropoietin in hypo- and hyperthyroidism. J Clin Endocrinol Metab 40:211–220, 1975.

87. Rogers JS, Shane SR, Jencks FS: Factor VIII activity and thyroid function. Ann Intern Med 97:713–716, 1982.

88. Hoogwerf BJ, Nuttal FQ: Long-term weight regulation in treated hyperthyroid and hypothyroid subjects. Am J Med 76:963–970, 1984.

89. Lenzen S, Bailey CJ: Thyroid hormones, gonadal and adrenocortical steroids and the function of the islets of Langerhans. Endocr Rev 5:411–434, 1984.

90. Valcavi R, Dieguez C, Preece M, et al: Effect of thyroxine replacement therapy on plasma insulin-like growth factor I levels and growth hormone responses to growth hormone releasing factor in hypothyroid patients. Clin Endocrinol 27:85–90, 1987

91. Chernausek SL, Turner R: Attenuation of spontaneous, nocturnal growth hormone secretion in children with primary hypothyroidism and its correlation with plasma insulin-like growth factor I concentrations. J Pediatrics 114:968–972, 1989.

92. Contreras P, Generini G, Michelsen H, et al: Hyperprolactinemia and galactorrhea: Spontaneous versus iatrogenic hypothyroidism. J Clin Endocrinol Metab 53:1036–1039, 1981.

93. Iranmanesh A, Lizarralde G, Veldhuis JD: Robustness of the male lactotropic axis to the hyperprolactinemic stimulus of primary thyroidal failure. J Clin Endocrinol Metab 74:559–564, 1992.

94. Iranmanesh A, Lizarralde G, Johnson ML, Veldhuis JD: Dynamics of 24-hour endogenous cortisol secretion and clearance in primary hypothyroidism assessed before and after partial thyroid hormone replacement. J Clin Endocrinol Metab 70:155–161, 1990.

95. Kamilaris TC, DeBold CR, Pavlou SN, et al: Effect of altered thyroid hormone levels on hypothalamic-pituitary-adrenal function. J Clin Endocrinol Metab 65:994–999, 1987.

96. Topliss DJ, White EL, Stockigt JR: Significance of thyrotropin excess in untreated primary adrenal insufficiency. J Clin Endocrinol Metab 50:52–56, 1980.

97. Levey GS: Catecholamine–thyroid hormone interactions and the cardiovascular manifestations of hyperthyroidism. Am J Med 88:642–646, 1990.

98. Polikar R, Kennedy B, Maisel A, et al: Decreased adrenergic sensitivity in patients with hypothyroidism. J Am Coll Cardiol 15:94–98, 1990.

99. Baran DT: The skeletal system in hypothyroidism. In Braverman LE, Utiger RD (eds): The Thyroid: A Fundamental and Clinical Text (ed 6). Philadelphia, JB Lippincott, 1991, pp 1056–1063.

100. Body J-J, DeMeester-Mirkine N, Borkowski A, et al: Calcitonin deficiency in primary hypothyroidism. J Clin Endocrinol Metab 62:700–703, 1986.

101. Thomas R, Reid RL: Thyroid disease and reproductive dysfunction: A review. Obstet Gynecol 70:789–798, 1987

102. Wortsman J, Rosner W, Dufau ML: Abnormal testicular function in men with primary hypothyroidism. Am J Med 82:207–212, 1987.

103. Davis LE, Leveno KJ, Cunningham FG: Hypothyroidism complicating pregnancy. Obstet Gynecol 72:108–112, 1988.

104. Klein RZ, Haddow JE, Faix JD, et al: Prevalence of thyroid deficiency in pregnant women. Clin Endocrinol 35:41–46, 1991.

105. Stagnaro-Green A, Roman SH, Cobin RH, et al: Detection of at-risk pregnancy by means of highly sensitive assays for thyroid autoantibodies. JAMA 264:1422–1425, 1990.
106. Shulkin BL, Utiger RD: Caloric restriction does not alter thyrotropin secretion in hypothyroidism. J Clin Endocrinol Metab 60:1076–1080, 1985.
107. Brent GA, Hershman JM, Braunstein GD: Patients with severe nonthyroidal illness and serum thyrotropin concentrations in the hypothyroid range. Am J Med 81:463–466, 1986.
108. Weinberg AD, Brennan MD, Gorman CA, et al: Outcome of anesthesia and surgery in hypothyroid patients. Arch Intern Med 143:893–897, 1983.
109. Ladenson PW, Levin AA, Ridgway EC, Daniels GH: Complications of surgery in hypothyroid patients. Am J Med 77:261–266, 1984.
110. Drucker DJ, Burrow GN: Cardiovascular surgery in the hypothyroid patient. Arch Intern Med 145:1585–1587, 1985.
111. Hamblin PS, Dyer SA, Mohr VS, et al: Relationship between thyrotropin and thyroxine changes during recovery from severe hypothyroxinemia of critical illness. J Clin Endocrinol Metab 62:717–722, 1986.
112. Kahn BB, Weintraub BD, Csako G, Zweig MH: Factitious elevation of thyrotropin in a new ultrasensitive assay: Implications for the use of monoclonal antibodies in "sandwich" immunoassay. J Clin Endocrinol Metab 66:526–533, 1988.
113. Spencer C, Eigen A, Shen D, et al: Specificity of sensitive assays of thyrotropin (TSH) used to screen for thyroid disease in hospitalized patients. Clin Chem 33:1391–1395, 1987.
114. Keating FR Jr, Parkin TW, Selby JB, Dickinson LS: Treatment of heart disease associated with myxedema. Prog Cardiovasc Dis 3:364–381, 1961.
115. Sherman SI, Ladenson PW: Percutaneous transluminal coronary angioplasty in hypothyroidism. Am J Med 90:367–370, 1991.
116. Polikar R, Feld GK, Dittrich HC, et al: Effect of thyroid replacement therapy on the frequency of benign atrial and ventricular arrhythmias. J Am Coll Cardiol 14:999–1002, 1989.
117. Fish LH, Schwartz HL, Cavanaugh J, et al: Replacement dose, metabolism, and bioavailability of levothyroxine in the treatment of hypothyroidism. Role of triiodothyronine in pituitary feedback in humans. N Engl J Med 316:764–770, 1987.
118. Saberi M, Utiger RD: Serum thyroid hormone and thyrotropin concentrations during thyroxine and triiodothyronine therapy. J Clin Endocrinol Metab 39:923–927, 1974.
119. Kabadi UM: Optimal daily levothyroxine dose in primary hypothyroidism. Its relation to pretreatment thyroid hormone indexes. Arch Intern Med 149:2209–2212, 1989.
120. Utiger RD: Therapy of hypothyroidism. When are changes needed? N Engl J Med 323:126–127, 1990.
121. Harmon SM, Seifert CF: Levothyroxine-cholestyramine interaction reemphasized. Ann Intern Med 115:658–659, 1991.
122. Havrankova J, Lahaie R: Levothyroxine binding by sucralfate. Ann Intern Med 117:445–446, 1992.
123. Campbell NRC, Hasinoff BB, Stalts H, et al: Ferrous sulfate reduces thyroxine efficacy in patients with hypothyroidism. Ann Intern Med 117:1010–1013, 1992.
124. Sperber AD, Liel Y: Evidence for interference with the intestinal absorption of levothyroxine sodium by aluminum hydroxide. Arch Intern Med 152:183–184, 1992.
125. Mandel SJ, Larsen PR, Seely EW, Brent GA: Increased need for thyroxine during pregnancy in women with primary hypothyroidism. N Engl J Med 323:91–96, 1990.
126. Kaplan MM: Monitoring thyroxine therapy during pregnancy. Thyroid 2:147–152, 1992.
127. Burger AG: Effects of pharmacologic agents on thyroid hormone metabolism. In Braverman LE, Utiger RD (eds): The Thyroid: A Fundamental and Clinical Text (ed 6). Philadelphia, JB Lippincott, 1991, pp 335–346.
128. Figge J, Dluhy RG: Amiodarone-induced elevation of thyroid stimulating hormone in patients receiving levothyroxine for primary hypothyroidism. Ann Intern Med 113:553–555, 1990.
129. Ain KB, Refetoff S, Fein HG, Weintraub BD: Pseudomalabsorption of levothyroxine. JAMA 266:2118–2120, 1991.
130. Bearcroft CP, Toms GC, Williams SJ, et al: Thyroxine replacement in post-radioiodine hypothyroidism. Clin Endocrinol 34:115–118 1991.
131. Griffin JE: Hypothyroidism in the elderly. Am J Med Sci 299:334–345, 1990.
132. England ML, Hershman JM: Serum TSH concentration as an aid to monitoring compliance with thyroid hormone therapy in hypothyroidism. Am J Med Sci 292:264–266, 1986.
133. Arem R, Patsch W: Lipoprotein and apolipoprotein levels in subclinical hypothyroidism. Arch Intern Med 150:2097–2100, 1990.
134. Greenspan SL, Greenspan FS, Resnick NM, et al: Skeletal integrity in premenopausal and postmenopausal women receiving long-term L-thyroxine therapy. Am J Med 91:5–14, 1991.
135. Franklyn JA, Betteridge J, Daykin J, et al: Long-term thyroxine treatment and bone mineral density. Lancet 340:9–13, 1992.
136. Leese GP, Jung RT, Guthrie C, et al: Morbidity in patients on L-thyroxine: A comparison of those with a normal TSH to those with a suppressed TSH. Clin Endocrinol 37:500–503, 1992.
137. Petersen K, Bengtsson C, Lapidus L, et al: Morbidity, mortality, and quality of life for patients treated with levothyroxine. Arch Intern Med 150:2077–2081, 1990.
138. Ross DS: Subclinical hypothyroidism. In Braverman LE, Utiger RD (eds): The Thyroid: A Fundamental and Clinical Text (ed 6). Philadelphia, JB Lippincott, 1991, pp 1256–1262.
139. Cooper DS, Halpern R, Wood LC, et al: L-Thyroxine therapy in subclinical hypothyroidism: A double-blind, placebo-controlled trial. Ann Intern Med 101:18–24, 1984.
140. Nystrom E, Caidahl K, Fager G, et al: A double-blind cross-over 12-month study of L-thyroxine treatment of women with 'subclinical' hypothyroidism. Clin Endocrinol 29:63–76, 1988.
141. Wartofsky L: Myxedema coma. In Braverman LE, Utiger RD (ed): The Thyroid: A Fundamental and Clinical Text (ed 6). Philadelphia, JB Lippincott, 1991, pp 1084–1091.
142. Hylander B, Rosenqvist U: Treatment of myxoedema coma—factors associated with fatal outcome. Acta Endocrinol (Copenh) 108:65–71, 1985.
143. Ridgway EC, McCammon JA, Benotti J, Maloof F: Acute metabolic responses in myxedema to large doses of intravenous L-thyroxine. Ann Intern Med 77:549–555, 1972.
144. Kaptein EM, Quion-Verde H, Swinney RS, et al: Acute hemodynamic effects of levothyroxine loading in critically ill hypothyroid patients. Arch Intern Med 146:662–666, 1986.
145. Arlot S, Debussche X, Lalau J-D, et al: Myxoedema coma: Response of thyroid hormones with oral and intravenous high-dose L-thyroxine treatment. Intensive Care Med 17:16–18, 1991.

46

Multinodular Goiter*

HUGO STUDER
HANS GERBER

DEFINITION AND FUNDAMENTAL CONSIDERATIONS

Nodular goiters result from focal hyperplasia of follicular cells at one site or, most often, at multiple sites within the thyroid gland. The basic process in goitrogenesis is the generation of new follicular cells, which are used either to form new follicles or to enlarge the size of the newly formed follicles.[1, 2] The sprouting of a capillary network, embedded in stromal cells, is a necessary secondary event.

The driving force behind multinodular goiter growth is an intrinsically abnormal growth potential of a small fraction of all thyroid cells[1-5] in much the same way as in other benign tumors. Extrathyroidal factors, such as thyroid-stimulating hormone (TSH), may act upon this basic process and thereby accelerate goiter growth.

Two types of nodular goiter may be distinguished. In the first type, the thyroid contains a single nodule or a limited number of well-encapsulated nodules embedded in an otherwise normal parenchyma. Such nodules, considered to be true adenomas or benign thyroid tumors grown from a single cell clone,[6, 7] are rare.[8] They are characterized by a thoroughly uniform structure and function and by an equally uniform growth pattern. In the second, much more common type of nodular goiter, the entire gland may be littered with nodules of widely varying size and structure. No morphological, functional, or biochemical characteristic clearly distinguishes these nodules from the extranodular tissue. Nor does any reliable criterion exist for unequivocally characterizing a true adenoma and delimiting it against focal hyperplasia except, by definition, demonstration of a clonal marker.[9-11b]

It has only recently been shown that even monoclonal adenomas may consist of morphologically and functionally heterogeneous follicles indistinguishable from those characterizing clonal nodules.[11a] Thus, clonal adenomas are un-doubtedly more common than hitherto thought on grounds of morphological criteria only.[2, 12, 13]

Multinodular goiters are invariably able to produce enough T_4 and T_3 to maintain euthyroidism. Excess hormone production with subsequent clinical hyperthyroidism is, however, a frequent complication.[1, 2, 14, 15]

MORPHOLOGICAL AND FUNCTIONAL HETEROGENEITY

The macroscopic, histological, and autoradiographic aspects of simple goiters are extremely variable. At one end of the large spectrum are scattered tiny nodules consisting of small clusters of morphologically normal but functionally abnormal follicles that take up iodide at a slower or faster rate than the surrounding normal tissue. These nodules may be embedded in a little-altered gland.[14] At the other end of the spectrum is the grossly enlarged thyroid containing numerous nodules of widely differing size, structure, and function. In fact, a considerable degree of regional heterogeneity, structural as well as functional, is—together with the invariable nodule formation—the most characteristic hallmark of simple goiters.[1-5, 8, 14-16]

The microscopic appearance of thyroid nodules has been well known since the early days of thyroid histology.[17-19] A nodule may consist either of small follicles or of solid tissue with little stored colloid and high cuboidal cells, or, on the contrary, it may be composed of large follicles containing huge amounts of colloid held together by a thin layer of flat cells. Many nodules contain small as well as large follicles side by side. In addition, varying amounts of hypocellular and/or edematous connective tissue may separate individual follicles or groups of follicles. Cyst formation, hemorrhage, fibrosis, and calcification are common.[6-8, 17-19]

In the normal thyroid gland, small follicles invariably have a more rapid iodine turnover than large ones.[20] In contrast, unordered interfollicular heterogeneity of iodine

*The research work from our own laboratory discussed in this chapter was supported by Swiss National Science Foundation Grant 32-30204.90.

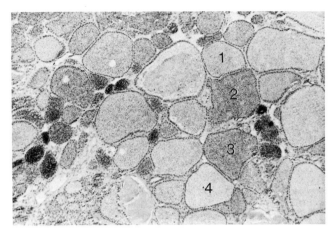

FIGURE 46–1. **Autoradiograph of a hot nodule illustrating interfollicular heterogeneity of iodine metabolism.** [125]I was given 14 days before surgery. (Magnification, ×88. Exposure time, 45 days. Staining, hematoxylin and eosin.) Many follicles of this active nodule escape the law of an inverse correlation between follicular size and relative velocity of intrafollicular iodine turnover characteristic of normal thyroid glands. For example, the follicles numbered 1 to 4 are morphologically similar. Nevertheless, grain density is considerably higher in follicles 2 and 3 than in the adjacent follicles 1 and 4. This is but one illustration of the fundamental functional differences between normal and goiter follicles. In addition, the autoradiograph demonstrates the nearly total lack of correlation between the morphology of a follicle and the intensity of its iodine turnover.

turnover independent of follicular size is the rule in multinodular goiter (Figs. 46–1 to 46–3). Other features of normal thyroid function, such as the finely tuned balance between thyroglobulin synthesis and resorption, resulting in a fairly comparable size of most follicles, are distorted in thyroid nodules.[21] A typical example is given in Figure 46–2: A small nodule consisting mainly of enormous follicles has grown among healthy but somewhat compressed tissue.

This nodule was recognized as being "hot" by its high ^{131}I uptake early after tracer application. Several other similar nodules in this large multinodular goiter illustrate the absence of any correlation between the size and shape of the follicular cells and their functional capacity in terms of iodine transport and organification.[1–4] The joint hormone production of the slowly growing number of all hot follicles causes the insidious appearance of thyrotoxicosis (i.e., Plummer's disease).[14] This was also true for the goiter illustrated in Figure 46–2. Thus, with endogenous thyrotropin (TSH) secretion suppressed, the giant follicles must be growing and functioning autonomously. Normal thyroid follicles were clearly less functional than the nodule, as illustrated by the low density of silver grains over their lumina.

An entirely different example morphologically of a hot nodule is depicted in Figure 46–3. It consists of a cohort of tiny follicles with intense iodine metabolism lying among morphologically identical follicles with very little iodine turnover. Some additional hot follicles are scattered all over. No capsule of connective tissue delimits hot from cold follicles.

Figure 46–4 illustrates that the amount of thyroglobulin stored in thyroid nodules has no correlation whatsoever with radioiodine metabolism. The finding confirms what morphology and autoradiography suggest: the lack of any correlation between morphology and function in many goitrous follicles.[1–4, 14]

In summary, morphological and autoradiographic studies of nodular goiter tissue fail to disclose structural features infallibly characteristic of either hyperfunction or hypofunction. This is particularly evident in autoradiographs from human goiter tissue transplanted to nude mice.[4] Another impressive illustration of functional heterogeneity is provided by the coexistence, within the same goiter, of cold follicles due to a trapping defect with morphologically

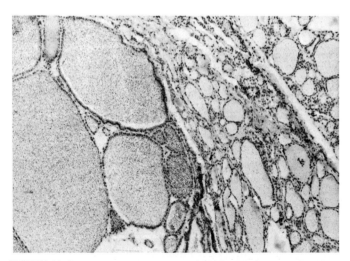

FIGURE 46–2. **Autoradiograph of one of several scintigraphically identified hot nodules in a multinodular toxic goiter.** [125]I was administered 25 days prior to surgery. (Exposure time, 13 days. Magnification, ×88. Staining, hematoxylin and eosin.) [125]I turnover is confined almost exclusively to the follicles within the nodule at left. This is true for all follicles irrespective of their size. Again, no correlation exists between structure and size of a follicle on the one hand and iodine turnover on the other. This nodule, in contrast to those illustrated in Figures 46–1 and 46–3, consists of a few enormously oversized follicles. In this case, newly generated follicular cells were not used to form a large number of microfollicles but, on the contrary, to enlarge the hull of the few new follicles.

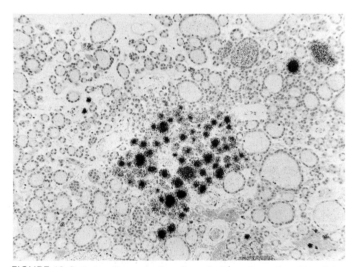

FIGURE 46–3. **Autoradiographed section of a large, hyperthyroid nodular goiter in a 70-year-old male patient.** [125]I was given 17 hours before surgery. (Magnification, ×110. Exposure time, 24 days. Staining, nuclear fast red.) A cohort of tiny follicles with intense iodine metabolism has grown amidst morphologically identical follicles with very little iodine turnover. Additional hot and intermediately active follicles are scattered all over. There is no capsule of connective tissue delimiting hot from cold follicles. Here, a large number of morphologically identical but functionally very heterogeneous microfollicles have been generated in the process of goitrogenesis.

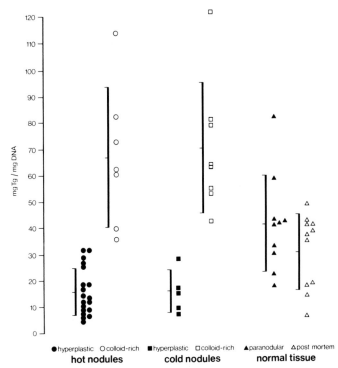

FIGURE 46–4. **Content of thyroglobulin (Tg) in relation to cellularity (expressed as mg of Tg per mg of DNA ± SD) in a series of hot and cold nodules,** identified by ^{131}I scintiscans and compared with normal tissue. Note that cold as well as hot nodules may contain any amount of thyroglobulin. In accordance with this finding, histological classification into hyperplastic and colloid-rich nodules has no relation to iodine metabolism.

identical follicles that are unable to organify the normally trapped iodide.[22] The unique heterogeneity of size, shape, and iodine turnover among the individual follicles is one of the most characteristic hallmarks of nodular goiter.

The autoradiographic findings reported above readily explain why a scintiscan of a nodular goiter with ^{131}I or ^{99m}Tc pertechnetate invariably shows a mottled aspect. This appearance may be caused by different mechanisms: (1) Smaller or larger clusters of hot and cold follicles are scattered throughout the entire goiter[1–4, 14–16, 23] (see Fig. 46–3); (2) the goiter contains hot nodules embedded within normal or suppressed paranodular tissue (see Fig. 46–2)[1–4, 14–16, 23]; and (3) it contains cysts and/or connective tissue in various states of degeneration.[8]

Considering the differences of iodide clearance and iodine discharge from one nodule to the other or even from one follicle to its neighbor, the appearance of a ^{131}I scintiscan is expected to vary considerably according to the time elapsed since administration of the tracer.[15, 16, 22, 24–27] Whereas one nodule may display a high tracer uptake within hours and an equally rapid discharge, other nodules still retain their peak radioactivity at a time when the more active nodule has lost most of its [131]I.[22, 26, 27]

If numerous active micronodules are scattered all over a multinodular goiter, the resulting scintiscan can closely resemble that of diffuse goiter. Therefore, such a micronodular goiter may be mistaken for a diffuse goiter of Graves' disease.[14, 28]

In single autonomous adenomas, the degree of suppression of surrounding tissue is believed to be inversely correlated with the amount of hormone produced by the nod-

ule. This rule, however, does not apply to goiters containing autonomously functioning micronodules scattered all over the gland.

If Graves' disease develops in an individual with pre-existing nodular goiter, the scintiscan shows patchy ^{131}I distribution indistinguishable from that in simple multinodular goiter. Correct diagnosis may require additional investigations such as determination of thyroid-stimulating immunoglobulins (TSI's). It may even be impossible without the rarely justified thyroid biopsy.

Studies of ^{131}I or ^{99m}Tc pertechnetate uptake are of limited value in the management of multinodular goiter, because roughly half of all benign thyroid nodules are altogether cold. Therefore, scintigraphy is of little help in deciding whether or not a growing nodule should be surgically explored.[29, 30]

BIOCHEMISTRY

Numerous reports have been made on the biochemistry of iodoproteins in nodular goiter. Most of them are concerned with nonthyroglobulin iodoproteins, which may be present in goiters with congenital defects of hormonogenesis.[31–32a] However, abnormal iodoproteins are not found in the overwhelming majority of endemic or sporadic multinodular goiters.[32–35] Iodoproteins of low molecular weight, different from normal thyroglobulin and resistant to enzymatic hydrolysis, may be intracellularly located, slowly metabolized breakdown products of thyroglobulin hydrolysis.[24, 36, 37] Intracellular iodine stores have recently been optically visualized by analytical ion microscopy.[38] They may be more relevant than the bulk of extracellularly located, thyroglobulin-bound iodine in explaining the pharmacological actions of iodine on thyroid function and growth.[25]

Thyroglobulin in endemic or sporadic nodular goiter is often poorly iodinated but can be readily iodinated in vitro.[33, 39, 40] The simplest explanation for the pathogenesis of poorly iodinated thyroglobulin in the absence of iodine shortage is the loss of normal synchronization, in goiter follicles, between the cellular processes of thyroglobulin synthesis and endocytosis on the one hand and iodide transport and organification on the other hand. This view is supported by the demonstration that the normal correlation between the number of cells per unit of thyroid weight and its thyroglobulin content is lost in many follicles of simple goiters (Fig. 46–4).[41] If thyroglobulin synthesis proceeds at a higher rate than endocytosis and iodide transport, storage of poorly iodinated thyroglobulin results.

Low iodination of thyroglobulin is a very serious handicap for hormone synthesis[25, 33, 35] and has a profound impact on thyroidal iodine turnover.[25] Indeed, iodine content is the most decisive single factor regulating the iodothyronine content of thyroglobulin. The ratio of iodothyronine to iodotyrosine residues is severely depressed in poorly iodinated thyroglobulin.[25, 35] Consequently, a larger fraction of poorly iodinated thyroglobulin must be broken down in order to produce the same amount of hormone.

Several intrathyroidal mechanisms are designed to optimize the efficiency of hormone synthesis. One is the particular structure of the thyroglobulin molecule itself, which contains distinct domains designed for optimal iodothyronine synthesis (see Ch. 34).[32a] Another, rarely considered but probably highly efficient mechanism is the rapidly changing colloid viscosity, depending on thyroglobulin iodination, which regulates the availability of thyroglobulin molecules at the apical cell border for further iodination and iodotyrosine coupling.[42–44] Eventually there may be a mechanism permitting the preferential endocytosis of higher iodinated thyroglobulin molecules.[45]

The concentration of total iodine per gram of wet tissue is low in most multinodular goiters, although this is not true for every single area within a goiter.[41] The total amount of iodine per goiter is, surprisingly enough, as high as or even higher than in normal glands but not all iodine stores may be available for hormone synthesis.[24, 25] Even within the lumen of goitrous follicles, thyroglobulin may become compartmentalized and, thus, unavailable to free diffusion and hormone synthesis.[24, 25, 43, 44, 46] Thyroglobulin storage and iodine uptake are—to a considerable extent—independent mechanisms. Highly iodinated thyroglobulin is characteristically found in hyperplastic hot nodules, whereas poorly iodinated thyroglobulin can be obtained from cold as well as from hot nodules[41] (Fig. 46–5). Moreover, even normal thyroid tissue may contain thyroglobulin embracing a large spectrum of different iodine concentrations.

PATHOGENESIS

Generation of Heterogeneity

In addition to somatic mutations leading to clonal tumor growth (see Ch. 50), three basically different phenomena are involved in the generation of the tremendous regional heterogeneity of growth, structure, and function[1–5, 12–16, 23, 47, 48] of multinodular human goiters. The first is the pre-existing constitutive heterogeneity of normal follicular epithelial cells, which accounts for the highly individual traits of the progenies of different epithelial cells generated during goitrogenesis.[1–5, 12–16, 47, 49, 50] The second process is the acquisition by replicating follicular cells of new inheritable qualities,[1–4, 23, 47, 51, 52] and the third is the appearance of secondary structural abnormalities in the newly generated goiter tissue. These three processes are considered separately.

CONSTITUTIVE HETEROGENEITY OF NORMAL FOLLICULAR CELLS. A normal follicle consists of a number of cell subsets with widely differing qualities. For instance, some normal follicular cells have a very high capacity to iodinate thyroglobulin whereas others nearly totally lack this quality.[1–4, 23, 53] Similarly, large differences in the peroxidase content may exist between different cell subpopulations within the same follicle.[1, 2, 28] Perhaps most impressive is the enormous variation in growth potential among the many cell families building up a single follicle.[1–5, 13, 23, 49, 50] Some of the cells may have constitutively active growth mechanisms enabling them to proliferate autonomously in much the same way as the cells of other benign tumors (Figs. 46–6 to 46–8).[1–5, 12, 13, 23, 54] This type of stable intercellular heterogeneity is not due to somatic mutations but to a number of epigenetic mechanisms, whose ability to stably change the phenotype and function of daughter cells and their progeny becomes increasingly known. (This important issue is discussed in

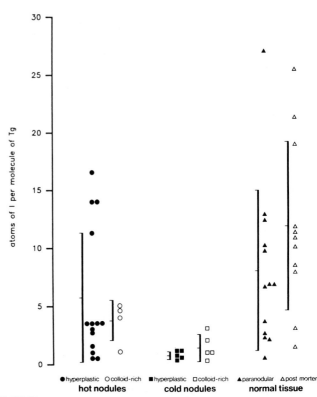

FIGURE 46–5. Degree of thyroglobulin (Tg) iodination in hot and cold nodules compared with normal thyroid tissue. Whereas poorly iodinated thyroglobulin occurs in hot nodules as well as in cold nodules or normal tissue, a high degree of iodination is not found in cold nodules. Again, the histological picture is not related to thyroglobulin iodination. Note that even thyroid glands considered to be normal contain thyroglobulin with extremely variable levels of iodination.

the following paragraph). Somatic mutations may of course occur in dividing cells in addition to their diversity caused by epigenetic events. A number of these genomic mutations produce changes in the structure of proteins involved in the control of cell growth such as the *ras*-oncogene

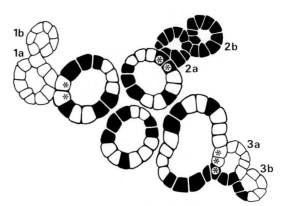

FIGURE 46–6. Generation of two consecutive progenies of heterogeneous daughter follicles from normal polyclonal mother follicles. Asterisks (*) indicate normal follicular cells with a high intrinsic growth potential transmissible to the offspring. The whole progeny therefore divides at a higher than average rate, either autonomously or in response to an extrathyroidal stimulus such as TSH. Solid black, high peroxidase content; solid white, low peroxidase content; 1, cold follicle; 2, hot follicle; 3, mixed follicle. (From Gerber H, Peter HJ, Ramelli F, et al: Autonomie und Heterogenität der Follikel in der euthyreoten und hyperthyreoten menschlichen Knotenstruma: Die Lösung alter Rätsel? Schweiz Med Wochenschr 113:1178, 1983.)

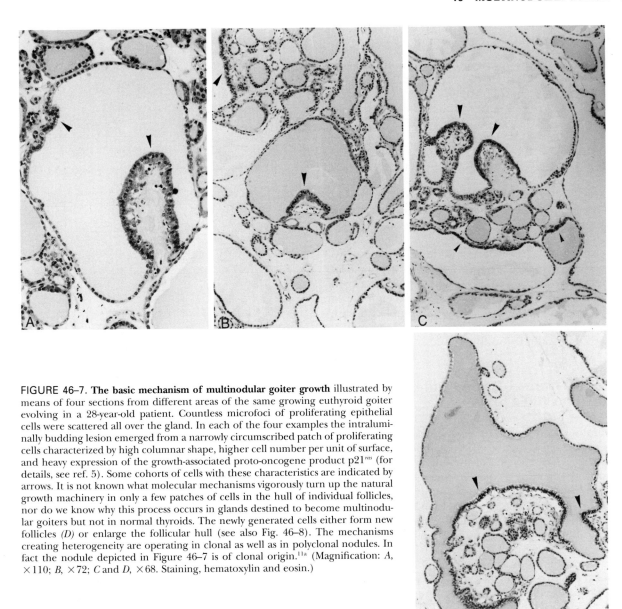

FIGURE 46–7. **The basic mechanism of multinodular goiter growth** illustrated by means of four sections from different areas of the same growing euthyroid goiter evolving in a 28-year-old patient. Countless microfoci of proliferating epithelial cells were scattered all over the gland. In each of the four examples the intraluminally budding lesion emerged from a narrowly circumscribed patch of proliferating cells characterized by high columnar shape, higher cell number per unit of surface, and heavy expression of the growth-associated proto-oncogene product p21^{ras} (for details, see ref. 5). Some cohorts of cells with these characteristics are indicated by arrows. It is not known what molecular mechanisms vigorously turn up the natural growth machinery in only a few patches of cells in the hull of individual follicles, nor do we know why this process occurs in glands destined to become multinodular goiters but not in normal thyroids. The newly generated cells either form new follicles (D) or enlarge the follicular hull (see also Fig. 46–8). The mechanisms creating heterogeneity are operating in clonal as well as in polyclonal nodules. In fact the nodule depicted in Figure 46–7 is of clonal origin.[11a] (Magnification: A, ×110; B, ×72; C and D, ×68. Staining, hematoxylin and eosin.)

products. This process may provide the cell with a powerful growth advantage that leads to clonal expansion and thus to the formation of true adenomas and, eventually, to carcinoma.[8–11] These mechanisms are fully considered in Chapter 50. (See also later section on Formation of Nodules, Adenomas, and Tumors.)

ACQUISITION OF NEW INHERITABLE QUALITIES BY REPLICATING EPITHELIAL CELLS. Modern molecular biology has recognized that gene expression of a cell is less uniform and immutable than hitherto thought and that newly generated cells may well acquire qualities not previously present in mother cells by mechanisms that do not involve genomic mutations.[2, 4, 47, 55–65] New qualities may also be passed on from mother to daughter cells by extrachromosomal mechanisms.[55] Although the appearance of entirely new cell qualities by mechanisms operating in addition to somatic mutation is well known in malignant tumors,[55–59] intercellular heterogeneity has rather recently been recognized to be a feature of normal cells as well.[2–4, 48, 60–65] Growing, simple goiters provide unique examples of the acqui-

sition of new inheritable properties by some cell sublines of autonomously replicating benign human tissue.[2, 4, 47] The most impressive example of this process is the abnormal growth pattern of all or part of the goitrous tissue that is faithfully reproduced when a tiny sample grows as a transplant in a nude mouse.[4, 54] Other regionally variable functional properties of human goitrous tissue, such as responsiveness to TSH,[2, 3, 41, 47, 48] may arise in the same way. Heterogeneity of growth and TSH dependence commonly arise in the subclones of a cloned rat thyroid FRTL-5 cell line, and their individual growth traits are stable in subsequent passages.[52] An in vivo example of autonomous replication of thyroid follicular cells is provided by nodular goiters in aging cats.[54] Follicles from these goiters grow autonomously when seeded into a defined medium not containing TSH.[66]

SECONDARY FUNCTIONAL AND STRUCTURAL ABNORMALITIES IN GROWING GOITERS. New follicles produced during goitrogenesis may have widely differing qualities depending on the individual mother cells from which they originate. Replicating follicular cells with a high thyroglobulin and colloid production rate but low capacity for endocytosis produce large follicles. Cells with a constitutively active endocytotic machinery[21] generate microfollicles, whereas some cells with a low morphogenetic potential[67] produce solid tissue when growing. In addition, morphological[68] and histochemical[69, 69a] evidence indicates that follicles of the second and subsequent generations, formed during goiter growth, are less perfectly built than their mother follicles. For instance, the highly sophisticated compartmentalization of key enzymes may become altered.[69] If so, the system of intercellular communication may be distorted, and the long chain of biochemical events linking TSH receptors to ultimate follicular response[31] may be disrupted.[41] As a consequence, the multiple coordinated functions of a single follicle, such as iodide transport, thyroglobulin synthesis, storage, endocytosis, and deiodination, may become desynchronized. A striking example of the impact of the secondary failure of a particular cell function comes from the conversion, in the aging mouse and hamster thyroid, of an ever-increasing number of follicles into oversized, colloid-stuffed, and functionless units.[70–73]

Growth of the Normal Thyroid and Its Transformation into a Goiter

TSH is undoubtedly by far the most important stimulator of thyroid growth and function under physiological in vivo conditions.[31, 74] However, experimental results, obtained mostly with cell cultures, have clearly established the growth-promoting effect of some ubiquitous cytokines such as insulin-like growth factor (IGF) I and II, epidermal growth factor, and perhaps fibroblast growth factor[75] and the growth-inhibiting action of others such as transforming growth factor (TGF)-β[75] (see also Ch. 35). Their role for in vivo growth remains to be clarified, but there is no doubt that the local production of such growth factors, including proto-oncogene products, is severely altered in nodular goiters.[5, 11a] This has been shown for IGF, which is produced in loco by autonomously growing thyroid nodules.[76–78] Although few authors doubt the decisive role of TSH in endemic goiter caused by iodine deficiency (see Ch. 49), multinodular goiter has a different pathogenesis in nonendemic areas. In this case, it is an intrinsic disease of the thyroid gland: To put it in the simplest terms, multinodular goiter is a multifocally growing benign tumor of the thyroid gland.[3, 5, 11a] Indeed, it has recently been demonstrated that growth of nodular goiter proceeds by episodic, autonomous replication of a multitude of cell cohorts scattered all over the single nodules and even over presumably normal extranodular tissue (see Fig. 46–7).[5]

It is on this substrate that extrathyroidal growth-stimulating agents such as TSH (in the case of iodine deficiency) or TSI's (in the case of Graves' disease) may come to act. Some authors have described "growth-stimulating immunoglobulins" (GSI) in patients with nodular goiters.[79–81] Whatever extrathyroidal stimulus may be present, the inevitable nodularity of a long-standing goiter can be understood only if the constitutive heterogeneity of the growth response between individual cells is taken into account.[1–5]

If thyroid-stimulating agents are present in the blood stream in high concentration, diffuse hyperplastic goiters

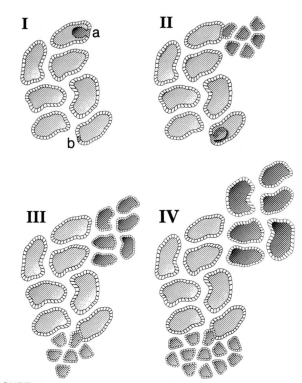

FIGURE 46–8. Diagrammatic illustration of the two most frequent variants in the natural evolution of autonomously growing microfoci (see Fig. 46–7) during goitrogenesis. Focus a first produces six new follicles (I). Thereafter, the newly generated cells are built into the steadily enlarging follicular monolayer, which may grow from a tiny paucicellular ball to a voluminous hull containing tens of thousands of cells (II to IV). This process of colloid goiter formation takes place whenever the newly produced cells belong to a progeny whose colloid-producing capacity prevails over its potential to engulf the colloid. Focus b continues to generate new microfollicles made up of cells that promptly resorb the colloid they produce. The natural history of nodular goiter demonstrates that growth can come to a halt at any time.

result. This is illustrated, on the one hand, by Graves' disease (see Ch. 41) and, on the other, by the TSH-induced thyroid hyperplasia in severe endemic goiter or in experimentally induced goiters in laboratory animals[21, 71, 82] (see Ch. 49). However, the evolution of an entirely different, intrinsic thyroid disease, namely simple nodular goiter, may be promoted if only small amounts of stimulating agents are circulating in the blood as in the case of slightly increased TSH or of the still controversial GSI.[83, 84] In this case, only the most sensitive of all follicular functions, which is the replication of a few cells with an unusually high growth potential, respond.[1–4] Thus, a weak growth stimulator, be it TSH, GSI, or any other growth factor, accelerates the preferential replication of a progeny of constitutively growth-prone cells. Because proliferation of these particular cells is stimulated without concomitant hypertrophy (which is produced by different mechanisms),[21, 85] gentle growth promotion acting for a long enough time period produces nodules consisting of a large number of new follicles lacking the morphological signs of acute hyperstimulation.[1–5, 23, 28] By the way, even longstanding Graves' goiters invariably become nodular with time.[86] A schematic illustration of the concept of generation of heterogeneity in multinodular goiters by amplification of the natural intercellular heterogeneity of growth and function is given in Figure 46–6. In any case, extrathyroidal stimuli only accelerate the process of goitrogenesis but do not alter the basically intrathyroidal, cellular pathophysiology.

Autonomy of Growth

Normal thyroid glands contain subpopulations of follicular cells with a constitutively high growth potential.[1–4, 49, 50] In the thyroid destined to become a goiter, a fraction of these cells may replicate autonomously, that is, by constitutive activation of the cell's own growth machinery. Some molecular mechanisms causing accelerated cell growth are about to be unraveled.[86a, 86b] These cells, scattered in multiple small foci all over the gland,[2, 5, 11a] divide at variable individual rates even in the absence of TSH,[52] which is the most potent physiological growth stimulator in vivo.[31, 74, 75] TSH may, however, still further accelerate the growth of cells with a high autonomous replication rate. Autonomously growing cells with short interdivision intervals steadily take a larger share of the entire follicular cell population. This process results in the growth of clinically apparent nodules. It may evolve at such a rate that rapidly growing polyclonal and widely heterogeneous nodules appear already in children and young adults.[87, 88] Once the autonomously growing and rapidly dividing cells are present in large enough numbers, the whole thyroid or parts thereof may autonomously grow in the absence of any further extrathyroidal stimulation.[1–4, 23, 28, 89]

Autonomously growing cells in the adult thyroid behave very much like the thyrocytes of fetal glands. Indeed, evidence suggests that these cells have failed to develop the receptor system transforming autonomously growing fetal cells into TSH-dependent adult cells.[51] Identical mechanisms may operate in other benign tumor cells. The largely autonomous, that is, TSH-independent, nature of nonendemic goiter is demonstrated by the common failure of TSH-suppressing doses of T_4 to stop progression of nodular growth, let alone to revert a nodular goiter into a normal thyroid (for a review of recent literature, see ref. 90). However, because TSH, even in low concentrations, is still one of many growth factors, a certain growth-retarding effect is often observed even in largely autonomous goiters.

Autonomy of Function

It has been mentioned before that the normal thyroid contains subsets of cells with constitutively higher than average iodinating capacity.[1–4, 20] If new follicles happen to arise from these cells, they have a high iodine turnover too (see Fig. 46–6). Their intrinsic metabolism is less suppressible by abolition of TSH secretion than that of the genuinely less active sister cells, although some degree of residual autonomous iodine turnover is present in most follicular cells.[1–4, 14–16, 23, 42, 91]

It is important to realize that autonomous function and autonomous growth are entirely unrelated qualities of individual thyroid cells.[4] This explains the common clinical observation that cold areas of a nodular goiter have exactly the same growth potential as hot ones. Similarly, they may both respond or be refractory to TSH-suppressing T_4 treatment.

Formation of Nodules, Adenomas, and Tumors

The pathogenetic concept of nodule formation in multinodular goiters may be summarized as follows: Three basically different processes may cause the nearly invariable nodularity of long-standing simple human goiters and even normal thyroids in aged persons.[1, 2, 8, 92] The first one is the regionally variable prevalence of epithelial cell subsets with high autonomous growth rates in a few follicles. Their growth advantage and their strong tendency to remain clustered after division necessarily cause focal hyperplasia appearing as nodules. Because rapidly replicating cells are otherwise identical with other follicular cells, it is not surprising that most thyroid nodules are functionally and structurally identical with extranodular tissue.[1–6, 8, 12, 23, 47]

The second mechanism of nodule formation is that operating in clonal tumor formation, thought to be due to an early somatic mutation conferring a heritable growth advantage to one single cell (see Ch. 50). Subsequent further mutation and/or chromosomal losses may secondarily alter tumor progression up to the appearance of malignant thyroid tumors. Indeed, clonal tumors, which may be called adenomas in the strict sense of the term, have commonly been observed within nodular goiters in many laboratories, including our own.[9–11a]

The third mechanism that imposes a nodular growth pattern on any slowly expanding goiter is the network of fibrous, inelastic strands of connective tissue woven throughout the goiter parenchyma, which are the late result of scarring of the multiple necroses and hemorrhages in single follicles or entire cohorts of follicles studding any goiter of a certain size. Necrosis occurs in any growing tissue when the sprouting of the newly growing capillary net cannot keep pace with the expansion of the parenchyma.[1, 8]

Excessive Hormone Production

Because the majority of all follicles have at least some degree of nonsuppressible iodine turnover and because many of the newly formed hot follicles have a much higher than average autonomous iodine turnover, the overall hormone production by any nodular goiter depends on the number of new follicles on the one hand and on the relative fraction of cold and hot follicles on the other. Because follicle neogeneration is a slow process, most nodular goiters are euthyroid, and thyrotoxicosis insidiously appears only in the course of many years.[1–4, 14, 28, 54] This is in sharp contrast to the stormy onset of Graves' thyrotoxicosis.[28] The pathogenetic concept of Plummer's disease (i.e. thyrotoxicosis caused by multinodular goiters) is, in essence, that originally proposed by Miller et al. some 30 years ago.[15, 16, 91]

ETIOLOGY

Worldwide the most frequent single cause of endemic multinodular goiter is still iodine deficiency[93, 94] (see Ch. 49). In areas where the iodine supply is scarce, a TSH-mediated compensatory mechanism is set into motion.[24] As a consequence, the thyroid gland diffusely enlarges and, as time passes by, gradually becomes nodular by mechanisms described in the previous section.

Iodine deficiency is not the only cause of endemic goiter, because a high prevalence of goiter has been reported from areas where iodine supply is abundant[95] (for a review, see ref. 93) and because multinodular goiter continues to be a highly prevalent disorder in areas, such as Switzerland, where iodine deficiency has long been eradicated.[96, 97]

The foregoing section on pathogenesis should make it clear that nonendemic nodular goiters are the late results of intrinsic disorders of intracellular growth-control mechanisms, just as in other clonal and polyclonal benign tumors.[5] The molecular basis of the disorder is currently being investigated.[86a, 86b] In clonal thyroid nodules, a somatic cell mutation activating an intrinsic growth control cascade is thought to be the initial culprit (see Ch. 50).

Whereas TSI's cause the goiter of Graves' disease (see Ch. 41), specific GSI's are considered by some authors to be a causative factor in a fraction of nodular goiters.[79–81] Even if the existence of GSI's should be established beyond any doubt,[84] they could only be considered auxiliary factors that accelerate clinical appearance of the intrinsic pathogenetic mechanisms causing regionally differing growth and function of nodular goiters. The same interaction holds true for the action of TSH secretion increased by iodine deficiency or goitrogenic agents.

Since the early work of Bray,[98] low intrathyroidal iodine concentration has episodically been claimed to enhance thyroid growth by itself.[99] Lately, low intrathyroidal stores have been shown to decrease the production of the growth-inhibiting cytokine TGF-β.[100] However, because the bulk of iodine is contained in extracellularly located thyroglobulin and because the extreme compartmentalization of extracellular as well as of intracellular iodocompounds[24, 25] is rarely ever taken into account, we do not think that global assessment of tissue iodine stores has a physiological meaning. A note of caution may also be added for the growth-inhibiting action of pharmacological doses of iodide,[101] because they occur only in a range barely obtained in vivo under physiological conditions.

HEREDITY

The clustering of thyroid diseases, including simple goiters, in some families or pedigrees has prompted a host of investigations on the possible role of hereditary factors in the genesis of euthyroid goiter. Existing evidence indicates that genetic factors help to determine the development of goiter, but no simple mode of inheritance can be postulated.[102] A possible hereditary factor is complex and unlikely to depend solely upon the effect of a single gene.[102]

Since the discovery of inherited disorders of thyroid hormone synthesis (see Ch. 52), the suspicion has arisen that in sporadic and possibly even in endemic goiter such a disorder could be at least an ancillary causative factor.[93, 94] However, up to now, none of the inherited disorders of thyroid hormone synthesis or action have been convincingly demonstrated to be responsible for the bulk of sporadic or endemic multinodular goiter. All abnormalities of iodine metabolism found in this disease may be explained as secondary events.[24] Recent advances in understanding the pathophysiology of nodular goiter growth suggest that

unraveling the hereditary basis of this disease may be a more remote goal than ever thought before. One would first have to understand why in goitrous glands not all cells, but just a tiny fraction of them, have a constitutively activated growth mechanism, brought about by a different setting of many interacting gene activities.

CLINICAL ASPECTS

Natural History

A diffuse enlargement of the thyroid gland is often found in children of both sexes at puberty. In areas with endemic goiter, it is almost invariably present. The diffuse goiter usually disappears in early adolescence. The higher the overall prevalence of simple goiter in a given area, the more frequent are childhood goiters and the more likely is their persistence into adult life, with the gradual appearance of nodularity. From adolescence to old age, there is always a three- to six-fold higher incidence of goiters in women than in men. In countries with high goiter prevalence, such as Switzerland, the percentage of individuals with nodular goiter increases steadily with age.[2, 97, 103] This means that a most common clinical course of multinodular goiter is slow growth extending over several decades. On the other hand, one or several nodules within a multinodular goiter may appear in children and young adults[87, 88] and grow at a very fast pace. Other nodules may apparently change their biological behavior and start growing at a fast pace later in life. This phenomenon may be more apparent than real, because the intrinsic replication rate of the cells is probably unaltered. As with all tumors, a doubling of the volume appears clinically as very rapid growth once the tumor first becomes palpable.[104] At surgery, such nodules may well have a structure similar to that of extranodular tissue.[5, 8] Another frequently observed behavior of nodular goiter is slow growth over several decades with no further changes thereafter. It is indeed very common to see elderly patients, aware of a nodular goiter since their 30s, who have never noticed a change in size or consistency of the enlarged gland. Finally, a large spectrum of retrogressive changes ranging from acute and painful hemorrhage to clinically silent cyst may occur within some or several nodules. In an individual case one cannot usually predict whether the nodules will remain quiet and stable or will keep growing steadily.[29, 30, 105–107]

With respect to iodine uptake and hormone formation, an autonomously functioning thyroid nodule usually retains its functional characteristics unless its follicles are destroyed by regressive changes. A cold thyroid nodule remains so throughout its life span, although it may or may not enlarge its volume. Because even cold nodules, just like normal thyroid follicles, retain a certain degree of TSH-independent iodine uptake and hormone production, it is not surprising that large goiters made up of poorly functioning nodules may eventually produce enough hormone to cause hyperthyroidism.[15] Careful epidemiological studies have established that the most common clinical course of multinodular goiter is a very slow autonomous growth over decades with insidiously increasing hormone production by the newly generated follicles, leading first to TSH suppression and later on to overt hyperthyroidism.[1–4, 14–16, 23, 28, 103, 108]

Thyrotoxicosis in Multinodular Goiter (Plummer's Disease)

A frequent complication of multinodular goiter is thyrotoxicosis, although in both endemic and sporadic goiter, the progression of a small, autonomously functioning thyroid nodule to a large, toxic nodule is the exception rather than the rule.[105, 107] Because Plummer's disease is due to slow multiplication of autonomous hot follicles, hyperthyroidism may be very difficult to recognize, particularly in older patients with accompanying nonthyroidal disease. Occasional laboratory checks of thyroid status are therefore mandatory in every patient with multinodular goiter. A suppressed TSH serum level (see Ch. 39) may point to subclinical thyrotoxicosis, which may or may not progress to overt clinical disease.[108, 109]

A different mechanism is responsible for excessive hormone production in thyrotoxicosis subsequent to exogenous iodide loads.[110–113] Although this mechanism was held responsible for hyperthyroidism in 50 per cent of the patients described in one report,[112] it is usually a much less frequent event.[107, 113] Experimentally, even the normal, slightly stimulated rat thyroid gland responds with a burst of hormone secretion to a small exogenous iodide load, although a considerable fraction of excess iodide is rejected by autoregulatory mechanisms.[24, 114] In multinodular goiter containing highly active autonomous follicles, autoadaptation may be less effective, so that excessive hormone production may be the response to increasing iodide load. An example is given in Figure 46–9.[110] In addition, unlike the normal gland, autonomous nodules fail to stop secreting hormones when TSH secretion is suppressed.

Clinical Signs and Symptoms (Table 46–1)

The overwhelming majority of patients with nontoxic nodular goiter present no signs and symptoms other than those of local growth of the thyroid gland. Very often, diffuse or nodular enlargement of the thyroid is unknown to the patient and is discovered at the time of a check-up for reasons unrelated to the thyroid. Sometimes a goiter is revealed by a chest radiograph.

Diffuse enlargement of the thyroid gland does not become palpable before the volume of the gland has doubled. A visibly diffusely enlarged goiter indicates at least three times the normal thyroid weight of 15 to 20 g. Detection of small nodules depends very much on the skill and training of the physician (see Ch. 50). The patient is usually unaware of the presence of a nodule smaller than 2 cm in diameter. Sometimes growth of a nodule or painful sensations due to hemorrhage into a nodule bring the

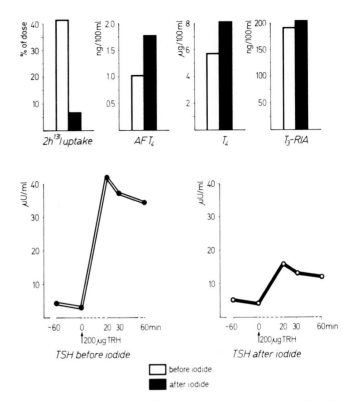

FIGURE 46–9. **Response of a patient with euthyroid multinodular goiter to 0.5 mg iodide given twice daily for four days.** Thyroid function tests were performed the day before exposure to iodide and at day 7. Note that free T_4 (AFT$_4$), total T_4, and, to a small extent, total T_3 increase, whereas the TSH response to TRH is blunted. The initially high ^{131}I uptake decreases, but the iodide clearance is not lowered far enough to prevent iodide from entering the pathway of iodothyronine synthesis[110] (see also ref. 114). This patient is probably prone to develop hyperthyroidism when exposed to iodide for longer periods of time.

goiter to attention. Even a large multinodular goiter causes remarkably little discomfort to its bearer. Compression of neck structures such as the trachea, the veins, or, very seldom, the recurrent laryngeal nerve is the exception rather than the rule. Such signs indicate that the goiter has plunged into the upper aperture of the thoracic cage, where it cannot expand externally, or that thyroid carcinoma, rather than benign multinodular goiter, is present.

Inspection and palpation of the neck, preferably done with the patient swallowing gulps of water, may reveal anything from a single, small nodule embedded in an otherwise normal, unpalpable thyroid to a large mass made up of multiple nodules. The consistency of the nodules varies widely even within a single gland, ranging from soft to stone-hard. Fluctuation in a cyst may be felt if it measures more than 2 cm in diameter. Nodules may be well delimited and clearly individualized from each other, or they may appear as smaller or larger lumps embedded in the body of an enlarged thyroid.

Although the clinical diagnosis of nodular goiter is usually very easy, it is often more difficult to establish, even using scintigraphy or ultrasonography, whether the gland contains more than one nodule (Table 46–2). In the overwhelming majority of all cases, histological work-up discloses multinodularity[1–5, 8, 92] or at least multiple foci of replicating follicular cells.[5] Detection of borderline but nevertheless clinically relevant hyperthyroidism requires laboratory tests (see Ch. 39). If some of the results are

TABLE 46–1. CLINICAL SIGNS OF MULTINODULAR GOITER

Slowly growing neck mass
Enlargement during pregnancy
Tracheal deviation or compression
Sudden pain or enlargement secondary to hemorrhage
Occasional cough and dysphagia
Gradually developing thyrotoxicosis
Iodide-induced thyrotoxicosis
Superior vena cava obstruction syndrome
Recurrent nerve palsy (rare)

TABLE 46–2. DIAGNOSIS OF MULTINODULAR GOITER

Multinodularity on examination
Asymmetry, tracheal deviation
No adenopathy
Ultrasound finding of nodularity
Scintiscan with hot and cold areas
Fine-needle aspiration of dominant nodules—benign
Free thyroxine index normal or increased, TSH normal or decreased, thyroglobulin elevated
Thyroid antibodies negative (usually)
CT scan evidence of nonhomogeneous mass

borderline, repetition at yearly intervals is recommended to detect early hyperthyroidism. In any patient with a euthyroid multinodular goiter, insidiously developing hyperthyroidism must be considered whenever the patient presents with otherwise unexplained illness. This is particularly true for patients presenting with cardiac failure and arrhythmias. Hyperthyroidism appearing very slowly in the course of many years is a frequent complication of long-standing goiters because the process of autonomous goiter growth may insidiously add new follicles—some "hot" and some "cold"—to the mass of pre-existing ones.[103] Transition from a euthyroid to a hyperthyroid state is heralded by suppressed serum TSH levels. It is only later that free T_3 and, often still later, free T_4 also rise into the frankly thyrotoxic range (see Chs. 39 and 41).

Once the diagnosis of euthyroid or hyperthyroid uninodular or multinodular goiter is established, ultrasonography is helpful in documenting the size and the structure of the goiter. It is mandatory, in our view, if an attempt is planned to make the goiter shrink by T_4 treatment (see below) because it provides an objective means of judging the effect of the treatment. Many clinicians also use scintigraphy, CT scans, or even PET scans to further document details of the goiter's size and function. However, these additional diagnostic maneuvers rarely yield information decisive for clinical management in an individual case. The one exception is fine-needle aspiration of clinically dominant nodules, which is very helpful in the case of a result indicating malignant growth (see Ch. 50) but less so in the large majority of benign nodules. For reasons explained in the section on "Morphological and Functional Heterogeneity," we do not recommend routine ^{99m}Tc-pertechnetate or iodine scans.

The only thyroid disease—besides carcinomas—that may be mistaken for simple multinodular goiter is thyroiditis and, in particular, Hashimoto's thyroiditis with abundant lymphocytic infiltration leading to nodular enlargement of the gland (see Ch. 43). Therefore, a complete work-up of a patient with nodular goiter must include a determination of antimicrosomal antibodies.

Treatment

Prevention and medical treatment of euthyroid multinodular goiter are based on suppression of TSH secretion. Considering the modest role of TSH, if any, in non-endemic, autonomous multinodular goiter growth (see "Pathogenesis") and its frequently low or suppressed level in large goiters,[1–4, 103, 111] it is not surprising that the outlook for a definite success is dim. In our own country, Switzer-land, as in many other areas (for review see refs. 90, 115, and 116), successful goiter treatment by T_4 has become exceptional since iodine deficiency has been eradicated.[96, 97] Even in areas where iodine-deficiency goiter is still endemic, half of all goiters may be caused by other factors.[117] However, in many centers around the world, a trial of T_4 treatment is still recommended in most patients with multinodular goiter.

The extent of decrease in goiter size achieved by T_4 treatment aimed at TSH suppression is quite variable and cannot be predicted.[90, 115, 116] It depends on such factors as the amount of autonomously growing parenchyma and the presence of connective tissue, with or without degenerative changes. In line with the pathogenetic concept outlined earlier is the fact that thyroid nodules that appear cold on scintiscans may still shrink to some extent after TSH suppression.[118] For all these reasons, neither a scintiscan nor ultrasonography is helpful for predicting the outcome of T_4 treatment. There is no effective substitute for an empirical trial. Complete regression of thyroid volume is unusual.[90, 115, 116, 119] Most authors consider a 30 per cent reduction of thyroid volume, confirmed by ultrasonography, to be a success, whereas others, including ourselves, do not share this view. In addition, there are several shortcomings in T_4 treatment: First, any persistence of one or several nodules requires long-time, cumbersome surveillance and continuous treatment, because most goiters regrow to their original size shortly after stopping treatment.[103, 115, 116, 119] Second, although some nodules may shrink under T_4 treatment, others may not. Eventually, if autonomous hormone secretion persists in part of the goiter, T_4 treatment even in modest doses may induce subclinical hyperthyroidism with unwanted side effects, for example, on bone mass.[120] Despite these limitations, T_4 treatment can safely be used as a first-line choice as long as close medical surveillance of the patient is ensured.

In the absence of signs of recent growth in a fortuitously discovered multinodular goiter in an elderly patient, no active treatment should be given, for in most of these patients goiter growth has come to a halt for unknown reasons. Establishment of euthyroidism and baseline ultrasonography are recommended. Follow-up is all that is required.

There is considerably more concern whenever one or more thyroid nodules remain unchanged or keep growing under T_4 treatment. This is true regardless of the result of fine-needle aspiration.[121] In these cases, we seriously consider surgical treatment. This somewhat aggressive approach—not shared by all thyroidologists—is chosen particularly in children and young adults, but also in patients younger than 50. It has evolved not so much because of fear of malignant growth, which is less than 15 per cent even in growing nodules[122, 123] (see Ch. 50), but because of the awareness that any persistent nodule in young patients is a problem of lasting concern that requires constant expensive follow-up unless it is removed.[121]

It has been shown that high circulating levels of thyroglobulin may be caused by follicular necroses in growing goiters.[124] Although the acute response of goiter size to T_4 treatment and the response of the serum thyroglobulin levels show no clinical correlation,[125] we personally believe, along with a minority of other authors,[126] that persistently high serum thyroglobulin levels indicate the presence of autonomously growing foci within a nodular goiter[124, 127] and that permanent normalization of elevated serum TSH levels is helpful in predicting treatment success. This view is supported by the demonstration that surgical removal of all nodular tissue normalizes elevated serum thyroglobulin levels.[128] Medical treatment aims at keeping serum TSH at low normal levels without suppressing secretion to avoid subclinical hyperthyroidism with possible side effects on the cardiovascular system in elderly patients[129] and on bone mineralization in younger patients.[120] A review of published studies[90, 103, 115, 116, 118, 119, 126] suggests the following facts:

1. Both thyroid hormones, T_4 as well as T_3, may be effective in reducing the size of euthyroid nodular goiter.

2. Although T_4 treatment is often considered to be successful if a 30 per cent reduction of goiter size is achieved or even if a goiter stops growing, a more impressive result, preferably disappearance of the goiter, is desirable in our mind, particularly in young patients. This goal is seldom obtained, except in severe iodine-deficiency goiters. A less ambitious attitude is perfectly acceptable as long as the patient's compliance and surveillance are ensured.

3. A rather moderate daily dose (50 μg T_3 or 100 to 150 μg T_4) is sufficient to achieve the therapeutic goal, provided that it is administered over months or years. A higher dose may bring more harm than benefit. Indeed, because the degree of suppression of autonomous thyroid tissue cannot be predicted before therapy is started, the potential risk exists of adding the exogenous T_3 or T_4 to an already borderline excessive and nonsuppressible endogenous hormone production. This may be dangerous, particularly in older patients with ischemic heart disease.[129]

4. A significant decrease in the size of multinodular goiter may initially be expected in more than 50 per cent of all patients. However, an initial success in reducing thyroid volume may not eliminate later goiter growth.

5. The degree of radioiodine uptake and its reduction during therapy are only loosely correlated with the response of the goiter to hormonal therapy.

6. The optimal duration of treatment is not known. We recommend assessment of failure or success after one year, followed by temporary cessation of therapy in the case of a clear success (including definite normalization of elevated serum thyroglobulin levels). Rapid regrowth of the goiter must raise the question whether a probably life-long treatment is feasible and desirable in an individual patient.

Overall, the enthusiasm for medical treatment of nodular goiters in nonendemic areas is on the wane. Once treatment has begun, correct guidance by measuring peripheral hormone concentration is difficult. It is best achieved by measuring serum TSH, which should be in the low normal range. The single most important sign that heralds failure of T_4 treatment and calls for considering the surgical approach is documented recent growth of any nodule.

If surgery is being considered for T_4-resistant, actually growing uninodular or multinodular goiter, three conditions have to be fulfilled: (1) Surgery must be carried out by highly trained surgeons; (2) facilities for admittedly very difficult intraoperative inspection of frozen sections from all solid nodules should be available; and (3) the operative procedure should be planned carefully in advance. Commonly the procedure is a bilateral subtotal thyroidectomy, and less commonly a near-total resection. In some centers the possibility is taken into account that the definitive postoperative histological work-up could reveal previously unsuspected follicular carcinoma in a removed lobe.[130] In this plan total lobectomy is done on one side, leaving the carefully weighed possibility of removing the remaining tissue in a second intervention within a few days and before scarring occurs. "Completion" of thyroidectomy can also be accomplished by ^{131}I therapy if only a small amount of tissue remains. Usually further resection is not advised if pathological evaluation reveals only incidentally a cancer less than 1 cm in size. (For further discussion the reader is referred to Ch. 50.) The goal of the surgical procedure is removal of all thyroid tissue of nodular appearance.[131–133] This is not primarily done for fear of carcinoma but because all nodules, whether hot or cold, may contain clusters of autonomously growing cells, causing late recurrence. Even paranodular tissue often harbors microscopic growth foci that may cause the reappearance of nodules within years or decades.[1, 2, 4, 5] Prophylactic surgery to avoid carcinoma is not justified in nodular goiter. However, surgery offers the optimal outlook, if neoplastic growth is detected. Morbidity is negligible in well-selected patients.

Most patients operated on for nodular goiter are placed on substitution therapy with T_4 to prevent recurrence by keeping TSH in the low normal range. However, some authors doubt whether this procedure is truly effective in autonomously growing nodular goiters.[134, 135] It can be speculated that most recurrences of nodules are due to autonomously replicating growth foci[5] not detected and therefore left behind at surgery. In euthyroid patients with all macroscopically diseased tissue removed at surgery and with normal circulating thyroglobulin levels, we refrain from prophylactic treatment.

Single or multiple hot nodules or disseminated hot follicles (see Fig. 46–2) may be eradicated with therapeutic doses of [131]I. This form of therapy is the treatment of choice in elderly patients. The incidence of late hypothyroidism is negligible because suppressed or inactive thyroid tissue takes over hormone production once the hot nodules are removed. In some centers, ^{131}I is also used to diminish the volume of large, euthyroid multinodular goiters.[136, 137] However, the results are rather unpredictable because the invariably coexistent cold nodules are not affected by the isotope and may go on growing. For this reason, the ^{131}I therapy of euthyroid multinodular goiter is only slowly gaining wider acceptance.[138, 139]

Available data on the natural history of hot nodules are rather scarce. Thyrotoxicosis is by no means an obligatory late complication of overactive autonomous clusters of follicles. On the contrary, standstill of evolution, spontaneous regression, involution, and degeneration have been documented.[105, 106] Therefore, whereas surveillance of hot nodules is mandatory, treatment with ^{131}I or surgery is not.

REFERENCES

1. Studer H, Ramelli F: Simple goiter and its variants: Euthyroid and hyperthyroid multinodular goiters. Endocr Rev 3:40–61, 1982.
2. Peter HJ, Studer H, Forster R, Gerber H: The pathogenesis of "hot" and "cold" follicles in multinodular goiters. J Clin Endocrinol Metab 55:941–946, 1982.
3. Studer H, Peter HJ, Gerber H: Natural heterogeneity of thyroid cells: The basis for understanding thyroid function and nodular goiter growth. Endocr Rev 10:125–135, 1989.
4. Peter HJ, Gerber H, Studer H, Smeds S: Pathogenesis of heteroge-

neity in human multinodular goiter. A study on growth and function of thyroid tissue transplanted onto nude mice. J Clin Invest 76:1992–2002, 1985.

5. Studer H, Gerber H, Zbären J, Peter HJ: Histomorphological and immunohistochemical evidence that human nodular goiters grow by episodic replication of multiple clusters of thyroid follicular cells. J Clin Endocrinol Metab 75:1151–1158, 1992.

6. Hedinger C, Williams ED, Sobin LH: Histological Typing of Thyroid Tumours (ed 2). International Histological Classification of Tumours, No 11. Berlin, Springer-Verlag, 1988.

7. LiVolsi VA: Surgical Pathology of the Thyroid. Major Problems in Pathology, Vol 22. Philadelphia, WB Saunders, 1990.

8. Ramelli F, Studer H, Bruggisser D: Pathogenesis of thyroid nodules in multinodular goiter. Am J Pathol 109:215–223, 1982.

9. Thomas GA, Williams D, Williams ED: The clonal origin of thyroid nodules and adenomas. Am J Pathol 134:141–147, 1989.

10. Namba H, Matsuo K, Fagin JA: Clonal composition of benign and malignant human thyroid tumors. J Clin Invest 86:120–125, 1990.

11. Fey MF, Peter HJ, Hinds HL, et al: Clonal analysis of human tumors with M27β, a highly informative polymorphic X chromosomal probe. J Clin Invest 89:1438–1444, 1992.

11a. Aeschimann S, Kopp PA, Kimura ET, et al: Morphological and functional polymorphism within clonal thyroid nodules. J Clin Endocrinol Metab, in press.

11b. Sobrinho-Simões M: Thyroid oncology: The end of the dogmas. Endocr Pathol 2:117–119, 1991.

12. Gerber H, Peter HJ, Studer H, Kaempf J: Apparently clonal thyroid adenomas may contain heterogeneously growing and functioning cell subpopulations. In Medeiros-Neto GA, Gaitan E (eds): Frontiers in Thyroidology. New York, Plenum Press, 1986, pp 901–905.

13. Smeds S, Peter HJ, Jörtsö E, et al: Naturally occurring clones of cells with high intrinsic proliferation potential within the follicular epithelium of mouse thyroids. Cancer Res 47:1646–1651, 1987.

14. Studer H, Hunziker HR, Ruchti C: Morphologic and functional substrate of thyrotoxicosis caused by nodular goiters. Am J Med 65:227–234, 1978.

15. Miller JM, Horn RC, Block MA: The autonomous functioning thyroid nodule in the evolution of nodular goiter. J Clin Endocrinol Metab 27:1264–1274, 1967.

16. Miller JM, Block MA: Relative function of the "hot" autonomous thyroid nodule: Double and single isotope autoradiographic studies. J Nucl Med 10:691–696, 1969.

17. Jackson AS: Goiter and other diseases of the thyroid gland. New York, Paul B. Hoeber, 1927.

18. Wegelin C: Schilddrüse. In Henke F, Lubarsch O (eds): Handbuch der Speziellen Pathologischen Anatomie und Histologie, Vol 8. Berlin, Springer, 1926, pp 170–239.

19. de Quervain F, Wegelin C: Der Endemische Kretinismus. In Aschoff L, Elias H, Eppinger H, et al (eds): Pathologie und Klinik, Vol 7. Berlin, Springer, 1936, pp 84–98.

20. Loewenstein JE, Wollman SH: Distribution of organic ^{125}I and ^{127}I in the rat thyroid gland during equilibrium labeling as determined by autoradiography. Endocrinology 81:1074–1085, 1967.

21. Gerber H, Studer H, Conti A, et al: Reaccumulation of thyroglobulin and colloid in rat and mouse thyroid follicles during intense thyrotropin stimulation: A clue to the pathogenesis of colloid goiters. J Clin Invest 68:1338–1347, 1981.

22. Schürch M, Peter HJ, Gerber H, Studer H: Cold follicles in a multinodular human goiter arise partly from a failing iodide pump and partly from deficient iodine organification. J Clin Endocrinol Metab 71:1224–1229, 1990.

23. Gerber H, Peter HJ, Ramelli F, et al: Autonomie und Heterogenität der Follikel in der euthyreoten und hyperthyreoten menschlichen Knotenstruma: Die Lösung alter Rätsel? Schweiz Med Wochenschr 113:1178–1187, 1983.

24. Studer H, Kohler H, Bürgi H: Iodine deficiency. In Greer MA, Solomon DH (eds): Handbook of Physiology. Section 7. Thyroid, Vol III. Baltimore, Williams & Wilkins, 1974, pp 303–328.

25. Studer H, Gerber H: Intrathyroidal iodine: Heterogeneity of iodocompounds and kinetic compartmentalization. Trends Endocrinol Metab 2:29–34, 1991.

26. Medeiros-Neto G, Ferraz A, Nicolau W, Kieffer J: Autonomous thyroid nodules. II. Double labeling with iodide isotopes and study of biochemical constituents of nodular and paranodular tissues. J Nucl Med 13:738–743, 1972.

27. Rösler H, Kinser J: The leakage phenomenon in thyroid nodules. Acta Endocrinol (Copenh) (Suppl) 179:80–81, 1973.

28. Studer H, Peter HJ, Gerber H: Toxic nodular goiter. Clin Endocrinol Metab 14: 351–372, 1985.

29. Ashcraft MW, Van Herle AJ: Management of thyroid nodules. II. Scanning techniques, thyroid suppressive therapy, and fine needle aspiration. Head Neck Surg 3:297–322, 1981.

30. Rojeski MT, Gharib H: Nodular thyroid disease. Evaluation and management. N Engl J Med 313:428–436, 1985.

31. Dumont JE, Vassart G, Refetoff S: Thyroid disorders. In Sciver CR, Beaudet AL, Sly WS, Valle D (eds): The Metabolic Basis of Inherited Disease. New York, McGraw-Hill, 1983, pp 1843–1879.

32. Stanbury JB: Inherited metabolic disorders of the thyroid system. In Braverman LE, Utiger R (eds): Werner and Ingbar's The Thyroid. Philadelphia, JB Lippincott, 1991, pp 934–941.

32a. Medeiros-Neto G, Targovnik HM, Vassart G: Defective thyroglobulin synthesis and secretion causing goiter and hypothyroidism. Endocr Rev 14:165–183, 1993.

33. Ermans AM, Kinthaert J, Camus M: Defective intrathyroidal iodine metabolism in non-toxic goiter: Inadequate iodination of thyroglobulin. J Clin Endocrinol Metab 28:1307–1316, 1968.

34. Rapoport B, Niepomniszcze H, Bigazzi M, et al: Studies on the pathogenesis of poor thyroglobulin iodination in non-toxic multinodular goiter. J Clin Endocrinol Metab 34:822–830, 1972.

35. Rolland M, Monfort MF, Valenta L, Lissitzky S: Iodoamino acid composition of the thyroglobulin of normal and diseased thyroid glands: Comparison with in vitro iodinated thyroglobulin. Clin Chim Acta 39:95–108, 1972.

36. Kohler H, Haeberli A, Binswanger CH, et al: Experimental procedures leading to a relative accumulation of non-thyroglobulin thyroidal iodocompounds in rat thyroid glands. Acta Endocrinol (Copenh) 67:216–224, 1971.

37. Haeberli A, Studer H, Kohler H, et al: Autoradiographic localization of slow-turnover iodocompounds in the follicular cells of the rat thyroid gland. Endocrinology 97:978–984, 1975.

38. Fragu P, Briançon C, Noel M, Halpern S: Imaging and relative quantification of ^{127}I in human thyroid follicles by analytical ion microscope: Characterization of benign thyroid epithelial tumors. J Clin Endocrinol Metab 69:304–309, 1989.

39. de Crombrugghe B, Edelhoch H, Beckers C, de Visscher M: Thyroglobulin from human goiters: Effects of iodination on sedimentation and iodoamino acid synthesis. J Biol Chem 242:5681–5685, 1967.

40. Wildberger E, von Grünigen C, Kohler J, et al: Regulation of enzymatic iodothyronine synthesis in thyroglobulin by low concentrations of iodide. Eur J Biochem 130:485–490, 1983.

41. Rentsch HP, Studer H, Frauchiger B, Siebenhüner L: Topographical heterogeneity of basal and thyrotropin-stimulated adenosine 3'5'-monophosphate in human nodular goiter. J Clin Endocrinol Metab 53:514–520, 1981.

42. Gerber H, Studer H, von Grünigen C: Paradoxical effects of TSH on diffusion of thyroglobulin in the colloid of rat thyroid follicles after long term thyroxine treatment. Endocrinology 116:303–310, 1985.

43. Studer H, von Grünigen C, Haeberli A, et al: Iodination of thyroglobulin molecules depends on their diffusion velocity in follicular colloid. Mol Cell Endocr 45:91–103, 1986.

44. Gerber H, Peter HJ, Studer H: Diffusion of thyroglobulin in the follicular colloid. Endocrinol Exp 20:23–33, 1986.

45. Van den Hove MF, Couvreur M, De Visscher M, Salvatore G: A new mechanism for the reabsorption of thyroid iodoproteins: Selective fluid pinocytosis. Eur J Biochem 122:415–422, 1982.

46. Ermans AM: Intrathyroid iodine metabolism in goiter. In Stanbury JB (ed): Endemic Goiter. Pan American Health Organization, Scientific Publication No. 193. Washington, DC, Pan American Regional Office of WHO, 1969, pp 1–18.

47. Gerber H, Peter HJ, Studer H: Goiter heterogeneity—a consequence of variable gene expression in growing human tissue. In Reinwein D, Scriba PC (eds): Treatment of Endemic and Sporadic Goiter. Stuttgart, Schattauer Verlag, 1985, pp 1–12.

48. Gerber H, Peter HJ, Bachmeier C, et al: Progressive recruitment of follicular cells with graded secretory responsiveness during stimulation of the thyroid gland by thyrotropin. Endocrinology 120:91–96, 1987.

49. Groch KM, Clifton KH: The plateau phase rat goiter contains a subpopulation of TSH-responsive follicular cells capable of proliferation following transplantation. Acta Endocrinol 126: 85–96, 1992.

50. Groch KM, Clifton KH: The effects of goitrogenesis, involution, and goitrogenic rechallenge on the clonogenic cell content of the rat thyroid. Acta Endocrinol 126:515–523, 1992.

51. Peter HJ, Studer H, Groscurth P: Autonomous growth, but not autonomous function, in embryonic human thyroids: A clue to understanding autonomous goiter growth? J Clin Endocrinol Metab 66:968–973, 1988.

52. Huber H, Derwahl M, Kaempf J, et al: Generation of intercellular heterogeneity of growth and function in cloned rat thyroid cells (FRTL–5). Endocrinology 126:1639–1645, 1990.

53. Wollman SH, Wodinsky I: Localization of protein-bound ^{131}I in the thyroid gland of the mouse. Endocrinology 56:9–20, 1955.

54. Peter HJ, Gerber H, Studer H, et al: Autonomy of growth and of iodine metabolism in hyperthyroid feline goiters transplanted onto nude mice. J Clin Invest 80:491–498, 1987.

55. Alberts B, Bray D, Lewis J, et al: Molecular Biology of the Cell (ed 2). New York, Garland Publishing, 1989.

56. Nicolson GL: Tumor cell instability, diversification, and progression to the metastatic phenotype: From oncogene to oncofetal expression. Cancer Res 47:1473–1487, 1987.

57. Faber E, Rubin H: Cellular adaptation in the origin and development of cancer. Cancer Res 51:2751–2761, 1991.

58. Heppner GH: Tumor heterogeneity. Cancer Res 44:2259–2265, 1984.

59. Medrano EE: A model for the study of cellular heterogeneity in human tumors. In Perspectives on Cellular Regulation: From Bacteria to Cancer. New York, Wiley-Liss, 1991, pp 213–223.

60. Bosco D, Chanson M, Bruzzone R, Meda P: Visualization of amylase secretion from individual pancreatic acini. Am J Physiol 254:G664–G670, 1988.

61. O'Sullivan AJ, Cheek TR, Moreton RB, et al: Localization and heterogeneity of agonist induced changes in cytosolic calcium concentration in single bovine adrenal chromaffin cells from video imaging. EMBO J 8:401–411, 1989.

62. Koury MJ, Bondurant MC, et al: Quantitation of erythropoietin-producing cells in kidneys of mice by in situ hybridization: Correlation with hematocrit, renal erythropoietin mRNA, and serum erythropoietin concentration. Blood 74:645–651, 1989.

63. Boockfor FR, Schwarz LK, Derick FC III: Sertoli cells in culture are heterogeneous with respect to transferrin release: Analysis by reverse hemolytic plaque assay. Endocrinology 125:1128–1133, 1989.

64. Scarbrough K, Weiland NG, Larson GH, et al: Measurement of peptide secretion and gene expression in the same cell. Mol Endocrinol 5:134–142, 1991.

65. Giordano E, Bosco D, Cirulli V, Meda P: Repeated glucose stimulation reveals distinct and lasting secretion patterns of individual rat pancreatic B cells. J Clin Invest 87:2178–2185, 1991.

66. Peter HJ, Gerber H, Studer H, et al: Autonomous growth and function of cultured thyroid follicles from cats with spontaneous hyperthyroidism. Thyroid 1:331–338, 1991.

67. Peter HJ, Gerber H, Studer H, et al: Thyroid cell lines forming follicle-like lumina in vitro. In Gordon A, Gross J, Hennemann G (eds): Progress in Thyroid Research. Rotterdam, Balkema, 1991, pp 579–582.

68. Sobrinho–Simões M, Johannessen JV: A scanning and transmission electron microscopic study of human nodular goitre. Histopathology 7:65–76, 1983.

69. Mizukami Y, Matsubara F, Matsukawa S: Localization of adenylate cyclase and 5'–nucleotidase activities in human thyroid follicular cells. Histochemistry 74:9–19, 1982.

69a. Vitale M, Bassi V, Fenzi G, et al: Integrin expression in thyroid cells from normal glands and nodular goiters. J Clin Endocrinol Metab 76:1575–1579, 1993.

70. Studer H, Forster R, Conti A, et al: Transformation of normal follicles into thyrotropin-refractory "cold" follicles in the aging mouse thyroid gland. Endocrinology 102:1576–1586, 1978.

71. Gerber H, Peter HJ, Studer H: Age-related failure of endocytosis may be the pathogenetic mechanism responsible for "cold" follicle formation in the aging mouse thyroid. Endocrinology 120:1758–1764, 1987.

72. Nève P, Authelet M, Golstein J: Effect of aging on the morphology and function of the thyroid gland of the cream hamster. Cell Tissue Res 220:499–509, 1981.

73. Mestdagh C, Many MC, Halpern S, et al: Correlated autoradiographic and ion-microscopic study of the role of iodine in the formation of "cold" follicles in young and old mice. Cell Tissue Res 260:449–457, 1990.

74. Dumont JE, Maenhaut C, Lamy F: Control of cell proliferation and goitrogenesis. Trends Endocrinol Metab 3:12–17, 1992.

75. Bidey SP: Control of thyroid cell and follicle growth. Recent advances and current controversies. Trends Endocrinol Metab 1:174–178, 1990.

76. Minuto F, Barreca A, Del Monte P, et al: Immunoreactive insulin-like growth factor I (IGF-1) and IGF-I-binding protein content in human thyroid tissue. J Clin Endocrinol Metab 68:621–626, 1989.

77. Williams DW, Williams ED, Wynford-Thomas D: Evidence for autocrine production of IGF-1 in human thyroid adenomas. Mol Cell Endocrinol 61:139–143, 1989.

78. Maciel RMB, Lopez MHC, Alberti VN: Insulin-like growth factor I (IGF–I). In Gordon A, Gross J, Hennemann G (eds): Progress in Thyroid Research. Rotterdam, Balkema, 1991, pp 627–630.

79. Drexhage HA, Bottazzo GF, Doniach D, et al: Evidence for thyroid-growth-stimulating immunoglobulins in some goitrous thyroid diseases. Lancet 2:287–291, 1980.

80. Smyth PPA, Neylan D, O'Donovan DK: The prevalence of thyroid-stimulating antibodies in goitrous disease assessed by cytochemical section bioassay. J Clin Endocrinol Metab 54:357–361, 1982.

81. Wilders–Truschnig MM, Drexhage HA, Leb G, et al: Chromatographically purified immunoglobulin G of endemic and sporadic goiter patients stimulates FRTL-5 cell growth in a mitotic arrest assay. J Clin Endocrinol Metab 70:444–452, 1990.

82. Correa P: Pathology of endemic goiter. In Stanbury JB, Hetzel BS (eds): Endemic Goiter and Endemic Cretinism. New York, John Wiley & Sons, 1980, pp 303–332.

83. Studer H, Gerber H, Peter HJ: Autoimmunity in nodular goiter? In Drexhage HA, Wiersinga WM (eds): The Thyroid and Autoimmunity. Amsterdam, Elsevier, 1986, pp 217–226.

84. Zakarija M, McKenzie JM: Do thyroid growth-promoting immunoglobulins exist? J Clin Endocrinol Metab 70:308–310, 1990.

85. Norman JT, Bohman RE, Fischman G, et al: Patterns of mRNA expression during early cell growth differ in kidney epithelial cells destined to undergo compensatory hypertrophy versus regenerative hyperplasia. Proc Natl Acad Sci 85:6768–6772, 1988.

86. Studer H, Huber, G, Derwahl M, Frey P: Die Umwandlung von Basedowstrumen in Knotenkröpfe: Ein Grund des Hyperthyreoserezidivs. Schweiz Med Wochenschr 119:203–208, 1989.

86a. Selzer E, Wilfing A, Schiferer A, et al: Stimulation of human thyroid growth via the inhibitory guanine nucleotide binding (G) protein G_i. Constitutive expression of the G-protein α subunit $G_{i\alpha-1}$ in autonomous adenoma. Proc Natl Acad Sci 90:1609–1613, 1993.

86b. Othsubo M, Roberts JM: Cyclin-dependent regulation of G_1 in mammalian fibroblasts. Science 259:1908–1912, 1993.

87. Namba H, Ross JL, Goodman D, Fagin JA: Solitary polyclonal autonomous thyroid nodule: A rare cause of childhood hyperthyroidism. J Clin Endocrinol Metab 72:1108–1112, 1991.

88. Aebi U, Gerber H, Studer H: Thyroid adenomas: A morphologically and functionally heterogeneous disease. In Gordon A, Gross J, Hennemann G (eds): Progress in Thyroid Research. Rotterdam, Balkema, 1991, pp 679–682.

89. Smeds S, Peter HJ, Gerber H, et al: Effects of thyroxine on cell proliferation in human multinodular goiter: A study on growth of thyroid tissue transplanted to nude mice. World J Surgery 12:241–245, 1988.

90. Reverter JL, Lucas A, Salinas I, et al: Suppressive therapy with levothyroxine for solitary thyroid nodules. Clin Endocrinol 36:25–28, 1992.

91. Miller JM, Kawas BS: The combined use of iodine-125 and iodine-131 in autoradiographic studies of nodular goiter. J Nucl Med 7:188–196, 1966.

92. Mortensen ID, Woolner LB, Bennet WA: Gross and microscopic findings in clinically normal thyroid glands. J Clin Endocrinol Metab 15:1270–1280, 1955.

93. Stanbury JB, Hetzel BS (eds): Endemic Goiter and Endemic Cretinism. Iodine Nutrition in Health and Disease. New York, John Wiley & Sons, 1980.

94. Dunn JT, Pretell EA, Daza CH, Viteri FE (eds): Towards the Eradication of Endemic Goiter, Cretinism, and Iodine Deficiency. Proceedings of the V Meeting of the PAHO/WHO Technical Group on Endemic Goiter, Cretinism, and Iodine Deficiency. Scientific Publication No. 502, Pan American Health Organization, 1986.

95. Gaitan E: Iodine-sufficient goiter and autoimmune thyroiditis: The Kentucky and Colombian experience. In Medeiros-Neto GA, Gaitan E (eds): Frontiers in Thyroidology. New York, Plenum Press, 1986, pp 19–25.

96. Mordasini C, Abetel G, Lauterburg H, et al: Untersuchungen zum Kochsalzkonsum und zur Jodversorgung der schweizerischen Bevölkerung. Schweiz Med Wochenschr 114:1924–1929, 1984.

97. Bürgi H, Supersaxo Z, Selz B: Iodine deficiency diseases in Switzerland one hundred years after Theodor Kocher's survey: A historical review with some new goitre prevalence data. Acta Endocrinol (Copenh) 123:577–590, 1990.

98. Bray GA: Increased sensitivity of the thyroid in iodine-depleted rats to the goitrogenic effects of thyrotropin. J Clin Invest 47:1640–1647, 1968.

99. Stübner D, Gärtner R, Greil W, et al: Hypertrophy and hyperplasia during goiter growth and involution in rats—separate bioeffects of TSH and iodine. Acta Endocrinol 116:537–548, 1987.

100. Grubeck-Loebenstein B, Buchan G, Sadeghi R, et al: Transforming growth factor beta regulates thyroid growth. J Clin Invest 83:764–770, 1989.

101. Beere HM, Tomlinson S, Bidey SP: Iodide autoregulation of functional and morphological differentiation events in the FRTL-5 rat thyroid cell strain. J Endocrinol 124:19–25, 1990.

102. Farid NR: Genetic factors in thyroid disease. *In* Braverman LE, Utiger RD (eds): Werner and Ingbar's The Thyroid. Philadelphia, JB Lippincott, 1991, pp 588–602.

103. Berghout A, Wiersinga WM, Smits NJ, Touber JL: Interrelationships between age, thyroid volume, thyroid nodularity, and thyroid function in patients with sporadic nontoxic goiter. Am J Med 89:602–608, 1990.

104. Gullino PM: Natural history of breast cancer: Progression from hyperplasia to neoplasia as predicted by angiogenesis. Cancer 39:2697–2703, 1977.

105. Blum M, Shenkman L, Hollander CH: The autonomous nodule of the thyroid: Correlation of patient age, nodule size and functional status. Am J Med Sci 269:43–50, 1975.

106. Hamburger JI: Solitary autonomously functioning thyroid lesions. Am J Med 58:740–748, 1975.

107. Silverstein GE, Burke G, Cogan R: The natural history of the autonomous hyperfunctioning thyroid nodule. Ann Intern Med 67:539–548, 1967.

108. Gemsenjäger E, Staub JJ, Girard J, Heitz PH: Preclinical hyperthyroidism in multinodular goiter. J Clin Endocrinol Metab 43:810–816, 1967.

109. Staub JJ, Gräni R, Birkhäuser M, et al: Evaluation of "preclinical hyperthyroidism" using oral TRH, metoclopramide, systolic time intervals, sex-hormone-binding globulin and T4-suppression test. J Mol Med 4:49–58, 1980.

110. Trost BN, Buchli R, Osterwalder HJ, et al: The handling of moderately excessive iodide loads by normal and goitrous human thyroid glands. J Mol Med 4:167–175, 1980.

111. Lima N, Medeiros-Neto G: Transient thyrotoxicosis in endemic goiter patients following exposure to a normal iodine intake. Clin Endocrinol (Oxf) 21:631–637, 1984.

112. Vagenakis AG, Wang C, Burger A, et al: Iodide induced thyrotoxicosis in Boston. N Engl J Med 287:523–527, 1972.

113. Fradkin JE, Wolff J: Iodide-induced thyrotoxicosis. Medicine 62:1–20, 1983.

114. Studer H, Bürgi H, Kohler H, et al: A transient rise of hormone secretion. A response of the stimulated rat thyroid gland to small increments of iodide supply. Acta Endocrinol (Copenh) 81:507–515, 1976.

115. Berghout A, Wiersinga WM, Drexhage HA, et al: Comparison of placebo with L-thyroxine alone or with carbimazole for treatment of sporadic non-toxic goitre. Lancet 336:193–197, 1990.

116. Edmonts C: Treatment of sporadic goitre with thyroxine. Clin Endocrinol (Oxf) 36:21–23, 1992.

117. Grubeck-Loebenstein B, Kletter K, Kiss A, et al: Endemische Struma in Oesterreich. Ist Jodmangel die primäre Kropfursache? Schweiz Med Wochenschr 112:1526–1530, 1982.

118. Shimaoka K, Sokal JE: Suppressive therapy of nontoxic goiter. Am J Med 57:576–583, 1974.

119. Perrild H, Hansen JM, Hegedüs L, et al: Triiodothyronine and thyroxine treatment of diffuse non-toxic goitre evaluated by ultrasonic scanning. Acta Endocrinol 100:382–387, 1982.

120. Baran DT: The skeletal system in thyrotoxicosis. *In* Braverman LE, Utiger RD (eds): Werner and Ingbar's The Thyroid. Philadelphia, JB Lippincott, 1991, pp 836–844.

121. Studer H: Diffuse nontoxic and multinodular goiter. *In* Bardin CW (ed): Current Therapy in Endocrinology and Metabolism. Philadelphia, BC Decker, 1991, pp 84–86.

122. Molitch ME, Beck JR, Dreisman M, et al: The cold thyroid nodule: An analysis of diagnostic and therapeutic options. Endocr Rev 5:185–199, 1984.

123. Franklyn JA, Sheppard MC: Thyroid nodules and thyroid cancer: Diagnostic aspects. Baillieres Clin Endocrinol Metab 2:761–775, 1988.

124. Gebel F, Ramelli F, Bürgi U, et al: The site of leakage of intrafollicular thyroglobulin into the blood stream in simple human goiter. J Clin Endocrinol Metab 57:915–919, 1983.

125. Feldt-Rasmussen U, Hegedüs L, Hansen JM, Perrild H: Relationship between thyroid volume and serum thyroglobulin during long-term suppression with triiodothyronine in patients with diffuse non-toxic goitre. Acta Endocrinol (Copenh) 105:184–189, 1984.

126. Morita T, Tamai H, Ohshima A, et al: Changes in serum thyroid hormone, thyrotropin and thyroglobulin concentrations during thyroxine therapy in patients with solitary thyroid nodules. J Clin Endocrinol Metab 69:227–230, 1989.

127. Bürgi U, Gebel F, Gerber H: Die diagnostische Bedeutung der Thyreoglobulinbestimmung im Blut. Schweiz Med Wochenschr 114:365–368, 1984.

128. Gemsenjäger E, Girard J, Martina B: Prä- und postoperative Thyreoglobulinabgabe in das Blut bei Knotenstruma. Schweiz Med Wochenschr 114:826–829, 1984.

129. Dillman WH: The cardiovascular system in thyrotoxicosis. *In* Braverman LE, Utiger RD (eds): Werner and Ingbar's The Thyroid. Philadelphia, JB Lippincott, 1991, pp 759–770.

130. Smeds S, Madsen M, Rüter A, Lennquist S: Evaluation of preoperative diagnosis and surgical management of thyroid tumours. Acta Chir Scand 150:513–519, 1984.

131. Gemsenjäger E, Heitz PU, Staub JJ, et al: Surgical aspects of thyroid autonomy in multinodular goiter. World J Surg 7:363–371, 1983.

132. Teuscher J, Peter HJ, Gerber H, et al: Pathogenesis of nodular goiter and its implications for surgical management. Surgery 103:87–93, 1988.

133. Röher HD, Goretzki PE: Management of goiter and thyroid nodules in an area of endemic goiter. Surg Clin North Am 67:233–249, 1987.

134. Geerdsen JP, Frolund L: Recurrence of nontoxic goiter with and without postoperative thyroxine medication. Clin Endocrinol (Oxf) 21:529–533, 1984.

135. Bang U, Blichert M, Petersen PH, et al: Thyroid function after resection for non-toxic goiter with special reference to thyroid lymphocytic aggregation and circulating thyroid autoantibodies. Acta Endocrinol (Copenh) 109:214–219, 1985.

136. Frey KW, Leisner B: Langzeitergebnisse der 131-Jodtherapie der blanden Struma im Kropfendemiegebiet. *In* Scriba PC, Rudorff KH, Weinheimer B (eds): Schilddrüse 1981. Stuttgart, Georg Thieme Verlag, 1982, pp 329–335.

137. Verelst J, Bonnyns M, Glinoer D: Radioiodine therapy in voluminous multinodular non-toxic goitre. Acta Endocrinol (Copenh) 122:417–421, 1990.

138. Hegedüs L, Hansen BM, Knudsen N, Hansen JM: Reduction of size of thyroid with radioactive iodine in multinodular non-toxic goitre. Br Med J 297:661–662, 1988.

139. Hegedüs L, Nygaard B, Hansen JM, et al: Long-term follow-up of thyroid volume and function in patients with nontoxic multinodular goitre treated with radioiodine. J Endocrinol Invest 16 (Suppl. 2 to no. 6):1993. Abstr. no. 81.

Thyroid Disease in the Fetus, Neonate, and Child

DELBERT A. FISHER
DANIEL H. POLK

Thyroid hormones exert important effects on energy metabolism and on the metabolism of lipids, carbohydrates, proteins, nucleic acids, vitamins, and inorganic ions. These actions of thyroid hormones, reviewed in earlier chapters, are qualitatively similar during childhood and adolescence and in adults. Thyroid hormones also exert profound effects on growth and differentiation, and, in contrast to the metabolic effects, these developmental actions of thyroid hormones are uniquely manifest during the first two decades of life.[1, 2] In addition, physical anomalies and genetic abnormalities involving thyroid hormone production or action are particularly prominent in the differential diagnosis of thyroid disorders during infancy. Previous chapters have dealt in depth with thyroid hormone biosynthesis, secretion, metabolism, actions, and control and with the pathogenesis, diagnosis, and management of thyroid-related diseases. In the present chapter, selected aspects of these topics particularly important or unique to fetal development and neonatal thyroid function as well as pathophysiology are reviewed.

MATURATION OF FETAL THYROID FUNCTION

Development of Thyroid System Control

The placenta is impermeable to thyrotropin (TSH), and although permeable to thyrotropin-releasing hormone (TRH), maternal TRH appears to play no role in the maturation of the fetal hypothalamic-pituitary axis. Thyroid function in the fetus develops largely autonomously of the maternal system. Maternally derived thyroid hormone is known to be present in fetal tissues during early development of the rat, but its significance is not yet clear.[3] T_4 is present at about one half of maternal concentration in cord blood of athyroid human fetuses, indicating some placental transfer of thyroid hormone.[4] T_4 and T_3 do not cross the placental barrier freely. However, both the placenta and the fetal membranes express an active inner ring iodothyronine monodeiodinase, which converts T_4 to reverse T_3 (rT_3) and T_3 to diiodothyronine (T_2).[5] This activity likely contributes to the low placental permeability to T_4 and T_3 and results in high levels of rT_3 in amniotic fluid.[5] T_4 and rT_3 concentrations in amniotic fluid peak near midgestation at roughly comparable levels, falling off toward term.[6] T_3 values in amniotic fluid are low, averaging about 2 per cent of the rT_3 concentration at midgestation. TSH concentrations in amniotic fluid also are low, averaging 0.44 and 0.27 mU/L during the second and third trimesters, respectively. These values are shown in Figure 47–1. Amniotic fluid iodothyronine levels are derived from both maternal and fetal sources and are not useful in determining the thyroid status of the fetus.[7] Fetal hepatic T_4 conversion probably accounts for most of the high circulating levels of rT_3 in fetal serum,[8, 9] but placental conversion of fetal and maternal T_4 may contribute.

The fetal hypothalamic-pituitary complex is capable of synthesizing TRH and TSH by 8 to 10 weeks, and vascular communications between the hypothalamus and pituitary appear as early as 11 to 12 weeks.[8–10] However, fetal serum TSH, T_4, and free T_4 levels remain low until midgestation, after which time there are progressive increases to term[9–11] (Fig. 47–2). Serum TSH concentrations increase to a mean value of 10 mU/L at term; T_4 levels plateau at a mean approximating 140 nmol/L after 35 weeks.[10, 12] Cord serum T_3 levels remain low until 30 to 32 weeks, when a gradual increase begins; by 40 weeks the mean concentration approximates 0.65 nmol/L (42 ng/dl, the prenatal T_3 surge). Free T_4 (FT_4) and free T_3 (FT_3) concentrations parallel the

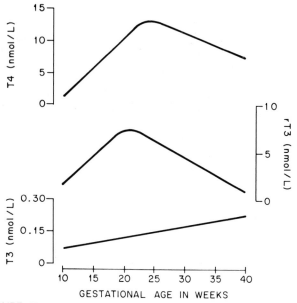

FIGURE 47–1. Amniotic fluid iodothyronine concentrations during gestation in the human. Values are reported as means from 10 weeks' gestation to term.

changes in total hormone levels. However, because of extensive tissue uptake of hormone, and local T_4 to T_3 deiodination, brain and liver T_3 levels in the human fetus are close to adult levels from the 20th week through term.[12a]

These progressive changes in fetal serum TSH and iodothyronine concentrations reflect maturational events at several levels of the hypothalamic-pituitary-thyroid (HPT) axis. Pituitary TRH receptors are present by midgestation, so that activation of the HPT axis at that time probably represents augmented TRH secretion and/or transport.[10] During the third trimester, the progressive increases in serum TSH and FT_4 levels reflect several simultaneous events, including (1) a progressive increase in TRH secretion, (2) a progressive maturation of pituitary T_3 negative feedback sensitivity, and (3) maturation of thyroid gland TSH responsiveness. Pituitary T_4 to T_3 conversion capacity and pituitary T_3 receptors probably are mature by midgestation.[9, 10] T_4 feedback modulation of TSH secretion is operative in small premature infants delivered early in the process of third trimester maturation.[13, 14] The third trimester maturation of pituitary negative feedback sensitivity seems to involve a T_3-induced decrease in TRH receptors and a T_3-induced augmentation of T_3 receptor binding. A maturation of the post-T_3 receptor response also may be involved.[10] The timing of these events of hypothalamic-pituitary maturation in the human fetus is noted in Table 47–1.

Thyroid Autoregulation

The mature thyroid follicular cell can modify plasma membrane iodine transport relative to iodine intake and exclusive of TSH levels.[15–17] This thyroid autoregulation develops only after 36 to 40 weeks' gestation in the human fetus and involves the capacity of thyroid follicular cells to increase iodide trapping in the presence of low plasma iodide levels and to decrease iodide trapping when prevailing iodide levels are increased.[18] Studies in the developing rabbit thyroid gland suggest that the failure of the imma-

TABLE 47–1. MATURATION OF HYPOTHALAMIC-PITUITARY CONTROL OF TSH SECRETION IN THE HUMAN FETUS

EVENT	TIME OF APPEARANCE*
TRH	<0.3
TSH synthesis	<0.3
TRH stimulation of TSH	0.5
TSH response to cold	<0.6
T_3 inhibition of TSH synthesis and release	<0.65
Dopamine inhibition of TSH secretion	>1.0

*Fractional proportion of thyroid system maturation; complete maturation time in man approximates 10 months of developmental age, and 10 months = 1.0.
Modified from Fisher DA: Ontogenesis of hypothalamic-pituitary-thyroid function in the human fetus. In Delange F, Fisher DA, Malvaux P (eds): Pediatric Thyroidology. Basel, Karger, 1985, pp 19–32.

ture gland to autoregulate relates to reduced or absent iodination of an 8000 to 10,000 MW protein that is a component of the thyroid follicular cell.[15, 16] The late maturation of fetal thyroid autoregulation accounts for the susceptibility of the preterm infant to iatrogenic iodine-induced hypothyroidism. Iodine overload in these infants may result from maternal iodine ingestion, intra-amniotic administration of radiographic contrast agents, or application of iodine compounds to the skin.

Maturation of Iodothyronine Deiodination Systems

As indicated, serum T_3 levels are very low or unmeasurable in the human fetus until about 30 weeks of gestation, after which time the concentration increases modestly to a mean level of about 0.65 nmol/L at term.[9, 10] Serum rT_3

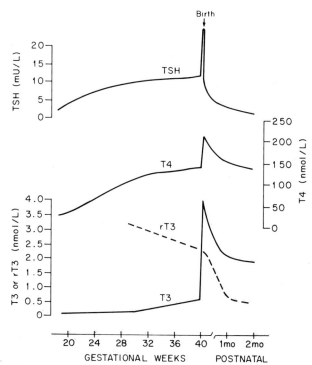

FIGURE 47–2. Ontogeny of serum thyrotropin (TSH), T_4, reverse T_3 (rT_3), and T_3 levels during human development and over the first two months of life.

concentrations exceed 3.25 nmol/L (211 ng/dl) early in the last trimester and decrease steadily to term (Fig. 47–2). Recent data also indicate relatively high concentrations of iodothyronine sulfate in fetal serum. T_4 sulfate (T_4S), rT_3S, and T_3S levels in newborn cord serum average 245, 684, and 164 nmol/L.[18a, 18b, 18c] Similar changes occur in the fetal-neonatal sheep, in which species the mechanism and significance of these changes have been studied.[19–21] In the middle third of ovine gestation, T_4 is monodeiodinated predominantly to the inactive metabolite rT_3; there is little or no deiodination to T_3.[20] In addition, there are relatively high levels of sulfated iodothyronines in fetal sheep serum. Circulating concentrations of T_4S, rT_3S, and T_3S peak at 125 to 130 days' gestation (term is 150 days), averaging 420, 210, and 200 ng/dl, respectively.[21a, 21b]

Fetal serum T_3 levels gradually increase during the week immediately preceding parturition (the prenatal T_3 surge) and then abruptly increase (the postnatal surge) during the early hours after birth.[10, 21, 22] This two-phase (prenatal and postnatal) increase in serum T_3 concentrations is associated with a progressive decrease in fetal serum rT_3 levels, as in the human fetus. The changes in serum T_3 before and after parturition are associated with parallel changes in iodothyronine production rates[23] and parallel increases in the capacity of hepatic tissue to monodeiodinate T_4 to T_3.

The three iodothyronine deiodinase (MDI) enzyme activities responsible for the progressive deiodination of thyroxine have been quantified in the sheep fetus. The levels are developmentally regulated and also influenced by the level of circulating T_4.[19, 24] The expression of type I MDI activity, which mediates T_4 to T_3 conversion and accounts for most of the circulating T_3, is low in most fetal tissues during the first two thirds of gestation. Activities are highest in liver, with lesser activities in kidney, brain cortex, thyroid, brown adipose tissue (BAT), and skin. Levels increase during the last third of gestation and particularly in the perinatal period. The most marked increases occur in liver and BAT.[19] Type II MDI activity is most prominent in brain, skin, and BAT in that order, and tissue activities increase during the perinatal period similarly to the type I MDI. Type III MDI activity is detectable in most fetal tissues during the middle third of gestation but is most prominent in placenta and liver. The type III MDI activity in fetal tissues allows for conversion of most of the available T_4 to inactive rT_3. Type II activity in brain appears to mediate local T_4 to T_3 conversion; this enzyme activity, which increases in the hypothyroid state, is believed to provide T_3 preferentially to brain tissue in the hypothyroid fetus.[19, 20] BAT also expresses type II activity, and thus T_3 generated locally in this tissue may be important to the onset of thermogenesis at birth.

The sulfation pathway in the fetus is active early in gestation; T_3S is present in human fetal blood by 19 weeks' gestation.[24a] Production rates of sulfated iodothyronines in fetal sheep are maximal during the latter third of gestation.[21b] However, the high serum levels are due both to increased production and decreased clearance.[21b, 24b] Available evidence suggests that the metabolism of thyroid hormones involves both sulfation and deiodination. Sulfation facilitates iodothyronine monodeiodination by type I MDI, and the relatively low activity of this enzyme in fetal tissues is largely responsible for the reduced clearance of the sulfated analogues.[21b, 24b] The sulfated iodothyronines appear to be biologically inactive, but desulfation of T_3S to T_3 in the fetus may be significant.[24b]

In the neonatal rat, the capacity for hepatic conversion of T_4 to T_3 also is very low in the fetus and increases markedly during the first week of postnatal life.[9, 10, 25] As expected, T_3 is undetectable in fetal rat serum and rT_3 concentrations are markedly elevated. The low serum T_3 levels at birth increase to adult values during the first two to three weeks of postnatal life, and the high rT_3 concentration falls to adult levels by one week. These data extend the observations in sheep and support the view that the ontogenic changes in iodothyronine β-ring monodeiodination of T_4 in hepatic tissue, and perhaps kidney, are predominantly responsible for the changes in serum T_3 observed during fetal and neonatal development.

Maturation of Thyroid Nuclear Receptors

Thyroid hormone receptor maturation has been most carefully investigated in fetal rats and sheep. In fetal sheep maximal binding capacities for T_3 in liver increase from a mean of 68 fmol/mg DNA at 80 days' gestation to 684 at term (150 days).[26] Specific saturable brain T_3 binding is apparent at 50 days, increases twofold by 80 days, and plateaus by 150 days at a mean level of 410 fmol/mg DNA.[26, 27] Similar results have been observed in developing rats; that is, brain receptor binding appears relatively early in development, whereas T_3 binding in liver matures relatively late in development.[28] Data in the human fetus are limited. Significant receptor binding in brain, lung, and liver has been measured in the second trimester of gestation.[29, 30] In a preliminary report, Su and co-workers noted a sixfold increase in T_3 receptor density in human cerebrum from 12 to 36 weeks' gestation.[31]

Several studies of thyroid receptor mRNA levels have been reported for developing rat brain.[32–34a] The two thyroid hormone receptor genes—α and β—are transcribed in most brain tissues and are developmentally regulated; peak levels are observed in the neonatal period. The α_1 mRNA levels are higher than β_1.[32–34a] However, the predominant mRNA species in developing brain are α receptor variants that arise via alternate splicing of the α gene. These mRNA variants code for receptors that do not bind T_3. These variant proteins can compete with the T_3-binding α_1 receptor for DNA binding. It has been postulated that the carboxy terminal–extended α gene variants may serve to modulate the biological responses to thyroid hormones in developing brain. Studies of T_3 receptor occupancy in developing rat brain have shown a positive correlation with serum T_3 concentrations with peak values at postnatal day 15.[35] Thus, rat brain T_3 receptor mRNA levels, T_3 receptor binding, and serum T_3 levels show co-ordinate developmental expression with peak values in the neonatal period.

Maturation of Thyroid Hormone Actions

The developmental effects of thyroid hormones are manifest in every organ and tissue. However, they can be classified clinically as effects on somatic growth, brain development, bone growth and maturation, dental development and eruption, metabolic systems, and hypothalamic-pituitary function, including pubertal development. The relative effects of thyroid hormones versus age on these broad categories of thyroid-dependent processes are summarized in Table 47–2.

It is now clear that thyroid hormone deficiency has minimal untoward effects in the human fetus when maternal thyroid function is normal. Although serum TSH levels are markedly elevated in the athyroid fetus, somatic growth and development proceed normally and linear bone growth is not inhibited. Bone maturation may be retarded; this is most evident in the distal femoral and proximal tibial epiphyses during the last two months of gestation.[36–39] In addition, brain growth, as assessed by head circumference measurements, is not abnormal; and any effects of thyroid hormone deficiency on brain maturation in the human fetus seem to be largely reversible by early postnatal thyroid hormone replacement. The mean IQ in reported series of infants with congenital hypothyroidism treated in the neonatal period is similar to that in control infants.[40–43] Data in pregnant rats indicate a significant contribution of maternal T_4 to fetal tissue T_4 levels and near normalization of fetal brain T_3 concentrations (via increased local T_4 to T_3 conversion) in the hypothyroid rat fetus.[3, 25, 44, 45, 45a] It has been suggested on the basis of these data as well as significant levels of T_4 (of presumed maternal origin) in athyroid human newborn cord sera, that the failure to observe brain damage in most treated infants with congenital hypothyroidism may be due, at least in part, to a protective effect of maternal thyroid hormone.[4, 44, 45, 45a] Thyroxine levels at birth in athyroid neonates are about half the maternal level, indicating a significant transfer of hormone from mother to fetus.[45b]

Progressive signs and symptoms of hypothyroidism appear during the early weeks of extrauterine life in the athyroid infant. By six to seven weeks the average growth rate has been reduced from 6 to 2 cm/month and an increasing variety of signs and symptoms of hypothyroidism become manifest, including myxedema, gastrointestinal hypofunction, nervous system hypofunction, decreased thermogenesis, hepatic dysfunction, and cardiovascular hypoactivity.[36–38] Thus, growth and metabolism clearly become thyroid hormone dependent soon after birth. The reason for the relative lack of thyroid hormone effect in the fetus is not clear. Several factors may contribute, including deficiency of nuclear T_3 receptors, and/or immaturity of T_3 responsiveness at the postreceptor level.[9, 46] Further, lack of hormone production by the [athyroid] fetus is partially compensated by transplacental passage of maternal hormone.

As the above data indicate, the developmental effects of thyroid hormones are most obvious during infancy and early childhood. Somatic growth, bone growth and maturation, and tooth development and eruption are critically thyroid dependent at this time. In addition, some two thirds of postnatal brain growth and differentiation occur during the first two years of life, the period during which brain thyroid dependency is most manifest.[47] Thyroid hormone replacement begun within one month after birth minimizes permanent brain damage.[42, 43] After three years of age thyroid hormone deficiency is not associated with mental retardation, but delayed somatic and linear growth and delayed eruption of permanent dentition are prominent.[1, 9] In hypothyroid children, bone maturation (measured as bone age) also is delayed, diaphyseal bone growth is reduced, and epiphyseal growth and mineralization largely cease.[1, 2]

MECHANISM OF DEVELOPMENTAL EFFECTS OF THYROID HORMONES

As discussed, growth and development of the human fetus are largely independent of thyroid status. Growth factors, including the somatomedins, probably modulate aspects of fetal growth but are not generally thyroid hormone dependent in the developing fetus.[1, 2, 48, 49] The actions of thyroid hormones become progressively more prominent in the perinatal period.[1, 2] Accumulating evidence supports the view that the effects of thyroid hormones on postnatal somatic and skeletal growth and differentiation are mediated, at least in part, via effects on growth hormone (GH) and somatomedin synthesis and action.[1, 49] A synergism between GH and thyroid hormones with regard to growth has long been recognized. Recent information indicates several mechanisms for this synergism. GH synthesis by pituitary cells is known to be thyroid hormone dependent. There is a marked reduction in pituitary GH content in hypothyroid animals, and investigations of GH synthesis in rat pituitary tumor cells have demonstrated a direct dependency on thyroid hormone.[50–53] This is likely conferred by thyroid hormone response elements located in the 5' promoter region of the GH gene.[54] GH in turn tends to increase the conversion of T_4 to T_3.[55, 56]

The growth effects of GH are mediated largely via somatomedins, a family of insulin-like hormones under GH control.[57] GH binding to hepatocytes and other cells stimulates somatomedin production,[57–61] which, in turn, stimulates anabolism and growth, particularly in bone and muscle tissues.[53–57] T_4 has been shown to increase serum somatomedin activity in hypopituitary mice incapable of synthesizing GH. Moreover, combined T_3 and GH therapy of hypophysectomized rats is necessary to normalize growth as well as serum somatomedin levels.[62] In addition, evidence suggests that thyroid hormones potentiate the actions of somatomedin on cartilage growth.[54] Thus, thyroid hormones appear to exert effects at several levels to stimulate skeletal and carcass growth. In rats, thyroid hormones stimulate GH synthesis by anterior pituitary cells, stimulate or potentiate stimulation of hepatic somatomedin production by GH, and potentiate the growth effects of somatomedins in cartilage (and perhaps other tissues). In man, a pituitary action is less obvious; thyroid hormones appear to poten-

TABLE 47–2. Relative Effects of Thyroid Hormones Versus Age on Development and Metabolism

	Fetus	0–3 yrs	3–12 yrs	12–20 yrs	>20 yrs
Somatic growth	0	4+	3+	2+	0
Brain development	±	4+	±	0	0
Bone growth, maturation	+	4+	3+	2+	0
Dental development	0	4+	2+	+	0
Hypothalamic-pituitary function	0	±	2+	3+	+
Metabolic effects	±	2+	3+	3+	4+

tiate GH stimulation of somatomedin production and actions.[63]

The precise mechanism of T_4 dependency on other growth and developmental processes is not as clear. Evidence suggests that other peptide growth factors mediate the thyroid hormone effects on specific target issues. In the mouse, the epidermal growth factor (EGF) content of various tissues has been shown to be thyroid hormone responsive,[64–67] and EGF has been shown to stimulate T_4-dependent eye opening and incisor eruption in hypothyroid neonatal mice.[50, 66] T_4 also increases EGF receptor binding in selected tissues.[68, 69] Erythropoietin synthesis by the kidney is thyroid hormone responsive, and there are known positive correlations between circulating erythropoietin levels, erythrocyte production, and hemoglobin concentrations in hypothyroidism and hyperthyroidism.[50] It has been suggested that nerve growth factor (NGF) or its variants mediate the effects of thyroid hormone on sympathetic nervous system development and may play a role in T_4 dependency of the developing CNS.[50]

These observations have suggested the hypothesis that thyroid hormones exert their developmental effects, at least in part, via stimulation of the production and/or effect of various tissue-specific growth factors. The extent, as well as the significance, of these pathways, however, is not yet clear. We do not know to what extent thyroid hormone effects on growth factor metabolism are due to direct effects on growth factor synthesis or growth factor receptor binding characteristics. Thyroid hormones have clear effects on both EGF synthesis and EGF receptor binding, but data are not yet available for other growth factors. It also is likely that non–growth factor–mediated direct tissue effects of thyroid hormones are involved in the regulation of organ growth and maturation. For example, in animal models, thyroid hormones increase mRNA levels of a variety of neuronal genes and modulate expression of genes for cardiac muscle myosin and several gene products influencing cellular metabolism.[70–73] Whatever the mechanism or mechanisms, growth and differentiation are important concerns of the physician during the diagnosis and treatment of thyroid disorders during childhood.

NEONATAL ADAPTATION

At the time of parturition, cutting the umbilical cord and cooling the neonate in the extrauterine environment evoke a marked, transient TSH secretion response maximal at 30 minutes[9, 10] (Fig. 47–2). A marked augmentation of hepatic T_4 to T_3 conversion capacity also occurs.[8, 9] The TSH surge stimulates T_4 secretion and thyroidal conversion of T_4 to T_3, and there is a concomitant further increase in hepatic T_3 production from T_4. As a result, in term infants, serum T_3 concentrations increase to peak values at 3 to 4 hours (the postnatal T_3 surge), fall slightly, and increase again at the time of the T_4 concentration peak 24 to 36 hours after birth.[8–10] TSH secretion decreases over the first two to three days of life. The transient neonatal hyperthyroid state disappears by 20 to 30 days[8, 9] (Fig. 47–3). The elevated levels of rT_3, T_4S, T_3S and rT_3S in fetal (cord) blood at term rapidly decrease, and these metabolites approximate adult levels by two to three weeks.[9, 10, 21b]

In the preterm infant the changes in thyroid function

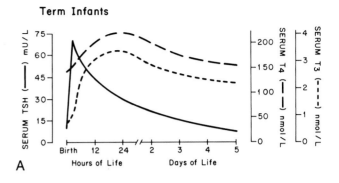

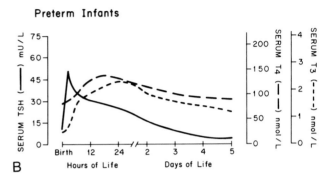

FIGURE 47–3. Patterns of serum thyrotropin (TSH), T_4, and T_3 levels in term infants (P*A*) and preterm infants (P*B*) during the first five days of life.

parameters in the neonatal period, although qualitatively similar, are relatively obtunded.[9, 10, 13] The early 30-minute peak of the TSH surge and the 24- to 36-hour T_4 peak decrease progressively in amplitude with decreasing gestational age. The early T_3 peak also is relatively reduced in amplitude, and in small premature infants serum T_3 levels reach values comparable to those in term infants only after several weeks. The high serum rT_3 values normalize by three to four weeks, as in term infants (Fig. 47–3).

TRANSIENT THYROID DYSFUNCTION IN PREMATURE INFANTS

Newborn screening for congenital hypothyroidism (CH) was begun in the mid-1970's and now is routine in North America, Europe, Scandinavia, Australia, Japan, New Zealand, and other selected areas of the world. This screening is conducted using measurements of T_4 and/or TSH in cord blood or on filter paper blood spots collected during the first few days of life. The screening programs have been highly successful in identifying infants with elevated levels of TSH at risk for the sequelae of CH. In addition, these programs have provided data to characterize a variety of previously unrecognized thyroid dysfunction syndromes in neonates, particularly in premature infants. These are reviewed briefly. For further information, consult the indicated references.

Transient Hypothyroxinemia

Cord serum total T_4 and FT_4 concentrations increase with gestational age, so that all premature infants have some degree of hypothyroxinemia.[10, 13, 14, 74] The prevalence of total serum T_4 concentrations less than 83 nmol/L (6.5 μg/dl) approximates 50 per cent in infants delivered before 30 weeks of gestation and 25 per cent in all premature infants.[74] FT_4 levels are proportionately reduced.[10, 13, 74] The low FT_4 levels in these infants are associated with normal or even low basal serum TSH values and normal TSH responses to TRH. These features characterize a state of hypothalamic (or tertiary) hypothyroidism, which represents a normal stage of thyroid system development. The hypothyroxinemia is transient, correcting spontaneously (over four to eight weeks) with progressive maturation. Current information suggests that this transient hypothyroxinemic state does not require treatment.[74, 75]

Transient Primary Hypothyroidism

In areas of environmental iodine deficiency, premature infants may develop marked hypothyroxinemia associated with reductions in FT_4 levels into the range observed in infants with congenital hypothyroidism.[76] In these infants, serum TSH concentrations increase into the primary hypothyroid range during the first postnatal weeks. Cord blood T_4 and TSH levels in these infants usually are in the normal range for premature infants. Thus, the primary hypothyroid state develops during the first one to two weeks of extrauterine life and is superimposed on the usual state of transient hypothyroxinemia (tertiary hypothyroidism) characteristic of prematurity.[76] Urinary iodine excretion and thyroid iodine content are relatively reduced in these infants, suggesting that the acquired primary hypothyroidism is the result of limited iodine substrate relative to the increased thyroid hormone needs of early infancy.[76]

The hypothyroidism is transient in these infants but may persist for two to three months. Thus, treatment is recommended. In the study of Delange and colleagues,[76] a series of such infants was treated with T_3 (5μg/kg/day in three divided doses); serum T_4 levels were observed to increase spontaneously during the T_3 treatment, indicating spontaneous recovery of thyroid functional capacity. The average time for recovery of function and discontinuation of treatment was 50 days.[76]

Premature infants also are particularly susceptible to iodine-induced hypothyroidism.[13, 77] This may develop in utero if the mother is given iodine-containing medication or is studied using iodine-containing contrast agents,[78] or hypothyroidism may develop after birth in infants with neonatal iodine exposure.[68] In utero iodine exposure may be associated with development of goiter. The hypothyroidism, with or without goiter, is characterized by low serum T_4 and FT_4 concentrations and high levels of TSH. Treatment of these infants is indicated and should be continued for two or three months or until the goiter disappears. Transient hypothyroidism also has been reported in term infants exposed to iodine in utero and term infants delivered in areas of iodine deficiency.[77-79] The latter manifest a transient primary hypothyroidism responsive to iodide treatment.[76, 79] In areas of severe endemic goiter, the infants with transient iodine-deficiency hypothyroidism may constitute several percent of the newborn population. In iodine-sufficient areas, including North America and Japan, the prevalence of transient hypothyroidism is low,

perhaps 1 in 50,000 infants.[79] In these areas the mechanism is likely to be iodine overload, exposure to antithyroid medications or substances, or placental transfer from mother to fetus of TSH receptor–blocking antibodies, which produce a hypothyroid state lasting until the maternal immunoglobulin is degraded.[80-84]

The prevalence of maternal TSH receptor antibody-induced transient hypothyroidism in the neonate is unclear. Antithyroglobulin, antimicrosomal, and/or antithyroperoxidase autoantibodies are present in as many as 10 per cent of women during pregnancy.[86] These antibodies do not typically affect either pregnancy or fetal outcome.[86] However, transient maternal hypothyroidism has been reported in 25 to 30 per cent of these women during the postpartum period.[85, 86] Maternal TSH receptor–blocking antibodies are detected much less frequently than common thyroid autoantibodies and often are associated with maternal atrophic thyroiditis.[84] The neonatal hypothyroid state induced by TSH receptor antibody may be severe, and the maternal blocking antibody may be detectable for many weeks in newborn serum.[82, 83] Treatment of such infants often is necessary. Careful observation of neonates born of women with Graves' disease or Hashimoto's thyroiditis and special attention to the routine hypothyroid screening results in such newborns are recommended.

Nonthyroidal Illness

Thyroid function in the newborn premature infant is relatively immature. The TSH and T_4 surges and the T_3 responses to extrauterine exposure are relatively obtunded (Fig. 47–3), and the degree of obtundation correlates with the degree of prematurity.[9, 13] The low postnatal serum T_3 levels in premature infants presumably reflect, in part, a reduced T_3 production rate due to a relatively reduced rate of T_4 to T_3 conversion. Premature infants have an increased susceptibility to neonatal morbidity of several varieties. Infants less than 34 weeks of gestation have a high incidence of respiratory distress, and premature infants, in general, have an increased risk of vascular accidents, hypoxia, hypoglycemia, hypocalcemia, and infection as well as relative malnutrition. All of these factors tend to inhibit T_4 to T_3 conversion further in the neonatal period and aggravate the extent of the low T_3 state. Serum T_3 values may remain low in these infants (<1.0 nmol/L; 80 ng/dl) for one to two months; T_4 given to such infants increases rT_3 but not T_3 concentrations.[87] Thus, characteristics of the low T_3 syndrome or sick euthyroid syndrome in the premature infant are similar to those in older children or adults.[87-89] These include a low serum T_3 concentration due to a decreased rate of conversion of T_4 to T_3 in nonthyroidal tissues and variable serum rT_3 levels; values may be equal to or lower than concentrations in "healthy" premature infants.[87-89] We have little information on rT_3 kinetics or production rates in sick premature infants so that the mechanism(s) of the marked variability in rT_3 levels is not clear. Infants with the sick euthyroid syndrome manifest normal or low total serum T_4 concentrations, with FT_4 levels usually in the range of values for healthy premature infants of matched gestational age and weight.[87, 89] In some of these infants serum thyroid-binding globulin (TBG) levels are low and in others there may be an inhibitor of T_4 binding to TBG as described in adults with the low T_3 syndrome. Finally, these infants typically demonstrate normal serum TSH concentrations. Treatment of these infants in the absence of elevated TSH levels is not indicated.

Idiopathic Transient Hyperthyrotropinemia

Transient hyperthyrotropinemia in the newborn may occur in response to intrauterine antithyroid drug exposure or to intrauterine iodine excess or deficiency, and it has been recorded as an assay artifact.[90] In Japan the prevalence of idiopathic hyperthyrotropinemia is 1 in 16,000 to 19,000 newborns.[90, 91] Thyroid function parameters are normal in these infants except for the serum TSH concentration, which remains elevated for three to nine months. Values usually fall in the 10 to 30 mU/L range but may be higher during the neonatal period. Affected infants do not require treatment, but prolonged follow-up is necessary to exclude the possibility of an ectopic thyroid or an inborn defect in thyroid hormonogenesis.[92] If there is doubt about the diagnosis and serum FT_4 concentrations fall within the lower half of the normal range, a trial of thyroxine therapy may be diagnostic.

CONGENITAL HYPOTHYROIDISM

Mass screening for congenital hypothyroidism during the past two decades has provided extensive data characterizing the prevalence and spectrum of congenital, permanent hypothyroidism and is available in infants and children.[93–96] A summary is shown in Table 47–3.

Thyroid Dysgenesis

Thyroid dysgenesis is responsible for decreased thyroid function in most infants with permanent congenital hypothyroidism detected in screening programs. The term *thyroid dysgenesis* applies to infants with ectopic or hypoplastic thyroid glands (or both) as well as those with total thyroid

TABLE 47–3. TYPES OF THYROID DISEASE IN NEONATES

Permanent
  Thyroid dysgenesis
    Athyreotic
    Hypoplastic
    Ectopic
    Eutopic
  Thyroid dyshormonogenesis (inborn defects)
    Iodide-trapping defect
    Organification defect
    Thyroglobulin abnormality
    Iodotyrosine deiodinase deficiency
    TSH response defect
  Hypothalamic-pituitary hypothyroidism
    TSH deficiency
    TRH deficiency
Transient
  Drug-induced
  TSH receptor–blocking antibody
  Iodine deficiency
  Idiopathic

agenesis. Some thyroid tissue is present in as many as 60 per cent of these infants, so that they represent a spectrum of severity of thyroid deficiency. Thyroid scanning and uptake tests may not be sensitive enough to detect small amounts of residual functioning thyroid tissue in some infants. Normal or nearly normal circulating levels of T_3 in the face of low T_4 values suggest the presence of residual thyroid tissue, even in the absence of detectable radioiodine uptake on scanning. Measurable levels of serum thyroglobulin also indicate the presence of thyroid tissue.[97]

Thyroid dysgenesis is more prevalent in female than in male infants; the female:male ratio approximates 2:1. Although the disorder usually is sporadic, familial cases have been described. Seasonal variation in the incidence of thyroid dysgenesis, with a peak during summer months, has been reported in Japan. The prevalence is increased somewhat in Hispanic and relatively decreased in black infants (unpublished data, California Screening Program). Infants with Down's syndrome have been reported to be at increased risk; thyroid dysgenesis has also been reported in infants born with a variety of congenital anomalies, including congenital heart disease, chromosomal abnormalities, and spina bifida.[98, 99] In rare instances thyroid dysgenesis has occurred in association with maternal autoimmune thyroiditis; the disorder in these instances has been attributed to transplacentally acquired antithyroid factors.[82–84] However, there usually is no correlation between thyroid dysgenesis and the presence of maternal autoimmune thyroiditis or circulating thyroid autoantibodies.[9] Immunoglobulins that block TSH-stimulated thyroid cell growth in vitro have been reported in 15 of 34 mothers of infants with sporadic congenital hypothyroidism and in 8 of 16 postpartum infant blood samples.[100] Thus, transplacental passage of maternal immunoglobulins inhibiting TSH-induced fetal thyroid growth may play a role in the pathogenesis of sporadic congenital hypothyroidism.

Intrauterine diagnosis of congenital thyroid dysgenesis is not usually possible because of the sporadic nature of the disease. Moreover, amniotic fluid iodothyronine concentrations are not altered significantly from normal in the presence of a hypothyroid fetus.[7] Recently, fetal hypothyroidism was diagnosed on the basis of an elevated amniotic fluid TSH level and presence of a fetal goiter in a single infant; however, this approach has not been standardized.[7] Fetal hypothyroidism is easily diagnosed by direct fetal cord blood sampling, and this approach is desirable in high-risk situations (maternal antithyroid drugs, maternal autoimmune thyroiditis, familial goiter).[11, 102] Most infants with thyroid dysgenesis are asymptomatic, and few have signs of hypothyroidism during the early weeks of life. Consequently, few infants are detected by clinical criteria before the chemical screening diagnosis. Most affected infants have low serum T_4 and high TSH concentrations in cord blood or in filter paper blood spots collected at two to five days of age. Two additional subgroups of infants have been identified: One group has T_4 levels in the low normal or normal range with increased TSH values; these infants usually have ectopic thyroid tissue on scanning and may constitute 10 to 15 per cent of infants with congenital thyroid dysgenesis. The second subgroup demonstrates low serum levels of T_4 and TSH at birth, with a delayed increase in TSH to primary hypothyroid levels during the early postnatal period. The prevalence of this subgroup of infants approximates 1 in 40,000 neonates, or 5 to 10 per cent of hypothyroid infants.

Thyroid Dyshormonogenesis

The second most frequent cause of permanent congenital hypothyroidism is thyroid dyshormonogenesis.[9, 96, 101] The several hereditary defects in thyroid hormone synthesis or metabolism are reviewed in Chapter 34. Female infants with this abnormality only slightly outnumber similarly affected males. Congenital goiter may occur at birth in association with thyroid dyshormonogenesis but more commonly develops during the early months and years of extrauterine life. Thyroid radioiodine uptake is normal or increased in these infants (except in infants with a defect in iodine-concentrating ability), in contrast to most infants with thyroid dysgenesis, and normal-appearing thyroid tissue has been visible on scans in the few cases examined. These infants usually also present with low T_4 and high serum TSH concentrations, but some may be partly compensated with low serum T_4, normal T_3, and elevated TSH values.[92] A few may have normal T_4 and T_3 concentrations maintained at the expense of an elevated TSH level.

TSH-Deficient Hypothyroidism

Permanent congenital hypothyroidism due to decreased effective TSH stimulation of thyroid hormone secretion can result from various abnormalities in TSH synthesis and metabolism. Affected infants may have anomalous hypothalamic or pituitary development or may manifest a sporadic or familial deficiency in TRH or TSH secretion, either alone or in association with other pituitary hormone deficiencies.[103] Several syndromes have been described and are reviewed in Chapter 7. These include hypothalamic hypothyroidism with TRH deficiency or insensitivity (or both), isolated TSH deficiency, familial panhypopituitarism, congenital absence of the pituitary, and panhypopituitarism with absence of the sella turcica. A mutation of the homeobox gene pit-I has been shown in a Japanese family with an autosomal recessive pattern of transmission of multiple pituitary hormone deficiencies, including TSH, GH, and prolactin.[104] The pit-I gene encodes a protein that normally activates a series of target genes programming pituitary gland development.

Infants with hypothalamic (tertiary) hypothyroidism due to TRH deficiency are suspected on the basis of persistently low serum T_4, T_3, and FT_4 values with variable serum TSH concentrations.[105] In addition, infants with hypothalamic hypothyroidism may have a normal or prolonged TSH response to exogenous TRH. Infants with pituitary TSH deficiency have low serum T_4, T_3, and FT_4 levels associated with normal or low serum TSH concentrations, and they do not manifest a normal TSH response to TRH. These infants usually are not detected in screening programs unless infants with low T_4 and low TSH levels are further examined.

EVALUATION AND TREATMENT OF INFANTS WITH SUSPECTED CONGENITAL HYPOTHYROIDISM

A positive screening report for CH (elevated serum TSH) in a newborn requires prompt evaluation of the infant, including a history, physical examination, and laboratory testing. A careful maternal history should be obtained. A history of autoimmune thyroid disease in the family suggests the possibility of transient CH, either drug or maternal TSH receptor autoantibody induced. Recurrent CH in the same sibship also suggests maternal autoantibody-mediated disease. A history of familial congenital thyroid disease suggests thyroid dyshormonogenesis, which usually is transmitted as an autosomal recessive trait.

Physical examination may reveal one of several early and subtle manifestations of hypothyroidism, including a large posterior fontanelle (>1 cm diameter), prolonged jaundice (hyperbilirubinemia >7 days), macroglossia, hoarse cry, distended abdomen, umbilical hernia, hypotonia, and goiter. The prevalence of congenital anomalies in infants screening positive for CH is increased. These include congenital heart disease, trisomy 18 or 21, spina bifida, Pierre Robin syndrome, spastic diplegia or quadriplegia, and metabolic disorders.[99]

The diagnosis of CH is confirmed by measurements of plasma or serum T_4 and TSH levels. In infants with proven CH, 90 per cent have TSH levels above 50 mU/L (50 μU/ml) and 75 per cent have T_4 concentrations below 84 nmol/L (6.5 μg/dl). Some 25 per cent of CH infants have T_4 levels in the 84 to 165 nmol/L range (6.5 to 13 μg/dl), usually with clearly elevated TSH concentrations (>30 mU/L; 30 μU/ml). A few infants manifest serum levels of T_4 in the low normal range (84 to 165 nmol/L) with only modest TSH elevations (10 to 30 mU/L). The latter infants may require repeated examinations in order to establish a firm diagnosis of CH.

All infants with abnormal test results should undergo radionuclide scanning if possible, using either technetium or ^{123}I.[103] Radioiodine-123 is preferred, if available; technetium is trapped by thyroid follicular cells but not organified. Use of radioiodine provides greater isotope concentration and allows later scanning (6 to 24 hours) with lower background radioactivity and improved discrimination. The confirmation of an ectopic thyroid gland provides a definitive diagnosis of thyroid dysgenesis. The absence of uptake of radioisotope suggests thyroid agenesis, but low radioisotope uptake may be due to a TSH receptor defect, an iodide trapping defect, or TSH receptor blockade by maternal TSH receptor–blocking antibody (TBA). These infants or their mothers should have blood drawn for measurement of TBA if there is a history of maternal autoimmune thyroid disease. Thyroid ultrasonography confirms thyroid gland agenesis.

A normal thyroid scan and/or an ultrasound-positive thyroid gland in the presence of hypothyroidism indicates impaired thyroid hormone synthesis.[103] This can be due to blockade by drugs, to a TSH or TSH receptor defect, or to an inborn defect in thyroid hormone synthesis. Infants with mild to moderate TBA-mediated transient CH may have normal thyroid scan results. Thyroid gland function in these infants is a function of the titer and affinity of the TSH receptor–blocking antibody. A serum thyroglobulin measurement may be helpful in infants with absent uptake or normal scans. A very low or absent serum thyroglobulin level indicates thyroid agenesis in an infant with absent radioisotope uptake and suggests a defect in thyroglobulin synthesis in infants with a normal imaging study. Infants with thyroid dysgenesis have elevated serum thyroglobulin levels that relate to the mass of residual thyroid tissue and the degree of TSH receptor stimulation. However, their levels usually do not exceed 1000 pmol/L (660 ng/ml).[4] Very high levels (>1000 pmol/L) may be observed in infants with CH due to defective T_4 synthesis not involving the capacity of thyroglobulin production.[4] Serum calcitonin levels also are low in CH infants with thyroid agenesis but offer no advantage over the thyroglobulin measurement in diagnosis. These approaches are summarized in Figure 47–4.

Treatment is begun promptly in all infants. The goal of newborn CH screening is the institution of early, adequate thyroid hormone replacement therapy. It is now clear from animal studies that most of the brain cell thyroid hormone is derived from local T_4 to T_3 conversion; approximately 70 per cent of the T_3 in the cerebral cortex of perinatal rats is derived via local T_4 monodeiodination.[43, 44] Thus, the preferred thyroid hormone preparation for treatment of infants with CH is sodium-L-thyroxine (Na-L-T_4).

To guarantee adequate hormone to all infants, it is desirable to maintain the serum T_4 in the upper half of the normal range during therapy. The 97 per cent upper limit of serum T_4 levels in hypothyroid infants often ranges to 130 nmol/L (10 μg/dl). For these reasons the target range for the total T_4 concentration is 130 to 206 nmol/L. This assumes a normal serum TBG concentration that can be confirmed by measuring a normal range T_3 resin uptake or TBG level at the time of the first post-treatment T_4 meas-

urement. Alternatively, a direct FT_4 measurement can be used and should be maintained in the upper half of the normal range for the method. To rapidly normalize the serum T_4 concentration in the CH infant, an initial dose of Na-L-T_4 of 10 to 15 μg/kg/day is recommended.[106, 107] For the average term infant an initial dose of 50 μg (0.050 mg) daily is recommended. This dose increases the total serum T_4 concentration to the upper half of the normal range within 1 to 2 weeks.[106] Individual T_4 doses are adjusted at four- to six-week intervals during the first six months and at two-month intervals during the next year to maintain serum T_4 levels in the 130 to 206 nmol/L (10 to 16 μg/dl) range.

Serum TSH concentrations in most treated infants with CH remain relatively high despite normalized levels of T_4 or FT_4.[108, 109] The relative elevation of serum TSH is more marked during the early months of therapy but can persist to some degree through the second decade of life.[109] Raising the total serum T_4 to 130 to 206 nmol/L (10 to 16 μg/dl) or the FT_4 to the upper half of the normal range during the first one to two years of treatment lowers the serum TSH concentration below 20 mU/L (20 μ U/ml) in most CH infants. In the remainder, raising the serum T_4 level to the 155 to 206 nmol/L (12 to 16 μg/dl) range usually lowers the TSH value to less than 20 mU/L. Untoward serum TSH elevations or thyrotoxic signs and symptoms should be avoided. The elevated serum TSH level relative to T_4 concentration in CH infants is due to a resetting of the feedback threshold for T_4 suppression of TSH release in infants with CH. This resetting occurs in utero, but the mechanism remains obscure.

Physical growth and development of infants with CH usually are normalized by early adequate therapy, and infants with a delay in bone maturation at the time of diag-

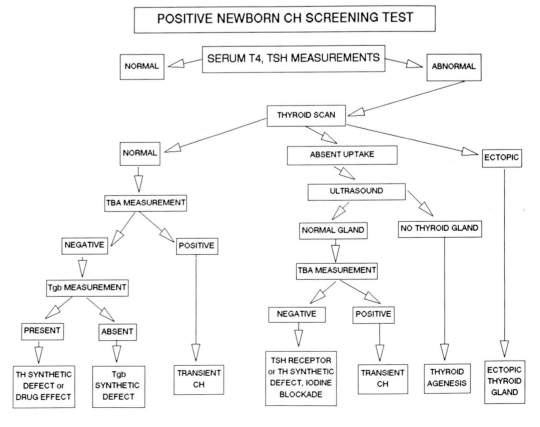

FIGURE 47–4. Suggested work-up of an infant with positive newborn congenital hypothyroidism screening results. Abbreviations: CH, congenital hypothyroidism; Tgb, thyroglobulin; TBA, thyroid blocking antibodies. See text for details.

nosis normalize their bone age by one to two years of age. IQ values and mental and motor development also are normalized in most infants with CH. However, low normal or occasionally low IQ values have been reported in a small subset of CH children with very low serum T_4 and delayed bone maturation at birth.[110-112] Many of these infants were treated with a relatively low dose of T_4. Rovet and colleagues[111] have observed that increasing the dose of replacement T_4 from 7 to 9 µg/kg day to 8 to 10 µg/kg day increases the childhood IQ of CH infants by four or five points. These investigators also have noted a significant 5- to 10-point lower mean IQ in infants in whom onset of treatment was delayed four weeks or more in association with more severe hypothyroidism manifested by a delayed bone age and/or higher serum TSH level at the time of diagnosis.[111] Thus, the most critical period of thyroid dependency of the human CNS is the first year of postnatal life. It is possible that this critical period extends for a few weeks in utero, but IQ values are normalized even in most athyroid infants by early adequate postnatal treatment.

A definitive cause of CH often can be established during the neonatal period. However, the specific defect (agenesis versus transplacentally acquired TBA versus inborn error) may not be resolved by the pretreatment assessment of many infants. In the absence of a definitive cause, the Na-L-T_4 treatment can be withdrawn for 30 days at two to three years of age without compromising brain maturation. After hormone withdrawal, persistence of the primary hypothyroid state can be confirmed by measurement of a low serum T_4 concentration and elevated TSH level. Appropriate scan, ultrasound, chemical, kinetic, and biopsy evaluation can be conducted at that time to determine the cause of the hypothyroid state. These approaches have been outlined in detail elsewhere (see Chapter 45).

NEONATAL GRAVES' DISEASE

Neonatal Graves' disease is uncommon, accounting for about 1 per cent of pediatric cases of Graves' disease. This presumably is due to the low incidence of thyrotoxicosis in pregnancy (1 to 2 cases per 1000 pregnancies) and the fact that neonatal disease occurs only in about 1 in 70 cases of thyrotoxic pregnancy.[113, 114] In most cases the disease is due to transplacental passage of maternal thyroid-stimulating antibody (TSA) from a mother with active or inactive Graves' disease or Hashimoto's thyroiditis.[115-120] Thus, prediction of neonatal Graves' disease from the maternal clinical status is not possible. However, it is possible to predict neonatal disease in offspring of women with high TSA titers.[115, 116, 119] TSA titers (measured by stimulation of cAMP in FRTL rat thyroid cells or human thyroid slices) exceeding 500 per cent of control values usually are associated with fetal and/or neonatal hyperthyroidism.[115] Neonatal hyperthyroidism is also more likely if cord blood TSH levels are suppressed (<2 mU/L) even in the presence of normal cord serum T_4 levels.[121] The presence of TSH receptor-binding inhibiting antibodies (TBIAb) also has been demonstrated in infants developing neonatal Graves' disease, and a high titer of TBIAb can transiently block the effect of TSAb, thus delaying the onset of neonatal thyrotoxicosis by several weeks.[116, 117] However, most infants with neonatal Graves' disease do not manifest blocking antibod-

ies, and the disease is manifest in utero or in the first week of life.

Graves' disease in the newborn is manifested by irritability, flushing, tachycardia, hypertension, poor weight gain or excessive weight loss, thyroid enlargement, and exophthalmos.[122-125] Thrombocytopenia with hepatosplenomegaly and jaundice and hypoprothrombinemia also have been observed. Arrhythmias, cardiac failure, and death may occur if the thyrotoxicity is severe and the treatment is inadequate. Mortality approaches 25 per cent in disease severe enough to be diagnosed. Although Graves' disease may be manifest at birth, in some infants the onset of symptoms and signs may be delayed as long as eight to 10 days. This is due to the postnatal depletion of transplacentally acquired blocking doses of antithyroid drugs and to the increase in hepatic conversion of T_4 to active T_3 at the time of birth.[9, 123] Most of the T_4 secreted in the fetus is converted to inactive rT_3. The diagnosis is confirmed by measuring high levels of T_4, FT_4, and T_3 in blood drawn postnatally. Cord blood values may be normal or nearly normal, whereas levels at two to five days may be markedly increased. The serum TSH is low in cord blood before the clinical manifestations of hyperthyroidism and remains low in the hyperthyroid state. Neonatal Graves' disease usually resolves spontaneously as maternal TSA in the newborn is degraded; the half-life approximates 21 days. The usual clinical course of neonatal Graves' disease extends 3 to 12 weeks.[120, 123]

The treatment of hyperthyroidism in the newborn includes sedatives and digitalis as necessary. Iodide or thionamide drugs are administered to decrease thyroid hormone secretion.[125] These drugs have additive effects with regard to inhibition of hormone synthesis; in addition, iodide rapidly inhibits hormone release. Lugol's solution (5 per cent iodine and 10 per cent potassium iodide; 126 mg of iodine per milliliter) is given in doses of one drop (about 8 mg) three times daily. Methimazole or propylthiouracil is administered in doses of 0.5 to 1 mg or 5 to 10 mg, respectively, per kilogram daily in divided doses at 8-hour intervals. A therapeutic response should be observed within 24 to 36 hours. If a satisfactory response is not observed, the dose of methimazole or propylthiouracil and iodide can be increased by 50 per cent. Treatment with sodium ipodate or sodium iopanoate may be useful.[120] Adrenal corticosteroids in anti-inflammatory doses and propranolol (1 to 2 mg/kg/day) also may be helpful.[123-125]

THYROID DISEASE IN CHILDHOOD AND ADOLESCENCE

Maturation of Thyroid Function

The thyroid gland during childhood is hyperactive relative to the adult, and a progressive decrease in activity occurs during the first two decades of life. With increasing age there is a decreasing oxygen consumption rate, a decrease in the percentage of protein-bound iodine-131 appearing in plasma 24 hours after administration of a tracer dose of ^{131}I, a decreasing serum thyroglobulin concentration, and a decreasing daily T_4 degradation rate. These changes are depicted in Figure 47–5. These changes are reflected in a decreasing oral replacement dose of T_4 with increasing age. Suggested doses are listed in Table 47–5. Serum total T_4 and T_3 concentrations also decrease progressively with age, largely owing to a decrease in TBG concentration during the first decade. These changes are outlined in Figure 47–4.

Hypothyroidism in Childhood

Differential Diagnosis

The differential diagnosis of hypothyroidism in childhood is summarized in Table 47–4. The prevalence of late-onset hypothyroidism in children with congenital thyroid dysgenesis who are not detected in the newborn period is not clear. It is clear that most infants with thyroid dysgenesis are detected at birth. However, it is possible that infants with a relatively large mass of residual thyroid tissue at birth many manifest hypothyroidism after age two or three years as the functioning thyroid tissue fails or is removed surgically.[92] In addition, infants with TSH deficiency or a delayed rise in serum TSH are not detected at birth and present with hypothyroidism in infancy or early childhood.[96, 103] Infants with peripheral thyroid hormone resistance usually are not detected at birth and present during childhood with clinical evidence of delayed growth and development. In most patients the hypothyroidism is mild to moderate in degree; however, the peripheral resistance syndrome is heterogeneous, with varying degrees of goiter, clinical hypothyroidism, modes of inheritance, and responsiveness to exogenous thyroid hormones (see Ch. 45).

Acquired drug-induced goiter may occur in patients taking iodides, cobalt-containing drugs, lithium salts, paraminosalicylic acid (PAS), aminoglutethimide, phenylbutazone, or antithyroid drugs (propylthiouracil, methimazole, perchlorate, thiocyanate).[126] Naturally occurring goitrogens have been reported in ground water, soybeans, and plant members of the genus *Brassicae* (such as cabbage). Acquired hypothalamic-pituitary hypothyroidism is uncommon. Perhaps the most common cause is surgery for CNS tumors, including craniopharyngiomas. Idiopathic cases have been reported to present with growth failure, and such cases may be difficult to distinguish from children with primary hypothyroidism.

The most common cause of acquired hypothyroidism in

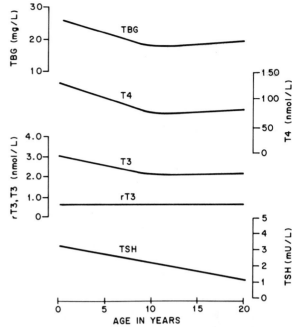

FIGURE 47–5. Variations in serum thyroxine binding globulin (TBG), T_4, T_3, reverse T_3 (rT_3), and TSH concentrations during the first 20 years of life.

children in North America after six years of age is Hashimoto's thyroiditis. The disorder was diagnosed in 1.3 per cent of a series of 5000 surveyed school children 11 to 18 years of age and may have a prevalence as high as 6 per cent in areas of Appalachia.[126, 127] The disease is similar in childhood and in adulthood, and children, like adults, usually are asymptomatic during the early stages of the disease, presenting with a euthyroid goiter.[126, 128, 129] The spectrum of the disease in children, as in adults, includes hypothyroid goiter, thyrotoxicosis, nodular goiter, thyroid antigen-antibody nephritis, and multiple endocrine deficiency disease. The latter includes diabetes mellitus, adrenal insufficiency, hypoparathyroidism, moniliasis, and, less commonly, pernicious anemia and thrombocytopenia.[130] Hashimoto's thyroiditis has been reported with increased frequency in children with gonadal dysgenesis, Down's syndrome, Klinefelter's syndrome, and Noonan's syndrome.[131] The mechanism is not clear.

Hypothyroidism, either compensated or overt, also is observed in association with nephropathic cystinosis or after treatment of brain tumors in children.[132, 133] In cystinosis the thyroid gland shows extensive destruction and infiltration of the epithelium with cystine crystals. The prevalence of goiter, cretinism, and hypothyroidism in children in endemic goiter areas is well known and is discussed in Chapter 49. Acquired hypothyroidism also is common after surgical or radioiodine treatment of thyrotoxicosis.

Clinical Manifestations

Somatic growth, bone growth and maturation, and tooth development and eruption are critically thyroid dependent. In addition, some two thirds of postnatal brain growth and differentiation occurs during the first two years of life, the period during which thyroid dependency is manifest. After three years of age thyroid hormone defi-

TABLE 47–4. CAUSES OF HYPOTHYROIDISM IN CHILDHOOD AND ADOLESCENCE: LATE-ONSET CONGENITAL DISEASE

1. Rudimentary thyroid in usual location, "cryptothyroidism"
2. Rudimentary ectopic thyroid
3. Inborn defect in thyroid metabolism—partially compensated goitrous hypothyroidism
4. Peripheral resistance to thyroid hormone action
5. Hashimoto's thyroiditis
   a. Isolated
   b. With other endocrine gland deficiencies
6. Hypothalamic-pituitary hypothyroidism
7. Drug-induced hypothyroidism
8. Endemic iodine deficiency
9. Miscellaneous
   a. Chromosomal disorders
   b. Cystinosis
   c. Thalassemia

ciency is not associated with mental retardation, but delayed somatic and linear bone growth and delayed eruption of permanent dentition are prominent.[126] Bone maturation, measured as bone age, also is delayed, diaphyseal bone growth is reduced, and epiphyseal growth and mineralization largely cease.

Hypothalamic–anterior pituitary function also may be abnormal in hypothyroid children. Although in most children thyroid hormone deficiency leads to delayed sexual development, occasional children manifest precocious sexual maturation[134–137]; increased levels of circulating gonadotropins have been measured in children of both genders with such manifestations. In girls, serum prolactin levels also tend to be increased, and galactorrhea may occur if serum estrogen levels are high enough to permit breast development and milk production. The mechanism of the precocious gonadotropin and prolactin hypersecretion is not clear. Hypertrichosis, muscular hypertrophy, and pituitary enlargement also may be observed.[126, 138, 139] These changes seem to occur in children with high serum TSH levels.

During childhood and adolescence and until epiphyseal closure, thyroid hormone deficiency leads to reduced somatic growth, reduced linear bone growth, and delayed bone maturation. This is depicted in Figure 47–6. In addition, epiphyseal dysgenesis is commonly observed. Reilly and Smyth in 1937 coined the term *cretinoid epiphyseal dysgenesis*[140] to characterize the stippled and scattered pattern of calcification in developing epiphyses of hypothyroid children. The effects of thyroid hormone deficiency on dental development are less profound, but delay in eruption of second dentition may occur. Abnormalities of hypothalamic-pituitary function secondary to hypothyroidism also are common in adolescence.[126] Puberty often is delayed or incomplete. In normal girls, menstrual cycling evolves gradually during adolescence so that early menstrual cycles commonly are nonovulatory and bleeding may be irregular. This pattern usually is more prolonged in

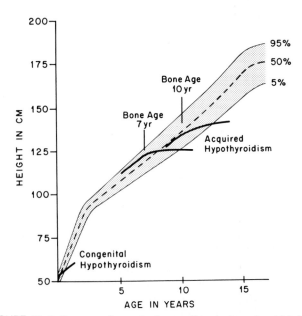

FIGURE 47–6. Patterns of growth abnormalities in hypothyroid infants and children. One of the most consistent manifestations is a decreased growth rate.

TABLE 47–5. RECOMMENDED REPLACEMENT DOSAGE OF NA-L-T₄ FOR HYPOTHYROIDISM IN CHILDHOOD

Age (years)	Dose of Na-L-T$_4$ (μg/kg/day)
0–1	5–15
1–5	6
6–10	4
11–20	3

hypothyroid female adolescents. In addition, menorrhagia or hypomenorrhea may occur.

Treatment

The treatment of juvenile hypothyroidism is accomplished using Na-L-T$_4$. The drug is usually given orally in a single daily dose. It is not necessary to begin treatment with a reduced dosage. After two to three years of age, the optimal maintenance dose is the dose that normalizes serum thyroxine (corrected thyroxine) to the midrange ($\pm$ 1 SD) for age and normalizes growth. Recent studies of replacement therapy for hypothyroidism suggest that the optimal dose of thyroxine is somewhat less than that recommended in the past. Currently recommended doses are shown in Table 47–5 and vary with age. In children with acquired hypothyroidism, in contrast to infants with congenital hypothyroidism, no pituitary "reset" of the feedback control of thyroid hormones occurs, so that serum TSH levels should be normal in optimally treated children.

Hyperthyroidism in Childhood

The predominant cause of hyperthyroidism in childhood and adolescence, as in adulthood, is Graves' disease. The disorder in children accounts for 1 to 5 per cent of all Graves' disease patients, 10 to 15 per cent of all pediatric thyroid disorders, and some 30 per cent of goiters observed in children.[126, 141–143] The disorder is rare before three years and increases progressively with age thereafter. The differential diagnosis of hyperthyroidism in childhood and adolescence includes hyperfunctioning thyroid adenoma or carcinoma, a TSH-secreting pituitary adenoma, inappropriate TSH secretion (pituitary T$_3$ resistance), subacute thyroiditis, and iatrogenic (factitious) hyperthyroidism. Diagnosis and management of these disorders are dealt with in Chapters 41 and 43.

Signs and symptoms of juvenile Graves' disease are generally similar to those in adults and include goiter (virtually 100 per cent, proptosis (70 to 80 per cent), sympathetic hyperactivity, myopathy, increased appetite, weight loss, heat intolerance, diarrhea, and emotional lability.[141–144] However, severe eye disease (stages 3 to 6) and pretibial myxedema are rare in childhood. Significant acceleration of growth and bone maturation also may occur. The mechanism is not clear; increased GH and somatomedin secretion or effect may be involved.

Treatment differs significantly in children and in adults. Surgery, although a viable option, is not commonly the initial treatment.[126, 141–143] A recent review of surgical complications in childhood showed a 3 per cent incidence of permanent hypoparathyroidism, an 8 per cent incidence of unilateral recurrent laryngeal nerve paralysis, and a 65 per cent incidence of permanent hypothyroidism.[141] These complications generally are inversely correlated with thyroid remnant size and can be minimized by an experienced surgeon.[145]

Radioiodine therapy also is avoided by most pediatric clinicians as the first choice of treatment. It now is clear that the risk of thyroid cancer in adult patients receiving radioiodine for therapy of Graves' disease is not increased above the risk in surgically treated patients (see Chapter 41). The number of Graves' disease patients treated with radioiodine between 10 and 20 years of age is limited, but available evidence suggests that in this group the cancer risk also is negligible. However, there is a high risk of permanent hypothyroidism and a significant risk of thyroid adenomas. Because of the long life expectancy of children and the long latency of late radiation effects, physicians are justifiably reluctant to use radioiodine as a first-line therapy in patients less than 15 years of age. However, radioiodine has become a preferred second treatment choice in older adolescents and has been proposed as an acceptable initial treatment alternative.[146] An ablative dose of radioiodine eliminates concerns about later neoplasia and multiple treatment doses. Moreover, cost and convenience favor this approach in all patients who do not respond to a single 6- to 12-month course of an antithyroid drug.[146]

The majority of juvenile Graves' disease patients are treated with antithyroid drugs. The use and complications of thionamide drug treatments are similar in adults and children. Two recent reviews document results of treatment with propylthiouracil or methimazole in 169 children.[141, 143] The usual dose is 150 to 300 mg daily of propylthiouracil or 15 to 30 mg daily of methimazole. The lower dose is used in smaller children. Maintenance doses were 100 to 150 or 10 to 15 mg daily, respectively, in either two or three doses.[141, 143] The average period from onset of therapy to euthyroidism was eight weeks. For long-term management, two types of drug management are used: propylthiouracil or methimazole alone, or an antithyroid drug plus supplemental Na-L-T$_4$. Some believe that with the latter approach higher doses of antithyroid drug can be given to assure continuing blockade of hormone synthesis while avoiding hypothyroidism and TSH-induced goiter. The adequacy of drug treatment can be monitored by serial measurements of serum T$_4$ and T$_3$ and on occasion TSH.[147] The disappearance of goiter has been found to correlate with the likelihood of a spontaneous remission.[141, 143] Some physicians have recommended using a perchlorate discharge test to assess the adequacy of the antithyroid drug blockade. However, TSA assays provide a more direct approach to monitor disease activity. The remission rate in children approximates 25 per cent each two years over a six-year follow-up period.

Drug toxicity occurs in 10 to 15 per cent of patients; about half of these manifest minor and half major problems. The latter include granulocytopenia, thrombocytopenia, erythema multiforme, and drug fever. Minor reactions (urticaria or generalized pruritus without rash) usually can be resolved with a change in drug. One quarter to one third of initially drug-treated patients are eventually treated surgically because of radioiodine reactions, noncompliance, or lack of remission with long-term drug treatment.[141, 143, 146]

REFERENCES

1. Fisher DA: Thyroid hormone effects on growth and development. In Delange F, Fisher DA, Malvaux P (eds): Pediatric Thyroidology. Basel, Karger, 1985, pp 75–89.
2. Schwartz HL: Effect of thyroid hormone on growth and development. In Oppenheimer JH, Samuels HH (eds): Molecular Basis of Thyroid Hormone Action. New York, Academic Press, 1983, pp 413–444.
3. Morreale de Escobar G, Pastor R, Obregon MJ, Escobar del Rey F: Effects of maternal hypothyroidism on the weight and thyroid hormone content of rat embryonic tissues before and after onset of fetal thyroid function. Endocrinology 117:1890–1896, 1985.
4. Vulsma T, Gons MH, De Vijlder JJM: Maternal fetal transfer of thyroxine in congenital hypothyroidism due to a total organification defect or thyroid agenesis. N Engl J Med 321:13–16, 1989.
5. Roti E, Gnudi A, Braverman LE: The placental transport, synthesis and metabolism of hormones and drugs which affect thyroid function. Endocrinol Rev 4:131–149, 1983.
6. Klein AH, Murphy BEP, Oddie TH, Fisher DA: Amniotic fluid thyroid hormone concentrations during human gestation. Am J Obstet Gynecol 136:626–630, 1980.
7. Kourides IA, Berkowitz RL, Pang S, et al: Antepartum diagnosis of goitrous hypothyroidism by fetal ultrasonography and amniotic fluid thyrotropin concentration. J Clin Endocrinol Metab 59:1016–1018, 1984.
8. Fisher DA, Dussault JH, Sack J, Chopra IJ: Ontogenesis of hypothalamic-pituitary-thyroid function and metabolism in man, sheep and rat. Recent Prog Horm Res 33:59–116, 1977.
9. Fisher DA, Klein AH: Thyroid development and disorders of thyroid function in the newborn. N Engl J Med 304:702–712, 1981.
10. Fisher DA: Ontogenesis of hypothalamic-pituitary-thyroid function in the human fetus. In Delange F, Fisher DA, Malvaux P (eds): Pediatric Thyroidology. Basel, Karger, 1985, pp 19–32.
11. Thorpe-Beeston JG, Nicolaides KH, Felton CV, et al: Maturation of the secretion of thyroid hormone and thyroid-stimulating hormone in the fetus. N Engl J Med 324:532–536, 1991.
12. Klein AH, Oddie TH, Parlow M, Fisher DA: Development changes in pituitary thyroid function in the human fetus and newborn. Early Human Develop 6:321–330, 1982.
12a. Costa A, Avisio R, Benedetto C, et al: Thyroid hormones in tissues from human embryos and fetuses. J Endocrinol Invest 14:559–568, 1991.
13. Delange F, Bourdous P, Ermans AM: Transient disorders of thyroid function and regulation in preterm infants. In Delange F, Fisher DA, Malvaux P (eds): Pediatric Thyroidology. Basel, Karger, 1985, pp 367–393.
14. Fuse Y, Shimizu M, Uga N, et al: Maturation of feedback control of thyrotropin in premature infants. J Dev Physiol 14:17–22, 1990.
15. Price DJ, Sherwin JR: Autoregulation of iodide transport in the rabbit: Absence of autoregulation in fetal tissue and comparison of maternal and fetal iodination products. Endocrinology 119:2547–2552, 1986.
16. Sherwin JR, Price DJ: Autoregulation of thyroid iodide transport: Evidence for the mediation of protein synthesis in iodide-induced suppression of iodide transport. Endocrinology 119:2553–2559, 1986.
17. Theodoropoulos T, Braverman LE, Vagenakis AG: Iodine-induced hypothyroidism: A potential hazard during perinatal life. Science 205:502–503, 1979.
18. Castaing H, Fournet LP, Leger FA, et al: Thyroid of the newborn and postnatal iodine overload. Arch Franc Pediatr 36:356–358, 1979.
18a. Wu SY, Huang WS, Polk D, et al: Identification of thyroxine sulfate (T$_4$S) in human serum and amniotic fluid by a novel T$_4$S radioimmunoassay. Thyroid 2:101–105, 1992.
18b. Chopra IJ, Wu SY, Chu A, et al: A radioimmunoassay for measurement of 3,5,3′ triiodothyronine sulfate: Studies in thyroidal and nonthyroidal disease, pregnancy, and neonatal life. J Clin Endocrinol Metab 75:189–194, 1992.
18c. Wu SY, Huang WS, Polk D, et al: The development of a radioimmunoassay for reverse triiodothyronine sulfate in human serum and amniotic fluid. J Clin Endocrinol Metab 76:1625–1630, 1983.
19. Wu SY, Fisher DA, Polk DH, Chopra IJ: Maturation of thyroid hormone metabolism. In Wu SY (ed): Thyroid Hormone Metabolism: Regulation and Clinical Implications. Cambridge, MA, Blackwell Scientific, 1991, pp 293–320.

20. Chopra IJ, Sack J, Fisher DA: 3,3',5' triiodothyronine (reverse T₃) and 3,5,3' triiodothyronine (T₃) in fetal and adult sheep: Studies of metabolic clearance rates, production rates, serum binding and thyroidal content relative to thyroxine. Endocrinology 97:1080–1088, 1975.

21. Klein AH, Oddie TH, Fisher DA: Effect of parturition in serum iodothyronine concentrations in fetal sheep. Endocrinology 103:1453–1457, 1978.

21a. Wu SY, Polk D, Wong S, et al: Thyroxine sulfate is a major thyroid hormone metabolite and a potential intermediate in the monodeiodination pathways in fetal sheep. Endocrinology 131:1751–1756, 1992.

21b. Polk D, Wu SY, Huang WS, et al: Kinetics of thyroid hormone sulfoconjugate metabolism in developing sheep. Proceedings of 66th Annual Mtng of the Am Thyroid Assoc, p 541, 1992.

22. Nivosu UC, Kaplan MM, Utiger RD, Delivoria-Papadopoulos M: Surge of fetal plasma triiodothyronine before birth in sheep. Am J Obstet Gynecol 132:489–494, 1978.

23. Klein AH, Oddie TH, Fisher DA: Iodothyronine kinetic studies in the newborn lamb. J Dev Physiol 2:29–35, 1980.

24. Polk DH, Wu SY, Wright C, et al: Ontogeny of thyroid hormone effect on tissue 5'monodeiodinase activity in fetal sheep. Am J Physiol 254:E337–E341, 1988.

24a. Santini F, Cortelazzi D, Baggiani AM, et al: A study of the serum 3,5,3' triiodothyronine sulfate concentration in normal and hypothyroid fetuses at various gestational stages. J Clin Endocrinol Metab 76:1583–1587, 1993.

24b. Santini F, Chopra IJ, Wu SY, et al: Metabolism of 3,5,3' triiodothyronine sulfate by tissues of the fetal rat: A consideration of the role of desulfation of 3,5,3' triiodothyronine sulfate as a source of T₃. Pediatr Res 31:541–544, 1992.

25. Ruiz de Ona C, Obregon MJ, Escobar del Rey F, Morreale de Escobar G: Developmental changes in rat brain 5'deiodinase and thyroid hormones during the fetal period: The effects of fetal hypothyroidism and maternal thyroid hormones. Pediatr Res 24:588–594, 1988.

26. Polk D, Cheromcha D, Reviczky A, Fisher DA: Nuclear thyroid hormone receptors: Ontogeny and thyroid hormone effects in sheep. Am J Physiol 256:E543–E549, 1989.

27. Ferreiro B, Bernal J, Potter BJ: Ontogenesis of thyroid hormone receptor in fetal lambs. Acta Endocrinol 116:205–210, 1987.

28. Perez-Castillo A, Bernal J, Ferreiro B, Pans T: The early ontogenesis of thyroid hormone receptor in the rat fetus. Endocrinology 117:2457–2461, 1985.

29. Bernal J, Pekonen F: Ontogenesis of the nuclear 3,5,3' triiodothyronine receptor in the human fetal brain. Endocrinology 114:667–679, 1984.

30. Gonzales LW, Ballard PL: Identification and characterization of nuclear T₃ binding sites in fetal human lung. J Clin Endocrinol Metab 53:21–28, 1981.

31. Su JH, Lung P, Yang RK, Chao HC: Ontogenesis of nuclear T₃ receptor in human fetal brain. In Delong GR, Robbins J, Condliffe PG (eds): Iodine and the Brain. New York, Plenum Press, 1989, p 358.

32. North D, Fisher DA: Thyroid hormone receptor and receptor related RNA levels in developing rat brain. Pediatr Res 28:622–625, 1990.

33. Wills KN, Zhang XK, Pfahl M: Coordinate expression of functionally distinct thyroid hormone receptor α isoforms during neonatal brain development. Molecular Endocrinol 5:1109–1119, 1991.

34. Millstrom B, Naranjo JR, Satos A, et al: Independent expression of the α and β c-erbA genes in developing rat brain. Mol Endocrinol 5:1339–1350, 1991.

34a. Strait KA, Schwartz HL, Perez Castillo A, Oppenheimer JH: Relationship of c-erbA mRNA content to tissue triiodothyronine nuclear binding capacity and function in developing and adult rat. J Biol Chem 265:10514–10521, 1990.

35. Ferreiro B, Pastor R, Bernal J: T₃ receptor occupancy and T₃ levels in plasma and cytosol during rat brain development. Acta Endocrinol 123:95–99, 1990.

36. Letarte J, Guyda H, Dussault JH: Clinical biochemical and radiological features of neonatal hypothyroid infants. In Burrow GN, Dussault JH (eds): Neonatal Screening. New York, Raven Press, 1980, pp 225–236.

37. Price DA, Ehrlich RM, Walfish PG: Congenital hypothyroidism, clinical and laboratory characteristics of infants detected by neonatal screening. Arch Dis Child 56:845–851, 1981.

38. Letarte J, LaFranchi S: Clinical features of congenital hypothyroidism. In Walker P, Dussault JH (eds): Congenital Hypothyroidism. New York, Marcel Dekker, 1983, pp 351–383.

39. Ilicki A, Larsson A, Mortensson W: Neonatal skeletal maturation in congenital hypothyroidism and its prognostic value for psychomotor development at 3 years in patients treated early. Horm Res 33:260–264, 1990.

40. Klein AH, Meltzer S, Kenny FN: Improved prognosis of congenital hypothyroidism treated before age 3 months. J Pediatr 81:912–915, 1972.

41. Raiti S, Newns GA: Cretinism: Early diagnosis and its relation to mental prognosis. Arch Dis Child 46:692–694, 1971.

42. Glorieux J, Dussault JH, Morissette J, et al: Follow-up at ages 5 and 7 years on mental development in children with hypothyroidism detected by Quebec screening program. J Pediatr 107:913–915, 1985.

43. New England Congenital Hypothyroidism Collaborative: Neonatal hypothyroidism screening: Status of patients at 6 years of age. J Pediatr 107:915–918, 1985.

44. Morreale de Escobar G, Calvo R, Obregon MJ, Escobar del Rey F: Contribution of maternal thyroxine to fetal thyroxine pools in normal rats near term. Endocrinology 126:2765–2767, 1990.

45. Ruiz de Ona C, Morreale de Escobar G, Calvo R, et al: Thyroid hormones and 5' deiodinase in the rat fetus late in gestation: Effects of maternal hypothyroidism. Endocrinology 128:422–432, 1991.

45a. Porterfield SP, Hendrich CE: The role of thyroid hormones in prenatal and neonatal neurological development: current perspectives. Endocr Rev 14:94–106, 1993.

45b. Vulsma T, Gons MH, DeViljder JJM: Maternal-fetal transfer of thyroxine in congenital hypothyroidism due to a total organification defect or thyroid agenesis. N Engl J Med 321:13–16, 1989.

46. Klein AH, Reviczky A, Padbury JF, Fisher DA: Effect of changes in thyroid status on tissue respiration in fetal and newborn sheep. Am J Physiol 244:E603–E606, 1983.

47. Dobbing J: The later growth of the brain and its vulnerability. J Pediatr 53:2–6, 1974.

48. D'Ercole AJ: Somatomedins, insulin-like growth factors and fetal growth. J Dev Physiol 9:481–495, 1987.

49. Fisher DA: The endocrinology of fetal development. In Wilson JD, Foster DW (eds): Textbook of Endocrinology (ed 8). Philadelphia, WB Saunders, 1992, pp 1049–1078.

50. Fisher DA, Hoath S, Lakshmanan J: The thyroid hormone effects on growth and development may be mediated by growth factors. Endocrinol Exp 16:259–271, 1982.

51. Hervas F, Morreale de Escobar G, Escobar del Rey F: Rapid effects of single small doses of L-thyroxine and triiodo-L-thyronine on growth hormone, as studied in the rat by radioimmunoassay. Endocrinology 97:91–101, 1975.

52. Samuels HH, Stanley F, Shapiro LE: Dose-dependent depletion of nuclear receptors for L-triiodothyronine: Evidence for a role in induction of growth hormone synthesis in cultured GH cells. Proc Natl Acad Sci USA 73:3877–3881, 1976.

53. Baxter JD, Eberhardt NL, Apriletti JW, et al: Thyroid hormone receptors and responses. Recent Prog Horm Res 35:97–154, 1979.

54. Brent GA, Harvey JW, Moore DD, Larsen PR: Multihormonal regulation of human, rat and bovine growth hormone promoters: differential effects of 3', 5' cyclic adenosine monophosphate, thyroid hormones and glucocorticoids. Mol Endocrinol 2:792–798, 1988.

55. Sato T, Suzuki Y, Taketani T, et al: Enhanced peripheral conversion of thyroxine to triiodothyronine during hGH therapy in GH deficient children. J Clin Endocrinol Metab 45:324–329, 1977.

56. Grunfeld C, Sherman BM, Cavalieri RR: The acute effects of human growth hormone and thyroid function in normal man. J Clin Endocrinol Metab 67:1111–1114, 1988.

57. VanWyk JJ, Underwood LE, Hintz RL, et al: The somatomedins: A family of insulin like hormones under growth hormone control. Recent Prog Horm Res 30:259–318, 1974.

58. Froesch ER, Zapf J, Audhya TK, et al: Nonsuppressible insulin-like activity and thyroid hormones: Major pituitary dependent sulfation factors for chick embryo cartilage. Proc Natl Acad Sci USA 73:2904–2908, 1976.

59. Holder AT, Wallis M: Actions of growth hormone, prolactin and thyroxine on serum somatomedin-like activity and growth in hypopituitary dwarf mice. J Endocrinol 74:223–229, 1977.

60. Hughes JP: Identification and characterization of high and low affinity binding sites for growth hormone in rabbit liver. Endocrinology 105:414–420, 1979.

61. Schalch DS, Udo EH, Draznin B, et al: Role of the liver in regulating somatomedin activity: Hormonal effects on the synthesis and release of insulin-like growth factor and its carrier protein by the isolated perfused rat liver. Endocrinology 104:1143–1151, 1979.

62. Glassock GF, Nicoll CS: Hormonal control of growth in the infant rat. Endocrinology 109:176–184, 1981.

63. Cavalieri H, Knobel M, Medeiros-Neto G: Effect of thyroid hormone therapy on plasma insulin-like growth factor I levels in normal subjects, hypothyroid patients and endemic cretins. Horm Res 25:132–139, 1987.

64. Walker P, Weichsel ME Jr, Hoath SB, et al: Effect of thyroxine, testosterone and corticosterone on nerve growth factor (NGF) and epidermal growth factor (EGF) concentrations in female mouse submaxillary gland: Dissociation of NGF and EGF responses. Endocrinology 109:582–587, 1981.

65. Hoath SB, Lakshmanan J, Scott SM, Fisher DA: Effect of thyroid hormones on epidermal growth factor concentration in neonatal mouse skin. Endocrinology 112:308–314, 1983.

66. Lakshmanan J, Perheentupa J, Hoath SB, et al: Epidermal growth factor in mouse ocular tissue: Effect of thyroxine and exogenous EGF. Pediatr Res 19:315–319, 1985.

67. Perheentupa J, Lakshmanan J, Fisher DA: Epidermal growth factor in mouse urine: Maturative effect of thyroxine. Pediatr Res 18:1080–1084, 1984.

68. Hoath SB, Lakshmanan J, Fisher DA: Epidermal growth factor binding to neonatal mouse skin explants and membrane preparations: effect of triiodothyronine. Pediatr Res 19:277–280, 1985.

69. Mukku VR: Regulation of epidermal growth factor receptor levels by thyroid hormone. J Biol Chem 259:6543–6547, 1984.

70. Munoz A, Rodriguez-Pena A, Perez-Castillo A, et al: Effects of neonatal hypothyroidism on rat brain gene expression. Mol Endocrinol 5:273–280, 1991.

71. Forsett A, Mitsuhashi T, DesVergue B, et al: Molecular basis of thyroid hormone regulation of myelin basic protein gene expression in rodent brain. J Biol Chem 266:23226–23232, 1991.

72. Izumo S, Nadal-Ginard B, Mahdavi V: All members of the myosin heavy chain multigene family respond to thyroid hormone in a highly tissue-specific manner. Science 231:597–600, 1986.

73. Samuels HH, Forman BM, Horowitz Z, Ye ZS: Regulation of gene expression by thyroid hormone. J Clin Invest 81:957–967, 1988.

74. Hadeed AJ, Asay LD, Klein AH, Fisher DA: Significance of transient hypothyroxinemia in premature infants with and without respiratory distress syndrome. Pediatrics 68:494–498, 1981.

75. Chowdhry P, Scanlon JW, Auerbach R, Abbassi V: Results of controlled double-blind study of thyroid replacement in very low birth weight premature infants with hypothyroxinemia. Pediatrics 73:301–304, 1984.

76. Delange F, Dalhem A, Bourdoux P, et al: Increased risk of hypothyroidism in preterm infants. J Pediatr 105:462–469, 1984.

77. Bongiovanni AM, Eberlein WR, Thomas PZ, Anderson WB: Sporadic goiter of the newborn. J Clin Endocrinol Metab 16:146–152, 1956.

78. Rodesch F, Camu M, Ermans AM, et al: Adverse effect of amniofetography on fetal thyroid function. Am J Obstet Gynecol 126:723–726, 1976.

79. Delange F, Bourdoux P, Ketelbant-Balasse P, et al: Transient primary hypothyroidism in the newborn. In Dussault JH, Walker P (eds): Congenital Hypothyroidism. New York, Marcel Dekker, 1983, pp 275–301.

80. Foley TP Jr: Sporadic congenital hypothyroidism. In Dussault JH, Walker P (eds): Congenital Hypothyroidism. New York, Marcel Dekker, 1983, pp 231–259.

81. Walfish PG: Drug and environmentally induced neonatal hypothyroidism. In Dussault JH, Walker P (eds): Congenital Hypothyroidism. New York, Marcel Dekker, 1983, pp 303–315.

82. Matsura N, Yamada Y, Nohara Y, et al: Familial neonatal transient hypothyroidism due to maternal TSH binding inhibitor immunoglobulins. N Engl J Med 303:738–741, 1980.

83. Zakarija M, McKenzie JM, Edison MS: Transient neonatal hypothyroidism: Characterization of maternal antibodies to the thyrotropin receptor. J Clin Metab 70:1239–1246, 1990.

84. Brown RS, Keating P, Mitchell E: Maternal thyroid-blocking immunoglobulins in congenital hypothyroidism. J Clin Endocrinol Metab 70:1341–1346, 1990.

85. Bech K, Hertel J, Rasmussen NG, et al: Effect of maternal thyroid autoantibodies and postpartum thyroiditis on the fetus and neonate. Acta Endocrinol 125:146–149, 1991.

86. Weetman AP, McGregor AM: Autoimmune thyroid disease: Developments in our understanding. Endocr Rev 5:309–355, 1984.

87. Eggermont E, Vanderschueren-Lodeweyckx M, De Nayer PH, et al: The thyroid system function in preterm infants of postmenstrual ages of 31 weeks or less: Evidence for a ''transient lazy thyroid system.'' Helv Paediatr Acta 39:209–222, 1984.

88. Franklin R, O'Grady C: Neonatal thyroid function: Effects of nonthyroidal illness. J Pediatr 107:599–602, 1985.

89. Fisher DA: Euthyroid low T_4 and T_3 states in prematures and sick infants. Pediatr Clin North Am 37:1297–1312, 1990.

90. Gendrel D, Feinstein MC, Grenier J, et al: Falsely elevated serum thyrotropin (TSH) in newborn infants: Transfer from mothers to infants of a factor interfering in the TSH radioimmunoassay. J Clin Endocrinol Metab 52:62–65, 1981.

91. Miki K, Nose O, Miyai K, et al: Transient infantile hyperthyrotropinemia. Arch Dis Child 64:1177–1182, 1989.

92. Tyfield LA, Abusrewil SSA, Jones SR, Savage DCL: Persistent hyperthyrotropinemia since the neonatal period in clinically euthyroid children. Eur J Pediatr 150:308–309, 1991.

93. Burrow GN, Dussault JH: Neonatal Thyroid Screening. New York, Raven Press, 1980, pp 1–322.

94. Fisher DA, Dussault JH, Foley TP, et al: Screening for congenital hypothyroidism: Results of screening one million North American infants. J Pediatr 94:700–705, 1979.

95. Delange F, Beckers C, Hofer B, et al: Progress report on neonatal screening for congenital hypothyroidism in Europe. In Burrow GN, Dussault JH (eds): Neonatal Thyroid Screening. New York, Raven Press, 1980, pp 107–131.

96. Fisher DA: Screening for congenital hypothyroidism. Trends Endocrinol 12:129–133, 1991.

97. Czernichow P, Schlumberger M, Pomarde R, Ragu P: Plasma thyroglobulin measurement helps determine the type of thyroid defect in congenital hypothyroidism. J Clin Endocrinol Metab 56:242–245, 1983.

98. Fort P, Lifshitz F, Bellisario R, et al: Abnormalities of thyroid function in infants with Down's syndrome. J Pediatr 104:545–549, 1984.

99. Delange F, Fisher DA, Glinoer D: Research in congenital hypothyroidism: NATO Advanced Science Institute Series. New York, Plenum Press, 1989.

100. Van Der Gaag RD, Drexhage HA, Dussault JA: Role of maternal immunoglobulins blocking TSH-induced thyroid growth in sporadic forms of congenital hypothyroidism. Lancet 1:246–250, 1985.

101. LaFranchi SH, Hanna CE, Krantz PL, et al: Screening for congenital hypothyroidism with specimen collection at two time periods: Results of the Northwest Regional Screening Program. Pediatrics 76:734–740, 1985.

102. Davidson KM, Richards DS, Shatz DA, Fisher DA: Successful in utero treatment of a large fetal goiter and hypothyroidism with intra-amniotic levothyroxine administration. N Engl J Med 324:543–546, 1991.

103. Fisher DA: Management of congenital hypothyroidism. J Clin Endocrinol Metab 72:523–529, 1991.

104. Tatsumi KI, Miyaki K, Notomi T, et al: Cretinism with combined hormone deficiency caused by a mutation in the pit-I gene. Nature Genet 1:56–62, 1992.

105. Foley TP Jr: Congenital hypothyroidism. In Dussault JH, Walker P (eds): Congenital Hypothyroidism. New York, Marcel Dekker, 1983, pp 331–348.

106. Fisher DA, Foley BL: Early treatment of congenital hypothyroidism. Pediatrics 83:785–789, 1989.

107. Germak JA, Foley TP Jr: Longitudinal assessment of L-thyroxine therapy for congenital hypothyroidism. J Pediatr 117:211–219, 1980.

108. Sato T, Suzuki Y, Taketani T, et al: Age related change in pituitary threshold for TSH release during thyroxine replacement therapy for cretinism. J Clin Endocrinol Metab 44:553–559, 1977.

109. McCrossin RB, Sheffield LJ, Robertson EF: Persisting abnormality in the pituitary-thyroid axis in congenital hypothyroidism. In Nagataki S, Stockigt JHR (eds): Thyroid Research VIII. Canberra, Australian Academy of Science, 1980, pp 37–40.

110. Glorieux J, DesJardins M, Letarte J, et al: Useful parameters to predict the eventual mental outcome of hypothyroid children. Pediatr Res 24:6–8, 1988.

111. Rovet J, Ehrlich R, Sorbara D: Intellectual outcome in children with fetal hypothyroidism. J Pediatr 110:700–704, 1987.

112. Heyerdahl S, Kase BJ, Lie S: Intellectual development in children with congenital hypothyroidism in relation to recommended thyroxine treatment. J Pediatr 118:850–857, 1991.

113. Harve P, Francis HH: Pregnancy and thyrotoxicosis. Br Med J 2:817–822, 1962.

114. Becks GP, Burrow GN: Thyroid disease and pregnancy. Med Clin North Am 75:121–150, 1991.

115. Zakarija M, McKenzie JM: Pregnancy-associated change in thyroid stimulating antibody of Graves' disease and the relationship to neonatal hyperthyroidism. J Clin Endocrinol Metab 57:1036–1040, 1983.

116. Zakarija M, McKenzie JM, Hoffman H: Prediction and therapy of intrauterine and late-onset neonatal hyperthyroidism. J Clin Endocrinol Metab 62:368–371, 1986.

117. Zakarija M, McKenzie JM, Munro DS: Immunoglobulin G inhibitor of thyroid-stimulating antibody as a cause of delay in the onset of neonatal Graves' disease. J Clin Invest 72:1352–1356, 1983.
118. Ten CS, Tong TC, Hutchinson JH, Yeung RTT: Thyroid stimulating immuno-globulin in neonatal Graves' disease. Arch Dis Child 55:896–906, 1980.
119. Fisher DA: Neonatal thyroid disease in the offspring of women with autoimmune thyroid disease. Thyroid Today 9:1–7, 1986.
120. Karpman BA, Rapaport B, Filetti G, Fisher DA: Treatment of neonatal hyperthyroidism due to Graves' disease with sodium ipodate. J Clin Endocrinol Metab 64:119–123, 1987.
121. Tamaki H, Amino N, Takeoka K, et al: Prediction of later development of thyrotoxicosis or central hypothyroidism from the cord serum thyroid stimulating hormone level in neonates born to mothers with Graves' disease. J Pediatr 115:318–321, 1989.
122. Hollingsworth DR, Mabry CC: Congenital Graves' disease. *In* Fisher DA, Burrow GN (eds): Perinatal Thyroid Physiology and Disease. New York, Raven Press, 1975, pp 163–183.
123. Smallridge RC, Wartofsky L, Chopra IJ, et al: Neonatal thyrotoxicosis: Alterations in serum concentrations in LATS-protector, T$_4$, T$_3$, reverse T$_3$ and 3, 3'T2. J Pediatr 93:118–120, 1978.
124. Eason E, Costom B, Papageorgiou AN: Hypertension in neonatal thyrotoxicosis. J Pediatr 100:766–768, 1982.
125. Fisher DA: Thyroid disease. *In* Gellis SS, Kagan BM (eds): Current Pediatric Therapy (ed 11). Philadelphia, WB Saunders, 1984, pp 288–293.
126. Fisher DA: The Thyroid. *In* Brook C (ed): Clinical Paediatric Endocrinology (ed 2). Oxford, Blackwell Scientific Publications, 1989, pp 309–337.
127. Rallison M, Dobyns BM, Keating FR, et al: Chronic thyroiditis: Occurrence and natural history of chronic lymphocytic thyroiditis in children. J Pediatr 86:675–682, 1975.
128. Greenberg AH, Czernichow P, Hung W, et al: Juvenile chronic lymphocytic thyroiditis: Clinical, laboratory, and histologic correlations. J Clin Endocrinol Metab 30:293–301, 1970.
129. Ling SM, Kaplan SA, Weitzman JJ, et al: Euthyroid goiters in children. Correlation of needle biopsy with other clinical and laboratory findings in chronic lymphocytic thyroiditis and simple goiter. Pediatrics 44:695–708, 1969.
130. Bright GM, Blizzard RM, Kaiser DL, Clarke WL: Organ specific autoantibodies in children with common endocrine diseases. J Pediatrics 100:8–14, 1982.
131. Fisher DA: Thyroid Disorders. *In* Emery AEH, Rimoin DL (eds): Principles and Practice of Medical Genetics (ed 2). Edinburgh, Churchill Livingstone, 1990, pp 1489–1502.
132. Lucky AW, Howley PM, Megyesi K, et al: Endocrine studies in cystinosis: Compensated primary hypothyroidism. J Pediatr 91:204–210, 1977.
133. Ogilvy Stuart AL, Shalet SM, Gattamaneni HR: Thyroid function after treatment of brain tumors in children. J Pediatr 119:733–737, 1991.
134. Van Wyk JJ, Grumbach MM: Syndrome of precocious menstruation and galactorrhea in juvenile hypothyroidism: An example of hormonal overlap in pituitary feedback. J Pediatr 57:416–435, 1960.
135. Costin G, Kershnar AK, Kogut MD, Turkington RW: Prolactin activity in juvenile hypothyroidism and precocious puberty. Pediatrics 50:881–889, 1972.
136. Lee PA, Blizzard RM: Serum gonadotropins in hypothyroid girls with and without sexual precocity. Johns Hopkins Med J 135:55–60, 1974.
137. Hemady ZS, Siler-Khodr TM, Najjar S: Precocious puberty in juvenile hypothyroidism. J Pediatr 92:55–59, 1978.
138. Nishi Y, Hamamoto K, Kajiyama M, et al: Pituitary enlargement, hypertrichosis and blunted growth hormone secretion in primary hypothyroidism. Acta Paediatr Scand 78:136–140, 1989.
139. Hung W, Fitz CR, Lee EDH: Pituitary enlargement due to lingual thyroid gland and primary hypothyroidism. Pediatr Neurol 6:60–62, 1990.
140. Reilly WA, Smyth FS: Cretinoid epiphyseal dysgenesis. J Pediatr 11:786–796, 1937.
141. Barnes V, Blizzard RM: Antithyroid drug therapy for toxic diffuse goiter (Graves' disease): Thirty years experience in children and adolescents. J Pediatr 91:313–320, 1977.
142. Maenpaa J, Kuusi A: Childhood hyperthyroidism. Acta Paediatr 60:137, 1980.
143. Collen RJ, Landau EM, Kaplan SA, Lippe PM: Remission rates of children and adolescents with thyrotoxicosis treated with antithyroid drugs. Pediatrics 65:550–556, 1980.
144. Howard CP, Hayles AB: Hyperthyroidism in childhood. Clin Endocrinol Metab 7:127–163, 1978.
145. Richie W, Beck JS, Pollet JE: Prevention and management of hypothyroidism after thyroidectomy for thyrotoxicosis. World J Surg 2:307–319, 1978.
146. Hamburger JI: Management of hyperthyroidism in children and adolescents. J Clin Endocrinol Metab 60:1019–1024, 1985.
147. Golden MP, Kaplan SA, Lippe BM, Lee WNP: Value of simultaneous T$_3$, T$_4$, and TSH measurements for management of Graves' disease in children. Pediatrics 59:762–767, 1977.

Diagnosis and Treatment of Thyroid Disease During Pregnancy

GREGORY P. BECKS
GERARD N. BURROW

BACKGROUND AND HISTORICAL PERSPECTIVE

Thyroid diseases occur commonly in women of reproductive age and are well described complications in reproductive dysfunction, pregnancy, and the puerperium.[1-6] Historically, an enlarging thyroid gland was viewed as a positive sign of pregnancy in younger women in Egyptian and Roman times,[7-9] but it remains controversial whether significant goiter is an acceptable physiological accompaniment of pregnancy. The spectrum of thyroid disease in pregnancy is similar to that in the normal female population (Table 48–1). Some cases of thyrotoxicosis are attributed to the thyroid-stimulating action of human chorionic gonadotropin (hCG) or related molecules.[10, 11] One in 20 women experiences postpartum thyroiditis.[12] The clinical manifestations of thyroid disease overlap those of normal pregnancy, and results of traditional tests of thyroid and metabolic status may be abnormal due to pregnancy itself.[13-15] Furthermore, fetal considerations influence thyroid diagnostic protocols and therapy for women of reproductive age and for the pregnant woman.[16] Fortunately, improved assays for free thyroid hormones and thyroid-stimulating hormone (TSH)[16-19] permit accurate assessment of thyroid status in pregnancy.[17-20] The availability of effective therapy, in conjunction with close clinical follow-up and monitoring, generally ensures a safe pregnancy for the mother and largely ameliorates fetal morbidity and mortality due to spontaneous abortion, intrauterine growth retardation, stillbirth, and neonatal deaths.[16]

Pregnancy itself may be viewed as a euthyroid state amid the complex changes in endocrine (including thyroid) and cardiovascular physiology that characterize gestation.[13, 14, 21-24] Pregnancy can have a favorable effect on the course of maternal autoimmune thyroid disorders, although there is a tendency to exacerbation postpartum.[25, 26] This favorable effect is due to the generalized suppression of humoral and cell-mediated immunity during gestation, which is itself an example of a successful allograft bearing a complement of maternal antigens.[27-31] The loss of immune suppression with delivery often results in a rebound during the postpartum period. Herein, we focus on thyroid problems in reproduction and of the mother during and after delivery, including the effects of thyroid disease and treatment on the fetus and changes in maternal thyroid function during normal pregnancy.

THYROID DISEASE AND REPRODUCTION

Thyroid disease has been implicated in several reproductive disorders including menstrual abnormalities, infertility, hyperprolactinemia, and pregnancy wastage.[1] Whether reproductive status has an effect on the risk of women developing thyroid disease is not clear.

Hypothyroidism

Menstruation and Fertility

Overt hypothyroidism (myxedema) may be accompanied by amenorrhea and anovulation and is sometimes associated with elevated prolactin (PRL), galactorrhea, or an enlarged sella turcica.[32-35a] Increased production of thyrotropin-releasing hormone (TRH) could account for TSH

TABLE 48–1. THYROID DISORDERS IN PREGNANCY

Goiter and thyroid nodules	Simple (nontoxic) goiter
	Thyroiditis
	Colloid nodular disease
	Iodine deficiency disorders
	Simple (true) cyst
	Papillary carcinoma
	Follicular neoplasms
Hyperthyroidism	Graves' diseases (autoimmune thyrotoxicosis)
	Subacute (painful) thyroiditis
	Lymphocytic (painless) thyroiditis
	Toxic adenoma
	Toxic multinodular goiter
	Inappropriate TSH secretion
	Metastatic follicular carcinoma (rare)
	Thyrotoxicosis factitia
	Iodine-induced thyrotoxicosis
	Gestational trophoblastic neoplasia
	Hyperemesis gravidarum (hCG-mediated)
	Hyperplacentosis
Hypothyroidism	Hashimoto's thyroiditis
	Primary myxedema
	Postablative hypothyroidism
	Surgical hypothyroidism
Postpartum thyroiditis	Thyrotoxicosis
	Hypothyroidism

and PRL hypersecretion. Another proposed mechanism is a defect in hypothalamic dopamine turnover that would also explain the observation of increased luteinizing hormone (LH) levels.[36-38] Ovulatory defects, increased PRL, and galactorrhea are thought to be reversible with thyroxine replacement therapy in severe hypothyroidism. Mild hypothyroidism may be associated with menorrhagia.[39] Anovulatory cycles and luteal phase dysfunction contribute to infertility and may accompany mild or subclinical hypothyroidism.[40-43] Subclinical hypothyroidism may also be associated with slight elevations in serum PRL or an excessive PRL response to TRH (latent hyperprolactinemia).[44-46] Studies in infertile women with mild hypothyroidism have also found increased PRL responses to metaclopramide challenge.[40, 45, 47]

A recent study from an iodine-deficient area of Germany identified 12 per cent of infertile women as having mild or subclinical hypothyroidism defined by TRH testing with excessive TSH and prolactin responses.[47] This approximated the prevalence of thyroid dysfunction in the general female population of Southern Germany. The authors indicated that previous suggestions of a major etiological role of thyroid dysfunction in infertile women may have been overestimated. A higher prevalence of abnormal postcoital tests was noted, along with a reduced number of spontaneous conceptions in the hypothyroid patients. Thyroxine therapy for hypothyroidism resulted in more pregnancies, while an equal percentage of women required thyroid hormone therapy plus clomiphene or gonadotropins for conception. Other female and male factors accounted for a high percentage of infertility, which persisted despite thyroxine or other hormone therapy. Contrary to earlier reports,[40, 44] treatment of latent hyperprolactinemia in hypothyroidism with dopamine agonists was not effective in improving pregnancy rates.[47] An ovarian hyperstimulation syndrome (multiple giant follicular cysts), with normal prolactin and gonadotropin levels has been reported in a patient with primary hypothyroidism.[48] Thyroxine therapy resulted in cyst involution.

Pregnancy Wastage

In some patients, recurrent abortions have been attributed to the presence of hypothyroidism.[49] An earlier study that assessed thyroid function by butanol extractable iodine reported a higher rate of spontaneous abortions in hypothyroidism than in pregnant euthyroid controls.[50] Up to a two-fold increase in abortions has been reported with overt hypothyroidism.[51] In some cases, lower serum thyroxine (T_4) levels may be due to a fall in thyroxine-binding globulin (TBG) associated with declining estrogen levels in a nonviable pregnancy rather than to the presence of hypothyroidism.[16] These and other studies suggest that thyroxine replacement therapy improves early pregnancy outcome when significant hypothyroidism is present.[49, 51-53] There was no difference in abortion rates among mildly hypothyroid subjects before or after thyroxine replacement therapy as compared with euthyroid individuals.[47] Two recent studies have separately reported a significantly increased risk of spontaneous abortion associated with the presence of maternal thyroid antibodies, independent of maternal age and thyroid function status.[54, 55] This may reflect an underlying generalized disorder of autoimmunity leading to increased fetal loss. Whether T_4 therapy is helpful in this situation is not known. However, the vast majority of women with recurrent miscarriages have no evidence of thyroid dysfunction or autoimmunity and are unlikely to benefit from thyroxine therapy.

Premenstrual Syndrome

It has been suggested that mild hypothyroidism, defined by isolated elevation in serum TSH levels or an exaggerated TSH response to TRH, is associated with premenstrual syndrome (PMS) in a significant proportion of cases.[56, 57] This was not confirmed is a prospective study in PMS patients and age-matched controls.[58] There would seem to be little basis now for associating PMS with thyroid dysfunction or in recommending thyroxine replacement therapy in this condition.

Thyrotoxicosis

Mild to moderate thyrotoxicosis does not necessarily affect fertility.[16] These thyrotoxic women remain ovulatory and are at normal risk for pregnancy.[32] Severe thyrotoxicosis may be accompanied by oligomenorrhea and amenorrhea.[1] The exact mechanism for this is not known. Hyperthyroidism is a hyperestrogenic state, in part caused by increased conversion of weak androgens to estrogen.[59] Gonadotropins may be elevated with loss of the midcycle LH surge[60] yet remain responsive to exogenous gonadotropin-releasing hormone (GnRH).[61, 62] There is no difference in estrogen levels despite variable gonadotropin responses to GnRH associated with menstrual disorders in hyperthyroidism, so the effects are probably due to the thyroid hormones themselves.[62] Nutritional, weight, and psychological changes in thyrotoxicosis may also contribute to menstrual dysfunction.[63] Only severe thyrotoxicosis is likely to be associated with an increased risk of spontaneous abortion.[64] Women with thyrotoxicosis in early pregnancy are usually already treated or will be treated, and there are really no adequate control data for untreated thyrotoxicosis during gestation. Adequate treatment of thyrotoxicosis should restore fertility and menstruation toward normal and reduce any early pregnancy wastage.

Reproductive Status and Thyroid Disease

Epidemiological studies of thyroid disease indicate a high prevalence among women, typically in late-reproductive or postreproductive years, including autoimmune thyroid disease, nodular thyroid disease, and thyroid carcinoma.[65, 66] This suggests possible influences of sex hormones on the development of thyroid disease. Experimentally, autoimmune thyroiditis in rats and chickens is modulated by exposure to estrogens and androgens, androgens having a protective effect.[67, 68] Estrogen exposure leads to a reduction in suppressor/cytotoxic T cells that may permit an increase in autoantibody synthesis.[69] A case-control study in 89 patients with autoimmune thyroiditis (Hashimoto's disease) found no association of thyroiditis with parity.[70] However, longer reproductive span (early menarche and/or late menopause) was associated with a two- to three-fold increased relative risk of developing euthyroid or hypothyroid Hashimoto's disease. A prospective study in pregnancy from an area of marginally low-iodine intake reported that a greater number of pregnancies and increased parity were associated with an increased prevalence of nodular thyroid disease and goiter in women with thyroid autoimmunity, or in women with a past history of thyroid disease compared with controls.[55] These changes were independent of maternal age, biochemical thyroid status, or evidence of thyroid autoimmunity. Iodide levels in the population may have played a role.

THYROID STATUS IN PREGNANCY

Thyroid Physiology

Basal Metabolic Rate

Basal metabolic rate increases 15 to 20 per cent between 4 and 8 months' gestation.[13] Most of this increase is due to oxygen consumption by the fetoplacental unit; the balance is accounted for by changes in cardiovascular physiology accompanying pregnancy.[23] Difficulties in distinguishing true basal metabolic rate, which could be a useful indicator of thyroid function status, from total metabolism in the setting of pregnancy mitigates against performing this procedure any longer.

Iodine Economy

Glomerular filtration rates increase 50 per cent in pregnancy, resulting in a sustained increase in iodide clearance.[13] Reduced tubular reabsorption of iodide by the kidneys may also contribute to increased renal clearance.[71] Plasma inorganic iodide (PII) levels may fall as a result. Similar changes in renal iodide clearance have been observed in women treated with diethylstilbestrol postpartum.[71] Additionally, iodide readily crosses the placenta (Table 48–2), with a reported fetal:maternal gradient of 5:1 suggesting an active transport process.[72, 73] Iodide accumulates in the fetal thyroid primarily after 90 days' gestation.[74–78] Lactation is another source of iodide loss in the mother.[79] This iodide loss during pregnancy has implications for maternal and fetal thyroid hormone economy considering the major problems still encountered with endemic iodine deficiency disorders on a global basis[80–82] and the existence of many geographic areas outside North America where iodide intake is marginal, that is, an average intake of less than 100 μg per day.[55, 71, 83] Goiter is unlikely to develop unless PII levels are less than 0.08 μg/dl.[84] Levels are considerably higher than this in North America with no differences in iodide balance reported in pregnant versus nonpregnant women.[85] Although such studies are now contraindicated, previous measurements of thyroid radioiodine uptake have shown increases in pregnancy dependent upon changes in PII and thyroid-stimulating activity.[13, 74–77, 86, 87] These studies used ^{132}I or in some cases ^{131}I treatment was inadvertently given to thyrotoxic pregnant women.

Serum Thyroid Hormones and Protein Binding

Circulating TBG concentrations double in pregnancy owing to estrogen stimulation of hepatic production[88] and a reduction in clearance of TBG owing to sialylation.[89] Transthyretin (prealbumin) and albumin levels are reduced.[90–92] As a result, total serum T_4, triiodothyronine (T_3), and reverse T_3 (rT_3) levels are frankly elevated in

TABLE 48–2. PLACENTAL TRANSFER AND FETAL THYROID FUNCTION

Without difficulty
Iodides
Thionamides
Thyroid autoantibodies
TRH
Some transfer
T_4
T_3
Little or no transfer
TSH

Modified from Burrow GN: Thyroid diseases in pregnancy. In Burrow GN et al (eds): Thyroid Function and Disease. Philadelphia, WB Saunders Co, 1989, p 292.

pregnancy due to increased hormone-TBG binding;[9, 90–99] binding to transthyretin and albumin is reduced.[91] As a consequence the percentage of free T_4 (FT_4) and free T_3 (FT_3) falls. Indirect estimates of free thyroid hormone status using the resin T_3 uptake test (T_3U) are typically reduced due to increased TBG and the free T_4 index (FTI) calculated from T_3U and total serum T_4 generally remains within normal limits.[17] However, this is not a particularly accurate estimate of free hormone status when TBG concentrations are increased.[100] Women with congenital TBG deficiency show little TBG rise or change in serum T_4 in pregnancy.[101, 102] At the same time, hypothyroid patients on low-dose replacement therapy fail to increase protein-bound iodine (T_4) following estrogen therapy even though T_4 binding capacity, i.e., TBG, is increased.[93] This indicates that an increase in T_4 production is required during normal pregnancy along with the increased binding capacity. It is now well recognized that many hypothyroid women require an increase of 25 to 40 per cent in T_4 dosage during pregnancy. However, studies of T_4 turnover in pregnant and estrogen-treated women have yielded normal results—around 90 µg per day.[103] Although fractional T_4 turnover is reduced, the absolute amount remains normal owing to the increase in total T_4. Glinoer and colleagues[104] recently observed that serum T_4 and T_3 concentrations failed to increase as much during pregnancy as predicted by the measured increase in serum TBG (Fig. 48–1). Thus, a state of relative hypothyroxinemia was observed, accompanied by a slight increase in serum TSH levels within the normal range in later pregnancy. Serum thyroglobulin (TG) levels also increased during pregnancy, returning to normal by 6 weeks postpartum.[55, 104, 105] These data represent one of the largest groups of pregnant women studied longitudinally and cross-sectionally during pregnancy, albeit in an area of marginal iodide intake.

Early studies of free thyroid hormone concentrations during pregnancy suggest that these remained within normal limits.[91, 98, 106, 107] Results from longitudinal studies reveal significant fluctuations in free thyroid hormone levels throughout pregnancy, although these too generally remain within normal reference limits.[19, 90–92, 104, 107–109] Free T_4 and FT_3 levels are normal or slightly increased in the first trimester between 6 and 12 weeks, fall progressively to lower normal or borderline low levels by the third trimester, and TBG saturation is reduced (Fig. 48–2). This is a consistent pattern regardless of the FT_4 assay method used (dialysis, ultrafiltration, gel filtration and adsorption, or free hormone immunoassay).[19, 110] Thus, reductions in free thyroid hormone levels in late pregnancy seem to be a real phenomenon, unaccountable for by changes in serum albumin, nonesterified fatty acids, or TBG.[19, 90, 92] The physiological relevance of these observations is unclear. The $T_3:T_4$ ratio is increased in the third trimester.[92] T_4 bound to transthyretin and albumin are possible precursors for T_3 production.[91] Increased binding of T_4 and T_3 to monocyte nuclear receptors has been reported in human pregnancy.[111] These changes may help to ensure adequate thyroid hormone action in maternal tissues. Alternatively, reduced FT_4 and FT_3 may be adaptive to energy conservation in pregnancy, which is characterized by an energy gap of approximately 600 kilojoules (KJ) per day after adjustments for changes in physical activity.[112] In support of this, reduced concentrations of T_4 and T_3 in peripheral tissues

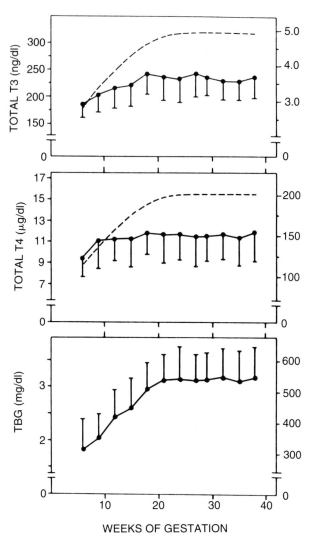

FIGURE 48–1. Serum T_4, T_3, and TBG as a function of gestational age. Each point gives the mean value ($\pm$ 1 SD) of determinations performed at the initial presentation, pooled for 3 weeks, between 5 and 28 weeks (n = 510), and again for samples obtained between 28 and 39 weeks (n = 355). The latter samples include both late initial evaluations and the second series of determinations at 30–33 weeks. Each point represents an average of 72 individual determinations. The dashed lines illustrate the theoretical curves of T_3 and T_4 concentrations required to yield the average molar ratios of T_4/TBG and T_3/TBG that correspond to nonpregnant reference subjects (0.37 for T_4/TBG and 0.0089 for T_3/TBG, using a mol wt of 57 kDa for TBG. (From Glinoer D, De Nayer P, Bourdoux P et al: Regulation of maternal thyroid during pregnancy. J Clin Endocrinol Metab 71:276, 1990. © The Endocrine Society.)

(excluding cerebral cortex) have been reported in pregnant rats near term.[113]

Thyroid Stimulation and Regulation

The histological picture of the thyroid gland during pregnancy is one of active stimulation. Columnar epithelium lining hyperplastic follicles can be seen.[114] Radioactive iodine uptake by the thyroid appears to be responsive to thyroid hormone administration in pregnancy as determined by T_3 suppression testing,[86, 87] although other studies suggest reduced sensitivity in terms of radioiodine suppression or reduction in serum protein bound iodine in late gestation following T_3 administration.[115, 116] TRH tests have been performed in pregnancy. In several studies normal

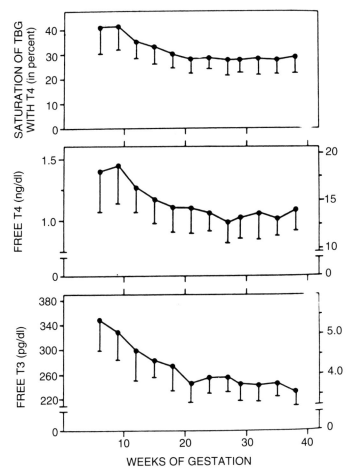

FIGURE 48-2. **Serum free T_4 and T_3 concentrations and TBG saturation as a function of gestational age.** TBG saturation by T_4 corresponds to the molar T_4/TBG ratio expressed as a percentage and was calculated from each individual set of data. Each point gives the mean values (± 1 SD) of determinations performed at the initial presentation, pooled as indicated in Figure 48-1. Each point represents an average of 72 individual determinations for TBG saturation, 64 for free T_4, and 24 for free T_3. (From Glinoer D, De Nayer P, Bourdoux P et al: Regulation of maternal thyroid during pregnancy. J Clin Endocrinol Metab 71:276, 1990. © The Endocrine Society.)

TSH responses were reported as measured by older radioimmunoassays.[117-119] We previously reported increased TSH responsiveness to TRH in women in the second trimester between 16 and 20 weeks' gestation compared with the first trimester.[120] Similar TSH responses were also seen in women taking oral contraceptives, suggesting a possible influence of estrogen. Among women undergoing first trimester therapeutic abortions, reduced TSH responses were observed in those with higher FT_4 concentrations as compared with the second trimester or normal controls.[91] The safety of TRH testing in pregnancy has been defended,[9] but TRH does the cross the placenta and it probably should not be used routinely.[72] Serum TSH levels measured by sensitive RIA or newer immunometric assays are normal to suppressed in early pregnancy and may increase within the normal range in the second and third trimester.[9, 90-92, 104-109, 121] These results are compatible with normal feedback responses at the hypothalamus and pituitary in accord with the reported changes in free thyroid hormone levels throughout pregnancy and with the presence of other thyroid stimulators, such as hCG, in early pregnancy.

hCG. With the recognition that trophoblastic hyperthyroidism is due to the thyromimetic actions of hCG,[11, 117, 122, 123] interest has focused recently on the possibility that hCG is a physiological regulator of thyroid function in early pregnancy.[91, 104, 106, 107, 124-127] Clinically, hCG levels peak in pregnancy at 50 to 100×10^3 IU/L between 6 and 12 weeks; this correlates with reduced TSH levels in the first trimester[104, 125] (Fig. 48-3). Levels decline thereafter and are undetectable by a few weeks postpartum. An overall increase in thyromimetic activity in the sera of women during early pregnancy may be due to hCG as determined by immunoadsorption studies employing hCG monoclonal antibodies.[126, 127]

Ekins[125, 128, 129] has effectively argued that an alternative control system such as hCG may regulate maternal thyroid activity in early pregnancy when the most important changes in TBG and T_4 secretion occur, ensuring an adequate supply of thyroid hormones to the placenta and embryo (Fig. 48-4B). This is compared to the conventional model of thyroid gland control which predicts a temporary decline in FT_4 during early pregnancy (Fig. 48-4A).

Experimentally, in vitro studies show that hCG binds to TSH receptors as assessed by radioreceptor assays using porcine and human thyroid membranes incubated with ^{125}I-TSH,[130-133] also stimulates adenylate cyclase activity and cAMP generation, and enhances T_3 secretion in human and porcine thyroid slices.[134] More recently hCG has been shown to stimulate growth, iodide uptake, and cAMP generation in the rat thyroid cell line FRTL5.[126, 127, 135-137] Species differences[138, 139] and microheterogeneity of hCG molecules through pregnancy and in gestational trophoblastic diseases may account for the variable thyrotropic activities reported.[125-127, 133-135, 140-142] However, with reported TSH bioactivity of up to 0.7 μU/U hCG,[133, 135] the hCG levels obtained in early pregnancy could produce a noticeable thyrotropic effect.

Thyroid Function and the Fetus

The fetal hypothalamic-pituitary-thyroid axis develops autonomously and has been extensively studied in the human, sheep, and rat.[72, 73, 143-145] A number of agents and maternal factors may affect fetal thyroid function depending on whether or not they cross the placenta (Table 48-2).

Placental Transfer

TRH/TSH. The placenta is impermeable to TSH but permeable to TRH, although endogenous maternal levels are probably too low to influence fetal thyroid function.[72] Pituitary and serum TSH in the fetus may be under control of pancreatic TRH prior to maturation of hypothalamic TRH after 20 weeks' gestation.[146-149] Injection of TRH in the mother is accompanied by increased cord serum TSH, T_4, and T_3 levels, indicating that endogenous TSH stimulates the fetal thyroid.[150] This action of TRH has been used in the prevention of respiratory distress syndrome (RDS) in the premature neonate.[151] Experimental human and animal data suggest a role of thyroid hormones in pulmonary surfactant synthesis.[152, 153]

THYROID HORMONES. Prior to the onset of human fetal

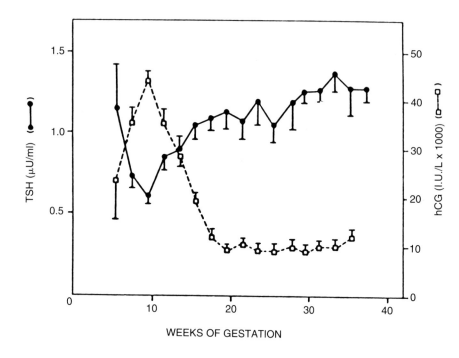

FIGURE 48–3. **Serum TSH and hCG as a function of gestational age.** Serum hCG was determined at initial evaluation and TSH at initial evaluation and during late gestation. The symbols give the mean value (± SE) for samples pooled for 2 weeks of gestation. Each point corresponds to the average of 33 determinations for hCG and 49 for TSH. (From Glinoer D, De Nayer P, Bourdoux P et al: Regulation of maternal thyroid during pregnancy. J Clin Endocrinol Metab 71:276, 1990. © The Endocrine Society.)

thyroid gland function after 10 to 12 weeks' gestation,[74–78] any requirement for thyroid hormone would be met from the maternal supply. This point is controversial. The appearance of human fetal tissue thyroid hormones and receptors before 12 to 18 weeks when fetal serum T_4 levels increase is consistent with an early requirement for thyroid hormones from the mother.[154] The placenta has generally been viewed as a substantial barrier to thyroid hormone transfer, in part owing to preferential 5-monodeiodination of T_4 to rT_3.[72, 144]

In rats there is good evidence for transfer of maternal thyroid hormones to the fetus in early and late pregnancy, which may be important for early brain development and later brain growth and neuronal differentiation.[155–160] T_4 is more important than T_3 although the latter remains the major biologically active hormone via local or systemic T_4 to T_3 conversion catalysed by 5'-monodeiodinase. In humans and sheep, maternal thyroid hormones have more limited access to the fetal circulation.[144] However, the apparent normality of sporadic congenitally hypothyroid infants at birth suggests a role of maternal thyroid hormones.[161] The devastating effects of maternal and fetal/neonatal thyroid hormone deficiency in endemic cretinism in humans underscores the overall importance of thyroid hormones to the fetus.[80–82] Fortunately, this does not seem to be a problem in areas where iodine intake is just marginal,[83] yet concern remains with respect to any effect of maternal hypothyroxinemia on early fetal brain development and the effects on progeny.[128, 129, 154, 162–164] Early studies suggested limited transfer of T_4 and T_3 across the placenta in humans in later pregnancy and at term.[116, 165–170] T_3 crosses more readily than does T_4. A recent report[171] in neonates born with a complete organification defect convincingly demonstrates maternal to fetal T_4 transfer, albeit with subnormal fetal T_4 values as compared with normals.[171]

The nonhalogenated thyroid hormone analogue 3,5 dimethyl-3'-isopropyl-L-thyroxine (DIMIT) crosses the placenta more readily than do T_4 and T_3 and has been shown to alleviate maternal and fetal hypothyroidism and goiter induced in rats and monkeys and hypothyroidism in pregnant ewes but not cretinism in the lambs.[81, 172, 173] On balance the evidence suggests at least some degree of placental transfer of thyroid hormones and that maternal thyroid hormones play a role in fetal development.

IODIDE. Iodide is actively transported to the fetus.[72] Fetal thyroid autoregulation does not develop until near term, meaning that the fetal and neonatal thyroid is susceptible to iodine-induced hypothyroidism and goiter with excessive exposure.[144, 174, 175] This can occur following intravenous, oral, mucosal or topical exposure and absorption in the mother,[176] amniography,[177] and postnatal topical absorption,[178] and can occur through breast milk.[179] A number of pregnant women have been treated with amiodarone, an antiarrhythmic drug containing 75 mg of iodine per 200 mg dose, which partially crosses the placenta and increases maternal and fetal iodide levels.[180] Although the thyroid function may remain normal, there are case reports of fetal or neonatal goiter, hypothyroidism, or hyperthyroxinemia associated with maternal amiodarone therapy.[181–183]

Diagnosis of Fetal Thyroid Disorders in Utero

The possibility of thyroid disease in the fetus is usually considered because of maternal thyroid disease. Hyperthyroidism is usually encountered in the setting of maternal Graves' disease, and hypothyroidism is associated with iodine deficiency disorders, thyroid autoimmunity, and maternal therapy.[184–186] In hypothyroidism, a fetal goiter may be visible on ultrasound,[187] or the radiographic appearance of distal femoral or proximal tibial epiphyses delayed.[188, 189] The latter has limited clinical application. Measurement of T_4 and TSH in serum collected by percutaneous umbilical cord sampling (cordocentesis)[145] is currently the most reliable means to diagnose in utero hypothyroidism[190] or hyperthyroidism.[191] This probably has advantages over the measurement of thyroid hormones or TSH in amniotic fluid,[192–194] although there is some risk to the fetus with the procedure. The fetus can absorb thyroid hormones injected into amniotic fluid and this has been used successfully in treatment of hypothyroidism and goiter in utero.[190, 195] Intramuscular thyroxine injections in utero have also been described in the treatment of hypothyroidism[196] but are probably less desirable than the amniotic fluid route.

Goiter and Pregnancy

Goiter has been historically associated with pregnancy, but its incidence and prevalence vary with geographic area and iodine status of the general population. Up to 70 per cent of pregnant women in Scotland and Ireland were considered to have a goiter on clinical grounds (visible and palpable thyroid gland) compared with 38 per cent of nonpregnant controls.[197, 198] No cumulative influence of successive pregnancies was observed as goiters were seen in 39 per cent of nulliparous women and 35 per cent of nonpregnant parous women. These studies are from areas of relatively low iodine intake. A comparative study in Iceland,[199] an area of iodine sufficiency, showed a lower basal prevalence of goiter (20 per cent) and no increase in pregnancy. Similar results are reported in studies from North America,[200, 201] leading some authors to suggest that goiter in pregnancy is a myth.[202] Most goiters during pregnancy in North America are related to autoimmune thyroid disease, colloid nodular disease, or thyroiditis. Ultrasonography has added a quantitative perspective to the assessment of goiter in pregnancy. In Denmark, an area of marginal iodine intake, a 30 per cent increase in thyroid volume has been documented between 18 and 36 weeks' gestation.[203] Volume returned to baseline postpartum and there was no evidence of thyroid dysfunction or thyroid autoimmunity. Only 25 per cent of the women actually had a goiter on clinical grounds. Serum TG levels were also increased during pregnancy.[204] Only a 13 per cent increase in thyroid volume was reported in a North American study.[205] The largest longitudinal and cross-sectional study of thyroid volume in pregnancy has been reported in over 600 women from Belgium, another area of marginal iodine intake.[104] Seventy per cent of women had a 20 per cent or greater increase in thyroid volume during pregnancy, although only 9 per cent had a significant goiter as defined by thyroid volume in excess of 23 ml. Thyroid volume showed positive correlations with higher serum TG levels and increased serum $T_3:T_4$ ratio. There was no correlation with urine iodide excretion and a negative correlation with serum TSH levels. The latter may have been due to the influence of hCG during pregnancy. The same authors from Belgium prospectively studied pre-existing mild thyroid abnormalities through pregnancy,[55] noting a significant goitrogenic effect and also an increase in the incidence and prevalence of thyroid nodules. Many of these nodules were subclinical and detected only on thyroid ultrasound. Serum TG levels were disproportionately increased in women with goiters and nodules as compared with controls, pregnant women with autoimmune thyroid disease or a history of previous thyroid abnormalities. They further suggested that previous pregnancies represented a significant risk factor for goiter and thyroid nodules. This

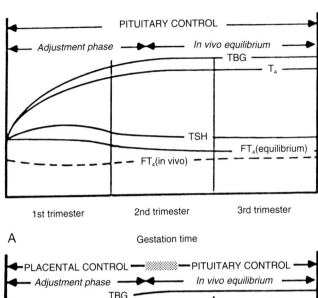

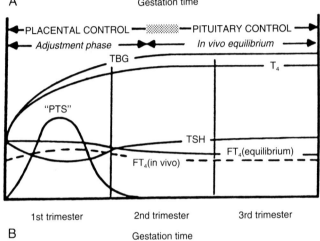

Figure 48–4. *A,* **Conventional model of maternal thyroid gland control.** Diagrammatic representation of concepts relating to maternal thyroid hormone function throughout pregnancy if based on the traditional hypothalamic/pituitary/feedback mechanism. **B, Hypothetical model of maternal thyroid gland control.** Diagrammatic representation of a hypothetical model of maternal thyroid hormone control throughout pregnancy if a putative "placental thyroid stimulator" (PTS), possibly hCG, assumes the regulatory control over maternal thyroid secretion. (From Ballabio M, Poshyachinda M, Ekins RP: Pregnancy-induced changes in thyroid function: role of human chorionic gonadotropin as a putative regulator of maternal thyroid. J Clin Endocrinol Metab 73:824, 1991. © The Endocrine Society.)

was also suggested in a study from the Netherlands.[206] It should be noted that an increase in thyroid volume during pregnancy does not necessarily denote increased mitotic activity; increased colloid volume, cell hypertrophy, inflammation, or increased thyroid blood flow could account for some of the enlargement.

There is no evidence of adverse effects on fetal development or neonatal thyroid function in these studies from areas of marginal iodine uptake.[55, 83, 104] Nor does there appear to be any increased risk of neonatal thyroid dysfunction in goitrous iodine sufficient areas.[207] This contrasts with studies from areas of endemic iodine deficiency.[80–82, 208] Maternal smoking has been shown to be a risk factor for neonatal thyroid enlargement as determined ultrasonographically.[209] Neonatal thyroid volume correlated with cord serum TG and thiocyanate levels, but there was no evidence of neonatal thyroid dysfunction.

THYROTOXICOSIS IN PREGNANCY

All forms of thyroid disease are more common in women than in men, and thyrotoxicosis is not a rare event during pregnancy, occurring in about two of every 1000 pregnancies. Thyrotoxicosis in the mother significantly increases the prevalence of low-birth-weight offspring with a trend toward increased neonatal mortality.[51, 210] Whether fetal wastage is increased in established pregnancy is not clear. In one study of 57 thyrotoxic pregnancies, the fetal wastage rate was 8.4 per cent, which compares favorably to an estimated overall fetal wastage of 17 per cent in normal women, including spontaneous abortion.[64] Very early spontaneous abortions could easily be missed in thyrotoxic women. The suggestion of a higher incidence of minor congenital malformations has been reported in the children of thyrotoxic women who were untreated during pregnancy.[210a] Down's syndrome has also been reported more frequently in children born to women with hyperthyroidism.[211] There have been reports of a greater prevalence of toxemia in thyrotoxic women, but the studies were not well-controlled.

Etiology

Autoimmune thyrotoxicosis, or Graves' disease, is the most common cause of thyrotoxicosis in the pregnant woman, accounting for about 90 per cent of cases. Toxic adenomas or nodular goiters are much less common in this age group. Other causes of thyrotoxicosis in pregnancy include gestational trophoblastic neoplasia[11, 122] and hyperemesis gravidarum (see Table 48–1).

HYPEREMESIS GRAVIDARUM. This is pernicious nausea and vomiting in pregnancy usually associated with weight loss, and fluid and electrolyte disturbances. The presentation and diagnosis can be complicated because other causes of severe nausea and vomiting in pregnancy must be excluded (Table 48–3), and thyrotoxicosis itself may be associated with hyperemesis.[212] As many as 50 per cent of cases of hyperemesis gravidarum have been reported to be hyperthyroxinemic, including increases in FT_4, FT_3, and T_3.[213, 213a] Clinical signs of thyrotoxicosis are uncommon, and the hyperthyroxinemia tends to return to normal with progression of the pregnancy and remission of the hyperemesis, or after delivery. If a goiter or thyroid antibodies are present, this suggests a primary thyroid problem. Serum TSH levels are suppressed in some but not all studies.[212–214] This may depend on the sensitivity of the TSH assays employed.

TABLE 48–3. CAUSES OF SEVERE NAUSEA AND VOMITING IN PREGNANCY

Hyperemesis gravidarum
Gastroenteritis
Gastroesophageal reflux disease
Peptic ulcer disease
Cholecystitis
Pancreatitis
Small bowel obstruction
Pyelonephritis
Thyrotoxicosis
Adrenal insufficiency
Diabetic ketoacidosis
Psychological disorders

In one study of women with hyperemesis gravidarum, 60 per cent had TSH values that were suppressed.[214, 214a] Serum hCG concentrations correlated with the FT_4 concentrations and inversely with serum TSH determinations,[214] suggesting that this may be a form of hCG-mediated thyrotoxicosis. Other investigators have postulated an increase in peripheral T_4 to T_3 conversion to account for the abnormal thyroid hormone values in cases in which TSH levels remain normal.[213a] Treatment with antithyroid medication in hyperemesis is controversial.[212, 215] Patients with hyperemesis who remain symptomatic after 20 weeks' gestation with elevated thyroid hormone concentrations and suppressed TSH levels should be considered for antithyroid drug therapy.

It has been suggested that women with hyperemesis gravidarum may be differentiated from those with Graves' disease on the basis of erythrocyte zinc levels.[216] Excessive thyroid hormone inhibits the synthesis of carbonic anhydrase, a zinc metalloenzyme. Consequently, changes in erythrocyte zinc concentrations tend to reflect the long-term influence of thyroid hormones. At the time of diagnosis, erythrocyte zinc values are low in women with Graves' disease and normal in patients with hyperemesis gravidarum. However, this observation is not of proven diagnostic value.

Diagnosis

The clinical diagnosis of mild to moderate hyperthyroidism is not easy and may be much more difficult during pregnancy. Hyperdynamic symptoms and signs are common in the normal pregnant woman, including anxiety, heat intolerance, tachycardia, and warm, moist skin. Laboratory tests may support a suspicion of thyrotoxicosis but confirmation can be difficult. The ocular changes of thyroid ophthalmopathy or pretibial myxedema do not indicate whether Graves' thyrotoxicosis is active. A resting pulse above 100, which is not decreased by a Valsalva maneuver, is strongly suggestive of thyrotoxicosis.

Despite the difficulty in interpretation of thyroid function tests because of the elevated TBG concentration during pregnancy, the diagnosis of hyperthyroidism in the pregnant woman depends on the laboratory. A sensitive TSH determination with a value less than 0.05 μU/ml with an elevated serum FT_4 or FT_3 concentration is diagnostic. The sensitive TSH assay is of particular importance because of the average decrease in FT_4 concentration of about 30 per cent during the second and third trimesters in normal pregnancy.[19, 90, 108, 109] During the first trimester the serum TSH determination may fall in response to increase in the hCG concentration.[104] The sensitive TSH determination appears to be the best laboratory indicator of thyroid function during pregnancy.[217, 218]

If the diagnosis is not clear-cut, one can usually wait three to four weeks and repeat the thyroid function tests because pregnant women tolerate mild to moderate thyrotoxicosis without difficulty in most instances. The determination of TSH receptor (TSH-R) antibodies can be helpful in a prognostic sense to alert the physician to the possibility of fetal or neonatal thyrotoxicosis. Determination of TSH-R antibodies has not been particularly helpful in the diagnosis of thyrotoxicosis in the mother during pregnancy.

Treatment

Once the diagnosis of thyrotoxicosis is established in the pregnant woman, therapy should be instituted. Preterm delivery, perinatal mortality, and maternal congestive heart failure were markedly increased in untreated and inadequately treated thyrotoxic patients in a retrospective study of 60 pregnant women with hyperthyroidism admitted to an inner city hospital over a 12-year period.[219] Women newly diagnosed as thyrotoxic during pregnancy had a higher incidence of morbidity and mortality compared with those women diagnosed and treated before conception. Socioeconomic conditions might have played a role in the severity of hyperthyroidism or poor outcomes, but treatment of thyrotoxicosis is indicated nonetheless. These patients are at risk to develop congestive heart failure because the hyperdynamic state of thyrotoxicosis is superimposed on the increased cardiac output of normal pregnancy.[220] The management of diseases such as diabetes mellitus is also complicated in the pregnant woman with thyrotoxicosis with erratic glycemic control and the need for increased insulin.[221] Treatment of thyrotoxicosis in the pregnant woman is limited to antithyroid drug therapy or surgery because radioactive iodine is contraindicated.[222–224] If ^{131}I treatment is inadvertently given to a woman in early pregnancy, the effects may be blocked with iodide administration. Because radiation doses to the fetus can approach threshold levels for malformations and mental retardation, pregnancy termination might be discussed with the patient. Maternal and fetal or neonatal hypothyroidism are also potential consequences of ^{131}I administration in pregnancy. Plasmapheresis has been used successfully in the treatment of thyrotoxicosis in pregnancy but is of limited value.[225]

THIONAMIDE THERAPY. The thiourea derivatives—propylthiouracil (PTU), methimazole (MMI), and carbimazole—are all prescribed in the treatment of thyrotoxicosis during pregnancy. Carbimazole, which is metabolized to MMI, is used mainly in Europe. All these agents cross the placenta and also are secreted in breast milk. MMI is transferred four times as well as PTU.[226] The serum half-lives of PTU and MMI are one hour and five hours, respectively, and are unaltered by either the thyrotoxicosis or the pregnancy.[227–231] These two antithyroid drugs have been used interchangeably. PTU does have the potential additional advantage of partially blocking the conversion of T_4 to T_3. Additionally, the possibility has been raised that MMI is associated with the development of aplasia cutis of the scalp in the treated mother's offspring.[232–236] However, no such association has been found in mothers receiving carbimazole.[234]

If minor drug reactions occur, the thionamides may be interchanged but cross-sensitivity is seen in about half the patients.[237] The most common reactions include fever, nausea, skin rash, pruritus, and metallic taste.[238] Transient leukopenia is not an uncommon reaction to thionamide therapy, occurring in about 12 per cent of adults.[238, 239] This association may be complicated because mild leukopenia is not uncommon in untreated Graves' disease.[227] This mild leukopenia is not a sign of agranulocytosis, which occurs in about 0.5 per cent of patients and usually develops within 12 weeks of the onset of therapy, and may be an autoimmune phenomenon.[240–243] Hepatitis and vasculitis have also been reported as side effects of thionamide therapy.[244–246]

Thionamides block the synthesis but not the release of thyroid hormone. The clinical response thus depends on the depletion of previously synthesized hormone. The typical patient will note some improvement after the first week or two and may approach euthyroidism after four to six weeks. The goal of antithyroid drug therapy is to gain control of the maternal thyrotoxicosis and maintain the maternal FT_4 concentration in the high normal range. This approach minimizes the incidence of transient hypothyroidism in newborns.[223]

PTU is usually started at doses of 100 to 150 mg every eight hours, but the dose may be increased after four weeks if necessary to gain control of the thyrotoxicosis. Some women require up to 600 to 900 mg/day of PTU for this purpose. The need for larger doses correlates with low serum concentrations of PTU[247] and could be caused by poor compliance with the medication. In one study serum PTU concentrations were consistently lower in thyrotoxic patients during the third trimester as compared with the postpartum period.[248] FT_4 or FT_3 and sensitive TSH determinations should be done monthly during pregnancy and the dose of thionamide decreased as control is achieved and maintained. If a requirement for higher doses of PTU continues and there is concern for effects on the fetus, thyroid surgery should be considered.

Combined thionamide-l-thyroxine therapy has been reported, but there is no apparent fetal or maternal advantage and this therapy may result in the use of higher doses of thionamides.[249] One report suggested that the addition of levothyroxine during antithyroid therapy in nonpregnant patients with Graves' disease decreased the production of thyroid-stimulating antibodies and the recurrence rate of thyrotoxicosis.[250] The same authors now suggest that T_4 therapy reduces postpartum relapses of Graves' thyrotoxicosis that remitted during pregnancy after antithyroid drug therapy.[250a] These studies in Japanese subjects require corroboration in the North American population.

BETA-ADRENERGIC BLOCKERS. If it is necessary to give drugs to a pregnant woman, they should be the least toxic agent possible. For this reason, the use of β-adrenergic blocking drugs has been advocated for the treatment of the pregnant woman with hyperthyroidism.[251] β-blockers have been used in large numbers of pregnant women to treat hypertension without apparent significant side effects.[252–254] However, intrauterine growth retardation with a small placenta, impaired response to anoxic stress, postnatal bradycardia, and hypoglycemia have been reported in the offspring of mothers receiving these agents.[255–257] They are particularly useful for rapid control of the β-adrenergic manifestations of thyrotoxicosis such as tremor and tachycardia. Propranolol, 20 to 40 mg three or four times a day, or atenolol, 50 to 100 mg/day, are usually adequate to control the maternal heart rate at 80 to 90 beats per minute. Esmolol, an ultrashort-acting cardioselective β-blocker given intravenously, controlled the heart rate in a pregnant woman with hyperthyroidism who required emergency surgery and was unresponsive to large doses of propranolol.[258] Current practice is to control hyperthyroidism with antithyroid drugs and to add β-blockers only in exceptional cases.

SURGERY. In pregnant thyrotoxic women with poor compliance or potential side effects, or if there is concern about maternal or fetal toxicity from antithyroid drug therapy, subtotal thyroidectomy may be advised.[259, 260] Thyrotoxicosis needs to be controlled medically before a subtotal thyroidectomy can be performed. This treatment includes antithyroid drugs, β-blockers, and possibly the short-term use of oral iodides.[260a] A useful clinical parameter of control is a resting heart rate of 80 to 90 beats per minute. Because of concern about spontaneous abortion, surgery is often delayed until after the first trimester. If surgery is indicated during the first trimester, there does not appear to be an increased risk greater than in other trimesters, although spontaneous abortion is more frequent during the first 12 weeks of gestation.[251] The small but real anesthetic and surgical risk is probably greater than the risks associated with thionamide therapy.[261, 262] Although the surgical complications of recurrent laryngeal nerve paralysis and hypoparathyroidism are rare in patients treated by an accomplished surgeon, they occasionally occur and are difficult to treat.

FETAL AND NEONATAL THYROTOXICOSIS. Pregnant women with Graves' disease have TSH-R–stimulating immunoglobulins that, like other immunoglobulins (IgG), cross the placenta[263] and in high enough concentrations may cause fetal or neonatal thyrotoxicosis. About 1 per cent of women with Graves' disease have offspring with neonatal thyrotoxicosis, but the condition may also occur in pregnant women with apparent Hashimoto's disease. Neonatal thyrotoxicosis may occur in women who have a history of Graves' disease but are euthyroid during the pregnancy. At present, TSH-R antibodies can be measured only by radioreceptor assay or in functional assays of biological stimulation.[144, 264] The TSH-R antibodies may have stimulating or blocking activity resulting in neonatal hyperthyroidism or hypothyroidism.[186, 265–267] Neonatal hyperthyroidism and hypothyroidism have been described in the same patient.[268] Because of this heterogeneity, the severity of thyrotoxicosis in the mother does not necessarily correlate with fetal or neonatal thyroid disease.[265, 269] A suppressed cord serum TSH determination may be predictive of neonatal thyrotoxicosis when the mother has Graves' disease.[270]

The fetal thyroid becomes susceptible to stimulation by maternal TSH-R–stimulating immunoglobulins about the 20th week of gestation and beyond. The pathology of fetal thyrotoxicosis includes goiter, visceromegaly, adenopathy, and pulmonary hypertension.[271] Fetal thyrotoxicosis may be treated unknowingly by placental transfer of thionamides used in treating thyrotoxicosis in the mother. Fetal thyrotoxicosis may also occur if the mother with Graves' is euthyroid following previous therapy.[272] In this situation the diagnosis of thyrotoxicosis is suggested by a fetal heart rate over 160 beats per minute, a fetal goiter visible on ultrasound, and elevated TSH-R antibodies in the mother; the condition should be treated by administration of thionamides to the mother.[273] Thyroxine therapy may be required to prevent hypothyroidism in the mother.

Neonatal thyrotoxicosis is frequently not clinically evident at birth if the mother has been receiving thionamides. The risk can be predicted to a certain extent on the basis of TSH-R antibody assay results in the mother.[274] Five to ten days after delivery the neonate may become irritable and develop feeding problems. Other manifestations include proptosis, goiter, and failure to thrive. In severe cases congestive heart failure, jaundice, and thrombocytopenia may occur and there can be a significant mortality.[275] Usually the disease runs a self-limited course over several months.[144] Treatment is indicated temporarily with iodides,

β-blockers, and antithyroid drugs. Overall, physicians caring for pregnant women and their offspring need to have a high index of suspicion for neonatal thyrotoxicosis when there is a maternal history of Graves' disease or Hashimoto's disease.

HYPOTHYROIDISM IN PREGNANCY

Maternal Hypothyroidism

INCIDENCE AND ETIOLOGY. Hypothyroidism is encountered more often in pregnancy than is hyperthyroidism.[9, 26, 51] The main causes are related to thyroid autoimmunity: Hashimoto's thyroiditis, primary myxedema, and postablative hypothyroidism in Graves' disease (Table 48–1). In most women the hypothyroidism has been already diagnosed and treated before pregnancy. A recent population survey identified 2.5 per cent of pregnant women as having compensated hypothyroidism based on elevated serum TSH levels, and 0.3 per cent were overtly hypothyroid with reduced FT_4 or T_4:TBG ratio.[276] Thyroid microsomal and peroxidase (TPO) antibodies were positive in 60 to 90 per cent of all the hypothyroid subjects compared with 11 per cent of controls. There was a positive correlation of serum TSH with thyroid antibody titers and maternal age. No data were available on pregnancy outcome. A similar prevalence of hypothyroidism and thyroid autoimmunity has been found in previous studies during pregnancy[51, 163, 164] and in a community survey in nonpregnant women.[277]

Evidence of thyroid autoimmunity is seen in other autoimmune endocrine disorders such as insulin-dependent (type I) diabetes mellitus,[278] including during pregnancy.[279] Up to 40 per cent of diabetic women are thyroid antibody positive and up to 10 per cent are mildly hypothyroid with elevated TSH levels. Hypothyroidism does not appear to progress in pregnancy unless proteinuria develops, in which case overt hypothyroidism may ensue.[280] The hypothyroidism may result from increased urinary losses of thyroid hormones with proteinuria in conjunction with the pre-existing impaired thyroid reserve.[281] Thyroxine therapy in this situation is appropriate but may result in an increase in insulin requirements. On the other hand, glucose intolerance is found more often in euthyroid pregnant women with thyroid antibodies.[282]

A significant proportion of patients with primary myxedema have TSH-R–blocking antibodies; these are thought to play an etiological role in the hypothyroidism.[283] Antibodies that stimulate TSH-R may be present in patients with postablative hypothyroidism in Graves' disease or in Hashimoto's thyroiditis, as discussed above.

DIAGNOSIS. Clinical assessment of thyroid status in pregnancy is imprecise. Normal pregnancy symptoms such as lethargy and weight gain may be suggestive of hypothyroidism. Paresthesias due to median nerve compression (carpal tunnel syndrome) are seen in both hypothyroidism and pregnancy. Delayed relaxation of deep tendon reflexes (pseudomyotonia) is a good clinical sign of hypothyroidism if present, but pregnancy is also listed as one of its causes.[284] Signs of myxedema such as decreased body temperature, periorbital edema, swelling, thick tongue, and hoarse voice should be apparent in pregnancy but can be confused with the presentation of pre-eclampsia leading to delayed diagnosis of the hypothyroidism.[285-287] Goiter may be present but its absence does not detract from a diagnosis of hypothyroidism. The most sensitive indicator of primary hypothyroidism in pregnancy is an elevated serum TSH level in conjunction with reduced FT_4 or T_4:TBG ratio.[9, 276] The presence of TPO antibodies indicates a likely autoimmune etiology. Hypothalamic or pituitary hypothyroidism is rarely encountered; its presence is suggested by low FT_4 with normal or slightly elevated TSH.[283]

TREATMENT. If hypothyroidism is diagnosed during pregnancy, thyroxine therapy should be initiated at a fairly full replacement dose, 0.1 mg per day, and this is usually well tolerated in these otherwise healthy individuals. Serum TSH and FT_4 should be repeated in a month's time and the T_4 dose adjusted accordingly, maintaining these parameters within normal limits for pregnancy. There is no good rationale for using T_3 replacement in this situation. In patients already receiving T_4 replacement, this should be continued throughout pregnancy with biochemical monitoring of the maternal TSH and FT_4 levels in each trimester. Up to a 30 per cent increase in T_4 dose requirements has been noted in some patients during pregnancy.[288-290, 290a] The reason for this is unclear but may reflect a discrepancy between increased TBG concentrations, the metabolic demands of pregnancy, and intake of a fixed T_4 replacement dose. This may be seen more frequently now that hypothyroidism is treated with relatively lower T_4 doses than in the past.[291] However, a similar increased T_4 requirement was also seen in pregnant patients with a history of thyroid carcinoma taking suppressive doses of thyroxine T_4.[292] T_4 replacement doses should be reassessed postpartum.

PREGNANCY OUTCOME. Although hypothyroidism has a negative impact on pregnancy, there are numerous reports over the last 100 years of hypothyroid women carrying their pregnancies to term.[293-302] In total, results of approximately 500 births in 250 pregnant hypothyroid women have been reviewed in the literature.[49-51, 163, 164, 301, 302] Early studies reported up to a 20 per cent incidence of perinatal mortality and congenital malformations associated with maternal hypothyroxinemia,[49-51] (that is, untreated or inadequately treated hypothyroidism), with up to 60 per cent of surviving children having evidence of impaired mental or physical development.[163, 164] An increase in congenital malformations was seen even in cases of patients considered to have adequate thyroxine replacement therapy. However, the biochemical assessment of thyroid hormone status in these studies was imprecise. In more recent studies, patients were well-characterized with respect to the degree of hypothyroidism and the adequacy of thyroxine replacement therapy.[301, 302] Still, untreated or inadequately treated overtly hypothyroid women experienced up to a 40 per cent incidence of anemia, pre-eclampsia, placental abruption, and postpartum hemorrhage; 30 per cent of neonates were small for gestational age and there was a 10 per cent incidence of perinatal mortality and congenital anomalies. Women with untreated subclinical hypothyroidism (elevated serum TSH only) had approximately one third the incidence of these problems and in both groups it appeared that maternal and fetal outcomes were improved with adequate thyroxine therapy.[301] A recent population-based case-control study found no overall relationship between a history of maternal hypothyroidism, thyroxine therapy, and total birth defects.[303] There was a weak associ-

ation of maternal hypothyroidism and thyroxine therapy with multiple anomalies associated with intestinal malrotation and single or multiple limb reduction defects (twofold relative risk, 2 per cent absolute risk) but no association with genetic trisomy syndromes. These results are at odds with the 10 to 20 per cent risk in the literature, cited above.

AUTOIMMUNE HYPOTHYROIDISM AND EFFECTS OF PREGNANCY. Serum immunoglobulin levels fall in pregnancy.[27] This is associated with an absolute or relative decrease in T-helper cell activity[304, 305] and is reflected by a progressive decline in thyroid antibody titers during pregnancy that increase again postpartum.[306] There are reports of remissions of goitrous Hashimoto's thyroiditis and hypothyroidism during pregnancy.[306-308] Maternal IgG antibodies, particularly subclasses 1 and 3, are able to cross the placenta after 20 weeks' gestation, including thyroid auto-antibodies.[263, 309] This occurs by micropinocytosis following IgG binding to Fc receptors on the syncytiotrophoblast. The role of TSH-R stimulating antibodies in fetal and neonatal hyperthyroidism has been discussed earlier. There is no evidence for a role of thyroid antibodies in placental pathology in women with autoimmune thyroid disease,[310] and it is debatable whether TPO and TG antibodies have any significant influence on fetal or neonatal growth and development or thyroid function.[185, 279, 311] The role of TSH-R–blocking antibodies is discussed later.

Neonatal Hypothyroidism

The incidence of congenital hypothyroidism is 1 per 4000 live births with most cases having primary hypothyroidism.[144, 161] Any delay in treatment with T_4 beyond two or three months reduces the chance of normal development and future intellectual performance.[188, 312-315] Since clinical diagnosis is imprecise, the solution has been mass neonatal screening programs to measure serum TSH levels in a heel prick blood sample drawn between three and five days postpartum.[313, 314, 316, 317] Maternal thyroid autoimmunity may play a role in transient neonatal hypothyroidism due to transplacental passage of TSH-R antibodies that block thyroid function or growth, or both, in utero or postpartum.[184-186, 318, 319, 319a] This transient hypothyroidism accounts for up to 10 per cent of congenital hypothyroidism. Familial forms are also recognized.[266, 267] The main risk seems to be a maternal history of primary myxedema rather than goitrous Hashimoto's disease.[185] However, the majority of cases of congenital hypothyroidism are considered sporadic and likely to be permanent. A proportion of these may also be due to maternal autoimmunization[320, 321] or may be associated with maternal TSH-R antibodies that inhibit thyroid growth or function[322-324] or with cytotoxic antibodies.[325, 326] Antibodies to TG or TPO are probably not causal in the hypothyroidism.[327] Endemic cretinism has also been associated with the finding of maternal thyroid growth-blocking antibodies,[328] but this has yet to be widely confirmed.

In any case, neonatal hypothyroidism must be treated with T_4,[315] including transient cases.[329] The risk of developmental problems may already be increased if there has been maternal hypothyroxinemia during pregnancy.[330, 331] Treatment may be withdrawn in cases of suspected tran-

TABLE 48–4. SUMMARY OF POSTPARTUM THYROIDITIS SURVEYS

	NO. (%) OF PATIENTS		
	Nikolai et al[345]	Jansson et al[353]	Amino et al[352]
No. screened	238	460	507
No. affected	16 (6.7)	30 (6.5)	28 (5.5)
Transient thyrotoxicosis	7 (2.9)	8 (1.7)	13 (2.6)
Followed by transient hypothyroidism	3 (1.3)	2 (0.2)	7 (1.4)
Transient hypothyroidism	3 (1.3)	20 (4.3)	7 (1.4)
Persistent hypothyroidism	3 (1.3)	0	1 (0.2)
Positive MCHA* titer			
Affected women	15/27 (56)	23/30 (77)	25/28 (89)
Unaffected women	4/40 (10)	21/430 (4.9)	37/479 (7.7)
Family history of thyroid disease			
Affected women	14/27 (52)†	ND‡	⋯§
Unaffected women	22/125 (18)†	ND‡	⋯§

*MCHA indicates microsomal hemagglutinin antibody
†Difference highly significant (P < .001)
‡ND indicates not done.
§Family history difference not significant; numbers not given
From Nikolai TF, Turney SL, Roberts RC: Postpartum lymphocytic thyroiditis. Prevalence, clinical course, and long-term follow up. Arch Intern Med 147:221, 1987. Copyright 1987, American Medical Association.

sient hypothyroidism after two or three years to assess for thyroid recovery.

POSTPARTUM THYROID DISEASE

Thyroid dysfunction is a well-recognized complication of the puerperium,[5, 6] and it follows that a close surveillance of the mother with thyroid disease, or a history of thyroid disease, should be continued after delivery. Whereas there is a tendency for Graves' thyrotoxicosis and Hashimoto's thyroiditis to improve in later pregnancy, there is often a relapse postpartum,[25, 26, 306–308, 332] which may be transient or protracted. The reason for relapse at this time is most likely the rebound in immune surveillance that occurs postpartum.[27–31] TPO antibodies often increase postpartum in Hashimoto's disease and Graves' disease, but there has been a relatively weak correlation of TSH-R antibody status and the onset or relapse of thyrotoxicosis.[333] Rarely postpartum thyroid dysfunction is associated with hypothalamic-pituitary disease as part of pituitary failure in Sheehan's syndrome or lymphocytic hypophysitis.[334–336] Transient isolated thyrotropin deficiency in the postpartum period has been described.[336] Most often thyroid dysfunction in the puerperium is part of the spectrum of postpartum thyroiditis, which differs significantly in terms of its pathogenesis, treatment, and outcome from the aforementioned disorders. Otherwise the diagnosis and treatment of thyroid disease in the postpartum period is as outlined above, employing the usual precautions relevant to pregnancy or breast feeding.

Postpartum Thyroiditis

Postpartum thyroiditis (PPT) is now well recognized as a distinct variant of silent (painless) thyroiditis[337] associated with thyroid autoimmunity and transient thyroid dysfunction, either hypothyroidism[338] or hyperthyroidism.[339] Since the first modern descriptions of PPT over 15 years ago, much has been learned about the pathophysiology, clinical course, treatment, and outcome of this disorder.[12, 340–354]

Clinical Features

The incidence of PPT averages 5 per cent,[12] ranging from as low as 1 to 2 per cent[343, 344, 354] to as high as 10 to 15 per cent.[345, 346] A summary of PPT surveys and the changes in thyroid antibody levels during and after pregnancy are shown in Table 48–4 and Figure 48–5, respectively. Diagnostic measures for PPT are highlighted in Table 48–5.

THYROTOXIC PHASE. Typically, 70 per cent of the women experience a transient period of thyrotoxicosis with onset between six weeks and three months postpartum, lasting one to two months before spontaneously resolving. A goiter develops in 50 per cent of cases. Thyrotoxic symptoms are usually milder than in Graves' disease and may be overlooked or attributed to the adjustment to motherhood. Fatigue and palpitations may be prominent. Hypertension is occasionally seen.[355, 356] Specific tests to detect biochemical thyrotoxicosis are the same as those usually employed in pregnancy. A caveat is that some patients who develop PPT have antibodies to T_4 and T_3, which may give spuriously high or low results for total or free thyroid hormone levels depending on the immunoassay method used.[357] TPO antibodies are usually present, higher titers being associated with more severe disease and a greater risk of subsequent hypothyroidism.[350]

It is important to distinguish between thyrotoxicosis due to PPT and Graves' disease. Radioactive iodine uptake and thyroid scan readily differentiates the two, being elevated in Graves' disease and reduced or absent in thyrotoxic PPT. Other causes of reduced radioactive iodine uptake and scan include iodine-induced thyrotoxicosis and iatrogenic thyrotoxicosis owing to thyroid hormone administration. Special consideration must be given to nursing mothers who should interrupt breast feeding, while continuing to express milk, for one to three days after tracer doses of Tc-99m or radioactive iodine.[358] [123]I may be preferable to ^{131}I, although this remains controversial.[359] In either case the use of nanocurie as opposed to microcurie doses of radioactivity will still provide an accurate assessment of thyroid gland activity.

When symptoms of PPT thyrotoxicosis are more severe,

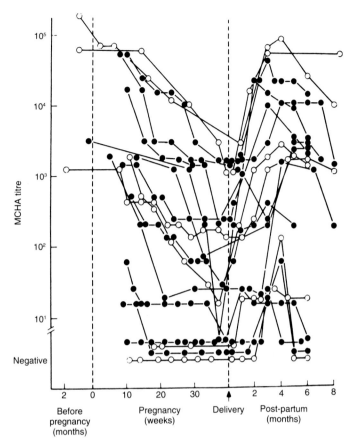

FIGURE 48–5. Sequential changes in serum antithyroid antibodies (MCHA) during pregnancy and after delivery in patients with Graves' disease *(black dot)* and autoimmune thyroiditis *(open dot).* (From Amino N, Kuro R, Tanizawa O et al: Changes in serum antithyroid antibodies during and after pregnancy in autoimmune thyroid diseases. Clin Exp Immunol 31:30, 1978.)

the differential diagnosis includes postpartum psychotic depression (postpartum psychosis). Typically this occurs earlier than PPT, one to two weeks following delivery, and is less common, 1 per 1000 deliveries.[360] Although hyperthyroxinemia and impaired TSH responses to TRH may be seen in patients with acute psychiatric disorders,[361] thyrotoxicosis has not been confirmed in postpartum psychosis.[362, 363] Thyroid antibodies are typically negative in postpartum psychosis.

HYPOTHYROID PHASE. Most commonly, with or without symptoms or documentation of a preceding episode of thyrotoxicosis, primary hypothyroidism presents three to six months postpartum. Symptoms of lethargy, cold intolerance, and impaired memory and concentration are typically mild. An increase in depressive symptomatology and

depression scores have been reported with PPT hypothyroidism as compared with euthyroid postpartum controls.[364–366] Up to 20 per cent of patients were considered to be mildly depressed based on symptom scores, although results did not achieve statistical significance.[365] Moreover, depressed mood related to the course of hypothyroidism and positive thyroid antibodies was seen more often in women with postpartum depression.[366, 366a] However, it is not yet proved that postpartum hypothyroidism is a major cause of postpartum depression. Hypothyroidism should be considered in patients presenting with later postpartum depression, because treatment with thyroid hormone may result in clinical improvement.

Although spontaneous recovery is usual by 10 to 12 month postpartum, 10 to 15 per cent of women remain permanently hypothyroid in the long-term.[367] There is a high prevalence of organification defects and susceptibility to iodine-induced hypothyroidism following PPT.[368] The risk of recurrence following subsequent pregnancies is up to 25 per cent.

Predisposing Factors

The major risk factor in development of PPT is of course the postpartum state; the condition may also occur after miscarriage or abortion.[341, 343, 352] Women with a personal or family history of thyroid disease are also at increased risk, specifically those with Hashimoto's thyroiditis. TPO antibody titer reflects disease risk when detected in the first trimester[311, 348, 351, 353, 369] or at the time of delivery.[364, 364a] The presence of other endocrine autoimmune disorders, particularly type I diabetes mellitus, is associated with an increase in thyroid autoimmunity and PPT.[278, 279] White and Asian women, as opposed to blacks, may be at increased risk of PPT,[364] as are cigarette smokers.[351] Maternal age, parity, presence of a goiter, breast feeding, and infant birth weight have not been associated with an increased risk of PPT.[351] It is controversial whether sex of the infant has any association with PPT.[351, 352] On the other hand, a lower ponderal index[279] and reduced early neonatal growth rate[311] have been reported in association with maternal thyroid antibody positivity in pregnancy and the subsequent development of PPT. Maternal thyroid function was normal in the women during these pregnancies. Iodide exposure may also be a risk factor for the development of PPT,[370, 371] although a similar incidence of PPT is seen in geographic areas of high[352] and low[353] iodine intake.

It has been suggested that all pregnant women be screened for thyroid antibodies during pregnancy to predict the risk of PPT.[348] Whether this would truly be cost effective is unclear.[364] It would seem reasonable to screen

TABLE 48–5. DIAGNOSTIC MEASURES IN POSTPARTUM THYROIDITIS (PPT)

INVESTIGATION	RESULTS
Thyroid function tests	TSH suppressed, FT_4, or FT_3 elevated in thyrotoxicosis; TSH increased, FT_4 normal or low in hypothyroidism
Thyroid autoantibodies	Positive result indicates autoimmune thyroid disorder; higher titers associated with hypothyroidism
Isotope uptake and scan (thyrotoxicosis only)	Low or absent uptake and scan in PPT; increased uptake and scan in Graves' disease
TSH-R antibodies (thyrotoxicosis only, not routine)	Negative in PPT; positive in Graves' disease

those with a previous episode of PPT, or other thyroid and autoimmune disorders, and women with a history of postpartum psychiatric disturbance.

Pathophysiology

The immune injury to the thyroid gland in PPT is mediated by humoral and cellular mechanisms. A rebound in the immune response is thought to exacerbate autoimmune thyroid disease postpartum.[27–31, 304–306] A decline in serum cortisol levels at this time may also be important.[372]

GENETICS. The risk of developing PPT has been associated with HLA haplotypes B8, DR3, 4 and 5, and DRW3, 8, and 9.[367, 373–377] The relative risk is increased two- to fivefold. The risk of PPT is reduced in association with HLA-DR2 haplotype.[367] The variability in HLA haplotypes associated with PPT risk may be due to geographic and population differences. Also, as proposed by DeGroot,[378] it is the interaction of genetics along with immune dysfunction and environmental factors that contributes to the clinical expression of autoimmune thyroid disorders.

HUMORAL MECHANISMS. TPO antibodies reflect disease activity in PPT. Total IgG concentrations are elevated in women with PPT.[379, 380] Thyroid antibodies are associated predominantly with IgG subclasses 1 and 4.[380–382] Nonspecific increase in anti-DNA antibodies is seen in postpartum relapses of thyroid autoimmune disorders, including the thyrotoxic phase of PPT.[383]

CELLULAR MECHANISMS. Thyroid cytolytic activity due to T-cell or killer cell attack[371, 378] may be important in the release of thyroid hormones in PPT, as opposed to thyroid antibodies that serve as markers of the disease process.[382] A significant increase in circulating large peripheral granular lymphocytes having killer-cell and cytotoxic activity has been reported in women with PPT compared with euthyroid controls or patients with Graves' disease.[384] Others found no differences in natural killer cell activity between postpartum euthyroid controls or PPT subjects,[385] although both groups showed a relative increase compared with reduced killer cell activity found immediately postpartum. Similarly, these and other investigators showed no change in antibody-dependent cell-mediated cytotoxicity in PPT.[384, 385] Analysis of circulating lymphocyte subsets showed an increase in activated T cells with helper-inducer activity in PPT,[386] opposite to the findings in Graves' thyrotoxicosis. Another study reported no change in peripheral blood lymphocytes in PPT but observed an increase in intrathyroidal activated B lymphocytes and T cells with helper-inducer activity.[387] Overall the cellular mechanisms involved in the pathogenesis of PPT, while undoubtedly important, remain relatively poorly defined.

Treatment

Treatment for PPT is often unnecessary. The thyrotoxicosis is typically mild and self-limited. In more severe cases, β-blockers may provide symptomatic relief of tremor, hyperkinesis, palpitations, and anxiety symptoms. Antithyroid drugs and radioactive iodine have little role in the treatment of PPT during the hyperthyroid phase, although some physicians advise therapy with PTU to decrease T_4 to T_3 conversion in patients with PPT who are severely thyrotoxic. Glucocorticoids or the oral contrast agents ipodate

and iopanoic acid could be used for this purpose as well. Symptomatic hypothyroidism may be treated with thyroid hormone replacement, but this can usually be withdrawn after six months or at a year postpartum, followed by reevaluation of thyroid function after six weeks with measurement of serum TSH. Thyroid hormone therapy may also be useful in patients with PPT and depression who have evidence of hypothyroidism.

THYROID NODULES AND CARCINOMA DURING PREGNANCY

There is a suggestion that thyroid nodules appear more frequently during pregnancy,[55, 206] although this is based on ultrasonographic data and disease may be subclinical. Thyroid scanning is contraindicated in the work-up of a patient with a thyroid nodule during pregnancy, and while ultrasound provides excellent definition of anatomy, it is relatively nonspecific in terms of thyroid histology or pathology. If a nodule is clinically palpable, the diagnosis can be made most specifically by fine-needle aspiration biopsy (FNAB),[388] including the diagnosis of papillary carcinoma.[389, 390] Surgery for nodules that arouse suspicion of or are diagnostic for thyroid cancer can be safely performed during pregnancy if the nodule is discovered during the first or second trimester, or can usually be delayed without concern until the postpartum period if discovered during the third trimester.[389, 391] In cases when surgery is delayed, attempted suppression with thyroid hormone may be employed.

Cancer per se is relatively uncommon in pregnancy; it is generally held that pregnancy has little effect on the development or progression of thyroid carcinoma or that thyroid carcinoma has any significant effect on pregnancy outcome.[392, 393] Not all authorities agree. Some authors have reported an increased prevalence of neoplasia in thyroid nodules initially discovered during pregnancy, assessed by FNAB as being suspicious or diagnostic for thyroid cancer, and subsequently operated on during or following pregnancy.[389] Forty per cent of these highly selected cases showed thyroid epithelial cell malignancy, and the total incidence of neoplasia (including follicular adenomas) was up to 80 per cent. There is an isolated report in pregnancy of an apparent exacerbation of quiescent follicular carcinoma with distant bone metastasis and hypercalcemia.[393] Recurrent laryngeal edema has been reported during pregnancy following remote successful surgical treatment of papillary carcinoma.[394] Other authors have recommended against pregnancy in women with residual thyroid cancer following primary therapy.[395] Although theoretically important, the roles of estrogens, thyroid stimulators and other growth factors, and immunosuppression on the development or progression of thyroid neoplasia during pregnancy remain largely unknown. Overall, there seems to be a small effect of pregnancy on the incidence or progression of thyroid cancer in women with a goiter, thyroid nodule, or history of upper body x-ray exposure.[396]

The diagnosis and treatment of clinically apparent thyroid nodules with FNAB, thyroid hormone suppression, and surgery may be pursued as aggressively in pregnant as nonpregnant women. It seems prudent to maintain close clinical follow-up and ensure adequate thyroid hormone replacement and suppression in patients with a history of thyroid carcinoma, and assess disease control and stability before pregnancy. Conception should be delayed for six months or more following high-dose radioactive iodine therapy for ablation of normal thyroid remnants or suspected residual disease.

REFERENCES

1. Thomas R, Reid RL: Thyroid disease and reproductive dysfunction: A review. Obstet Gynecol 70:789, 1987.
2. Crotti A: Simple goiter and pregnancy. *In* Thyroid and Thymus, Philadelphia, Lea & Febiger, 1918, p 170.
3. Crotti A: Exophthalmic goiter in pregnancy. *In* Thyroid and Thymus. Philadelphia, Lea & Febiger, 1918, p 367.
4. Seitz L: Trans Dtsch Ges Gynecol 1:213, 1913.
5. Gull W: On a cretinoid state supervening in adult life in women. Trans Clin Soc London 7:180, 1874.
6. Robertson HEW: Lassitude, coldness, and hair changes following pregnancy, and their response to thyroid extract. Br Med J 2:93, 1948.
7. Medvei VC: A History of Endocrinology. Boston, MTP Press, 1982, p 58.
8. Belchetz PE: Thyroid disease in pregnancy. Br Med J 294:264, 1987.
9. Rodin A, Rodin A: Thyroid disease in pregnancy. Br J Hosp Med 41:234, 1989.
10. Lazarus JH, Othman S: Thyroid disease in relation to pregnancy. Clin Endocrinol 34:91, 1991.
11. Rajatanavin R, Chailurkit L, Srisupandit S, et al: Trophoblastic hyperthyroidism: Clinical and biochemical features in five cases. Am J Med 85:237, 1988.
12. Gerstein HC: How common is postpartum thyroiditis? A methodological overview of the literature. Arch Intern Med 150:1397, 1990.
13. Abdoul-Khair SA, Crooks J, Turnbull AC, et al: The physiologic changes in thyroid function during pregnancy. Clin Sci 27:195, 1964.
14. Mussey RD: The thyroid in gland and pregnancy. Am J Obstet Gynecol 36:529, 1938.
15. Smith SCH, Bold AM: Interpretation of in vitro thyroid function tests in pregnancy. Br J Obstet Gynecol 90:532, 1983.
16. Burrow GN: Thyroid diseases in pregnancy. *In* Burrow GN, Oppenheimer JH, Volpé R (eds): Thyroid Function and Disease. Philadelphia, WB Saunders Co, 1989, p 292.
17. Becks GP, Burrow GN: Thyroid function tests—recent developments. Med N Am 3:2503, 1987.
18. Ekins R: Measurement of free hormones in blood. Endocr Rev 11:5, 1990.
19. Wiersinga WM, Vet T, Berghout A, et al: Serum free thyroxine during pregnancy: A meta-analysis. *In* Beckers C, Reinwein D (eds) The Thyroid and Pregnancy. Stuttgart, Shattauer, 1991, p 79.
20. Nicoloff JT, Spencer CA: The use and misuse of sensitive thyrotropin assays. J Clin Endocrinol Metab 72:553, 1990.
21. Kalkhoff RK, Kissebah AH, Kim HJ: Carbohydrate and lipid metabolism during normal pregnancy: relation to gestational hormone faction. *In* Merkoty IR, Adam PAF (eds) The Diabetic Pregnancy: A Perinatal Perspective. New York, Grune and Stratton, 1979.
22. Burrow GN: Pituitary and adrenal disorders. *In* Burrow GN, Ferris TF (eds) Medical Complications During Pregnancy, 3rd ed. Philadelphia, WB Saunders, 1988, p 254.
23. McAnultry JH, Metcalfe J, Ueland K: 1988–Cardiovascular disease. *In* Burrow GN, Ferris TF (eds) Medical Complications During Pregnancy, 3rd ed. Philadelphia, WB Saunders, 1988, p 180.
24. Burwell CS: Circulating adjustments to pregnancy. Am J Obstet Gynecol 36:529, 1954.
25. Salvi M, How J: Pregnancy and autoimmune thyroid disease. Endocrinol Metab Clin N Am 16:431, 1987.
26. Amino N, Tanizawa O, Mori H, et al: Aggravation of thyrotoxicosis in early pregnancy and after delivery in Graves' disease. J Clin Endocrinol Metab 55:108, 1982.
27. Amino N, Tanizawa O, Miyai K, et al: Changes in serum immunoglobulins during pregnancy. Obstet Gynecol 52:115, 1978.
28. Beer AE, Billingham RE: Immunobiology of mammalian reproduction. Adv Immunol 14:1, 1971.
29. Froelich CJ, Goodwin JS, Bankhurst AD, et al: Pregnancy, a temporary fetal graft of suppressor cells in autoimmune disease? Am J Med 69:329, 1980.
30. Lewis JE, Coulam CB, Moore SB: Immunologic mechanisms in the maternal-fetal relationship. Mayo Clin Proc 61:655, 1986.
31. Scott RM, How J, Gerrie LM, et al: Serum levels of pregnancy α2-glycoprotein during pregnancy in autoimmune thyroid disease. Clin Exp Immunol 59:564, 1985.
32. Goldsmith R, Sturgis S, Lerman J, et al: Menstrual pattern in thyroid disease. J Clin Endocrinol Metab 12:846, 1952.
33. Honbo KS, VanHerle AJ, Kellet KA: Serum prolactin in untreated primary hypothyroidism. Am J Med 64:782, 1978.
34. Kleinberg DL, Noel G, Frantz AG: Galactorrhea: A study of 235 cases. N Engl J Med 296:589, 1977.
35. Yamada T, Tsuki T, Ikerjiri K, et al: Volume of sella turcica in normal patients and in patients with primary hypothyroidism. J Clin Endocrinol Metab 42:817, 1976.
35a. Heyburn PJ, Gibby OM, Hourihan M, et al: Primary hypothyroidism presenting as amenorrhea and galactorrhea with hyperprolactinemia and pituitary enlargement. Br Med J 292:1660, 1986.
36. Feek CM, Sawers JSA, Brown NS, et al: Influence of thyroid status on dopaminergic inhibition of thyrotropin and prolactin secretion. J Clin Endocrinol Metab 51:585, 1980.
37. Kramer M, Kauschansky A, Genel M: Adolescent secondary amenorrhea: association with hypothalamic hypothyroidism. Pediatrics 94:300, 1979.
38. Scanlon MF, Chan V, Heath M, et al: Dopaminergic control of thyrotropin a-subunit, thyrotropin B-subunit and prolactin in euthyroidism and hypothyroidism. J Clin Endocrinol Metab 53:360, 1981.
39. Willansky DL, Greisman B: Early hypothyroidism in patients with menorrhagia. Am J Obstet Gynecol 160:673, 1989.
40. Bohnet HG, Fieldlerk, Leidenberger FA: Subclinical hypothyroidism and infertility. Lancet 2:1278, 1981.
41. Del Pozo E, Wyss H, Tolis G, et al: Prolactin and deficient luteal function. Obstet Gynecol 53:282, 1979.
42. Gerhard I, Becker T, Eggert-Kruse W, et al: Thyroid and ovarian function in infertile women. Hum Reprod 6:338, 1991.
43. Louvet JP, Gouarre M, Saladin AM, et al: Hypothyroidism and anovulation. Lancet 1:1032, 1979.
44. Peillon F, Vincens M, Cesselin F, et al: Exaggerated prolactin response to thyrotropin-releasing hormone in women with anovulatory cycles: Possible role of endogenous estrogen and effect of bromocriptine. Fertil Steril 37:530, 1982.
45. Lombardi G, Iodice M, Miletto P, et al: Prolactin and TSH-response to TRH and metoclopramide before and after therapy in subclinical hypothyroidism. Neuroendocrinology 43:676, 1986.
46. Seki K, Kato K: Increased thyroid-stimulating hormone response to thyrotropin-releasing hormone in hyperprolactinemic women. J Clin Endocrinol Metab 61:1138, 1985.
47. Gerhard I, Eggert-Kruse W, Merzoug K, et al: Thyrotropin-releasing hormone (TRH) and metoclopramide testing in infertile women. Gynecol Endocrinol 5:15, 1991.
48. Rotmensch S, Scommegna A: Spontaneous ovarian hyperstimulation syndrome associated with hypothyroidism. Am J Obstet Gynecol 160:1220, 1989.
49. Greenman GW, Gabrielson MA, Howard-Flanders I, et al: Thyroid dysfunction in pregnancy: fetal loss and follow-up of evaluation of surviving infants. N Engl J Med 267:426, 1962.
50. Jones W, Man E: Thyroid function in human pregnancy. VI. Premature deliveries and reproduction failure of pregnant women with low serum-butanol extractable iodines. Am J Obstet Gynecol 104:909, 1969.
51. Niswander KR, Gordon M, Berendes HW: The women and their pregnancies. *In* The Collaborative Perinatal Study of the National Institutes of Neurological Disease and Stroke. Philadelphia, WB Saunders, 1972, p 239.
52. Winikoff D, Malinek M: The predictive value of thyroid test profile in habitual abortion. Br J Obstet Gynecol 82:760, 1975.
53. White A: The effect of thyroid and ovarian gland extracts in cases of previous miscarriage and stillbirth. Br Med J 1:90, 1924.
54. Stagnaro-Green A, Roman SH, Cobin R, et al: Detection of at-risk pregnancy by means of highly sensitive assays for thyroid autoantibodies. JAMA:264, 1422, 1990.
55. Glinoer D, Fernandez Soto M, Bourdoux P, et al: Pregnancy in patients with mild thyroid abnormalities: Maternal and neonatal repercussions. J Clin Endocrinol Metab 73:421, 1991.
56. Brayshaw ND, Brayshaw DD: Thyroid hypofunction in premenstrual syndrome. N Engl J Med 315:1486, 1986.

57. Roy-Byrne PP, Rubinow DR, Hoban MC, et al: TSH and prolactin response to TRH in patients with premenstrual syndrome. Am J Psychiatry 144:480, 1987.

58. Casper RF, Patel-Christopher A, Powell AM: Thyrotropin and prolactin responses to thyrotropin releasing hormone in premenstrual syndrome. J Clin Endocrinol Metab 68:608, 1989.

59. Southern AL, Olivio J, Gorelon GG, et al: The conversion of androgens to estrogen in hyperthyroidism. J Clin Endocrinol Metab 38:207, 1974.

60. Akande E, Hockaday T: Plasma luteinizing hormone levels in women with thyrotoxicosis. J Endocrinol 53:173, 1972.

61. Distiller L, Sayel J, Morley J: Assessment of pituitary gonadotropin reserve using luteinizing releasing hormone in states of altered thyroid function. J Clin Endocrinol Metab 40:512, 1975.

62. Tanaka T, Tamai H, Kuma K, et al: Gonadotropin response to luteinizing hormone releasing hormone in hyperthyroid patients with menstrual disturbances. Metabolism 30:323, 1981.

63. Roger J: Menstruation and systemic disease. N Engl J Med 259:676, 1958.

64. Mussey RD: Hyperthyroidism complicating pregnancy. Mayo Clin Proc 14:205, 1939.

65. Amino N: Autoimmunity and hypothyroidism. In Lazarus JH, Hall R (eds) Hypothyroidism and Goiter. London, WB Saunders, 1988, p591.

66. Rojeski MT, Gharib H: Nodular thyroid disease: evaluation and management. N Engl Med 313:428, 1985.

67. Gause WC, Marsh JA: Effects of testosterone on the development of autoimmune thyroiditis in two strains of chicken. Clin Immunol Immunopathol 36:10, 1985.

68. Ansar Ahmed S, Young PR, Penhale WJ: Beneficial effect of testosterone in the treatment of chronic autoimmune thyroiditis in rats. J Immunol 136:143, 1986.

69. Talal N, Ansar Ahmed S: Immunomodulation by hormones—an area of growing importance. J Rheumatol 14:191, 1987.

70. Phillips DIW, Lazarus JH, Butland BK: The influence of pregnancy and reproductive span on the occurrence of autoimmune thyroiditis. Clin Endocrinol 32:301, 1990.

71. Beckers C: Iodine economy in and around pregnancy. In Beckers C, Reinwein D (eds) The Thyroid and Pregnancy. Stuttgart, Schattauer 1991, p 25.

72. Roti E, Gnudi A, Braverman LE: The placental transport, synthesis and metabolism of hormones and drugs which affect thyroid function. Endocr Rev 4:131, 1983.

73. Roti E: Regulation of thyroid-stimulating hormone (TSH) secretion in the fetus and neonate. J Endocrinol Invest 11:145, 1988.

74. Evans TC, Kretschmar RM, Hodges RE, et al: Radioiodine uptake studies of the human fetal thyroid. J Nucl Med 8:157, 1967.

75. Johnson JR: Fetal thyroid dose from intake of radioiodine by the mother. Health Physics 43:573, 1955.

76. Hodges RE, Evans TC, Bradbury JT, et al: The accumulation of radioactive iodine by human fetal thyroid. J Clin Endocrinol Metab 15:661, 1955.

77. Chapman EM, Corner GW, Robinson D, et al: The collection of radioactive iodine by human fetal thyroid. J Clin Endocrinol 8:717, 1948.

78. Fisher DA, Dussault J: Development of the mammalian thyroid gland. In Greer MA, Solomon DH (eds) Handbook of Physiology: Endocrinology. III. Baltimore, Williams and Wilkins, 1974, p 21.

79. Gushurst CA, Mueller JA, Green JA, et al: Breast milk iodide: Reassessment in 1980. Pediatrics 73:354, 1984.

80. Hetzel BS: Progression in the prevention and control of iodine deficiency disorders. Lancet 2:266, 1987.

81. Hetzel BS, Mano MT: A review of experimental studies of iodine deficiency in fetal development. J Nutr 119:145, 1989.

82. Hetzel BS: Iodine deficiency disorders and their eradication. Lancet 2:1136, 1983.

83. Delange F, Bürgi H: Iodine deficiency disorders in Europe. Bull WHO 67:317, 1989.

84. Alexander WD, Koutras DA, Crooks J, et al: Quantitative studies of iodine metabolism in thyroid disease. Q J Med 31:281, 1966.

85. Dworkin HJ, Jacquez JA, Beirewaltes WH: Relationship of iodine ingestion to iodine excretion in pregnancy. J Clin Endocrinol Metab 26:1329, 1966.

86. Halnan KE: Radioiodine uptake of the human thyroid in pregnancy. Clin Sci 17:281, 1958.

87. Pochin EE: The iodine uptake of the human thyroid throughout the menstrual cycle and in pregnancy. Clin Sci 11:441, 1952.

88. Glinoer D, Gershengorn MC, Dubois A et al: Stimulation of thyroxine-binding globulin synthesis by isolated rhesus monkey hepatocytes after in vivo β-estradiol administration. Endocrinology 100:807, 1977.

89. Ain KB, Mori Y, Refetoff S: Reduced clearance of thyroxine binding globulin (TBG) with increased sialylation: A mechanism for estrogen-induced elevation of serum TBG concentration. J Clin Endocrinol Metab 65:686, 1987.

90. Ball R, Freeman DB, Holmes JC et al: Low-normal concentrations of free thyroxine in late pregnancy; physiological fact, not technical artefact. J Clin Chem 35:1891, 1989.

91. Guillaume J, Schussler GC, Goldman J, et al: Components of the total serum thyroxine during pregnancy. High free thyroxine and blunted thyrotropin (TSH) response to TSH-releasing hormone in the first trimester. J Clin Endocrinol Metab 60:678, 1985.

92. Price A, Griffiths H, Morris BW: A longitudinal study of thyroid function in pregnancy. Clin Chem 35:275, 1989.

93. Engbring NH, Engstrom WW: Effects of estrogen and testosterone on circulating thyroid hormone. J Clin Endocrinol Metab 19:783, 1959.

94. Robbins J, Nelson JH: Thyroxine-binding by serum protein in pregnancy and in the newborn. J Clin Invest 37:153, 1958.

95. Sköldebrand L, Brundin J, Carlström A, et al: Thyroid associated components in serum during normal pregnancy. Acta Endocrinol 100:504, 1982.

96. Man EB, Reid WA, Hellegers AE, et al: Thyroid function in human pregnancy. III. Serum thyroxine-binding prealbumin (TBPA) and thyroxine-binding globulin (TBG) of pregnant women aged 14 through 43 years. Am J Obstet Gynecol 103:338, 1969.

97. Oppenheimer JH: Role of plasma proteins in the binding, distribution and metabolism of thyroid hormones. N Engl J Med 278:1153, 1968.

98. Osathanondh R, Tulchinsky D, Chopra IJ: Total and free thyroxine and triiodothyronine in normal and complicated pregnancy. J Clin Endocrinol Metab 42:98, 1976.

99. Whitworth AS, Midgley JEM, Wilkins TA: A comparison of free T4 and the ratio of total T4 to T4-binding globulin in serum through pregnancy. Clin Endocrinol 17:307, 1982.

100. Wilke TJ: A challenge of several concepts of free thyroxine index for assessing thyroid status in patients with altered thyroid-binding protein capacity. Clin Chem 29:56, 1983.

101. Nikolai TF, Seal US: X-chromosome linked familial decrease in thyroxine binding globulin activity. J Clin Endocrinol Metab 26:835, 1966.

102. Premachandra BN, Gossain VV, Perlstein IB: Effect of pregnancy on thyroxine binding globulin (TBG) in partial TBG deficiency. Am J Med Sci 274:189, 1977.

103. Dowling JT, Appleton WG, Nicoloff JT: Thyroxine turnover during human pregnancy. J Clin Endocrinol Metab 27:1749, 1967.

104. Glinoer D, De Nayer P, Bourdoux P, et al: Regulation of maternal thyroid during pregnancy. J Clin Endocrinol Metab 71:276, 1990.

105. Rasmussen NG, Hornnes PJ, Hegedus L, et al: Serum thyroglobulin during the menstrual cycle, pregnancy and postpartum. Acta Endocrinol 121:168, 1989.

106. Harada A, Hershman JM, Reed AW, et al: Comparison of thyroid stimulators and thyroid hormone concentrations in the sera of pregnant women. J Clin Endocrinol Metab 48:793, 1979.

107. Yamamoto T, Amino N, Tanizawa O, et al: Longitudinal study of serum thyroid hormones, chorionic gonadotropin and thyrotropin during and after normal pregnancy. Clin Endocrinol 10:459, 1979.

108. Pachiarotti A, Martino E, Bartalena L, et al: Serum thyrotropin by ultrasensitive immunoradiometric assay and free thyroid hormones in pregnancy. J Endocrinol Invest 9:185, 1986.

109. Weeke J, Dybkjaer L, Granlie K, et al: A longitudinal study of serum TSH, and total and free iodothyronines during normal pregnancy. Acta Endocrinol 101:531, 1982.

110. Gow SM, Kellett HA, Seth J, et al: Limitations of new thyroid function tests in pregnancy. Clin Chim Acta 152:325, 1985.

111. Kventy J, Poulsen HK: Nuclear thyroxine and 3,5,3'-triiodothyronine receptors in human mononuclear blood cells during pregnancy. Acta Endocrinol 105:19, 1984.

112. VanRaaij JMA, Vermatta-Miedema SH, Schonk CM, et al: Energy requirements of pregnancy in the Netherlands. Lancet 2:953, 1987.

113. Calvo R, Obregon MJ, Riuz de Ona C, et al: Thyroid hormone economy in pregnant rats near term: A physiological animal model of non-thyroidal illness? Endocrinology 126:10, 1990.

114. Stoffer RP, Koeneke IA, Chesky VE et al: The thyroid in pregnancy. Am J Obstet Gynecol 74:300, 1957.

115. Werner SC: The effect of triiodothyronine administration on the elevated protein-bound iodine level in human pregnancy. Am J Obstet Gynecol 75:1193, 1958.

116. Raiti S, Holsman GB, Scott RL et al: Evidence for placental transfer of triiodothyronine in human beings. N Engl J Med 277:456, 1967.

117. Kenimer JC, Hershman JM, Higgins HP: The thyrotropin in hydatidiform moles in human chorionic gonadotropin. J Clin Endocrinol Metab 40:482, 1975.

118. Valdalem JL, Pirens G, Hennen G, et al: Thyroliberin and gonadoliberin tests during pregnancy and the puerperium. Acta Endocrinol 86:695, 1977.

119. Ylikorkala O, Kivinen S, Reinilä MI: Serial prolactin and thyrotropin responses to thyrotropin-releasing hormone throughout normal human pregnancy. J Clin Endocrinol Metab 48:288, 1979.

120. Burrow GN, Polackwich R, Donabedian R: The hypothalamic-pituitary-thyroid axis in normal pregnancy. In Fisher DA, Burrow GN (eds): Perinatal Thyroid Physiology and Disease. New York, Raven Press, 1975, p 1.

121. Chan BY, Swaminanthan R: Serum thyrotropin concentration measured by sensitive assays in normal pregnancy. Br J Obstet Gynecol 95:1332, 1988.

122. Desai RK, Norman RJ, Jialal I, et al: Spectrum of thyroid function abnormalities in gestational trophoblastic neoplasia. Clin Endocrinol 29:583, 1988.

123. Cave Jr WT, Dunn JT: Choriocarcinoma with hyperthyroidism: Probable identity of the thyrotropin with human chorionic gonadotropin. Ann Intern Med 85:60, 1976.

124. Pekonen F, Alfthan H, Stenman UH, et al: Human chorionic gonadotropin (hCG) and thyroid function in early human pregnancy: Circadian variation and evidence for intrinsic thyrotropic activity of hCG. J Clin Endocrinol Metab 66:853, 1988.

125. Ballabio M, Poshyachinda M, Ekins RP: Pregnancy-induced changes in thyroid function: Role of human chorionic gonadotropin as a putative regulator of maternal thyroid. J Clin Endocrinol Metab 73:824, 1991.

126. Yoshikawa N, Nishikawa M, Horimoto M, et al: Thyroid stimulating activity in sera of normal pregnant women. J Clin Endocrinol Metab 69:891, 1989.

127. Kinmura M, Amino N, Tamaki H, et al: Physiologic thyroid activation in normal pregnancy is induced by circulating hCG. Obstet Gynecol 75:775, 1990.

128. Ekins R: Roles of serum thyroxine binding proteins and maternal thyroid hormones in fetal development. Lancet 1:1129, 1985.

129. Ekins R, Sinha A, Ballabio M, et al: Role of maternal carrier proteins in the supply of thyroid hormones to the feto-placental unit: Evidence of a feto-placental requirement for thyroxine. In Delange F, Fisher DA, Glinoer D (eds): Research in Congenital Hypothyroidism. New York, Plenum Press, 1989, p 45.

130. Carayon P, Lefort G, Nisula B: Interaction of human chorionic gonadotropin and human luteinizing hormone with human thyroid membranes. Endocrinology 106:1907, 1980.

131. Davies TF, Taliadouros GS, Catt KJ, et al: Assessment of urinary thyrotropin-completing activity in choriocarcinoma and thyroid disease: Further evidence for human chorionic gonadotropin interacting at the thyroid cell membrane. J Clin Endocrinol Metab 49:353, 1979.

132. Silverberg J, O'Donnel J, Sugenaya A, et al: Effect of human chorionic gonadotropin on human thyroid tissue in vitro. J Clin Endocrinol Metab 46:420, 1978.

133. Carayon P, Amir S, Nisula B, et al: Effect of carboxypeptidase digestion of the human chorionic gonadotropin molecule on its thyrotropic activity. Endocrinology 108:1891, 1981.

134. Mann K, Schneider N, Hoermann R: Thyrotropic activity of acidic isoelectric variants of human chorionic gonadotropin from trophoblastic tumors. Endocrinology 118:1558, 1986.

135. Hershman JM, Lee HY, Sugawara M, et al: Human chorionic gonadotropin stimulates iodide uptake, adenylate cyclase and deoxyribonucleic acid synthesis in cultured rat thyroid cells. Endocrinology 67:74, 1988.

136. Davies TF, Platzer M: hCG-induced TSH receptor activation and growth acceleration in FRTL-5 cells. Endocrinology 118:2149, 1986.

137. Ballabio M, Sinha AK, Ekins RP: Thyrotropic activity of crude hCG in FRTL-5 rat thyroid cells. Acta Endocrinol 116:479, 1987.

138. Amir SM, Eudo K, Osathanoudh R, et al: Divergent responses by human and mouse thyroids to human chorionic gonadotropin in vitro. Mol Cell Endocrinol 39:31, 1985.

139. Pekary AE, Azukizawa M, Hershman JM: Thyroidal responses to human chorionic gonadotropin in the chicken and rat. Horm Res 17:36, 1983.

140. Uchimura H, Nagataki S, Ito K, et al: Inhibition of the thyroid adenylate cyclase response to thyroid-stimulating immunoglobulin G by crude and asailo-human choriogonadotropin. J Clin Endocrinol Metab 55:347, 1982.

141. Amir S, Shimohigashi Y, Carayon P, et al: Role of carbohydrate moiety of the human chorionic gonadotropin molecule in its thyrotropic activity. Arch Biochem Biophys 229:170, 1984.

142. Fein HG, Rosen SW, Weintraub BD: Increased glycosylation of serum human chorionic gonadotropin and subunits from eutopic and ectopic sources: Comparison with placental and urinary forms. J Clin Endocrinol Metab 50:1111, 1980.

143. Fisher DA, Dussault JH, Sack J et al: Ontogenesis of hypothalamic-pituitary—thyroid function in man, sheep and rat. Recent Prog Horm Res 33:59, 1977.

144. Fisher DA, Polk DH: Development of the thyroid. Baillieres Clin Endocrinol Metab 3:627, 1989.

145. Thorpe-Beeston JG, Nicolaides KH, Felton CV, et al: Maturation of the secretion of thyroid hormone and thyroid-stimulating hormone in the fetus. N Engl J Med 324:532, 1991.

146. Greenberg AH, Czernichow P, Reba RC, et al: Observations on the maturation of thyroid function in early fetal life. J Clin Invest 49:1790, 1970.

147. Koivusalo F: Evidence of thyrotropin releasing hormone activity in autopsy pancreata from newborns. J Clin Endocrinol Metab 5:734, 1981.

148. Leduque P, Aratan-Spire S, Czernichow P, et al: Ontogenesis of thyrotropin releasing hormone in human fetal pancreas. J Clin Invest 78:1028, 1986.

149. Polk DH, Reviczky AL, Lam RW et al: Thyrotropin releasing hormone: Effect of thyroid status on tissue concentrations in fetal sheep. Clin Res 36:203, 1988.

150. Roti E, Gundi A, Braverman LE et al: Human cord blood concentrations of thyrotropin, thyroglobulin and iodothyronines after maternal administration of thyrotropin-releasing hormone. J Clin Endocrinol Metab 53:813, 1981.

151. Robertson B: Pathology and pathophysiology of neonatal surfactant deficiency ("respiratory distress syndrome," "hyaline membrane disease"). In Robertson B, van Golde LMG, Batenburg JJ (eds): Pulmonary surfactant. Amsterdam, Elsevier Science, 1984, p 383.

152. Smith BT: Pulmonary surfactant during fetal development and neonatal adaptation: Hormonal control. In Robertson B, van Golde LMG, Batenburg JJ (eds) Pulmonary surfactant. Amsterdam, Elsevier Science, 1984, p 357.

153. Devaskar U, Nitta K, Szewczyk K, et al: Transplacental stimulation of functional morphological fetal rabbit lung maturation: Effect of thyrotropin-releasing hormone. Am J Obstet Gynecol 1567:460, 1987.

154. Bernal J, Pekonen F: Ontogenesis of nuclear 3,5,3' triiodothyronine receptors in human fetal brain. Endocrinology 114:677, 1984.

155. Calvo R, Obregon MJ, Ruiz de Ona C, et al: Congenital hypothyroidism as studied in rats: crucial role of maternal thyroxine but not 3,5,3'-triiodothyronine in the protection of the fetal brain. J Clin Invest 86:889, 1990.

156. Morreale de Escobar G, Obregon MJ, Escobar del Rey F: Maternal-fetal thyroid hormone relationships and the fetal brain. Acta Med Austriaca 15:66, 1988.

157. Morreale de Escobar G, Obregon MJ, Ruiz de Ona C, et al: Comparison of maternal to fetal transfer of 3,5,3'-triiodothyronine versus thyroxine in rats. Acta Endocrinol 120:20, 1989.

158. Ruiz de Ona C, Obregon MJ, Escobar del Rey F, et al: Developmental changes in rat brain 5'-deiodinase and thyroid hormones in the fetal period. Pediatr Res 24:588, 1988.

159. Vaccari A: Teratogenic mechanisms of dysthyroidism in the central nervous system. Prog Brain Res 73:71, 1988.

160. Morreale de Escobar G, Calvo R, Obregon MJ, et al: Contribution of maternal thyroxine to fetal thyroxine pools in normal rats near term. Endocrinology 126:2765, 1990.

161. Illig R: Congenital hypothyroidism. J Clin Endocrinol Metab 8:49, 1979.

162. Ferreiro B, Bernal J, Goodyear G, et al: Estimation of nuclear thyroid hormone receptor saturation in human fetal brain and lung during early gestation. Endocrinology 5667:853, 1988.

163. Man EB, Jones WS, Holden RH, et al: Thyroid function in human pregnancy. VIII. Retardation of progeny aged 7 years: Relationships to maternal age and maternal thyroid function. Am J Obstet Gynecol 111:905, 1971.

164. Man EB, Brown JF, Serunian SA: Maternal hypothyroxinemia: Psychoneurological deficits of progeny. Ann Clin Lab Sci 21:227, 1991.

165. Dussault J, Row VV, Lickrish G, et al: Studies of serum triiodothyronine concentration in maternal and cord blood. J Clin Endocrinol Metab 29:595, 1969.

166. Fisher DA, Lehman H, Lackey C: Placental transport of thyroxine. J Clin Endocrinol Metab 24:393, 1964.

167. Grumbach MM, Werner SC: Transfer of thyroid hormones across the human placenta at term. J Clin Endocrinol Metab 16:1392, 1956.

168. Carr EA, Bierwaltes WH, Raman G, et al: The effect of maternal thyroid function on fetal thyroid function and development. J Clin Endocrinol Metab 19:1, 1959.

169. Kearns JE, Hutson W: Tagged isomers and analogs of thyroxine: their transmission across the human placenta and other studies. J Nucl Med 4:453, 1963.

170. Myant NB: Passage of thyroxine and triiodothyronine from mother to fetus in pregnant women. Clin Sci 17:75, 1958.

171. Vulsma T, Gous MH, De Vijlder JJM: Maternal-fetal transfer of thyroxine in congenital hypothyroidism due to a total organification defect or thyroid agenesis. N Engl J Med 321:13, 1989.

172. Comite F, Burrow GN, Jorgensen EC: Thyroid hormone analogues and fetal goiter. J Clin Endocrinol Metab 102:1670, 1978.

173. Bachrach LK, Kudlow JE, Silverberg JDH, et al: Treatment of ovine cretinism in utero with 3′5-dimethyl-3′-isopropyl-L-thyroxine. Endocrinology 111:132, 1982.

174. Penel C, Rognoni JB, Pastiani P: Thyroid autoregulation. Am J Physiol 16:E165, 1987.

175. Theodoropoulos T, Braverman LE, Vagenakis AG: Iodine-induced hypothyroidism. Science 205:502, 1979.

176. Mahillon I, Peers W, Bourdoux P, et al: Effects of vaginal douching with povidone-iodine during early pregnancy on the iodine supply to mother and fetus. Biol Neonate 56:210, 1989.

177. Stubbe P, Heidemann P, Schurnbrand P, et al: Transient congenital hypothyroidism after amniofetography. Eur J Pediatr 135:97, 1980.

178. Smerdley P, Boyages SC, Wu D, et al: Topical iodine-containing antiseptics and neonatal hypothyroidism in very low birth weight infants. Lancet 2:661, 1989.

179. Danziger Y, Pertzelan A, Mimouni M: Transient congenital hypothyroidism after topical iodine in pregnancy and lactation. Arch Dis Child 62:295, 1987.

180. Rey E, Bachrach LK, Burrow GN: Effects of amiodarone during pregnancy. Can Med Assoc J 136:959, 1987.

181. DeWolf D, DeSchepper J, Verhaaren H, et al: Congenital hypothyroid goiter and amiodarone. Acta Pediatr Scand 77:616, 1988.

182. Tubman R, Jenkins J, Lim J: Neonatal hyperthyroxinemia associated with maternal amiodarone therapy. Irish J Med Sci 157:243, 1988.

183. Widehorn J, Bhandari AK, Bughi S, et al: Fetal and neonatal adverse effects profile of amiodarone treatment during pregnancy. Am Heart J 122:1162, 1991.

184. Dussault JH, Rousseau F: Immunologically mediated hypothyroidism. Endocrinol Metab Clin N Am 16:417, 1987.

185. Tamaki H, Amino N, Aozasa M, et al: Effective method for prediction of transient neonatal hypothyroidism in infants born to mothers with chronic thyroiditis. Am J Perinatol 6:296, 1989.

186. Matsuura N, Konishi J: Transient hypothyroidism in infants born to mothers with chronic thyroiditis. A nationwide study of twenty-three cases. Endocrinol Jpn 37:369, 1990.

187. Perelman AH, Johnston RL, Clemons RD, et al: Intrauterine diagnosis and treatment of fetal goitrous hypothyroidism. J Clin Endocrinol Metab 71:618, 1990.

188. Glorieux J, Desjardins M, Letarte J, et al: Useful parameters to predict eventual mental outcome of hypothyroid children. Pediatr Res 24:6, 1988.

189. Virtanen M, Perheentupa J: Bone age at birth: Method and effect of hypothyroidism. Acta Pediatr Scand 78:412, 1989.

190. Davidson KM, Richards DS, Schatz DA, et al: Successful in utero treatment of fetal goiter and hypothyroidism. N Engl J Med 324:543, 1991.

191. Wenstrom KD, Weiner CP, Williamson RA, et al: Prenatal diagnosis of fetal hyperthyroidism using funipuncture. Obstet Gynecol 76:513, 1990.

192. Chopra IJ, Crandall BF: Thyroid hormones and thyrotropin in amniotic fluid. N Engl J Med 293:740, 1975.

193. Yoshida K, Sakurada T, Takahashi T, et al: Measurement of TSH in human amniotic fluid. Clin Endocrinol 25:313, 1986.

194. Hollingsworth DR, Alexander NM: Amniotic fluid concentrations of iodothyronines and thyrotropin do not reliably predict fetal thyroid status in pregnancies complicated by maternal thyroid disorders or anencephaly. J Clin Endocrinol Metab 57:349, 1983.

195. Lightner ES, Fisher DA, Giles H, et al: Intra-amniotic injections of thyroxine to a human fetus. Am J Obstet Gyn 127:487, 1977.

196. VanHerle AJ, Young RT, Fisher DA, et al: Intrauterine treatment of a hypothyroid fetus. J Clin Endocrinol Metab 40:474, 1975.

197. Crooks J, Abdoul-Khair SA, Turnbull AC, et al: The incidence of goiter during pregnancy. Lancet 2:334, 1966.

198. Drury MI: Hyperthyroidism in pregnancy. J R Soc Med 79:317, 1986.

199. Crooks J, Tulloch MI, Turnbull AC, et al: Comparative incidence of goiter in pregnancy in Iceland and Scotland. Lancet 2:625, 1964.

200. Long TJ, Felice ME, Hollingsworth DR: Goiter in pregnant teenagers. Am J Obstet Gynecol 152:670, 1985.

201. Murray TK: Goiter in Canada. Can J Public Health 68:431, 1977.

202. Levy RP, Newman DM, Rejali LS, et al: The myth of goiter in pregnancy. Am J Obstet Gynecol 137:701, 1980.

203. Rasmussen NG, Hornnes PJ, Hegedus L: Ultrasonographically determined thyroid size in pregnancy and postpartum. Am J Obstet Gynecol 160:1216, 1989.

204. Pedersen KM, Börlum KG, Knudson PR, et al: Urinary iodine excretion is low and serum thyroglobulin high in pregnant women on parts of Denmark. Acta Obstet Gynecol Scand 67:413, 1988.

205. Nelson M, Wickus GG, Caplan RH et al: Thyroid gland size in pregnancy. J Reprod Med 32:888, 1987.

206. Struve C, Ohlen S: The influence of previous pregnancies on the prevalence of goitre and thyroid nodules in women without clinical evidence of thyroid disease. Dtsch Med Wschr 115:1050, 1990.

207. Gaitan E, Cooksey RC, Meydrech EF, et al: Thyroid function in neonates from goitrous and non-goitrous iodine-sufficient areas. J Clin Endocrinol Metab 69:359, 1989.

208. Liu JL, Zhuang ZJ, Cao XM: Changes in thyroid, cerebral cortex and bones of therapeutically aborted fetuses from endemic goiter region supplied with iodized salt for 5 years. Chin Med J 101:133, 1988.

209. Chanoine JP, Toppet V, Bourdoux P, et al: Smoking during pregnancy: A significant cause of neonatal thyroid enlargement. Br J Obstet Gynecol 98:65, 1991.

210. Mitsuda N, Tamaki H, Amino N, et al: Risk factors for developmental disorders in infants born to women with Graves' disease. Obstet Gynecol 80:359, 1992.

210a. Momotani N, Ito K, Hamada N, et al: Maternal hyperthyroidism and congenital malformation in the offspring. Clin Endocrinol 20:695, 1984.

211. Dinani S, Carpenter S: Down's syndrome and thyroid disorder. J Mental Deficiency Res 34:187, 1990.

212. Dozeman R, Kaiser FE, Case O, et al: Hyperthyroidism appearing as hyperemesis gravidarum. Arch Intern Med 143:2202, 1983.

213. Chin RKH, Lao TTH: Thyroxine concentration and outcome of hyperemetic pregnancies. Br J Obstet Gynecol 95:507, 1988.

213a. Lao TT, Chin RKH, Panesar NS, et al: Observations on thyroid hormones in hyperemesis gravidarum. Asia-Oceania J Obstet Gynecol 14:449, 1988.

214. Goodwin TM, Montoro M, Mestman JH, et al: The role of chorionic gonadotropin in transient hyperthyroidism of hyperemesis gravidarum. J Clin Endocrinol Metab 75:1333, 1992.

214a. Goodwin TM, Montoro M, Mestman JH: Transient hyperthyroidism and hyperemesis gravidarum: Clinical aspects. Am J Obstet Gynecol 167:648, 1992.

215. Kirshon B, Lee W, Cotton DB: Prompt resolution of hyperthyroidism and hyperemesis gravidarum after delivery. Obstet Gynecol 71:1032, 1988.

216. Chin RKH, Lao TT, Swaminathan R, et al: A longitudinal study of changes in erythrocyte zinc concentration in hyperemesis gravidarum. Gynecol Obstet Invest 29:22, 1990.

217. de los Santos ET, Mazzaferri EL: Sensitive thyroid-stimulating hormone assays: Clinical applications and limitations. Compr Ther 14:26, 1988.

218. Bassett F, Cresswell J, Eastman CJ, et al: Diagnostic value of thyrotropin concentrations in serum as measured by a sensitive immunoradiometric assay. Clin Chem 32:461, 1986.

219. Davis LE, Lucas MJ, Hankins GDV, et al: Thyrotoxicosis complicating pregnancy. Am J Obstet Gynecol 160:63, 1989.

220. Easterling TR, Schmucker BC, Carlson KL, et al: Maternal hemodynamics in pregnancies complicated by hyperthyroidism. Obstet Gynecol 78:348, 1991.

221. Bruner JP, Landon MB, Gabbe SG: Diabetes mellitus and Graves' disease complicated by maternal allergies to antithyroid drugs. Obstet Gynecol 72:443, 1988.

222. Burrow GN: The management of thyrotoxicosis in pregnancy. N Engl J Med 313:562, 1985.
223. Momotani N, Noh J, Oyanagi H, et al: Antithyroid drug therapy for Graves' disease during pregnancy, optimal regimen for fetal thyroid status. N Engl J Med 315:24, 1986.
224. Pekonen F, Lamberg B-A: Thyrotoxicosis during pregnancy. Ann Chir Gynaecol 67:165, 1978.
225. Derksen RHWM, van de Wiel A, Poortman J et al: Plasma-exchange in the treatment of severe thyrotoxicosis in pregnancy. Eur J Obstet Gynaecol Reprod Biol 18:139, 1984.
226. Mutjaba Q, Burrow GN: Treatment of hyperthyroidism in pregnancy with propylthiouracil and methimazole. Obstet Gynecol 46:282, 1975.
227. Cooper DS, Saxe VC, Meskell M, et al: Acute effects of propylthiouracil (PTU) on thyroidal iodide organification and peripheral iodothyronine deiodination: Correlation with serum PTU levels measured by radioimmunoassay. J Clin Endocrinol Metab 54:101, 1982.
228. Cooper DS, Bode HH, Nath B, et al: Methimazole pharmacology in man: Studies using a newly developed radioimmunoassay for methimazole. J Clin Endocrinol Metab 58:473, 1984.
229. Sitar DS, Abu-Bakare A, Gardiner RJ: Propylthiouracil disposition in pregnancy and postpartum women. Pharmacology 25:57, 1982.
230. Skellern GG, Knight BI, Otter M, et al: The pharmacokinetics of methimazole in pregnant patients after oral administration of carbimazole. Br J Clin Pharmacol 9:145, 1980.
231. Marchant B, Brownlie BEW, Hart DM, et al: The placental transfer of propylthiouracil, methimazole and carbimazole. J Clin Endocrinol Metab 45:1187, 1977.
232. Milham S: Scalp defects in infants of mothers treated for hyperthyroidism with methimazole or carbimazole during pregnancy. Teratology 32:231, 1985.
233. Stephan MJ, Smith DW, Ponzi JW, et al: Origin of scalp vertex aplasia cutis. J Pediatr 101:850, 1982.
234. Van Dijke CP, Heydendael RJ, De Kleine MJ: Methimazole, carbimazole and congenital skin defects. Ann Intern Med 106:60, 1987.
235. Bachrach LK, Burrow GN: Aplasia cutis congenita and methimazole. Can Med Assoc J 130:1264, 1984.
236. Frieden IJ: Aplasia cutis congenita: A clinical review and proposal for classification. J Am Acad Dermatol 14:646, 1986.
237. Amrhein JA, Kenny FM, Ross D: Granulocytopenia, lupus-like syndrome, and other complications of propylthiouracil therapy. J Pediatr 76:54, 1970.
238. Jackson IMD: Management of thyrotoxicosis. J Maine Med Assoc 66:224, 1975.
239. Wing ES Jr, Asper SP Jr: Observations on the use of propylthiouracil in hyperthyroidism with special reference to long-term treatment. Bull Johns Hopkins Hosp 90:152, 1952.
240. Bilezikian SB, Lalei U, Tsan M-F, et al: Immunological reactions involving leukocytes. III. Agranulocytosis induced by antithyroid drugs. Johns Hopkins Med J 138:124, 1976.
241. Wall JR, Fang SL, Kuroki T, et al: In vitro immunoactivity to propylthiouracil, methimazole, and carbimazole in patients with Graves' disease: A possible cause of antithyroid drug-induced agranulocytosis. J Clin Endocrinol Metab 58:868, 1984.
242. Weitzman SA, Stossel TP, Desmond M: Drug-induced immunological neutropenia. Lancet 1:1068, 1978.
243. Tajiri J, Noguchi S, Murakami T, et al: Antithyroid drug-induced agranulocytosis. Arch Intern Med 150:621, 1990.
244. Romaldini JH, Bromberg N, Werner RS, et al: Comparison of effects of high and low dosage regimens of antithyroid drugs in the management of Graves' hyperthyroidism. J Clin Endocrinol Metab 57:563, 1983.
245. Safani MM, Tatro DS, Rudd P: Fatal propylthiouracil-induced hepatitis. Arch Intern Med 142:838, 1982.
246. Vasily DB, Tyler WB: Propylthiouracil-induced cutaneous vascutitis: Case presentation and review of the literature. JAMA 23:458, 1980.
247. Sato K, Mimura H, Kato S, et al: Serum propylthiouracil concentration in patients with Graves' disease with various clinical courses. Acta Endocrinol 104:189, 1983.
248. Gardner DF, Cruikshank DP, Hays PM, et al: Pharmacology of propylthiouracil (PTU) in pregnant hyperthyroid women: Correlation of maternal PTU concentrations with cord serum thyroid function tests. J Clin Endocrinol Metab 62:217, 1986.
249. Ramsay I, Kaur S, Krassas G: Thyrotoxicosis in pregnancy: Results of treatment by antithyroid drugs combined with T_4. Clin Endocrinol 18:73, 1983.
250. Hashizume K, Ichikawa K, Sakurai A, et al: Administration of thyroxine in treated Graves' disease. N Engl J Med 324:947, 1991.
250a. Hashizume K, Ichikawa K, Nishii Y, et al: Effect of administration of thyroxine on the risk of postpartum recurrence of hyperthyroid Graves' disease. J Clin Endocrinol Metab 75:6, 1992.
251. Bullock JL, Harris RL, Young R: Treatment of thyrotoxicosis during pregnancy with propranolol. Am J Obstet Gynecol 121:242, 1975.
252. Rubin PB: Beta-blockers in pregnancy. N Engl J Med 18:73, 1983.
253. Rubin PC, Butters L, Clark DM, et al: Placebo-controlled trial of atenolol in treatment of pregnancy-associated hypertension. Lancet 1:431, 1983.
254. Sandstrom BL: Antihypertensive treatment with the adrenergic beta-receptor blocker metroprolol during pregnancy. Gynecol Invest 9:195, 1978.
255. Gladstone GR, Hordof A, Gersony WM: Propranolol administration during pregnancy: Effects on the fetus. J Pediatr 86:962, 1975.
256. Habib A, McCarthy JS: Effects on the neonate of propranolol administration during pregnancy. J Pediatr 91:808, 1977.
257. Pruyn SC, Phelan JP, Buchanan GC: Long-term propranolol therapy in pregnancy: Maternal and fetal outcome. Am J Obstet Gynecol 135:485, 1979.
258. Isley WL, Dahl S, Gibbs H: Use of esmolol in managing a thyrotoxic patient needing emergency surgery. Am J Med 89:122, 1990.
259. Worley RJ, Crosby WM: Hyperthyroidism during pregnancy. Am J Obstet Gynecol 119:150, 1974.
260. Innerfield R, Hollander CS: Thyroidal complications of pregnancy. Med Clin North Am 61:67, 1977.
260a. Momotani N, Hisaoka T, Noh J, et al: Effects of iodine on thyroid status of fetus versus mother in treatment of Graves' disease complicated by pregnancy. J Clin Endocrinol Metab 75:738, 1992.
261. Brodsky JF, Cohen EN, Brown BW Jr, et al: Surgery during pregnancy and fetal outcome. Am J Obstet Gynecol 138:1165, 1980.
262. Weingold AB: Surgical diseases in pregnancy. Clin Obstet Gynecol 26:793, 1983.
263. Pitcher-Willmott RW, Hindocha P, Wood CBS: The placental transfer of IgG subclasses in human pregnancy. Clin Exp Immunol 41:308, 1980.
264. McKenzie JM, Zakarija M: The clinical use of thyrotropin receptor antibody measurements. J Clin Endocrinol Metab 69:1093, 1989.
265. Clavel S, Madec AM, Bornet H, et al: Anti-TSH-receptor antibodies in pregnant patients with autoimmune thyroid disorder. Br J Obstet Gynaecol 97:1003, 1990.
266. Matsuura N, Yamada Y, Nohara Y, et al: Familial neonatal transient hypothyroidism due to maternal TSH-binding inhibitor immunoglobulins. N Engl J Med 303:738, 1980.
267. Iseki M, Shimizu YM, Oikawa T, et al: Sequential serum measurements of thyrotropin binding inhibition immunoglobulin G in transient familial neonatal hypothyroidism. J Clin Endocrinol Metab 57:384, 1983.
268. Zakarija M, McKenzie JM, Hoffman WH: Prediction and therapy of intrauterine and late onset neonatal hyperthyroidism. J Clin Endocrinol Metab 62:368, 1986.
269. Mortimer RH, Tyack SA, Galligan JP, et al: Graves' disease in pregnancy: TSH receptor binding inhibiting immunoglobulins and maternal and neonatal thyroid function. Clin Endocrinol 32:141, 1990.
270. Tamaki H, Amino N, Takeoka K, et al: Prediction of later development of thyrotoxicosis or central hypothyroidism from the cord serum TSH level in neonates born to mothers with Graves' disease. J Pediatr 115:318, 1989.
271. Page DV, Brady K, Mitchell J, et al: The pathology of intrauterine thyrotoxicosis: Two case reports. Obstet Gynecol 72:479, 1988.
272. Houck JA, Davis RE, Sharma HM: Thyroid stimulating immunoglobulin as a cause of recurrent intrauterine fetal death. Obstet Gynecol 71:1018, 1988.
273. Bruinse HW, Vermeulen-Meiners C, Wit JM: Fetal therapy for thyrotoxicosis in nonthyrotoxic pregnant women. Fetal Ther 3:152, 1988.
274. Tamaki H, Amino N, Aozasa M, et al: Universal predictive criteria for neonatal overt thyrotoxicosis requiring treatment. Am J Perinatol 5:152, 1988.
275. Delange F: Effect of maternal thyroid function during pregnancy on fetal development. In Beckers C, Reinwein D (eds): The Thyroid and Pregnancy. Stuttgart, Schattauer, 1991, p 7.
276. Klein RZ, Haddow JE, Faix JD, et al: Prevalence of thyroid deficiency in pregnant women. Clin Endocrinol 35:41, 1991.
277. Tunbridge WMG, Evered D, Hall R, et al: The spectrum of thyroid disease in a community: the Wickham survey. Clin Endocrinol 7:481, 1977.

278. Gray RS, Dorsey DQ, Seth J, et al: Prevalence of subclinical thyroid failure in insulin dependent diabetes. J Clin Endocrinol Metab 50:1034, 1980.

279. Bech K, Hoier-Madsen M, Feldt-Rasmussen U, et al: Thyroid function and autoimmune manifestations in insulin-dependent diabetes mellitus during and after pregnancy. Acta Endocrinol 124:534, 1991.

280. Jovanovic-Peterson L, Peterson CM: De novo clinical hypothyroidism in pregnancies complicated by type I diabetes, subclinical hypothyroidism and proteinuria. Am J Obstet Gynecol 104:909, 1989.

281. Gavin LA, McMahon FA, Laske JN, et al: Alterations in serum thyroid hormones and thyroxine binding globulin in patients with nephrosis. J Clin Endocrinol Metab 46:125, 1978.

282. Hornnes PJ, Rasmussen N, Hegedus L, et al: Glucose tolerance and incidence of pancreatic islet cell antibodies in pregnancy in women with thyroid autoantibodies. Horm Metab Res 23:122, 1991.

283. Amino N: Autoimmunity and hypothyroidism. Clin Endocrinol Metab 2:591, 1988.

284. Dillon RS: Disorders of the thyroid gland. In Dillon RS (ed) Handbook of Endocrinology–2. Philadelphia, Lea and Febiger, 1980, p 297.

285. Mizgala L, Lao TT, Hannah ME: Hypothyroidism presenting as hypothermia following pre-eclampsia at 23 weeks gestation. Case report and review of the literature. Br J Obstet Gynecol 98:221, 1991.

286. Patel S, Robinson S, Bidgood RJ, et al: A pre-eclampsia-like syndrome associated with hypothyroidism during pregnancy. Q J Med 79:435, 1991.

287. Lao TT, Chin RHK, Swaminanthan R: Thyroid function in pre-eclampsia. Br J Obstet Gynecol 95:880, 1988.

288. Mandel SJ, Larsen PR, Seely EW, et al: Increased need for thyroxine during pregnancy in women with primary hypothyroidism. N Engl J Med 323:91, 1990.

289. Pekonen F, Teramo K, Ikonen E, et al: Women on thyroid hormone therapy: Pregnancy course, fetal outcome and amniotic fluid thyroid hormone level. Obstet Gynecol 63:635, 1984.

290. Reinwein D, Jaspers C, Kirbas C, et al: Thyroxine substitution during pregnancy. In Beckers C, Reinwein D (eds): The Thyroid and Pregnancy. Schattauer, Stuttgart, 1991, p 115.

290a. Kaplan MM: Monitoring thyroxine treatment during pregnancy. Thyroid 2:147, 1992.

291. Stock JM, Surks MI, Oppenheimer JH: Replacement dosage of L-thyroxine in hypothyroidism. A re-evaluation. N Engl J Med 290:529, 1974.

292. Tamaki H, Amino N, Takeoka K, et al: Thyroxine requirement during pregnancy for replacement therapy of hypothyroidism. Obstet Gynecol 76:230, 1990.

293. Townsend CW: A pregnant cretin. Arch Pediatr 14:20, 1897.

294. Hodges RE, Hamilton HE, Keitel WC: Pregnancy in myxedema. Arch Intern Med 90:863, 1952.

295. Echt CR, Doss JF: Myxedema in pregnancy report of 3 cases. Obstet Gynecol 22:615, 1963.

296. Lachelin GCL: Myxedema and pregnancy: A case report. J Obstet Gynecol Br Commonw 7:77, 1970.

297. Anderson MM, Beales DL: Myxedema in pregnancy. J Obstet Gynecol Br Commonw 7:74, 1970.

298. Baylan P, Frury MI: Pregnancy in untreated hypothyroidism. Irish J Med Sci 148:10, 1979.

299. Kennedy AL, Montgomery DAD: Hypothyroidism in pregnancy. Review. Br J Obstet Gynecol 85:225, 1978.

300. Balen AH, Kurtz AB: Successful outcome of pregnancy with severe hypothyroidism. Case report and literature review. Br J Obstet Gynecol 97:536, 1990.

301. Davis LE, Leveno KJ, Cunningham FG: Hypothyroidism complicating pregnancy. Obstet Gynecol 72:108, 1988.

302. Montoro M, Collea JV, Frasier SD, et al: Successful outcome of pregnancy in hypothyroid women. Ann Intern Med 94:31, 1986.

303. Khoury MJ, Becerra JE, d'Almada PJ: Maternal thyroid disease and risk of birth defects in offspring: A population-based case-control study. Pediatr Perinat Epidemiol 3:402, 1989.

304. Sridama V, Pacini F, Yan SL, et al: Decreased levels of helper T cells: A possible cause of immunodeficiency in pregnancy. N Engl J Med 307:352, 1982.

305. Tallon DF, Corcoran DJD, O'Dwyer EM, et al: Circulating lymphocyte subpopulations in pregnancy: A longitudinal study. J Immunol 132:1784, 1984.

306. Amino N, Kuro R, Tanizawa O, et al: Changes in serum antithyroid antibodies during tand after pregnancy in autoimmune thyroid diseases. Clin Exp Immunol 31:30, 1978.

307. Parker RH, Bierwaltes WH, Elzinga KF, et al: Thyroid antibodies during pregnancy and in the newborn. J Clin Endocrinol Metab 21:792, 1961.

308. Nelson JC, Palmer FJ: A remission of goitrous hypothyroidism during pregnancy. J Clin Endocrinol Metab 40:383, 1975.

309. Ewin DL, McGregor AM: Pregnancy and autoimmune thyroid disease. Trend Endocrinol Metab 1:296, 1990.

310. Labarrere CA, Catoggio LJ, Mullen EG, et al: Placental lesions in maternal autoimmune diseases. Am J Reprod Immuno Micro 12:78, 1986.

311. Bech K, Hertel J, Rasmussen NG, et al: Effect of maternal thyroid autoantibodies and postpartum thyroiditis on the fetus and neonate. Acta Endocrinol 125:146, 1991.

312. Rovet J, Ehrilich R, Sorbara D: Intellectual outcome in children with fetal hypothyroidism. J Pediatr 110:700, 1987.

313. New England Congenital Hypothyroidism Collaborative: Neonatal hypothyroidism screening: status of patients at six years of age. J Pediatr 107:915, 1985.

314. New England Congenital Hypothyroidism Collaborative: Elementary school performance of children with congenital hypothyroidism. J Pediatr 116:27, 1990.

315. Fisher DA, Foley BL: Early treatment of congenital hypothyroidism. Pediatrics 83:785, 1989.

316. New England Congenital Hypothyroidism Collaborative: Characteristics of infantile hypothyroidism discovered on neonatal screening. J Pediatr 104:539, 1984.

317. Coakley JC, Francis I, Gold H, et al: Transient primary hypothyroidism in the newborn: Experience of the Victorian neonatal thyroid screening program. Aust J Pediatr 25:25, 1989.

318. Cho BY, Shong YK, Lee HK, et al: Transient neonatal hypothyroidism due to transplancentral transfer of maternal immunoglobulins that inhibit TSH binding, TSH-induced cAMP increases and cell growth. Endocrinol Jpn 35:819, 1988.

319. Takasu N, Mori T, Koizumi Y, et al: Transient neonatal hypothyroidism due to maternal immunoglobulins that inhibit thyrotropin-binding and post-receptor processes. J Clin Endocrinol Metab 59:142, 1984.

319a. Root AW: The role of maternal autoimmune thyroid disease in neonatal hypothyroidism. Am J Dis Child 146:1029, 1992.

320. Blizzard RM, Chandler RW, Landing BH, et al: Maternal autoimmunization to thyroid as a probable cause of athyreotic cretinism. N Engl J Med 263:327, 1960.

321. Sutherland JM, Esselborn VM, Burket RL, et al: Familial non-goitrous cretinism apparently due to maternal antithyroid antibody. N Engl J Med 263:336, 1960.

322. Van der Gaag RD, Drexhage HA, Dussault JH: Role of maternal immunoglobulin blocking TSH-induced growth in sporadic forms of congenital hypothyroidism. Lancet 1:246, 1985.

323. Dussault JH, Bernier D: ^{125}I uptake by FRTL5 cells: A screening test to detect pregnant women at risk of giving birth to hypothyroid infants. Lancet 2:1029, 1985.

324. Brown RS, Keating P, Mitchell E: Maternal thyroid-blocking immunoglobulins in congenital hypothyroidism. J Clin Endocrinol Metab 70:1341, 1990.

325. Bogner U, Graters Ah, Sigle B, et al: Cytotoxic antibodies in congenital hypothyroidism. J Clin Endocrinol Metab 68:671, 1989.

326. Orgiazzi J, Rodien P, Morel Y, et al: Thyroid autoimmune disorders and pregnancy. In Beckers C, Reinwein D (eds): The Thyroid and Pregnancy. Stuttgart, Schattauer, 1991, p 45.

327. Dussault JH, Letarte J, Guyda H, et al: Lack of influence of thyroid antibodies on thyroid function in the newborn and on a mass screening program. J Pediatr 96:385, 1980.

328. Boyages SC, Halpern JP, Maberly GF, et al: Endemic cretinism: Possible role for thyroid autoimmunity. Lancet 2:529, 1989.

329. Francis G, Riley W: Congenital familial transient hypothyroidism secondary to transplacental thyrotropin-blocking autoantibodies. Am J Dis Child 141:1081, 1987.

330. Pharoah POD, Conolly KJ, Ekins RP, et al: Maternal thyroid hormone levels in pregnancy and the subsequent cognitive and motor performance of the children. Clin Endocrinol 21:265, 1984.

331. Bonet B, Herrera E: Differential response to maternal hypothyroidism during the first and second half of gestation in the rat. Endocrinology 122:450, 1986.

332. Jansson R, Dahlberg PA, Winsa B, et al: The postpartum period constitutes an important risk for the development of clinical Graves' disease in young women. Acta Endocrinol 116:321, 1987.

333. Tamaki H, Amino N, Aozasa M, et al: Serial changes in thyroid-

stimulating antibody and thyrotropin binding inhibitor immunoglobulin at the time of postpartum occurrence of thyrotoxicosis in Graves' disease. J Clin Endocrinol Metab 65:324, 1988.

334. Asa SL, Bilbao JM, Kovacs K, et al: Lymphocytic hypophysitis of pregnancy resulting in hypopituitarism: A distinct clinicopathologic entity. Ann Intern Med 96:166, 1981.

335. Kumar S: Isolated thyroid stimulating hormone deficiency following childbirth. Proc R Soc Med 59:1281, 1966.

336. Merenich JA, McDermott MT, Kidd GS: Transient isolated thyrotropin deficiency in the postpartum period. Am J Med 86:361, 1989.

337. Papetrou PD, Jackson IMD: Thyrotoxicosis due to silent thyroiditis. Lancet I:361, 1975.

338. Amino N, Miyai K Onishi I, et al: Transient hypothyroidism after delivery in autoimmune thyroiditis. J Clin Endocrinol Metab 42:296, 1976.

339. Ginsberg J, Walfish PG: Post-partum transient thyrotoxicosis with painless thyroiditis. Lancet 1:1125, 1977.

340. Singer PA, Gorsky JE: Familial postpartum transient hyperthyroidism. Arch Intern Med 145:240, 1985.

341. Amino N, Miyai K, Kuro R, et al: Transient postpartum hypothyroidism: Fourteen cases with autoimmune thyroiditis. Ann Intern Med 87:155, 1977.

342. Fein HG, Goldman JM, Weintraub BD: Postpartum lymphocytic thyroiditis in American women: a spectrum of thyroid dysfunction. Am J Obstet Gynecol 138:504, 1980.

343. Freeman R, Rosen H, Thysen B: Incidence of thyroid dysfunction in an unselected postpartum population. Arch Intern Med 146:1361, 1986.

344. Lervang HH, Pryds O, Ostergaard Kristensen HP: Thyroid dysfunction after delivery: Incidence and clinical course. Acta Med Scand 222:369, 1987.

345. Nikolai TF, Turney SL, Roberts RC: Postpartum lymphocytic thyroiditis. Prevalence, clinical course, and long-term follow-up. Arch Intern Med 147:221, 1987.

346. Dailey GE: Recurrent postpartum transient hyperthyroidism. Ann Intern Med 90:719, 1979.

347. Walfish PG, Chan JYC: Postpartum hyperthyroidism. Clin Endocrinol Metab 14:417, 1985.

348. Ramsay I: Postpartum thyroiditis—an underdiagnosed disease. Br J Obstet Gynecol 93:1121, 1986.

349. Goldman JM: Postpartum thyroid dysfunction. Arch Intern Med 146:1296, 1986.

350. Jansson R, Dahlberg PA, Karlsson F: Postpartum thyroiditis. Baillieres Clin Endocrinol Metab 2:619, 1988.

351. Fung HYM, Kologlu M, Collison K, et al: Postpartum thyroid dysfunction in Mid Glamorgan. Br Med J 296:241, 1988.

352. Amino N, Mori H, Iwatani Y, et al: High prevalence of transient postpartum thyrotoxicosis and hypothyroidism. N Engl J Med 306:849, 1982.

353. Jansson R, Bernander S, Karlsson A, et al: Autoimmune thyroid dysfunction in the postpartum period. J Clin Endocrinol Metab 58:681, 1984.

354. Wilson R, McKillop JH, Walker JJ, et al: The incidence of clinical thyroid dysfunction in an unselected group of pregnant and postpartum women. Scot Med J 35:170, 1990.

355. White WB, Andreoli JW: Painless postpartum thyroiditis seen initially as severe hypertension. Am J Obstet Gynecol 148:346, 1984.

356. White WB, Andreoli JW: Severe, accelerated postpartum hypertension associated with hyperthyroxinemia. Br J Obstet Gynecol 93:1297, 1986.

357. Rhys J, Othman S, Parkes AB, et al: Interference in thyroid function tests in postpartum thyroiditis. Clin Chem 37:1397, 1991.

358. Romney BM, Nickoloff EL, Esser PD, et al: Radionuclide administration to nursing mothers: mathematically derived guidelines. Radiology 160:549, 1986.

359. Dydek GJ, Blue PW: Human breast milk excretion of iodine-131 following diagnostic and therapeutic administration to a lactating patient with Graves' disease. J Nucl Med 29:407, 1988.

360. Robinson GE, Stewart DE: Postpartum psychiatric disorders. Can Med Assoc J 134:31, 1986.

361. Spratt DI, Pont A, Miller MB, et al: Hyperthyroxinemia in patients with acute psychiatric disorders. Am J Med 74:41, 1982.

362. Stewart DE, Addison AM, Robinson GE, et al: Thyroid function in psychosis following childbirth. Am J Psychiatry 145:1579, 1988.

363. Jansson R: Autoimmune thyroiditis—a clinical epidemiological and immunological study with special reference to transient aggravation

in the postpartum period (Thesis). Acta Univ Upsaliensis 492:1, 1984.

364. Hayslip CC, Fein HG, O'Donnell VM, et al: The value of serum antimicrosomal antibody testing in screening for symptomatic postpartum thyroid dysfunction. Am J Obstet Gynecol 159:203, 1989.

364a. Solomon BL, Fein HG, Smallridge RC: Usefulness of antimicrosomal antibody titers in the diagnosis and treatment of postpartum thyroiditis. J Fam Pract 36:177, 1993.

365. Harris B, Fung H, Johns S, et al: Transient post-partum thyroid dysfunction and postnatal depression. J Affect Disord 17:243, 1989.

366. Pop VJM, de Rooy HAM, Vadar HL, et al: Postpartum thyroid dysfunction and depression in an unselected population. N Engl J Med 324:1815, 1991.

366a. Harris B, Othman S, Davies JA, et al: Association between postpartum thyroid dysfunction and thyroid antibodies and depression. Br Med J 305:152, 1992.

367. Tachi J, Amino N, Tamaki H, et al: Long-term follow-up and HLA association in patients with postpartum hypothyroidism. J Clin Endocrinol Metab 66:480, 1988.

368. Roti E, Minelli R, Gardini E, et al: Impaired intrathyroidal organification and iodine-induced hypothyroidism in euthyroid women with a previous episode of postpartum thyroiditis. J Clin Endocrinol Metab 73:958, 1991.

369. Feldt-Rasmussen U, Hoier-Madsen M, Rasmussen NG, et al: Antithyroid peroxidase antibodies during pregnancy and postpartum. Relation to postpartum thyroiditis. Autoimmunity 6:211, 1990.

370. Kampe O, Jansson R, Karlsson FA: Effects of L-thyroxine and iodide on the development of autoimmune postpartum thyroiditis. J Clin Endocrinol Metab 70:1014, 1990.

371. Bech K: Importance of cytolytic activity and dietary iodine in the pathogenesis of postpartum thyroiditis. Allergy 43:161, 1988.

372. Takasu N, Komiya I, Nagasawa Y, et al: Exacerbation of autoimmune thyroid dysfunction after unilateral adrenalectomy in patients with Cushing's syndrome due to an adrenocortical adenoma. N Engl J Med 322:1708, 1990.

373. Thompson C, Farid NR: Postpartum thyroiditis and goitrous Hashimoto's thyroiditis are associated with HLA-DR4. Immunol Lett 11:301, 1985.

374. Vargas MT, Briones-Urbina R, Gladman D, et al: Antithyroid microsomal autoantibodies and HLA-DR5 are associated with postpartum thyroid dysfunction: Evidence supporting an autoimmune pathogenesis. J Clin Endocrinol Metab 67:327, 1988.

375. Kologlu M, Fung H, Darke C, et al: Postpartum thyroid dysfunction and HLA status. Eur J Clin Invest 20:56, 1990.

376. Jansson R, Safwenberg J, Dahlberg PA: Influence of the HLA-DR4 antigen and iodine status on the development of autoimmune postpartum thyroiditis. J Clin Endocrinol Metab 60:168, 1985.

377. Pryds O, Lervang HH, Ostergaard-Kristensen HP, et al: HLA-DR factors associated with postpartum hypothyroidism: An early manifestation of Hashimoto's thyroiditis? Tissue Antigens 30:34, 1987.

378. DeGroot LJ, Quintans J: The causes of autoimmune thyroid disease. Endocr Rev 10:537, 1989.

379. Jansson R, Karlsson FA, Linde A, et al: Postpartum activation of autoimmunity: Transient increase of total IgG levels in normal women and in women with autoimmune thyroiditis. Clin Exp Immunol 70:68, 1987.

380. Weetman AP, Fung HYM, Richards CJ, et al: IgG subclass distribution and relative functional affinity of thyroid microsomal antibodies in postpartum thyroiditis. Eur J Clin Invest 20:133, 1990.

381. Jansson R, Thompson PM, McLachlan FC, et al: Association between thyroid microsomal antibodies of subclass IgG-1 and hypothyroidism in autoimmune postpartum thyroiditis. Clin Exp Immunol 63:80, 1986.

382. Briones-Urbina R, Parkes AB, Bogner U, et al: Increase in antimicrosomal antibody-related IgG1 and IgG4 and titers of antithyroid peroxidase antibodies but not antibody dependent cell-mediated cytotoxicity in post-partum thyroiditis with transient hyperthyroidism. J Endocrinol Invest 13:879, 1990.

383. Tachi J, Amino N, Iwatani Y, et al: Increase in antideoxyribonucleic acid antibody titer in postpartum aggravation of autoimmune thyroid disease. J Clin Endocrinol Metab 67:1049, 1988.

384. Iwatani Y, Amino N, Tamaki H, et al: Increase in peripheral large granular lymphocytes in postpartum autoimmune thyroiditis. Endocrinol Jpn 35:447, 1988.

385. Hayslip CC, Baker JR, Wartofsky L, et al: Natural killer cell activity and serum autoantibodies in women with postpartum thyroiditis. J Clin Endocrinol Metab 66:1089, 1988.

386. Chan JYC, Walfish PG: Activated (Ia+) T-lymphocytes and their subsets in autoimmune thyroid diseases: Analysis by dual laser flow microfluorocytometry. J Clin Endocrinol Metab 62:403, 1986.
387. Jansson R, Totterman TH, Sallstrom J, et al: Intrathyroidal and circulating lymphocyte subsets in different stages of autoimmune postpartum thyroiditis. J Clin Endocrinol Metab 58:942, 1984.
388. Goldman MH, Tisch B, Chattock AG: Fine needle biopsy of a solitary thyroid nodule arising during pregnancy. J Med Soc NJ 80:525, 1986.
389. Rosen IB, Walfish PG: Pregnancy as a predisposing factor in thyroid neoplasia. Arch Surg 121:1287, 1986.
390. Fukada K, Hachisuga T, Sugimori H, et al: Papillary carcinoma of the thyroid occurring during pregnancy. Acta Cytol 35:725, 1991.
391. Rosen IB, Walfish PG, Nikore V: Pregnancy and surgical thyroid disease. Surgery 98:1135, 1985.
392. Orr JW, Shingleton A: Cancer in pregnancy. Curr Probl Cancer 8:3, 1983.
393. Hod M, Sharony R, Friedman S, et al: Pregnancy and thyroid carcinoma: A review of incidence, course and prognosis. Obstet Gynecol Surv 44:774, 1989.
394. Laitinen K: Life-threatening laryngeal edema in a pregnant woman previously treated for thyroid carcinoma. Obstet Gynecol 78:937, 1991.
395. Asteris GT, DeGroot L: Thyroid cancer: Relationship to radiation exposure and to pregnancy. J Reprod Med 4:209, 1976.
396. McTiernan AM, Weiss NS, Daling JR: Incidence of thyroid cancer in women in relation to reproductive and hormonal factors. Am J Epidemiol 120:423, 1984.
397. Balan KK, Critchley M: Outcome of pregnancy following treatment of well-differentiated thyroid cancer with [131]iodine. Br J Obstet Gynecol 99:1021, 1992.

Iodide Deficiency Disorders

GERALDO MEDEIROS-NETO

Iodide deficiency disorders (IDD) remain a major health problem in the world. More than one billion people in the world today live in iodide-deficient areas and consequently are at risk to a wide spectrum of iodide deficiency-induced ill effects on growth and development (Table 49–1, Fig. 49–1). For many years it has been recognized that there is usually, if not always, a close and inverse relationship between iodide in the soil and water and the appearance of endemic goiter and allied diseases. Nevertheless, it cannot be said as of this writing that the cause of IDD has been completely determined in all cases, or even in any case, because nutritional, constitutional, genetic, or immunological factors may be additive in the sum total of causes that lead to the appearance of these diseases. Therefore, iodide deficiency is a *necessary* cause, although it may not always be a *sufficient* cause. The role of the iodide deficiency as the main etiological factor in endemic goiter and cretinism has been extensively confirmed by the success of iodide prophylaxis programs in several countries, although iodide deficiency has persisted despite readily available means of supplementation, such as iodized salt and iodized oil.[1–12] In 1960 Kelly and Snedden[1] estimated that there were 200 million goitrous persons worldwide. Twenty years later Matovinovic's[6] figure for the less-developed regions of the world was 320 million, and this is probably an underestimate. Thus, even at present, IDD continue to play the same role in a large part of the world that they have for centuries.

One important factor in the failure to apply available knowledge is the geographical isolation of iodide-deficient communities. A second and special reason for the social and political neglect of these disorders is their designation simply as *goiter*. Goiter is often a cause of disfigurement, may be associated with increased incidence of an aggressive type of anaplastic thyroid carcinoma, and may produce obstruction of the trachea, but it is less serious than other health problems in developing countries. However, the impact of iodide deficiency on brain function in the fetus, the newborn baby, and the child have remained unchanged or have even worsened in most of the so-called Third World, especially in remote areas of countries with recent statehood and difficult environmental conditions. Thus, the effects of iodide deficiency extend far beyond goiter and may well constitute a barrier to the social development of people living in communities with a very low iodide intake. Hetzel[7] makes a strong case for this spectrum of ill effects, and he favors the term *iodide deficiency disorders* for endemic goiter, cretinism, and associated diseases.

IODIDE SUPPLY

Iodide is found in relative abundance in marine plants and animals, in the thyroid gland of vertebrates, in deposits of organic origin, in certain natural mineral water, in sedimentary phosphate rock, and in association with certain mineral deposits. Most of the iodide ingested by humans comes from food of animal and plant origin. This iodide, in turn, is derived from the soil. Only a relatively small fraction is derived from drinking water. A most important factor in the depletion of iodide has been glaciation, which removes old soil and scrapes bare the virgin rocks, which have iodide concentrations far lower than those of covering soil. This situation is found in regions that remained longest under Quaternary glaciers and that lost their iodide when the ice thawed (Fig. 49–1).

Much effort has been expended to determine the minimal daily requirements for iodide.[8–11] One can estimate with reasonable certainty that a mean daily intake of at least 50 μg/day is needed. There are indications of an

TABLE 49–1. THE SPECTRUM OF IODIDE-DEFICIENCY DISORDERS (IDD)

Fetus	Abortions
	Stillbirths
	Congenital anomalies
	Increased perinatal mortality
	Increased infant mortality
	Neurological cretinism: mental deficiency, deaf-mutism, spastic diplegia
	Myxedematous cretinism: dwarfism, mental deficiency
	Psychomotor defects
Neonate	Neonatal goiter
	Neonatal hypothyroidism
Child and Adolescent	Goiter
	Juvenile hypothyroidism
	Impaired mental function
	Retarded physical development
Adult	Goiter with its complications
	Hypothyroidism
	Impaired mental function

Adapted from Hetzel BS, Dunn JT, Stanbury JB: The Prevention and Control of Iodide Deficiency Disorders. Amsterdam, Elsevier, 1987.

upward trend in iodide consumption above these limits in certain countries (United States, Canada, and Japan), causing daily urinary excretion of iodide in excess of 800 μg/g creatinine.[8-10]

PREVALENCE

Goiter prevalence (percentage) rates in various segments of the population, determined by the modified World Health Organization (WHO) classification of thyroid size grading and the thyroid surface outline (TSO) measurements, are good indicators of ID severity and its response to iodide prophylaxis and control programs.[11] Elimination of iodide deficiency disorders (to 0 to 5 per cent endemic goiter prevalence) has been achieved in practically all the economically developed countries of North America, Europe, Asia (Japan), and Oceania (New Zealand and Australia).[9-11] Recent reports on goiter and iodide deficiency in Europe[13-15] indicated, however, that goiter persists in adults (but is seldom seen in children) in Bulgaria, Czechoslovakia, The Netherlands, Switzerland, and Belgium. Substantial areas of high goiter prevalence persist in Austria, Hungary, Romania, Poland, Yugoslavia, and West Russia. In other countries (Southwestern Germany, Greece, Italy, Portugal, Romania, Spain, and Turkey) iodide prophylaxis is not mandatory, and goiter and even endemic cretinism continue to be major problems, either nationally or regionally (goiter prevalence rates of 18 to 22 per cent). The overall results of this study give grounds for concern and point to the need for a comprehensive iodination program in Europe.

Goiter prevalence is high in some South American countries, especially in the mountainous ranges of the Andes (Ecuador, Peru, and Bolivia) as well as in the central part of South America (Paraguay).[8] In these countries goiter prevalence is still high in school children.[9-11] In the sub-Himalayan area of Pakistan, the overall prevalence of goiter is 39.7 per cent, and endemic cretinism is common.[16] The Himalayas of India, Nepal, Buthan, and Southern China, as well as the mountains extending into Northern Burma, Thailand, Laos, and Vietnam, have long been known as goitrous areas. The Philippines and Indonesia are also severely iodide deficient. Worse conditions persist in the remote regions of African countries,[17-19] some with recent statehood (Zaire, Nigeria, Senegal, Tanzania), where pioneering surveys and experimental investigation of endemic goiter and cretinism have been carried out by investigators from Belgium.[18] In Papua-New Guinea there

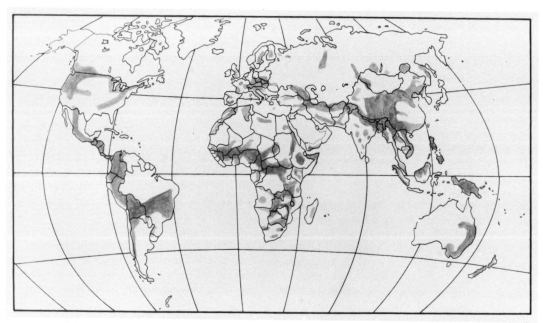

FIGURE 49–1. Map showing areas of geological iodide deficiency (ID) indicated by shading. In some of the areas ID has been eliminated through an effective and successful iodination program. See text to locate areas where ID is extremely severe or moderate to severe. (From Infant and Young Child Nutrition, Report by the Director-General, World Health Organization, Forty-third World Health Assembly, Geneva, 7–17 May 1990, Geneva, World Health Organization, 1990 (WHA43/1990/REC/1), Annex 1, Figure 2, p 45.)

is goiter and cretinism of a severity similar to that of some provinces of the Republic of Zaire.[20] It is estimated that there are 30 million Chinese with goiter and possibly 200,000 suffering from the consequences of endemic cretinism.[21] An intensive program of salt iodization and administration of iodized oil (orally and intramuscularly), however, has reduced the prevalence of goiter and endemic cretinism in China.[12] With the increase in the world population, IDD may become worse and spread further unless a program of world public health and welfare is found that will eliminate iodide deficiency (Fig. 49–1).

ETIOLOGY

Absolute and chronic ID is the principal cause of endemic goiter and allied disorders. It is entirely possible that in certain limited situations other etiological factors such as genetic predisposition in highly inbred and isolated groups, the presence of effective goitrogens in unusual dietary situations (Table 49–2), and autoimmune phenomena may be considered as contributing factors to local endemics. The argument supporting iodide deficiency as the cause of endemic goiter is threefold:

1. There is an association between a low iodide content in soil and water and the appearance of the disease in the population.
2. A reduction in goiter incidence occurs when iodide is added to the diet.
3. It has been demonstrated that the metabolism of iodide by patients with endemic goiter fits the pattern that is produced in animals submitted to a low-iodine diet.

Some observations, however, suggest that iodide deficiency may be present in populations (notably Indians from the upper Orinoco River in Venezuela), in which no abnormal prevalence of goiter was noticed.[22] Another example is the wide prevalence of goiter in an island of Lake Kivu in Zaire.[18] Here northern villages show a prevalence of more than 60 per cent, but the incidence of goiter is limited to 10 per cent in the southwest part of the island. The degree of iodide deficiency, as assessed by iodide urinary excretion and ^{131}I thyroid uptake, was found to be nearly identical in the two populations. The areas also have very homogeneous ethnic, nutritional, and socioeconomic patterns. The *geological nature of soils* might be responsible

TABLE 49–2. Goitrogenic Factors Associated with Endemic Goiter

Bacterial pollution	Progoitrin	Inhibits organification
	Thyroid-stimulating factor	Promotes growth
Millet	Thiocyanate phenolics	Inhibits I⁻ uptake
Cassava	Thiocyanate	Inhibits iodide transport
Babassu coconut	Flavonoids	Inhibits thyroperoxidase
Brassica genus	Goitrin (VTO)	Inhibits organification
Water borne	Disulfides	Inhibits organification
Soybean	Unknown	Fecal loss of T4
Seaweed (kelp)	Iodide excess	Inhibits release of hormones
Malnutrition	Vitamin A deficiency	Abnormal Tg structure

Data from references 25–35.

for the difference in goiter prevalence between the two populations, or, alternatively, geological differences, soil characteristics, trace elements in drinking water, and bacterial pollution could act in association with iodide deficiency to increase goiter prevalence in one population.[23, 24]

A possible connection between *bacterial pollution* in the drinking water and endemic prevalence has been raised by several investigators.[25–27] Supporting evidence for this concept is available. Cultures of *Escherichia coli* contain an antithyroid compound that diminishes the iodide uptake of the murine thyroid.[25] Bacteria from a *Paracolobactrum* genus produce myrosinase, an enzyme that converts the naturally occurring progoitrin into the active thyroid blocker goitrin.[26] Also, *Clostridium perfringens* produces a substance that has a strong thyroid-stimulating activity.[27]

Natural goitrogens (i.e., organic and microbial water pollutants) (Table 49–2) may be considered significant determinants in the prevalence of endemic goiter, either in iodine-deficiency areas or in localities where iodide intake is abundant. This finding was very well documented in studies conducted by Gaitan and others in Colombia[28] and, more recently, in the coal-rich Appalachian area of eastern Kentucky.[29] Goitrogenic effects[28–37] may be related to the consumption of certain foodstuffs (cassava, millet, Babassu coconut, piñon, and vegetables from the genus *Brassica*). The goitrogenic factor in cassava is related to hydrocyanic acid, liberated from the cyanogenic glucoside (linamarin) and endogenously changed to thiocyanate, which competitively inhibits trapping and promotes efflux of intrathyroidal iodide.[30, 31] *Pearl millet* is one of the most important food crops in the semiarid tropics (large portions of Africa and Asia). Millet porridge is rich in C-gluycosylflavones and has also thiocyanate.[32] Both are additive in their antithyroid effects. *Babassu coconut* is largely consumed in Northern Brazil, and recent studies[33] have demonstrated the possible presence of flavonoids in the edible part of the nut. Thus in areas where millet and Babassu coconut are a major component of the diet, their ingestion may contribute to the genesis of goiter. Furthermore, flavonoids, besides being potent inhibitors of thyroid peroxidase, also interact with thyroid hormone at the peripheral level.[11] From turnips the compound 1-5-vinyl-2-thiooxazolidone (VTO, goitrin) was isolated; it is similar in action and potency to synthetic antithyroid drugs.[36] Soybean-based foods and soybean milk formulas increase the loss of T4 from the blood via bile into the gut.[37] Disulfides of aliphatic hydrocarbons from sedimentary rock drained by waters into deep wells are believed to be the cause of the incomplete reduction of endemic goiter following use of iodized salt in Colombia.[29] Excess consumption of iodine-rich kelp (dry seaweed, 80 to 200 mg iodide/day) has caused sporadic and even endemic goiter in humans.[38] In this case goiter is common in some families and more frequent in girls at puberty, suggesting possible influences of additional genetic and hormonal factors. The organification of iodide and, consequently, synthesis of T4 and T3 were lower than normal, and an iodine-rich colloid goiter was observed in patients submitted to thyroidectomy from the endemic coast goiter of Hokkaido, Japan.[38]

Generalized malnutrition (protein-calorie deprivation) has been recognized as an additive factor in the prevalence of endemic goiter in afflicted populations.[39] On the basis of epidemiological data recorded in goitrous patients living in Senegal, it was recently observed that goiter correlated with vitamin A deficiency.[40] Also vitamin A deficiency was reported to alter thyroglobulin (Tg) structure, with poorly mannosylated Tg and abnormal spatial rearrangement of tyrosyl residues. This incorrect alignment increases the distance separating tyrosyl residues and hampers the normal closure of several disulfide linkages, rendering the tyrosine-to-thyronine coupling reactions less efficient. Thus the hormonogenic potency of Tg is severely depressed and, in combination with iodide deficiency, could be considered one explanation for the additional effects of prolonged malnutrition in areas of endemic goiter.

Abnormal immunological phenomena have been associated with sporadic and endemic goiter.[41-58] Thyrotropin (TSH) receptor autoantibodies have been described in multinodular euthyroid goiters, either as TSH-binding inhibiting immunoglobulins (TSBAb) or as thyroid-stimulating immunoglobulins (TSAb).[41, 43] Later it was reported that patients with endemic goiter showed high immunoglobulin A (IgA) levels and positive responses to thyroid antigen in the leukocyte migration inhibition test.[46] It was also found that IgG isolated from patients with large goiters (some recurring after partial thyroidectomy) increases DNA synthesis in guinea pig thyroid cell cultures.[47] This finding was interpreted as the effect of a distinct type of autoantibody (thyroid growth-promoting IgG, TGI) that promotes thyroid cell growth without stimulation of function.[42] The same group of investigators reported that 67 per cent of euthyroid patients with nonendemic goiter had a positive cytochemical bioassay for thyroid growth–stimulating immunoglobulins, and values tended to be high in diffuse goiter, nodular goiters recurring after partial thyroidectomy, and those with recent growth.[48] These studies were confirmed by observing ³H-thymidine incorporation in cultivated porcine thyroid follicles[50, 51] and raise the question of whether thyroid growth in sporadic and endemic goiter could be partially dependent on an autoimmune mechanism.[42, 54, 57] Growth-promoting activity was found in IgGs prepared from sera of 24 of 42 goitrous subjects from a region of severe iodide deficiency in northern Brazil.[51, 53] In the later patients, treatment with iodized oil injection resulted after one year in loss of positive growth values in every case, simultaneously with considerable reduction in goiter size.

Some doubt has been raised about the value of TGI studies.[54] Particularly the methods to measure cell growth and the methods to prepare IgGs have been criticized.[54, 55] More recently TGI activity was evaluated using purified IgG preparations and measuring thyrocyte replication as the end-point parameter.[56] A positive growth stimulation index was found in IgG preparations of 65 of 71 patients with endemic goiter and in 9 of 14 IgG preparations of patients with sporadic goiter (Fig. 49–2). The functional rat thyroid (cell) line 5 (FRTL5) cultured cell growth stimulation with those IgGs could be detected only when IgG was tested in combination with a small dose of TSH. These findings suggest that autoimmunity growth mechanisms may be involved in the pathogenesis of both endemic and sporadic goiters.

PATHOPHYSIOLOGY

The theoretical basis for human adaptation to iodide deficiency was enunciated by Stanbury and co-workers in

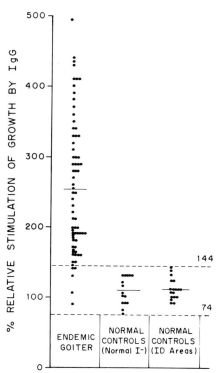

FIGURE 49–2. Autoimmune growth mechanisms may be involved in the pathogenesis of endemic goiter. In this figure percentage relative stimulation indicates the ratio (times 100) between the percentage of mitotic cells in cultures driven by (1) IgG plus 50 μU TSH/mL and (2) that in cultures driven by this dose of TSH alone. The latter was taken as 100 per cent. Samples of IgG (n = 71) from endemic goiter patients gave a mean relative stimulation of 255 per cent. IgG preparations of control subjects from areas with normal iodide intake or from iodide-deficient areas gave a mean relative stimulation of 110 percent (74 - 144, dashed lines). This study would favor the presence of autoimmune mechanisms in iodide-deficient goiters. (Adapted from Wilders-Truschmig MM, Drexhage HA, Leb G, et al: Chromatographically purified immunoglobulin G of endemic and sporadic goiter patients stimulates FRTL 5 cell growth in a mitotic arrest assay. J Clin Endocrinol Metab 70:444–452, 1990, © The Endocrine Society.)

classic field studies in Mendonza, Argentina.[4] Goiter was regarded as an obligatory response to prolonged and severe iodide deficiency, and an increase in thyroid iodide clearance was shown to be the basic mechanism of iodide conservation. Subsequently, a shift in thyroid hormone synthesis in favor of T_3 indicated an additional mechanism.[59, 60] Concepts have improved our understanding of how humans cope with a low iodide intake as well as of the effects that both the lack of iodide and the adaptation mechanisms have on thyroid physiology.[60-73] Thus adaptation to iodide deficiency involves a number of biochemical and physiological adjustments that ultimately result in the maintenance of the intracellular concentration of T_3 within normal limits. These mechanisms are listed in Table 49–3.

Increase in Thyroid Clearance of Plasma Inorganic Iodide

An increase in the thyroid clearance of plasma inorganic iodide (PII) is the fundamental adaptive mechanism by which the thyroid gland maintains a constant concentration of accumulated iodide, in the presence of chronic iodide deficiency. A clear inverse relationship between PII

TABLE 49–3. MECHANISMS INVOLVED IN THE ADAPTATION TO IODIDE DEFICIENCY

1. Increased thyroid clearance of plasma inorganic iodide (PII)
2. Hyperplasia of the thyroid and morphological abnormalities
3. Changes in the iodide stores and in thyroglobulin (Tg) synthesis
4. Modifications of the iodoamino acid content of the gland
5. Enrichment of thyroid secretion in triiodothyronine (T_3)
6. Enhanced T_4 to T_3 peripheral conversion in some tissues
7. Increased thyroid-stimulating hormone (TSH) production

concentration and thyroid clearance was found by several authors.[59, 60] The relationship is such that the product of thyroid clearance and iodide concentration is constant within the observed range of serum iodide concentration. This product represents the absolute iodide uptake (AIU), which is the mass of iodide available to the gland per unit of time. Despite the elevated clearance, the value of AIU tends to be lower in iodine-deficiency areas, indicating that the compensatory mechanism is neither perfect nor complete.[59] Inability to compensate fully for the low PII with an appropriate increase in thyroid clearance probably accounts for the fall in iodide concentration in endemic goiter. The increased iodide trapping reflects TSH stimulation but also an intrinsic autoregulatory mechanism dependent on intrathyroidal iodide concentration.

Hyperplasia of the Thyroid

Although thyroid clearance may be increased without demonstrable goiter, the anatomical accompaniment of the functional activity is an increase in gland mass.[61] Another interesting point is that iodide-concentrating ability is not uniformly distributed among follicular cells, even in normal glands. A certain level of TSH-dependent, autonomous iodide trapping is a feature of normal thyroid follicles, and generation of new follicles from mother cells with inherently high capacity for iodide trapping could well explain the heterogeneity of iodide metabolism among the follicles of glands affected by endemic goiter.[66] Also, partial autonomy of iodide trapping could account for the persistently high uptake after the administration of iodide supplements.[61] Deficiency of cytosolic superoxide dismutase in endemic goiter tissues has been claimed to cause a more prolonged exposure to oxygen-free radicals and contribute to degenerative changes found in these tissues.[99]

Changes in Iodide Stores and Thyroglobulin Synthesis

A constant finding reported in endemic goiter is a drastic reduction of the iodide concentration expressed in iodide per gram of tissue. The organic iodide in the thyroid affected by endemic goiter may range from 1.0 to 2.5 mg, in contrast with values of 10 mg obtained in normal control glands.[62, 63] Concomitantly, thyroid iodide turns over much faster, as shown by an increase in the release rate of ^{131}I from the gland. Ermans[59] postulated the presence of two compartments of organic iodide in the iodine-deficient gland: a slow- and a fast-releasing compartment of differing sizes. The fast-release pattern is seen in children and ado-

lescents with small, diffuse goiters and is associated with a rapid rise of plasma-bound ^{131}I. (PB^{131}I). In most adult goitrous patients, there is a slow-release pattern, with normal or low PB^{131}I and a prolonged biological half-life of the thyroid ^{131}I. These observations suggest that intrathyroidal iodide in these long-standing multinodular glands is turning over at a subnormal rate. Slow secretion of the tracer is apparently due to dilution in a large endogenous pool of stable iodide, largely as monoiodotyrosine (MIT) and diiodotyrosine (DIT), present to an excessive degree in the poorly iodinated Tg.

Modification of the Iodoamino Acid Content of the Gland

Experimental studies in the rat show that thyroid hyperplasia induced by iodide deficiency is associated with an altered pattern of iodide distribution within the gland.[64, 65] An increase in labeled MIT and a decrease in the concentration of DIT, as well as a progressive increase in the ratio of T_3 to T_4, are the main changes in the thyroid gland occurring during prolonged iodide deficiency and are directly related to the degree of iodide depletion of the gland. These alterations caused by iodide deficiency appear to be associated with a structural change in the Tg. Experimental studies have shown a greater degree of heterogeneity of the Tg molecule. Its altered sedimentation peak, significantly lower than 19 S, indicates a failure of maturation of Tg.[63] In large human goiters, as the concentration of iodide is reduced, the MIT:DIT ratio increases and the fraction of the tracer found in the form of T_4 and T_3 is markedly reduced. Possibly many of the iodotyrosyl groups do not have the spatial configuration favoring the normal coupling process, and therefore only a small fraction of the iodide accumulated is actually incorporated into the normal pathway of hormone synthesis and secretion. A significant amount of iodide seems to be wasted by incorporation into iodo compounds that are clearly different from Tg, that are resistant to hydrolysis, and that have a very long half-life and low molecular weight. These iodo compounds are, at least in part, fragments of Tg.[65, 66]

Preferential Secretion of Triiodothyronine

The enhanced synthesis and release of T_3 at the expense of T_4 constitute an additional adaptive mechanism entirely different from those described above. T_3 contains one iodide atom less than T_4, and its biological activity is greater. Therefore, increasing the T_3:T_4 ratio of the hormones actually secreted by the thyroid makes the secretion biologically more active while it contains less iodide. Data obtained on thyroidal and extrathyroidal iodide kinetics in experimental models and in humans with goiter have suggested preferential T_3 release.[67-79] Coupling of MIT and DIT seems to be favored over that of two DIT molecules and is directly related to the decreasing levels of Tg iodination.[60, 62] A low level of Tg iodination and intense TSH stimulation are necessary conditions for increasing T_3 biosynthesis and release (Fig. 49–3).

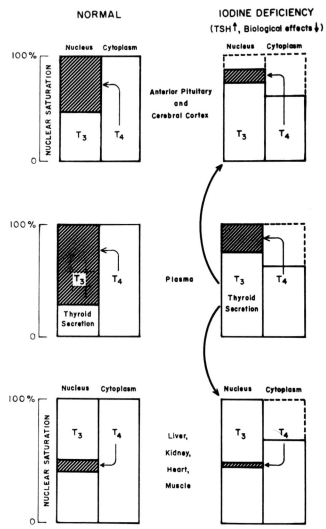

FIGURE 49–3. Normally half of the pituitary nuclear T_3 is produced locally from T_4 deiodination, and the remainder is from blood (via plasma as shown on the left side). In other tissues 25 per cent or less of T_3 is produced locally; the remainder exchanges actively with plasma T_3. Plasma T_3 is mostly produced (3/4). From T_4 but in iodide deficiency, as a consequence of TSH stimulation and low iodide concentration, the thyroid secretion shifts to a preferential T_3 secretion. Tissues other than the pituitary have almost a normal supply of T_3, but the pituitary is significantly depleted of T_3 because of the shortage of T_4. (From Silva JE: Adaptation to iodine deficiency in the light of some newer concepts of thyroid physiology. *In* Soto R, Sartorio E, Forteza I (eds): New Concepts in Thyroid Disease. New York, Alan R. Liss, 1983, pp 75–104).

Enhanced Peripheral Thyroxine to Triiodothyronine Conversion

A compensatory increase in T_4 to T_3 peripheral conversion can take place in a condition of chronic iodide deficiency. It was recently demonstrated in iodide-deficient animals that a striking increase in T_4 to T_3 conversion is observed in the cerebral cortex, whereas the liver showed a change in the opposite direction.[60, 67] Thus tissues highly dependent on T_4 for their intracellular content of T_3, such as the brain, undergo a significant increase in T_4 to T_3 conversion in the presence of a chronic deficiency of iodide, and this may prevent harmful consequences for brain development in early stages of life.[79]

Increased Thyrotropin Production

In iodide deficiency, as in other thyroid conditions with a limited glandular reserve, subjects with normal serum T_3 and low T_4 levels may have elevated levels of serum TSH, although they are clinically euthyroid. A clear-cut increase in the mean level of serum TSH was found in subjects living in areas where the iodide supply was reduced and no difference was evident between individuals with and without goiter.[76, 78, 79] Also, it has been demonstrated that serum TSH levels correlate much better with serum T_4 than with serum T_3. When T_4 is low, the pituitary seems to be hypothyroid, whereas most other tissues are not metabolically affected, provided that the serum T_3 level is normal or elevated.[60, 73] The most elevated TSH values have been observed in newborns and young adults living in areas with severe endemic goiter, whereas in long-standing multinodular goiters the increased thyroid mass and the presence of autonomous areas may bring serum TSH levels toward the normal range.[76-81] An increased sensitivity of endemic goiter tissue to TSH has been proposed as an additional factor for continuous goiter growth.[81] Both thyroid peroxidase activity and 5'-deiodinase activity are elevated in the presence of normal serum TSH,[98] and this has been claimed to be related to increased tissue sensitivity to TSH. In an attempt to delineate further the role of TSH in the pathogenesis of goiter, various investigators have administered thyrotropin-releasing hormone (TRH) to goitrous patients.[81-83, 87] An exaggerated and sustained TSH response to TRH was observed in most studies, indicating an increase in pituitary TSH reserve and less than optimal T_4-induced TSH suppression at the pituitary level. This finding further documents the role in the pituitary of intracellular T_3 generated from T_4 in suppressing TSH.

CLINICAL AND LABORATORY DIAGNOSIS

The clinical picture of endemic goiter is identical to that of sporadic or simple goiter, the difference being only an epidemiological one. Classically, infants and children up to school age have only a diffuse enlargement of the thyroid gland. Further thyroid growth is often observed, mostly in girls, until puberty, constituting what is commonly called *diffuse colloid goiter*. After adolescence the gland becomes more nodular and grows in size as the adult ages. A few patients (less than 15 per cent of the adult goitrous population) may exhibit very large multinodular glands, with total mass estimated to be over 150 g. Age and gender influence the prevalence of goiter, females being more often affected than males.[84]

The presence of endemic goiter occasions no other recognized changes in the body, unless the patient is hypothyroid, which is unusual. Goitrous individuals in areas of endemic goiter seem to feel perfectly good, are able to perform hard work, and show no signs of intellectual or physical impairment. A few patients with very large goiters may show symptoms of tracheal compression, with dyspnea or other symptoms due to compression of jugular veins. The intensity of symptoms and signs of compression on structures surrounding the goiter is not necessarily dependent on goiter size. Large, pendulous goiters can be seen in patients who do not have any other complaint. On the other hand, relatively small goiters enclosed in the upper thoracic region can generate signs of tracheal obstruction.

A frequent complication in large multinodular goiters is hemorrhage or infarction of a thyroid nodule, often accompanied by an inflammatory reaction and an abrupt rise of the serum Tg level. Hyperthyroidism, often due to an autonomously functioning adenoma, is frequently observed if the patients have access to even a small iodide load.[89] Thyroiditis, a rare complication, is often subacute and sometimes focal in type. The pathological features of endemic goiter do not differ materially from those of simple nodular goiter. These pathological changes have been described in detail in an excellent review by Studer and Ramelli.[61] Follicular and anaplastic carcinomas and especially sarcomas are more frequent in regions of endemic goiter. The prevalence of these tumor types means that highly aggressive thyroid cancer prevails in countries with endemic goiter, whereas relatively benign forms (papillary carcinomas) are less frequently recognized.[85] The prognosis of thyroid cancer in regions of endemic goiter is worse than in goiter-free areas because most of the patients are first seen in a tumor stage in which no cure by surgery can be expected.[85, 86] Table 49–4 shows the incidence and survival rate of thyroid cancer in an area of endemic goiter and in a goiter-free region. Highly aggressive, prognostically poor types of thyroid malignancy prevail in association with endemic goiter. Iodide supplementation results in a relative decrease of these tumor types, and the incidence shifts toward a better prognosis.

A large number of laboratory tests have been applied to the study and evaluation of chronic iodide deficiency and its consequences.[87, 88] Test results are substantially altered after iodide supplementation (iodized salt or iodized oil).[91] The radioiodine uptake determination is usually high (>50 per cent per 24 h), but some subjects may have a normal uptake. An inverse correlation is found between the urinary ^{127}I excretion (μg of I per 24 h) and the ^{131}I uptake. An appreciable number of subjects show a high radioactive iodide uptake, a low PB^{131}I formation, and a long biological half-life of the tracer within the gland. This finding suggests that some glands affected by endemic goiter may retain incoming iodide in compartments with slowly labeled pools.[59]

Serum T_3 levels in inhabitants of regions where goiter is endemic are typically normal or moderately elevated at a time when serum T_4 is below normal or low.[69, 71, 76] Elevated serum T_3 levels provide an explanation for the apparent paradox of clinical euthyroidism despite subnormal T_4 levels. Serum TSH is elevated in goitrous patients with low T_4 and correlates better with serum T_4 than with serum T_3

levels. The serum $T_3:T_4$ ratio is commonly used to express the adaptive processes that are described above. Euthyroid subjects living in areas where iodide is abundant have a mean ratio of 15:1, whereas in areas of endemic goiter the mean $T_3:T_4$ ratios reach values of 29 to 34:1.[69] Following treatment with iodized oil there is a progressive fall in this ratio.[87] Serum reverse T_3 (rT_3) tends to follow the direction of serum T_4, but in pregnant women from areas of endemic goiter serum rT_3 is significantly higher than rT_3 levels in nonpregnant subjects from the same region.[75] Increased binding capacity of thyroxine-binding globulin (TBG) is observed and may be related to the elevated serum T_3 concentrations. This could play an important role in the maintenance of a normal level of free T_3.[88]

Subjects with goiter have significantly higher peak TSH values than normal individuals without goiter, after a provocative test with TRH. The exaggerated and sustained TSH response to TRH may be seen in spite of normal serum T_4 concentration and normal or elevated serum T_3 levels.[80–83] When goitrous patients move to an urban area where iodide supply is more abundant, a blunted TSH response to TRH is often observed,[89] and this has been attributed to a significantly higher production of both T_3 and T_4 from autonomous nodules within the multinodular gland. A third of these patients may also show signs of a mild, transient form of thyrotoxicosis.

Serum Tg levels are often elevated in patients with endemic goiter.[92–97] Serum Tg correlates positively with log TSH, but factors other than TSH might also be operative in the release of Tg. Other investigators have concluded that circulating Tg values, although elevated, are not dependent on TSH stimulation but rather correlate significantly with goiter size.[95] Varying elevated concentrations of Tg in the serum of patients with endemic goiter may result from leakage via intercellular junctions and from episodic necrosis of follicles, which allows Tg to be taken up by the lymph channels.[96] Others had reported that the increased serum Tg concentrations in endemic goiter could be partly related to the reduced concentration of iodide in goiter tissues and the intrathyroidal metabolic changes secondary to persistent and chronic iodide deficiency.[97]

Serum basal and the peak Tg response to bovine TSH are elevated in untreated endemic goiter, and it was found that both values slowly returned to the normal range at 30 months after treatment with iodized oil.[94]

PRINCIPLES OF TREATMENT

Treatment of endemic goiter can be carried out by oral administration of L-thyroxine (0.15 to 0.20 mg/day) for a

TABLE 49-4. INCIDENCE AND 5-YEAR SURVIVAL RATES OF DIFFERENT CANCER TYPES IN CHRONIC IODIDE DEFICIENCY AREAS AND NORMAL IODIDE INTAKE AREAS

	DIFFERENTIATED		UNDIFFERENTIATED†		OTHERS‡	
	Incidence %	5 yr (%)	Incidence (%)	5 yr %	Incidence %	5 yr %
Iodine-deficient area (n = 202)	56.2	69	28.4	14	15.4	0
Normal iodide intake (n = 1456)	72.8	75	1.9	16	25.3	3.1

Adapted from Riccabona G: Thyroid cancer and endemic goiter. *In* Stanbury JB, Hetzel BS (eds): Endemic Goiter and Endemic Cretinism. New York, John Wiley, 1980, p 333.

†In iodine-deficient area: mostly solid anaplastic carcinomas.

‡Medullary carcinomas, lymphomas, and not clearly classified carcinomas.

prolonged period of time. This suppressive therapy induces, through a decrease in TSH and the TSH response to TRH, functional atrophy of the goiter. Results are often satisfactory in relatively small colloid goiters but less effective in large multinodular glands. Iodide administration is equally effective when introduced intramuscularly as iodized oil. The increased thyroidal secretion of thyroid hormones will suppress pituitary TSH, and more than half of the treated population will experience a remarkable reduction in goiter size. Surgery should be considered when the goiter is very large, when there is an impairment of the tracheal lumen of more than one third of its normal width, and when malignancy is suspected. In patients who have had thyroid surgery previously, the possibility of shrinking the gland with radioiodine should be considered. Also, ^{131}I treatment can be used in patients in whom surgery is not an option because of an increased risk. The goal of ^{131}I treatment is to reduce the thyroid size, and this can be achieved only by large doses (12,000 to 15,000 rads) of the isotope. A rather high percentage (32 per cent) of the patients will become hypothyroid years after treatment, as also noted in subjects treated with radioiodine for Graves' disease.[85] Prophylactic L-thyroxine treatment in these patients could be instituted to prevent recurrence of the goiter and/or hypothyroidism.

ENDEMIC CRETINISM

Endemic cretinism is now largely a disease in remote, underdeveloped areas of the Third World (Fig. 49–4). It occurs when the iodide intake is below a critical level of 25 µg/day and may affect up to 10 per cent of populations living under conditions of severe iodide deficiency.[99, 100] The disorder is found in India, Indonesia, China, Oceania (Papua-New Guinea), Africa (Zaire), and South America (Ecuador, Peru, Bolivia). In all these locations, with the exception of Zaire, neurological features are predominant.[101, 102] Endemic cretinism may be defined as irreversible changes in mental development in individuals born in an area of endemic goiter, who exhibit a combi-

nation of some of the following characteristics not explained by other causes: (1) a predominant neurological syndrome consisting of defects of hearing and speech, associated or not with characteristic disorders of stance and gait of varying degree; (2) stunted growth; (3) mental deficiency; and (4) hypothyroidism. In its most common form, mental deficiency, deaf-mutism, and spastic diplegia are associated with or without goiter. This is referred to as the *neurological form* of endemic cretinism,[101, 102] in contrast to the *myxedematous* form.[18] It should be made clear, however, that the two types of endemic cretinism represent polar opposites of a wide spectrum of clinical abnormalities.[101-106] Although the myxedematous type is more common in Zaire, the condition may be found in the Himalayas, in the Hetian and Luopu districts of Xing-Jiang (China), in Sicily (Italy), and in South America (Bolivia and Peru).

In Central Africa (Zaire) the severity of cretinism was found to be proportional to the degree of hypothyroidism but also to be correlated with selenium deficiency.[116, 119, 126] The hypothesis was put forth that defective glutathione peroxidase caused by selenium deficiency resulted in lack of protection against peroxidative damage induced by high levels of H_2O_2 in the thyroid cell. Glutathione peroxidase activity was found to be decreased in selenium-deficient areas in Zaire and Ubangi, and the enzyme activity in cretins half the level in normal subjects.[116, 119] Selenium supplementation for two months corrected the enzyme levels in both normal subjects and endemic cretins.[121, 124] However, this treatment also produced decreases in serum T_4 and T_3 and an increase in TSH.[121a] In view of these findings it is advisable to supplement with iodide before administration of selenium in populations deficient in both of these elements.

Thyroid growth-inhibiting immunoglobulins (TGII) have been found in myxedematous endemic cretins with thyroid atrophy.[128, 130, 132, 134] In these patients purified IgG fractions inhibited thyrotrophin-induced DNA synthesis in Guinea pig thyroid segments in a sensitive cytochemical bioassay[128] and also had an inhibiting effect in the cellular growth expressed by a diminished incorporation of 3H-

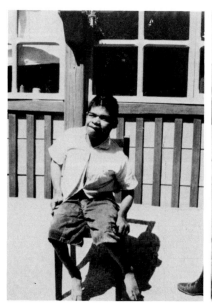
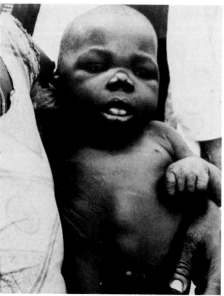

FIGURE 49–4. *Left,* A typical *neurological* endemic cretin from South America with deaf mutism, spastic diplegia, goiter, and mental retardation. Although thyroid hormone levels are usually normal, an exaggerated and sustained TSH response to TRH is frequently observed, suggesting a low thyroid reserve. *Right,* A *myxedematous cretin* from Zaire with all the features of severe hypothyroidism and markedly delayed bone maturation, but with a thyroid normal in size and position (courtesy of F. Delange). Thyroid atrophy is commonly found later in life of myxedematous cretins and has been attributed to environmental agents and/or blocking autoantibodies.

thymidine into the DNA of TSH-stimulated FRTL5 cells.[132] The thyroid-blocking antibodies are believed to be directed against the thyrotropin receptor and may inhibit thyroid cell growth.

Deaf-Mutism and Endemic Cretinism

The endemic cretin is frequently partially or completely deaf. The cause of deafness is uncertain. Lesions can be produced experimentally in the organ of Corti in the chick by injecting an antithyroid drug into the yolk sac.[107] Also, antithyroid drug (propylthiouracil, PTU) administered to pregnant mice or to pups after birth causes abnormalities in the tectorial membrane of the organ of Corti and results in deafness.[108, 109] These experiments strongly suggest that intrauterine hypothyroidism somehow damages the developing auditory system, causing deafness as well as other neurological defects. The absence of deafness in severely hypothyroid endemic cretins from Central Africa remains unexplained. Its absence in sporadic congenital hypothyroidism may be the result of protective action of thyroid hormone passing to the fetus from the mother.

Diagnosis of Endemic Cretinism

The differentiation between sporadic congenital hypothyroidism and endemic cretinism is important both clinically and etiologically. The former is the result of hypothyroidism caused by developmental anomalies or metabolic defects, whereas the latter is associated with severe iodide deficiency in the maternal-fetal unit. Thus the common form of endemic cretinism, during childhood or in adults, unlike untreated sporadic congenital hypothyroidism, is often not associated with severe clinical hypothyroidism,[110a] although a decreased thyroid reserve and an exaggerated TSH response to TRH are often found in neurological cretins.[110, 111] Mixed forms with both neurological and myxedematous features occur. Important studies from South America, Papua-New Guinea, and Indonesia reveal subnormal coordination in otherwise normal children whose mothers were iodide deficient during pregnancy.[113, 114] This neurological defect indicates that the effect of fetal iodide deficiency extends beyond the full clinical picture of endemic cretinism and has been described as endemic mental retardation.[112]

Neonatal Hypothyroidism in Iodide-Deficiency Areas

A serious consequence of chronic iodide deficiency is a higher incidence of neonatal hypothyroidism. In India and Zaire it has been reported that this condition is 200- to 500-fold higher than that observed in countries with adequate iodide intake.[115, 117, 118, 120] In iodine-deficient areas of India, as many as 4 per cent of newborn babies have a cord blood serum thyroxine level below 2 μg/dl,[115] and in Zaire low T_4 concentrations have been observed in up to 10 per cent.[118] A further deterioration of thyroid function occurred in Zaire in children between two and four years, followed by a pronounced prevalence of hypothyroidism

between five and seven years. This is linked to persistent iodide deficiency accompanied by an increase in thiocyanate load, originating from a very high consumption of cassava.[118]

Experimental work has confirmed that severe iodide deficiency affects brain development by reducing both maternal and fetal thyroid function. When sheep or marmosets are kept on a severely iodine-deficient diet for 6 to 12 months before pregnancy and also during pregnancy, reduced brain weight and low DNA content of the fetal cerebral cortex occur as early as day 70 of gestation.[99]

Similarly, the number of spines on the shafts of pyramidal neurons from the visual cortex of iodine-deficient rats is lower than in animals supplemented with iodide.[122] This finding supports the concept that thyroid hormone affects brain maturation through specific effects on cell differentiation. The severe neurological damage found in endemic cretinism is probably due to thyroid hormone deficiency early in pregnancy (first trimester), and it might have become irreversible by birth, at which time thyroid hormones reverse the hypothyroidism, if present, but not the neurological deficits. Both forms of the syndrome, however, can be prevented by correction of severe iodide deficiency before pregnancy by iodized oil injections. When given in the first trimester, however, the iodized oil does not prevent the syndrome of endemic cretinism, suggesting that these effects of maternal iodide deficiency arise very early.[123] Thus elemental iodide, apart from its hormonal role, may be essential for normal neural tube development, but the mechanism responsible for this action is not known.

PROPHYLAXIS AND TREATMENT OF IODIDE DEFICIENCY DISORDERS

Prevention of endemic goiter and cretinism by the addition of supplements of iodide to the daily diet has been accepted and widely employed since the beginning of the twentieth century. The main resources for mass correction of iodide deficiency are iodized salt and iodized oil.

Iodized Salt

The sources of most common salt are solar evaporation of sea water and salt mines.[4] Sea salt as usually produced does not contain enough iodide to meet minimal human needs, as the average iodide content of the ocean salts is approximately 2 parts/million. Human salt consumption (5 to 15 g/day) varies widely among cultures and with climatic conditions. Thus the level of iodization of salt may be varied in order to conform to regional condition (1:25,000 to 1:100,000). It is accepted that 30 parts per million (30 mg of potassium iodate/kg of salt) is the lowest level that will ensure the provision of 100 μg of iodide/day. Many local problems confound the program of iodination of salt for the many millions of people at risk.[129] Inadequate iodinate of the salt, difficulties in importing potassium iodate, problems of transportation and coordination of distribution efforts, and the consumption of poorly iodinated "cattle" salt, by the rural population are the main problems that have obstructed the efforts of effective iodination prophylaxis. Successful salt iodination programs have been implemented in many countries and are highly dependent on continuous surveillance of the iodized salt produced and consumed.[129]

An increase in the incidence of thyrotoxicosis has been reported after the institution of iodized salt programs in Europe and South America and the introduction of iodized bread in Holland and Tasmania.[131, 133, 138] Thyrotoxicosis was more frequently seen in patients older than age 40 and was closely associated with increasing weight and nodularity of the goiter and with the existence of nonhomogeneity on the thyroid scan.[90] A mild and transient form of thyrotoxicosis or a prethyrotoxic state characterized by a blunted TSH response to TRH is frequently observed in endemic goiter patients moving to urban areas, where iodized salt is commonly used.[89] These large multinodular goiters, adapted to chronic iodide deficiency, exhibit autonomous areas particularly susceptible to small loads of iodide with generation of excessive amounts of T_3 or T_4. This situation is often transient, and hormone production will eventually decrease in 6 to 12 months without need for therapy unless cardiovascular disease and related complications are present.

Water Iodination

Reduction in goiter rate from 61 per cent to 30 per cent, with 70 per cent of goiters showing visible reduction, has been demonstrated following water iodination.[125, 127] The introduction of an iodide filter in the wells used in small villages provided an accessible and simple method for control of iodide deficiency disorders.[106] It was also suggested that iodinated water may be more convenient than iodized salt, and there may be less likelihood of iodide-induced thyrotoxicosis, but this method is appropriate at village level only if a specific source of drinking water can be identified.

Iodized Oil

The iodized ethylesters of fatty acids of poppyseed, walnut, and soybean oil (475 to 540 mg iodide/ml) have been used by means of intramuscular injection or oral administration for prevention of endemic goiter and cretinism.[135, 136, 139–145] The doses used have varied from 0.5 to 1.0 ml in infants and young children to 0.5 to 2.0 ml for adults. The oil is stored in the muscle and intermuscular fibrous tissue. This mode of administration was started in Papua-New Guinea and extended to South America, Zaire, Nepal, Sudan, Indonesia, India, and China. Oral administration of iodized soybean oil was extensively studied in China and reported to be effective in a mass population program to control endemic goiter.[135, 144]

There is a large breakdown of the iodinated compounds during the first few months (1 to 5 mg iodide excreted/day), and the urine may contain more than 50 μg iodide/day for two to five years. Although oral administration of iodized oil is cheaper, safer, and simpler, its effective duration is considerably shorter than that of the injected form. From the data with urinary iodide, levels were always satisfactory six months after the oral administration and frequently for two years.[136] After the injection of iodized

oil, the serum T_4 and T_3 increase to normal or elevated levels, with a concomitant decrease of serum TSH and the TSH peak response to TRH and a sharp decline in the previously elevated serum Tg levels.[139, 140] A recent report mentions the reversibility of severe hypothyroidism following treatment with iodized oil in children with endemic cretinism. This was more evident in younger children than in older groups.[136] In a few patients, a lowering of serum thyroid hormones and an increase of TSH suggest an acute Wolff-Chaikoff effect.

After iodized oil administration, there have been a few cases of thyrotoxicosis reported in South America, but none so far in Papua-New Guinea, India, or Zaire.[90, 131] This condition, called *jodbasedow*, is largely confined to people over 40 years of age, who constitute a relatively small proportion of the population in developing countries. This complication may be minimized by restricting administration of iodized oil to those under age 40. An autoimmune reaction, characterized by the development of anti-Tg and mainly antimicrosomal antibodies, was reported in 42.8 per cent of patients treated with iodized oil and was associated with glandular necrosis caused by the large dose of iodide.[57] This finding was not confirmed, however, in other studies in Indonesia and China involving a larger number of patients.[143, 144] Also, a controlled study recently reported indicated that anti-Tg or antimicrosomal antibodies were not found in a group of individuals who received iodized oil during the following five years of observation.[58]

The use of iodized oil has proved to be effective not only in reducing the frequency of endemic goiter but also in reducing the size of established goiters and in preventing the major neuromotor, physical, and mental deficits that are found in association with endemic goiter and endemic cretinism.[137] Iodized oil provides effective, safe, and economically sound prophylaxis against endemic goiter and related disabilities in those situations in which salt iodation is not feasible for economic or political reasons.

REFERENCES

1. Kelly FC, Snedden WW: Prevalence and geographical distribution of endemic goitre. *In* Endemic Goitre. WHO Monograph Series 44. Geneva, WHO, 1960.
2. Dunn JT, Mederiros-Neto GA: Endemic Goiter and Cretinism: Continuing Threats to World Health. Washington, DC, Pan American Health Organization Publication 292, 1974.
3. Ibbertson HK: Endemic goitre and cretinism. Clin Endocrinol Metab 8:97–128, 1979.
4. Stanbury JB, Hetzel BS: Endemic Goiter and Endemic Cretinism. New York, John Wiley, 1980.
5. Dunn JT, Pretell EA, Daza CH, Viteri FE (eds): Towards Eradication of Endemic Goiter, Cretinism and Iodine Deficiency. Washington, DC, Pan American Health Organization Publication 502, 1986.
6. Matovinovic J: Endemic goiter and cretinism at the dawn of the Third Millennium. Annu Rev Nutr 3:341–412, 1983.
7. Hetzel BS: Iodine deficiency disorders (IDD) and their eradication. Lancet 2:1126–1129, 1983.
8. Hetzel BS, Dunn JT, Stanbury JB (eds): The Prevention and Control of Iodine Deficiency Disorders. Amsterdam, Elsevier Science Publishers, 1987.
9. Medeiros-Neto GA: Iodine deficiency disorders. Thyroid 1:73–82, 1990.
10. Gaitan E, Nelson NC, Poole GV: Endemic goiter and endemic thyroid disorders. World J Surg 15:205–215, 1991.
11. Gaitan E, Dunn JT: Epidemiology of iodine deficiency. Trends Endocrinol Metab 3:170–175, 1992.

12. Dunn JT: Iodine deficiency, the next target for elimination? N Engl J Med 326:267–268, 1992.
13. Scriba P, Wood WC, Evered DC: Goiter and iodine deficiency in Europe: Report of the Subcommittee for the Study of Endemic Goitre and Iodine Deficiency of the European Thyroid Association. Lancet 1:1289–1293, 1985.
14. Delange F, Burgi H: Iodine deficiency in Europe. Bull WHO 67:317–325, 1989.
14a. Delange F, Dunn JT, Glinoer D (eds): Iodine Deficiency in Europe: A Continuing Concern. NATO ASI Series A, Life Sciences, Vol 241, 1993.
15. Burgi H, Supersaxo Z, Selz B: Iodine deficiency diseases in Switzerland one hundred years after Theodor Kocher's survey: A historical review with some new goitre prevalence data. Acta Endocrinol (Copenh) 123:577–590, 1990.
16. Subramian P: Goiter and iodine deficiency disorders control through universal iodination of salt in India. IDD Newsletter 3:12–16, 1987.
17. Wachter W, Mvungi MG, Triebel E, et al: Iodine deficiency, hypothyroidism and endemic goiter in Southern Tanzania. J Epidemiol Community Health 39:263–270, 1985.
17a. Aquaron R, Zarrouck K, El Jarabi M, et al: Endemic goiter in Morocco: Skoura-Toundoute areas in the high Atlas. J Endocrinol Invest 16:9–13, 1993.
18. Delange F: Endemic Goiter and Thyroid Function in Central Africa. Monographs in Pediatrics 2. Basel, Karger, 1974.
18a. Das SS, Isichei UP: The feto-maternal thyroid function interrelationships in an iodine-deficient region in Africa: The role of T3 in possible fetal defense. Acta Endocrinol 128:116–120, 1993.
19. Eastman CJ, Phillips DIW: Endemic goitre and iodine deficiency disorders: aetiology, epidemiology and treatment. In Lazarus JH, Hall R (eds): Hypothyroidism and Goitre. Clin Endocrinol Metab. London, Baillière Tindall-Saunders, 1988, pp 719–735.
20. Buttfield IH, Hetzel BS: Endemic goiter in eastern New Guinea with special reference to the use of iodized oil in prophylaxis and treatment. Bull WHO 36:243–262, 1967.
21. Ma T, Lu TZ: Iodine deficiency disorders in China: Current state, control measures, and future strategy. IDD Newsletter 1:4–5, 1985.
22. Roche M: Elevated thyroidal ^{131}I uptake in the absence of goiter in isolated Venezuelan Indians. J Clin Endocrinol Metab 19:1440–1446, 1959.
23. Delange F, Thilly CH, Ermans AM: Iodine deficiency: A permissive condition in development of endemic goiter. J Clin Endocrinol Metab 28:114–116, 1968.
24. Koutras DA: Trace elements, genetic and other factors. In Stanbury JB, Hetzel BS (eds): Endemic Goiter and Endemic Cretinism. New York, John Wiley, 1980, pp 255–268.
25. Vought RL, Brown FA, Sibinivic KH: Antithyroid compound(s) produced by E. coli: Preliminary report. J Clin Endocrinol Metab 38:861–865, 1974.
26. Oginsky EL, Stein AE, Greer MA: Myrosinase activity in bacteria as demonstrated by the conversion of progoitrin into goitrin. Proc Soc Exp Biol 119:360–364, 1965.
27. Macchia V, Bates RW, Pastan I: The purification and properties of a thyroid stimulating factor isolated from Clostridium perfringens. J Biol Chem 242:3726–2738, 1967.
28. Gaitan E: Goitrogens in the etiology of endemic goiter. In Stanbury JB, Hetzel BS (eds): Endemic Goiter and Endemic Cretinism. New York, John Wiley, 1980, pp 219–236.
29. Gaitan E: Iodine-sufficient goiter and autoimmune thyroiditis: The Kentucky and Colombian experience. In Medeiros-Neto G, Gaitan E (eds): Frontiers in Thyroidology. New York, Plenum Press, 1986, pp 19–26.
30. Bourdoux P, Delange F, Gerard M, et al: Evidence that cassava ingestion increases thiocyanate formations: A possible etiologic factor in endemic goiter. J Clin Endocrinol Metab 46:613–621, 1978.
31. Delange F, Alhuwalia R: Cassava Toxicity and Thyroid: Research and Public Health Issues. Ottawa, International Development Research Centre, IDRC 207e, 1983.
32. Osman AK, Basu TK, Dickerson JWT: A goitrogenic agent from millet in Darfur province, Western Sudan. Ann Nutr Metab 27:14–18, 1983.
33. Gaitan E, Cooksey RC, Legan J, et al: Antithyroid effects in vivo of babassu and mandioca: A staple food in endemic goiter areas of Brazil. In Gordon A, Gross J, Hennemann G (eds): Progress in Thyroid Research. Rotterdam, A.A. Balkema Publ., 1991, pp 647–650.
34. Eltom M, Salih MAM, Bostrom H, Dahlberg PA: Differences in etiology and thyroid function in endemic goitre between rural and urban areas of the Darfur region of the Sudan. Acta Endocrinol (Copenh) 108:356–360, 1985.
35. Greer MA: The natural occurrence of goitrogenic agents. Recent Prog Horm Res 18:187–193, 1962.
36. Krusius FE, Reltola P: The goitrogenic effect of naturally occurring L-5-vinyl and L-5-phenyl-2-thiooxazolidone in rats. Acta Endocrinol 53:342–347, 1966.
37. Von Wykj J, Arnold MB, Wynn J, Pepper F: The effects of a soybean product on thyroid function in humans. Pediatrics 24:752–760, 1959.
38. Suzuki H: Etiology of endemic goiter and iodide excess. In Stanbury JB, Hetzel BS (eds): Endemic Goiter and Endemic Cretinism. New York, John Wiley, 1980, pp 237–253.
39. Medeiros-Neto GA: General nutrition and endemic goiter. In Stanbury JB, Hetzel BS (eds): Endemic Goiter and Endemic Cretinism. New York, John Wiley, 1980, pp 269–283.
40. Ingenbleek Y: Vitamin A deficiency impairs the normal mannosylation conformation and iodination of thyroglobulin: A new etiological approach to endemic goitre. In Mauron J (ed): Nutritional Adequacy, Nutrient Availability and Needs. Basel, Birkhauser Verlag, 1983, pp 264–297.
41. Brown RS, Jackson IMD, Pohl S, Reichlin S: Do thyroid stimulating immunoglobulins cause nontoxic and toxic multinodular goitre? Lancet 1:904–906, 1978.
42. Doniach D: Les immunoglobulines stimulantes de croissance (TGI): Peuvent-elles expliquer certains goitres sporadiques euthyroidiens? Ann Endocrinol (Paris) 43:534–547, 1982.
43. Knobel M, Medeiros-Neto G: TSH-binding inhibiting immunoglobulins in endemic goiter. IRCS Med Sci 14:366–367, 1986.
44. Smyth PPA, Neylan D, O'Donovan DK: Association of thyroid-stimulating immunoglobulins and thyrotropin-releasing hormone responsiveness in women with euthyroid goiter. J Clin Endocrinol Metab 57:1001–1006, 1983.
45. Smyth PPA, McMullan NM, Grubeck-Loebenstein B, O'Donovan DK: Thyroid growth-stimulating immunoglobulins in goitrous disease: Relationship to thyroid-stimulating immunoglobulins. Acta Endocrinol 111:321–330, 1986.
46. Moto NGS, Kiy Y, Iwasso MTR, Peracoli MTS: Tumoral and cell-mediated immunity in large non-toxic multinodular goitre. Clin Endocrinol (Oxf) 13:173–180, 1980.
47. Drexhage H, Botazzo GF, Doniach D: Evidence for thyroid growth stimulating immunoglobulins in some goitrous thyroid diseases. Lancet 2:287–292, 1980.
48. Van der Gaag RD, Drexhage HA, Wiersinga WM, et al: Further studies on thyroid growth stimulating immunoglobulins in euthyroid nonendemic goiter. J Clin Endocrinol Metab 60:972–979, 1985.
49. Schatz H, Beckman FH, Floren H: Radioassay for thyroid growth stimulating immunoglobulins (TCI) with cultivated porcine thyroid follicles. Horm Metab Res 15:627–628, 1983.
50. Schatz H, Pschierer-Berg K, Nickel JA, et al: Assay for thyroid growth stimulating immunoglobulins: Stimulation of (3H) thymidine incorporation into isolated thyroid follicles by TSH, EGF, and immunoglobulins from goitrous patients in an iodine-deficient region. Acta Endocrinol 112:253–530, 1986.
51. Medeiros-Neto GA, Halpern A, Cozzi Z, et al: Thyroid growth immunoglobulins (TGI) in large multinodular endemic goiter. Effect of iodized oil. J Clin Endocrinol Metab 63:644–650, 1986.
52. Wadeleux PA, Winand RJ: Thyroid growth modulating factors in the sera of patients with simple non-toxic goitre. Acta Endocrinol 112:502–508, 1986.
53. Halpern A, Medeiros-Neto GA: The significance of immunoglobulins related to stimulation of thyroid growth in patients with endemic goiter. In Pinchera A, Ingbar S, MacKenzie J (eds): Thyroid Autoimmunity, New York, Plenum Press, pp 359–362.
54. Dumont JE, Roger PP, Ludgate M: Assays for thyroid growth immunoglobulins and their clinical implications, methods, concepts, and misconceptions. Endocr Rev 8:448–452, 1987.
55. Zakarija M, McKenzie JM: Do thyroid growth-promoting immunoglobulins exist? J Clin Endocrinol Metab 70:308–310, 1990.
56. Wilders-Truschnig MM, Drexhage HA, Leb G, et al: Chromatographically purified immunoglobulin G of endemic and sporadic goiter patients stimulates FRTL 5 cell growth in a mitotic arrest assay. J Clin Endocrinol Metab 70:444–452, 1990.
57. Boukis MA, Koutras DA, Souvatzoglou A, et al: Thyroid hormones and immunological studies in endemic goiter. J Clin Endocrinol Metab 57:859–862, 1983.
58. Knobel M, Medeiros-Neto G: Iodized oil treatment for endemic goiter does not induce the surge of positive serum concentrations of anti-thyroglobulin or antimicrosomal autoantibodies. J Endocrinol Invest 9:321–324, 1986.
59. Ermans AM: Etiopathogenesis of endemic goiter. In Stanbury JB,

Hetzel BS (eds): Endemic Goiter and Endemic Cretinism. New York, John Wiley, 1980, pp 287–301.

60. Silva JE: Adaptation to iodine deficiency in the light of some newer concepts of thyroid physiology. *In* Soto R, Sartorio E, Forteza J (eds): New Concepts in Thyroid Disease. New York, Alan R. Liss, 1983, pp 75–104.

61. Studer H, Ramelli F: Simple goiter and its variants: Euthyroid and hyperthyroid multinodular goiters. Endocr Rev 3:40–61, 1982.

62. Ermans AM, Kinthaert J, Camus M: Defective intrathyroidal metabolism in nontoxic goiter: Inadequate iodination of thyroglobulin. J Clin Endocrinol Metab 28:1307–1316, 1968.

63. Camus M, Ermans AM: Relation between the coefficient of sedimentation of human thyroglobulin and its iodination level. Horm Metab Res 3:423–429, 1971.

64. Riesco G, Taurog A, Larsen PR, Krulich L: Acute and chronic responses to iodine deficiency in rats. Endocrinology 100:303–308, 1977.

65. Kohler H, Haeberli A, Biswanger CH, et al: Experimental procedures leading to a relative accumulation of nonthyroglobulin thyroidal iodo compounds in rat thyroid glands. Acta Endocrinol (Copenh) 67:216–224, 1971.

66. Medeiros-Neto GA, Nicolau W, Cintra ABU: Studies in the concentration of particular iodoprotein, RNA and DNA in normal and endemic goiter glands. *In* Stanbury JB (ed): Endemic Goiter. Washington DC, Pan American Health Organization Publication 193, 1969, pp 183–193.

67. Silva JE, Larsen PR: Contributions of plasma triiodothyronine and local thyroxine monodeiodination to triiodothyronine to nuclear triiodothyronine receptor saturation in pituitary, liver and kidney of hypothyroid rats. J Clin Invest 61:1247–1259, 1978.

68. Santisteban P, Obregon MJ, Rodrigues-Pena A, et al: Are iodine-deficient rats euthyroid? Endocrinology 110:1780–1786, 1982.

69. Delange F, Camus M, Ermans AM: Circulating thyroid hormones in endemic goiter. J Clin Endocrinol Metab 34:891–895, 1972.

70. Vagenakis AG, Koutras DA, Burger A, et al: Studies of serum triiodothyronine, thyroxine and thyrotropin concentrations in endemic goiter in Greece. J Clin Endocrinol Metab 37:485–489, 1973.

71. Patel YC, Pharoah POD, Hornabrook RW, Hetzel BS: Serum triiodothyronine, thyroxine, and thyroid-stimulating hormone in endemic goitre: A comparison of goitrous and nongoitrous subjects in New Guinea. J Clin Endocrinol Metab 37:783–789, 1973.

71a. Weber P, Krause U, Gaffga G, et al: Unaltered pulsatile and circadian TSH release in euthyroid patients with endemic goitre. Acta Endocrinol 124:386–390, 1991.

72. Pharoah POD, Lawton NF, Elles SM, et al: The role of triiodothyronine in the maintenance of euthyroidism in endemic goitre. Clin Endocrinol (Oxf) 2:193–199, 1973.

73. Larsen PR, Silva JE, Kaplan MM: Relationship between circulating and intracellular thyroid hormones: Physiological and clinical implications. Endocr Rev 2:87–102, 1981.

74. Sugawara M, Kita T, Lee ED, et al: Deficiency of superoxide dismutase in endemic goiter tissue. J Clin Endocrinol Metab 67:1156–1161, 1988.

75. Medeiros-Neto GA, Walfish PH, Almeida F, et al: 3 3′ 5′ Triiodothyronine thyroxine, triiodothyronine and thyrotropin levels in maternal and cord blood sera from endemic goiter regions of Brazil. J Clin Endocrinol Metab 47:508–511, 1976.

76. Hershman JM, Due DT, Sharp B, et al: Endemic goiter in Vietnam. J Clin Endocrinol Metab 57:243–249, 1983.

77. Morreale de Escobar G, Escobar del Rey F, Ruiz-Marcos A: Thyroid hormone and the developing brain. *In* Dussault JH, Walker P (eds): Congenital Hypothyroidism. New York, Marcel Dekker Inc, 1983.

78. Delange F, Hershman JM, Ermans AM: Relationship between the serum thyrotropin level, the prevalence of goiter and the pattern of iodine metabolism in Idjwi Island. J Clin Endocrinol Metab 33:261–268, 1971.

79. Kochupillai N, Karmakar MC, Weightman D, et al: Pituitary-thyroid axis in Himalayan endemic goiter. Lancet 1:1021–1024, 1973.

80. Bachtarzi H, Benmiloud M: TSH-regulation and goitrogenesis in severe iodine deficiency. Acta Endocrinol (Copenh) 103:21–29, 1983.

81. Medeiros-Neto GA: TSH secretion and regulation in endemic goiter and endemic cretinism. *In* Soto R, Sartorio G, Forteza I (eds): Concepts in Thyroid Diseases. New York, Alan R. Liss, 1983, pp 119–130.

82. Rothenbuchner G, Koutras DA, Raptis S, et al: The effect of TRH on serum TSH levels in non-toxic goiter. Horm Metab Res 6:501–505, 1974.

83. Medeiros-Neto GA, Penna M, Monteiro K, et al: The effect of iodized

84. Freire Maia DV, Freire Maia A: Sex and age prevalence of endemic goitre: An epidemiological study. J Hyg Epidemiol Microbiol Immunol 25:401–406, 1981.

85. Riccabona G: Thyroid cancer and endemic goiter. *In* Stanbury JB, Hetzel BS (eds): Endemic Goiter and Endemic Cretinism. New York, John Wiley, 1980, p 333.

86. Harach HR, Escalante DA, Onativia A, et al: Thyroid carcinoma and thyroiditis in an endemic goiter region before and after iodine prophylaxis. Acta Endocrinol (Copenh) 108:55–60, 1985.

87. Medeiros-Neto G: Laboratory evaluation in iodine deficiency disorders. Arq Bras Endocrinol Metab 29:100–113, 1984.

88. Glinoer D, Fernandez-Deville M, Ermans AM: Use of direct TBG measurements in the evaluation of thyroid function. J Endocrinol Invest 1:329–335, 1978.

89. Lima N, Medeiros-Neto GA: Transient thyrotoxicosis in endemic goiter patients following exposure to a normal iodine intake. Clin Endocrinol (Oxf) 21:631–637, 1984.

90. Martins MC, Lima N, Knobel M, Medeiros-Neto GA: Natural course of iodine-induced thyrotoxicosis (Jod-Basedow) in endemic goiter area: a 5 year follow-up. J Endocrinol Invest 12:239–244, 1989.

91. Kiy Y, Lima N, Medeiros-Neto GA: Effective salt iodination changes in the pattern of the TSH response to TRH in endemic goiter patients. Med Sci Res 15:849–850, 1987.

92. Van Herle AJ, Chopra IJ, Hershman JM, Hornabrook RW: Serum thyroglobulin in inhabitants of an endemic goiter region of New Guinea. J Clin Endocrinol Metab 43:512–516, 1976.

93. Pezzino V, Vigneri R, Squatrito S, et al: Increased serum thyroglobulin levels in patients with nontoxic goiter. J Clin Endocrinol Metab 46:653–657, 1978.

94. Lima N, Knobel M, Medeiros-Neto GA: Long term effect of iodized oil on serum thyroglobulin levels in endemic goitre patients. Clin Endocrinol 24:635–641, 1986.

95. Macchia E, Fenzi GF, Monzani F, et al: Relationship between serum thyroglobulin, serum TSH and goiter size in an endemic area. Ann Endocrinol (Paris) 44:53A, 1983.

96. Gebel F, Ramelli F, Burgi U, et al: The site of leakage of intrafollicular thyroglobulin into the blood stream in simple human goiter. J Clin Endocrinol Metab 57:915–919, 1983.

97. Unger J, de Maertelaer V, Golstein J, et al: Relationship between serum thyroglobulin and intrathyroidal stable iodine in human simple goiter. Clin Endocrinol (Oxf) 23:1–6, 1985.

98. Sugawara M, Summer CN, Kobayashi A, et al: Thyroid peroxidase in endemic goiter tissue. J Endocrinol Invest 13:893–899, 1990.

99. Hetzel BS, Potter BJ: Iodine deficiency and the role of thyroid hormones in brain development. *In* Dreosti JE, Smith RM (eds). Neurobiology of the Trace Elements. Clifton, NJ, Humana Press, 1983, pp 83–133.

100. Stanbury JB, Kroc RL: Human Development and the Thyroid Gland: Relation to Endemic Cretinism. New York, Plenum Press, 1972.

101. DeLong GR, Stanbury JB, Fierro-Benitez R: Neurological signs in congenital iodine deficiency disorders (endemic cretinism). Div Med Child Neurol 27:317–322, 1985.

102. Halpern JP, Boyages SC, Maberly GF, et al: The neurology of endemic cretinism: a study of two endemias. Brain 114:825–841, 1991.

102a. Boyages SC, Halpern JP: Endemic cretinism: Toward a unifying hypothesis. Thyroid 3:59–71, 1993.

103. Delong GR: The effect of iodine deficiency on neuromuscular development. IDD Newsletter 6:1–9, 1990.106.

104. Shenkman L, Medeiros-Neto GA, Mitsuma T, et al: Evidence for hypothyroidism in endemic cretinism in Brazil. Lancet 2:67–70, 1973.

105. Fierro-Benitez R, Penafiel W, DeGroot LJ, Ramirez I: Endemic goiter and endemic cretinism in the Andean Region. N Engl J Med 280:296–302, 1969.

106. Squatrito S, Delange F, Trimarchi F, et al: Endemic cretinism in Sicily. J Endocrinol Invest 4:295–302, 1981.

107. Doel MS: An experimental approach to the understanding and treatment of hereditary syndrome with congenital deafness and hypothyroidism. J Med Genet 10:235–243, 1973.

108. Van Middleworth L, Norris CH: Audiogenic seizures and cochlear damages in rats after perinatal antithyroid treatment. Endocrinology 106:1686–1690, 1980.

109. Uziel A, Legrand C, Ohresser M, Marot M: Maturational and degenerative processes in the organ of Corti after neonatal hypothyroidism. Horm Res 11:203–218, 1983.

110. Medeiros-Neto GA, Hollander CS, Knobel M, et al: Effects of iodides

on the hypothalmic-pituitary-thyroid axis in neurological endemic cretinism: Evidence for compensated thyroidal failure in adult life. Clin Endocrinol (Oxf) 8:213–218, 1978.

110a. Cavaliere H, Knobel M, Medeiros-Neto G: Effect of thyroid hormone therapy on plasma insulin-like growth factor I levels in normal subjects, hypothyroid patients and endemic cretins. Horm Res 25:132–139, 1987.

111. Medeiros-Neto GA, Kourides IA, Almeida F, et al: Enlargement of the sella turcica in some patients with longstanding untreated endemic cretinism: Serum TSH, alpha, TSH-beta and prolactin responses to TRH. J Endocrinol Invest 4:303–307, 1981.

112. Fierro-Benitez R, Cazar R, Stanbury JB: The effect of iodine deficiency correction by iodized oil on endemic mental retardation of the Andean Rural Communities endemized by goiter. In Medeiros-Neto G, Gaitan E (eds): Frontiers in Thyroidology. New York, Plenum Press, 1986, pp 1051–1054.

113. Connolly KC, Pharoah POD, Hetzel BS: Fetal iodine deficiency and motor performance during childhood. Lancet 2:1149–1151, 1979.

114. Bleichrodt N, Drenth PJD, Querido A: Effects of iodine deficiency on mental and psychomotor abilities. Am J Phys Anthropol 53:55–67, 1980.

115. Pandav CS, Kochupillai N, Godbole MM, Karmakar MC: Iodine deficiency and neonatal hypothyroidism in India. Ann Endocrinol (Paris) 44:20A, 1983.

116. Goyens P, Golstein J, Nsombola B, Vis H, Dumont JE: Selenium deficiency as a possible factor in the pathogenesis of myxedematous endemic cretinism. Acta Endocrinol (Copenh) 114:497–502, 1987.

117. Kochupillai N, Godbole MM, Pandav CS, et al: Severity of environmental iodine deficiency and incidence of neonatal hypothyroidism. In Medeiros-Neto G, Gaitan E (eds): Frontiers in Thyroidology. New York, Plenum Press, 1986.

118. Vanderpass J, Bourdoux P, Lagasse R, et al: Endemic infantile hypothyroidism in severe endemic goitre area of Central Africa. Clin Endocrinol 20:327–340, 1984.

119. Vanderpas JB, Contempre B, Duale NL, et al: Iodine and selenium deficiency associated with cretinism in Northern Zaire. Am J Clin Nutr 52:1087–1093, 1990.

120. Sava L, Delange F, Belfiore A, et al: Transient impairment of thyroid function in newborn from an area of endemic goiter. J Clin Endocrinol Metab 59:90–95, 1984.

121. Contempre B, Dumont J, Bebe N, et al: Effect of selenium supplementation in hypothyroid subjects of an iodine and selenium deficient area: the possible danger of indiscriminate supplementation of iodine-deficient subjects with selenium. J Clin Endocrinol Metab 73:213–215, 1991.

121a. Berry MJ, Reed Larsen P: The role of selenium in thyroid hormone action. Endocr Rev 13:207–219, 1992.

122. Obregon MJ, Santisteban P, Rodriquez-Pena A, et al: Cerebral hypothyroidism in rats with adult-onset iodine deficiency. Endocrinology 115:614–624, 1984.

123. Pharoah POD, Buttfield IH, Hetzel BS: Neurological damage to the fetus resulting from severe iodine deficiency during pregnancy. Lancet 1:308–310, 1971.

124. Contempre B, Duale NL, Dumont JE, Ngo B, Diplock AT, Vanderpas J: Effect of selenium supplementation on thyroid hormone metabolism in an iodine selenium deficient population. Clin Endocrinol 36:579–583, 1992.

125. Maberly G, Eastman CJ, Corcoran J: Effect of iodination of a village water-supply on goitre size and thyroid function. Lancet 2:1270–1272, 1981.

126. Berry MJ, Larsen PR: The role of selenium in thyroid hormone action. Endocr Rev 13:207–219, 1992.

127. Squatrito S, Vigneri R, Runelo F, et al: Prevention and treatment of endemic iodine deficiency goiter by iodination of a municipal water supply. J Clin Endocrinol Metab 63:368–375, 1986.

128. Boyages SC, Maberly GF, Chen J, et al: Endemic cretinism: possible role for thyroid autoimmunity. Lancet 2:529–531, 1989.

129. Medeiros-Neto GA: Towards the eradication of iodine-deficiency disorders in Brazil through a salt iodination programme. Bull WHO 66:637–642, 1988.

130. Medeiros-Neto GA, Tsuboi K, Lima N: Thyroid autoimmunity and endemic cretinism. Lancet 335:111, 1990.

131. Fradkin JE, Wolf J: Iodide-induced thyrotoxicosis. Medicine 62:1–20, 1983.

132. Tsuboi K, Lima N, Ingbar SH, Medeiros-Neto G: Thyroid atrophy in myxedematous endemic cretinism: Possible role for growth blocking immunoglobulins. Autoimmunity 9:201–206, 1991.

133. Van Leewen E: Eon vorm van genuine hyperthyreose (M. Basedow zonder exophthalmus) na Gebruik van geojodeerd brood. Tijdschr Geneeskd 98:81–85, 1954.

134. Tang T, Wang YG, Tsuboi K, et al: Blocking type immunoglobulins in patients with non-goitrous primary hypthyroidism in area of iodine deficiency Japan 38:661–665, 1991.

135. Lu TZ, Ma T: A clinical investigation in China on the use of oral versus intramuscular iodized oil in the treatment of endemic goiter. In Medeiros-Neto G, Maciel RMB, Halpern A (eds): Iodine Deficiency Disorders and Congenital Hypothyroidism. Sao Paulo, Brazil, Aché, 1986.

136. Tonglet R, Bourdoux P, Munga T, Ermans AM: Efficacy of low oral doses of iodized oil in the control of iodine deficiency in Zaire. N Engl J Med 326:236–241, 1992.

137. Vanderpas JB, Rivera-Vanderpas MT, Bourdoux P, et al: Reversibility of severe hypothyroidism with supplementary iodine in patients with endemic cretinism. N Engl J Med 315:791–795, 1986.

138. Vidor CI, Stewart JC, Wall JR, et al: Pathogenesis of iodine induced thyrotoxicosis studies in Northern Tasmania. J Clin Endocrinol Metab 37:901–909, 1973.

139. Pretell E, Moncloa F, Salinas R, et al: Prophylaxis and treatment of endemic goiter in Peru with iodized oil. J Clin Endocrinol Metab 29:1586–1594, 1969.

140. Fierro-Benitez R, Ramirez I, Estrella E, et al: The effect of goitre prophylaxis with iodized oil on the prevention of endemic cretinism. In Fellinger K, Hofer R (eds): Further Advances in Thyroid Research. Vienna, Verlagder Wiener Med Akad, 1971, pp 61–77.

141. Medeiros-Neto GA, Nicolau W, Takeda A, Cintra ABU: Effect of iodized oil on iodine content, thyroglobulin maturation and on biochemical constituents of endemic goitre in Brazil. Acta Endocrinol (Copenh) 79:439–450, 1975.

142. Thilly CH, Delange F, Coldstein-Golaire J, Ermans AM: Endemic goiter prevention by iodized oil: A reassessment. J Clin Endocrinol Metab 36:1196–1203, 1973.

143. Djokomoeljanto R, Tarwotjo IG, Maspaitella F: Goiter control program in Indonesia. In Ui N, Torizuka K, Nagataki S, Miyai K (eds): Current Problems in Thyroid Research. ICS 605. Amsterdam, Excerpta Medica, 1984, pp 403–405.

144. Ouyang A, Wang O, Liu ZT, et al: Progress in the prevention and treatment of endemic goiter with iodized oil in China. In Ui N, Torizuka K, Nagataki S, Miyai K (eds): Current Problems in Thyroid Research. ICS 605. Amsterdam, Excerpta Medica, 1984, pp 403–405.

145. Lazarus JH, Parkes AB, John R, N'Diaye M, Prysor-Jones SG: Endemic goitre in Senegal, thyroid function etiological factors and treatment with oral iodized oil. Acta Endocrinol (Copenh) 126:149–154, 1992.

50

Thyroid Neoplasia

LESLIE J. DeGROOT

Thyroid cancer is statistically a minor health problem, since it accounts for 0.4 per cent of all cancer deaths and kills only 8 in 1 million people per year in the United States. Its clinical importance, however, is much greater, because up to 4 per cent of the population harbor clinically detectable nodular thyroids, and any clinical consideration of the nodular thyroid must raise the possible diagnosis of thyroid cancer. This discussion evaluates the problem of the thyroid nodule and, subsequently, the management of diagnosed thyroid cancer.

THYROID ADENOMAS AND THE "SOLITARY NODULE"

A thyroid adenoma can be defined as a benign neoplastic growth, usually contained within a capsule. The terms "adenoma" and "nodule" are used interchangeably but perhaps imprecisely. *Adenoma* implies a specific new tissue growth, while a *nodule* could be a carcinoma, lobule of normal gland, or any other focal lesion. Data on prevalence comes from the population sampled in Framingham, Massachusetts, where 4 per cent were found to have a palpable thyroid nodule (or nodules). Of these lesions, one-half were considered multinodular and one-half solitary. New nodules appeared with an incidence of 1 per 1000 per year.[1] A study from Connecticut indicates a prevalence of 2 per cent of nodular glands in an adult population.[2]

Studies on consecutive autopsy series indicate that many more glands harbor nodules when the glands are carefully examined. In a series reported in 1955, half of the thyroids contained one or more nodules, and in 12 per cent there was a solitary nodule. There was an age-related increase in thyroid weight and nodularity.[3] A recent study of autopsy cases from Italy recorded a 38 per cent incidence of nodular goiter, 4.3 per cent incidence of adenomas, and 2.3 per cent incidence of carcinomas.[4] Thus the prevalence of clinically detectable nodules is 1 to 3 per cent, but many more are present if autopsy data are considered. Recent widespread use of thyroid ultrasonography has also shown that many glands that are normal on palpation contain small nodules detectable by ultrasound. In addition, it should be noted that multinodular goiters, both in endemic and nonendemic areas, contain adenomas that are in all ways histologically similar to those appearing as isolated examples in the single nodule.

Pathology

A classification of thyroid tumors is given in Table 50–1. Most adenomas are follicular and have a histological appearance characteristic of thyroid tissue. Many look almost like a normal gland. There is a uniform architecture, few mitoses, no capsular or lymphatic invasion, and usually a

TABLE 50–1. PATHOLOGICAL CLASSIFICATION OF THYROID
NEOPLASMS

BENIGN	MALIGNANT
A. Adenoma	A. Carcinoma
1. Follicular	1. Papillary adenocarcinoma
a. Colloid variant	a. Pure papillary adenocarcinoma
b. Embryonal	b. Mixed papillary and follicular carcinoma
c. Fetal	c. Papillary microcarcinoma
d. Hürthle cell variant	d. Diffuse sclerosing carcinoma
2. Papillary (perhaps always malignant)	2. Follicular carcinoma
	a. Pure follicular carcinoma
	b. Clear cell carcinoma
	c. Hürthle (oxyphil) cell carcinoma
	3. Insular carcinoma
	4. Medullary carcinoma
	a. Mixed medullary–follicular carcinoma
	5. Undifferentiated carcinoma
B. Teratoma	B. Other malignant tumors
	1. Lymphoma
	2. Sarcoma
	3. Fibrosarcoma
	4. Epidermoid carcinoma
	5. Mucoepidermoid carcinoma
	6. Metastatic tumor

discrete fibrous capsule. Fetal and embryonal adenomas show a progressively less "adult" structure (Fig. 50–1, A to E). In the fetal adenoma, sheets of large cells may be present. Hürthle cell adenomas have an eosinophilic liver cell–like appearance. Tumors, classified initially as embryonal, fetal, or Hürthle cell adenoma, occasionally recur as invasive carcinomas, indicating that histological classification of these lesions is difficult. Most pathologists classify all papillary lesions as carcinomas, although others state that some may be adenomas. Similarly, the difficulty in defining the malignant potential of Hürthle cell lesions on histological grounds has led to the current designation of "Hürthle cell tumor" with the implication that it may behave as either a benign or malignant lesion. About half of all single nodules show, on sectioning, a gelatinous appearance and have large, colloid-filled follicles within a poorly demarcated capsule. These are classified by some pathologists as follicular adenomas and by others as "colloid nodules," suggesting a focal process that is different from development of a true adenoma.

Etiology

This is discussed below in the section on thyroid carcinoma. It has been established that most if not all adenomas are clonal, that is, made up of one unique type of cell. This probably indicates that an adenoma develops from one unique cell that has undergone a somatic mutation.[5]

Course and Symptomatology

Adenomas grow slowly, remain dormant for years, must reach a size of 0.5 to 1 cm before they can be palpated, and typically are asymptomatic. Thus they are often discovered accidentally by the patient or physician and rarely produce local symptoms of dysphagia, dysphonia, stridor, or pain. Occasionally bleeding into a tumor causes local pain and tenderness and, very rarely, transient thyrotoxicosis. Such bleeding may be followed by spontaneous regression of the nodule but more likely results in cyst formation.

About 70 per cent of thyroid nodules or adenomas are hypofunctional in terms of accumulation of radioactive iodide and are "cold" on isotope scans. About 20 per cent may be borderline in function and appear to have uptake on isotope scan equivalent to the remainder of the thyroid. One in 10 (or less) is hyperfunctional, concentrates iodide avidly, may suppress the function of the remainder of the gland, and may even produce thyrotoxicosis. This typically occurs when the functioning nodule has grown larger than 3 cm in diameter, and in older patients. Usually an adenoma once formed seems committed to this "lifestyle" indefinitely, although, rarely, pathological evidence suggests that adenomas can transform into invasive carcinoma. Sequential change from hyperplasia to adenoma formation to invasive carcinoma has been found in patients with congenital goitrous hypothyroidism and can be produced experimentally in animals.

Interesting studies have been reported on the metabolic function of nodules. Cold nodules typically have an inability to transport iodide into the thyroid as a result of a specific deletion of the transport mechanism. They are not able to maintain a concentration gradient for iodide between thyroid cell and serum, although peroxidase function may be intact in the tissue.[6] In such adenomas thyrotropin (TSH) is able to bind to the cell membrane and activate adenyl cyclase, but subsequent metabolic steps are lacking. Since other factors related to transport such as Na^+, K^+ ATPase levels are normal, it appears that there is a specific deletion of the iodide transport mechanism. Other "cold nodules" have been shown to lack peroxidase enzyme. These studies suggest that adenoma formation is associated with genetic mutational events causing loss or dysfunction of specific enzymes in the iodide metabolic pathway.

Diagnosis and Differential Diagnosis

The differential diagnosis to be considered in examining a patient with a nodule includes thyroid carcinoma, adenoma, multinodular goiter, or more rarely, thyroiditis, an irregular regrowth of tissue following prior surgery, thyroid hemiagenesis, and cysts (Table 50–2). The incidence of cancer among thyroid nodules has been reported from 6.5 to 28 per cent[7, 8] and is of course the main concern when a nodule is detected.

The adenoma is usually felt as a discrete lump in an otherwise normal gland, moving with the thyroid and movable over the trachea. The patient is most often euthyroid. Occasionally, signs of thyrotoxicosis are present, and then T_3 and T_4 may be elevated or selective T_3 toxicosis may be present.

Factors that should be considered in reaching a decision on management include the history of growth, the presence of pain or other local symptoms, age, sex, family history of the patient, history of exposure to irradiation, physical characteristics of the gland, and laboratory studies. Obviously, enlarged nodes near the thyroid, the supraclavicular areas, or cervical chains suggest malignant disease.

Since the ratio of malignant to benign lesions is higher in young people, nodules in patients under 25 or 30 years

TABLE 50–2. THYROID LESIONS THAT MAY PRESENT AS A "SINGLE NODULE"

Adenoma
Cyst
Acute hemorrhage into thyroid
Carcinoma
Multinodular goiter
Hashimoto's thyroiditis
Subacute thyroiditis
Effect of prior operation or ^{131}I therapy
Thyroid hemiagenesis
Metastasis
Parathyroid cysts or adenoma
Thyroglossal cyst
Nonthyroidal lesions
   Inflammatory or neoplastic nodes
   Cystic hygroma
   Aneurysm
   Bronchocele
   Laryngocele
   Thyroglossal duct cyst
   Parathyroid cyst

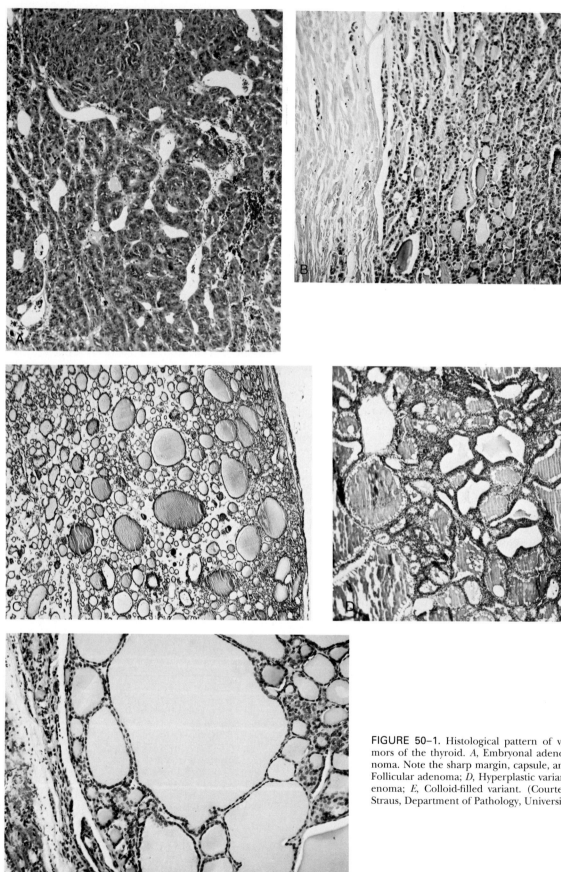

FIGURE 50–1. Histological pattern of various benign tumors of the thyroid. *A*, Embryonal adenoma; *B*, Fetal adenoma. Note the sharp margin, capsule, and tiny follicles. *C*, Follicular adenoma; *D*, Hyperplastic variant of follicular adenoma; *E*, Colloid-filled variant. (Courtesy of Dr. Francis Straus, Department of Pathology, University of Chicago.)

are considered more likely to be malignant. Benign nodules are much less common in men than in women; thus, nodules in males are more highly suspected of being malignant. Some patients present with multifocal medullary carcinomas as part of the familial multiple endocrine tumor syndromes (types II and III), which include pheochromocytoma and hyperparathyroidism.[9] Six per cent of our patients with differentiated thyroid cancer had a family history of malignant thyroid neoplasm. Thus, family history is relevant.

Changes noted on physical examination are important. Fixation of the nodule to strap muscles or to the trachea is alarming. Pain or tenderness usually indicates hemorrhage into a nodule but can indicate invasive malignancy. If the problem is due to hemorrhage into a benign lesion, the symptoms pass in a few days or weeks. Hoarseness suggests invasive disease but can arise from pressure on the recurrent nerve by a benign lesion. Deviation of the trachea or compression of the trachea may be visualized, especially if the lesion is more than 3 or 4 cm in diameter. Soft tissue x-rays may bring out the fine stippled calcification typical of the psammoma bodies present in papillary adenocarcinomas. "Signet ring" calcification and large streaks and flecks of calcium are usually typical of multinodular goiter. Dense calcification and calcified nodes suggest medullary cancer.

The presence of a multinodular gland, as ascertained either on the basis of physical examination or ultrasonography, is usually interpreted as a sign of safety. It is true that a significant proportion (4 to 17 per cent) of operated multinodular goiters are found to harbor carcinoma, but this is probably due to selection of patients.[10, 11] If there is one area within a multinodular gland that seems entirely different from the remainder of the gland ("dominant nodule") or has undergone recent change or growth, one should consider a malignant rather than a benign process. This also holds true in glands involved with Hashimoto's disease, since lymphoma may develop in this substrate.

As discussed below, a history of prior irradiation to the head or neck during infancy or childhood is strongly associated with subsequent occurrence of carcinoma.[12] History of such radiation exposure and the presence of a palpable nodule or nodules must raise the possibility of thyroid cancer and requires a cytological diagnosis. Occasionally a nodule is detected in a gland with the characteristics of thyroiditis, including diffuse enlargement, a palpable pyramidal lobe, and positive thyroid autoantibodies. This may indicate the coincidence of two diseases; the physician should not be dissuaded by this from independent evaluation of the significance of the nodule.

Isotope scintiscans provide some help but are relatively less important if cytologic study is done (see below)[8, 10] (Fig. 50–1). Nodules that are hyperfunctional and produce hyperthyroidism are rarely malignant, and those that accumulate iodide in concentrations equal to the surrounding normal thyroid tissue are usually, but not always, benign (Fig. 50–2).[13, 14] Cold nodules are also typically benign, but when viewed the other way, most thyroid cancers do present as inactive areas on thyroid scan. In practice, except for the specific case of the toxic nodule, scans probably aid little in the differential diagnosis, and there is a growing tendency to omit scanning from diagnostic maneuvers. The scintiscans can confirm the diagnosis of multinodular

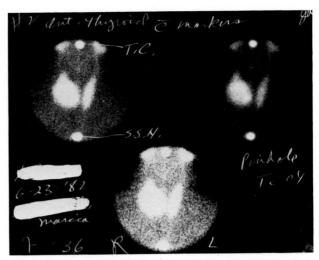

FIGURE 50–2. Scintillation scan view of a functioning nodule in a 36-year-old female. At operation the nodule proved to be a mixed papillary-follicular neoplasm.

goiter and can show the presence of diffuse disease (such as Hashimoto's thyroiditis) in some patients when nodularity is suspected.

Newer scanning techniques have been developed that show promise for differential diagnosis. Lesions that concentrate radioactive phosphorus or selenomethionine but do not concentrate iodide are said to be usually malignant. Differentiated cancers can usually be visualized by [201]Th-chloride scanning, and anaplastic cancers usually accumulate ^{67}Ga-citrate. However, these techniques have not found a place in routine preoperative evaluation. Fluorescent thyroid scanning allows one to quantitate the distribution of stable iodide in thyroid nodules[15] and has been reported to allow differentiation of benign from malignant lesions.[16] Our own studies do not support this contention. Echo imaging using ultrasound can delineate cystic structures, which are usually associated with a benign process[17] (Fig. 50–3). Unfortunately this fact aids little in managing an individual patient. Thyroid thermography, thyroidography using injections of contrast media directly into the substance of the gland, and thyroid arteriography have also been utilized. CT scanning is expensive but occasionally useful, especially in unusually large substernal glands. MRI scanning is rarely necessary but is occasionally useful in identifying abnormal nodes.

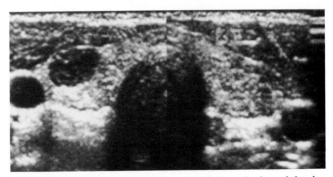

FIGURE 50–3. Sagittal echo scan of a palpable 2-cm single nodule, showing a lesion in the R lobe. On aspiration 2 ml of brownish colloid was obtained. The few cells present showed Hürthle cell changes.

Needle biopsy for diagnosis of thyroid nodules was formerly frowned upon, on the assumption that it might spread the lesion or provide an inadequate diagnostic specimen for the pathologist. This attitude has radically changed with growing experience and the shift from core biopsy to the fine-needle aspiration (FNA) techniques (Fig. 50–4). During the last two decades, FNA biopsy has been used on a large number of patients with a high degree of accuracy.[18–23] In centers that have an experienced cytologist and good aspiration technique, a low percentage of false-positives (about 1 per cent) and false-negatives (less than 5 per cent)[18, 19] can be achieved. These findings are comparable to results of needle biopsy by the Tru-Cut needle or Vim-Silverman method,[24] but with less trauma and almost no complications. Diagnostic sensitivity and specificity are superior to isotope scanning and ultrasound examination. Material obtained by FNA, as well as Tru-Cut biopsy, is inadequate to differentiate between a hypercellular follicular adenoma and a follicular carcinoma. The fixed tissue sections from a thyroidectomy are required to demonstrate capsular, vascular, or nerve invasion. Biopsy data offer important assistance in most cases. Patients with lesions diagnosed as malignant or suspicious of malignancy should be sent to surgery, as are those with hypercellular follicular lesions. Patients with benign aspirates are followed at 6 to 12-month intervals, usually on thyroxine suppression. Obviously, growth of the lesion or development of other clinical signs, such as adenopathy, suggesting the presence of malignancy requires reaspiration and/or surgery.

Another advantage of FNA is the therapeutic aspiration of cystic thyroid nodules. The vast majority of cystic lesions are benign, and single or multiple aspirations may satisfactorily reduce the size of at least a third of cysts.[25] Intracystic injection of tetracycline (1 ml containing 100 mg) is reported to inhibit recurrence of cysts. Leakage of tetracycline out of the cyst can cause temporary pain. Although this technique has been reported for several years, it has not been widely adopted.

Potential Value of Surgery

It is probable that a high degree of selection is involved in the processing of patients with thyroid nodules and that

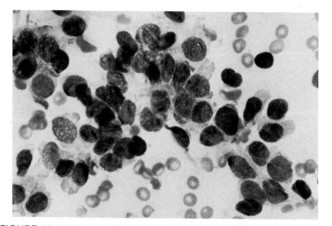

FIGURE 50–4. Fine-needle aspiration cytologic specimen. Epithelial cells in a papillary formation from a papillary thyroid carcinoma. (Courtesy of Dr. Marluce Bibbo.)

the operative results reflect this selection process rather than the histology and course of all thyroid nodules in the population. In the past, perhaps 30 per cent of patients with nodules presenting to physicians were ultimately operated upon, and in most series, from 8 to 20 per cent of the nodules examined after surgery were malignant. From 10 to 50 per cent of patients had, in fact, multinodular goiters. In recent experience, since introduction of FNA cytologic examination, the proportion of patients having surgery has dropped to 15 to 20 per cent, and 30 to 40 per cent of nodules removed are diagnosed by the pathologist as malignant. FNA has thus profoundly improved our ability to target surgery to dangerous lesions.

Therapeutic Approaches

All patients should receive a thorough history and physical examination, with particular emphasis on the points discussed above as well as a laboratory evaluation including serum T_4 and thyroid autoantibody measurements, and usually an ultrasound scan. Scintiscans are frequently omitted in patients in whom the physical findings clearly indicate a single nodule in an otherwise normal gland (Table 50–3). Because of the strong association of exposure to x-ray with multicentric malignant lesions, patients having this history are usually scanned. If in the irradiated patient there is a clearly defined single nodule, it is subjected to FNA and therapy is determined by the result, much as with other nodules. Usually there are multiple nodules in irradiated glands, and it is not possible to sample all nodules by FNA. If the abnormalities cannot be explained on the basis of some other condition such as thyroiditis or Graves' disease, the patient is usually referred for operation.

Patients with presumed multinodular goiter but no history of irradiation are usually followed on replacement therapy with thyroid hormone.

Patients with cystic lesions are treated by diagnostic and therapeutic aspiration, and cysts are reaspirated as needed. Up to 50 per cent of these patients have a dramatic reduction in the size of the cystic nodule without recurrence after one or more aspiration.[25, 26] In 20 to 30 per cent of cases, recurrence of the cyst leads to its resection at a later time. The aspirated fluid is subjected to cytologic examination. Commonly the fluid contains only degenerate cells, but occasionally the cytology provides useful support for a benign or malignant diagnosis. Thyroid hormone therapy has not proved effective in reducing the recurrence of cystic nodules after aspirations.[26] Since mixed solid and cystic lesions are alleged to be more frequently malignant than "pure" cysts, the presence of a significant residual mass after aspiration must be viewed with caution and may be reason for resection. Rarely aspiration of a cyst appears to cause release of thyroid hormone and transient thyrotoxicosis.

Patients with toxic adenomas are treated by surgery or with radioactive iodide. We generally prefer surgery because it offers a resolution of the problem and because it leaves normal tissue in situ. Radioactive iodide ablation of a toxic nodule usually requires administration of a high dose of ^{131}I such as 20 to 60 mCi, giving significant radiation exposure to the individual. It may cause hypothyroidism by damage to the remainder of the gland.[27] It leaves an

TABLE 50–3. FACTORS IN MANAGEMENT OF COLD NODULES

HISTORY	PHYSICAL EXAMINATION	LABORATORY TESTS
Radiation	Size	Free thyroxine index (FTI)
Age	Fixation	Antithyroid antibodies
Sex	Cystic nature	
Duration	Tenderness	TG
Local symptoms	Adenopathy	Chest x-ray film
Growth	Diffuse/local process	Ultrasound scan(?)
Multiple endocrine neoplasia (MEN) syndrome	Cord paralysis	Scan(?)
Thyrotoxicity	Single versus multiple nodules	X-ray of soft tissues of the neck(?)
Geographic residence		
Family history		

MANAGEMENT

inactive hard nodule in the thyroid gland of half the patients, which may be disconcerting during the rest of the patient's life. It is, however, a common mode of treatment and is especially useful in older individuals or patients with high surgical risk. Injection of ethanol has been introduced as therapy for patients with toxic adenomas. Repeated injections under ultrasound guidance reduce functioning tissue to a level compatible with euthyroidism.[28]

Patients with solid, nontoxic thyroid nodules are subjected to FNA to determine the nature of the nodules. Patients with malignant or suspicious cytology are advised to have surgical resection of the lesions. Patients with benign cytology are observed on thyroid hormone suppressive therapy. Repeat FNA within 6 to 12 months is recommended for patients with a history or physical examination suggestive of higher risk for thyroid malignancy. When there is a strong clinical suspicion of malignancy despite a negative cytological diagnosis, surgical exploration is still recommended.

We believe it is crucial to work in conjunction with a surgeon who has frequent and continuous experience in thyroid surgery, if good results are to be obtained. This is not to say that resection of a thyroid lobe for a nodule is a difficult procedure. However, if more extensive surgery is required, and especially if total or near-total thyroidectomy and lymph node resections are indicated, it is imperative that the surgeon have the proper knowledge and experience to reduce the possibility of damage to the recurrent laryngeal nerves and parathyroid glands. The usual procedure is a lobectomy, which is relatively harmless, with an incidence of complications approaching zero. Usually patients are discharged within two to three days. Complications are more common if more extensive dissection is done, as discussed below. The thyroid specimen itself, any abnormal areas in the gland, and any abnormal-appearing lymph nodes should be immediately examined by frozen

section. Differentiating benign from malignant thyroid lesions is admittedly difficult, especially using frozen sections, but experienced pathologists can make the distinction with a high degree of reliability. Occasionally, follicular lesions are believed by the pathologist to be benign at surgery, but permanent sections reveal changes that indicate malignancy. Reoperation and near-total thyroidectomy is probably desirable in these patients, since up to one third can be expected to have residual tumor in the contralateral lobe.[29] To avoid these second operations, we recommend lobectomy and contralateral subtotal resection for very cellular follicular lesions as the initial procedure. Occasionally a small papillary or follicular cancer is found in the pathological specimen after conclusion of the operation. If this is less than 1 cm, a well-demarcated single focus, and the patient is under 45, nothing further need be done. After operation, all patients are placed on replacement thyroxine therapy in the hope that this will prevent the recurrence of other nodules.

Although the simplicity of FNA cytology currently dominates decision making in regard to thyroid nodules, it has been argued that all nodules should be treated simply by suppressive therapy with thyroid hormone.[30, 31] It is true that the vast majority are benign, that the cancers present are usually of a low degree of malignancy and can be controlled to some extent by suppressive hormone treatment, and that the anaplastic and undifferentiated lesions are readily recognized but almost uniformly fatal, even if surgery is performed. Occasionally we give thyroid hormone for a period of one to three months before operation on nodules in an effort to shrink the gland and make the differentiation of benign and abnormal tissue easier for the surgeon. Our results with long-term replacement therapy of nodules have not been as satisfactory as those described by others. The majority of single adenomas do not disappear, although sometimes they appear to shrink a bit as the normal tissue around them is made atrophic. Ramacciotti et al. found that 12 per cent of nodules disappeared on suppression, and 10 per cent were significantly reduced in size.[19] It is well known that a decrease in size does not certify the benign nature of the lesion, since proven cancers have been shown to decrease in size during administration of thyroid hormone.[32, 33]

The role of administration of "suppressive" doses of thyroid hormone and its potential adverse effects have been much debated in recent years.[34] Thyroxine treatment shrinks only a minority of nodules, although it may also inhibit growth of others. Excessive T_4 given over years is known to promote osteoporosis and can cause cardiac arrhythmias. We believe administration of T_4 in dosages to keep the TSH by sensitive assay in the range of 0.3 to 0.6 $\mu U/ml$ will shrink some nodules and prevent growth of others, and that administration of T_4 in this dosage has not been proved to decrease bone mass.[35] Serum TG characteristically declines in patients who respond to T_4 treatment, and the decrease can be used to predict the response.[36]

THYROID CARCINOMA

Incidence and Distribution

Thyroid carcinoma has occurred in the United States during the past 20 years with an incidence of about 40 new cases per million people per year[37] and has been associated with a death rate of approximately 8 in 1 million per year (Fig. 50–5). The ratio of females to males with the disease is 2:1. Studies from the Mayo Clinic suggest that the incidence of thyroid cancer is about 36 in 1 million cases per year, or possibly 60 in 1 million if small, occult tumors are included in the statistics.[38] Tumors are rare in children and increase in frequency with age. As noted below the tumor type distribution is age-related. It is not certain that carci-

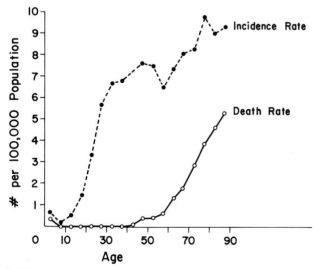

FIGURE 50–5. The incidence rate of thyroid carcinoma and death rate from thyroid cancer are diagramed in relation to the experience per 100,000 population in each decade. The sharply increasing mortality occurring after age 50 is evident. (Data obtained from Young JL Jr, Percy CL, Astaire AJ, (eds.): Surveillance, Epidemiology, and End Results: Incidence and Mortality Data, 1973–77. National Cancer Institute Monograph 57, NIH Publication No. 81-2330, 1981.)

noma occurs with increased frequency in areas of endemic goiter, although there is a clear increase in the relative proportion of anaplastic neoplasms. The prevalence of neoplasms at autopsy is highly variable, depending on the population selected and the care of the survey. Prevalence ranges from 0.1 to 2.7 per cent.[39, 40] Two studies of consecutive autopsies of patients dying in hospitals found that 2.7 per cent of thyroids harbored unsuspected thyroid cancer and that an equivalent percentage had metastatic carcinoma in the gland.[4, 40] A significant proportion of thyroid cancers are not diagnosed during life and are not the cause of death of the patients. These data are in accord with the leisurely growth of the majority of thyroid tumors.

Studies by Sampson and co-workers[41] and Fukunaga and Yatani[42] indicate that a high prevalence (up to 5.7 per cent) of unsuspected microcarcinomas may exist in adults. These lesions are mostly below 0.5 cm in their greatest dimension, are usually papillary in nature, and are believed to behave in a relatively benign manner. They are, effectively, detected only by a pathologist. Recognition of such "minimal thyroid cancers" does not demand the same therapeutic response as does the discovery of a larger tumor, although small tumors certainly can metastasize and occasionally are fatal.

Etiology

Iodide deficiency,[43] long-term administration of goitrogenic drugs,[44] exposure of the thyroid to external irradiation or radioactive iodide[45] alone or in combination is known to produce thyroid hyperplasia, adenoma formation, and ultimately malignancy in experimental animals. Irradiation causes damage to the DNA, and this presumably leads to carcinomatous changes. Also the irradiation damages the cell, reducing its ability to produce thyroid hormone. This leads to chronic TSH stimulation, a common factor in all of the experimental conditions. Usually, experimental tumors are at first TSH-dependent, but with serial passage through thyroidectomized animals they ultimately become autonomous and will grow in a normal host.

Radiation exposure to the head and neck in childhood was first related to subsequent thyroid cancer in the report of Duffy and Fitzgerald four decades ago.[46] These children were treated primarily for enlargement of the thymus in infancy or for enlargement of the tonsils and adenoids in early childhood. The radiation dose to the thyroid gland was from 200 to 700 rads. As many as 80 per cent of children with thyroid carcinoma were found to have a history of prior x-ray treatment, but the relationship is less constant in patients who are beyond the age of 35.[47, 48] The frequency of thyroid cancer may be increased 100-fold after significant x-ray exposure,[49, 50] and the incidence has been reported to reach 2 per cent with doses of about 500 rads[51] (Fig. 50–6). Our own study[52] indicated an incidence of proved thyroid cancer of 5 per cent in patients given irradiation primarily for enlargement of the tonsils or adenoids and possibly a higher level in those treated with higher doses for acne. The peak incidence was 20 to 25 years after irradiation (Fig. 50–7). In addition to malignancies, benign nodules also occur with perhaps 10 times the frequency of cancers. Thyroid irradiation is also associated

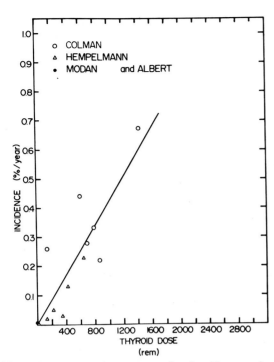

FIGURE 50-6. Estimated dose response for thyroid cancer in humans from external irradiation. The incidence of carcinomas each year is plotted against the original thyroid radiation dose. (From Maxon H, Thomas SR, Saenger EL, et al: Ionizing irradiation and the induction of clinically significant disease in the human thyroid gland. Am J Med 63:967, 1977.)

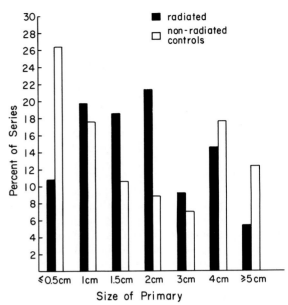

FIGURE 50-8. Comparison of the distribution of the size of primary tumors among 100 non–radiation-associated thyroid malignancies and an equal number of radiation-associated tumors. All were differentiated thyroid carcinomas. The distribution of sizes was not statistically different, although the radiation-associated tumors were slightly larger on average in this comparison than the tumors lacking association with prior x-ray treatment.

with a 7 to 20 times increased incidence of Graves' disease and increased incidence of ophthalmopathy and thyroiditis.[53] X-ray exposure of the adult thyroid gland probably also has some carcinogenic potential, as seen from the results of studies on survivors of the Nagasaki and Hiroshima atomic bomb explosions, although it is less carcinogenic in adults than in children.[54] The lesions associated with radiation exposure usually occur in young adults, are multicentric in half of the cases, are rarely undifferentiated, and infrequently cause death. Their size distribution (Fig. 50–8) and clinical behavior are essentially identical to those of all thyroid cancers in young people. X-ray–induced lesions are not more aggressive than other thyroid cancers.[55]

There has been a striking lack of cancer among patients treated with radioactive iodide for Graves' disease.[56, 57] This may be because the treatment was given primarily to older adults, because the period of follow-up has been inadequate, because of the much slower rate of irradiation delivered by ^{131}I, because more than half the patients had totally ablated thyroid glands, or because the high dose of irradiation given may effectively preclude cell division.

Thyroid hyperplasia in humans, induced by congenital metabolic defects and the resultant elevation in TSH levels, can lead to carcinomatous degeneration if the subclinical hypothyroidism is unrecognized and untreated for decades.[58] Abnormalities in TSH receptors have been sought in tumor cells. It appears that differentiated tumors have normal receptors, presumably explaining their TSH-dependent growth, whereas anaplastic cancers lack high affinity receptors and thus respond poorly to TSH.[59] Thyroid stimulating immunoglobulins (TSI) that are present in sera of patients who have coincident autoimmune thyroid disease may cause tumor growth and occasionally appear to make the tumors behave more aggressively, but usually co-occurrence of Graves' disease does not worsen the prognosis.[60] While there is no evidence that TSI causes malignancy, it is of interest that up to 6 per cent of thyroid glands removed because of Graves' disease harbor a carcinoma.[61, 62] It has also been reported that positive associations exist between Hashimoto's thyroiditis (or multinodular goiter) and thyroid cancer. A similar association has been reported with parathyroid adenomas.[63] Other data suggest that there is no increased incidence of neoplasms in these patients.[64] An association with parathyroid adenomas probably could be explained by co-occurrence of radiation-associated parathyroid adenomas and thyroid tumors.

Genetic factors influencing the development of thyroid cancer have been reported, including chromosome insta-

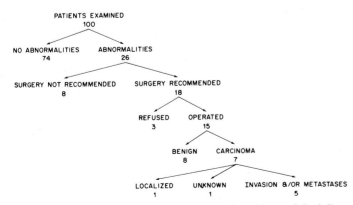

FIGURE 50-7. Relation of physical findings to disposition and final diagnosis after operation in 100 patients with a history of thyroid irradiation and no previously known thyroid disease. Of 15 who came to surgery, 7 had thyroid carcinoma.

bility in patients with medullary thyroid carcinoma.[65] An increased incidence of HLA-DR1 in differentiated thyroid carcinoma that was reported by one group[66] was not found by others.[67] We recently detected an association of HLA-DR7 with differentiated follicular thyroid cancer in patients without previous history of irradiation to the head and neck, but not in irradiation-associated thyroid cancer.[68]

Thyroid carcinomas are present in several familial syndromes, including Cowden's disease (hamartomas, multinodular goiters, and thyroid, breast, colon, and lung cancers),[69] familial adenomatous polyposis,[70, 71] Gardner's syndrome,[72] and familial chemodectomas.[73] The incidence of thyroid cancer is estimated to be increased 100-fold above baseline in patients with intestinal polyposis.[70, 71]

The most interesting new concept in tumor etiology relates to the role played by oncogenes and tumor-suppressor genes. Oncogenes are usually silent unless activated by chromosomal translocation, mutations, or deletions, and then "transform" cells into a state of uncontrolled growth. Expression of C-myc and C-fos is stimulated in normal thyroid tissue by TSH and occurs in adenomas and carcinomas,[74] perhaps as a consequence of the neoplastic phenotype. Ras, activated by mutations of specific codons, is found expressed in nodular goiters, indicating that it may be an early factor in oncogenesis and is expressed in up to 45 per cent of benign and malignant tumors[75, 76]; Ras mutations do not seem to correlate specifically with the pathology or behavior of the tumor. Oncogene Gsp is activated in adenomas and carcinomas.[76a] A specific oncogene (a rearranged ret oncogene) has been found in many papillary cancers.[77] The papillary thyroid carcinoma (PTC) oncogene is generated by fusion of the tyrosine kinase domain of the ret proto-oncogene on chromosome 10 to the first exon of "H4," an unknown gene. Another oncogene, trk, is also found in papillary cancers, and is formed by rearrangement of the trk proto-oncogene.[78] Loss of tumor suppressor genes present on chromosomes 11q13[79] and 10[80] appears to be the etiological factor in multiple endocrine neoplasia (MEN) I and MEN II syndromes. Recent data indicate that the tumor suppressor gene at the 11q13 locus is lost in some follicular adenomas and carcinomas.[81] The p53 tumor suppressor gene is mutated in poorly differentiated thyroid cancers, and Farid and coworkers have found that the RB tumor suppressor gene is also mutated or deleted in a high proportion of thyroid tumors. Thus accumulating data strongly indicate that a series of mutations activating ras, possibly myc, and including PTC/ret, trk, and the tumor suppressor genes p53 and RB is fundamental in the progression of tumorigenesis from normal cell growth to adenoma or carcinoma.

Pathology

Histologic diagnosis of malignancy is usually very simple, but in some tumors it is difficult. Increased nuclear area, enlarged vesicular nuclei, increased mitoses, hyperchromasia, invasion of thyroid tumor capsule, thyroid tissue or surrounding tissue, blood vessels and lymph channels, and loss of the normal follicular architecture are important characteristics. Examples of the histological patterns are given in Figure 50–9. Papillary lesions tend to be infiltrative and multicentric; they have little tendency to invade blood vessels and may contain psammoma bodies. The nuclei are characteristically vesicular (or "open"), often grooved, and often have cytoplasmic inclusions. Diffuse sclerosing, tall cell and macrofollicular variants are described. Follicular carcinomas are more frequently encapsulated, but vessel and capsule invasion is typical. Hyalinizing, clear cell, mucin-containing, and insular variants are noted. The majority of lesions have a mixture of papillary and follicular elements. Perhaps 15 to 20 per cent can be classified as pure papillary, up to 60 per cent as mixed papillary and follicular, 15 to 20 per cent as pure follicular, and the remainder as undifferentiated or poorly differentiated tumors. Hürthle cell carcinomas grow as follicles or solid sheets of eosinophilic granular cells and are usually a variety of follicular cancer, although some appear to be papillary. Multicentricity occurs especially in lesions of young individuals and is reported to exist in from 20 to 80 per cent of cancers.[82] Occasionally, both papillary and follicular tumors occur as small, less than 0.5-cm lesions, surrounded by a dense fibrotic reaction. These "occult sclerosing" lesions are usually benign, but lymph node and distant metastases may occur.[83] Medullary tumors occur as solid masses of spindle or rounded cells with large nuclei, much fibrosis, and deposits of amyloid.[84] These tumors do not originate from thyroid follicular cells but are derived from the calcitonin-secreting "C cells" present in the thyroid. In the familial syndromes MEN IIA and IIB, C-cell hyperplasia precedes the cancer and is typically present in the gland.

Immunochemical staining for thyroglobulin (TG), thyroid peroxidase (TPO), calcitonin (CT), and keratin are useful in differentiating thyroid tumors from other histological types, especially when the origin of metastatic adenocarcinoma is being considered.

Clinical Presentation and Course

The clinical presentation is usually that described above for the single nodule, a thyroid mass that is asymptomatic and found incidentally. Occasionally, a neoplasm presents as an enlarging painful mass with concurrent local symptoms and rarely as a diffuse goiter.[85] Sometimes patients first are seen with metastatic nodules elsewhere in the body (especially in the lung), with pathological fractures caused by osseous metastasis, and rarely because of hyperthyroidism. Fixation of the mass to the trachea, unusual firmness, recent growth, symptoms of dysphagia, dysphonia, or hoarseness, and presence of enlarged lymph nodes clearly suggest the possibility of malignancy.

Papillary carcinomas occur in children and increase in frequency to have highest incidence in the third and fourth decades.[86] They remain in the thyroid gland for a long period of time, and multicentric lesions are present in half the patients. One third present with nodal metastases, about 10 per cent with extrathyroidal invasion, and 7.5 per cent with distant metastasis.[87, 88] These tumors may exist for decades without producing serious symptoms or causing death.[89] The tumors tend to metastasize to cervical lymph nodes and ultimately to the lungs. It is an especially benign process in young adults and rarely causes death under age 40. In older patients the disease is more invasive and behaves in some instances like undifferentiated carci-

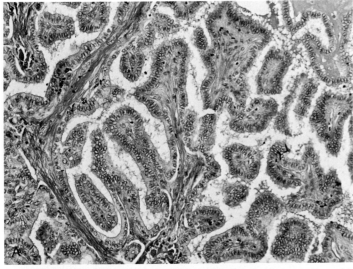

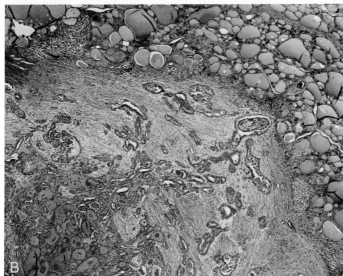

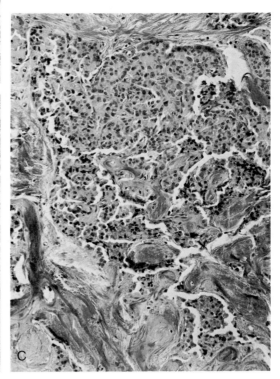

FIGURE 50–9. *A,* Histologic pattern of malignant tumors of the thyroid—papillary carcinoma. Note the tall cells and the fibrovascular core of the papillae. *B,* Follicular adenocarcinoma showing fair preservation of architecture, active colloid resorption, and vesicular nuclei. *C,* Medullary carcinoma, with sheets of large cells, fibrosis, and amyloid visible with Congo red stain. (Courtesy of Dr. Francis Straus.)

noma.[90] Positive cervical nodes do not seem to carry an adverse risk in young individuals but do imply a worse prognosis in patients over 40 (Fig. 50–10). Pulmonary metastasis may present as large "snowballs" or may give a diffuse mottling appearance on the chest x-ray. Almost all papillary cancer metastases have some ability to take up[131]I when first diagnosed. Occasionally, these lesions produce large amounts of thyroid hormone. Patients with extensive pulmonary metastases tend to gradually develop obstructive pulmonary disease, arteriovenous shunting, hypoxia, and cyanosis. The primary lesions are, as noted above, commonly found to have areas of both papillary and follicular patterns, and the metastatic deposits may be of either variety. Lesions with mixed papillary and follicular elements in the primary tumor behave more or less like papillary cancers, but in our experience they tend to be more malignant, with a greater incidence of recurrence, invasion, and death, than lesions with a purely papillary histology.

The mortality due to papillary cancer is 8 to 20 per cent, mainly among patients who have fixed or invasive cervical lesions or distant metastases at the time of diagnosis[91] (Fig. 50–11). About half the patients dying of this disease succumb because of local invasion.

Papillary carcinoma occurs in children and tends to be aggressive in preteenagers. Children more frequently have lymph node or pulmonary metastases than do adults,[92] and the tumor causes death in 10 per cent or more of the patients. Treatment is essentially as outlined for adults, but long-term follow-up is stressed because of the continued occurrence of relapses.

As noted previously, differentiated cancer is believed by some investigators to occur with increased frequency in Graves' disease and may progress more rapidly.[93, 94] Presumably, TSI produces this effect.[95] Thus, near-total thyroidectomy,[131]I ablation, and careful follow-up are especially important in these patients.

Follicular cancers occur in an older age group, with peak incidence in the fifth decade of life. They frequently present as a slowly growing thyroid mass: about 25 per cent with extrathyroidal invasion, 5 to 10 per cent with local nodes, and 10 to 20 per cent with distant metastases. The histological pattern ranges from an almost normal-appearing thyroid tissue to rather anaplastic-looking sheets of cells. Direct invasion of strap muscles and trachea is characteristic, and resectability depends upon this feature. These lesions tend to metastasize to lungs and bone. The

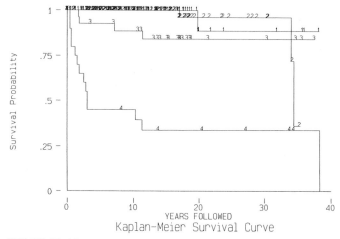

FIGURE 50–10. Deaths from papillary thyroid carcinoma in relation to clinical class, as defined in Table 50–5. Patients with extrathyroidal invasion (class III) have a significantly worse prognosis, and those with distant metastasis at diagnosis (class IV) have a >50 per cent mortality in four years, although some survive for four decades. The numbers above each line refer to the time individual surviving patients were followed.

bone metastases are usually osteolytic. Commonly the lesions retain the ability to accumulate radioactive iodide and are thus theoretically susceptible to ^{131}I treatment. The results, which are not so satisfactory, are discussed below. Follicular cancers are more lethal than papillary tumors, and the mortality, over 10 or 15 years after diagnosis, is 10 to 50 per cent, again primarily in patients with fixed or invasive disease or distant metastases at the time of initial diagnosis.[91]

Hürthle cell carcinomas behave much like the other follicular tumors.[96] They have a pronounced tendency to recur in the neck many years after the original resection and to cause death by local invasion. Hürthle cell carcinomas usually accumulate ^{131}I poorly and are not amenable to this therapy.

Medullary thyroid cancer was first described as a unique tumor of the thyroid characterized by sheets of cells with large nuclei, fibrosis, multicentricity, and extensive amyloid deposits with an unexpectedly benign course.[84] These tumors account for 2 to 4 per cent of thyroid cancers, and are now known to be derived from the C cells, or parafollicular cells, which are of ultimobranchial origin. About 70 per cent occur alone, and 30 per cent as part of type II MEN in association with pheochromocytoma parathyroid adenoma, and adrenal adenoma, or type III in association with unilateral or bilateral pheochromocytomas, mucosal neuromas, neurofibromas, café au lait spots, and possibly Gardner's syndrome.[97–99] Hyperplasia of the C cells precedes development of cancer.[99] Medullary tumors secrete CT and carcinoembryonic antigen, which allows for their diagnosis and, in addition, can produce serotonin, prostaglandins, ACTH, histaminase, and other peptides.[100–102] CT is produced in excess, but the patients are typically eucalcemic. The associated parathyroid hyperplasia and adenomas probably represent a pleomorphic genetic effect rather than a response to thyrocalcitonin excess. Diagnosis can be achieved by measuring CT levels after a provocative stimulus with calcium infusion[103] or pentagastrin stimulation. The tumors follow a course almost like that of follic-

ular cancer[104] and can often be controlled by surgery. This tumor is discussed more fully in Chapter 51.

Undifferentiated tumors occur with various configurations giving rise to terms such as *small cell, giant cell, carcinosarcoma,* and *epidermoid carcinoma.* They behave much as do invasive tumors elsewhere, tending to cause local invasion and compression of structures in the neck, and they metastasize to nodes and lungs. Perhaps 10 per cent are resectable when first discovered; the remainder are rapidly and uniformly lethal within six months to one year. A variety of evidence suggests that many anaplastic cancers originate from long-existing differentiated thyroid cancers.[105] A subgroup of tumors usually classified as anaplastic, having characteristic islands of cells, has been designated as *insular carcinomas.* These tumors are less aggressive than the usual anaplastic cancers; because they often collect therapeutically useful quantities of ^{131}I, their recognition is important.[106]

Lymphoma may originate in the thyroid gland. In 30 to 80 per cent of these cases the thyroid gland is also extensively involved with Hashimoto's thyroiditis, and hypothyroidism may be present. It appears probable that the lymphomas arise from the lymphocytes associated with thyroiditis. The lymphomas are typically of the diffuse, large cell variety. The clinical picture usually is that of a rapidly enlarging neck mass producing symptoms from pressure on contiguous structures in an adult. The lesion spreads to adjacent lymph node clusters. The lesion enlarges rapidly and often is painful. Confusion with thyroiditis or small cell carcinoma is common on biopsy unless appropriate tumor cell markers are identified. Although the incidence is low, Hashimoto's disease definitely is a risk factor for lymphoma.

Metastatic carcinomas occur in a significant proportion of patients dying of other malignancies. These come from melanomas, breast tumors, pulmonary carcinomas, gastric, pancreatic, and intestinal carcinomas, lymphomas, cervical carcinomas, and renal cancers. It is sometimes difficult to differentiate these lesions from primary thyroid cancer. Rarely, thyroidectomy is needed for this purpose.

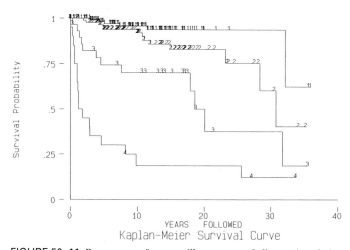

FIGURE 50–11. Recurrences from papillary cancer of all types in relation to clinical class. See description in Table 50–5 and in legend for Figure 50–10. Each increasing clinical class carries a significantly increased risk of recurrence. It is of interest that recurrences continued to occur throughout the entire period of observation, even up to >30 years after initial treatment.

Diagnosis and Differential Diagnosis

The possibility of thyroid carcinoma arises whenever a discrete nodule is found in the thyroid gland. The steps used in evaluating the patients and the differential diagnostic points were discussed above in association with thyroid nodules. We have listed the criteria used to decide whether operation is indicated. Differential diagnosis includes consideration of any cause of a single "nodule" in the thyroid gland and differentiation from multinodular goiter. Diffuse nodularity of the thyroid or the presence of a mottled uptake of radioiodide uptake on thyroid scan is suggestive of the diagnosis of multinodular goiter and usually dictates a conservative course. However, this diagnosis cannot be made with certainty, and if other observations indicate that cancer may be present, operation is indicated. Similarly, concurrence of Hashimoto's thyroiditis or Graves' disease does not exclude the possibility of thyroid carcinoma if other indications on physical examination or scan suggest the presence of such a lesion. Occasionally, youngsters with Hashimoto's thyroiditis will have an unusually firm area in one portion of the gland or clusters of lymph nodes around the upper poles of the thyroid gland. With time and replacement hormone therapy the whole process may subside, and thus it is safe to observe events for several months. If the lymph nodes do not disappear with treatment, biopsy or operation is indicated.

Factors in Selecting Therapy

The variables to be considered in choice of therapy for thyroid cancer include the extent of the initial thyroid resection, the extent of lymph node dissection, prophylactic and therapeutic use of radioactive iodide, postoperative replacement therapy, and the use of ancillary treatments (e.g., chemotherapy and radiotherapy). Although the histopathology of the tumor has some influence on therapeutic decisions, most treatment plans for differentiated cancer rest primarily on the clinical stage of the cancer, as determined by a combination of the findings obtained before operation, observations of the pathologist and surgeon, final histological diagnosis, and subsequent scans. A useful method of clinical staging is the following:

1. Class I: Tumors with single or multiple intrathyroidal foci.
2. Class II: Tumors with cervical metastases, which are not fixed and without invasion.
3. Class III: Thyroid tumors with local cervical invasion or fixed cervical metastases.
4. Class IV: Lesions metastatic outside of the neck.

More thorough staging is possible using the TNM classification[107] but is not of practical value (Tables 50–4 and 50–5).

During the past few years much information has been collected on the natural history of differentiated thyroid cancer and its treatment. Basically these data show that the risk of recurrence and death is very low for patients having papillary or follicular cancers under 2.5 cm in size, in individuals under age 45, and in those without local invasion or distant metastases.[87, 88, 108–110] The prognosis is influenced adversely by increasing age (past 45 years), increasing size

TABLE 50–4. TNM CLINICAL CLASSIFICATION OF THYROID CANCER

T—Primary tumor
 T_0 —No evidence of primary tumor
 T_1 —Single tumor < 1 cm confined to the gland
 T_2 —Single tumor 1–4 cm confined to the gland
 T_3 —tumor > 4 cm confined to the thyroid
 T_4 —Tumor extending beyond the thyroid capsule
N—Regional lymph nodes
 N_0 —No regional node metastasis
 N_{1a} —Regional homolateral node metastasis
 N_{1b} —Regional contralateral or bilateral node metastasis or mediastinal nodes
M—Distant metastasis
 M_0 —No evidence of distant metastases
 M_1 —Distant metastases present

(over 3 to 4 cm), incomplete surgery, poorly differentiated histology, and especially by local invasion and distant metastases.[108–115] Male gender and positive neck nodes have a weak adverse effect.[111] These observations have been used to develop scoring systems—AGES,[88] AJC[116], EORTC,[117, 118] and AMES,[119]—used to segregate the large proportion of low-risk patients from those few at high risk.[120–122] In theory, this knowledge allows prediction of outcome and thus possibly selection of limited therapy (lobectomy and no ^{131}I ablation) for those at low risk versus more aggressive treatment (near-total thyroidectomy and ^{131}I ablation[123]) for patients at high risk. This should, if the logic is correct, reduce the complications from surgery, the dependence on T_4 therapy, the exposure to ^{131}I, and the need for close follow-up for many patients.

We find that the distinction between low- and high-risk groups is clearly reflected in the simple clinical staging just described—the high-risk patients are mainly those with invasive or metastatic disease. Further, it is in many instances impossible to stage correctly at the time of operation, since final pathological review, node status, and results of ^{131}I scanning are unavailable. Some "low-risk" tumors unfortunately behave as if they were "high-risk," and this difference cannot be predicted.[124, 125] Complications of surgery are minimal in the hands of an experienced surgeon.[87, 123] Thyroxine replacement is probably indicated in every patient who has had thyroid cancer, regardless of the extent of surgery. The radiation exposure from ^{131}I scanning and ablation is equal to that of one CT scan and is probably inconsequential. More complete thyroid surgery (at least a lobectomy plus contralateral subtotal thyroidectomy, or near-total thyroidectomy) improves the overall prognosis even for low-risk patients with tumors over 1 cm in size in clinical classes I and II.[87, 126] [131]I ablation decreases recurrences and may[87, 126, 127] or may not[88] decrease deaths, but it clearly improves the value of postablation whole-body scans and makes serial TG measurements useful. Further study is

TABLE 50–5. COMPARISON OF TWO CLINICAL STAGING SYSTEMS

CLINICAL STAGE		COMPARABLE TNM CLASSIFICATION
I.	Intrathyroidal	$T_0, T_1, T_2, T_3, N_0, M_0$
II.	Cervical adenopathy	T_0–T_3, N_1, M_0
III.	Locally invasive disease	T_3, N_0–N_1, M_0
IV.	Distant metastases	M_1

needed to prove the value of routine postoperative ^{131}I ablation.[112] For these reasons, we believe that the patient's best interest is served in most cases by more complete surgery, postoperative ^{131}I ablation, T[4] replacement, and careful follow-up, as described below.

Class I Differentiated (Papillary and Follicular) Neoplasms

Intrathyroidal lesions are treated by lobectomy and contralateral subtotal lobectomy by many surgeons, and this operation is probably appropriate, especially if the surgeon is not a specialist in this area. If the lesion is larger than a "minimal" 1-cm lesion, we usually prefer a near-total thyroidectomy and biopsy of nodes in the adjacent tracheoesophageal groove (Table 50–6). This operation is a planned attempt to take out most of the thyroid without damaging the recurrent laryngeal nerves or parathyroid glands. These structures are carefully identified, and portions of the thyroid (especially the posterior capsule on the contralateral side) are left behind, if necessary, to prevent damage. No attempt is made to remove every piece of thyroid tissue. In lesions that are found to be multicentric on the basis of observations by the surgeon or pathologist, a greater effort is made to do a total thyroidectomy, so long as this can be done without compromise of the parathyroid glands. After surgery, as described below, residual thyroid tissue is ablated by ^{131}I administration in most cases, and especially in patients who have either multicentric foci or a history of irradiation. All patients are given replacement therapy with thyroid hormone. The dosage should be sufficient to reduce TSH to a level slightly below normal. This approach is probably the most widely accepted throughout the world.[108]

Our own experience[87] and a long-term follow-up of 576 cases with papillary thyroid cancer by Mazzaferri et al. appear to support this approach.[127, 128] Patients with near-total thyroidectomy and postoperative ablation had a significantly improved prognosis, especially when follow-up extended over 10 to 15 years. Massin and co-workers[129] also found that "complete thyroidectomy" and ^{131}I ablation gave the lowest incidence of late metastatic recurrence, as did Samaan et al.[126] Samaan et al. found that ^{131}I treatment was the most important influence on recurrence and survival.

It must be noted that different opinions exist in regard to the appropriate operation for this lesion. Perhaps the most common alternative is to do a lobectomy on the involved side if there is no evidence of multicentricity.[117, 130, 131] Several surgical studies support this position and indicate that a more limited operation minimizes damage to the parathyroid glands and recurrent laryngeal nerves and that survival using lobectomy is nearly equal to that for the general population and comparable to results obtained by more extensive surgical procedures.[132] Most series reporting on the results of total or near-total thyroidectomy indicate that hypoparathyroidism occurs in from 1 to 15 per cent of patients, recurrent unilateral nerve damage in 2 to 5 per cent, but fortunately bilateral nerve injury is rare.[133] It is because of these complications, and the apparently satisfactory results with lobectomy, that some investigators prefer the simpler procedure. On the other hand, from 20 to 80 per cent of stage I thyroid cancers are multicentric.[82, 134] It is clear that not all of these foci are of clinical importance, but the recurrence rate of cancer in the contralateral lobe following unilateral lobectomy is at least 6 per cent, and some patients with recurrence eventually die of their lesion.[129, 135, 136] Because of known multicentricity, the ability of our collaborating surgeons to avoid hypoparathyroidism, and the associated improved prognosis,[87] we prefer the more extensive resection. Surgeons who are especially skilled in doing thyroidectomies can hold the incidence of hypoparathyroidism to about 1 per cent and have an equally low incidence of recurrent nerve damage.

In past years, more radical procedures, including prophylactic radical neck dissection, were advocated for thyroid carcinomas. Forty-six per cent of patients with presumed stage I disease were found, in fact, to have lymph node involvement when specimens were thoroughly studied after prophylactic neck dissections.[137] Apparently, however, these lymph node metastases, when not clinically detectable, are in some way controlled by the body's defense mechanisms and rarely lead to death of the patient. Thus, recent opinion is strongly against prophylactic node dissection and against radical or en bloc neck dissection.

Since follicular lesions tend to be more directly invasive and lethal than papillary lesions,[138] many surgeons pursue a more aggressive operative approach with stage I follicular cancer than with papillary cancer and do routine near-total thyroidectomies in patients with the former lesion.[139] Postoperative ^{131}I thyroid ablation and continuous thyroid hormone administration are considered essential.[140]

Up to 20 per cent of low-grade follicular neoplasms are misdiagnosed on operative frozen sections as benign, with the diagnosis achieved 1 to 3 days later after review of

TABLE 50–6. SUGGESTED SURGICAL PROCEDURES IN THYROID CANCER

TYPE	CLINICAL CLASS	OPERATION
Papillary, follicular	I: <1 cm	Lobectomy + contralateral STT* (if detected in a resected specimen, do not reoperate)
Papillary, follicular	I: >1 cm, or multicentric or postradiation	NTT*, or lobectomy + contralateral subtotal
Papillary, follicular	II	NTT + MND* dissection
Papillary, follicular	III	Resection without mutilation
Papillary, follicular	IV	Resection without mutilation
Medullary	Any	NTT; MND as needed
Anaplastic	Any	NTT or tumor resection if possible

*STT, Subtotal thyroidectomy; NTT, Near-total thyroidectomy; MND, Modified neck dissection.

permanent sections. If the lesion is less than 1 cm, unicentric, intrathyroidal, and the patient is under the age of 45, no further surgery is required, and as indicated before, some physicians accept lobectomy as a definitive procedure. In general, in patients with lesions over 1 cm who are over 45 or with multifocality, we would prefer reoperation to achieve near-total thyroidectomy and subsequent ^{131}I therapy. In an analysis of patients who have undergone a second operation, we found that in 31 per cent of the operations residual cancer was recovered on the remaining lobe.[28] This problem is best avoided by doing at least a lobectomy plus contralateral subtotal thyroidectomy if there is any question at operation about the benignity of the "adenoma."

The use of radioactive iodide, as described above, can also be questioned because the ablative dosage exposes the patients, who are frequently young, to 10 or 15 rads of whole-body radiation. While the genetic and carcinogenic risk of this radiation dosage cannot be completely ignored, it is minimally different from the average background whole-body radiation exposure that individuals normally receive by age 30 and is most likely not a significant hazard.

Ten to twenty per cent of patients who undergo an initial near-total thyroidectomy for stage I cancer will later have cervical lymph node recurrence. These patients ultimately require a neck dissection or simple node removal.

Class II Differentiated Thyroid Cancer

There is less disagreement on how to manage class II disease. The usual procedure is a near-total or total thyroidectomy.[129, 132, 141] Small portions of the gland may be left in situ (for later radioiodide ablation), if necessary to preserve recurrent laryngeal nerves or viability of the parathyroid glands. A modified neck dissection is also performed to remove involved nodes. An attempt is made to retain the jugular vein and sternocleidomastoid muscles, and an en bloc resection is not attempted, except occasionally in patients with metastatic follicular cancer. If both sides of the neck are involved, the resections usually are staged, since otherwise the incidence of tracheal edema requiring tracheostomy is significant. A radical neck dissection with removal of the jugular vein and sternocleidomastoid muscle is not favored since the disease usually can be managed by the less mutilating procedure, and uninvolved nodes that become apparent at a later date can usually be successfully resected. Patients are given ^{131}I to ablate residual thyroid tissue after surgery and to treat functioning metastases found on scanning.

Class III Differentiated Carcinoma

Patients with class III disease should receive a near-total or total thyroidectomy, appropriate lymph node dissection, and resection of all possible invading neoplasm. There is a tendency at present to avoid mutilating surgery in patients under age 45 in the effort to resect all cancerous tissue, because less extensive surgery, ^{131}I treatment, and suppressive thyroid hormone therapy usually lead to prolonged survival or cure, even if complete excision of the tumor is impossible.[142] [131]I therapy is given as discussed below. Exter-

nal irradiation may be useful in preventing recurrence.[143] However, since most cases appear to be controlled by surgery and ^{131}I and definitive experience with supplemental prophylactic irradiation is not available, the usual course is to withhold irradiation until recurrence is seen in younger patients but to advise prophylactic treatment in patients over 45 to 50 years of age.

Management of Class IV Differentiated Disease

Patients with a thyroid mass and solitary metastasis in lung or bone probably should have thyroidectomy and excision of the single metastasis, because cure or prolonged survival may be obtained. If there are multiple metastases, thyroidectomy is probably the quickest way to achieve hypothyroidism, in order that uptake of radioactive iodide in the metastases, and possible therapy, can be evaluated. Occasionally it is appropriate, in the presence of complicating illness, to achieve thyroid ablation by administration of 50 mCi [131]I.

Hürthle Cell Carcinoma

It is clear that Hürthle cell tumors range in invasiveness from none to an aggressively locally invading lesion or a tumor with rapidly growing pulmonary metastases. These variations result in a wide range of opinion on therapy.[144–146] We advocate treatment as described for follicular cancers, of which these are a subgroup. Postoperative ^{131}I ablation is carried out, although its value may be restricted, since many Hürthle cell tumors fail to accumulate [131]I. Invasive tumors (class III) should be treated by mantle irradiation. [131]I treatment is attempted for class III or IV tumors but usually is not possible despite the presence of functioning metastases as proved by elevated TG levels.

Lymphomas

Staging should include neck, chest, and abdominal CT scans, and bone marrow biopsy. If the disease appears limited to the thyroid gland and contiguous lymph nodes, thyroidectomy is advised, although occasionally only biopsy is possible. Patients with intrathyroidal lymphoma, or disease limited to the neck and upper mediastinum, have conventionally been treated by mantle irradiation to about 45 gy over three to four weeks.[147] Because overall survival at five years has been about 50 per cent,[147–149] patients are increasingly being treated primarily by chemotherapy. Patients with more extensive disease and those who have relapse are given chemotherapy.

Undifferentiated Lesions

The surgical approach is total thyroidectomy, en bloc dissection of the tumor, and neck dissection, in an attempt to totally remove the disease if this seems feasible.[150] Frequently it is obvious that complete resection is not possible and operation is limited to partial resection or simply to biopsy. After this procedure, we have routinely studied such patients for possible radioactive iodide accumulation and ^{131}I therapy, although the expected results are negative. All patients are given radiotherapy to the neck and upper mediastinum. Coincident low-dose Adriamycin therapy given during radiotherapy is apparently advantageous. Chemotherapy is discussed below.

Thyroxine Therapy

Because TSH does induce growth of some thyroid cancers, it appears logical to treat all patients having this disease with T_4, although the proof of universal efficacy is lacking. Clearly replacement is needed in thyroidectomized patients. However, suppression of TSH to low levels by supraphysiological doses of T_4 is associated with osteoporosis,[151] and often cardiac arrhythmias. The perfect answer to this therapeutic dilemma is uncertain. We advise initial replacement T_4 in all patients who have had thyroid cancer to produce a TSH of 0.2 to 0.4 μU/ml.[151] Patients with proved active cancer should be treated with higher dosages to suppress TSH to 0 to 0.1 μU/ml if this is not associated with adverse cardiac, or other side effects.

In patients who, during progressive follow-up, can be reasonably assumed to have been cured of their cancers (most patients in classes I and II), it is reasonable to alter T_4 dosage gradually to a replacement level producing a TSH in the 0.4 to 1 μU/ml range.

Radioactive Iodide Therapy

Radioiodine ablation of residual thyroid tissue is attempted in most patients with class I disease, especially those with multicentric lesions or a history of radiation, and in patients in clinical classes II, III, and IV. We do not routinely ablate individuals with lesions less than 1 cm in size who are under age 30 unless they have a history of x-ray exposure, because their prognosis is excellent and their life expectancy is essentially "normal." Radioiodide therapy of metastatic disease is attempted, so long as significant accumulation of the isotope occurs in the lesions.[152, 153]

Patients are placed on suppressive hormone therapy immediately after surgery and are maintained on this for a period of approximately eight weeks, because we prefer not to have high circulating TSH levels in these patients at a time when implants of thyroid tumor cells may be present, scattered throughout the neck or elsewhere in the body. About eight weeks after surgery, suppressive therapy is changed to T_3 (25 μg bid) for three weeks and then discontinued, and two to three weeks later the patients are studied. It is advantageous that patients take T_3 for three weeks before discontinuation of hormone treatment because this hormone will disappear from circulation more rapidly and this procedure allows more rapid TSH response. Two weeks after T_3 withdrawal, TSH levels usually have risen to 40 to 60 U/ml, and adequate stimulation of ^{131}I uptake in thyroid tissue or tumor cells can be anticipated. If possible, TSH levels should be obtained before completion of the scan in order to ensure that the level is greater than 25 μU/ml and adequate stimulation of [131]I

uptake is present. Patients are given a 2-mCi dose of ^{131}I for scans, and uptake is quantitated using the gamma camera for each area of the body. Even when total thyroidectomy is attempted, more than 80 per cent of the patients will have residual thyroid tissue in the neck, and often the uptake will be 2 to 5 per cent of the "tracer." Thirty to fifty mCi of ^{131}I is administered as an ablative dose, and this may have to be repeated once more, after six months, to achieve total destruction of residual thyroid tissue. While 50 mCi or larger doses of ^{131}I provides more certain ablation,[154] the lower 30 mCi dose can be given on an outpatient basis, with less expense and lower whole-body radiation dose.[155] If on the initial scan evidence of isotope accumulation is found outside of the thyroid bed, the patient is treated for metastatic thyroid cancer, as described below. Otherwise patients are placed back on replacement therapy for another six to nine months, at which time replacement is discontinued using the same procedure, and the 2-mCi ^{131}I scan is repeated (Fig. 50–12). Scans are obtained at 48 and 72 hours, since at this time body isotope background has been greatly reduced, and it is possible to clearly detect lesions accumulating as little as 0.1 per cent of the isotope dose.

Patients with significant uptake of radioactive iodide in definable metastatic foci, usually collecting above 0.2 per cent of the test dose, are considered for ^{131}I therapy. No attempt is made to measure secretion of radioactive iodide–labeled organic compounds into blood, or excretion of the isotope in the urine. Patients with significant retention of ^{131}I in metastatic deposits in the neck are given 75 to 100 mCi, and if metastases are present elsewhere, they are routinely given 150 to 250 mCi of radioactive iodide. This dose can be tolerated without acute radiation sickness and is below that which would, in almost all instances, produce excessive irradiation to any structure, including the lungs if diffuse pulmonary metastases are present. If radioactive iodide uptake in metastatic deposits in the lung exceeds 50 per cent, appropriate reductions in the total dosage should be made so that the ^{131}I deposit in the lungs never exceeds 60 to 75 mCi. The day after ^{131}I is administered, the patients are placed back on suppressive doses of thyroid hormone, and the cycle is repeated at six- to nine-month intervals so long as evidence of significant tumor

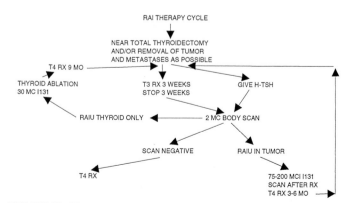

FIGURE 50–12. RAI therapy cycle showing the program for ablation of residual thyroid tissue and subsequent treatment of patients with repetitive doses of 75 to 200 mCi RA[131]I.

uptake of isotope is noted and no adverse effects of radioactive iodide administration are detected (Fig. 50–13). If uptake does not occur after hormone withdrawal, TSH (5 U subcutaneously daily for three days), can be given in an attempt to stimulate uptake, and isotope administration is repeated if uptake is achieved. After ^{131}I therapy, TSH can be suppressed rapidly by administering supraphysiological doses of T_3, but it is uncertain that this is clinically important.

Maxon et al. advocate careful evaluation of ^{131}I accumu-

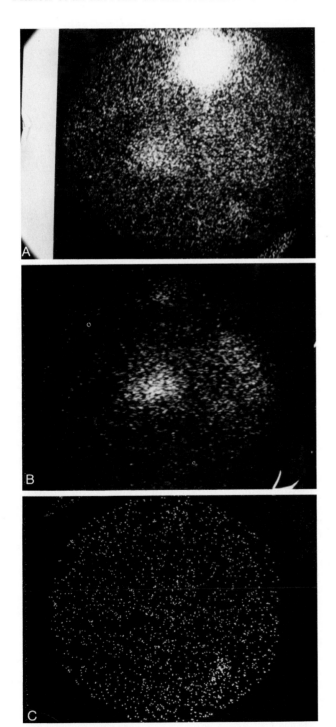

FIGURE 50–13. Serial anterior views of lung fields during a 1 mCi ^{131}I whole-body scan, in a patient with metastatic papillary carcinoma (A) before, (B) during, and (C) after completion of ^{131}I therapy. There was no recurrence throughout the subsequent 18 years.

lation by metastatic deposits and administration of larger doses designed to deliver, if possible, 80 gy to the lesions.[156] Unfortunately, it is usually impossible to calculate the radiation dose achieved in metastatic deposits, since one almost never knows the actual size or geometry of the lesions. However, it can be calculated that patients with small deposits weighing fractions of a gram can readily be given doses in the order of 10,000 to 15,000 rads through such treatments, and presumably this should be cancerocidal. When uptake falls below 0.2 per cent, when there are large extensive metastases with small uptake, or when minimal uptake is scattered throughout lung fields, the effectiveness of ^{131}I treatment is greatly reduced and probably should be abandoned. Some physicians advocate treatment with 100-mCi doses of ^{131}I, even if uptake cannot be detected by the 2-mCi scanning dose studies, and suggest this may lower TG levels, but the effect on survival is unknown.[157] [131]I treatment is repeated if there is evidence of functional tumor, unless adverse effects occur, as noted below. Therapy is limited most frequently by failure of ^{131}I uptake in tumor or by bone marrow suppression.

Adverse effects of radiation usually are minimal. Obviously patients should be screened for pregnancy; even possible pregnancy, or lactation, is an absolute contraindication to therapy. Patients having ingested radioactive iodide must be hospitalized until the body burden is less than 30 mCi, and appropriate arrangements must be made for disposal of urine and feces and any contaminated material. The patient is kept in a private room and personnel must be instructed in proper precautions. Whole-body radiation is approximately one third to one half rad/mCi administered, and comes primarily from the "iodide phase" exposure, since little radioactive hormone is formed in most patients. Mild nausea occasionally occurs, and radiation to the salivary glands may produce a metallic taste or dry mouth for some weeks. Repeated ^{131}I treatment may reduce salivary flow and produce dental problems. Transient alterations in liver function have been reported, and treatment of functioning pelvic metastases may provide a sterilizing dose to the gonads.[158]

A dose-dependent depression of spermatogenesis following ^{131}I therapy for thyroid cancer was reported by Handelsman and Turtle.[159] A clinically significant testicular damage was found in patients who received more than 100 mCi of ^{131}I; however, the effect was reversible during two years of follow-up. Excessive ^{131}I deposition in lung metastases has caused fatal pulmonary fibrosis and death. Leukopenia is seen after each radiation exposure but rapidly clears.[160] If bone marrow metastases are present, progressive marrow destruction may occur, with leukopenia, thrombocytopenia, and anemia, and this may limit further dosage. Leukemia occurs with increased frequency in patients who receive multiple large doses of radioactive iodide,[161] and there is evidence for a minimal increase in the incidence of tumors of salivary glands and gonads.[162, 163]

The overall effectiveness of this treatment is variable. Mazzaferri and Young's study clearly shows that, overall, ^{131}I ablation and therapy greatly improves prognosis in differentiated cancers.[128] In children with functioning metastases, sometimes complete ablation of the lesions occurs, and it seems certain from studies of Varma et al.[164] and Leeper[165] that radioactive iodide treatment in patients under age 40 is distinctly beneficial. In older patients less effect is seen, but the course of follicular cancers is probably favorably altered. Most patients with metastases accumulate iodide in sufficient dosage to warrant a serious therapeutic trial, and sometimes extensive deposits can be ablated. Soft tissue lesions respond best to radioactive iodide. Osseous lesions often function but can rarely be destroyed. However, it appears that only a fraction of these patients are actually cured of their lesions. Multiple periods of exposure of the metastases to high levels of TSH during thyroid hormone withdrawal preceding ^{131}I scanning may actually lead to acceleration of tumor growth in some instances. Over years a proportion of patients gradually develops tumor foci that do not accumulate ^{131}I, and eventually these tumors are lethal.

Radiolabeled antithyroglobulin scanning is currently being evaluated for detection of thyroid tumor.[166] It is reported to be more sensitive than conventional ^{131}I scanning. Positive results can be obtained while patients continue to take thyroid hormone, and this could avoid the inconvenience and potential risks of hypothyroidism.

Long-Term Follow-up

Patients in class I given ^{131}I ablation are rescanned at six to nine months, then at approximately 18 months, three years, and five years. At each interval, physical examination, chest radiograph, and serum TG determination are performed. Patients in classes II to IV are followed similarly after completion of ^{131}I therapy. Serial bone scans or skeletal radiographs are not cost-effective procedures in following patients without known metastatic disease[167] (Table 50–7).

Although serum TG levels are not useful in preoperative differentiation of thyroid cancer from other non-neoplastic thyroid disease,[168] the measurement is useful in the follow-up of thyroid cancer after surgical and radioactive iodide ablation.[169, 170] Elevated TG levels in this circumstance is a useful indicator of the presence of metastatic disease, whereas TG levels below 3 ng/ml are more or less reliable indicators of the absence of metastasis. Assay of TG while patients are on replacement hormone leads to a correct interpretation of status in about 90 per cent of patients. However, in some patients, TG is suppressed by thyroid hormone therapy, and thus for best results patients should be hypothyroid before TG assay is obtained (Fig. 50–14). An elevated TG level does not uniformly predict treatable ^{131}I uptake. Thus the TG assay supplements but does not replace ^{131}I whole-body scans in managing these patients. Since most TG assays are invalidated by the presence of TG

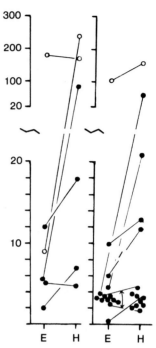

FIGURE 50–14. Serum TG (Y axis) levels in patients with and without replacement therapy. E = euthyroid, H = hypothyroid. The majority of patients with low or high serum TG levels are not moved from one category to the other after thyroid hormone withdrawal and subsequent TSH stimulation. However, some patients have TG suppressed into the normal range while taking replacement therapy but have elevated TG levels when hypothyroid.

autoantibodies, samples should be routinely screened for their presence.

RECOMBINANT HUMAN TSH. TSH is currently in clinical trial and presumably will be available for clinical use within a year.[171] TSH will alter for the better the postoperative management of patients with thyroid carcinoma. The drug is very effective; one or two daily injections of 10 to 20 units stimulate thyroidal ^{131}I uptake in patients starting with suppressed TSH levels (<0.1 μU/ml) to a degree equal to 2 to 3 weeks of hormone withdrawal. Side effects appear to be minimal, although long-term studies of possible antibody formation are not yet available. Thus it will be possible to stimulate ^{131}I uptake and TG secretion without induction of hypothyroidism. This will make ^{131}I whole-body scanning and TG testing more acceptable to patients and doctors. It is not clear exactly how this will alter the pattern of scanning or testing during follow-up, but it is likely that ^{131}I postoperative ablation will be more routine, that scans will be somewhat more frequent, that yearly stimulated TG

TABLE 50–7. MEDICAL MANAGEMENT AFTER SURGERY

PATIENT CATEGORY	PHYSICAL EXAMINATION, CHEST X-RAY FILM, FTI	REPEAT ^{131}I BODY SCAN	SERUM THYROGLOBULIN (DESIRED LEVEL)
I. Tumor removed, residual thyroid in situ	Annually		Below 5 ng/ml while receiving therapy
II. Tumor ± nodes removed, thyroid ablated by surgery or [131]I	At least annually	At 6–9 months after ablation, then at 1, 3, and 5 years	Below 3 ng/ml when not taking hormone
III. Tumor removed, thyroid ablated, metastatic disease treated	At 3–6 months, then at least annually	At 3–6 months after therapy, and annually for 3–5 years	Below 3 ng/ml when not taking hormone

TABLE 50–8. INDICATIONS FOR RADIATION THERAPY

TUMOR	STAGE	TREATMENT (15–20 MV ELECTRONS OR ^{60}CO)
Papillary or follicular	Invasive, patient under age 45	Possibly 4000 rads at 2–3 cm depth to thyroid bed after radioactive iodine (RAI) treatment; value uncertain in this instance
	Invasive or possible residual, patient over 45	5000 rads* to thyroid bed after RAI treatment
	Recurrent, patient any age	5000 rads* to thyroid bed after RAI treatment
	Isolated lesion in bone	5000–6000 rads, as required for symptoms after RAI treatment
Medullary	Stage III	4000–5000 rads** to thyroid bed
	Abnormal or increasing thyrocalcitonin (TCT)	5000 rads** to mantle
	Recurrent tumor, isolated metastasis	5000–6000 rads* to area
		5000–6000 rads for symptoms
Lymphoma	All	5000 rads** to thyroid and mantle
Anaplastic	All	4500–5500 rads** to thyroid and mantle

Note: Spinal cord dosage does not exceed 3000* rads or 3500** rads.

testing will be more common, and that ^{131}I therapy may be more effective.

Radiation Therapy

Radiation therapy is appropriate for any class III differentiated tumor not responding to ^{131}I therapy or hormone suppression, for class III Hürthle cell tumors and follicular cancers in older patients, for any expanding class IV lesion, for painful osseous metastases, and for lymphomas and undifferentiated tumors.[172] Unfortunately, no results from adequate study are available to assess prophylactic radiation after resection of class III tumors. Prophylactic mantle radiotherapy may be useful in medullary thyroid cancer patients who have residual hypercalcitoninemia after surgery in the absence of detectable lesions (Table 50–8), but the value of this treatment is debated.[173]

Chemotherapy

A variety of chemotherapeutic approaches have been attempted with uncertain success. The overall response rate of thyroid cancer to various chemotherapeutic agents, including the alkylating agents 5-fluorouracil and methotrexate, is estimated to be 10 to 15 per cent, which was comparable to that for other solid tumors.[174] Bleomycin, and especially doxorubicin (Adriamycin),[174–180] have been reported to provide a higher percentage of remission (20 to 33 per cent). However, the response to these chemotherapeutic agents is partial and of short duration with limitation imposed by toxicity of the medication. Chemotherapeutic agents given in combination appear to be slightly more effective than doxorubicin alone.[174–180] Che-

TABLE 50–9. CHEMOTHERAPY FOR THYROID CARCINOMA

PRIMARY TUMOR
Progressive differentiated thyroid cancer, symptomatic medullary cancer, anaplastic cancer; two programs have been proposed:
Doxorubicin (Adriamycin) + *cis*-diamine-dichloroplatinum + Vp-16
Doxorubicin (Adriamycin) + *cis*-diamine-dichloroplatinum

SECONDARY THERAPY FOR FAILURE OF PRIMARY TREATMENT
Differentiated cancer: bleomycin + cyclophosphamide
Medullary cancer: 5-fluorouracil + streptozocin
Anaplastic cancer: bleomycin + hydroxyurea

motherapy in differentiated thyroid carcinoma, preferably doxorubicin, is warranted in class III and IV lesions after other modalities of therapy have been exhausted and tumor growth is certain (Table 50–9). Chemotherapy may be used in treatment of anaplastic thyroid carcinoma after surgery in combination with external radiation. Kim and Leeper[178] report that doxorubicin (10 mg/m^2/week) given concurrently with hyperfractionated radiation produced much enhanced local control with acceptable morbidity.

REFERENCES

1. Vander JB, Gaston EA, Dawber TR: The Significance of Nontoxic Thyroid Nodules. Final Report of a 15-Year Study of the Incidence of Thyroid Malignancy. Ann Intern Med 69:537, 1968.
2. Baldwin DB, Rowett D: Incidence of thyroid disorders in Connecticut. JAMA 239:742–744, 1978.
3. Mortensen JD, Woolner LB, Bennett WA: Gross and microscopic findings in clinically normal thyroid glands. J Clin Endocrinol Metab 15:1270, 1955.
4. Bisi H, Fernandes VSO, Asato de Camargo RY, et al: The prevalence of unsuspected thyroid pathology in 300 sequential autopsies, with special reference to the incidental carcinoma. Cancer 64:1888–1893, 1989.
5. Namba H, Matsuo K, Fagin JA: Clonal composition of benign and malignant human thyroid tumors. J Clin Invest 86:120–125, 1990.
6. DeGroot LJ: Lack of iodide trapping in "cold" thyroid nodules. Acta Endo Panam 1:27, 1970.
7. Werk EE Jr, Vernon BM, Gonzalez JJ, et al: Cancer in thyroid nodules. A community hospital survey. Arch Intern Med 144:474–476, 1984.
8. Rojeski MT, Gharib H: Nodular thyroid disease: Evaluation and management. N Engl J Med 313:428–436, 1985.
9. Schimke RN, Hartmann WH, Prout TE, Rimoin DL: Syndrome of bilateral pheochromocytoma, medullary thyroid carcinoma, and multiple neuromas. N Engl J Med 279:1, 1968.
10. Sokal JE: The problem of malignancy in nodular goiter—recapitulation and a challenge. JAMA 170:61, 1959.
11. Ott RA, Calandra DB, McCall A, et al: The incidence of thyroid carcinoma in patients with Hashimoto's thyroiditis and solitary cold nodules. Surgery 98:1202–1206, 1985.
12. Refetoff S, Harrison J, Karanfilski BT, et al: Continuing occurrence of thyroid carcinoma after irradiation to the neck in infancy and childhood. N Engl J Med 292:171, 1975.
13. Van Herle AJ, Rich P, Ljung BM, et al: The thyroid nodule. Ann Intern Med 96:221–232, 1982.
14. Kendall LW, Condon RE: Prediction of malignancy in solitary thyroid nodules. Lancet 1:1071, 1969.
15. Hoffer PB, Gottschalk A, Refetoff S: Thyroid scanning techniques: The old and the new. Curr Probl Radiol 2:5, 1972.
16. Hollifield JW, Patton JA, Lee GS, Brill AB: Differentiation of malignant from benign thyroid nodules by fluorescent thyroid scanning. J Nucl Med 17:17–21, 1976.

17. Thijs LJ: Diagnostic ultrasound in clinical thyroid investigation. J Clin Endocrinol Metab 32:709, 1971.

18. Lowhagen T, Granberg PO, Lundell G, et al: Aspiration biopsy cytology (ABC) in nodules of the thyroid gland suspected to be malignant. Surg Clin North Am 59:3–18, 1979.

19. Ramacciotti CE, Pretorius HT, Chu EW, et al: Diagnostic accuracy and use of aspiration biopsy in the management of thyroid nodules. Arch Intern Med 144:1169–1173, 1984.

20. Gharib H, Goellner JR, Zinsmeister AR, et al: Fine-needle aspiration biopsy of the thyroid: The problem of suspicious cytologic findings. Ann Intern Med 101:25–28, 1984.

21. Hamberger B, Gharib H, Melton LJ, et al: Fine-needle aspiration biopsy of thyroid nodules: Impact on thyroid practice, and cost of care. Am J Med 73:381–384, 1982.

22. Miller TR, Abele JS, Greenspan FS: Fine needle aspiration biopsy in the management of thyroid nodules. West J Med 134:198–205, 1981.

23. Walfish PG, Hazani B, Strawbridge HTG, et al: Combined ultrasound and needle aspiration cytology in the assessment and management of hypofunctioning thyroid nodule. Ann Intern Med 87:270, 1977.

24. Ridgway EC: Clinical review 30. Clinician's evaluation of a solitary thyroid nodule. J Clin Endocrinol Metab 74:231–235, 1992.

25. Miller JM, Zafar SU, Karo JJ: The cystic thyroid nodule: Recognition and management. Radiology 110:257–261, 1974.

26. McCowen KD, Reed JW, Fariss BL: The role of thyroid therapy in patients with thyroid cysts. Am J Med 68:853–855, 1980.

27. Goldstein R, Hart IR: Follow-up of solitary autonomous thyroid nodules treated with 131-I. N Engl J Med 309:1473–1476, 1983.

28. Paracchi A, Ferrari C, Livraghi T, et al: Percutaneous intranodular ethanol injection: A new treatment for autonomous thyroid adenoma. J Endocrinol Invest 15:353–362, 1992.

29. DeGroot LJ, Kaplan EL: Second operations for "completion" of thyroidectomy in treatment of differentiated thyroid cancer. Surgery 110:936–940, 1991.

30. Greer MA, Astwood EB: Treatment of simple goiter with thyroid. J Clin Endocrinol Metab 13:1312, 1953.

31. Astwood EB, Cassidy CE, Auerbach GD: Treatment of goiter and thyroid nodules with thyroid. JAMA 174:459, 1960.

32. Glassford GH, Fowler EF, Cole WH: The treatment of nontoxic nodular goiter with desiccated thyroid: Results and evaluation. Surgery 58:621, 1965.

33. Hill LD, Beebe HG, Hipp R, Jones HW: Thyroid suppression. Arch Surg 108:403, 1974.

34. Baran DT, Braverman LE: Editorial: Thyroid hormones and bone mass. J Clin Endocrinol Metab 72:1182–1183, 1991.

35. Muller C, Bayley TA, Harrison JE, Tsang R: Suppressive thyroxine therapy does not affect bone mass. Thyroid 2:S–13, 1992.

36. Morita T, Tamai H, Ohshima A, et al: Changes in serum thyroid hormone, thyrotropin and thyroglobulin concentrations during thyroxine therapy in patients with solitary thyroid nodules. J Clin Endocrinol Metab 69:227, 1989.

37. National Institutes of Health Publication No. 88–2789, Annual Cancer Statistical Review, 1987.

38. Verby JE, Woolner LB, Nobrega FT, et al: Thyroid cancer in Olmsted County, 1935–1965. J Nat Can Inst 43:813, 1969.

39. Vanderlaan WP: The occurrence of carcinoma of the thyroid gland in autopsy material. N Engl J Med 237:221, 1947.

40. Silverberg SG, Vidone RA: Carcinoma of the thyroid in surgical and postmortem material. Ann Surg 164:291, 1966.

41. Sampson RJ, Woolner LB, Bahn RC, Kurland LT: Occult thyroid carcinoma in Olmsted County, Minnesota: Prevalence at autopsy compared with that in Hiroshima and Nagasaki, Japan. Cancer 34:2072, 1974.

42. Fukunaga FH, Yatani R: Geographic pathology of occult thyroid carcinomas. Cancer 36:1095, 1975.

43. Schaller RT, Stevenson JK: Development of carcinoma of the thyroid in iodine-deficient mice. Cancer 19:1063, 1966.

44. Money WL, Rawson RW: The experimental production of thyroid tumors in the rat exposed to prolonged treatment with thiouracil. Cancer 3:321, 1950.

45. Doniach I: The effect of radioactive iodine alone and in combination with methylthiouracil upon tumor production in the rat's thyroid gland. Br J Cancer 7:181, 1953.

46. Duffy BJ Jr, Fitzgerald PJ: Cancer of the thyroid in children: A report of 28 cases. J Clin Endocrinol 10:1296, 1950.

47. Clark DE: Association of irradiation with cancer of the thyroid in children and adolescents. JAMA, 159:1007, 1955.

48. DeGroot LJ, Paloyan E: Thyroid carcinoma and radiation. A Chicago endemic. JAMA 225:487, 1973.

49. Saenger EL, Silverman FN, Sterling TD, Turner ME: Neoplasia following therapeutic irradiation for benign conditions in childhood. Radiology 74:889, 1960.

50. Shore RE, Woodard E, Hildreth N, et al: Thyroid tumors following thymus irradiation. J Natl Cancer Inst 74:1177–1184, 1985.

51. Maxon H, Thomas SR, Saenger EL, et al: Ionizing irradiation and the induction of clinically significant disease in the human thyroid gland. Am J Med 63:967, 1977.

52. DeGroot LJ, Reilly M, Pinnameneni K, Refetoff S: Retrospective and prospective study of radiation-induced thyroid disease. Am J Med 74:852–862, 1983.

53. Hancock SL, Cox RS, McDougall IR: Thyroid diseases after treatment of Hodgkin's disease. N Engl J Med 325:599–605, 1991.

54. Socolow EL, Hashizume A, Neriishi S, Nitani R: Thyroid carcinoma in man after exposure to ionizing radiation: A summary of the findings in Hiroshima and Nagasaki. N Engl J Med 268:406, 1963.

55. Roudebush CP, Asteris GT, DeGroot LJ: Natural history of radiation-associated thyroid cancer. Arch Intern Med 138:1631–1634, 1978.

56. Dobyns, PM, Sheline GE, Workman, JB, et al: Malignant and benign neoplasms of the thyroid in patients treated for hyperthyroidism: A report of the Cooperative Thyrotoxicosis Therapy Follow-up Study. J Clin Endocrinol Metab 38:973, 1974.

57. Holm L-E, Dahlqvist I, Israelsson A, Lundell G: Malignant thyroid tumors after iodine-131 therapy. N Engl J Med 303:188, 1980.

58. Cooper DS, Axelrod L, DeGroot LJ, et al: Congenital goiter and the development of metastatic follicular carcinoma with evidence for a leak of nonhormonal iodide: Clinical, pathological, kinetic, and biochemical studies and a review of the literature. J Clin Endocrinol Metab 52:294–303, 1981.

59. Abe Y, Ichikawa Y, Muraki T, et al: Thyrotropin (TSH) receptor and adenylate cyclase activity in human thyroid tumors: Absence of high affinity receptor and loss of TSH responsiveness in undifferentiated thyroid carcinoma. J Clin Endocrinol Metab 52:23–28, 1981.

60. Hales IB, McElduff A, Crummer P, et al: Does Graves' disease or thyrotoxicosis affect the prognosis of thyroid cancer? J Clin Endocrinol Metab 75:886–889, 1992.

61. Pacini F, Elisei R, Di Coscio GC, et al: Thyroid carcinoma in thyrotoxic patients treated by surgery. J Endocrinol Invest 11:107, 1988.

62. Behar R, Arganini M, Wu T-C, et al: Graves' disease and thyroid cancer. Surgery 100:1121–1127, 1986.

63. Ellenberg AH, Goldman L, Gordan GS, Lindsay S: Thyroid carcinoma in patients with hyperparathyroidism. Surgery 51:708–717, 1962.

64. Lever EG, Refetoff S, Straus FH, et al: Coexisting thyroid and parathyroid disease—Are they related? Surgery 94:893–900, 1983.

65. Hsu TC, Pathak S, Samaan N, Hickey RC: Chromosome instability in patients with medullary carcinoma of the thyroid. JAMA 246:2046–2048, 1981.

66. Panza N, Vecchio LD, Maio M, et al: Strong association between an HLA-DR antigen and thyroid carcinoma. Tissue Antigen 20:155–158, 1982.

67. Weissel M, Kainz H, Hoefer R, Mayr WR: HLA-DR and differentiated thyroid cancer. Lack of association with the nonmedullary types and possible association with the medullary type. Cancer 62:2486–2488, 1988.

68. Sridama V, Hara Y, Fauchet R, DeGroot LJ: Association of differentiated thyroid carcinoma with HLA-DR7 antigen. Fifty-ninth Meeting of the American Thyroid Association, New Orleans, LA, Oct. 1983, No. 24 (abstract).

69. Lloyd KM II, Dennis M: Cowden's disease. A possible new symptom complex with multiple system involvement. Ann Intern Med 58:136–142, 1963.

70. de Mestier P: Thyroid cancer and familial rectocolonic polyposis. Chirurgie 116:514–516, 1990.

71. Plail RO, Bussey HJ, Glazer G, Thomson JP: Adenomatous Polyposis: An association with carcinoma of the thyroid. Br J Surg 74:377–380, 1987.

72. Camiel MR, Mule JE, Alexander LL, Benninghoff DL: Association of thyroid carcinoma with Gardner's syndrome in siblings. N Engl J Med 278:1056, 1968.

73. Albores-Saavedra J, Duran ME: Association of thyroid carcinoma in chemodectoma. Am J Surg 116:887–890, 1968.

74. Yamashita S, Ong J, Fagin JA, Melmed S: Expression of the *myc* cellular proto-oncogene in human thyroid tissue. J Clin Endocrinol Metab 63:1170, 1986.

75. Namba H, Gutman RA, Matsuo K, et al: H-*ras* proto-oncogene mutations in human thyroid neoplasms. J Clin Endocrinol Metab 71:223–229, 1990.

76. Namba H, Rubin SA, Fagin JA: Point mutations of *ras* oncogenes are an early event in thyroid tumorigenesis. Mol Endocrinol 4:1474–1479, 1990.

76a. Suarez HG, du Villard JA, Caillou B, et al: Gsp mutations in human thyroid tumors. Oncogene 6:677–679, 1991.

77. Donghi R, Sozzi G, Pierotti MA, et al: The oncogene associated with human papillary thyroid carcinoma (PTC) is assigned to chromosome 10q11-q12 in the same region as multiple endocrine neoplasia type 2A (MEN2A). Oncogene 4:521–523, 1989.

78. Schlumberger M, Suarez H, Caillou B, Bressac B: Thyroid oncogenes and anti-oncogenes. J Endocrinol Invest 15:35, 1992.

79. Thakker RV, Bouloux P, Wooding C, et al: Association of parathyroid tumors in multiple endocrine neoplasia type I with loss of alleles on chromosome 11. N Engl J Med 321:218–224, 1989.

80. Mathew CG, Chin KS, Easton DF, et al: A linked genetic marker for multiple endocrine neoplasia type 2A on chromosome 10. Nature 328:527–528, 1987.

81. Matsuo K, Tang S-H, Fagin JA: Allelotype of human thyroid tumors: Loss of chromosome 11q13 sequences in follicular neoplasms. Mol Endocrinol 5:1873–1879, 1991.

81a. Fagin JA, Matsuo K, Karmarkar A, et al: High prevalence of mutations of p53 gene in poorly differentiated thyroid carcinomas. J Clin Invest 91:179–184, 1993.

82. Iida F, Yonekura M, Miyakawa M: Study of intraglandular dissemination of thyroid cancer. Cancer 24:764, 1969.

83. Hazard JB: Small papillary carcinoma of the thyroid. Lab Invest 9:86, 1960.

84. Hazard JB, Hawk WA, Crile G Jr: Medullary (solid) carcinoma of the thyroid: A clinicopathologic entity. J Clin Endocrinol Metab 19:152, 1959.

85. Wu P S-C, Leslie PJ, McLaren KM, Toft AD: Diffuse sclerosing papillary carcinoma of thyroid: A wolf in sheep's clothing. Clin Endocrinol 31:535–540, 1989.

86. McDermott WV Jr, Morgan WS, Hamlin E Jr, Cope O: Cancer of the thyroid. J Clin Endocrinol Metab 14:1336, 1954.

87. DeGroot LJ, Kaplan EL, McCormick M, Straus FH: Natural history, treatment, and course of papillary thyroid carcinoma. J Clin Endocrinol Metab 71:414–424, 1990.

88. Hay ID: Papillary thyroid carcinoma. Endocrinol Metab Clin North Am 19:545–576, 1990.

89. Woolner LB, Lemmon ML, Beahrs OH, et al: Occult papillary carcinoma of the thyroid: Study of 140 cases observed in a 30-year period. J Clin Endocrinol Metab 20:89, 1960.

90. Franssila K: Value of histologic classification of thyroid cancer. Acta Pathol Micro Scand, Section A. Supplement No. 225, 1971, pp. 1–76.

91. McConahey WM, Hay ID, Woolner LB, et al: Papillary thyroid cancer treated at the Mayo Clinic, 1946 through 1970: Initial manifestations, pathologic findings, therapy, and outcome. Mayo Clin Proc 61:978–996, 1986.

92. Schlumberger M, De Vathaire F, Travagli JP, et al: Differentiated thyroid carcinoma in childhood: Long-term follow-up of 72 patients. J Clin Endocrinol Metab 65:1088–1094, 1987.

93. Belfiore A, Garofalo MR, Giuffrida D, et al: Increased aggressiveness of thyroid cancer in patients with Graves' disease. J Clin Endocrinol Metab 70:830–835, 1990.

94. Mazzaferri EL: Editorial: Thyroid cancer and Graves' disease. J Clin Endocrinol Metab 70:826–829, 1990.

95. Filetti S, Belfiore A, Amir SM, et al: The role of thyroid-stimulating antibodies of Graves' disease in differentiated thyroid cancer. N Engl J Med 318:753–759, 1988.

96. Har-El G, Hadar T, Segal K, et al: Hürthle cell carcinoma of the thyroid gland. Cancer 57:1613–1617, 1986.

97. Sipple JH: The association of pheochromocytoma with carcinoma of the thyroid gland. Am J Med 31:163–166, 1961.

98. Camiel MR, Mule JE, Alexander LL, Benninghoff DL: Association of thyroid carcinoma with Gardner's syndrome in siblings. N Engl J Med 278:1056, 1968.

99. Wolfe HJ, Melvin KEW, Cervi-Skinner SJ, et al: C-cell hyperplasia preceding medullary thyroid carcinoma. N Engl J Med 289:437, 1973.

100. Donahower GF, Schumacher OP, Hazard JB: Medullary carcinoma of the thyroid—A cause of Cushing's syndrome: Report of two cases. J Clin Endocrinol Metab 28:1199, 1968.

101. Baylin SB, Beaven MA, Engelman K, Sjoerdsma A, et al: Elevated histaminase activity in medullary carcinoma of the thyroid gland. N Engl J Med 283:1239, 1970.

102. Graze K, Spiler IJ, Tashjian AH Jr, et al: Natural history of familial medullary thyroid carcinoma. Effect of a program for early diagnosis. N Engl J Med 299:980–985, 1978.

103. Melvin KEW, Miller HH, Tashjian AH: Early diagnosis of medullary carcinoma of the thyroid gland by means of calcitonin assay. N Engl J Med 285:1115, 1971.

104. Halnan KE: Perspectives and Prospects in Thyroid Cancer. *In* Duncan, W. (ed): Recent Results in Cancer Research, Vol. 73, New York, Springer-Verlag, 1980, pp 129–137.

105. Harada T, Ito K, Shimaoka K, et al: Fatal thyroid carcinoma. Anaplastic transformation of adenocarcinoma. Cancer 39:2588–2596, 1977.

106. Justin EP, Seabold JE, Robinson RA, et al: Insular carcinoma: A distinct thyroid carcinoma with associated iodine-131 localization. J Nucl Med 32:1358–1363, 1991.

107. Harmer MH: Application of TNM classification rules to malignant tumors of the thyroid gland. *In* Hedlinger CE (ed): Thyroid Cancer. UICC Monograph Series 12:64, Berlin, Springer, 1969.

108. Baldet L, Manderscheid J-C, Glinoer D, et al: The management of differentiated thyroid cancer in Europe in 1988. Results of an international survey. Acta Endocrinol (Copenh) 120:547–558, 1989.

109. McConahey WM, Hay ID, Woolner LB, et al: Papillary thyroid cancer treated at the Mayo Clinic, 1946 through 1970: Initial manifestations, pathologic findings, therapy, and outcome. Mayo Clin Proc 61:978–996, 1986.

110. Simpson WJ, McKinney SE, Carruthers JS, et al: Papillary and follicular thyroid cancer. Prognostic factors in 1,578 patients. Am J Med 83:479–488, 1987.

111. Cady B, Rossi R, Silverman M, Wool M: Further evidence of the validity of risk group definition in differentiated thyroid carcinoma. Surgery 98:1171–1178, 1985.

112. Snyder J, Gorman C, Scanlon P: Thyroid remnant ablation: Questionable pursuit of an ill-defined goal. J Nucl Med 24:659–665, 1983.

113. Thoresen SO, Akslen LA, Glattre E, et al: Survival and prognostic factors in differentiated thyroid cancer—a multivariate analysis of 1,055 cases. Br J Cancer 59:231–235, 1989.

114. Beenken S, Guillamondegui O, Shallenberger R, et al: Prognostic factors in patients dying of well-differentiated thyroid cancer. Arch Otolaryngol Head Neck Surg 115:326–330, 1989.

115. Hamming JF, Van de Velde CJH, Goslings BM, et al: Prognosis and morbidity after total thyroidectomy for papillary, follicular, and medullary thyroid cancer. Eur J Cancer Clin Oncol 25:1317–1323, 1989.

116. Jensen MH, Davis RK, Derrick L: Thyroid cancer: A computer-assisted review of 5287 cases. Otolaryngol Head Neck Surg 102:51–65, 1990.

117. Tennvall J, Biorklund A, Moller T, et al: Is the EORTC prognostic index of thyroid cancer valid in differentiated thyroid carcinoma? Retrospective multivariate analysis of differentiated thyroid carcinoma with long follow-up. Cancer 57:1405–1414, 1986.

118. Byar DP, Green SB, Dor P, et al: A prognostic index for thyroid carcinoma. A study of the E.O.R.T.C. thyroid cancer cooperative group. Eur J Cancer 15:1033–1041, 1979.

119. Cady B, Rossi R: An expanded view of risk-group definition in differentiated thyroid carcinoma. Surgery 104:947–953, 1988.

120. Andry G, Chantrain G, Van Glabbeke M, Dor P: Papillary and follicular thyroid carcinoma. Individualization of the treatment according to the prognosis of the disease. Eur J Cancer Clin Oncol 24:1641–1646, 1988.

121. Schelfhout LJDM, Creutzberg CL, Hamming JF, et al: Multivariate analysis of survival in differentiated thyroid cancer: The prognostic significance of the age factor. Eur J Cancer Clin Oncol 24:331–337, 1988.

122. Hamming JF, Van de Velde CJH, Fleuren GJ, Goslings BM: Differentiated thyroid cancer: A stage adapted approach to the treatment of regional lymph node metastases. Eur J Cancer Clin Oncol 24:325–330, 1988.

123. Clark OH, Levin K, Zeng Q-H, et al: Thyroid cancer: The case for total thyroidectomy. Eur J Cancer Clin Oncol 24:305–313, 1988.

124. Harness JK, McLeod MK, Thompson NW, et al: Deaths due to differentiated thyroid cancer. A 46-year perspective. World J Surg 12:623–629, 1988.

125. Allo MD, Christianson W, Koivunen D: Not all "occult" papillary carcinomas are "minimal." Surgery 104:971–976, 1988.

126. Samaan NA, Schultz PN, Hickey RC, et al: The results of various modalities of treatment of well differentiated thyroid carcinoma: A retrospective review of 1,599 patients. J Clin Endocrinol Metab 75:714–720, 1992.

127. Mazzaferri EL: Treating differentiated thyroid carcinoma: Where do we draw the line? Mayo Clin Proc 66:105–111, 1991.

128. Mazzaferri EL, Young RL: Papillary thyroid carcinoma: A ten-year

follow-up report of the impact of therapy in 576 patients. Am J Med 70:511–518, 1981.

129. Massin J-P, Savoie J-C, Garnier H, et al: Pulmonary metastases in differentiated thyroid carcinoma. Study of 58 cases with implications for the primary tumor treatment. Cancer 53:982–992, 1984.

130. Andry G, Chantrain G, Van Glabbeke M, Dor P: Papillary and follicular thyroid carcinoma. Individualization of the treatment according to the prognosis of the disease. Eur J Cancer Clin Oncol 24:1641–1646, 1988.

131. Brennan MD, Bergstralh EJ, van Heerden JA, McConahey WM: Follicular thyroid cancer treated at the Mayo Clinic, 1946 through 1970: Initial manifestations, pathologic findings, therapy, and outcome. Mayo Clin Proc 66:11–22, 1991.

132. Buckwalter JA, Thomas CG: Selection of surgical treatment for well-differentiated thyroid carcinomas. Ann Surg 176:565, 1972.

133. Rustad WH, Lindsay S, Dailey ME: Comparison of the incidence of complications following total and subtotal thyroidectomy for thyroid carcinoma. Surg Gynec Obstet 116:109, 1963.

134. Black B, Yadeau R, Woolner L: Surgical treatment of thyroid carcinomas. Arch Surg 88:610, 1964.

135. Shands WC, Gatling RR: Cancer of the thyroid: Review of 109 cases. Ann Surg 171:735, 1970.

136. Tollefsen HR, Shah JP, Huvos AG: Papillary carcinoma of the thyroid. Recurrence in the thyroid gland after initial surgical treatment. Am J Surg 124:468, 1972.

137. Tollefson H, DeCosse J: Papillary carcinoma of the thyroid: The case for radical neck dissection. Am J Surg 108:547, 1964.

138. Lang W, Choritz H, Hundeshagen H: Risk factors in follicular thyroid carcinomas. A retrospective follow-up study covering a 14-year period with emphasis on morphological findings. Am J Surg Pathol 10:246–255, 1986.

139. Duffield RGM, Lowe D, Burnand KG: Treatment of well-differentiated carcinoma of the thyroid based on initial staging. Br J Surg 69:426–428, 1982.

140. Young RL, Mazzaferri EL, Rahe AJ, Dorfman SG: Pure follicular thyroid carcinoma: Impact of therapy in 214 patients. J Nucl Med 21:733–737, 1980.

141. Block GE, Wilson SM: A modified neck dissection for carcinoma of the thyroid. Surg Clin North Am 51:139, 1971.

142. Mustard RA: Treatment of papillary carcinoma of the thyroid with emphasis on conservative neck dissection. Am J Surg 120:697, 1970.

143. Simpson WJ, Panzarella T, Carruthers JS, et al: Papillary and follicular thyroid cancer: Impact of treatment in 1578 patients. Int J Radiation Oncol Biol Phys 14:1063–1075, 1988.

144. Watson RG, Brennan MD, Goellner JR, et al: Invasive Hürthle cell carcinoma of the thyroid: Natural history and management. Mayo Clin Proc 59:851–855, 1984.

145. Watson RG, Brennan MD, Goellner JR, et al: Invasive Hürthle cell carcinoma of the thyroid. Natural history and management. Mayo Clin Proc 59:851–855, 1984.

146. Har-El G, Hadar T, Segal K, et al: Hürthle cell carcinoma of the thyroid gland: A tumor of moderate malignancy. Cancer 57:1613–1617, 1986.

147. Devine RM, Edis AJ, Banks PM: Primary lymphoma of the thyroid: A review of the Mayo Clinic experience through 1978. World J Surg 5:33–38, 1981.

148. Butler JS, Jr, Brady LW, Amendola BE: Lymphoma of the thyroid. Report of five cases and review. Am J Clin Oncol 13:64–69, 1990.

149. Leedman PJ, Sheridan WP, Downey WF, et al: Combination chemotherapy as single modality therapy for stage IE and IIE thyroid lymphoma. Med J Aust 152:40–43, 1990.

150. Nel CJC, van Heerden JA, Goellner JR, et al: Anaplastic carcinoma of the thyroid. A clinicopathologic study of 82 cases. Mayo Clin Proc 60:51–58, 1985.

151. Gam AN, Jensen GF, Hasselstrom K, et al: Effect of thyroxine therapy on bone metabolism in substituted hypothyroid patients with normal or suppressed levels of TSH. J Endocrinol Invest 14:451–455, 1991.

152. Tubiana M, Schlumberger M, Rougier P, et al: Long-term results and prognostic factors in patients with differentiated thyroid carcinoma. Cancer 55:794–804, 1985.

153. Samaan NA, Schultz PN, Haynie TP, Ordonez, NG: Pulmonary metastasis of differentiated thyroid carcinoma: Treatment results in 101 patients. J Clin Endocrinol Metab 65:376–380, 1985.

154. Beierwaltes WH, Rabbani R, Dmuchowski C, et al: An analysis of "ablation of thyroid remnants" with ^{131}I in 511 patients from 1947–

1984: Experience at University of Michigan. J Nucl Med 25:1287–1293, 1984.

155. DeGroot LJ, Reilly M: Comparison of 30- and 50-mCi doses of iodine-131 for thyroid ablation. Ann Intern Med 96:51–53, 1982.

156. Maxon HR III, Smith HS: Radioiodine-131 in the diagnosis and treatment of metastatic well-differentiated thyroid cancer. Endocrinol Metab Clin North Am 19:685–718, 1990.

157. Pacini F, Lippi F, Formica N, et al: Therapeutic doses of iodine-131 reveal undiagnosed metastases in thyroid cancer patients with detectable serum thyroglobulin levels. J Nucl Med 28:1888–1891, 1987.

158. Dobyns B, Maloof F: Study and treatment of 119 cases of carcinoma of the thyroid with radioactive iodine. J Clin Endocrinol 11:1323, 1951.

159. Handelsman DJ, Turtle JR: Testicular damage after radioactive iodine (I-131) therapy for thyroid cancer. Clin Endocrinol 18:465–472, 1983.

160. Keldsen N, Mortensen BT, Hansen HS: Hematological effects from radioiodine treatment of thyroid cancer. Acta Oncolog 29:1035, 1990.

161. Pochin EE: Leukemia following radioiodine treatment of thyrotoxicosis. Br Med J 2:1545, 1960.

162. Edmonds CJ, Smith T: The long-term hazards of the treatment of thyroid cancer with radioiodine. Br J Radiol 59:45–51, 1986.

163. Hall P, Holm L-E, Lundell G, et al: Cancer risks in thyroid cancer patients. Br J Cancer 64:159–163, 1991.

164. Varma VM, Beierwaltes WH, Nofal MM, et al: Treatment of thyroid cancer. Death rates after surgery and after surgery followed by sodium iodide I-131. JAMA 214:1437, 1970.

165. Leeper RD: The effect of 131-I therapy on survival of patients with metastatic papillary or follicular thyroid carcinoma. J Clin Endocrinol Metab 36:1143, 1973.

166. Fairweather DS, Bradwell AR, Watson-James SF, et al: Detection of thyroid tumors using radio-labelled anti-thyroglobulin. Clin Endocrinol 18:563–570, 1983.

167. DeGroot LJ, Reilly M: Use of isotope bone scans and skeletal survey X-rays in the follow-up of patients with thyroid carcinoma. J Endocrinol Invest 7:175, 1984.

168. DeGroot LJ, Hoye K, Refetoff S, et al: Serum antigens and antibodies in the diagnosis of thyroid cancer. J Clin Endocrinol Metab 45:1220–1223, 1977.

169. Barsano CP, Skosey C, DeGroot LJ, Refetoff S: Serum thyroglobulin in the management of patients with thyroid cancer. Arch Intern Med 142:763–767, 1982.

170. Gerfo PL, Stillman T, Colacchio D, Feind C: Serum thyroglobulin and recurrent thyroid cancer. Lancet 1:881–882, 1977.

171. Meier CA, Braverman LE, Ebner SA, et al: Diagnostic use of recombinant human thyrotropin in patients with thyroid carcinoma. Thyroid 2:S–35, 1992.

172. Simpson WJ, Carruthers JS: The role of external radiation in the management of papillary and follicular thyroid cancer. Am J Surg 136:457–460, 1978.

173. Grauer A, Raue F, Gagel RF: Changing concepts in the management of hereditary and sporadic medullary thyroid carcinoma. Endocrinol Metab Clin North Am 19:613–635, 1990.

174. Shimaoka K: Adjunctive management of thyroid cancer: Chemotherapy. J Surg Oncol 15:283–286, 1980.

175. Bukowski RM, Brown L, Weick JK, et al: Combination chemotherapy of metastatic thyroid cancer. Phase II study. Am J Clin Oncol 6:579–581, 1983.

176. De Besi P, Busnardo B, Toso S, et al: Combined chemotherapy with bleomycin, Adriamycin, and platinum in advanced thyroid cancer. J Endocrinol Invest 14:475–480, 1991.

177. Droz J-P, Schlumberger M, Rougier P, et al: Chemotherapy in metastatic nonanaplastic thyroid cancer: Experience at the Institut Gustave-Roussy. Tumori 76:480–483, 1990.

178. Kim JH, Leeper RD: Treatment of anaplastic giant and spindle cell carcinoma of the thyroid gland with combination Adriamycin and radiation therapy. A new approach. Cancer 52:954–957, 1983.

179. Gottlieb JA, Hill CS: Adriamycin (NSC-123127) therapy in thyroid carcinoma. Cancer Chemotherapy Reports, Part 3, Vol. 6:283–296, 1975.

180. Hill CS: Chemotherapy of thyroid cancer. In Kaplan EL (ed): Surgery of the Thyroid and Parathyroid Glands. Edinburgh, Churchill Livingstone, 1983, pp. 120–126, 1983.

Medullary Carcinoma of the Thyroid

E. DILLWYN WILLIAMS

Medullary carcinoma of the thyroid was recognized as a separate type of thyroid carcinoma derived from thyroid C cells about 30 years ago.[1] It is now clearly established as a distinct entity defined as a malignant tumor showing evidence of C-cell differentiation.[2] It can occur either as part of a group of dominantly inherited cancer syndromes in which the tumor is associated with C-cell hyperplasia or as a sporadically occurring tumor. Whether genetically determined or sporadic, it may be associated with a variety of humorally mediated syndromes. The different embryological origins of C and follicular cells were apparently paralleled by complete separation of the tumors derived from them. The description over the last few years of a tumor showing evidence of both C-cell and follicular-cell differentiation, the mixed medullary follicular carcinoma, has lead to a reappraisal of the origins of the C cell.

The first observations that established the existence of a second type of epithelial cell in the thyroid were those of Baber in 1876.[3] His work in the dog was confirmed and extended to other species by numerous observers. The study of the morphology of these cells was helped by the discovery that they could be distinguished from the follicular cells by silver impregnation techniques.[4] We currently recognize that there are two morphologically quite separate types of epithelial cells in the mammalian thyroid— the follicular cell and the C, or parafollicular, cell. The C cell usually lies between the follicular cell and the basement membrane (Fig. 51–1) or forms small solid nests of cells in an apparent interfollicular position. Electron microscopy shows that it lacks the distended cisternae of the follicular cell and contains electron-dense secretory granules of the type seen in polypeptide hormone–producing endocrine cells. Getzowa[5] suggested that the embryological origin of these cells was different from that of the thyroid follicular cell as long ago as 1907. Her suggestion that these cells were derived from the ultimobranchial body was sup-

ported in 1937 by Godwin.[6] Pearse and Carvalheira[7] demonstrated by cytochemical techniques in the rodent that these cells were carried to the thyroid by the ultimobranchial body, but the quail chick transplant work of Le Douarin and Le Lievre[8] showed that precursor cells reached the ultimobranchial body from the neural crest. The mammalian thyroid is thus clearly established as a dual endocrine gland. The usually accepted view is that the major component is formed by the follicular cells, which are derived from the thyroglossal duct, and can be regarded as modified intestinal cells, secreting into and absorbing from a lumen. The minor component is formed by the C cells, which are derived from the neural crest, secrete calcitonin (Figs. 51–2, 3), and are true endocrine cells.

The embryology of the thyroid is more complex than was at first thought. The simple proposal that the thyroglossal duct gives rise to follicular cells concerned with thyroid hormone synthesis and the neural crest gives rise to C cells that reach the thyroid via the ultimobranchial body and are concerned with calcitonin and related peptide production remains accepted but is incomplete. Studies of patients with maldescent of the central thyroid anlage found that the ultimobranchial body had not fused with the inadequately descended thyroglossal duct thyroid and contained C cells, recognized by their morphology and calcitonin content.[9] This demonstrated that in humans the C cells reach the thyroid via the ultimobranchial body. However, a small number of thyroglobulin-containing follicles also were described in ultimobranchial tissue, and thyroglobulin also has been found in the branchial cleft mucosa.[10] Thyroid follicles may therefore be derived from both the central and lateral anlages. C cells have not been shown to arise from thyroglossal duct tissue, but the work of Le Douarin and Le Lievre, which clearly demonstrates that C-cell precursors are derived from the neural crest in the quail, does not prove that all C cells in humans are of neural crest derivation.

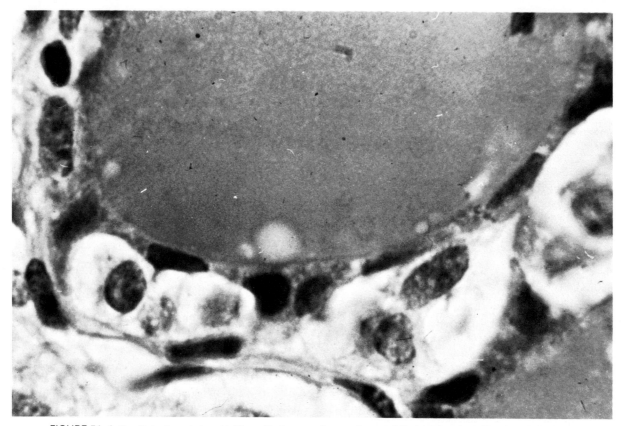

FIGURE 51–1. C cells in the rat thyroid. The cells show a pale cytoplasm and lie between the follicular cells and the basement membrane. They are unusually numerous in this photomicrograph (PAS stain; × 900).

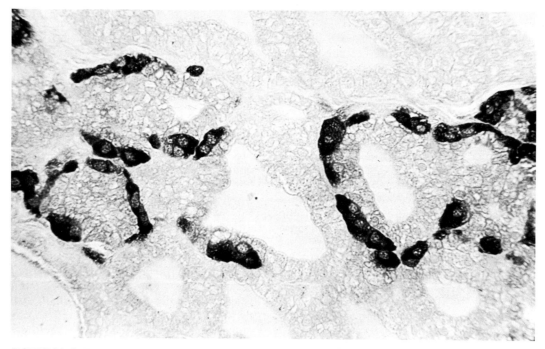

FIGURE 51–2. Calcitonin in rat C cells. This immunoperoxidase technique uses an antibody to human calcitonin. The C cells are darkly staining with relatively unstained nuclei. The follicular cells can just be distinguished (peroxidase stain; × 350).

INCIDENCE

Medullary carcinoma has been reported to comprise between 1.4 and 10 per cent of all thyroid carcinomas,[11, 12] with a mean figure of 6.8 per cent. Several factors may influence this variation in reported incidence. First, the incidence of either medullary carcinoma or thyroid carcinomas derived from the follicular cell may be influenced by racial or environmental factors. Second, the diagnostic criteria or the accuracy of their application for both C-cell and follicular-cell tumors may well vary in different areas. Third, the existence of a large family with many affected members in one area will lead to a considerable increase in frequency of occurrence of this tumor in the hospital serving that population. Finally, the figures quoted are for relative, not absolute, incidence.

Despite the importance of these factors, it seems likely that there is a geographical variation in the incidence of sporadic medullary carcinoma. A study of the incidence of medullary carcinoma in two well-defined populations—Iceland and northeast Scotland—has shown that it accounted for 5 per cent of all thyroid cancers in Iceland, an area with an unusually high incidence of papillary carcinomas, but that no cases occurred in a 20-year period in a population of 500,000 people in northeast Scotland.[13] Although the numbers in this study were small, the Icelandic incidence is similar to the 3.6 per cent incidence reported in a large recent study in Norway,[14] and the incidence in northeast Scotland confirmed previous personal communications that this tumor is rare in Scotland. In Japan, a country like Iceland with a high iodine intake and a high incidence of papillary carcinoma, medullary carcinoma accounted for only 1.4 per cent of over 10,000 registered cases of thyroid carcinoma.[12] Absolute rather than relative figures for the incidence of medullary carcinoma of the thyroid are available for several tumor registries; for Connecticut and Sweden, it is approximately 2 per million per year; for Norway, approximately 1.5 new cases per million per year.[14–16]

In contrast to the other types of thyroid cancer and to most thyroid disease, the incidence in males and females is almost equal. In sporadic cases, the female-to-male ratio is 1.3:1; in genetically determined cases, it is 1:1. The age at presentation varies widely from infancy to old age, with the majority of sporadic cases presenting in the fourth, fifth, and sixth decades.

PATHOLOGY

The classic histopathological features of this tumor have been described in detail elsewhere.[11, 17] The tumor is a solid, often hard mass, well circumscribed but not encapsulated. At a light-microscope level, it is composed of sheets of cells with abundant granular cytoplasm. Typically, it contains irregular masses of amyloid and often much collagen, and it lacks papillary or follicular differentiation (Fig. 51–4). On electron microscopy, characteristic small electron-dense membrane-limited secretory granules can be seen (Fig. 51–5). The tumor may be composed of fusiform cells forming a whorling pattern, and rarely the more rapidly growing forms may show a pattern reminiscent of an oat-cell carcinoma. While the tumor was originally recognized by its amyloid content, the definition of medullary carcinoma as a calcitonin-secreting tumor and the use of calcitonin immunocytochemistry to recognize the tumor content of calcitonin has greatly broadened the spectrum of tumors recognized as medullary carcinoma. Glandular, papillary, small-cell, and anaplastic variants have all been described,[18–22] and in about 20 per cent of cases, no amyloid can be detected histochemically.[23] Although normal C cells in humans do not form glandular structures, these may be found in ultimobranchial glands of lower vertebrates. The variant patterns may be found together with the classic pattern or may be uniform. Their recognition implies that in any histologically puzzling thyroid tumor it is necessary to use calcitonin immunohistochemistry before a medullary carcinoma can be excluded. Very rarely, medullary carcinoma of the thyroid also may be associated with melanin production, and the same tumor cell has been shown to contain both melanin and calcitonin.[24]

No single histological feature of the tumor can be used reliably to distinguish genetically determined from sporadic medullary carcinoma. The major microscopic differences are that the genetically determined tumors may show multifocality and especially that they are associated with C-cell hyperplasia in the normal background thyroid. The histological features of a tumor are linked to its clinical behavior, with the more slowly growing tumors showing regular polygonal cells with abundant granular cytoplasm often with abundant stromal amyloid, few mitoses, and a well-delimited, rounded tumor and the more rapidly growing tumors showing spindle cells, little or no amyloid, frequent mitoses, and wide infiltration of the gland, often including vascular infiltration. The calcitonin content of tumor cells broadly correlates with the degree of differentiation. Interestingly, the calcitonin mRNA content shown by in situ hybridization (Fig. 51–6) may still be high at a time when peptide storage shown by immunohistochemistry is greatly reduced.[25]

CLINICAL PRESENTATION AND SPREAD

The majority of patients who present with sporadic tumors are found to have a thyroid mass, often with palpable

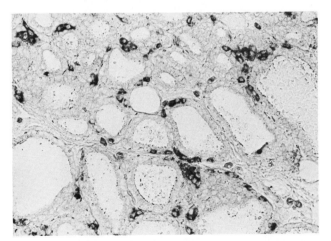

FIGURE 51–3. Localization of calcitonin mRNA in normal rat thyroid using a digoxigenin-labeled oligoprobe and alkaline phosphatase detection system (× 175).

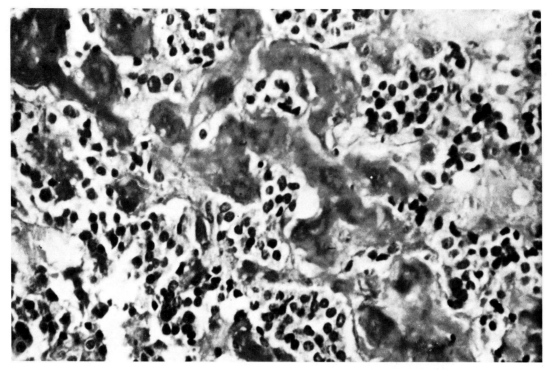

FIGURE 51–4. Typical histological appearance of medullary carcinoma of the thyroid. The amorphous amyloid lies between solid groups of regular tumor cells (H&E stain; × 200).

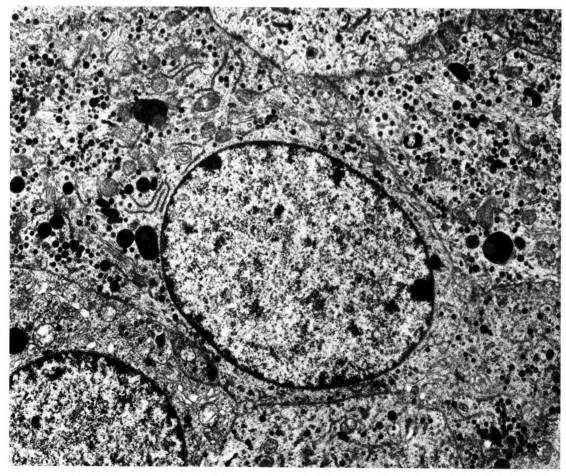

FIGURE 51–5. Electron micrograph of medullary carcinoma showing a light cell with numerous small electron-dense secretory granules (× 14,000).

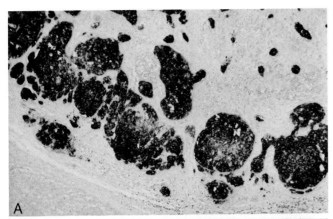

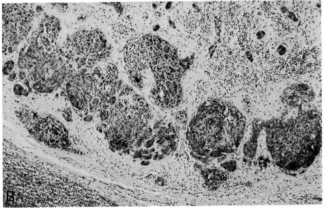

FIGURE 51–6. Comparison of localization of calcitonin mRNA by in situ hybridization with localization of calcitonin peptide by immunocytochemistry in a medullary carcinoma metastatic to lymph node. Note relative uniformity of mRNA distribution in these serial sections. (*A*) In situ hybridization using a digoxigenin-labeled calcitonin oligoprobe and alkaline phosphatase detection system. (*B*) Immunocytochemistry using polyclonal antibody to human calcitonin and peroxidase detection system.

cervical lymph nodes. The diagnosis, as with any thyroid tumor, is commonly established by fine-needle aspiration and can be confirmed by plasma calcitonin assay. At operation, involved cervical lymph nodes are found in two thirds of the patients.[11] The other common site for early extrathyroid tumor spread is the upper mediastinum, where massive secondary tumor deposits may be found (Fig. 51–7). Spread beyond the neck and mediastinum usually occurs late in the natural history of the disease, with the lungs, liver, and bones being the most common sites. Metastases to bone are sometimes osteoblastic, although lytic metastasis to the spine with paralysis due to cord compression is not infrequent in disseminated medullary carcinoma. In one autopsy study, all cases were found to show involvement of cervical lymph nodes, with 75 per cent showing mediastinal involvement. Lungs were involved in 85 per cent, liver in 69 per cent, and bones in 54 per cent. All other sites occurred in less than a third of the cases.[26] Among the various sites, it is worth mentioning skin, which is very uncommonly involved in other types of thyroid carcinoma but occasionally involved by metastatic medullary carcinoma.[27] Of the various hormonally mediated syndromes associated with medullary carcinoma, diarrhea is the most prominent clinically. It is present in about one quarter of all patients and may be the presenting complaint. The presence of diarrhea in a patient with

a thyroid mass, clinically a neoplasm, should raise the suspicion of medullary carcinoma.

CALCITONIN AND OTHER SECRETORY PRODUCTS

Calcitonin

Calcitonin is consistently produced by medullary carcinoma of the thyroid (Fig. 51–8). The tumor, like the normal C cell, contains electron-dense membrane-limited secretory granules, which are the site of calcitonin storage. The chemistry and action of calcitonin are discussed elsewhere.

The measurement of serum calcitonin is of value in establishing the diagnosis of medullary carcinoma, in establishing the presence of metastases, and in following the effects of treatment.[28, 29] It has been of particular value in family studies on the genetic group, especially if stimulation tests such as calcium infusion, pentagastrin infusion, or alcohol are used.

Excess calcitonin may be found in association with other tumors, particularly oat cell carcinoma of the lung, carci-

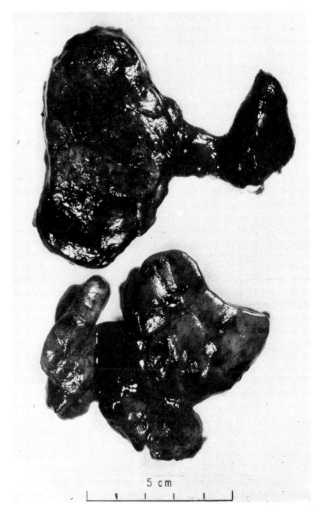

5 cm

FIGURE 51–7. Macroscopic appearance of medullary carcinoma of the thyroid. The greater part of the right lobe of the thyroid is replaced by a solid tumor. The lower mass of tumor was removed from the upper anterior mediastinum.

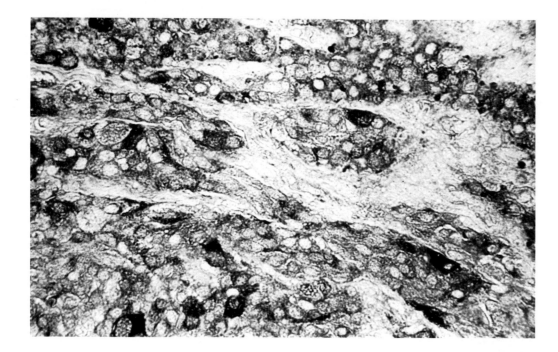

FIGURE 51–8. Calcitonin in medullary carcinoma. The cords of tumor cells show a variable content of calcitonin, demonstrated with an immunoperoxidase technique (× 400).

noids, and carcinoma of the breast,[30, 31] and in patients with the Zollinger-Ellison syndrome.[32] In most of these cases it can be shown that the calcitonin is being produced by the tumor itself, and in some cases, patients with nonmedullary carcinomas have been shown to have both elevated circulating levels of calcitonin and an increase following pentagastrin stimulation.[33] The finding of a high circulating level of calcitonin is therefore not in itself proof of the presence of medullary carcinoma. In one survey, thyroid tumors were responsible for elevated calcitonin only in a minority of cases. A number of nonmalignant causes for elevated circulating calcitonin levels have been described. These include diseases with elevated levels of gut hormones such as gastrin or glucagon, which are known to stimulate calcitonin release.

Calcitonin Gene Products

The product of the calcitonin gene, which in humans lies on chromosome 11,[34] is complex, and as well as two flanking peptides, a quite separate peptide, calcitonin gene–related peptide (CGRP), is known to exist. The C-terminal flanking peptide katacalcin has no known function, although it was at first thought to share the hypocalcemic property of calcitonin. It is produced in equimolar amounts with calcitonin and can be localized to normal C cells and to the cells of medullary carcinoma.[35] CGRP is produced by differential RNA processing from the calcitonin gene and is present in normal C cells, although in much reduced amounts by comparison with calcitonin. The calcitonin gene is active in the cells of the nervous system, where it produces CGRP rather than calcitonin.[36] CGRP is a highly potent vasoactive peptide with no known effect on calcium metabolism. It is present in medullary carcinoma; immunohistochemistry commonly shows strongly positive scattered large tumor cells with elongated processes and in a generally weak or negative tumor.[37] CGRP may be produced by other tumors; for example, like

calcitonin, it is secreted by some oat-cell carcinomas of the lung.[38, 39]

Recently the synthesis of calcitonin and CGRP has been shown to be more complex. CGRP may be produced by a second gene, and a novel carboxy-terminal peptide encoding calcitonin has been described in both medullary carcinoma and normal thyroid tissue. Most calcitonin mRNA is produced by splicing the first three exons to the fourth polyadenylated exon, while CGRP results from splicing the first three exons to the fifth and the sixth polyadenylated exon. The second type of calcitonin mRNA results from splicing all six exons, excluding part of exon four. The resulting peptides are calcitonin and a newly recognized 21-amino acid carboxy-terminal peptide.[40, 41]

ACTH and Corticotropin-Releasing Hormone

Cushing's syndrome has been recorded on a number of occasions with medullary carcinoma.[42] In most cases, ectopic production of ACTH by the tumor is the cause of the Cushing's syndrome. Production of both calcitonin and ACTH by the same tumor has been demonstrated, and removal of the thyroid carcinoma has led to regression of the Cushing's syndrome.[42–44] Other products of the proopiomelanocortin gene also have been described as being produced by medullary carcinoma; for example, B melanocyte–stimulating hormone[45] and proopiomelanocortin mRNA has been found in metastases of two patients with medullary carcinoma.[46]

Ectopic production of corticotropin-releasing hormone (CRH) also may be the cause of the Cushing's syndrome in some cases of medullary carcinoma. CRH and ACTH may be present in the same tumor[47] or CRH alone may be found,[48] and as with ACTH, removal of a CRH-containing medullary carcinoma has led to cure of the associated Cushing's syndrome.[49]

Other Regulatory Peptides

A number of other regulatory peptides have been found in medullary carcinoma, including somatostatin, β-endorphin, leuenkephalin, bombesin, substance P, vasoactive intestinal peptide (VIP), and neurotensin. Of these, somatostatin is found in the normal C cell, where it co-localizes with calcitonin in a subpopulation of C cells in the rat thyroid.[50] It is possible that one or more of the regulatory peptides are involved in the pathogenesis of the diarrhea associated with medullary carcinoma, but proof is lacking. It also has been suggested that bombesin secretion may on rare occasions be the cause of an associated Cushing's syndrome through potentiation of the secretion of CRH.[51] Somatostatin is often found in scattered single cells in medullary carcinoma, the positive cells sometimes showing elongated processes. Between 70 and 100 per cent of tumors contain immunoreactive somatostatin, but only 10 per cent show elevated serum levels.[52, 53] It has been suggested that somatostatin-rich tumors are associated with a better survival than tumors with little or no detectable somatostatin.[53, 54] Regulatory peptides also occur in the nerve fibers in the thyroid and may, together with some of the peptides produced by C cells, play a role in modulating thyroid follicular cell function.

Biogenic Amines

It has been known for many years that the thyroid in some species has a high content of 5-hydroxytryptamine (5-HT).[55] Falck et al.[56] showed that in the sheep thyroid, the amine was confined to the parafollicular (C) cells. It also has been shown that C cells contain dopa decarboxylase and are able to take up dopa and 5-hydroxytryptophan and decarboxylate them, respectively, to dopamine and 5-HT.[57, 58] It is therefore not surprising that some patients with medullary carcinoma show a raised urinary excretion of 5-hydroxyindoleacetic acid, although the majority do not show elevated levels.[59, 60] High levels of 5-HT have been recorded in the tumor itself,[59, 61] which also has been shown to have a high dopa decarboxylase content.[61, 62] It is rather more surprising that high levels of histaminase have been found in both tumor and serum in patients with medullary carcinoma.[63, 64] The flare response after intradermal histamine injection may be absent in patients with medullary carcinoma of the thyroid.[65, 66] While there has been speculation that this may be related to the raised levels of histaminase, the patients reported with absent flare also have had multiple mucosal neuromas. It seems likely that the abnormal response to histamine is due to a neural abnormality leading to an abnormal axon reflex.

Tumor Markers and Other Humoral Factors

Calcitonin is of course the main tumor marker for medullary carcinoma, although it must always be remembered that it may be produced by nonthyroid tumors. Katacalcin and CGRP assays add little information to that given by measurement of the serum calcitonin level. The second major tumor marker is carcinoembryonic antigen (CEA). Elevated levels of plasma CEA are found in the majority of cases of medullary carcinoma and only rarely in other types of thyroid carcinoma.[67, 68] There is a broad inverse relationship between measurable levels of serum calcitonin and CEA in relation to the degree of malignancy of the medullary carcinoma such that calcitonin levels are higher in the better-differentiated tumors and CEA levels are more consistently abnormal and also higher in the more malignant tumors.[29, 69, 70] While CEA measurements can therefore be used to define a high-risk group of patients with medullary carcinoma, it also has been suggested that cellular heterogeneity for dopa decarboxylase, histaminase, and calcitonin in the tumor is linked to poor prognosis.[71]

Some medullary carcinomas contain and secrete prostaglandins E_2 and F_2,[72–76] and prostaglandin production has been shown in tissue culture.[77] It is not consistently present, however,[78] and its significance in various tumor syndromes remains uncertain. A number of less clearly defined factors have occasionally been found in medullary carcinoma. A substance with prolactin-stimulating activity has been found in one patient, associated with galactorrhea.[47] Gynecomastia was recorded in one other case.[79] An osteoblast-stimulating factor has been described in the parafollicular cells of "gray lethal" mice,[80] and it is of interest that osteopetrosis has been described in the children of a patient with medullary carcinoma of the thyroid.[81] Finally, high levels of nerve growth factor have been found in the plasma of a patient with medullary carcinoma of the thyroid.[82]

Amyloid

The initial recognition of medullary carcinoma as a separate entity was based on the presence of amyloid. Clarification of its histogenesis has redefined the tumor as one showing C-cell differentiation. A significant minority of tumors lack any demonstrable amyloid, but it remains a common finding.[23]

The amyloid is produced by the tumor cells themselves, as has been shown by morphological and tissue culture studies. The first indication that the amyloid from medullary carcinoma of the thyroid differs from the amyloid associated with chronic infections came from a study by Benditt and Eriksen,[83] who found that the amino acid composition of amyloid from several patients with chronic infections was consistent and was different from that found in a case of medullary carcinoma. Pearse et al.,[84] using histochemical techniques, found that the amyloid associated with endocrine tumors differed from that associated with chronic infections in its negative reaction to tyrosine and tryptophan—although Benditt and Eriksen had found little difference in tyrosine content.

Tashjian et al.[85] found that antibodies to calcitonin reacted with the amyloid in sections of medullary carcinoma, although the interpretation of this observation is made more difficult by the finding that the amyloid may contain cellular fragments, including secretory granules.[86] Sletten et al.,[87] however, have prepared and partially characterized amyloid fibril proteins from medullary carcinoma. The main fibril component was found to differ from other known amyloid proteins, and the AA and light-chain variable fragments found in other amyloids were not present in medullary carcinoma amyloid. The amino acid composition of the amyloid protein from medullary carcinoma differed considerably from calcitonin, but it contained an amino acid sequence identical to residues 9–19 in human calcitonin. The β-pleated sheet structure characteristic of amyloid has been shown to exist also in the amyloid associated with medullary carcinoma,[88] and the amyloid has been shown to take up bone-seeking phosphonates in vivo.[89]

It can be concluded, then, that as with other endocrine tumor amyloid, the amyloid found in medullary carcinoma is related to the peptide hormone product of the cell and is in a β-pleated sheet configuration. The AA protein typical of the amyloid associated with chronic inflammation and the immunoglobulin light chain typical of the amyloid associated with myeloma are absent.

Cutaneous lichen amyloidosis has been recorded in some families with MEN IIA. It is unrelated to the amyloid production by the tumor and forms part of a clearly defined autosomal dominant syndrome.[90–92]

HUMORALLY MEDIATED SYNDROMES

The range of substances secreted by medullary carcinoma of the thyroid is considerable, and it is not surprising that a variety of clinical syndromes due to humoral factors may be found in association with this tumor, whether sporadic or genetic. The most common of these is diarrhea. Williams[59] found that severe diarrhea was relatively common in patients with medullary carcinoma and that it was very frequent in patients with widespread tumors. These findings have been confirmed on a number of occasions, and the combined results of two large series show that diarrhea was present in about 20 per cent of all patients with medullary carcinoma and in about half the patients with disseminated carcinoma.[17, 35] It is surprising that although the diarrhea has been known to be associated with the tumor for over 25 years, the humoral factor concerned is not yet identified with certainty. There is no doubt that the diarrhea is humorally mediated, since resection of tumor may lead to great improvement in the diarrhea.[59, 93–95] One reason that the humoral factor has not yet been identified may be because several of the factors that medullary carcinoma may produce are likely to increase in gut motility. Certainly, prostaglandins may lead to hypermotility, and calcitonin itself may lead to borborygmi and increased jejunal secretion of water and electrolytes.[96, 97] It also has been shown to stimulate intestinal alkaline phosphatase activity.[98] Some of the other regulatory peptides that are produced by medullary carcinoma also may be associated with increased intestinal activity, as may 5-HT, although in the carcinoid syndrome kinins also may be involved.

The diarrhea is characterized by intestinal hypermotility, which may be extreme, with undigested food in the very frequent watery stools. Bernier et al.[94] found that steatorrhea was mild or absent and that there was excessive loss of water and electrolytes in the stools. Jejunal absorption is normal, but in the ileum, Na^+, Cl^-, and water were secreted into the lumen, while bicarbonate was absorbed—the reverse of normal.[73] These findings, and the abnormalities in intestinal transit, have been reported after administration of prostaglandin $F_{2\alpha}$. Nutmeg, which contains a prostaglandin synthetase inhibitor, given orally leads to improvement in the diarrhea.[76, 99] While prostaglandins seem

most consistently implicated, they have not always been demonstrable in patients with diarrhea,[78] and a multifactorial cause still seems likely.

This conclusion is supported by the variable occurrence of the other symptoms which may be associated with diarrhea. Flushing is the most common of these, occurring in one third of the patients with diarrhea; in some cases, there is pronounced episodic flushing, which, as in the carcinoid syndrome, may be induced by alcohol ingestion.[59, 60] Of the various substances produced by medullary carcinoma, CGRP, which is an extremely powerful peripheral vasodilator, is the most likely mediator.

Cushing's syndrome is another important humorally mediated complication of medullary carcinoma; it is found in approximately 5 per cent of cases.[100] In many examples of the ectopic ACTH syndrome, some of the typical clinical features are absent, probably because of the combination of the severity of the continual overproduction, the rapidity of onset, and the co-existence of a rapidly growing carcinoma with its accompanying weight loss. When Cushing's syndrome occurs with medullary carcinoma of the thyroid, it may show all the classic features, or it may resemble the atypical Cushing's syndrome found with tumors such as oat cell carcinoma of the lung. The cause of the Cushing's syndrome in these cases is almost always production of ACTH by the tumor, although, as has been mentioned above, CRH or bombesin, both of which possess CRH-releasing activity, also may be implicated. Treatment, as for other tumors that produce ectopic ACTH, is resection of tumor where possible and otherwise adrenalectomy.

Hypocalcemia is a major effect of the acute administration of calcitonin, but surprisingly, hypocalcemia does not appear to be a humoral effect of the chronic hypercalcitoninemia associated with medullary carcinoma of the thyroid in humans. Hypocalcemia has, however, been recorded as a humoral effect of C-cell tumors in dogs.[101]

The frequency of occurrence of diarrhea and Cushing's syndrome appears to be similar in both genetic and sporadic medullary carcinoma. Paraneoplastic eosinophilia has been described with metastatic medullary carcinoma.[102]

GENETICALLY MEDIATED SYNDROMES

One of the most interesting features of medullary carcinoma is the part it plays in a variety of genetically determined syndromes. Williams[103] and Schimke and Hartmann[104] pointed out that the link, reviewed by Sipple,[105] between pheochromocytoma and thyroid carcinoma was specifically with medullary carcinoma of the thyroid and that the condition was inherited. It is now evident that medullary carcinoma may be inherited without pheochromocytoma, that it may be inherited together with pheochromocytoma, or that it may be inherited with multiple mucosal neuromas, pheochromocytomas, ganglioneuromatosis of the gastrointestinal tract, or a number of associated abnormalities. Each of these three syndromes is usually separately inherited, and together they comprise about 20 per cent of all cases of medullary carcinoma.[106–109]

In these inherited syndromes, the development of medullary carcinoma is preceded by C-cell hyperplasia,[110] and it appears that the sequence of events is diffuse hyperplasia followed by nodular hyperplasia and then carcinoma—commonly bilateral (Fig. 51–9). Growth stimulation of endocrine cells is an important factor in endocrine tumor development generally, and the observed situation could arise through an inherited mutation causing a defect in a tissue-specific growth control mechanism. Prolonged C-cell growth will increase the chance of somatic mutation, causing subsequent progression through nodular hyperplasia to carcinoma. In theory, the inherited defect could be in one copy of a tumor suppressor gene with development of a neoplasm resulting in part from loss of heterozygosity so that both copies of the gene are ineffective and clonal growth results. The gene for inherited medullary carcinoma has been located to the pericentromeric region of chromosome 10, where at least one growth control gene—the *ret* oncogene—is known to be sited. Studies of familial medullary carcinoma have not shown loss of heterozygosity for chromosome 10,[111] suggesting that the gene involved is unlikely to be a tumor suppressor gene. In an interesting contrast, the gene for MEN I lies on chromosome 11, and loss of heterozygosity of chromosome 11 is commonly involved in the tumors in that condition.[112] In MEN II, there have been suggestions that chromosome 1 also may be involved, and loss of heterozygosity for this chromosome has been found in medullary carcinoma.[113] The molecular basis for inherited medullary carcinoma is therefore likely to be a mutation in an oncogene located on chromosome 10 which leads to hyperplasia of C cells with the subsequent development of tumors related to loss of a suppressor gene, possibly on chromosome 1. The *ret* oncogene, located within the relatively small region of chromosome 10 where the MEN II gene is known to be located, is expressed in medullary carcinoma and pheochromocytoma.[114] It is therefore a prime candidate to be the gene which is mutated in the MEN II syndromes. Very recent work has identified a mutation in the *ret* gene in a series of family members with MEN IIA.[115]

The reason for the different phenotypes in the inherited syndromes will become clear when the gene responsible is identified in all the syndromes involved but could involve point mutations, small deletions, or translocations conferring tissue-specific activity on the gene. The specificity of activity is likely to reflect a normally tissue-specific growth mechanism, as has been shown for some G proteins. Tissue-specific mechanisms also can occur through translocation of an oncogene to a tissue-specific promotor, as in some parathyroid adenomas, where a cyclin-related gene

has been shown to be translocated to the PTH promotor region.[116] When pheochromocytomas also form part of the inherited syndrome, it has been shown that these are associated with adrenal medullary hyperplasia so that the inherited component is again leading to tissue-specific cell growth out of which tumors arise, presumably through somatic mutation.

The patterns in which medullary carcinoma is inherited form three major groups and several subgroups. The nomenclature used here conforms with that suggested at an international workshop on MEN II in Heidelberg in 1989.[117] The main abnormalities that may be associated with the inherited MCT are parathyroid hyperplasia or tumors, adrenal medullary hyperplasia or tumors, multiple mucosal neuromas, a marfanoid phenotype with muscular weakness, a variety of musculoskeletal defects, and cutaneous lichen amyloidosis. The abnormalities group themselves into medullary carcinoma,[118] medullary carcinoma with parathyroid lesions,[119] medullary carcinoma with pheochromocytomas (classical MEN IIA), medullary carcinoma with pheochromocytomas and parathyroid lesions, medullary carcinoma with pheochromocytomas, multiple mucosal neuromas, and marfanoid phenotype (MEN IIB), and classical MEN IIA with lichen amyloidosis. The main groups defined by occurrence within a family, not an individual, are medullary carcinoma without pheochromocytoma, MEN IIA with or without parathyroid disease or cutaneous lichen amyloidosis, and MEN IIB. Each of these has been shown to be inherited, giving a consistent phenotype over several generations. There are, however, variations in particular within MEN IIA families. There is great variation in the frequency of pheochromocytomas, with pheochromocytomas being very frequent in some families (75 per cent of affected members) and uncommon in others.[120] The gene in each of the three main types (medullary carcinoma only, MEN IIA, and MEN IIB) has been located to the same region on the short arm of chromosome 10 near the centromere,[112, 119-121] so the differences may reflect the effect of modifying genes, differing mutations within the *ret* gene conferring different effects in different tissues, or mutations in closely linked genes forming part of a specific neuroendocrine growth pathway.

The different syndromes differ in ways other than the tissues involved. The medullary carcinoma in the medullary carcinoma only group is the least aggressive, with a mean age of diagnosis after screening of 43 years compared with 21 years for MEN IIA.[118] None of the affected members of two large kindreds was known to have died from medullary carcinoma. In contrast, the medullary carcinoma in MEN IIB is the most aggressive, with the tumors presenting at a much younger age than MEN IIA, with a higher percentage involvement of regional nodes at thyroidectomy, and with a poor survival.[112] These differences between MEN IIA and IIB appear to correlate with the degree of C-cell hyperplasia, which is commonly much more obvious in the individuals with MEN IIB than in those with MEN IIA.

Inherited Medullary Carcinoma (Without Pheochromocytomas)

This syndrome is much less common than MEN IIA despite being the least likely to lead to death before the end

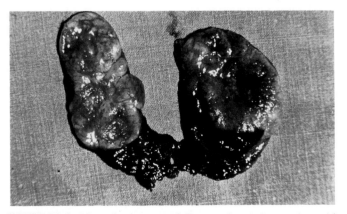

FIGURE 51–9. Bilateral primary medullary carcinoma in a patient with genetically determined disease.

of the reproductive age. Among 15 kindreds with inherited medullary carcinoma studied by Farndon et al.[118] in 1986, 2 showed no evidence of any other inherited endocrine tumor or of neuromas. A total of 178 members of these two kindreds were screened. No member of either family was known to have died of medullary carcinoma, and a comparison of the ages at which the tumor was detected by screening showed that this was 43 for these kindreds and 21 for MEN IIA. One kindred covering seven generations included two consanguineous marriages in which both parents had proven or suspected medullary carcinoma. In contrast to the involvement in this kindred of approximately a third of those at risk in generations 4 and 5 and approximately a tenth in generations 6 and 7, 12 of 13 members of the two sibships born to consanguineous parents were affected. Their tumors developed at an earlier mean age and were associated with much higher stimulated plasma calcitonin values and more frequent metastases. The likely explanation is the presence of homozygous mutations in a proportion of these children. Twenty-five per cent of the children would be expected to be homozygous, possibly more, since one parent was himself born of a consanguineous marriage and therefore possibly homozygous.

Medullary carcinoma and parathyroid tumors were inherited in one family studied by Carson et al.[119] in 1990, who showed that the gene responsible was in the same region of the chromosome as the gene for classical MEN IIA. Thirty affected members of this family showed either C-cell hyperplasia or medullary carcinoma. Seven have developed parathyroid tumors, and none has developed pheochromocytomas. Other studies also point to a good prognosis for families with inherited medullary carcinoma without pheochromocytoma,[122, 123] but few have studied enough family members to be certain of the family classification.

Multiple Endocrine Neoplasia Type IIA

The most common pattern of inherited medullary carcinoma is MEN IIA, in which the affected members are liable to develop medullary carcinomas and pheochromocytomas. In a 20-year French study of medullary carcinoma, over 800 cases of medullary carcinoma were identified. Thirty per cent were familial forms of the disease, including 53 who proved to belong to MEN IIA families and 26 to families with medullary carcinoma but in whom none of the affected members had pheochromocytoma.[124] It is likely that some of the latter families will be reclassified as MEN IIA, because the mean number of affected members was only 3.5 per family, too small to exclude a low incidence of pheochromocytoma. In this study, the mean age of presentation (clinical not screening) was 47 years for the inherited medullary carcinoma without pheochromocytoma families compared with 39 years for the MEN IIA families and 48 years for the apparently nonhereditary MTC's. Overall, 82 per cent of the 837 patients presented with goiter, 34 per cent had palpable cervical lymph nodes, 28 per cent had diarrhea, and 25 per cent evidenced flushing. In the MEN IIA patients, the tumors were almost always bilateral, and palpable cervical lymph nodes and diarrhea were much less common than in the sporadic patients, reflecting a lower total tumor burden and possibly

a slower growth rate of the tumor. MEN IIA patients show a better prognosis than those with sporadic tumors, with 90 per cent surviving 10 years compared with 55 per cent.[123] In this study, the 10-year survival of 17 cases of familial disease diagnosed by screening was 100 per cent. In MEN IIA, the medullary carcinoma more often presents before the pheochromocytoma than the reverse. The frequency of detectable pheochromocytomas in the families is very variable. In one study of six families with inherited medullary carcinoma thought through linkage analysis to have a common ancestral origin, the incidence of pheochromocytomas in the carriers varied between 0 and 74 per cent. It therefore seems likely that additional factors modify the expression of the MEN IIA gene.[125] The incidence of parathyroid disease is similarly variable, ranging from 15 per cent in a study reported by Vasen et al.[126] to 92 per cent in early observations by Melvin et al.[127] The majority of cases show hyperplasia with adenoma in a minority.

Multiple Endocrine Neoplasia Type IIB

The third inherited form is the association of medullary carcinoma with pheochromocytomas, multiple mucosal neuromas, intestinal ganglioneuromatosis, marfanoid habitus, muscular weakness, high arched palate, pes cavus, and a number of other abnormalities. This syndrome was first defined by Williams and Pollock,[128] who reported two cases, one of which was known to be familial, and reviewed the earlier literature. Since then, there have been a considerable number of individual case reports and a number of families affected by this syndrome. The majority present in their teens with medullary carcinoma, and the prognosis is in most cases less good than for MEN IIA (59 per cent 10-year survival versus 90 per cent for MEN IIA).[123]

These patients have very characteristic facies (Fig. 51–10) with thick, nodular, rather everted lips, thickened eyelids with small polypoid grayish tumors on the contact margins, usually near the inner canthus (Fig. 51–11), and similar small polypoid lesions in the anterior third of the tongue, particularly near the tip and lateral border (Fig. 51–12). These lesions are usually present at birth, although in a minority of cases they appear to arise in adult life. Histologically, they are pure neuromas (Fig. 51–13). Ganglioneuromatosis of the intestine probably occurs in the majority of the patients and may be associated with the presence of diverticulosis in childhood or with areas of megacolon.[129]

Histologically, it is important to separate the intestinal lesion found in MEN IIB, which is a transmural ganglioneuromatosis with particular involvement of the myenteric plexus (Fig. 51–14), from mucosal ganglioneuromatosis not involving the myenteric plexus. The latter has been found in association with a variety of conditions, including lipomatosis, megacolon, multinodular goiter, and neurofibromatosis, but not medullary carcinoma.[130, 131]

The variability in the behavior of medullary carcinoma between those families with multiple mucosal neuromas and those without is important not only when discussing the prognosis but also in relation to treatment. In addition, it is relevant to the frequency of occurrence of isolated cases. One striking finding on reviewing the literature is the high proportion of reports of individual cases of mul-

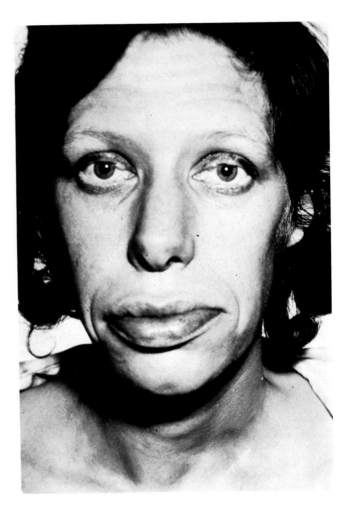

FIGURE 51–10. Facial appearance of the fully developed syndrome of multiple mucosal neuromas. Note the eyelid neuromas and the thickened "bumpy" lips. (Case 2, from Williams and Pollock, 1959.)

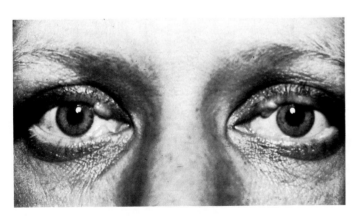

FIGURE 51–11. Eyes in a patient with multiple mucosal neuromas (same case as in Figure 51–10). (Case 2, from Williams and Pollock, 1959.)

FIGURE 51–12. Tongue in a patient with multiple mucosal neuromas.

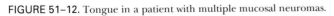

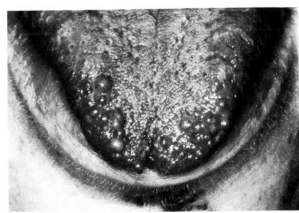

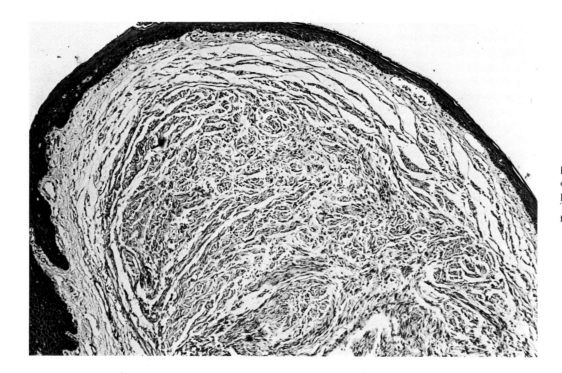

FIGURE 51–13. Histology of one of the mucosal neuromas from the patient shown in Figure 51–12. The lesion is composed of nerve fibers (H&E stain; × 75).

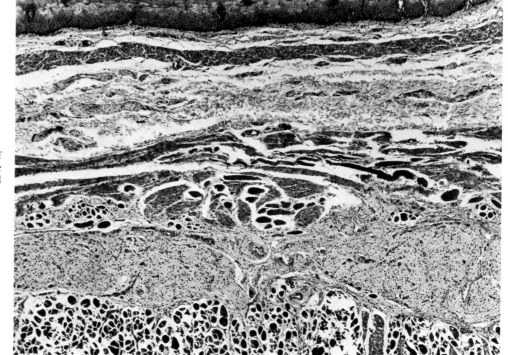

FIGURE 51–14. Ganglioneuromatosis of the esophagus in a patient with multiple mucosal neuromas. A greatly enlarged Auerbach plexus is shown (H&E stain; × 3).

tiple mucosal neuromas with medullary carcinoma and pheochromocytoma without a family history and the high proportion of reports of cases of medullary carcinoma and pheochromocytoma with a family history. Obviously, severe facial disfigurement, present in some cases with mucosal neuromas, may militate against the likelihood of having children. When to this is added the earlier age of presentation of medullary carcinoma and the frequency of death before the end of the reproductive period in those cases with multiple mucosal neuromas, it is obvious that fertility in patients with this syndrome is likely to be considerably reduced. Under these circumstances, the maintenance of a constant gene pool in the population requires a relatively high proportion of cases due to spontaneous mutation as compared with inheritence.

MANAGEMENT

It is clear that it is essential to establish whether a patient with medullary carcinoma belongs to the sporadic or genetic group. Obviously, if a patient shows the multiple mucosal neuromas syndrome, then the medullary carcinoma is genetically determined, whether or not a family history is present—and, as discussed above, in many cases it will not be present. In the absence of mucosal neuromas, a patient is more likely to belong to the genetic group if the medullary carcinoma is bilateral, if he or she belongs to a young age group, if there are symptoms suggestive of pheochromocytoma or hyperparathyroidism, if C-cell hyperplasia is found in the resected thyroid, or if there is a family history of medullary carcinoma, pheochromocytomas, or hyperparathyroidism. Irrespective of these findings, however, it is advisable to screen for pheochromocytoma before any operations are undertaken on a patient with medullary carcinoma. Obviously, pheochromocytoma, if present, should be dealt with first. Because of the high proportion of epinephrine produced by these tumors, it has been suggested that β-adrenergic blockade should be used as well as α-adrenergic blockade during surgery.[140]

In the absence of any clinical or biochemical finding in the patient or clinical findings in the family suggesting that the disease is genetically determined, it is still necessary to investigate for the possibility of a familial tumor. The clinical penetrance is incomplete, with only 60 per cent of gene carriers presenting with symptoms by the age of 70 in one study.[141] Screening using calcitonin assay after pentagastrin stimulation detects 93 per cent of carriers by age 31. Identification of the gene involved clearly radically changes management of familial cases. When the mutation in the family is known, all potentially affected family members can be offered screening for the mutation followed by the possibility of total thyroidectomy if the mutation is present and reassurance where it is not. When the mutation is not known, biochemical screening can still be carried out. For the apparently sporadic cases, the ret mutations commonly found in MEN IIA should be sought in the index case. These account for the majority of inherited cases. MEN IIB can be identified by its phenotype, and inherited medullary carcinoma without pheochromocytoma is an extremely slowly growing tumor. It therefore remains debatable whether all clinically normal first-degree relatives in cases without an identifiable ret mutation and without any other indication that the tumor is genetically determined should be screened.

Surgical Treatment

The definitive treatment for medullary carcinoma, whether sporadic or genetically determined, is surgery while the disease is confined to the neck. Total thyroidectomy is generally recommended, since it is extremely difficult to exclude preoperatively the possibility of bilateral disease, whether due to bilateral primary disease in genetically determined cases or direct spread in sporadic cases.[142] The lymph nodes from the central compartment of the neck are generally removed. Some surgeons advise careful search for and removal of any enlarged cervical nodes. Surgery is also the treatment for children with C-cell hyperplasia or medullary carcinoma detected by screening. Here the preoperative level of plasma calcitonin has been shown to correlate with the extent of the disease, so patients with high basal and particularly high stimulated levels showed more metastases than patients with normal basal and abnormal but not greatly elevated stimulated plasma calcitonin levels.[143] The extent of surgery carried out in these children will be determined in part by the surgical findings, but metastases have been found even when the primary tumor was less than 5 mm in diameter,[140, 144] and in general, total thyroidectomy with a search for involved nodes is the minimum reasonable therapy for cases identified by biochemical screening. The recognition of the mutation in MEN IIA families means that elective surgery can be carried out before any detectable rise in basal or stimulated calcitonin levels. The age at which surgery should be carried out and its extent remain to be determined, since previous studies have only carried out surgery on MEN IIA patients when screening was positive. One such study from the Mayo Clinic found that in 33 children operated on at the age of 15 or less, metastatic disease was found only in those aged 12 years or over. The youngest patient with MEN IIA and a medullary carcinoma was age 3.[145] Metastatic disease has been reported in children as young as 7 in other studies of MEN IIA. It may therefore be appropriate to offer thyroidectomy at the age of 2 or 3 for children shown to carry the MEN IIA gene. For children with the MEN IIB phenotype, it is generally accepted that thyroidectomy should be carried out as soon as the condition is recognized. There is no good evidence for the existence of mutiple mucosal neuromas without associated medullary carcinoma of the thyroid, and medullary carcinoma has been recognized in a child of 6 months of age with MEN IIB.[145]

MIXED MEDULLARY FOLLICULAR CARCINOMA

It is now established that a minority of thyroid tumors show signs of dual differentiation, recognized by the tumor content of both thyroglobulin and calcitonin and the structural pattern of the tumor. This is follicular in the areas containing thyroglobulin and resembles medullary carcinoma in the areas containing calcitonin.[2] Care must be taken to distinguish the true mixed tumor from tumors where thyroglobulin in the tumor cells arises from phagocytosis of thyroglobulin released from non-neoplastic follicles trapped within the tumor. In the true mixed tumor, the morphology and the peptide content correlate, and in a number of instances, both peptides have been present in metastatic lesions.[132, 133] The lesion is rare but of interest from a variety of standpoints. It is the likely explanation of earlier reports of radioiodine uptake by medullary carcinoma.[132, 134, 135] It has been described as a familial tumor.[136] It is possible that it is derived from follicular cells if these, like other endodermally derived cells, retain the possibility of true endocrine differentiation. It is also possible that it is derived from C cells, perhaps from a subgroup that is not neural crest in origin but which comes from the endodermal component of the ultimobranchial body and retains the capacity of differentiation into both C and follicular cells. It is also possible that it might be derived from fusion of C and follicular cells. The occurrence of mixed medullary follicular tumors on a familial basis is of particular interest, since the *ret* oncogene which is mutated in MEN IIA is also involved in papillary carcinoma of the thyroid. In the latter tumor, the tyrosine kinase portion of the *ret* gene is translocated, coming to lie next to the *H4* gene through inversion. The lesion appears to be specific to papillary carcinoma.[137] The familial mixed tumor was described as follicular, but a number of mixed medullary/papillary carcinomas have been described.[138, 139] It will be important to see if the *ret* gene is involved in both components of the tumor.

REFERENCES

1. Williams ED: Histogenesis of medullary carcinoma of the thyroid. J Clin Pathol 19:114, 1966.
2. Hedinger C, Williams ED, Sobin LH: Histological typing of thyroid tumours. *In* WHO International Histological Classification of Tumours. Berlin, Springer-Verlag, 1988.
3. Baber ED: Contributions to the minute anatomy of the thyroid gland of the dog. Philos Trans R Soc Lond Biol 166:557, 1876.
4. Nonidez JF: Further observations on parafollicular cells of mammalian thyroid. Anat Rec 53:339, 1932.
5. Getzowa S: Über die Glandula parathyroidea, intrathyroideale Zellhaufen derselben und Reste des postbranchialen Korpers. Virchows Arch Pathol Anat 188:181, 1907.
6. Godwin MC: Complex IV in the dog with special emphasis on the relation of the ultimobranchial body to interfollicular cells in the postnatal thyroid gland. Am J Anat 60:299, 1937.
7. Pearse AGE, Carvalheira AF: Cytochemical evidence for an ultimobranchial origin of rodent thyroid C cells. Nature 214:929, 1967.
8. Le Douarin N, Le Lievre CH: Démonstration de l'origine neurale des cellules a calcitonine du corps ultimobranchial chez l'embryon de poulet. C R Acad Sci 270:2857, 1970.
9. Williams ED, Toyn CE, Harach HR: The ultimobranchial gland and congenital thyroid abnormalities in man. J Pathol 159:135–141, 1989.
10. Parham DM: Laterally situated neck cysts derived from the embryological remnants of thyroid development. Histopathology 12:95–104, 1988.
11. Williams ED, Brown CL, Doniach I: Pathological and clinical findings in a series of 67 cases of medullary carcinoma of the thyroid. J Clin Pathol 19:103, 1966.
12. Ezaki H, Ebihara, S, Fujimoto Y, et al: Analysis of thyroid carcinoma based on material registered in Japan during 1977–1986 with special reference to predominance of papillary type. Cancer 70:808–814, 1992.
13. Williams ED, Doniach L, Bjarnson O, Michie W: Thyroid cancer in an iodide rich area—A histopathological study. Cancer 39:215, 1977.
14. Hie J, Jorgensen OG, Stenwig AE, Langmark F: Medullary thyroid cancer in Norway: A 30-year experience. Acta Chir Scand 154(5–6):339–343, 1988.
15. Ron E, Kleinerman RA, Boice JD, et al: A population-based case-control study of thyroid cancer. J Natl Cancer Inst 79:1–12, 1987.
16. Bergholm U: Selected studies on etiology and epidemiology. Diss Abstr Int [C] 50(4):686, 1989.
17. Williams ED: Medullary carcinoma of the thyroid. *In* Harrison CV, Weinbren K (eds): Recent Advances in Pathology (ed 9). Edinburgh, Churchill Livingstone, 1975, pp 156–182.
18. Harach HR, Williams ED: Glandular variants of medullary carcinoma of the thyroid. Histopathology 102(Suppl 252):11, 1983.
19. Kaudo K, Miyauchi A, Takai S, et al: C cell carcinoma of the thyroid. Acta Pathol Jpn 29:653, 1979.
20. Mendelsohn G, Bigner SH, Eggleston JC, et al: Anaplastic variants of medullary thyroid carcinoma. Am J Surg Pathol 4:333, 1980.
21. Martinelli G, Bazzocchi F, Govoni E, Santini D: Anaplastic type of medullary thyroid carcinoma. Virchows Arch [A] 400:61, 1983.
22. Harach HR, Bergholm U: Small cell variant of medullary carcinoma of the thyroid with neuroblastoma-like features. Histopathology 21:378–380, 1992.
23. Harach HR, Wilander E, Gimelius L, et al: Chromogranin A immunoreactivity compared with argyrophilia, calcitonin immunoreactivity, and amyloid as tumour markers in the histopathological diagnosis of medullary (C-cell) thyroid carcinoma. Pathol Res Pract 188:123–130, 1992.
24. Beerman H, Rigaud C, Bogomoletz WV, et al: Melanin production in black medullary thyroid carcinoma (MTC). Histopathology 16:227–233, 1990.
25. Boultwood J, Wynford-Thomas D, Richards GP, et al: In-situ analysis of calcitonin and CGRP expression in medullary thyroid carcinoma. Clin Endocrinol 33:381–390, 1990.
26. Kakudo K: Subclassification and prognostic factors of medullary (C cell) carcinoma of the thyroid. *In* Lechago J, Kameya T (eds): Endocrine Pathology Update. Field and Wood, 1990.
27. Ordonez NG, Samaan NA: Medullary carcinoma of the thyroid metastatic to the skin: report of two cases. J Cutan Pathol 14(4):251–254, 1987.
28. Goltzman D, Potts JT Jr, Ridgway EC, Maloof F: Calcitonin as a tumor marker. N Engl J Med 290:1035, 1974.
29. Rougier P, Calmettes C, LaPlanche A, et al: The values of calcitonin and carcinoembryonic antigen in the treatment and management of nonfamilial medullary thyroid carcinoma. Cancer 51:855, 1983.
30. Milhaud G, Calmette C, Faboulet J, et al: Hypersecretion of calcitonin in neoplastic conditions. Lancet 1:462, 1974.
31. Coombes RD, Hillyard C, Greenberg PB, MacIntyre I: Plasma-immunoreactive calcitonin in patients with non-thyroid tumours. Lancet 1:1080, 1974.
32. Sizemore GW, Go VLW, Kaplan EL, et al: Relations of calcitonin and gastrin in the Zollinger-Ellison syndrome and medullary carcinoma of the thyroid. N Engl J Med 288:641, 1973.
33. McLeod MK, Vinik AI: Calcitonin immunoreactivity and hypercalcitoninemia in two patients with sporadic, nonfamilial, gastroenteropancreatic neuroendocrine tumors. Surgery 111:484–488, 1992.
34. Hoppener JWB, Steenbergh PH, Zandberg J, et al: Localization of the polymorphic human calcitonin gene on chromosome II. Hum Genet 66:309, 1984.
35. Ali-Rachedi A, Varndell IM, Facer P, et al: Immunocytochemical localisation of katacalcin, a calcium-lowering hormone cleaved from the human calcitonin precursor. J Clin Endocrinol Metab 57:680, 1983.
36. Amara SG, Jonas V, Rosenfeld MG: Alternative RNA processing in calcitonin gene expression generates mRNAs encoding different polypeptide products. Nature 298:240, 1982.
37. Williams ED, Ponder B, Craig RK: Immunohistochemical study of CGRP in human medullary carcinoma and C cell hyperplasia: An immunohistochemical study. Clin Endocrinol 27:107–114, 1987.
38. Edbrooke MR, Parker D, McVey JH, et al: Expression of the human calcitonin/CGRP gene in lung and thyroid carcinoma. EMBO J 4:715, 1985.
39. Nelkin BD, Rosenfeld KI, de Bustros A, et al: Structure and expression of a gene encoding human calcitonin and calcitonin gene related peptide. Biochem Biophys Res Commun 123:648, 1984.
40. Minvielle S, Giscard-Dartevelle S, Cohen R, et al: A novel calcitonin carboxyl-terminal peptide produced in medullary thyroid carcinoma by alternative RNA processing of the calcitonin/calcitonin gene-related peptide gene. J Biol Chem 266(36):24627–24631, 1991.

41. Adema GJ, Baas PD: A novel calcitonin-encoding mRNA is produced by alternative processing of calcitonin/calcitonin gene-related peptide-1 pre-mRNA. J Biol Chem 267(11):7943–7948, 1992.

42. Williams ED, Morales AM, Horn RD: Thyroid carcinoma and Cushing's syndrome. J Clin Pathol 21:129, 1968.

43. Donahower GF, Schumacher OP, Hazard JB: Medullary carcinoma of the thyroid—A cause of Cushing's syndrome. Report of two cases. J Clin Endocrinol 28:1199, 1968.

44. Melvin KEW, Tashjian AH Jr, Cassidy CE, Givens JR: Cushing's syndrome caused by ACTH- and calcitonin-secreting medullary carcinoma of the thyroid. Metabolism 19:831, 1970.

45. Deftos JL, Bone HG III, Parthemore JG: Immunohistological studies on medullary thyroid carcinoma and C cell hyperplasia. J Clin Endocrinol Metab 51:857, 1980.

46. Steenbergh PH, Hoppener JWM, Zandberg J, et al: Expression of the proopiomelanocortin gene in human medullary thyroid carcinoma. J Clin Endocrinol Metab 58:904, 1984.

47. Birkenhager JC, Upton GV, Seldenrath JH, et al: Medullary thyroid carcinoma: Ectopic production of peptides with ACTH-like, corticotrophin releasing factor-like and prolactin production-stimulating activities. Acta Endocrinol (Copenh) 83:280, 1976.

48. Belsky JL, Cuello B, Swanson LW, et al: Cushing's syndrome due to ectopic production of corticotrophin-releasing factor. J Clin Endocrinol Metab 60:496, 1985.

49. Tourniaire J, Rebattu B, Conte-Devolx B, et al: Cushing's syndrome caused by ectopic production of CRF by a medullary carcinoma of the thyroid body. Ann Endocrinol (Paris) 49(1):61–67, 1988.

50. van Noorden S, Polak JM, Pearse ACE: Single cellular origin of somatostatin and calcitonin in the rat thyroid gland. Histochemistry 53:243, 1977.

51. Howlett TA, Price J, Hale AC, et al: Pituitary ACTH-dependent Cushing's syndrome due to ectopic production of a bombesin-like peptide by a medullary carcinoma of the thyroid. Clin Endocrinol (Oxf) 22:91, 1985.

52. Modigliani E, Alamowitch C, Cohen R, et al: The intratumoral immunoassayable somatostatin concentration is frequently elevated in medullary thyroid carcinoma: Results in 34 cases. Cancer 65(2):224–228, 1990.

53. Scopsi L, Ferrari C, Pilotti S, et al: Immunocytochemical localization and identification of prosomatostatin gene products in medullary carcinoma of human thyroid gland. Hum Pathol 21:820–830, 1990.

54. Pacini F, Basolo F, Elisei R, et al: Medullary thyroid cancer: An immunohistochemical and humoral study using six separate antigens. Am J Clin Pathol 95(3):300–308, 1991.

55. Paasonen MK: 5-Hydroxytryptamine in mammalian thyroid gland. Experientia 14:95, 1958.

56. Falck B, Larson B, von Mecklenburg C, et al: On the presence of a second specific cell system in mammalian thyroid gland. Acta Physiol Scand 62:491, 1964.

57. Hakanson R, Owman C, Sunler F: Aromatic L-amino acid decarboxylase in calcitonin-producing cells. Biochem Pharmacol 20:2187, 1971.

58. Pearse AGE: 5-Hydroxytryptophan uptake by dog thyroid "C" cells, and its possible significance in polypeptide hormone production. Nature 211:598, 1966.

59. Williams ED: Diarrhoea and thyroid carcinoma. Proc R Soc Med 59:602, 1966.

60. Steinfeld CM, Moertel CG, Woolner LB: Diarrhea and medullary carcinoma of the thyroid. Cancer 31:1237, 1973.

61. Falck B, Ljungberg O, Rosengren E: On the occurrence of monoamines and related substances in familial medullary thyroid carcinoma with phaeochromocytoma. Acta Pathol Microbiol Scand 74:1, 1968.

62. Atkins FL, Beaven MA, Keisner HR: Dopa decarboxylase in medullary carcinoma of the thyroid. N Engl J Med 289:545, 1973.

63. Baylin SB, Beaven MA, Engelman K, Sjoersdma A: Elevated histaminase activity in medullary carcinoma of the thyroid gland. N Engl J Med 283:1239, 1970.

64. Baylin SB, Beaven MA, Keiser HR, et al: Serum histaminase and calcitonin levels in medullary carcinoma of the thyroid. Lancet 1:455, 1972.

65. Baum JL: Abnormal intradermal histamine reaction in the syndrome of pheochromocytoma, medullary carcinoma of the thyroid gland and multiple mucosal neuromas. N Engl J Med 284:963, 1971.

66. Gorlin RJ: Skin test for medullary thyroid carcinoma. N Engl J Med 284:963, 1971.

67. Ishikawa N, Hamada S: Association of medullary carcinoma of the thyroid with carcinoembryonic antigen. Br J Cancer 34:111, 1976.

68. Cimitan M, Busnardo B, Girelli ME, et al: Carcinoembryonic antigen in thyroid cancer. J Endocrinol Invest 2:241, 1979.

69. Busnardo B, Girelli ME, Simioni N, et al: Nonparallel patterns of calcitonin and carcinoembryonic antigen levels in the follow-up of medullary thyroid carcinoma. Cancer 53:278, 1984.

70. Mendelsohn G, Wells SA, Baylin SB: Relationship of tissue carcinoembryonic antigen and calcitonin to tumor virulence in medullary thyroid carcinoma. Cancer 54:657, 1984.

71. Lippman SM, Mendelsohn G, Trump DL, et al: The prognostic and biological significance of cellular heterogeneity in medullary thyroid carcinoma: A study of calcitonin, L-dopa decarboxylase, and histaminase. Clin Endocrinol Metab 54:233, 1982.

72. Williams ED, Karim SMM, Sandler M: Prostaglandin secretion by medullary carcinoma of the thyroid. Lancet 1:22, 1968.

73. Isaacs P, Whittaker S, Turnberg LA: The mechanisms for the diarrhea associated with medullary thyroid carcinoma. Eur J Clin Invest 3:240, 1973.

74. Levin DL, Perlia C, Tashjian AJ Jr: Medullary carcinoma of the thyroid gland: The complete syndrome in a child. Pediatrics 52:192, 1973.

75. Schaison G, Nathan C, Gilbert-Dreyfus: Exploration biologique dans trois cas de cancers médullaires de al thyroïde. Ann Endocrinol (Paris) 35:291, 1974.

76. Barrowman JA, Bennett A, Hillenbrand P, et al: Diarrhoea in thyroid medullary carcinoma: Role of prostaglandins and therapeutic effect of nutmeg. Br Med J 3:11, 1975.

77. Grimley PM, Deftos LJ, Weeks JR, Rabson AS: Growth in vitro and ultrastructure of cells from a medullary carcinoma of the human thyroid gland: Transformation by simian virus 40 and evidence of thyrocalcitonin and prostaglandins. J Natl Cancer Inst 42:663, 1969.

78. Ménage JJ, Besnard JB, Guilmot JL, et al: Preuves de l'absence de sécrétion de prostaglandines par un carcinome médullaire de la thyroïde avec diarrhé motrice. Nouv Presse Med 4:2862, 1975.

79. Baum JL, Adler ME: Pheochromocytoma, medullary thyroid carcinoma, multiple mucosal neuroma. Arch Ophthalmol 87:574, 1972.

80. Marks SC: The parafollicular cell of the thyroid gland as the source of an osteoblast-stimulating factor. J Bone Joint Surg 51A:875, 1969.

81. Verdy M, Beaulieu R, Demers L, et al: Plasma calcitonin activity in a patient with thyroid medullary carcinoma and her children with osteopetrosis. J Clin Endocrinol Metab 32:216, 1971.

82. Bigazzi M, Revoltella R, Casciano S, Vigneti E: High level of a nerve growth factor in the serum of a patient with medullary carcinoma of the thyroid gland. Clin Endocrinol 6:105, 1977.

83. Benditt EP, Eriksen N: Chemical classes of amyloid substance. Am J Pathol 65:231, 1971.

84. Pearse AGE, Ewen SWB, Polak JM: The genesis of apudamyloid in endocrine polypeptide tumours: Histochemical distinction from immunamyloid. Virchows Arch [B] 10:93, 1972.

85. Tashjian AJ Jr, Wolfe HJ, Voelkel EF: Human calcitonin: Immunologic assay, cytologic localization and studies on medullary thyroid carcinoma. Am J Med 56:840, 1974.

86. Newman GR, Williams ED: Electron microscopic findings in medullary carcinoma of the thyroid. Unpublished observations.

87. Sletten K, Westermark P, Natvig JB: Characterization of amyloid fibril proteins from medullary carcinoma of the thyroid. J Exp Med 143:993, 1976.

88. O'Leary TJ, Levin IW: Secondary structure of endocrine amyloid: infrared spectroscopy of medullary carcinoma of the thyroid. Lab Invest 53(2):240, 1985.

89. Reuter E, Bethge N, Matthes M, Koppenhagen K: ^{99m}Tc-phosphonates for imaging of amyloid in C-cell carcinoma. Eur J Nucl Med 8:398, 1983.

90. Nunziate V, Giannattasio R, Di Giovanni G, et al: Hereditary localized pruritus in affected members of a kindred with multiple endocrine neoplasia type 2A (Sipple's syndrome). Clin Endocrinol (Oxf) 30(1):57–63, 1989.

91. Gagel RF, Levy ML, Donovan DT, et al: Multiple endocrine neoplasia type 2a associated with cutaneous lichen amyloidosis. Ann Intern Med 111:802–806, 1989.

92. Ferrer JP, Halperin I, Palou J: Cutaneous lichen amyloidosis and familial medullary thyroid carcinoma. Ann Intern Med 112:551–552, 1990.

93. Bernier JJ, Bouvry M, Cattan D, Prost A: Diarrhée motrice par cancer médullaire thyroidien. Presse Med 75:593, 1967.

94. Bernier JJ, Rambaud JC, Cattan D, Prost A: Diarrhea associated with medullary carcinoma of the thyroid. Gut 10:980, 1969.

95. Debray C, Leymarios J, Tourneur R, Chariot J: Les cancers thyroïdiens médullaires diarrhéogenes. Ann Intern Med 120:73, 1969.

96. Edwards IR, Smith AH: The mechanisms of the diuretic response to porcine calcitonin in normal subjects. Clin Sci 42:5P, 1972.

97. Gray TK, Bieberdorf FA, Fortran JS: Thyrocalcitonin and the jejunal absorption of calcium, water and electrolytes in normal subjects. J Clin Invest 52:3084, 1973.

98. Lechi C, De Bastiani G, Zatti M: In vitro stimulation of apparent intestinal alkaline phosphatase activity by thyrocalcitonin. Clin Chim Acta 57:171, 1974.

99. Fawell WN, Thompson G: Nutmeg for diarrhea of medullary carcinoma of the thyroid. N Engl J Med 289:108, 1973.

100. Melvin KEW, Tashjian AH Jr, Miller HH: Studies in familial (medullary) thyroid carcinoma. Recent Prog Horm Res 28:399, 1972.

101. Williams ED: Endocrine tumours of the thyroid. In Nagasawa H, Abe K (eds): Hormone Related Tumours. Tokyo, Japan Scientific Societies Press, 1981, pp 87–100.

102. Balducci L, Chapman SW, Little DD, Hardy CL: Paraneoplastic eosinophilia: Report of a case with in vitro studies of hemopoiesis. Cancer 64:2250–2253, 1989.

103. Williams ED: A review of 17 cases of carcinoma of the thyroid and pheochromocytoma. J Clin Pathol 18:288, 1965.

104. Schimke RN, Hartmann WH: Familial amyloid-producing medullary thyroid carcinoma of pheochromocytoma. Ann Intern Med 63:1027, 1965.

105. Sipple JH: The association of pheochromocytoma with carcinoma of the thyroid gland. Am J Med 31:163, 1961.

106. Chong GC, Beahrs HO, Sizemore GW, Woolner LH: Medullary carcinoma of the thyroid gland. Cancer 35:695, 1975.

107. Dunn EL, Nishiyama RH, Thompson NW: Medullary carcinoma of the thyroid gland. Surgery 73:848, 1973.

108. Gordon PR, Huvos AG, Strong EW: Medullary carcinoma of the thyroid gland—A clinicopathologic study of 40 cases. Cancer 31:915, 1973.

109. Beaugie JM, Brown CL, Doniach I, Richardson JE: Primary malignant tumours of the thyroid: The relationship between histological classification and clinical behaviour. Br J Surg 63:173, 1976.

110. Wolfe HJ, Melvin KEW, Cervi-Skinner SJ, et al: C-cell hyperplasia preceding medullary thyroid carcinoma. N Engl J Med 289:437, 1973.

111. Ponder BAJ, Smith BA, Marcus EM, et al: Genetic events in tumorigenesis in multiple endocrine neoplasia type 2. Cancer Cells 7:219–221, 1989.

112. Thakker RV: The molecular genetics of the multiple endocrine neoplasia syndromes. Clin Endocrinol (Oxf) 38:1–14, 1993.

113. Mathew CGP, Smith BA, Thorpe K: Deletion of genes on chromosome 1 in endocrine neoplasia. Nature 328:524–526, 1987.

114. Santoro M, Rosati R, Grieco M: The ret proto-oncogene is consistently expressed in human pheochromocytomas and thyroid medullary carcinomas. Oncogene 5:1595–1598, 1990.

115. Mulligan LM, Kowk JBJ, Healey CS, et al: Germ line mutations of the ret proto-oncogene in multiple endocrine neoplasia type IIa (MEN 2a). Nature 363:458–460, 1993.

116. Motokura T, Bloom T, Kim HG: A novel cyclin encorded by a bcl1-linked candidate oncogene. Nature 350:512–515, 1991.

117. Ponder B: Multiple endocrine neoplasia type 2. Br Med J 300:484–485, 1990.

118. Farndon JR, Leight GS, Dilley WG, et al: Familial medullary thyroid carcinoma without associated endocrinopathies: A distinct clinical entity. Br J Surg 73:278–281, 1986.

119. Carson NL, Wu J, Jackson CE, et al: The mutation for medullary thyroid carcinoma with parathyroid tumors (MTC with PTs) is closely linked to the centromeric region of chromosome 10. Am J Hum Genet 47:946–951, 1990.

120. Narod SA, Sobol H, Nakamura Y, et al: Linkage analysis of hereditary thyroid carcinoma with and without pheochromocytoma. Hum Genet 83(4):53–58, 1989.

121. Lichter JB, Wu J, Brooks Wilson Ar, et al: A new polymorphic marker (D10S97) tightly linked to the multiple endocrine neoplasia type 2A (MEN2A) locus. Hum Genet 5:516, 1993.

122. Kakudo K, Carney A, Sizemore GW: Medullary carcinoma of the thyroid: Biologic behavior of the sporadic and familial neoplasm. Cancer 55:2818–2821, 1985.

123. Parmentier C, Gardet P, de Vathaire F, et al: Prognostic factors in medullary thyroid carcinoma (MTC): A study based on 207 patients treated at the Institut Gustave Roussy. In Calmettes C, Colloque JMG (eds): Medullary Thyroid Carcinoma. Paris, John Libbey Eurotext, 1991, pp 193–198.

124. Rosenberg-Bourgin M, Farkas D, Calmettes C, et al: Epidemiologic and genetic analysis of medullary thyroid carcinoma in France. In Calmettes C, Colloque JMG (eds): Medullary Thyroid Carcinoma. Paris, John Libbey Eurotext, 1991, pp 149–157.

125. Narod SA, Lavoue MF, Morgan K, et al: Genetic analysis of 24 French families with multiple endocrine neoplasia type 2A. Am J Hum Genet 51:469–477, 1992.

126. Vasen HFA, Nieuwenhuijzen Kruseman AC, Berkel H: Multiple endocrine neoplasia syndrome type 2: The value of screening and central registration. A study of 15 kindreds in the Netherlands. Am J Med 83:847–852, 1987.

127. Melvin KEW, Tashjian AH Jr, Miller HH: Studies in familial (medullary) thyroid carcinoma. Recent Prog Horm Res 28:399, 1972.

128. Williams ED, Pollock DJ: Multiple mucosal neuromata with endocrine tumours: A syndrome allied to von Recklinghausen's disease. J Pathol Bacteriol 91:71, 1966.

129. Carney JA, Go VLW, Sizemore GW, Hayes AB: Alimentary-tract ganglioneuromatosis. N Engl J Med 295:1287, 1976.

130. Hegstrom JL, Kircher T: Alimentary tract ganglioneuromatosis-lipomatosis, adrenal myelolipomas, pancreatic telangiectasia, and multinodular thyroid goiter: A possible neuroendocrine syndrome. Am J Clin Pathol 83(6):744–747, 1985.

131. d'Amore ESG, Manivel JC, Pettinato G, et al: Intestinal ganglioneuromatosis: Mucosal and transmural types. A clinicopathologic and immunohistochemical study of six cases. Hum Pathol 22(3):276–286, 1991.

132. Hales M, Rosenau W, Okerlund MD, Galante M: Carcinoma of the thyroid with a mixed medullary and follicular pattern: Morphologic, immunohistochemical and clinical laboratory studies. Cancer 50:1352–1359, 1982.

133. Holm R, Sobrinho-Simoes M, Nesland JM, et al: Medullary thyroid carcinoma with thyroglobulin immunoreactivity: A special entity? Lab Invest 57(3):258–268, 1987.

134. Nusynowitz ML, Pollard E, Benedetto AR, et al: Treatment of medullary carcinoma of the thyroid with I-131. J Nucl Med 23:143, 1982.

135. Parthasarathy KL, Shimaoka K, Bakshi SP, Razack MS: Radiotracer uptake in medullary carcinoma of the thyroid. Clin Nucl Med 5:45–48, 1980.

136. Noel M, Delehaye MC, Segond N, et al: Study of calcitonin and thyroglobulin gene expression in human mixed follicular and medullary thyroid carcinoma. Thyroid 13:249–256, 1991.

137. Santora M, Carlomagno F, Hay ID, et al: Ret oncogene activation in human thyroid neoplasms is restricted to the papillary cancer subtype. J Clin Invest 89(5):1517–1522, 1992.

138. Parker LN, Kollin J, Wu S-Y, et al: Carcinoma of the thyroid with a mixed medullary, papillary, follicular and undifferentiated pattern. Arch Intern Med 145:1507–1509, 1985.

139. Albores-Saavedra J, Gorraez de la Mora T, de la Torre-Rendon F, Gould E: Mixed medullary-papillary carcinoma of the thyroid: A previously unrecognized variant of thyroid carcinoma. Hum Pathol 21:1151–1155, 1990.

140. Gagel RF, Melvin KEW, Tashjian AH Jr, et al: Natural history of the familial medullary thyroid carcinoma—Pheochromocytoma syndrome and the identification of preneoplastic stages by screening studies: A five-year report. Trans Assoc Am Physicians 88:177, 1975.

141. Easton DF, Ponder MA, Cummings T, et al: The clinical and screening age-at-onset distribution for the MEN-2 syndrome. Am J Hum Genet 44(2):208–215, 1989.

142. Russell CF, Van Heerden JA, Sizemore GW, et al: The surgical management of medullary thyroid carcinoma. Ann Surg 101:941, 1982.

143. Wells SA, Baylin SB, Leight GS, et al: The importance of early diagnosis in patients with hereditary medullary thyroid carcinoma. Ann Surg 195:595, 1982.

144. Telenius-Berg M, Berg B, Hamerger B, et al: Impact of screening of prognosis in the multiple endocrine neoplasia type 2 syndromes: Natural history and treatment results in 105 patients. Henry Ford Hosp Med J 32:225, 1984.

145. Telander RL, Zimmerman D, Sizemore GW, et al: Medullary carcinoma in children: Results of early detection and surgery. Arch Surg 124(7):841–843, 1989.

52

Congenital Defects in Thyroid Hormone Formation and Action

LESLIE J. DeGROOT

In this chapter, we describe a group of inherited disorders of thyroid metabolism. Since the initial descriptions of inherited goiter by Osler[1] and Pendred[2] more than 80 years ago, our understanding of inborn errors of thyroid metabolism has grown tremendously; at present nine major biochemical defects, consisting of more than 20 heterogeneous subgroups, have been identified (Table 52–1). These congenital disorders result from mutations of genes involved in any step of thyroid hormone synthesis, storage, secretion, delivery, or utilization.

The disorders are probably inherited according to classic Mendelian rules. Autosomal recessive patterns of inheritance have been postulated or proven for most of these syndromes, with the exception of some families with generalized resistance to thyroid hormone and those with goiter and intrathyroidal calcification, for whom autosomal dominant modes have been suggested. In addition, an X-linked dominant pattern in inherited thyroxine-binding globulin (TBG) deficiency and excess has been demonstrated.

Because the study of these conditions has provided a wealth of information about normal thyroid function, these disorders are of great interest and significance despite the small number of reported cases. We review each of the categories listed in Table 52–1 and end with a general approach to the clinical and biochemical investigation of the inherited disorders.

UNRESPONSIVENESS TO THYROTROPIN

Thyrotropin (TSH) interacts with and activates a thyroid cell surface receptor. This activated receptor binds to a regulatory protein, which in turn binds guanosine triphosphate (GTP); the activated regulatory protein can then bind to and activate adenyl cyclase, which in turn catalyzes the generation of cAMP from adenosine triphosphate (ATP). cAMP is thought to mediate most effects of TSH by the activation of protein kinases with subsequent phosphorylation of specific protein substrates in the cell. Thy-rotropin also appears to stimulate via its receptor the activation of phospholipase C, leading to augmented levels of inositol triphosphate and diacylglycerol, increased Ca^{2+}, and activation of protein kinase C. Through these regulatory proteins, intrathyroidal mRNA and protein synthesis is stimulated, iodide transport and hormone secretion are augmented, and division of thyroid cells is promoted. A failure of the thyroid cell to respond to TSH could theoretically occur because of an abnormality of TSH or of the membrane receptor, an inhibitor of TSH binding, a defective GTP regulatory protein, defective adenylate cyclase, an abnormality in the action of cAMP, or abnormalities in the phospholipase C pathway.

Congenital cretinism due to isolated TSH deficiency has been reported by several authors. In the family studied by Miyai et al,[3] the two subjects had no TSH in their blood, although other pituitary glycoprotein hormones were present. Thyrotropin-releasing hormone (TRH) administration caused secretion of TSH α but no TSH or free TSH β subunit. Subsequently, Hayashizaki et al[4] cloned and sequenced portions of the TSH β subunit gene from several families and demonstrated in those families a single base substitution in the codon for the 29th amino acid (glycine-GGA to arginine-AGA). This mutation produces a partially unfolded protein that is thought to be responsible for the failure to form normal TSH α/β dimers (Fig. 52–1). Another occurrence of familial hypothyroidism due to a G94T transversion and formation of a truncated peptide was reported by Dacou-Voutetakis et al.[5]

Three patients have been reported with defects in TSH responsiveness.[6–13] The following case was reported by Codaccioni and colleagues.[13]

Congenital hypothyroidism was suspected in an 18-month-old boy with growth and mental retardation. His grandparents were first cousins. His serum protein bound iodine was low, and treatment with desiccated thyroid was begun. The patient was re-evaluated at age 17, and thyroid replacement was discontinued. His mental development and physical development had been satisfactory since treatment was initiated. Thyroid scan was normal. Serum triio-

TABLE 52–1. BIOCHEMICAL CLASSIFICATION OF INHERITED DISORDERS OF THYROID METABOLISM

MAIN DEFECT	SUBGROUPS
1. Unresponsiveness to TSH	a. Abnormal TSH† b. TSH receptor defect* c. Regulatory protein abnormality* d. Adenyl cyclase abnormality* e. cAMP action blocked*
2. Iodide transport defect	a. Complete b. Partial
3. Organification defect	a. Quantitative deficiency of peroxidase b. Apoenzyme defect with defective heme binding c. Inhibitor of TPO† d. Abnormal intracellular location of TPO e. Inadequate substrate Tg† f. Abnormality in binding substrate g. Other mutational defects in TPO gene h. H_2O_2 generation defect i. Abnormality in the iodine acceptor - Tg†
4. Pendred's syndrome	
5. "Coupling" defect	
6. Tg defect	a. Abnormal mRNA/reduced quantity/abnormal location of mRNA b. Tg transport defect† c. Abnormal glycosylation d. Qualitative defects: subunit lability, inaccessible tyrosyl residues, iodohistidine formation
7. Iodotyrosine dehalogenase deficiency	a. Generalized b. Isolated thyroidal deficiency c. Only diiodotyrosine dehalogenase deficiency
8. Thyroid transport protein defect	a. Familial TBG excess† b. TBG deficiency† c. Analbuminemia d. Familial dysalbuminemic hyperthyroxinemia e. Familial excess thyroxine-binding prealbumin f. Qualitative abnormalities of TBG due to gene mutations†
9. Resistance to thyroid hormone	a. Generalized b. Isolated pituitary defect (?) c. Isolated peripheral defect (?)
10. Others	a. Multinodular goiter (see Ch. 46) b. Intrathyroidal calcification c. I⁻ leak

*Hypothetical.
†TSH, thyroid-stimulating hormone; TPO, thyroid peroxidase; Tg, thyroglobulin; TBG, thyroxine-binding globulin.

mg/kg/min for 1 hour). A thyroid biopsy specimen revealed follicles of small and medium sizes, with lumen generally devoid of colloid. On electron microscopy, abnormal membranes with extensive increases in the surface and width of the basal plasma membrane and basal lamina were demonstrated. TSH binding kinetics were normal. Adenyl cyclase activity in these membranes was stimulated by fluoride but not by exogenous TSH.

In vitro studies in this patient suggest, therefore, that an abnormality is present in the coupling of the TSH receptor with cAMP generation. Two other patients similarly had normal bioassayable TSH and failed to respond to exogenous TSH.[6–12] Histological examination showed thyroid hyperplasia with no detectable thyroglobulin (Tg). All three patients were mentally retarded and hypothyroid and did not have goiters at the time of diagnosis.

Decreased responsiveness to TSH has also been described and characterized in the familial disorder, Type 1a pseudohypoparathyroidism, in which a defect in expression of the α subunit of G_s protein (coupling receptor to cyclase) is present.[8] Along with the characteristics of pseudohypoparathyroidism and Albright's hereditary osteodystrophy, these patients tend to have mild clinical evidence of hypothyroidism with slightly decreased free thyroxine index (FTI), elevated TSH, and exaggerated TRH responsiveness.[9] The thyroid is usually not enlarged. Gonadal function may also be abnormal. A related defect in the TSH receptor–G protein complex is responsible for hypothyroidism in the *hyt/hyt* mouse.[10] Although defects in TSH production may not be totally within the purview of this chapter, it is of interest to note another recently recognized cause of reduced production of growth hormone, prolactin, and TSH. Pit-1 is a protein causing tissue-specific expression of the genes coding for these proteins. Mutations have been found in this protein, making it unable to bind to the specific response element in the promoter for the genes and leading to deficient expression of the mRNA's and proteins.[11, 12]

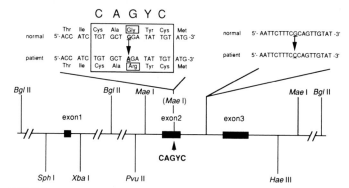

FIGURE 52–1. **Physical map of the normal TSH β-subunit gene and the gene from a family with a nonfunctional β subunit.** Some restriction sites and part of the nucleotide sequence are shown. Sequences and cleavage sites with DNA's from the patients in three families were identical, showing nucleotide substitutions in exon 2 and intron 2. The former substitution lying in the CAGYC region has generated a new cleavage site for Mae I. Substitution of arginine for glycine produced a β subunit that could not combine with the α subunit to form the normal TSH molecule. Solid black areas indicate the exons. (Modified from Hayashizaki Y, Hiraoka Y, Tatsumi K, et al: Deoxyribonucleic acid analyses of five families with familial inherited thyroid stimulating hormone deficiency. J Clin Endocrinol Metab 71:792–796, © by the Endocrine Society, 1990.)

dothyronine (T_3) was 5 ng/dl. Thyroxine (T_4) was 1 μg/dl, thyroglobulin was 1 ng/ml, and TSH was 385 μU/ml by radioimmunoassay (RIA) and 400 μU/ml by the McKenzie bioassay. Uptake of ^{131}I by the thyroid was similar under basal conditions and after TSH stimulation (10 IU/day intramuscularly for 6 days), but a substantial increase was observed after the infusion of dibutyryl cAMP (0.1

DIAGNOSIS. Diagnostic criteria for this group of patients are not well formulated. In general patients would be expected to demonstrate variable degrees of hypothyroidism, usually small thyroids with low radioactive iodine uptake (RAIU), and low serum T_4 and T_3 levels. Patients with defective TSH[3] have been hypothyroid cretins and have had absent serum TSH. Patients with defective TSH receptors have had elevated TSH, small or normal thyroids, low or normal RAIU, and poor response to injected TSH. In vitro studies of thyroid slices show no response to TSH, that is, no cAMP formation, protein iodination, or glucose oxidation (^{14}C-labeled glucose), and demonstrate normal responses to sodium fluoride and dibutyryl cAMP.

GENETICS. Some of the patients were products of consanguineous marriages, and a recessive inheritance pattern is most probable for some of the traits, including the TSH mutation.

THERAPY. Thyroxine therapy is indicated as soon as possible to avoid neurological damage.

IODIDE TRANSPORT DEFECT

The first step in the synthesis of the thyroid hormones is the transport of inorganic iodide from the extracellular fluid into the thyroid. Active transport of iodide occurs against an electrical and concentration gradient.[14] The bulk of the energy for this process derives from oxidative metabolism. It is inhibited by agents that impair aerobic metabolism, such as cyanide. It fails at low temperatures and in the presence of agents that uncouple oxidative phosphorylation, such as dinitrophenol. Transport is also inhibited by ouabain, which inhibits the Na^+,K^+-linked adenosine triphosphatase (ATPase). The process presumably involves a membrane-bound iodide carrier. The process is carried out by a membrane Na^+/I^- "symporter." Although not so far cloned, the mRNA of the symporter has been identified by expression in oocytes.[15]

A selective iodide concentration gradient of 20 or more is normally maintained and regulated at least in part by TSH. Hypophysectomy decreases I^- transport in rats, and exogenous TSH restores it after a six- to eight-hour delay.[17] TSH causes a biphasic response—an initial efflux of iodide from the gland followed by an influx of iodide.[18] The TSH action on iodide uptake is blunted by inhibitors of protein synthesis, such as puromycin and cycloheximide.[19]

Iodide transport is reversibly inhibited by other monovalent ions of similar molecular size and shape, such as perchlorate and pertechnetate. Thiocyanate also inhibits iodide transport, although it is not itself concentrated within the thyroid, as are perchlorate and pertechnetate.

Similar iodide transport systems are present in salivary glands, gastric mucosa, mammary glands, ciliary body, placenta, choroid plexus, and small intestine.[20] These are not TSH responsive.

CLINICAL PRESENTATION. More than 30 cases of iodide transport defects have been reported in the literature.[21–36] A representative case has been studied in some detail by Saito and colleagues.[21]

> A 32-year-old man was studied because of goiter. His early development had been moderately delayed and school performance was poor. At the age of 15 years he was found to

have a goiter, and a left hemithyroidectomy was performed. Hypothyroidism was suspected at 22 years of age, and he began taking desiccated thyroid extract irregularly at that time. At the time of the study he was only 144.8 cm tall and weighed 64.5 kg. His face was puffy. The right thyroid lobe was an elastic soft mass with a hard nodule. Serum T_3 was 39 ng/dl, T_4 was 1.0 µg/dl, and TSH was 217 µU/ml. The thyroidal ^{131}I uptake was 0.05% at 24 hours. The saliva to serum ratio of [131]I 2 h after injection was 0.95:1. The gastric juice to serum ratio of ^{131}I was 0.97:1. Kinetic analysis revealed absence of a significant pool of iodine in the gland. Study of a biopsy specimen disclosed intense hyperplasia. When the patient was given iodide, a euthyroid state was quickly established.

This patient has a defect of the iodide transport system, which is common to the transport systems of the thyroid, the salivary gland, and the gastric mucosa. It is a "complete" defect with a saliva/plasma ^{131}I concentration gradient less than 1. Concentration gradients greater than 1 but less than 20 have been reported in other patients[25, 27–29, 31, 32] and are termed "incomplete" defects; concentration gradients greater than 20 are considered normal. Hypothyroidism associated with pronounced goiter and low 24-hour iodine uptake characterize most of the cases, although patients with partial or incomplete transport defects are reported to have small goiters.[27, 32] The age at which patients present has ranged between birth and 50 years. Hypothyroidism may be recognized late, as in this case, and physical and mental retardation may or may not be present. Other patients with complete transport defects have not been permanently retarded. Nine of the cases are reported from Japan, and, interestingly, some of these cases are milder in clinical presentation. This finding may reflect an incomplete defect of transport that is partially compensated by large iodine intakes characteristic of the Japanese diet.[32]

DIAGNOSIS. In the neonatal period infants with a transport defect are found to have a normal-size thyroid by ultrasonography and very elevated serum Tg levels.[33] A low 24-hour RAIU in the presence of a goiter is necessary to make a diagnosis of a transport defect. Usually this study is deferred until the infant is 6 to 36 months old. Other causes of decreased RAIU, such as iodide administration or thyroiditis, must be excluded. Also suggestive of the diagnosis is a 24-hour RAIU that does not increase with TSH stimulation. Measurement of saliva to plasma, gastric juice to plasma, or CSF to plasma ^{131}I ratio is necessary to confirm the diagnosis. The normal ratio of saliva or gastric juice iodide to plasma iodide is greater than 20:1; CSF to plasma iodide is normally approximately 0.04:1 because the choroid plexus transports iodide out of the CSF into the blood. CSF to plasma ratios of iodide are not, however, necessary to make the diagnosis. Additional confirmation of the diagnosis has been obtained by showing that thyroid biopsy slices failed to accumulate ^{131}I in vitro.[21, 23, 28] Histological examination of the thyroid may show hyperplasia, but this is not pathognomonic; measurement of low thyroid iodine content may also provide confirmatory evidence, as does inability of the salivary glands to concentrate thiocyanate. Final confirmation is obtained by successful response to iodide therapy.

GENETICS. Consanguinity is reported in the parents of 6 of 21 reported cases. Because the disease is present in male and female siblings and not in the parents, it is thought to be autosomal recessive in inheritance pattern. At present there is no test for heterozygous carriers, and unaffected parents and siblings have normal 24-hour RAIU.

THERAPY. A satisfactory response to oral potassium iodide (KI) therapy (1 to 5 mg every day initially) remains one of the most useful diagnostic criteria. Larger doses (up to 189 mg/day) have been used. The chronic effects of KI therapy are satisfactory, but T_4 administration is probably to be preferred after the initial response to KI has been established. It is the drug of choice in pregnancy to avoid the goitrogenic effect on the fetus of large doses of KI.

ORGANIFICATION DEFECT

After iodide is transported into the thyroid gland, it is oxidized and bound to tyrosyl residues present in thyroglobulin. This step in thyroid hormonogenesis depends upon intact thyroid peroxidase (TPO) activity, generation of an oxidizing agent (presumably H_2O_2), availability of iodide and Tg, and correct spatial organization of these components.

TPO is a heme-containing enzyme and is membrane-bound. It is active only in the presence of H_2O_2; there are at least two reactive sites on the enzyme, one for tyrosine and one for iodide. The iodide and tyrosine are thought to be oxidized in adjacent enzyme sites; the product of this oxidation reaction is uncertain. Either a free radical of iodine[37] or the iodinium ion (I^+) is formed. The active iodine intermediate and the tyrosine are then covalently bound by TPO to form iodotyrosine. TPO also catalyzes the peroxidative reaction leading to coupling of two iodotyrosines to form T_4 or T_3. The reactions catalyzed by TPO are inhibited by antithyroid drugs, and, under some conditions, by high iodide concentration (Wolff-Chaikoff block). TPO was identified as a protein present in two forms of 102 and 107 kDa and identical to the "microsomal antigen" of the thyroid.[38, 39] The cDNA has been cloned and sequenced in several laboratories.[40]

Hydrogen peroxide functions as the oxidant of iodide, but the nature of the H_2O_2-generating system is not well understood. Nicotinamide-adenine dinucleotide phosphate (NADPH) oxidation by NADPH–cytochrome C reductase has been proposed to account for the source of H_2O_2,[41] but studies by Virion et al.[42] indicate that the NADPH oxidase in thyroid cell membranes is a different Ca^{2+}-activated protein. Additionally, other mechanisms involving the reduced form of nicotinamide-adenine dinucleotide (NADH)–cytochrome b_5 reductase, monoamine oxidase, and xanthine oxidase have also been proposed.

At present five subgroups of defects are reported in the organification process:

1. Quantitative deficiency of TPO enzyme[43–48]
2. Qualitative abnormalities of TPO enzyme
   a. Apoenzyme defect with defective heme binding[49, 50]
   b. Inhibitor of TPO[51, 52]
   c. Possible abnormal intracellular location of TPO[50, 53, 54]
   d. Abnormality in binding substrate[55, 56]
   e. Other mutational defects in the TPO gene[61]
3. Deficiency of H_2O_2 generation[57]

4. Abnormality of iodine acceptor-Tg[59, 60]
5. Pendred's syndrome (see below)

Additional case reports have been published, but the cases cannot be classified biochemically.[68–78]

CLINICAL PRESENTATION. A patient with a quantitative deficiency of peroxidase was described by Pommier and colleagues.[43]

> A 17-year-old man was seen for goiter. He was noted at 6 months of age to be hypothyroid, and treatment with T_4 was begun, although the dose was insufficient. At the time of admission (at 17 years old), he appeared to be clinically euthyroid, with normal physical development, but had mild mental deficiency. His height was 170 cm, weight 52 kg; serum cholesterol was 315 mg/dl; serum protein-bound iodine (PBI) was 1 μg/dl, serum total T_4 was 1.2 μg/dl, serum TSH 165 μU/ml, and the ^{131}I thyroid uptake was 26 per cent at 2 h and 7 per cent at 24 h. Administration of 400 mg of potassium perchlorate one hour after a tracer dose of ^{131}I resulted in discharge of 90 per cent of the thyroid radioactivity within 45 minutes. After administration of 100 μg of TRH, the TSH level reached 250 μU/ml. A right lobectomy was performed. The lobe weight was 50 g. Macroscopic examination revealed colloid goiter without any nodules and without fibrous and hemorrhagic areas. No peroxidase activity could be demonstrated, either before or after solubilization with trypsin and digitonin, when tested by guaiacol peroxidation, by iodination using poorly iodinated thyroglobulin as substrate, or by the $I^- \rightarrow I_2$ reaction. Activity was not enhanced by preincubation with hematin. This case is an example of complete absence of peroxidase activity.

A number of other cases of complete or partial absence of TPO activity have been reported.[44–48] Direct assays of TPO activity utilizing triiodide formation,[61] guaiacol peroxidation,[63] or tyrosine iodination[63] reveal no TPO activity or poorly efficient TPO activity. Peroxidase activity cannot be normalized in these cases by solubilization with digitonin[64] or with trypsin and deoxycholate[65, 66] or by the addition of hematin, H_2O_2, or Tg (Fig. 52–2).

In addition to quantitative deficiencies of TPO enzyme, qualitative abnormalities have been reported. Two cases of prosthetic group defects have been reported by Niepomniszcze and colleagues.[49, 50] In these patients, thyroid tissue had negligible peroxidase activity in the tyrosine-iodinase, triiodide, and guaiacol assays, but preincubation of subcellular fractions with hematin restored activity (Fig. 52–2).

Other qualitative abnormalities of TPO have been demonstrated. Pommier et al.[51, 52] reported one case in which a dialyzable inhibitor of iodination by peroxidase was found in association with high peroxidase concentration. Several cases of possible abnormal intracellular locations of TPO have been reported.[50, 53, 54] In one case,[50] peroxidase activity in the goiter tissue was quantitatively decreased but kinetically normal with respect to apparent K_m for H_2O_2. Peroxidase activity had abnormal subcellular distribution because pellets sedimenting between 39,000 and 105,000 g contained most of the activity. In normal glands, the bulk of peroxidase is present in fractions sedimenting between 700 and 39,000 g. How this abnormal location contributes to decreased TPO activity is unclear.

An additional qualitative abnormality of TPO enzyme is an abnormality in binding substrate. Two such cases have

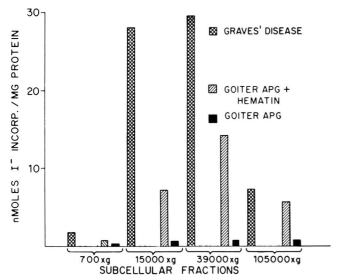

FIGURE 52–2. Peroxidase activity of the subcellular fractions of goiter from a patient who demonstrated prosthetic group defect of TPO. Following preincubation with 10^{-4} M hematin, activity in the tyrosine iodinase assay was augmented. Also illustrated is peroxidase activity in a Graves' disease gland. Results are expressed as nanomoles of iodide incorporated into tyrosine per milligram of particulate protein. (From Niepomniszcze H, Rosenbloom AL, DeGroot LJ, et al: Differentiation of two abnormalities in thyroid peroxidase causing organification defect and goitrous hypothyroidism. Metabolism 24:57, 1975.)

been described.[55, 56] In one patient, Medeiros-Neto and associates[56] demonstrated extremely low TPO activity, which could be increased from 2.6 per cent to 40 per cent of normal by incubating TPO with higher concentrations of I^- substrate (100 μM to 12 mM), suggesting an abnormality in the binding of I^- rather than a quantitative deficiency of the enzyme.

In addition to quantitative and qualitative TPO defects, two cases of deficiency of H_2O_2 generation have been reported.[57, 58]

A 37-year-old woman was noted to have a goiter after her first pregnancy. The goiter steadily increased in size. Thyroxine was normal, TSH was elevated at 17.8 μU/ml, and the RAI uptake at 24 hours was 81.4 per cent. Within 1 h after oral administration of 1 g potassium thiocyanate, 67.8% of ^{131}I was discharged. In vitro organification of iodide in the thyroid homogenate from the patient was impaired, and it was restored to normal by the addition of H_2O_2, glucose and glucose oxidase system, flavin adenine dinucleotide (FAD), or reduced cytochrome b_5. The microsomal NADPH–cytochrome b_5 reductase activity was definitely low in the patient's thyroid. The defect was reversed by preincubation of microsomes with FAD, and administration of high doses of FAD (250 mg/day) led to the restoration of thyroidal iodide organification with increased thyroid hormone production and a marked decrease of the goiter.[57]

Finally, four cases of organification defect related to diminished iodine "acceptor," that is, a Tg abnormality, have been reported.[59, 60] Niepomniszcze and colleagues[60] studied thyroid tissue specimens obtained from three sisters with congenital goiter. Peroxidase and NADPH–cytochrome C reductase levels were elevated. Tg, however, was totally absent. The thyroid cytosol contained iodoalbumin and other iodinated proteins, and trapped iodide was perchlorate-dischargeable. It is believed that a deficiency in normal substrate leads to a functional defect in iodination.

Abramowicz et al[61] have recently identified a TPO defect at the molecular level for the first time. Their patient was a hypothyroid individual, the product of a consanguineous marriage. TPO mRNA was reverse-transcribed, and the cDNA was sequenced. A duplication of four base pairs —GGCC— was found in exon 8. This led to a frameshift and should have caused a severely truncated protein. Interestingly, use of a cryptic acceptor splice-site in exon 9 led to elimination of 124 bp of message but restored the open reading frame. This mRNA is thought to code for a protein with partial peroxidase function (Fig. 52–3).

As these cases illustrate, considerable clinical and biochemical heterogeneity exists among the various defects of organification. Most of the untreated patients with complete defects are hypothyroid, have large goiters, and have physical and mental retardation. Those with partial defects may be euthyroid or compensated hypothyroid and have no physical or mental retardation. Available reports provide data from clinical or biochemical studies, but details at the molecular genetic level are lacking, except in one case.[61]

DIAGNOSIS. The major criterion for impaired iodide organification in these patients is the rapid discharge of iodide on administration of perchlorate.[67] No drop is usually detectable in labeled iodine after administration of perchlorate or thiocyanate in the normal person because trapped iodide is immediately bound to Tg. A defect in organification is thought to be present if 10 per cent or more of labeled iodide is discharged into the plasma within two hours of oral or intravenous administration of perchlorate or thiocyanate (Fig. 52–4). Perchlorate discharge is incomplete in patients with partial defects of organification. This test has certain problems. Impaired absorption of the thiocyanate or perchlorate invalidates the test. In addition, high background extrathyroidal neck tissue radioactivity can obscure results. Rapid turnover of radioactive iodine (RAI) by a small gland can produce a fall in counts over the thyroid and be misinterpreted as an iodide discharge. This problem can be circumvented by simultaneously serially measuring the appearance of protein-bound ^{131}I in serum, which should increase if no organification defect is present and hormone is rapidly released from the gland. Finally, if the defect in organification is partial, the time of administration of thiocyanate or perchlorate may influence the result. Usually perchlorate is administered two hours after the oral or intravenous iodide tracer is given. The greater the delay in administering thiocyanate or perchlorate after RAI, the less dischargeable iodide is still present in the gland.

Further diagnostic criteria include the rapid accumulation and release of radioiodine and a thyroid biopsy that reveals hyperplasia, low thyroidal iodine content, and little, if any, organic iodine. As already described, peroxidase enzyme activity may be absent or low and may or may not be restored by hematin addition or H_2O_2 addition. In vivo iodine kinetics are consistent with an expanded inorganic iodide pool.

GENETICS. In family studies, the organification defect occurs in both genders and in siblings but not in parents. Therefore, an autosomal recessive inheritance pattern is most likely.

THERAPY. For patients with hypothyroidism, T_4 replacement therapy is indicated. Thyroidectomy may be neces-

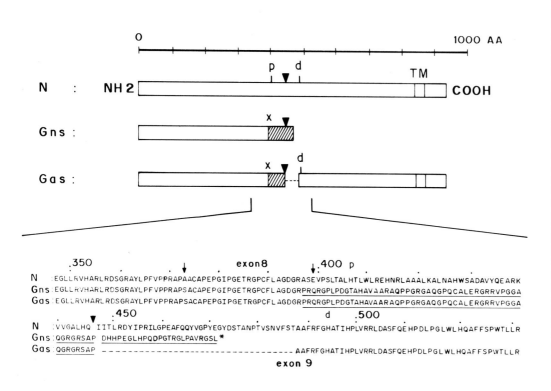

FIGURE 52–3. **Effects of mutations and splicing on TPO protein sequence.** Primary structures of the proteins deduced from cDNA sequences are compared. N, normal gene product; Gns, product of goiter gene and normal splicing; Gas, product of goiter gene and alternative splicing as observed in goiter mRNA from patient DM. p and d, putative proximal and distal heme-binding histidine residues, respectively. TM, transmembrane domain. X, GGCC duplication. Asterisk, stop codon. Amino acids are in the one-letter code. The mutated region is cross-hatched in the upper panel and underlined in the lower panel. Arrows indicate the point mutations. The arrowhead indicates the exon 8/exon 9 junction. The dashed line denotes deleted amino acids. The insertion at codon 397 altered the reading frame and produced a truncated protein (Gns) or, with alternate splicing, a longer TPO protein presumed to have some residual activity. (From Abramowicz M, Targovnik H, Cochaux P, Vassart G: Identification of a mutation in the coding sequence of the human thyroid peroxidase gene causing congenital goiter. J Clin Invest 90:1200–1204, 1992, by copyright permission of the American Society for Clinical Investigation.)

sary for large goiters that do not decrease sufficiently with therapy.

PENDRED'S SYNDROME

A disorder related to organification defect is Pendred's syndrome,[2] initially described in 1896. Patients with this

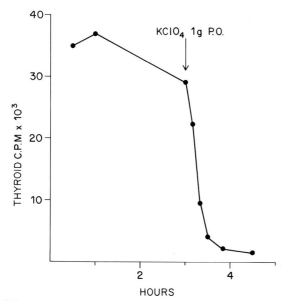

FIGURE 52–4. **Perchlorate test.** Rapid discharge of labeled iodide after perchlorate administration in a patient with impaired organification.

syndrome have congenital sensorineural deafness of variable severity, goiter, variable degrees of hypothyroidism, and a positive perchlorate discharge test. The biochemical abnormality responsible for the organification defect is unknown. Peroxidase activity, when measured, is normal in vitro.[79–81] The production of H_2O_2 may be abnormal, although NADPH–cytochrome C reductase activity has been found to be normal.[79] An abnormality in Tg synthesis has been postulated by Medeiros-Neto and colleagues,[82] who found a large fraction of the iodine in thyroid specimens to be present in a particulate non-Tg iodoprotein, and less than 15 per cent of total soluble protein in the 19S thyroglobulin peak. Shane and co-workers[83] found suggestive evidence for a partial coupling defect; chromatography of an extract of thyroid tissue from a patient with Pendred's syndrome demonstrated monoiodotyrosine (MIT) and diiodotyrosine (DIT), but no T_3 or T_4. This particular patient was clinically euthyroid, however, which indicates a partial rather than complete coupling defect. Also, the changes observed could be secondary to decreased iodination activity. Other reports have shown deficient but qualitatively normal Tg,[79, 81] although Cave and Dunn[81] reported heterogeneity in the composition of amino acids in the protein of Tg from a patient with Pendred's syndrome. Niepomniszcze and colleagues[84] postulated a cytostructural defect that precluded the normal function of the iodination site. Finally, Abdelmoumene and associates[85] reported an abnormal TPO with low K_m for the oxidation of iodide to I_2 and with little activity toward Tg iodination. Thus the biochemical abnormality responsible for the thyroidal defect in patients with Pendred's syndrome is uncertain at present.

The cause of sensorineural hearing loss is a congenitally malformed cochlea (Mondini's cochlea).[86–88] Whether this is a separate expression of a pleomorphic genetic trait or is in some way related to hypothyroidism is less certain. Injections of propylthiouracil (PTU) into the yolk sacs of developing chicks can induce changes in the cochlea.[89] Pregnant mice, when made hypothyroid with PTU, produce offspring with hair cell and tectorial membrane changes in the inner ear. Administration of T_4 can prevent the appearance of these changes in the litter.[80] However, the relationship of these findings in animals to Pendred's syndrome is unclear, because patients with Pendred's syndrome are generally not hypothyroid in utero or at birth. Interestingly, sensorineural hearing loss is common in iodine-deficient endemic cretinism, whereas athyreotic cretins are usually not deaf. Possibly maternal hormones partially protect the fetus in individuals with Pendred's syndrome or in those who are athyreotic.

CLINICAL PRESENTATION. Several hundred patients with Pendred's syndrome have been reported in the literature,[2, 79–85, 91–96] and the clinical presentations are fairly similar. Sensorineural deafness is usually evident at birth, and goiter may be present at birth or develop during childhood. In some cases, patients are only partially deaf or the deafness is more severe on one side than the other. The patients are either euthyroid or mildly hypothyroid and usually have a normal IQ and normal growth, although cases of mental retardation have been reported.[97] The goiters are generally small to moderate in size.

DIAGNOSIS. In addition to goiter and nerve deafness in the presence of normal dietary intake of iodide, the diagnosis of Pendred's syndrome depends on a partial discharge of ^{131}I following perchlorate or thiocyanate administration. There is a suggestion of hypersensitivity to perchlorate in that an abnormal prolongation of inhibition of radioiodine uptake following perchlorate administration has been observed.[95] Mild hypothyroidism or compensated hypothyroidism, as manifested by an exaggerated response to TRH,[98] may be present. A familial history is helpful. CT scans of the cochlea give a typical picture of the Mondini cochlea.[86–88]

GENETICS. In most cases, the pattern of inheritance is autosomal recessive with tight concordance between goiter and deafness. However, families in which goiter and deafness are dissociated have been reported, and one family with goiter and deafness but a normal perchlorate discharge test has been noted.[81]

THERAPY. Thyroxine replacement therapy is necessary if patients are clinically or borderline hypothyroid or if goiters are large. However, most patients do not require T_4 therapy.

"COUPLING" DEFECT

Patients with an inability to form adequate amounts of iodothyronines but with adequate formation of iodotyrosines in Tg have, by definition, a defect in coupling. However, coupling requires the adequate function of all parts of the iodination sequence and is deranged secondarily in any gland stressed by other primary abnormalities. It is convenient to refer to certain cases as representative of a "coupling defect," but this implies a set of biochemical findings that are not necessarily related to a separate specific enzymatic defect.[99, 100]

The synthesis of T_4 from two molecules of DIT or T_3 from DIT and MIT is termed the coupling reaction. The manner in which this reaction proceeds is uncertain. Peroxidase and a source of H_2O_2 are necessary for the coupling of precursors into hormones,[99] and thus TPO is the "coupling enzyme." The reaction proceeds entirely as an intramolecular rearrangement of specific iodotyrosyl residues within the peptide chain of Tg. In the current view, two iodotyrosines, both of which are held in peptide bond within the Tg molecule, are coupled to form iodothyronine.[101] A free radical mechanism is thought to be involved; a quinol ether intermediate formed by the coupling of two DIT's is split to form T_4 and a dehydroalanine residue that has been identified in Tg. This oxidative reaction is catalyzed by TPO. Although, in a sense, a deficiency in TPO is synonymous with a decrease in coupling, it remains possible that an abnormal TPO molecule is able to carry out one function (iodination) but not another (coupling). In this situation, a specific "coupling defect" might occur.

CLINICAL PRESENTATION. The following case was described by Stanbury and colleagues.[102]

A 25-year-old mentally retarded woman was first noted to be hypothyroid at age 4. Thyroid hormone therapy was initiated, and some improvement was noted. Hormone was given intermittently, however. At age 17, the patient's gland was noted to be enlarged. At 22, her PBI was 3.5 μg/dl. There was no abnormal discharge of ^{131}I from the gland following thiocyanate administration. Radioiodine uptake was very rapid, with a maximum of 99.3 per cent in the first 24 hours, and thereafter slowly dropped at a rate of 3 per cent per day. With the administration of methimazole, the rate increased to 7.3 per cent per day. Iodine clearance by the kidney was normal. Chromatographic analysis of blood samples 7 to 79 hours after the tracer dose of ^{131}I revealed small amounts of T_4 and T_3 present in all samples of peripheral blood. A total thyroidectomy was performed. Extreme hyperplasia was noted on histologic examination. It was possible to demonstrate only a trace of T_4 and T_3 in thyroid tissue specimens at the time of operation (79 hours after ^{131}I administration), although abundant MIT, DIT, and iodide were demonstrated.

The authors proposed that organic binding of iodine by the gland was enhanced but that enzymatically controlled hormone synthesis from iodinated tyrosine was impaired. The data suggest a limited ability of the thyroid to couple MIT and DIT into T_3 and T_4. The T_4 that was formed, however, was rapidly secreted, but only a small fraction of the iodine leaving the gland could have been in the form of thyroid hormone, because otherwise the patient would have been thyrotoxic.

In a number of other reported cases,[103–111] increased MIT and DIT and almost complete absence of T_3 and T_4 have been demonstrated on chromatographic analysis of in vivo labeled thyroidal iodoproteins (Fig. 52–5). Abnormalities that could produce a coupling defect include deficiency of the hypothetical coupling site in peroxidase enzyme; a defect in the activation by the enzyme of iodide or DIT; an error in the structure of the receptor protein of iodination (Tg) such that steric arrangements would impair coupling of the involved tyrosyl groups; and other abnormalities not yet identified.

DIAGNOSIS. Reported patients with a coupling defect

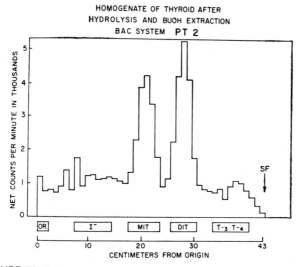

HOMOGENATE OF THYROID AFTER
HYDROLYSIS AND BUOH EXTRACTION
BAC SYSTEM **PT 2**

FIGURE 52–5. **Chromatographic analysis of in vivo labeled thyroidal iodoproteins in a patient with a "coupling" defect.** Homogenate of thyroid after hydrolysis and butanol extraction reveals large amounts of MIT and DIT and small amounts of T_3 and T_4, consistent with defective coupling of iodotyrosines. (From Morris JH: Defective coupling of iodotyrosines in familial goiters. Arch Intern Med 114:417, 1964, copyright by The American Medical Association.)

have usually been hypothyroid with a goiter with or without mental retardation. Rapid uptake of radioiodine, negative perchlorate discharge test, decreased production of thyroid hormones, and exclusion of other recognized defects are necessary for diagnosis. Thyroid biopsy four or more days after radioiodine administration reveals hyperplasia, abnormally high levels of labeled MIT and DIT, and almost total absence of labeled intrathyroidal T_3 and T_4. Kinetic studies demonstrate rapid recirculation of iodine through an intrathyroidal organic pool. At present, no rigid criteria exist for diagnosis of patients with a coupling defect, and the differentiation of Tg defects from coupling defects is uncertain.

GENETICS. Inheritance appears to follow an autosomal recessive pattern.

THERAPY. Thyroid hormone replacement is indicated for hypothyroidism and/or goiter.

ABNORMALITIES OF THYROGLOBULIN SYNTHESIS AND SECRETION

Thyroglobulin is a high molecular weight glycoprotein of complex structure. It is composed of two identical 12S subunits comprising 2748 amino acids and has a molecular weight of 650 kDa and a sedimentation coefficient of 19S. The subunits are synthesized by polyribosomes bound to the endoplasmic reticulum. After discharge of Tg into the cisternae of the endoplasmic reticulum, glycosylation of Tg occurs in the rough endoplasmic reticulum (RER) during its transfer to the Golgi apparatus. Tg is transported into the colloid space by fusion of exocytotic vesicles with the apical membrane of the cell. Most of the iodination takes place in or near the apical membrane. Tg is the storage form of thyroid hormone, and subsequent hydrolysis of Tg, with liberation of T_4 and T_3, completes the process of hormone formation.

Recent work has demonstrated variations in the structure of Tg from both normal and goitrous human thyroids. "Normal" Tg has been demonstrated to vary in content of iodine, monosaccharides, and amino acids, and this variability is greater in goitrous Tg.[112] Only about 7 per cent of the tyrosine residues contained in the Tg molecule are involved in hormone formation. Recent work[113] has identified specific peptides that are the major hormonogenic sites in the Tg molecule. Interestingly, the primary structure of the hormone-forming site is remarkably similar in several animal species.

A number of quantitative and qualitative abnormalities in Tg formation and processing have been described in animals and humans and reflect defects at a number of levels of gene expression. A defective DNA code for Tg has been suggested by findings in sheep,[114–117] cattle,[118–121] goats,[122, 123] a rat tumor line,[125] and humans.[126–135] In congenitally goitrous goats from the Netherlands,[122, 123] only a trace of Tg can be identified in the thyroid glands. By utilizing DNA complementary to the beef Tg gene as a probe, a decreased quantity of Tg messenger (mRNA) sequences (2.5 to 10 per cent of normal) was shown. Subsequently, a mutation was found in exon 8 which caused early termination of the message.[124] In addition, the intracellular location of mRNA was abnormal, with a disproportionate concentration in the nuclei. Thus an error in the rate of synthesis of Tg mRNA or abnormal processing or transport to the endoplasmic reticulum could account for the nearly absent Tg in these animals.

Studies of a strain of cattle from South Africa with congenital goiter have revealed an abnormal Tg that reacts with anti-Tg antibody.[118–121] These animals had complete absence of the 19S species of Tg, and only a 12S species could be demonstrated. The amino acid composition of the 12S component resembled that of Tg. In addition, the RER appeared poorly developed. It was postulated that a post-translational defect was present in these animals, with a possible defect in transport across the poorly developed endoplasmic reticulum. However, a recent study in this strain of cattle has revealed an abnormal Tg mRNA, which is present in decreased amount and is slightly smaller than the mRNA from normal bovine thyroid tissue.[136] The genetic lesions underlying the biochemical defect in these animals have been shown by Ricketts et al.[137] to be a mutation in exon 9 causing a stop codon. In some transcripts, this mutation is removed by splicing out of exon 9, producing a translatable but shorter mRNA coding for a protein of 2400 residues (Fig. 52–6).

Studies in humans have revealed a number of possible abnormalities.[127–132] A patient with a large congenital goiter, reported by Medeiros-Neto and Stanbury,[138] was found to have large amounts of a particulate or membrane-linked thyroidal iodoprotein, which differed from Tg in salting-out characteristics and contained MIT and DIT but no detectable iodothyronine. An abnormality in the tertiary structure of Tg was suggested in a goitrous patient reported by Kusakabe.[135] In this patient's Tg, the majority of diiodotyrosyl and thyroxyl residues, as well as tyrosyl and monoiodotyrosyl residues, appeared to be strongly buried inside the protein molecule. A report by Silva and colleagues[139] of a 12-year-old goitrous girl demonstrated an abnormal Tg that had a low molecular weight, was well iodinated, formed thyroid hormones poorly, and was prob-

FIGURE 52–6. **Diagram of the defect recognized in hTG gene in a patient with goitrous hypothyroidism and deficient Tg.** cDNA sequences and the derived amino acid sequence corresponding to full length (a) and 171 nt deleted (b) Tg transcripts from C (multinodular simple goiter) and JNA (congenital goiter). The Taq I site and the tyrosine residue in position 1509 are indicated by solid and dotted lines, respectively. The arrow points to the mutation (C to T), and the generated termination codon at position 1510 is indicated by "stop." The leucine residue resulting from the deletion is boxed. nt numbering starts at nt 1 of Tg mRNA. (From Targovnik HM, Medeiros-Neto G, Varela V, et al: A nonsense mutation causes human hereditary congenital goiter with preferential production of a 171 nt deleted thyroglobulin RNA messenger. J Clin Endocrinol Metab 77:210, 1993. © by The Endocrine Society.)

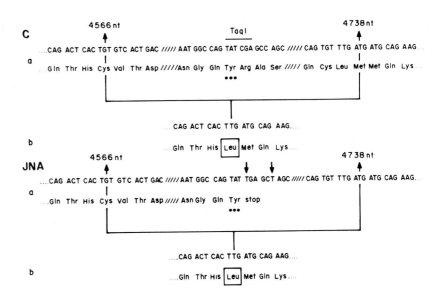

ably resistant to hydrolysis. Further qualitative abnormalities include those described by Lissitzky et al.[140] Two goitrous brothers were found to have overdistended endoplasmic reticulum cisternae containing Tg-related iodoproteins. Incomplete glycosylation of Tg was found, although there was evidence for normal sialyltransferase and galactosyltransferase activities, and a Tg transport defect from the cisternae into the thyroid follicular lumen was suggested. A case described by Monaco et al[141] was shown to have an increase in the membrane-bound 19S component of Tg and decreased sialic acid moieties.

Studies by Medeiros-Neto and collaborators[142] have demonstrated specific mutational defects in several hypothyroid individuals with deficient Tg production. In one patient, a C to G transversion upstream of the acceptor splice site of intron 3 apparently led to removal of exon 4 and thus an altered Tg molecule with probable shorter half-life and lacking the hormonogeneic tyrosine in exon 4.[143] Targovnik et al[144] reported another patient in whom a C to T transition introduced a stop codon at position 1510. The point mutation is removed from some transcripts by a 171-bp deletion, which maintains the reading frame, presumably by splicing out one exon.[144]

A mis-sense mutation within thyroglobulin gene exon 10, causing a glutamine to histidine substitution, has been recognized in three families with "simple" goiter. The association was by genetic analysis, with a lod score of 3.9. This mutation, of unknown significance, can be recognized on Southern blots of DNA.[144a]

Abnormal iodoproteins have replaced Tg in the thyroids of a number of other patients. Iodoalbumin was the predominant iodoprotein in a case described by Lizarralde and colleagues,[126] as well as a number of other cases,[127, 134, 141, 145–154] and other abnormal iodoproteins were identified in a patient reported by Riesco and co-workers[155] and in three patients reported by Michel and associates[156] and others.[150] Abnormal iodoproteins are found in a number of other conditions, including Graves' disease, Hashimoto's thyroiditis,[145] multinodular goiter, endemic goiter,[146] and thyroid carcinoma,[148] and the presence of abnormal iodoproteins therefore cannot be considered pathognomonic of defects in Tg synthesis or secretion.

Thus this category of inherited disorders of Tg synthesis is heterogeneous and may include an abnormal gene, abnormal mRNA processing, abnormal intracellular processing of Tg with defective glycosylation, transport, and exocytosis, and most likely, a number of other unestablished abnormalities.

CLINICAL PRESENTATION. The clinical presentation in the reported cases is variable. All patients have goiters, but hypothyroidism and mental retardation may or may not be present. The serum T_4, FTI, PBI, and non–butanol-extractable iodine vary from high to low. The RAIU has been elevated in almost all cases reported. In some patients, thyroidal iodide turnover is accelerated, and the perchlorate discharge test may be positive. In many cases serum Tg levels have been low.

DIAGNOSIS. The simultaneous serum measurement of PBI and butanol-extractable iodide (BEI) or T_4 iodine by RIA usually reveals abnormal iodoproteins because they are measured in the PBI but not in the BEI or T_4 RIA. Thus PBI would be greater than BEI or the T_4 RIA. As mentioned earlier, however, the detection of abnormal circulating iodoprotein does not in itself indicate an inborn error of the thyroid because such circulating proteins are present in a number of conditions, particularly those with hyperplastic glands. A low serum Tg in the presence of a goiter and elevated TSH is strong indication of a defect, but serum Tg has varied from absent to elevated. There may be diminished increment in serum Tg after injections of TSH.[147]

Thyroid biopsy is necessary to confirm Tg defect. Cell hyperplasia should be evident; 19S Tg and iodine content are low, although 3S to 12S Tg subunits may be demonstrated. Hybridization with a Tg cDNA may reveal abnormal total content or subcellular localization of the Tg mRNA, and ideally examination of the cloned cDNA may identify defects in the gene. Electron microscopy may reveal distended cisternae or abnormal RER membranes. Abnormal iodoproteins may be present as well.

GENETICS. A positive family history for goiter is obtained in approximately 50 per cent of cases. Both genders are affected, and an autosomal recessive pattern of inheritance is most likely.

THERAPY. As with all defects considered thus far, T_4 replacement is necessary if hypothyroidism or goiter is present.

IODOTYROSINE DEHALOGENASE DEFICIENCY

Iodotyrosines liberated from Tg are subject to deiodination by the action of an iodotyrosine dehalogenase. This enzyme is NADPH-dependent and is found in the thyroid particulate fraction. FAD may function as a co-factor in the deiodination.[157, 158] TSH enhances the activity of this enzyme system, perhaps by increasing NADPH production. Following the deiodination of MIT and DIT, some of the released iodide is secreted into the blood, but most is reused in hormone synthesis. Approximately 80 per cent of iodine present in Tg is recirculated in this way. In addition, deiodinase is present in other tissues, and thus iodine economy is facilitated. If iodotyrosines are not deiodinated, they are excreted in the urine. This causes a very large loss of iodine from the body each day, leading to iodine deficiency, hypothyroidism, and goiter.[159, 160]

CLINICAL PRESENTATION. The following case was reported by Stanbury and colleagues.[161, 162]

A 27-year-old man had a goiter at birth that slowly increased in size despite intermittent therapy with desiccated thyroid. At the time of study, the serum concentration of PBI was 0.5 μg/dl. The patient's parents were not consanguine, but a younger brother also had a goiter at birth and had mental and physical retardation. RAI uptake was rapid and reached a maximum observed value of 74% of the administered dose within 2 1/2 hours. This was followed by a rapid release of labeled iodine from the gland; by 48 hours, only 25 per cent of the administered dose remained in the gland. Chromatographic analysis of serial specimens of blood revealed labeled MIT and DIT within 2 hours after administration of ^{131}I. Levels increased in concentration and then decreased until they were not detectable at 72 hours. Thyroidectomy was performed because of pressure symptoms. Histological study revealed primarily hyperplasia, although some areas resembled colloid goiter, and other areas showed fibrosis; 3.4 per cent was recoverable as T_4. An approximately equal amount was T_3. The remainder consisted of a small amount of iodide and large amounts of MIT and DIT. Intravenous administration of labeled MIT or DIT[163] resulted in excretion of primarily unchanged organic iodine as MIT or DIT (Fig. 52–7). Only a small fraction of the label was excreted as inorganic iodide.

This case is an example of combined thyroidal and peripheral deiodinase defects. This abnormality was first reported by Hutchison and McGirr[163] in 1954. Four siblings from a closely inbred family were affected. All were goitrous and hypothyroid and demonstrated a rapid uptake of RAI. Similar case reports of a total body deiodinase defect have been reported[164–167]; in such cases, in addition to an absence of thyroidal deiodinase, a peripheral tissue deiodinase defect can be demonstrated by the fact that intravenously administered labeled iodotyrosines are not deiodinated. Isolated thyroidal deiodinase deficiency was reported by Kusakabe and Miyake[168] in 1964. In three goitrous sisters, thyroid tissue was nearly inactive in deiodination of ^{131}I-labeled L-DIT in vitro, whereas the rate of deiodination of ^{131}I-labeled L-DIT administered intravenously was normal. Thus, defective deiodinating activity of

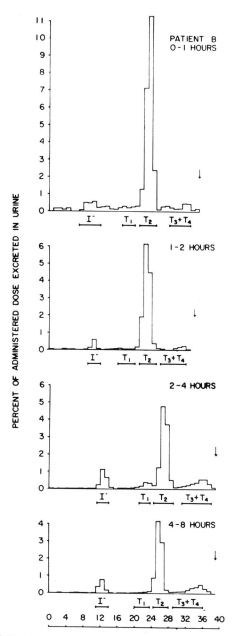

FIGURE 52–7. **Chromatograms of urine specimens obtained at various intervals after administration of labeled diiodotyrosine to a patient with total dehalogenase deficiency.** A butanol–acetic acid solvent system was employed. The labeled diiodotyrosine is excreted unchanged as DIT (indicated by T_2). The x axis represents centimeters from origin. (From Stanbury JB, Meijer JWA, Kassenaar AAH. The metabolism of iodotyrosines. II. The metabolism of mono- and diiodotyrosine in certain patients with familial goiter. J Clin Endocrinol Metab 16:848. Copyright by the Endocrine Society, 1956.)

the thyroid was demonstrated, but peripheral activity remained intact.

An additional variant of deiodinase defect was described by Ismail-Beigi and Rahimifar.[169] Three siblings, products of a consanguineous marriage, demonstrated significant ability to deiodinate intravenously injected L-MIT but not L-DIT.

Patients with reported cases of total body deiodinase defect are goitrous, generally hypothyroid, and sometimes severely retarded. The 24-hour RAI uptake and turnover are rapid, and serum chromatography reveals low levels of labeled T_3 and T_4 and elevated levels of labeled DIT and MIT. An increased incidence of thyroid carcinoma and Werdnig-Hoffmann's paralysis has been associated with this defect. Patients with isolated intrathyroidal defects are goitrous but euthyroid, and 24-hour RAIU is also rapid.

DIAGNOSIS. The diagnosis is confirmed by detecting large amounts of labeled DIT and MIT in serum following RAIU. After injection of labeled DIT or MIT, excretion of unchanged ^{131}I-DIT or MIT in the urine confirms a peripheral tissue defect. In vitro studies of thyroid slices incubated with ^{131}I-DIT or MIT reveal failure to release free iodide. Thyroid biopsy reveals abundant MIT and DIT but little or no iodothyronine, confirming an intrathyroidal defect. Correction of hypothyroidism by administration of iodine supplements is also a diagnostically valuable maneuver.

GENETICS. The family history of the original family investigated by Hutchison and McGirr revealed close intermarriage.[170-172] Thirteen goitrous cretins were known to have appeared among 31 persons in four sets of siblings. This form of goitrous cretinism behaves as a simple autosomal recessive trait. Relatives of some of these patients are euthyroid but demonstrate abnormal DIT deiodinase activity. These patients are presumably heterozygote carriers and have been shown to be less efficient in deiodinating injected labeled DIT.[162]

THERAPY. Either thyroid hormone or oral iodide is indicated. Thyroid hormone administration is generally more convenient.

DISORDERS OF THYROID HORMONE TRANSPORT

The thyroid hormones are bound to three transport proteins in the circulation: TBG, serum albumin (SA), and thyroxine-binding prealbumin (TBPA). Only a small fraction of the total T_4 (0.03 per cent) or T_3 (0.3 per cent) circulates in the free (unbound) form. Sixty per cent of circulating T_4 is bound to TBG, 30 per cent to TBPA, and 10 per cent to SA. T_3 is predominantly transported by TBG, and the remainder is transported by serum albumin.

Abnormalities of thyroid hormone transport are primarily quantitative in nature, but qualitative abnormalities have recently been described. The genetic alterations in transport proteins described include (1) familial deficiency or absence of TBG,[174-202] (2) familial excess of TBG,[188, 203-209] (3) analbuminemia,[210] (4) familial excess albumin binding (or familial dysalbuminemic hyperthyroxinemia),[211-217] (5) familial excess TBPA binding,[218, 219] and (6) qualitative variants of TBG.[220-224] These syndromes are described in Chapter 36.

In general, patients with abnormalities of transport proteins are clinically euthyroid. Free hormone levels are normal, and patients do not require therapy. The abnormalities of thyroid hormone transport are discussed more extensively in Chapter 36.

SYNDROMES OF THYROID HORMONE RESISTANCE

Since 1967, when the first three cases of thyroid hormone resistance were described by Refetoff et al.,[225] more than 200 cases have been documented with general thyroid hormone resistance.[226-253] In addition, some patients are reported to have selective pituitary resistance to the effects of thyroid hormone,[254-256, 257] and some cases of apparent isolated peripheral resistance have been reported.[244] One patient has been reported who appears to have a general hypersensitivity to the effects of thyroid hormone.[258]

The peripheral effects and mechanism of action of thyroid hormone are discussed in Chapter 37. This information is very briefly reviewed here in relation to thyroid hormone resistance. Thyroid hormone enters the cells by active transport and probably passive diffusion. Inside the cells it is bound to specific proteins that may control its transport to the nucleus, and in the extranuclear compartment, T_4 undergoes deiodination to T_3. T_3 and to some extent T_4 then enter the nucleus, possibly by active transport against a gradient, and there bind to thyroid hormone receptor (TR) proteins, which may already be bound to response elements on DNA. There are three active forms of receptor and one receptor-related control protein. TRβ1 is widely distributed in tissues, and the related form TRβ2 is present in the pituitary, and to a lesser extent, in some other areas of the brain. TRα1 is also widely distributed throughout the body and is closely related to the non-T_3 binding TRvα2. The receptors function by binding to response elements in the promoter area of responsive genes. The basic response element appears to be a six-nucleotide sequence such as AGGTCA, or variations on this theme, and exists commonly as two "half-sites" forming a palindromic sequence, as two half-sites forming a direct repeat separated by four nucleotides, or as an inverted palindrome. The receptors appear to bind to the response elements (TRE's) weakly as monomers, or more strongly, as dimers. The dimers may arise from homodimerization with an identical receptor or other form of receptor, or with a variety of other proteins (thyroid receptor accessory proteins—TRAP's). Heterodimerization with retinoid acid receptor X may be a common phenomenon and most important in activation. Possibly heterodimers are formed with several different TRAP's. Thyroid hormone receptors also bind to retinoic acid response elements and cause activation of transcription and may bind nonproductively to estrogen response elements. Unliganded receptor, occupying the response elements, typically has a negative effect on transcription. The non-T_3 binding form of the receptor, TRvα2, in some way inhibits transcriptional activation by the T_3-binding TR's, α1 and β. The mechanism of this inhibition is uncertain. The mutant receptors, described below, form heterodimers with the normal functional receptors or TRAP's and inhibit their action.

After initial definition of the clinical syndrome, defective function of receptor was identified in studies of lymphocytes and fibroblasts derived from affected patients.[246] However, in many studies no clear abnormality was identified. In 1989,[259] we reported a patient with clinical signs of generalized resistance to thyroid hormone (GRTH) action who had a mutation in the ligand-binding domain of TRβ (Fig. 52–8). This mutation caused the receptor to be unable to bind T_3, although it bound normally to DNA (Fig. 52–9). The abnormal receptor inhibited the function of normal hTRβ1 or hTRα1 in a co-transfection system, akin to the inhibitory action of the non-T_3 binding receptor—

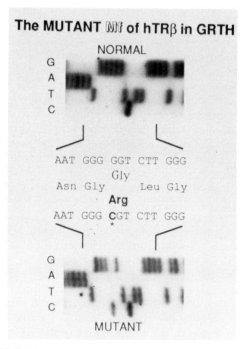

The MUTANT Mf of hTRβ in GRTH

FIGURE 52–8. **Mutation in the hTRβ1 gene.** cDNA's from the normal gene and the mutant were cloned and sequenced. The tracks for guanosine (G), adenosine (A), thymidine (T), and cytosine (C) are shown. Replacement of a G by a C in the mutant changed the codon to arginine, which produces a difference in the ligand-binding area and presumably makes the thyroid hormone receptor unable to bind T_3.

like molecule, hTRvα2 (Fig. 52–10). Subsequently, many more mutations have been detected, almost all located within the ligand-binding domain of hTRβ.[260] One infant has been reported with a homozygous mutation, producing a severe defect.[261] In one family a deletion of hTRβ has been found.[262] In the heterozygous state, this is inconse-

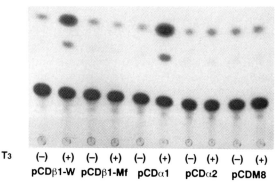

FIGURE 52–9. **Transcriptional regulation by various TR's.** Two micrograms of plasmid vector containing either the normal "wild" type TRβ1 (pCDβ1-W) or the normal hTRα1 (pCDα1) were co-transfected into COS-7 cells along with 2 or 10 μg pCDβ1-Mf containing the mutant receptor or 10 μg pCDM8 (vector alone), and 4 μg pUrGH(S). pUrGH(S) is a reporter plasmid expressing chloramphenicol acetyl transferase activity when activated. CAT activity was determined in cell extracts by chromatography. The lower spots indicate the original chloramphenicol, and the upper spots indicate the acetylated product. The addition of T_3 activated transcription by pCDβ1-W and caused strong acetylation. hTRα1 was also active, but the vector containing TRβ1-Mf was completely inactive. The non–T_3-binding receptor-related protein hTRvα2 also, as expected, produced no response. (From Sakurai A, Miyamoto T, Refetoff S, et al: Dominant negative transcriptional regulation by a mutant thyroid hormone receptor-beta in a family with generalized resistance to thyroid hormone. Mol Endocrinol 4:1988–1994, 1990.)

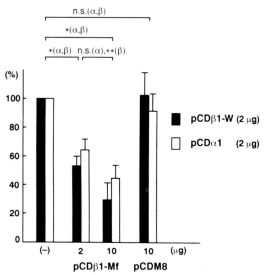

FIGURE 52–10. **Negative transcriptional regulation by hTRβ, cloned from a subject heterozygous for GRTH due to a mutational defect.** Two micrograms of each expression vector for hTRβ1-W, wild type, or TRα1, increasing amounts of a vector pCDβ1-Mf, and a control plasmid (pCDM8) were transfected into COS-7 cells along with 4 μg of the reporter plasmid pUrGH(S). After 48-hour incubation in the absence (−) or presence (+) of 5 nM T_3, cells were collected and CAT activities were estimated. CAT activity in COS-7 cells transfected with either pCDβ1-W or pCDα1 and pUrGH(S), in the presence of 5 nM T_3, was normalized to 100 per cent. Statistical significance was examined for the effect of pCDβ1-Mf on pCDβ1 and pCDα1 by t test. (*, $P < 0.01$; **, $P < 0.05$; n.s., not significant.) Addition of the nonfunctional mutant receptor inhibited function of both the normal hTRβ1 and normal hTRα1, presumably by competition for binding to the DNA or by forming inactive dimers with the normal receptor or auxiliary proteins.

quential, but homozygous subjects have evidence of severe thyroid hormone resistance.

The clinical findings in these patients are heterogeneous but fit within certain broad categories. Individuals who are heterozygous for deletion of a β receptor have a normal phenotype. Apparently having two normal α receptors and one normal β receptor allows normal function. Individuals who are heterozygous for a mutation in the ligand-binding domain of TRβ constitute the bulk of reported cases. These patients have typical GRTH with elevated thyroid hormone levels in the presence of (usually) normal TSH, but few physical stigmata. Many appear to have a hyperactivity-associated learning disability, and some may have mild mental deficiency and evidence of hypothyroidism. Presumably, in this instance, the expressed mutated receptor, which cannot bind T_3, forms inactive heterodimers with normal receptors or TRAP's and in some way limits their function. In response to diminished feedback signal at the pituitary level, because the mutation affects the hTRβ2 as well as hTRβ1, increased levels of TSH and thus T_4 are produced. The effect of this may be to normalize hormone responses in many tissues but may produce hypernormal levels of thyroid hormone and thyroid hormone activity in certain tissues, especially those in which TRα may be dominant, such as the brain and heart. Some of these patients are born with significantly elevated TSH, suggesting that they are hypothyroid, but in later childhood and in adult life the patients are characteristically euthyroid unless they have received some treatment to lower the

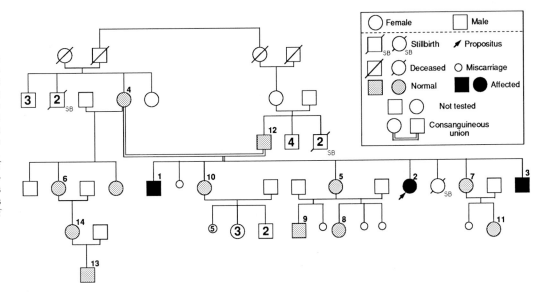

FIGURE 52–11. **Pedigree of the G family.** ID numbers are at the upper right of symbols. Numbers within the symbols indicate the number of siblings of the same gender. The significance of high frequency of miscarriage (9 of a total of 17 pregnancies) in the three normal female siblings (nos. 10, 5, and 7), who are products of the consanguineous union, is unclear. The heterozygous carriers are normal. Three homozygous children are evident. (Courtesy of Dr. Samuel Refetoff.)

thyroid hormone level based on the false assumption that they were hyperthyroid.[260]

Homozygous deletion of the β receptor has been identified in the original sibship, described below, and causes the classic form of GRTH associated with deaf-mutism, retarded bone development, and abnormal growth[262] (Figs.

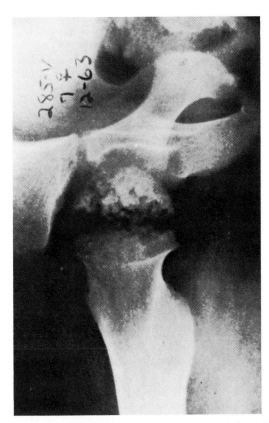

FIGURE 52–12. **Roentgenogram of the proximal end of the right femur of a patient with thyroid hormone resistance.** Mottled areas of increased density are present throughout the ossification centers of the head of the femur. The appearance is that of an epiphysis formed from multiple minute centers that have coalesced to a degree. The gross outline of the epiphysis is normal. (From Refetoff S, DeWind LT, DeGroot LJ: Familial syndrome combining deaf-mutism, stippled epiphyses, goiter, and abnormally high PBI: Possible target organ refractoriness to thyroid hormone. J Clin Endocrinol Metab 27:279. Copyright by the Endocrine Society, 1967.)

52–11 to 52–13). These patients have two functional α receptor genes and no β receptors and have the functional inhibitory form of α, hTRvα2. This defect proves that hTRα is sufficient for supporting life, although not normality. In the absence of hTRβ receptors, hTRvα2 appears to exert a derogatory inhibitory effect on the function of hTRα1, or perhaps hTRα1 alone does not provide enough receptor function to cause normal tissue thyroid hormone responses. In any event, the patients appear to have a mixture of tissue effects, including some tissues that are apparently hypothyroid and others that appear to be hypermetabolic. Presumably this is because the deficient feedback on the pituitary allows elevated levels of thyroid hormone to exist in compensation. The elevated T_4 level may hypersaturate α receptors, which predominate in some tissues

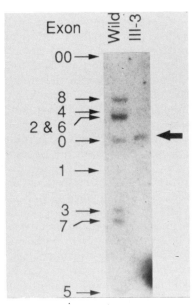

FIGURE 52–13. **Genomic DNA from a normal subject and a patient were digested with TAQ 1 enzyme.** Fragments were separated by electrophoresis and transferred to nitrocellulose paper. Probing with ^{32}P-labeled hTRβ1 recognized eight fragments, corresponding to the numbered exons, in the DNA from the normal subject, but only a small portion of the gene was present in the genomic DNA from this patient with GRTH.

such as brain and heart. Other tissues lack sufficient receptor function in the absence of hTRβ.

The presence of homozygosity for a mutation of the β receptor in the ligand-binding domain has been reported in one unfortunate individual with severe mental and physical retardation. Thus the presence of two normal α receptors is unable to overcome the negative effect of two receptor forms that can bind to DNA but cannot bind T_3.[261]

Almost all mutations identified so far have been in the ligand-binding domain of hTRβ and are generally, as indicated above, partially compensated by increasing T_4 levels. No α receptor mutations have been described so far, possibly because this represents a lethal effect. No mutational defects have been defined in areas other than those that affect ligand binding, possibly because of the method of detecting the abnormalities through elevated thyroid hormone levels. No strict correlation exists between the deficiency in binding T_3 and the abnormality produced by a mutated receptor present in a heterozygous state, suggesting that mutations may interfere with a variety of receptor functions such as dimerization with accessory proteins or other receptors, in addition to binding T_3 ligand.

Studies on patients with presumed selective pituitary resistance to thyroid hormone are less advanced. In theory this syndrome should produce peripheral hyperthyroidism, but it is often difficult to differentiate true tissue hypermetabolism from the tissue and clinical abnormalities found in generalized resistance to thyroid hormone. This is especially true because only imperfect markers are available for determining "tissue hyperthyroidism." Recent studies prove that some of these patients actually have generalized resistance to thyroid hormone associated with a mutation in TRβ.[260] Perhaps others have an abnormality in the pituitary, possibly due to a mutation in the amino-terminal portion of hTRβ which is specific for the pituitary form of this protein. Although the amino-terminal portion of the β receptor, hTRβ2, may determine tissue specificity, the remainder of the molecule is identical to hTRβ1.[263] Thus, mutations in the DNA-binding domain or ligand-binding domains of the receptor would be evident in both peripheral tissues and pituitary and would not confer selective pituitary resistance. In summary, no clear concept has been formulated of how a mutation in the amino terminal domain of hTRβ2 would produce selective pituitary thyroid hormone resistance, and little evidence indicates that the syndrome exists.

Selective peripheral resistance to thyroid hormone action has also been reported but not documented fully by metabolic studies, and again it is uncertain that this syndrome actually exists.[264] The one patient reported with alleged increased sensitivity to thyroid hormone action has not been carefully studied clinically or biochemically.[258]

In addition to abnormalities in the receptor, there obviously could be syndromes of thyroid hormone resistance due to a variety of mechanisms controlling receptor turnover or postreceptor mechanisms such as functionally abnormal TRAP's. Also, thyroid hormone resistance due to selective decrease of T_4 plasma membrane transport was reported and confirmed by in vitro study of erythrocytes.[264] This syndrome differs from conventional thyroid hormone resistance in that elevations in serum T_4, free T_4, and reverse T_3 (rT_3) are present with only minimally increased levels of T_3. Hypothetically, defective conversion of T_4 to T_3

could also be a cause of thyroid hormone resistance, as could selective hypermetabolism of T_4 and/or T_3.

CLINICAL PRESENTATION. The first patient with thyroid hormone resistance was described by Refetoff et al.[225] in 1967.

A 6-year-old girl, deaf from birth, on skeletal roentgenographic survey had stippling of the major secondary ossification centers (Fig. 52–12). The epiphyses appeared to have developed from multiple centers. The child had no symptoms or signs of hyper- or hypothyroidism. Her thyroid gland was diffusely enlarged on palpation. She exhibited certain striking morphologic characteristics that were also present in two of her brothers, that is, bird-like facies, pigeon breast, and winged scapulae. A brisk Achilles reflex, elevated pulse rate, and slight hyperactivity were the sole physical findings compatible with hyperthyroidism. There was a striking discrepancy between the euthyroid clinical state and the clinical laboratory evidence consistent with hyperthyroidism. The initial mean PBI levels in the patient and her two brothers were 14.0, 20.8, and 19.3 μg/dl, respectively. The 24-hour uptake of ^{131}I fell within the hyperthyroid range in one of the siblings (70%) and was borderline for the other two (49 and 51%, respectively). This finding was a reflection of rapid iodine turnover within the gland. Serum TSH levels, basal metabolic rate, serum lipids, cholesterol, enzymes, tyrosine, and TBG levels were normal.

Further studies were done to investigate the cause of this resistance to thyroid hormone. The glands of these subjects secreted approximately 5 times the normal amount of T_4 daily. T_4 and free T_3 levels in blood were in the hyperthyroid range. The T_4 in blood was identified as normal L-T_4 by several tests. Administration of 1 mg/day of L-T_4 or 375 μg/day L-T_3 partially suppressed the elevated RAIU and increased the initially depressed creatinine and hydroxyproline secretion. β-Adrenergic blockade and 45 days of PTU therapy failed to produce detectable effects. TSH responded normally to the administration of TRH despite the presence in serum of T_4, free T_4, and T_3 in concentrations threefold above the mean normal range.[251] Cortisone suppressed TSH release, as in normal subjects. Studies with labeled hormone showed that the patient's lymphocyte nuclear receptors bound T_3 with a lower affinity and higher capacity than normal lymphocyte nuclear receptors.[245]

These cases demonstrate an elevation of circulating levels of free thyroid hormone in the face of a euthyroid or mildly hypothyroid state. This is characteristic of all cases of generalized thyroid hormone resistance. In addition, goiter and inappropriately detectable or elevated TSH are typical. The somatic abnormalities present in these three cases—abnormal facies, winged scapulae, and pigeon breast—have not been present in other cases. A number of other major or minor somatic defects, such as scaphocephaly,[233] short fourth metacarpals,[233] and Besnier's prurigo,[264] have been reported, but the relation to thyroid hormone deprivation is unclear. Neuropsychiatric defects including mental retardation, learning disabilities, hearing defects, nystagmus, and emotional disturbances have been present and may be related to tissue deprivation of thyroid hormone. The presence of stippled epiphyses is variable and probably reflects the age of presentation of the patient because epiphyseal fusion and even disappearance of stippling have been observed with advancing age of the subjects.[250] Many patients have had previous therapy with antithyroid medication, thyroidectomy, or RAI before the diagnosis of resistance was made.

Patients with alleged selective pituitary resistance, in contrast, present with elevated free thyroid hormone levels, inappropriately elevated TSH, and symptoms of hyperthyroidism. The peripheral tissues are sensitive to the effects of elevated circulating thyroid hormone, in contrast to those with generalized resistance. A number of cases of selective pituitary resistance associated with cystinosis have been reported.[265] Finally, cases of isolated peripheral resistance have been reported.[244, 264] These patients' hypothalamic-pituitary axes were normally suppressed with physiological doses of the hormone, although larger doses were required to achieve a eumetabolic state. Thus all hormone tests of thyroid function were normal, but tests measuring the action of thyroid hormone on peripheral tissues, such as oxygen consumption, were abnormal.

DIAGNOSIS. High serum T_4 and T_3 levels and inappropriately elevated or detectable TSH are found in all cases of generalized resistance. Thyroid hormone transport defects and anti-T_4 antibodies must be ruled out, and the presence of common thyroid diseases must be excluded. TRH stimulation should produce an inappropriate increase in TSH for the level of circulating thyroid hormone. Administration of pharmacological doses of T_4 or T_3 should produce an inadequate metabolic response in those patients with peripheral tissue resistance to thyroid hormone action. A spectrum of tests, including assay of creatine phosphokinase, cholesterol, testosterone-estradiol–binding globulin (TEBG), ferritin, calorie consumption, and basal metabolic rate, should ideally be employed to monitor the response to thyroid hormone. Most important, the TSH response to TRH should be preserved or only partially suppressed during the administration of supraphysiological doses of thyroid hormone. In the method reported by Sarne et al.,[266] patients are given increments of T_3 orally every three days (50, 75, and 100 μg twice a day) and TRH tests are performed serially at the end of each period. Normal subjects are suppressed by 50 μg twice a day. Normal suppression of the TSH response to TRH during the administration of glucocorticoids or dopaminergic drugs should be demonstrated. Measurement of ferritin, cholesterol, TBG, TEBG, urinary creatine, and creatinine, should produce data typical of euthyroidism.

In patients who have strong evidence of GRTH, the final diagnosis rests on sequencing the cDNA for hTRβ and/or hTRα and further studies including in vitro expression and study of function in transfection assays.[259]

Patients reported with isolated "pituitary" resistance have similarly high serum levels of T_4 and T_3 and elevated levels of TSH but are clinically hyperthyroid, in contrast to patients with generalized resistance. In patients with isolated pituitary resistance, autonomous hypersecretion of TSH by a pituitary adenoma must be ruled out by MR imaging or CT scan, measurements of TSH α, and possibly measurements of other pituitary function. TRH stimulation should produce an inappropriate increase in TSH for the level of circulating thyroid hormone, in contrast to typically depressed responses in patients with TSH-producing adenomas.

Resistance to thyroid hormone action selective to peripheral tissues is the most difficult to diagnose. All hormone tests of thyroid function are normal because of the normal sensitivity of the pituitary feedback regulation to physiological levels of thyroid hormone. TSH secretion is not elevated despite apparent hypometabolism at the tissue level. Until methods improve for measuring hypometabolism at the tissue level, selective peripheral resistance to thyroid hormone will be difficult to diagnose, and the syndrome remains indefinite.

GENETICS. The abnormality is usually inherited, although many sporadic cases have been reported. Consanguinity has been established in many families. The defect has occurred in one set of identical twins, and in another instance, only one fraternal twin was affected. The male:female ratio is equal. Inheritance is by an autosomal gene, but expression may be dominant in the case of a mutated receptor or recessive in the case of the deleted receptor gene.

THERAPY. At present no adequate treatment exists for an adult with generalized resistance. Therapy with RAI, thyroidectomy, or antithyroid drugs is obviously contraindicated. Exogenous thyroid hormone may be indicated only if certain peripheral tissues are still relatively deficient in thyroid hormone action despite the elevated circulating levels of hormone. Infants and children with generalized resistance, on the other hand, may benefit from supraphysiological doses of T_4 or T_3 to maintain normal growth, bone maturation, anabolic state, and mental development.

Selective "pituitary" resistance to thyroid hormone is also difficult to treat. RAI, thyroidectomy, or antithyroid drugs lower the circulating thyroid hormone levels, but at the risk of producing further TSH secretion and possible pituitary hyperplasia or pituitary tumors. In addition, goiter size increases with antithyroid drugs. Some success in suppressing TSH production has been reported using dopamine agonists, such as bromocriptine[267, 268] or pergolide,[269] but experience with this use of the drugs is limited. The hormone analogue 3,5,3′-triiodothyroacetic acid (TRIAC) was reported in one case to lower TSH secretion effectively.[270] In one kindred serum TSH could be suppressed to normal by T_3 administration (25 to 50 μg/d), with resultant normal circulating thyroid hormone levels and no symptoms of hyperthyroidism.[271] Pituitary ablation is effective but introduces its own complications.

Selective peripheral thyroid hormone resistance may be treated with thyroid hormone. Tests of peripheral thyroid hormone action and subjective responses to therapy are necessary to titrate the dose.

MISCELLANEOUS CONDITIONS

Intrathyroidal Calcification and Goiter

Nontoxic goiter associated with patchy intrathyroidal calcification was reported to occur in five generations of a family.[272] Despite extensive investigations, none of the recognized thyroid dyshormonogenetic abnormalities was detected. In vivo ^{131}I tracer studies showed a pattern of increased thyroid iodine avidity and rapid turnover, but the defect underlying this syndrome is as yet unrecognized.

Dyshormonogenetic Goiter and Abnormal Iodide Leak

A large kindred with familial goiter and a leak of nonhormonal iodide from the thyroid was reported by Cooper

42. Virion A, Michot JL, Deme D, et al: NADPH-dependent H_2O_2 generation and peroxidase activity in thyroid particulate fraction. Mol Cell Endocrinol 36:95–105, 1984.

43. Pommier J, Tourniaire J, Rahmoun B, et al: Thyroid iodine organification defects: A case with lack of thyroglobulin iodination and a case without any peroxidase activity. J Clin Endocrinol Metab 42:319, 1976.

44. Valenta LJ, Bode H, Vickery AL, et al: Lack of thyroid peroxidase activity as the cause of congenital goitrous hypothyroidism. J Clin Endocrinol Metab 36:830, 1973.

45. Eggo MC, Burrow GN, Alexander NM, Gordon JH: Iodination and the structure of human thyroglobulin. J Clin Endocrinol Metab 51:7, 1980.

46. Medeiros-Neto GA, Knobel M, Yamamoto K, et al: Deficient thyroid peroxidase causing organification defect and goitrous hypothyroidism. J Endocrinol Invest 2:353, 1979.

47. Niepomniszcze H, Degrossi OJ, Scavini LM, Curutchet HP: Familial goiter with partial iodine incorporation block and euthyroidism due to the deficient peroxidase defect. *In* Thyroid Research, 7th International Thyroid Conference. New York, Excerpta Medica, 1976, p 470.

48. Nunez J, Pommier J, Dominici R, et al: Peroxidase and thyroglobulins from different goiters. *In* Thyroid Research, 7th International Thyroid Conference. New York, Excerpta Medica, 1976, p 467.

49. Niepomniszcze H, DeGroot LJ, Hagen GA: Abnormal thyroid peroxidase causing iodide organification defect. J Clin Endocrinol Metab 34:607, 1972.

50. Niepomniszcze H, Rosenbloom AL, DeGroot LJ, et al: Differentiation of two abnormalities in thyroid peroxidase causing organification defect and goitrous hypothyroidism. Metabolism 24:57, 1975.

51. Pommier J, Tourniaire J, Deme D, et al: A defective thyroid peroxidase solubilized from a familial goiter with iodine organification defect. J Clin Endocrinol Metab 39:69, 1974.

52. Pommier J, Dominici R, Bougneres P, et al: A dialyzable inhibitor bound to thyroglobulins from four simple goiters and from two goiters with iodine organification defect. J Mol Med 2:169, 1977.

53. Niepomniszcze H, Castells S, DeGroot LJ, et al: Peroxidase defect in congenital goiter with complete organification block. J Clin Endocrinol Metab 36:347, 1973.

54. Medeiros-Neto GA, Nakashima T, Taurog A, et al: Congenital goiter and hypothyroidism with impaired iodide organification and high thyroid peroxidase concentration. Clin Endocrinol 11:123, 1979.

55. Niepomniszcze H, Coleoni AH, Targovnik HM, et al: Congenital goiter due to thyroid peroxidase-iodinase defect. Acta Endocrinol 93:25, 1980.

56. Medeiros-Neto GA, Okamura K, Cavaliere H, et al: Familial thyroid peroxidase defect. Clin Endocrinol 17:1, 1982.

57. Kusakabe T: Deficient cytochrome b reductase activity in nontoxic goiter with iodide organification defect. Metabolism 24:1103, 1975.

58. Niepomniszcze H, Targovnik HM, Gluzman BE, Curutchet P: Abnormal H_2O_2 supply in the thyroid of a patient with goiter and iodine organification defect. J Clin Endocrinol Metab 65:344–348, 1987.

59. Kusakabe T: A goitrous subject with defective synthesis of diiodotyrosine due to thyroglobulin abnormalities. J Clin Endocrinol Metab 37:317, 1973.

60. Niepomniszcze H, Medeiros-Neto GA, Refetoff S, et al: Familial goiter with partial iodine organification defect, lack of thyroglobulin, and high levels of thyroid peroxidase. Clin Endocrinol 6:27, 1977.

61. Abramowicz M, Targovnik H, Cochaux P, Vassart G: Identification of a mutation in the coding sequence of the human thyroid peroxidase gene causing congenital goiter. J Clin Invest 90:1200–1204, 1992.

62. Hosoya T: Effect of various reagents including antithyroid compounds upon the activity of thyroid peroxidase. J Biochem 53:381, 1963.

63. DeGroot LJ, Davis AM: Studies on the biosynthesis of iodotyrosines: A soluble thyroidal iodide-peroxidase tyrosine-iodinase system. Endocrinology 70:492, 1962.

64. Pommier J, de Prailauné S, Nunez J: Peroxydase particulaire thyroidienne. Biochimie 54:483, 1972.

65. DeGroot LJ, Davis AM: Studies on the biosynthesis of iodotyrosines: The relationship of peroxidase, catalase, and cytochrome oxidase. Endocrinology 70:505, 1962.

66. Alexander NM, Burrow GN: Thyroxine biosynthesis in human goitrous cretinism. J Clin Endocrinol Metab 30:308, 1970.

67. Stewart RDH, Murray IPC: An evaluation of the perchlorate discharge test. J Clin Endocrinol Metab 26:1050, 1966.

68. Perez-Cuvit E, Crigler JF Jr, Stanbury JB: Partial and total iodide organification defect in different sibships in a kindred. Am J Hum Genet 29:142, 1977.

69. Haddad HM, Sidbury JB Jr: Defect of the iodinating system in congenital goitrous cretinism: Report of a case with biochemical studies. J Clin Endocrinol Metab 19:1446, 1959.

70. Schultz A, Flink EB, Kennedy BJ, Zieve L: Exchangeable character of accumulated ^{131}I in the thyroid gland of a goitrous cretin. J Clin Endocrinol Metab 17:441, 1957.

71. Clayton GW, Smith JD, Leiser A: Familial goiter with defect in intrinsic metabolism of thyroxine without hypothyroidism. J Pediatr 52:129, 1958.

72. Furth ED, Carvalho M, Vianna B: Familial goiter due to an organification defect in euthyroid siblings. J Clin Endocrinol Metab 27:1137, 1967.

73. Lelong M, Joseph R, Canlorbe P, et al: L'hypothyroidie par anomalie congenitale de l'hormonogenese (cinq observations). Arch Fr Pediatr 13:341, 1956.

74. Mouriz J, Riesco G, Usobiaga P: Thyroid proteins in a goitrous cretin with iodide organification defect. J Clin Endocrinol Metab 29:942, 1969.

75. Gardner JU, Hayles AB, Woolner LB, Owen CA: Iodine metabolism in goitrous cretins. J Clin Endocrinol Metab 19:638, 1959.

76. Konig MP, Baumann T, Scharer K, Herren C: Familiare kongenitale storung der schilddrusenhormonsynthese: Fehlerhafte oxydation von anorganischem zu organischem jod. Schweiz Med Wochenschr 94:319, 1964.

77. Jackson ADM: Non-endemic goitrous cretinism. Arch Dis Child 29:571, 1954.

78. Pena J, Belmonte AV, Tojo R: Hipotiroidismo bocioso por defecto en el proceso de organificacion del iodo: Una observacion en gemelos. Rev Esp Pediatr 21:103, 1965.

79. Burrow GN, Spaulding SW, Alexander NM, Bower BF: Normal peroxidase activity in Pendred's syndrome. J Clin Endocrinol Metab 36:522, 1973.

80. Ljunggren J-G, Lindstrom H, Hjern B: The concentration of peroxidase in normal and adenomatous human thyroid tissue with special reference to patients with Pendred's syndrome. Acta Endocrinol 72:272, 1973.

81. Cave WT Jr, Dunn JT: Studies on the thyroidal defect in an atypical form of Pendred's syndrome. J Clin Endocrinol Metab 41:590, 1975.

82. Medeiros-Neto GA, Nicolau W, Kieffer J, Ulhoa-Cintra AB: Thyroidal iodoproteins in Pendred's syndrome. J Clin Endocrinol Metab 28:1205, 1968.

83. Shane SR, Jones JE, Flink EB: Familial goiter and congenital nerve deafness. J Clin Endocrinol Metab 25:1085, 1965.

84. Niepomniszcze H, Coleoni AH, Degrossi OJ, et al: Biochemical studies on the iodide organification defect of Pendred's syndrome. Acta Endocrinol 89:70, 1978.

85. Abdelmoumene N, Gavaret JM, Pommier J, Nunez J: A defective thyroid peroxidase in a case of Pendred's syndrome. J Molec Med 3:305, 1978.

86. Johnsen T, Larsen C, Friis J, Hougaard-Jensen F: Pendred's syndrome. Acoustic, vestibular and radiological findings in 17 unrelated patients. J Laryngol Otol 101:1187–1192, 1987.

87. Friis J, Johnsen T, Feldt-Rasmussen U, et al: Thyroid function in patients with Pendred's syndrome. J Endocrinol Invest 11:97–101, 1988.

88. Johnsen T, Videbaek H, Olesen KP: CT-scanning of the cochlea in Pendred's syndrome. Clin Otolaryngol 14:389–393, 1989.

89. Bargman GJ, Gardner LI: Otic lesions and congenital hypothyroidism in the developing chick. J Clin Invest 46:1828, 1967.

90. Deol MS: Congenital deafness and hypothyroidism. Lancet 2:105, 1973.

91. Fraser GR, Morgans ME, Trotter WR: The syndrome of sporadic goiter and congenital deafness. Q J Med 53:279, 1960.

92. Elman DS: Familial association of nerve deafness with nodular goiter and thyroid carcinoma. N Engl J Med 259:219, 1958.

93. Thould AK, Scowen EF: The syndrome of congenital deafness and simple goiter. *In* Pitt-Rivers R (ed): Advances in Thyroid Research. New York, Pergamon Press, 1961, p 22.

94. Nilsson LR, Borgfors N, Gamstorp I, et al: Nonendemic goiter and deafness. Acta Pediatr 53:117, 1964.

95. Milutinovic PS, Stanbury JB, Wicken JV, Jones EW: Thyroid function in a family with the Pendred syndrome. J Clin Endocrinol Metab 29:962, 1969.

96. Almeida F, Temporal A, Cavalcanti N, et al: Pendred's syndrome in an area of endemic goiter in Brazil. *In* Dunn JT, Medeiros-Neto GA

(eds): Genetic and Metabolic Studies in Endemic Goiter and Cretinism. Washington, DC, WHO, 1974.
97. Thompson J, Maguire NC, Hurwitz LJ: A family with deafness, goiter, epilepsy, and low intelligence segregating independently. Ir J Med Sci 3:427, 1970.
98. Gomez-Pan A, Evered DC, Hall R: Pituitary-thyroid function in Pendred's syndrome. BMJ 2:152, 1974.
99. Pommier J, Deme D, Fimiani E, et al: Mechanism of thyroid peroxidase catalysis of thyroid hormone synthesis [abstract 54]. International Congress Series No. 361. Amsterdam, Excerpta Medica, 1975.
100. Mallet E, Carayon P, Amr S, et al: Coupling defect of thyrotropin receptor and adenylate cyclase in a pseudohypoparathyroid patient. J Clin Endocrinol Metab 54:1028, 1982.
101. Gavaret J-M, Cahnmann HJ, Nunez J: Thyroid hormone synthesis in thyroglobulin: The mechanism of the coupling reaction. J Biol Chem 256:9167, 1981.
102. Stanbury JB, Ohela K, Pitt-Rivers R: The metabolism of iodine in two goitrous cretins compared with that in two patients receiving methimazole. J Clin Endocrinol Metab 15:54, 1955.
103. Jacobsen BB: Normal serum T$_3$ value in one of two siblings with goitrous hypothyroidism and dyshormonogenesis. Dan Med Bull 20:192, 1973.
104. Morris JH: Defective coupling of iodotyrosine in familial goiters. Arch Intern Med 114:417, 1964.
105. Choufoer JC, Kassenaar AAH, Querido A: The syndrome of congenital hypothyroidism with defective dehalogenation of iodotyrosines: Further observations and discussion of pathophysiology. J Clin Endocrinol Metab 20:983, 1960.
106. Mosier HD, Blizzard RM, Wilkins L: Congenital defects in the biosynthesis of thyroid hormones: Report of two cases. Pediatrics 21:248, 1958.
107. Joseph R, Job J-C: Les hypothyroidies par troubles congenitaux de l'hormonogenese. Vie Med Can Fr 42:1259, 1961.
108. Werner SC, Block RJ, Mandl RH, Kassenaar AAH: Pathogenesis of a case of congenital goiter with abnormally high levels of SPI and with mono- and diiodotyrosine in the serum. J Clin Endocrinol Metab 17:817, 1957.
109. Leszynsky HE: Metabolic defects of thyroid hormone synthesis in a case of infantilism without clinical evidence of thyroid pathology (thyrogenic infantilism). Acta Endocrinol 36:221, 1961.
110. Whitelaw MJ, Thomas S, Reilly WA: A nongoitrous cretin with a high level of serum PBI and thyroidal ^{131}I uptake. J Clin Endocrinol Metab 16:983, 1956.
111. Cooper DS, Axelrod L, DeGroot LJ, et al: Congenital goiter and the development of metastatic follicular carcinoma with evidence for a leak of nonhormonal iodide: Clinical, pathological, kinetic, and biochemical studies and a review of the literature. J Clin Endocrinol Metab 52:294, 1981.
112. Dunn JT, Ray SC: Variations in the structure of thyroglobulins from normal and goitrous human thyroids. J Clin Endocrinol Metab 47:861, 1978.
113. Lejeune PJ, Marriq C, Rolland M, Lissitzky S: Amino acid sequence around a hormonogenic tyrosine residue in the N-terminal region of human thyroglobulin after in vivo and in vitro iodination. Biochem Biophys Res Commun 114:73, 1983.
114. Falconer IR: Studies of the congenitally goitrous sheep: The iodinated compounds of serum and circulating thyroid-stimulating hormone. Biochem J 100:190, 1966.
115. Falconer IR: Studies of the congenitally goitrous sheep: Composition and metabolism of goitrous thyroid tissue. Biochem J 100:197, 1966.
116. Falconer IR, Roitt I, Scamark RF, Torrigiani G: Studies of the congenitally goitrous sheep: Iodoproteins of the goiter. Biochem J 117:417, 1970.
117. Rac R, Hill GN, Pain RW, Mulhearn CJ: Congenital goiter in merino sheep due to an inherited defect in the biosynthesis of thyroid hormone. Vet Sci 9:209, 1968.
118. Pammenter MD: The biochemical nature of the primary defect in the genetically determined goiter of Afrikander cattle [thesis]. University of Stellenbosch, South Africa, 1978.
119. Van Jaarsveld PP, Sena L, Van der Walt B, Van Zyl A: Abnormal iodoproteins in a congenital bovine goiter. In Fellinger K, Hofer R (eds): Further Advances in Thyroid Research. Wien, G Gistel & Cie, 1971, pp 465–479.
120. Van Jaarsveld P, Van der Walt B, Theron CN: Afrikander cattle congenital goiter: Purification and partial identification of the complex iodoprotein pattern. Endocrinology 91:470, 1972.
121. Van Zyl A, Schulz K, Wilson B, Pansegrouw D: Thyroidal iodine and

enzymatic defects in cattle with congenital goiter. Endocrinology 76:353, 1965.
122. De Vijlder JJM, van Voorthuizen WF, van Dijk JE, et al: Hereditary congenital goiter with thyroglobulin deficiency in a breed of goats. Endocrinology 102:1214, 1978.
123. Rijnberk A, De Vijlder JJM, Van Dijk JE, et al: Congenital defect in iodothyronine synthesis: Clinical aspects of iodine metabolism in goats with congenital goiter and hypothyroidism. Br Vet J 133:495, 1977.
124. Veenboer GJM, de Vijlder JJM: Molecular basis of the thyroglobulin synthesis defect in Dutch goats. Endocrinology 132:377–381, 1993.
125. Monaco F, Robbins J: Defective thyroglobulin synthesis in an experimental rat thyroid tumor. J Biol Chem 248:2328, 1973.
126. Lizarralde G, Jones B, Seal US, Jones JE: Goitrous cretinism with chromosomal aberration and defect in thyroglobulin synthesis. J Clin Endocrinol Metab 26:1227, 1966.
127. Sulton C, Bismuth J, Castay M, et al: Hypothyroidie par anomalie congenitale de synthese de la thyroglobuline. Arch Fr Pediatr 31:11, 1974.
128. De Luca F, Michel R, Salabe GB, Baschieri L: Cretinismo sporadico congenito con gozzo da alterata structura della tireoglobulina. Folia Endocrinol 16:141, 1963.
129. Lelong M, Canlorbe P, Michel R, et al: Un cas d'hypothyroidie par anomalie de l'hormonogénèse: Présence dans la thyroid d'une thyroglobuline anormale. Arch Fr Pediatr 17:164, 1960.
130. Roche J, Michel R, Tubiana M: Caractéres de la thyroglobuline anormale extraite de certains goitres congenitauz avec trouble de l'hormonogénèse. Revue Fr Clin Biol 4:1051, 1959.
131. Tubiana M, Mozziconacci P, Attal C, et al: Goitre simple avec trouble de l'hormonogénèse. Ann Endocrinol (Paris) 26:109, 1965.
132. Tubiana M, Vignalou J, Nataf B, et al: Goiter avec troubles de formation des iodothyronines et présence d'iodoprotéines anormales. Ann Endocrinol (Paris) 29:313, 1968.
133. Torresani J, Lissitzky S: Further studies on abnormal thyroglobulin from congenital goitres likely related to defective thyroglobulin export. In Robbins J, Braverman LE (eds): Advances in Thyroid Research. New York, Excerpta Medica, American Elsevier, 1976, p 453.
134. Wagar G, Lamberg BA, Saarinen P: Congenital goitre with thyroglobulin deficiency. In Robbins J, Braverman LE (eds): Advances in Thyroid Research. New York, Excerpta Medica, American Elsevier, 1976, p 463.
135. Kusakabe T: A goitrous subject with structural abnormality of thyroglobulin. J Clin Endocrinol Metab 35:785, 1972.
136. Tassi VPN, Di Lauro R, Van Jaarsveld P, Alvino CG: Two abnormal thyroglobulin-like polypeptides are produced from Afrikander cattle congenital goiter mRNA. J Biol Chem 259:10507, 1984.
137. Ricketts MH, Simons JH, Parma J, et al: A nonsense mutation causes hereditary goiter in the Afrikander cattle and unmasks alternative splicing of thyroglobulin transcripts. Proc Natl Acad Sci 84:3181–3184, 1987.
138. Medeiros-Neto GA, Stanbury JB: Particulate iodoprotein in abnormal thyroid glands. J Clin Endocrinol Metab 26:23, 1966.
139. Silva JE, Santelices R, Kishihara M, Schneider A: Low molecular weight thyroglobulin leading to a goiter in a 12-year-old girl. J Clin Endocrinol Metab 58:526, 1984.
140. Lissitzky S, Torresani J, Burrow GN, et al: Defective thyroglobulin export as a cause of congenital goiter. Clin Endocrinol 4:363, 1975.
141. Monaco F, Andreoli M, Beretta-Anguissola A: Isolation and characterization of soluble and particulate thyroid iodoproteins in human congenital goiter. Horm Res 5:141, 1974.
142. Medeiros-Neto G, Targovnik HM, Vassart G: Defective thyroglobulin synthesis and secretion causing goiter and hypothyroidism. Endocr Rev 14:165, 1993.
143. Ieiri T, Cochaux P, Targovnik HM, et al: A 3′ splice site mutation in the thyroglobulin gene responsible for congenital goiter with hypothyroidism. J Clin Invest 88:1901–1905, 1991.
144. Targovnik HM, Medeiros-Neto G, Varela V, et al: A nonsense mutation causes human hereditary congenital goiter with preferential production of a 171 nt deleted thyroglobulin RNA messenger. J Clin Endocrinol Metab 77:210, 1993.
144a. Corral J, Martin C, Pérez R, et al: Thyroglobulin gene mutation associated with non-endemic simple goiter. Lancet 341:462, 1993.
145. DeGroot LJ, Hall R, McDermott WV, Davis AM: Hashimoto's thyroiditis: A genetically conditioned disease. N Engl J Med 267:267, 1962.
146. Lamberg BA, Hintze G, Karlsson R: Non-butanol extractable iodine in the serum of eumetabolic adult goiter patients. Acta Endocrinol 44:291, 1963.

147. Leite Z, Carneiro P, Halpern A, Medeiros-Neto G: Reduced serum thyroglobulin response to bovine TSH in malignant hypofunctioning solid thyroid nodules: Comparison to benign nodular disease. J Endocrinol Invest 10:255–259, 1987.

148. Tata JR, Rall JE, Rawson RW: Studies on an iodinated protein in the serum of subjects with cancer of the thyroid. J Clin Endocrinol Metab 16:1554, 1956.

149. Riddick FA Jr, Desai KB, Stanbury JB, Murison PJ: Familial goiter with diminished synthesis of thyroglobulin. Z Exp Med 150:203, 1969.

150. Mouriz J, Riesco G, Usobiaga P: Thyroid proteins in a goitrous cretin with iodide organification defect. J Clin Endocrinol Metab 29:942, 1969.

151. DeGroot LJ, Stanbury JB: The syndrome of congenital goiter with butanol-insoluble serum iodine. Am J Med 27:586, 1959.

152. Lissitzky S, Bismuth J, Codaccioni J, Cartouzou G: Congenital goiter with iodoalbumin replacing thyroglobulin. J Clin Endocrinol Metab 28:1797, 1968.

153. McGirr EM, Hutchison JH, Clement WE, et al: Goiter and cretinism due to the production of an abnormal iodinated thyroid compound. Scott Med J 5:189, 1960.

154. Pittman CS, Pittman JA Jr: A study of the thyroglobulin, thyroidal protease, and iodoproteins in two congenital goitrous cretins. Am J Med 40:49, 1966.

155. Riesco G, Bernal J, Sanchez-Franco F: Thyroglobulin defect in a human congenital goiter. J Clin Endocrinol Metab 38:33, 1974.

156. Michel R, Rall JE, Roche J, Tubiana M: Thyroidal iodoproteins in patients with goitrous hypothyroidism. J Clin Endocrinol Metab 24:352, 1964.

157. Rosenberg IN, Ahn CS: Enzymatic deiodination of diiodotyrosine: Possible mediation by reduced flavin nucleotide. Endocrinology 84:727, 1969.

158. Goswami A, Rosenberg IN: Ferredoxin and ferredoxin reductase activities in bovine thyroid: Possible relationship to iodotyrosine deiodinase. J Biol Chem 256:893, 1981.

159. Laurberg P: The effect of propylthiouracil on thyroid stimulating hormone–induced alterations in iodothyronine secretion from perfused dog thyroids. Biochim Biophys Acta 588:351, 1979.

160. Vague J, Codaccioni JL: Bilan de 7 ans de traitement par l'iode d'un premier cas d'hypothyroidie infantile par defaut de desiodation des iodotyrosines. Ann Endocrinol (Paris) 31:1156, 1970.

161. Stanbury JB, Kassenaar AAH, Meijer JWA, Terpstra J: The occurrence of mono- and diiodotyrosine in the blood of a patient with congenital goiter. J Clin Endocrinol Metab 15:1216, 1955.

162. Stanbury JB, Meijer JWA, Kassenaar AAH: The metabolism of iodotyrosines: II. The metabolism of mono- and diiodotyrosine in certain patients with familial goiter. J Clin Endocrinol Metab 16:848, 1956.

163. Hutchison JH, McGirr EM: Hypothyroidism as an inborn error of metabolism. J Clin Endocrinol Metab 14:869, 1954.

164. Kusakabe T, Miyake T: Defective deiodination of ^{131}I labeled L-diiodotyrosine in patients with simple goiter. J Clin Endocrinol Metab 23:132, 1963.

165. Choufoer JC: Further observations on congenital hypothyroidism with defective dehalogenation of iodotyrosines. In Pitt-Rivers R (ed): Advances in Thyroid Research, New York, Pergamon, 1961, p 36.

166. Codaccioni JL, Pierron H, Rouault F, et al: Hypothyroidie infantile par defaut d'iodotyrosine-deshalogenase: I. Quatre nouveaux cas. Ann Endocrinol (Paris) 31:1161, 1970.

167. Rochiccioli P, Dutau G: Trouble de l'hormonosynthese thyroidienne par déficit en iodotyrosine-déshalogenase. Arch Fr Pediatr 31:25, 1974.

168. Kusakabe T, Miyake T: Thyroidal deiodination defect in three sisters with simple goiter. J Clin Endocrinol Metab 24:456, 1964.

169. Ismail-Beigi F, Rahimifar M: A variant of iodotyrosine-dehalogenase deficiency. J Clin Endocrinol Metab 44:499, 1977.

170. Hutchison JH, McGirr EM: Sporadic nonendemic goitrous cretinism. Lancet 1:1035, 1956.

171. McGirr EM, Hutchison JH, Clement WE: Sporadic goitrous cretinism: Dehalogenase deficiency in the thyroid gland of a goitrous cretin and in heterozygous carriers. Lancet 2:823, 1959.

172. Murray P, Thomson JA, McGirr EM, et al: Absent and defective iodotyrosine deiodination in a family, some of whose members are goitrous cretins. Lancet 1:183, 1965.

173. Borst GC, Eil C, Burman KD: Euthyroid hyperthyroxinemia. Ann Intern Med 98:366, 1983.

174. Sakurada T, Yamaguchi T, Yamamoto M, et al: Effect of estrogen on serum total and free thyroxine and triiodothyronine in a thyroxine-binding globulin deficient family. Tohuku J Exp Med 112:35, 1974.

175. Marshall JS, Levy RP, Steinberg AG: Human thyroxine-binding globulin deficiency: A genetic study. N Engl J Med 274:1469, 1966.

176. Nikolai TF, Seal US: X-chromosome-linked familial decrease in thyroxine-binding globulin activity. J Clin Endocrinol Metab 26:835, 1966.

177. Nikolai TF, Seal US: X-chromosome-linked inheritance of thyroxine-binding globulin deficiency. J Clin Endocrinol Metab 27:1515, 1967.

178. Refetoff S, Selenkow HA: Familial thyroxine-binding globulin deficiency in a patient with Turner's syndrome (XO): Genetic study of a kindred. N Engl J Med 278:1081, 1968.

179. Kraemer E, Wiswell JG: Familial thyroxine-binding globulin deficiency. Metabolism 17:260, 1968.

180. Shishiba Y, Shimizu T, Yoshimura S, Shizume K: One family with thyroxine-binding globulin deficiency (in Japanese). Folia Endocrinol Jpn 46:28, 1970.

181. Torkington P, Harrison RJ, Maclagan NF, Burston D: Familial thyroxine-binding globulin deficiency. BMJ 3:27, 1970.

182. Nusynowitz ML, Clark RF, Strader WJ III, et al: Thyroxine-binding globulin deficiency in three families and total deficiency in a normal woman. Am J Med 50:458, 1971.

183. AvRuskin TW, Braverman LE, Crigler JF Jr: Thyroxine-binding globulin deficiency and associated neurological deficit. Pediatrics 50:638, 1972.

184. Kato K, Takakura I, Kuno Y, Ishikawa K: Familial thyroxine binding globulin deficiency. Acta Paediatr Jpn 14:1, 1972.

185. Sakurada T, Yamaguchi T, Yoshida K, et al: Metabolism of thyroxine and triiodothyronine in one case of thyroxine-binding globulin deficiency associated with hypothyroidism (in Japanese). Folia Endocrinol Jpn 49:1354, 1973.

186. Leiba S, Landau B, Ber A, et al: Thyroxine binding-globulin (T.B.G.) deficiency and glucose-6-phosphate dehydrogenase (G-6-PD) deficiency in the same family. J Clin Endocrinol Metab 38:569, 1974.

187. Grant DB, Minchin-Clarke HG, Putman D: Familial thyroxine-binding globulin deficiency: Search for linkage with Xg blood groups. J Med Genet 11:271, 1974.

188. Refetoff S, Robin NI, Alper CA: Study of four new kindreds with inherited thyroxine-binding globulin abnormalities: Possible mutations of single gene locus. J Clin Invest 51:848, 1972.

189. Nicoloff JT, Dowling JT, Patton DD: Inheritance of decreased thyroxine-binding by the thyroxine-binding globulin. J Clin Endocrinol Metab 24:294, 1964.

190. Gerversman DAPS, Bottema JK: Hereditair tekort aan thyroxine-bindende globuline. Ned Tijdschr Geneeskd 112:1408, 1968.

191. Bayley TA, Higgins HP, Row VV, et al: The metabolic significance of thyroxine-binding globulin: Studies in a family with decreased thyroxine-binding globulin. Acta Endocrinol 61:137, 1969.

192. Moloshok RE, Hsu LYF, Seal US, and Hirschhorn K: Partial thyroxine-binding globulin deficiency in a family. Pediatrics 44:518, 1969.

193. Roberts RC, Nikolai TF, Lohrenz FN: A TBG-deficient family with a male exhibiting decreased but not zero TBG levels. J Clin Endocrinol Metab 30:131, 1970.

194. Heinonen OP, Lamberg B-A, Virtamo J: Inherited decrease of the binding capacity of thyroxine-binding globulin (TBG). Acta Endocrinol 64:171, 1970.

195. Barbosa JJ, Rivas ML, Merritt AD, Oliner L: Observations on the varying genetic transmission of thyroxine-binding globulin deficiency: Abstracts of the 44th Meeting of the American Thyroid Association. Washington, DC, 1968, p 41.

196. Hennemann G, Docter R, Dolman A: Relationship between total thyroxine and absolute free thyroxine and the influence of absolute free thyroxine on thyroxine disposal in humans. J Clin Endocrinol Metab 33:63, 1971.

197. DeNayer PH, Oei LS, Broeckk J, DeVisscher M: Familial partial thyroxine-binding globulin deficiency. Ann Endocrinol 32:617, 1971.

198. Malvaux P, DeNayer P: X-chromosome-linked inheritance of decreased thyroxine-binding globulin. Arch Dis Child 47:635, 1972.

199. Bode HH, Rothman KJ, Danon M: Linkage of thyroxine-binding globulin deficiency to other X-chromosome loci. J Clin Endocrinol Metab 37:25, 1973.

200. Wallace EZ, Kapoor S, Veleanu M: Study of a kindred with thyroxine-binding globulin deficiency and oligomenorrhea. Am J Obstet Gynecol 122:79, 1975.

201. Niimi H, Sasaki N: Familial thyroxine-binding globulin deficiency in a patient with congenital hypothyroidism. Endocrinol Jpn 22:35, 1975.

202. Horwitz DL, Refetoff S: Graves' disease associated with familial deficiency of thyroxine-binding globulin. J Clin Endocrinol Metab 44:242, 1977.

203. Beierwaltes WH, Carr EA Jr, Hunter RL: Hereditary increase in the thyroxine-binding sites in the serum-globulin. Trans Assoc Am Physicians 74:170, 1961.

204. Florsheim WH, Dowling JT, Meister L, Bodfish RE: Familial elevation of serum thyroxine-binding capacity. J Clin Endocrinol Metab 22:735, 1962.

205. Jones JE, Seal US: X-chromosome-linked inheritance of elevated thyroxine-binding globulin. J Clin Endocrinol Metab 27:1521, 1967.

206. Siersbaek-Nielsen K, Hansen JM, Hippe E: Familial elevation of serum thyroxine-binding globulin capacity. Acta Endocrinol (Copenh) 60:130, 1969.

207. Fialkow PJ, Giblett ER, Musa B: Increased serum thyroxine-binding globulin capacity: Inheritance and linkage relationships. J Clin Endocrinol Metab 30:66, 1970.

208. Shane SR, Seal US, Jones JE: X-chromosome-linked inheritance of elevated thyroxine-binding globulin in association with goiter. J Clin Endocrinol Metab 32:587, 1971.

209. Thomson JA, Meredith EM, Baird SG, et al: Raised free thyroxine values in patients with familial elevation of thyroxine binding globulin. Q J Med 41:49, 1972.

210. Hollander CS, Bernstein G, Oppenheimer JH: Abnormalities of thyroxine binding in analbuminemia. J Clin Endocrinol Metab 28:1064, 1968.

211. Ruiz M, Rajatanavin R, Young RA, et al: Familial dysalbuminemic hyperthyroxinemia. N Engl J Med 306:635, 1982.

212. Lee WNP, Golden MP, VanHerle AJ, et al: Inherited abnormal thyroid hormone-binding protein causing selective increase of total serum thyroxine. J Clin Endocrinol Metab 49:292, 1979.

213. Stockigt JR, Topliss DC, Barlou JW, et al: Familial euthyroid thyroxine excess: An appropriate response to abnormal thyroxine binding associated with albumin. J Clin Endocrinol Metab 53:353, 1981.

214. Docter R, Bos G, Krenning EP, et al: Inherited thyroxine excess: A serum abnormality due to an increased affinity for modified albumin. Clin Endocrinol 15:363, 1981.

215. Silverberg JDH, Premachandra BN: Familial hyperthyroxinemia due to abnormal thyroid hormone binding Ann Intern Med 96:183, 1982.

216. Borst GC, Eil C, Burman KD: Euthyroid familial hyperthyroxinemia due to abnormal thyroid hormone-binding protein. Am J Med 73:366, 1982.

217. Lalloz MRA, Byfield PGH, Himsworth RL: Hyperthyroxinemia: Abnormal binding of T_4 by an inherited albumin variant. Clin Endocrinol 18:11, 1983.

218. Moses AC, Lawlor J, Haddow J, Jackson IMD: Familial euthyroid hyperthyroxinemia resulting from increased thyroxine binding to thyroxine-binding prealbumin. N Engl J Med 306:966, 1982.

219. Byfield PGH, et al: Variant prealbumin: Another cause of euthyroid hyperthyroxinemia [abstract 539]. 7th International Congress of Endocrinology, Quebec, 1984.

220. Daiger SP, Rummel DP, Wang L, et al: Detection of genetic variation with radioactive ligands: IV. X-linked, polymorphic genetic variation of thyroxine-binding globulin (TBG). Am J Hum Genet 33:640, 1981.

221. Himsworth RL, et al: Inherited low-T_4 syndrome: Defective autosomal structural gene for thyroxine-binding globulin [abstract 1091]. 7th International Congress of Endocrinology, Quebec, 1984.

222. Dick M, Watson F: A possible variant of thyroxine-binding globulin in Australian Aborigines. Clin Chim Acta 116:361, 1981.

223. Refetoff S, Murata Y: X-Chromosome–linked inheritance of the variant thyroxine-binding globulin in Australian Aborigines. J Clin Endocrinol Metab 60:356, 1985.

224. Yabu Y, Amir SY, Ruiz M, et al: Heterogeneity of thyroxine binding by serum albumins in normal subjects and patients with familial dysalbuminemic hyperthyroxinemia. J Clin Endocrinol Metab 60:451, 1985.

225. Refetoff S, DeWind LT, DeGroot LJ: Familial syndrome combining deaf-mutism, stippled epiphyses, goiter, and abnormally high PBI: Possible target organ refractoriness to thyroid hormone. J Clin Endocrinol Metab 27:279, 1967.

226. Bode HH, Danon M, Weintraub BD, et al: Partial target organ resistance to thyroid hormone. J Clin Invest 52:776, 1973.

227. Schneider G, Keiser HR, Bardin CW: Peripheral resistance to thyroxine: A cause of short stature in a boy without goiter. Clin Endocrinol 4:111, 1975.

228. Agerbaek H: Congenital goiter presumably resulting from tissue resistance to thyroid hormone. Isr J Med Sci 8:1859, 1972.

229. Seif FJ, Scherbaum W, Klingler W: Syndrome of elevated thyroid hormones and TSH blood levels: A case report. Acta Endocrinol (Suppl)215:81, 1978.

230. Elewaut A, Mussche M, Vermeulen A: Familial partial target organ resistance to thyroid hormones. J Clin Endocrinol Metab 43:575, 1976.

231. Tamagna EI, Carlson HE, Hershman JM, Reed AW: Pituitary and peripheral resistance to thyroid hormone. Clin Endocrinol 10:431, 1979.

232. Daubresse JC, Dozin-Van Roye B, DeNayer P, DeVisscher M: Partial resistance to thyroid hormones: Reduced affinity of lymphocyte nuclear receptors for T_3 in two siblings. In Stockigt JR, Nagataki S (eds): Thyroid Research VIII. Canberra, Australian Academy of Science, 1980, p 295.

233. Maenpaa J, Liewendahl K: Peripheral insensitivity to thyroid hormones in a euthyroid girl with goiter. Arch Dis Child 55:207, 1980.

234. Brooks MH, Barbato AL, Collins S, et al: Familial thyroid hormone resistance. Am J Med 71:414, 1981.

235. Kaplowitz PB, D'Ercole AJ, Utiger RD: Peripheral resistance to thyroid hormone in an infant. J Clin Endocrinol Metab 53:958, 1981.

236. Oseki T, Egawa M, Egi S, Yamori K: Brother and sister with presumed thyroid hormone resistance [abstract 69]. Proceedings of the 13th Annual Meeting of the Japanese Society for Pediatric Endocrine Research, Hamamatsu, Japan, 1979.

237. Vandalem JL, Pirens G, Hennen G: Partial resistance to thyroid hormone and TSH hypersecretion: A familial syndrome [abstract]. RIA 80 International Symposium on Recent Progress in Radioimmunoassay of Hormones, Proteins, and Enzymes, Brescia, Italy, 1980.

238. Linde R, Alexander N, Island DP, Rabin D: Familial insensitivity of the pituitary and periphery to thyroid hormone: A case report in two generations and a review of the literature. Metabolism 31:510, 1982.

239. Chait A, Kanter R, Green W, Kenny M: Defective thyroid hormone action in fibroblasts cultured from subjects with the syndrome of resistance to thyroid hormones. J Clin Endocrinol Metab 54:767, 1982.

240. Kasai Y, Utsunomiya S, Matsunobu M, et al: Refetoff syndrome in two siblings. Folia Endocrinol Jpn (Suppl)57:1397, 1981.

241. Lakka-Papadodima E, Souvatzoglon A, Pandos PG, et al: Two cases of peripheral tissue resistance to thyroxine of different mechanism. Ann Endocrinol (Suppl)38:17A, 1977.

242. Salazar A, Refetoff S, Smith TJ, et al: Studies on a new case of resistance to the action of thyroid hormone. Endocrinology (Suppl)208:265, 1981.

243. Meier CA, Dickstein BM, Ashizawa K, et al: Variable transcriptional activity and ligand binding of mutant β1 3,5,3'-triiodothyronine receptors from four families with generalized resistance to thyroid hormone. Mol Endocrinol 6:248–258, 1992.

244. Kaplan MM, Swartz SL, Larsen PR: Partial peripheral resistance to thyroid hormone. Am J Med 70:1115, 1981.

245. Bernal J, Refetoff S, DeGroot LJ: Abnormalities of triiodothyronine binding to lymphocyte and fibroblast nuclei from a patient with peripheral tissue resistance to thyroid hormone action. J Clin Endocrinol Metab 47:1266, 1978.

246. Ichikawa K, Hughes IA, Horwitz AL, DeGroot LJ: Characterization of nuclear thyroid hormone receptors of cultured skin fibroblasts from patients with resistance to thyroid hormone. Metabolism 36:392–399, 1987.

247. Eil C, Fein HG, Smith TJ, et al: Nuclear binding of [^{125}I]-triiodothyronine in dispersed cultured skin fibroblasts from patients with resistance to thyroid hormone. J Clin Endocrinol Metab 55:502, 1982.

248. Liewendahl K, Rosengard S, Lamberg B-A: Nuclear binding of triiodothyronine and thyroxine in lymphocytes from subjects with hyperthyroidism, hypothyroidism, and resistance to thyroid hormones. Clin Chim Acta 83:41, 1978.

249. Maxon HR, Burman KD, Premachandra BN: Euthyroid, familial hyperthyroxinemia. N Engl J Med 302:1263, 1980.

250. Refetoff S, DeGroot LJ, Benard B, DeWind LT: Studies of a sibship with apparent hereditary resistance to the intracellular action of thyroid hormone. Metabolism 21:723, 1972.

251. Refetoff S, DeGroot LJ, Barsano CP: Defective thyroid hormone feedback regulation in the syndrome of peripheral resistance to thyroid hormone. J Clin Endocrinol Metab 51:41, 1980.

252. Gheri RG, Bianchi R, Mariani G, et al: A new case of familial partial generalized resistance to thyroid hormones: Study of 3,5,3'-triiodothyronine (T_3) binding to lymphocyte and skin fibroblast nuclei and

in vivo conversion of thyroxine to T$_3$. J Clin Endocrinol Metab 58:563, 1984.

253. Refetoff S: Syndromes of resistance to thyroid hormone. Endocr Rev 14:348, 1993.

254. Gershengorn MC, Weintraub BD: Thyrotropin-induced hyperthyroidism caused by selective pituitary resistance to thyroid hormone: A new syndrome of "inappropriate secretion of TSH." J Clin Invest 56:633, 1975.

255. Emerson CH, Utiger RD: Hyperthyroidism and excessive thyrotropin secretion. N Engl J Med 287:328, 1972.

256. Novogroder M, Utiger R, Boyar R, Levine LS: Juvenile hyperthyroidism with elevated thyrotropin (TSH) and normal 24 hour FSH, LH, GH, and prolactin secretory patterns. J Clin Endocrinol Metab 45:1053, 1977.

257. Rosler A, Litvin Y, Hage C, et al: Familial hyperthyroidism due to inappropriate thyrotropin secretion successfully treated with triiodothyronine. J Clin Endocrinol Metab 54:76, 1982.

258. Jaffiol C, Baldet L, Torresani J, et al: A case of hypersensitivity to thyroid hormones with normally functioning thyroid gland and increased nuclear triiodothyronine receptors: Case report. J Endocrinol Invest 13:839–845, 1990.

259. Sakurai A, Takeda K, Ain K, et al: Generalized resistance to thyroid hormone associated with a mutation in the ligand-binding domain of the human thyroid hormone receptor beta. Proc Natl Acad Sci USA 86:8977–8981, 1989.

260. DeGroot LJ, Nakai A, Sakurai A, Macchia E: The molecular basis of thyroid hormone action. J Endocrinol Invest 12:843–861, 1989.

261. Usala SJ, Menke JB, Watson TL, et al: A homozygous deletion in the c-erbA-beta thyroid hormone receptor gene in a patient with generalized thyroid hormone resistance: Isolation and characterization of the mutant receptor. Mol Endocrinol 5:327–335, 1991.

262. Takeda K, Sakurai A, DeGroot LJ, Refetoff S: Recessive inheritance of thyroid hormone resistance caused by complete deletion of the protein-coding region of the thyroid hormone receptor beta gene. J Clin Endocrinol Metab 74:49–55, 1991.

263. Hodin RA, Lazar MA, Wintman BI, et al: Identification of a thyroid hormone receptor that is pituitary specific. Science 244:76–79, 1989.

264. Wortsman J, Premachandra BN, Williams K, et al: Familial resistance to thyroid hormone associated with decreased transport across the plasma membrane. Ann Intern Med 98:904, 1983.

265. Bercu BB, Orloff S, Schulman JD: Pituitary resistance to thyroid hormone in cystinosis. J Clin Endocrinol Metab 51:1262, 1980.

266. Sarne DH, Swobieszcyzy S, Ain KB, Refetoff S: Serum thyrotropin and prolactin in the syndrome of generalized resistance to thyroid hormone: Responses to thyrotropin-releasing hormone stimulation and short term triiodothyronine suppression. J Clin Endocrinol Metab 70:1305–1311, 1990.

267. Connell JMC, McCruden DC, Davies DL, Alexander WD: Bromocriptine for inappropriate thyrotropin secretion. Ann Intern Med 96:251, 1982.

268. Bajorunas DR, Rosner W, Kourides IA: Use of bromocriptine in a patient with generalized resistance to thyroid hormone. J Clin Endocrinol Metab 58:731, 1984.

269. Sriwatanakul K, McCormick K, Woolf P: Thyrotropin (TSH)-induced hyperthyroidism: Response of TSH to dopamine and its agonists. J Clin Endocrinol Metab 58:255, 1984.

270. Beck-Peccoz P, Piscitelli G, Cattaneo MG, Faglia G: Effectiveness of 3,5,3'-triiodothyroacetic acid (TRIAC), but not bromocriptine, in lowering TSH secretion in one hyperthyroid patient with non-neoplastic pituitary TSH hypersecretion [abstract 59]. Annual Meeting of the European Thyroid Association, Madrid, 1983.

271. Rosler A, Litvin Y, Hage C, et al: Familial hyperthyroidism due to inappropriate thyrotropin secretion successfully treated with triiodothyronine. J Clin Endocrinol Metab 54:76, 1982.

272. Murray IPC, Thomson JA, McGirr EM, et al: Unusual familial goiter associated with intrathyroidal calcification. J Clin Endocrinol Metab 26:1039, 1966.

273. de Zegher F, Vanderschueren-Lodeweyckx M, Heninrichs C, et al: Thyroid dyshormonogenesis: Severe hypothyroidism after normal neonatal thyroid stimulating hormone screening. Acta Pediatr 81:274–276, 1992.

274. Germak JA, Foley TP Jr: Longitudinal assessment of L-thyroxine therapy for congenital hypothyroidism. J Pediatr 117:211–219, 1990.

275. Lever EG, Medeiros-Neto GA, DeGroot LJ: Inherited disorders of thyroid metabolism. Endocr Rev 4:213, 1983.

53

Developmental Abnormalities of the Thyroid

EDWIN L. KAPLAN
MANAN SHUKLA
HISATO HARA
KOICHI ITO

In order to understand the different thyroid anomalies, it is important to review briefly the normal development of this gland. The thyroid is embryologically an offshoot of the primitive alimentary tract, from which it later becomes separated[1, 2] (Figs. 53–1 and 53–2). During the third to fourth week in utero, a median anlage of epithelium arises from the pharyngeal floor in the region of the foramen cecum of the tongue, that is, at the junction of the anterior two thirds and the posterior third of the tongue. The main body of the thyroid, referred to as the median lobe or median thyroid component, follows the descent of the heart and great vessels and moves caudally into the neck from this origin. It divides into an isthmus and two lobes, and by seven weeks it forms a "shield" over the front of the trachea and thyroid cartilage. It is joined by a pair of lateral thyroid lobes originating from the fourth and fifth branchial pouches[3, 4] (Fig. 53–3). From these lateral thyroid components, now frequently called the ultimobranchial bodies, the C cells (parafollicular cells) enter the thyroid lobes. C cells contain and secrete calcitonin and are the cells that give rise to a medullary carcinoma of the thyroid gland. Williams and associates[5] have described cystic structures in the neck near the upper parathyroid glands in cases in which thyroid tissue was totally lingual in location. These cysts contained both cells staining for calcitonin and others staining for thyroglobulin. This study, they believe, offers conclusive evidence that the ultimobranchial body contributes both C cells and follicular cells to the thyroid gland of man.

As the gland moves downward, it leaves behind a trace of epithelial cells known as the thyroglossal tract. From this structure both thyroglossal duct cysts and the pyramidal lobe of the thyroid develop. The eventual mature thyroid gland takes on many different configurations owing to the embryological development of the thyroid and its descent (Fig. 53–4).

Thyroid Abnormalities

The median thyroid anlage may rarely fail to develop, causing *athyreosis*, that is, absence of the thyroid gland, which is associated with cretinism, or it may differentiate in locations other than the isthmus and lateral lobes. The most common developmental abnormality, if looked upon as such, is the *pyramidal lobe*, which has been reported to be present in as many as 80 per cent of patients in whom the gland was surgically exposed. Usually the pyramidal lobe is small; however, in Graves' disease or lymphocytic thyroiditis, it is often enlarged and is frequently clinically palpable. The pyramidal lobe usually lies in the midline but can arise from either lobe. An origin from the left lobe is more common than from the right lobe.[6]

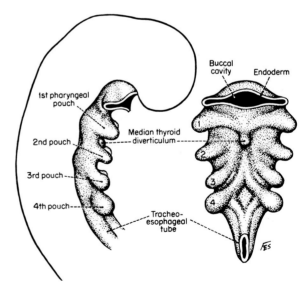

FIGURE 53–1. **Early embryological development of the pharyngeal anlage in a 4-mm embryo.** Note the beginning of thyroid development in the median thyroid diverticulum. (From Sedgwick CE, Cady B: Surgery of the Thyroid and Parathyroid Glands (ed 2). Philadelphia, WB Saunders Company, 1980, p 7. Adapted from Weller GL: Development of the thyroid, parathyroid and thymus glands in man. Contrib Embryol Carnegie Inst Wash 24:93–142, 1933.)

Supported in part by a generous grant from the Nathan and Frances Goldblatt Society for Cancer Research.

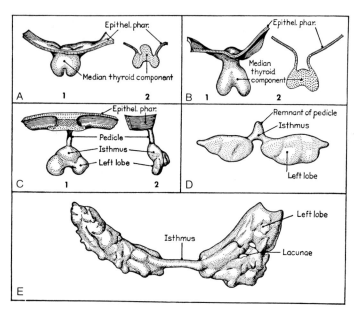

FIGURE 53–2. **Stages in the development of the thyroid gland.** *A*, 1, Thyroid primordium and pharyngeal epithelium of a 4.5-mm human embryo; 2, section through the same structure, showing raised central portion. *B*, 1, Thyroid primordium of a 6.5-mm embryo; 2, section through the same structure. *C*, 1, Thyroid primordium of an 8.2-mm embryo, beginning to descend; 2, lateral view of the same structure. *D*, Thyroid primordium of an 11-mm embryo. The connection with the pharynx is broken, and the lobes are beginning to grow laterad. *E*, Thyroid gland of a 13.5-mm embryo. The lobes are thin sheets curving around the carotid arteries. Several lacunae, which are not to be confused with follicles, are present in the sheets. (From Weller GL: Development of the thyroid, parathyroid and thymus glands in man. Contrib Embryol Carnegie Inst Wash 24:93–142, 1933.)

Thyroid Hemiagenesis

More than 100 cases have been reported in which only one lobe of the thyroid is present.[7] The left lobe is absent in 80 per cent of cases. Often the thyroid lobe that is present is enlarged. Both hyperthyroidism and hypothyroidism have been reported at times. Females are affected three times as often as males. Both benign and malignant nodules have been reported in this condition.[8]

Other variations involving the median thyroid anlage represent an arrest in the usual descent of part or all of the thyroid-forming material along the normal pathway. *Ectopic thyroid development* can result in a lingual thyroid or in thyroid tissue in a suprahyoid, infrahyoid, or intratracheal location. The persistence of the thyroglossal duct as a sinus tract or cyst called a *thyroglossal duct cyst* is the most common of the clinically important anomalies of thyroid development. Finally, the entire gland or part of it may descend more caudally, which results in thyroid tissue located in the superior mediastinum behind the sternum, adjacent to the aortic arch or between the aorta and pulmonary trunk, within the upper portion of the pericardium, and even within the interventricular septum of the

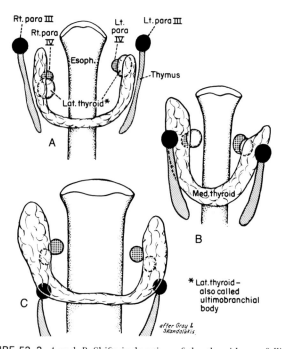

FIGURE 53–3. *A* and *B*, Shifts in location of the thyroid, parafollicular, and parathyroid tissues. *C* approximates the adult location. Note that what has been called the lateral thyroid is now commonly referred to as the ultimobranchial body, which contains both C cells and follicular elements. (From Sedgwick CE, Cady B: Surgery of the Thyroid and Parathyroid Glands (ed 2). Philadelphia, WB Saunders Company, 1980. Adapted from Norris EH: Parathyroid glands and lateral thyroid in man: Their morphogenesis, histogenesis, topographic anatomy and prenatal growth. Contrib Embryol Carnegie Inst Wash 26:247–294, 1937.)

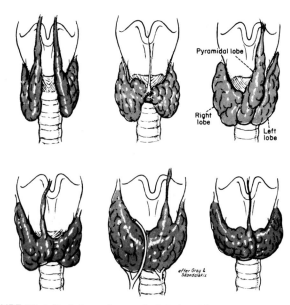

FIGURE 53–4. Variations of normal adult thyroid anatomy resulting from the embryological descent and division of the thyroid gland. (From Sedgwick CE, Cady B: Surgery of the Thyroid and Parathyroid Glands (ed 2). Philadelphia, WB Saunders Company, 1980. Adapted from Gray SW, Skandalakis JE: Embryology for Surgeons. Philadelphia, WB Saunders Company, 1972.)

heart. Most *intrathoracic goiters*, however, are not true anomalies but rather are extensions of pathological elements of a normally situated gland into the anterior or posterior mediastinum. Each of these abnormalities is discussed in greater depth.

ECTOPIC THYROID

Lingual Thyroid

Lingual thyroid is relatively rare, estimated to occur in 1 in 3000 cases of thyroid disease. However, it represents the most common location for functioning ectopic thyroid tissue. Lingual thyroid tissue is associated with an absence of the normal cervical thyroid in 70 per cent of cases. It occurs much more commonly in women than in men.

The diagnosis is usually made by the discovery of an incidental mass on the back of the tongue in an asymptomatic patient (Fig. 53–5). The mass may enlarge and cause dysphagia, dysphonia, dyspnea, or a sensation of choking.[9] Hypothyroidism is frequently present and may cause the mass to enlarge and become symptomatic, but hyperthyroidism is very unusual. In women, symptomatic lingual thyroid glands develop during puberty or early adulthood in the majority of cases. Buckman,[10] in his review of 140 cases of symptomatic lingual thyroids in females, reported that 30 per cent occurred in puberty, 55 per cent between the ages of 18 and 40 years, 10 per cent at menopause, and 5 per cent in old age. He attributed this distribution to hormonal disturbances, which are more apparent in female subjects during puberty and may be precipitated by pregnancy. The incidence of malignancy in lingual thyroid glands is low.[11] The diagnosis of lingual thyroid should be suspected when a mass is detected in the region of the foramen cecum of the tongue and is established definitively by radioisotope scanning (Fig. 53–5).

The usual treatment for this condition is thyroid hormone therapy to suppress the lingual thyroid and reduce its size. Only rarely is surgical excision necessary. Indications for extirpation are failure of suppressive therapy to reduce the size, ulceration, hemorrhage, or suspicion of malignancy.[12] Autotransplantation of thyroid tissue has rarely been tried when no other thyroid tissue is present and has apparently been successful. Recently, lingual thyroid was reported in two natural brothers, suggesting that this condition may be inherited.[13]

Suprahyoid and Infrahyoid Thyroid

In these cases thyroid tissue is present in a midline position above or below the hyoid bone. Hypothyroidism with elevation of thyrotropin (TSH) secretion is commonly present because of the absence of a normal thyroid gland in most instances. An enlarging mass commonly occurs during infancy, childhood, or later life. Often this mass is mistaken for a thyroglossal duct cyst, for it is usually located in the same anatomical position.[14] If it is removed, all thyroid tissue may be ablated, a consequence that has definite physiological as well as possible medicolegal implications. In order to prevent this from happening, many recommend that a thyroid scan be performed in all cases of a thyroglossal duct cyst before its removal to be certain that a normal thyroid gland is present. Furthermore, before removing what appears to be a thyroglossal duct cyst, the prudent surgeon should be certain that no solid areas are present. If any doubt exists, the normal thyroid gland should be explored and palpated. Finally, if ectopic thyroid tissue rather than a thyroglossal duct cyst is encountered at operation, its blood supply should be preserved and the ectopic gland should be divided vertically and each half translocated laterally, deep to the strap muscles, where it no longer presents as a mass. If normal thyroid tissue is

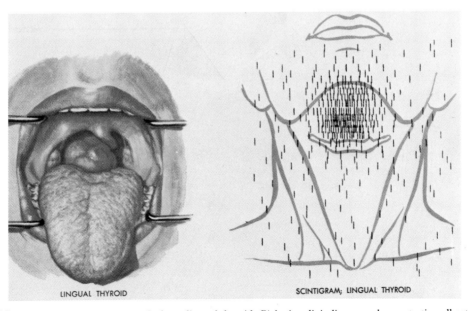

LINGUAL THYROID

SCINTIGRAM; LINGUAL THYROID

FIGURE 53–5. *Left*, The appearance of a large lingual thyroid. *Right*, A radioiodine scan demonstrating all activity to be above the hyoid bone, with no evidence of the presence of normally placed thyroid tissue. (From Netter RA: Endocrine system and selected metabolic diseases. Ciba Collection of Medical Illustrations. Ciba-Geigy Corporation, 1974, p 45.)

demonstrated to be present elsewhere, it may be better to remove the ectopic tissue rather than transplant it because carcinoma arising from these developmental abnormalities, although rare, has been reported.

THYROGLOSSAL DUCT CYSTS

Both cysts and fistulas can develop along the course of the thyroglossal duct[15] (Fig. 53–6). These cysts are the most common anomaly in thyroid development in clinical practice.[16] Normally the thyroglossal duct becomes obliterated early in embryonic life, but occasionally it persists as a cyst. Such lesions occur equally in males and females. They present at birth in about 25 per cent of cases, most appear in early childhood, and the final third become apparent only after age 30.[17] Cysts usually appear in the midline or just off the midline between the isthmus of the thyroid and the hyoid bone. They frequently become repeatedly infected and may rupture spontaneously. When this occurs, a sinus tract or fistula persists. Removal of a thyroglossal cyst or fistula requires excision of the central part of the hyoid bone and dissection of the thyroglossal tract to the base of the tongue if recurrence is to be minimized (the Sistrunk procedure). This procedure is necessary because the thyroglossal duct is intimately associated with the central part of the hyoid bone (Fig. 53–7). Recurrent cysts are very common if this operative procedure is not followed.

At least 115 cases of thyroid carcinoma have been reported to originate from the thyroglossal duct.[16] Not infrequently, there is an association with low-dose external irradiation to the head and neck given in infancy or childhood in such cases. Almost all carcinomas have been papillary, and their prognosis is excellent. If a carcinoma is recognized at the time of operation, the thyroid gland should be inspected for evidence of other tumor nodules, and lateral lymph nodes should be sampled. Whether or not a routine thyroidectomy should be performed in each of these indi-

viduals remains to be clarified. However, in one series of 35 patients with papillary carcinoma arising in a thyroglossal duct cyst, the thyroid gland of 4 patients (11.4 per cent) also contained papillary cancer.[16] In such a situation a total or near-total thyroidectomy and appropriate neck dissections are also mandatory. Of interest is the fact that about 5 per cent of all carcinomas arising from a thyroglossal duct cyst are squamous, although rare cases of Hürthle cell and anaplastic cancers have been reported. Finally, three families have been reported in which a total of 11 members had a thyroglossal duct cyst.[18]

Lateral Aberrant Thyroid

Small amounts of histologically normal thyroid tissue are rarely found during surgery along the course of the internal carotid artery, in the supraclavicular fossa, or in the mediastinum, entirely separate from the thyroid. If these tissue elements are near the thyroid, not in lymph nodes, and entirely normal histologically, it is possible that they represent developmental abnormalities. True lateral aberrant thyroid tissue or embryonic rests of thyroid tissue in lymph nodes of the lateral neck are very rare. Most agree that an overwhelming number of cases of what was called "lateral aberrant thyroid" in the past actually represent well-differentiated, metastatic thyroid cancer within cervical lymph nodes rather than an embryonic rest. In such cases, we favor a near-total or total thyroidectomy with a modified radical neck dissection, probably followed by radioiodine therapy.

Several lateral thyroid masses have been reported that are said to be benign adenomas in lateral ectopic sites.[19, 20] The authors of these studies suggest that they may develop ectopically because of a failure of fusion of the lateral thyroid component with the median thyroid. However, before accepting this explanation, it is important to be certain that each of these lesions does not represent a well-

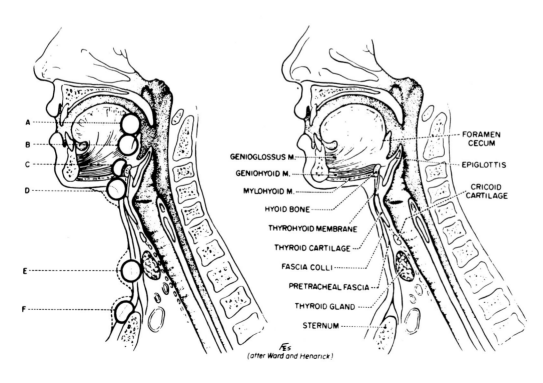

GENIOGLOSSUS M.

GENIOHYOID M.

MYLOHYOID M.

HYOID BONE

THYROHYOID MEMBRANE

THYROID CARTILAGE

FASCIA COLLI

PRETRACHEAL FASCIA

THYROID GLAND

STERNUM

FORAMEN CECUM

EPIGLOTTIS

CRICOID CARTILAGE

(after Ward and Hendrick)

FIGURE 53–6. **Location of thyroglossal cysts.** *A*, In front of foramen cecum; *B*, at foramen cecum; *C*, suprahyoid; *D*, infrahyoid; *E*, area of thyroid gland; *F*, suprasternal. (From Sedgwick CE, Cady B: Surgery of the Thyroid and Parathyroid Glands (ed 2). Philadelphia, WB Saunders Company, 1980.)

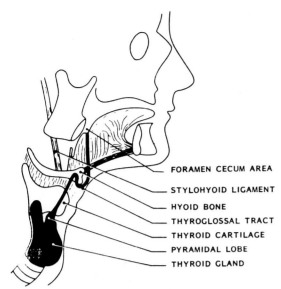

FORAMEN CECUM AREA
STYLOHYOID LIGAMENT
HYOID BONE
THYROGLOSSAL TRACT
THYROID CARTILAGE
PYRAMIDAL LOBE
THYROID GLAND

FIGURE 53–7. **Diagram of the course of the thyroglossal tract.** Note its proximity to the hyoid bone. (From Allard RHB: The thyroglossal cyst. Head Neck Surg 5:134–146, 1982.)

differentiated metastasis that has totally replaced a lymph node, in which the primary thyroid carcinoma is small or even microscopic and was not recognized.

SUBSTERNAL GOITERS

Developmental abnormalities may lead to the finding of thyroid tissue in the mediastinum, rarely even within the tracheal or esophageal wall. However, undoubtedly, most substernal goiters originate in the neck and "fall" or are "swallowed" into the mediastinum and are not embryologically determined at all.

Intrathoracic goiters have been reported to occur in 0.1 to 21 per cent of patients in whom thyroidectomies were performed. This large variability undoubtedly is due partly to a difference of classification among the authors but may also be due to the incidence of endemic goiter. The more recent series report an incidence of 2 per cent or less.[21]

Many substernal goiters are found on routine chest radiography in patients who are completely asymptomatic.

Other patients may have dyspnea or dysphagia due to tracheal or esophageal compression or displacement. Superior vena caval obstruction can occasionally occur.[22] In these instances, edema and cyanosis of the face and venous engorgement of the arms and face are present (Fig. 53–8). Most individuals with substernal goiters are euthyroid or hypothyroid; however, occasionally hyperthyroidism is present. Although the goiters of Graves' disease are rarely intrathoracic, single or multiple "hot" nodules may occur within an intrathoracic goiter and result in hyperthyroidism as part of a toxic nodular goiter.

Intrathoracic goiters are usually found in the anterior mediastinum and less commonly in the posterior mediastinum. In either instance the diagnosis is suggested if a goiter can be palpated in the neck and appears to continue below the sternum. Rarely, however, no thyroid enlargement in the cervical area is present, and, instead of being in continuity, the intrathoracic component may be attached to the cervical thyroid only by a narrow bridge of thyroid or of fibrous tissue. The diagnosis of an intrathoracic thyroid mass can be made with certainty by use of a thyroid isotope scan; however, CT scan or MR imaging may also be helpful.

Regarding therapy, I generally agree with the recommendation made by Lahey and Swinton more than 50 years ago that goiters that are definitely intrathoracic should usually be removed if the patient is a good operative risk.[23] Because of the cone-shaped anatomy of the upper thoracic outlet, once part of a thyroid goiter has passed into the superior mediastinum, it can increase its size only by descending further into the chest. Thus, delay in surgical management may lead to an increased size of the lesion, a greater degree of symptoms, and perhaps a more difficult or hazardous operative procedure.

Substernal goiters should be operated upon initially through a cervical incision because the blood supply to the substernal thyroid almost always originates in the neck and can be readily controlled in this area. Only rarely does an intrathoracic goiter receive its blood supply from mediastinal vessels; however, such a finding favors a developmental cause. Thus, in most instances, good hemostasis can be obtained by control of the superior and inferior thyroid arteries in the neck. The thyroid gland is carefully dissected along its capsule by blunt dissection into the superior mediastinum. While gentle traction is exerted from

FIGURE 53–8. **Large substernal goiter resulting in superior vena caval syndrome.** *Left*, A venogram demonstrated complete obstruction to the superior vena cava, displacement of the innominate veins, and marked collateral circulation. *Right*, Three weeks after thyroidectomy, patency of the vena cava was restored. Some displacement of the innominate veins remained at that time. (From Lesavoy MA, Norberg HP, Kaplan EL: Substernal goiter with superior vena caval obstruction. Surgery 77:325–329, 1975.)

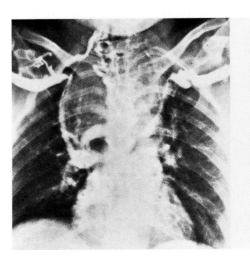
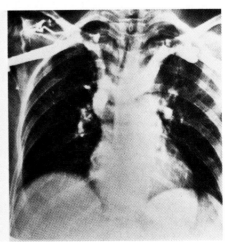

above, the mass is elevated by the surgeon's fingers or blunt, curved clamps (Fig. 53–9). Frequently, these maneuvers suffice to permit extraction of a mass from the mediastinum and into the neck area. Any fluid-filled cysts may be aspirated to reduce the size of the mass and to permit its egress through the thoracic outlet. Piecemeal morcellation of the thyroid gland should not be practiced, for this occasionally has led to severe bleeding. Furthermore, several substernal goiters have been found to contain carcinoma, and this technique violates all principles of cancer surgery.

With the use of this method, the great majority of substernal thyroid glands can be removed. If the thyroid gland cannot be easily extracted from the mediastinum, however, a partial or complete sternotomy should be performed. This procedure affords direct control of any mediastinal vessels and permits the resection of the thyroid gland to be carried out safely.

As in all thyroid surgery, the recurrent laryngeal nerves must be preserved and treated with care. The parathyroid glands should be identified and preserved, and the inferior thyroid artery's branches should be ligated close to the thyroid capsule to prevent ischemia to the parathyroid glands, which might result in hypoparathyroidism.

STRUMA OVARII

Ectopic development of thyroid tissue far from the neck area can also lead to difficulties in rare instances. Dermoid cysts or teratomata are rare ovarian germ-cell tumors that occur in female subjects of all age groups. About 3 per cent of these can be classified as an ovarian struma on the basis of the presence of functionally significant thyroid tissue or thyroid tissue occupying more than 50 per cent of the volume of the tumor. Many more have some small element of thyroid tissue. Some strumae ovarii are associated with carcinoid-appearing tissue. These strumal carcinoid tumors secrete or contain thyroid hormones as well as somatostatin, chromogranin, serotonin, glucagon, insulin, gastrin, or calcitonin.[24] Some are associated with carcinoid syndromes.

The struma may present as an abdominal mass lesion, often with peritoneal or pleural effusion, which may be bloody. Most of these lesions synthesize and iodinate thyroglobulin poorly, and thus, despite growth of the mass, patients do not develop thyrotoxicosis. However, a significant proportion, perhaps one fourth to one third of ovarian strumae, are associated with thyrotoxicosis.[25, 26] Many of these lesions may be contributing to autoimmune hyperthyroidism in response to a common stimulator such as long-acting thyroid stimulator (LATS) or thyroid-stimulating immunoglobulins (TSI's). In others instances, the struma alone clearly is responsible for the thyrotoxicity. An elevated free thyroxine index (FTI), a suppressed TSH value, and uptake of radioiodine in a mass in the pelvis are the obvious prerequisites for making the diagnosis.[27] Often in ovarian struma, symptoms and findings of thyrotoxicosis are present in patients who have a low uptake of radioiodine in their thyroid gland. Of course, a "high index of suspicion" is most important. Usually operative resection of the ovarian tumor is indicated. Following this, transient postoperative hypothyroidism and "thyroid storm" have been occasionally reported to occur.

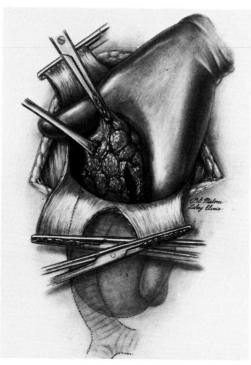

FIGURE 53–9. **Finger dissection of substernal goiter.** Note that the index finger is inserted into the mediastinum outside the thyroid capsule and is swept around until the gland is freed from the pleura and other tissue in the mediastinum. Occasionally, despite traction, the substernal goiter does not pass out through the superior thoracic outlet because of its size. In such cases, it may be necessary to evacuate some of the colloid material from within the goiter. Then, with gentle upward traction on the capsule, the mass can be elevated into the neck wound and resected. (From Sedgwick CE, Cady B: Surgery of the Thyroid and Parathyroid Glands (ed 2). Philadelphia, WB Saunders Company, 1980.)

Benign thyroid adenomas in strumae are common. About 5 per cent manifest evidence of carcinoma.[28] Usually, these are resectable, but radiation therapy and/or ^{131}I ablation has been advised after resection of the tumors in order to avoid the tendency for late recurrence or metastatic disease, which sometimes has been fatal. Metastatic disease occurs in about 5 per cent of malignant tumors. It is best treated with ^{131}I therapy, and TSH suppression should be given as for thyroid cancer originating in the usual location.

STRUMA CORDIS

Functioning apparently "normal" intracardiac thyroid tissue has been reported a few times, and has been visualized by radioiodine imaging.[29] The clinical presentation usually is a right ventricular mass, and the diagnosis has typically been made after operative removal.

ACKNOWLEDGMENT: We thank Kim Maddy for her expert assistance.

REFERENCES

1. Sedgwick CE, Cady B: Surgery of the Thyroid and Parathyroid Glands (ed 2). Philadelphia, WB Saunders Company, 1980.

2. Weller GL: Development of the thyroid, parathyroid and thymus glands in man. Contrib Embryol Carnegie Inst Wash 24:93–142, 1933.
3. Gray SW, Skandalakis JE: Embryology for Surgeons. Philadelphia, WB Saunders Company, 1972.
4. Norris EH: Parathyroid glands and lateral thyroid in man: Their morphogenesis, histogenesis, topographic anatomy and prenatal growth. Contrib Embryol Carnegie Inst Wash 26:247–294, 1937.
5. Williams ED, Toyn CE, Harach HR: The ultimobranchial gland and congenital thyroid abnormalities in man. J Pathol 159:135–141, 1989.
6. Siraj QH, Aleem N, Inam-Ur-Rehman A, et al: The pyramidal lobe: A scintigraphic assessment. Nucl Med Commun 10:685–693, 1989.
7. Vasquez-Chavez C, Acevedo-Rivera K, Sartorius C, Espinosa-Said L: Thyroid hemiagenesis: Report of 3 cases and review of the literature. Gac Med Mex 125:395–399, 1989.
8. Khatri VP, Espinosa MH, Harada WA: Papillary adenocarcinoma in thyroid hemiagenesis. Head Neck 14:312–315, 1992.
9. Netter RA: Endocrine System and Selected Metabolic Diseases. Ciba Collection of Medical Illustration. Summit, NJ, Ciba Pharmaceutical Company, 1974, p 45.
10. Buckman LT: Lingual thyroid. Laryngoscope 46:765–784, 878–897, 935–955, 1936.
11. Zink A, Rave F, Hoffmann R, Ziegler R: Papillary carcinoma in ectopic thyroid. Horm Res 35:86–88, 1991.
12. Elprana D, Manni JJ, Smals AGH: Lingual thyroid. ORL J Otorhinolaryngol Relat Spec 46:147–152, 1984.
13. Defoer FY, Mahler C: Lingual thyroid in two natural brothers. J Endocrinol Invest 13:65–67, 1990.
14. Conklin WT, Davis RM, Dabb RW, Reilly CM: Hypothyroidism following removal of a "thyroglossal duct cyst." Plast Reconstr Surg 68:930–932, 1981.
15. Allard RHB: The thyroglossal cyst. Head Neck 5:134–146, 1982.
16. Weiss SD, Orlich CC: Primary papillary carcinoma of a thyroglossal duct cyst: Report of a case and review of the literature. Br J Surg 78:87–89, 1991.
17. Katz AD, Hachigian M: Thyroglossal duct cysts: A thirty year experience with emphasis on occurrence in older patients. Am J Surg 155:741–744, 1988.
18. Issa MM, de Vries P: Familial occurrence of thyroglossal duct cyst. J Pediatr Surg 26:30–31, 1991.
19. Helidonis E, Dokianakis G, Papazoglou G, et al: Ectopic thyroid gland in the submandibular region. J Laryngol Otol 94:219–224, 1980.
20. Stanton A, Allen-Mersh TG: Is laterally situated ectopic thyroid tissue always malignant? J R Soc Med 77:333–334, 1984.
21. Wychulis AR, Payne WS, Clagett OT, et al: Surgical treatment of mediastinal tumors. J Thorac Cardiovasc Surg 62:379, 1971.
22. Lesavoy MA, Norberg HP, Kaplan EL: Substernal goiter with superior vena caval obstruction. Surgery 77:325–329, 1975.
23. Lahey FH, Swinton NW: Intrathoracic goiter. Surg Gynecol Obstet 59:627, 1934.
24. Stagno PA, Petras RE, Hart WR: Strumal carcinoids of the ovary: An immunohistologic and ultrastructural study. Arch Pathol Lab Med 111:440–446, 1987.
25. Ramagopal E, Stanbury JB: Studies of the distribution of iodine and protein in a struma ovarii. J Clin Endocrinol Metab 25:526, 1965.
26. Kempers RD, Dockerty MB, Hoffman DL, Bartholomew LG: Struma ovarii—ascitic, hyperthyroid, and asymptomatic syndromes. Ann Intern Med 72:883, 1970.
27. March DE, Desai AG, Park CH, et al: Struma ovarii: Hyperthyroidism in a postmenopausal woman. J Nucl Med 29:263–265, 1988.
28. Thomas RD, Batty VB: Metastatic malignant struma ovarii: Two case reports. Clin Nucl Med 17:577–578, 1992.
29. Rieser GD, Ober KP, Cowan RJ, Cordell AR: Radioiodide imaging of struma cordis. Clin Nucl Med 13:421, 1988.

54

Surgery of the Thyroid

EDWIN L. KAPLAN
HISATO HARA
KOICHI ITO

Modern thyroid surgery, as we know it today, began in the 1860's in Vienna with the school of Billroth.[1] The mortality of thyroidectomy was high, recurrent laryngeal nerve injuries were common, and tetany was thought to be due to "hysteria." The parathyroid glands in humans were not discovered by Sandström until 1880,[2] and the fact that hypocalcemia was the definitive cause of tetany was not wholly accepted until several decades into the 20th century. Kocher, a master thyroid surgeon who operated in the late 19th and early 20th centuries in Bern, practiced meticulous surgical technique and greatly reduced the mortality and operative morbidity of thyroidectomy for goiter. He described "cachexia strumipriva" in patients years after thyroidectomy[3] (Fig. 54–1). He recognized that only those patients who had total thyroidectomy developed this dreaded syndrome. As a result, he stopped performing total resection of the thyroid. We now know, of course, that cachexia strumipriva was surgical hypothyroidism. Kocher received the Nobel Prize for this very important contribution, which proved beyond a doubt the physiological importance of the thyroid gland.

By 1920, advances in thyroid surgery had reached the point that Halsted[1] referred to this operation as a "feat which today can be accomplished by any competent operator without danger of mishap." Unfortunately, decades later, complications still occur. In the best of hands, however, thyroid surgery can be performed today with a mortality that varies little from the risk of general anesthesia alone, and with a low morbidity as well. In order to obtain such enviable results, however, the surgeon must have a thorough understanding of the pathophysiology of thyroid disorders, be versed in the preoperative and postoperative care of patients, have a clear knowledge of the anatomy of the neck region, and, finally, use an unhurried, careful, meticulous operative technique.

IMPORTANT SURGICAL ANATOMY

The thyroid gland, which means "shield," is composed of two lobes connected by an isthmus that lies on the trachea approximately at the level of the second tracheal ring (Fig. 54–2). The gland is enveloped by the deep cervical fascia and is attached firmly to the trachea by the ligament of Berry. Each lobe resides in a bed between the trachea and larynx medially and the carotid sheath and sternocleidomastoid muscles laterally. The strap muscles are anterior to the thyroid lobes, and the parathyroid glands and recurrent laryngeal nerves are associated with the posterior surface of each lobe. A pyramidal lobe is often present. This is a long, narrow projection of thyroid tissue extending upward from the isthmus lying on the surface of the thyroid cartilage. It represents a vestige of the embryonic thyroglossal duct and often becomes palpable in cases of thyroiditis or Graves' disease. The normal thyroid varies in size in different parts of the world, depending upon the iodine content in the diet. In the United States it weighs about 15 g.

Vascular Supply

The thyroid has an abundant blood supply. The arterial supply to each thyroid lobe is two-fold. The *superior thyroid*

Supported in part by a generous grant from the Nathan and Frances Goldblatt Society for Cancer Research.

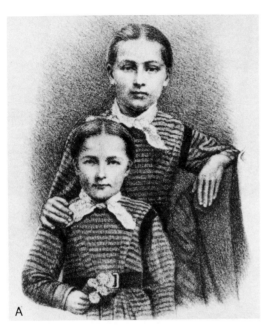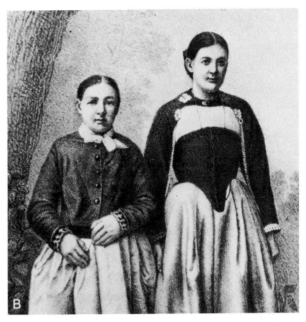

FIGURE 54–1. The dramatic case of Maria Richsel, the first patient to have come to Kocher's attention with postoperative myxedema. *A*, The child and her younger sister before the operation. *B*, The changes nine years after the operation. The younger sister, now fully grown, contrasts vividly with the dwarfed and stunted patient. Also note Maria's thickened face and fingers, which are typical of myxedema. (From Kocher T: Uber Kropfextirpation und ihre Folgen. Arch Klin Chir 29:254, 1883.)

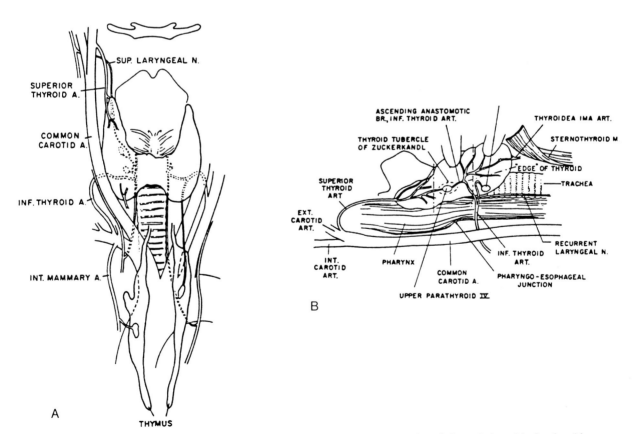

FIGURE 54–2. **Anatomy of the thyroid and parathyroid glands.** *A*, Anterior view. *B*, Lateral view with the thyroid retracted anteriorly and medially to show the surgical landmarks (the head of the patient is to the left). (From Kaplan EL: Thyroid and parathyroid. *In* Schwartz SI (ed): Principles of Surgery (ed 5). New York, McGraw-Hill Book Company, 1989, pp 1613–1685.)

artery arises from the external carotid artery on each side and descends several centimeters in the neck to reach the upper poles of each thyroid lobe where they branch. The *inferior thyroid arteries*, each of which arises from the thyrocervical trunk of the subclavian artery, cross beneath the carotid sheath and enter the lower or midpart of the thyroid lobe. The *thyroidea ima* is sometimes present; it arises from the arch of the aorta and enters the thyroid in the midline. A venous plexus forms under the thyroid capsule. Each lobe is drained by the *superior thyroid vein* at the upper pole, which flows into the internal jugular vein, and the *middle thyroid vein* at the middle part of the lobe, which enters either the internal jugular or innominate vein. Arising from each lower pole is the *inferior thyroid vein*, which drains directly into the innominate vein.

Nerves

The thyroid gland's relation to the *recurrent laryngeal nerve* and to the *external branch of the superior laryngeal nerve* is of major surgical significance, because damage to these nerves leads to a disability of phonation or to difficulty in breathing.[4] Both nerves are branches of the vagus nerve.

Recurrent Laryngeal Nerve

The *right recurrent laryngeal nerve* loops posteriorly around the subclavian artery and ascends behind the right lobe of the thyroid (Fig. 54–3). It enters the larynx behind the cricothyroid muscle and the inferior cornu of the thyroid

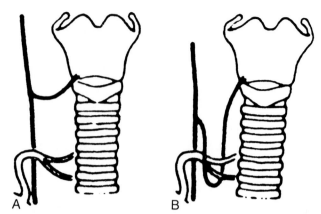

FIGURE 54–4. **"Nonrecurrent" right recurrent laryngeal nerves,** coursing near the superior pole vessels *(A)* or around the inferior thyroid artery *(B)*. Because of the abnormal location of "nonrecurrent" nerves, they are much more likely to be damaged during operation. (From Skandalakis JE, Droulis C, Harlaftis N, et al: The recurrent laryngeal nerve. Am Surg 42:629–634, 1976.)

cartilage and innervates all of the intrinsic laryngeal muscles except the cricothyroid. The left recurrent laryngeal nerve loops posteriorly around the arch of the aorta and ascends in the tracheoesophageal groove posterior to the left lobe of the thyroid, entering the larynx and innervating the musculature in a similar fashion as the right nerve. Several factors make the recurrent laryngeal nerve vulnerable to injury, especially in the hands of inexperienced surgeons.[4]

1. The presence of nonrecurrent laryngeal nerves (Fig. 54–4). Nonrecurrent nerves occur more on the right side (0.6 per cent) than on the left (0.04 per cent).[5] They are associated with vascular anomalies—an aberrant take-off of the right subclavian artery from the descending aorta (on the right) or a right-sided aortic arch (on the left). In this setting the nerve is at greater risk of being divided.

2. Proximity of the recurrent nerve to the thyroid gland (Fig. 54–5). The recurrent nerve is not always in the tracheoesophageal groove where it is expected to be. It can

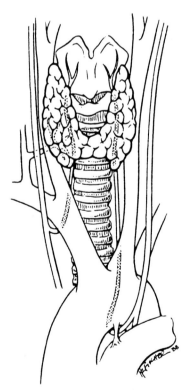

FIGURE 54–3. Anatomy of the recurrent laryngeal nerves. (From Thompson NW, Demers M: Exposure is not necessary to avoid the recurrent laryngeal nerve during thyroid operations. *In* Simmons RL, Udekwu AO (eds): Debates in Clinical Surgery. Chicago, Year Book Medical Publishers, 1990.)

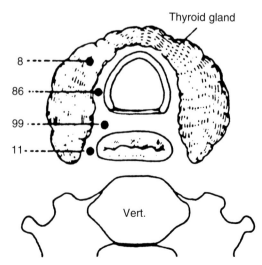

FIGURE 54–5. The location of 204 recurrent laryngeal nerves in dissections from 102 cadavers. (From Skandalakis JE, Droulias C, Harlaftis N, et al: The recurrent laryngeal nerve. Am Surg 42:629–634, 1976.)

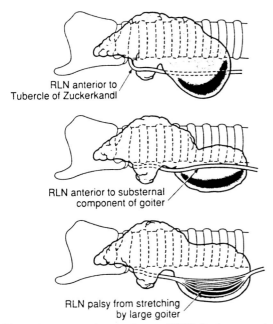

FIGURE 54–6. **Recurrent laryngeal nerve (RLN) displacements by cervical and substernal goiters.** Such nerves are at risk during lobectomy unless anticipated at possible locations. Rarely the nerves are so stretched that a spontaneous palsy results. After careful dissection and preservation, functional recovery may occur postoperatively. (From Thompson NW, Demers M: Exposure is not necessary to avoid the recurrent laryngeal nerve during thyroid operations. *In* Simmons RL, Udekwu AO (eds): Debates in Clinical Surgery. Chicago, Year Book Medical Publishers, 1990.)

often be posterior or anterior to this or may even be within the thyroid parenchyma. Thus the nerve is vulnerable to injury if it is not visualized and traced up to the larynx during thyroidectomy.

3. Relationship of the nerve to the inferior thyroid artery. The nerve frequently passes anterior, posterior, or through the branches of the inferior thyroid artery. Medial traction of the lobe often lifts the nerve anteriorly, making it more vulnerable. Likewise, ligation of this artery, prac-

ticed by many surgeons, is dangerous if the nerve is not identified first.

4. Deformities due to large thyroid nodules.[6] In the presence of large nodules the right laryngeal nerve may not be anatomically in its "correct" location but may be found even anterior to the thyroid (Fig. 54–6). Once more, there is no substitute for identification of the nerve in a gentle and careful manner.

External Branch of the Superior Laryngeal Nerve

On each side, the *external branch of the superior laryngeal nerve* innervates the cricothyroid muscle. In most cases, these nerves lie close to the vascular pedicles of the superior poles of the thyroid glands,[7] requiring that the vessels be ligated with care to avoid their injury (Fig. 54–7). In 21 per cent these nerves are intimately associated with the superior thyroid vessels. In only 15 per cent of cases is the superior laryngeal nerve sufficiently distant from the superior pole vessels to be protected from manipulation by the surgeon. Unfortunately, many surgeons do not even attempt to identify this nerve prior to ligation of the upper pole of the thyroid.[8]

Parathyroid Glands

The parathyroids are small glands that secrete parathyroid hormone, the major hormone that controls serum calcium homeostasis in humans. Usually four glands are present, but three to six glands have been found. Each gland normally weighs 30 to 40 mg but may be heavier if more fat is present. Because of their small size, their delicate blood supply, and their usual anatomical position adjacent to the thyroid gland, these structures are at risk of being accidentally removed, traumatized, or devascularized during thyroidectomy.[9]

The upper parathyroid glands arise embryologically

FIGURE 54–7. Proximity of the external branch of the superior laryngeal nerve to the superior thyroid vessels. (From Moosman DA, DeWeese MS: The external laryngeal nerve as related to thyroidectomy. Surg Gynecol Obstet 127:1101, 1968.)

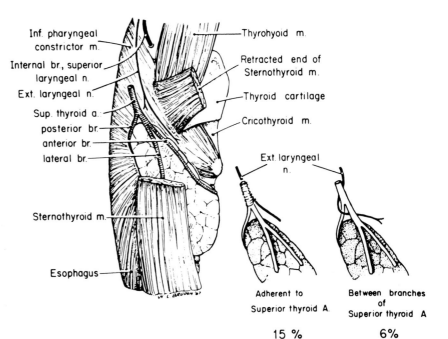

from the fourth pharyngeal pouch (see Fig. 53–3). They descend only slightly during embryological development, and their position in adult life remains quite constant.[10] This gland is usually found adjacent to the posterior surface of the middle part of the thyroid lobe, often just anterior to the recurrent laryngeal nerve as it enters the larynx.

The lower parathyroid glands arise from the third pharyngeal pouch along with the thymus (see Fig. 53–3). Hence, they often descend with the thymus. Because they travel so far in embryological life, they have a wide range of distribution in the adult, from just beneath the mandible to the anterior mediastinum[10] (Fig. 54–8). Usually, however, these glands are found on the lateral or posterior surface of the lower part of the thyroid gland or within several centimeters of the lower thyroid pole within the thymic tongue.

Parathyroid glands can be recognized by their tan appearance, their small vascular pedicle, the fact that they bleed freely when a biopsy is performed, as opposed to fatty tissues, and their darkening color of hematoma formation when they are traumatized. With experience, one becomes much more adept in recognizing these very important structures and in differentiating them from either lymph nodes or fat. Frozen section examination during operation can be helpful for their identification.

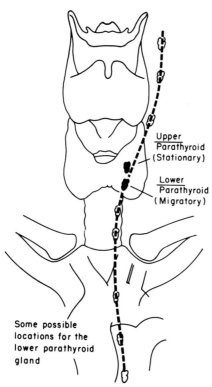

FIGURE 54–8. **Descent of the lower parathyroid.** While the upper parathyroid occupies a relatively constant position in relation to the middle or upper third of the lateral thyroid lobe, the lower parathyroid normally migrates in embryonic life and may end up anywhere along the course of the dotted line. When this gland is in the chest, it is nearly always in the anterior mediastinum. (From Kaplan EL: Thyroid and parathyroid. *In* Schwartz SI (ed): Principles of Surgery (ed 5). New York, McGraw-Hill Book Company, 1989, pp 1613–1685.)

Lymphatics

A practical description of the lymphatic drainage of the thyroid gland for the thyroid surgeon has recently been proposed by Taylor.[11] The results of his studies, which are clinically very relevant to the lymphatic spread of thyroid carcinoma, are summarized below.

Central Compartment of the Neck

1. The most constant site to which dye goes when injected into the thyroid is the trachea, the wall of which contains a rich network of lymphatics. This fact probably accounts for the frequency with which the trachea is involved by thyroid carcinoma, especially when it is anaplastic. This involvement is sometimes the limiting factor in surgical excision.

2. A chain of lymph nodes lies in the groove between the trachea and the esophagus.

3. Lymph can always be shown to drain toward the mediastinum and to the nodes intimately associated with the thymus.

4. A group of nodes lying above the isthmus and therefore in front of the larynx is sometimes involved. These have been called the *delphian nodes* (named for the oracle of Delphi) because it has been said that, if palpable, they are diagnostic of carcinoma. However, this clinical sign is often misleading. A *central lymph node dissection* clears out all of these lymph nodes from one carotid artery to the other carotid artery and down into the superior mediastinum as far as possible.

Lateral Compartment of the Neck

A constant group of nodes lies along the jugular vein on each side of the neck. The lymph glands found in the supraclavicular fossae may also be involved in the more distant spread of malignant disease from the thyroid gland. Finally, it should not be forgotten that the thoracic duct on the left side of the neck is a lymph vessel of considerable size, arching up out of the mediastinum and passing forward and laterally to drain into the left subclavian vein, usually just lateral to its junction with the internal jugular vein. If the thoracic duct is damaged, the wound is likely to fill with lymph; in this case, the duct should always be sought and tied. A wound that discharges lymph postoperatively should always raise the suspicion of damage to the thoracic duct or a major tributary. A *lateral lymph node dissection* encompasses removal of these lateral lymph nodes.

INDICATIONS FOR THYROIDECTOMY

Thyroidectomy is usually performed for the following reasons:

1. As therapy for some individuals with thyrotoxicosis, both those with Graves' disease and others with hot nodules.

2. To establish the definitive diagnosis of a mass within the thyroid gland, especially when the cytological analysis after fine-needle aspiration (FNA) is either nondiagnostic or equivocal.

3. To treat benign and malignant thyroid tumors.

4. To alleviate pressure symptoms or respiratory difficulties associated with a benign or malignant process.

5. To remove an unsightly goiter.

SOLITARY THYROID NODULES

Solitary thyroid nodules are clinically present in 4 to 6 per cent of patients in the United States, and most are benign. Therefore, rather than operating on every patient with a thyroid nodule, the physician or surgeon should select patients for operation who are at high risk for thyroid cancer. Furthermore, each surgeon must know the complications of thyroidectomy and be able to perform a proper operation for thyroid cancer in a safe and effective manner or refer the patient to a center where this can be done.

Low-dose External Irradiation to the Head and Neck

A history of *low-dose external irradiation* to the head or neck is probably the most important historical fact that can be obtained because it indicates that a cancer of the thyroid is more likely (about 35 per cent of cases) even if the gland is multinodular.[12, 13] Low-dose irradiation and its implications are discussed in Chapter 50.

High-dose External Irradiation Therapy

Recently, we and others[14] have documented that *high-dose external irradiation therapy*—that is, more than 2000 rads—does not confer safety from thyroid carcinoma, as was previously thought. Rather, an increased prevalence of thyroid carcinoma, usually papillary cancer, has been found, particularly in patients with Hodgkin's disease and other lymphomas who received upper mantle irradiation that included the thyroid gland. Usually a dose of about 4000 rads was given. Both benign and malignant thyroid nodules are beginning to be recognized now that these persons have survived for longer periods of time. If a thyroid mass appears,

it should be treated aggressively. These patients should also be observed carefully for the development of hypothyroidism.

Diagnosis of Thyroid Nodules

A number of diagnostic modalities have been used in the past, but currently most have been superseded by FNA of the mass with *cytological analysis.*[15] In the hands of a good thyroid cytologist, about 90 per cent of nodules can be categorized histologically. Approximately 65 per cent are found to be compatible with a colloid nodule. Twenty per cent demonstrate sheets of follicular cells, 5 per cent are malignant, and 10 per cent are nondiagnostic.

All patients who have *malignant* cytological results should be operated on. False-positive diagnoses are rare. All patients with *sheets of follicular cells* should also be operated on. Most nodules exhibiting sheets of follicular cells on cytological examination are benign follicular adenomas. However, follicular carcinomas exhibit the same cytological characteristics and cannot be differentiated by this technique. Only by careful histological examination after operative removal can follicular carcinoma and adenoma be differentiated.

When the diagnosis of *colloid nodule* is made cytologically, the patient can be observed and not operated upon unless severe compression symptoms or substernal goiters are present. Finally, if an *inadequate specimen* is obtained, the needle aspiration of the nodule with cytological examination can be repeated. Thus, FNA with cytology is the most powerful tool in our armamentarium for the diagnosis of a thyroid nodule.[16]

In summary, the algorithm for the diagnosis of a thyroid nodule using isotope scintigraphy and ultrasonography as initial steps (Fig. 54–9) is being replaced in many hospitals, including our own, by emphasizing the importance of the early use of needle aspiration with cytological examination (Fig. 54–10). Far fewer isotope scans are currently being done because carcinomas represent only 10 per cent of all cold nodules. Furthermore, far fewer ultrasonographic examinations of the thyroid are being done, because with needle aspiration a cystic lesion can be recognized immediately.

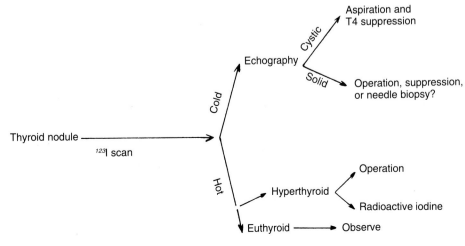

FIGURE 54–9. Algorithm for the diagnosis of a thyroid nodule, which utilizes isotope scanning and ultrasound examination (echography) as primary modalities. Needle aspiration with cytology is performed on selected nodules.

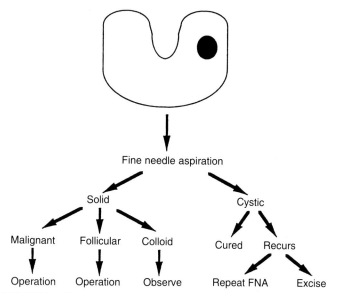

FIGURE 54–10. Algorithm for the diagnosis of a thyroid nodule, which uses needle aspiration with cytological examination of each nodule. Greater accuracy is obtained by using this diagnostic scheme. (Courtesy of Dr. Jon van Heerden.)

PREPARATION FOR OPERATION

Most patients undergoing thyroid operations are euthyroid and require no specific preoperative preparation related to their thyroid gland. A serum calcium level should be determined in all individuals, and indirect laryngoscopy should be performed, possibly in all patients but certainly in those who have had a prior thyroid or parathyroid operation in order to detect the possibility of a recurrent laryngeal nerve injury.

Hypothyroidism

Severe hypothyroidism can be diagnosed clinically by myxedema, as well as slowness of affect, speech, and reflexes.[17] The circulating T_4 and free thyroxine index (FTI) values are low. The serum thyroid-stimulating hormone (TSH) level is high in all cases of hypothyroidism which are not due to pituitary insufficiency. In the presence of severe hypothyroidism, both the morbidity and the mortality of operation are increased as a result of the effects of both the anesthesia and the operation. Such patients have a higher incidence of perioperative hypotension, gastrointestinal hypomotility, prolonged anesthetic recovery, and neuropsychiatric disturbances. They metabolize drugs slowly and are very sensitive to all medications. Therefore, when severe myxedema is present, it is preferable to defer elective surgery if possible until a euthyroid state is achieved. However, if urgent surgery is necessary, it should not be postponed simply for repletion of thyroid hormone. Endocrine consultation is imperative, and an excellent anesthesiologist is mandatory for success. In most cases, intravenous T_4 can be started preoperatively and continued thereafter. In general, small doses of T_4 are first given to patients who are severely hypothyroid and then the dose is gradually increased.

Hyperthyroidism

In the United States, most patients with thyrotoxicosis have Graves' disease. Persons with Graves' disease or other thyrotoxic states should be treated preoperatively in order to restore a euthyroid state and to prevent *thyroid storm*, a severe accentuation of the symptoms and signs of hyperthyroidism which can occur during or after operation. Thyroid storm results in tachycardia or cardiac arrhythmias, fever, disorientation, coma, and even death. In the early days of thyroid surgery, operations on the toxic gland were among the most dangerous surgical procedures because of the frequent occurrence of severe bleeding and all the symptoms and signs already described. Now, with proper preoperative preparation,[18] operations on the thyroid gland in Graves' disease can be performed with about the same degree of safety as with other thyroid conditions.

In mild cases of thyrotoxicosis, iodine therapy alone can be used for preoperative preparation, although we do not recommend this approach.[17] Lugol's solution or a saturated solution of potassium iodide (SSKI) is given for several weeks. Although only several drops per day is needed to block the release of T_4 from the toxic thyroid gland, it is our practice to administer three drops three times daily. This medication is taken in milk or orange juice to make it palatable.

Most of our patients with Graves' disease are treated initially with the antithyroid drugs, propylthiouracil (PTU) or methimazole (Tapazole), until they approach a euthyroid state. Then iodine is added to the regimen for 10 to 14 days before operation. The iodine decreases the vascularity and increases the firmness of the gland. Sometimes T_4 is added to this regimen to prevent hypothyroidism and to decrease the size of the gland.

The β-adrenergic blocker propranolol (Inderal) has increased the safety of thyroidectomy for Graves' disease.[18] We use it frequently with antithyroid drugs to block β-adrenergic receptors and ameliorate the major signs of Graves' disease by decreasing the patient's pulse rate and eliminating the tremor. Some surgeons recommend the use of propranolol alone or with iodine and consider the gland to be less friable.[19] These regimens, they believe, shorten the preparation time of patients with Graves' disease for operation and make the operation easier because the thyroid gland is smaller and less friable than it would otherwise be.[19] We do not favor these regimens as our *routine* preparation, for they do not appear to offer the same degree of safety as do preoperative programs that restore a euthyroid state before operation. Several instances of fever and tachycardia have been reported in persons with Graves' disease who were taking only propranolol. We have used propranolol therapy alone or with iodine without difficulty in some patients who are allergic to antithyroid medications. In such patients it is essential to *continue the propranolol for one to two weeks postoperatively.* Remember that they are still thyrotoxic immediately after operation, although the peripheral manifestations of their disease have been blocked.

The advantages and disadvantages of radioiodine versus thyroidectomy as definitive treatment of Graves' disease are listed in Table 54–1. In our patients we have never had a death from operation in over 20 years. Surgical resection

TABLE 54–1. ABLATIVE TREATMENT OF GRAVES' DISEASE WITH THYROTOXICOSIS

METHOD	DOSE OR EXTENT OF SURGERY	ONSET OF RESPONSE	COMPLICATIONS*	REMARKS
Surgery	Subtotal (90–95%) excision of gland	Immediate	Mortality: <1% Perm hypothyroidism: 20–30% Recur hyperthyroidism: <15% Vocal cord paralysis: ~1% Hypoparathyroidism: ~1%	Applicable in younger patients and pregnant women
Radioiodine	5–10 mCi	Several weeks to months	Perm hypothyroidism: 50–70% often with delayed onset; multiple treatments sometimes necessary; recurrence possible	Potential risks require ongoing study; close long-term follow-up needed; avoid in children or pregnant women

*Perm, permanent; recur, recurrent.

involves either subtotal thyroidectomy (see Fig. 54–11) or lobectomy with contralateral subtotal lobectomy. Currently we leave about 4 to 5 g of thyroid tissue in the neck at the end of the operative procedure. Leaving more leads to a higher rate of recurrence.[20] In children and adolescents, one should consider leaving smaller remnants because the incidence of recurrence of thyrotoxicosis appears to be greater in this group. The major benefits of thyroidectomy appear to be the speed with which normalization is achieved and the lesser rate of hypothyroidism.

SURGICAL APPROACH TO THYROID NODULES

Nonirradiated Patients

Any nodule suspected of being a carcinoma should be completely removed, along with surrounding tissue, which means that a total lobectomy (or lobectomy with isthmusectomy) is the initial operation of choice in most patients (Fig. 54–11). A frozen section should be obtained intra-

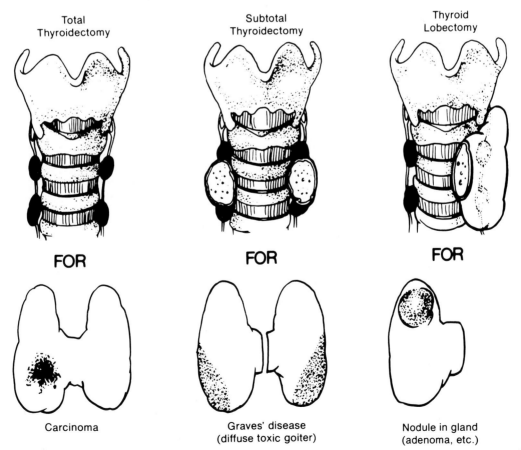

FIGURE 54–11. **Common operations on the thyroid.** In near-total thyroidectomy a small amount of thyroid tissue is left to protect the recurrent laryngeal nerve and upper parathyroid gland. (From Kaplan EL: Surgical endocrinology. *In* Polk HC, Stone HH, and Gardner B (eds): Basic Surgery (ed 4). St. Louis, Quality Medical Publishing, 1993, pp 162–195.)

operatively. If a diagnosis of a *colloid nodule* is made, the operation is terminated. When a diagnosis of an *adenoma* is made, the treatment is more controversial. Differentiating a follicular adenoma from a follicular carcinoma or a benign Hürthle cell tumor from a Hürthle cell carcinoma on frozen section is usually very difficult. These diagnoses require the careful assessment of cellular morphology as well as capsular and vascular invasion, which are often difficult to evaluate on frozen section. To aid in the diagnosis, enlarged lymph nodes of the central compartment are sampled, and a biopsy of the jugular nodes is also performed. If the result is negative, there are two options: stopping the operation after lobectomy, with the understanding that a second operation may be necessary to complete the thyroidectomy if a carcinoma is ultimately diagnosed, or performing a subtotal resection on the contralateral side. We favor this latter approach if the patient consents, particularly when a preoperative needle aspiration suggests that a follicular lesion will be encountered intraoperatively, or if examination of frozen sections identifies a follicular lesion. We treat most patients with benign neoplasms with thyroxine replacement anyway, even if only one lobe has been removed. Furthermore, a second operation is eliminated if the lesion is later diagnosed as malignant, for the remaining small thyroid remnant can be ablated with radioiodine therapy.

Irradiated Patients

In patients who have been exposed to low-dose, external irradiation to the head and neck during infancy, childhood, or adolescence, because of the frequency of bilaterality of the disease, the known coincidence of benign and malignant nodules in the same gland, and the prevalence of papillary carcinoma in 35 to 40 per cent, a near-total resection of the thyroid gland with a biopsy of the jugular nodes usually is performed, even if a frozen section of the dominant nodule is benign.[13] This therapy is thought to be advantageous because the remaining thyroid remnant of these patients usually can be ablated with one 30-mCi dose of radioiodine given on an outpatient basis if a carcinoma is found on permanent section analysis. In any event, these patients require therapy with thyroid hormone.

Patients who have received high-dose radiation to their thyroid bed, such as those treated with mantle radiation for Hodgkin's disease, are also at greater risk for developing thyroid carcinomas years later and should be followed carefully.[14] Once more, if they are operated upon, most of the thyroid tissue should be removed even if the dominant mass is thought to be benign.

SURGICAL APPROACH TO THYROID CANCER

Papillary Carcinoma

The surgical treatment of papillary carcinoma is best divided into two groups, based on the clinical characteristics and virulence of these lesions.

Minimal Papillary Carcinoma

The term *minimal papillary carcinoma* refers to a small papillary tumor, less than 1 cm in diameter, that demonstrates no local invasiveness through the thyroid capsule, is not associated with lymph node metastases, and is often found in a young person as an occult lesion when thyroidectomy has been done for another benign condition. In such instances, especially when the cancer is unicentric and 5 mm or less in size, lobectomy is sufficient and reoperations are unnecessary. Thyroid hormone is given to suppress serum TSH levels, and the patient is followed at regular intervals.

Standard Treatment of Most Papillary Carcinomas

Most papillary carcinomas are neither minimal nor occult. These tumors are known to be microscopically multicentric in up to 80 per cent of cases, occasionally to invade locally into the trachea or esophagus, to metastasize commonly to lymph nodes and later to the lungs and other tissues, and to recur clinically in the other thyroid lobe in 7 to 18 per cent of patients if treated only by thyroid lobectomy.[21]

The authors firmly believe that the best treatment for papillary cancer is near-total or total thyroidectomy (Fig. 54-11), with appropriate central and lateral neck dissections when nodes are involved. The so-called cherry-picking operations, which remove only the enlarged lymph nodes, should not be performed. Rather, when tumor is found in the lateral triangle, a modified radical neck dissection should be performed[22] (Fig. 54-12). At the conclusion of a modified radical neck dissection, the lymph node–bearing tissue from the lateral triangle is removed while the carotid artery, jugular vein, phrenic nerve, sympathetic ganglia, brachial plexus, and spinal accessory nerve are spared and are left in place. Prophylactic neck dissections of the lateral triangle should not be performed for papillary cancer, and these dissections should be done only when enlarged nodes with tumor are found.

The surgeon with limited experience should probably not perform total or near-total thyroidectomy unless he or she is capable of doing so with a low incidence of recurrent laryngeal nerve injuries and permanent hypoparathyroidism because these are serious complications. Otherwise, it may be advisable to refer these patients to a major medical center where such expertise is available.

Following operation, radioiodine scanning and treatment are frequently utilized.[23] [131]I is taken up by most metastatic papillary cancers, but only if the TSH level is very high and almost all normal thyroid tissue has been removed. If all or most of a lobe of normal thyroid remains, radioiodine scanning and treatment of metastases cannot be performed effectively.

Recent studies have attempted to predict the potential aggressiveness of a given papillary carcinoma by nuclear DNA measurements as well as by formulations of a set of risk factors, including age of the patient, size of the tumor, presence or absence of local invasion or distant metastases, and change in tumor grade (the AGES[24] and AMES[25] clas-

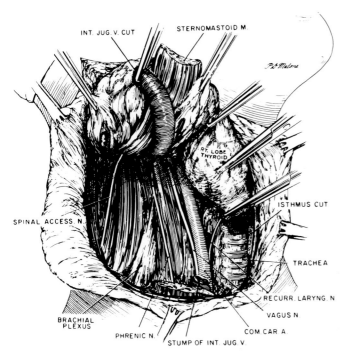

FIGURE 54–12. **Lateral neck dissection.** Note that during this procedure the vagus nerve, sympathetic ganglia, phrenic nerve, brachial plexus, and spinal accessory nerve are preserved. In a modified neck dissection the sternocleidomastoid muscle is usually not divided and the jugular vein is not removed unless lymph nodes with tumor are adherent to it. (From Sedgwick CE, Cady B: *In* Surgery of the Thyroid and Parathyroid Glands. Philadelphia, WB Saunders, 1980, p 180.)

sifications). Perhaps in the future, the extent of treatment for each patient will be individualized according to such criteria as they become more exact.

Follicular Carcinoma

True follicular carcinomas are far less common than papillary cancers. Remember that the "follicular variant" of papillary cancer should be classified and treated as a papillary carcinoma. Patients with follicular carcinoma are usually older than those with papillary cancer, and, once more, females predominate. Microscopically, follicular lesions that demonstrate vascular and/or capsular invasion are present. Multicentricity of tumor and lymph node metastases are far less common than with papillary carcinoma. Metastatic spread of tumor occurs by hematogenous dissemination to the lungs, bones, and other peripheral tissues.

A single tumor that demonstrates only *microinvasion* of the capsule has a very good prognosis. In this situation, perhaps an ipsilateral lobectomy is sufficient. However, for most patients with follicular cancer that demonstrates gross capsular invasion or vascular invasion, the ideal operation is similar to that for papillary cancer, although the rationale for its performance differs. Near-total or total thyroidectomy should be performed not because of multicentricity but rather to facilitate a later total-body scan with radioiodine. If peripheral metastases are detected (Fig. 54–13), they should be treated with high-dose radioiodine therapy. Although lymph node metastases in the lateral neck are

not commonly found, a modified radical neck dissection should be performed if they are present.

Finally, regardless of the operation, all patients with papillary or follicular cancer should be treated with L-thyroxine therapy for life in sufficient doses to suppress the TSH level to near zero. Care should be taken not to cause cardiac problems from thyrotoxicosis, however.

Hürthle Cell Tumors and Cancer

Hürthle cell tumors are thought to be variants of follicular neoplasms. They are more difficult to treat than the usual follicular neoplasms, however, for several reasons[26]: (1) The incidence of carcinoma varies from 5.3 to 62 per cent in different clinical series. (2) Benign-appearing tumors have later metastasized in 2.5 to 11.5 per cent of patients. (3) Hürthle cell cancers are far less likely to concentrate radioiodine than the usual follicular neoplasms, which makes treatment of metastatic disease particularly difficult.

Of 54 patients with Hürthle cell tumors whom we treated,[26] 4 had grossly malignant lesions, 10 had questionable diagnoses ("intermediate" lesions) because of partial penetration of their capsule by tumor, and 40 (75 per cent) had lesions that were thought to be benign. About half of the patients had a history of low-dose external radiation. Many had separate papillary or follicular cancers of the thyroid.

During a mean follow-up period of 8.4 years, three additional Hürthle cell tumors were recognized as malignant after metastases were discovered: Two were originally classified as intermediate lesions, and one was in the benign-appearing group. Thus, 7 of 54 of our patients (13 per cent) had Hürthle cell carcinomas. One of the seven patients with Hürthle cell cancer died of widespread metastases after 35 years, and the other six are currently free of disease.

We believe that therapy of these lesions should be individualized.[26] Total thyroid ablation is appropriate for frankly malignant Hürthle cell cancers, for all Hürthle cell tumors in patients who received low-dose childhood irradiation, for patients with associated papillary or follicular carcinomas, for all large tumors, and for patients who exhibit partial capsular invasion. On the other hand, single, well-encapsulated, benign-appearing Hürthle cell tumors that are small may be treated by lobectomy and careful follow-up, because the chance that they will later exhibit malignant behavior is low (2.5 per cent in our series and 1.5 per cent among patients described in the recent literature).[26] Nuclear DNA analysis may aid the surgeon in recognizing tumors that are potentially aggressive, because such tumors usually demonstrate aneuploidy.[27]

Anaplastic Carcinoma

Anaplastic thyroid carcinoma remains one of the most virulent of all cancers in humans. The tumor grows very rapidly, and systemic symptoms are common. Survival for most patients is measured in months. The previously so-called "small cell type" is now considered to be a lymphoma by most pathologists and is treated by a combina-

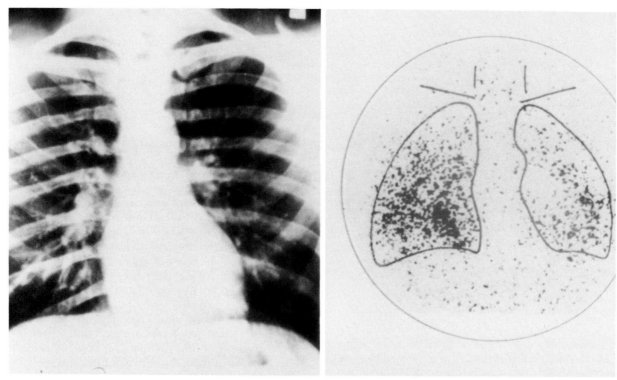

FIGURE 54–13. Despite the fact that the chest radiograph was read as normal, a total-body scan using radioiodine demonstrated uptake in both lung fields, thus signifying the presence of unknown metastatic disease. Note that the thyroid has been removed surgically because no uptake of isotope is present in the neck.

tion of surgery, external radiation, and/or chemotherapy. The "large cell type" may present as a solitary thyroid nodule early in its clinical course. If it is operated on at that time, a near-total or total thyroidectomy should be performed, with appropriate central and lateral neck dissections. However, almost always the tumor is advanced when the patient is first evaluated. In these patients, surgical cure is unlikely no matter how aggressively it is pursued. In particularly advanced cases, diagnosis by needle biopsy or by small open biopsy may be all that is appropriate. Sometimes, the isthmus must be divided to relieve tracheal compression, or a tracheostomy might be beneficial. Most treatment, however, is by external radiation therapy, chemotherapy, or both. Hyperfractionation external radiation therapy that uses several treatments per day has some enthusiasts. Radioiodine treatment is almost always ineffective because tumor uptake is absent. Although some success has been observed with doxorubicin, prolonged remissions are rarely achieved, and multidrug regimens and combinations of chemotherapy with radiation therapy are being tried.[28, 29] Although remissions do occur, cures have rarely if ever been achieved in advanced cases.

Medullary Thyroid Carcinoma

Medullary thyroid carcinoma is a C-cell, calcitonin-producing tumor that contains amyloid or an amyloid-like substance. In addition to calcitonin, it may elaborate or secrete other peptides and amines such as carcinoembryonic antigen (CEA), serotonin, neurotensin, and a high molecular weight ACTH-like peptide. These may result in a carcinoid-like syndrome with diarrhea, as well as Cushing's syndrome, especially when widely metastatic tumor is present. Most medullary cancer of the thyroid is sporadic, but it can also be transmitted in a familial pattern. This tumor, or its precursor, C-cell hyperplasia, occurs as a part of the MEN IIA and MEN IIB syndromes[30] (Table 54–2, Fig. 54–14). The MEN II syndromes are transmitted as an autosomal dominant trait, so that 50 per cent of the offspring would be expected to have this disease.

Hence, all patients with medullary thyroid carcinoma should be screened for hyperparathyroidism and pheochromocytoma. If a pheochromocytoma or adrenal medullary hyperplasia is present, this should be operated upon *first* because it represents the greatest immediate risk to the patient. The family members of patients with medullary cancer of the thyroid should also be screened for medullary cancer of the thyroid by serum calcitonin and CEA determinations. When basal levels of serum calcitonin are borderline, provocative testing with calcium, pentagastrin, or both should be performed. Family members should be screened for the MEN II syndrome as well.

Medullary cancer spreads to lymph nodes of the neck and mediastinum and later disseminates to the lungs,

TABLE 54–2. DISEASES INCLUDED IN THE MEN II SYNDROMES

MEN IIA	MEN IIB
Medullary carcinoma	Medullary carcinoma
Pheochromocytoma	Pheochromocytoma
Hyperparathyroidism	Hyperparathyroidism (rarely)
	Ganglioneuroma phenotype

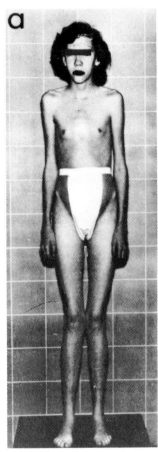
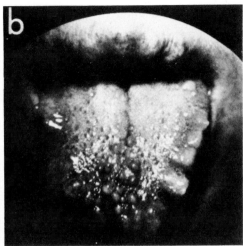

FIGURE 54–14. An 18-year-old girl, who demonstrates the appearance typically associated with multiple endocrine neoplasia, type IIB (MEN IIB), was found to have bilateral medullary carcinoma of the thyroid gland at operation. *A*, The Marfan-like body habitus and facial features typically present in patients with MEN IIB are clearly seen. *B*, Multiple neuromas of the tongue and lips are demonstrated. (Courtesy of Glen W. Sizemore.)

bone, liver, and elsewhere. The tumor is relatively radioresistant, does not take up radioiodine, and is not responsive to thyroid hormone suppression. Hence, an aggressive surgical approach is mandatory. The operation of choice for medullary cancer is total thyroidectomy coupled with an *aggressive* resection of central and mediastinal lymph nodes.[31] If lymph nodes of the lateral neck contain tumor, careful and extensive modified radical neck dissections are required. Reoperations for metastatic tumor rarely were rewarding until the work of Tisell and Jansson.[31] Their work demonstrated that some patients with elevated circulating calcitonin levels postoperatively could be rendered normocalcitoninemic by extensive, meticulous, *reoperative* neck dissections using magnification to remove all of the tiny lymph nodes. In other patients, CT and MR imaging have localized tumor recurrence. Furthermore, thallium or metaiodobenzylguanidine (MIBG) isotope scanning has sometimes localized metastatic deposits of tumor, which have later been successfully removed. Recently ⁹⁹ᵐTc-SestaMIBI scanning has been successful in some patients.

Cure is most likely in young patients who are found by calcitonin screening. Patients with MEN IIA syndrome have a better prognosis than those with sporadic tumor.[30] Patients with MEN IIB syndrome have very aggressive tumors and rarely survive to middle age. In some patients, postoperative radiation therapy has been used. Recent long-term studies of medullary cancer from the Mayo Clinic group[32] demonstrate that in patients without initial distant metastatic involvement and with complete resection of tumor, 20-year survival free of distant metastatic lesions was 81 per

cent. Overall 10- and 20-year survival rates were 63 per cent and 44 per cent, respectively. Thus, early diagnosis and thorough initial resection of tumor are very important. The treatment of pheochromocytomas and hyperparathyroidism is discussed elsewhere.

Finally, in recent years, the site of the gene for the MEN II syndromes has been localized to chromosome 10.[33] This is a potentially great advance, because in the future it may be possible to screen families by genetic methods to determine with certainty which patients are at risk of getting the disease.

Lymphoma of the Thyroid

The usefulness of thyroid resection in the management of primary thyroid lymphoma has been debated for years. In the past, some investigators claimed that resection, followed by radiation therapy, was more effective than radiation therapy alone. The tendency was to attempt resection whenever a tumor was small or confined to the thyroid and to resort to radiation therapy alone only when the lymphoma was of the inoperable extrathyroidal type. Today most investigators agree that no significant survival advantage is afforded by combining resection with radiation therapy to treat lymphoma, because most cases are advanced and extrathyroidal at the time of diagnosis.[34]

In the usual case today, lymphoma can be diagnosed by either an open biopsy or a core-needle biopsy. Some pathologists make the diagnosis by FNA with cytological testing, although most require more tissue for study. Following diagnosis, clinical staging is done to rule out local invasion, regional metastases, or distant metastases. Then radiation therapy is performed when disease is limited to the thyroid. Combination regimens of chemotherapy and radiation therapy are used frequently for local and regional spread, and chemotherapy is used in rare instances of distant metastases.

The overall five-year survival rates were 50 per cent and 54 per cent in several large series. Survival was not significantly different by histological type but related primarily to the stage of the disease at the time of diagnosis.

Extrathyroidal spread of tumor, either by direct soft tissue invasion or by regional lymph node involvement, has a distinctly adverse effect on prognosis. The five-year survival rate for patients in whom lymphoma had spread beyond the confines of the thyroid capsule was 38 per cent, in contrast to 86 per cent for those in whom the tumor was still confined to the thyroid.

OPERATIVE TECHNIQUE FOR THYROIDECTOMY

Under general endotracheal anesthesia, the patient is placed in a supine position with the neck extended. A low collar incision, approximately 9 cm long, is made and is carried down through the subcutaneous tissue and platysma muscle (Fig. 54–15). Superior and inferior subplatysmal flaps are developed, and the strap muscles are divided vertically in the midline and retracted laterally.

Lobectomy or Total Thyroidectomy

The thyroid lobe is bluntly dissected free from its investing fascia and rotated medially. The middle thyroid vein is ligated. The superior pole of the thyroid is dissected free, and care is taken to identify and preserve the external branch of the superior laryngeal nerve (see Fig. 54–7). The superior pole vessels are ligated adjacent to the thyroid lobe, rather than cephalic to it, to prevent damage to this

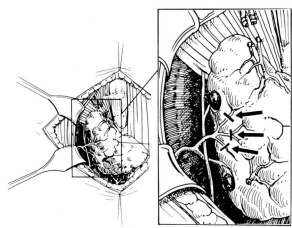

FIGURE 54–16. The thyroid lobe is retracted medially and, by careful blunt dissection, the recurrent laryngeal nerve, the inferior thyroid artery, and the parathyroid glands are identified. The inferior thyroid artery is not ligated laterally as a single trunk. Rather, each small branch is ligated and divided at a point distal to the parathyroid glands (*arrows*) to preserve their blood supply. Then the thyroid lobe can be removed from its tracheal attachments if a lobectomy is to be performed. (From Kaplan EL: Surgery of the thyroid glands. *In* DeGroot LS, Larsen PR, Refetoff S, Stanbury JB (eds): The Thyroid and Its Diseases. New York, John Wiley & Sons, 1984, p 851.)

nerve. The inferior thyroid artery and recurrent laryngeal nerve are identified. To preserve the blood supply to the parathyroid glands, the inferior thyroid artery should not be ligated laterally; rather, its branches should be ligated individually on the capsule of the lobe after they have supplied the parathyroid glands (Fig. 54–16). The parathyroid glands are identified, and an attempt is made to leave each with an adequate blood supply. Any parathyroid gland that appears to be devascularized can be minced and implanted into the sternocleidomastoid muscle after a frozen section biopsy confirms that it is in fact a parathyroid gland. Care is taken to identify the recurrent laryngeal nerve along its entire course if a total lobectomy is to be done. The nerve is gently unroofed from surrounding tissue, with care taken to avoid trauma to it. The nerve is in greatest danger near the junction of the trachea with the larynx, where it is adjacent to the thyroid gland. Once the nerve and parathyroid glands have been identified and preserved, the thyroid lobe can be removed from its tracheal attachments by dividing the ligament of Berry. The contralateral thyroid lobe is removed in a similar manner when a total thyroidectomy is performed. A near-total thyroidectomy means that a small amount of thyroid tissue is left on the contralateral side to protect the parathyroid glands and recurrent nerve. Careful hemostasis and visualization of all important anatomical structures are mandatory for success.

When closing, we do not tightly approximate the strap muscles in the midline but, rather, use only one or two sutures to prevent a hematoma in the deep space. Furthermore, we obtain better cosmesis by not approximating the platysmal muscle. The dermis is approximated by subcuticular interrupted 5-0 sutures, and the epithelial edges are approximated with sterile paper tapes (Steri-Strips). A small suction catheter is usually inserted through a stab wound and is generally removed within 24 hours.

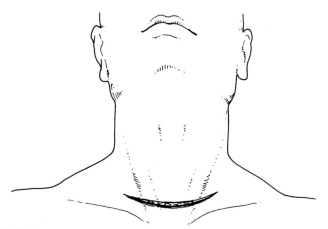

FIGURE 54–15. **Incision for thyroidectomy.** The neck is extended and a symmetrical, gently curved incision is made 1 to 2 cm above the clavicle.

Subtotal Thyroidectomy

Subtotal thyroidectomy is used to treat Graves' disease. About 2 g of thyroid tissue should be left on each side to attain satisfactory postoperative thyroid function without a high incidence of recurrent thyrotoxicosis. An alternative operation, which is equally good, is a lobectomy on one side and a subtotal lobectomy on the other side. Once more, the parathyroid glands and recurrent nerves should be identified and preserved. Great care should be taken not to damage the recurrent laryngeal nerve when cutting across or suturing the thyroid lobe.

POSTOPERATIVE COMPLICATIONS

Wound Hemorrhage

Wound hemorrhage with hematoma is an uncommon complication, reported in 0.3 to 1.0 per cent of patients in most large series. However, it is a well-recognized and potentially lethal complication. A small hematoma deep to the strap muscles can compress the trachea and cause respiratory distress. A small suction drain placed in the wound is not adequate for decompression if bleeding occurs from an arterial vessel. Swelling of the neck and bulging of the wound can be quickly followed by respiratory impairment. Treatment consists of immediately opening the wound and evacuating the clot, even at the bedside. Pressure should be applied with a sponge and the patient returned to the operating room. Later, the bleeding vessel can be ligated in a careful and more leisurely manner under optimal conditions with good lighting in the operating room. The urgency of treating this condition as soon as it occurs cannot be overemphasized.

Injury to the Recurrent Laryngeal Nerve

Injuries to the recurrent laryngeal nerve occur in 1 to 2 per cent of thyroid operations, especially those performed for malignant disease. The injuries can be unilateral or bilateral, temporary or permanent, and can be deliberate or accidental. Loss of function can be caused by transection, ligation, traction, or handling of the nerve. Tumor invasion can also involve the nerve. Occasionally, vocal cord impairment occurs as a result of pressure from an endotracheal tube. In *unilateral* recurrent nerve injuries, the voice becomes husky because the vocal cords do not approximate one another. Usually, vocal cord function returns within several months but certainly within six to nine months if it is to return. If no function returns by that time, the voice can be improved by injection of the paralyzed vocal cord with collagen or Teflon, which usually helps by bringing it to the midline.

Bilateral recurrent laryngeal nerve damage is much more serious because both vocal cords may assume a median or paramedian position, resulting in airway obstruction and difficulty with respiratory toilet. Often, tracheostomy is required. In the author's experience, permanent injuries to the recurrent laryngeal nerve are best avoided by identifying and carefully tracing the path of the nerve. Accidental transection occurs most often at the level of the upper two tracheal rings, where the nerve closely approximates the thyroid lobe in the area of Berry's ligament. If recognized, the transected nerve should be reapproximated by microsurgical techniques. A number of procedures to reinnervate the laryngeal muscles have been attempted with variable success.

Injury to the *external branch of the superior laryngeal nerve* may occur when the upper pole vessels are divided (see Fig. 54–7) if the nerve is not visualized.[8] This injury results in an inability to forcefully project one's voice or to sing high notes. Often, this disability improves during the first three months after surgery.

Hypoparathyroidism[9]

The incidence of hypoparathyroidism has been reported to be as high as 20 per cent when a total thyroidectomy and radical neck dissection are performed and as low as 0.9 per cent for subtotal thyroidectomy. Postoperative hypoparathyroidism is rarely the result of inadvertent removal of all parathyroid glands but, more commonly, is due to disruption of their blood supply. Devascularization can be minimized during thyroid lobectomy by carefully ligating the branches of the inferior thyroid artery on the thyroid capsule distal to their supply of the parathyroid glands (Fig. 54–16) and by treating the parathyroids with great care. If a parathyroid gland is recognized to be nonviable during operation, after identification by frozen section, it can be autotransplanted at that time. The gland is minced into 1- to 2-mm cubes and placed into pockets in the sternocleidomastoid muscle.

Postoperative hypoparathyroidism results in hypocalcemia and hyperphosphatemia and is manifested by circumoral numbness, tingling, and intense anxiety during the first few days after operation. Chvostek's sign appears early, and carpopedal spasm can occur. Symptoms develop in most patients when the serum calcium level is between 7.5 and 8 mg/dl.

Routinely, we measure the serum calcium level every 12 hours for the first few days. Patients with symptomatic hypocalcemia may be given 1 g (10 ml) of 10 per cent calcium gluconate intravenously over several minutes, and then several grams of this calcium solution should be placed in each 500-ml intravenous bottle to run continuously during each eight-hour period. If necessary, several more grams can be added to each bottle. Oral calcium, usually as calcium carbonate (3 to 4 g in divided doses), should be started. On this treatment regimen, most patients become asymptomatic, and therapy usually can be stopped within a few days if *transient* hypoparathyroidism is present.

The management of more persistent severe hypocalcemia requires the addition of a vitamin D preparation to facilitate absorption of oral calcium. We prefer the use of 1,25-dihydroxyvitamin D (Rocaltrol) because this is the active metabolite of vitamin D and has the most rapid action. Rocaltrol (0.5 μg) with oral calcium carbonate therapy are given four times daily for the first several days. Then this priming dose of vitamin D is reduced. The usual maintenance dose for most patients with permanent hypoparathyroidism is Rocaltrol (0.25 to 0.5 μg daily) along with calcium carbonate (500 mg Ca^{2+} once or twice daily). The serum calcium levels must be monitored carefully and the doses of the medications adjusted promptly to prevent hypercalcemia as well as hypocalcemia. Finally, the serum parathyroid hormone level should be analyzed periodically to determine whether permanent hypoparathyroidism is truly present, because we and others have seen cases of postoperative tetany, perhaps due to "bone hunger," which later resolved completely. Remember that in bone hunger, both the serum calcium and phosphorus values are low.

ACKNOWLEDGMENT: We thank Kim Maddy and Noreen Fulton for their assistance.

REFERENCES

1. Halsted WS: The operative story of goitre. Johns Hopkins Hosp Rep 19:71, 1920.
2. Thompson NW: The history of hyperparathyroidism. Acta Chir Scand 156:5–21, 1990.
3. Kocher T: Uber Kropfextirpation und ihre Folgen. Archiv fur klinische Chirurgie 29:254, 1883.
4. Kaplan EL, Kadowaki MH, Schark C: Routine exposure of the recurrent laryngeal nerve is important during thyroidectomy. *In* Simmons RL, Udekwu AO (eds): Debates in Clinical Surgery, vol 1. Chicago, Year Book Medical Publishers, 1990, pp 191–206.
5. Henry JF, Audriffe J, Denizot A, et al: The non-recurrent inferior laryngeal nerve: Review of 33 cases including 2 on the left side. Surgery 104:977–984, 1988.
6. Thompson NW, Demers M: Exposure is not necessary to avoid the recurrent laryngeal nerve during thyroid operations. *In* Simmons RL, Udekwu AO (eds): Debates in Clinical Surgery, vol 1. Chicago, Year Book Medical Publishers, 1990, pp 207–219.
7. Moosman DA, DeWeese JS: The external laryngeal nerve as related to thyroidectomy. Surg Gynecol Obstet 127:1011, 1968.
8. Lennquist S, Cahlin C, Smeds S: The superior laryngeal nerve in thyroid surgery. Surgery 102:999, 1987.
9. Kaplan EL, Sugimoto J, Yang H, Fredland A: Postoperative hypoparathyroidism: Diagnosis and management. *In* Kaplan EL (ed): Surgery of the Thyroid and Parathyroid Glands. New York, Churchill Livingstone, 1983, pp 262–274.
10. Gilmour JR: The embryology of the parathyroid glands, the thymus and certain associated rudiments. J Pathol 45:507, 1937.
11. Taylor S: Surgery of the thyroid gland. *In* DeGroot LJ, Stanbury JB: The Thyroid and Its Diseases (ed 4). New York, John Wiley & Sons, 1975, pp 776–779.
12. DeGroot LJ: Clinical features and management of radiation-associated thyroid carcinoma. *In* Kaplan EL (ed): Surgery of the Thyroid and Parathyroid Glands. Edinburgh, Churchill Livingstone, 1983, p 940.
13. Kaplan EL: An operative approach to the irradiated thyroid gland with possible carcinoma: Criteria technique and results. *In* DeGroot LJ, Frohman LA, Kaplan EL, Refetoff S (eds): Radiation Associated Carcinoma of the Thyroid. New York, Grune and Stratton, 1977, p 371.
14. Naunheim KS, Kaplan EL, Straus FH II, et al: High dose external radiation to the neck and subsequent thyroid carcinoma. *In* Kaplan EL (ed): Surgery of the Thyroid and Parathyroid Glands. New York, Churchill Livingstone, 1983, pp 51–62.
15. Backdahl M, Wallin G, Lowhagen T, et al: Fine needle biopsy cytology and DNA analysis. Surg Clin North Am 67:197, 1987.
16. Grant CS, van Heerden JA, Goellner JR: New diagnostic techniques in endocrine surgery. Prob Gen Surg 1:141–153, 1984.
17. Becker C: Hypothyroidism and atherosclerotic heart disease: Pathogenesis, medical management, and the role of coronary artery bypass surgery. Endocr Rev 6:432, 1985.
18. Klementschitsch P, Shen K-L, Kaplan EL: Reemergence of thyroidectomy as treatment for Graves' disease. Surg Clin North Am 59:35, 1979.
19. Lennquist S, Jortso E, Anderberg B, Smeds S: Beta-blockers compared with antithyroid drugs as preoperative treatment of hyperthyroidism: Drug tolerance, complications and postoperative thyroid function. Surgery 98:1141, 1985.
20. Sridama V, Reilly M, Kaplan EL, et al: Long term follow-up study of compensated low dose ^{131}I therapy for Graves' disease. N Engl J Med 311:426, 1984.
21. Clark OH: Total thyroidectomy: The treatment of choice for patients with differentiated thyroid cancer. Ann Surg 196:361–370, 1982.
22. Attie JN: Modified neck dissection in treatment of thyroid cancer: A safe procedure. Eur J Cancer Clin Oncol 2:315–324, 1988.
23. Beierwaltes WH: Treatment of metastatic thyroid cancer with radioiodine and external radiation therapy. *In* Kaplan EL (ed): Surgery of the Thyroid and Parathyroid Glands, Clinical Surgery International, vol 4. Edinburgh, Churchill Livingstone, 1983, p 103.
24. Hay ID, Grant CS, Taylor WF, et al: Ipsilateral lobectomy versus bilateral lobar resection in papillary thyroid carcinoma: A retrospective analysis of surgical outcome using a novel prognostic scoring system. Surgery 102:1088, 1988.
25. Cady B, Rossi R: An expanded view of risk-group definition in differentiated thyroid carcinoma. Surgery 104:947, 1988.
26. Arganini M, Behar R, Wu FL, et al: Hürthle cell tumors: A twenty-five year experience. Surgery 100:1108, 1986.
27. Schark C, Fulton N, Yashiro T, et al: The value of measurement of *ras* oncogenes and nuclear DNA analysis in the diagnosis of Hürthle cell tumors of the thyroid. World J Surg 16:745–752, 1992.
28. Hill SC Jr: Chemotherapy of thyroid cancer. *In* Kaplan EL (ed): Surgery of the Thyroid and Parathyroid Glands, Clinical Surgery International, vol 4. Edinburgh, Churchill Livingstone, 1983, p 103.
29. Kim JH, Leeper RD: Treatment of anaplastic and spindle cell carcinoma of the thyroid with combination Adriamycin and radiation therapy. Cancer 52:954, 1983.
30. Sizemore GW, van Heerden JA, Carney JA: Medullary carcinoma of the thyroid gland and the multiple endocrine neoplasia type 2 syndrome. *In* Kaplan EL (ed): Surgery of the Thyroid and Parathyroid Glands, Clinical Surgery International, vol 4. Edinburgh, Churchill Livingstone, 1983, p 75.
31. Tisell LE, Jansson S: Recent results of reoperative surgery in medullary carcinoma of the thyroid. Wien Klin Wochenschr 100:347–348, 1988.
32. Gharib H, McConahey WM, Tiego RD, et al: Medullary thyroid carcinoma: Clinicopathologic features and long-term follow-up of 65 patients treated during 1946 through 1970. Mayo Clin Proc 67:934–940, 1992.
33. Lairmore TC, Howe JR, Korte JA, et al: Familial medullary thyroid carcinoma and multiple endocrine neoplasia type 2B map to the same region of chromosome 10 as multiple endocrine neoplasia type 2A. Genomics 9:181–192, 1991.
34. Rasbach DA, Mondschein MS, Harris NL, et al: Malignant lymphoma of the thyroid gland: A clinical and pathological study of twenty cases. Surgery 98:1166, 1985.

Index

Note: Page numbers in *italics* refer to illustrations; page numbers followed by t refer to tables.

Choriocarcinoma, hyperthyroidism in, 676–677, 2780–2781
ovarian, 2121
testicular, 2442, *2443*, 2444
Chorion frondosum, 2173, *2173, 2175*
Chorion laeve, endocrine activity of, 2196
structure of, *2173*, 2175, *2175*
Chorionic corticotropin, human, synthesis of, 2242
Chorionic gonadotropin, human, 2177t, *2178*, 2178–2182
actions of, 230, 803, 2181, 2242
alpha-subunit of, *2178–2179*, 2178–2180
as tumor marker, 2181
clearance of, 2181
antibodies to, 2182
as tumor marker, 2182, 2444, 2777–2780
assays for, 237, 2181–2182, 2182t
beta-core fragment of, 230–231
beta-subunit of, *2178–2179*, 2178–2180
clearance of, 2181
clearance of, 2180–2181
clinical uses of, 231
distribution of, 2778–2779
excess of, gynecomastia in, 2479
hypogonadism in, 2383
genes of, 231, *2178*, 2178–2179
glycosylation of, 2178, *2179*
half-life of, 233
hyperandrogenism related to, 2103
in cryptorchidism, 2389–2390, 2390t
in fetus, 244–245, 2179
in follicular stimulation, for oocyte retrieval, 2038
in immunoregulation, 2967t, 2978
in luteoma stimulation, 2125
in mammary growth, 2226
in nonpregnant subjects, 2182
in obesity treatment, 2654
in ovarian tumor stimulation, 2120–2121
in ovulation induction, 2068–2070, *2069–2070*, 2082, 2082t
in hyperandrogenism, 2106
in pituitary function testing, 491
in testosterone synthesis regulation, 2316
in thyroid stimulation, 548, 611, *612*, 677, 2780–2781
in trophoblastic disease, 2182, 2183t
interference of, with thyroid-stimulating hormone assay, 2294
levels of, vs. fetal steroid levels, 1895–1896
vs. gestational age, 803, *804*, 2179, 2179–2180
metabolism of, 230–231, 2180–2181
oligosaccharides of, 2178–2179, *2179*
receptor for, 231, 237–238
cross-reactivity of, 58, 59t
secretion of, 236, *2179*, 2179–2180
after menopause, 2129, *2130*
from tumors, 1968, 2121, 2123, 2777–2780
in paraneoplastic syndromes, 2757t
stimulation test with, in delayed puberty evaluation, 1964
in sexual differentiation disorders, 1927
structure of, 231–232, *232–234*, 2178–2179, *2178–2179*
subunits of, 2178–2179, *2178–2179*
in tumors, 2780
synthesis of, in placenta, 2242
regulation of, 2180
therapy with, in hypogonadotropic hypogonadism, 2384–2386, *2385–2386*
thyromimetic properties of, 803, *804–805*

Chorionic gonadotropin (*Continued*)
vs. molar thyroid-stimulating hormone, 677
Chorionic plate, 2173, *2175*
Chorionic proopiomelanocortin peptides, *2178*, 2189, *2189*
Chorionic somatomammotropin (placental lactogen), human, 369–370, 370t, 2183–2186, 2289–2290, *2290*
actions of, 2184–2186, *2185*, 2242
as fetal growth hormone, 2186
assays for, 2187
big, 2777
deficiency of, 2186
gene of, 2183, *2184*
evolution of, 303, *304*, 368–369, *369*
mutations of, 2186
in carbohydrate metabolism, 2185–2186
in lactation, 2229–2230
in lipid metabolism, 2185
in mammary gland function, 2186
in mammary gland growth, 2226
insulin response to, 1355
secretion of, 2183–2184
ectopic, 2776–2777
in paraneoplastic syndromes, 2757t
structure of, 303, 2183, *2185*
synthesis of, 2183–2184, 2242
Choristoma, pituitary, 462
Chromaffin cells, 1860–1861, *1860–1861*
tumors of. See also *Pheochromocytoma.*
extra-adrenal, 1853
Chromaffin reaction, in pheochromocytoma, 1859
Chromatin, structure of, 7
nuclear receptors and, 108, *109*
thyroid hormone receptor association with, 586
Chromogens, Porter-Silber, measurement of, 1735, *1735–1736*
Chromogranin A, 1311–1312
in carcinoid tumor, 2804, 2807
in parathyroid hormone secretion regulation, 940
in pheochromocytoma, 1861, 1867
measurement of, 1867
physiology of, 2878
Chromogranin B, physiology of, 2878
Chromophobe adenoma, 166, *166*
Chromosomal analysis, in sexual differentiation disorders, 1926
Chromosomal walking, in mutation detection, 133
Chvostek's sign, in hypocalcemia, 1124
Chylomicron(s), metabolism of, 2732, *2733*
Chylomicronemia syndrome, 2737–2739, *2738*
Chymotrypsin, in thyroglobulin degradation, 534
Ciliary neurotrophic factor, *2611*, 2611–2612
Cimetidine, antiandrogen activity of, 2343, 2397
in hyperprolactinemia diagnosis, 398
in prolactin secretion, 186
in Zollinger-Ellison syndrome, 2817
structure of, *2343*
testicular function and, 2397
Circadian rhythms, 2488–2512
abnormal, 2505–2510, *2506, 2509–2510*
affective disorders and, 2508, 2510, *2510*
aging effects on, 2499, *2500*, 2501
amplitude of, 2489–2490, *2490*
blindness and, 2508
clinical implications of, 2510–2512, *2511*
definition of, 2488–2489
endogenous nature of, 2488–2489

Circadian rhythms (*Continued*)
entrainment of, *2490–2491*, 2490–2492, 2495, 2497
functional significance of, 2492
generation of, 2495, 2497
genetic basis for, 2497–2498, *2498*
in free-running conditions, 2489, *2489*, 2501, 2501–2502
in seasonal rhythm timing, 2518–2519
jet lag and, 439–440, 2505–2507, *2506*
manipulation of, 439–441, *440*
measurement of, methods for, 2421, 2520, *2521*
of ACTH secretion, 183, 365
of aldosterone secretion, in aldosteronism, 1783, *1784*
of androstenedione secretion, 2525, *2526*
of body temperature, *2502*, 2502–2503
of cortisol secretion, 2487–2488, *2488*, 2498, *2499*, 2503, 2525–2526, *2526–2527*
age-related changes in, *2500*
of dehydroepiandrosterone secretion, 2525, *2526*
of follicle-stimulating hormone secretion, 2530–2532
of growth hormone secretion, 306, *306*, 495, 2487–2488, *2488*, 2502–2504, 2527–2529, *2528*
age-related changes in, *2500*
of hormone secretion, 4
of hydroxyandrostenedione secretion, 2525, *2526*
of insulin secretion, 1360–1361, 2533–2536, *2534–2535*
of luteinizing hormone secretion, 2530–2532
of melatonin secretion, 433–437, *434, 436*, 2503, 2505, 2536–2538
age-related changes in, *2500*
of prolactin secretion, 378, 2487–2488, *2488*, 2529–2530
age-related changes in, *2500*
of testosterone secretion, 2510, *2511*, 2531–2532
of thyroid-stimulating hormone, *2500*, 2503
of thyroid-stimulating hormone secretion, 211, *2504*, 2504, 2532–2533, *2533*
of thyrotropin-releasing hormone secretion, 197, 2487–2488, *2488*
of thyroxine secretion, 2533
of triiodothyronine secretion, 2533, *2533*
ontogeny of, 2498–2501, *2500*
period of, 2489, *2490*
phase of, 2489–2490, *2490*
shifting of, *2504*, 2504–2505
quantification of, procedures for, 2421
seasonal rhythm interactions with, 2493
shift work and, 2507–2508
sleep and, *2502–2503*, 2502–2504, 2508, 2516
suprachiasmatic nucleus in, 2493–2497, *2496*
synchronization of, *2490–2491*, 2490–2492, *2504*, 2504–2505
transmeridian flights and, 439–440, 2505–2507, *2506*
ultradian rhythm interactions with, 2492–2493
vs. diurnal rhythms, 2489
Circannual rhythms, 4, 2518
Circatrigantan rhythms, 4
Circhoral rhythms, 4, 2512
Circulating growth factor, in multiple endocrine neoplasia, 2826–2827
Cirrhosis, edema in, 1704
insulin-like growth factor levels in, 315
thyroid hormone levels in, 671

β-Endorphin *(Continued)*
  synthesis of, 13, *13, 359,* 359–360
    in placenta, 2242
Endorphin(s), in immunoregulation, 2967t,
    2972
  measurement of, in pheochromocytoma,
    1867
  neuronal pathways for, *182*
  secretion of, in paraneoplastic syndromes,
    2757t
  synthesis of, 2755, *2755*
Endosomes, in insulin degradation, 1383
  in receptor-mediated endocytosis, 32–33, *33*
  in thyroglobulin transport, *509,* 513, 533
Endostyle, in thyroid development, 518
Endothelial growth factor, 2592
Endothelins, 2907–2912
  actions of, 2911–2912
    intracellular, 2909–2910, *2910*
  distribution of, 2909
  gene of, 2909
  in aldosterone secretion, 1673
  in parturition, 2214
  isoforms of, *2908,* 2908–2909
  levels of, 2910–2911
  metabolism of, 2910
  physiology of, 2882
  precursors of, *2908,* 2908–2909
  receptors for, 2909–2910
  secretion of, 2909
    in postural change, 2935
    inhibition of, 2902
  structure of, *2908,* 2908–2909
  synthesis of, *2908,* 2908–2909, *2910*
Endothelium-derived relaxing factor, 2907,
    2909–2910, *2910*
  osteoclast activity and, 982, *982*
Endotoxemia, hypothalamic-pituitary-adrenal
    axis response in, *345*
Endotoxin. See *Lipopolysaccharide.*
End-stage renal disease, in diabetes mellitus,
    1574
  prevalence of, 1570
  treatment of, 1580–1586, *1580–1586,*
    1581t–1583t
  in diabetic nephropathy, 1574
Endurance training, adaptation to, *2698,* 2698–
    2699
Energy/fuel. See also *Carbohydrates; Glucose;
    Lipid(s); Protein.*
  distribution of, 1390–1391
  expenditure of, 1397, 1397t
    components of, *2636*
    in hypothyroidism, 760
    in obesity, 2637
    in starvation, 2667
    individual variation in, 2648
    measurement of, 2634–2637, *2636*
  intake of, determination of, 2637
  metabolism of, 1389–1390, 1390t
  requirements of, in nutritional therapy plan-
    ning, *2672,* 2672–2673, 2673t
    in weight loss diet, 2649, 2649t
  sources of, 1389–1390, 1390t
  storage of, 1389–1390
    in adipose tissue, 2631, *2632*
  transport of, placental, 2258–2261, *2259*
Engorgement, breast, in lactation, 2234
Enhancer(s), in gene expression, 8, 8–9, *10*
Enhancer-binding proteins, as transcription
    factors, 126, *126*
Enkephalin(s), in ACTH regulation, 364
  in gonadotropin-releasing hormone secre-
    tion, 2000

Enkephalin(s) *(Continued)*
  in immunoregulation, 2967t, 2972
  in reproductive behavior, 453–455, *455*
  neuronal pathways for, *182*
  physiology of, 2880–2881
  secretion of, ectopic, 2775
    in obesity, 2642
    in paraneoplastic syndromes, 2757t
  vs. endorphins, 362
Enkephalinase, in atrial natriuretic peptide
    metabolism, 2900
Enteral nutrition, 2675–2676
  complications of, 2673–2674
Enteric hyperoxaluria, 1187
Enteritis, regional, growth attenuation in, 2578,
    2578
Enterochromaffin cells, in carcinoid tumor,
    2804
Enterogastrone, 2873
Enteroglucagon, physiology of, 2875
Enteroglucagonoma, 2886
Enteroinsular axis, 1278, 1344
Enteropathy, gluten (celiac disease),
    gastrointestinal hormone action in, 2883
Enterostatin, in appetite control, 2632–2633
Entrainment, of circadian rhythms, *2490–2491,*
    2490–2492, 2495, 2497
Entrapment neuropathy, in diabetes mellitus,
    1555
Environmental factors, in diabetes mellitus,
    1426t, 1426–1427
  in polyglandular failure syndromes, 3018
  in spermatogenesis, 2409
Enzyme(s). See also specific enzyme.
  genes of, mutations in, detection of, 134–135
    diseases caused by, 130t, 139–140
  inhibitors of, in obesity treatment, 2654
  placental, 2197
Enzyme-linked immunosorbent assay, for
    thyroid hormones, 623
Enzyme-multiplied immunoassay technique, for
    thyroid hormones, 623
Eosinophil granule major basic protein,
    placental, 2197t
Eosinophilic granuloma, delayed puberty in,
    1961
  of hypothalamus, 486
Ependymal zone, of median eminence, 153
Ependymoma, precocious puberty in, 1969
Ephedrine, in obesity, 2654
Epidermal growth factor, 2600–2603
  actions of, 2602–2603
    intra-ovarian, 2024
  gene of, 2601, *2601*
  heparin-binding, 2600, *2601*
  in adrenal androgen control, 1841
  in benign prostatic hyperplasia, 2466t, 2466–
    2467, *2467*
  in fetus, 2251
  in lactation, 2230
  in mammary growth, 2226
  in ovary, 2024
  in parathyroid hormone-related protein/pep-
    tide gene expression, 970
  in placental growth, 2176
  in prolactin gene regulation, 375
  in Sertoli cells, 2325
  in steroid synthesis, 2095
  in thyroid hormone mediation, 787
  in thyroid regulation, 543t, 544
    of cell growth and differentiation, *553,*
    553–554, *555*
  nomenclature of, 2600
  placental transport of, 2240, 2240t

Epidermal growth factor *(Continued)*
  precursors of, 2601, *2601*
  receptor for, 2602
    activation of, 41–42
    in fetus, 2251
    oncogenes and, 59, 59t
    serine phosphorylation of, 45
    structure of, 28, *28, 2597*
  secretion of, ectopic, 2792
  structure of, 2600–2601, *2601*
Epidermoid cyst, parasellar, 462, 482, *485*
Epididymis, examination of, 2410, *2410*
  obstruction of, infertility in, 2418–2419
  surgery on, 2419
Epinephrine, actions of, 1854, 1858, 1859t
  drug effects on, 180t
    on adrenergic receptors, 1856t
  deficiency of, in diabetes mellitus, 1554
  distribution of, 157
  in ACTH regulation, 363
  in aging, 2714
  in corticotropin-releasing hormone regula-
    tion, 343
  in exercise, *2695,* 2698
  in fetus, 2248, *2248,* 2267
  in gluconeogenesis, 2267
  in glucose metabolism, 1394, 1409, 1607–
    1608, *1608*
  in glycogen metabolism, 47
  in gonadotropin secretion, 1993, *1994*
  in gonadotropin-releasing hormone secre-
    tion, *1999,* 1999–2000
  in hypoglycemia, 1607–1608, *1608*
  in ketoacidosis, 1511, 1511t
  in lipolysis, 2667
  in parathyroid hormone secretion, 940
  in prolactin secretion, 185
  insulin response to, 1356
  localization of, 157
  measurement of, in plasma, 1866–1867
    in urine, 1865–1866, 1866t
  placental transport of, 2240–2241
  secretion of, from pheochromocytoma, 1853,
    2834, *2835*
    thyroid hormone effects on, *194*
  structure of, *1855*
  synthesis of, *179,* 1854, *1855*
Epiphysis, growth abnormalities of, in
    hypothyroidism, 794
Epiphysis cerebri. See *Pineal gland.*
Epithelial cells, thyroid, abnormal replication
    of, 773
Epostane, in progesterone synthesis inhibition,
    2210
Equilibrium dialysis, isotopic, in free thyroid
    hormone measurement, 626–627
Ergocalciferol. See *Vitamin D_2.*
Ergolines. See also *Bromocriptine.*
  in acromegaly, 324–325, *325*
Ergosterol. See *Provitamin D_2* (ergosterol).
Ergot derivatives, in orthostatic hypotension,
    2940
  in prolactinoma, 189
ERK. See *Mitogen-activated protein kinase.*
Erythema, in glucagonoma, 2885–2886
Erythema gyratum repens, as paraneoplastic
    syndrome, 2761
Erythroblastosis fetalis, growth disorders in,
    2567
  hypoglycemia in, 2273
Erythrocytes, glucose levels in, 1390–1391
  glucose metabolism in, 1395–1396, 1396t
  Graves' disease effects on, 688

Gastrin-releasing peptide. See *Bombesin (gastrin-releasing peptide)*.
Gastro-entero-pancreatic system, development of, 1278, 1280
Gastrointestinal tract, adrenergic receptors in, 1857t
　bleeding from, somatostatin therapy in, 274
　bypass procedures on, in obesity, 2655–2657, *2656*
　corticotropin-releasing hormone in, 349, 351
　disorders of, in diabetes mellitus, 1549–1550
　octreotide in, 275
　fistula of, nutrition support in, 2675
　Graves' disease effects on, 688
　hormones of. See also specific hormones, e.g., *Gastrin;* specific tumor, e.g., *Glucagonoma.*
　　cells producing, *2870,* 2870–2871
　　historical aspects of, 2870
　　in colon carcinoma, 2884
　　in gastric pathology, 2882–2883
　　in inflammatory diarrhea, 2884
　　in intestinal surgery, 2883
　　in irritable bowel syndrome, 2884
　　in malabsorption, 2883
　　in neural disorders, 2883–2884
　　tumors secreting, 2884–2886, 2885t
　hyperparathyroidism effects on, 1052–1053
　hypocalcemia effects on, 1124
　hypothyroidism effects on, 760
　manipulation of, vasopressin secretion in, 410–411
　pheochromocytoma effects on, 1863
　prolactin in, osmoregulatory action of, 387
　protection of, in nutrition support, 2675
　somatostatin effects on, 268, 268t, 273–274
　somatostatin in, 270t, 271
　somatostatinoma of, 273
Gastroparesis, in diabetes mellitus, 1549, 1559–1560
Gemfibrozil, in dyslipoproteinemia, 2749t–2750t
Gender, aldosteronism and, 1779
　assignment of, in adrenal hyperplasia, 1828–1829
　diabetes mellitus incidence and, 1426
　diabetic retinopathy and, 1526
　differentiation of. See *Sexual differentiation.*
　growth hormone-releasing hormone secretion and, 283
　reassignment of, in transsexualism, 1981
Gender dysphoria, 1981
Gender identity, 1981
Gender role, 1981
Gene(s). See also under specific hormone or protein.
　alternate splicing in, 121
　cloning of, 121–123, *122–123*
　deletions from, identification of, 131t, 131–135, *132–135,* 134t
　eukaryotic vs. prokaryotic, 7–8, *7–8*
　expression of, analysis of, 123–124, *124,* 124t
　　enhancers in, 8, 8–9, *10*
　　for housekeeping proteins, 6
　　mRNA maturation in, 10–11, *10–11*
　　mRNA translation in, 11–12, *12*
　　pathways for, 6–7, *7*
　　post-translational events in, 12–13, *13*
　　promoters in, 8, *8*
　　protein precursor processing in, 12–13, *13*
　　regulation of, *10–14,* 10–15
　　　receptors in, *49,* 49–50
　　　sites for, *14,* 15
　　　structural aspects of, *8–9,* 8–10

Gene(s) *(Continued)*
　thyroid hormone receptors in, *585–588,* 585–589, 587t
　tissue-specific, 6
　transcription in. See *Gene(s), transcription of.*
　transient, 125, *125*
　in sexual differentiation, 1881–1886, *1883–1886,* 1891, *1891*
　knockout of, in animals, 129, *129*
　LOD score of, 2821
　mapping of, 2819
　mutation of. See *Mutation.*
　post-transcriptional regulation of, analysis of, 124–125
　recombinant, 8
　recombination factor of, 2821
　regulatory (flanking) region of, *7–8,* 8–10
　reporter, 8, 125, *125*
　structural region of, *7–8,* 8
　structure of, *7–9,* 7–10, 121
　　analysis of, molecular biology techniques in, 119–123, *120–123*
　thrifty, in diabetes mellitus, 1570
　transcription of, *120,* 120–121. See also *Transcription factors.*
　　analysis of, 124–125, *124–125*
　　glucocorticoid receptor, 1657, *1657, 1660,* 1660–1663
　　hormone response elements in, 103–104
　　modification after, in receptors, 111
　　promoters for, 107, *107*
　　protein kinase A in, 87–89, *88*
　　regulation of, 10, *10,* 13–14, *14*
　　structural aspects of, 8–9, *8–9*
　transfection of, 125, *125*
　transfer of, 128–129, *129*
　translation of, 6, *7,* 120, *120*
　tumor suppressor (antioncogenes), 2769
　　in multiple endocrine neoplasia, 141, 2819–2820, *2819–2920*
　　in parathyroid adenoma, 1046, *1046*
　　loss of, thyroid carcinoma in, 842
　tumor-promoting. See *Oncogenes.*
Genetic counseling, in sexual differentiation disorders, 1930, 1930t
Genetic factors, in diabetic retinopathy, 1526
　in glucocorticoid resistance, 1771
　in obesity, 2646t, 2646–2647
　in polyglandular failure syndromes, 3018
　in puberty timing, 1956
　in sexual differentiation, 1881–1886, *1883–1886,* 1891, *1891*
Geniculohypothalamic tract, in circadian rhythm synchronization, 2494
Genitalia, ambiguous, degenerative renal disease with, 1922
　enzyme defects in, 130t, 140
　gender assignment in, 1828–1829
　in androgen insensitivity/resistance, 1919–1921, 1979
　in dysgenetic male pseudohermaphroditism, 1904–1905
　in hermaphroditism, 1910–1911
　in hyperandrogenism, 1815–1816, *1816*
　in mixed gonadal dysgenesis, 1903–1904, *1904*
　in pregnenolone synthesis impairment, 1913
　in 5α-reductase deficiency, 1979–1980, 2342
　multiple congenital anomalies with, 1922–1923, 1923t
　development of, 1938, 1938t
　differentiation of. See *Sexual differentiation.*

Genitalia *(Continued)*
　17α-hydroxylase/17,20 lyase deficiency effects on, 1825
　3β-hydroxysteroid dehydrogenase deficiency effects on, 1823–1824
　hyperandrogenism effects on, 1815–1816, *1816–1817*
Genitourinary tract, adrenergic receptors in, 1857t
　thyrotropin-releasing hormone in, 198–199
Germ cell(s), aplasia of, 2391, *2391*
　in embryo, 1888, *1889*
　Sertoli cell interactions with, 2322–2324
Germ cell tumors, hypothalamic, 463
　ovarian, gonadoblastoma as, 2119–2120
　mixed primitive, 2121
　parasellar, imaging of, 482, *484*
　testicular, 2442–2444, *2443*
Germinoma, ovarian, gonadoblastoma as, 2120
Gestation. See also *Pregnancy.*
　melatonin effects on, 435
Gestational diabetes. See *Diabetes mellitus, gestational.*
Gestational trophoblastic disease. See *Trophoblastic disease.*
Gestodene, in oral contraceptives, 2144–2145, *2145*
GH. See *Growth hormone.*
GHF-1. See *Pit-1 gene and protein.*
GHRH. See *Growth hormone-releasing hormone.*
GH-RIH (growth hormone release-inhibiting hormone). See *Somatostatin.*
Giant cell(s), in subacute thyroiditis, *743,* 743–744
Giant cell tumors, in Paget's disease, 1265–1266
　osteomalacia with, 1218, *1218*
GIFT (gamete intrafallopian transfer), 2091
Gigantism, *320,* 320–322, 2580
　cerebral, 321, 2567
　hypertrophic neuropathy in, 323
　in pituitary adenoma, 166, 169
　infant, 2567
　mitochondrial, in acidophil stem-cell adenoma, 169, *170*
　treatment of, 324
Glaucoma, in diabetes mellitus, 1530
Glial cell growth factors, 2602
Glicentin, 1315–1316, *1316, 1338,* 1338–1339
　in glucagonoma, 1349, *1349*
　synthesis of, *2874, 2875*
Glioma, hypothalamic, imaging of, 479, *482*
　optic, 463
　optic chiasmal, imaging of, 479, 482, *483*
Glipizide, pharmacology of, 1493–1494, 1494t
　structure of, *1493*
Globus hystericus, vs. subacute thyroiditis, 746
Glomerular filtration rate, atrial natriuretic peptide effects on, 2901
　in diabetic nephropathy, *1571–1572,* 1571–1576
　in pregnancy, 2287
　sodium excretion and, 1686–1687, *1687,* 1687t
Glomerulosclerosis, in diabetic nephropathy, 1573–1574
Glomerulotropic factor, in aldosterone secretion regulation, 1697
Glomerulotubular balance, sodium excretion and, 1686–1687, *1687,* 1687t
Glomerulus, lesions of, in diabetic nephropathy, *1572,* 1572–1573, *1575,* 1575–1576
GLP fragments, of proglucagon, 1316, *1316,* 1337–1338, *1338*

Growth hormone-releasing hormone *(Continued)*
  secretion of, age-related changes in, 283
    ectopic, 283, 2776
    eutopic, 285
    excessive, 283, 319
    from lymphocytes, 2974–2975
    from tumors, 284–285, 319
    gender-dependent differences in, 283
    neurotransmitter effects on, 182t
    regulation of, 283
    somatostatin effects on, 268
  structure of, 280, 281t
  synthesis of, in placenta, 2243
  therapy with, 292–295, *293*, 294t–295t
    in aging, 2707
    in growth hormone deficiency, 337
  tumors secreting, 2886
Growth plate, rickets effects on, 1208, *1209*
Growth without growth hormone syndrome, 2551
gsp oncogene, in thyroid carcinoma, 842
GTPase, oncogenes as, 59, 59t
GTPase-activating protein, in signal transduction, *44*, 1380
Guanabenz, action of, on adrenergic receptors, 1856
Guanethidine, thyroid function effects of, 649
Guanine, in DNA structure, 119–120, *120*
  in RNA structure, 120
Guanine nucleotide(s), ras gene product binding to, 43, *44*
Guanine nucleotide-releasing factor, 43, *44*, 1380
Guanine-binding proteins/guanine nucleotide-binding proteins. See *G proteins.*
Guanosine triphosphate-binding proteins, in thyroid regulation, *544*, 544–545
Guanyl nucleotide-binding proteins, in thyroid-stimulating hormone synthesis, 209, *209*
Guanylate cyclase, in protein kinase activation, *46*
  receptors for, 23t, 25t, 29
Gubernaculum testis, 1893
Gusducin, properties of, 37
Gustatory sweating, in diabetes mellitus, 1553
Gut glucagon. See *Glicentin.*
Gynandroblastoma, 2118
Gynecomastia, 2474–2484
  adult, 2475, *2475–2476*
  androgen-induced, 2480, 2480t
  causes of, 2476–2481, *2479*, 2480t
  estrogen levels and, 2476–2477, *2479*
  evaluation of, 2481, *2481*
  familial, *2478*, 2480
  familial idiopathic, precocious puberty and, 1970
  from cimetidine, 2397
  from drugs, 2397–2398
  idiopathic, 2481
  in chemotherapy, 2397
  in ectopic chorionic somatomammotropin secretion, 2777
  in ectopic gonadotropin secretion, 2777–2779
  in Graves' disease, 689–690
  in hypergonadotropic disorders, 254
  in infertility, 2409
  in kidney failure, 2395
  in Klinefelter's syndrome, 1906–1907, 2387, *2387*
  in testicular tumors, 2443–2444, *2444*
  newborn, 2474
  pathological forms of, 2475–2480, *2476*, 2477t, *2478–2479*

Gynecomastia *(Continued)*
  physiological, 2474–2475, *2475–2476*
  pubertal, 2474–2475, 2480
  traumatic, 2480
  treatment of, 2481–2482, 2482t
  vs. body mass index, 2475, *2475–2476*
  vs. pseudogynecomastia, 2475, *2476*

Hair, excess of. See *Hirsutism.*
  Graves' disease effects on, 687
  hypocalcemia effects on, 1124
  pubic, development of, in females, 1940–1941, *1941–1942*, 1942t
    in males, 1938, 1939t, *1939–1940*
    premature appearance of, 1816, 1818, 2097
  sexual, development of, 2096, *2096*
    evaluation of, 2104, *2104*
    premature appearance of, 2097
  terminal, 2096, *2096*
  vellus, 2096, *2096*
    in Cushing's syndrome, 1744, *1744*
HAIR-AN acronym, in hyperandrogenism, 2097, 2103
Half-site, in TSH DNA sequence, 208
Haloperidol, action of, on adrenergic receptors, 1858
Hamartoblastoma, of hypothalamus, 463
Hamartoma, hypothalamic, 463
  imaging of, 482, *484*
  precocious puberty in, 1969, *1972–1973*
Ham's F-10 solution, in sperm separation, 2090
Hand-Schüller-Christian disease, delayed puberty in, 1961
Harris-Benedict formula, for energy requirements, 2672
Hashimoto's disease. See *Thyroiditis, autoimmune (Hashimoto's disease).*
Head, circumference of, standards for, 2556, *2557*
  injury of, diabetes insipidus in, 413
Headache, in acromegaly, 323
  in hypoglycemia, *1611*
  in pheochromocytoma, 1862
  in pituitary tumor, 396, 459
Hearing loss, in Paget's disease, 1264
Heart. See also *Cardiovascular; Cardiac* entries.
  adrenergic receptors in, 1857t
  calcification of, in Paget's disease, 1268
  glucose metabolism in, *1395*, 1396t
  palpitations of, in pheochromocytoma, 1862
  thyroid tissue in, 898
Heart rate, abnormalities of, in diabetes mellitus, 1551–1552
  variation of, tests for, 1552
Heat, intolerance of, in Graves' disease, 687
  testicular damage from, 2409
Heat shock proteins, Graves' ophthalmopathy and, 714, *717*
  in androgen receptor activation, 2344
  in glucocorticoid receptor binding, 1656, *1657*
  receptors associated with, 97–98, *97–98*, 110–111, *111*, 113, 2338, *2338*
Height. See also *Stature.*
  measurement of, 2562
  midparental, 1956
  prediction of, from bone age, 2557, 2558t–2560t, *2559–2560*
  rate of increase of, vs. age, 1944, *1945*
  vs. weight, standards for, 2627–2628, 2628t, 2719–2720, 2720t
Height age, 2562
Height velocity, error of, 332

Helper T lymphocytes, 2992–2993, 3002
Hemagglutination test, for thyroglobulin antibodies, 728, *729*, 729t
  for thyroid antibodies, 634, 636
Hemangioblastomatosis, cerebelloretinal, pheochromocytoma in, 1863t, 1864
Hematologic system, function of, phosphate in, 1026
Hematoma, after thyroid surgery, 913
Hematopoiesis, disorders of, anabolic steroids in, 2366–2367
  hypothyroidism effects on, 760
  regulation of, 2943–2945, *2943–2945*, 2944t
    colony-stimulating factors in. See *Colony-stimulating factor(s).*
    erythropoietin in. See *Erythropoietin.*
    interleukins in, 2943–2944, *2944*, 2944t
    leukemia inhibitory factor in, 2944, *2944*, 2944t
    stem cell factor in, *2944*, 2944t, 2944–2945
Hematopoietic growth factor, receptor for, 30
Hematopoietin receptor superfamily, 308, *309*, 382–383, *383*
Hemianopsia, in pituitary tumor, 459
Hemihypertrophy, congenital, 2581–2582
Hemihypophysectomy, in Cushing's disease, 1758
Hemochromatosis, hypoparathyroidism in, 1127
  of adrenal gland, imaging of, 1721, *1722*
  testicular function in, 2396, 2396t
  vs. polyglandular failure syndrome, 3020
Hemodialysis, aluminum intoxication in, 1087
  hypercalcemia in, 1086–1087
  in diabetic nephropathy, *1580*, 1580–1581, 1581t, *1582*
  renal osteodystrophy in, 1086–1087
Hemoglobin, glycosylated, measurement of, 1487, 1488t
  in diabetes mellitus, 1421
  in pregnancy, 1470
  production of, anabolic steroid effects on, 2366–2367
Hemoglobinopathy, delayed puberty in, 1959
Hemolytic plaque assay, for prolactin, 375, *376*
Hemophilia, anabolic steroids in, 2367
Hemorrhage, adrenal, imaging of, 1721, *1722*
  after thyroid surgery, 913
  as paraneoplastic syndrome, 2761
  gastrointestinal, somatostatin therapy in, 274
  in pituitary adenoma, 472, *474*
  orthostatic hypotension in, 2936–2937, *2937*
  pituitary, 165, 458
    imaging of, 398
Henle, loop of, vasopressin action in, 411–412
Heparin, hypoaldosteronism from, 1807
Heparin-binding epidermal growth factor, 2600, *2601*
Hepatic. See also *Liver.*
Hepatic artery, embolization of, in carcinoid tumor, 2810
Hepatic lipase, in lipoprotein metabolism, 2732
Hepatic osteodystrophy, 1216
Hepatitis, alcoholic, anabolic steroids in, 2368
  testicular function in, 2395–2396, 2396t
Hepatocellular neoplasia, from anabolic steroids, 2371
Hepatocyte growth factor, 2612–2613, *2613*
  in thyroid regulation, 544
  receptor for, 29, 42
Hepatoma, hypoglycemia in, 1617
Hereditary angioneurotic edema, anabolic steroids in, 2367
Heregulins, 2602

In situ hybridization, in gene expression analysis, 124, *124*
In vitro fertilization, with embryo transfer, 2090–2092
  ovulation induction for, 2037–2041, 2039t, *2039–2041*
Incidentaloma (silent adenoma), 171–172, *172*, 500
  imaging of, 1724, 1726, *1726*
Incontinence, fecal, in diabetes mellitus, 1550
Incretin effect, 1354, 2721, 2873–2874
Indapamide, in nephrolithiasis, 1184
Index methods, for free thyroid hormone measurement, 627
Indomethacin, in hypercalcemia, 1098
Infancy, idiopathic hypercalcemia of, 1084–1085
Infant(s), breastfeeding of. See *Breastfeeding; Lactation.*
  diencephalic syndrome in, 461, 461t
  hypoglycemia in, 1618
  inhibin in, 2012
  newborn. See *Neonates.*
  of diabetic mothers, 2271–2272, 2272t
    congenital malformations in, *1468*, 1468–1469, 1474–1475
    growth disorders in, 2567
    long-term development of, *1475*, 1475–1476
    macrosomia in, 1473, 1475
    morbidities in, 1475
  premature. See *Neonates, premature.*
  small-for-gestational-age, hyperglycemia in, 2270–2271, *2271*
    hypoglycemia in, 2269–2270, *2270*
  thyroid function in, 610
Infantilism, sexual, in gonadal dysgenesis, 1911t
  in Turner's syndrome, 1908
Infarction, pituitary, 165, 458, 2069
Infection, as Graves' disease trigger, 685
  from intrauterine device, 2163–2165, *2165*
  genital, infertility in, 2408
  in ketoacidosis, 1515
  in parenteral nutrition, 2674
  in vitamin D deficiency, 1006
  pituitary, 458
  preterm labor in, 2219
  testicular failure in, 2391–2392
  urinary tract, in diabetic nephropathy, 1579
Infertility, definition of, 2405
  female, 2080–2092. See also *Amenorrhea; Anovulation; Ovarian failure.*
    after oral contraceptive discontinuation, 2150
    assisted reproductive technologies for, 2090–2092
      ovulation induction in, 2037–2041, 2039t, *2039–2041*
    causes of, 2080
    cervical factors in, 2082–2084, 2083t
    epidemiology of, 2080
    evaluation of, 2081–2084
      in endometriosis, 2087–2088
      in tubal disease, 2084–2085
    hyperprolactinemia in, 395, 398–399
    idiopathic, 2080
    immunologic factors in, 2088–2089
    in depo-medroxyprogesterone acetate use, 2156
    in diabetes mellitus, 1466
    in endometriosis, 2086–2088
    in hyperprolactinemia, 396
    in hypothyroidism, 762, 799–800, 2090
    luteal phase defects in, 2075, 2089–2090

Infertility *(Continued)*
  male factors with, 2406
  mycoplasmal infections in, 2089
  ovulation documentation in, 2081
  ovulation induction in. See *Ovulation, induction of.*
  pelvic factors in, 2084–2088
  postcoital test in, 2083t, 2083–2084
  spontaneous conception in, 2080–2081
  tubal disease in, 2084–2086
  vs. age, 2080
  vs. normal conception rate, 2080
  male, 2404–2433. See also *Testicular failure.*
    classification of, 2406–2407, 2407t
    definitions of, 2405–2506
    distribution of, 2506
    donor insemination and, 2427–2428
    duration of, 2406
    etiology of, 2406–2407, 2407t
    evaluation of, clinical, 2407t, 2407–2411, *2410*
      genetic studies in, 2415
      history in, 2407–2409
      hormone assessment in, 2414
      laboratory, 2411–2416, *2412*, 2413t, *2415–2416*
      physical examination in, 2409–2411, *2410*
      semen analysis in, 2411–2414, *2412*, 2413t
      testicular biopsy in, 2415–2416, *2415–2416*
    familial factors in, 2406
    female factors interacting with, 2506
    historical aspects of, 2405
    hyperprolactinemia in, 395
    iatrogenic, 2408–2409
    in kidney failure, 2395
    in vitro fertilization for, 2424–2427
    incidence of, 2506
    management of, *2423*, 2423–2424
      androgens in, 2355
      empirical, 2424, *2424*
      in coital disorders, 2419–2421, 2438–2439
      in genital tract inflammation, 2421
      in genital tract obstruction, 2418–2419
      in sperm autoimmunity, 2416–2418
      in varicocele, 2421–2423
      prognosis for, 2423, *2423*
      psychological aspects of, 2423
    prevention of, 2428–2429
    semen examination in, 2082, 2082t
  patient education on, 1983–1984
  primary, definition of, 2080
  relative, 2080
  vaginal factor in, 2083
Inflammation. See also *Cytokines.*
  glucocorticoid action in, 1643–1644, 1647–1648, *1648*
  growth factors produced in, 2608, *2608*
  nerve growth factors in, 2610
  with intrauterine devices, 2160
Inflammatory bowel disease, gastrointestinal hormone action in, 2884
Infrahyoid thyroid, 895–896
Infundibulum. See also *Median eminence.*
  granulomatous disease of, *485*, 486
  imaging of, *471*, *472*, *476*
  tumors of, imaging of, 482
Infusion pump, for insulin delivery, 1497
Inhibins, 2604, *2604*
  actions of, 250, 1993, *1994*, 2008–2009, 2023
  assays for, 250, 2011, 2014–2015, *2015*

Inhibins *(Continued)*
  clinical significance of, 2014–2015, *2015*
  discovery of, 2008
  forms of, 2008, *2009*
  genes of, *124*, 2008
  in chorionic gonadotropin synthesis, 2180
  in fetus, 244–245, 2012
  in follicle-stimulating hormone secretion regulation, 2320–2321, *2321*
  in gonadotropin secretion, 1993, *1994*, 1997
  in gonadotropin-releasing hormone action, 2003–2004
  in infants, 2012
  in lactation, 2014
  in menopause, 2014
  in menstrual cycle, 2012–2014, *2013*
  in pregnancy, 2014
  in puberty, 2012
  in testicular failure, 2386
  in testis, 2320–2321, 2323
  physiology of, 2012–2014, *2013*
  placental, 2190, *2191*
  secretion of, 2010
    vs. menstrual cycle phase, 2046–2047, *2047*, *2049*
  species differences in, 2008
  structure of, 2008–2009, *2009*, 2023
  synthesis of, 2023
Initiator, in gene expression, 8, *8–9*
Injury. See *Stress and injury.*
Inositol bisphosphates, in phosphoinositide cycle, 68
Inositol hexakisphosphate, in phosphoinositide cycle, 68, 70
Inositol pentakisphosphate, in phosphoinositide cycle, 68, 70
Inositol tetrakisphosphate, in phosphoinositide cycle, 68, 70
Inositol triphosphates, actions of, 39–40, *40*, 40t
  in aldosterone secretion, 1673, *1674*
  in arachidonic acid cascade, 2215, 2215–2216
  in calcium mobilization, 71–73
  in glucagon action, 1345
  in phosphoinositide cycle, 68, 70
  in thyroid regulation, *544*, 545–546, *546*
  metabolism of, 68, 69–70
  receptors for, 39–40, *40*, 40t, 71–72
Insemination, cervical cup in, 2083–2084
  intrauterine, 2083–2084, 2091
  transcervical intratubal, 2092
  with donor sperm, 2427–2428
  with husband's sperm, 2421
Insomnia, advanced sleep phase, 2508
  delayed sleep phase, 2508
    melatonin in, 440
  in hypothalamic lesions, 461
Insular carcinoid, ovarian, 2122
Insulin, absorption of, 1497–1498
  action of. See also *Insulin receptor.*
    age-related changes in, 2721
    cellular defects in, insulin resistance in, *1443*, 1443–1445, *1445–1446*
    glucose transport and, 1380–1383, *1381–1382*, 1382t
    immediate effects of, 1373, *1374*
    insulin resistance and, 1593–1594
    intermediate effects of, 1373, *1374*
    kinetics of, 19
    levels of, 1373, *1374*
    long-term effects of, 1373, *1374*
    on other islet hormones, 1340–1341
    opposing glucagon action, *1344–1345*, 1345
    overview of, 1373, *1374*

Insulin (*Continued*)

species variation in, 1297
time course of, 1496
turning off, 1383–1384, *1384*
vs. insulin-like growth factor action, 317
allergy to, 1498
antagonists of, 1442–1443
  insulin resistance in, 1595
antibodies to, hypoglycemia from, 1616–1617, 3007
  insulin action affected by, 1442–1443
  insulin resistance from, 1595
assays for, 1297–1298, 1421
autoantibodies to, 1285, 1287
binding of, to receptor, 1375–1376, 1443–1445, *1445*
  unpredictable release from, 3007
characterization of, 1297–1298
crystallization of, 1307
deficiency of. See *Diabetes mellitus.*
degradation of, 1357–1358, 1383–1384, 1595
distribution of, insulin resistance and, 1443
edema induced by, 1499–1500
evolution of, 1299
excess of. See *Hyperinsulinemia.*
gene of, 1309–1311, *1310*
  defects in, 1310–1311, *1311*, 1442
  mutation of, 130t, 1601t–1602t, 1601–1602
  structure of, 1309–1310, *1310*
glucose transporters and, 1396–1397
historical aspects of, 1296, *1297*
impurities of, in extracted preparations, 1297
in adrenal androgen control, 1840
in amino acid metabolism, 1406, *1407*
in androgen synthesis, *2094*, 2095
in bone resorption, 1199
in calcium reabsorption, 1023
in endurance-trained athletes, 2699
in exercise, 1357, *2695–2696*, 2696–2697
in fasting, *1392–1394*, 1392–1395
in fatty acid metabolism, 1403–1406, *1404–1406*
in fetus, 1475, 2248, 2261–2264
  growth and, 2251
in futile cycles, 1397–1398
in glucagon synthesis, 1339, 1341–1342, *1341–1342*
in glucose metabolism, 1400–1403, *1400–1403*, 1605–1607, *1606*
in glucose regulation, 1343–1344
in glucose transport, 48–49, 1444, 2260
in glucose uptake, 1455
in glycogenesis, 47, 1402, *1402–1403*
in glycogenolysis, 1392–1393, *1393–1394*
in hepatic glucose metabolism, *1400*, 1400–1402
in hyperglycemia, in small-for-gestational-age infant, 2271
in insulinoma, 1612, *1612–1614*, 1613t
in ketoacidosis, 1511t
in ketone metabolism, 1407
in lactation, 2230
in lipid synthesis, 1406–1407
in muscle glucose metabolism, 1402–1403, *1402–1403*
in obesity, 1362, *1363*, 1441, *1442*
in parathyroid hormone action, 951
in parenteral nutrition, 2674
in peripheral glucose metabolism, *1400–1401*, 1400–1402
in phosphate reabsorption, 1033
in placental glucose transport, 2260
in pregnancy, 1464–1465
in prolactin regulation, 380

Insulin (*Continued*)

in protein synthesis, 2666, *2666*
in stress, 1343, 2670
injection of, 1497
intermediate-acting, 1496
isolation of, 1296–1298, *1297*
levels of, chorionic somatomammotropin effects on, 2185–2186
  excessive. See *Hyperinsulinemia.*
lipoatrophy and lipohypertrophy from, 1498
long-acting, 1496
measurement of, 1297–1298, 1421
metabolism of, 1357–1358, 1383–1384
orthostatic hypotension from, 1551
placental transport of, 2240, 2240t
porcine, structure of, 1298–1299, *1299*
precursors of, 1300–1303, *1301–1303*
preparations of, impurities in, 1297
receptor for. See *Insulin receptor.*
receptor-binding region of, 1299–1300, *1300*
resistance to. See *Insulin resistance.*
retroendocytosis of, 1384
secretion of, after islet-cell transplantation, 1365–1366
  after pancreas transplantation, 1365
  aging effects on, 1363–1364
  alterations of, 1362–1366, *1363–1366*
  amino acids and, 1355
  amylin effects on, 987
  anomeric specificity in, 1355
  circadian rhythms of, 1360–1361, 2533–2536, *2534–2535, 2537*
  cytokine effects on, 2982–2983
  ectopic, 2783t, 2783–2785
  excessive. See *Hyperinsulinemia.*
  exercise and, 1357
  first-phase, in diabetes mellitus, 1438–1440, *1439*
  gastric inhibitory polypeptide in, 2873–2874
  glucose levels and, 1354–1355
  granule formation in, 1306–1307, *1307*
  high-frequency oscillations in, 2517, *2518*
  in B cells, 1279, *1280*
  in diabetes mellitus, 1363–1365, *1365–1366*
    non-insulin-dependent (type II), 1436, *1437*, 1438–1441, *1439–1440, 1442*
  in glucose abundance, 1344
  in impaired glucose tolerance, 1441
  in insulinoma, 1366
  incretin effect in, 1354, 2721, 2873–2874
  insulin therapy effects on, 1455–1456, *1455–1456*
  lipids and, 1355
  neurotransmitters in, 1343
  oscillatory, 1361, *1361–1362*
  postprandial, 1360–1361
  protein effects on, *1342*, 1342–1343
  pulsatile, 2514, *2515, 2524*
    impaired, 1454
  quantitation of, 1398–1399, *1399*
  regulation of, 271t, 1309–1311, *1309–1311*, 2262–2264
    glucoreceptor theory of, 1329
    glucose metabolism and, 1329–1335, *1331–1332, 1334*
    hormonal, 1355–1357, *1356*
    physiological, 1354–1357, *1356*
  schematic model of, *1303*
  second-phase, in diabetes mellitus, 1438–1439, *1439*
  sleep and, 2534, *2535*
  somatostatin effects on, 268

Insulin (*Continued*)

substances promoting, 1329, 1332
sulfonylurea effects on, 1493
ultradian rhythm of, 2534, 2536
vitamin D effects on, 1007
vs. sensitivity, 1399–1400, *1400*
sensitivity to, decreased, 1445, *1446.* See also *Insulin resistance.*
  quantitation of, 1398–1399, *1399*
  vs. secretion, 1399–1400, *1400*
short acting, 1496
species variation in, 1297–1299
storage of, in granules, 1306–1307, *1307*
structure of, 1298–1299, *1298–1299*
synthesis of, 1300–1309
  beta granule formation in, 1306–1307, *1307*
  C-peptide accumulation in, 1307–1309, *1308*
  in B cells, 1279, *1280*
  morphologic aspects of, 1302–1303, *1303*
  precursors in, 1300–1303, *1301–1303*
  proinsulin-to-insulin conversion in, 1303–1306, *1304–1305*
  regulation of, 1309–1311, *1309–1311*
  schematic model of, *1303*
therapy with. See *Insulin therapy.*
transcytosis of, 1383–1384
turnover of, in pregnancy, 1464–1465
types of, for therapy, 1496
variants of, 1310–1311, *1311*, 1601t–1602t, 1601–1602
vasoconstrictor effect of, 2931, *2932*
Insulin glucose clamp technique, 1398–1399, *1399*
Insulin neuritis, 1546
Insulin receptor, activation of, 41–42, 1376–1377
affinity of, 20, *22*
antibodies to, 57, *57*–58, 58t
  hypoglycemia in, 1617
  insulin resistance from, 1443, 1595t, 1595–1596
  properties of, 1595
cross-reactivity of, 58, *58*, 58t–59t
defects of, 55, *55*, 55t, *56*
  in leprechaunism, *1598*, 1598–1599
  in Rabson-Mendenhall syndrome, 1599
  insulin resistance in, *1443*, 1443–1445, *1445–1446*, 1592–1594
deficiency of, 1375, 1444, *1445*
dephosphorylation of, in insulin action turn-off, 1384, *1384*
function of, signaling mechanisms in, 1452–1453, *1452–1453*
gene of, 1374
  mutations of, 130t, 137, 1374, *1376, 1597*, 1597t, 1597–1598
  structure of, 1449, *1449*
hybrid with insulin-like growth factor receptor, 315, 1377, 1593–1594
in fetus, 2248
in insulin metabolism, 1358–1359, 1383
in signal transduction, 44, *44*, 1377–1380, *1378–1380*
insulin binding to, 1374–1375, 1443–1445, *1445*
number of, 1374
phosphorylation of, 45, 1376–1377, 1452–1453, *1452–1453*
post-binding defect of, 1444–1445, 1447–1448, 1456
regulatory region of, 1377

Insulinopathies, gene defects in, 1310–1311, *1311*
Insulitis, 1284, 1287
    in diabetes mellitus, 1428
    in polyglandular failure syndrome, 3013
int-2 oncogene, 59, 59t
Intercalated cells, in electrolyte transport, 1689
Intercellular adhesion molecules, in Graves' ophthalmopathy, 716, *716–717*
    in T lymphocyte activation, *2997*, 2998, 2998t
Intercourse. See *Sexual intercourse.*
Interferon(s), in carcinoid syndrome, 2809
    in thyroid regulation, *555*
    receptors for, 30, 382, *383*
Interferon regulatory factor 1, synthesis of, prolactin effects on, 2973
Interferon-alpha, hypothyroidism from, 756–757
Interferon-gamma, glucocorticoid regulation of, 1647–1648, *1648*
    in autoimmune thyroiditis, 732–733, 733t
    in Graves' ophthalmopathy, 716
    in Leydig cell inflammation, 2325
    in thyroid regulation, 543t
Interferon-stimulated gene factor-3, in gene expression regulation, 49
Intergeniculate leaflet, in circadian rhythm synchronization, 2494
Interleukin(s). See also specific interleukin, e.g., *Interleukin-1.*
    in bone resorption regulation, 1199–1200
    in corticotropin-releasing hormone regulation, 2189
    in growth hormone secretion, 2981
    in hematopoiesis, 2943–2944, *2944*, 2944t
    in hypothalamic-pituitary-adrenal axis regulation, 1645
    receptors for, 308, *309*, 382, *383*, 2949
        structures of, 30, *30*
    synthesis of, in estrogen deficiency, 1236
        in testis, 2982
Interleukin-1, actions of, *2968*
    on brain, 2979
    on Leydig cells, 2326–2327
    on ovary, 2982
    on pancreatic islets, 2982–2983
    on pituitary, 2979–2981
    on testis, 2982
    on thyroid, 2983
    in ACTH secretion, 365–366
    in Alzheimer's disease, 2979–2980
    in autoimmune disease, 733, 733t, 3008
    in corticotropin-releasing hormone regulation, 345, *345–346*
    in diabetes mellitus, 1284–1285
    in Graves' ophthalmopathy, 716
    in hypoaldosteronism, 1805
    in Leydig cell inflammation, 2325
    in nonthyroidal illness, 2980
    in paraneoplastic syndromes, 2756
    in stress, 2670
    in thyroid regulation, 543t, *555*
    properties of, 2966t
    secretion of, vs. estrogen levels, 2977
    synthesis of, in exercise, 2394
        in ovary, 2982
Interleukin-1α, actions of, 2326
    in pituitary hormone regulation, 187t
Interleukin-1β, actions of, 2326–2327
    in pituitary hormone regulation, 187t
Interleukin-1–like factor, in seminiferous tubules, 2323
Interleukin-1 receptor antagonist, 2966
Interleukin-2, actions of, *2968*

Interleukin-2 *(Continued)*
    on pituitary-adrenal axis, 2979
    in ACTH secretion, 365–366
    in autoimmune thyroiditis, 732–733, 733t
    in corticotropin-releasing hormone regulation, 345, *346*
    in hypothyroidism, 756–757
    in T lymphocyte activation, 2997
    properties of, 2966t
    receptor for, levels of, vs. thyroid hormone levels, 2978
        prolactin effects on, 387
    synthesis of, 2973
Interleukin-3. See *Colony-stimulating factor(s), multipotential (interleukin-3).*
Interleukin-4, properties of, 2966t
Interleukin-6, actions of, *2968*
    on ovary, 2982
    on pituitary, 2979, 2981
    in ACTH secretion, 365–366
    in autoimmune disease, 733, 733t, 3008
    in corticotropin-releasing hormone regulation, 345, *346*
    properties of, 2966t
    receptor for, 2611, *2611*
    secretion of, in ovary, 2982
Interleukin-8, in parturition, 2213
Intersex disorders. See *Pseudohermaphroditism; Sexual differentiation, disorders of.*
Interstitial cells, of testis, 2314
Interstitial fluid, in steroidogenesis regulation, 2327
Intertubular tissue, between seminiferous tubules, *2313*, 2313–2314. See also *Leydig cells.*
Intervening sequences (introns), 7, *7–8*, *120*, 121
    removal of, *10*, 11
Intestinal bypass surgery, osteomalacia in, 1211–1212
Intestine. See also *Colon.*
    calcium absorption in. See *Calcium, absorption of.*
    dysfunction of, in diabetes mellitus, 1550
    ganglioneuromatosis of, in multiple endocrine neoplasia, 864
    glucagon synthesis in, 1315–1316, *1316*, 1337–1339, *1338*
    glucose metabolism in, 1395, *1395*, 1396t, 1397
    motility of, motilin in, 2876
    phosphate absorption in, 1027–1208
    surgery on, hormone action after, 2883
    vitamin D action in, 1003–1004
Intracavernosal vasodilator injection, in impotence, 2438–2439
Intracellular signaling, growth hormone-releasing hormone in, 282
Intracrine action, definition of, 2592
Intramembranous ossification, 1194–1195, *1195*
Intraocular pressure, measurement of, 719
Intrauterine devices, 2160–2165
    adverse effects of, 2161–2163, 2162t
    benefits of, 2160
    efficacy of, 2160
    failure of, 2141t–2142t
    infection with, 2154–2155
    insertion of, 2161
    mechanism of action of, 2160
    postcoital, 2159, 2159t
    pregnancy complications with, 2163–2164
    safety record of, 2165
    types of, 2160–2161, *2161*
    use of, statistics on, 2141t

Intrauterine growth. See *Growth, intrauterine.*
Introns, 7, *7–8*, *120*, 121
    removal of, *10*, 11
Iodination, in thyroid hormone synthesis, 511–512, *512*, 522, 522–523, *524*, 526–532, 549–550
    compounds I, II, and III formation in, 529, *529–530*
    hydrogen peroxide in, 528–529, *529–531*, 531–532, 546, *546*, 549–550
    in multinodular goiter, 771–772, *771–772*
    inhibition of, 531–532
    iodine supply for, 526
    iodine transport in, 526–527
    molecular mechanism of, 529, *530–531*, 531
    organification process in. See *Iodine and iodide, organification of.*
    site of, 525–526
    thyroid peroxidase in, 527–529, *529–531*, 549–550
    of water supply, 830
Iodine and iodide, absorption of, 511
    as goitrogen, 613, *613*
    as iodination inhibitor, 531–532
    clearance of, in deficiency, 824–825
    daily requirements for, 821–822
    deficiency of, 526, 821–842
        adaptation to, 824–826, 825t, *826*
        cretinism in. See *Cretinism.*
        disorders caused by, diagnosis of, 826–827, 827t
            etiology of, 823t, 823–824, *824*
            pathophysiology of, 824–826, 825t, *826*
            prophylaxis of, 829–830
            treatment of, 827–828, 829–830
            types of, 821, 822t
        geographic considerations in, *822*, 822–823, 828–829
        goiter in. See *Goiter, in iodine deficiency.*
        hypothyroidism in, 756
            in premature infants, 788
        in fetus, 829
        in neonates, 829
        in pregnancy, 611, 2292
        iodotyrosine coupling in, 550
        stores in, 825
        thyroglobulin synthesis in, 825
        thyroid clearance in, 824–825
        thyroid hormone ratio in, 535
        thyroid hormone secretion in, 825, *826*
        thyroid hyperplasia in, 825
        thyroid regulation in, 608
        thyroid-stimulating hormone secretion in, 826
        thyroxine-to-triiodothyronine conversion in, 826
    dietary intake of, 526
    excess of, Graves' disease in, 684
        hypothyroidism in, 756
            in premature infants, 788
        thyroid hormone synthesis and release in, *608*, 608–609
    excretion of, 822
    fetal, 804
    food supplementation with, 829–830
    hyperthyroidism from, 677–678
        in Graves' disease, neonatal, 792
        in hyperthyroidism therapy, 698–701
            before thyroid surgery, 906
        in thyroid hormone synthesis, 529–530, *529–530*
        in thyroid regulation, 543t, 546, *546*, *608*, 608–609

Sleep *(Continued)*
  growth hormone secretion and, 488, 2527–2529, *2528*
  hormone secretion and, experimental studies of, 2520, *2520*
  insulin secretion and, 2534, *2535*
  length of, seasonal rhythms of, 2519, *2519*
  melatonin secretion and, 437, 2536–2538
  prolactin secretion and, 2529–2530
  stages of, hormone release and, 2516–2517, *2517*
  thyroid-stimulating hormone secretion and, 2532–2533, *2533*
  ultradian rhythms in, 2512, 2516–2517, *2517*
Sleep apnea, in acromegaly, 323
  in diabetes mellitus, 1552
  in obesity, 2639
Slipped capital femoral epiphysis, in growth hormone therapy, 336
Small intestine, dysfunction of, in diabetes mellitus, 1550
Small nuclear riboprotein complexes, in gene expression, 11
Small-for-gestational-age infants, hyperglycemia in, 2270–2271, *2271*
  hypoglycemia in, 2269–2270, *2270*
Smith-Lemli-Opitz syndrome, 2571t
Smoking, diabetic retinopathy and, 1528t, 1529–1530
  Graves' ophthalmopathy and, 713
  in oral contraceptive use, cardiovascular risks of, 2149–2150, 2150t
Smooth muscle, parathyroid hormone-related protein effects on, 971–972
  prostaglandins effects on, 2218
SMS 201–995. See *Octreotide.*
Sodium. See also *Salt.*
  abnormal levels of. See *Hypernatremia; Hyponatremia.*
  depletion of, in aldosterone deficiency, 1701–1702
    orthostatic hypotension in, *2936*, 2937
  dietary, aldosterone secretion and, 1670–1672, *1671*, 2917–2918, *2919*
    calcium reabsorption and, 1023
    in nonmodulating hypertension, 2925–2929, *2926–2929*
    insulin resistance and, 2930–2931, *2931*
    kidney stone formation and, 1180, 1180t
    plasma renin activity and, 2919–2920, *2920*
    recommended daily intake of, 1491
    renal response to, 1686, *1686*
  excretion of. See also *Natriuretic peptides.*
    glucocorticoids in, 1649
    mechanisms of, 1686–1688, 1687t, *1687–1688*
    regulation of, 1688–1693, *1689, 1691–1692*, 1692t
    volume regulation and, 1693–1694, *1694*
    vs. intake, 1686, *1686*
  fluid homeostasis and, 1685–1686, *1686*
  homeostasis of, glucocorticoids in, 1649
  in ketoacidosis, 1511t, 1512
  in phosphate transport, 1029
  in vasopressin regulation, 409–410, *409–410*
  reabsorption of, 1686–1688, 1687t, *1687–1688*
    in mineralocorticoid excess, 1700, *1700*
  regulation of, aldosterone in, 1668–1672, *1669*, 1670t, *1671*
  restriction of, aldosterone secretion in, 1670–1671, *1671*
    in aldosteronism, 1788
  retention of, edema in, 1704–1705

Sodium *(Continued)*
  escape from, 1671–1672, 1700, *1700*
    growth hormone in, 311
    in pregnancy, 1703–1704
    transport of, aldosterone in, 1679–1681
      sodium-potassium ATPase in, 1690, *1691*
Sodium channels, aldosterone activation of, 1679–1680
Sodium-calcium exchange, in calcium flux, 70, *71*
  parathyroid hormone effects on, 929
Sodium-glucose transporters, 1381–1382, 2260
Sodium/hydrogen ion antiporter, activity of, 1687, *1688*
  aldosterone effects on, 1678, 1681
  parathyroid hormone effects on, 930–931
Sodium-L-thyroxine, in hypothyroidism, in children, 794, 794t
  in neonates, 791–792
Sodium-phosphorus cotransporters, parathyroid hormone effects on, 929–930
Sodium-potassium ATPase, deficiency of, diabetic neuropathy and, 1540
  in aldosterone action, 1690, *1691*
  in calcium flux, 70
  in iodine transport, 527
  in sodium transport, 1687
  ouabain-like factor inhibition of, 1693
  synthesis of, aldosterone effects on, 1680–1681
Solitary central maxillary incisor syndrome, growth hormone deficiency in, 331
Somatic growth. See *Growth.*
Somatic mutation, endocrine neoplasia in, 140–143, *143*
Somatocrinin. See *Growth hormone-releasing hormone.*
Somatolactin, gene of, 369, *369*
Somatomammotrophs. See *Mammosomatotrophs (somatomammotrophs).*
Somatomammotropin, chorionic. See *Chorionic somatomammotropin (placental lactogen).*
Somatomedins. See also *Insulin-like growth factor(s); Proinsulin.*
  actions of, *2598–2599*, 2598–2600
  binding proteins for, 2596–2598
  in tumors, 1617
  secretion of, in paraneoplastic syndromes, 2757t
Somatosensory evoked potentials, in diabetic neuropathy, 1557
Somatostatin, 266–279
  actions of, 267–269, 268t, 1317, 2876–2877
    mechanism of, 269
    on other islet hormones, 1340–1341
    vs. structure, 269
  analogues of, 269. See also *Octreotide.*
    clinical uses of, 274–275, *274–275*
    in acromegaly, 325–326
    in hyperandrogenism, 2106
  assays for, 269–270
  clinical uses of, 274–275, *274–275*
  deficiency of, hyperinsulinemia in, 2273–2274
  discovery of, 152
  distribution of, *155*, 155–156, 266–267, 270t, 270–271, 271t
  evolution of, 266
  excess of, causes of, 2885t
  forms of, 267
  gastrointestinal effects of, 268, 268t, 273–274
  gene of, 2876
  half-life of, 272
  heterogeneity of, 267

Somatostatin *(Continued)*
  hormonal effects of, 268
  in acromegaly, 325
  in carcinoid syndrome, 2808–2809
  in Cushing's disease, 1756–1757
  in gastrin secretion regulation, 2871
  in gastrointestinal disease, 274
  in growth hormone secretion, 184, 272, 305, 2550, *2550*
  in immunoregulation, 2967t
  in neurological disease, 272–273
  in pancreatic disease, 273, 273t
  in pituitary regulation, 272
  in prolactin secretion, 381
  in thyroid-stimulating hormone secretion, 209, *209*, 211–212, 272
  in thyrotropin-releasing hormone secretion, 604–605
  insulin response to, 1355
  isolation of, 266
  localization of, *155*, 155–156, 270t–271t, 270–271
  measurement of, 269–270
  metabolism of, 272
  native, clinical uses of, 274
  neurologic effects of, 268, 272–273
  neuronal pathways for, 182
  neurotransmitter function of, 272–273
  pancreatic effects of, 267–268, 273
  peptides related to, 266, 267t
  phylogeny of, 266
  physiology of, 272–274, 273t, 2876, 2876–2877
  pituitary effects of, 267–268, 272
  precursors of, 271–272
  receptor for, 269, 1317, 2877
  secretion of, 1317, 2876–2877
    neurotransmitter effects on, 182t
    pulsatile, 2514
    regulatory factors for, 270, 271t
    thyroid hormone effects on, *194*
    thyrotropin-releasing hormone in, *193*
  side effects of, 274
  structure of, 266–267, *267*, 267t, *1317*, 1317–1318, 2876, *2876*
    vs. activity, 269
  synthesis of, 271–272, 1317–1318
    cells for, 1339–1340, *1340*
    in placenta, 2243
    in thyroid medullary carcinoma, 861
  thyrotropin-releasing hormone interaction with, 196–197, *197*
  transport of, 272
Somatostatin-28 (larger form), 1317–1318
Somatostatinoma, 2886
  gastrointestinal, 273
  in multiple endocrine neoplasia, 2818
  pancreatic, 273, 273t
Somatotrophs, 162, *162*
  adenoma of, 166–168, *167*
    clonality of, 319
    growth hormone-releasing hormone and, 285
    mixed, 169, *169*
  growth hormone-releasing hormone in, 281, 284
  hyperplasia of, 162
  interconvertible with lactotrophs, 376
  Pit-1 protein in, 373, *374*
Somatotropic axis, biological rhythms in, 2527–2529, *2528*
Somatotropin. See *Somatostatin.*
Somatotropin release-inhibiting factor. See *Somatostatin.*

ISBN 0-7216-4263-2

90038